IV Inco[mpatibilities]
Compat[ibilities]
important
IV drugs.

D0285147

5

rigidity, peripheral circulatory collapse, cardiac arrest, anaphylactoid effects).
Storage • Store at room temperature.

Epidural, Liposomal
• May give either diluted or undiluted. • Do not use an in-line filter. • Store solution in refrigerator/do not freeze. May store at room temperature for 7 days. • Following withdrawal from vial, use within 4 hrs. • Gently invert vial to resuspend drug; avoid aggressive agitation.

IV INCOMPATIBILITIES

Amphotericin B complex (Abelcet, AmBisome, Amphotec), cefepime (Maxipime), doxorubicin (Doxil), lipids, phenytoin (Dilantin), thiopental.

IV COMPATIBILITIES

Amiodarone (Cordarone), atropine, bumetanide (Bumex), bupivacaine (Marcaine, Sensorcaine), diltiazem (Cardizem), diphenhydramine (Benadryl), dobutamine (Dobutrex), dopamine (Intropin), glycopyrrolate (Robinul), heparin, hydroxyzine (Vistaril), lidocaine, lorazepam (Ativan), magnesium, midazolam (Versed), milrinone (Primacor), nitroglycerin, potassium, propofol (Diprivan), total parenteral nutrition (TPN).

INDICATIONS/ROUTES/DOSAGE

◄**ALERT►** Dosage should be titrated to desired effect.
Analgesia
PO (IMMEDIATE-RELEASE): ADULTS, ELDERLY: 10–30 mg q3–4h as needed. **CHILDREN:** 0.15–0.3 mg/kg q3–4h as needed.
PO (EXTENDED-RELEASE [AVINZA]): ADULTS, ELDERLY: Dosage requirement should be established using prompt-release formulations and is based on total daily dose. Avinza is given once a day only.
PO (EXTENDED-RELEASE [KADIAN]): ADULTS, ELDERLY: Dosage requirement should be established using prompt-release formulations and is based on total daily dose. Dose is given once a day or divided and given q12h.

Patient-Controlled Analgesia (PCA)
IV: ADULTS, ELDERLY: Loading dose: 5–10 mg. **Intermittent bolus:** 0.5–3 mg. **Lockout interval:** 5–12 min. **Continuous infusion:** 1–10 mg/hr. **4-hr limit:** 20–30 mg.

SIDE EFFECTS

Frequent: Sedation, decreased B/P (including orthostatic hypotension), diaphoresis, facial flushing, constipation, dizziness, drowsiness, nausea, vomiting. **Occasional:** Allergic reaction (rash, pruritus), dyspnea, confusion, palpitations, tremors, urinary retention, abdominal cramps, vision changes, dry mouth, headache, decreased appetite, pain/burning at injection site. **Rare:** Paralytic ileus.

**ADVERSE EFFECTS/
TOXIC REACTIONS**

Overdose results in respiratory depression, skeletal muscle flaccidity, cold/clammy skin, cyanosis, extreme drowsiness progressing to seizures, stupor, coma. Tolerance to analgesic effect, physical dependence may occur with repeated use.

NURSING CONSIDERATIONS

BASELINE ASSESSMENT
Pt should be in recumbent position before drug is given by parenteral route. Assess onset, type, location, duration of pain.

INTERVENTION/EVALUATION
Monitor vital signs 5–10 min after IV administration, 15–30 min after subcutaneous, IM. Be alert for decreased respirations, B/P. Check for adequate voiding. Monitor daily pattern of bowel activity and stool consistency. Avoid constipation.

PATIENT/FAMILY TEACHING
• Discomfort may occur with injection. • Change positions slowly to avoid orthostatic hypotension. • Avoid tasks that require alertness, motor skills until response to drug is established. • Avoid alcohol, CNS depressants.

M

Side Effects section in each drug monograph specifies the frequency of particular side effects.

Adverse Reactions highlight the particularly dangerous side effects.

✦ Canadian trade name   ▧ Non-Crushable Drug   ▦ High Alert drug

High Alert drugs are shaded in blue for easy identification.

New to this Edition!
• 26 drugs recently approved by the FDA
• Hundreds of updates and revisions
• More than 300 Black Box Alerts

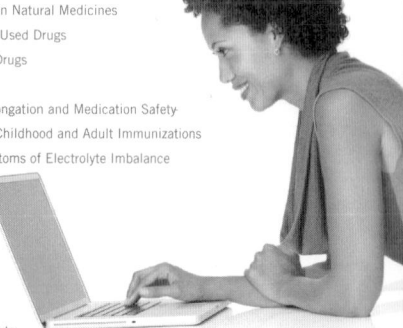

CONTENTS

AUTHOR BIOGRAPHIES

Robert (Bob) J. Kizior, BS, RPh

Bob graduated from the University of Illinois School of Pharmacy and is licensed to practice in the state of Illinois. He has worked as a hospital pharmacist for more than 40 years at Alexian Brothers Medical Center in Elk Grove Village, Illinois—a suburb of Chicago. Bob is the Pharmacy Surgery Coordinator for the Department of Pharmacy, where he participates in educational programs for pharmacists, nurses, physicians, and patients. He plays a major role in coordinating pharmacy services in the OR satellite. Bob is a former adjunct faculty member at William Rainey Harper Community College in Palatine, Illinois. It was there that Bob first met Barbara and commenced their long-standing professional association.

An avid fan of Big Ten college athletics, Bob also has eclectic tastes in music that range from classical, big band, rock 'n' roll, and jazz to country and western. Bob spends much of his free time reviewing the professional literature to stay current on new drug information.

Barbara B. Hodgson, RN, OCN

Born and raised in Michigan, Barbara was married and raising a young family in Chicago when she decided to fulfill a lifelong dream and become a nurse. After graduation, she started her own business as author and publisher of **Medcards, The Total Medication Reference Guide,** the first of its kind. These drug cards were designed to assist nursing students in understanding drug information to give knowledgeable care to their patients.

In 1981, she met co-author Robert (Bob) Kizior, who was teaching a pharmacology class. After class, Barbara approached him and asked if he would be interested in working on **Medcards** with her. He agreed, and together they became so successful that a few years later Barbara was able to fulfill another dream and move to Florida.

By 1987, Barbara was approached by W.B. Saunders and asked to author the **Saunders Nursing Drug Handbook.** Since then, Barbara and Bob have worked together on this handbook and on two more drug resources, the **Saunders Electronic Nursing Drug Cards** and the **Saunders Drug Handbook for Health Professions.**

Barbara specialized in oncology at the Cancer Institute, St. Joseph's Hospital, in Tampa, Florida, and at Morton Plant Mease Northbay Hospital in New Port Richey, Florida. Barbara's daughter Lauren is a nurse manager, and her daughter Kathryn, her son Keith, and her son-in-law Jim are all nurses, working in their respective fields of patient care.

Keith J. Hodgson, RN, BSN, CCRN

Keith was born into a loving family in Chicago, Illinois. His mother, Barbara B. Hodgson, was an author and publisher of several medication products, and her work has been a part of his life since he was a child. By the time he was four years old, Keith was already helping his mother with the drug cards by stacking the draft pages that were piled up throughout their home.

Because of his mother's influence, Keith contemplated becoming a nurse in college, but his mind was fully made up after he shadowed his sister in the Emergency Department. Keith received his Associates Degree in Nursing from Hillsborough Community College and his Bachelor of Science in Nursing from the University of South Florida in Tampa, Florida. Keith started his career in the Emergency Department and now works in the Trauma/Neurological/Surgical Intensive Care Unit at St. Joseph's Hospital in Tampa, Florida.

Keith's favorite interests include music, reading, Kentucky basketball, and, if he gets the chance, watching every minute of the Olympic Games.

REVIEWERS

Reamer L. Bushardt, PharmD, PA-C
Professor and Chair, Department of
    Physician Assistant Studies
Wake Forest University School of Medicine
Winston-Salem, North Carolina

Sarah E. Heeter, RN, BSN
Barnes-Jewish St. Peters Hospital
St. Peters, Missouri

Joshua J. Neumiller, PharmD, CDE, FASCP
Assistant Professor
Department of Pharmacotherapy
College of Pharmacy
Washington State University
Spokane, Washington

CONSULTANTS*

Katherine B. Barbee, MSN, ANP, F-NP-C
Kaiser Permanente
Washington, DC

Lisa Brown
Jackson State Community College
Jackson, Tennessee

Marla J. DeJong, RN, MS, CCRN, CEN, Capt
Wilford Hall Medical Center
Lackland Air Force Base, Texas

Diane M. Ford, RN, MS, CCRN
Andrews University
Berrien Springs, Michigan

Denise D. Hopkins, PharmD
College of Pharmacy
University of Arkansas
Little Rock, Arkansas

Barbara D. Horton, RN, MS
Arnot Ogden Medical Center School
    of Nursing
Elmira, New York

Mary Beth Jenkins, RN, CCRN, CAPA
Elliott One Day Surgery Center
Manchester, New Hampshire

Kelly W. Jones, PharmD, BCPS
McLeod Family Medicine Center
McLeod Regional Medical Center
Florence, South Carolina

Autumn E. Korson
Western Michigan University
    Bronson School of Nursing
Kalamazoo, Michigan

Linda Laskowski-Jones, RN, MS, CS, CCRN, CEN
Christiana Care Health System
Newark, Delaware

Jessica K. Leet, RN, BSN
Cardinal Glennon Children's Hospital
St. Louis, Missouri

Denise Macklin, BSN, RNC, CRNI
President, Professional Learning Systems,
    Inc.
Marietta, Georgia

Nancy L. McCartney
Valencia Community College
Orlando, Florida

Judith L. Myers, MSN, RN
Health Sciences Center
St. Louis University School of Nursing
St. Louis, Missouri

Kimberly R. Pugh, MSEd, RN, BS
Nurse Consultant
Baltimore, Maryland

Regina T. Schiavello, BSN, RNC
Wills Eye Hospital
Philadelphia, Pennsylvania

Gregory M. Susla, PharmD, FCCM
National Institutes of Health
Bethesda, Maryland

Elizabeth Taylor
Tennessee Wesleyan College of Nursing
Fort Saunders Regional
Knoxville, Tennessee

---

*The author acknowledges the work of the consultants in previous edition(s).

v

ACKNOWLEDGMENTS

I would like to thank my co-author Bob Kizior for his knowledge, experience, support, and friendship. We would like to give special thanks to Lauren Lake, Kari Terwelp, Robin Carter, Lisa Bushey, and the entire Elsevier team for their superior dedication, hard work, and belief in us. We gratefully acknowledge Amy Simpson and the staff at Graphic World for their tenacious detail and work. We would also like to thank Jim Witmer, RN, BSN, for his support, attention to detail, and knowledge. Without this wonderful team, none of this would be possible.

Keith J. Hodgson, RN, BSN, CCRN

DEDICATION

I dedicate my work on this edition in fond memory to my former student and longtime friend and co-author Barbara B. Hodgson. Our partnership spanned three decades and was hallmarked by our common goal to write a drug handbook that was current, complete, and accurate. Always compatible and mutually supportive, I will miss you, Barb.

Bob Kizior, BS, RPh

I dedicate this work to my sister, Lauren, a foundation for our family; my sister, Kathryn, for her love and support; my father, David Hodgson, the best father a son could have; my brothers-in-law, Andy and Jim, great additions to the family; the grandchildren, Paige Olivia, Logan James, Ryan James, and Dylan Boyd; to Jen Nicely for always being there; and to my band of brothers, Peter, Jamie, Miguel, Ritch, George, Jon, Domingo, Ben, Craig, Pat, and Shay.

We also make a special dedication to Barbara B. Hodgson, RN, OCN. She truly was a piece of something wonderful. Barbara often gave her love and support without needing any in return, and would do anything for a smile. Not only was she a colleague and a friend, she was also a small business owner, an artist, a dreamer, and an innovator. We hope the pride we offer in her honor comes close to what she always gave us. Her dedication and perseverance lives on.

Keith J. Hodgson, RN, BSN, CCRN

BIBLIOGRAPHY

Briggs GG, Freeman RK, Yaffe SJ: *Drugs in Pregnancy and Lactation: A Reference Guide to Fetal and Neonatal Risk*, ed 9, Philadelphia, 2011, Lippincott Williams & Wilkins.
Drug Facts and Comparisons 2013, Philadelphia, 2013, Lippincott Williams & Wilkins.
Generali J, Paxton L: *Black Box Warnings Study Guide 2013*, Black Box Rx LLC.
Lacy CF, Armstrong LL, Goldman MP, Lance LL: *Lexi-Comp's Drug Information Handbook*, ed 22, Hudson, OH, 2013–2014, Lexi-Comp.
Lexi-Comp's Drug Information Handbook for Oncology, ed 9, Hudson, OH, 2011, Lexi-Comp.
Natural Medicines Comprehensive Database, 2009.
Takemoto CK, Hodding JH, Kraus DM: *Lexi-Comp's Pediatric Dosage Handbook*, ed 20, Hudson, OH, 2013–2014, Lexi-Comp.
Trissel LA: *Handbook of Injectable Drugs*, ed 17, Bethesda, MD, 2013, American Society of Health-System Pharmacists.

ILLUSTRATION CREDITS

Kee JL, Hayes ER, McCuiston LE (eds): *Pharmacology: A Nursing Process Approach*, ed 7, Philadelphia, 2012, Saunders.
Mosby's GenRx, ed 12, St. Louis, 2004, Mosby.

PREFACE

Nurses are faced with the ever-challenging responsibility of ensuring safe and effective drug therapy for their patients. Not surprisingly, the greatest challenge for nurses is keeping up with the overwhelming amount of new drug information, including the latest FDA-approved drugs and changes to already approved drugs, such as new uses, dosage forms, warnings, and much more. Nurses must integrate this information into their patient care quickly and in an informed manner.

Saunders Nursing Drug Handbook 2015 is designed as an easy-to-use source of current drug information to help the busy nurse meet these challenges. What separates this book from others is that it guides the nurse through patient care to better practice and better care.

This handbook contains the following:

1. **An IV compatibility chart.** This handy chart is bound into the handbook to prevent accidental loss.
2. **The Drug Classifications section.** The action and uses for some of the most common clinical and pharmacotherapeutic classes are presented. Unique to this handbook, each class provides an at-a-glance table that compares all the generic drugs within the classification according to product availability, dosages, side effects, and other characteristics. Its half-page color tab ensures you can't miss it!
3. **An alphabetical listing of drug entries by generic name.** Blue letter thumb tabs help you page through this section quickly. Information on medications that contain a Black Box Alert is an added feature of the drug entries. This alert identifies those medications for which the FDA has issued a warning that the drugs may cause serious adverse effects. Tall Man lettering, with emphasis on certain syllables to avoid confusing similar sounding/looking medications, is shown in slim blue capitalized letters (e.g., *aceta**ZOLAMIDE***). High Alert drugs with a blue icon ▇▇▇ are considered dangerous by The Joint Commission and the Institute for Safe Medication Practices (ISMP) because if they are administered incorrectly, they may cause life-threatening or permanent harm to the patient. The entire High Alert generic drug entry sits on a blue-shaded background so that it's easy to spot! To make scanning pages easier, each new entry begins with a shaded box containing the generic name, pronunciation, trade name(s), fixed-combination(s), and classification(s).
4. **A comprehensive reference section.** Appendixes include vital information on calculation of doses; controlled drugs; chronic wound care; drugs of abuse; equianalgesic dosing; FDA pregnancy categories; herbals: common natural medicines; lifespan, cultural aspects, and pharmacogenomics of drug therapy; normal laboratory values; cytochrome P450 enzymes; poison antidotes; preventing medication errors; and parenteral fluid administration.
5. **Drugs by Disorder.** You'll find Drugs by Disorder in the front of the book for easy reference. It lists common disorders and the drugs most often used for treatment.
6. **The index.** The comprehensive index is located at the back of the book on light blue pages. Undoubtedly the best tool to help you navigate the handbook, the comprehensive index is organized by showing generic drug names in **bold,** trade names in regular type, classifications in *italics,* and the page number of the main drug entry listed first and in **bold.**

A DETAILED GUIDE TO THE SAUNDERS NURSING DRUG HANDBOOK

An intensive review by consultants and reviewers helped us to revise the **Saunders Nursing Drug Handbook** so that it is most useful in both educational and clinical practice. The main objective of the handbook is to provide essential drug information in a user-friendly format. The bulk of the handbook contains an alphabetical listing of drug entries by generic name.

To maintain the portability of this handbook and meet the challenge of keeping content current, we have also included additional information for some medications on the Evolve® Internet site. Users can also choose from 200 monographs for the most commonly used medications and customize and print drug cards. Evolve® also includes drug alerts (e.g., medications removed from the market) and drug updates (e.g., new drugs, updates on existing entries). Information is periodically added, allowing the nurse to keep abreast of current drug information.

You'll also notice that some entries for infrequently used medications are condensed to reflect only the absolutely essential points the nurse should know when called on to administer them.

We have incorporated the IV Incompatibilities/Compatibilities 🖼 heading. The drugs listed in this section are compatible or incompatible with the generic drug when administered directly by IV push, via a Y-site, or via IV piggyback. We have highlighted the intravenous drug administration and handling information with a special heading icon 🖋 and have broken it down by Reconstitution, Rate of Administration, and Storage.

We present entries in an order that follows the logical thought process the nurse undergoes whenever a drug is ordered for a patient:

- What is the drug?
- How is the drug classified?
- What does the drug do?
- What is the drug used for?
- Under what conditions should you **not** use the drug?
- How do you administer the drug?
- How do you store the drug?
- What is the dose of the drug?
- What should you monitor the patient for once he or she has received the drug?
- What do you assess the patient for?
- What interventions should you perform?
- What should you teach the patient?

The following are included within the drug entries:

Generic Name, Pronunciation, Trade Names. Each entry begins with the generic name and pronunciation, followed by the U.S. and Canadian trade names. Exclusively Canadian trade names are followed by a blue maple leaf 🍁. Trade names that were most prescribed in the year 2013 are underlined in this section.

Black Box Alert. This feature highlights drugs that carry a significant risk of serious or life-threatening adverse effects. Black Box Alerts are ordered by the FDA.

Do Not Confuse With. Drug names that sound similar to the generic and/or trade names are listed under this heading to help you avoid potential medication errors.

Fixed-Combination Drugs. Where appropriate, fixed-combinations, or drugs made up of two or more generic medications, are listed with the generic drug.

Pharmacotherapeutic and Clinical Classification Names. Each full entry includes both the pharmacotherapeutic and clinical classifications for the generic drug.

The page number of the classification description in the front of the book is provided in this section as well.

Action/Therapeutic Effect. This section describes how the drug is predicted to behave, with the expected therapeutic effect(s) under a separate heading.

Pharmacokinetics. This section includes the absorption, distribution, metabolism, excretion, and half-life of the medication. The half-life is bolded in blue for easy access.

Uses/Off-Label. The listing of uses for each drug includes both the FDA uses and the off-label uses. The off-label heading is shown in bold blue for emphasis.

Precautions. This heading incorporates a discussion about when the generic drug is contraindicated or should be used with caution. The cautions warn the nurse of specific situations in which a drug should be closely monitored.

Lifespan Considerations ⚥. This section includes the pregnancy category and lactation data and age-specific information concerning children and elderly people.

Interactions. This heading enumerates drug, food, and herbal interactions with the generic drug. As the number of medications a patient receives increases, awareness of drug interactions becomes more important. Also included is information about therapeutic and toxic blood levels in addition to the altered lab values that show what effects the drug may have on lab results.

Product Availability. Each drug monograph gives the form and availability of the drug. The icon 🗑 identifies non-crushable drug forms.

Administration/Handling. Instructions for administration are given for each route of administration (e.g., IV, IM, PO, rectal). Special handling, such as refrigeration, is also included where applicable. The routes in this section are always presented in the order IV, IM, Subcutaneous, and PO, with subsequent routes in alphabetical order (e.g., Ophthalmic, Otic, Topical). **IV administration** 🗑 is broken down by reconstitution, rate of administration (how fast the IV should be given), and storage (including how long the medication is stable once reconstituted).

IV Incompatibilities/IV Compatibilities 🖾. These sections give the nurse the most comprehensive compatibility information possible when administering medications by direct IV push, via a Y-site, or via IV piggyback.

Indications/Routes/Dosage. Each full entry provides specific dosing guidelines for adults, elderly people, children, and patients with renal and/or hepatic impairment. Dosages are clearly indicated for each approved indication and route.

Side Effects. Side effects are defined as those responses that are usually predictable with the drug, are **not** life-threatening, and may or may not require discontinuation of the drug. Unique to this handbook, side effects are grouped by frequency listed from highest occurrence percentage to lowest so that the nurse can focus on patient care without wading through myriad signs and symptoms of side effects.

Adverse Effects/Toxic Reactions. Adverse effects and toxic reactions are very serious and often life-threatening undesirable responses that require prompt intervention from a health care provider.

Nursing Considerations. Nursing considerations are organized as care is organized. That is:

- What needs to be assessed or done before the first dose is administered? (Baseline Assessment)
- What interventions and evaluations are needed during drug therapy? (Intervention/Evaluation)
- What explicit teaching is needed for the patient and family? (Patient/Family Teaching)

Saunders Nursing Drug Handbook is an easy-to-use source of current drug information for nurses, students, and other health care providers. It is our hope that this handbook will help you provide quality care to your patients.

We welcome any comments you may have that would help us to improve future editions of the handbook. Please contact us via the publisher at *http://evolve.elsevier.com/SaundersNDH.*

Robert J. Kizior, BS, RPh
Keith J. Hodgson, RN, BSN, CCRN

NEWLY APPROVED MEDICATIONS

Name	Indication
Ado-trastuzumab (Kadcyla)	*HER2*-targeted antibody and microtubule inhibitor conjugate indicated for treatment of *HER2*-positive metastatic breast cancer
Afatinib (Gilotrif)	Kinase inhibitor for certain types of metastatic non–small cell lung cancer
Alogliptin (Nesina)	DDP-4 inhibitor indicated as an adjunct to diet and exercise to improve glycemic control in adults with type 2 diabetes
Canagliflozin (Invokana)	Sodium glucose co-transporter 2 inhibitor indicated as adjunct to diet and exercise to improve glycemic control in adults with type 2 diabetes
Crofelemer (Fuilyzaq)*	Antidiarrheal for symptomatic relief of noninfectious diarrhea in adult patients with HIV on antiretroviral therapy
Cysteamine (Procsybi)*	Cysteine-depleting agent for management of nephropathic cystinosis
Dabrafenib (Tafinlar)	Kinase inhibitor indicated for treatment of unresectable or metastatic melanoma with *BRAF V600E* mutation
Dimethyl fumarate (Tecfidera)	Fumaric acid ester for the treatment of relapsing-remitting multiple sclerosis
Dolutagravir (Tivicay)	Integrase strand transfer inhibitor for HIV-1 infection
Ferric carboxymaltose (Injectafer)	Injectable iron replacement formulation for iron deficiency anemia
Ibrutinib (Imbruvica)	Oral tyrosine kinase inhibitor for the treatment of mantle cell lymphoma
Levomilnacipram (Fetzima)	SNRI for depression
Macitentan (Opsumit)	Endothelin receptor antagonist for pulmonary arterial hypertension
Mipomersen (Kynamro)	Oligonucleotide inhibitor indicated as an adjunct to diet and medications to reduce LDL-C, apo-B, total cholesterol and non–HDL-C in patients with homozygous familial hypercholesterolemia
Obinutuzumab (Gazyva)	CD20-directed cytolytic antibody for treatment of chronic lymphocytic leukemia

continued

*Selected new drugs approved by the FDA in late 2013. Monographs for these drugs are on *Evolve*.

xi

Name	Indication
Ospemifene (Osphena)	Estrogen agonist/antagonist indicated for treatment of moderate to severe dyspareunia due to menopause
Pegaspargase (Oncaspar)	Treatment of ALL
Pomalidomide (Pohmalyst)	Thalidomide analogue indicated for patients with multiple myeloma
Prothrombin complex concentrate (Kcentra)	Indicated for urgent reversal of acquired coagulation factor deficiency induced by vitamin K antagonist therapy in adults with acute major bleeding
Riociguat (Adempax)	Guanylate cyclase stimulator for pulmonary hypertension
Simeprevir (Olysio)	Protease inhibitor for the treatment of chronic hepatitis C virus infection
Sofosbuvir (Sovaldi)	Oral nucleotide analogue for treatment of chronic hepatitis C virus infection
Sucroferric oxyhydroxide (Velphoro)	Chewable, iron-based phosphate binder for the control of serum phosphorus levels in patients with chronic kidney disease on dialysis
Taliglucerase alfa (Elelyso)*	Lysosomal enzyme for long-term replacement for adults with confirmed diagnosis of type 1 Gaucher disease
Trametinib (Mekinest)	Kinase inhibitor indicated for treatment of unresectable or metastatic melanoma with *BRAF V600E* mutation
Vortioxetene (Brintellix)	Indicated for the treatment of major depression

*Selected new drugs approved by the FDA in late 2013. Monographs for these drugs are on *Evolve*.

DRUGS BY DISORDER

Note: Not all medications appropriate for a given condition are listed, nor are those not listed inappropriate.
Generic names appear first, followed by brand names in parentheses.

Alcohol dependence
Acamprosate (Campral)
Disulfiram (Antabuse)
Naltrexone (Depade, ReVia, Vivitrol)

Allergic rhinitis
Azelastine (Astepro)
Azelastine/fluticasone (Dymista)
Beclomethasone (Beconase AQ)
Budesonide (Rhinocort Aqua)
Ciclesonide (Omnaris)
Flunisolide (Nasarel)
Fluticasone (Flonase)
Mometasone (Nasonex)
Olopatadine (Patanase)
Triamcinolone (Nasacort)

Allergy
Beclomethasone (Beclovent, Vanceril)
Betamethasone (Celestone)
Brompheniramine (Dimetane)
Budesonide (Pulmicort, Rhinocort)
Cetirizine (Zyrtec)
Chlorpheniramine (Chlor-Trimeton)
Clemastine (Tavist)
Cyproheptadine (Periactin)
Desloratadine (Clarinex)
Dexamethasone (Decadron)
Dimenhydrinate (Dramamine)
Diphenhydramine (Benadryl)
Epinephrine (Adrenalin)
Fexofenadine (Allegra)
Flunisolide (AeroBid, Nasalide)
Fluticasone (Flovent)
Hydrocortisone (Solu-Cortef)
Levocetirizine (Xyzal)
Loratadine (Claritin)
Prednisolone (Prelone)
Prednisone (Deltasone)
Promethazine (Phenergan)
Triamcinolone (Kenalog)

Alzheimer's disease
Donepezil (Aricept, Aricept ODT)
Galantamine (Razadyne, Razadyne ER)
Memantine (Namenda)
Rivastigmine (Exelon, Exelon Patch)

Angina
Amlodipine (Norvasc)
Atenolol (Tenormin)
Diltiazem (Cardizem, Dilacor)
Isosorbide (Imdur, Isordil)
Metoprolol (Lopressor)
Nadolol (Corgard)
Nicardipine (Cardene)
Nifedipine (Adalat, Procardia)
Nitroglycerin
Propranolol (Inderal)
Verapamil (Calan, Isoptin)

Anxiety
Alprazolam (Xanax)
Buspirone (BuSpar)
Diazepam (Valium)
Hydroxyzine (Atarax, Vistaril)
Lorazepam (Ativan)
Oxazepam (Serax)
Paroxetine (Paxil)
Trazodone (Desyrel)
Venlafaxine (Effexor)

Arrhythmias
Acebutolol (Sectral)
Adenosine (Adenocard)
Amiodarone (Cordarone, Pacerone)
Digoxin (Lanoxin)
Diltiazem (Cardizem, Dilacor)
Disopyramide (Norpace)
Dofetilide (Tikosyn)
Dronedarone (Multaq)
Esmolol (Brevibloc)
Flecainide (Tambocor)

Ibutilide (Corvert)
Lidocaine
Magnesium sulfate
Metoprolol (Lopressor)
Mexiletine (Mexitil)
Procainamide (Procan, Pronestyl)
Propafenone (Rythmol)
Propranolol (Inderal)
Quinidine
Sotalol (Betapace)
Tocainide (Tonocard)
Verapamil (Calan, Isoptin)

Arthritis, rheumatoid (RA)
Abatacept (Orencia)
Adalimumab (Humira)
Anakinra (Kineret)
Aspirin
Auranofin (Ridaura)
Aurothioglucose (Solganal)
Azathioprine (Imuran)
Capsaicin (Zostrix)
Celecoxib (Celebrex)
Certolizumab (Cimzia)
Cyclosporine (Sandimmune)
Diclofenac (Cataflam, Voltaren)
Diflunisal (Dolobid)
Etanercept (Enbrel)
Golimumab (Simponi)
Hydroxychloroquine (Plaquenil)
Infliximab (Remicade)
Leflunomide (Arava)
Methotrexate
Penicillamine (Cuprimine)
Prednisone (Deltasone)
Rituximab (Rituxan)
Sulfasalazine (Azulfidine-EN)
Tocilizumab (Actemra)
Tofacitinib (Xeljanz)

Asthma
Albuterol (Proventil, Ventolin)
Aminophylline (Theophylline)
Arformoterol (Brovana)
Beclomethasone (Beclovent, Vanceril)
Budesonide (Pulmicort)
Ciclesonide (Alvesco)
Cromolyn (Crolom, Intal)
Epinephrine (Adrenalin)
Flunisolide (AeroBid)
Fluticasone (Flovent)
Formoterol (Foradil)
Hydrocortisone (Solu-Cortef)
Ipratropium (Atrovent)

Levalbuterol (Xopenex)
Metaproterenol (Alupent)
Methylprednisolone (Solu-Medrol)
Mometasone (Asmanex)
Montelukast (Singulair)
Nedocromil (Tilade)
Prednisolone (Prelone)
Prednisone (Deltasone)
Salmeterol (Serevent)
Terbutaline (Brethine)
Theophylline (SloBid)
Zafirlukast (Accolate)
Zileuton (Zyflo, Zyflo CR)

Attention-deficit hyperactivity disorder (ADHD)
Atomoxetine (Strattera)
Bupropion (Wellbutrin)
Clonidine (Catapres, Kapvay)
Desipramine (Norpramin)
Dexmethylphenidate (Focalin, Focalin XR)
Dextroamphetamine (Dexedrine, Dextrostat)
Guanfacine (Intuniv)
Imipramine (Tofranil)
Lisdexamfetamine (Vyvanse)
Methylphenidate (Concerta, Daytrana, Focalin, Methylin, Ritalin)
Mixed amphetamine (dextroamphetamine and amphetamine salts) (Adderall, Adderall XR)
Modafinil (Provigil)
Nortriptyline (Aventyl, Pamelor)
Venlafaxine (Effexor)

Benign prostatic hypertrophy (BPH)
Alfuzosin (Uroxatral)
Doxazosin (Cardura)
Dutasteride (Avodart)
Finasteride (Proscar)
Mirabegron (Myrbetriq)
Silodosin (Rapaflo)
Tadalafil (Cialis)
Tamsulosin (Flomax)
Terazosin (Hytrin)

Bipolar disorder (mania)
Carbamazepine (Tegretol)
Lamotrigine (Lamictal)
Lithium (Lithobid)
Oxcarbazepine (Trileptal)
Quetiapine (Seroquel)
Valproic acid (Depakene, Depakote)

Bladder hyperactivity
Darifenacin (Enablex)
Oxybutynin (Ditropan, Gelnique)
Solifenacin (VESIcare)
Tolterodine (Detrol)
Trospium (Sanctura)

Bronchospasm
Albuterol (Proventil, Ventolin)
Bitolterol (Tornalate)
Levalbuterol (Xopenex)
Metaproterenol (Alupent)
Salmeterol (Serevent)
Terbutaline (Brethine)

Cancer
Abarelix (Plenaxis)
Abiraterone (Zytiga)
Ado-trastuzumab (Kadeyla)
Afatinib (Gilotrif)
Aldesleukin (Proleukin)
Alemtuzumab (Campath)
Alitretinoin (Panretin)
Altretamine (Hexalen)
Anastrozole (Arimidex)
Arsenic trioxide (Trisenox)
Asparaginase (Elspar)
Axitinib (Inlyta)
Azacitidine (Vidaza)
BCG (TheraCys, Tice BCG)
Bendamustine (Treanda)
Bevacizumab (Avastin)
Bexarotene (Targretin)
Bicalutamide (Casodex)
Bleomycin (Blenoxane)
Bortezomib (Velcade)
Bosutinib (Bosulif)
Brentuximab (Adcetris)
Busulfan (Myleran)
Cabazitaxel (Jevtana)
Cabozantinib (Cometriq)
Capecitabine (Xeloda)
Carboplatin (Paraplatin)
Carfilzomib (Kyprolis)
Carmustine (BiCNU)
Cetuximab (Erbitux)
Chlorambucil (Leukeran)
Cisplatin (Platinol)
Cladribine (Leustatin)
Clofarabine (Clolar)
Crizotinib (Xalkori)
Cyclophosphamide (Cytoxan)
Cytarabine (Ara-C, Cytosar)

Dabrafenib (Tafinlar)
Dacarbazine (DTIC)
Dactinomycin (Cosmegen)
Dasatinib (Sprycel)
Daunorubicin (Cerubidine, DaunoXome)
Degarelix (Firmagon)
Denileukin (Ontak)
Docetaxel (Taxotere)
Doxorubicin (Adriamycin, Doxil)
Enzalutamide (Xtandi)
Epirubicin (Ellence)
Eribulin (Halaven)
Erlotinib (Tarceva)
Estramustine (Emcyt)
Etoposide (VePesid)
Everolimus (Afinitor)
Fludarabine (Fludara)
Fluorouracil
Flutamide (Eulexin)
Fulvestrant (Faslodex)
Gefitinib (Iressa)
Gemcitabine (Gemzar)
Goserelin (Zoladex)
Hydroxyurea (Hydrea)
Ibritumomab (Zevalin)
Ibrutinib (Imbruvica)
Idarubicin (Idamycin)
Ifosfamide (Ifex)
Imatinib (Gleevec)
Interferon alfa-2b (Intron A)
Ipilimumab (Yervoy)
Irinotecan (Camptosar)
Ixabepilone (Ixempra)
Lapatinib (Tykerb)
Letrozole (Femara)
Leuprolide (Lupron)
Lomustine (CeeNU)
Mechlorethamine (Mustargen)
Megestrol (Megace)
Melphalan (Alkeran)
Mercaptopurine (Purinethol)
Methotrexate
Mitomycin (Mutamycin)
Mitotane (Lysodren)
Mitoxantrone (Novantrone)
Nelarabine (Arranon)
Nilotinib (Tasigna)
Nilutamide (Nilandron)
Obinutuzumab (Gazyva)
Ofatumumab (Arzerra)
Omacetaxine (Synribo)
Oxaliplatin (Eloxatin)
Paclitaxel (Taxol)
Panitumumab (Vectibix)

Pazopanib (Votrient)
Pegaspargase (Oncaspar)
Pemetrexed (Alimta)
Pentostatin (Nipent)
Pertuzumab (Perjeta)
Plicamycin (Mithracin)
Pomalidomide (Pohmalyst)
Ponatinib (Iclusig)
Pralatrexate (Folotyn)
Procarbazine (Matulane)
Rasburicase (Elitek)
Regorafenib (Stivarga)
Rituximab (Rituxan)
Romidepsin (Istodax)
Sipuleucel-T (Provenge)
Sorafenib (Nexavar)
Streptozocin (Zanosar)
Sunitinib (Sutent)
Tamoxifen (Nolvadex)
Temozolomide (Temodar)
Temsirolimus (Torisel)
Teniposide (Vumon)
Thioguanine
Thiotepa (Thioplex)
Tipifarnib (Zarnestra)
Topotecan (Hycamtin)
Toremifene (Fareston)
Tositumomab (Bexxar)
Trametinib (Mekinest)
Trastuzumab (Herceptin)
Tretinoin (ATRA, Vesanoid)
Valrubicin (Valstar)
Vandetanib (Caprelsa)
Vemurafenib (Zelboraf)
Vinblastine (Velban)
Vincristine (Oncovin)
Vinorelbine (Navelbine)
Vismodegib (Erivedge)
Vorinostat (Zolinza)

Cerebrovascular accident (CVA)
Aspirin
Clopidogrel (Plavix)
Heparin
Nimodipine (Nimotop)
Prasugrel (Effient)
Ticlopidine (Ticlid)
Warfarin (Coumadin)

Chronic obstructive pulmonary disease (COPD)
Aclidinium (Tudorza)
Albuterol (Proventil HFA, Ventolin HFA)

Aminophylline (Theophylline)
Arformoterol (Brovana)
Budesonide (Pulmicort)
Budesonide/formoterol (Symbicort)
Formoterol (Foradil)
Indacaterol (Arcapta)
Ipratropium (Atrovent HFA)
Levalbuterol (Xopenex)
Pirbuterol (Maxair)
Roflumilast (Daliresp)
Salmeterol (Serevent)
Salmeterol/fluticasone (Advair)
Theophylline (Theochron, Theo ZY)
Tiotropium (Spiriva)

Constipation
Bisacodyl (Dulcolax)
Docusate (Colace)
Lactulose (Kristalose)
Lubiprostone (Amitiza)
Methylcellulose (Citrucel)
Milk of magnesia (MOM)
Polyethylene glycol (MiraLax)
Psyllium (Metamucil)
Senna (Senokot)
Tegaserod (Zelnorm)

Crohn's disease
Adalimumab (Humira)
Azathioprine (Azasan)
Budesonide (Entocort EC)
Certolizumab (Cimzia)
Hydrocortisone (Cortenema)
Infliximab (Remicade)
Mesalamine (Asacol, Pentasa)
Natalizumab (Tysabri)
Sulfasalazine (Azulfidine)

Deep vein thrombosis (DVT)
Dalteparin (Fragmin)
Enoxaparin (Lovenox)
Heparin
Tinzaparin (Innohep)
Warfarin (Coumadin)

Depression
Amitriptyline (Elavil, Endep)
Bupropion (Wellbutrin)
Citalopram (Celexa)
Clomipramine (Anafranil)
Desipramine (Norpramin)
Desvenlafaxine (Pristiq)
Doxepin (Sinequan)

Duloxetine (Cymbalta)
Escitalopram (Lexapro)
Fluoxetine (Prozac)
Fluvoxamine (Luvox)
Ievomilnacipram (Fetzima)
Imipramine (Tofranil)
Maprotiline (Ludiomil)
Mirtazapine (Remeron)
Nortriptyline (Aventyl, Pamelor)
Paroxetine (Paxil)
Phenelzine (Nardil)
Selegiline (Emsam)
Sertraline (Zoloft)
Tranylcypromine (Parnate)
Trazodone (Desyrel)
Venlafaxine (Effexor)
Vilazodone (Viibryd)
Vortioxetene (Brintellix)

Diabetes mellitus
Acarbose (Precose)
Alogliptin (Nesina)
Bromocriptine (Cycloset)
Canaglifozin (Invokana)
Colesevelam (Welchol)
Exenatide (Byetta)
Glimepiride (Amaryl)
Glipizide (Glucotrol)
Glyburide (Micronase)
Insulin preparations
Linagliptin (Tradjenta)
Liraglutide (Victoza)
Metformin (Glucophage)
Miglitol (Glyset)
Nateglinide (Starlix)
Pioglitazone (Actos)
Pramlintide (Symlin)
Repaglinide (Prandin)
Rosiglitazone (Avandia)
Saxagliptin (Onglyza)
Sitagliptin (Januvia)

Diabetic peripheral neuropathy
Amitriptyline (Elavil)
Bupropion (Wellbutrin)
Capsaicin (Trixaicin)
Carbamazepine (Tegretol)
Citalopram (Celexa)
Desipramine (Norpramin)
Duloxetine (Cymbalta)
Gabapentin (Neurontin)
Lamotrigine (Lamictal)
Lidocaine patch (Lidoderm)

Nortriptyline (Pamelor)
Oxcarbazepine (Trileptal)
Oxycodone (OxyContin)
Paroxetine (Paxil)
Pregabalin (Lyrica)
Tramadol (Ultram)
Valproic acid (Depakote)
Venlafaxine, extended-release
(Effexor XR)

Diarrhea
Bismuth subsalicylate (Pepto-Bismol)
Diphenoxylate and atropine (Lomotil)
Fidaxomicin (Dificid)
Kaolin-pectin (Kaopectate)
Loperamide (Imodium)
Octreotide (Sandostatin)
Rifaximin (Xifaxan)

Duodenal, gastric ulcer
Cimetidine (Tagamet)
Esomeprazole (Nexium)
Famotidine (Pepcid)
Lansoprazole (Prevacid)
Misoprostol (Cytotec)
Nizatidine (Axid)
Omeprazole (Prilosec)
Pantoprazole (Protonix)
Rabeprazole (Aciphex)
Ranitidine (Zantac)
Sucralfate (Carafate)

Edema
Amiloride (Midamor)
Bumetanide (Bumex)
Chlorthalidone (Hygroton)
Ethacrynic acid (Edecrin)
Furosemide (Lasix)
Hydrochlorothiazide (HydroDIURIL)
Indapamide (Lozol)
Metolazone (Zaroxolyn)
Spironolactone (Aldactone)
Torsemide (Demadex)
Triamterene (Dyrenium)

Epilepsy
Acetazolamide (Diamox)
Carbamazepine (Tegretol)
Clobazam (Onfi)
Clonazepam (Klonopin)
Clorazepate (Tranxene)
Diazepam (Valium)
Eslicarbazepine (Aptiom)

Ezogabine (Potiga)
Fosphenytoin (Cerebyx)
Gabapentin (Neurontin)
Lamotrigine (Lamictal, Lamictal ODT,
    Lamictal XR)
Levetiracetam (Keppra)
Lorazepam (Ativan)
Oxcarbazepine (Trileptal)
Perampanel (Fycompa)
Phenobarbital
Phenytoin (Dilantin)
Primidone (Mysoline)
Tiagabine (Gabitril)
Topiramate (Topamax)
Valproic acid (Depakene, Depakote)
Vigabatrin (Sabril)
Zonisamide (Zonegran)

Esophageal reflux, esophagitis
Cimetidine (Tagamet)
Dexlansoprazole (Kapidex)
Esomeprazole (Nexium)
Famotidine (Pepcid)
Lansoprazole (Prevacid)
Nizatidine (Axid)
Omeprazole (Prilosec)
Pantoprazole (Protonix)
Rabeprazole (Aciphex)
Ranitidine (Zantac)

Fever
Acetaminophen (Tylenol)
Aspirin
Ibuprofen (Advil, Caldolor, Motrin)
Naproxen (Aleve, Anaprox, Naprosyn)

Fibromyalgia
Acetaminophen (Tylenol)
Amitriptyline (Elavil)
Carisoprodol (Soma)
Citalopram (Celexa)
Cyclobenzaprine (Flexeril)
Duloxetine (Cymbalta)
Fluoxetine (Prozac)
Gabapentin (Neurontin)
Milnacipran (Savella)
Paroxetine (Paxil)
Pregabalin (Lyrica)
Tramadol (Ultram)
Venlafaxine (Effexor)

Gastritis
Cimetidine (Tagamet)
Famotidine (Pepcid)

Nizatidine (Axid)
Ranitidine (Zantac)

Gastroesophageal reflux disease (GERD)
Cimetidine (Tagamet)
Dexlansoprazole (Kapidex)
Esomeprazole (Nexium)
Famotidine (Pepcid)
Lansoprazole (Prevacid)
Metoclopramide (Metozolv ODT, Reglan)
Nizatidine (Axid)
Omeprazole (Prilosec)
Pantoprazole (Protonix)
Rabeprazole (Aciphex)
Ranitidine (Zantac)

Glaucoma
Acetazolamide (Diamox)
Apraclonidine (Iopidine)
Betaxolol (Betoptic)
Bimatoprost (Lumigan)
Brimonidine (Alphagan)
Brinzolamide (Azopt)
Carbachol
Carteolol (Ocupress)
Dipivefrin (Propine)
Dorzolamide (Trusopt)
Echothiophate iodide (Phospholine)
Latanoprost (Xalatan)
Levobunolol (Betagan)
Metipranolol (OptiPranolol)
Pilocarpine (Isopto Carpine)
Timolol (Timoptic)
Travoprost (Travatan)
Unoprostone (Rescula)

Gout
Allopurinol (Zyloprim)
Colchicine (Colcrys)
Febuxostat (Uloric)
Ibuprofen (Motrin)
Indomethacin (Indocin)
Naproxen (Naprosyn)
Pegloticase (Krystexxa)
Piroxicam (Feldene)
Probenecid (Benemid)
Sulindac (Clinoril)

Heart failure (HF)
Bisoprolol (Zebeta)
Bumetanide (Bumex)
Candesartan (Atacand)
Captopril (Capoten)

Carvedilol (Coreg)
Digoxin (Lanoxin)
Dobutamine (Dobutrex)
Dopamine (Intropin)
Enalapril (Vasotec)
Eplerenone (Inspra)
Fosinopril (Monopril)
Furosemide (Lasix)
Hydralazine (Apresoline)
Isosorbide (Isordil)
Lisinopril (Prinivil, Zestril)
Losartan (Cozaar)
Metoprolol (Lopressor)
Milrinone (Primacor)
Nitroglycerin
Quinapril (Accupril)
Ramipril (Altace)
Spironolactone (Aldactone)
Torsemide (Demadex)
Valsartan (Diovan)

Hepatitis B
Adefovir (Hepsera)
Entecavir (Baraclude)
Lamivudine (Epivir)
Peginterferon alpha-2a (Pegasys)
Telbivudine (Tyzeka)
Tenofovir (Viread)

Hepatitis C
Boceprevir (Victrelis)
Interferon alfa-2b (Intron-A)
Interferon alfacon-1 (Infergen)
Peginterferon alfa-2a (Pegasys)
Peginterferon alfa-2b (Pegintron)
Ribavirin (Copegus)
Simeprevir (Olysio)
Sofosbuvir (Sovaldi)
Telaprevir (Incivek)

Human immunodeficiency virus (HIV)
Abacavir (Ziagen)
Atazanavir (Reyataz)
Darunavir (Prezista)
Delavirdine (Rescriptor)
Didanosine (Videx)
Dolutegravir (Tivicay)
Efavirenz (Sustiva)
Emtricitabine (Emtriva)
Enfuvirtide (Fuzeon)
Etravirine (Intelence)
Fosamprenavir (Lexiva)
Indinavir (Crixivan)

Lamivudine (Epivir)
Lopinavir/ritonavir (Kaletra)
Maraviroc (Selzentry)
Nelfinavir (Viracept)
Nevirapine (Viramune)
Raltegravir (Isentress)
Rilpivirine (Edurant)
Ritonavir (Norvir)
Saquinavir (Invirase)
Stavudine (Zerit)
Stribild (cobicistat, elvitagravir,
    emtricitabine, tenafovir)
Tenofovir (Viread)
Tesamorelin (Egrifta)
Tipranavir (Aptivus)
Zidovudine (AZT, Retrovir)

Hypercholesterolemia
Atorvastatin (Lipitor)
Cholestyramine (Questran)
Colesevelam (Welchol)
Colestipol (Colestid)
Ezetimibe (Zetia)
Fenofibrate (Antara, Lofibra, Tricor)
Fish oil (Lovaza)
Fluvastatin (Lescol)
Gemfibrozil (Lopid)
Lomitapide (Juxapid)
Lovastatin (Altoprev, Mevacor)
Mipomersen (Kynamro)
Niacin (Niaspan, Slo-Niacin)
Pitavastatin (Livalo)
Pravastatin (Pravachol)
Rosuvastatin (Crestor)
Simvastatin (Zocor)

Hyperphosphatemia
Aluminum salts
Calcium salts
Lanthanum (Fosrenol)
Sevelamer (Renagel)

Hypertension
Aliskiren (Tekturna)
Amlodipine (Norvasc)
Atenolol (Tenormin)
Azilsartan (Edarbi)
Benazepril (Lotensin)
Bisoprolol (Zebeta)
Candesartan (Atacand)
Captopril (Capoten)
Clevidipine (Cleviprex)
Clonidine (Catapres)

Diltiazem (Cardizem, Dilacor)
Doxazosin (Cardura)
Enalapril (Vasotec)
Eplerenone (Inspra)
Eprosartan (Teveten)
Felodipine (Plendil)
Fosinopril (Monopril)
Hydralazine (Apresoline)
Hydrochlorothiazide (HydroDIURIL)
Indapamide (Lozol)
Irbesartan (Avapro)
Isradipine (DynaCirc)
Labetalol (Normodyne, Trandate)
Lisinopril (Prinivil, Zestril)
Losartan (Cozaar)
Methyldopa (Aldomet)
Metolazone (Diulo, Zaroxolyn)
Metoprolol (Lopressor)
Minoxidil (Loniten)
Moexipril (Univasc)
Nadolol (Corgard)
Nebivolol (Bystolic)
Nicardipine (Cardene)
Nifedipine (Adalat, Procardia)
Nitroglycerin
Nitroprusside (Nipride)
Olmesartan (Benicar)
Perindopril (Aceon)
Pindolol (Visken)
Prazosin (Minipress)
Propranolol (Inderal)
Quinapril (Accupril)
Ramipril (Altace)
Spironolactone (Aldactone)
Telmisartan (Micardis)
Terazosin (Hytrin)
Timolol (Blocadren)
Trandolapril (Mavik)
Valsartan (Diovan)
Verapamil (Calan, Isoptin)

Hypertriglyceridemia
Atorvastatin (Lipitor)
Colesevelam (Welchol)
Fenofibrate (Tricor)
Fluvastatin (Lescol)
Gemfibrozil (Lopid)
Icosapent (Vascepa)
Lovastatin (Mevacor)
Niacin (Niaspan)
Omega-3 acid ethyl esters (Lovaza)
Pravastatin (Pravachol)
Rosuvastatin (Crestor)
Simvastatin (Zocor)

Hyperuricemia
Allopurinol (Zyloprim)
Febuxostat (Uloric)
Pegloticase (Krystexxa)
Probenecid (Benemid)

Hypotension
Dobutamine (Dobutrex)
Dopamine (Intropin)
Ephedrine
Epinephrine
Norepinephrine (Levophed)
Phenylephrine (Neo-Synephrine)

Hypothyroidism
Levothyroxine (Levoxyl, Synthroid)
Liothyronine (Cytomel)
Thyroid

Idiopathic thrombocytopenic purpura (ITP)
Cyclophosphamide (Cytoxan)
Dexamethasone (Decadron)
Hydrocortisone (Solu-Cortef)
Immune globulin intravenous
Methylprednisolone (Solu-Medrol)
Prednisone
$Rh_o(D)$ immune globulin (RhoGam)
Rituximab (Rituxan)

Insomnia
Diphenhydramine (Benadryl)
Estazolam (ProSom)
Eszopiclone (Lunesta)
Flurazepam (Dalmane)
Ramelteon (Rozerem)
Temazepam (Restoril)
Zaleplon (Sonata)
Zolpidem (Ambien, Edluar)

Migraine headaches
Almotriptan (Axert)
Amitriptyline (Elavil, Endep)
Diclofenac (Cambia)
Dihydroergotamine
Eletriptan (Relpax)
Ergotamine (Ergomar)
Frovatriptan (Frova)
Naratriptan (Amerge)
Propranolol (Inderal)
Rizatriptan (Maxalt)
Sumatriptan (Imitrex)
Zolmitriptan (Zomig)

Multiple sclerosis (MS)
Dalfampridine (Ampyra)
Dimethyl fumarate (Tecfidera)
Fingolimod (Gilenya)
Glatiramer (Copaxone)
Interferon beta-1a (Avonex, Rebif)
Interferon beta-1b (Betaseron, Extavia)
Mitoxantrone (Novantrone)
Natalizumab (Tysabri)
Teriflunomide (Aubagio)

Myelodysplastic syndrome
Azacitidine (Vidaza)
Clofarabine (Clolar)
Decitabine (Dacogen)
Lenalidomide (Revlimid)

Myocardial infarction (MI)
Alteplase (Activase)
Aspirin
Atenolol (Tenormin)
Captopril (Capoten)
Clopidogrel (Plavix)
Dalteparin (Fragmin)
Diltiazem (Cardizem, Dilacor)
Enalapril (Vasotec)
Enoxaparin (Lovenox)
Heparin
Lidocaine
Lisinopril (Prinivil, Zestril)
Metoprolol (Lopressor)
Morphine
Nitroglycerin
Propranolol (Inderal)
Quinapril (Accupril)
Ramipril (Altace)
Reteplase (Retavase)
Streptokinase
Timolol (Blocadren)
Warfarin (Coumadin)

Nausea
Aprepitant (Emend)
Chlorpromazine (Thorazine)
Dexamethasone (Decadron)
Dimenhydrinate (Dramamine)
Dolasetron (Anzemet)
Dronabinol (Marinol)
Droperidol (Inapsine)
Fosaprepitant (Emend)
Granisetron (Kytril)
Hydroxyzine (Vistaril)
Lorazepam (Ativan)
Meclizine (Antivert)

Metoclopramide (Reglan)
Nabilone (Cesamet)
Ondansetron (Zofran)
Palonosetron (Aloxi)
Prochlorperazine (Compazine)
Promethazine (Phenergan)
Trimethobenzamide (Tigan)

Obesity
Benzphetamine (Didrex)
Bupropion (Wellbutrin)
Diethylpropion (Tenuate)
Exenatide (Bydureon, Byetta)
Lorcaserin (Belviq)
Methamphetamine (Desoxyn)
Orlistat (Alli, Xenical)
Phendimetrazine (Bontril)
Phentermine (Ionamin)
Phentermine and topiramate (Qsymia)

Obsessive-compulsive disorder (OCD)
Citalopram (Celexa)
Clomipramine (Anafranil)
Escitalopram (Lexapro)
Fluoxetine (Prozac)
Fluvoxamine (Luvox)
Paroxetine (Paxil)
Sertraline (Zoloft)

Organ transplant, rejection prophylaxis
Azathioprine (Imuran)
Basiliximab (Simulect)
Belatacept (Nulojix)
Cyclophosphamide (Cytoxan, Neosar)
Cyclosporine (Sandimmune)
Daclizumab (Zenapax)
Everolimus (Zortress)
Mycophenolate (CellCept)
Sirolimus (Rapamune)
Tacrolimus (Prograf)

Osteoarthritis
Acetaminophen (Tylenol)
Celecoxib (Celebrex)
Diclofenac (Cataflam, Pennsaid, Voltaren)
Etodolac (Lodine)
Flavocoxid (Limbrel)
Flurbiprofen (Ansaid)
Ibuprofen (Motrin)
Ketoprofen (Orudis)
Meloxicam (Mobic)
Nabumetone (Relafen)
Naproxen (Naprosyn)

Oxaprozin (Daypro)
Piroxicam (Feldene)
Salicylates (Aspirin)
Sulindac (Clinoril)
Tramadol (Ultram)

Osteoporosis
Alendronate (Fosamax)
Calcitonin (Miacalcin)
Calcium salts
Denosumab (Prolia)
Ibandronate (Boniva)
Raloxifene (Evista)
Risedronate (Actonel)
Teriparatide (Forteo)
Vitamin D
Zoledronic acid (Reclast)

Paget's disease
Alendronate (Fosamax)
Calcitonin (Miacalcin)
Etidronate (Didronel)
Pamidronate (Aredia)
Risedronate (Actonel)
Tiludronate (Skelid)
Zoledronic acid (Reclast)

Pain, mild to moderate
Acetaminophen (Tylenol)
Aspirin
Celecoxib (Celebrex)
Codeine
Diclofenac (Cataflam, Voltaren, Zipsor)
Diflunisal (Dolobid)
Etodolac (Lodine)
Flurbiprofen (Ansaid)
Ibuprofen (Advil, Caldolor, Motrin)
Ketorolac (Toradol)
Naproxen (Anaprox, Naprosyn)
Salsalate (Disalcid)
Tramadol (Ultram)

Pain, moderate to severe
Butorphanol (Stadol)
Fentanyl (Onsolis, Sublimaze)
Hydromorphone (Dilaudid)
Meperidine (Demerol)
Methadone (Dolophine)
Morphine (MS Contin)
Morphine/naltrexone (Embeda)
Nalbuphine (Nubain)
Oxycodone (OxyFast, Roxicodone)
Oxymorphone (Opana)
Ziconotide (Prialt)

Panic attack disorder
Alprazolam (Xanax)
Clonazepam (Klonopin)
Paroxetine (Paxil)
Sertraline (Zoloft)
Venlafaxine (Effexor)

Parkinsonism
Amantadine (Symmetrel)
Apomorphine (Apokyn)
Bromocriptine (Parlodel)
Carbidopa/levodopa (Sinemet, Sinemet CR)
Diphenhydramine (Benadryl)
Entacapone (Comtan)
Pramipexole (Mirapex)
Rasagiline (Azilect)
Ropinirole (Requip)
Rotigotine (Neupro)
Selegiline (Eldepryl, Zelapar)
Tolcapone (Tasmar)

Peptic ulcer disease
Cimetidine (Tagamet)
Esomeprazole (Nexium)
Famotidine (Pepcid)
Lansoprazole (Prevacid)
Misoprostol (Cytotec)
Nizatidine (Axid)
Omeprazole (Prilosec)
Pantoprazole (Protonix)
Rabeprazole (Aciphex)
Ranitidine (Zantac)
Sucralfate (Carafate)

Pneumonia
Amoxicillin (Amoxil)
Amoxicillin/clavulanate (Augmentin)
Ampicillin (Polycillin)
Azithromycin (Zithromax)
Cefaclor (Ceclor)
Cefpodoxime (Vantin)
Ceftriaxone (Rocephin)
Cefuroxime (Kefurox, Zinacef)
Clarithromycin (Biaxin)
Co-trimoxazole (Bactrim, Septra)
Erythromycin
Gentamicin (Garamycin)
Levofloxacin (Levaquin)
Linezolid (Zyvox)
Moxifloxacin (Avelox)
Piperacillin/tazobactam (Zosyn)
Tobramycin (Nebcin)
Vancomycin (Vancocin)

Pneumonia, *Pneumocystis jiroveci*
Atovaquone (Mepron)
Clindamycin (Cleocin)
Co-trimoxazole (Bactrim, Septra)
Pentamidine (Pentam)
Trimethoprim (Proloprim)

Post-traumatic stress disorder
Amitriptyline (Elavil)
Aripiprazole (Abilify)
Citalopram (Celexa)
Escitalopram (Lexapro)
Fluoxetine (Prozac)
Imipramine (Tofranil)
Lamotrigine (Lamictal)
Olanzapine (Zyprexa)
Paroxetine (Paxil)
Phenelzine (Nardil)
Prazosin (Minipress)
Propranolol (Inderal)
Quetiapine (Seroquel)
Risperidone (Risperdal)
Sertraline (Zoloft)
Topiramate (Topamax)
Valproic acid (Depakote)
Venlafaxine (Effexor)
Ziprasidone (Geodon)

Pruritus
Amcinonide (Cyclocort)
Brompheniramine (Dimetane)
Cetirizine (Zyrtec)
Chlorpheniramine (Dimetane)
Clemastine (Tavist)
Clobetasol (Temovate)
Cyproheptadine (Periactin)
Desloratadine (Clarinex)
Desonide (Tridesilon)
Desoximetasone (Topicort)
Diphenhydramine (Benadryl)
Fluocinolone (Synalar)
Fluocinonide (Lidex)
Halobetasol (Ultravate)
Hydrocortisone (Cort-Dome, Hytone)
Hydroxyzine (Atarax, Vistaril)
Prednisolone (Prelone)
Prednisone (Deltasone)
Promethazine (Phenergan)

Psychosis
Aripiprazole (Abilify)
Asenapine (Saphris)
Chlorpromazine (Thorazine)
Clozapine (Clozaril)
Fluphenazine (Prolixin)
Haloperidol (Haldol)
Iloperidone (Fanapt)
Loxapine (Adasuve)
Lurasidone (Latuda)
Olanzapine (Zyprexa)
Perphenazine (Trilafon)
Quetiapine (Seroquel, Seroquel XR)
Risperidone (Risperdal)
Thioridazine (Mellaril)
Thiothixene (Navane)
Ziprasidone (Geodon)

Pulmonary arterial hypertension
Ambrisentan (Letairis)
Bosentan (Tracleer)
Epoprostenol (Flolan)
Iloprost (Ventavis)
Macitentan (Opsumit)
Riociguat (Adempax)
Sildenafil (Revatio)
Tadalafil (Adcirca)
Treprostinil (Remodulin, Tyvaso)

Respiratory distress syndrome (RDS)
Beractant (Survanta)
Calfactant (Infasurf)
Poractant alfa (Curosurf)

Restless legs syndrome
Cabergoline (Dostinex)
Carbidopa/levodopa (Sinemet)
Clonazepam (Klonopin)
Gabapentin (Horizant, Neurontin)
Levodopa
Oxycodone (Roxicodone)
Pramipexole (Mirapex)
Ropinirole (Requip)
Rotigotine (Neupro)
Tramadol (Ultram)
Zaleplon (Sonata)
Zolpidem (Ambien)

Schizophrenia
Aripiprazole (Abilify)
Asenapine (Saphris)
Chlorpromazine (Thorazine)
Clozapine (Clozaril)
Fluphenazine (Prolixin)
Haloperidol (Haldol)
Iloperidone (Fanapt)
Lurasidone (Latuda)

Olanzapine (Zyprexa)
Paliperidone (Invega, Invega Sustenna)
Perphenazine (Trilafon)
Quetiapine (Seroquel, Seroquel XR)
Risperidone (Risperdal)
Thioridazine (Mellaril)
Thiothixene (Navane)
Ziprasidone (Geodon)

Smoking cessation
Bupropion (Zyban)
Clonidine (Catapres)
Nicotine (Nicoderm, Nicotrol)
Nortriptyline (Pamelor)
Varenicline (Chantix)

Thrombosis
Apixaban (Eliquis)
Dalteparin (Fragmin)
Enoxaparin (Lovenox)
Fondaparinux (Arixtra)
Heparin
Tinzaparin (Innohep)
Warfarin (Coumadin)

Thyroid disorders
Levothyroxine (Levoxyl, Synthroid)
Liothyronine (Cytomel)
Thyroid

Transient ischemic attack (TIA)
Aspirin
Clopidogrel (Plavix)
Prasugrel (Effient)
Ticlopidine (Ticlid)
Warfarin (Coumadin)

Tremor
Atenolol (Tenormin)
Chlordiazepoxide (Librium)
Diazepam (Valium)
Lorazepam (Ativan)
Metoprolol (Lopressor)
Nadolol (Corgard)
Propranolol (Inderal)

Tuberculosis (TB)
Bedaquiline (Sirturo)
Cycloserine (Seromycin)
Ethambutol (Myambutol)
Isoniazid (INH)
Pyrazinamide
Rifabutin (Mycobutin)

Rifampin (Rifadin)
Rifapentine (Priftin)
Streptomycin

Urticaria
Cetirizine (Zyrtec)
Cimetidine (Tagamet)
Clemastine (Tavist)
Cyproheptadine (Periactin)
Diphenhydramine (Benadryl)
Hydroxyzine (Atarax, Vistaril)
Loratadine (Claritin)
Promethazine (Phenergan)
Ranitidine (Zantac)

Vertigo
Dimenhydrinate (Dramamine)
Diphenhydramine (Benadryl)
Meclizine (Antivert)
Scopolamine (Trans-Derm Scop)

Vomiting
Aprepitant (Emend)
Chlorpromazine (Thorazine)
Dexamethasone (Decadron)
Dimenhydrinate (Dramamine)
Dolasetron (Anzemet)
Dronabinol (Marinol)
Droperidol (Inapsine)
Fosaprepitant (Emend)
Granisetron (Kytril)
Hydroxyzine (Vistaril)
Lorazepam (Ativan)
Meclizine (Antivert)
Metoclopramide (Reglan)
Nabilone (Cesamet)
Ondansetron (Zofran)
Palonosetron (Aloxi)
Prochlorperazine (Compazine)
Promethazine (Phenergan)
Scopolamine (Trans-Derm Scop)
Trimethobenzamide (Tigan)

Zollinger-Ellison syndrome
Aluminum salts
Cimetidine (Tagamet)
Esomeprazole (Nexium)
Famotidine (Pepcid)
Lansoprazole (Prevacid)
Omeprazole (Prilosec)
Pantoprazole (Protonix)
Rabeprazole (Aciphex)
Ranitidine (Zantac)

DRUG CLASSIFICATION CONTENTS

Allergic Rhinitis Nasal Preparations

USES	ACTION
Relieves symptoms associated with allergic rhinitis. These symptoms include rhinorrhea, nasal congestion, pruritus, sneezing, postnasal drip, nasal pain. Allergic rhinitis or hay fever is an inflammation of the nasal airways occurring when an allergen (e.g., pollen) is inhaled. This triggers antibody production. The antibodies bind to mast cells, which contain histamine. Histamine is released, causing symptoms of allergic rhinitis.	**Intranasal corticosteroids:** Depresses migration of polymorphonuclear leucocytes and fibroblasts, reverses capillary permeability, and stabilizes nasal membranes to prevent/control inflammation. **Intranasal antihistamines:** Reduces histamine mediated symptoms of allergic rhinitis, including pruritus, sneezing, rhinorrhea, watery eyes.	**Intranasal mast cell stabilizers:** Inhibits the mast cell release of histamine and other inflammatory mediators. **Intranasal anticholinergics:** Blocks acetylcholine in the nasal mucosa. Effective in treating rhinorrhea associated with allergic rhinitis. **Intranasal decongestants:** Vasoconstricts the respiratory mucosa, provides short-term relief of nasal congestion.

CORTICOSTEROIDS

Generic (Brand)	Adult Dose	Pediatric Dose	Side Effects
Beclomethasone (p. 119) (Beconase AQ) (Qnasi)	Beconase AQ: 1–2 sprays in each nostril 2 times/day Qnasi: 2 sprays in each nostril once daily	Beconase AQ: 5–11 yrs: 1–2 sprays in each nostril 2 times/day	Altered taste and smell, epistaxis, burning, stinging, headache, nasal septum perforation
Budesonide (p. 159) (Rhinocort Aqua)	1 spray in each nostril daily	6–11 yrs: 1 spray in each nostril daily	Bronchospasm, cough, epistaxis, nasal/throat irritation
Ciclesonide (p. 245) (Omnaris, Zetonna)	Omnaris: 2 sprays in each nostril daily Zetonna: 1 spray in each nostril daily	Omnaris: 2–11 yrs: 1–2 sprays in each nostril daily	Fever, headache, nausea, cough, epistaxis, nasal septum disorder
Flunisolide (p. 501) (Nasalide)	2 sprays in each nostril 2 or 3 times/day (maximum: 8 sprays in each nostril daily)	6–14 yrs: 2 sprays in each nostril 2 times/day or 1 spray in each nostril 3 times/day (maximum: 4 sprays in each nostril daily)	Nasal burning/stinging, nasal dryness/irritation

	Adult Dose	Pediatric Dose	Side Effects
Fluticasone (p. 510) (Flonase)	2 sprays in each nostril daily or 1 spray in each nostril twice daily	4–17 yrs: 1–2 sprays in each nostril daily	Dizziness, fever, headache, nausea, cough, epistaxis
Fluticasone/Azelastine (Dymista)	1 spray in each nostril 2 times/day	Not indicated in children younger than 12 yrs	Same as fluticasone and azelastine
Fluticasone (p. 510) (Veramyst)	1–2 sprays in each nostril daily	2–11 yrs: 1–2 sprays in each nostril once daily	Same as fluticasone
Mometasone (p. 806) (Nasonex)	2 sprays in each nostril daily	2–11 yrs: 1 spray in each nostril daily	Headache, nasopharyngitis, sinusitis
Triamcinolone (p. 1232) (Nasacort AQ)	1–2 sprays in each nostril daily	2–5 yrs: 1 spray in each nostril once daily 6–11 yrs: 1–2 sprays in each nostril daily	Bronchitis, chest congestion, cough, epistaxis, pharyngitis, sinusitus

ANTIHISTAMINES

Generic (Brand)	Adult Dose	Pediatric Dose	Side Effects
Azelastine (p. 108) (Astelin) Astepro 0.15%	Astelin: 1–2 sprays in each nostril 2 times/day Astepro 0.15%: 1–2 sprays in each nostril two times/day or 2 sprays each nostril once daily	Astelin: 5–11 yrs: 1 spray in each nostril 2 times/day	Sedation, epistaxis, nasal irritation
Azelastine/Fluticasone (p. 108, 000) (Dymista)	1 spray in each nostril 2 times/day	Not approved for children younger than 12 yrs	Same as azelastine and fluticasone
Olopatadine (Patanase)	2 sprays in each nostril 2 times/day	6–11 yrs: 1 spray in each nostril 2 times/day	Same as azelastine

(continued)

MAST CELL STABILIZERS

Generic (Brand)	Adult Dose	Pediatric Dose	Side Effects
Cromolyn (Nasalcrom)	1 spray in each nostril 3–6 times/day	2–11 yrs: 1 spray in each nostril 3–6 times/day	Nasal irritation, unpleasant taste

ANTICHOLINERGICS

Generic (Brand)	Adult Dose	Pediatric Dose	Side Effects
Ipratropium (p. 637) (Atrovent) 0.03%	2 sprays in each nostril 2–3 times/day	6–11 yrs: 2 sprays in each nostril 2–3 times/day	Nasal irritation, epistaxis, dizziness, headache, blurry vision
Ipratropium (p. 637) (Atrovent) 0.06%	2 sprays in each nostril 4 times/day	5–11 yrs: 2 sprays in each nostril 4 times/day	Same as ipratropium 0.03%

DECONGESTANTS

Generic (Brand)	Adult Dose	Pediatric Dose	Side Effects
Oxymetazoline (Afrin)	2–3 drops or sprays 2 times/day	2–3 drops or sprays 2 times/day	Insomnia, tachycardia, nervousness, nausea, vomiting, transient burning, headache, rebound congestion if used longer than 72 hrs
Phenylephrine (p. 956) (Neo-Synephrine)	2–3 drops or 1–2 sprays q4h as needed (0.25% or 0.5%)	6–11 yrs: 2–3 drops (0.25%) q4h as needed 1–5 yrs: 2–3 drops (0.125%) q4h as needed	Restlessness, nervousness, headache, rebound nasal congestion, burning, stinging, dryness

Anesthetics: General

USES

IV anesthetic agents are used to induce general anesthesia. The general anesthetic state consists of unconsciousness, amnesia, analgesia, immobility, and attenuation of autonomic responses to noxious stimuli.

Volatile inhalation agents produce all the components of the anesthetic state but are administered through the lungs via an anesthesia machine. Agents for use include desflurane, sevoflurane, isoflurane, enflurane, and halothane.

General anesthetics are medications producing unconsciousness and a lack of response to all painful stimuli.

ACTION

IV anesthetic agents: Most agents produce CNS depression by action on the gamma-aminobutyric acid (GABA) receptor complex. GABA is the primary inhibitory neurotransmitter in the CNS. Ketamine produces dissociation between the thalamus and the limbic system.

Volatile inhalation agents: The action of these agents is not fully understood, but they may disrupt neuronal transmission throughout the CNS. These agents may either block excitatory or enhance inhibitory transmission through axons or synapses.

ANESTHETICS: GENERAL

Name	Availability	Uses	Dosage Range	Side Effects
Etomidate (Amidate)	**I:** 2 mg/ml	IV induction	0.2–0.6 mg/kg	Myoclonus, pain on injection, nausea, vomiting, respiratory depression
Ketamine (Ketalar)	**I:** 10 mg/ml, 50 mg/ml, 100 mg/ml	Analgesia, sedation, IV induction	1–4.5 mg/kg	Delirium, euphoria, nausea, vomiting
Methohexital (Brevital)	**Powder for injection:** 500 mg	IV induction, sedation	50–120 mg	Cardiovascular depression, myoclonus, nausea, vomiting, respiratory depression

(continued)

ANESTHETICS: GENERAL   *(continued)*

Name	Availability	Uses	Dosage Range	Side Effects
Midazolam (p. 784) (Versed)	I: 1 mg/ml, 5 mg/ml	Anxiolytic, amnesic, sedation	1–5 mg titrated slowly	Respiratory depression
Propofol (p. 1007) (Diprivan)	I: 10 mg/ml	Sedation IV induction Maintenance	0.5 mg/kg 2–2.5 mg/kg 100–200 mcg/kg/min	Cardiovascular depression, delirium, euphoria, pain on injection, respiratory depression

I, Injection.

Anesthetics: Local

USES

Local anesthetics suppress pain by blocking impulses along axons. Suppression of pain does not cause generalized depression of the entire nervous system. Local anesthetics may be given topically and by injection (local infiltration, peripheral nerve block [axillary], IV regional [Bier block], epidural, and spinal).

ACTION

Most local anesthetics fall into one of two groups: esters or amides. Both provide anesthesia and analgesia by reversibly binding to and blocking sodium (Na) channels. This slows the rate of depolarization of the nerve action potential; thus, propagation of the electrical impulses needed for nerve conduction is prevented.

ANESTHETICS: LOCAL

Name	Uses	Onset (min)	Duration (hrs)	Side Effects
Esters				
Chloroprocaine (Nesacaine)	Local infiltrate, nerve block, spinal	6–12	0.5–1	Seizures, bradycardia, cardiac arrest, hypotension, arrhythmias, anxiety, dizziness, restlessness, erythema, pruritus, urticaria, blurred vision, allergic reaction
Procaine (Novocaine)	Local infiltrate, nerve block, spinal	2–5	0.5–1.5	Burning sensation/pain at injection site, tissue irritation, CNS stimulation followed by CNS depression, chills
Amides				
Bupivacaine (Marcaine, Sensorcaine)	Local infiltrate, nerve block, epidural, spinal	5	2–9	Cardiac arrest, hypotension, bradycardia, palpitations, seizures, restlessness, anxiety, dizziness, nausea, vomiting, blurred vision, weakness, tinnitus, apnea
Lidocaine (p. 697)	Local infiltrate, nerve block, spinal, epidural, topical, IV regional	Less than 2	0.5–1	Bradycardia, hypotension, arrhythmias, agitation, anxiety, dizziness, seizures, pruritus, rash, nausea, vomiting, altered taste, visual changes, tinnitus, respiratory depression, allergic reaction
Mepivacaine (Carbocaine, Polocaine)	Local infiltrate, nerve block, epidural	3–20	2–2.5	Bradycardia, syncope, arrhythmias, anxiety, seizures, dizziness, restlessness, chills, pruritus, urticaria, nausea, vomiting, incontinence, blurred vision, tinnitus, allergic reaction
Ropivacaine (Naropin)	Local infiltrate, nerve block, epidural, spinal	1–15	3–15	Hypotension, bradycardia, headache, pruritus, nausea, vomiting, dizziness, anxiety, tinnitus, dyspnea, cardiac arrest, arrhythmias, seizures, syncope, chills

Note: Most side effects are manifestations of excessive plasma concentrations.

Anesthetics: Local Topical

ANESTHETICS: LOCAL TOPICAL

Name	Indications	Peak Effect (min)	Duration (min)
Amides			
Dibucaine (Nupercainal)	Skin	Less than 5	15–45
Lidocaine (p. 697)	Skin, mucous membranes	2–5	15–45
Esters			
Benzocaine	Skin, mucous membranes	Less than 5	15–45
Cocaine	Mucous membranes	2–5	30–60
Tetracaine (Pontocaine)	Skin, mucous membranes	3–8	30–60

Angiotensin-Converting Enzyme (ACE) Inhibitors

USES

Treatment of hypertension (HTN), adjunctive therapy for HF.

ACTION

Antihypertensive: Exact mechanism unknown. May be related to competitive inhibition of angiotensin I converting enzyme (ACE) activity causing decreased conversion of angiotensin I to angiotensin II, a potent vasoconstrictor. Reduces peripheral arterial resistance. *HF:* Decreases peripheral vascular resistance (afterload), pulmonary capillary wedge pressure (preload); improves cardiac output, exercise tolerance.

ACE INHIBITORS

Name	Availability	Uses	Dosage Range (per day)	Side Effects
Benazepril (p. 126) (Lotensin)	**T:** 5 mg, 10 mg, 20 mg, 40 mg	HTN	**HTN:** 5–80 mg in 1 or 2 doses	Headaches, dizziness, fatigue, cough
Captopril (p. 186) (Capoten)	**T:** 12.5 mg, 25 mg, 50 mg, 100 mg	HTN HF	**HTN:** 12.5–150 mg in 2–3 doses **HF:** 12.5–450 mg	Insomnia, headaches, dizziness, fatigue, GI complaints, cough, rash
Enalapril (p. 415) (Vasotec)	**T:** 2.5 mg, 5 mg, 10 mg, 20 mg **IV:** 1.25 mg/ml	HTN HF	**HTN:** 2.5–40 mg in 1 or 2 doses; (**IV:** 1.25 mg q6h) **HF:** 5–20 mg	Chest pain, hypotension, headaches, fatigue, dizziness
Fosinopril (p. 524) (Monopril)	**T:** 10 mg, 20 mg, 40 mg	HTN HF	**HTN:** 10–80 mg in 1 or 2 doses **HF:** 20–40 mg	Hypotension, nausea, vomiting, cough
Lisinopril (p. 707) (Prinivil, Zestril)	**T:** 2.5 mg, 5 mg, 10 mg, 20 mg, 40 mg	HTN HF	**HTN:** 5–40 mg **HF:** 5–20 mg	Chest pain, hypotension, headaches, dizziness, fatigue, diarrhea
Moexipril (Univasc)	**T:** 7.5 mg, 15 mg	HTN	**HTN:** 7.5–30 mg in 1 or 2 doses	Dizziness, fatigue, diarrhea, cough
Perindopril (Aceon)	**T:** 2 mg, 4 mg, 6 mg	HTN	**HTN:** 4–8 mg in 1 or 2 doses	Hypotension, dizziness, fatigue, syncope, cough
Quinapril (p. 1025) (Accupril)	**T:** 5 mg, 10 mg, 20 mg, 40 mg	HTN HF	**HTN:** 10–80 mg in 1 or 2 doses **HF:** 10–40 mg	Chest pain, hypotension, headaches, dizziness, fatigue, diarrhea, nausea, vomiting, cough

(continued)

ACE INHIBITORS   *(continued)*

Name	Availability	Uses	Dosage Range (per day)	Side Effects
Ramipril (p. 1034) (Altace)	**C:** 1.25 mg, 2.5 mg, 5 mg, 10 mg	HTN HF	**HTN:** 2.5–20 mg in 1 or 2 doses **HF:** 1.25–10 mg	Hypotension, headaches, dizziness, cough
Trandolapril (Mavik)	**T:** 1 mg, 2 mg, 4 mg	HTN HF	**HTN:** 1–8 mg in 1 or 2 doses **HF:** 1–4 mg	Dizziness, dyspepsia, cough, asthenia (loss of strength, energy), syncope, myalgia

C, Capsules; *HF,* heart failure; *HTN,* hypertension; *IV,* intravenous; *T,* tablets.

Angiotensin II Receptor Antagonists

USES

Treatment of hypertension (HTN) alone or in combination with other antihypertensives. Treatment of heart failure (HF).

ACTION

Angiotensin II receptor antagonists (AIIRA) block vasoconstrictor and aldosterone-secreting effects on angiotensin II by selectively blocking the binding of angiotensin II to AT_1 receptors in vascular smooth muscle and adrenal gland, causing vasodilation and a decrease in aldosterone effects.

ANGIOTENSIN II RECEPTOR ANTAGONISTS

Name	Availability	Uses	Dosage Range (per day)	Side Effects
Azilsartan (Edarbi) (p. 109)	**T:** 40 mg, 80 mg	HTN	40–80 mg once daily	Diarrhea, hypotension, muscle spasms, weakness
Candesartan (p. 183) (Atacand)	**T:** 4 mg, 8 mg, 16 mg, 32 mg	HTN HF	8–32 mg in 1–2 divided doses 4–32 mg once daily	Headaches, upper respiratory tract infection, pain, dizziness

Eprosartan (p. 434) (Teveten)	**T:** 400 mg, 600 mg	HTN	400–800 mg in 1–2 divided doses	Headaches, upper respiratory tract infection, myalgia
Irbesartan (p. 639) (Avapro)	**T:** 75 mg, 150 mg, 300 mg	HTN Nephropathy	150–300 mg once daily 300 mg once daily	Headaches, upper respiratory tract infection
Losartan (p. 723) (Cozaar)	**T:** 25 mg, 50 mg, 100 mg	HTN Nephropathy	25–100 mg in 1–2 divided doses 100 mg once daily	Dizziness, headaches, upper respiratory tract infection, diarrhea, fatigue, cough
Olmesartan (p. 881) (Benicar)	**T:** 5 mg, 20 mg, 40 mg	HTN	20–40 mg once daily	Headaches, upper respiratory tract infection, flu-like symptoms, dizziness, bronchitis, rhinitis, back pain, pharyngitis, sinusitis, diarrhea, peripheral edema
Telmisartan (p. 1156) (Micardis)	**T:** 40 mg, 80 mg	HTN CV risk reduction	20–80 mg once daily 80 mg once daily	Upper respiratory tract infection, dizziness, back pain, sinusitis, diarrhea
Valsartan (p. 1250) (Diovan)	**T:** 80 mg, 160 mg	HTN HF Post MI	80–320 mg once daily 40–160 mg twice daily 20–160 mg twice daily	Dizziness, headaches, upper respiratory tract infection, diarrhea, fatigue

CV, Cardiovascular; *HF,* heart failure; *HTN,* hypertension; *MI,* myocardial infarction; *T,* tablets.

Antacids

USES

Relief of symptoms associated with hyperacidity (e.g., heartburn, acid indigestion, sour stomach), hyperacidity associated with gastric/duodenal ulcers, treatment of pathologic gastric hypersecretion associated with Zollinger-Ellison syndrome, symptomatic treatment of gastroesophageal reflux disease (GERD), prevention and treatment of upper GI stress-induced ulceration and bleeding (esp. in ICU). Aluminum hydroxide in conjunction with a low-phosphate diet to reduce elevated phosphate in pts with renal insufficiency. Calcium for calcium deficiency; magnesium for magnesium deficiency.

ACTION

Antacids act primarily in the stomach to neutralize gastric acid (increase pH). Antacids do not have a direct effect on acid output. The ability to increase pH depends on the dose, dosage form used, presence or absence of food in the stomach, and acid-neutralizing capacity (ANC). ANC is the number of mEq of hydrochloric acid that can be neutralized by a particular weight or volume of antacid.

Antacids reduce elevated phosphate by binding with phosphate in the intestine to form an insoluble complex, which is then eliminated.

ANTACIDS

Antacid	Brand Names	Availability	Dosage Range	Side Effects
Aluminum				
Hydroxide	Amphojel, Alu-Tab, Dialume	**T:** 300 mg, 500 mg, 600 mg **C:** 500 mg	500–1,500 mg 3–6 times/day	Chalky taste, mild constipation, abdominal cramps *Long-term use:* Neurotoxicity in dialysis pts, hypercalcemia, osteoporosis *Large doses:* Fecal impaction, peripheral edema

Calcium

Carbonate (p. 178)	Tums, Caltrate 600, Oyst-Cal 500	**T (chewable):** 500 mg, 750 mg, 1,000 mg **T:** 1,250 mg	500–1,500 mg as needed (**Maximum:** 7,000 mg in 24 hrs)	Chalky taste *Large doses:* Fecal impaction, peripheral edema, metabolic alkalosis *Long-term use:* Difficult/painful urination
Citrate	Calcitrate	**C:** 225 mg **T:** 200 mg	500–2,000 mg	Constipation, nausea, vomiting

Magnesium

Hydroxide (p. 734)	Milk of Magnesia	**T (chewable):** 311 mg **L:** 400 mg/5 ml, 800 mg/5 ml	**T:** 622–1,244 mg up to 4 times/day **L:** 2.5–7.5 ml up to 4 times/day	Chalky taste, diarrhea, laxative effect, electrolyte imbalance (dizziness, irregular heartbeat, fatigue)
Oxide (p. 734)	Mag-Ox 400	**T:** 400 mg, 420 mg, 500 mg	400–800 mg/day	Same as above

C, Capsules; *L,* liquid; *T,* tablets.

Antianxiety Agents

USES

Treatment of anxiety including generalized anxiety disorder (GAD), panic disorder, obsessive-compulsive disorder (OCD), social anxiety disorder (SAD), post-traumatic stress disorder (PTSD), and acute stress disorder. In addition, some benzodiazepines are used as hypnotics, anticonvulsants to prevent delirium tremors during alcohol withdrawal, and as adjunctive therapy for relaxation of skeletal muscle spasms. Midazolam, a short-acting benzodiazepine, is used for preop sedation and relief of anxiety for short diagnostic/endoscopic procedures (see individual monograph for midazolam).

ACTION

Benzodiazepines are the largest and most frequently prescribed group of antianxiety agents. The exact mechanism is unknown, but they may increase the inhibiting effect of gamma-aminobutyric acid (GABA), which inhibits nerve impulse transmission by binding to specific benzodiazepine receptors in various areas of the central nervous system (CNS).

◀**ALERT**▶ Refer to individual entries of nonbenzodiazepine drugs for more information on uses and actions.

ANTIANXIETY AGENTS

Name	Availability	Uses	Dosage Range (per day)	Side Effects
Benzodiazepine				
Alprazolam (p. 42) (Xanax)	**T:** 0.25 mg, 0.5 mg, 1 mg, 2 mg **S:** 0.5 mg/5 ml, 1 mg/ml **ER:** 0.5 mg, 1 mg, 2 mg, 3 mg **ODT:** 0.25 mg, 0.5 mg, 1 mg, 2 mg	Anxiety, panic disorder	0.75–10 mg	Drowsiness, weakness, fatigue, ataxia, slurred speech, confusion, lack of coordination, impaired memory, paradoxical agitation, dizziness, nausea
Chlordiazepoxide (p. 240) (Librium)	**C:** 5 mg, 10 mg, 25 mg **T:** 10 mg, 25 mg **I:** 100 mg	Anxiety, alcohol withdrawal	5–100 mg	Drowsiness, fatigue, ataxia, memory impairment

Name	Availability	Uses	Dosage Range	Side Effects
Clorazepate (p. 277) (Tranxene)	**C:** 3.75 mg, 7.5 mg, 15 mg **SD:** 11.25 mg, 22.5 mg	Anxiety, alcohol withdrawal, anticonvulsant	7.5–90 mg	Hypotension, drowsiness, fatigue, ataxia, memory impairment, headache, nausea
Diazepam (p. 352) (Valium)	**T:** 2.5 mg, 5 mg, 10 mg **S:** 5 mg/5 ml, 5 mg/ml **I:** 5 mg/ml	Anxiety, alcohol withdrawal, anticonvulsant, muscle relaxant	2–40 mg	Hypotension, ataxia, drowsiness, fatigue, vertigo
Lorazepam (p. 720) (Ativan)	**T:** 0.5 mg, 1 mg, 2 mg **S:** 2 mg/ml **I:** 2 mg/ml, 4 mg/ml	Anxiety	0.5–10 mg	Sedation, respiratory depression, ataxia, dizziness, headache
Nonbenzodiazepine				
Buspirone (p. 167) (BuSpar)	**T:** 5 mg, 10 mg, 15 mg, 30 mg	Anxiety	7.5–60 mg	Dizziness, light-headedness, headaches, nausea, restlessness
Hydroxyzine (p. 585) (Atarax, Vistaril)	**T:** 10 mg, 25 mg, 50 mg, 100 mg	Anxiety, rhinitis, pruritus, urticaria, nausea or vomiting	100–400 mg	Drowsiness; dry mouth, nose, and throat
Paroxetine (p. 924) (Paxil)	**S:** 10 mg/5 ml **T:** 10 mg, 20 mg, 30 mg, 40 mg **T (CR):** 12.5 mg, 25 mg, 37.5 mg	Anxiety, depression, obsessive-compulsive disorder, panic disorder	10–50 mg	Drowsiness, dry mouth, nose, and throat; dizziness; diarrhea; diaphoresis; constipation; vomiting; tremors
Trazodone (p. 1226) (Desyrel)	**T:** 50 mg, 100 mg, 150 mg, 300 mg	Anxiety, depression	100–400 mg	Drowsiness, dizziness, headaches, dry mouth, nausea, vomiting, unpleasant taste
Venlafaxine (p. 1261) (Effexor)	**C (ER):** 37.5 mg, 75 mg, 150 mg **T (ER):** 37.5 mg, 75 mg, 150 mg **T:** 25 mg, 37.5 mg, 50 mg, 75 mg, 150 mg	Anxiety, depression	37.5–225 mg	Drowsiness, nausea, headaches, dry mouth

C, Capsules; *CR,* controlled-release; *ER,* extended-release; *I,* injection; *ODT,* orally disintegrating tablet; *S,* solution; *SD,* single dose; *T,* tablets.

Antiarrhythmics

USES

Prevention and treatment of cardiac arrhythmias, such as premature ventricular contractions, ventricular tachycardia, premature atrial contractions, paroxysmal atrial tachycardia, atrial fibrillation and flutter.

ACTION

The antiarrhythmics are divided into four classes based on their effects on certain ion channels and/or receptors located on the myocardial cell membrane. Class I is further divided into three subclasses (IA, IB, IC) based on electrophysiologic effects.

Class I: Blocks cardiac sodium channels and slows conduction velocity, prolonging refractory period and decreasing automaticity of sodium-dependent tissue.

Class IA: Blocks sodium and potassium channels.

Class IB: Shortens the repolarization phase.

Class IC: No effect on repolarization phase, but slows conduction velocity.

Class II: Slows sinus and atrioventricular (AV) nodal conduction.

Class III: Blocks cardiac potassium channels, prolonging the repolarization phase of electrical cells.

Class IV: Inhibits the influx of calcium through its channels, causing slower conduction through the sinus and AV nodes.

ANTIARRHYTHMICS

Name	Availability	Uses	Dosage Range	Side Effects
Class IA				
Disopyramide (Norpace, Norpace CR)	**C:** 100 mg, 150 mg **C (ER):** 100 mg, 150 mg	AF, WPW, PSVT, PVCs, VT	400–800 mg/day	Dry mouth, blurred vision, urinary retention, HF, proarrhythmia, heart block, nausea, vomiting, diarrhea, hypoglycemia, nervousness
Procainamide (p. 996) (Procan-SR, Pronestyl)	**T:** 250 mg, 375 mg, 500 mg **C:** 250 mg, 375 mg, 500 mg **T (SR):** 250 mg, 500 mg, 750 mg, 1,000 mg **I:** 100 mg/ml, 500 mg/ml	AF, WPW, PVCs, VT	**A (PO):** 250–500 mg q3h; **(ER):** 250–750 mg q6h	Hypotension, fever, agranulocytosis, SLE, headaches, proarrhythmia, confusion, disorientation, GI symptoms, hypotension

Quinidine (Quinaglute, Quinidex)	**T:** 200 mg, 300 mg **T (ER):** 300 mg, 324 mg **I:** 80 mg/ml	AF, WPW, PVCs, VT	**A (PO):** 200–600 mg q2–4h; **(ER):** 300–600 mg q8h	Diarrhea, hypotension, nausea, vomiting, cinchonism, fever, bitter taste, heart block, thrombocytopenia, proarrhythmia
Class IB				
Lidocaine (p. 697) (Xylocaine)	**I:** 300 mg for IM **IV Infusion:** 2 mg/ml, 4 mg/ml	PVCs, VT, VF	**IV:** 50–100 mg bolus, then 1–4 mg/min infusion	Drowsiness, agitation, muscle twitching, seizures, paresthesia, proarrhythmia, slurred speech, tinnitus, cardiac depression, bradycardia, asystole
Mexiletine (Mexitil)	**C:** 150 mg, 200 mg, 250 mg	PVCs, VT, VF	**A:** 600–1,200 mg/day	Drowsiness, agitation, muscle twitching, seizures, paresthesia, proarrhythmia, nausea, vomiting, blood dyscrasias, hepatitis, fever
Tocainide (Tonocard)	**T:** 400 mg, 600 mg	PVCs, VT, VF	**A:** 1,200–1,800 mg/day	Drowsiness, agitation, muscle twitching, seizures, paresthesia, proarrhythmia, nausea, vomiting, diarrhea, agranulocytosis
Class IC				
Flecainide (Tambocor)	**T:** 50 mg, 100 mg, 150 mg	AF, PSVT, life-threatening ventricular arrhythmias	**A:** 200–400 mg/day	Dizziness, tremors, bradycardia, heart block, heart failure, GI upset, neutropenia, flushing, blurred vision, metallic taste, proarrhythmia
Propafenone (p. 1005) (Rythmol)	**T:** 150 mg, 225 mg, 300 mg	PAF, WPW, life-threatening ventricular arrhythmias	**A:** 450–900 mg/day	Dizziness, blurred vision, altered taste, nausea, exacerbation of asthma, proarrhythmia, bradycardia, heart block, heart failure, GI upset, bronchospasm, hepatotoxicity

(continued)

ANTIARRHYTHMICS   *(continued)*

Name	Availability	Uses	Dosage Range	Side Effects
Class II (Beta-Blockers)				
Acebutolol (Sectral)	**C:** 200 mg, 400 mg	Ventricular arrhythmias	**A:** 600–1,200 mg/day	Bradycardia, hypotension, depression, nightmares, fatigue, sexual dysfunction, SLE, arthritis, myalgia
Esmolol (p. 446) (Brevibloc)	**I:** 10 mg/ml, 20 mg/ml	Supraventricular tachycardia	**A:** 50–200 mcg/kg/min	Hypotension, heart block, heart failure, bronchospasm
Propranolol (p. 1009) (Inderal)	**T:** 10 mg, 20 mg	Tachyarrhythmias	**A:** 10–30 mg 3–4 times/day	Bradycardia, hypotension, depression, nightmares, fatigue, sexual dysfunction, heart block, bronchospasm
Class III				
Amiodarone (p. 54) (Cordarone, Pacerone)	**T:** 200 mg, 400 mg **I:** 50 mg/ml	AF, PAF, PSVT, life-threatening ventricular arrhythmias	**A (PO):** 800–1,600 mg/day for 1–3 wks, then 600–800 mg/day **(IV):** 150 mg bolus, then IV infusion	Blurred vision, photophobia, constipation, ataxia, proarrhythmia, pulmonary fibrosis, bradycardia, heart block, hyperthyroidism or hypothyroidism, peripheral neuropathy, GI upset, blue-gray skin, optic neuritis, hypotension
Dofetilide (p. 383) (Tikosyn)	**C:** 125 mcg, 250 mcg, 500 mcg	AF, A flutter	**A:** Individualized	Torsade de pointes, hypotension
Dronedarone (p. 402) (Multaq)	**T:** 400 mg	AF, A flutter	**A (PO):** 400 mg 2 times/day	Diarrhea, nausea, abdominal pain, vomiting, asthenia (loss of strength, energy)
Ibutilide (Corvert)	**I:** 0.1 mg/ml	AF, A flutter	**A (greater than 60 kg):** 1 mg over 10 min; **(less than 60 kg):** 0.01 mg/kg over 10 min	Torsade de pointes

Sotalol (p. 1124) (Betapace)	T: 80 mg, 120 mg, 160 mg, 240 mg		AF, PAF, PSVT, life-threatening ventricular arrhythmias	A: 160–640 mg/day	Fatigue, dizziness, dyspnea, bradycardia, proarrhythmia, heart block, hypotension, bronchospasm
Class IV (Calcium Channel Blockers)					
Diltiazem (p. 366) (Cardizem)	I: 25 mg/ml vials Infusion: 1 mg/ml		AF, A flutter, PSVT	A (IV): 20–25 mg bolus, then infusion of 5–15 mg/hr	Hypotension, bradycardia, dizziness, headaches, heart block, asystole, heart failure
Verapamil (p. 1263) (Calan, Isoptin)	I: 5 mg/2 ml		AF, A flutter, PSVT	A (IV): 5–10 mg	Hypotension, bradycardia, dizziness, headaches, constipation, heart block, heart failure, asystole, fatigue, edema, nausea

A, Adults; *AF,* atrial fibrillation; *A flutter,* atrial flutter; *C,* capsules; *HF,* heart failure; *ER,* extended-release; *I,* injection; *PAF,* paroxysmal atrial fibrillation; *PSVT,* paroxysmal supraventricular tachycardia; *PVCs,* premature ventricular contractions; *SLE,* systemic lupus erythematosus; *SR,* sustained-release; *T,* tablets; *VT,* ventricular tachycardia; *WPW,* Wolff-Parkinson-White syndrome.

Antibiotics

USES	ACTION
Treatment of wide range of gram-positive or gram-negative bacterial infections, suppression of intestinal flora before surgery; control of acne, prophylactically to prevent rheumatic fever, prophylactically in high-risk situations (e.g., some surgical procedures or medical conditions) to prevent bacterial infection.	Antibiotics are natural or synthetic compounds that have the ability to kill or suppress the growth of microorganisms.
	One means of classifying antibiotics is by their antimicrobial spectrum. Narrow-spectrum agents are effective against few microorganisms (e.g., aminoglycosides are effective against gram-negative aerobes), whereas broad-spectrum agents are effective against a wide variety of microorganisms (e.g., fluoroquinolones are effective against gram-positive cocci and gram-negative bacilli).
	Antimicrobial agents may also be classified based on their mechanism of action.
	• Agents that inhibit cell wall synthesis or activate enzymes that disrupt the cell wall, causing a weakening in the cell, cell lysis, and death. Include penicillins, cephalosporins, vancomycin, imidazole antifungal agents.
	• Agents that act directly on the cell wall, affecting permeability of cell membranes, causing leakage of intracellular substances. Include antifungal agents amphotericin and nystatin, polymyxin, colistin.
	• Agents that bind to ribosomal subunits, altering protein synthesis and eventually causing cell death. Include aminoglycosides.
	• Agents that affect bacterial ribosome function, altering protein synthesis and causing slow microbial growth. Do not cause cell death. Include chloramphenicol, clindamycin, erythromycin, tetracyclines.
	• Agents that inhibit nucleic acid metabolism by binding to nucleic acid or interacting with enzymes necessary for nucleic acid synthesis. Inhibit DNA or RNA synthesis. Include rifampin, metronidazole, fluoroquinolones (e.g., ciprofloxacin).
	• Agents that inhibit specific metabolic steps necessary for microbial growth, causing a decrease in essential cell components or synthesis of nonfunctional analogues of normal metabolites. Include trimethoprim, sulfonamides.
	• Agents that inhibit viral DNA synthesis by binding to viral enzymes necessary for DNA synthesis, preventing viral replication. Include acyclovir, vidarabine.

SELECTION OF ANTIMICROBIAL AGENTS

The goal of therapy is to achieve antimicrobial action at the site of infection sufficient to inhibit the growth of the microorganism. The agent selected should be the most active against the most likely infecting organism, least likely to cause toxicity or allergic reaction. Factors to consider in selection of an antimicrobial agent include the following:

- Sensitivity pattern of the infecting microorganism
- Location and severity of infection (may determine route of administration)
- Pt's ability to eliminate the drug (status of renal and hepatic function)
- Pt's defense mechanisms (includes both cellular and humoral immunity)
- Pt's age, pregnancy status, genetic factors, allergies, CNS disorder, preexisting medical problems

CATEGORIZATION OF ORGANISMS BY GRAM STAINING

Gram-Positive Cocci	Gram-Negative Cocci	Gram-Positive Bacilli	Gram-Negative Bacilli
Aerobic	**Aerobic**	**Aerobic**	**Aerobic**
Staphylococcus aureus	Neisseria gonorrhoeae	Listeria monocytogenes	Escherichia coli
Staphylococcus epidermidis	Neisseria meningitidis	Bacillus anthracis	Klebsiella pneumoniae
Streptococcus pneumoniae	Moraxella catarrhalis	Corynebacterium diphtheriae	Proteus mirabilis
Streptococcus pyogenes		**Anaerobic**	Serratia marcescens
Viridans streptococci		Clostridium difficile	Acinetobacter spp.
Enterococcus faecalis		Clostridium perfringens	Pseudomonas aeruginosa
Enterococcus faecium		Clostridium tetani	Enterobacter spp.
Anaerobic		Actinomyces spp.	Haemophilus influenzae
Peptostreptococcus spp.			Legionella pneumophila
Peptococcus spp.			**Anaerobic**
			Bacteroides fragilis
			Fusobacterium spp.

Antibiotic: Aminoglycosides

USES

Treatment of serious infections when other less toxic agents are not effective, are contraindicated, or require adjunctive therapy (e.g., with penicillins or cephalosporins). Used primarily in the treatment of infections caused by gram-negative microorganisms, such as those caused by *Proteus*, *Klebsiella*, *Pseudomonas*,

Escherichia coli, *Serratia*, and *Enterobacter*. Inactive against most gram-positive microorganisms. Not well absorbed systemically from GI tract (must be administered parenterally for systemic infections). Oral agents are given to suppress intestinal bacteria.

ACTION

Bactericidal. Transported across bacterial cell membrane; irreversibly bind to specific receptor proteins of bacterial ribosomes. Interfere with protein synthesis, preventing cell reproduction and eventually causing cell death.

ANTIBIOTIC: AMINOGLYCOSIDES

Name	Availability	Dosage Range	Side Effects
Amikacin (p. 52) (Amikin)	**I:** 50 mg/ml, 250 mg/ml	**A:** 7.5 mg/kg q12h or 15–20 mg/kg once daily **C:** 7.5 mg/kg q12h	Nephrotoxicity, neurotoxicity, ototoxicity (both auditory and vestibular), hypersensitivity (skin itching, redness, rash, swelling)
Gentamicin (p. 545) (Garamycin)	**I:** 10 mg/ml, 40 mg/ml	**A:** 5–7 mg/kg once daily or 1–2.5 mg/kg q8h **C:** 1–2.5 mg/kg q8h	Same as amikacin
Neomycin	**T:** 500 mg	**A:** 1 g for 3 doses as preop	Nausea, vomiting, diarrhea
Tobramycin (p. 1200) (Nebcin)	**I:** 10 mg/ml, 40 mg/ml	**A:** 5–7 mg/kg once daily or 1–2.5 mg/kg q8h **C:** 1–2.5 mg/kg q8h	Same as amikacin

A, Adults; *C (dosage),* children; *I,* injection; *T,* tablets.

Antibiotic: Cephalosporins

USES

Broad-spectrum antibiotics, which, like penicillins, may be used in a number of diseases, including respiratory diseases, skin and soft tissue infection, bone/joint infections, GU infections, prophylactically in some surgical procedures.

First-generation cephalosporins have activity against gram-positive organisms (e.g., streptococci and most staphylococci) and activity against most gram-negative organisms, including *Escherichia coli, Klebsiella pneumoniae, Proteus mirabilis, Salmonella,* and *Shigella.*

ACTION

Second-generation cephalosporins have same effectiveness as first-generation and increased activity against gram-negative organisms, including *H. influenzae, Neisseria, Enterobacter,* and several anaerobic organisms.

Third-generation cephalosporins are less active against gram-positive organisms but more active against the Enterobacteriaceae with some activity against *Pseudomonas aeruginosa, Serratia* spp., and *Acinetobacter* spp.

Fourth-generation cephalosporins have good activity against gram-positive organisms (e.g., *Staphylococcus aureus*) and gram-negative organisms (e.g., *Pseudomonas aeruginosa, E. coli, Klebsiella,* and *Proteus*).

Fifth-generation cephalosporins have good activity against gram-positive organisms (e.g., *Staphylococcus aureus, Streptococcus* spp.) and gram-negative organisms (e.g., *E. coli, Klebsiella* spp.).

Cephalosporins inhibit cell wall synthesis or activate enzymes that disrupt the cell wall, causing cell lysis and cell death. May be bacteriostatic or bactericidal. Most effective against rapidly dividing cells.

ANTIBIOTIC: CEPHALOSPORINS

Name	Availability	Dosage Range	Side Effects
First-Generation			
Cefadroxil (p. 205) (Duricef)	**C:** 500 mg **T:** 1 g **S:** 125 mg/5 ml, 250 mg/5 ml, 500 mg/5 ml	**A:** 500 mg–1 g q12h **C:** 15 mg/kg q12h	Abdominal cramps/pain, fever, nausea, vomiting, diarrhea, headaches, oral/vaginal candidiasis

(continued)

ANTIBIOTIC: CEPHALOSPORINS   *(continued)*

Name	Availability	Dosage Range	Side Effects
Cefazolin (p. 207) (Ancef)	**I:** 500 mg, 1 g, 2 g	**A:** 500 mg–2 g q6–8h **C:** 25–100 mg/kg/day divided q6–8h	Fever, rash, diarrhea, nausea, pain at injection site
Cephalexin (p. 232) (Keflex, Keftab)	**C:** 250 mg, 500 mg **T:** 250 mg, 500 mg, 1 g	**A:** 250 mg–1 g q6–12h **C:** 25–100 mg/kg/day divided q6–8h	Headache, abdominal pain, diarrhea, nausea, dyspepsia
Second-Generation			
Cefaclor (p. 204) (Ceclor)	**C:** 250 mg, 500 mg **T (ER):** 500 mg **S:** 125 mg/5 ml, 187 mg/5 ml, 250 mg/5 ml, 375 mg/5 ml	**A:** 250–500 mg q8h **C:** 20–40 mg/kg/day q8–12h	Rash, diarrhea, increased transaminases May have serum sickness–like reaction
Cefotetan	**I:** 1 g, 2 g	**A:** 500 mg–3 g q12h **C:** 20–50 mg/kg q12h	Diarrhea, increased AST, ALT, hypersensitivity reactions
Cefoxitin (p. 216) (Mefoxin)	**I:** 1 g, 2 g	**A:** 1–2 g q6–8h **C:** 80–160 mg/kg/day divided q6h	Diarrhea
Cefprozil (p. 220) (Cefzil)	**T:** 250 mg, 500 mg **S:** 125 mg/5 ml, 250 mg/5 ml	**A:** 500 mg q12–24h **C:** 7.5–15 mg/kg q12h	Dizziness, abdominal pain, diarrhea, nausea, increased AST, ALT
Cefuroxime (p. 229) (Ceftin, Kefurox, Zinacef)	**T:** 125 mg, 250 mg, 500 mg **S:** 125 mg/5 ml, 250 mg/5 ml **I:** 750 mg, 1.5 g	**A (PO):** 125–500 mg q12h **(IM/IV):** 750 mg–1.5 g q8–12h **C (PO):** 10–15 mg/kg q12h **(IM/IV):** 50–150 mg/kg/day divided q8h	Diarrhea, nausea, vomiting, thrombophlebitis, increased AST, ALT

Third-Generation

Drug	Forms	Dosage	Side Effects
Cefdinir (p. 209) (Omnicef)	C: 300 mg S: 125 mg/5 ml	A: 300 mg q12h or 600 mg once daily C: 7 mg/kg q12h or 14 mg/kg once daily	Headache, hyperglycemia, abdominal pain, diarrhea, nausea
Cefditoren (Spectracef)	T: 200 mg	A: 200–400 mg q12h C: (>11 yrs): 200–400 mg q12h	Diarrhea, nausea
Cefotaxime (p. 214) (Claforan)	I: 500 mg, 1 g, 2 g	A: 1–2 g q4–12h C: 50–200 mg/kg/day divided q4–6h	Rash, diarrhea, nausea, pain at injection site
Cefpodoxime (p. 218) (Vantin)	T: 100 mg, 200 mg S: 50 mg/5 ml, 100 mg/5 ml	A: 100–400 mg q12h C: 5 mg/kg q12h	Rash, diarrhea, nausea
Ceftazidime (p. 223) (Fortaz, Tazicef, Tazidime)	I: 500 mg, 1 g, 2 g	A: 500 mg–2 g q8–12h C: 30–100 mg/kg q8h	Diarrhea, pain at injection site
Ceftibuten (p. 225) (Cedax)	C: 400 mg S: 90 mg/5 ml, 180 mg/5 ml	A: 400 mg once daily C: 4.5 mg/kg bid or 9 mg/kg once daily	Headache, nausea, diarrhea
Ceftriaxone (p. 226) (Rocephin)	I: 250 mg, 500 mg, 1 g, 2 g	A: 1–2 g q12–24h C: 50–100 mg/kg/day divided q12–24h	Rash, diarrhea, eosinophilia, increased AST, ALT

Fourth-Generation

Drug	Forms	Dosage	Side Effects
Cefepime (p. 210) (Maxipime)	I: 500 mg, 1 g, 2 g	A: 1–2 g q8–12h C: 50 mg/kg q8–12h	Rash, diarrhea, nausea; increased AST, ALT

Fifth-Generation

Drug	Forms	Dosage	Side Effects
Ceftaroline (p. 221) (Teflaro)	I: 400 mg, 600 mg	A: 600 mg q12h	Headache, insomnia, rash, pruritus, diarrhea, nausea

A, Adults; *C,* capsules; *C (dosage),* children; *ER,* extended-release; *I,* injection; *S,* suspension; *T,* tablets.

Antibiotic: Fluoroquinolones

USES

Fluoroquinolones act against a wide range of gram-negative and gram-positive organisms. They are used primarily in the treatment of lower respiratory infections, skin/skin structure infections, UTIs, and sexually transmitted diseases.

ACTION

Bactericidal. Inhibit DNA gyrase in susceptible microorganisms, interfering with bacterial DNA replication and repair.

ANTIBIOTIC: FLUOROQUINOLONES

Name	Availability	Dosage Range	Side Effects
Ciprofloxacin (p. 252) (Cipro)	**T:** 100 mg, 250 mg, 500 mg, 750 mg **S:** 250 mg/5 ml, 500 mg/5 ml **I:** 200 mg, 400 mg	**A (PO):** 250–750 mg q12h; **(IV):** 200–400 mg q12h	Dizziness, headaches, anxiety, drowsiness, insomnia, abdominal pain, nausea, diarrhea, vomiting, phlebitis (parenteral)
Gemifloxacin (p. 544) (Factive)	**T:** 320 mg	**A:** 320 mg once daily	Headache, dizziness, rash, diarrhea, nausea
Levofloxacin (p. 691) (Levaquin)	**T:** 250 mg, 500 mg, 750 mg **I:** 250 mg, 500 mg, 750 mg **OS:** 250 mg/10 ml	**A (PO/IV):** 250–750 mg/day as single dose	Headache, insomnia, dizziness, rash, nausea, diarrhea, constipation
Moxifloxacin (p. 813) (Avelox)	**T:** 400 mg **I:** 400 mg	**A:** 400 mg/day	Headache, dizziness, insomnia, nausea, diarrhea
Norfloxacin (p. 865) (Noroxin)	**T:** 400 mg	**A:** 400 mg q12h	Same as ciprofloxacin
Ofloxacin (p. 876)	**T:** 200 mg, 300 mg, 400 mg	**A:** 200–400 mg q12h	Dizziness, headache, insomnia, abdominal cramps, diarrhea, nausea

A, Adults; *I,* injection; *OS,* oral solution; *S,* suspension; *T,* tablets.

Antibiotic: Macrolides

USES

Macrolides act primarily against most gram-positive microorganisms and some gram-negative cocci. Azithromycin and clarithromycin appear to be more potent than erythromycin. Macrolides are used in the treatment of pharyngitis/tonsillitis, sinusitis, chronic bronchitis, pneumonia, uncomplicated skin/skin structure infections.

ACTION

Bacteriostatic or bactericidal. Reversibly binds to the P site of the 50S ribosomal subunit of susceptible organisms, inhibiting RNA-dependent protein synthesis.

ANTIBIOTIC: MACROLIDES

Name	Availability	Dosage Range	Side Effects
Azithromycin (p. 110) (Zithromax)	**T:** 250 mg, 600 mg **S:** 100 mg/5 ml, 200 mg/5 ml, 1-g packet **I:** 500 mg	**A (PO):** 500 mg once, then 250 mg once daily (**IV):** 500 mg/day **C (PO/IV):** 5–10 mg/kg once daily	**PO:** Nausea, diarrhea, vomiting, abdominal pain **IV:** Pain, redness, swelling at injection site
Clarithromycin (p. 261) (Biaxin)	**T:** 250 mg, 500 mg **T (XL):** 500 mg **S:** 125 mg/5 ml	**A:** 250–500 mg q12h **C:** 7.5 mg/kg q12h	Headaches, loss of taste, nausea, vomiting, diarrhea, abdominal pain/discomfort
Erythromycin (p. 442) (EES, Eryc, EryPed, Ery-Tab, Erythrocin, PCE)	**T:** 200 mg, 250 mg, 333 mg, 400 mg, 500 mg **C:** 250 mg **S:** 100 mg/2.5 ml, 125 mg/5 ml, 200 mg/5 ml, 250 mg/5 ml, 400 mg/5 ml	**A (PO):** 250–500 mg q6h (**IV):** 500 mg–1 g q6h **C (PO):** 7.5 mg/kg q6h (**IV):** 15–50 mg/kg/day in divided doses q6h	**PO:** Nausea, vomiting, diarrhea, abdominal pain **IV:** Inflammation, phlebitis at injection site

A, Adults; *C (dosage),* children; *I,* injection; *S,* suspension; *T,* tablets; *XL,* long-acting.

Antibiotic: Penicillins

USES

Penicillins (also referred to as beta-lactam antibiotics) may be used to treat a large number of infections, including pneumonia and other respiratory diseases, UTIs, septicemia, meningitis, intra-abdominal infections, gonorrhea and syphilis, bone/joint infection.

Penicillins are classified based on an antimicrobial spectrum:

Natural penicillins are very active against gram-positive cocci but ineffective against most strains of *Staphylococcus aureus* (inactivated by enzyme penicillinase).

Penicillinase-resistant penicillins are effective against penicillinase-producing *Staphylococcus aureus* but are less effective against gram-positive cocci than the natural penicillins.

Broad-spectrum penicillins are effective against gram-positive cocci and some gram-negative bacteria (e.g., *Haemophilus influenzae, Escherichia coli, Proteus mirabilis, Salmonella,* and *Shigella*).

Extended-spectrum penicillins are effective against gram-negative organisms, including *Pseudomonas aeruginosa, Enterobacter, Proteus* spp, *Klebsiella, Serratia* spp., and *Acinetobacter* spp.

ACTION

Penicillins inhibit cell wall synthesis or activate enzymes, which disrupt the bacterial cell wall, causing cell lysis and cell death. May be bacteriostatic or bactericidal. Most effective against bacteria undergoing active growth and division.

ANTIBIOTIC: PENICILLINS

Name	Availability	Dosage Range	Side Effects
Natural			
Penicillin G benzathine (p. 940) (Bicillin, Bicillin LA)	**I:** 600,000 units, 1.2 million units, 2.4 million units	**A:** 1.2–2.4 million units as single dose **C:** 25,000–50,000 units/kg as single dose	Mild diarrhea, nausea, vomiting, headaches, sore mouth/tongue, vaginal itching/discharge, allergic reaction (including anaphylaxis, skin rash, urticaria, pruritus)
Penicillin G potassium (p. 941) (Pfizerpen)	**I:** 1, 2, 3, 5 million-unit vials	**A:** 2–4 million units q4h **C:** 100,000–250,000 units/kg/day divided q4–6h	Rash, injection site reaction, phlebitis

Penicillin V potassium (p. 943) (Apo-Pen-VK)	**T:** 250 mg, 500 mg **S:** 125 mg/5 ml, 250 mg/5 ml	**A:** 250–500 mg q6–8h **C:** 25–50 mg/kg/day in divided doses q6–8h	Diarrhea, nausea, vomiting
Penicillinase-Resistant			
Dicloxacillin (Dynapen, Pathocil)	**C:** 125 mg, 250 mg, 500 mg **S:** 62.5 mg/5 ml	**A:** 125–500 mg q6h **C:** 25–50 mg/kg/day divided q6h	Abdominal pain, diarrhea, nausea
Nafcillin (p. 822) (Unipen)	**I:** 500 mg, 1 g, 2 g	**A (IV):** 500 mg–2 g q4–6h **C (IV):** 50–150 mg/kg/day in divided doses q4–6h	Inflammation, pain, phlebitis Increased risk of interstitial nephritis
Oxacillin (Bactocill)	**C:** 250 mg, 500 mg **S:** 250 mg/5 ml **I:** 250 mg, 500 mg, 1 g, 2 g	**A (IV):** 1–2 g q4–6h **C (IV):** 25–50 mg/kg q6h	Diarrhea, nausea, vomiting Increased risk of hepatotoxicity, interstitial nephritis
Broad-Spectrum			
Amoxicillin (p. 60) (Amoxil, Trimox)	**T:** 125 mg, 250 mg, 500 mg, 875 mg **C:** 250 mg, 500 mg **S:** 50 mg/ml, 125 mg/5 ml, 250 mg/5 ml	**A:** 250–500 mg q8h or 500–875 g q12h **C:** 20–90 mg/kg/day divided q8–12h	Diarrhea, colitis, nausea
Amoxicillin/clavulanate (p. 62) (Augmentin)	**T:** 250 mg, 500 mg, 875 mg **T (chewable):** 125 mg, 200 mg, 250 mg, 400 mg **S:** 125 mg/5 ml, 200 mg/5 ml, 250 mg/5 ml, 400 mg/5 ml	**A:** 875 mg q12h or 250–500 mg q8h **C:** 25–90 mg/kg/day divided q12h	Diarrhea, rash, nausea, vomiting

(continued)

ANTIBIOTIC: PENICILLINS   *(continued)*

Name	Availability	Dosage Range	Side Effects
Ampicillin (p. 66) (Principen)	**C:** 250 mg, 500 mg **S:** 125 mg/5 ml, 250 mg/5 ml **I:** 125 mg, 250 mg, 500 mg, 1 g, 2 g	**A: (PO):** 250–500 mg q6h **(IV):** 500 mg–2 g q6h **C (PO):** 12.5–50 mg/kg q6h **(IV):** 25–50 mg/kg q6h	Nausea, vomiting, diarrhea
Ampicillin/sulbactam (p. 68) (Unasyn)	**I:** 1.5 g, 3 g	**A:** 1.5–3 g q6h **C:** 25–50 mg/kg q6h	Local pain at injection site, rash, diarrhea
Extended-Spectrum			
Piperacillin/tazobactam (p. 964) (Zosyn)	**I:** 2.25 g, 3.375 g, 4.5 g	**A:** 3.375 g q6h or 4.5 g q6–8h **C:** 240–300 mg/kg/day divided q8h	Diarrhea, insomnia, headache, fever, rash
Ticarcillin/clavulanate (Timentin)	**I:** 3.1 g	**A:** 3.1 g q4–6h **C:** 200–300 mg/kg/day divided q4–6h	Colitis, nausea, vomiting, diarrhea

A, Adults; *C,* capsules; *C (dosage),* children; *I,* injection; *S,* suspension; *T,* tablets.

Anticoagulants/Antiplatelets/Thrombolytics

USES	ACTION
Treatment and prevention of venous thromboembolism, acute MI, acute cerebral embolism; reduce risk of acute MI; reduction of total mortality in pts with unstable angina; prevent occlusion of saphenous grafts following open heart surgery; prevent embolism in select pts with atrial fibrillation, prosthetic heart valves, valvular heart disease, cardiomyopathy. Heparin also used for acute/chronic consumption coagulopathies (disseminated intravascular coagulation).	*Anticoagulants:* Inhibits blood coagulation by preventing the formation of new clots and extension of existing ones *but do not dissolve formed clots.* Anticoagulants are subdivided into three classes. *Heparin* (including low molecular weight heparin): Indirectly interferes with blood coagulation by blocking the conversion of prothrombin to thrombin and fibrinogen to fibrin. *Coumarin:* Acts indirectly to prevent synthesis in the liver of vitamin K–dependent clotting factors. *Direct Thrombin Inhibitors:* Inhibits thrombin from converting fibrinogen to fibrin. *Antiplatelets:* Interferes with platelet aggregation. Effects are irreversible for life of platelet. Medications in this group act by different mechanisms. Aspirin irreversibly inhibits cyclo-oxygenase, irreversibly inhibits formation of thromboxane A$_2$. Clopidogrel, dipyridamole, prasugrel, and ticlopidine have similar effects as aspirin and are known as adenosine diphosphate (ADP) inhibitors. Abciximab, eptifibatide, and tirofiban block binding of fibrinogen to the glycoprotein IIb/IIIa receptor on platelet surface (known as platelet glycoprotein IIb/IIIa receptor antagonists). *Thrombolytics:* Acts directly or indirectly on fibrinolytic system to dissolve clots (converting plasminogen to plasmin, an enzyme that digests fibrin clot).

ANTICOAGULANTS/ANTIPLATELETS/THROMBOLYTICS

Name	Availability	Uses	Side Effects
Anticoagulants			
Direct Thrombin Inhibitors			
Argatroban (p. 79)	I: 100 mg/ml	Prevent/treat VTE in pts with HIT or at risk for HIT undergoing PCI	Bleeding, hypotension, hematuria
Bivalirudin (p. 144) (Angiomax)	I: 250-mg vials	Pts with unstable angina undergoing PTCA	Bleeding, hypotension, pain, headache, nausea, back pain
Dabigatran (p. 305) (Pradaxa)	C: 75 mg, 150 mg	Reduce risk for stroke/embolism with nonvalvular atrial fibrillation	Bleeding, gastritis, dyspepsia
Desirudin (Iprivask)	I: 15 mg	Hip surgery	Bleeding
Heparin, Low Molecular Weight Heparins			
Dalteparin (p. 310) (Fragmin)	I: 2,500 units, 5,000 units, 7,500 units, 10,000 units	Hip surgery, abdominal surgery, unstable angina or non–Q-wave MI	Bleeding, hematoma, increased ALT, AST, pain at injection site, bruising
Enoxaparin (p. 419) (Lovenox)	I: 30 mg, 40 mg, 60 mg, 80 mg, 100 mg, 120 mg, 150 mg	Hip surgery, knee surgery, abdominal surgery, unstable angina or non–Q-wave MI, acute illness	Bleeding, thrombocytopenia, hematoma, increased ALT, AST, nausea, bruising
Heparin (p. 568)	I: 1,000 units/ml, 2,500 units/ml, 5,000 units/ml, 7,500 units/ml, 10,000 units/ml, 20,000 units/ml	Prevent/treat VTE	Bleeding, thrombocytopenia, skin rash, itching, burning
Tinzaparin (p. 1194) (Innohep)	I: 20,000 units/ml vials	Treatment of VTE (with warfarin)	Bleeding, thrombocytopenia, increased ALT, injection site hematoma

Factor Xa Inhibitor

Drug	Form	Uses	Side Effects
Apixaban (p. 76) (Eliquis)	**T:** 2.5 mg, 5 mg	Reduce risk of stroke/embolism in nonvalvular atrial fibrillation	Bleeding, nausea, anemia
Fondaparinux (p. 517) (Arixtra)	**I:** 2.5 mg	Hip surgery, knee surgery, DVT	Bleeding, thrombocytopenia, hematoma, fever, nausea, anemia
Rivaroxaban (p. 1067) (Xarelto)	**T:** 10 mg	Prevent DVT post knee, hip replacement Prevent thromboembolism in atrial fibrillation	Bleeding

Coumarin

Drug	Form	Uses	Side Effects
Warfarin (p. 1289) (Coumadin)	**PO:** 1 mg, 2 mg, 2.5 mg, 3 mg, 4 mg, 5 mg, 6 mg, 7.5 mg, 10 mg **I:** 5 mg	Prevent/treat VTE in pts; prevent systemic embolism in pts with heart valve replacement, valve heart disease, MI, atrial fibrillation	Bleeding, skin necrosis, anorexia, nausea, vomiting, diarrhea, rash, abdominal cramps, purple toe syndrome, drug interactions (see individual monograph)

Antiplatelets

Drug	Form	Uses	Side Effects
Abciximab (p. 4) (ReoPro)	**I:** 2 mg/ml	Adjunct to PCI to prevent acute cardiac ischemic complications (with heparin and aspirin)	Bleeding, hypotension, nausea, vomiting, back pain, allergic reactions, thrombocytopenia
Aspirin (p. 89)	**PO:** 81 mg, 165 mg, 325 mg, 500 mg, 650 mg	TIA Prevention of reinfarction and thromboembolism post MI	Tinnitus, dizziness, hypersensitivity, dyspepsia, minor bleeding, GI ulceration
Clopidogrel (p. 276) (Plavix)	**PO:** 75 mg	Reduce risk of stroke, MI, or vascular death in pts with recent MI, noncardioembolic stroke, peripheral artery disease. Reduce CV death, MI, stroke, reinfarction in pts with non-STEMI/STEMI	Bleeding, rash, pruritus, bruising, epistaxis

HIT, Heparin-induced thrombocytopenia; *I,* injection; *MI,* myocardial infarction; *PCI,* percutaneous coronary intervention; *PO,* oral; *PTCA,* percutaneous transluminal coronary angioplasty; *T,* tablet; *VTE,* venous thromboembolism.

(continued)

ANTICOAGULANTS/ANTIPLATELETS/THROMBOLYTICS　*(continued)*

Name	Availability	Uses	Side Effects
Dipyridamole (p. 377) (Persantine)	**PO:** 25 mg, 50 mg, 75 mg	Prevent postop thromboembolic complications following cardiac valve replacement	Dizziness, GI distress
Eptifibatide (p. 435) (Integrilin)	**I:** 0.75 mg/ml, 2 mg/ml	Treatment of acute coronary syndrome	Bleeding, hypotension
Prasugrel (p. 983) (Effient)	**PO:** 5 mg, 10 mg	Reduce thrombotic cardiovascular events in pts with ACS to be managed with PCI (including stenting)	Bleeding, hypotension
Ticagrelor (p. 1187) (Brilinta)	**PO:** 90 mg	Reduce thrombotic cardiovascular events in pts with ACS	Bleeding, dyspnea
Ticlopidine (p. 1189) (Ticlid)	**PO:** 250 mg	Reduce risk stroke in pts with CVA precursors, TIA Prevention of stent thrombosis	Neutropenia, agranulocytosis, thrombocytopenia, aplastic anemia, increased serum cholesterol/triglycerides, rash, diarrhea, nausea, vomiting, GI pain
Tirofiban (Aggrastat)	**I:** 50 mcg/ml, 250 mcg/ml	Treatment of acute coronary syndrome	Bleeding, thrombocytopenia, bradycardia, pelvic pain
Thrombolytics			
Alteplase (p. 46) (Activase)	**I:** 50 mg, 100 mg	Acute MI, acute ischemic stroke, pulmonary embolism	Bleeding, epistaxis
Reteplase (p. 1046) (Retavase)	**I:** 10.4 units	Acute MI	Bleeding, injection site bleeding, anemia
Tenecteplase (p. 1162) (TNKase)	**I:** 50 mg	Acute MI	Bleeding, hematuria

ACS, Acute coronary syndrome; *CVA,* cerebrovascular attack; *I,* injection; *MI,* myocardial infarction; *PCI,* percutaneous coronary intervention; *PO,* oral; *TIA,* transient ischemic attack.

Anticonvulsants

USES

Anticonvulsants are used to treat seizures. Seizures can be divided into two broad categories: partial seizures and generalized seizures. *Partial seizures* begin focally in the cerebral cortex, undergoing limited spread. Simple partial seizures do not involve loss of consciousness but may evolve secondarily into generalized seizures. Complex partial seizures involve impairment of consciousness.

Generalized seizures may be convulsive or nonconvulsive and usually produce immediate loss of consciousness.

ACTION

Anticonvulsants can prevent or reduce excessive discharge of neurons with seizure foci or decrease the spread of excitation from seizure foci to normal neurons. The exact mechanism is unknown but may be due to (1) suppressing sodium influx, (2) suppressing calcium influx, or (3) increasing the action of gamma-aminobutyric acid (GABA), which inhibits neurotransmitters throughout the brain.

ANTICONVULSANTS

Name	Availability	Uses	Dosage Range	Side Effects
Carbamazepine (p. 188) (Carbatrol, Tegretol, Tegretol XR)	**S:** 100 mg/5 ml **T (chewable):** 100 mg **T:** 200 mg **T (ER):** 100 mg, 200 mg, 400 mg **C (ER):** 200 mg, 300 mg	Complex partial, tonic-clonic, mixed seizures; trigeminal neuralgia	**A:** 800–1,600 mg/day in 2–3 doses **C:** 400–800 mg/day in 3–4 doses	Dizziness, diplopia, leukopenia, drowsiness, blurred vision, headache, ataxia, nausea, vomiting, hyponatremia
Clonazepam (p. 271) (Klonopin)	**T:** 0.5 mg, 1 mg, 2 mg	Petit mal, akinetic, myoclonic, absence seizures	**A:** 1.5–8 mg/day in 2–3 doses	CNS depression, sedation, ataxia, confusion, depression, behavior disorders, respiratory depression
Ezogabine (p. 469) (Potiga)	**T:** 50 mg, 200 mg, 300 mg, 400 mg	Partial onset seizures	**A:** 600–1,200 mg/day in 3 doses	Dizziness, somnolence, fatigue, confusion, vertigo, tremor, diplopia, blurred vision, balance disorder

(continued)

ANTICONVULSANTS *(continued)*

Name	Availability	Uses	Dosage Range	Side Effects
Fosphenytoin (p. 526) (Cerebyx)	**I:** 50 mg PE/ml	Status epilepticus, seizures occurring during neurosurgery	**A:** 15–20 mg PE/kg bolus, then 4–6 mg PE/kg/day maintenance	Burning, itching, paresthesia, nystagmus, ataxia
Gabapentin (p. 533) (Neurontin)	**C:** 100 mg, 300 mg, 400 mg	Partial seizures with and without secondary generalization	**A:** 1,800–3,600 mg/day in 3 doses	CNS depression, fatigue, drowsiness, dizziness, ataxia, nystagmus, blurred vision, confusion
Lacosamide (p. 665) (Vimpat)	**T:** 50 mg, 100 mg, 150 mg, 200 mg **S:** 10 mg/ml **I:** 10 mg/ml	Adjunctive therapy, partial seizures	**A:** 200–400 mg/day in 2 doses	Diplopia, headache, dizziness, nausea
Lamotrigine (p. 670) (Lamictal)	**T:** 25 mg, 100 mg, 150 mg, 200 mg **T (ER):** 25 mg, 50 mg, 100 mg, 200 mg **T (ODT):** 25 mg, 50 mg, 100 mg, 200 mg	Partial seizures, primary generalized tonic-clonic seizures, generalized seizures of Lennox-Gastaut syndrome	**A:** 100–600 mg/day in 2 doses	Dizziness, ataxia, drowsiness, diplopia, nausea, rash, headache, vomiting, insomnia, incoordination
Levetiracetam (p. 688) (Keppra)	**T:** 250 mg, 500 mg, 750 mg, 2,000 mg **S:** 100 mg/ml	Adjunctive therapy, partial seizures, primary tonic-clonic seizures, myoclonic seizures	**A:** 1,000–3,000 mg/day in 2 doses	Dizziness, drowsiness, weakness, irritability, hallucinations, psychosis
Oxcarbazepine (p. 900) (Trileptal)	**T:** 150 mg, 300 mg, 600 mg	Partial seizures	**A:** 1,200–2,400 mg/day in 2 doses	Drowsiness, dizziness, headaches, diplopia, ataxia, nausea, vomiting
Phenobarbital (p. 952)	**T:** 30 mg, 60 mg, 100 mg **I:** 65 mg, 130 mg	Tonic-clonic, partial seizures; status epilepticus	**A (PO):** 100–300 mg/day; **(IM/IV):** 200–600 mg **C (PO):** 3–5 mg/kg/day; **(IM/IV):** 100–400 mg	CNS depression, sedation, paradoxical excitement and hyperactivity, rash

Drug	Forms	Uses	Dosage	Side Effects
Phenytoin (p. 958) (Dilantin)	**C:** 100 mg **T (chewable):** 50 mg **S:** 125 mg/5 ml **I:** 50 mg/ml	Tonic-clonic, psychomotor seizures	**A (PO):** 300–600 mg/day in 1–3 doses; **IV:** 150–250 mg **C (PO):** 4–8 mg/kg/day in 1–3 doses; **(IV):** 10–15 mg/kg	Nystagmus, ataxia, hypertrichosis, gingival hyperplasia, rash, osteomalacia, lymphadenopathy
Pregabalin (p. 991) (Lyrica)	**C:** 25 mg, 50 mg, 75 mg, 100 mg, 150 mg, 200 mg, 225 mg, 300 mg	Adjunctive therapy, partial seizures	**A:** 150–600 mg/day in 2 or 3 doses	Confusion, drowsiness, dizziness, ataxia, weight gain, dry mouth, blurred vision, peripheral edema
Primidone (p. 993) (Mysoline)	**T:** 50 mg, 250 mg **S:** 250 mg/5 ml	Complex partial, akinetic, tonic-clonic seizures	**A:** 750–1250 mg/day in 3–4 doses **C:** 10–25 mg/kg/day	CNS depression, sedation, paradoxical excitement and hyperactivity, rash, dizziness, ataxia
Tiagabine (p. 1186) (Gabitril)	**T:** 4 mg, 12 mg, 16 mg, 20 mg	Partial seizures	**A:** Initially, 4 mg up to 56 mg/day in 2–4 doses **C:** Initially, 4 mg up to 32 mg/day in 2–4 doses	Dizziness, asthenia (loss of strength, energy), nervousness, anxiety, tremors, abdominal pain
Topiramate (p. 1210) (Topamax)	**T:** 25 mg, 100 mg, 200 mg	Partial seizures	**A:** 200–400 mg/day in 2 doses **C:** 1–9 mg/kg/day in 2 divided doses	Drowsiness, dizziness, headache, ataxia, confusion, weight loss, diplopia
Valproic acid (p. 1247) (Depakene, Depakote)	**C:** 250 mg **S:** 250 mg/5 ml **Sprinkles:** 125 mg **T:** 125 mg, 250 mg, 500 mg **T (ER):** 500 mg **I:** 100 mg/ml	Complex partial, absence seizures	**A, C:** 15–60 mg/kg/day in 2–3 doses	Nausea, vomiting, tremors, thrombocytopenia, hair loss, hepatic dysfunction, weight gain, decreased platelet function

(continued)

ANTICONVULSANTS   (continued)

Name	Availability	Uses	Dosage Range	Side Effects
Vigabatrin (Sabril)	**T:** 500 mg **PS:** 500 mg	Infantile spasms, refractory complex partial seizures	**A:** 3 g/day in 2 divided doses **C:** 40–100 mg/kg/day in 2 divided doses	Vision changes, eye pain, abdominal pain, agitation, confusion, mood/mental changes, abnormal coordination
Zonisamide (p. 1303) (Zonegran)	**C:** 100 mg	Partial seizures	**A:** 100–400 mg/day in 1 or 2 doses	Drowsiness, dizziness, anorexia, diarrhea, weight loss, agitation, irritability, rash, nausea

A, Adults; *C,* capsules; *C (dosage),* children; *ER,* extended-release; *I,* injection; *ODT,* orally disintegrating tablets; *PE,* phenytoin equivalent; *PS,* powder sachet; *S,* suspension; *T,* tablets.

Antidepressants

USES

Used primarily for the treatment of depression. Depression can be a chronic or recurrent mental disorder presenting with symptoms such as depressed mood, loss of interest or pleasure, guilt feelings, disturbed sleep/appetite, low energy, and difficulty in thinking. Depression can also lead to suicide.

ACTION

Antidepressants include tricyclics, monoamine oxidase inhibitors (MAOIs), selective serotonin reuptake inhibitors (SSRIs), serotonin-norepinephrine reuptake inhibitors (SNRIs), and other antidepressants. Depression may be due to reduced functioning of monoamine neurotransmitters (e.g., norepinephrine, serotonin [5-HT],

dopamine) in the CNS (decreased amount and/or decreased effects at the receptor sites). Antidepressants block metabolism, increase amount/effects of monoamine neurotransmitters, and act at receptor sites (change responsiveness/sensitivities of both presynaptic and postsynaptic receptor sites).

ANTIDEPRESSANTS

Name	Availability	Uses	Dosage Range (per day)	Side Effects
Tricyclics				
Amitriptyline (p. 57) (Elavil)	**T:** 10 mg, 25 mg, 50 mg, 75 mg, 100 mg, 150 mg	Depression, neuropathic pain	50–150 mg	Drowsiness, blurred vision, constipation, confusion, postural hypotension, cardiac conduction defects, weight gain, seizures, dry mouth
Clomipramine (p. 270) (Anafranil)	**C:** 25 mg, 50 mg, 75 mg	OCD	25–250 mg	Dizziness, somnolence, drowsiness, headache, xerostomia, constipation, nausea
Desipramine (p. 336) (Norpramin)	**T:** 10 mg, 25 mg, 50 mg, 75 mg, 100 mg, 150 mg	Depression, neuropathic pain	50–150 mg	Dizziness, drowsiness, fatigue, headache, anorexia, diarrhea, nausea
Imipramine (p. 609) (Tofranil)	**T:** 10 mg, 25 mg, 50 mg **C:** 75 mg, 100 mg, 125 mg, 150 mg	Depression, enuresis, neuropathic pain, panic disorder, ADHD	25–100 mg	Dizziness, fatigue, headache, vomiting, xerostomia
Nortriptyline (p. 866) (Aventyl, Pamelor)	**C:** 10 mg, 25 mg, 50 mg, 75 mg **S:** 10 mg/5 ml	Depression, neuropathic pain, smoking cessation	75–150 mg	Dizziness, fatigue, headache, anorexia, xerostomia
Monoamine Oxidase Inhibitors				
Phenelzine (p. 951) (Nardil)	**T:** 15 mg	Depression	45–60 mg	Sedation, hypertensive crisis, weight gain, orthostatic hypotension
Tranylcypromine (p. 1223) (Parnate)	**T:** 10 mg	Depression	10–60 mg	Same as phenelzine

(continued)

ANTIDEPRESSANTS (continued)

Name	Availability	Uses	Dosage Range (per day)	Side Effects
Selective Serotonin Reuptake Inhibitors				
Citalopram (p. 258) (Celexa)	**T:** 20 mg, 40 mg **S:** 10 mg/5 ml	Depression, OCD, panic disorder	20–40 mg	Insomnia or sedation, nausea, agitation, headaches
Escitalopram (p. 444) (Lexapro)	**T:** 5 mg, 10 mg, 20 mg	Depression, GAD	10–20 mg	Insomnia or sedation, nausea, agitation, headaches
Fluoxetine (p. 504) (Prozac)	**C:** 10 mg, 20 mg, 40 mg **T:** 10 mg **S:** 20 mg/5 ml	Depression, OCD, bulimia, panic disorder, anorexia, bipolar disorder, premenstrual syndrome	10–80 mg	Akathisia, sexual dysfunction, skin rash, urticaria, pruritus, decreased appetite, asthenia (loss of strength, energy), diarrhea, drowsiness, headaches, diaphoresis, insomnia, nausea, tremors
Fluvoxamine (p. 514) (Luvox, Luvox CR)	**T:** 25 mg, 50 mg, 100 mg **C (SR):** 100 mg, 150 mg	OCD, SAD	100–300 mg	Sexual dysfunction, fatigue, constipation, dizziness, drowsiness, headaches, insomnia, nausea, vomiting
Paroxetine (p. 924) (Paxil)	**T:** 10 mg, 20 mg, 30 mg, 40 mg **S:** 10 mg/5 ml	Depression, OCD, panic attack, SAD	20–50 mg	Asthenia (loss of strength, energy), constipation, diarrhea, diaphoresis, insomnia, nausea, sexual dysfunction, tremors, vomiting, urinary frequency or retention
Sertraline (p. 1096) (Zoloft)	**T:** 25 mg, 50 mg, 100 mg **S:** 20 mg/ml	Depression, OCD, panic attack	50–200 mg	Sexual dysfunction, dizziness, drowsiness, anorexia, diarrhea, nausea, dry mouth, abdominal cramps, decreased weight, headaches, increased diaphoresis, tremors, insomnia

Serotonin-Norepinephrine Reuptake Inhibitors

Drug	Dose Forms	Uses	Dosage Range	Side Effects
Desvenlafaxine (p. 341) (Pristiq)	**T:** 50 mg, 100 mg	Depression	50–100 mg	Nausea, dizziness, insomnia, hyperhidrosis, constipation, drowsiness, decreased appetite, anxiety, male sexual function disorders
Duloxetine (p. 404) (Cymbalta)	**C:** 20 mg, 30 mg, 60 mg	Depression, fibromyalgia, neuropathic pain	40–60 mg	Nausea, dry mouth, constipation, decreased appetite, fatigue, diaphoresis
Venlafaxine (p. 1261) (Effexor)	**T:** 25 mg, 37.5 mg, 50 mg, 75 mg, 100 mg **T (ER):** 37.5 mg, 75 mg, 150 mg	Depression, anxiety	75–375 mg	Increased blood pressure, agitation, sedation, insomnia, nausea
Other				
Bupropion (p. 165) (Wellbutrin)	**T:** 75 mg, 100 mg **SR:** 100 mg, 150 mg	Depression, smoking cessation, ADHD, bipolar disorder	150–450 mg	Insomnia, irritability, seizures
Mirtazapine (p. 798) (Remeron)	**T:** 15 mg, 30 mg, 45 mg	Depression	15–45 mg	Sedation, dry mouth, weight gain, agranulocytosis, hepatic toxicity
Trazodone (p. 1226) (Desyrel)	**T:** 50 mg, 100 mg, 150 mg, 300 mg	Depression	50–600 mg	Sedation, orthostatic hypotension, priapism
Vilazodone (p. 1266) (Viibyrd)	**T:** 10 mg, 20 mg, 40 mg	Depression	10–40 mg	Diarrhea, nausea, dizziness, dry mouth, insomnia, vomiting, decreased libido

ADHD, Attention-deficit hyperactivity disorder; *C*, capsules; *ER*, extended-release; *GAD*, generalized anxiety disorder; *OC*, oral concentrate; *OCD*, obsessive-compulsive disorder; *S*, suspension; *SAD*, social anxiety disorder; *SR*, sustained-release; *T*, tablets.

Antidiabetics

USES	ACTION
Insulin: Treatment of insulin-dependent diabetes (type 1) and non–insulin-dependent diabetes (type 2). Also used in acute situations such as ketoacidosis, severe infections, major surgery in otherwise non-insulin-dependent diabetics. Administered to pts receiving parenteral nutrition. Drug of choice during pregnancy. All insulins, including long-acting insulins, can cause hypoglycemia and weight gain.	*Insulin:* A hormone synthesized and secreted by beta cells of Langerhans' islet in the pancreas. Controls storage and utilization of glucose, amino acids, and fatty acids by activated transport systems/enzymes. Inhibits breakdown of glycogen, fat, protein. Insulin lowers blood glucose by inhibiting glycogenolysis and gluconeogenesis in liver; stimulates glucose uptake by muscle, adipose tissue. Activity of insulin is initiated by binding to cell surface receptors.
Alpha-glucosidase inhibitors: Adjunct to diet and exercise for management of type 2 diabetes mellitus.	*Alpha-glucosidase inhibitors:* Works locally in small intestine, slowing carbohydrate breakdown and glucose absorption.
Biguanides: Adjunct to diet and exercise for management of type 2 diabetes mellitus.	*Biguanides:* Inhibits hepatic gluconeogenesis, glycogenolysis; enhance insulin sensitivity in muscle and fat.
Dipeptidyl peptidase 4 inhibitors (DPP-4): Adjunct to diet and exercise for management of type 2 diabetes mellitus.	*DPP-4:* Inhibits degradation of endogenous incretins, which increases insulin secretion, decreases glucagon secretion.
Meglitinide: Adjunct to diet and exercise for management of type 2 diabetes mellitus.	*Meglitinide:* Stimulates pancreatic insulin secretion.
Sulfonylureas: Adjunct to diet and exercise for management of type 2 diabetes mellitus.	*Sulfonylureas:* Stimulates release of insulin from beta cells of the pancreas.
Thiazolidinediones: Adjunct to diet and exercise for management of type 2 diabetes mellitus.	*Thiazolidinediones:* Enhances insulin sensitivity in muscle and fat.

ANTIDIABETICS

INSULIN (p. 622)

Type	Onset	Peak	Duration	Comments
Rapid-Acting				
Apidra, glulisine	10–15 min	1–1.5 hrs	3–5 hrs	Stable at room temp for 28 days Can mix with NPH
Humalog, lispro	15–30 min	0.5–2.5 hrs	6–8 hrs	Stable at room temp for 28 days Can mix with NPH
Novolog, aspart	10–20 min	1–3 hrs	3–5 hrs	Stable at room temp for 28 days Can mix with NPH
Short-Acting				
Humulin R, Novolin R, regular	30–60 min	1–5 hrs	6–10 hrs	Stable at room temp for 28 days Can mix with NPH
Intermediate-Acting				
Humulin N, Novolin N, NPH	1–2 hrs	6–14 hrs	16–24 hrs	Stable at room temp for 28 days Can mix with aspart, lispro, glulisine
Long-Acting				
Lantus, glargine	1.1 hrs	No significant peak	24 hrs	Do NOT mix with other insulins Stable at room temp for 28 days
Levemir, detemir	0.8–2 hrs	No significant peak	12–24 hrs (dose dependent)	Do NOT mix with other insulins Stable at room temp for 42 days

(continued)

ANTIDIABETICS   *(continued)*

ORAL AGENTS

Sulfonylureas

Name	Availability	Dosage Range	Side Effects
Glimepiride (p. 549) (Amaryl)	**T:** 1 mg, 2 mg, 4 mg	1–8 mg/day	Hypoglycemia, dizziness, headache, nausea, flu-like syndrome
Glipizide (p. 551) (Glucotrol)	**T:** 5 mg, 10 mg **T (XL):** 5 mg	**T:** 2.5–40 mg/day **XL:** 5–20 mg/day	Dizziness, nervousness, anxiety, diarrhea, tremor
Glyburide (p. 554) (DiaBeta, Micronase)	**T:** 1.25 mg, 2.5 mg, 5 mg **PT:** 1.5 mg, 3 mg	**T:** 1.25–20 mg/day **PT:** 1.5–12 mg/day	Dizziness, headache, nausea

Alpha-Glucosidase Inhibitors

Name	Availability	Dosage Range	Side Effects
Acarbose (Precose)	**T:** 25 mg, 50 mg, 100 mg	75–300 mg/day	Flatulence, diarrhea, abdominal pain, increased risk of hypoglycemia when used with insulin or sulfonylureas
Miglitol (Glyset)	**T:** 25 mg, 50 mg, 100 mg	75–300 mg/day	Flatulence, diarrhea, abdominal pain, rash

Dipeptidyl Peptidase Inhibitors

Name	Availability	Dosage Range	Side Effects
Linagliptin (p. 701) (Tradjenta)	**T:** 5 mg	5 mg/day	Arthralgia, back pain, headache
Saxagliptin (p. 1090) (Onglyza)	**T:** 2.5 mg, 5 mg	2.5–5 mg/day	Upper respiratory tract infection, urinary tract infection, headache
Sitagliptin (p. 1109) (Januvia)	**T:** 25 mg, 50 mg, 100 mg	25–100 mg/day	Nasopharyngitis, upper respiratory infection, headaches, modest weight gain, increased incidence of hypoglycemia when added to a sulfonylurea

Biguanides

Name	Availability	Dosage Range	Side Effects
Metformin (p. 758) (Glucophage)	**T:** 500 mg, 850 mg **XR:** 500 mg	**T:** 0.5–2.5 g/day **XR:** 1,500–2,000 mg/day	Nausea, vomiting, diarrhea, loss of appetite, metallic taste, lactic acidosis (rare but potentially fatal complication)

Glucagon-Like Peptide-1 (GLP-1)			
Exenatide (p. 466) (Byetta)	I: 5 mcg, 10 mcg	5–10 mcg 2 times/day	Diarrhea, dizziness, dyspnea, headaches, nausea, vomiting
Exenatide extended-release (p. 466) (Bydureon)	I: 2 mg	2 mg once weekly	Diarrhea, nausea, headache
Liraglutide (p. 704) (Victoza)	I: 0.6 mg, 1.2 mg, 1.8 mg (6 mg/ml)	0.6–1.8 mg/day	Headache, nausea, diarrhea
Meglitinides			
Nateglinide (p. 833) (Starlix)	T: 60 mg, 120 mg	60–120 mg 3 times/day	Hypoglycemia, upper respiratory infection, dizziness, back pain, flu-like syndrome
Repaglinide (p. 1044) (Prandin)	T: 0.5 mg, 1 mg, 2 mg	0.5–1 mg with each meal (**Maximum:** 16 mg/day)	Headache, hypoglycemia, upper respiratory infection
Thiazolidinediones			
Pioglitazone (p. 962) (Actos)	T: 15 mg, 30 mg, 45 mg	15–45 mg/day	Mild to moderate peripheral edema, weight gain, increased risk of HF, associated with reduced bone mineral density and increased incidence of fractures
Rosiglitazone (p. 1078) (Avandia)	T: 2 mg, 4 mg, 8 mg	4–8 mg/day	Increased cholesterol, wgt gain, back pain, upper respiratory tract infection
Miscellaneous			
Bromocriptine (p. 157) (Cycloset)	T: 0.8 mg	1.6–4.8 mg/day	Nausea, fatigue, dizziness, vomiting
Colesevelam (p. 284) (Welchol)	T: 625 mg S: 1.875 g, 3.75 g packet	3.75 g/day	Constipation, dyspepsia, nausea
Pramlintide (p. 982) (Symlin)	I: 0.6 mg/ml	15–60 mcg immediately prior to meals	Abdominal pain, anorexia, headaches, nausea, vomiting, severe hypoglycemia may occur when used in combination with insulin (reduction in dosages of short-acting, including premixed, insulins recommended)

HF, Heart failure; *I,* injection; *PT,* prestab; *S,* suspension; *T,* tablets; *XL,* extended-release; *XR,* extended-release.

Antidiarrheals

USES

	ACTION
Acute diarrhea, chronic diarrhea of inflammatory bowel disease, reduction of fluid from ileostomies.	*Systemic agents:* Acts as smooth muscle receptors (enteric) disrupting peristaltic movements, decreasing GI motility; increasing transit time of intestinal contents. *Local agents:* Adsorbs toxic substances and fluids to large surface areas of particles in the preparation. Some of these agents coat and protect irritated intestinal walls. May have local anti-inflammatory action.

ANTIDIARRHEALS

Name	Availability	Type	Dosage Range
Bismuth (p. 142) **(Pepto-Bismol)**	**T:** 262 mg **C:** 262 mg **L:** 130 mg/15 ml, 262 mg/15 ml, 524 mg/15 ml	Local	**A:** 2 T or 30 ml **C (9–12 yrs):** 1 T or 15 ml **C (6–8 yrs):** 2/3 T or 10 ml **C (3–5 yrs):** 1/3 T or 5 ml
Diphenoxylate with atropine (p. 375) **(Lomotil)**	**T:** 2.5 mg **L:** 2.5 mg/5 ml	Systemic	**A:** 5 mg 4 times/day **C:** 0.3–0.4 mg/kg/day in 4 divided doses **(L)**
Loperamide (p. 715) (Imodium)	**C:** 2 mg **T:** 2 mg **L:** 1 mg/5 ml, 1 mg/ml	Systemic	**A:** Initially, 4 mg **(Maximum:** 16 mg/day) **C (9–12 yrs):** 2 mg 3 times/day **C (6–8 yrs):** 2 mg 2 times/day **C (2–5 yrs):** 1 mg 3 times/day **(L)**

A, Adults; *C*, capsules; *C (dosage)*, children; *L*, liquid; *S*, suspension; *T*, tablets.

Antifungals: Systemic Mycoses

Systemic mycoses are subdivided into opportunistic infections (candidiasis, aspergillosis, cryptococcosis, and mucormycosis) that are seen primarily in debilitated or immunocompromised hosts and nonopportunistic infections (blastomycosis, histoplasmosis, and coccidioidomycosis) that occur in any host. Treatment can be difficult because these infections often resist treatment and may require prolonged therapy.

ANTIFUNGALS: SYSTEMIC MYCOSES

Name	Indications	Side Effects
Amphotericin B (p. 64)	Potentially life-threatening fungal infections, including aspergillosis, blastomycosis, coccidioidomycosis, cryptococcosis, histoplasmosis, systemic candidiasis	Fever, chills, headache, nausea, vomiting, nephrotoxicity, hypokalemia, hypomagnesemia, hypotension, dyspnea, arrhythmias, abdominal pain, diarrhea, increased hepatic function tests
Amphotericin B lipid complex (Abelcet) (p. 64)	Invasive fungal infections	Chills, fever, hypotension, headache, nausea, vomiting
Amphotericin B liposomal (AmBisome) (p. 64)	Empiric therapy for presumed fungal infections in febrile neutropenic pts, treatment of cryptococcal meningitis in HIV-infected pts, treatment of *Aspergillus, Candida, Cryptococcus* infections, treatment of visceral leishmaniasis	Peripheral edema, tachycardia, hypotension, chills, insomnia, headache
Amphotericin colloidal dispersion (Amphotec) (p. 64)	Invasive *Aspergillus*	Hypotension, tachycardia, chills, fever, vomiting

(continued)

ANTIFUNGALS: SYSTEMIC MYCOSES   *(continued)*

Name	Indications	Side Effects
Anidulafungin (Eraxis) (p. 73)	Candidemia, esophageal candidiasis	Diarrhea, hypokalemia, increased hepatic function tests, headache
Caspofungin (Cancidas) (p. 202)	Candidemia, invasive aspergillosis, empiric therapy for presumed fungal infections in febrile neutropenic pts	Headache, nausea, vomiting, diarrhea, increased hepatic function tests
Fluconazole (Diflucan) (p. 496)	Treatment of vaginal candidiasis; oropharyngeal, esophageal candidiasis; and cryptococcal meningitis. Prophylaxis to decrease incidence of candidiasis in pts undergoing bone marrow transplant receiving cytotoxic chemotherapy and/or radiation	Nausea, vomiting, abdominal pain, diarrhea, dysgeusia, increased hepatic function tests, liver necrosis, hepatitis, cholestasis, headache, rash, pruritus, eosinophilia, alopecia
Itraconazole (Sporanox) (p. 651)	Blastomycosis, histoplasmosis, aspergillosis, onychomycosis, empiric therapy of febrile neutropenic pts with suspected fungal infections, treatment of oropharyngeal and esophageal candidiasis	Congestive heart failure, peripheral edema, nausea, vomiting, abdominal pain, diarrhea, increased hepatic function tests, liver necrosis, hepatitis, cholestasis, headache, rash, pruritus, eosinophilia
Ketoconazole (Nizoral) (p. 657)	Candidiasis, chronic mucocutaneous candidiasis, oral thrush, candiduria, blastomycosis, coccidioidomycosis	Nausea, vomiting, abdominal pain, diarrhea, gynecomastia, increased hepatic function tests, liver necrosis, hepatitis, cholestasis, headache, rash, pruritus, eosinophilia
Micafungin (Mycamine) (p. 782)	Esophageal candidiasis, *Candida* infections, prophylaxis in pts undergoing hematopoietin stem cell transplantation	Fever, chills, hypokalemia, hypomagnesemia, hypocalcemia, myelosuppression, thrombocytopenia, nausea, vomiting, abdominal pain, diarrhea, increased hepatic function tests, dizziness, headache, rash, pruritus, pain or inflammation at injection site, fever
Posaconazole (Noxafil) (p. 974)	Prevent invasive aspergillosis and *Candida* infections in pts 13 yrs and older who are immunocompromised, treatment of oropharyngeal candidiasis	Fever, headaches, nausea, vomiting, diarrhea, abdominal pain, hypokalemia, cough, dyspnea
Voriconazole (Vfend) (p. 1283)	Invasive aspergillosis, candidemia, esophageal candidiasis, serious fungal infections	Visual disturbances, nausea, vomiting, abdominal pain, diarrhea, increased hepatic function tests, liver necrosis, hepatitis, cholestasis, headache, rash, pruritus, eosinophilia

Antifungals: Topical

USES

Treatment of tinea infections, cutaneous candidiasis (moniliasis) due to *Candida albicans*.

ACTION

Exact mechanism unknown. May deplete essential intracellular components by inhibiting transport of potassium, other ions into cells; alter membrane permeability, resulting in loss of potassium, other cellular components.

ANTIFUNGALS: TOPICAL

Name	Availability	Dosage Range	Side Effects
Butenafine (Mentax)	**C:** 1%	2 times/day	Burning, stinging, pruritus, contact dermatitis, erythema
Ciclopirox (Loprox)	**C:** 1% **L:** 1%	2 times/day	Irritation, pruritus, redness
Clioquinol (Vioform)	**C:** 3% **O:** 3%	2–3 times/day	Irritation, stinging, swelling
Clotrimazole (Lotrimin, Mycelex)	**C:** 1% **L:** 1% **S:** 1%	2 times/day	Erythema, stinging, blistering, edema, pruritus
Econazole (Spectazole)	**C:** 1%	1–2 times/day	Burning, stinging, irritation, erythema
Ketoconazole (p. 657) (Nizoral)	**C:** 2%	1–2 times/day	Irritation, pruritus, stinging
Miconazole (p. 783) (Micatin, Monistat)	**C:** 2% **P:** 2%	2 times/day	Irritation, burning, allergic contact dermatitis

(continued)

ANTIFUNGALS: TOPICAL   *(continued)*

Name	Availability	Dosage Range	Side Effects
Nystatin (p. 868) (Mycostatin, Nilstat)	**C:** 100,000 g **O:** 100,000 g **P:** 100,000 g	2–3 times/day	Irritation
Oxiconazole (Oxistat)	**C:** 1% **L:** 1%	1–2 times/day	Pruritus, burning, stinging, irritation, pain, tingling
Sertaconazole (Ertaczo)	**C:** 2%	2 times/day	Dry skin, burning, pruritus, erythema
Terbinafine (p. 1167) (Lamisil)	**C:** 1% **G:** 10 mg	1–2 times/day	Irritation, burning, pruritus, dryness
Tolnaftate (Tinactin)	**C:** 1% **G:** 1% **S:** 1%	2 times/day	Mild irritation
Triacetin (Fungoid)	**C:** 1% **S:** 1%	3 times/day	Irritation
Undecylenic acid (Caldesene, Cruex, Desenex)	**C:** 8%, 20% **P:** 10%, 12%, 15%, 19%, 25% **O:** 25%	As needed	None significant

C, Cream; *G,* gel; *L,* lotion; *O,* ointment; *P,* powder; *S,* solution.

Antiglaucoma Agents

USES

Reduction of elevated intraocular pressure (IOP) in pts with open-angle glaucoma and ocular hypertension.

ACTION

Medications decrease IOP by two primary mechanisms: decreasing aqueous humor (AH) production or increasing AH outflow.

- *Miotics (direct acting and indirect acting):* Constricts pupils, opening channels in the trabecular meshwork, reducing resistance to outflow of AH.
- *Alpha₂-agonists:* Activates receptors in ciliary body, inhibiting aqueous secretion and increasing uveoscleral aqueous outflow.
- *Beta-blockers:* Reduces production of aqueous humor.
- *Carbonic anhydrase inhibitors:* Decrease production of AH by inhibiting enzyme carbonic anhydrase.
- *Prostaglandins:* Increases outflow of aqueous fluid through uveoscleral route.

ANTIGLAUCOMA AGENTS

Name	Availability	Dosage Range	Side Effects
Miotics			
Carbachol (Isopto-Carbachol)	**S:** 1.5%, 3%	1 drop qid	Brow ache, corneal toxicity, conjunctival inflammation, transient myopia, blurred vision, retinal detachment
Pilocarpine (Isopto Carpine Pilopine HS [Gel])	**G:** 4% **S:** 1%, 2%, 4%	**S:** 1 drop qid **G:** 1 drop HS	Same as carbachol

(continued)

ANTIGLAUCOMA AGENTS   *(continued)*

Name	Availability	Dosage Range	Side Effects
Alpha₂-Agonists			
Apraclonidine (Iopidine)	**S:** 0.5%, 1%	1 drop tid	Fatigue, somnolence, local allergic reaction, dry eyes, stinging
Brimonidine (Alphagan HP)	**S:** 0.1%, 0.15%, 0.2%	1 drop tid	Same as apraclonidine
Prostaglandins			
Bimatoprost (Lumigan)	**S:** 0.01%	1 drop daily in evening	Conjunctival hyperemia; darkening of iris, eyelids; increase in length, thickness, and number of eyelashes; local irritation; itching; dryness; blurred vision
Latanoprost (Xalatan)	**S:** 0.005%	1 drop daily in evening	See bimatoprost
Tafluprost (Zioptan)	**S:** 0.0015%	1 drop daily in evening	See bimatoprost
Travoprost (Travatan)	**S:** 0.004%	1 drop daily in evening	See bimatoprost
Unoprostone (Rescula)	**S:** 0.15%	1 drop bid	See bimatoprost
Beta-Blockers			
Betaxolol (Betoptic, Betoptic-S)	**Suspension (Betoptic-S):** 0.25% **S (Betoptic):** 0.5%	Betoptic-S: 1 drop 2 times/day Betoptic: 1–2 drops 2 times/day	Fatigue, dizziness, bradycardia, respiratory depression, mask symptoms of hypoglycemia, block effects of beta-agonists in treatment of asthma

Levobunolol (Betagan)	**S:** 0.25%, 0.5%	1 drop 1–2 times/day	Same as betaxolol
Timolol (p. 1193) (Betimol, Istalol, Timoptic, Timoptic XE)	**S:** 0.25%, 0.5% **G, Timoptic XE:** 0.25%, 0.5%	**S:** 1 drop 2 times/day (Istalol): 1 drop daily **G:** 1 drop daily	Same as betaxolol
Carbonic Anhydrase Inhibitors			
Brinzolamide (Azopt)	**Suspension:** 1%	1 drop 3 times/day	Bitter taste, stinging, redness, burning, conjunctivitis, dry eyes, blurred vision
Dorzolamide (Trusopt)	**S:** 2%	1 drop 3 times/day	Same as brinzolamide
Combinations			
Brimonidine/timolol (Combigan)	0.2%/0.5%	1 drop bid	See individual agents
Brinzolamide/ brimonidine (Simbrinza)	1%/0.2%	1 drop tid	See individual agents
Timolol/dorzolamide (Cosopt)	0.5%/2%	1 drop bid	See individual agents

C, Capsules; *G*, gel; *O*, ointment; *S*, solution; *T*, tablets.

Antihistamines

USES	ACTION
Symptomatic relief of upper respiratory allergic disorders. Allergic reactions associated with other drugs respond to antihistamines, as do blood transfusion reactions. Used as a second-choice drug in treatment of angioneurotic edema. Effective in treatment of acute urticaria and other dermatologic conditions. May also be used for preop sedation, Parkinson's disease, and motion sickness.	Antihistamines (H_1 antagonists) inhibit vasoconstrictor effects and vasodilator effects on endothelial cells of histamine. They block increased capillary permeability, formation of edema/wheal caused by histamine. Many antihistamines can bind to receptors in CNS, causing primarily depression (decreased alertness, slowed reaction times, drowsiness) but also stimulation (restlessness, nervousness, inability to sleep). Some may counter motion sickness.

ANTIHISTAMINES

Name	Availability	Dosage Range	Side Effects
Cetirizine (p. 236) **(Zyrtec)**	**T:** 5 mg, 10 mg **C:** 5 mg, 10 mg **T (chew):** 5 mg/10 mg **S:** 5 mg/5 ml	**A:** 5–10 mg/day **C (6–12 yrs):** 5–10 mg/day **C (2–5 yrs):** 2.5–5 mg/day	Headache, somnolence, fatigue, abdominal pain, dry mouth
Desloratadine (p. 338) **(Clarinex)**	**T:** 5 mg **ODT:** 2.5 mg, 5 mg **S:** 0.5 mg/ml	**A, C (12 yrs and older):** 5 mg/day **C (6–11 yrs):** 2.5 mg/day **C (1–5 yrs):** 1.25 mg/day **C (6–11 mos):** 1 mg/day	Dizziness, fatigue, headache, nausea

Dimenhydrinate (p. 369) (Dramamine)	**T:** 50 mg **T (chew):** 25 mg, 50 mg	**A:** 50–100 mg q4–6h **C:** 12.5–50 mg q6–8h	Dizziness, drowsiness, headache, nausea
Diphenhydramine (p. 373) (Benadryl)	**T:** 25 mg, 50 mg **C:** 25 mg, 50 mg **L:** 12.5 mg/5 ml	**A:** 25–50 mg q6–8h **C (6–11 yrs):** 12.5–25 mg q4–6h **C (2–5 yrs):** 6.25 mg q4–6h	Chills, confusion, dizziness, fatigue, headache, sedation, nausea
Fexofenadine (p. 489) (Allegra)	**T:** 30 mg, 60 mg, 180 mg **ODT:** 30 mg **S:** 30 mg/5 ml	**A:** 60 mg q12h or 180 mg/day **C (2–11 yrs):** 30 mg q12h, **(6–23 mos):** 15 mg bid	Headache, vomiting, fatigue, diarrhea
Hydroxyzine (p. 585) (Atarax)	**T:** 10 mg, 25 mg, 50 mg **C:** 25 mg, 50 mg, 100 mg **S:** 10 mg/5 ml	**A:** 25 mg q6–8h **C:** 2 mg/kg/day in divided doses q6–8h	Dizziness, drowsiness, fatigue, headache
Levocetirizine (p. 690) (Xyzal)	**T:** 5 mg **S:** 2.5 mg/ml	**A, C (12 yrs and older):** 5 mg once daily in evening **C (6–11 yrs):** 2.5 mg once daily in evening **(6 mos–5 yrs):** 1.25 mg once daily	Fatigue, fever, somnolence, vomiting
Loratadine (p. 718) (Claritin)	**ODT:** 10 mg **T (chew):** 5 mg **T:** 10 mg **S:** 1 mg/ml	**A:** 10 mg/day **C (6–12 yrs):** 10 mg/day **(2–5 yrs):** 5 mg/day	Fatigue, headache, malaise, somnolence, abdominal pain
Promethazine (p. 1003) (Phenergan)	**T:** 12.5 mg, 25 mg, 50 mg **S:** 6.25 mg/5 ml	**A:** 25 mg at bedtime or 12.5 mg q8h **C:** 0.5 mg/kg at bedtime or 0.1 mg/kg q6–8h	Confusion, dizziness, drowsiness, fatigue, constipation, nausea, vomiting

A, Adults; *C,* capsules; *C (dosage),* children; *L,* liquid; *ODT,* orally disintegrating tablet; *S,* syrup; *SR,* sustained-release; *T,* tablets.

Antihyperlipidemics

USES	ACTION
Cholesterol management.	*Bile acid sequestrants:* Binds bile acids in the intestine; prevent active transport and reabsorption and enhance bile acid excretion. Depletion of hepatic bile acid results in the increased conversion of cholesterol to bile acids. *HMG-CoA reductase inhibitors (statins):* Inhibits HMG-CoA reductase, the last regulated step in the synthesis of cholesterol. Cholesterol synthesis in the liver is reduced. *Niacin (nicotinic acid):* Reduces hepatic synthesis of triglycerides and secretion of VLDL by inhibiting the mobilization of free fatty acids from peripheral tissues. *Fibric acid:* Increases the oxidation of fatty acids in the liver, resulting in reduced secretion of triglyceride-rich lipoproteins, and increases lipoprotein lipase activity and fatty acid uptake. *Cholesterol absorption inhibitor:* Acts in the gut wall to prevent cholesterol absorption through the intestinal villi. *Omega fatty acids:* Exact mechanism unknown. Mechanisms may include inhibition of acyl-CoA, decreased lipogenesis in liver; increased lipoprotein lipase activity.

ANTIHYPERLIPIDEMICS

Name	Primary Effect	Dosage	Comments/Side Effects
Bile Acid Sequestrants			
Cholestyramine (Prevalite, Questran) (p. 244)	Decreases LDL Increases HDL, TG	4 g once or twice daily or 8 g once daily	May bind drugs given concurrently. Take at least 1 hr before or 4–6 hrs after cholestyramine. **Side Effects:** Constipation, heartburn, nausea, vomiting, stomach pain
Colesevelam (p. 284) (Welchol)	Decreases LDL Increases HDL, TG	6–7 625-mg tablets once daily or 2 divided doses with meals	Take with food. **Side Effects:** Constipation, dyspepsia, weakness, myalgia, pharyngitis

Colestipol (Colestid)	Decreases LDL Increases TG	10 g once daily or 5 g twice daily	Do not crush tablets. May bind drugs given concurrently. Take at least 1 hr before or 4–6 hrs after colestipol. **Side Effects:** Constipation, headache, dizziness, anxiety, vertigo, drowsiness, nausea, vomiting, diarrhea, flatulence
Cholesterol Absorption Inhibitor			
Ezetimibe (Zetia) (p. 468)	Decreases LDL Increases HDL Decreases TG	10 mg once daily	Administer at least 2 hrs before or 4 hrs after bile acid sequestrants. **Side Effects:** Dizziness, headache, fatigue, diarrhea, abdominal pain, arthralgia, sinusitis, pharyngitis
Fibric Acid			
Fenofibrate (Antara, Lofibra, Tricor, Triglide) (p. 478)	Decreases TG Decreases LDL Increases HDL	Antara: 43–130 mg/day Lofibra: 67–200 mg/day Tricor: 48–145 mg/day Triglide: 50–160 mg/day	May increase levels of ezetimibe. Concomitant use of statins may increase rhabdomyolysis, elevate CPK levels, and cause myoglobinuria. **Side Effects:** Abdominal pain, constipation, diarrhea, respiratory complaints, headache, fever, flu-like syndrome, asthenia (loss of strength, energy)
Fenofibric acid (p. 480) (Fibricor, Trilipix)	Decreases TG, LDL Increases HDL	45–135 mg/day	May give without regard to meals. Concomitant use of statins may increase rhabdomyolysis. **Side Effects:** Headache, upper respiratory tract infection, pain, nausea, dizziness, nasopharyngitis
Gemfibrozil (Lopid) (p. 542)	Decreases TG Increases HDL	600 mg 2 times/day	Give 30 min before breakfast and dinner. Concomitant use of statins may increase rhabdomyolysis, elevate CPK levels, and cause myoglobinuria. **Side Effects:** Fatigue, vertigo, headache, rash, eczema, diarrhea, abdominal pain, nausea, vomiting, constipation

(continued)

ANTIHYPERLIPIDEMICS *(continued)*

Name	Primary Effect	Dosage	Comments/Side Effects
Niacin			
Niacin, nicotinic acid (Niacor, Niaspan) (p. 843)	Decreases LDL, TG Increases HDL	**Regular-release (Niacor):** 1 g tid **Extended-release (Niaspan):** 1 g at bedtime	Diabetics may experience a dose-related elevation in glucose. **Side Effects:** Increased hepatic function tests, hyperglycemia, dyspepsia, itching, flushing, dizziness, insomnia
Statins			
Atorvastatin (Lipitor) (p. 96)	Decreases LDL, TG Increases HDL	10–80 mg/day	May interact with CYP3A4 inhibitors (e.g., amiodarone, diltiazem, cyclosporine, grapefruit juice) increasing risk of myopathy. **Side Effects:** Myalgia, myopathy, rhabdomyolysis, headache, chest pain, peripheral edema, dizziness, rash, abdominal pain, constipation, diarrhea, dyspepsia, nausea, flatulence, increased hepatic function tests, back pain, sinusitis
Fluvastatin (Lescol) (p. 513)	Decreases LDL, TG Increases HDL	20–80 mg/day	Primarily metabolized by CYP2C9 enzyme system. May increase levels of phenytoin, rifampin. May lower fluvastatin levels. **Side Effects:** Headache, fatigue, dyspepsia, diarrhea, nausea, abdominal pain, myalgia, myopathy, rhabdomyolysis
Lovastatin (Mevacor) (p. 725)	Decreases LDL, TG Increases HDL	20–80 mg/day	May interact with CYP3A4 inhibitors (e.g., amiodarone, diltiazem, cyclosporine, grapefruit products) increasing risk of myopathy. **Side Effects:** Increased CPK levels, headache, dizziness, rash, constipation, diarrhea, abdominal pain, dyspepsia, nausea, flatulence, myalgia, myopathy, rhabdomyolysis
Pitavastatin (p. 967) (Livalo)	Decreases LDL, TG Increases HDL	1–4 mg/day	Erythromycin, rifampin may increase concentration. **Side Effects:** Myalgia, back pain, diarrhea, constipation, pain in extremities

Pravastatin (Pravachol) (p. 985)	Decreases LDL, TG Increases HDL	20–80 mg/day	May be less likely to be involved in drug interactions. Cyclosporine may increase pravastatin levels. **Side Effects:** Chest pain, headache, dizziness, rash, nausea, vomiting, diarrhea, increased hepatic function tests, cough, flu-like symptoms, myalgia, myopathy, rhabdomyolysis
Rosuvastatin (Crestor) (p. 1079)	Decreases LDL, TG Increases HDL	5–40 mg/day	May be less likely to be involved in drug interactions. Cyclosporine may increase rosuvastatin levels. **Side Effects:** Chest pain, peripheral edema, headache, rash, dizziness, vertigo, pharyngitis, diarrhea, nausea, constipation, abdominal pain, dyspepsia, sinusitis, flu-like symptoms, myalgia, myopathy, rhabdomyolysis
Simvastatin (Zocor) (p. 1105)	Decreases LDL, TG Increases HDL	5–80 mg/day	May interact with CYP3A4 inhibitors (e.g., amiodarone, diltiazem, cyclosporine, grapefruit products) increasing risk of myopathy. **Side Effects:** Constipation, flatulence, dyspepsia, increased hepatic function tests, increased CPK, upper respiratory tract infection

Omega Fatty Acids

Icosapent (p. 598) (Vascepa)	Decreases TG	2 g twice daily	**Side Effects:** Arthralgia
Lovaza (p. 887)	Decreases TG Increases LDL, HDL	2 g twice daily or 4 g once daily	Use with caution with fish or shellfish allergy. **Side Effects:** Eructation, dyspepsia, taste perversion

CPK, Creatine phosphokinase; *G*, granules; *HDL*, high-density lipoprotein; *LDL*, low-density lipoprotein; *T*, tablets; *TG*, triglycerides.

Antihypertensives

USES

Treatment of mild to severe hypertension.

ACTION

Many groups of medications are used in the treatment of hypertension.

ACE inhibitors: Decreases conversion of angiotensin I to angiotensin II, a potent vasoconstrictor, reducing peripheral vascular resistance and B/P.

Alpha-agonists (central action): Stimulates alpha₂-adrenergic receptors in the cardiovascular centers of the CNS, reducing sympathetic outflow and producing an antihypertensive effect.

Alpha-antagonists (peripheral action): Blocks alpha₁-adrenergic receptors in arterioles and veins, inhibiting vasoconstriction and decreasing peripheral vascular resistance, causing a fall in B/P.

Angiotensin receptor blockers: Blocks vasoconstrictor effects of angiotensin II by blocking the binding of angiotensin II to AT1 receptors in vascular smooth muscle, helping blood vessels to relax and reduce B/P.

Beta-blockers: Decreases B/P by inhibiting beta₁-adrenergic receptors, which lowers heart rate, heart workload, and the heart's output of blood.

Calcium channel blockers: Reduces B/P by inhibiting flow of extracellular calcium across cell membranes of vascular tissue, relaxing arterial smooth muscle.

Diuretics: Inhibits sodium (Na) reabsorption, increasing excretion of Na and water. Reduce plasma, extracellular fluid volume, and peripheral vascular resistance.

Renin inhibitors: Directly inhibits renin, decreasing plasma renin activity (PRA), inhibiting conversion of angiotensinogen to angiotensin, producing antihypertensive effect.

Vasodilators: Directly relaxes arteriolar smooth muscle, decreasing vascular resistance. Exact mechanism unknown.

ANTIHYPERTENSIVES

Name	Availability	Dosage Range	Side Effects
(ACE) Inhibitors			
Benazepril (p. 126) (Lotensin)	**T:** 5 mg, 10 mg, 20 mg, 40 mg	20–80 mg/day as single or 2 divided doses	Postural dizziness, headache, cough

Enalapril (p. 415) (Vasotec)	**T:** 2.5 mg, 5 mg, 10 mg, 20 mg	2.5–40 mg/day in 1–2 divided doses	Hypotension, chest pain, syncope, headache, dizziness, fatigue
Lisinopril (p. 707) (Prinivil, Zestril)	**T:** 2.5 mg, 5 mg, 10 mg, 20 mg, 30 mg, 40 mg	10–40 mg/day	Hypotension, headache, fatigue, dizziness, hyperkalemia, cough
Quinapril (p. 1025)	**T:** 5 mg, 10 mg, 20 mg, 40 mg	10–40 mg/day	Hypotension, dizziness, fatigue, headache, myalgia, hyperkalemia
Ramipril (p. 1034) (Altace)	**T or C:** 1.25 mg, 2.5 mg, 5 mg, 10 mg	2.5–20 mg/day	Cough, hypotension, angina, headache, dizziness, hyperkalemia
Alpha-Agonists: Central Action			
Clonidine (p. 273) (Catapres)	**T:** 0.1 mg, 0.2 mg, 0.3 mg **P:** 0.1 mg/hr, 0.2 mg/hr, 0.3 mg/hr	**PO:** 0.1–0.8 mg/day **Topical:** 0.1–0.6 mg/wk	Sedation, dry mouth, constipation, sexual dysfunction, bradycardia, xerostomia, drowsiness, headache
Methyldopa (Aldomet)	**T:** 125 mg, 250 mg, 500 mg	**PO:** 250–1,000 mg/day in 2 divided doses	Nausea, vomiting, weight gain, impaired memory, depression, nasal congestion
Alpha-Agonists: Peripheral Action			
Doxazosin (p. 392) (Cardura)	**T:** 1 mg, 2 mg, 4 mg, 8 mg	**PO:** 2–16 mg/day	Dizziness, vertigo, headaches
Prazosin (p. 986) (Minipress)	**C:** 1 mg, 2 mg, 5 mg	**PO:** 6–20 mg/day	Dizziness, light-headedness, headaches, drowsiness
Terazosin (p. 1165) (Hytrin)	**C:** 1 mg, 2 mg, 5 mg, 10 mg	**PO:** 1–20 mg/day	Dizziness, headaches, asthenia (loss of strength, energy)
Angiotensin Receptor Blockers			
Azilsartan (p. 109) (Edarbi)	**T:** 40 mg, 80 mg	40–80 mg/day	Diarrhea, hypotension, nausea, cough
Candesartan (p. 183) (Atacand)	**T:** 4 mg, 8 mg, 16 mg, 32 mg	8–32 mg/day	Hypotension, dizziness, headache, hyperkalemia

(continued)

ANTIHYPERTENSIVES   (continued)

Name	Availability	Dosage Range	Side Effects
Losartan (p. 723) (Cozaar)	**T: 25 mg, 50 mg, 100 mg**	25–100 mg/day	Chest pain, fatigue, hypoglycemia, weakness, cough, hypotension
Olmesartan (p. 881) (Benicar)	**T: 5 mg, 20 mg, 40 mg**	20–40 mg/day	Dizziness, headache, diarrhea, flu-like symptoms
Valsartan (Diovan)	**T: 80 mg, 160 mg, 320 mg**	80–320 mg/day	Dizziness, fatigue, increased BUN
Beta-Blockers			
Atenolol (p. 93) (Tenormin)	**T: 25 mg, 50 mg, 100 mg**	25–100 mg/day	Fatigue, bradycardia, reduced exercise tolerance, increased triglycerides, bronchospasm, sexual dysfunction, masked hypoglycemia
Bisoprolol (Zebeta)	**T: 5 mg, 10 mg**	2.5–10 mg/day	Fatigue, insomnia, diarrhea, arthralgia, upper respiratory infections
Metoprolol (p. 777) (Lopressor)	**T: 25 mg, 50 mg, 100 mg**	50–100 mg/day	Hypotension, bradycardia, fatigue, 1st degree heart block, dizziness
Metoprolol XL (p. 777) (Toprol XL)	**T: 25 mg, 50 mg, 100 mg, 200 mg**	50–100 mg/day	Same as metoprolol
Calcium Channel Blockers			
Amlodipine (p. 59) (Norvasc)	**T: 2.5 mg, 5 mg, 10 mg**	2.5–10 mg/day	Headache, fatigue, peripheral edema, flushing, worsening heart failure
Diltiazem CD (p. 366) (Cardizem CD)	**C: 120 mg, 180 mg, 240 mg, 300 mg**	180–420 mg/day	Dizziness, headache, bradycardia, heart block, worsening heart failure, edema, constipation
Felodipine (p. 477) (Plendil)	**T: 2.5 mg, 5 mg, 10 mg**	2.5–20 mg/day	Headache, flushing, peripheral edema

Nifedipine XL (p. 849) (Adalat CC, Procardia XL)	**T:** 30 mg, 60 mg, 90 mg	90–120 mg/day	Flushing, peripheral edema, headache, dizziness, nausea
Verapamil SR (p. 1263) (Calan SR)	**T:** 120 mg, 180 mg, 240 mg **T (Sustained-Release):** 120 mg, 180 mg	**T (Immediate-Release):** 80–320 mg/day **T (Sustained-Release):** 120–480 mg/day	Headache, gingival hyperplasia, constipation
Diuretics			
Chlorthalidone (Hygroton)	**T:** 25 mg, 50 mg	12.5–25 mg/day	Same as hydrochlorothiazide
Hydrochlorothiazide (p. 572) (Hydrodiuril)	**T:** 25 mg, 50 mg	12.5–50 mg/day	Hypokalemia, hyperuricemia, hypomagnesemia, hyperglycemia
Renin Inhibitor			
Aliskiren (p. 36) (Tekturna)	**T:** 150 mg, 300 mg	**PO:** 150–300 mg/day	Diarrhea, dyspepsia, headache, dizziness, fatigue, upper respiratory tract infection
Vasodilators			
Hydralazine (p. 570) (Apresoline)	**T:** 10 mg, 25 mg, 50 mg, 100 mg	**PO:** 40–300 mg/day	Anorexia, nausea, diarrhea, vomiting, headaches, palpitations
Minoxidil (p. 793) (Loniten)	**T:** 2.5 mg, 10 mg	**PO:** 10–40 mg/day	Rapid/irregular heartbeat, hypertrichosis, peripheral edema

C, Capsules; *P,* patch; *T,* tablets.

Antimigraine (Triptans)

USES

Treatment of migraine headaches with or without aura in adults 18 yrs and older.

ACTION

Triptans are selective agonists of the serotonin (5-HT) receptor in cranial arteries, which cause vasoconstriction and reduce inflammation associated with antidromic neuronal transmission correlating with relief of migraine headache.

TRIPTANS

Name	Availability	Dosage Range	Contraindications	Side Effects
Almotriptan (p. 39) (Axert)	**T:** 6.25 mg, 12.5 mg	6.25–12.5 mg; may repeat after 2 hrs	Ischemic heart disease, angina pectoris, arrhythmias, previous MI, uncontrolled hypertension, hemiplegic or basilar migraine, peripheral vascular disease	Drowsiness, dizziness, fatigue, hot flashes, chest pain/discomfort, paresthesia, nausea, vomiting
Eletriptan (p. 411) (Relpax)	**T:** 20 mg, 40 mg	**A:** 20–40 mg; may repeat after 2 hrs (**Maximum:** 60 mg/day)	Same as almotriptan	Asthenia (loss of strength, energy), nausea, dizziness, drowsiness
Frovatriptan (p. 527) (Frova)	**T:** 2.5 mg	2.5 mg; may repeat after 2 hrs; no more than 3 **T**/day	Same as almotriptan	Hot/cold sensations, dizziness, fatigue, headaches, chest pain, skeletal pain, dry mouth, dyspepsia, flushing
Naratriptan (p. 831) (Amerge)	**T:** 1 mg, 2.5 mg	1–2.5 mg; may repeat once after 4 hrs	Same as almotriptan plus severe renal/hepatic disease	Atypical sensations, pain, nausea, fatigue

Rizatriptan (p. 1071) (Maxalt, Maxalt-MLT)	T: 5 mg, 10 mg; DT: 5 mg, 10 mg	5 or 10 mg; may repeat after 2 hrs	Same as almotriptan	Atypical sensations, pain, nausea, dizziness, drowsiness, asthenia (loss of strength, energy), fatigue
Sumatriptan (p. 1139) (Imitrex, Sumavel DosePro)	T: 25 mg, 50 mg, 100 mg NS: 5 mg, 20 mg I: 4 mg, 6 mg	PO: 25–100 mg; may repeat after 2 hrs NS: 5–20 mg; may repeat after 2 hrs Subcutaneous: 4–6 mg; may repeat after 1 hr	Same as almotriptan plus severe hepatic dysfunction	*Oral:* Atypical sensations, pain, malaise, fatigue *Injection:* Atypical sensations, flushing, chest pain/discomfort, injection site reaction, dizziness, vertigo *Nasal:* Discomfort, nausea, vomiting, altered taste
Zolmitriptan (p. 1299) (Zomig, Zomig-ZMT)	T: 2.5 mg, 5 mg DT: 2.5 mg, 5 mg NS: 5 mg/0.1 ml	2.5–5 mg; may repeat after 2 hrs NS: 1 spray (5 mg) at onset of migrane headache	Same as almotriptan plus symptomatic Wolff-Parkinson White syndrome	Atypical sensations, pain, nausea, dizziness, asthenia (loss of strength, energy), drowsiness

A, Adults; *DT,* disintegrating tablets; *I,* injection; *NS,* nasal spray; *T,* tablets.

Antipsychotics

USES

Primarily used in managing psychotic illness (esp. in pts with increased psychomotor activity). Also used to treat the manic phase of bipolar disorder, behavioral problems in children, nausea and vomiting, intractable hiccups, anxiety and agitation, as adjunct in treatment of tetanus, and to potentiate effects of narcotics.

ACTION

Effects of these agents occur at all levels of the CNS. Antipsychotic mechanism unknown but may antagonize dopamine action as a neurotransmitter in basal ganglia and limbic system. Antipsychotics may block postsynaptic dopamine receptors, inhibit dopamine release, increase dopamine turnover. These medications can be divided into the phenothiazines and nonphenothiazines (miscellaneous). In addition to their use in the symptomatic treatment of psychiatric illness, some have antiemetic, antinausea, antihistamine, anticholinergic, and/or sedative effects.

ANTIPSYCHOTICS

Name	Availability	Dosage	Relative Side Effect Profile				
			EPS	Anticholinergic	Sedation	Hypotension	
Aripiprazole (p. 80) (Abilify)	**T:** 2 mg, 5 mg, 10 mg, 15 mg, 20 mg, 30 mg **DT:** 10 mg, 15 mg **I:** 9.75 mg **S:** 1 mg/ml	**PO:** 15–30 mg/day **I:** Up to 30 mg/day	Low	Very low	Very low	Low	
Chlorpromazine (p. 241) (Thorazine)	**T:** 10 mg, 25 mg, 50 mg, 100 mg, 200 mg **SR:** 30 mg, 75 mg, 100 mg **OC:** 30 mg/ml, 100 mg/ml	30–800 mg/day in 1–4 divided doses	Moderate	Moderate	High	High	
Clozapine (p. 279) (Clozaril, FazaClo)	**T:** 25 mg, 50 mg, 100 mg, 200 mg **DT:** 12.5 mg, 25 mg, 100 mg	75–900 mg/day	Very low	High	High	High	
Fluphenazine (p. 506) (Prolixin)	**T:** 1 mg, 2.5 mg, 5 mg, 10 mg **I:** 25 mg/ml **OC:** 5 mg/ml	**PO:** 2–40 mg/day **I:** 12.5–75 mg q2–4wks	High	Low	Low	Low	
Haloperidol (p. 566) (Haldol)	**T:** 0.5 mg, 1 mg, 2 mg, 5 mg, 10 mg, 20 mg **I:** 5 mg/ml **OC:** 2 mg/ml	0.5–5 mg 2–3 times/day	High	Low	Low	Low	
Iloperidone (p. 602) (Fanapt)	**T:** 1 mg, 2 mg, 4 mg, 6 mg, 8 mg, 10 mg, 12 mg	6–12 mg 2 times/day	Low	Very low	Low	Low/moderate	

Loxapine (Adasuve)	C: 5 mg, 10 mg, 25 mg, 50 mg OC: 25 mg/ml I: 50 mg/ml	60–100 mg/day in 2–4 divided doses	Moderate	Low	Moderate	Low
Olanzapine (p. 878) (Zyprexa)	T: 2.5 mg, 5 mg, 7.5 mg, 10 mg, 15 mg, 20 mg DT: 5 mg, 10 mg, 15 mg, 20 mg I: 10 mg	10–20 mg once daily	Low	Moderate	Moderate/high	Moderate
Paliperidone (p. 914) (Invega)	T: 1.5 mg, 3 mg, 6 mg, 9 mg I: 39 mg, 78 mg, 117 mg, 234 mg	3–12 mg once daily IM: Initially, 234 mg once, then 156 mg 1 wk later, then 39–234 mg monthly	Low	Very low	Low/moderate	Moderate
Quetiapine (p. 1023) (Seroquel)	T: 25 mg, 50 mg, 100 mg, 200 mg, 300 mg, 400 mg ER: 50 mg, 150 mg, 200 mg, 300 mg, 400 mg	300–800 mg/day in 2–3 divided doses ER: 400–800 mg once daily	Very low	Moderate	Moderate/high	Moderate
Risperidone (p. 1061) (Risperdal)	T: 0.25 mg, 0.5 mg, 1 mg, 2 mg, 3 mg, 4 mg OC: 1 mg/ml I: 12.5 mg, 25 mg, 37.5 mg, 50 mg	4–8 mg/day in 1–2 divided doses IM: 25–50 mg q2wks	Low	Very low	Low/moderate	Moderate
Thioridazine (p. 1181) (Mellaril)	T: 10 mg, 15 mg, 25 mg, 50 mg, 100 mg, 150 mg, 200 mg	150–800 mg/day in 2–4 divided doses	Low	High	High	Moderate/high
Thiothixene (p. 1185) (Navane)	C: 1 mg, 2 mg, 5 mg, 10 mg	10–60 mg/day in 2 divided doses	High	Low	Low	Low/moderate
Trifluoperazine (p. 1235) (Stelazine)	T: 1 mg, 2 mg, 5 mg, 10 mg	2–20 mg/day in 2 divided doses	High	Low	Low	Low

(continued)

ANTIPSYCHOTICS   *(continued)*

Name	Availability	Dosage	Relative Side Effect Profile			
			EPS	Anticholinergic	Sedation	Hypotension
Ziprasidone (p. 1296) (Geodon)	**C:** 20 mg, 40 mg, 60 mg, 80 mg **I:** 20 mg	20–100 mg twice daily **IM:** 10 mg q2h or 20 mg q4h (**Maximum:** 40 mg/day)	Low	Very low	Low to moderate	Low to moderate

C, Capsules; *DT*, disintegrating tablets; *EPS*, extrapyramidal symptoms; *ER*, extended-release; *I*, injection; *OC*, oral concentrate; *SR*, sustained-release; *T*, tablets; *TSL*, sublingual tablets.

Antivirals

USES

Treatment of HIV infection. Treatment of cytomegalovirus (CMV) retinitis in pts with AIDS, acute herpes zoster (shingles), genital herpes (recurrent), mucosal and cutaneous herpes simplex virus (HSV), chickenpox, and influenza A viral illness.

ACTION

Effective antivirals must inhibit virus-specific nucleic acid/protein synthesis. Possible mechanisms of action of antivirals used for non-HIV infection may include interference with viral DNA synthesis and viral replication, inactivation of viral DNA polymerases, incorporation and termination of the growing viral DNA chain, prevention of release of viral nucleic acid into the host cell, or interference with viral penetration into cells.

ANTIVIRALS

Name	Availability	Uses	Side Effects
Abacavir (p. 1) (Ziagen)	**T:** 300 mg **OS:** 20 mg/ml	HIV infection	Nausea, vomiting, loss of appetite, diarrhea, headaches, fatigue, hypersensitivity reactions
Acyclovir (p. 16) (Zovirax)	**T:** 400 mg, 800 mg **C:** 200 mg **I:** 50 mg/ml	Mucosal/cutaneous HSV-1 and HSV-2, varicella-zoster (shingles), genital herpes, herpes simplex, encephalitis, chickenpox	Malaise, anorexia, nausea, vomiting, light-headedness
Adefovir (p. 21) (Hepsera)	**T:** 10 mg	Chronic hepatitis B	Asthenia (loss of strength, energy), headaches, abdominal pain, nausea, diarrhea, flatulence, dyspepsia
Amantadine (p. 49) (Symmetrel)	**T:** 100 mg **C:** 100 mg **S:** 50 mg/5 ml	Influenza A	Anxiety, dizziness, headaches, nausea, loss of appetite
Cidofovir (p. 247) (Vistide)	**I:** 75 mg/ml	CMV retinitis	Decreased urination, fever, chills, diarrhea, nausea, vomiting, headaches, loss of appetite
Darunavir (p. 319) (Prezista)	**T:** 75 mg, 150 mg, 400 mg, 600 mg, 800 mg	HIV infection	Diarrhea, nausea, vomiting, headaches, skin rash, constipation
Delavirdine (p. 332) (Rescriptor)	**T:** 100 mg, 200 mg	HIV infection	Diarrhea, fatigue, rash, headaches, nausea
Didanosine (p. 359) (Videx)	**C:** 125 mg, 200 mg, 250 mg, 400 mg **Powder for suspension:** 2 g, 4 g	HIV infection	Peripheral neuropathy, anxiety, headaches, rash, nausea, diarrhea, dry mouth
Efavirenz (p. 409) (Sustiva)	**C:** 50 mg, 200 mg **T:** 600 mg	HIV infection	Diarrhea, dizziness, headaches, insomnia, nausea, vomiting, drowsiness

(continued)

ANTIVIRALS   *(continued)*

Name	Availability	Uses	Side Effects
Etravirine (p. 462) (Intelence)	**T:** 25 mg, 100 mg, 200 mg	HIV infection	Rash, nausea, abdominal pain, vomiting
Famciclovir (p. 472) (Famvir)	**T:** 125 mg, 250 mg, 500 mg	Herpes zoster, genital herpes, herpes labialis, mucosal/cutaneous herpes simplex	Headaches, nausea
Foscarnet (p. 522) (Foscavir)	**I:** 24 mg/ml	CMV retinitis, HSV infections	Decreased urination, abdominal pain, nausea, vomiting, dizziness, fatigue, headaches
Ganciclovir (p. 536) (Cytovene)	**I:** 500 mg	CMV retinitis, CMV disease	Sore throat, fever, unusual bleeding/bruising
Indinavir (p. 616) (Crixivan)	**C:** 200 mg, 400 mg	HIV infection	Blood in urine, weakness, nausea, vomiting, diarrhea, headaches, insomnia, altered taste
Lamivudine (p. 668) (Epivir)	**T:** 100 mg, 150 mg, 300 mg **OS:** 5 mg/ml, 10 mg/ml	HIV infection, chronic hepatitis B	Nausea, vomiting, abdominal pain, paresthesia
Lopinavir/ritonavir (p. 717) (Kaletra)	**T:** 100 mg/25 mg, 200 mg/50 mg **OS:** 80 mg/20 mg per ml	HIV infection	Diarrhea, nausea
Maraviroc (p. 739) (Selzentry)	**T:** 150 mg, 300 mg	HIV infection	Cough, pyrexia, upper respiratory tract infection, rash, musculoskeletal symptoms, abdominal pain, dizziness
Nelfinavir (p. 837) (Viracept)	**T:** 250 mg, 625 mg	HIV infection	Diarrhea
Oseltamivir (p. 894) (Tamiflu)	**C:** 30 mg, 45 mg, 75 mg **S:** 6 mg/ml	Influenza A or B	Diarrhea, nausea, vomiting
Raltegravir (p. 1031) (Isentress)	**T:** 400 mg **T (chew):** 25 mg, 100 mg	HIV infection	Nausea, headache, diarrhea, pyrexia

Ribavirin (p. 1049) (Virazole)	**Aerosol:** 6 g **OS:** 40 mg/ml **T:** 200 mg, 400 mg, 600 mg	Lowers respiratory infections in infants, children due to respiratory syncytial virus (RSV), chronic hepatitis C	Anemia
Ritonavir (p. 1064) (Norvir)	**C:** 100 mg **T:** 100 mg **OS:** 80 mg/ml	HIV infection	Weakness, diarrhea, nausea, decreased appetite, vomiting, altered taste
Saquinavir (p. 1086) (Invirase)	**C:** 200 mg **T:** 500 mg	HIV infection	Weakness, diarrhea, nausea, oral ulcers, abdominal pain
Stavudine (p. 1127) (Zerit)	**C:** 15 mg, 20 mg, 30 mg, 40 mg **OS:** 1 mg/ml	HIV infection	Paresthesia, decreased appetite, chills, fever, rash
Tenofovir (p. 1164) (Viread)	**T:** 150 mg, 200 mg, 250 mg, 300 mg **Powder (oral):** 40 mg/g	HIV infection	Diarrhea, nausea, pharyngitis, headaches
Valacyclovir (p. 1244) (Valtrex)	**T:** 500 mg, 1 g	Herpes zoster, genital herpes, herpes labialis, chickenpox	Headaches, nausea
Valganciclovir (p. 1245) (Valcyte)	**T:** 450 mg, **OS:** 50 mg/ml	CMV retinitis	Anemia, abdominal pain, diarrhea, headaches, nausea, vomiting, paresthesia
Zanamivir (p. 1293) (Relenza)	**Inhalation:** 5 mg	Influenza A and B	Cough, diarrhea, dizziness, headaches, nausea, vomiting
Zidovudine (p. 1294) (Retrovir)	**C:** 100 mg **S:** 50 mg/5 ml **I:** 10 mg/ml	HIV infection	Fatigue, fever, chills, headaches, nausea, muscle pain

C, Capsules; *I,* injection; *OS,* oral solution; *S,* syrup; *T,* tablets.

Beta-Adrenergic Blockers

USES

Management of hypertension, angina pectoris, arrhythmias, hypertrophic subaortic stenosis, migraine headaches, MI (prevention), glaucoma.

ACTION

Beta-adrenergic blockers competitively block beta$_1$-adrenergic receptors, located primarily in myocardium, and beta$_2$-adrenergic receptors, located primarily in bronchial and vascular smooth muscle. By occupying beta-receptor sites, these agents prevent naturally occurring or administered epinephrine/norepinephrine from exerting their effects. The results are basically opposite to those of sympathetic stimulation.

Effects of beta$_1$-blockade include slowing heart rate, decreasing cardiac output and contractility; effects of beta$_2$-blockade include bronchoconstriction, increased airway resistance in pts with asthma or COPD. Beta-blockers can affect cardiac rhythm/automaticity (decrease sinus rate, SA/AV conduction; increase refractory period in AV node). Decreases systolic and diastolic B/P; exact mechanism unknown but may block peripheral receptors, decrease sympathetic outflow from CNS, or decrease renin release from kidney. All beta-blockers mask tachycardia that occurs with hypoglycemia. When applied to the eye, reduce intraocular pressure and aqueous production.

BETA-ADRENERGIC BLOCKERS

Name	Availability	Indication	Dosage Range
Acebutolol (Sectral)	**C:** 200 mg, 400 mg	HTN, arrhythmias	**HTN:** 400–1,200 mg/day in 1–2 divided doses **Arrhythmia:** 300–600 mg BID
Atenolol (p. 93) (Tenormin)	**T:** 25 mg, 50 mg, 100 mg	HTN, angina, MI	**Angina:** 50–100 mg once daily **HTN:** 50–100 mg once daily **MI:** 50 mg bid or 100 mg once daily
Bisoprolol (p. 143) (Zebeta)	**T:** 5 mg, 10 mg	HTN	2.5–20 mg once daily

Carvedilol (p. 200) (Coreg)	**T:** 3.125 mg, 6.25 mg, 12.5 mg, 25 mg **C (SR):** 10 mg, 20 mg, 40 mg, 80 mg	HF, LVD after MI, HTN	**Immediate-Release HF:** 3.125–50 mg BID **LVD after MI:** 6.25–25 mg BID **HTN:** 6.25–25 mg BID **Extended-Release HF:** 10–80 mg once daily **LVD after MI:** 10–80 mg once daily **HTN:** 20–80 mg once daily
Labetalol (p. 663) (Trandate)	**T:** 100 mg, 200 mg, 300 mg **I:** 5 mg/ml	HTN	200–2,400 mg/day in 2–3 divided doses **I:** 20–80 mg at 10-min intervals (**Maximum:** 300 mg)
Metoprolol (p. 777) (Lopressor [IR], Toprol XL [SR])	**T (IR):** 50 mg, 100 mg **I:** 1 mg/ml **T (SR):** 25 mg, 50 mg	HTN, angina, HF, MI	**IR:** **Angina:** 100–400 mg bid **HTN:** 100–450 mg once daily or BID **Post-MI:** 100 mg bid **SR:** **Angina:** 100–400 mg once daily **HF:** 12.5–200 mg once daily **HTN:** 25–400 mg once daily
Nadolol (p. 820) (Corgard)	**T:** 20 mg, 40 mg, 80 mg	HTN, angina	40–320 mg once daily
Nebivolol (p. 835) (Bystolic)	**T:** 2.5 mg, 5 mg, 10 mg, 20 mg	HTN	5–40 mg once daily
Pindolol (Visken)	**T:** 5 mg, 10 mg	HTN	10–60 mg bid

BETA-ADRENERGIC BLOCKERS (continued)

Name	Availability	Indication	Dosage Range
Propranolol (p. 1009) (Inderal)	**T (IR):** 10 mg, 20 mg, 40 mg, 60 mg, 80 mg **C (SR):** 60 mg, 80 mg, 120 mg, 160 mg **S:** 4 mg/ml, 8 mg/ml **I:** 1 mg/ml	HTN, angina, MI, arrhythmias, migraine, essential tremor, hypertrophic subaortic stenosis	**IR:** **Angina:** 80–320 mg/day in 2–4 divided doses **Arrhythmias:** 10–30 mg bid or tid **HTN:** 40 mg bid up to 240 mg/day in 2–3 divided doses **Hypertrophic subaortic stenosis:** 20–40 mg 3–4 times/day **Post-MI:** 180–240 mg/day in 2–4 divided doses **Migraine:** 80–240 mg/day in divided doses **Tremor:** 80–120 mg/day in divided doses **SR:** **Angina:** 80–320 mg once daily **HTN:** 80–120 mg once daily **Migraine:** 80–240 mg once daily **Hypertrophic subaortic stenosis:** 80–160 mg once daily
Timolol (p. 1193) (Blocadren)	**T:** 5 mg, 10 mg, 20 mg	HTN, post-MI, migraine prevention	**HTN:** 10–20 mg bid **Post-MI:** 10 mg bid **Migraine:** 10 mg bid or 20 mg once daily

C, Capsules; *HF,* heart failure; *HTN,* hypertension; *I,* injection; *LVD,* left ventricular dysfunction; *MI,* myocardial infarction; *S,* solution; *SR,* sustained-release; *T,* tablets.

USES

Relief of bronchospasm occurring during anesthesia and in bronchial asthma, bronchitis, emphysema.

ACTION

Inhaled corticosteroids: Exact mechanism unknown. May act as anti-inflammatories, decrease mucus secretion.

Beta₂-adrenergic agonists: Stimulate beta-receptors in lung, relax bronchial smooth muscle, increase vital capacity, decrease airway resistance.

Anticholinergics: Inhibit cholinergic receptors on bronchial smooth muscle (block acetylcholine action).

Leukotriene modifiers: Decrease effect of leukotrienes, which increase migration of eosinophils, producing mucus/edema of airway wall, causing bronchoconstriction.

Methylxanthines: Directly relax smooth muscle of bronchial airway, pulmonary blood vessels (relieve bronchospasm, increase vital capacity). Increase cyclic 3,5-adenosine monophosphate.

BRONCHODILATORS

Name	Availability	Dosage Range	Side Effects
Anticholinergics			
Aclidinium (p. 15) (Tudorza)	**Inhalation powder:** 400 mcg/actuation	**A:** 400 mcg twice daily	Headache, nasopharyngitis, cough
Ipratropium (p. 637) (Atrovent)	**NEB:** 0.02% (500 mcg) **MDI:** 18 mcg/actuation	**A (NEB):** 500 mcg q6–8h **A (MDI):** 2 puffs 4 times/day	Upper respiratory tract infection, bronchitis, sinusitis, headache, dyspnea
Tiotropium (p. 1196) (Spiriva)	**Inhalation powder:** 18 mcg/capsule	**A:** Once/day (inhaled twice)	Xerostomia, upper respiratory tract infection, sinusitis, pharyngitis

(continued)

BRONCHODILATORS *(continued)*

Name	Availability	Dosage Range	Side Effects
Bronchodilators			
Albuterol (p. 29) (AccuNeb, ProAir HFA, Proventil HFA, Ventolin HFA)	**MDI:** 90 mcg/actuation **NEB:** 2.5 mg/3 ml, 2.5 mg/0.5 ml, *(AccuNeb):* 0.63–1.25 mg/3 ml	**MDI:** 2 inhalations q4–6h as needed **NEB:** 1.25–5 mg q4–6h as needed	Tachycardia, skeletal muscle tremors, muscle cramping, palpitations, insomnia, hypokalemia, increased serum glucose
Albuterol/ipratropium (pp. 00, 29) (Combivent, DuoNeb)	**MDI:** 90 mcg albuterol/ 18 mcg ipratropium/ actuation **NEB:** 2.5 mg albuterol/ 0.5 mg ipratropium/3 ml	**MDI:** 2 inhalations 4 times/day as needed **NEB:** 2.5 mg/0.5 mg 4 times/day as needed	Same as individual listing for albuterol and ipratropium
Arformoterol (Brovana)	**NEB:** 15 mcg/2 ml	**NEB:** 15 mcg 2 times/day	Same as formoterol
Formoterol (p. 519) (Foradil, Perforomist)	**DPI:** 12 mcg/capsule **NEB:** 20 mcg/2 ml	**DPI:** 12 mcg q12h **NEB:** 20 mcg q12h	Diarrhea, nausea, asthma exacerbation, bronchitis, infection
Formoterol/budesonide (p. 519) (Symbicort)	**MDI:** 80, 160 mcg/ 4.5 mcg/inhalation	**MDI:** 2 inhalations 2 times/day	Same as individual listing for formoterol and budesonide
Formoterol/mometasone (p. 519) (Dulera)	**MDI:** 5 mcg/100 mcg, 5 mcg/200 mcg	**MDI:** 2 inhalations 2 times/day	Same as individual listing for formoterol and beclomethasone
Indacaterol (p. 613) (Arcapta)	**DPI:** 75 mcg/capsule	**DPI:** 75–300 mcg once/day	Cough, oropharyngeal pain, nasopharyngitis, headache, nausea
Levalbuterol (p. 686) (Xopenex)	**MDI:** 45 mcg/actuation **NEB:** 0.31, 0.63, 1.25 mg/3 ml	**MDI:** 2 inhalations q4–6h as needed **NEB:** 0.63–1.25 mg q6-8h	Tremor, rhinitis, viral infection, headache, nervousness, asthma, pharyngitis, rash

Salmeterol (p. 1085) (Serevent Diskus)	**DPI:** 50 mcg/blister	**DPI:** 50 mcg q12h	Headache, pain, throat irritation, nasal congestion, bronchitis, pharyngitis
Salmeterol/fluticasone (pp. 510, 1085) (Advair Diskus, Advair HFA)	**DPI:** 100, 250, 500 mcg/ 50 mcg/blister **MDI:** 45, 115, 230 mcg/ 21 mcg/inhalation	**DPI:** 1 inhalation 2 times/day **MDI:** 2 inhalations 2 times/day	Same as individual listing for salmeterol and fluticasone
Inhaled Corticosteroids			
Beclomethasone (p. 119) (Qvar)	**MDI:** 40, 80 mcg/inhalation	**MDI:** 40–320 mcg 2 times/day	Cough, hoarseness, headache, pharyngitis
Budesonide (p. 159) (Pulmicort Flexhaler, Pulmicort Respules)	**DPI: (Flexhaler):** 90, 180 mcg/inhalation **DPI: (Turbuhaler):** 200 mcg/inhalation **NEB: (Respules):** 0.25, 0.5 mg/2 ml	**DPI: (Flexhaler):** 180–720 mcg 2 times/day **DPI: (Turbuhaler):** 400–2,400 mcg/day in 2–4 divided doses **NEB: (Respules):** 250–500 mcg 1–2 times/day or 1 mg once daily	Headache, nausea, respiratory infection, rhinitis
Ciclesonide (p. 245) (Alvesco HFA)	**HFA:** 80, 160 mcg/inhalation	**HFA:** 80–320 mcg 2 times/day	Headache, nasopharyngitis, upper respiratory infection, epistaxis, nasal congestion, sinusitis
Fluticasone (p. 510) (Flovent Diskus, Flovent HFA)	**DPI: (Flovent Diskus):** 50, 100, 250 mcg/blister **MDI: (Flovent HFA):** 44, 110, 220 mcg/inhalation	**DPI: (Flovent Diskus):** 100–1,000 mcg 2 times/day **MDI: (Flovent HFA):** 88–880 mcg 2 times/day	Headache, nasal congestion, pharyngitis, sinusitis, respiratory infections
Formoterol/budesonide (p. 519) (Symbicort)	**MDI:** 80, 160 mcg/4.5 mcg/ inhalation	**MDI:** 2 inhalations 2 times/day	Same as individual listing for formoterol and budesonide

(continued)

BRONCHODILATORS   *(continued)*

Name	Availability	Dosage Range	Side Effects
Mometasone (p. 806) (Asmanex Twisthaler)	**DPI:** 110–220 mcg/inhalation	**DPI:** 220–880 mcg once daily in evening or 220 mcg bid	Same as beclomethasone
Salmeterol/fluticasone (pp. 510, 1085) (Advair Diskus, Advair HFA)	**DPI:** 100, 250, 500 mcg/50 mcg/blister **MDI:** 45, 115, 230 mcg/21 mcg/inhalation	**DPI:** 1 inhalation 2 times/day **MDI:** 2 inhalations 2 times/day	Same as individual listing for salmeterol and fluticasone
Leukotriene Modifiers			
Montelukast (p. 808) (Singulair)	**T:** 4 mg, 5 mg, 10 mg	**A:** 10 mg/day **C (6–14 yrs):** 5 mg/day **C (2–5 yrs):** 4 mg/day	Dyspepsia, increased hepatic function tests, cough, nasal congestion, headache, dizziness, fatigue
Zafirlukast (p. 1291) (Accolate)	**T:** 10 mg, 20 mg	**A, C (12 yrs and older):** 20 mg 2 times/day **C (5–11 yrs):** 10 mg 2 times/day	Headache, nausea, diarrhea, infection
PDE-4 Inhibitor			
Roflumilast (p. 1072) (Daliresp)	**T:** 500 mcg	**A:** 500 mcg once daily	Headache, dizziness, insomnia

A, Adults; *C (dosage),* children; *DPI,* dry powder inhaler; *HFA,* hydrofluoroalkane; *MDI,* metered dose inhaler; *NEB,* nebulization; *T,* tablets.

Calcium Channel Blockers

USES

Treatment of essential hypertension, treatment of and prophylaxis of angina pectoris (including vasospastic, chronic stable, unstable), prevention/control of supraventricular tachyarrhythmias, prevention of neurologic damage due to subarachnoid hemorrhage.

ACTION

Calcium channel blockers inhibit the flow of extracellular Ca^{2+} ions across cell membranes of cardiac cells, vascular tissue. They relax arterial smooth muscle, depress the rate of sinus node pacemaker, slow AV conduction, decrease heart rate, produce negative inotropic effect (rarely seen clinically due to reflex response). Calcium channel blockers decrease coronary vascular resistance, increase coronary blood flow, reduce myocardial oxygen demand. Degree of action varies with individual agent.

CALCIUM CHANNEL BLOCKERS

Name	Availability	Dosage Range	Side Effects	Indications
Amlodipine (p. 59) (Norvasc)	**T:** 2.5 mg, 5 mg, 10 mg	**HTN:** 2.5–10 mg once daily **Angina:** 10 mg once daily	Abdominal pain, flushing, headaches, peripheral edema	HTN, angina
Diltiazem (p. 366) (Cardizem)	**T:** 30 mg, 60 mg, 90 mg **T (SR):** 120 mg, 180 mg, 240 mg **C (SR):** 60 mg, 90 mg, 120 mg, 180 mg, 240 mg, 300 mg, 360 mg **I:** 5 mg/ml	**HTN:** 120–540 mg/day **Angina:** 120–480 mg/day **I:** 20–25 mg IV bolus, then 5–15 mg/hr infusion	Dizziness, drowsiness, edema, headache	**PO:** HTN, Angina **IV:** Arrhythmias
Felodipine (p. 477) (Plendil)	**T:** 2.5 mg, 5 mg, 10 mg	2.5–20 mg once daily	Peripheral edema, headaches	HTN
Isradipine (p. 650) (DynaCirc)	**C:** 2.5 mg, 5 mg	2.5–10 mg/day in 2 divided doses	Headaches	HTN
Nicardipine (p. 845) (Cardene)	**C (IR):** 20 mg, 30 mg **C (ER):** 30 mg, 45 mg, 60 mg **I:** 2.5 mg/ml	**HTN (IR):** 20–40 mg tid or **(ER):** 30–60 mg bid **Angina (IR):** 20–40 mg tid	Flushing, peripheral edema, headache, dizziness	HTN, angina

(continued)

CALCIUM CHANNEL BLOCKERS   *(continued)*

Name	Availability	Dosage Range	Side Effects	Indications
Nifedipine (p. 849) (Adalat, Procardia)	**C (IR):** 10 mg, 20 mg **T (ER):** 30 mg, 60 mg, 90 mg	**HTN (ER):** 90–120 mg once daily **Angina (IR):** 10–20 mg tid or **(ER):** 120–180 mg once daily	Peripheral edema, dizziness, flushed face, headaches, nausea	HTN, angina
Nimodipine (p. 853) (Nimotop)	**C:** 30 mg	60 mg q4h for 21 days	Nausea, reduced B/P, headache, rash, diarrhea	Prevent neurologic damage following subarachnoid hemorrhage
Verapamil (p. 1263) (Calan, Isoptin)	**T (IR):** 40 mg, 80 mg, 120 mg **T (SR):** 120 mg, 180 mg, 240 mg	**Angina (IR):** 80–160 mg tid or **(SR):** 180–480 mg once daily **HTN (IR):** 80–320 mg/day in 2 divided doses or **(SR):** 120–480 mg/day in 2 divided doses	Nausea, gingival hyperplasia, headache, fatigue, dizziness	HTN, angina

C, Capsules; *CR,* controlled-release; *ER,* extended-release; *HTN,* hypertension; *I,* injection; *SR,* sustained-release; *T,* tablets.

Chemotherapeutic Agents

USES

Treatment of a variety of cancers; may be palliative or curative. Treatment of choice in hematologic cancers. Often used as adjunctive therapy (e.g., with surgery or irradiation); most effective when tumor mass has been removed or reduced by radiation. Often used in combinations to increase therapeutic results, decrease toxic effects. Certain agents may be used in nonmalignant conditions: polycythemia vera, psoriasis, rheumatoid arthritis, or immunosuppression in organ transplantation (used only in select cases that are severe and unresponsive to other forms of therapy). Refer to individual monographs.

ACTION

Most antineoplastics can be divided into alkylating agents, antimetabolites, anthracyclines, plant alkaloids, and topoisomerase inhibitors. These agents affect cell division or DNA synthesis. Newer agents (monoclonal antibodies and tyrosine kinase inhibitors) directly target a molecular abnormality in certain types of cancer. Hormones modulate tumor cell behavior without directly attacking those cells. Some agents are classified as miscellaneous.

CHEMOTHERAPEUTIC AGENTS

Name	Availability	Category	Side Effects
Abiraterone (p. 6) (Zytiga)	**T:** 250 mg	Antiandrogen	Joint swelling, hypokalemia, edema, muscle discomfort, hot flashes, diarrhea, UTI, cough, hypertension, arrhythmia, dyspepsia, upper respiratory tract infection
Aldesleukin (p. 632) (Proleukin)	**I:** 22 million units	Biologic response modifier	Hypotension, sinus tachycardia, nausea, vomiting, diarrhea, renal impairment, anemia, rash, fatigue, agitation, pulmonary congestion, dyspnea, fever, chills, oliguria, weight gain, dizziness
Alemtuzumab (p. 31) (Campath)	**I:** 30 mg/3 ml	Monoclonal antibody	Rigors, fever, fatigue, hypotension, neutropenia, anemia, sepsis, dyspnea, bronchitis, pneumonia, urticaria

(continued)

CHEMOTHERAPEUTIC AGENTS   (continued)

Name	Availability	Category	Side Effects
Anastrozole (p. 71) (Arimidex)	T: 1 mg	Aromatase inhibitor	Peripheral edema, chest pain, nausea, vomiting, diarrhea, constipation, abdominal pain, anorexia, pharyngitis, vaginal hemorrhage, anemia, leukopenia, rash, weight gain, diaphoresis, increased appetite, pain, headaches, dizziness, depression, paresthesia, hot flashes, increased cough, dry mouth, asthenia (loss of strength, energy), dyspnea, phlebitis
Arsenic trioxide (p. 84) (Trisenox)	I: 10 mg/ml	Miscellaneous	AV block, GI hemorrhage, hypertension, hypoglycemia, hypokalemia, hypomagnesemia, neutropenia, oliguria, prolonged QT interval, seizures, sepsis, thrombocytopenia
Asparaginase (p. 87) (Elspar)	I: 10,000 units	Miscellaneous	Anorexia, nausea, vomiting, hepatic toxicity, pancreatitis, nephrotoxicity, clotting factor abnormalities, malaise, confusion, lethargy, EEG changes, respiratory distress, fever, hyperglycemia, depression, stomatitis, allergic reactions, drowsiness
Axitinib (p. 102) (Inlyta)	T: 1 mg, 5 mg	Kinase inhibitor	Diarrhea, hypertension, fatigue, decreased appetite, nausea, dysphonia, vomiting, asthenia (loss of strength, energy), constipation
Azacitidine (p. 104) (Vidaza)	I: 100 mg	DNA methylation inhibitor	Edema, hypokalemia, weight loss, myalgia, cough, dyspnea, upper respiratory tract infection, back pain, pyrexia, weakness
BCG (TheraCys, Tice BCG)	I: 50 mg, 81 mg	Biologic response modulator	Nausea, vomiting, anorexia, diarrhea, dysuria, hematuria, cystitis, urinary urgency, anemia, malaise, fever, chills
Bendamustine (p. 128) (Treanda)	I: 100 mg	Alkylating agent	Neutropenia, pyrexia, thrombocytopenia, nausea, anemia, leukopenia, vomiting
Bevacizumab (p. 136) (Avastin)	I: 25 mg/ml	Monoclonal antibody	Increased B/P, fatigue, blood clots, diarrhea, decreased WBCs, headaches, decreased appetite, stomatitis
Bexarotene (p. 138) (Targretin)	C: 75 mg Gel: 1%	Miscellaneous	Anemia, dermatitis, fever, hypercholesterolemia, infection, leukopenia, peripheral edema

Drug		Classification	Adverse Effects
Bicalutamide (p. 139) (Casodex)	T: 50 mg	Antiandrogen	Gynecomastia, hot flashes, breast pain, nausea, diarrhea, constipation, nocturia, impotence, pain, muscle pain, asthenia (loss of strength, energy), abdominal pain
Bleomycin (p. 146) (Blenoxane)	I: 15 units, 30 units	Antibiotic	Nausea, vomiting, anorexia, stomatitis, hyperpigmentation, alopecia, pruritus, hyperkeratosis, urticaria, pneumonitis progression to fibrosis, weight loss, rash
Bortezomib (p. 150) (Velcade)	I: 3.5 mg	Proteasome inhibitor	Anxiety, dizziness, headaches, insomnia, peripheral neuropathy, pruritus, rash, abdominal pain, decreased appetite, constipation, diarrhea, dyspepsia, nausea, vomiting, arthralgia, dyspnea, asthenia (loss of strength, energy), edema, pain
Bosutinib (p. 153) (Bosulif)	T: 100 mg, 500 mg	Kinase inhibitor	Nausea, diarrhea, thrombocytopenia, vomiting, abdominal pain, anemia, fever, fatigue
Brentuximab (p. 155) (Adcetris)	I: 50 mg	Miscellaneous	Neutropenia, peripheral sensory neuropathy, fatigue, nausea, anemia, upper respiratory tract infection, diarrhea, pyrexia, thrombocytopenia, cough, vomiting
Busulfan (p. 168) (Myleran)	T: 2 mg	Alkylating agent	Nausea, vomiting, hyperuricemia, myelosuppression, skin hyperpigmentation, alopecia, anorexia, weight loss, diarrhea, stomatitis
Cabazitaxel (p. 171) (Jevtana)	I: 60 mg/1.5 ml	Microtubule inhibitor	Neutropenia, anemia, leukopenia, thrombocytopenia, diarrhea, fatigue, nausea, vomiting, constipation, asthenia (loss of strength, energy), abdominal pain, hematuria, anorexia, peripheral neuropathy, dyspnea, alopecia
Capecitabine (p. 185) (Xeloda)	T: 150 mg, 300 mg	Antimetabolite	Nausea, vomiting, diarrhea, stomatitis, myelosuppression, palmar-plantar erythrodysesthesia syndrome, dermatitis, fatigue, anorexia
Carboplatin (p. 193) (Paraplatin)	I: 50 mg, 150 mg, 450 mg	Alkylating agent	Nausea, vomiting, nephrotoxicity, myelosuppression, alopecia, peripheral neuropathy, hypersensitivity, ototoxicity, asthenia (loss of strength, energy), diarrhea, constipation
Carfilzomib (p. 195) (Kyprolis)	I: 60 mg	Proteasome inhibitor	Anemia, fatigue, nausea, thrombocytopenia, dyspnea, diarrhea, pyrexia
Carmustine (p. 198) (BiCNU)	I: 100 mg	Alkylating agent	Anorexia, nausea, vomiting, myelosuppression, pulmonary fibrosis, pain at injection site, diarrhea, skin discoloration
Cetuximab (p. 237) (Erbitux)	I: 2 mg/ml	Monoclonal antibody	Dyspnea, hypotension, acne-like rash, dry skin, weakness, fatigue, fever, constipation, abdominal pain

(continued)

CHEMOTHERAPEUTIC AGENTS *(continued)*

Name	Availability	Category	Side Effects
Chlorambucil (p. 239) (Leukeran)	**T:** 2 mg	Alkylating agent	Myelosuppression, dermatitis, nausea, vomiting, hepatic toxicity, anorexia, diarrhea, abdominal discomfort, rash
Cisplatin (p. 256) (Platinol-AQ)	**I:** 50 mg, 100 mg	Alkylating agent	Nausea, vomiting, nephrotoxicity, myelosuppression, neuropathies, ototoxicity, anaphylactic-like reactions, hyperuricemia, hypomagnesemia, hypophosphatemia, hypokalemia, hypocalcemia, pain at injection site
Cladribine (p. 259) (Leustatin)	**I:** 1 mg/ml	Antimetabolite	Nausea, vomiting, diarrhea, myelosuppression, chills, fatigue, rash, fever, headaches, anorexia, diaphoresis
Crizotinib (p. 292) (Xalkori)	**C:** 200 mg, 250 mg	Tyrosine kinase inhibitor	Vision disorders, nausea, vomiting, diarrhea, edema, constipation
Cyclophosphamide (p. 297) (Cytoxan)	**I:** 100 mg, 200 mg, 500 mg, 1 g, 2 g **T:** 25 mg, 50 mg	Alkylating agent	Nausea, vomiting, hemorrhagic cystitis, myelosuppression, alopecia, interstitial pulmonary fibrosis, amenorrhea, azoospermia, diarrhea, darkening skin/fingernails, headaches, diaphoresis
Cytarabine (p. 302) (Ara-C, Cytosar)	**I:** 100 mg, 500 mg, 1 g, 2 g	Antimetabolite	Anorexia, nausea, vomiting, stomatitis, esophagitis, diarrhea, myelosuppression, alopecia, rash, fever, neuropathies, abdominal pain
Dacarbazine (p. 308) (DTIC)	**I:** 200 mg	Alkylating agent	Nausea, vomiting, anorexia, hepatic necrosis, myelosuppression, alopecia, rash, facial flushing, photosensitivity, flu-like symptoms, confusion, blurred vision
Dasatinib (p. 321) (Sprycel)	**T:** 20 mg, 50 mg, 70 mg	Tyrosine kinase inhibitor	Pyrexia, pleural effusion, febrile neutropenia, GI bleeding, pneumonia, thrombocytopenia, dyspnea, anemia, cardiac failure, diarrhea
Daunorubicin (p. 322) (Cerubidine)	**I:** 20 mg	Anthracycline	HF, nausea, vomiting, stomatitis, mucositis, diarrhea, hematuria, myelosuppression, alopecia, fever, chills, abdominal pain
Daunorubicin liposomal (p. 322) (DaunoXome)	**I:** 50 mg	Anthracycline	Nausea, diarrhea, abdominal pain, anorexia, vomiting, stomatitis, myelosuppression, rigors, back pain, headaches, neuropathy, depression, dyspnea, fatigue, fever, cough, allergic reactions, diaphoresis
Denileukin (p. 334) (Ontak)	**I:** 300 mcg/2 ml	Miscellaneous	Hypersensitivity reaction, back pain, dyspnea, rash, chest pain, tachycardia, asthenia (loss of strength, energy), flu-like symptoms, chills, nausea, vomiting, infection

Name	Dosage	Classification	Side Effects
Docetaxel (p. 379) (Taxotere)	I: 20 mg, 80 mg	Antimicrotubular	Hypotension, nausea, vomiting, diarrhea, mucositis, myelosuppression, rash, paresthesia, hypersensitivity, fluid retention, alopecia, asthenia (loss of strength, energy), stomatitis, fever
Doxorubicin (p. 396) (Adriamycin)	I: 10 mg, 20 mg, 50 mg, 75 mg, 150 mg, 200 mg	Anthracycline	Cardiotoxicity, including HF; arrhythmias, nausea, vomiting, stomatitis, esophagitis, GI ulceration, diarrhea, anorexia, hematuria, myelosuppression, alopecia, hyperpigmentation of nail beds and skin, local inflammation at injection site, rash, fever, chills, urticaria, lacrimation, conjunctivitis
Doxorubicin liposomal (p. 396) (Doxil)	I: 20 mg, 50 mg	Anthracycline	Neutropenia, palmar-plantar erythrodysesthesia syndrome, cardiomyopathy, HF
Enzalutamide (Xtandi)	C: 40 mg	Antiandrogen	Fatigue, weakness, back pain, diarrhea, tissue swelling, musculoskeletal pain, headache, upper respiratory tract infections, blood in urine, spinal cord compression
Epirubicin (p. 428) (Ellence)	I: 2 mg/ml	Anthracycline	Anemia, leukopenia, neutropenia, infection, mucositis
Erlotinib (p. 438) (Tarceva)	T: 25 mg, 100 mg, 150 mg	Tyrosine kinase inhibitor	Diarrhea, rash, nausea, vomiting
Estramustine (p. 452) (Emcyt)	C: 140 mg	Alkylating agent	Increased risk of thrombosis, gynecomastia, nausea, vomiting, diarrhea, thrombocytopenia, peripheral edema
Etoposide (p. 460) (VePesid)	I: 20 mg/ml C: 50 mg	Podophyllotoxin derivative	Nausea, vomiting, anorexia, myelosuppression, alopecia, diarrhea, drowsiness, peripheral neuropathies
Everolimus (p. 463) (Afinitor, Zortress)	T (Afinitor): 5 mg, 10 mg T (Zortress): 0.25 mg, 0.5 mg, 0.75 mg	mTOR kinase inhibitor	Stomatitis, infections, asthenia (loss of strength, energy), fatigue, cough, diarrhea
Exemestane (p. 465) (Aromasin)	T: 25 mg	Aromatase inactivator	Dyspnea, edema, hypertension, mental depression

(continued)

CHEMOTHERAPEUTIC AGENTS (continued)

Name	Availability	Category	Side Effects
Fludarabine (p. 499) (Fludara)	I: 50 mg	Antimetabolite	Nausea, diarrhea, stomatitis, bleeding, anemia, myelosuppression, skin rash, weakness, confusion, visual disturbances, peripheral neuropathy, coma, pneumonia, peripheral edema, anorexia
Fluorouracil (p. 502) (Adrucil, Efudex)	I: 50 mg/ml Cream: 1%, 5% Solution: 1%, 2%, 5%	Antimetabolite	Nausea, vomiting, stomatitis, GI ulceration, diarrhea, anorexia, myelosuppression, alopecia, skin hyperpigmentation, nail changes, headaches, drowsiness, blurred vision, fever
Flutamide (p. 509) (Eulexin)	C: 125 mg	Antiandrogen	Hot flashes, nausea, vomiting, diarrhea, hepatitis, impotence, decreased libido, rash, anorexia
Fulvestrant (p. 529) (Faslodex)	I: 125 mg/2.5 ml, 250 mg/5 ml syringes	Estrogen receptor antagonist	Asthenia (loss of strength, energy), pain, headaches, injection site pain, flu-like symptoms, fever, nausea, vomiting, constipation, anorexia, diarrhea, peripheral edema, dizziness, depression, anxiety, rash, increased cough, UTI
Gefitinib (p. 539) (Iressa)	T: 250 mg	Tyrosine kinase inhibitor	Diarrhea, rash, acne, nausea, dry skin, vomiting, pruritus, anorexia
Gemcitabine (p. 540) (Gemzar)	I: 200 mg, 1 g	Antimetabolite	Increased hepatic function tests, nausea, vomiting, diarrhea, stomatitis, hematuria, myelosuppression, rash, mild paresthesia, dyspnea, fever, edema, flu-like symptoms, constipation
Goserelin (p. 558) (Zoladex)	I: 3.6 mg, 10.8 mg	Hormone agonist	Hot flashes, sexual dysfunction, erectile dysfunction, gynecomastia, lethargy, pain, lower urinary tract symptoms, headaches, nausea, depression, diaphoresis
Hydroxyurea (p. 583) (Hydrea)	C: 500 mg	Antimetabolite	Anorexia, nausea, vomiting, stomatitis, diarrhea, constipation, myelosuppression, fever, chills, malaise
Ibritumomab (p. 590) (Zevalin)	Injection kit	Monoclonal antibody	Neutropenia, thrombocytopenia, anemia, infection, asthenia (loss of strength, energy), abdominal pain, fever, pain, headaches, nausea, peripheral edema, allergic reaction, GI hemorrhage, apnea

Idarubicin (p. 599) (Idamycin PFS)	**I:** 5 mg, 10 mg, 20 mg	Anthracycline	HF, arrhythmias, nausea, vomiting, stomatitis, myelosuppression, alopecia, rash, urticaria, hyperuricemia, abdominal pain, diarrhea, esophagitis, anorexia
Ifosfamide (p. 601) (Ifex)	**I:** 1 g, 3 g	Alkylating agent	Nausea, vomiting, hemorrhagic cystitis, myelosuppression, alopecia, lethargy, drowsiness, confusion, hallucinations, hematuria
Imatinib (p. 605) (Gleevec)	**C:** 100 mg	Tyrosine kinase inhibitor	Nausea, fluid retention, hemorrhage, musculoskeletal pain, arthralgia, weight gain, pyrexia, abdominal pain, dyspnea, pneumonia
Interferon alfa-2b (p. 626) (Intron-A)	**I:** 3 million units, 5 million units, 10 million units, 18 million units, 25 million units, 50 million units	Miscellaneous	Mild hypotension, hypertension, tachycardia with high fever, nausea, diarrhea, altered taste, weight loss, thrombocytopenia, myelosuppression, rash, pruritus, myalgia, arthralgia associated with flu-like symptoms
Ipilimumab (p. 634) (Yervoy)	**I:** 5 mg/ml	Miscellaneous	Fatigue, diarrhea, pruritus, rash, colitis
Irinotecan (p. 640) (Camptosar)	**I:** 40 mg, 100 mg	Camptothecin	Diarrhea, nausea, vomiting, abdominal cramps, anorexia, stomatitis, increased AST, severe myelosuppression, alopecia, diaphoresis, rash, weight loss, dehydration, increased serum alkaline phosphatase, headaches, insomnia, dizziness, dyspnea, cough, asthenia (loss of strength, energy), rhinitis, fever, back pain, chills
Ixabepilone (p. 654) (Ixempra)	**I:** 15 mg, 45 mg	Antimicrotubular	Peripheral sensory neuropathy, fatigue, myalgia, alopecia, nausea, vomiting, stomatitis, diarrhea, anorexia, abdominal pain
Lapatinib (p. 675) (Tykerb)	**T:** 250 mg	Tyrosine kinase inhibitor	Diarrhea, palmar-plantar erythrodysesthesia, nausea, rash, vomiting, fatigue
Letrozole (p. 681) (Femara)	**T:** 2.5 mg	Aromatase inhibitor	Hypertension, nausea, vomiting, constipation, diarrhea, abdominal pain, anorexia, rash, pruritus, musculoskeletal pain, arthralgia, fatigue, headaches, dyspnea, coughing, hot flashes
Leuprolide (p. 684) (Lupron)	**I:** 3.75 mg, 5 mg, 7.5 mg, 11.25 mg, 15 mg, 22.5 mg, 30 mg	Hormone agonist	Hot flashes, gynecomastia, nausea, vomiting, constipation, anorexia, dizziness, headaches, insomnia, paresthesia, bone pain

(continued)

CHEMOTHERAPEUTIC AGENTS   *(continued)*

Name	Availability	Category	Side Effects
Lomustine (p. 714) (CeeNU)	**C:** 10 mg, 40 mg, 100 mg	Alkylating agent	Anorexia, nausea, vomiting, stomatitis, hepatotoxicity, nephrotoxicity, myelosuppression, alopecia, confusion, slurred speech
Mechlorethamine (Mustargen)	**I:** 10 mg/ml	Alkylating agent	Severe nausea and vomiting, metallic taste, diarrhea, myelosuppression, alopecia, phlebitis, vertigo, tinnitus, hyperuricemia, infertility, azoospermia, anorexia, headaches, drowsiness, fever
Megestrol (p. 744) (Megace)	**T:** 20 mg, 40 mg **Suspension:** 40 mg/ml	Hormone	Deep vein thrombosis, Cushing-like syndrome, alopecia, carpal tunnel syndrome, weight gain, nausea
Melphalan (p. 746) (Alkeran)	**T:** 2 mg	Alkylating agent	Anorexia, nausea, vomiting, myelosuppression, diarrhea, stomatitis
Mercaptopurine (Purinethol)	**T:** 50 mg	Antimetabolite	Anorexia, nausea, vomiting, stomatitis, hepatic toxicity, myelosuppression, hyperuricemia, diarrhea, rash
Methotrexate (p. 763) (Rheumatrex)	**T:** 2.5 mg, 5 mg, 7.5 mg, 10 mg, 15 mg **I:** 5 mg, 50 mg, 100 mg, 200 mg, 250 mg	Antimetabolite	Nausea, vomiting, stomatitis, GI ulceration, diarrhea, hepatic toxicity, renal failure, cystitis, myelosuppression, alopecia, urticaria, acne, photosensitivity, interstitial pneumonitis, fever, malaise, chills, anorexia
Mitomycin (p. 801) (Mutamycin)	**I:** 20 mg, 40 mg	Antibiotic	Anorexia, nausea, vomiting, stomatitis, diarrhea, renal toxicity, myelosuppression, alopecia, pruritus, fever, hemolytic uremic syndrome, weakness
Mitotane (Lysodren)	**T:** 500 mg	Miscellaneous	Anorexia, nausea, vomiting, diarrhea, skin rashes, depression, lethargy, drowsiness, dizziness, adrenal insufficiency, blurred vision, impaired hearing
Mitoxantrone (p. 803) (Novantrone)	**I:** 20 mg, 25 mg, 30 mg	Anthracenedione	HF, tachycardia, ECG changes, chest pain, nausea, vomiting, stomatitis, mucositis, myelosuppression, rash, alopecia, urine discoloration (bluish green), phlebitis, diarrhea, cough, headaches, fever

Drug	Form/Dose	Classification	Side Effects
Nelarabine (p. 836) (Arranon)	I: 5 mg/ml	Antimetabolite	Anemia, neutropenia, thrombocytopenia, nausea, vomiting, diarrhea, fatigue, fever, dyspnea, severe neurologic events (convulsions, peripheral neuropathy)
Nilotinib (p. 851) (Tasigna)	C: 200 mg	Tyrosine kinase inhibitor	Rash, pruritus, nausea, fatigue, headache, constipation, diarrhea, vomiting, thrombocytopenia, neutropenia
Nilutamide (p. 852) (Nilandron)	T: 50 mg	Antiandrogen	Hypertension, angina, hot flashes, nausea, anorexia, increased hepatic enzymes, dizziness, dyspnea, visual disturbances, impaired adaptation to dark, constipation, decreased libido
Oxaliplatin (p. 897) (Eloxatin)	I: 50 mg, 100 mg	Alkylating agent	Fatigue, neuropathy, abdominal pain, dyspnea, diarrhea, nausea, vomiting, anorexia, fever, edema, chest pain, anemia, thrombocytopenia, thromboembolism, altered hepatic function tests
Paclitaxel (p. 910) (Taxol)	I: 30 mg, 100 mg	Antimicrotubular	Hypertension, bradycardia, ECG changes, nausea, vomiting, diarrhea, mucositis, myelosuppression, alopecia, peripheral neuropathies, hypersensitivity reaction, arthralgia, myalgia
Panitumumab (p. 920) (Vectibix)	I: 20 mg/ml	Monoclonal antibody	Pulmonary fibrosis, severe dermatologic toxicity, infusion reactions, abdominal pain, nausea, vomiting, constipation, skin rash, fatigue
Pegaspargase (p. 927) (Oncaspar)	I: 750 international units/ml	Miscellaneous	Hypotension, anorexia, nausea, vomiting, hepatotoxicity, pancreatitis, depression of clotting factors, malaise, confusion, lethargy, EEG changes, respiratory distress, hypersensitivity reaction, fever, hyperglycemia, stomatitis
Pemetrexed (p. 937) (Alimta)	I: 500 mg	Antimetabolite	Anorexia, constipation, diarrhea, neuropathy, anemia, chest pain, dyspnea, rash, fatigue
Pentostatin (Nipent)	I: 10 mg	Antibiotic	Nausea, vomiting, hepatic disorders, elevated hepatic function tests, leukopenia, anemia, thrombocytopenia, rash, fever, upper respiratory infection, fatigue, hematuria, headaches, myalgia, arthralgia, diarrhea, anorexia
Pertuzumab (p. 948) (Perjeta)	I: 420 mg/14 ml	HER2/neu receptor antagonist	Alopecia, diarrhea, nausea, neutropenia, rash, fatigue, peripheral neuropathy

(continued)

CHEMOTHERAPEUTIC AGENTS   *(continued)*

Name	Availability	Category	Side Effects
Procarbazine (p. 998) (Matulane)	**C:** 50 mg	Alkylating agent	Nausea, vomiting, stomatitis, diarrhea, constipation, myelosuppression, pruritus, hyperpigmentation, alopecia, myalgia, paresthesia, confusion, lethargy, mental depression, fever, hepatic toxicity, arthralgia, respiratory disorders
Rituximab (p. 1065) (Rituxan)	**I:** 100 mg, 500 mg	Monoclonal antibody	Hypotension, arrhythmias, peripheral edema, nausea, vomiting, abdominal pain, leukopenia, thrombocytopenia, neutropenia, rash, pruritus, urticaria, angioedema, myalgia, headaches, dizziness, throat irritation, rhinitis, bronchospasm, hypersensitivity reaction
Sipuleucel-T (Provenge)	**I:** Minimum of 50 million autologous CD54+ cells in lactated Ringer's	Miscellaneous	Chills, fatigue, fever, back pain, nausea, headache, joint ache
Sorafenib (p. 1122) (Nexavar)	**T:** 200 mg	Tyrosine kinase inhibitor	Fatigue, alopecia, nausea, vomiting, anorexia, constipation, diarrhea, neuropathy, dyspnea, cough, asthenia (loss of strength, energy), pain
Sunitinib (p. 1141) (Sutent)	**C:** 12.5 mg, 25 mg, 50 mg	Tyrosine kinase inhibitor	Hypotension, edema, fatigue, headache, fever, dizziness, rash, hyperpigmentation, diarrhea, nausea, dyspepsia, altered taste, vomiting, neutropenia, thrombocytopenia, increased ALT/AST
Tamoxifen (p. 1147) (Nolvadex-D)	**T:** 10 mg, 20 mg	Estrogen receptor antagonist	Skin rash, nausea, vomiting, anorexia, menstrual irregularities, hot flashes, pruritus, vaginal discharge or bleeding, myelosuppression, headaches, tumor or bone pain, ophthalmic changes, weight gain, confusion
Temozolomide (p. 1159) (Temodar)	**C:** 5 mg, 20 mg, 100 mg, 250 mg	Alkylating agent	Amnesia, fever, infection, leukopenia, neutropenia, peripheral edema, seizures, thrombocytopenia
Temsirolimus (p. 1161) (Torisel)	**I:** 25 mg/ml	mTOR kinase inhibitor	Rash, asthenia (loss of strength, energy), mucositis, nausea, edema, anorexia, thrombocytopenia, leukopenia
Thioguanine (Tabloid)	**T:** 40 mg	Antimetabolite	Anorexia, stomatitis, myelosuppression, hyperuricemia, nausea, vomiting, diarrhea

(continued)

Drug	Classification	Dose	Adverse Effects
Thiotepa (p. 1183) (Thioplex)	Alkylating agent	I: 15 mg	Anorexia, nausea, vomiting, mucositis, myelosuppression, amenorrhea, reduced spermatogenesis, fever, hypersensitivity reactions, pain at injection site, headaches, dizziness, alopecia
Topotecan (p. 1213) (Hycamtin)	Camptothecin	I: 4 mg	Nausea, vomiting, diarrhea, constipation, abdominal pain, stomatitis, anorexia, neutropenia, leukopenia, thrombocytopenia, anemia, alopecia, headaches, dyspnea, paresthesia
Toremifene (p. 1215) (Fareston)	Estrogen receptor antagonist	T: 60 mg	Elevated hepatic function tests, nausea, vomiting, constipation, skin discoloration, dermatitis, dizziness, hot flashes, diaphoresis, vaginal discharge or bleeding, ocular changes, cataracts, anxiety
Trastuzumab (p. 1224) (Herceptin)	Monoclonal antibody	I: 440 mg	HF, heart murmur (S_3 gallop), nausea, vomiting, diarrhea, abdominal pain, anorexia, rash, peripheral edema, back or bone pain, asthenia (loss of strength, energy), headaches, insomnia, dizziness, cough, dyspnea, rhinitis, pharyngitis
Tretinoin (p. 1229) (Vesanoid)	Miscellaneous	C: 10 mg	Flushing, nausea, vomiting, diarrhea, constipation, dyspepsia, mucositis, leukocytosis, dry skin/mucous membranes, rash, pruritus, alopecia, dizziness, anxiety, insomnia, headaches, depression, confusion, intracranial hypertension, agitation, dyspnea, shivering, fever, visual changes, earaches, hearing loss, bone pain, myalgia, arthralgia
Valrubicin (Valstar)	Anthracycline	I: 200 mg/5 ml	Dysuria, hematuria, urinary frequency/incontinence/urgency
Vandetanib (p. 1253) (Caprelsa)	Tyrosine kinase inhibitor	T: 100 mg, 300 mg	Diarrhea, rash, acne, nausea, hypertension, headache, fatigue, decreased appetite, abdominal pain
Vinblastine (p. 1267) (Velban)	Vinca alkaloid	I: 10 mg	Nausea, vomiting, stomatitis, constipation, myelosuppression, alopecia, peripheral neuropathy, loss of deep tendon reflexes, paresthesia, diarrhea
Vincristine (p. 1269) (Oncovin)	Vinca alkaloid	I: 1 mg, 2 mg, 3 mg	Nausea, vomiting, stomatitis, constipation, pharyngitis, polyuria, myelosuppression, alopecia, numbness, paresthesia, peripheral neuropathy, loss of deep tendon reflexes, headaches, abdominal pain
Vincristine liposomal (p. 1269) (Marqibo)	Vinca alkaloid	I: 5 mg/31 ml	Constipation, nausea, pyrexia, fatigue, peripheral neuropathy, febrile neutropenia, diarrhea, anemia, reduced appetite, insomnia

CHEMOTHERAPEUTIC AGENTS   *(continued)*

Name	Availability	Category	Side Effects
Vinorelbine (p. 1271) (Navelbine)	*I:* 10 mg, 50 mg	Vinca alkaloid	Elevated hepatic function tests, nausea, vomiting, constipation, ileus, anorexia, stomatitis, myelosuppression, alopecia, vein discoloration, venous pain, phlebitis, interstitial pulmonary changes, asthenia (loss of strength, energy), fatigue, diarrhea, peripheral neuropathy, loss of deep tendon reflexes
Vismodegib (p. 1274) (Erivedge)	*C:* 150 mg	Hedgehog pathway inhibitor	Alopecia, muscle spasms, dysgensia, weight loss, fatigue, nausea, diarrhea, reduced appetite, vomiting, arthralgia
Vorinostat (p. 1285) (Zolinza)	*C:* 100 mg	Histone deacetylase inhibitor	Diarrhea, fatigue, nausea, thrombocytopenia, anorexia, dysgeusia
ziv-aflibercept (Zaltrap)	*I:* 25 mg/ml	Miscellaneous	Leukopenia, neutropenia, diarrhea, proteinuria, increased ALT/AST, stomatitis, thrombocytopenia, hypertension, epistaxis, headache, abdominal pain

C, Capsules; *I,* injection; *T,* tablets.

Contraception

ACTION

Combination oral contraceptives decrease fertility primarily by inhibition of ovulation. In addition, they can promote thickening of the cervical mucus, thereby creating a physical barrier for the passage of sperm. Also, they can modify the endometrium, making it less favorable for nidation.

CLASSIFICATION

Oral contraceptives either contain both an estrogen and a progestin (combination oral contraceptives) or contain only a progestin (progestin-only oral contraceptives). The combination oral contraceptives have three subgroups:

Monophasic: Daily estrogen and progestin dosage remains constant.

Biphasic: Estrogen remains constant, but the progestin dosage increases during the second half of the cycle.

Triphasic: Progestin changes for each phase of the cycle.

Over the past several years, options have expanded to include a combined hormonal patch (Ortho Evra), vaginal ring (NuvaRing), and extended cycle contraceptives (e.g., Loestrin-24 FE, Seasonale, Seasonique, Yaz). The latest oral contraceptive, Natazia, is a four-phase dosing regimen (estradiol steps down and dienogest, a progestin, steps up during the cycle to help avoid breakthrough bleeding).

COMMON COMPLAINTS WITH ORAL CONTRACEPTIVES

Too much estrogen	Nausea, bloating, breast tenderness, increased B/P, melasma, headache
Too little estrogen	Early or midcycle breakthrough bleeding, increased spotting, hypomenorrhea
Too much progestin	Breast tenderness, headache, fatigue, changes in mood
Too little progestin	Late breakthrough bleeding
Too much androgen	Increased appetite, weight gain, acne, oily skin, hirsutism, decreased libido, increased breast size, breast tenderness, increased LDL cholesterol, decreased HDL cholesterol

(continued)

CONTRACEPTIVES

Name	Estrogen Content	Progestin Content
Low-Dose Monophasic Pills		
Aviane-28 Lessina Lutera Sronyx	EE 20 mcg	Levonorgestrel 0.1 mg
Junel 1/20 Junel Fe 1/20 Loestrin Fe 1/20 Microgestin Fe 1/20	EE 20 mcg	Norethindrone 1 mg
Levora Nordette-28 Portia-28	EE 30 mcg	Levonorgestrel 0.15 mg
Cryselle-28 Lo/Ovral-28 Low-Ogestrel-21, -28	EE 30 mcg	Norgestrel 0.3 mg
Junel 1.5/30 Junel Fe 1.5/30 Loestrin Fe 1.5/30 Microgestin 1.5/30 Microgestin Fe 1.5/30	EE 30 mcg	Norethindrone acetate 1.5 mg
Apri Desogen Ortho-Cept Reclipsen Solia	EE 30 mcg	Desogestrel 0.15 mg

Yasmin Ocella	EE 30 mcg	Drospirenone 3 mg
Kelnor 1/35 Zovia 1/35	EE 35 mcg	Ethynodiol diacetate 1 mg
Ortho-Cyclen-28 Mononessa Previfem Sprintec	EE 35 mcg	Norgestimate 0.25 mg
Necon 1/50 Norinyl 1+50	Mestranol 50 mcg	Norethindrone 1 mg
Balziva Femcon Fe Ovcon-35 Zenchent	EE 35 mcg	Norethindrone 0.4 mg
	EE 35 mcg	Norethindrone 0.5 mg (total of 10.5 mg/cycle)
Brevicon-28 Modicon-28 Necon 0.5/35 Nortrel 0.5/35	EE 35 mcg	
Necon 1/35-28 Norinyl 1+35-28 Nortrel 1/35-28 Ortho-Novum 1/35-28	EE 35 mcg	Norethindrone 1 mg (total of 21 mg/cycle)
High-Dose Monophasic Pills		
Zovia 1/50-28	EE 50 mcg	Ethynodiol diacetate 1 mg
Ogestrel 0.5/50-28	EE 50 mcg	Norgestrel 0.5 mg
Ovcon-50	EE 50 mcg	Norethindrone 1 mg

(continued)

CONTRACEPTIVES   *(continued)*

Name	Estrogen Content	Progestin Content
Biphasic Pills		
Azurette Kariva Mircette	EE 20 mcg × 21 days, placebo × 2 days, 10 mcg × 5 days	Desogestrel 0.15 mg × 21 days
Necon 10/11	EE 35 mcg	Norethindrone 0.5 mg × 10 days, 1 mg × 11 days
Triphasic Pills		
Estrostep Fe Tilia Tilia Fe Tri-Legest Fe	EE 20 mcg × 5 days, 30 mcg × 7 days, 35 mcg × 9 days	Norethindrone 1 mg × 21 days
Ortho Tri-Cyclen Lo Tri Lo Sprintec	EE 25 mcg × 21 days	Norgestimate 0.18 mg × 7 days, 0.215 mg × 7 days, 0.25 mg × 7 days
Caziant Cesia Cyclessa Velivet	EE 25 mcg × 21 days	Desogestrel 0.1 mg × 7 days, 0.125 mg × 7 days, 0.15 mg × 7 days
Enpresse Trivora	EE 30 mcg × 6 days, 40 mcg × 5 days, 30 mcg × 10 days	Levonorgestrel 0.05 mg × 6 days, 0.075 mg × 5 days, 0.125 mg × 10 days
Ortho Tri-Cyclen Trinessa Tri-Previfem Tri-Sprintec	EE 35 mcg × 21 days	Norgestimate 0.18 mg × 7 days, 0.215 mg × 7 days, 0.25 mg × 7 days
Aranelle Leena Tri-Norinyl	EE 35 mcg × 21 days	Norethindrone 0.5 mg × 7 days, 1 mg × 9 days, 0.5 mg × 5 days

Ortho-Novum 7/7/7 Nortrel 7/7/7 Necon 7/7/7	EE 35 mcg × 21 days	Norethindrone 0.5 mg × 7 days, 0.75 mg × 7 days, 1 mg × 7 days
Four Phasic		
Natazia	Estradiol 3 mg × 2 days, then 2 mg × 22 days, then 1 mg × 2 days, then 2-day pill-free interval	Dienogest none × 2 days, then 2 mg × 5 days, then 3 mg × 17 days, then none for 4 days
Extended-Cycle Pills		
Loestrin-24 FE	EE 20 mcg × 24 days	Norethindrone 1 mg × 24 days
Jolessa	EE 30 mcg × 84 days	Levonorgestrel 0.15 mg × 84 days
Quartette Quasense Seasonale	EE 20 mcg × 42 days, 25 mcg × 21 days, 30 mcg × 21 days, then 10 mcg × 7 days	Levonorgestrel 0.15 mg × 84 days
Seasonique	EE 30 mcg × 84 days, 10 mcg × 7 days	Levonorgestrel 0.15 mg × 84 days
Yaz Gianvi	EE 20 mcg × 24 days	Drospirenone 3 mg × 24 days
Continuous Cycle Pill		
Lybrel	EE 20 mcg	Levonorgestrel 90 mcg
Progestin-Only Pills		
Camilia Errin Jolivette Micronor Nor-QD Nora-BE	N/A	Norethindrone 0.35 mg

(continued)

CONTRACEPTIVES   *(continued)*

Name	Estrogen Content	Progestin Content
Emergency Contraception		
Plan B Next Choice	N/A	Levonorgestrel 0.75-mg tablets taken 12 hrs apart
Ella (Ulipristal)	N/A	Ulipristal 30 mg one time within 5 days after unprotected intercourse
Hormonal Alternative to Oral Contraception		
Depo-Provera Cl Medroxyprogesterone Acetate	None	Medroxyprogesterone 150 mg
Depo-SubQ Provera 104	None	Medroxyprogesterone 104 mg
Implanon	None	Etonogestrel (release rate varies over time)
Mirena	None	Levonorgestrel 20 mcg/day for 5 yrs
NuvaRing	Ethinyl estradiol 15 mcg/day	Etonogestrel 0.12 mg/day
Ortho Evra	Ethinyl estradiol 20 mcg/day	Norelgestromin 150 mcg/day

Corticosteroids

USES

Replacement therapy in adrenal insufficiency, including Addison's disease. Symptomatic treatment of multi-organ disease/conditions. Rheumatoid arthritis (RA), osteoarthritis, severe psoriasis, ulcerative colitis, lupus erythematosus, anaphylactic shock, acute exacerbation of asthma, status asthmaticus, organ transplant.

ACTION

Suppresses migration of polymorphonuclear leukocytes (PML) and reverses increased capillary permeability by their anti-inflammatory effect. Suppresses immune system by decreasing activity of lymphatic system.

CORTICOSTEROIDS

Name	Availability	Route of Administration	Side Effects
Beclomethasone (p. 119) (Beconase, Qnasl, QVAR)	**Aerosol (oral inhalation), QVAR:** 40 mcg/inhalation, 80 mcg/inhalation **Aerosol (spray, intranasal), Qnasl:** 80 mcg/inhalation **Suspension (intranasal), Beconase:** 42 mcg/inhalation	Inhalation, intranasal	**I:** Cough, dry mouth/throat, headaches, throat irritation, increased blood glucose **Nasal:** Headaches, sore throat, intranasal ulceration, increased blood glucose
Betamethasone (p. 133) (Celestone)	**I:** 6 mg/ml	IV, intralesional, intra-articular	Nausea, vomiting, increased appetite, weight gain, insomnia, increased blood glucose
Budesonide (p. 159) (Pulmicort, Rhinocort)	**Nasal:** 32 mcg/spray **Suspension for nebulization:** 250 mcg, 500 mcg	Intranasal	Headaches, sore throat, intranasal ulceration, increased blood glucose
Cortisone (p. 290) (Cortone)	**T:** 5 mg, 10 mg, 25 mg	PO	Insomnia, nervousness, increased appetite, indigestion, increased blood glucose

(continued)

CORTICOSTEROIDS (continued)

Name	Availability	Route of Administration	Side Effects
Dexamethasone (p. 343) (Decadron)	**T:** 0.5 mg, 1 mg, 4 mg, 6 mg **OS:** 0.5 mg/5 ml **I:** 4 mg/ml, 10 mg/ml	PO, parenteral	Insomnia, weight gain, increased appetite, increased blood glucose
Fludrocortisone (Florinef)	**T:** 0.1 mg	PO	Edema, headache, peptic ulcer, increased blood glucose
Flunisolide (p. 501) (Nasalide)	**Nasal:** 25 mcg/spray	Inhalation, intranasal	Headache, nasal congestion, pharyngitis, upper respiratory infections, altered taste/smell, increased blood glucose
Fluticasone (p. 510) (Flonase, Flovent)	**Inhalation:** 44 mcg, 110 mg, 220 mcg **Nasal:** 50 mg, 100 mcg	Inhalation, intranasal	Headache, burning/stinging, nasal congestion, upper respiratory infections, increased blood glucose
Hydrocortisone (p. 577) (Solu-Cortef)	**T:** 5 mg, 10 mg, 25 mg **I:** 100 mg, 250 mg, 500 mg, 1 g	PO, parenteral	Insomnia, headache, nausea, vomiting, increased blood glucose
Methylprednisolone (p. 771) (Solu-Medrol)	**T:** 4 mg **I:** 40 mg, 125 mg, 500 mg, 1 g, 2 g	PO, parenteral	Headache, insomnia, nervousness, increased appetite, nausea, vomiting, increased blood glucose
Prednisolone (p. 988) (Prelone)	**T:** 5 mg **OS:** 5 mg/5 ml, 15 mg/5 ml	PO	Headache, insomnia, weight gain, nausea, vomiting, increased blood glucose
Prednisone (p. 990)	**T:** 1 mg, 2.5 mg, 5 mg, 10 mg, 20 mg, 50 mg	PO	Headache, insomnia, weight gain, nausea, vomiting, increased blood glucose
Triamcinolone (p. 1232) (Kenalog, Nasacort AQ)	**Injection, suspension:** 10 mg/ml, 40 mg/ml **Intranasal, suspension:** 55 mcg/inhalation	IM, inhalation (nasal)	**PO:** Insomnia, increased appetite, nausea, vomiting, increased blood glucose **I:** Cough, dry mouth/throat, headaches, throat irritation, increased blood glucose

I, Injection; *OS,* oral suspension; *T,* tablets.

Corticosteroids: Topical

USES

Provide relief of inflammation/pruritus associated with corticosteroid-responsive disorders (e.g., contact dermatitis, eczema, insect bite reactions, first- and second-degree localized burns/sunburn).

ACTION

Diffuse across cell membranes, form complexes with cytoplasm. Complexes stimulate protein synthesis of inhibitory enzymes responsible for anti-inflammatory effects (e.g., inhibit edema, erythema, pruritus, capillary dilation, phagocytic activity).

Topical corticosteroids can be classified based on potency:

May use for facial and intertriginous application for only limited time.

High potency: For more severe inflammatory conditions (e.g., lichen simplex chronicus, psoriasis). May use for facial and intertriginous application for short time only. Used in areas of thickened skin due to chronic conditions.

Low potency: Modest anti-inflammatory effect, safest for chronic application, facial and intertriginous application, with occlusion, for infants/young children.

Medium potency: For moderate inflammatory conditions (e.g., chronic eczematous dermatoses).

Very high potency: Alternative to systemic therapy for local effect (e.g., chronic lesions caused by psoriasis). Increased risk of skin atrophy. Used for short periods on small areas. Avoid occlusive dressings.

CORTICOSTEROIDS: TOPICAL

Name	Availability	Potency	Side Effects
Alclometasone (Aclovate)	C, O: 0.05%	Low	Skin atrophy, contact dermatitis, stretch marks on skin, enlarged blood vessels in the skin, hair loss, pigment changes, secondary infections
Amcinonide (Cyclocort)	C, O, L: 0.1%	High	Same as alclometasone
Betamethasone dipropionate (p. 133)	C, O, G, L: 0.05%	High	Same as alclometasone

(continued)

CORTICOSTEROIDS: TOPICAL (continued)

Name	Availability	Potency	Side Effects
Betamethasone valerate (p. 133)	**C:** 0.01%, 0.05%, 0.1% **O:** 0.1% **L:** 0.1%	High	Same as alclometasone
Clobetasol (Temovate)	**C, O:** 0.05%	High	Same as alclometasone
Desonide (Tridesilon)	**C, O, L:** 0.05%	Low	Same as alclometasone
Desoximetasone (Topicort)	**C:** 0.25%, 0.5% **O:** 0.25% **G:** 0.05%	High	Same as alclometasone
Dexamethasone (p. 343) (Decadron)	**C:** 0.1%	Medium	Same as alclometasone
Fluocinolone (Synalar)	**C:** 0.01%, 0.025%, 0.2% **O:** 0.025%	High	Same as alclometasone
Fluocinonide (Lidex)	**C, O, G:** 0.05%	High	Same as alclometasone
Flurandrenolide (Cordran)	**C, O, L:** 0.025%, 0.05%	Medium	Same as alclometasone
Fluticasone (p. 510) (Cutivate)	**C:** 0.05% **O:** 0.005%	Medium	Same as alclometasone
Halobetasol (Ultravate)	**C, O:** 0.05%	High	Same as alclometasone
Hydrocortisone (p. 577) (Hytone)	**C, O:** 0.5%, 1%, 2.5%	Medium	Same as alclometasone
Mometasone (p. 806) (Elocon)	**C, O, L:** 0.1%	Medium	Same as alclometasone
Prednicarbate (Dermatop)	**C:** 0.1%	—	Same as alclometasone
Triamcinolone (p. 1232) (Aristocort, Kenalog)	**C, O, L:** 0.025%, 0.1%, 0.5%	Medium	Same as alclometasone

C, Cream; *G,* gel; *L,* lotion; *O,* ointment.

Diuretics

USES

Thiazides: Management of edema resulting from a number of causes (e.g., HF, hepatic cirrhosis); hypertension either alone or in combination with other antihypertensives.
Loop: Management of edema associated with HF, cirrhosis of the liver, and renal disease. Furosemide used in treatment of hypertension alone or in combination with other antihypertensives.
Potassium-sparing: Adjunctive treatment with thiazides, loop diuretics in treatment of HF and hypertension.

ACTION

Increases the excretion of water/sodium and other electrolytes via the kidneys. Exact mechanism of antihypertensive effect unknown; may be due to reduced plasma volume or decreased peripheral vascular resistance. Subclassifications of diuretics are based on their mechanism and site of action.
Thiazides: Acts at cortical diluting segment of nephron, block reabsorption of Na, Cl, and water; promote excretion of Na, Cl, K, and water. *Loop:* Acts primarily at the thick ascending limb of Henle's loop to inhibit Na, Cl, and water absorption.

Potassium-sparing: Spironolactone blocks aldosterone action on distal nephron (causes K retention, Na excretion). Triamterene, amiloride act on distal nephron, decreasing Na reuptake, reducing K secretion.

DIURETICS

Name	Availability	Dosage Range	Side Effects
Thiazide, Thiazide-related			
Chlorothiazide (Diuril)	**T:** 250 mg, 500 mg **S:** 250 mg/5 ml **I:** 500 mg	**Edema:** 500–1,000 mg 1–2 times/day **HTN:** 500–2,000 mg/day in 1–2 divided doses	Confusion, fatigue, muscle cramps, abdominal discomfort
Chlorthalidone (Hygroton)	**Hygroton:** 25 mg, 50 mg	**Edema:** 50–200 mg/day **HTN:** 12.5–100 mg/day	Same as chlorothiazide

(continued)

DIURETICS   *(continued)*

Name	Availability	Dosage Range	Side Effects
Hydrochlorothiazide (p. 572) (HydroDIURIL)	**T:** 12.5 mg, 25 mg, 50 mg **C:** 12.5 mg	**Edema:** 25–100 mg/day in 1–2 divided doses **HTN:** 12.5/50 mg once daily	Orthostatic hypotension, photosensitivity, hypokalemia, anorexia, epigastric distress, increased blood glucose
Indapamide (p. 615) (Lozol)	**T:** 1.25 mg, 2.5 mg	**Edema:** 2.5–5 mg once daily **HTN:** 1.25–5 mg once daily	Loss of appetite, diarrhea, headaches, dizziness, light-headedness, insomnia, upset stomach
Metolazone (p. 775) (Zaroxolyn)	**T:** 2.5 mg, 5 mg, 10 mg	**Edema:** 2.5–20 mg once daily **HTN:** 2.5–5 mg once daily	Orthostatic hypotension, dizziness, hypokalemia, nausea, diarrhea, abdominal pain
Loop			
Bumetanide (p. 161) (Bumex)	**T:** 0.5 mg, 1 mg, 2 mg **I:** 0.25 mg/ml	**Edema:** 1–10 mg/day	Orthostatic hypotension, cramps or pain, hypokalemia (dry mouth, fatigue, muscle cramps), blurred vision, headaches
Furosemide (p. 530) (Lasix)	**T:** 20 mg, 40 mg, 80 mg **OS:** 10 mg/ml, 40 mg/5 ml **I:** 10 mg/ml	**HTN:** 20–80 mg/day in 2 divided doses **Edema:** Up to 600 mg/day	Orthostatic hypotension, cramps or pain, hypokalemia (dry mouth, fatigue, muscle cramps), blurred vision, headaches
Torsemide (p. 1216) (Demadex)	**T:** 5 mg, 10 mg, 20 mg, 100 mg **I:** 10 mg/ml	**Edema:** 10–200 mg/day **HTN:** 5–10 mg/day	Constipation, dizziness, upset stomach, headache, hypokalemia (dry mouth, fatigue, muscle cramps)

Potassium-sparing			
Amiloride (Midamor)	**T:** 5 mg	**Edema:** 5–20 mg/day **HTN:** 5–10 mg/day in 1–2 divided doses	Hyperkalemia, nausea, abdominal pain, diarrhea
Eplerenone (p. 430) (Inspra)	**T:** 25 mg, 50 mg	**Heart Failure:** 25–50 mg/day **HTN:** 50–100 mg/day	Hyperkalemia, hypertriglyceridemia
Spironolactone (p. 1125) (Aldactone)	**T:** 25 mg, 50 mg, 100 mg	**Edema:** 100 mg/day **HTN:** 50–200 mg/day **Hypokalemia:** 25–100 mg/day **Heart Failure:** 25–50 mg/day	Hyperkalemia, nausea, vomiting, abdominal cramps, diarrhea
Triamterene (p. 1233) (Dyrenium)	**C:** 50 mg, 100 mg	**Edema, HTN:** 100–300 mg/day in 1–2 divided doses	Same as amiloride

C, Capsules; *HTN,* hypertension; *I,* injection; *OS,* oral solution; *S,* suspension; *T,* tablets.

Fertility Agents

Infertility is defined as unsuccessful conception after 12 months of attempting to conceive, as opposed to *sterility*, the inability to reproduce. Infertility may be due to reproduction dysfunction of the male, female, or both.

Female infertility can be due to disruption of any phase of the reproductive process. The most critical phases include follicular maturation, ovulation, transport of the ovum through the fallopian tubes, fertilization of the ovum, nidation, and growth/development of the conceptus. Causes of infertility include the following:

Anovulation, failure of follicular maturation: Absence of adequate hormonal stimulation; ovarian follicles do not ripen, and ovulation will not occur.

Unfavorable cervical mucus: Normally the cervical glands secrete large volumes of thin, watery mucus, but if the mucus is unfavorable (scant, thick, or sticky), sperm is unable to pass through to the uterus.

Hyperprolactinemia: Excessive prolactin secretion may cause amenorrhea, galactorrhea, and infertility.

Luteal phase defect: Progesterone secretion by the corpus luteum is insufficient to maintain endometrial integrity.

Endometriosis: Endometrial tissue is implanted in abnormal locations (e.g., uterine wall, ovary, extragenital sites).

Androgen excess: May decrease fertility (most common condition is polycystic ovary).

Male infertility is due to decreased density or motility of sperm or semen of abnormal volume or quality. The most obvious manifestation of male infertility is impotence (inability to achieve erection). Whereas in female infertility an identifiable endocrine disorder can be found, most cases of male infertility are not associated with an identifiable endocrine disorder.

ACTION

Antiestrogens: Nonsteroidal estrogen antagonist that increases follicle-stimulating hormone (FSH) and leutinizing hormone (LH) levels by blocking estrogen-negative feedback at the hypothalamus.

Gonadotropins: Produce ovulation induction in women with hypogonadotropic hypogonadism and polycystic ovary syndrome (PCOS). Ovaries must be able to respond normally to FSH and LH stimulation.

Gonadotropin-releasing hormone (GnRH) agonists: Causes down-regulation of endogenous FSH and LH levels. GnRH agonists stimulate release of pituitary gonadotropins. Suppression of endogenous LH can decrease number of oocytes released prematurely, improve oocyte quality, and increase pregnancy rates.

Gonadotropin-releasing hormone (GnRH) antagonists: Suppresses endogenous LH surges during ovarian stimulation. GnRH antagonists avoid initial flare-up seen with GnRH agonists, shortening the number of days needed for LH suppression and allowing ovarian stimulation to begin within the spontaneous cycle.

MEDICATIONS TO INDUCE OVULATION

Name	Category	Availability	Uses	Side Effects
Cetrorelix (Cetrotide)	GnRH antagonist	**I:** 0.25 mg, 3 mg	Inhibition of premature LH surges in women undergoing ovarian hyperstimulation	OHSS (ovarian hyperstimulation syndrome): Abdominal pain, indigestion, bloating, decreased urinary output, nausea, vomiting, diarrhea, rapid weight gain, dyspnea, peripheral/dependent edema; headaches, pain/redness at injection site, mood swings, hot flashes, insomnia, vaginal dryness
Chorionic gonadotropin (Novarel, Ovidrel, Pregnyl)	Gonadotropin	**I:** 5,000 units, 10,000 units, 20,000 units **Ovidrel:** 250 mcg/ 0.5 ml	In conjunction with clomiphene, human menotropins or urofolitropin to stimulate ovulation	OHSS (ovarian hyperstimulation syndrome): Abdominal pain, indigestion, bloating, decreased urinary output, nausea, vomiting, diarrhea, rapid weight gain, dyspnea, peripheral/dependent edema; ovarian enlargement, ovarian cyst formation, headache, pain at injection site
Clomiphene (Clomid, Milophene, Serophene)	Antiestrogen	**T:** 50 mg	Anovulation, oligo-ovulation with intact pituitary/ovarian response and endogenous estrogen	Ovarian cyst formation, ovarian enlargement, visual disturbances, premenstrual syndrome, hot flashes, headaches, blurred vision, nausea, breast tenderness

(continued)

MEDICATIONS TO INDUCE OVULATION *(continued)*

Name	Category	Availability	Uses	Side Effects
Follitropin alpha (Gonal-F)	Gonadotropin	**Injection, powder:** 75 units, 450 units, 1,050 units **Injection, solution:** 300 units/0.5 ml, 450 units/0.75 ml, 900 units/15 ml	In conjunction with human chorionic gonadotropin to stimulate ovarian follicular development in pts with ovulatory dysfunction not due to primary ovarian failure (e.g., anovulation, oligo-ovulation)	OHSS (ovarian hyperstimulation syndrome): Abdominal pain, indigestion, bloating, decreased urinary output, nausea, vomiting, diarrhea, rapid weight gain, dyspnea, peripheral/dependent edema; flu-like symptoms, upper respiratory tract infections, bleeding between menstrual periods, nausea, ovarian enlargement, ovarian cysts, acne, breast pain/tenderness, mood swings
Follitropin beta (Follistim AQ)	Gonadotropin	**I:** 75, 350, 650, 975 international units FSH	In conjunction with human chorionic gonadotropin to stimulate ovarian follicular development in patients with ovulatory dysfunction not due to primary ovarian failure (e.g., anovulation, oligo-ovulation)	OHSS (ovarian hyperstimulation syndrome): Abdominal pain, indigestion, bloating, decreased urinary output, nausea, vomiting, diarrhea, rapid weight gain, shortness of breath, peripheral/dependent edema; flu-like symptoms, breast tenderness, dry skin, rash, dizziness, fever, headaches, nausea, fatigue, mood swings
Goserelin (p. 558) (Zoladex)	GnRH agonist	**Implant:** 3.6 mg, 10.8 mg	Endometriosis, adjunct to menotropins for ovulation induction	Hot flashes, amenorrhea, blurred vision, edema, headaches, nausea, vomiting, breast tenderness, weight gain, mood swings, insomnia, vaginal dryness

Name	Class	Dose/Form	Indications	Side Effects
Leuprolide (p. 684) (Eligard, Lupron)	GnRH agonist	**Injection, Solution:** 5 mg/ml for subcutaneous injection **Injection, powder:** 3.75 mg, 7.5 mg, 11.25 mg, 15 mg, 22.5 mg, 30 mg	Endometriosis, adjunct to menotropins/human chorionic gonadotropin for ovulation induction	Hot flashes, amenorrhea, blurred vision, edema, headaches, nausea, vomiting, breast tenderness, weight gain, mood swings, insomnia, vaginal dryness
Menotropins (Menopur, Repronex)	Gonadotropin	75 units FSH, 75 units LH activity	In conjunction with chorionic gonadotropin for ovulation stimulation in pts with ovulatory dysfunction due to primary ovarian failure	OHSS (ovarian hyperstimulation syndrome): Abdominal pain, indigestion, bloating, decreased urinary output, nausea, vomiting, diarrhea, rapid weight gain, dyspnea, edema of lower extremities; ovarian enlargement, ovarian cyst formation, breast tenderness, mood swings
Nafarelin (Synarel)	GnRH	2 mg/ml nasal spray (200 mcg/spray)	Endometriosis, adjunct to menotropins/human chorionic gonadotropin for ovulation induction	Loss of bone mineral density, breast enlargement, bleeding between regular menstrual periods, acne, mood swings, seborrhea, hot flashes, headache, insomnia, vaginal dryness
Urofollitropin (Bravelle)	Gonadotropin	75 units FSH activity	In conjunction with human chorionic gonadotropin for ovulation stimulation in pts with polycystic ovary syndrome who have elevated LH:FSH ratio and have failed clomiphene therapy	OHSS (ovarian hyperstimulation syndrome): Abdominal pain, indigestion, bloating, decreased urinary output, nausea, vomiting, diarrhea, rapid weight gain, shortness of breath, edema of lower extremities; ovarian enlargement, ovarian cyst formation, pain/redness at injection site, breast tenderness, nausea, vomiting, diarrhea, mood swings

I, Injection; *T,* tablets.

H₂ Antagonists

USES

Short-term treatment of duodenal ulcer (DU), active benign gastric ulcer (GU), maintenance therapy of DU, pathologic hypersecretory conditions (e.g., Zollinger-Ellison syndrome), gastroesophageal reflux disease (GERD), and prevention of upper GI bleeding in critically ill pts.

ACTION

Inhibits gastric acid secretion by interfering with histamine at the histamine H_2 receptors in parietal cells. Also inhibit acid secretion caused by gastrin. Inhibition occurs with basal (fasting), nocturnal, food-stimulated, or fundic distention secretion. H_2 antagonists decrease both the volume and H_2 concentration of gastric juices.

H₂ ANTAGONISTS

Name	Availability	Dosage Range	Side Effects
Cimetidine (p. 249) (Tagamet)	**T:** 200 mg, 300 mg, 400 mg, 800 mg **L:** 300 mg/5 ml **I:** 150 mg/ml	**Treatment of DU:** 800 mg at bedtime, 400 mg 2 times/day or 300 mg 4 times/day **Maintenance of DU:** 400 mg at bedtime **Treatment of GU:** 800 mg at bedtime or 300 mg 4 times/day **GERD:** 1,600 mg/day **Hypersecretory:** 1,200–2,400 mg/day	Headaches, fatigue, dizziness, confusion, diarrhea, gynecomastia

Drug	Forms	Dosage	Side Effects
Famotidine (p. 473) (Pepcid)	**T:** 10 mg, 20 mg, 40 mg **T (chewable):** 10 mg **DT:** 20 mg, 40 mg **Gelcap:** 10 mg **OS:** 40 mg/5 ml **I:** 10 mg/ml	**Treatment of DU:** 40 mg/day **Maintenance of DU:** 20 mg/day **Treatment of GU:** 40 mg/day **GERD:** 40–80 mg/day **Hypersecretory:** 80–640 mg/day	Headaches, dizziness, diarrhea, constipation, abdominal pain, tinnitus
Nizatidine (p. 862) (Axid)	**OS:** 15 mg/ml **C:** 150 mg, 300 mg	**Treatment of DU:** 300 mg/day **Maintenance of DU:** 150 mg/day	Fatigue, urticaria, abdominal pain, constipation, nausea
Ranitidine (p. 1036) (Zantac)	**T:** 75 mg, 150 mg, 300 mg **C:** 150 mg, 300 mg **Syrup:** 15 mg/ml **I:** 25 mg/ml	**Treatment of DU:** 300 mg/day **Maintenance of DU:** 150 mg/day **Treatment of GU:** 300 mg/day **GERD:** 300 mg/day **Hypersecretory:** 0.3–6 g/day	Blurred vision, constipation, nausea, abdominal pain

C, Capsules; *DT,* disintegrating tablets; *I,* injection; *L,* liquid; *OS,* oral suspension; *T,* tablets.

Hematinic Preparations

USES

Prevention or treatment of iron deficiency resulting from improper diet, pregnancy, impaired absorption, or prolonged blood loss.

ACTION

Iron supplements are provided to ensure adequate supplies for the formation of hemoglobin, which is needed for erythropoiesis and O_2 transport.

HEMATINIC (IRON) PREPARATIONS

Name	Availability	Side Effects
Ferrous fumarate (p. 486) (Femiron, Feostat)	**T:** 63 mg, 200 mg, 324 mg	Constipation, nausea, vomiting, diarrhea, abdominal pain/cramps
Ferrous gluconate (p. 486) (Fergon)	**T:** 240 mg, 325 mg	Same as ferrous fumarate
Ferrous sulfate (Fer-In-Sol)	**T:** 325 mg **Liquid:** 300 mg/5 ml **E:** 220 mg/5 ml **D:** 75 mg/ml	Same as ferrous fumarate
Ferrous sulfate exsiccated (Slow-Fe)	**T:** 200 mg	Same as ferrous fumarate

C, Caplets; *D,* drops; *E,* elixir; *ER,* extended-release; *S,* suspension; *SR,* sustained-release; *T,* tablets.

Hormones

USES

Functions of the body are regulated by two major control systems: the nervous system and the endocrine (hormone) system. Together they maintain homeostasis and control different metabolic functions in the body.

Hormones are concerned with control of different metabolic functions in the body (e.g., rates of chemical reactions in cells, transporting substances through cell membranes, cellular metabolism [growth/secretions]). By definition, a hormone is a chemical substance secreted into body fluids by cells and has control over other cells in the body.

Hormones can be local or general:

• *Local hormones* have specific local effects (e.g., acetylcholine, which is secreted at parasympathetic and skeletal nerve endings).

ACTION

- *General hormones* are mostly secreted by specific endocrine glands (e.g., epinephrine/norepinephrine are secreted by the adrenal medulla in response to sympathetic stimulation), transported in the blood to all parts of the body, causing many different reactions.

Some general hormones affect all or almost all cells of the body (e.g., thyroid hormone from the thyroid gland increases the rate of most chemical reactions in almost all cells of the body); other general hormones affect only specific tissue (e.g., ovarian hormones are specific to female sex organs and secondary sexual characteristics of the female).

Endocrine hormones almost never directly act intracellularly affecting chemical reactions. They first combine with hormone receptors either on the cell surface or inside the cell (cell cytoplasm or nucleus). The combination of hormone and receptors alters the function of the receptor, and the receptor is the direct cause of the hormone effects. Altered receptor function may include the following:

Altered cell permeability, which causes a change in protein structure of the receptor, usually opening or closing a channel for one or more ions. The movement of these ions causes the effect of the hormone.

Activation of intracellular enzymes immediately inside the cell membrane (e.g., hormone combines with receptor that then becomes the activated enzyme adenyl cyclase, which causes formation of cAMP).

◀ALERT▶ cAMP has effects inside the cell. It is not the hormone but cAMP that causes these effects.

Regulation of hormone secretion is controlled by an internal control system, the negative feedback system:

- Endocrine gland oversecretes.
- Hormone exerts more and more of its effect.

- Target organ performs its function.
- Too much function in turn feeds back to endocrine gland to decrease secretory rate.

The endocrine system contains many glands and hormones. A summary of the important glands and their hormones secreted are as follows:

The pituitary gland (hypophysis) is a small gland found in the sella turcica at the base of the brain. The pituitary is divided into two portions physiologically; the anterior pituitary (adenohypophysis) and the posterior pituitary (neurohypophysis). Six important hormones are secreted from the anterior pituitary and two from the posterior pituitary.

Anterior pituitary hormones:

- Growth hormone (GH)
- Adrenocorticotropin (corticotropin)
- Thyroid-stimulating hormone (thyrotropin) (TSH)
- Follicle-stimulating hormone (FSH)
- Luteinizing hormone (LH)
- Prolactin

Hormones   *(continued)*

ACTION *(cont.)*

Posterior pituitary hormones:

- Antidiuretic hormone (vasopressin)
- Oxytocin

Almost all secretions of the pituitary hormones are controlled by hormonal or nervous signals from the hypothalamus. The hypothalamus is a center of information concerned with the well-being of the body, which in turn is used to control secretions of the important pituitary hormones just listed. Secretions from the posterior pituitary are controlled by nerve signals originating in the hypothalamus; anterior pituitary hormones are controlled by hormones secreted within the hypothalamus. These hormones are as follows:

- Thyrotropin-releasing hormone (TRH) releasing thyroid-stimulating hormone
- Corticotropin-releasing hormone (CRH) releasing adrenocorticotropin
- Growth hormone-releasing hormone (GHRH) releasing growth hormone and growth hormone inhibitory hormone (GHIH) (same as somatostatin)
- Gonadotropin-releasing hormone (GnRH) releasing the two gonadotropic hormones LH and FSH
- Prolactin inhibitory factor (PIF) causing inhibition of prolactin and prolactin-releasing factor

Anterior Pituitary Hormones

All anterior pituitary hormones (except growth hormone) have as their principal effect stimulating target glands.

Growth Hormone (GH)

Growth hormone affects almost all tissues of the body. GH (somatotropin) causes growth in almost all tissues of the body (increases cell size, increases mitosis with increased number of cells, and differentiates certain types of cells). Metabolic effects include increased rate of protein synthesis, mobilization of fatty acids from adipose tissue, decreased rate of glucose utilization.

Thyroid-Stimulating Hormone (TSH)

Thyroid-stimulating hormone controls secretion of the thyroid hormones. The thyroid gland is located immediately below the larynx on either side of and anterior to the trachea and secretes two significant hormones, thyroxine (T_4) and triiodothyronine (T_3), which have a profound effect on increasing the metabolic rate of the body. The thyroid also secretes calcitonin, an important hormone for calcium metabolism. Calcitonin promotes deposition of calcium in the bones, which decreases calcium concentration in the extracellular fluid.

Adrenocorticotropin

Adrenocorticotropin causes the adrenal cortex to secrete adrenocortical hormones. The adrenal glands lie at the superior poles of the two kidneys. Each gland is composed of two distinct parts: the adrenal medulla and the cortex. The adrenal medulla, related to the sympathetic nervous system, secretes the hormones epinephrine and norepinephrine. When stimulated, they cause constriction of blood vessels, increased activity of the heart, inhibitory effects on the GI tract, and dilation of the pupils. The adrenal cortex secretes corticosteroids, of which there are two major types: mineralocorticoids and glucocorticoids. Aldosterone, the principal mineralocorticoid, primarily affects electrolytes of the extracellular fluids. Cortisol, the principal glucocorticoid, affects glucose, protein, and fat metabolism.

Luteinizing Hormone (LH)

Luteinizing hormone plays an important role in ovulation and causes secretion of female sex hormones by the ovaries and testosterone by the testes.

Follicle-Stimulating Hormone (FSH)

Follicle-stimulating hormone causes growth of follicles in the ovaries before ovulation and promotes formation

ACTION *(cont.)*

Ovarian sex hormones are estrogens and progestins. Estradiol is the most important estrogen; progesterone is the most important progestin.

Estrogens mainly promote proliferation and growth of specific cells in the body and are responsible for development of most of the secondary sex characteristics. Primarily cause cellular proliferation and growth of tissues of sex organs/other tissue related to reproduction. Ovaries, fallopian tubes, uterus, vagina increase in size. Estrogen initiates growth of breast and milk-producing apparatus, external appearance.

Progesterone stimulates secretion of the uterine endometrium during the latter half of the female sexual cycle, preparing the uterus for implantation of the fertilized ovum. Decreases the frequency of uterine contractions (helps prevent expulsion of the implanted ovum). Progesterone promotes development of breasts and alveolar cells to proliferate, enlarge, and become secretory in nature.

Testosterone is secreted by the testes and formed by the interstitial cells of *Leydig*. Testosterone production increases under the stimulus of the anterior pituitary gonadotropic hormones. It is responsible for distinguishing characteristics of the masculine body (stimulates the growth of male sex organs and promotes the development of male secondary sex characteristics, e.g., distribution of body hair, effect on voice, protein formation, and muscular development).

Prolactin

Prolactin promotes the development of breasts and secretion of milk.

POSTERIOR PITUITARY HORMONES

Antidiuretic Hormone (ADH) (Vasopressin)

ADH can cause antidiuresis (decreased excretion of water by the kidneys). In the presence of ADH, the permeability of the renal-collecting ducts and tubules to water increases, which allows water to be absorbed, conserving water in the body. ADH in higher concentrations is a very potent vasoconstrictor, constricting arterioles everywhere in the body, increasing B/P.

Oxytocin

Oxytocin contracts the uterus during the birthing process, esp. toward the end of the pregnancy, helping expel the baby. Oxytocin also contracts myoepithelial cells in the breasts, causing milk to be expressed from the alveoli into the ducts so that the baby can obtain it by suckling.

PANCREAS

The pancreas is composed of two tissue types: *acini* (secrete digestive juices in the duodenum) and *islets of Langerhans* (secrete insulin/glucagons directly into the blood). The islets of Langerhans contain three cells: alpha, beta, and delta. Alpha cells secrete glucagon, beta cells secrete insulin, and delta cells secrete somatostatin.

Insulin promotes glucose entry into most cells, thus controlling the rate of metabolism of most carbohydrates. Insulin also affects fat metabolism.

Glucagon effects are opposite those of insulin, the most important of which is increasing blood glucose concentration by releasing it from the liver into the circulating body fluids.

Somatostatin (same chemical as secreted by the hypothalamus) has multiple inhibitory effects: depresses secretion of insulin and glucagon, decreases GI motility, decreases secretions/absorption of the GI tract.

Human Immunodeficiency Virus (HIV) Infection

USES	ACTION
Antiretroviral agents are used in the treatment of HIV infection.	Seven classes of antiretroviral agents are used in the treatment of HIV disease. *Nucleoside reverse transcriptase inhibitors (NRTIs)* compete with natural substrates for formation of proviral DNA by reverse transcriptase inhibiting viral replication.
	Nucleotide reverse transcriptase inhibitors (NtRTIs) inhibits reverse transcriptase by competing with the natural substrate deoxyadenosine triphosphate and by DNA chain termination.
	Non-nucleoside reverse transcriptase inhibitors (NNRTIs) directly bind to reverse transcriptase and block RNA-dependent and DNA-dependent DNA polymerase activities by disrupting the enzyme's catalytic site.
	Protease inhibitors (PIs) binds to the active site of HIV-1 protease and prevent the processing of viral gag and gag-pol polyprotein precursors resulting in immature, noninfectious viral particles.
	Fusion inhibitors interfere with the entry of HIV-1 into cells by inhibiting fusion of viral and cellular membranes.
	CCR5 co-receptor antagonist selectively binds to human chemokine receptor CCR5 present on cell membrane preventing HIV-1 from entering cells.
	Integrase inhibitor inhibits catalytic activity of HIV-1 integrase, an HIV-1 encoded enzyme required for viral replication.

ANTIRETROVIRAL AGENTS FOR TREATMENT OF HIV INFECTION

Name	Availability	Dosage Range	Side Effects
Nucleoside Analogues			
Abacavir (p. 1) (Ziagen)	**T:** 300 mg **OS:** 20 mg/ml	**A:** 300 mg 2 times/day or 600 mg once/day	Nausea, vomiting, malaise, rash, fever, headaches, asthenia (loss of strength, energy), fatigue, hypersensitivity reactions
Abacavir/lamivudine (Epzicom)	**T:** 600 mg abacavir/300 mg lamivudine	**A:** 600 mg/300 mg once/day	Allergic reaction, insomnia, headaches, depression, dizziness, fatigue, diarrhea, fever, abdominal pain, anxiety
Didanosine (p. 359) (Videx EC)	**DR:** 125 mg, 200 mg, 250 mg, 400 mg **OS:** 2 g/bottle, 4 g/bottle	**DR (weighing 60 kg or more):** 400 mg once/day; **(weighing 25–59 kg):** 250 mg once/day; **(weighing 20–24 kg):** 200 mg once/day **OS (weighing more than 60 kg):** 200 mg q12h or 400 mg once/day; **(weighing less than 60 kg):** 125 mg q12h or 250 mg once/day	Peripheral neuropathy, pancreatitis, diarrhea, nausea, vomiting, headaches, insomnia, rash, hepatitis, seizures
Emtricitabine (p. 414) (Emtriva)	**C:** 200 mg **OS:** 10 mg/ml	**A:** 200 mg/day **(C)** 240 mg/day **(OS)**	Headaches, insomnia, depression, diarrhea, nausea, vomiting, rhinitis, asthenia (loss of strength, energy), rash
Emtricitabine/efavirenz/ tenofovir (Atripla)	**T:** 200 mg emtricitabine/ 600 mg efavirenz/ 300 mg tenofovir	**A:** 200 mg/600 mg/300 mg once/day	Lactic acidosis, headaches, dizziness, abdominal pain, nausea, vomiting, rash
Emtricitabine/rilpivirine/ tenofovir (Complera)	**T:** 200 mg emtricitabine/ 25 mg rilpivirine/300 mg tenofovir	**A:** 200 mg/25 mg/300 mg once daily with food	Insomnia, headache, diarrhea, nausea, fatigue, dizziness, depression, rash

(continued)

ANTIRETROVIRAL AGENTS FOR TREATMENT OF HIV INFECTION   *(continued)*

Name	Availability	Dosage Range	Side Effects
Emtricitabine/tenofovir (Truvada)	**T:** 200 mg emtricitabine/ 300 mg tenofovir	**A:** 200 mg/300 mg once daily with food	Dizziness, diarrhea, headaches, rash, belching/ flatulence, skin discoloration
Emtricitabine/ elvitegravir/cobicistat/ tenofovir (Stribild)	**T:** 200 mg emtricitabine 150 mg elvitegravir 150 mg cobicistat 300 mg tenofovir	**A:** 200 mg/150 mg/150 mg/300 mg once daily with food	Nausea, diarrhea
Lamivudine (p. 668) (Epivir)	**T:** 100 mg, 150 mg, 300 mg **OS:** 5 mg/ml, 10 mg/ml	**A:** 150 mg 2 times/day or 300 mg once/day **C:** 4 mg/kg 2 times/day	Diarrhea, malaise, fatigue, headaches, nausea, vomiting, abdominal pain, peripheral neuropathy, arthralgia, myalgia, skin rash
Stavudine (p. 1127) (Zerit)	**C:** 15 mg, 20 mg, 30 mg, 40 mg **OS:** 1 mg/ml	**A (weighing more than 60 kg):** 40 mg 2 times/day (20 mg 2 times/day if peripheral neuropathy occurs); **(weighing 60 kg or less):** 30 mg 2 times/day (15 mg 2 times/day if peripheral neuropathy occurs)	Peripheral neuropathy, anemia, leukopenia, neutropenia
Zidovudine (p. 1294) (Retrovir)	**C:** 100 mg **T:** 300 mg **Syrup:** 50 mg/5 ml, 10 mg/ml	**A:** 300 mg 2 times/day	Anemia, granulocytopenia, myopathy, nausea, malaise, fatigue, insomnia
Zidovudine/lamivudine (AZT/3TC) (Combivir)	**C:** 300 mg AZT/150 mg 3TC	**A:** 300 mg/150 mg 2 times/day	Myelosuppression, peripheral neuropathy, pancreatitis
Zidovudine/lamivudine/ abacavir (AZT/3TC/ABC) (Trizivir)	**C:** 300 mg AZT/150 mg 3TC/ 300 mg ABC	**A:** 300 mg/150 mg/300 mg 2 times/day	Myelosuppression, peripheral neuropathy, anaphylactic reaction

Nucleotide Analogues

Drug	Availability	Dosage	Side Effects
Tenofovir (Viread) (p. 1164)	T: 300 mg	A: 300 mg once daily	Nausea, vomiting, diarrhea, headache, fatigue
Tenofovir/elvitegravir/cobicistat/emtricitabine (Stribild)	T: 300 mg tenofovir 150 mg elvitegravir 150 mg cobicistat 200 mg emtricitabine	A: 300 mg/150 mg/150 mg/200 mg once daily with food	Nausea, diarrhea

Non-nucleoside Analogues

Drug	Availability	Dosage	Side Effects
Delavirdine (Rescriptor) (p. 332)	T: 100 mg, 200 mg	A: 200 mg 3 times/day for 14 days, then 400 mg 3 times/day	Rash, nausea, headaches, elevated hepatic function tests
Efavirenz (Sustiva) (p. 409)	C: 50 mg, 200 mg T: 600 mg	A: 600 mg/day C: 200–600 mg/day based on weight	Headaches, dizziness, insomnia, fatigue, rash, nightmares
Etravirine (Intelence) (p. 462)	T: 100 mg, 200 mg	A: 200 mg 2 times/day	Skin reactions (e.g., Stevens-Johnson syndrome, erythema multiforme), nausea, abdominal pain, vomiting
Nevirapine (Viramune, Viramune XR) (p. 842)	T: 200 mg T (ER): 400 mg S: 50 mg/ml	A: 200 mg/day for 14 days, then (if no rash) 200 mg 2 times/day	Rash, nausea, fatigue, fever, headaches, abnormal hepatic function tests
Rilpivirine (Edurant) (p. 1055)	T: 25 mg	A: 25 mg once/day with a meal	Depression, insomnia, headache, rash

Protease Inhibitors

Drug	Availability	Dosage	Side Effects
Atazanavir (Reyataz) (p. 91)	C: 100 mg, 150 mg, 200 mg, 300 mg	A: 400 mg/day or 300 mg (with 100 mg ritonavir) once/day	Headaches, diarrhea, abdominal pain, nausea, rash
Darunavir (Prezista) (p. 319)	T: 400 mg, 600 mg	A: 600 mg 2 times/day (with ritonavir 100 mg) or 800 mg once/day with ritonavir 100 mg	Diarrhea, nausea, vomiting, headaches, skin rash, constipation

(continued)

ANTIRETROVIRAL AGENTS FOR TREATMENT OF HIV INFECTION *(continued)*

Name	Availability	Dosage Range	Side Effects
Fosamprenavir (p. 520) (Lexiva)	T: 700 mg OS: 50 mg/ml	A: 1,400–2,800 mg/day with 100 mg ritonavir	Headaches, fatigue, rash, nausea, diarrhea, vomiting, abdominal pain
Indinavir (p. 616) (Crixivan)	C: 200 mg, 400 mg	A: 800 mg q8h or 800 mg 2 times/day with ritonavir 100 mg	Nephrolithiasis, hyperbilirubinemia, abdominal pain, asthenia (loss of strength, energy), fatigue, flank pain, nausea, vomiting, diarrhea, headaches, insomnia, dizziness, altered taste
Lopinavir/ritonavir (p. 717) (Kaletra)	C: 133/33 mg OS: 80/20 mg	A: 400 mg/100 mg 2 times/day or 800 mg/200 mg once/day C (4–12 yrs): 10–13 mg/kg 2 times/day	Diarrhea, nausea, vomiting, abdominal pain, headaches, rash
Nelfinavir (p. 837) (Viracept)	T: 250 mg Oral Powder: 50 mg/g	A: 750 mg q8h or 1,250 mg 2 times/day C: 20–25 mg/kg q8h	Diarrhea, fatigue, asthenia (loss of strength, energy), headaches, hypertension, impaired concentration
Ritonavir (p. 1064) (Norvir)	C: 100 mg OS: 80 mg/ml	A: Titrate up to 800 mg/day based on protease inhibitor	Nausea, vomiting, diarrhea, altered taste, fatigue, elevated hepatic function tests and triglyceride levels
Saquinavir (p. 1086) (Invirase)	C: 200 mg T: 500 mg	A: 1,000 mg 2 times/day with ritonavir 100 mg	Diarrhea, elevated hepatic function tests, hypertriglycerides, cholesterol, abnormal fat accumulation, hyperglycemia
Tipranavir (p. 1197) (Aptivus)	C: 250 mg OS: 100 mg/ml	A: 500 mg (with 200 mg ritonavir) 2 times/day	Diarrhea, nausea, fatigue, headaches, vomiting
Fusion Inhibitors			
Enfuvirtide (p. 418) (Fuzeon)	I: 108 mg (90 mg when reconstituted)	Subcutaneous: 90 mg 2 times/day	Insomnia, depression, peripheral neuropathy, decreased appetite, constipation, asthenia (loss of strength, energy), cough

CCR5 Antagonists			
Maraviroc (p. 739) (Selzentry)	T: 150 mg, 300 mg	**A:** 300 mg 2 times/day **CYP3A4 inducers:** 600 mg 2 times/day **CYP3A4 inhibitors:** 150 mg 2 times/day	Cough, pyrexia, upper respiratory tract infections, rash, musculoskeletal symptoms, abdominal pain, dizziness
Integrase Inhibitor			
Raltegravir (p. 1031) (Isentress)	T: 400 mg	**A:** 400 mg 2 times/day	Nausea, headache, diarrhea, pyrexia
Dolutegravir (p. 386) (Tivicay)	T: 50 mg	**A:** 50 mg once daily or 50 mg bid (with CYP3A inducers or resistance)	Insomnia, headache

A, Adults; *C,* capsules; *C (dosage),* children; *DR,* delayed-release; *ER,* extended-release; *I,* injection; *OS,* oral solution; *S,* suspension; *T,* tablets.

Immunosuppressive Agents

USES	ACTION
Improvement of both short- and long-term allograft survivals.	*Basiliximab:* An interleukin-2 (IL-2) receptor antagonist inhibiting IL-2 binding. This prevents activation of lymphocytes, and the response of the immune system to antigens is impaired. *Cyclosporine:* Inhibits IL-2 production and release of IL-2. *Daclizumab:* An IL-2 receptor antagonist inhibiting IL-2 binding. *Mycophenolate:* A prodrug that reversibly binds and inhibits inosine monophosphate dehydrogenase (IMPD), resulting in inhibition of purine nucleotide synthesis, inhibiting DNA and RNA synthesis and subsequent synthesis of T and B cells. *Sirolimus:* Inhibits IL-2–stimulated T-lymphocyte activation and proliferation, which may occur through formation of a complex. *Tacrolimus:* Inhibits IL-2–stimulated T-lymphocyte activation and proliferation, which may occur through formation of a complex.

IMMUNOSUPPRESSIVE AGENTS

Name	Availability	Dosage	Side Effects
Basiliximab (p. 117) (Simulect)	**I:** 10 mg, 20 mg	20 mg for 2 doses (on day of transplant, then 4 days after transplantation)	Abdominal pain, asthenia (loss of strength, energy), cough, dizziness, dyspnea, dysuria, edema, hypertension, infection, tremors
Cyclosporine (p. 299) (Neoral, Sandimmune)	**C:** 25 mg, 50 mg, 100 mg **S:** 100 mg/ml **I:** 50 mg/ml	Dose dependent on type of transplant and formulation	Hypertension, hyperkalemia, nephrotoxicity, coarsening of facial features, hirsutism, gingival hyperplasia, nausea, vomiting, diarrhea, hepatotoxicity, hyperuricemia, hypertriglyceridemia, hypercholesterolemia, tremors, paresthesia, seizures, risk of infection/malignancy
Mycophenolate (p. 816) (CellCept)	**C:** 250 mg **I:** 500 mg **S:** 200 mg/ml **T:** 500 mg	1–1.5 g 2 times/day based on type of transplant	Diarrhea, vomiting, leukopenia, neutropenia, infections
Sirolimus (p. 1107) (Rapamune)	**S:** 1 mg/ml **T:** 0.5 mg, 1 mg, 2 mg	2–6 mg/day	Dyspnea, leukopenia, thrombocytopenia, hyperlipidemia, abdominal pain, acne, arthralgia, fever, diarrhea, constipation, headaches, vomiting, weight gain
Tacrolimus (p. 1143) (Prograf)	**C:** 0.5 mg, 1 mg, 5 mg **I:** 5 mg/ml	**Heart:** 0.075 mg/kg/day in 2 divided doses q12h **Kidney:** 0.1–0.2 mg/kg/day in 2 divided doses q12h **Liver:** 0.1–0.15 mg/kg/day in 2 divided doses q12h	Nephrotoxicity, neurotoxicity, hyperglycemia, nausea, vomiting, photophobia, infections, hypertension, hyperlipidemia

C, Capsules; *I,* injection; *S,* oral solution or suspension; *T,* tablets.

Laxatives

USES

Short-term treatment of constipation; colon evacuation before rectal/bowel examination; prevention of straining (e.g, after anorectal surgery, MI); to reduce painful elimination (e.g., episiotomy, hemorrhoids, anorectal lesions); modification of effluent from ileostomy, colostomy; prevention of fecal impaction; removal of ingested poisons.

ACTION

Laxatives ease or stimulate defecation. Mechanisms by which this is accomplished include (1) attracting, retaining fluid in colonic contents due to hydrophilic or osmotic properties; (2) acting directly or indirectly on mucosa to decrease absorption of water and NaCl; or (3) increasing intestinal motility, decreasing absorption of water and NaCl by virtue of decreased transit time.

Bulk-forming: Acts primarily in small/large intestine. Retain water in stool, may bind water, ions in colonic lumen (soften feces, increase bulk); may increase colonic bacteria growth (increases fecal mass). Produces soft stool in 1–3 days.

Osmotic agents: Acts in colon. Similar to saline laxatives. Osmotic action may be enhanced in distal ileum/colon by bacterial metabolism to lactate, other organic acids. This decrease in pH increases motility, secretion. Produce soft stool in 1–3 days.

Saline: Acts in small/large intestine, colon (sodium phosphate). Poorly, slowly absorbed; causes hormone cholecystokinin release from duodenum (stimulates fluid secretion, motility); possesses osmotic properties; produces watery stool in 2–6 hrs (small doses produce semifluid stool in 6–12 hrs).

Stimulant: Acts in colon. Enhances accumulation of water/electrolytes in colonic lumen, enhances intestinal motility. May act directly on intestinal mucosa. Produces semifluid stool in 6–12 hrs.

◀ALERT▶ Bisacodyl suppository acts in 15–60 min.

Stool softener: Acts in small/large intestine. Hydrates and softens stools by its surfactant action, facilitating penetration of fat and water into stool. Produces soft stool in 1–3 days.

LAXATIVES

Name	Onset of Action	Uses	Side Effects/Precautions
Bulk-forming			
Methylcellulose (Citrucel)	12–24 hrs up to 3 days	Treatment of constipation for postpartum women, elderly, pts with diverticulosis, irritable bowel syndrome, hemorrhoids	Gas, bloating, esophageal obstruction, colonic obstruction, calcium and iron malabsorption
Psyllium (p. 1017) (Metamucil)	Same as methylcellulose	Treatment of chronic constipation and constipation associated with rectal disorders; management of irritable bowel syndrome	Diarrhea, constipation, abdominal cramps, esophageal/colon obstruction, bronchospasm
Stool Softener			
Docusate (p. 382) (Colace, Surfak)	1–3 days	Treatment of constipation due to hard stools, in painful anorectal conditions, and for those who need to avoid straining during bowel movements	Stomachache, mild nausea, cramping, diarrhea, irritated throat (with liquid and syrup dose forms)
Saline			
Magnesium citrate (p. 734) (Citrate of Magnesia, Citro-Mag)	30 min–3 hrs	Bowel evacuation prior to certain surgical and diagnostic procedures	Hypotension, abdominal cramping, diarrhea, gas formation, electrolyte abnormalities
Magnesium hydroxide (p. 734)	30 min–3 hrs	Short-term treatment of occasional constipation	Electrolyte abnormalities can occur; use caution in pts with renal or cardiac impairment; diarrhea, abdominal cramps, hypotension

(continued)

LAXATIVES *(continued)*

Name	Onset of Action	Uses	Side Effects/Precautions
Sodium phosphate (Fleet Phospho-Soda)	2–15 min	Relief of occasional constipation; bowel evacuation prior to certain surgical and diagnostic procedures	Electrolyte abnormalities; do not use for pts with HF, severe renal impairment, ascites, GI obstruction, active inflammatory bowel disease
Osmotic			
Lactulose (p. 666) (Kristalose)	24–48 hrs	Short-term relief of constipation	Nausea, vomiting, diarrhea, abdominal cramping, bloating, gas
Polyethylene glycol (p. 970) (MiraLax)	24–48 hrs	Short-term relief of constipation	Bitter taste, diarrhea
Stimulant			
Bisacodyl (p. 140) (Dulcolax)	**PO:** 6–12 hrs **Rectal:** 15–60 min	Short-term relief of constipation	Electrolyte imbalance, abdominal discomfort, gas, potential for overuse/abuse
Senna (p. 1094) (Senokot)	6–12 hrs	Short-term relief of constipation	Abdominal discomfort, cramps

Nitrates

USES

Sublingual: Acute relief of angina pectoris.

Oral, topical: Long-term prophylactic treatment of angina pectoris.

Intravenous: Adjunctive treatment in HF associated with acute MI. Produce controlled hypotension during surgical procedures; control B/P in perioperative hypertension, angina unresponsive to organic nitrates or beta-blockers.

ACTION

Relaxes most smooth muscles, including arteries and veins. Effect is primarily on veins (decrease left/right ventricular end-diastolic pressure). In angina, nitrates decrease myocardial work and O_2 requirements (decrease preload by venodilation and afterload by arteriodilation). Nitrates also appear to redistribute blood flow to ischemic myocardial areas, improving perfusion without increasing coronary blood flow.

NITRATES

Name	Availability	Dosage Range	Side Effects
Isosorbide dinitrate (p. 646) **(Isordil)**	**T:** 5 mg, 10 mg, 20 mg, 30 mg, 40 mg **T (ER):** 40 mg **SL:** 2.5 mg, 5 mg **C (SR):** 40 mg	**SL:** 2.5–5 mg **PO:** 10–40 mg 2–3 times/day **PO (SR):** 40 mg 1–2 times/day	Flushing, headaches, nausea, vomiting, orthostatic hypotension, restlessness, tachycardia
Isosorbide mononitrate (p. 646) **(Imdur, ISMO)**	**T:** 30 mg, 60 mg, 120 mg	**PO:** 30–240 mg once/day	Same as isosorbide dinitrate

(continued)

NITRATES   *(continued)*

Name	Availability	Dosage Range	Side Effects
Nitroglycerin (p. 857) (Minitran, Nitro-Bid, Nitro-Dur, Nitrostat)	**SL:** 0.4 mg **C (SR):** 2.5 mg, 6.5 mg, 9 mg **Topical:** 2% ointment **Trans:** 0.1 mg/hr, 0.2 mg/hr, 0.3 mg/hr, 0.4 mg/hr, 0.6 mg/hr, 0.8 mg/hr **I:** 5 mg/ml **Infusion:** 100 mcg/ml, 200 mcg/ml	**SL:** 0.4 mg up to 3 times q15min **SR:** 2.5–26 mg 3–4 times/day **Trans:** 0.1–0.8 mg/hr **T:** 1–2 inches up to 4–5 inches q4h	Flushing, hypotension, tachycardia, headache, dizziness, nausea, dyspnea

C, Capsules; *ER,* extended-release; *I,* injection; *SL,* sublingual; *SR,* sustained-release; *T,* tablets; *Trans,* transdermal.

Nonsteroidal Anti-Inflammatory Drugs (NSAIDs)

USES

Provide symptomatic relief from *pain/inflammation* in the treatment of musculoskeletal disorders (e.g., rheumatoid arthritis [RA], osteoarthritis, ankylosing spondylitis), *analgesic* for low to moderate pain, *reduction in fever* (many agents not suited for routine/prolonged therapy due to toxicity). By virtue of its action on platelet function, aspirin is used in treatment or prophylaxis of diseases associated with hypercoagulability (reduces risk of stroke/heart attack).

ACTION

Exact mechanism for anti-inflammatory, analgesic, antipyretic effects unknown. Inhibition of enzyme cyclooxygenase, the enzyme responsible for prostaglandin synthesis, appears to be a major mechanism of action. May inhibit other mediators of inflammation (e.g., leukotrienes). Direct action on hypothalamus heat-regulating center may contribute to antipyretic effect.

NSAIDs

Name	Availability	Dosage Range	Side Effects
Aspirin (p. 89)	**Caplet:** 500 mg **Suppository:** 300 mg, 600 mg **T:** 325 mg **T (EC):** 81 mg, 325 mg **T (chew):** 81 mg	**Analgesic/antipyretic:** 325–650 mg q4–6h prn **Anti-inflammatory:** 2.4–3.6 g/day	GI discomfort, dizziness, headaches, increased risk of bleeding
Celecoxib (p. 231) (Celebrex)	**C:** 50 mg, 100 mg, 200 mg, 400 mg	200 mg q12h (**Maximum:** 600 mg day 1, then 400 mg/day)	Diarrhea, back pain, dizziness, heartburn, headaches, nausea, abdominal pain
Diclofenac (p. 355) (Voltaren)	**T:** 25 mg, 50 mg, 75 mg	50 mg tid	Indigestion, constipation, diarrhea, nausea, headaches, fluid retention, abdominal cramps
Diflunisal (Dolobid)	**T:** 500 mg	**Arthritis:** 0.5–1 g/day in 2 divided doses **P:** 250–500 mg q8–12h	Headaches, abdominal cramps, indigestion, diarrhea, nausea
Etodolac (p. 458) (Lodine)	**T:** 400 mg, 500 mg **T (ER):** 400 mg, 500 mg, 600 mg **C:** 200 mg, 300 mg	**Arthritis:** 600–1,000 mg/day in divided doses **P:** 200–400 mg q6–8h as needed	Indigestion, dizziness, headaches, bloated feeling, diarrhea, nausea, weakness, abdominal cramps
Fenoprofen (Nalfon)	**C:** 200 mg, 400 mg **T:** 600 mg	**Arthritis:** 300–600 mg 3–4 times/day **P:** 200 mg q4–6h as needed	Nausea, indigestion, anxiety, constipation, shortness of breath, heartburn
Ibuprofen (p. 594) (Advil, Caldolor, Motrin)	**I:** 100 mg/ml **T:** 100 mg, 200 mg, 400 mg, 600 mg, 800 mg **C:** 200 mg **T (chewable):** 50 mg, 100 mg **S:** 100 mg/5 ml, 100 mg/2.5 ml	**Inflammatory disease:** 400–800 mg/ dose 3–4 times/day **Pain:** 200–400 mg/dose q4–6h as needed	Dizziness, abdominal cramps, abdominal pain, heartburn, nausea

(continued)

NSAIDs   (continued)

Name	Availability	Dosage Range	Side Effects
Indomethacin (p. 618) (Indocin)	**C:** 25 mg, 50 mg **C (SR):** 75 mg **S:** 25 mg/5 ml	**Arthritis:** 25–50 mg/dose 2–3 times/day **Bursitis/tendonitis:** 75–150 mg/day **GA:** 150 mg/day	Fluid retention, dizziness, headaches, abdominal pain, indigestion, nausea
Ketoprofen (p. 658) (Orudis KT)	**C:** 25 mg, 50 mg **C (ER):** 200 mg	**Arthritis:** 50 mg 4 times/day or 75 mg 3 times/day **P:** 25–50 mg q6–8h as needed	Headaches, anxiety, abdominal pain, bloated feeling, constipation, diarrhea, nausea
Ketorolac (p. 660) (Toradol)	**T:** 10 mg **I:** 15 mg/ml, 30 mg/ml	**P: (PO):** 10 mg q4–6h as needed; **(IM/IV):** 60–120 mg/day in divided doses	Fluid retention, abdominal pain, diarrhea, dizziness, headaches, nausea
Meloxicam (p. 745) (Mobic)	**C:** 7.5 mg, 15 mg **S:** 7.5 mg/5 ml	**Arthritis:** 7.5–15 mg once daily	Heartburn, indigestion, nausea, diarrhea, headaches
Nabumetone (p. 819) (Relafen)	**T:** 500 mg, 750 mg	**Arthritis:** 1–2 g/day in 1–2 divided doses	Fluid retention, dizziness, headaches, abdominal pain, constipation, diarrhea, nausea
Naproxen (p. 828) (Anaprox, Naprosyn)	**T:** 250 mg, 375 mg, 500 mg **T (CR):** 375 mg, 500 mg **S:** 125 mg/5 ml	**Arthritis:** 500–1,000 mg/day in 2 divided doses **P:** 250 mg q6–8h as needed	Tinnitus, fluid retention, shortness of breath, dizziness, drowsiness, headaches, abdominal pain, constipation, heartburn, nausea
Oxaprozin (p. 899) (Daypro)	**C:** 600 mg **T:** 600 mg	**Arthritis:** 600–1,200 mg once daily	Constipation, diarrhea, nausea, indigestion
Piroxicam (p. 966) (Feldene)	**C:** 10 mg, 20 mg	**Arthritis:** 10–20 mg/day in 1–2 divided doses	Abdominal pain, stomach pain, nausea
Sulindac (p. 1137) (Clinoril)	**T:** 150 mg, 200 mg	**Arthritis:** 150 mg bid **GA:** 200 mg bid	Dizziness, abdominal pain, constipation, diarrhea, nausea

A, Adults; *C,* capsules; *C (dosage),* children; *CR,* controlled-release; *ER,* extended-release; *FAP,* familial adenomatous polyposis; *GA,* gouty arthritis; *I,* injection; *JA,* juvenile arthritis; *JRA,* juvenile rheumatoid arthritis; *MI,* myocardial infarction; *OA,* osteoarthritis; *P,* pain; *RA,* rheumatoid arthritis; *RF,* rheumatic fever; *S,* suspension; *SR,* sustained-release; *T,* tablets; *TIA,* transient ischemic attack.

Nutrition: Enteral

Enteral nutrition (EN), also known as *tube feedings*, provides food/nutrients via the GI tract using special formulas, delivery techniques, and equipment. All routes of EN consist of a tube through which liquid formula is infused.

INDICATIONS

Tube feedings are used in pts with major trauma, burns; those undergoing radiation and/or chemotherapy; pts with hepatic failure, severe renal impairment, physical or neurologic impairment; preop and postop to promote anabolism; prevention of cachexia, malnutrition; dysphagia, pts requiring mechanical ventilation.

ROUTES OF ENTERAL NUTRITION DELIVERY

NASOGASTRIC (NG):

INDICATIONS: Most common for short-term feeding in pts unable or unwilling to consume adequate nutrition by mouth. Requires at least a partially functioning GI tract.

ADVANTAGES: Does not require surgical intervention and is fairly easily inserted. Allows full use of digestive tract. Decreases abdominal distention, nausea, vomiting that may be caused by hyperosmolar solutions.

DISADVANTAGES: Temporary. May be easily pulled out during routine nursing care. Has potential for pulmonary aspiration of gastric contents, risk of reflux esophagitis, regurgitation.

NASODUODENAL (ND), NASOJEJUNAL (NJ):

INDICATIONS: Pts unable or unwilling to consume adequate nutrition by mouth. Requires at least a partially functioning GI tract.

ADVANTAGES: Does not require surgical intervention and is fairly easily inserted. Preferred for pts at risk for aspiration. Valuable for pts with gastroparesis.

Nutrition: Enteral

ROUTES OF ENTERAL NUTRITION DELIVERY *(cont.)*

DISADVANTAGES: Temporary. May be pulled out during routine nursing care. May be dislodged by coughing, vomiting. Small lumen size increases risk of clogging when medication is administered via tube, more susceptible to rupturing when using infusion device. Must be radiographed for placement, frequently extubated.

GASTROSTOMY:

INDICATIONS: Pts with esophageal obstruction or impaired swallowing; pts in whom NG, ND, or NJ not feasible; when long-term feeding indicated.

ADVANTAGES: Permanent feeding access. Tubing has larger bore, allowing noncontinuous (bolus) feeding (300–400 ml over 30–60 min q3–6h). May be inserted endoscopically using local anesthetic (procedure called *percutaneous endoscopic gastrostomy* [PEG]).

DISADVANTAGES: Requires surgery; may be inserted in conjunction with other surgery or endoscopically (see ADVANTAGES). Stoma care required. Tube may be inadvertently dislodged. Risk of aspiration, peritonitis, cellulitis, leakage of gastric contents.

JEJUNOSTOMY:

INDICATIONS: Pts with stomach or duodenal obstruction, impaired gastric motility; pts in whom NG, ND, or NJ not feasible; when long-term feeding indicated.

ADVANTAGES: Allows early postop feeding (small bowel function is least affected by surgery). Risk of aspiration reduced. Rarely pulled out inadvertently.

DISADVANTAGES: Requires surgery (laparotomy). Stoma care required. Risk of intraperitoneal leakage. Can be dislodged easily.

INITIATING ENTERAL NUTRITION

With continuous feeding, initiation of isotonic (about 300 mOsm/L) or moderately hypertonic feeding (up to 495 mOsm/L) can be given full strength, usually at a slow rate (30–50 ml/hr) and gradually increased (25 ml/hr q6–24h). Formulas with osmolality greater than 500 mOsm/L are generally started at half strength and gradually increased in rate, then concentration. Tolerance is increased if the rate and concentration are not increased simultaneously.

SELECTION OF FORMULAS

Protein: Has many important physiologic roles and is the primary source of nitrogen in the body. Provides 4 kcal/g protein. Sources of protein in enteral feedings: sodium caseinate, calcium caseinate, soy protein, dipeptides.

Carbohydrate (CHO): Provides energy for the body and heat to maintain body temperature. Provides 3.4 kcal/g carbohydrate. Sources of CHO in enteral feedings: corn syrup, cornstarch, maltodextrin, lactose, sucrose, glucose.

Fat: Provides concentrated source of energy. Referred to as *kilocalorie dense* or *protein sparing.* Provides 9 kcal/g fat. Sources of fat in enteral feedings: corn oil, safflower oil, medium-chain triglycerides.

Electrolytes, vitamins, trace elements: Contained in formulas (not found in specialized products for renal/hepatic insufficiency).

All products containing protein, fat, carbohydrate, vitamin, electrolytes, trace elements are nutritionally complete and designed to be used by pts for long periods.

COMPLICATIONS

MECHANICAL: Usually associated with some aspect of the feeding tube.

Aspiration pneumonia: Caused by delayed gastric emptying, gastroparesis, gastroesophageal reflux, or decreased gag reflex. May be prevented or treated by reducing infusion rate, using lower-fat formula, feeding beyond pylorus, checking residuals, using small-bore feeding tubes, elevating head of bed 30°–45° during and for 30–60 min after intermittent feeding, and regularly checking tube placement.

Esophageal, mucosal, pharyngeal irritation, otitis: Caused by using large-bore NG tube. Prevented by use of small-bore whenever possible.

Irritation, leakage at ostomy site: Caused by drainage of digestive juices from site. Prevented by close attention to skin/stoma care.

Tube, lumen obstruction: Caused by thickened formula residue, formation of formula-medication complexes. Prevented by frequently irrigating tube with clear water (also before and after giving formulas/medication), avoiding instilling medication if possible.

GASTROINTESTINAL: Usually associated with formula, rate of delivery, unsanitary handling of solutions or delivery system.

Diarrhea: Caused by low-residue formulas, rapid delivery, use of hyperosmolar formula, hypoalbuminemia, malabsorption, microbial contamination, or rapid GI transit time. Prevented by using fiber supplemented formulas, decreasing rate of delivery, using dilute formula, and gradually increasing strength.

Cramps, gas, abdominal distention: Caused by nutrient malabsorption, rapid delivery of refrigerated formula. Prevented by delivering formula by continuous methods, giving formulas at room temperature, decreasing rate of delivery.

Nausea, vomiting: Caused by rapid delivery of formula, gastric retention. Prevented by reducing rate of delivery, using dilute formulas, selecting low-fat formulas.

Nutrition: Enteral   *(continued)*

COMPLICATIONS   *(cont.)*

Constipation: Caused by inadequate fluid intake, reduced bulk, inactivity. Prevented by supplementing fluid intake, using fiber-supplemented formula, encouraging ambulation.

METABOLIC: Fluid/serum electrolyte status should be monitored. Refer to monitoring section. In addition, the very young and very old are at greater risk of developing complications such as dehydration or overhydration.

MONITORING

Daily: Estimate nutrient intake, fluid intake/output, weight of pt, clinical observations.

Weekly: Serum electrolytes (potassium, sodium, magnesium, calcium, phosphorus), blood glucose, BUN, creatinine, hepatic function tests (e.g., AST, ALT, alkaline phosphatase), 24-hr urea and creatinine excretion, total iron-binding capacity (TIBC) or serum transferrin, triglycerides, cholesterol.

Monthly: Serum albumin.

Other: Urine glucose, acetone (when blood glucose is greater than 250), vital signs (temperature, respirations, pulse, B/P) q8h.

DRUG THERAPY: DOSAGE FOR SELECTION/ADMINISTRATION:

Drug therapy should not have to be compromised in pts receiving enteral nutrition:

- Temporarily discontinue medications not immediately necessary.
- Consider an alternate route for administering medications (e.g., transdermal, rectal, intravenous).
- Consider alternate medications when current medication is not available in alternate dosage forms.

ENTERAL ADMINISTRATION OF MEDICATIONS:

Medications may be given via feeding tube with several considerations:

- Tube type
- Tube location in the GI tract
- Site of drug action
- Site of drug absorption
- Effects of food on drug absorption
- Use of liquid dosage forms is preferred whenever possible; many tablets may be crushed; contents of many capsules may be emptied and given through large-bore feeding tubes.
- Many oral products should not be crushed (e.g., sustained-release, enteric coated, capsule granules).
- Some medications should not be given with enteral formulas because they form precipitates that may clog the feeding tube and reduce drug absorption.
- Feeding tube should be flushed with water before and after administration of medications to clear any residual medication.

Nutrition: Parenteral

Parenteral nutrition (PN), also known as *total parenteral nutrition* (TPN) or *hyperalimentation* (HAL), provides required nutrients to pts by IV route of administration. The goal of PN is to maintain or restore nutritional status caused by disease, injury, or inability to consume nutrients by other means.

INDICATIONS

Conditions when pt is unable to use alimentary tract via oral, gastrostomy, or jejunostomy route. Impaired absorption of protein caused by obstruction, inflammation, or antineoplastic therapy. Bowel rest necessary because of GI surgery or ileus, fistulas, or anastomotic leaks. Conditions with increased metabolic requirements (e.g., burns, infection, trauma). Preserve tissue reserves (e.g., acute renal failure). Inadequate nutrition from tube feeding methods.

COMPONENTS OF PN

To meet IV nutritional requirements, six essential categories in PN are needed for tissue synthesis and energy balance.

Protein: In the form of crystalline amino acids (CAA), primarily used for protein synthesis. Several products are designed to meet specific needs for pts with renal failure (e.g., NephrAmine), hepatic disease (e.g., HepatAmine), stress/trauma (e.g., Aminosyn HBC), use in neonates and pediatrics (e.g., Aminosyn PF, TrophAmine). Calories: 4 kcal/g protein.

Energy: In the form of dextrose, available in concentrations of 5%–70%. Dextrose less than 10% may be given peripherally; concentrations greater than 10% must be given centrally. Calories: 3.4 kcal/g dextrose.

IV fat emulsion: Available in 10% and 20% concentrations. Provides a concentrated source of energy/calories (9 kcal/g fat) and is a source of essential fatty acids. May be administered peripherally or centrally.

Nutrition: Parenteral *(continued)*

COMPONENTS OF PN *(cont.)*	ROUTE OF ADMINISTRATION

PN is administered via either peripheral or central vein.

Electrolytes: Major electrolytes (calcium, magnesium, potassium, sodium; also acetate, chloride, phosphate). Doses of electrolytes are individualized, based on many factors (e.g., renal/hepatic function, fluid status).

Vitamins: Essential components in maintaining metabolism and cellular function; widely used in PN.

Trace elements: Necessary in long-term PN administration. Trace elements include zinc, copper, chromium, manganese, selenium, molybdenum, iodine.

Miscellaneous: Additives include insulin, albumin, heparin, and histamine₂ blockers (e.g., cimetidine, ranitidine, famotidine). Other medication may be included, but compatibility for admixture should be checked on an individual basis.

Peripheral: Usually involves 2–3 L/day of 5%–10% dextrose with 3%–5% amino acid solution along with IV fat emulsion. Electrolytes, vitamins, trace elements are added according to pt needs. Peripheral solutions provide about 2,000 kcal/day and 60–90 g protein/day.

ADVANTAGES: Lower risks vs. central mode of administration.

DISADVANTAGES: Peripheral veins may not be suitable (esp. in pts with illness of long duration); more susceptible to phlebitis (due to osmolalities over 600 mOsm/L); veins may be viable only 1–2 wks; large volumes of fluid are needed to meet nutritional requirements, which may be contraindicated in many pts.

Central: Usually utilizes hypertonic dextrose (concentration range of 15%–35%) and amino acid solution of 3%–7% with IV fat emulsion. Electrolytes, vitamins, trace elements are added according to pt needs. Central solutions provide 2,000–4,000 kcal/day. Must be given through large central vein with high blood flow, allowing rapid dilution, avoiding phlebitis/thrombosis (usually through percutaneous insertion of catheter into subclavian vein then advancement of catheter to superior vena cava).

ADVANTAGES: Allows more alternatives/flexibility in establishing regimens; allows ability to provide full nutritional requirements without need of daily fat emulsion; useful in pts who are fluid restricted (increased concentration), those needing large nutritional requirements (e.g., trauma, malignancy), or those for whom PN indicated more than 7–10 days.

DISADVANTAGES: Risk with insertion, use, maintenance of central line; increased risk of infection, catheter-induced trauma, and metabolic changes.

MONITORING

May vary slightly from institution to institution.

Baseline: CBC, platelet count, PT, weight, body length/head circumference (in infants), serum electrolytes, glucose, BUN, creatinine, uric acid, total protein, cholesterol, triglycerides, bilirubin, alkaline phosphatase, LDH, AST, albumin, prealbumin, other tests as needed.

Daily: Weight, vital signs (temperature, pulse, respirations [TPR]), nutritional intake (kcal, protein, fat), serum electrolytes (potassium, sodium chloride), glucose (serum, urine), acetone, BUN, osmolarity, other tests as needed.

2–3 times/wk: CBC, coagulation studies (PT, PTT), serum creatinine, calcium, magnesium, phosphorus, acid-base status, other tests as needed.

Weekly: Nitrogen balance, total protein, albumin, prealbumin, transferrin, hepatic function tests (AST, ALT), serum alkaline phosphatase, LDH, bilirubin, Hgb, uric acid, cholesterol, triglycerides, other tests as needed.

COMPLICATIONS

Mechanical: Malfunction in system for IV delivery (e.g., pump failure; problems with lines, tubing, administration sets, catheter). Pneumothorax, catheter misdirection, arterial puncture, bleeding, hematoma formation may occur with catheter placement.

Infectious: Infections (pts often more susceptible to infections), catheter sepsis (e.g., fever, shaking, chills, glucose intolerance where no other site of infection is identified).

Metabolic: Includes hyperglycemia, elevated serum cholesterol and triglycerides, abnormal serum hepatic function tests.

Fluid, electrolyte, acid-base disturbances: May alter serum potassium, sodium, phosphate, magnesium levels.

Nutritional: Clinical effects seen may be due to lack of adequate vitamins, trace elements, essential fatty acids.

DRUG THERAPY/ADMINISTRATION METHODS: Compatibility of other intravenous medications pts may be administered while receiving parenteral nutrition is an important concern.

Intravenous medications usually are given as a separate admixture via piggyback to the parenteral nutrition line, but in some instances may be added directly to the parenteral nutrition solution. Because of the possibility of incompatibility when adding medication directly to the parenteral nutrition solution, specific criteria should be considered:

• Stability of the medication in the parenteral nutrition solution

• Properties of the medication, including pharmacokinetics that determine if the medication is appropriate for continuous infusion

• Documented chemical and physical compatibility with the parenteral nutrition solution

In addition, when medication is given via piggyback using the parenteral nutrition line, important criteria should include:

• Stability of the medication in the parenteral nutrition solution

• Documented chemical and physical compatibility with the parenteral nutrition solution

Obesity Management

138C   Obesity Management

USES

Adjunct to diet and physical activity in the treatment of chronic, relapsing obesity.

ACTIONS

Two categories of medications are used for weight control.

Appetite suppressants: Block neuronal uptake of norepinephrine, serotonin, dopamine, causing a feeling of fullness or satiety.

Digestion inhibitors: Reversible lipase inhibitors that block the breakdown and absorption of fats, decreasing appetite and reducing calorie intake.

ANOREXIANTS

Name	Availability	Dosage	Side Effects
Diethylpropion (Tenuate, Tenuate Dospan)	**T:** 25 mg, **T (CR):** 75 mg	25 mg 3–4 times/day or 75 mg once/day in midmorning	Headaches, insomnia, nervousness, anxiety, irritability, dry mouth, constipation, euphoria, palpitations, pulmonary hypertension, valvular heart disease, seizures, bone marrow depression
Lorcaserin (p. 722) **(BelViq)**	**C:** 10 mg	10 mg twice daily	Nausea, headache, dizziness, fatigue, dry mouth, diarrhea, constipation, hypoglycemia, hallucinations, decreased white/red blood cells
Orlistat (p. 893) **(Alli, Xenical)**	**C:** 60 mg, 120 mg	**Alli:** 60 mg up to tid with meals **Xenical:** 120 mg tid with each meal containing fat	Flatulence, rectal incontinence, oily stools, cholelithiasis, abdominal/rectal pain, hepatitis, pancreatitis
Phenteramine (Apidex-P)	**C:** 15 mg, 30 mg, 37.5 mg **T:** 37.5 mg **T (ODT):** 15 mg, 30 mg	15–37.5 mg/day in 1 or 2 divided doses **ODT:** 15–30 mg once daily in morning	Headaches, insomnia, nervousness, anxiety, irritability, dry mouth, constipation, euphoria, palpitations, hypertension, pulmonary hypertension, valvular heart disease, tremor
Phenteramine/ topiramate (Qsymia)	**C:** 13.75 mg/ 23 mg	3.75 mg/23 mg to 15 mg/92 mg once daily in the morning	Paresthesia, dizziness, insomnia, depression, tachycardia, cognitive impairment, angle-closure glaucoma, hypokalemia, metabolic acidosis

AS, Appetite suppressant; *C,* capsules; *CR,* controlled-release; *DI,* digestion inhibitor; *ODT,* orally disintegrating tablets; *T,* tablets.

Ophthalmic Medications for Allergic Conjunctivitis

Ophthalmic products used for allergic conjunctivitis include antihistamines, mast cell stabilizing agents, combination antihistamine/decongestants, and corticosteroids. **Antihistamines** selectively inhibit the H_1 histamine receptor, thus antagonizing histamine-stimulated vascular permeability in the conjunctiva.

Mast cell stabilizing agents block the release of mediators of hypersensitivity reactions from mast cells, eosinophils, neutrophils, macrophages, monocytes, and platelets. They inhibit the release of histamine from mast cells. **Combination antihistamine/decongestants** are used only for a short time because the regular use of a decongestant may cause rebound congestion.

Mast cell stabilizers/antihistamine combinations provide both the quick action of the antihistamine and more delayed action of the mast cell stabilizer. This latter combination is used for mild to moderately severe allergic conjunctivitis. **Corticosteroids**, although having no definite mechanism of action, exert their effect by controlling the biosynthesis of potent mediators of inflammation.

ANTIHISTAMINE

Names	Dosage	Comments/Side Effects
Alcaftadine 0.25% (Lastacaft)	One drop each eye once daily	Eye irritation, burning/stinging on instillation, eye redness/pruritus, nasopharyngitis, headache, influenza

ANTIHISTAMINE/DECONGESTANTS

Names	Dosage	Comments/Side Effects
Naphazoline/pheniramine (Naphcon-A, Opcon-A, Visine-A)	One or two drops into affected eye(s) up to 4 times/day	Remove contact lenses prior to using Do not use for more than 3 days Not for use in pts with heart disease, enlarged prostate, high blood pressure, and/or glaucoma Side effects: headache, mydriasis, pain in eye

(continued)

MAST CELL STABILIZER

Names	Dosage	Comments/Side Effects
Lodoxamine 0.1% (Alomide)	One to two drops in affected eye(s) 4 times/day	Avoid wearing contact lenses during treatment Side effects: burning, stinging, or irritation of eyes; watery, itching eyes; blurred vision; headache; dizziness; nausea or stomach discomfort
Nedocromil 2% (Alocril)	One or two drops in affected eye(s) 2 times/day	Remove contact lenses prior to using; may reinsert after 15 min if eyes are not red Side effects: headache, dizziness, blurring sensation in eye, light intolerance
Pemirolast 0.1% (Alamast)	One or two drops in affected eye(s) 4 times/day	Avoid wearing contact lenses if eyes are red Remove contact lenses prior to using; may reinsert after 10 min if eyes are not red Side effects: foreign body sensation, headache, dry eyes, burning sensation

ANTIHISTAMINE/MAST CELL STABILIZER

Names	Dosage	Comments/Side Effects
Azelastine 0.05% (p. 108) (Optivar)	One drop in affected eye(s) 2 times/day	Avoid wearing contact lenses if eyes are red Remove soft contact lenses prior to using; may reinsert after 10 min if eyes are not red Side effects: headache, drowsiness, burning sensation in eye
Epinastine 0.05% (Elestat)	One drop in affected eye(s) 2 times/day	Avoid wearing contact lenses if eyes are red Remove soft contact lenses prior to using; may reinsert after 10 min if eyes are not red Side effects: headache, burning sensation in eye
Ketotifen 0.025% (Alaway, Zaditor)	One drop in affected eye(s) 2 times/day	Avoid wearing contact lenses if eyes are red Remove soft contact lenses prior to using; may reinsert after 10 min if eyes are not red Side effects: headache, dry eyes, eye irritation, pain in eye

	Dosage	Comments/Side Effects
Olopatadine 0.1% (Patanol)	One drop in affected eye(s) 2 times/day	Avoid wearing contact lenses if eyes are red Remove soft contact lenses prior to using; may reinsert after 10 min if eyes are not red Side effects: headache, burning sensation in eye

CORTICOSTEROIDS

Names	Dosage	Comments/Side Effects
Loteprednol 0.2% (Alrex)	One drop in affected eye(s) 4 times/day	Recommended for short-term use only Remove soft contact lenses prior to using; may reinsert after 10 min if eyes are not red Side effects: abnormal vision, blurred vision, burning sensation in eye, itching in eye, light intolerance
Loteprednol 0.5% (Lotemax)	One or two drops in affected eye(s) 4 times/day	Recommended for short-term use only Remove soft contact lenses prior to using; may reinsert after 10 min if eyes are not red Side effects: abnormal vision, blurred vision, burning sensation in eye, itching in eye, light intolerance
Prednisolone 1% (p. 988) (AK-Pred)	Two drops in affected eye(s) 2–4 times/day	Recommended for short-term use only Remove soft contact lenses prior to using; may reinsert after 10 min if eyes are not red Side effects: blurred vision, burning sensation or irritation in eye, pain in eye

Osteoporosis

HISTORY

Osteoporosis is a bone disease that can lead to fractures. Bone mineral density (BMD) is reduced, bone microarchitecture is disrupted, and the amount and variety of proteins in bone are altered. Osteoporosis primarily affects women after menopause (postmenopausal osteoporosis) but may develop in men, in anyone in the presence of particular hormonal disorders (e.g., parathyroid glands), after overconsumption of dietary proteins, or as a result of medications (e.g., glucocorticoids). Several pharmacologic options, along with lifestyle changes, that can be used to prevent and/or treat osteoporotic fractures include bisphosphonates, selective estrogen receptor modulator (SERM), parathyroid hormone (PTH), calcitonin, and monoclonal antibodies.

ACTION

Bisphosphonates: Inhibits bone resorption via actions on osteoclasts or osteoclast precursors, decreases rate of bone resorption, leading to an indirect increase in BMD.

Selective estrogen receptor modulator (SERM): Decreases bone resorption, increasing BMD and decreasing the incidence of fractures.

Parathyroid hormone: Stimulates osteoblast function, increasing gastrointestinal calcium absorption and increasing renal tubular reabsorption of calcium. This increases BMD, bone mass, and strength, resulting in a decrease in osteoporosis-related fractures.

Calcitonin: Inhibitor of bone resorption. Efficacy not observed in early postmenopausal women and is used only in women with osteoporosis who are at least 5 yrs beyond menopause.

Monoclonal antibody: Inhibits the RANK ligand (RANKL), a cytokine member of the tumor necrosis factor family. This inhibits osteoclast formation, function, and survival, which decreases bone resorption and increases bone mass and strength in cortical and trabecular bone.

BISPHOSPHONATES

Name	Availability	Dosage	Side Effects
Alendronate (p. 33) (Binosto, Fosamax)	**T:** 5 mg, 10 mg, 35 mg, 40 mg, 70 mg **S:** 70 mg/75ml	**Prevention:** 5 mg/day or 35 mg/wk **Treatment:** 10 mg/day or 70 mg/wk	Transient, mild hypocalcemia, hypophosphatemia, dysphagia, esophagitis, esophageal and gastric ulcer, abdominal pain, diarrhea, musculoskeletal pain
Ibandronate (p. 589) (Boniva)	**T:** 150 mg **I:** 1 mg/ml	**Prevention and treatment:** 150 mg/mo **IV Injection: Treatment:** 3 mg/3 mos	Dyspepsia, back pain, dysphagia, esophagitis, esophageal and gastric ulcer, abdominal pain, diarrhea, musculoskeletal pain

I, injection; *IM,* intramuscular; *IV,* intravenous; *S,* solution (oral); *T,* tablet

Name	Availability	Dosage	Side Effects
Risedronate (p. 1060) (Actonel)	**T:** 5 mg, 30 mg, 35 mg, 150 mg, **T (DR):** 35 mg	**Prevention and treatment:** 5 mg/day, 35 mg/wk, or 150 mg/month	Hypertension, headache, rash, dysphagia, esophagitis, esophageal and gastric ulcer, abdominal pain, diarrhea, musculoskeletal pain
Zoledronic acid (p. 1298) (Reclast)	**I:** 5 mg	**Prevention: IV:** 5 mg every 2 yrs **Treatment: IV:** 5 mg every yr	Hypertension, pain, fever, headache, chills, fatigue, nausea, musculoskeletal pain

SERM

Name	Availability	Dosage	Side Effects
Raloxifene (p. 1030) (Evista)	**T:** 60 mg	**Prevention and treatment:** 60 mg/day	Peripheral edema, hot flashes, arthralgia, leg cramps, muscle spasms, flu syndrome, infection

PARATHYROID HORMONE

Name	Availability	Dosage	Side Effects
Teriparatide (p. 1171) (Forteo)	**I:** 250 mcg/ml syringe delivers 20 mcg/dose	**Treatment:** 20 mcg subcutaneously once daily	Hypercalcemia, muscle cramps, nausea, dizziness, headache

CALCITONIN

Name	Availability	Dosage	Side Effects
Calcitonin (p. 176) (Fortical, Miacalcin)	**I (Miacalcin):** 200 units/ml **Nasal (Fortical, Miacalcin):** 200 units/activation	**Treatment: IM/Subcutaneous (Miacalcin):** 100 units every other day **Nasal:** 200 units in 1 nostril daily	Rhinitis, local nasal irritation. **Injection:** nausea, local inflammation, flushing of face, hands

MONOCLONAL ANTIBODY RANKL INHIBITOR

Name	Availability	Dosage	Side Effects
Denosumab (p. 335) (Prolia)	**I:** 60 mg/ml	**Subcutaneous:** 60 mg once every 6 mos	Back pain, pain in extremity, hypercholesterolemia, musculoskeletal pain, cystitis

DR, delayed-release; *I,* injection; *IM,* intramuscular; *IV,* intravenous; *S,* solution (oral); *T,* tablet.

Parkinson's Disease Treatment

USES	ACTION
To slow or stop clinical progression of Parkinson's disease and to improve function and quality of life in pts with Parkinson's disease, a progressive neurodegenerative disorder.	Normal motor function is dependent on the synthesis and release of dopamine by neurons projecting from the substantia nigra to the corpus striatum. In Parkinson's disease, disruption of this pathway results in diminished levels of the neurotransmitter dopamine. Medication is aimed at providing improved function using the lowest effective dose.

TYPES OF MEDICATIONS FOR PARKINSON'S DISEASE
DOPAMINE PRECURSOR

Levodopa/carbidopa:

Levodopa: Dopamine precursor supplementation to enhance dopaminergic neurotransmission. A small amount of levodopa crosses the blood-brain barrier and is decarboxylated to dopamine, which is then available to stimulate dopaminergic receptors.

Carbidopa: Inhibits peripheral decarboxylation of levodopa, decreasing its conversion to dopamine in peripheral tissues, which results in an increased availability of levodopa for transport across the blood-brain barrier.

COMT INHIBITORS

Entacapone, tolcapone: Reversible inhibitor of catechol-*O*-methyltransferase (COMT). COMT is responsible for catalyzing levodopa. In the presence of a decarboxylase inhibitor (carbidopa), COMT becomes the major metabolizing enzyme for levodopa in the brain and periphery. By inhibiting COMT, higher plasma levels of levodopa are attained, resulting in more dopaminergic stimulation in the brain and lessening the symptoms of Parkinson's disease.

DOPAMINE RECEPTOR AGONISTS

Bromocriptine: Stimulates postsynaptic dopamine type 2 receptors in the neostriatum of the CNS.

Pramipexole: Stimulates dopamine receptors in the striatum of the CNS.

Ropinirole: Stimulates postsynaptic dopamine D2 type receptors within the caudate putamen in the brain.

MONOAMINE OXIDASE B INHIBITORS

Rasagiline, Selegiline: Increase dopaminergic activity due to irreversible inhibition of monoamine oxidase type B (MAO B). MAO B is involved in the oxidative deamination of dopamine in the brain.

Parkinson's Disease Treatment

MEDICATIONS FOR TREATMENT OF PARKINSON'S DISEASE

Name	Type	Availability	Dosage	Side Effects
Bromocriptine (p. 157) **(Parlodel)**	Dopamine agonist	**T:** 2.5 mg **C:** 5 mg	1.25 mg bid, increase by 2.5 mg/dose in 2–4 wk intervals (**Maximum:** 100 mg/day)	Nausea, drowsiness, lower extremity edema, postural hypotension, confusion, toxic psychosis (avoid use in pts with dementia)
Carbidopa/levodopa (p. 191) **(Parcopa, Sinemet, Sinemet CR)**	Dopamine precursor	**Orally disintegrating (Parcopa):** 10/100 mg, 25/100 mg, 25/250 mg **Immediate-release (Sinemet):** 10/100 mg, 25/100 mg, 25/250 mg **Controlled-release (Sinemet CR):** 25/100 mg, 50/200 mg	**Parcopa:** 300–1,500 mg levodopa in divided doses **Sinemet:** 300–1,500 mg levodopa in divided doses **Sinemet CR:** 400–1,600 mg levodopa in divided doses	Anorexia, nausea, vomiting, orthostatic hypotension initially; vivid dreams, hallucinations, delusions, confusion, and sleep disturbances with chronic use
Entacapone (p. 421) **(Comtan)**	COMT inhibitor	**T:** 200 mg	200 mg 3–4 times/day up to **maximum** of 8 times/day (1,600 mg)	Dyskinesias, nausea, diarrhea, urine discoloration
Pramipexole (p. 980) **(Mirapex, Mirapex ER)**	Dopamine agonist	**T:** 0.125 mg, 0.25 mg, 0.5 mg, 1 mg, 1.5 mg **ER:** 0.375 mg, 0.75 mg, 1.5 mg, 2.25 mg, 3 mg, 3.75 mg, 4.5 mg	**T:** 0.5–1.5 mg 3 times/day **ER:** 0.375–4.5 mg/day	Nausea, drowsiness, lower extremity edema, postural hypotension, confusion, toxic psychosis (avoid use in pts with dementia)

(continued)

Parkinson's Disease Treatment   *(continued)*

Name	Type	Availability	Dosage	Side Effects
Rasagiline (p. 1039) (Azilect)	MAO B inhibitors	**T:** 0.5 mg, 1 mg	0.5–1 mg once daily	Nausea, orthostatic hypotension
Ropinirole (p. 1076) (Requip, Requip XL)	Dopamine agonist	**T:** 0.25 mg, 0.5 mg, 1 mg, 2 mg, 3 mg, 4.5 mg **XL:** 2 mg, 4 mg, 6 mg, 8 mg, 12 mg	**T:** 3–8 mg 3 times/day **XL:** Up to 24 mg/day	Nausea, drowsiness, lower extremity edema, postural hypotension, confusion, toxic psychosis (avoid use in pts with dementia)
Selegiline (p. 1092) (Eldepryl, Zelapar)	MAO B inhibitor	**C (Eldepryl):** 5 mg **OD (Zelapar):** 1.25 mg	**C:** 5 mg with breakfast and lunch **OD:** 1.25–2.5 mg daily in the morning	Nausea, orthostatic hypotension
Tolcapone (Tasmar)	COMT inhibitor	**T:** 100 mg, 200 mg	100–200 mg 3 times/day	Dyskinesias, nausea, diarrhea, urine discoloration

C, Capsules; *COMT,* catechol-*O*-methyltransferase; *ER,* extended-release; *I,* injection; *MAO B,* monoamine oxidase B; *OD,* orally disintegrating; *T,* tablets; *XL,* extended-release.

Proton Pump Inhibitors

USES

Treatment of various gastric disorders, including gastric and duodenal ulcers, gastroesophageal reflux disease (GERD), pathologic hypersecretory conditions.

ACTION

Suppresses gastric acid secretion by specific inhibition of the hydrogen-potassium-adenosine triphosphatase (H^+/ K^+ ATPase) enzyme system, which transports the acid at the gastric parietal cells. These agents do not have anticholinergic or histamine receptor antagonistic properties.

PROTON PUMP INHIBITORS

Name	Availability	Indications	Usual Dosage	Side Effects
Dexlansoprazole (p. 345) **(Dexilant)**	**C:** 30 mg, 60 mg	Erosive esophagitis, heartburn associated with nonerosive GERD	30 mg/day	Diarrhea, abominal pain, nausea, upper respiratory tract infection, vomiting, flatulence
Esomeprazole (p. 447) **(Nexium)**	**C:** 20 mg, 40 mg **I:** 20 mg	*H. pylori* eradication, GERD, erosive esophagitis	20–40 mg/day	Headaches, diarrhea, abdominal pain, nausea
Lansoprazole (p. 672) **(Prevacid)**	**C:** 15 mg, 30 mg **I:** 30 mg **T (ODT):** 15 mg, 30 mg	Duodenal ulcer, gastric ulcer, NSAID-associated gastric ulcer, hypersecretory conditions, *H. pylori* eradication, GERD, erosive esophagitis	15–30 mg/day	Diarrhea, skin rash, pruritus, headaches
Omeprazole (p. 888) **(Prilosec)**	**C:** 10 mg, 20 mg, 40 mg	Duodenal ulcer, gastric ulcer, hypersecretory conditions, *H. pylori* eradication, GERD, erosive esophagitis	20–40 mg/day	Headaches, diarrhea, abdominal pain, nausea
Omeprazole and Sodium Bicarbonate (p. 888) **(Zegerid)**	**C:** 20 mg, 40 mg **P:** 20 mg, 40 mg	Duodenal ulcer, benign gastric ulcer, GERD, erosive esophagitis	20–40 mg/day	Headaches, abdominal pain, diarrhea, nausea
Pantoprazole (p. 922) **(Protonix)**	**T:** 20 mg, 40 mg **I:** 40 mg	Erosive esophagitis, hypersecretory conditions	40 mg/day	Diarrhea, headaches
Rabeprazole (p. 1029) **(Aciphex)**	**T:** 20 mg	Duodenal ulcer, hypersecretory conditions, *H. pylori* eradication, GERD, erosive esophagitis	20 mg/day	Headaches

C, Capsules; *GERD,* gastroesophageal reflux disease; *I,* injection; *NSAID,* nonsteroidal anti-inflammatory drug; *ODT,* orally disintegrating tablets; *P,* powder for suspension; *T,* tablets.

Sedative-Hypnotics

USES

Treatment of insomnia (i.e., difficulty falling asleep initially, frequent awakening, awakening too early).

ACTION

Benzodiazepines are the most widely used agents and largely replace barbiturates due to greater safety, lower incidence of drug dependence. Benzodiazepines nonselectively bind to at least three receptor subtypes accounting for sedative, anxiolytic, relaxant, and anticonvulsant properties. Benzodiazepines enhance the effect of the inhibitory neurotransmitter gamma-aminobutyric acid (GABA), which inhibits impulse transmission in the CNS reticular formation in brain. Benzodiazepines decrease sleep latency, number of nocturnal awakenings, and time spent in awake stage of sleep; increase total sleep time. The *nonbenzodiazepines* zaleplon and zolpidem preferentially bind with one receptor subtype, reducing sleep latency and nocturnal awakenings and increasing total sleep time. Ramelteon is a selective agonist of melatonin receptors (responsible for determining circadian rhythms and synchronizing sleep-wake cycles).

SEDATIVE-HYPNOTICS

Name	Availability	Dosage Range	Side Effects
Benzodiazepines			
Estazolam (ProSom)	**T:** 1 mg, 2 mg	**A:** 1–2 mg **E:** 0.5–1 mg	Daytime sedation, memory and psychomotor impairment, tolerance, withdrawal reactions, rebound insomnia, dependence
Flurazepam (p. 508) (Dalmane)	**C:** 15 mg, 30 mg	**A/E:** 15–30 mg	Headaches, unpleasant taste, dry mouth, dizziness, anxiety, nausea
Quazepam (Doral)	**T:** 15 mg	**A:** 7.5–15 mg **E:** 7.5 mg	Same as flurazepam
Temazepam (p. 1158) (Restoril)	**C:** 7.5 mg, 15 mg, 30 mg	**A:** 15–30 mg **E:** 7.5–15 mg	Same as flurazepam

Nonbenzodiazepines

Eszopiclone (p. 453) (Lunesta)	T: 1 mg, 2 mg, 3 mg	A: 2–3 mg E: 1–2 mg	Headaches, unpleasant taste, dry mouth, dizziness, anxiety, nausea
Ramelteon (p. 1033) (Rozerem)	T: 8 mg	A, E: 8 mg	Headaches, dizziness, fatigue, nausea
Zaleplon (p. 1292) (Sonata)	C: 5 mg, 10 mg	A: 5–20 mg E: 5 mg	Headaches, dizziness, myalgia, drowsiness, asthenia (loss of strength, energy), abdominal pain
Zolpidem (p. 1301) (Ambien, Ambien CR, Edluar, Zolpimist)	T: 5 mg, 10 mg CR: 6.25 mg, 12.5 mg SL: 5 mg, 10 mg OS: 5 mg/actuation	OS, T, SL: 5 mg (females); 5–10 mg (males) CR: 6.25 mg (females); 6.25–12.5 mg (males)	Dizziness, daytime drowsiness, headaches, confusion, depression, hangover, asthenia (loss of strength, energy)

A, Adults; *C,* capsules; *CR,* controlled-release; *E,* elderly; *OS,* oral solution; *SL,* sublingual; *T,* tablets.

Skeletal Muscle Relaxants

USES

Central acting muscle relaxants: Adjunct to rest, physical therapy for relief of discomfort associated with acute, painful musculoskeletal disorders (i.e., local spasms from muscle injury).

Baclofen, dantrolene, diazepam: Treatment of spasticity characterized by heightened muscle tone, spasm, loss of dexterity caused by multiple sclerosis, cerebral palsy, spinal cord lesions, CVA.

ACTION

Central acting muscle relaxants: Exact mechanism unknown. May act in CNS at various levels to depress polysynaptic reflexes; sedative effect may be responsible for relaxation of muscle spasm.

Baclofen, diazepam: May mimic actions of gamma-aminobutyric acid on spinal neurons; does not directly affect skeletal muscles.

Dantrolene: Acts directly on skeletal muscle, relieving spasticity.

SKELETAL MUSCLE RELAXANTS

Name	Indication	Dosage Range	Side Effects/Comments
Baclofen (p. 116) (Lioresal)	Spasticity associated with multiple sclerosis, spinal cord injury	Initially 5 mg 3 times/day Increase by 5 mg 3 times/day q3days **Maximum:** 20 mg 4 times/day	Drowsiness, dizziness, GI effects Caution with renal impairment, seizure disorders Withdrawal syndrome (e.g., hallucinations, psychosis, seizures)

(continued)

Carisoprodol (p. 197) (Rela)	Discomfort due to acute, painful, musculoskeletal conditions	250–350 mg 4 times/day	Drowsiness, dizziness, GI effects Hypomania at higher than recommended doses Withdrawal syndrome Hypersensitivity reaction (skin reaction, bronchospasm, weakness, burning eyes, fever) or idiosyncratic reaction (weakness, visual or motor disturbances, confusion) usually occurring within first 4 doses
Chlorzoxazone (Lorzone)	Discomfort due to acute, painful, musculoskeletal conditions	Initially 250–500 mg 3–4 times/day **Maximum:** 750 mg 3–4 times/day	Drowsiness, dizziness, GI effects, rare hepatotoxicity Hypersensitivity reaction (urticaria, itching) Urine discoloration to orange, red, or purple
Cyclobenzaprine (p. 295) (Flexeril)	Muscle spasm, pain, tenderness, restricted movement due to acute, painful, musculoskeletal conditions	Initially 5–10 mg 3 times/day	Drowsiness, dizziness, GI effects Anticholinergic effects (dry mouth, urinary retention) Quinidine-like effects on heart (QT prolongation) Long half-life
Dantrolene (p. 312) (Dantrium)	Spasticity associated with multiple sclerosis, cerebral palsy, spinal cord injury	Initially 25 mg/day for 1 week, then 25 mg 3 times/day for 1 week, then 50 mg 3 times/day for 1 week, then 100 mg 3 times/day **Maximum:** 100 mg 4 times/day	Drowsiness, dizziness, GI effects Contraindicated with hepatic disease Dose-dependent hepatotoxicity Diarrhea that is dose dependent and may be severe, requiring discontinuation
Diazepam (p. 352) (Valium)	Spasticity associated with cerebral palsy, spinal cord injury; reflex spasm due to muscle, joint trauma or inflammation	2–10 mg 3–4 times/day	Drowsiness, dizziness, GI effects Abuse potential
Metaxalone (p. 757) (Skelaxin)	Discomfort due to acute, painful, musculoskeletal conditions	800 mg 3–4 times/day	Drowsiness (low risk), dizziness, GI effects Paradoxical muscle cramps Mild withdrawal syndrome Contraindicated in serious hepatic or renal disease

SKELETAL MUSCLE RELAXANTS   *(continued)*

Name	Indication	Dosage Range	Side Effects/Comments
Methocarbamol (p. 762) (Robaxin)	Discomfort due to acute, painful, musculoskeletal conditions	Initially 1,500 mg 4 times/day **Maintenance: 1,000 mg 4 times/day**	Drowsiness, dizziness, GI effects Urine discoloration to brown, brown-black, or green
Orphenadrine (Norflex)	Discomfort due to acute, painful, musculoskeletal conditions	100 mg 2 times/day	Drowsiness, dizziness, GI effects Long half-life Anticholinergic effects (dry mouth, urinary retention) Rare aplastic anemia Some products may contain sulfites
Tizanidine (p. 1199) (Zanaflex)	Spasticity	Initially 4 mg q6–8h (**Maximum** 3 times/day), may increase by 2–4 mg as needed/tolerated **Maximum: 36 mg** (limited information on doses greater than 24 mg)	Drowsiness, dizziness, GI effects Hypotension (20% decrease in B/P) Hepatotoxicity (usually reversible) Withdrawal syndrome (hypertension, tachycardia, hypertonia) Effect is short lived (3–6 hrs) Dose cautiously with creatinine clearance less than 25 ml/min

Smoking Cessation Agents

Tobacco smoking is associated with the development of lung cancer and chronic obstructive pulmonary disease. Smoking is harmful not just to the smoker but also to family members, coworkers, and others breathing cigarette smoke.

Quitting smoking decreases the risk of developing lung cancer, other cancers, heart disease, stroke, and respiratory illnesses. Several medications have proved useful as smoking cessation aids. Nausea and light-headedness are possible signs of overdose of nicotine warranting a reduction in dosage.

SMOKING CESSATION AGENTS

Name	Availability	Dose Duration	Cautions/Side Effects	Comments
Bupropion (p. 165) **(Zyban)**	**T:** 150 mg	150 mg every morning for 3 days, then 150 mg 2 times/day Start 1–2 wks before quit date **Duration:** 7–12 wks up to 6 mos for maintenance	History of seizure, eating disorder, use of MAOI within previous 14 days, bipolar disorder **Side Effects:** Insomnia, dry mouth, tremor, rash	Stop smoking during second wk of treatment and use counseling support services along with medication
Clonidine (p. 273) **(Catapres, Catapres-TTS)**	**T:** 0.1 mg, 0.2 mg **Patch:** 0.1 mg/24 hrs, 0.2 mg/24 hrs, 0.3 mg/24 hrs	**Oral:** 0.15–0.75 mg/day **Patch:** 0.1–0.2 mg daily **Duration:** 3–10 weeks	Rebound hypertension. **Side Effects:** Dry mouth, drowsiness, dizziness, sedation, constipation	Abrupt discontinuation can result in anxiety, agitation, headaches, tremors accompanied or followed by rapid rise in B/P

(continued)

SMOKING CESSATION AGENTS   *(continued)*

Name	Availability	Dose Duration	Cautions/Side Effects	Comments
Nicotine gum (p. 847) (Nicorette, Thrive)	**Squares:** 2 mg, 4 mg	1 gum q1–2h for 6 wks, then q2–4h for 3 wks then q4–8h for 3 wks **Maximum:** 24 pieces/day **Duration:** up to 12 wks	Recent MI (within 2 wks), serious arrhythmias, serious or worsening angina pectoris **Side Effects:** Dyspepsia, mouth soreness, hiccups	2 mg recommended for pts smoking less than 25 cigarettes/day, 4 mg for pts smoking 25 or more cigarettes/day Chew until a peppery or minty taste emerges and then "park" between cheek and gums to facilitate nicotine absorption through oral mucosa Chew slowly and intermittently to avoid jaw ache and achieve maximum benefit Only water should be taken 15 min before and during chewing
Nicotine inhaler (p. 847) (Nicotrol)	**Cartridge:** 10 mg (delivers 4 mg nicotine)	6–16 cartridges daily; taper frequency of use over the last 6–12 wks **Duration:** up to 6 mos	Recent MI (within 2 wks), serious arrhythmias, serious or worsening angina pectoris **Side Effects:** Local irritation of mouth and throat, coughing, rhinitis	Use at or above room temperature (cold temperatures decrease amount of nicotine inhaled)
Nicotine lozenge (p. 847) (Commit)	**Lozenges:** 2 mg, 4 mg	One lozenge q1–2h for 6 wks, then q2–4h for 3 wks, then q4–8h for 3 wks **Duration:** 12 wks	Recent MI (within 2 wks), serious arrhythmias, serious or worsening angina pectoris **Side Effects:** Local skin reaction, insomnia, nausea, sore throat	First cigarette smoked within 30 min of waking, use 4 mg; after 30 min of waking, use 2 mg Use at least 9 lozenges/day first 6 wks Only 1 lozenge at a time, 5 per 6 hrs and 20 per 24 hrs Do not chew or swallow

Nicotine nasal spray (p. 847) (Nicotrol NS)	10 mg/ml (delivers 0.5 mg/spray)	8–40 doses/day A dose consists of one 0.5 mg delivery to each nostril; initial dose is 1–2 sprays/hr, increasing as needed **Duration:** 3–6 mos	Recent MI (within 2 wks), serious arrhythmias, serious or worsening angina pectoris **Side Effects:** Nasal irritation	Do not sniff, swallow, or inhale through nose while administering nicotine doses (may increase irritation) Tilt head back slightly for best results
Nicotine patch (p. 847) (NicoDerm CQ)	**Nicoderm CQ:** 7 mg/24 hrs, 14 mg/24 hrs, 21 mg/24 hrs **Nicotrol:** 5 mg/16 hrs, 10 mg/16 hrs, 15 mg/16 hrs	Apply upon waking on quit date: **Nicoderm CQ (greater than 10 cigarettes/day):** 21 mg/24 hrs for 4 wks, then 14 mg/24 hrs for 2 wks, then 7 mg/24 hrs for 2 wks **(10 or fewer cigarettes/day):** 14 mg/24 hrs for 6 wks, then 7 mg/24 hrs for 2 wks	Recent MI (within 2 wks), serious arrhythmias, serious or worsening angina pectoris **Side Effects:** Local skin reaction, insomnia	The 16- and 24-hr patches are of comparable efficacy Begin with a lower-dose patch in pts smoking 10 or fewer cigarettes/day Place new patch on relatively hair-free location, usually between neck and waist, in the morning If insomnia occurs, remove the 24-hr patch prior to bedtime or use the 16-hr patch Rotate patch site to diminish skin irritation
Nortriptyline (p. 866) (Pamelor)	**T:** 25 mg, 50 mg, 75 mg, 100 mg	Initially 25 mg/day, increasing gradually to target dose of 75–100 mg/day 10–28 days prior to selected "quit" date, continue for 12 wks or more after "quit" day **Duration:** up to 12 wks	Risk of arrhythmias **Side Effects:** Sedation, dry mouth, blurred vision, urinary retention, light-headedness, shaky hands	Initiate therapy 10–28 days before the quit date to allow steady state of nortriptyline at target dose

(continued)

SMOKING CESSATION AGENTS   *(continued)*

Name	Availability	Dose Duration	Cautions/Side Effects	Comments
Varenicline (p. 1257) (Chantix)	**T:** 0.5 mg, 1 mg	**Days 1–3:** 0.5 mg daily; **days 4–7:** 0.5 mg 2 times/day; **day 8 to end of treatment:** 1 mg 2 times/day **Duration:** begin 1 wk before set quit date, continue for 12 wks. May use additional 12 wks if failed to quit after first 12 wks	**Side Effects:** Nausea; sleep disturbances; headaches; may impair ability to drive, operate machinery; depressed mood; altered behavior; suicidal ideation reported	Use lower dosage if not able to tolerate nausea and vomiting Use counseling support services along with medication

MAOI, Monoamine oxidase inhibitor; *MI,* myocardial infarction; *T,* tablets.

Vitamins

INTRODUCTION

Vitamins are organic substances required for growth, reproduction, and maintenance of health and are obtained from food or supplementation in small quantities (vitamins cannot be synthesized by the body or the rate of synthesis is too slow/inadequate to meet metabolic needs). Vitamins are essential for energy transformation and regulation of metabolic processes. They are catalysts for all reactions using proteins, fats, carbohydrates for energy, growth, and cell maintenance.

WATER SOLUBLE

Water-soluble vitamins include vitamin C (ascorbic acid), B₁ (thiamine), B₂ (riboflavin), B₃ (niacin), B₅ (pantothenic acid), B₆ (pyridoxine), folic acid, B₁₂ (cyanocobalamin). Water-soluble vitamins act as coenzymes for almost every cellular reaction in the body. B-complex vitamins differ from one another in both structure and function but are grouped together because they first were isolated from the same source (yeast and liver).

FAT SOLUBLE

Fat-soluble vitamins include vitamins A, D, E, and K. They are soluble in lipids and are usually absorbed into the lymphatic system of the small intestine and then into the general circulation. Absorption is facilitated by bile. These vitamins are stored in the body tissue when excessive quantities are consumed. May be toxic when taken in large doses (see sections on individual vitamins).

VITAMINS

Name	Uses	Deficiency	Side Effects
Vitamin A (p. 1275) **(Aquasol A)**	Required for normal growth, bone development, vision, reproduction, maintenance of epithelial tissue	Dry skin, poor tooth development, night blindness	**High dosages:** Hepatotoxicity, cheilitis, facial dermatitis, photosensitivity, mucosal dryness
Vitamin B₁ (p. 1180) **(thiamine)**	Important in red blood cell formation, carbohydrate metabolism, neurologic function, myocardial contractility, growth, energy production	Fatigue, anorexia, growth retardation	**Large parenteral doses:** May cause pain on injection
Vitamin B₂ (riboflavin)	Necessary for function of coenzymes in oxidation-reduction reactions, essential for normal cellular growth, assists in absorption of iron and pyridoxine	Numbness in extremities, blurred vision, photophobia, cheilosis	Orange-yellow discoloration in urine

(continued)

VITAMINS *(continued)*

Name	Uses	Deficiency	Side Effects
Vitamin B₃ (niacin) (p. 843)	Coenzyme for many oxidation-reduction reactions	Pellegra, headache, anorexia, memory loss, insomnia	**High dosage (over 500 mg):** Nausea, vomiting, diarrhea, gastritis, hepatotoxicity, skin rash, facial flushing, headaches
Vitamin B₅ (pantothenic acid)	Precursor to coenzyme A; important in synthesis of cholesterol, hormones, fatty acids	Natural deficiency unknown	Occasional GI disturbances (e.g., diarrhea)
Vitamin B₆ (pyridoxine) (p. 1021)	Enzyme cofactor for amino acid metabolism, essential for erythrocyte production, Hgb synthesis	Neuritis, anemia, lymphopenia	**High dosages:** May cause sensory neuropathy
Vitamin B₁₂ (cyanocobalamin) (p. 294)	Coenzyme in cells, including bone marrow, CNS, and GI tract, necessary for lipid metabolism, formation of myelin	Gastrointestinal disorders, anemias, poor growth	Skin rash, diarrhea, pain at injection site
Vitamin C (ascorbic acid) (p. 85)	Cofactor in various physiologic reactions, necessary for collagen formation, acts as antioxidant	Poor wound healing, bleeding gums, scurvy	**High dosages:** May cause calcium oxalate crystalluria, esophagitis, diarrhea
Vitamin D (Calciferol) (p. 1276)	Necessary for proper formation of bone, calcium, mineral homeostasis, regulation of parathyroid hormone, calcitonin, phosphate	Rickets, osteomalacia	Hypercalcemia, kidney stones, renal failure, hypertension, psychosis, diarrhea, nausea, vomiting, anorexia, fatigue, headaches, altered mental status
Vitamin E (Aquasol E) (p. 1280)	Antioxidant, promotes formation, functioning of red blood cells, muscle, other tissues	Red blood cell breakdown	**High dosages:** GI disturbances, malaise, headaches

F, Females; *M,* males.

abacavir

a-**bak**-a-veer
(Ziagen)

BLACK BOX ALERT Serious, sometimes fatal hypersensitivity reactions, lactic acidosis, severe hepatomegaly with steatosis (fatty liver) have occurred.

FIXED-COMBINATION(S)

Epzicom: abacavir/lamivudine (antiretroviral): 600 mg/300 mg. **Trizivir:** abacavir/lamivudine (antiretroviral)/zidovudine (antiretroviral): 300 mg/150 mg/300 mg.

◆CLASSIFICATION

PHARMACOTHERAPEUTIC: Antiretroviral agent. **CLINICAL:** Antiviral (see pp. 69C, 117C).

ACTION

Inhibits activity of HIV-1 reverse transcriptase by competing with natural substrate dGTP and by its incorporation into viral DNA. **Therapeutic Effect:** Inhibits viral DNA replication.

PHARMACOKINETICS

Rapidly and extensively absorbed after PO administration. Protein binding: 50%. Widely distributed, including to cerebrospinal fluid (CSF) and erythrocytes. Metabolized in liver to inactive metabolites. Primarily excreted in urine. Unknown if removed by hemodialysis. **Half-life:** 1.5 hrs.

USES

Treatment of HIV infection, in combination with other agents.

PRECAUTIONS

Contraindications: Hypersensitivity to abacavir (do **not** rechallenge). Moderate or severe hepatic impairment. **Cautions:** Mild hepatic disease. Pts at risk for coronary heart disease (e.g., hypertension, hyperlipidemia, diabetes, smoking).

⧖ LIFESPAN CONSIDERATIONS

Pregnancy/Lactation: Unknown if excreted in breast milk. Breast-feeding not recommended (may increase potential for HIV transmission, adverse effects). **Pregnancy Category C. Children:** Safety and efficacy not established in those less than 3 mos of age. **Elderly:** No age-related precautions noted.

INTERACTIONS

DRUG: Alcohol may increase concentration, risk of toxicity. **HERBAL:** None significant. **FOOD:** None known. **LAB VALUES:** May increase serum AST, ALT, CPK, GGT, blood glucose, triglycerides. May decrease Hgb, leukocytes, lymphocytes.

AVAILABILITY (Rx)

Solution, Oral: 20 mg/ml. **Tablets:** 300 mg.

ADMINISTRATION/HANDLING

PO
• May give without regard to food. • Oral solution may be refrigerated. Do not freeze.

INDICATIONS/ROUTES/DOSAGE

HIV Infection (in Combination with Other Antiretrovirals)
PO: ADULTS: 300 mg twice a day or 600 mg once a day. **CHILDREN 3 MOS–16 YRS:** 8 mg/kg twice a day. **Maximum:** 300 mg twice a day.

Dosage in Hepatic Impairment
Mild impairment: 200 mg twice a day (oral solution recommended). **Moderate to severe impairment:** Not recommended (contraindicated by manufacturer).

SIDE EFFECTS

Adult: Frequent: Nausea (47%), nausea with vomiting (16%), diarrhea (12%), decreased appetite (11%). **Occasional:** Insomnia (7%). **Children: Frequent:** Nausea with vomiting (39%), fever (19%), headache, diarrhea (16%), rash

(11%). **Occasional:** Decreased appetite (9%).

ADVERSE EFFECTS/
TOXIC REACTIONS

Hypersensitivity reaction may be life-threatening. Signs and symptoms include fever, rash, fatigue, intractable nausea/vomiting, severe diarrhea, abdominal pain, cough, pharyngitis, dyspnea. Life-threatening hypotension may occur. Lactic acidosis, severe hepatomegaly may occur.

NURSING CONSIDERATIONS

BASELINE ASSESSMENT

Question for possibility of pregnancy. Obtain baseline laboratory testing, esp. CBC, hepatic function tests, before beginning therapy and at periodic intervals during therapy. Increased risk of sensitivity (cutaneous, GI, pulmonary) in those with positive HLA-B 5701 genotype status. Offer emotional support.

INTERVENTION/EVALUATION

Assess for nausea, vomiting. Monitor daily pattern of bowel activity, stool consistency. Assess dietary pattern; monitor for weight loss. Monitor lab values carefully, particularly hepatic function. Stop abacavir if 3 or more of the following occur: rash, fever, GI disturbances (diarrhea, nausea, vomiting), flu-like symptoms, respiratory difficulty.

PATIENT/FAMILY TEACHING

• Do not take any medications, including OTC drugs, without consulting physician. • Small, frequent meals may offset anorexia, nausea. • Abacavir is not a cure for HIV infection, nor does it reduce risk of transmission to others. • Pt must continue practices to prevent HIV transmission.

abatacept

a-**bay**-ta-sept
(Orencia)
Do not confuse Orencia with Oracea.

◆CLASSIFICATION

PHARMACOTHERAPEUTIC: Selective T-cell costimulation modulator. **CLINICAL:** Rheumatoid arthritis agent.

ACTION

Inhibits T-lymphocyte activation, necessary in the inflammatory cascade leading to joint inflammation and destruction. **Therapeutic Effect:** Induces major clinical response in adult pts with moderate to severely active rheumatoid arthritis (RA).

PHARMACOKINETICS

Higher clearance with increasing body weight. Age, gender do not affect clearance. **Half-life:** 8–25 days.

USES

Reduction of signs and symptoms, progression of structural damage in adults with moderate to severe rheumatoid arthritis (RA) alone or in combination with other disease-modifying antirheumatic medications. Treatment of moderate to severe active polyarticular juvenile idiopathic arthritis in pts 6 yrs and older. May use alone or in combination with methotrexate (do not use with anakinra or tumor necrosis factor [TNF] antagonists).

PRECAUTIONS

Contraindications: None known. **Cautions:** Chronic, latent, or localized infection, COPD (higher incidence of adverse effects), elderly.

⧗ LIFESPAN CONSIDERATIONS

Pregnancy/Lactation: Crosses placenta; unknown if distributed in breast milk. **Pregnancy Category C. Children:** Safety and efficacy not established in pts younger than 6 yrs. **Elderly:** Cautious use due to increased risk of serious infection and malignancy.

INTERACTIONS

DRUG: May increase risk of infection, decrease efficacy of immune response associated with **live vaccines. Tumor necrosis factor (TNF) antagonists (adalimumab, etanercept, infliximab)** may increase risk of infection. **HERBAL:** **Echinacea** may decrease concentration/effects. **FOOD:** None known. **LAB VALUES:** None significant.

AVAILABILITY (Rx)

Injection, Powder for Reconstitution: 250 mg. Injection, Solution: 125 mg/ml single-dose prefilled syringe.

ADMINISTRATION/HANDLING

 IV

Reconstitution • Reconstitute powder in each vial with 10 ml Sterile Water for Injection using the silicone-free syringe provided with each vial and an 18- to 21-gauge needle. • Rotate solution gently to prevent foaming until powder is completely dissolved. • From a 100-ml 0.9% NaCl infusion bag, withdraw and discard an amount equal to the volume of the reconstituted vials (for 2 vials remove 20 ml, for 3 vials remove 30 ml, for 4 vials remove 40 ml). • Slowly add the reconstituted solution from each vial into the infusion bag using the same syringe provided with each vial. • Concentration in the infusion bag will be 10 mg/ml or less abatacept.

Rate of Administration • Infuse over 30 min using a 0.2- to 1.2-micron low protein-binding filter.

Storage • Store vials in refrigerator. • Any reconstitution that has been prepared by using siliconized syringes will develop translucent particles and must be discarded. • Solution should appear clear and colorless to pale yellow. Discard if solution is discolored or contains precipitate. • Solution is stable for up to

24 hrs after reconstitution. • Reconstituted solution may be stored at room temperature or refrigerated.

Subcutaneous
• Store prefilled syringes in refrigerator. • Inject in front of thigh, outer areas of upper arms, or abdomen. • Avoid areas that are tender, bruised, red, scaly, or hard. • Do not rub injection site.

▩ IV INCOMPATIBILITIES

Do not infuse concurrently in same IV line as other agents.

INDICATIONS/ROUTES/DOSAGE

Rheumatoid Arthritis (RA)
IV: BODY WEIGHT 101 KG OR MORE: 1 g (4 vials) given as a 30-min infusion. Following initial therapy, give at 2 wks and 4 wks after first infusion, then q4wks thereafter. **BODY WEIGHT 60–100 KG:** 750 mg (3 vials) given as a 30-min infusion. Following initial therapy, give at 2 wks and 4 wks after first infusion, then q4wks thereafter. **BODY WEIGHT 59 KG OR LESS:** 500 mg (2 vials) given as a 30-min infusion. Following initial therapy, give at 2 wks and 4 wks after first infusion, then q4wks thereafter.

Subcutaneous: Following a single IV infusion, 125 mg given within a day, then 125 mg once a week.

Juvenile Idiopathic Arthritis
IV: CHILDREN 6 YRS AND OLDER, WEIGHING LESS THAN 75 KG: 10 mg/kg. **CHILDREN WEIGHING 75 KG OR MORE:** Refer to adult dosing. **Maximum:** 1,000 mg. Following initial therapy, give 2 wks and 4 wks after first infusion, then q4wks thereafter.

SIDE EFFECTS

Frequent (18%): Headache. **Occasional (9%–6%):** Dizziness, cough, back pain, hypertension, nausea.

ADVERSE EFFECTS/ TOXIC REACTIONS

Upper respiratory tract infection, nasopharyngitis, sinusitis, UTI, influenza, bronchitis occur in 5% of pts. Serious infections manifested as pneumonia, cellulitis, diverticulitis, acute pyelonephritis occur in 3% of pts. Hypersensitivity reaction (rash, urticaria, hypotension, dyspnea) occurs rarely.

NURSING CONSIDERATIONS

BASELINE ASSESSMENT

Assess onset, type, location, duration of pain/inflammation. Inspect appearance of affected joint for immobility, deformities, skin condition. Screen for latent TB infection prior to initiating therapy.

INTERVENTION/EVALUATION

Assess for therapeutic response: relief of pain, stiffness, swelling; increased joint mobility; reduced joint tenderness; improved grip strength. Monitor for hypersensitivity reaction (headache, B/P change, light-headedness).

PATIENT/FAMILY TEACHING

• Consult physician if infection, hypersensitivity reaction, infusion-related reaction occurs. • Do not receive live vaccines during treatment or within 3 mos of its discontinuation. • COPD pts must report worsening of respiratory symptoms.

---

abciximab   HIGH ALERT

ab-**sik**-si-mab
(c7E3 Fab, <u>ReoPro</u>)

◆ CLASSIFICATION

PHARMACOTHERAPEUTIC: Glycoprotein IIb/IIIa receptor inhibitor. **CLINICAL:** Antiplatelet; antithrombotic (see p. 33C).

ACTION

Rapidly inhibits platelet aggregation by preventing the binding of fibrinogen to GP IIb/IIIa receptor sites on platelets. **Therapeutic Effect:** Prevents occlusion of treated coronary arteries. Prevents acute cardiac ischemic complications.

PHARMACOKINETICS

Rapidly cleared from plasma. Initial-phase half-life is less than 10 min; second-phase half-life is 30 min.

USES

Adjunct to aspirin and heparin therapy to prevent cardiac ischemic complications in pts undergoing percutaneous coronary intervention (PCI) and those with unstable angina not responding to conventional medical therapy when PCI is planned within 24 hrs. **OFF-LABEL:** Support PCI during ST-segment elevation myocardial infarction (STEMI); STEMI as adjunct to half-dose thrombolytics.

PRECAUTIONS

Contraindications: Active internal bleeding, arteriovenous malformation or aneurysm, CVA with residual neurologic deficit, history of CVA (within the past 2 yrs) or oral anticoagulant use within the past 7 days unless PT is less than 1.2× control, history of vasculitis, hypersensitivity to murine proteins, intracranial neoplasm, prior IV dextran use before or during percutaneous transluminal coronary angioplasty (PTCA), recent surgery or trauma (within the past 6 wks), recent GI or GU bleeding (within the past 6 wks), thrombocytopenia (less than 100,000 cells/mcl), and severe uncontrolled hypertension. Concomitant use of another glycoprotein IIb/IIIa inhibitor. **Cautions:** Pts who weigh less than 75 kg; those older than 65 yrs; those with history of GI disease; those receiving thrombolytics; PTCA in less than 12 hrs of onset of symptoms for acute MI; prolonged PTCA (longer than 70 min); failed PTCA.

LIFESPAN CONSIDERATIONS

Pregnancy/Lactation: Unknown if distributed in breast milk. **Pregnancy Category C. Children:** Safety and efficacy not established. **Elderly:** Increased risk of major bleeding.

INTERACTIONS

DRUG: Antiplatelet medications, heparin, other anticoagulants, thrombolytics, NSAIDs, direct factor Xa inhibitors, thrombin inhibitors may increase risk of bleeding. **HERBAL:** None significant. **FOOD:** None known. **LAB VALUES:** Increases activated clotting time (ACT), prothrombin time (PT), activated partial thromboplastin time (aPTT); decreases platelet count.

AVAILABILITY (Rx)

Injection Solution: 2 mg/ml (5-ml vial).

ADMINISTRATION/HANDLING

 IV

Reconstitution • Bolus dose: Withdraw bolus dose into syringe using a 0.2- or 0.5-micron low protein-binding filter. • **Continuous infusion:** Withdraw dose through a 0.2- or 0.5-micron low protein-binding filter and further dilute into 250 ml D₅W or 0.9% NaCl.
Rate of Administration • Bolus given over 1 min.
Administration Precautions • Give in separate IV line; do not add any other medication to infusion. • For bolus injection and continuous infusion, use sterile, nonpyrogenic, low protein-binding 0.2- or 0.22-micron filter. • While vascular sheath is in position, maintain pt on complete bed rest with head of bed elevated at 30°. • Maintain affected limb in straight position. • After sheath removal, apply femoral pressure for 30 min, either manually or mechanically, then apply pressure dressing.
Storage • Store vials in refrigerator. • Solution appears clear, colorless. • Do not shake. • Prepared solution is stable for 12 hrs. Discard any unused portion left in vial or if preparation contains *any* opaque particles.

IV INCOMPATIBILITY

Administer in separate line; no other medication should be added to infusion solution.

IV COMPATIBILITIES

Adenosine (Adenocard), argatroban, atropine sulfate, bivalirudin (Angiomax), diphenhydramine (Benadryl), fentanyl (Sublimaze), metoprolol (Lopressor), midazolam (Versed).

INDICATIONS/ROUTES/DOSAGE

Percutaneous Coronary Intervention (PCI)
IV Bolus: ADULTS: 0.25 mg/kg 10–60 min before PCI, then 12-hr IV infusion of 0.125 mcg/kg/min. **Maximum:** 10 mcg/min.

PCI (Unstable Angina)
IV Bolus: ADULTS: 0.25 mg/kg, followed by 18- to 24-hr infusion of 10 mcg/min, ending 1 hr after procedure.

SIDE EFFECTS

Frequent: Nausea (16%), hypotension (12%). **Occasional (9%):** Vomiting. **Rare (3%):** Bradycardia, confusion, dizziness, pain, peripheral edema, UTI.

ADVERSE EFFECTS/ TOXIC REACTIONS

Major bleeding complications may occur; stop infusion immediately. Hypersensitivity reaction (rash, urticaria, hypotension, dyspnea) may occur. Atrial fibrillation or flutter, pulmonary edema, complete AV block occur occasionally.

NURSING CONSIDERATIONS

BASELINE ASSESSMENT

Heparin should be discontinued 4 hrs before arterial sheath removal. Maintain pt on bed rest for 6–8 hrs following sheath removal or drug discontinuation, whichever is later. Check platelet count, PT, aPTT, PFA, before infusion (assess for preexisting blood abnormalities), 2–4 hrs following treatment, and at 24 hrs or before discharge, whichever is first. Check insertion site, distal pulse of affected limb while femoral artery sheath is in place, and then routinely for 6 hrs following femoral artery sheath removal. Minimize need for injections, blood draws, catheters, other invasive procedures.

INTERVENTION/EVALUATION

Stop abciximab and/or heparin infusion if serious bleeding occurs that is uncontrolled by pressure. Observe for mental status changes. Assess skin for ecchymosis, petechiae, particularly at femoral arterial access, also at catheter insertion, arterial and venous puncture, cutdown, needle sites. Handle pt carefully and as infrequently as possible to prevent bleeding. Do not obtain B/P in lower extremities (possible deep vein thrombi). Assess for decrease in B/P, increase in pulse rate, complaint of abdominal or back pain, severe headache, evidence of GI hemorrhage. Monitor ACT, PT, aPTT, platelet count, Hgb, Hct. Question for increase in discharge during menses. Assess urinary output for hematuria. Monitor for hematoma. Use care in removing any dressing, tape.

PATIENT/FAMILY TEACHING

• Assess skin for bruising up to 3 days after infusion. • Report signs of bleeding.

---

abiraterone

a-bir-a-ter-one
(Zytiga)
Do not confuse Zytiga with Zetia or Zyrtec.

◆CLASSIFICATION

PHARMACOTHERAPEUTIC: Androgen biosynthesis inhibitor. **CLINICAL:** Testosterone inhibition agent (see p. 81C).

ACTION

Inhibits androgen production in adrenal gland, testes, and prostate tumors. **Therapeutic Effect:** Lowers serum testosterone to castrate levels.

PHARMACOKINETICS

Protein binding: 99%. Primarily excreted in feces. **Peak plasma concentration:** 2 hrs. **Half-life:** 12 hrs (up to 19 hrs with hepatic impairment).

USES

Treatment of metastatic castration-resistant prostate cancer in combination with prednisone in pts who have received prior chemotherapy containing docetaxel.
◀ALERT▶ Must be given on empty stomach. No food is to be consumed 2 hrs before or 1 hr after each dose. Food may increase absorption up to 10 times normal limit. Sexually active men must wear condoms during and for 1 wk after treatment due to potential risks to fetus.

PRECAUTIONS

Contraindications: Use in women who are pregnant or may become pregnant. **Cautions:** History of cardiovascular disease, arrhythmia, hypertension, hypokalemia, fluid retention, heart failure, moderate hepatic impairment, adrenal insufficiency.

⧗ LIFESPAN CONSIDERATIONS

Pregnancy/Lactation: Contraindicated in women who are or may become pregnant. **Pregnancy Category X. Children:** Safety and efficacy not established. **Elderly:** No age-related precautions noted.

INTERACTIONS

DRUG: May increase concentration/toxicity of **silodosin, tamoxifen, thioridazine, topotecan.** May decrease effect of **clopidogrel, tramadol. CYP3A4 inhibitors (e.g., clarithromycin, ketoconazole)** may increase concentration. **CYP3A4 inducers (e.g., carbamazepine)** may decrease concentration. **HERBAL:** None significant. **FOOD:** Do not give with **food** (no **food** should be consumed for at least 2 hrs before or 1 hr after giving abiraterone). **LAB VALUES:** May increase serum AST, ALT, bilirubin, triglycerides. May decrease potassium, phosphorus.

AVAILABILITY (Rx)

📎 **Tablets:** 250 mg.

ADMINISTRATION/HANDLING

PO

• Give on empty stomach only. • Give with water. • Swallow whole. Do not break, crush, dissolve, or divide tablets.

INDICATIONS/ROUTES/DOSAGE

◄ALERT► Consider increased dosage of prednisone during unusual stress or infection. Interrupting prednisone therapy may induce adrenocorticoid insufficiency.

Metastatic Castration-Resistant Prostate Cancer
PO: **ADULTS, ELDERLY:** 1,000 mg once daily. Coadminister with prednisone, 5 mg PO twice daily.

Dosage Modification
Hepatic Enzymes Greater Than Upper Limit of Normal (ULN)

Lab Values	Recommendation
AST, ALT elevations greater than 5 × ULN or bilirubin greater than 3 × ULN with 1,000 mg	Interrupt treatment and restart at 750 mg once AST, ALT less than 2.5 × ULN or bilirubin less than 1.5 × ULN.
AST, ALT elevations greater than 5 × ULN or bilirubin greater than 3 × ULN with 750 mg	Interrupt treatment and restart at 500 mg once AST, ALT less than 2.5 × ULN or bilirubin less than 1.5 × ULN.

If hepatotoxicity occurs at reduced dose of 500 mg daily, discontinue treatment. **Mild hepatic impairment:** No dosage adjustment necessary. **Moderate hepatic impairment:** Reduce dose to 250 mg daily. Discontinue if AST/ALT greater than 5 times ULN or bilirubin greater than 3 times ULN. **Severe hepatic impairment:** Contraindicated.

SIDE EFFECTS

Frequent (30%–26%): Joint swelling/discomfort, peripheral edema, muscle spasm, musculoskeletal pain, hypokale-mia. Occasional (19%–6%): Hot flashes, diarrhea, UTI, cough, hypertension, urinary frequency, nocturia. Rare (less than 6%): Heartburn, upper respiratory tract infection.

ADVERSE EFFECTS/ TOXIC REACTIONS

Mineralocorticoid excess (severe fluid retention, hypokalemia, hypertension) may compromise pts with prior cardiovascular history. Safety not established in pts with left ventricular ejection fraction less than 50%. Tachycardia, atrial fibrillation, supraventricular tachycardia, atrial flutter, complete AV block, bradyarrhythmia reported in 7% of pts. Chest pain, unstable angina, CHF reported in less than 4% of pts. Stress, infection, or interruption of daily steroids may cause adrenocortical insufficiency. Hepatotoxicity (AST/ALT greater than 5 times ULN) reported in 2% of pts. Pts with hepatic impairment are more likely to develop hepatotoxicity.

NURSING CONSIDERATIONS

BASELINE ASSESSMENT

Evaluate history of heart failure, myocardial infarction, arrhythmias, angina pectoris, peripheral edema, hepatic impairment, adrenal or pituitary abnormalities, left ventricular ejection fraction if applicable. Obtain baseline ALT/AST, alkaline phosphatase, bilirubin, BMP. Question possibility of pregnancy before treatment (Pregnancy Category X). Question history of corticosteroid intolerance if applicable.

INTERVENTION/EVALUATION

Assess for peripheral edema behind medial malleolus (sacral area in bedridden patients). Monitor BMP, hepatic function. Monitor for mineralocorticoid excess (hypokalemia, hypertension, fluid retention) at least once monthly. Assess for cardiac arrhythmia if hypokalemia occurs. Obtain EKG for palpitations, dyspnea, dizziness. Monitor for signs and symptoms of adrenocortical insufficiency during prednisone interruption, periods of stress, infection. Measure AST/ALT, alkaline phosphatase, bilirubin every 2 wks for 3 mos, then monthly. If hepatotoxicity occurs, dosage modification will be necessary. Pts with moderate hepatic impairment must have hepatic function tests every wk for first month, then every 2 wks for 2 mos, then monthly. If AST/ALT above 5 times ULN or bilirubin above 3 times ULN, treatment should be discontinued.

PATIENT/FAMILY TEACHING

• Must be taken on empty stomach (no food 2 hrs before and 1 hr after dose). • If taken with food, toxic levels may result. • Sexually active men must wear condom during treatment and for 1 wk after treatment. • Women who are pregnant or are planning pregnancy may not touch medication without gloves. • Dizziness, palpitations, headache, confusion, muscle weakness, leg swelling/discomfort may become more apparent during periods of unusual stress, infection, or interruption of prednisone therapy. • Blood test will be performed routinely. • Report signs of liver problems (yellowing of skin, bruising, light-colored stool, right upper quadrant pain), chest pain, palpitations. • An increase in urinary frequency or nocturia is expected as treatment becomes therapeutic.

TOP 200

acetaminophen

a-**seet**-a-**min**-oh-fen
(Abenol ✦, Acephen, Apo-Acetaminophen ✦, Atasol ✦, Feverall, Mapap, Ofirmev, Tempra ✦, Tylenol, Tylenol Arthritis Pain, Tylenol Children's Meltaways, Tylenol Junior Meltaways, Tylenol Extra Strength)

BLACK BOX ALERT Potential for severe liver injury.

Do not confuse Acephen with Aciphex, Feverall with Fiberall, Fioricet with Fiorinal, Percocet with Percodan, Tylenol with atenolol, timolol, Tylenol PM, or Tylox, or Vicodin with Hycodan.

FIXED-COMBINATION(S)

Note: The amount of acetaminophen in combination products will be limited to no more than 325 mg per FDA mandate.
Capital with Codeine, Tylenol with Codeine: acetaminophen/codeine: 120 mg/12 mg per 5 ml. **Endocet:** acetaminophen/oxycodone: 325 mg/5 mg, 325 mg/7.5 mg, 325 mg/10 mg, 500 mg/7.5 mg, 650 mg/10 mg. **Fioricet:** acetaminophen/caffeine/butalbital: 325 mg/40 mg/50 mg. **Hycet:** acetaminophen/hydrocodone: 325 mg/7.5 mg per 15 ml. **Lortab:** acetaminophen/hydrocodone: 500 mg/5 mg, 500 mg/7.5 mg. **Lortab Elixir:** acetaminophen/hydrocodone: 167 mg/2.5 mg per 5 ml. **Norco:** acetaminophen/hydrocodone: 325 mg/5 mg, 325 mg/7.5 mg, 325 mg/10 mg. **Percocet, Roxicet:** acetaminophen/oxycodone: 325 mg/5 mg. **Tylenol with Codeine:** acetaminophen/codeine: 300 mg/15 mg, 300 mg/30 mg, 300 mg/60 mg. **Tylox:** acetaminophen/oxycodone: 500 mg/5 mg. **Ultracet:** acetaminophen/tramadol: 325 mg/37.5 mg. **Vicodin:** acetaminophen/hydrocodone: 300 mg/5 mg. **Vicodin ES:** acetaminophen/hydrocodone: 300 mg/7.5 mg. **Vicodin HP:** acetaminophen/hydrocodone: 300 mg/10 mg. **Xodol:** acetaminophen/hydrocodone: 300 mg/5 mg, 300 mg/7.5 mg, 300 mg/10 mg. **Zydone:** acetaminophen/hydrocodone: 400 mg/5 mg, 400 mg/7.5 mg, 400 mg/10 mg.

◆CLASSIFICATION

PHARMACOTHERAPEUTIC: Central analgesic. **CLINICAL:** Non-narcotic analgesic, antipyretic.

ACTION

Appears to inhibit prostaglandin synthesis in the CNS and, to a lesser extent, block pain impulses through peripheral action. Acts centrally on hypothalamic heat-regulating center, producing peripheral vasodilation (heat loss, skin erythema, diaphoresis). **Therapeutic Effect:** Results in antipyresis. Produces analgesic effect.

PHARMACOKINETICS

Route	Onset	Peak	Duration
PO	Less than 60 min	1–3 hrs	4–6 hrs

Rapidly, completely absorbed from GI tract; rectal absorption variable. Protein binding: 20%–50%. Widely distributed to most body tissues. Metabolized in liver; excreted in urine. Removed by hemodialysis. **Half-life:** 1–4 hrs (increased in those with hepatic disease, elderly, neonates; decreased in children).

USES

Relief of mild to moderate pain, fever. **IV:** (Additional) Management of moderate to severe pain when combined with opioid analgesia.

PRECAUTIONS

Contraindications: Severe hepatic impairment or severe active liver disease (Ofirmev). **Cautions:** Sensitivity to acetaminophen; severe renal impairment; alcohol dependency, hepatic impairment, or active hepatic disease; chronic malnutrition and hypovolemia (Ofirmev); G6PD deficiency. Limit dose to less than 4 g/day.

⧖ LIFESPAN CONSIDERATIONS

Pregnancy/Lactation: Crosses placenta; distributed in breast milk. Routinely used in all stages of pregnancy, appears safe for short-term use. **Preg-**nancy Category B. **Children/Elderly:** No age-related precautions noted.

INTERACTIONS

DRUG: Alcohol (chronic use), **hepatotoxic medications** (e.g., **phenytoin**), **hepatic enzyme inducers** (e.g., **phenytoin, rifampin**) may increase risk of hepatotoxicity with prolonged high dose or single toxic dose. May increase risk of bleeding with **warfarin** with chronic, high-dose use. **HERBAL: St. John's wort** may decrease blood levels. **FOOD:** Food may decrease rate of absorption. **LAB VALUES:** May increase serum AST, ALT, bilirubin, prothrombin levels (may indicate hepatotoxicity).

AVAILABILITY (OTC)

Caplets (Tylenol): 500 mg. **Elixir:** 160 mg/5 ml. **Injection, Solution (Ofirmev):** 1,000 mg/100 ml glass vial. **Liquid (Oral [Tylenol Extra Strength]):** 160 mg/5 ml, 500 mg/5 ml, 500 mg/15 ml. **Solution (Oral Drops [Mapap]):** 80 mg/0.8 ml. **Suppository (Acephen, Feverall):** 120 mg, 325 mg, 650 mg. **Suspension (Mapap):** 160 mg/5 ml. **Tablets (Mapap, Tylenol):** 325 mg, 500 mg. **Tablets (Chewable [Mapap]):** 80 mg. **Tablets (Orally Disintegrating):** 80 mg, 160 mg.

🔖 **Caplets:** (Extended-Release [Tylenol Arthritis Pain]): 650 mg.

ADMINISTRATION/HANDLING

💧 IV

Reconstitution • Does not require further dilution. • Store at room temperature. • Withdraw doses less than 1,000 mg. • Place in separate empty, sterile container. **Rate of Administration** • Infuse over 15 min. **Stability** • Once opened or transferred, stable for 6 hrs at room temperature.

PO
• Give without regard to meals. • Tablets may be crushed. • Do not crush extended-release caplets. • Suspension: Shake well before use. • Take with full glass of water.

Rectal
• Moisten suppository with cold water before inserting well up into rectum.
• Do not freeze suppositories.

INDICATIONS/ROUTES/DOSAGE

Analgesia and Antipyresis

IV: ADULTS, ADOLESCENTS WEIGHING 50 KG OR MORE: 1,000 mg q6h or 650 mg q4h. **Maximum single dose:** 1,000 mg; **maximum total daily dose:** 4,000 mg. **ADULTS, ADOLESCENTS WEIGHING LESS THAN 50 KG:** 15 mg/kg q6h or 12.5 mg/kg q4h. **Maximum single dose:** 750 mg; **maximum total daily dose:** 75 mg/kg/day (3,750 mg). **CHILDREN 2–12 YRS:** 15 mg/kg q6h or 12.5 mg/kg q4h. **Maximum:** 75 mg/kg/day, not to exceed 3,750 mg/day. **INFANTS AND CHILDREN LESS THAN 2 YRS:** 7.5–15 mg/kg q6h. **Maximum:** 60 mg/kg/day. **NEONATES:** Loading dose: 20 mg/kg. **PMA 37 or greater than 37 wks:** 10 mg/kg/dose q6h. **Maximum:** 40 mg/kg/day. PMA 33–36 wks: 10 mg/kg/dose q8h. **Maximum:** 40 mg/kg/day. **PMA 28–32 wks:** 10 mg/kg/dose q12h. **Maximum:** 22.5 mg/kg/day. **PO: ADULTS, ELDERLY, CHILDREN 13 YRS AND OLDER:** 325–650 mg q4–6h or 1 g 3–4 times a day. **Maximum:** 4 g/day. **CHILDREN 12 YRS AND YOUNGER:** 10–15 mg/kg/dose q4–6h as needed. **Maximum:** 5 doses/24 hrs. **NEONATES:** Term: Initially, 30 mg/kg/once, then 20 mg/kg/dose q6–8h. **Maximum:** 90 mg/kg/day. **GA 33–37 wks or term less than 10 days:** Initially, 30 mg/kg once, then 15 mg/kg/dose q8h. **Maximum:** 60 mg/kg/day. **GA:** 28–32 wks: 20 mg/kg/dose q12h. **Maximum:** 40 mg/kg/day. **Rectal: ADULTS:** 325–650 mg q4–6h. **Maximum:** 4 g/24 hrs. **CHILDREN:** 10–20 mg/kg/dose q4–6h as needed. **Maximum:** 5 doses/24 hrs. **NEONATES:** Term: Initially, 30 mg/kg/once, then 20 mg/kg/dose q6–8h. **Maximum:** 90 mg/kg/day. **GA 33–37 wks or term less than 10 days:** Initially, 30 mg/kg once, then 15 mg/kg/dose q8h. **Maximum:** 60 mg/kg/day. **GA:** 28–32 wks: 20 mg/kg/dose q12h. **Maximum:** 40 mg/kg/day.

Dosage in Renal Impairment

Creatinine Clearance	Frequency
ORAL	
10–50 ml/min	q6h
Less than 10 ml/min	q8h
Continuous renal replacement therapy	q8h
IV	
30 ml/min or less (use caution, decrease daily dose, extend dosing interval)	

SIDE EFFECTS

Rare: Hypersensitivity reaction.

ADVERSE EFFECTS/ TOXIC REACTIONS

Early Signs of Acetaminophen Toxicity: Anorexia, nausea, diaphoresis, fatigue within first 12–24 hrs. **Later Signs of Toxicity:** Vomiting, right upper quadrant tenderness, elevated hepatic function tests within 48–72 hrs after ingestion. **Antidote:** Acetylcysteine (see Appendix K for dosage).

NURSING CONSIDERATIONS

BASELINE ASSESSMENT

If given for analgesia, assess onset, type, location, duration of pain. Effect of medication is reduced if full pain response recurs prior to next dose. Assess for fever. Assess alcohol usage.

INTERVENTION/EVALUATION

Assess for clinical improvement and relief of pain, fever. **Therapeutic serum level:** 10–30 mcg/ml; **toxic serum level:** greater than 200 mcg/ml. Do not exceed maximum daily recommended dose: 4 g/day.

PATIENT/FAMILY TEACHING

• Consult physician for use in children younger than 2 yrs, oral use longer than 5 days (children) or longer than 10 days (adults), or fever lasting longer than 3 days. • Severe/recurrent pain or high/continuous fever may indicate serious illness. • Advise not to take more than 4 g/24-hr period. Many nonprescription combination products contain acetaminophen. Avoid alcohol.

*acetaZOLAMIDE

a-seet-a-**zole**-a-myde
(Acetazolam ♣, Diamox ♣, Diamox Sequels)
Do not confuse Diamox with Trimox.

◆CLASSIFICATION

PHARMACOTHERAPEUTIC: Carbonic anhydrase inhibitor. **CLINICAL:** Antiglaucoma, anticonvulsant, diuretic, urinary alkalinizer.

ACTION

Reduces formation of hydrogen and bicarbonate ions by inhibiting the enzyme carbonic anhydrase. **Therapeutic Effect:** Increases excretion of sodium, potassium, bicarbonate, water in kidney; decreases formation of aqueous humor in eye; delays abnormal discharge from CNS neurons.

PHARMACOKINETICS

Well absorbed from GI tract. Protein binding: 90%. Excreted unchanged in urine. **Half-life:** Tablets: 10–15 hrs.

USES

Treatment of glaucoma; control of IOP before surgery; adjunct in management of seizures; edema (drug-induced or associated with CHF); decreases or prevents incidence/severity of symptoms associated with acute altitude sickness. **OFF-LABEL:** Urine alkalinization, respiratory stimulant in COPD, metabolic alkalosis.

PRECAUTIONS

Contraindications: Hypersensitivity to sulfonamides, severe renal/hepatic disease, adrenal insufficiency, hypochloremic acidosis, hypokalemia, hyponatremia, long-term administration in pts with chronic noncongestion angle-closure glaucoma. **Cautions:** Diabetes mellitus, gout, obstructive pulmonary disease, respiratory acidosis, moderate renal impairment. **Pregnancy Category C.**

INTERACTIONS

DRUG: May increase levels/effects of **anticonvulsants (barbituates, hydantoins), antihypertensives, carbamazepine, memantine, cyclosporine, amphetamines.** **HERBAL:** Licorice retains sodium; increases potassium. **FOOD:** None known. **LAB VALUES:** May increase serum ammonia, bilirubin, glucose, calcium, uric acid, chloride; may decrease serum bicarbonate, potassium.

AVAILABILITY (Rx)

Injection, Powder for Reconstitution: 500 mg. **Tablets:** 125 mg, 250 mg.

 Capsules (Extended-Release [Diamox Sequels]): 500 mg.

ADMINISTRATION/HANDLING

IV

Reconstitution • Reconstitute with at least 5 ml Sterile Water for Injection to provide concentration not more than 100 mg/ml.
Rate of Administration • Maximum rate: 500 mg/min.
Storage • Following reconstitution, stable for 12 hrs at room temperature, 1 wk if refrigerated.

PO

• Give with food. • May crush tablets. • Do not break, crush, chew, divide extended-release capsule. • May open, sprinkle on food.

IV INCOMPATIBILITY

Diltiazem (Cardizem).

IV COMPATIBILITIES

Pantoprazole (Protonix), ranitidine (Zantac).

INDICATIONS/ROUTES/DOSAGE

Open-Angle Glaucoma

IV: ADULTS, ELDERLY: 250–500 mg; may repeat in 2–4 hrs to a maximum of 1 g/day. **CHILDREN:** 5–10 mg/kg q6h. **Maximum:** 1 g a day.

PO: ADULTS, ELDERLY: 250 mg 1–4 times a day. **CHILDREN:** 8–30 mg/kg/day in divided doses q8h.

PO *(Extended-Release)*: **ADULTS, ELDERLY:** 500 mg twice a day.

Edema

PO, IV: ADULTS: 250–375 mg once daily. **CHILDREN:** 5 mg/kg/dose once a day.

Epilepsy

PO: ADULTS, ELDERLY, CHILDREN: 8–30 mg/kg/day in up to 4 divided doses. **Maximum:** 30 mg/kg/day or 1 g/day. Extended-release formulation not recommended for epilepsy.

Altitude Sickness

PO: ADULTS: 500–1,000 mg/day as 250 mg immediate-release q8–12h or 500 mg extended-release capsule q12–24h. Begin 24–48 hrs before and continue during ascent and for at least 48 hrs following arrival at high altitude.

Dosage in Renal Impairment

Creatinine Clearance	Dosage Interval
10–50 ml/min	q12h
Less than 10 ml/min	Not recommended

SIDE EFFECTS

Frequent: Fatigue, diarrhea, increased urination/frequency, decreased appetite/weight, dysgeusia (metallic), nausea, vomiting, paresthesia, circumoral numbness. **Occasional:** Depression, drowsiness. **Rare:** Headache, photosensitivity, confusion, tinnitus, severe muscle weakness, loss of taste.

ADVERSE EFFECTS/ TOXIC REACTIONS

Long-term therapy may result in acidotic state. Nephrotoxicity/hepatotoxicity occurs occasionally, manifested as dark urine/stools, pain in lower back, jaundice, dysuria, crystalluria, renal colic/calculi. Bone marrow depression may occur manifested as aplastic anemia, thrombocytopenia, thrombocytopenic purpura, leukopenia, agranulocytosis, hemolytic anemia.

NURSING CONSIDERATIONS

BASELINE ASSESSMENT

Glaucoma: Assess affected pupil for dilation, response to light. Question potential for eye discomfort, decrease in visual acuity. **Epilepsy:** Obtain history of seizure disorder (length, intensity, duration of seizure, presence of aura, level of consciousness [LOC]).

INTERVENTION/EVALUATION

Monitor for acidosis (headache, lethargy progressing to drowsiness, CNS depression, Kussmaul's respiration).

PATIENT/FAMILY TEACHING

• Report tingling/tremor in hands or feet, unusual bleeding or bruising, unexplained fever, sore throat, flank pain. • Avoid tasks that require alertness, motor skills until response to drug is established. • Use sunscreen, wear protective clothing.

acetylcysteine (N-acetylcysteine)

a-**seet**-il-**sis**-teen
(Acetadote, Mucomyst ✿,
Parvolex ✿)
Do not confuse acetylcysteine with acetylcholine, or Mucomyst with Mucinex.

◆CLASSIFICATION

PHARMACOTHERAPEUTIC: Respiratory inhalant, intratracheal. **CLINICAL:** Mucolytic, antidote.

ACTION

Splits linkage of mucoproteins, reducing viscosity of pulmonary secretions. **Therapeutic Effect:** Facilitates removal of pulmonary secretions by coughing, postural drainage, mechanical means. Protects against acetaminophen overdose-induced hepatotoxicity.

USES

Inhalation: Adjunctive treatment for abnormally viscid mucous secretions present in acute and chronic bronchopulmonary disease and pulmonary complications of cystic fibrosis and surgery, diagnostic bronchial studies. **Injection, PO:** Antidote in acute acetaminophen toxicity. **OFF-LABEL:** Prevention of contrast-induced renal dysfunction from dyes given during certain diagnostic tests (such as CT scans). Treatment of distal intestinal obstruction syndrome.

PRECAUTIONS

Contraindications: None known. **Cautions:** Systemic effects may occur in pts with bronchial asthma; debilitated pts with severe respiratory insufficiency. **Pregnancy Category B.**

INTERACTIONS

DRUG: None significant. **HERBAL:** None significant. **FOOD:** None known. **LAB VALUES:** None significant.

AVAILABILITY (Rx)

Inhalation Solution (Mucomyst): 10% (100 mg/ml), 20% (200 mg/ml). **Injection Solution (Acetadote):** 20% (200 mg/ml).

ADMINISTRATION/HANDLING

 IV

The total dose is 300 mg/kg administered over 21 hrs. Dose preparation is based on pt weight. Total volume administered should be adjusted for pts less than 40 kg and for those requiring fluid restriction. Store unopened vials at room temperature. Following dilution in D₅W, stable for 24 hrs at room temperature. Color change of opened vials may occur (does not affect potency).

Three-Bag Method (as Antidote): Loading, Second, and Third Doses
Pts Greater Than or Equal to 40 kg:
Loading dose: 150 mg/kg in 200 ml of diluent administered over 60 min.
Second dose: 50 mg/kg in 500 ml of diluent administered over 4 hrs.
Third dose: 100 mg/kg in 1,000 ml of diluent administered over 16 hrs.

Pts Greater Than 20 kg but Less Than 40 kg:
Loading dose: 150 mg/kg in 100 ml of diluent administered over 60 min.
Second dose: 50 mg/kg in 250 ml of diluent administered over 4 hrs.
Third dose: 100 mg/kg in 500 ml of diluent administered over 16 hrs.

Pts Less Than or Equal to 20 kg:
Loading dose: 150 mg/kg in 3 ml/kg of body weight of diluent administered over 60 min.
Second dose: 50 mg/kg in 7 ml/kg of body weight of diluent administered over 4 hrs.
Third dose: 100 mg/kg in 14 ml/kg of body weight of diluent administered over 16 hrs.

PO
• For treatment of acetaminophen overdose. • Give as 5% solution. • Dilute 20% solution 1:3 with cola, orange juice, other soft drink. • Give within 1 hr of preparation.

Inhalation, Nebulization
• May administer either undiluted or diluted with 0.9% NaCl; 10% solution may be undiluted; 20% solution can be diluted with D₅W or 0.9% NaCl.

IV COMPATIBILITIES

Cefepime (Maxipime), ceftazidime (Fortaz).

INDICATIONS/ROUTES/DOSAGE

Bronchopulmonary Disease
Inhalation, Nebulization

◄ALERT► Bronchodilators should be given 10–15 min before acetylcysteine. **ADULTS, ELDERLY, CHILDREN:** 3–5 ml (20% solution) 3–4 times a day or 6–10 ml (10% solution) 3–4 times a day. Range: 1–10 ml (20% solution) q2–6h or 2–20 ml (10% solution) q2–6h. **INFANTS:** 1–2 ml (20%) or 2–4 ml (10%) 3–4 times a day.

Intratracheal: ADULTS, CHILDREN: 1–2 ml of 10% or 20% solution instilled into tracheostomy q1–4h.

Acetaminophen Overdose

◄ALERT► It is essential to initiate treatment as soon as possible after overdose and, in any case, within 24 hrs of ingestion.

PO *(Oral Solution 5%)*: **ADULTS, ELDERLY, CHILDREN:** Loading dose of 140 mg/kg, followed in 4 hrs by maintenance dose of 70 mg/kg q4h for 17 additional doses (or until acetaminophen assay reveals nontoxic level). Repeat dose if emesis occurs within 1 hr of administration. **IV: ADULTS, ELDERLY, CHILDREN:** 150 mg/kg infused over 60 min, then 50 mg/kg infused over 4 hrs, then 100 mg/kg infused over 16 hrs (see Administration/Handling for dilution). Duration of administration may vary depending on acetaminophen levels and hepatic function tests obtained during treatment. Pts who still have detectable levels of acetaminophen or elevated hepatic function test results continue to benefit from additional acetylcysteine administration beyond 24 hrs.

Prevention of Contrast-Induced Nephropathy

PO: ADULTS, ELDERLY: 600–1,200 mg twice a day for 4 doses starting the day before the procedure. Hydrate pt with 0.9% NaCl concurrently.

Diagnostic Bronchial Studies
Inhalation, Nebulization: ADULTS:
1–2 ml of 20% solution or 2–4 ml of 10% solution 2–3 times before the procedure.

SIDE EFFECTS

IV: (7%–6%): Acute flushing, erythema. **(4%):** Pruritus. **Frequent: Inhalation:** Stickiness on face, transient unpleasant odor. **Occasional: Inhalation:** Increased bronchial secretions, throat irritation, nausea, vomiting, rhinorrhea. **Rare: Inhalation:** Rash. **PO:** Facial edema, bronchospasm, wheezing, nausea, vomiting.

ADVERSE EFFECTS/ TOXIC REACTIONS

Large doses may produce severe nausea/ vomiting. **(Less than 2%):** Serious anaphylactoid reactions including cough, wheezing, stridor, respiratory distress, bronchospasm, hypotension, and death have been known to occur with IV administration.

NURSING CONSIDERATIONS

BASELINE ASSESSMENT

Mucolytic: Assess pretreatment respirations for rate, depth, rhythm. **IV antidote:** Obtain baseline labs, including serum AST, ALT, bilirubin, PT/INR, BUN, creatinine, glucose, and drug screen. For use as antidote, obtain acetaminophen level to determine need for treatment with acetylcysteine.

INTERVENTION/EVALUATION

If bronchospasm occurs, discontinue treatment, notify physician; bronchodilator may be added to therapy. Monitor rate, depth, rhythm, type of respiration (abdominal, thoracic). Check sputum for color, consistency, amount. **IV antidote:** Administer within 8 hrs of acetaminophen ingestion for maximal hepatic protection; ideally, within 4 hrs after immediate-release and 2 hrs after liquid acetaminophen formulations.

PATIENT/FAMILY TEACHING

• Slight, disagreeable sulfuric odor from solution may be noticed during initial administration but disappears quickly. • Adequate hydration is important part of therapy. • Follow guidelines for proper coughing and deep breathing techniques.

aclidinium

a-kli-**din**-ee-um
(Tudorza)

◆CLASSIFICATION

PHARMACOTHERAPEUTIC: Long-acting antimuscarinic, anticholinergic. **CLINICAL:** Bronchodilator (see p. 75C).

ACTION

Inhibits M_1 to M_5 muscarinic receptors in smooth muscle of airway, preventing acetylcholine-induced bronchospasm. **Therapeutic Effect:** Bronchodilation.

PHARMACOKINETICS

Peak plasma levels noted within 10 min following inhalation. Extensively metabolized via hydrolysis, both chemically and enzymatically by esterases. Primarily eliminated in urine, with a smaller amount excreted in feces. **Half-life:** 5–8 hrs.

USES

Long-term maintenance treatment of airflow obstruction in pts with chronic obstructive pulmonary disease (COPD), including chronic bronchitis and emphysema.

PRECAUTIONS

◀**ALERT**▶ Not indicated for use as a rescue medication. Contact physician if paradoxical bronchospasm, worsening of narrow-angle glaucoma, urinary retention, or immediate hypersensitivity occurs. **Contraindications:** None known. **Cautions:** Prostatic hyperplasia, bladder-neck obstruction, narrow-angle glaucoma, hypersensitivity to milk proteins, atropine.

⌛ LIFESPAN CONSIDERATIONS

Pregnancy/Lactation: May produce teratogenic effects. May be excreted in breast milk; do not breastfeed. **Pregnancy Category C. Children:** Safety and efficacy not established. **Elderly:** No age-related precautions noted.

INTERACTIONS

DRUG: May increase effect of **anticholinergic agents. HERBAL:** None significant. **FOOD:** None known. **LAB VALUES:** None known.

AVAILABILITY (Rx)

Powder for Inhalation: 400 mcg/inhalation.

ADMINISTRATION/HANDLING

Inhalation
• Remove inhaler from pouch; allows 60 doses for oral inhalation. • The inhaler is a white and green device with a dose indicator, a storage unit containing drug product formulation, and a mouthpiece covered by a green protective cap. • Each actuation delivers 375 mcg of medication from the mouthpiece. • Follow manufacturer guidelines for assembly of plastic dosing mechanism and proper use of inhaler.
Storage • Store pouch at room temperature; inhaler should be stored inside the sealed pouch and only be opened immediately before use. • Discard inhaler 45 days after opening the pouch, after the marking "0" with a red background shows in middle of dose indicator, or when the device locks out, whichever comes first.

INDICATIONS/ROUTES/DOSAGE

Maintenance Therapy:
Inhalation: ADULTS, ELDERLY: 400 mcg twice daily.

SIDE EFFECTS

Occasional (7%–3%): Headache, nasopharyngitis, cough, diarrhea. **Rare (2%–1%):** Sinusitis, rhinitis, toothache, vomiting.

ADVERSE EFFECTS/ TOXIC REACTIONS

Severe dyspnea may indicate paradoxical bronchospasm. Acute narrow-angle glaucoma (eye pain or discomfort, blurred vision, visual halos, or colored images in association with red eyes from conjunctival congestion and corneal edema) occur rarely. Signs and symptoms of prostatic hyperplasia or bladder-neck obstruction (difficulty passing urine, painful urination) have been observed. Hypersensitivity reaction has been noted rarely.

NURSING CONSIDERATIONS

BASELINE ASSESSMENT

Assess rate, depth, rhythm, type of respirations. Monitor EKG, serum potassium, ABG determinations, O_2 saturation, pulmonary function test. Assess lung sounds for wheezing (bronchoconstriction), rales. Receive full medication history and screen for possible drug interactions.

INTERVENTION/EVALUATION

Monitor lung sounds. Observe for sudden shortness of breath, wheezing (pulmonary bronchospasm). Routinely monitor BMP, blood glucose, O_2 saturation. Evaluate EKG for palpitation, tachycardia. Monitor hypokalemia results. Monitor for acute urinary retention. Question for eye pain or discomfort, changes in vision, conjunctival congestion (worsening of narrow-angle glaucoma).

PATIENT/FAMILY TEACHING

• Discard pouch after 45 days, after the marking "0" with a red background shows in the middle of the dose indicator, or when device locks out, whichever comes first. • The inhaler contains 60 doses of medication, with the number 60 on dose indicator. • As each dose is used, the dose indicator will display down in intervals of 10. • The marking "0" with a red background shows in the middle of the dose indicator. • Increase fluid intake (decreases lung secretion viscosity). • Report difficulty breathing, painful or difficulty passing urine, visual changes.

acyclovir

a-**sye**-klo-veer
(Apo-Acyclovir ✦,
Novo-Acyclovir ✦, Zovirax)
Do not confuse acyclovir with ganciclovir, Retrovir, or valacyclovir, or Zovirax with Doribax, Valtrex, Zithromax, Zostrix, Zyloprim, or Zyvox.

FIXED-COMBINATION(S)

Liposivir: acyclovir/hydrocortisone (a steroid): 5%/1%.

◆CLASSIFICATION

PHARMACOTHERAPEUTIC: Synthetic nucleoside. **CLINICAL:** Antiviral (see p. 69C).

ACTION

Converts to acyclovir triphosphate, becoming part of DNA chain. **Therapeutic Effect:** Interferes with DNA synthesis and viral replication. Virustatic.

PHARMACOKINETICS

Poorly absorbed from GI tract; minimal absorption following topical application. Protein binding: 9%–36%. Widely distributed. Partially metabolized in liver. Excreted primarily in urine. Removed by hemodialysis. **Half-life:** 2.5 hrs (increased in renal impairment).

USES

Parenteral

Treatment of initial and prophylaxis of recurrent mucosal and cutaneous herpes simplex (HSV 1 and HSV 2) in immunocompromised pts. Treatment of severe initial episodes of herpes genitalis in immunocompetent pts. Treatment of herpes simplex encephalitis including neonatal herpes simplex virus. Treatment of varicella-zoster virus (VZV) infections in immunocompetent pts.

Oral
Treatment of initial episodes and prophylaxis of recurrent herpes simplex (HSV 2 genital herpes). Treatment of chickenpox (varicella). Acute treatment of herpes zoster (shingles).

Topical
Cream: Treatment of recurrent herpes labialis (cold sores). **Ointment:** Treatment of mucocutaneous HSV in immunocompromised pts. **OFF-LABEL:** Prevention of HSV reactivation in HIV-positive pts; hematopoietic stem cell transplant (HSCT); during periods of neutropenia in pts with cancer; prevention of VZV reactivation in allogenic HSCT; treatment of disseminated HSC or VZV in immunocompromised pts with cancer; empiric treatment of suspected encephalitis in immunocompromised pts with cancer; treatment of initial and prophylaxis of recurrent mucosal and cutaneous herpes simplex infections in immunocompromised pts.

PRECAUTIONS

Contraindications: Use in neonates when acyclovir is reconstituted with Bacteriostatic Water for Injection containing benzyl alcohol. Hypersensitivity to valacyclovir. **Cautions:** Renal/hepatic impairment, dehydration, fluid/electrolyte imbalance, concurrent use of nephrotoxic agents, neurologic abnormalities, immunocompromised pts, elderly, substantial hypoxia.

LIFESPAN CONSIDERATIONS

Pregnancy/Lactation: Crosses placenta; distributed in breast milk. **Pregnancy Category B. Children:** Safety and efficacy not established in those younger than 2 yrs (younger than 1 yr for IV use). **Elderly:** Age-related renal impairment may require decreased dosage. May experience more neurologic effects (e.g., agitation, confusion, hallucinations).

INTERACTIONS

DRUG: None significant. **HERBAL:** None significant. **FOOD:** None known. **LAB VALUES:** May increase BUN, serum creatinine concentrations, hepatic function tests.

AVAILABILITY (Rx)

Cream: 5%. **Injection, Powder for Reconstitution:** 500 mg, 1,000 mg. **Injection, Solution:** 50 mg/ml. **Ointment:** 5%. **Suspension, Oral:** 200 mg/5 ml. **Tablets:** 400 mg, 800 mg.

Capsules: 200 mg.

ADMINISTRATION/HANDLING
IV

Reconstitution • Add 10 ml Sterile Water for Injection to each 500-mg vial (50 mg/ml). Do not use Bacteriostatic Water for Injection containing benzyl alcohol or parabens (will cause precipitate). • Shake well until solution is clear. • Further dilute with at least 100 ml D$_5$W or 0.9 NaCl. Final concentration should be 7 mg/ml or less. (Concentrations greater than 10 mg/ml increase risk of phlebitis.)
Rate of Administration • Infuse over at least 1 hr (renal tubular damage may occur with too-rapid rate). • Maintain adequate hydration during infusion and for 2 hrs following IV administration.
Storage • Store vials at room temperature • Solutions of 50 mg/ml stable for 12 hrs at room temperature; may form precipitate if refrigerated. Potency not affected by precipitate and redissolution. • IV infusion (piggyback) stable for 24 hrs at room temperature. Yellow discoloration does not affect potency.

PO
• May give without regard to food. • Do not crush/break capsules. • Store capsules at room temperature.

Topical
• Avoid contact with eye. • Use finger cot/rubber glove to prevent autoinoculation.

 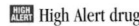

▦ IV INCOMPATIBILITIES

Aztreonam (Azactam), diltiazem (Cardizem), dobutamine (Dobutrex), dopamine (Intropin), levofloxacin (Levaquin), meropenem (Merrem IV), ondansetron (Zofran), piperacillin and tazobactam (Zosyn).

▦ IV COMPATIBILITIES

Allopurinol (Alloprim), amikacin (Amikin), ampicillin, cefazolin (Ancef), cefotaxime (Claforan), ceftazidime (Fortaz), ceftriaxone (Rocephin), cimetidine (Tagamet), clindamycin (Cleocin), diphenhydramine (Benadryl), famotidine (Pepcid), fluconazole (Diflucan), gentamicin, heparin, hydromorphone (Dilaudid), imipenem (Primaxin), lorazepam (Ativan), magnesium sulfate, methylprednisolone (Solu-Medrol), metoclopramide (Reglan), metronidazole (Flagyl), morphine, multivitamins, potassium chloride, propofol (Diprivan), ranitidine (Zantac), vancomycin.

INDICATIONS/ROUTES/DOSAGE

Genital Herpes (Initial Episode)
IV: ADULTS, ELDERLY, CHILDREN 12 YRS AND OLDER: 5 mg/kg q8h for 5–7 days.
PO: ADULTS, ELDERLY, CHILDREN 12 YRS AND OLDER: 200 mg q4h 5 times a day for 10 days or 400 mg 3 times a day for 7–10 days. **CHILDREN YOUNGER THAN 12 YRS:** 40–80 mg/kg/day in 3–4 divided doses for 5–10 days. **Maximum:** 1 g/day.
Topical: ADULTS: (Ointment) ½ inch for 4-inch square surface q3h (6 times a day) for 7 days.

Genital Herpes (Recurrent)
Intermittent Therapy
PO: ADULTS, ELDERLY, CHILDREN 12 YRS AND OLDER: 200 mg q4h 5 times a day for 5 days or 400 mg 3 times a day for 5–10 days.
Chronic Suppressive Therapy
PO: ADULTS, ELDERLY, CHILDREN 12 YRS AND OLDER: 400 mg twice a day or 200 mg 3–5 times a day for up to 12 mos. **CHILDREN YOUNGER THAN 12 YRS:** 80 mg/kg/day in 3 divided doses. **Maximum:** 1 g/day.

Herpes Simplex Mucocutaneous
PO: ADULTS, ELDERLY: 400 mg 5 times a day for 7–14 days.
IV: ADULTS, ELDERLY, CHILDREN 12 YRS AND OLDER: 5 mg/kg/dose q8h for 7–14 days. **CHILDREN YOUNGER THAN 12 YRS:** 10 mg/kg q8h for 7 days.
Topical: ADULTS: (Ointment) ½ inch for 4-inch square surface q3h (6 times a day) for 7 days.

Herpes Simplex Encephalitis
IV: ADULTS, ELDERLY, CHILDREN 12 YRS AND OLDER: 10 mg/kg q8h for 10 days. **CHILDREN 3 MOS–YOUNGER THAN 12 YRS:** 20 mg/kg q8h for 10 days.

Herpes Zoster (Shingles)
IV: ADULTS, CHILDREN 12 YRS AND OLDER: (immunocompromised) 10 mg/kg/dose q8h for 7 days. **CHILDREN YOUNGER THAN 12 YRS:** (immunocompromised) 20 mg/kg/dose q8h for 7 days.
PO: ADULTS, ELDERLY, CHILDREN 12 YRS AND OLDER: 800 mg q4h 5 times a day for 7–10 days.

Herpes Labialis (Cold Sores)
Topical: ADULTS, ELDERLY, CHILDREN 12 YRS AND OLDER: Apply to affected area 5 times a day for 4 days.

Varicella-Zoster (Chickenpox)
◄ALERT► Begin treatment within 24 hrs of onset of rash.
IV: ADULTS, ELDERLY, CHILDREN 12 YRS AND OLDER: 10 mg/kg/dose q8h for 7 days. **CHILDREN LESS THAN 12 YRS:** 20 mg/kg/dose q8h for 7 days.
PO: ADULTS, ELDERLY, CHILDREN OLDER THAN 12 YRS AND CHILDREN 2–12 YRS, WEIGHING 40 KG OR MORE: 800 mg 4 times a day for 5 days. **CHILDREN 2–12 YRS, WEIGHING LESS THAN 40 KG:** 20 mg/kg 4 times a day for 5 days. **Maximum:** 800 mg/dose.

Usual Neonatal Dosage
HSV (treatment) (IV): 20 mg/kg/dose q8h for 14–21 days.

HSV (chronic suppression) (PO): 300 mg/m²/dose q8h following IV therapy for 6 mos.

Varicella-Zoster (IV): 10–15 mg/kg/dose q8h for 5–10 days.

Dosage in Renal Impairment

Dosage and frequency are modified based on severity of infection and degree of renal impairment.

PO: Normal dose 200 mg q4h, 200 mg q8h, or 400 mg q12h.
Creatinine clearance 10 ml/min and less: 200 mg q12h.

PO: Normal dose 800 mg q4h.
Creatinine clearance greater than 25 ml/min: Give usual dose and at normal interval, 800 mg q4h. **Creatinine clearance 10–25 ml/min:** 800 mg q8h. **Creatinine clearance less than 10 ml/min:** 800 mg q12h.

IV:

Creatinine Clearance	Dosage
Greater than 50 ml/min	100% of normal q8h
25–50 ml/min	100% of normal q12h
10–24 ml/min	100% of normal q24h
Less than 10 ml/min	50% of normal q24h
Hemodialysis (HD)	2.5–5 mg/kg q24h (give after HD)
Peritoneal dialysis (PD)	50% normal dose q24h
Continuous renal replacement therapy (CRRT)	5–10 mg/kg q12–24h (q12h for viral meningoenphalitis/VZV infection)

SIDE EFFECTS

Frequent: Parenteral (9%–7%): Phlebitis or inflammation at IV site, nausea, vomiting. **Topical (28%):** Burning, stinging. **Occasional: Parenteral (3%):** Pruritus, rash, urticaria. **PO (12%–6%):** Malaise, nausea. **Topical (4%):** Pruritus. **Rare: PO (3%–1%):** Vomiting, rash, diarrhea, headache. **Parenteral (2%–1%):** Confusion, hallucinations, seizures, tremors. **Topical (less than 1%):** Rash.

ADVERSE EFFECTS/ TOXIC REACTIONS

Rapid parenteral administration, excessively high doses, or fluid and electrolyte imbalance may produce renal failure (abdominal pain, decreased urination, decreased appetite, increased thirst, nausea, vomiting). Toxicity not reported with oral or topical use.

NURSING CONSIDERATIONS

BASELINE ASSESSMENT

Question for history of allergies, esp. to acyclovir. Assess herpes simplex lesions before treatment to compare baseline with treatment effect.

INTERVENTION/EVALUATION

Assess IV site for phlebitis (heat, pain, red streaking over vein). Evaluate cutaneous lesions. Ensure adequate ventilation. Manage chickenpox and disseminated herpes zoster with strict isolation. Provide analgesics and comfort measures; esp. exhausting to elderly. Encourage fluids.

PATIENT/FAMILY TEACHING

• Drink adequate fluids. • Do not touch lesions with bare fingers to prevent spreading infection to new site. • **Genital Herpes:** Continue therapy for full length of treatment. • Space doses evenly. • Use finger cot/rubber glove to apply topical ointment. • Avoid sexual intercourse during duration of lesions to prevent infecting partner. • Acyclovir does not cure herpes infections. • Pap smear should be done at least annually due to increased risk of cervical cancer in women with genital herpes.

adalimumab
TOP 200

a-da-**lim**-ue-mab
(Humira)

BLACK BOX ALERT Tuberculosis, invasive fungal infections, other opportunistic infections have occurred. Test for tuberculosis prior to and during treatment. Lymphoma, other malignancies reported in children/adolescents. Lymphoma, other malignancies reported primarily in pts with Crohn's disease or ulcerative colitis and concomitant azathioprine or mercaptopurine.

Do not confuse Humira with Humalog or Humulin.

◆CLASSIFICATION

PHARMACOTHERAPEUTIC: Monoclonal antibody. **CLINICAL:** Rheumatoid arthritis agent.

ACTION

Binds specifically to tumor necrosis factor (TNF) alpha cell, blocking its interaction with cell surface TNF receptors. **Therapeutic Effect:** Reduces inflammation, tenderness, swelling of joints; slows or prevents progressive destruction of joints in rheumatoid arthritis (RA).

PHARMACOKINETICS

Half-life: 10–20 days.

USES

Reduces signs/symptoms, progression of structural damage and improves physical function in adults with moderate to severe RA. May be used alone or in combination with other disease-modifying antirheumatic drugs. First-line treatment of moderate to severe RA, treatment of psoriatic arthritis, treatment of ankylosing spondylitis, to induce/maintain remission of moderate to severe active Crohn's disease, moderate to severe plaque psoriasis, reduce signs and symptoms of moderate to severe active polyarticular juvenile rheumatoid arthritis in pts 4 yrs and older.

PRECAUTIONS

Contraindications: (Canada labeling) Severe infections (e.g., sepsis, TB). **Cautions:** Pts with chronic infections, predisposition to infections, decreased left ventricular function, CHF, demyelinating disorders, invasive fungal infections.

⌛ LIFESPAN CONSIDERATIONS

Pregnancy/Lactation: Unknown if distributed in breast milk. **Pregnancy Category B. Children:** Safety and efficacy not established. **Elderly:** Cautious use due to increased risk of serious infection and malignancy.

INTERACTIONS

DRUG: Abatacept, anakinra, immunosuppressive therapy may increase risk of infections. May decrease efficacy of immune response with **live vaccines. HERBAL: Echinacea** may decrease effects. **FOOD:** None known. **LAB VALUES:** May increase serum cholesterol, other lipids, alkaline phosphatase.

AVAILABILITY (Rx)

Injection Solution: 20 mg/0.4 ml, 40 mg/0.8 ml in prefilled syringes.

ADMINISTRATION/HANDLING

Subcutaneous
• Refrigerate; do not freeze. • Discard unused portion. • Rotate injection sites. Give new injection at least 1 inch from an old site and never into area where skin is tender, bruised, red, or hard.

INDICATIONS/ROUTES/DOSAGE

Rheumatoid Arthritis (RA)
Subcutaneous: ADULTS, ELDERLY: 40 mg every other wk. Dose may be increased to 40 mg/wk in those not taking methotrexate.

Ankylosing Spondylitis, Psoriatic Arthritis
Subcutaneous: ADULTS, ELDERLY: 40 mg every other wk.

Crohn's Disease
Subcutaneous: ADULTS, ELDERLY: Initially, 160 mg given as 4 injections on day 1 or 2 injections/day over 2 days, then 80 mg 2 wks later (day 15). Maintenance: 40 mg every other wk beginning at day 29.

Plaque Psoriasis
Subcutaneous: ADULTS, ELDERLY: Initially, 80 mg, then 40 mg every other wk starting 1 wk after initial dose.

Juvenile Rheumatoid Arthritis
Subcutaneous: CHILDREN 4 YRS AND OLDER, WEIGHING 15–29 KG: 20 mg every other wk. **WEIGHING 30 KG OR MORE:** 40 mg every other wk.

SIDE EFFECTS

Frequent (20%): Injection site erythema, pruritus, pain, swelling. **Occasional (12%–9%):** Headache, rash, sinusitis, nausea. **Rare (7%–5%):** Abdominal or back pain, hypertension.

ADVERSE EFFECTS/ TOXIC REACTIONS

Hypersensitivity reactions (rash, urticaria, hypotension, dyspnea), infections (primarily upper respiratory tract, bronchitis, urinary tract) occur rarely. More serious infections (pneumonia, tuberculosis, cellulitis, pyelonephritis, septic arthritis) also occur rarely.

NURSING CONSIDERATIONS

BASELINE ASSESSMENT

Assess onset, type, location, duration of pain or inflammation. Inspect appearance of affected joints for immobility, deformities, skin condition. If pt is to self-administer, instruct on subcutaneous injection technique, including areas of the body acceptable for injection sites.

INTERVENTION/EVALUATION

Monitor lab values, particularly CBC. Assess for therapeutic response: relief of pain, stiffness, swelling; increased joint mobility; reduced joint tenderness; improved grip strength.

PATIENT/FAMILY TEACHING

• Injection site reaction generally occurs in first month of treatment and decreases in frequency during continued therapy. • Do not receive live vaccines during treatment. Report rash, nausea.

adefovir

a-**def**-o-veer
(Hepsera)

BLACK BOX ALERT May cause HIV resistance in unrecognized or untreated HIV infection. Lactic acidosis, severe hepatomegaly with steatosis (fatty liver), acute exacerbation of hepatitis have occurred. Use with caution in pts with renal dysfunction or in pts at risk for renal toxicity.

◆CLASSIFICATION

PHARMACOTHERAPEUTIC: Antiviral. **CLINICAL:** Hepatitis B agent (see p. 69C).

ACTION

Inhibits DNA polymerase, an enzyme, causing DNA chain termination after its incorporation into viral DNA. **Therapeutic Effect:** Prevents viral cell replication.

PHARMACOKINETICS

Rapidly converted to adefovir in intestine. Binds to proteins after PO administration. Protein binding: less than 4%. Excreted in urine. **Half-life:** 7 hrs (increased in renal impairment).

USES

Treatment of chronic hepatitis B in adults with evidence of active viral replication based on persistent elevations of serum AST or ALT or histologic evidence.

PRECAUTIONS

Contraindications: None known. **Cautions:** Pts with known risk factors for hepatic disease, renal impairment, elderly. Concurrent administration with tenofovir-containing products.

⏳ LIFESPAN CONSIDERATIONS

Pregnancy/Lactation: Unknown if drug crosses placenta or is distributed in

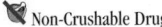

breast milk. **Pregnancy Category C. Children:** Safety and efficacy not established. **Elderly:** Age-related renal impairment, decreased cardiac function requires cautious use.

INTERACTIONS

DRUG: May increase effects of **tenofovir. HERBAL:** None significant. **FOOD:** None known. **LAB VALUES:** May increase serum ALT, AST, amylase.

AVAILABILITY (Rx)

Tablets: 10 mg.

ADMINISTRATION/HANDLING

PO
• Give without regard to food. • Avoid alcohol (increased risk of hepatotoxicity).

INDICATIONS/ROUTES/DOSAGE

Chronic Hepatitis B (Normal Renal Function)
PO: ADULTS, ELDERLY: 10 mg once a day.

Chronic Hepatitis B (Impaired Renal Function)
PO: ADULTS, ELDERLY WITH CREATININE CLEARANCE 30–49 ML/MIN: 10 mg q48h. **ADULTS, ELDERLY WITH CREATININE CLEARANCE 10–29 ML/MIN:** 10 mg q72h. **ADULTS, ELDERLY ON HEMODIALYSIS:** 10 mg every 7 days following dialysis.

SIDE EFFECTS

Frequent (13%): Asthenia (loss of strength, energy). Occasional (9%–4%): Headache, abdominal pain, nausea, flatulence. Rare (3%): Diarrhea, dyspepsia.

ADVERSE EFFECTS/ TOXIC REACTIONS

Nephrotoxicity, characterized by increased serum creatinine and decreased serum phosphorus levels, is treatment-limiting toxicity of adefovir therapy. Lactic acidosis, severe hepatomegaly occur rarely, particularly in female pts.

NURSING CONSIDERATIONS

BASELINE ASSESSMENT

Obtain baseline renal function lab values before therapy begins and routinely thereafter. Pts with renal insufficiency, preexisting or during treatment, may require dose adjustment. HIV antibody testing should be performed before therapy begins (unrecognized or untreated HIV infection may result in emergence of HIV resistance).

INTERVENTION/EVALUATION

Monitor I&O, serum creatinine; AST, ALT, alkaline phosphatase, phosphorus levels. Closely monitor for adverse reactions in those taking other medications that are excreted renally or with other drugs known to affect renal function.

PATIENT/FAMILY TEACHING

• Report nausea, vomiting, abdominal pain. • Avoid alcohol.

---

adenosine

ah-**den**-oh-seen
(Adenocard, Adenoscan)

◆**CLASSIFICATION**
PHARMACOTHERAPEUTIC: Cardiac agent, diagnostic aid. **CLINICAL:** Antiarrhythmic.

ACTION

Slows impulse formation in SA node and conduction time through AV node. Acts as a diagnostic aid in myocardial perfusion imaging or stress echocardiography. **Therapeutic Effect:** Depresses left ventricular function, restores normal sinus rhythm.

USES

Adenocard: Treatment of paroxysmal supraventricular tachycardia (PSVT), including those associated with accessory bypass tracts (Wolff-Parkinson-White syndrome). **Adenoscan:** Adjunct in diagnosis in myocardial perfusion imaging or stress echo-cardiography. **OFF-LABEL:** Stable and unstable narrow complex regular tachycardia; stable regular monomorphic wide complex tachycardia; acute vasodilator testing in pulmonary artery hypertension.

PRECAUTIONS

Contraindications: Atrial fibrillation/flutter, second- or third-degree AV block, symptomatic bradycardia, sick sinus syndrome (except in pts with functioning pacemaker). Atrial fibrillation/flutter with underlying Wolff-Parkinson-White syndrome, bronchoconstrictive or bronchospastic lung disease, asthma. **Cautions:** Underlying dysfunction of sinus or AV node, obstructive lung disease, elderly, concurrent use of digoxin or verapamil. **Pregnancy Category C.**

INTERACTIONS

DRUG: Methylxanthines (e.g., theophylline) may decrease effect. **Dipyridamole, nicotine** may increase effect. **Carbamazepine** may increase degree of heart block caused by adenosine. **HERBAL:** None significant. **FOOD:** Avoid **caffeine** (may decrease effect). **LAB VALUES:** None significant.

AVAILABILITY (Rx)

Injection Solution (Adenocard): 3 mg/ml in 2-ml, 4-ml vials. **Injection Solution (Adenoscan):** 3 mg/ml in 20-ml, 30-ml vials.

ADMINISTRATION/HANDLING

 IV

Rate of Administration • Administer very rapidly (over 1–2 sec) undiluted directly into vein, or if using IV line, use closest port to insertion site. If IV line is infusing any fluid other than 0.9% NaCl, flush line first. • After rapid bolus injection, follow with 0.9% NaCl flush. **Storage** • Store at room temperature. Solution appears clear. • Crystallization occurs if refrigerated; if crystallization occurs, dissolve crystals by warming to room temperature. • Discard unused portion.

⊞ IV INCOMPATIBILITIES

Any drug or solution other than 0.9% NaCl, D_5W, Ringer's lactate, or abciximab.

INDICATIONS/ROUTES/DOSAGE

Paroxysmal Supraventricular Tachycardia (PSVT) (Adenocard)

Rapid IV Bolus: ADULTS, ELDERLY, CHILDREN WEIGHING 50 KG OR MORE: Initially, 6 mg given over 1–2 sec. If first dose does not convert within 1–2 min, give 12 mg; may repeat 12-mg dose in 1–2 min if no response has occurred. Follow each dose with 20 ml 0.9% NaCl by rapid IV push. **CHILDREN WEIGHING LESS THAN 50 KG:** Initially 0.05–0.1 mg/kg. If first dose does not convert within 1–2 min, may increase dose by 0.05–0.1 mg/kg. May repeat until sinus rhythm is established or up to a maximum single dose of 0.3 mg/kg or 12 mg. Follow each dose with 5–10 ml 0.9% NaCl by rapid IV push.

Diagnostic Testing (Adenoscan)

IV Infusion: ADULTS: 140 mcg/kg/min for 6 min using syringe or infusion pump. Total dose: 0.84 mg/kg. Thallium is injected at midpoint (3 min) of infusion.

SIDE EFFECTS

Frequent (18%–12%): Facial flushing, dyspnea. **Occasional (7%–2%):** Headache, nausea, light-headedness, chest pressure. **Rare (1% or less):** Paresthesia, dizziness, diaphoresis, hypotension, palpitations; chest, jaw, or neck pain.

ADVERSE EFFECTS/TOXIC REACTIONS

Frequently produces transient, short-lasting heart block.

NURSING CONSIDERATIONS

BASELINE ASSESSMENT

Identify arrhythmia per cardiac monitor, 12-lead EKG, and assess apical pulse.

INTERVENTION/EVALUATION

Assess cardiac performance per continuous EKG. Monitor B/P, apical pulse (rate, rhythm, quality). Auscultate pt breath sounds for clarity. Monitor respiratory rate. Monitor I&O; assess for fluid retention. Check electrolytes.

PATIENT/FAMILY TEACHING
• May induce feelings of impending doom, which resolves quickly. • Flushing/headache may occur temporarily following drug administration. • Report continued chest pain, light-headedness, head or neck pain, difficulty breathing.

ado-trastuzumab

ado-tras-**tooz**-oo-mab
(Kadcyla)

BLACK BOX ALERT Do not substitute ado-trastuzumab for trastuzumab. Hepatotoxicity, hepatic failure may lead to death. Monitor hepatic function prior to each dose. May decrease left ventricular ejection fraction (LVEF). Embryo-fetal toxicity may result in birth defects and/ or fetal demise.
Do not confuse ado-trastuzumab with trastuzumab.

◆ CLASSIFICATION

PHARMACOTHERAPEUTIC: HER2-targeted antibody and microtubule inhibitor conjugate. **CLINICAL:** Antineoplastic.

ACTION

Inhibits proliferation of tumor cells that overexpress human epidermal growth factor receptor 2 (HER2). Promotes cellular death (apoptosis) by mediating release of cytotoxic catabolytes. Disrupts cellular microtubule networks. **Therapeutic Effect:** Inhibits tumor cell survival in HER2-positive breast cancer.

PHARMACOKINETICS

Metabolized in liver. Protein binding: 93%. Peak plasma concentration: 30–90 min. **Half-life:** 4 days.

USES

Treatment of HER2-positive, metastatic breast cancer in pts who have previously received trastuzumab and a taxane agent separately or in combination, or pts who have developed recurrence within 6 mos of completing adjuvant therapy.

PRECAUTIONS

Contraindications: None known. **Cautions:** History of cardiomyopathy, HF, MI, arrhythmias, hepatic disease, thrombocytopenia, pulmonary disease, peripheral neuropathy, pregnancy.

⧖ LIFESPAN CONSIDERATIONS

Pregnancy/Lactation: May cause fetal harm. Use contraception during treatment and up to 6 mos after discontinuation. Unknown if distributed in breast milk. Do not breast-feed. **Pregnancy Category D. Children:** Safety and efficacy not established. **Elderly:** No age-related precautions noted.

INTERACTIONS

DRUG: CYP3A4 inhibitors (e.g., ketoconazole, ritonavir) may increase concentration/effect. **HERBAL:** None significant. **FOOD:** None known. **LAB VALUES:** May increase serum AST, ALT, bilirubin. May decrease platelets, serum potassium.

AVAILABILITY (Rx)

Lyophilized Powder for Injection: 100-mg vial, 160-mg vial.

ADMINISTRATION/HANDLING

◀ALERT▶ Use 0.22-micron in-line filter. Do not administer IV push or bolus.

 IV

Reconstitution • Use proper chemotherapy precautions. • Slowly inject 5 ml of Sterile Water for Injection into 100 mg vial or 8 ml Sterile Water for Injection for 160 mg vial. • Final concentration: 20 mg/ml. • Gently swirl until completely dissolved. • Do not shake. • Inspect for particulate matter/discoloration. • Calculate dose from 20 mg/ml vial. • Further dilute in 250 ml of 0.9% NaCl only. • Invert bag to avoid foaming.

Rate of Administration • Infuse initial dose over 90 min. • Infuse subsequent doses over 30 min. • Slow or interrupt infusion rate if hypersensitivity reaction occurs.

Storage • Solution should be slightly opalescent and clear to pale brown. Do not use if cloudy. • Diluted infusion solution may be refrigerated for up to 4 hrs prior to use.

▦ IV INCOMPATIBILITIES

Do not use dextrose-containing solutions.

INDICATIONS/ROUTES/DOSAGE

Metastatic Breast Cancer
IV Infusion: ADULTS/ELDERLY: 3.6 mg/kg every 3 wks.

Dose Modification
Reduction Schedule for Adverse Effects:
Initial dose: 3.6 mg/kg. First reduction: 3 mg/kg. Second reduction: 2.4 mg/kg. **Increased AST, ALT:** If less than 5 times upper limit normal (ULN), continue same dose. If 5–20 times ULN, hold until less than 5 times ULN and reduce by one dose level. If greater than 20 times ULN, discontinue. **Increased Bilirubin:** Hold until less than 1.5 times ULN, then continue same dose. If 3–10 times ULN, hold until less than 1.5 times ULN, then reduce by one dose level. If greater than 10 times ULN, discontinue. **Left Ventricular Dysfunction:** If LVEF greater than 45%, continue same dose. If LVEF 40%–45% with a decrease less than 10% from baseline, continue dose (or reduce) and repeat LVEF in 3 wks. If LVEF 40%–45% with decrease greater than 10% from baseline, hold and repeat assessment in 3 wks. Discontinue therapy if no recovery within 10% of baseline, LVEF less than 40%, or symptomatic CHF. **Thrombocytopenia:** If platelet count is 25,000 mm³–50,000 mm³, hold until level

greater than 75,000 mm³ and then continue same dose. If platelet count is less than 25,000 mm³, hold until level greater than 75,000 mm³ and reduce one dose level.

SIDE EFFECTS

Frequent (40%–21%): Nausea, fatigue, musculoskeletal pain, headache, constipation, diarrhea. **Occasional (19%–7%):** Abdominal pain, vomiting, pyrexia, arthralgia, asthenia, cough, dry mouth, stomatitis, myalgia, insomnia, rash, dizziness, dyspepsia, chills, dysgeusia, peripheral edema. **Rare (6%–3%):** Pruritus, blurry vision, dry eye, conjunctivitis, lacrimation.

ADVERSE EFFECTS/TOXIC REACTIONS

Hepatotoxicity may include elevated transaminase, nodular regenerative hyperplasia, portal hypertension. Left ventricular dysfunction reported in 1.8% of pts. Interstitial lung disease (ILD), including pneumonitis, may lead to ARDS. Hypersensitivity reactions (flushing, chills, pyrexia, dyspnea, hypotension, wheezing, bronchospasm, tachycardia) reported in 1.4% of pts. Thrombocytopenia (34% of pts) may increase risk of bleeding. Peripheral neuropathy (hypoesthesia, hyperesthesia, paresthesia, burning sensation, neuropathic pain or weakness) observed rarely. Approx. 5.3% of pts tested positive for anti–ado-trastuzumab antibodies (immunogenicity).

NURSING CONSIDERATIONS

BASELINE ASSESSMENT

Obtain baseline CBC, serum chemistries, PT/INR if on anticoagulants. Confirm HER2-positive titer. Screen for baseline HF, hepatic impairment, peripheral edema, pulmonary disease, thrombocytopenia. Obtain negative urine pregnancy test before initiating treatment. Question current breast-feeding status. Obtain baseline echocardiogram for LVEF status.

INTERVENTION/EVALUATION

Monitor for hypersensitivity reactions during infusion. Monitor hepatic function tests, potassium levels before and during treatment. Obtain LVEF q3mos or with any dose reduction regarding LVEF status. Assess for bruising, jaundice, right upper quadrant (RUQ) abdominal pain. Obtain anti–ado-trastuzumab antibody titer if immunogenicity suspected. Obtain stat EKG for palpitations or irregular pulse, chest x-ray for difficulty breathing, cough, fever. Monitor for neurotoxicity (peripheral neuropathy).

PATIENT/FAMILY TEACHING

• Blood levels will be monitored routinely. • Avoid pregnancy. • Contraception should be used during treatment and up to 6 mos after discontinuation. • Report any black/tarry stools, RUQ abdominal pain, nausea, bruising, yellowing of skin or eyes, difficulty breathing, palpitations, bleeding of any kind. • Avoid alcohol. • Treatment may reduce the heart's ability to pump; expect routine echocardiograms. • Report bleeding of any kind or extremity numbness, tingling, weakness, pain.

---

afatinib

a-**fa**-ti-nib
(Gilotrif)

◆ **CLASSIFICATION**

PHARMACOTHERAPEUTIC: Kinase inhibitor. **CLINICAL:** Antineoplastic.

ACTION

Inhibits tyrosine kinase activity in tumor cells by inhibiting autophosphorylation of cell lines with mutation-specific expression. **Therapeutic Effect:** Inhibits lung cancer growth and metastasis.

PHARMACOKINETICS

Readily absorbed following PO administration. Enzymatic metabolism is minimal. Protein binding: 95%. Peak plasma concentration: 2–5 hrs. Excreted in feces (85%), urine (4%). **Half-life:** 37 hrs.

USES

First-line treatment of metastatic non–small cell lung cancer (NSCLC) in pts with epidermal growth factor (EDGF) exon 19 deletions or exon 21 (L858R) substitution mutations.

PRECAUTIONS

Contraindications: None known. **Cautions:** Liver impairment, hypovolemia, pulmonary disease, ulcerative lesions.

⧗ LIFESPAN CONSIDERATIONS

Pregnancy/Lactation: May cause fetal harm. Unknown if distributed in breast milk. Must either discontinue drug or discontinue breastfeeding. Contraception recommended during treatment and up to 2 wks after discontinuation. **Pregnancy Category D. Children:** Safety and efficacy not established. **Elderly:** No age-related precautions noted.

INTERACTIONS

DRUG: P-glycoprotein inhibitors (e.g., amiodarone, cyclosporine, ketoconazole) may increase concentration/effect. **P-glycoprotein inducers (e.g., carbamazepine, rifampin)** may decrease concentration/effect. **HERBAL: St. John's wort** may decrease concentration/effect. **FOOD:** High-fat meals may decrease absorption. **LAB VALUES:** May increase serum ALT, AST. May decrease serum potassium.

AVAILABILITY (Rx)

Tablets: 20 mg, 30 mg, 40 mg.

ADMINISTRATION/HANDLING

PO
• Give at least 1 hr before or 2 hrs after meal.

INDICATIONS/ROUTES/DOSAGE

Non–Small Cell Lung Cancer

PO: ADULTS/ELDERLY: Initially, 40 mg once daily until disease progression or no longer tolerated.

Dose Modification

Chronic Use of P-glycoprotein (P-gp) Inhibitors: Reduce daily dose by 10 mg if tolerated. Resume previous dose after discontinuation of inhibitor if tolerated. **Chronic Use of P-glycoprotein Inducers:** Increase daily dose by 10 mg if tolerated. May resume initial dose 2–3 days after discontinuation of P-gp inducer. **Moderate to Severe Diarrhea (more than 48 hrs):** Withhold dose until resolution to mild diarrhea. **Moderate Cutaneous Skin Reaction (more than 7 days):** Withhold dose until reaction resolves, then reduce dose appropriately. **Suspected Keratitis:** Withhold until appropriately ruled out. If keratitis confirmed, continue only if benefits outweigh risks.

Permanent Discontinuation

Persistent severe diarrhea, respiratory distress, severe dry eye, or life-threatening bullous, blistering, exfoliating lesions.

SIDE EFFECTS

Frequent (96%–58%): Diarrhea, rash, dermatitis, stomatitis, paronychia (nail infection). **Occasional (31%–11%):** Dry skin, decreased appetite, pruritus, epistaxis, weight loss, cystitis, pyrexia, cheilitis (lip inflammation), rhinorrhea, conjunctivitis.

ADVERSE EFFECTS/ TOXIC REACTIONS

Diarrhea may lead to severe, sometimes fatal, dehydration or renal impairment. Bullous and exfoliative skin lesions occur rarely. Rash, erythema, acneiform lesions occur in 90% of pts. Palmar-plantar erythrodysesthesia syndrome (PPES), a chemotherapy-induced skin condition that presents with redness, swelling, numbness, skin sloughing of the hands and feet, has been reported. Interstitial lung disease (ILD), including pulmonary infiltration, pneumonitis, ARDS, allergic alveolitis, reported in 2% of pts. Hepatotoxicity reported in 10% of pts. Keratitis such as eye inflammation, lacrimation,

light sensitivity, blurred vision, red eye occur in 1% of pts.

NURSING CONSIDERATIONS

BASELINE ASSESSMENT

Obtain baseline CBC, serum chemistries, visual acuity. Obtain negative pregnancy test before initiating therapy. Question current breastfeeding status. Screen for history/co-morbidities, contact lens use. Receive full medication history including vitamins, herbal products. Assess skin for lesions, ulcers, open wounds.

INTERVENTION/EVALUATION

Monitor renal/hepatic function tests, urine output. Encourage PO intake. Assess for hydration status. Offer antidiarrheal medication for loose stool. Report oliguria, dark or concentrated urine. Immediately report skin lesion, vision changes, dry eye, severe diarrhea. Obtain chest x-ray if ILD suspected.

PATIENT/FAMILY TEACHING

• Most pts experience diarrhea and severe cases may lead to dehydration or kidney failure; maintain adequate hydration. • Avoid pregnancy; contraception should be used during treatment and up to 2 wks after discontinuation. • Report any yellowing of skin or eyes, abdominal pain, bruising, black/tarry stools, dark urine, decreased urine output. • Minimize exposure to sunlight. • Immediately report eye problems (pain, swelling, blurred vision, vision changes) or skin blistering/redness. • Do not eat 1 hr before or 2 hrs after dose. • Do not wear contact lenses (may increase risk of keratitis).

albumin, human

al-**bue**-min
(Albuminar-5, Albuminar-25, AlbuRx, Albutein, Buminate, Flexbumin, Plasbumin)

Do not confuse albumin with albuterol, or Buminate with bumetanide.

◆CLASSIFICATION

PHARMACOTHERAPEUTIC: Plasma protein fraction. **CLINICAL:** Blood derivative.

ACTION

Blood volume expander. **Therapeutic Effect:** Provides temporary increase in blood volume, reduces hemoconcentration and blood viscosity.

PHARMACOKINETICS

Route	Onset	Peak	Duration
IV	15 min (in well-hydrated pt)	N/A	Dependent on initial blood volume

Distributed throughout extracellular fluid. **Half-life:** 15–20 days.

USES

Used for plasma volume expansion, maintenance of cardiac output in treatment of shock or impending shock. May be useful in treatment of severe burns, adult respiratory distress syndrome (ARDS), cardiopulmonary bypass, hemodialysis. **OFF-LABEL:** Large-volume paracentesis. In cirrhotics, with diuretics to help facilitate diuresis; volume expansion in dehydrated, mildly hypotensive cirrhotics. Used for prevention of renal impairment; reduced mortality associated with spontaneous bacterial peritonitis.

PRECAUTIONS

Contraindications: Heart failure, severe anemia. **Cautions:** Pts for whom sodium restriction is necessary, hepatic/renal failure. Avoid 25% concentration in preterm infants.

⌛ LIFESPAN CONSIDERATIONS

Pregnancy/Lactation: Unknown if drug crosses placenta or is distributed in breast milk. **Pregnancy Category C. Children/Elderly:** No age-related precautions noted.

INTERACTIONS

DRUG: None significant. **HERBAL:** None significant. **FOOD:** None known. **LAB VALUES:** May increase serum alkaline phosphatase.

AVAILABILITY (Rx)

Injection Solution: (5%): 50 ml, 250 ml, 500 ml. **(25%):** 20 ml, 50 ml, 100 ml.

ADMINISTRATION/HANDLING
🖐 IV

Reconstitution • A 5% solution may be made from 25% solution by adding 1 volume 25% to 4 volumes 0.9% NaCl (NaCl preferred). Do not use Sterile Water for Injection (life-threatening hemolysis, acute renal failure can result).
Rate of Administration • Give by IV infusion. Rate is variable, depending on use, blood volume, concentration of solute. 5%: Do not exceed 2–4 ml/min in pts with normal plasma volume, 5–10 ml/min in pts with hypoproteinemia. 25%: Do not exceed 1 ml/min in pts with normal plasma volume, 2–3 ml/min in pts with hypoproteinemia. 5% is administered undiluted; 25% may be administered undiluted or diluted. • May give without regard to pt blood group or Rh factor.
Storage • Store at room temperature. Appears as clear, brownish, odorless, moderately viscous fluid. • Do not use if solution has been frozen, appears turbid, contains sediment, or if not used within 4 hrs of opening vial.

🖼 IV INCOMPATIBILITIES

Lipids, micafungin (Mycamine), midazolam (Versed), vancomycin (Vancocin), verapamil (Isoptin).

🖼 IV COMPATIBILITIES

Diltiazem (Cardizem), lorazepam (Ativan).

INDICATIONS/ROUTES/DOSAGE

◀ **ALERT** ▶ 5% should be used in hypovolemic or intravascularly depleted pts. 25% should be used in pts in whom fluid and sodium intake must be minimized.

Usual Dosage
IV: ADULTS, ELDERLY: Initially, 25 g; may repeat in 15–30 min. **Maximum:** 250 g within 48 hrs.

Hypovolemia
IV: ADULTS, ELDERLY: 5% albumin: 0.5–1 g/kg/dose, repeat as needed. **CHILDREN:** 0.5–1 g/kg/dose (10–20 ml/kg/dose of 5% albumin). **Maximum:** 6 g/kg/day.

Hypoproteinemia
IV: ADULTS, ELDERLY, CHILDREN: 0.5–1 g/kg/dose, repeat every 1–2 days as needed to replace ongoing losses.

Hemodialysis
IV: ADULTS, ELDERLY: 50–100 ml (12.5–25 g) of 25% albumin as needed.

SIDE EFFECTS

Occasional: Hypotension. **Rare:** High dose in repeated therapy: altered vital signs, chills, fever, increased salivation, nausea, vomiting, urticaria, tachycardia.

ADVERSE EFFECTS/ TOXIC REACTIONS

Fluid overload may occur, marked by increased B/P, distended neck veins. Pulmonary edema may occur, evidenced by labored respirations, dyspnea, rales, wheezing, coughing. Neurologic changes that may occur include headache, weakness, blurred vision, behavioral changes, incoordination, isolated muscle twitching.

NURSING CONSIDERATIONS

BASELINE ASSESSMENT
Obtain B/P, pulse, respirations immediately before administration. Adequate hydration required before albumin is administered.

INTERVENTION/EVALUATION
Monitor B/P for hypotension/hypertension. Monitor Hgb, Hct, urine specific gravity. Assess frequently for evidence of fluid overload, pulmonary edema (see Adverse Effects/Toxic Reactions). Check skin for flushing, urticaria. Monitor I&O ratio (watch for decreased output). Assess for therapeutic response (increased B/P, decreased edema).

---

albuterol
TOP 200

al-**bue**-ter-ol
(AccuNeb, Airomir ♣, Apo-Salvent ♣, PMS-Salbutamol ♣, ProAir HFA, Proventil HFA, Ventolin HFA, VoSpire ER)
Do not confuse albuterol with Albumin or atenolol, Proventil with Bentyl, Prilosec, or Prinivil, or Ventolin with Benylin or Vantin.

FIXED-COMBINATION(S)

Combivent: albuterol/ipratropium (a bronchodilator): 103 mcg/18 mcg per actuation. **DuoNeb:** albuterol/ipratropium 3 mg/0.5 mg.

◆CLASSIFICATION

PHARMACOTHERAPEUTIC: Sympathomimetic (adrenergic agonist). **CLINICAL:** Bronchodilator (see p. 76C).

ACTION

Stimulates beta$_2$-adrenergic receptors in lungs, resulting in relaxation of bronchial smooth muscle. **Therapeutic Effect:** Relieves bronchospasm and reduces airway resistance.

PHARMACOKINETICS

Route	Onset	Peak	Duration
PO	15–30 min	2–3 hrs	4–6 hrs
PO (extended-release)	30 min	2–4 hrs	12 hrs
Inhalation	5–15 min	0.5–2 hrs	2–5 hrs

♣ Canadian trade name   🗡 Non-Crushable Drug   🟥 High Alert drug

Rapidly, well absorbed from GI tract; rapidly absorbed from bronchi after inhalation. Metabolized in liver. Primarily excreted in urine. **Half-life:** 3.8–6 hrs.

USES

Relief of bronchospasm due to reversible obstructive airway disease, prevention of exercise-induced bronchospasm.

PRECAUTIONS

Contraindications: History of hypersensitivity to sympathomimetics. **Cautions:** Hypertension, cardiovascular disease, hyperthyroidism, diabetes mellitus, heart failure, convulsive disorders, glaucoma, hypokalemia, arrhythmias.

⌛ LIFESPAN CONSIDERATIONS

Pregnancy/Lactation: Appears to cross placenta; unknown if distributed in breast milk. May inhibit uterine contractility. **Pregnancy Category C. Children:** Safety and efficacy not established in those younger than 2 yrs (syrup) or younger than 6 yrs (tablets). **Elderly:** May be more sensitive to tremor or tachycardia due to age-related increased sympathetic sensitivity.

INTERACTIONS

DRUG: Beta-adrenergic blocking agents (beta-blockers) antagonize effects. May produce bronchospasm. **Atomoxetine, MAOIs, tricyclic antidepressants** may potentiate cardiovascular effects. May increase effects of **loop diuretics** (produce hypokalemia), **sympathomimetics** (increase CNS stimulation). **HERBAL: St. John's wort** may decrease levels/effects. **Ephedra, yohimbe** may cause CNS stimulation. **FOOD:** Limit caffeine (may cause CNS stimulation). **LAB VALUES:** May increase blood glucose level. May decrease serum potassium level.

AVAILABILITY (Rx)

Inhalation Aerosol (ProAir HFA, Proventil HFA, Ventolin HFA): 90 mcg/spray. **Solution for Nebulization: AccuNeb:** 0.63 mg/3 ml (0.021%), 1.25 mg/3 ml (0.042%). **Proventil:** 2.5 mg/3 ml (0.084%), 5 mg/ml (0.5%). **Syrup:** 2 mg/5 ml. **Tablets (Proventil, Ventolin):** 2 mg, 4 mg.

🔖 **Tablets (Extended-Release [VoSpire ER]):** 4 mg, 8 mg.

ADMINISTRATION/HANDLING

PO
• Do not break, chew, crush, or divide extended-release tablets. • Administer with food.

Inhalation
• Shake container well before inhalation.
• Wait 2 min before inhaling second dose (allows for deeper bronchial penetration). • Rinse mouth with water immediately after inhalation (prevents mouth/throat dryness).

Nebulization
• Administer over 5–15 min. • Nebulizer should be used with compressed air or O_2 at rate of 6–10 L/min.

INDICATIONS/ROUTES/DOSAGE

Acute Bronchospasm
Inhalation: ADULTS, ELDERLY, CHILDREN OLDER THAN 12 YRS: 4–8 puffs q20min up to 4 hrs, then q1–4h as needed. **CHILDREN 12 YRS AND YOUNGER:** 4–8 puffs q20min for 3 doses, then q1–4h as needed.
Nebulization: ADULTS, ELDERLY, CHILDREN OLDER THAN 12 YRS: 2.5–5 mg q20min for 3 doses, then 2.5–10 mg q1–4h or 10–15 mg/hr continuously. **CHILDREN 12 YRS AND YOUNGER:** 0.15 mg/kg q20min for 3 doses (minimum: 2.5 mg), then 0.15–0.3 mg/kg q1–4h as needed. **Maximum:** 10 mg q1–4h as needed or 0.5 mg/kg/hr by continuous infusion.

Chronic Bronchospasm
PO: ADULTS, CHILDREN OLDER THAN 12 YRS: 2–4 mg 3–4 times a day. **Maximum:** 8 mg 4 times a day. **ELDERLY:** 2 mg 3–4 times a

day. **Maximum:** 8 mg 4 times a day. **CHILDREN 6–12 YRS:** 2 mg 3–4 times a day. **Maximum:** 24 mg/day. **CHILDREN 2–5 YRS:** 0.1–0.2 mg/kg/dose 3 times a day. **Maximum:** 4 mg 3 times a day.

PO *(Extended-Release)*: **ADULTS, CHILDREN OLDER THAN 12 YRS:** 4–8 mg q12h. **Maximum:** 32 mg/day. **CHILDREN 6–12 YRS:** 4 mg q12h. **Maximum:** 24 mg/day. **Nebulization: ADULTS, ELDERLY, CHILDREN 5 YRS AND OLDER:** 1.25–5 mg q4–8h as needed. **CHILDREN 4 YRS AND YOUNGER:** 0.63–2.5 mg q4–6h as needed. **Inhalation: ADULTS, ELDERLY, CHILDREN 4 YRS AND OLDER:** 1–2 puffs q4–6h. **Maximum:** 12 puffs per day.

Exercise-Induced Bronchospasm
Inhalation: ADULTS, ELDERLY, CHILDREN 5 YRS AND OLDER: 2 puffs 5–30 min before exercise. **CHILDREN 4 YRS AND YOUNGER:** 1–2 puffs 5 min before exercise.

Usual Neonatal Dosage
Nebulization: 1.25–2.5 mg q8h. **Inhalation:** (mechanically ventilated) 90 mcg/spray, 1–2 sprays q6h.

SIDE EFFECTS

Frequent: Headache (27%); restlessness, nervousness, tremors (20%); nausea (15%); dizziness (less than 7%); throat dryness and irritation, pharyngitis (less than 6%); B/P changes, including hypertension (5%–3%); heartburn, transient wheezing (less than 5%). **Occasional (3%–2%):** Insomnia, asthenia (loss of strength, energy), altered taste. **Inhalation:** Dry, irritated mouth or throat; cough; bronchial irritation. **Rare:** Drowsiness, diarrhea, dry mouth, flushing, diaphoresis, anorexia.

ADVERSE EFFECTS/TOXIC REACTIONS

Excessive sympathomimetic stimulation may produce palpitations, exectopy, tachycardia, chest pain, slight increase in B/P followed by substantial decrease, chills, diaphoresis, blanching of skin. Too-frequent or excessive use may lead to decreased bronchodilating effectiveness and severe, paradoxical bronchoconstriction.

NURSING CONSIDERATIONS

BASELINE ASSESSMENT

Assess lung sounds, pulse, B/P, color, character of sputum noted. Offer emotional support (high incidence of anxiety due to difficulty in breathing and sympathomimetic response to drug).

INTERVENTION/EVALUATION

Monitor rate, depth, rhythm, type of respiration; quality and rate of pulse; EKG; serum potassium, glucose; ABG determinations. Assess lung sounds for wheezing (bronchoconstriction), rales.

PATIENT/FAMILY TEACHING

• Follow guidelines for proper use of inhaler. • Increase fluid intake (decreases lung secretion viscosity). • Do not take more than 2 inhalations at any one time (excessive use may produce paradoxical bronchoconstriction or decreased bronchodilating effect). • Rinsing mouth with water immediately after inhalation may prevent mouth/throat dryness. • Avoid excessive use of caffeine derivatives (chocolate, coffee, tea, cola, cocoa).

alemtuzumab HIGH ALERT

al-em-**tooz**-ue-mab
(MabCampath ✦)
BLACK BOX ALERT Serious infections (bacterial, viral, fungal, protozoal) have been reported. Potentially fatal infusion-related reactions (respiratory distress, cardiac arrest, hypotension) may occur. Profound myelosuppression (autoimmune hemolytic anemia, thrombocytopenia) has occurred.

◆CLASSIFICATION

PHARMACOTHERAPEUTIC: Monoclonal antibody. **CLINICAL:** Antineoplastic (see p. 81C).

✦ Canadian trade name   🗲 Non-Crushable Drug   **HIGH ALERT** High Alert drug

ACTION

Binds to CD52, cell surface glycoprotein, found on surface of all B- and T-lymphocytes, most monocytes, macrophages, natural killer cells, granulocytes. **Therapeutic Effect:** Produces cytotoxicity, reducing tumor size.

PHARMACOKINETICS

Half-life: About 12 days. Peak and trough levels rise during first few wks of therapy and approach steady state by about wk 6.

USES

Treatment of B-cell chronic lymphocytic leukemia (B-CLL). **OFF-LABEL:** Treatment of refractory, cutaneous, peripheral T-cell leukemia; autoimmune cytopenia; preconditioning regimen for stem cell transplantation, renal and liver transplantation, relapsing-remitting multiple sclerosis.

PRECAUTIONS

Contraindications: None known. **Cautions:** Ischemic heart disease or those taking antihypertensive medications.

⏳ LIFESPAN CONSIDERATIONS

Pregnancy/Lactation: Has potential to cause fetal B- and T-lymphocyte depletion. Breast-feeding not recommended during treatment and for at least 3 mos after last dose. **Pregnancy Category C. Children:** Safety and efficacy not established. **Elderly:** No age-related precautions noted.

INTERACTIONS

DRUG: May increase levels/effects of **clozapine, natalizumab, vaccines (live). Pimecrolimus, tacrolimus** may decrease levels/effect. **HERBAL: Echinacea** may decrease effect. **FOOD:** None known. **LAB VALUES:** May decrease Hgb, platelet count, WBC count.

AVAILABILITY (Rx)

Injection Solution: 30 mg/ml.

ADMINISTRATION/HANDLING

 IV

◀**ALERT**▶ Do not give by IV push or bolus.

Reconstitution • Withdraw needed amount from ampule into a syringe. • Using a low protein-binding, non–fiber-releasing 5-micron filter, inject into 100 ml 0.9% NaCl or D$_5$W. • Invert bag to mix; do not shake.
Rate of Administration • Give the 100 ml solution as a 2-hr IV infusion.
Storage • Refrigerate undiluted ampules; do not freeze. (If frozen, may be thawed in refrigerator.) • Use within 8 hrs after dilution. Diluted solution may be stored at room temperature or refrigerated. • Discard if particulate matter is present or if solution is discolored.

🧫 IV INCOMPATIBILITIES

Do not mix with any other medications.

INDICATIONS/ROUTES/DOSAGE

◀**ALERT**▶ Pretreatment with acetaminophen 500–1,000 mg and diphenhydramine 50 mg before each infusion may prevent infusion-related side effects.

Chronic Lymphocytic Leukemia
◀**ALERT**▶ Dose escalation required. Do not exceed single doses greater than 30 mg or cumulative doses more than 90 mg/wk.
IV: ADULTS, ELDERLY: Initially, 3 mg/day as a 2-hr infusion. When tolerated (with only low-grade or no infusion-related toxicities), increase daily dose to 10 mg. When the 10 mg/day dose is tolerated, maintenance dose may be initiated. Maintenance: 30 mg/day 3 times a wk on alternate days (such as Monday, Wednesday, and Friday or Tuesday, Thursday, and Saturday) for up to 12 wks. The increase to 30 mg/day is usually achieved in 3–7 days. Adjust dosage for hematologic toxicity (severe neutropenia or thrombocytopenia).

SIDE EFFECTS

Frequent: Rigors, tremors (86%), fever (85%), nausea (54%), vomiting (41%), rash (40%), fatigue (34%), hypotension (32%), urticaria (30%), pruritus, skeletal pain, headache (24%), diarrhea (22%), anorexia (20%). **Occasional (less than 10%):** Myalgia, dizziness, abdominal pain, throat irritation, vomiting, neutropenia, rhinitis, bronchospasm, urticaria.

ADVERSE EFFECTS/ TOXIC REACTIONS

Neutropenia occurs in 85% of pts, anemia occurs in 80% of pts, and thrombocytopenia occurs in 72% of pts. Rash occurs in 40% of pts. Respiratory toxicity, manifested as dyspnea, cough, bronchitis, pneumonitis, and pneumonia, occurs in 26%–16% of pts. Serious, sometimes fatal bacterial, viral, fungal, and protozoan infections have been reported.

NURSING CONSIDERATIONS

BASELINE ASSESSMENT

Pretreatment with acetaminophen and diphenhydramine before each infusion may prevent infusion-related side effects. CBC, platelet count should be obtained frequently during and after therapy to assess for neutropenia, anemia, thrombocytopenia.

INTERVENTION/EVALUATION

Monitor for infusion-related symptoms complex consisting mainly of rigors, fever, chills, hypotension, generally occurring within 30 min–2 hrs of beginning of first infusion. Slowing infusion rate resolves symptoms. Monitor for hematologic toxicity (fever, sore throat, signs of local infection, unusual bleeding/bruising from any site), symptoms of anemia (excessive fatigue, weakness).

PATIENT/FAMILY TEACHING

• Avoid crowds, those with known infection. • Avoid contact with those who recently received live virus vaccine; do not receive vaccinations. • Report dyspnea, fever, chills, rash, nausea.

alendronate TOP 200

a-**len**-dro-nate
(Apo-Alendronate ✦, Binosto, Fosamax)
Do not confuse alendronate with risedronate, or Fosamax with Flomax.

FIXED-COMBINATION(S)

Fosamax Plus D: alendronate/cholecalciferol (vitamin D analogue): 70 mg/2,800 international units, 70 mg/5,600 international units.

◆CLASSIFICATION

PHARMACOTHERAPEUTIC: Bisphosphonate. **CLINICAL:** Bone resorption inhibitor, calcium regulator (see p. 142C).

ACTION

Inhibits normal and abnormal bone resorption, without retarding mineralization. **Therapeutic Effect:** Leads to significantly increased bone mineral density; reverses progression of osteoporosis.

PHARMACOKINETICS

Poorly absorbed after PO administration. Protein binding: 78%. After PO administration, rapidly taken into bone, with uptake greatest at sites of active bone turnover. Excreted in urine, feces (as unabsorbed drug). **Terminal half-life:** Greater than 10 yrs (reflects release from skeleton as bone is resorbed).

USES

Treatment of osteoporosis in men. Treatment of glucocorticoid-induced osteoporosis in men and women with low bone mineral density who are receiving at least 7.5 mg prednisone (or equivalent), treatment and prevention of osteoporosis in postmenopausal women, treatment of Paget's disease. **Binosto:** Treatment of osteoporosis in post-menopausal women. Increase bone mass in men with osteoporosis.

✦ Canadian trade name 🚫 Non-Crushable Drug 🔺 High Alert drug

PRECAUTIONS

Contraindications: Hypocalcemia, abnormalities of the esophagus, inability to stand or sit upright for at least 30 min, sensitivity to alendronate or other bisphosphonates; oral solution should not be used in pts at risk for aspiration. **Cautions:** Renal impairment, dysphagia, esophageal disease, gastritis, ulcers, or duodenitis.

⌛ LIFESPAN CONSIDERATIONS

Pregnancy/Lactation: Possible incomplete fetal ossification, decreased maternal weight gain, delay in delivery. Unknown if distributed in breast milk. Breastfeeding not recommended. **Pregnancy Category C. Children:** Safety and efficacy not established. **Elderly:** No age-related precautions noted.

INTERACTIONS

DRUG: Calcium, antacids may decrease absorption. **Aspirin, NSAIDs** may increase risk of ulcers, upper GI adverse effects. **HERBAL:** None significant. **FOOD:** Concurrent **beverages, dietary supplements, food** may interfere with alendronate absorption. **Caffeine** may reduce efficacy. **LAB VALUES:** Reduces serum calcium, phosphate concentrations. Significant decrease in serum alkaline phosphatase noted in those with Paget's disease.

AVAILABILITY (Rx)

Tablets: 5 mg, 10 mg, 35 mg, 40 mg, 70 mg. **Tablets, Effervescent: (Binosto):** 70 mg.

ADMINISTRATION/HANDLING

PO

• Give at least 30 min before first food, beverage, or medication of the day. • **Tablets:** Give with 6–8 oz plain water only (mineral water, coffee, tea, juice will decrease absorption). • **Tablets, Effervescent:** Dissolve in 4 oz water. Wait at least 5 min after effervescence stops. Stir for 10 sec and take.

INDICATIONS/ROUTES/DOSAGE

Osteoporosis (in Men)
PO: ADULTS, ELDERLY: 10 mg once a day in the morning or 70 mg weekly.

Glucocorticoid-Induced Osteoporosis
PO: ADULTS, ELDERLY: 5 mg once a day in the morning. **POSTMENOPAUSAL WOMEN NOT RECEIVING ESTROGEN:** 10 mg once a day in the morning.

Postmenopausal Osteoporosis
PO *(Treatment)*: **ADULTS, ELDERLY:** 10 mg once a day in the morning or 70 mg weekly.
PO *(Prevention)*: **ADULTS, ELDERLY:** 5 mg once a day in the morning or 35 mg weekly.

Paget's Disease
PO: ADULTS, ELDERLY: 40 mg once a day in the morning for 6 mos.

Dosage in Renal Impairment
Not recommended with creatinine clearance less than 35 ml/min.

SIDE EFFECTS

Frequent (8%–7%): Back pain, abdominal pain. **Occasional (3%–2%):** Nausea, abdominal distention, constipation, diarrhea, flatulence. **Rare (less than 2%):** Rash; severe bone, joint, muscle pain.

ADVERSE EFFECTS/ TOXIC REACTIONS

Overdose produces hypocalcemia, hypophosphatemia, significant GI disturbances. Esophageal irritation occurs if not given with 6–8 oz of plain water or if pt lies down within 30 min of administration.

NURSING CONSIDERATIONS

BASELINE ASSESSMENT

Hypocalcemia, vitamin D deficiency must be corrected before therapy. Check serum chemistries (esp. calcium, phosphorus, alkaline phosphatase serum levels).

INTERVENTION/EVALUATION

Monitor chemistries (esp. serum calcium, phosphorus, alkaline phosphatase levels).

PATIENT/FAMILY TEACHING

• Expected benefits occur only when medication is taken with full glass (6–8 oz) of plain water, first thing in the morning and at least 30 min before first food, beverage, or medication of the day is taken. Any other beverage (mineral water, orange juice, coffee) significantly reduces absorption of medication. • Do not lie down for at least 30 min after taking medication (potentiates delivery to stomach, reducing risk of esophageal irritation). • Report if swallowing difficulties develop, pain when swallowing, chest pain, new/worsening heartburn. • Consider weight-bearing exercises, modify behavioral factors (e.g., cigarette smoking, alcohol consumption). • Supplemental calcium and vitamin D should be taken if dietary intake inadequate.

---

alfuzosin

al-fue-**zoe**-sin
(Apo-Alfuzosin ✲, Uroxatral,
Xatral ✲)

◆CLASSIFICATION

PHARMACOTHERAPEUTIC: Alpha$_1$-adrenergic blocker. **CLINICAL:** Benign prostatic hyperplasia agent.

ACTION

Targets receptors around bladder neck and prostate capsule. **Therapeutic Effect:** Relaxes smooth muscle; improves urinary flow, symptoms of prostatic hyperplasia.

PHARMACOKINETICS

Readily absorbed (decreased under fasting conditions). Protein binding: 90%. Metabolized in liver. Primarily excreted in urine. **Half-life:** 10 hrs.

USES

Treatment of signs and symptoms of benign prostatic hyperplasia (BPH).

PRECAUTIONS

Contraindications: Moderate to severe hepatic impairment; concurrent use of strong CYP3A4 inhibitors (e.g., ketoconazole). **Cautions:** Pts with known QT prolongation. Severe renal or mild hepatic impairment.

⌛ LIFESPAN CONSIDERATIONS

Pregnancy/Lactation: Not indicated for use in this pt population. **Pregnancy Category B. Children:** Not indicated for use in this pt population. **Elderly:** No age-related precautions noted.

INTERACTIONS

DRUG: Other alpha-blocking agents (doxazosin, prazosin, tamsulosin, terazosin) may have additive effect. **CYP3A4 inhibitors (e.g., ritonavir, ketoconazole) PDE5 inhibitors (e.g., sildenafil)** may increase levels/effects. **HERBAL: St. John's wort** may decrease levels/effect. **FOOD: Food** increases absorption. **LAB VALUES:** None significant.

AVAILABILITY (Rx)

🗲 Tablets (Extended-Release): 10 mg.

ADMINISTRATION/HANDLING

PO
• Give immediately after the same meal each day. • Swallow whole; do not break, chew, crush, or dissolve extended-release tablets.

INDICATIONS/ROUTES/DOSAGE

Benign Prostatic Hyperplasia
PO: ADULTS: 10 mg once a day, after same meal each day.

SIDE EFFECTS

Frequent (7%–6%): Dizziness, headache, malaise. **Occasional (4%):** Dry mouth. **Rare (3%–2%):** Nausea, dyspepsia (heartburn, epigastric discomfort), diarrhea,

---

orthostatic hypotension, tachycardia, drowsiness.

ADVERSE EFFECTS/ TOXIC REACTIONS

Ischemia-related chest pain may occur rarely (2%). Priapism has been reported.

NURSING CONSIDERATIONS

BASELINE ASSESSMENT

Question for sensitivity to alfuzosin, use of other alpha-blocking agents (doxazosin, prazosin, tamsulosin, terazosin). Obtain B/P.

INTERVENTION/EVALUATION

Assist with ambulation if dizziness occurs. Report headache. Monitor for hypotension. Question for improvement in urine flow, hesitancy.

PATIENT/FAMILY TEACHING

• Take after the same meal each day.
• Avoid tasks that require alertness, motor skills until response to drug is established. • Do not break, chew, crush, or dissolve extended-release tablets.

---

aliskiren   TOP 200   HIGH ALERT

a-lis-**kye**-ren
(Rasilez ❋, Tekturna)

BLACK BOX ALERT May cause fetal injury, mortality if used during second or third trimester of pregnancy. **Do not confuse Tekturna with Valturna.**

FIXED-COMBINATION(S)

Amturnide: aliskiren/amlodipine (a calcium channel blocker)/hydrochlorothiazide (a diuretic): 150 mg/ 5 mg/12.5 mg, 300 mg/5 mg/12.5 mg, 300 mg/5 mg/25 mg, 300 mg/ 10 mg/12.5 mg, 300 mg/10 mg/ 25 mg. **Tekamlo:** aliskiren/amlodipine (a calcium channel blocker): 150 mg/5 mg, 150 mg/10 mg, 300

mg/5 mg, 300 mg/10 mg. **Tekturna HCT:** aliskiren/hydrochlorothiazide (a diuretic): 150 mg/12.5 mg, 150 mg/25 mg, 300 mg/12.5 mg, 300 mg/25 mg. **Valturna:** aliskiren/valsartan (an angiotensin II receptor antagonist): 150 mg/160 mg, 300 mg/320 mg.

◆CLASSIFICATION

PHARMACOTHERAPEUTIC: Renin-angiotensin system antagonist. **CLINICAL:** Antihypertensive (see p. 63C).

ACTION

Direct renin inhibitor. Decreases plasma renin activity (PRA), inhibiting the conversion of angiotensinogen to angiotensin I, blocking the effect of increased renin levels. **Therapeutic Effect:** Reduces B/P.

PHARMACOKINETICS

Peak plasma concentration reached within 1–3 hrs. Protein binding: 49%. Metabolized in liver. Minimally excreted in urine. Peak plasma steady-state levels reached in 7–8 days. **Half-life:** 24 hrs.

USES

Treatment of hypertension. May be used alone or in combination with other antihypertensives. **OFF-LABEL:** Treatment of persistent proteinuria in pts with type 2 diabetes, hypertension, nephropathy.

PRECAUTIONS

Contraindications: Concurrent use with ACE inhibitor or Angiotensin II Receptor Blockers in pts with diabetes. **Cautions:** Severe renal impairment. History of angioedema, dialysis, nephrotic syndrome, renovascular hypertension. Concurrent use with P-glycoprotein inhibitors (e.g., cyclosporine).

LIFESPAN CONSIDERATIONS

Pregnancy/Lactation: Carcinogenic potential to fetus. May cause fetal/neonatal morbidity, mortality. Unknown if distributed in breast milk. **Pregnancy Cate-**

gory C (**D if used in second or third trimester**). **Children:** Safety and efficacy not established. **Elderly:** No age-related precautions noted.

INTERACTIONS

DRUG: Cyclosporine, itraconazole may increase levels. **HERBAL: Ephedra, ginseng, yohimbe** may worsen hypertension. **Garlic, black cohosh** may increase antihypertensive effect. **FOOD: High-fat meals** substantially decrease absorption. **Grapefruit** may reduce antihypertensive effects. Separate by 4 hrs. **LAB VALUES:** May increase BUN, serum creatinine, uric acid, creatinine kinase, potassium. May decrease Hgb, Hct.

AVAILABILITY (Rx)

⬛ Tablets, Film-Coated: 150 mg, 300 mg.

ADMINISTRATION/HANDLING

PO
• High-fat meals substantially decrease absorption. • Consistent administration with regard to meals is recommended. • Do not crush film-coated tablets.

INDICATIONS/ROUTES/DOSAGE

Hypertension
PO: ADULTS, ELDERLY: Initially, 150 mg/ day. May increase to 300 mg/day.

SIDE EFFECTS

Rare (2%–1%): Diarrhea, particularly in women, elderly (older than 65 yrs), gastroesophageal reflux, cough, rash.

ADVERSE EFFECTS/ TOXIC REACTIONS

Angioedema, periorbital edema, edema of hands, generalized edema have been reported.

NURSING CONSIDERATIONS

BASELINE ASSESSMENT

Correct hypovolemia in pts on concurrent diuretic therapy. Obtain B/P and apical pulse immediately before each dose, in addition to regular monitoring (be alert to fluctuations). If excessive reduction in B/P occurs, place pt in supine position, feet slightly elevated.

INTERVENTION/EVALUATION

Assess for edema. Monitor I&O; weigh daily. Monitor daily pattern of bowel activity, stool consistency. Monitor B/P, renal function tests, potassium, Hgb, Hct.

PATIENT/FAMILY TEACHING

• Pregnant pts should avoid second- and third-trimester exposure to aliskiren.
• Report if diarrhea, swelling of face/lips/ tongue, difficulty breathing occurs. • Avoid strenuous exercise during hot weather (risk of dehydration, hypotension).

allopurinol   TOP 200

al-oh-**pure**-i-nole
(Aloprim, Apo-Allopurinol ✦, Novo-Purol ✦, Zyloprim)
Do not confuse allopurinol with Apresoline or haloperidol, or Zyloprim with Zorprin or Zovirax.

◆**CLASSIFICATION**

PHARMACOTHERAPEUTIC: Xanthine oxidase inhibitor. **CLINICAL:** Antigout.

ACTION

Decreases uric acid production by inhibiting xanthine oxidase, an enzyme. **Therapeutic Effect:** Reduces uric acid concentrations in serum and urine.

PHARMACOKINETICS

Route	Onset	Peak	Duration
PO, IV	2–3 days	1–3 wks	1–2 wks

Well absorbed from GI tract. Widely distributed. Protein binding: less than 1%. Metabolized in liver to active metabolite. Excreted primarily in urine. Removed by hemodialysis. **Half-life:** 1–3 hrs; metabolite, 12–30 hrs.

USES

PO: Management of primary or secondary gout (e.g., acute attack, nephropathy). Treatment of secondary hyperuricemia that may occur during cancer treatment. Management of recurrent uric acid and calcium oxalate calculi. **Injection:** Management of elevated uric acid in cancer treatment for leukemia, lymphoma, or solid tumor malignancies. **OFF-LABEL:** In mouthwash following fluorouracil therapy to prevent stomatitis.

PRECAUTIONS

Contraindications: None known. **Cautions:** Renal/hepatic impairment, pts taking diuretics, mercaptopurine or azathioprine, other drugs causing myelosuppression. Do not use in asymptomatic hyperuricemia.

⧖ LIFESPAN CONSIDERATIONS

Pregnancy/Lactation: Unknown if drug crosses placenta or is distributed in breast milk. **Pregnancy Category C. Children/Elderly:** No age-related precautions noted.

INTERACTIONS

DRUG: Thiazide diuretics may increase effect. May increase effect of **oral anticoagulants.** May increase concentration, toxicity of **azathioprine, mercaptopurine. Amoxicillin, ampicillin** may increase incidence of rash. **HERBAL:** None significant. **FOOD:** None known. **LAB VALUES:** May increase BUN, serum alkaline phosphatase, AST, ALT, creatinine.

AVAILABILITY (Rx)

Injection, Powder for Reconstitution (Aloprim): 500 mg. **Tablets (Zyloprim):** 100 mg, 300 mg.

ADMINISTRATION/HANDLING
💧 IV

Reconstitution • Reconstitute 500-mg vial with 25 ml Sterile Water for Injection, giving a clear, almost colorless solution (concentration of 20 mg/ml). • Further dilute with 0.9% NaCl or D₅W (50–100 ml) to a concentration of 6 mg/ml or less. **Rate of Administration •** Infuse over 15–60 min. Daily doses can be given as a single infusion or in equally divided doses at 6-, 8-, or 12-hr intervals.

Storage • Store unreconstituted vials at room temperature. • Do not refrigerate reconstituted and/or diluted solution. Must administer within 10 hrs of preparation. • Do not use if precipitate forms or solution is discolored.

PO

• Give after meals with plenty of fluid. • Fluid intake should yield slightly alkaline urine and output of approximately 2 L in adults. • Dosages greater than 300 mg/day to be administered in divided doses.

🚫 IV INCOMPATIBILITIES

Amikacin (Amikin), carmustine (BiCNU), cefotaxime (Claforan), clindamycin (Cleocin), cytarabine (Ara-C), dacarbazine (DTIC), diphenhydramine (Benadryl), doxorubicin (Adriamycin), doxycycline (Vibramycin), gentamicin, haloperidol (Haldol), hydroxyzine (Vistaril), idarubicin (Idamycin), imipenem-cilastatin (Primaxin), methylprednisolone (Solu-Medrol), metoclopramide (Reglan), ondansetron (Zofran), streptozocin (Zanosar), tobramycin, vinorelbine (Navelbine).

🚫 IV COMPATIBILITIES

Bumetanide (Bumex), calcium gluconate, furosemide (Lasix), heparin, hydromorphone (Dilaudid), lorazepam (Ativan), morphine, potassium chloride.

INDICATIONS/ROUTES/DOSAGE

◀ **ALERT** ▶ Doses greater than 300 mg given in divided doses.

Gouty Arthritis
PO: ADULTS, CHILDREN OLDER THAN 10 YRS: (Mild): 200–300 mg/day. **(Moderate to severe):** 400–600 mg/day in 2–3 divided doses. **Maximum:** 800 mg/day.

Secondary Hyperuricemia Associated with Chemotherapy
PO: ADULTS, CHILDREN OLDER THAN 10 YRS: 600–800 mg/day in 2–3 divided doses for 2–3 days starting 1–2 days before chemotherapy. **CHILDREN 6–10 YRS:** 300 mg/day in 2–3 divided doses. **CHILDREN YOUNGER THAN 6 YRS:** 150 mg/day in 3 divided doses.
◀ALERT▶ **IV:** Daily dose can be given as single infusion or at 6-, 8-, or 12-hr intervals.
IV: ADULTS, ELDERLY, CHILDREN 10 YRS OR OLDER: 200–400 mg/m^2/day beginning 24–48 hrs before initiation of chemotherapy. **CHILDREN YOUNGER THAN 10 YRS:** 200 mg/m^2/day. **Maximum:** 600 mg/day.

Recurrent Uric Acid Calcium Oxalate Calculi
PO: ADULTS: 200–300 mg/day in single or divided doses.

Usual Elderly Dosage
PO: Initially, 100 mg/day; gradually increase until optimal uric acid level is reached.

Dosage in Renal Impairment
Dosage is modified based on creatinine clearance. **PO:** Removed by hemodialysis, adult maintenance doses based on creatinine clearance. Administer dose posthemodialysis or administer 50% supplemental dose.

IV/PO

Creatinine Clearance	Dosage
10–20 ml/min	200 mg/day
3–9 ml/min	100 mg/day
Less than 3 ml/min	100 mg at extended intervals
HD	100 mg q48h (increase cautiously to 300 mg)

SIDE EFFECTS

Occasional: PO: Drowsiness, unusual hair loss. **IV:** Rash, nausea, vomiting. **Rare:** Diarrhea, headache.

ADVERSE EFFECTS/TOXIC REACTIONS

Pruritic maculopapular rash possibly accompanied by malaise, fever, chills, joint pain, nausea, vomiting should be considered a toxic reaction. Severe hypersensitivity (hypotension, wheezing, dyspnea) may follow appearance of rash. Bone marrow depression, hepatotoxicity, peripheral neuritis, acute renal failure occur rarely.

NURSING CONSIDERATIONS

BASELINE ASSESSMENT
Obtain baseline serum chemistries, hepatic function tests. Instruct pt to drink minimum of 2,500–3,000 ml of fluid daily while taking medication.

INTERVENTION/EVALUATION
Discontinue medication immediately if rash or other evidence of allergic reaction appears. Monitor I&O (output should be at least 2,000 ml/day). Assess serum chemistries, uric acid, hepatic function levels. Assess urine for cloudiness, unusual color, odor. **Gout:** Assess for therapeutic response: relief of pain, stiffness, swelling; increased joint mobility; reduced joint tenderness; improved grip strength.

PATIENT/FAMILY TEACHING
• May take 1 wk or longer for full therapeutic effect. • Maintain adequate hydration; drink 2,500–3,000 ml of fluid daily while taking medication. • Avoid tasks that require alertness, motor skills until response to drug is established. • Avoid alcohol (may increase uric acid).

almotriptan

al-moe-**trip**-tan
(Axert)
Do not confuse almotriptan with alvimopan, or Axert with Antivert.

◆CLASSIFICATION

PHARMACOTHERAPEUTIC: Serotonin receptor agonist (5-HT$_{1B}$). **CLINICAL:** Antimigraine (see p. 64C).

ACTION

Binds selectively to vascular receptors, producing a vasoconstrictive effect on cranial blood vessels. **Therapeutic Effect:** Produces relief of migraine headache.

PHARMACOKINETICS

Well absorbed after PO administration. Protein binding: 35%. Metabolized by liver to inactive metabolite, primarily excreted in urine. **Half-life:** 3–4 hrs.

USES

Acute treatment of migraine headache with or without aura in adults. Acute treatment of migraine headache in adolescents 12–17 yrs with history of migraine with or without aura and having attacks usually lasting 4 or more hrs when left untreated.

PRECAUTIONS

Contraindications: Cerebrovascular disease (e.g., stroke, transient ischemic attacks), peripheral vascular disease (e.g., ischemic bowel disease), hemiplegic or basilar migraine, ischemic heart disease (including angina pectoris, history of MI, silent ischemia, and Prinzmetal's angina), uncontrolled hypertension, use within 24 hrs of ergotamine-containing preparations or another 5-HT$_{1B}$ agonist. **Cautions:** Mild to moderate renal or hepatic impairment, pt profile suggesting cardiovascular risks, controlled hypertension, history of CVA, sulfonamide allergy.

⌛ LIFESPAN CONSIDERATIONS

Pregnancy/Lactation: Unknown if distributed in breast milk. **Pregnancy Category C. Children:** Safety and efficacy not established in those younger than 12 yrs. **Elderly:** No age-related precautions noted.

INTERACTIONS

DRUG: Ergotamine-containing drugs may produce vasospastic reaction. **MAOIs** may increase concentration. Combined use of **SSRIs** or **SNRIs (e.g., fluoxetine, fluvoxamine, paroxetine, sertraline)** may produce weakness, hyperreflexia, incoordination. **CYP3A4 inhibitors (e.g., erythromycin, itraconazole, ketoconazole, ritonavir)** may increase plasma concentration/effect. **HERBAL:** None significant. **FOOD:** None known. **LAB VALUES:** None significant.

AVAILABILITY (Rx)

📋 **Tablets:** 6.5 mg, 12.5 mg.

ADMINISTRATION/HANDLING

PO
• Swallow tablets whole. • Take with full glass of water. • May give without regard to food.

INDICATIONS/ROUTES/DOSAGE

Migraine Headache
PO: ADULTS, ELDERLY, ADOLESCENTS 12–17 YRS: Initially, 6.25–12.5 mg as a single dose. If headache returns, dose may be repeated after 2 hrs. **Maximum:** 2 doses/24 hrs (25 mg).

Dosage in Renal/Hepatic Impairment
For adult and elderly pts, recommended initial dose is 6.25 mg, maximum daily dose is 12.5 mg.

SIDE EFFECTS

Rare (2%–1%): Nausea, dry mouth, headache, dizziness, somnolence, paresthesia, flushing.

ADVERSE EFFECTS/ TOXIC REACTIONS

Excessive dosage may produce tremor, redness of extremities, decreased respirations, cyanosis, seizures, chest pain. Serious arrhythmias occur rarely but particularly in pts with hypertension, diabetes, obesity, smokers, and those with strong family history of coronary artery disease.

NURSING CONSIDERATIONS

BASELINE ASSESSMENT

Question for history of peripheral vascular disease, cardiac conduction disorders. Question pt regarding onset, location, duration of migraine, and possible precipitating factors.

INTERVENTION/EVALUATION

Evaluate for relief of migraine headache and associated photophobia, phonophobia (sound sensitivity), nausea, vomiting.

PATIENT/FAMILY TEACHING

• Take a single dose as soon as symptoms of an actual migraine attack appear. • Medication is intended to relieve migraine, not to prevent or reduce number of attacks. • Lie down in quiet, dark room for additional benefit after taking medication. • Avoid tasks that require alertness, motor skills until response to drug is established. • Report immediately if palpitations, pain or tightness in chest or throat, or pain or weakness of extremities occurs.

alogliptin

al-oh-**glip**-tin
(Nesina)
Do not confuse alogliptin with linagliptin saxagliptin, or sitagliptin.

FIXED COMBINATION(S)

Kazano: alogliptin/metformin (an antidiabetic): 12.5 mg/500 mg, 12.5 mg, 1,000 mg. **Oseni:** alogliptin/pioglitazone (an antidiabetic): 12.5 mg/15 mg, 12.5 mg/30 mg, 12.5 mg/45 mg, 25 mg/15 mg, 25 mg/30 mg, 25 mg/45 mg.

◆CLASSIFICATION

PHARMACOTHERAPEUTIC: Dipeptidyl peptidase-4 (DDP-4) inhibitor. **CLINICAL:** Antidiabetic.

ACTION

Slows inactivation of incretin hormones by inhibiting DDP-4 enzyme. **Therapeutic Effect:** Incretin hormones increase insulin synthesis/release from pancreas and decrease glucagon secretion. Lowers serum glucose levels.

PHARMACOKINETICS

Rapidly absorbed following PO administration. Metabolized in liver. Protein binding: 20%. Minimal metabolism (60%–70% excreted unchanged). Peak plasma concentration: 1–2 hrs. Primarily excreted in urine. **Half-life:** 21 hrs.

USES

Adjunctive treatment to diet and exercise to improve glycemic control in pts with type 2 diabetes mellitus.

PRECAUTIONS

Contraindications: Type I diabetes, diabetic ketoacidosis, history of hypersensitivity to DD4 inhibitors. **Cautions:** Concurrent use of other hypoglycemic medication, cholelithiasis, hepatic or renal impairment.

☒ LIFESPAN CONSIDERATIONS

Pregnancy/Lactation: Unknown if distributed in breast milk. **Pregnancy Category B. Children:** Safety and efficacy not established. **Elderly:** May have increased risk of hypoglycemia.

INTERACTIONS

DRUG: Insulin, oral hypoglycemics may increase risk of hypoglycemia. **HERBAL:** Herbal supplements having hypoglycemic effects may increase risk of hypoglycemia. **FOOD:** None known. **LAB VALUES:** May decrease serum glucose. May increase serum AST, ALT.

AVAILABILITY (Rx)

Tablets: 6.25 mg, 12.5 mg, 25 mg.

ADMINISTRATION/HANDLING

PO

• May give without regard to food.

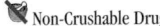 ◆ Canadian trade name   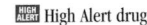 Non-Crushable Drug   🔲 High Alert drug

INDICATIONS/ROUTES/DOSAGE

Type 2 Diabetes Mellitus
PO: ADULTS/ELDERLY: 25 mg once daily.

Renal Impairment
Creatinine clearance 30–59 ml/min: 12.5 mg once daily. **Creatinine clearance less than 30 ml/min:** 6.25 mg once daily.

SIDE EFFECTS

Occasional (4%): Nasopharyngitis, cough, headache, upper respiratory tract infections.

ADVERSE EFFECTS/ TOXIC REACTIONS

Hypoglycemia reported in 1.5% of pts (5% specifically in elderly). Concomitant use of hypoglycemic medication may increase hypoglycemic risk. Pancreatitis reported in less than 1%. Hypersensitivity reactions including angioedema (tongue/ lip swelling), urticaria, bronchospasm occur rarely. Hepatic failure (fatal vs. nonfatal) reported in less than 2% of pts.

NURSING CONSIDERATIONS

BASELINE ASSESSMENT

Obtain baseline serum chemistries, capillary blood glucose, hemoglobin A1C level. Assess pt's understanding of diabetes management, routine home glucose monitoring. Receive full medication history, including vitamins, minerals, herbal products. Question history of co-morbidities, esp. alcohol dependency, renal or hepatic impairment.

INTERVENTION/EVALUATION

Monitor blood glucose, hemoglobin A1C level, hepatic/renal function tests. Assess for hypoglycemia (diaphoresis, tremors, dizziness, anxiety, headache, tachycardia, perioral numbness, hunger, diplopia, difficulty concentrating), hyperglycemia (polyuria, polyphagia, polydipsia, nausea, vomiting, fatigue, Kussmaul breathing), hypersensitivity reaction. Screen for glucose-altering conditions: fever, increased activity or stress, surgical procedures. Obtain dietary consult for nutritional education. Severe abdominal pain, nausea may indicate pancreatitis.

PATIENT/FAMILY TEACHING

• Diabetes mellitus requires lifelong control. Diet and exercise are principal parts of treatment; do not skip or delay meals. • Test blood glucose regularly. • When taking combination drug therapy or when glucose demands are altered (e.g., by fever, infection, trauma, stress, heavy physical activity), have hypoglycemic treatment (glucagon, oral dextrose) available. • Report suspected pregnancy or plans of breast-feeding. • Monitor daily calorie intake. • Avoid alcohol. • Report any abdominal pain, yellowing of the skin or eyes, fatigue, loss of appetite, dark urine, or decreased urine output.

---

alprazolam

al-**praz**-oh-lam
(Alprazolam Intensol, Apo-Alpraz ✦, Niravam, Novo-Alprazol ✦, Xanax, Xanax XR)
Do not confuse alprazolam with lorazepam, or Xanax with Tenex, Tylox, Xopenex, Zantac, or Zyrtec.

◆CLASSIFICATION

PHARMACOTHERAPEUTIC: Benzodiazepine **(Schedule IV). CLINICAL:** Antianxiety (see p. 14C).

ACTION

Enhances the action of the neurotransmitter gamma-aminobutyric acid in the brain. **Therapeutic Effect:** Produces anxiolytic effect due to CNS depressant action.

PHARMACOKINETICS

Well absorbed from GI tract. Protein binding: 80%. Metabolized in liver. Primarily excreted in urine. Minimal removal by hemodialysis. **Half-life:** 6–27 hrs.

USES

Management of anxiety disorders (with or without agoraphobia), anxiety associated with depression, panic disorder. **OFF-LABEL:** Anxiety in children.

PRECAUTIONS

Contraindications: Acute narrow angle-closure glaucoma, concurrent use with ketoconazole or itraconazole. **Cautions:** Renal/hepatic impairment, predisposition to urate nephropathy, obese pts. Concurrent CYP3A4 inhibitors/inducers and major CYP3A4 substrates; debilitated pt, respiratory disease, depression (esp. suicidal risk).

LIFESPAN CONSIDERATIONS

Pregnancy/Lactation: Crosses placenta; distributed in breast milk. Chronic ingestion during pregnancy may produce withdrawal symptoms, CNS depression in neonates. **Pregnancy Category D. Children:** Safety and efficacy not established. **Elderly:** Use small initial doses with gradual increase to avoid ataxia (muscular incoordination) or excessive sedation.

INTERACTIONS

DRUG: Potentiated effects when used with **other CNS depressants (including alcohol). CYP3A4 inhibitors:** (e.g., **antifungal agents [azole], olanzapine, protease inhibitors, SSRIs)** may increase CNS effects. **CYP3A4 inducers** (e.g., **carbamazepine, rifampin)** may decrease effects. **HERBAL: Gotu kola, kava kava, St. John's wort, valerian** may increase CNS depressant effect. **St. John's wort, yohimbe** may decrease effectiveness. **FOOD: Grapefruit juice** may increase level, effects. **LAB VALUES:** None significant.

AVAILABILITY (Rx)

Solution, Oral (Alprazolam Intensol): 1 mg/ml. **Tablets (Orally Disintegrating [Nira-**

vam]): 0.25 mg, 0.5 mg, 1 mg, 2 mg. **Tablets (Immediate-Release [Xanax]):** 0.25 mg, 0.5 mg, 1 mg, 2 mg.

Tablets (Extended-Release [Xanax XR]): 0.5 mg, 1 mg, 2 mg, 3 mg.

ADMINISTRATION/HANDLING

PO, Immediate-Release
• May give without regard to meals.
• Tablets may be crushed. • Orally disintegrating tablets may be given sublingually.

PO, Extended-Release
• Administer once daily. • Do not crush, chew, break extended-release tablets. Swallow whole.

PO, Orally Disintegrating
• Place tablet on tongue, allow to dissolve. • Swallow with saliva. • Administration with water not necessary. • If using 1/2 tab, discard remaining 1/2 tab.

INDICATIONS/ROUTES/DOSAGE

Anxiety Disorders
PO *(Immediate-Release)*: **ADULTS:** Initially, 0.25–0.5 mg 3 times a day. May titrate q3–4days. **Maximum:** 4 mg/day in divided doses. **CHILDREN, YOUNGER THAN 18 YRS:** 0.125 mg 3 times a day. May increase by 0.125–0.25 mg/dose. **Maximum:** 0.06 mg/kg/day.
PO *(Orally Disintegrating)*: **ADULTS:** 0.25–0.5 mg 3 times a day. **Maximum:** 4 mg/day in divided doses. **ELDERLY, DEBILITATED PTS, PTS WITH HEPATIC DISEASE OR LOW SERUM ALBUMIN:** Initially, 0.25 mg 2–3 times a day. Gradually increase to optimum therapeutic response.

Anxiety with Depression
PO: ADULTS: (average dose required) 2.5–3 mg/day in divided doses.

Panic Disorder
PO *(Immediate-Release)*: **ADULTS:** Initially, 0.5 mg 3 times a day. May increase at 3- to 4-day intervals in increments of 1 mg or less a day. Range: 5–6 mg/day. **Maximum:** 10 mg/day. **ELDERLY:** Initially,

 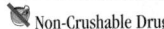

0.125–0.25 mg twice a day. May increase in 0.125-mg increments until desired effect attained.

PO (Extended-Release):

◄ **ALERT** ► To switch from immediate-release to extended-release form, give total daily dose (immediate-release) as a single daily dose of extended-release form.

ADULTS: Initially, 0.5–1 mg once a day. May titrate at 3- to 4-day intervals. Range: 3–6 mg/day. **Maximum:** 10 mg/day. **ELDERLY:** Initially, 0.5 mg once a day.

PO (Orally Disintegrating): **ADULTS:** Initially, 0.5 mg 3 times a day. May increase at 3- to 4-day intervals. Range: 5–6 mg/day. **Maximum:** 10 mg/day.

SIDE EFFECTS

Frequent (41%–20%): Ataxia, light-headedness, drowsiness, slurred speech (particularly in elderly or debilitated pts). **Occasional (15%–5%):** Confusion, depression, blurred vision, constipation, diarrhea, dry mouth, headache, nausea. **Rare (4% or less):** Behavioral problems such as anger, impaired memory; paradoxical reactions (insomnia, nervousness, irritability).

ADVERSE EFFECTS/ TOXIC REACTIONS

Abrupt or too-rapid withdrawal may result in pronounced restlessness, irritability, insomnia, hand tremors, abdominal/ muscle cramps, diaphoresis, vomiting, seizures. Overdose results in drowsiness, confusion, diminished reflexes, coma. Blood dyscrasias noted rarely. **Antidote:** Flumazenil (see Appendix K for dosage).

NURSING CONSIDERATIONS

BASELINE ASSESSMENT

Assess degree of anxiety; assess for drowsiness, dizziness, light-headedness. Assess motor responses (agitation, trembling, tension), autonomic responses (cold/clammy hands, diaphoresis).

INTERVENTION/EVALUATION

For those on long-term therapy, perform hepatic/renal function tests, blood counts periodically. Assess for paradoxical reaction, particularly during early therapy. Evaluate for therapeutic response: calm facial expression, decreased restlessness, insomnia. Monitor respiratory and cardiovascular status.

PATIENT/FAMILY TEACHING

• Drowsiness usually disappears during continued therapy. • If dizziness occurs, change positions slowly from recumbent to sitting position before standing. • Avoid tasks that require alertness, motor skills until response to drug is established. • Smoking reduces drug effectiveness. • Sour hard candy, gum, sips of tepid water may relieve dry mouth. • Do not abruptly withdraw medication after long-term therapy. • Avoid alcohol. • Do not take other medications without consulting physician.

alprostadil (prostaglandin E₁; PGE₁)

al-**pros**-ta-dil
(Prostin VR Pediatric)

BLACK BOX ALERT Apnea may occur in 10%–12% of neonates with congenital heart defects, esp. in those weighing less than 4.4 lb.

◆CLASSIFICATION

PHARMACOTHERAPEUTIC: Prostaglandin. **CLINICAL:** Patent ductus arteriosus agent.

ACTION

Direct effect on vascular and ductus arteriosus smooth muscle; relaxes trabecular smooth muscle. **Therapeutic Effect:** Causes vasodilation.

USES

Temporarily maintains patency of ductus arteriosus until surgery is performed in those with congenital heart defects and dependent on patent ductus for survival (e.g., pulmonary atresia or stenosis). **OFF-LABEL:** Treatment of pulmonary hypertension in infants, children.

PRECAUTIONS

Contraindications: Respiratory distress syndrome (hyaline membrane disease). **Cautions:** Neonates with bleeding tendencies. **Pregnancy Category:** Not indicated for use in pregnant women.

INTERACTIONS

DRUG: None significant. **HERBAL:** None significant. **FOOD:** None known. **LAB VALUES:** May increase serum bilirubin. May decrease serum glucose, potassium.

AVAILABILITY (Rx)

Injection, Solution (Prostin VR Pediatric): 500 mcg/ml.

ADMINISTRATION/HANDLING

🔲 **IV (Prostin VR Pediatric)**

Reconstitution • Dilute 500-mcg ampule with D$_5$W or 0.9% NaCl to volume depending on infusion pump capabilities. • **Maximum concentration:** 20 mcg/ml.

Rate of Administration • Infuse into a large vein or through an umbilical artery catheter placed at ductal opening. • Infuse for shortest time, lowest dose possible. • If significant decrease in arterial pressure is noted via umbilical artery catheter, auscultation, or Doppler transducer, decrease infusion rate immediately. • Discontinue infusion immediately if apnea or bradycardia occurs (overdosage).

Storage • Store parenteral form in refrigerator. • Must dilute before use. • Prepare fresh q24h. • Discard unused portions.

🔳 IV INCOMPATIBILITIES

No information available.

INDICATIONS/ROUTES/DOSAGE

Maintain Patency of Ductus Arteriosus
IV Infusion: NEONATES: Initially, 0.05–0.1 mcg/kg/min. Maintenance: 0.01–0.4 mcg/

kg/min. **Maximum:** 0.4 mcg/kg/min. Therapeutic response is indicated by increased pH in pts with acidosis or increase in oxygenation (usually seen within 30 min).

SIDE EFFECTS

Frequent: Systemic (greater than 1%): Fever, flushing, bradycardia, hypotension, tachycardia, diarrhea. **Occasional: Systemic (less than 1%):** Anxiety, lethargy, myalgia, arrhythmias, respiratory depression, anemia, bleeding, hematuria.

ADVERSE EFFECTS/ TOXIC REACTIONS

◀**ALERT**▶ Apnea experienced by 10%–12% of neonates with congenital heart defects.
Overdose manifested as apnea, flushing of the face/arms, bradycardia. Cardiac arrest, sepsis, seizures, thrombocytopenia occur rarely.

NURSING CONSIDERATIONS

INTERVENTION/EVALUATION

Monitor arterial pressure by umbilical artery catheter, auscultation, Doppler transducer. Monitor for symptoms of hypotension. If significant decrease in arterial pressure occurs, decrease infusion rate immediately. Maintain continuous cardiac monitoring. Assess heart sounds, femoral pulse (circulation to lower extremities), arterial blood gases, respiratory status frequently. If apnea or bradycardia occurs, discontinue infusion and notify physician. In infants with restricted systemic blood flow, efficacy should be measured by monitoring improvement of systemic B/P and blood pH.

PATIENT/FAMILY TEACHING

• Therapy maintains patency of ductus arteriosus until surgery is performed.

---

alteplase

al-te-plase
(<u>Activase</u>, Cathflo Activase)
**Do not confuse alteplase or
Activase with Altace, or Activase
with Cathflo Activase.**

◆CLASSIFICATION

PHARMACOTHERAPEUTIC: Tissue
plasminogen activator (tPA). **CLINI-
CAL:** Thrombolytic (see p. 34C).

ACTION

Binds to fibrin in a thrombus and converts entrapped plasminogen to plasmin,
initiating fibrinolysis. **Therapeutic Effect:** Degrades fibrin clots, fibrinogen,
other plasma proteins.

PHARMACOKINETICS

Rapidly metabolized in liver. Primarily
excreted in urine. **Half-life:** 35 min.

USES

Treatment of acute MI for lysis of
thrombi in coronary arteries, acute
ischemic stroke, acute massive pulmonary embolism. Treatment of occluded
central venous catheters. **OFF-LABEL:**
Acute peripheral occlusive disease,
basilar artery occlusion, cerebral infarction, deep vein thrombosis, femoro-
popliteal artery occlusion, mesenteric
or subclavian vein occlusion, pleural
effusion (parapneumonic). Acute ischemic stroke presenting 3–4½ hrs after
onset of symptoms.

PRECAUTIONS

Contraindications: Active internal bleeding, AV malformation or aneurysm,
bleeding diathesis, intracranial neoplasm, intracranial or intraspinal surgery
or trauma, recent (within past 2 mos)
CVA, severe uncontrolled hypertension,
suspected aortic dissection. **Cautions:** Recent (within 10 days) major surgery or
GI bleeding, OB delivery, organ biopsy,
recent trauma or CPR, left heart thrombus, endocarditis, severe hepatic disease,
pregnancy, elderly, cerebrovascular disease, diabetic retinopathy, thrombophlebitis, occluded AV cannula at infected
site.

⌛ LIFESPAN CONSIDERATIONS

Pregnancy/Lactation: Use only when
benefit outweighs potential risk to fetus.
Unknown if drug crosses placenta or is
distributed in breast milk. **Pregnancy Category C. Children:** Safety and efficacy
not established. **Elderly:** Risk of bleeding with thrombolytic therapy increases;
careful pt selection, monitoring recommended.

INTERACTIONS

DRUG: **Heparin,** **low molecular
weight heparins, medications altering platelet function (e.g., clopidogrel, NSAIDs, thrombolytics), oral
anticoagulants** increase risk of hemorrhage. **HERBAL:** **Cat's claw, dong quai,
evening primrose, feverfew, garlic,
ginkgo, ginseng, green tea, horse
chestnut, red clover** may increase risk
of bleeding due to antiplatelet activity.
FOOD: None known. **LAB VALUES:** Decreases plasminogen, fibrinogen levels
during infusion, decreases clotting time
(confirms the presence of lysis). Decreases Hgb, Hct.

AVAILABILITY (Rx)

Injection, Powder for Reconstitution: 2 mg
(Cathflo Activase), 50 mg (Activase), 100
mg (Activase).

ADMINISTRATION/HANDLING

 IV

Reconstitution • Activase: Reconstitute immediately before use with Sterile
Water for Injection. • Reconstitute 100-
mg vial with 100 ml Sterile Water for Injection (50-mg vial with 50 ml sterile
water) without preservative to provide a
concentration of 1 mg/ml. **Activase
Cathflo:** Add 2.2 ml Sterile Water for

Injection to provide concentration of 1 mg/ml. • Avoid excessive agitation; gently swirl or slowly invert vial to reconstitute. **Rate of Administration** • **Activase:** Give by IV infusion via infusion pump (see Indications/Routes/Dosage). • If minor bleeding occurs at puncture sites, apply pressure for 30 sec; if unrelieved, apply pressure dressing. • If uncontrolled hemorrhage occurs, discontinue infusion immediately (slowing rate of infusion may produce worsening hemorrhage). • Avoid undue pressure when drug is injected into catheter (can rupture catheter or expel clot into circulation). **Activase Cathflo:** Instill dose into occluded catheter. • After 30 min, assess catheter function by attempting to aspirate blood. • If still occluded, let dose dwell an additional 90 min. • If function not restored, a second dose may be instilled.

Storage • **Activase:** Store vials at room temperature. • After reconstitution, solution appears colorless to pale yellow. • Solution is stable for 8 hrs after reconstitution. Discard unused portions. • **Activase Cathflo:** Refrigerate vials.

🔲 IV INCOMPATIBILITIES

Dobutamine (Dobutrex), dopamine (Intropin), heparin.

🔲 IV COMPATIBILITIES

Lidocaine, metoprolol (Lopressor), morphine, nitroglycerin, propranolol (Inderal).

INDICATIONS/ROUTES/DOSAGE

Acute MI
IV Infusion: ADULTS WEIGHING MORE THAN 67 KG: Total dose: 100 mg over 90 min, starting with 15-mg bolus over 1–2 min, then 50 mg over 30 min, then 35 mg over 60 min. **ADULTS WEIGHING 67 KG OR LESS: Total dose:** Start with 15-mg bolus over 1–2 min, then 0.75 mg/kg over 30 min (**maximum:** 50 mg), then 0.5 mg/kg over 60 min (**maximum:** 35 mg). **Maximum total dose:** 100 mg.

Acute Pulmonary Emboli
IV Infusion: ADULTS: 100 mg over 2 hrs. May give as a 10-mg bolus followed by 90 mg over 2 hrs. Institute or reinstitute heparin near end or immediately after infusion when activated partial thromboplastin time (aPTT) or thrombin time (TT) returns to twice normal or less.

Acute Ischemic Stroke
◀**ALERT**▶ Dose should be given within the first 3 hrs of the onset of symptoms. Recommended total dose: 0.9 mg/kg. **Maximum:** 90 mg.
IV Infusion: ADULTS WEIGHING 100 KG OR LESS: 0.09 mg/kg as IV bolus over 1 min, then 0.81 mg/kg as continuous infusion over 60 min. **WEIGHING GREATER THAN 100 KG:** 9 mg bolus over 1 min, then 81 mg as continuous infusion over 60 min.

Central Venous Catheter Clearance
IV: ADULTS, ELDERLY: Up to 2 mg; may repeat after 2 hrs. If catheter functional, withdraw 4–5 ml blood to remove drug and residual clot.

Usual Neonatal Dosage
Occluded IV Catheter: Use 1 mg/ml conc (**maximum:** 2 mg/2 ml) leave in lumen up to 2 hrs, then aspirate.
Systemic Thrombosis: 0.1–0.6 mg/kg/hr for 6 hrs.

SIDE EFFECTS

Frequent: Superficial bleeding at puncture sites, decreased B/P. **Occasional:** Allergic reaction (rash, wheezing, bruising).

ADVERSE EFFECTS/ TOXIC REACTIONS

Severe internal hemorrhage may occur. Lysis of coronary thrombi may produce atrial or ventricular arrhythmias or stroke.

NURSING CONSIDERATIONS

BASELINE ASSESSMENT

Assess for contraindications to therapy. Obtain baseline B/P, apical pulse. Record weight. Evaluate 12-lead EKG, cardiac enzymes, electrolytes. Assess Hct, platelet count, thrombin time (TT), prothrombin time (PT), activated partial thromboplastin time (aPTT), fibrinogen level before therapy is instituted. Type and crossmatch, hold blood.

INTERVENTION/EVALUATION

Perform continuous cardiac monitoring for arrhythmias. Check B/P, pulse, respirations q15min until stable, then hourly. Check peripheral pulses, heart and lung sounds. Monitor for chest pain relief and notify physician of continuation or recurrence (note location, type, intensity). Assess for bleeding: overt blood, occult blood in any body substance. Monitor aPTT per protocol. Maintain B/P; avoid any trauma that might increase risk of bleeding (e.g., injections, shaving). Assess neurologic status frequently.

---

alvimopan

al-vi-moe-pan
(Entereg)
BLACK BOX ALERT Available only for short-term (15 doses) use in hospitalized pts. Only hospitals that have registered in and met all requirements for Entereg Access Support and Education (E.A.S.E.) program may use this medication.
Do not confuse alvimopan with almotriptan.

◆CLASSIFICATION

PHARMACOTHERAPEUTIC: Peripherally acting mu-opioid receptor antagonist. **CLINICAL:** Anti-ileus agent.

ACTION

Binds to opioid receptors in GI tract. **Therapeutic Effect:** Accelerates GI recovery period as defined by time to first bowel movement or flatus.

PHARMACOKINETICS

Protein binding: 80%–90%. Undergoes no significant hepatic metabolism but is metabolized by intestinal flora. Excreted 50% by biliary route. Unabsorbed and unchanged alvimopan resulting from biliary excretion is hydrolyzed to its metabolite by gut microflora. Metabolite eliminated in feces and urine as unchanged. **Half-life:** 10–17 hrs.

USES

Accelerates time to upper and lower GI recovery following partial large or small bowel resection surgery with primary anastomosis.

PRECAUTIONS

Contraindications: Pts who have taken therapeutic doses of opioids for more than 7 consecutive days prior to initiation (recent exposure to opioids heightens pt's sensitivity to drug's effects, increasing susceptibility to abdominal pain, nausea, vomiting, diarrhea). **Cautions:** Complete bowel obstruction, hepatic/renal impairment, recent exposure to opioids.

⧗ LIFESPAN CONSIDERATIONS

Pregnancy/Lactation: Unknown if drug crosses placenta or is distributed in breast milk. **Pregnancy Category B. Children:** Safety and efficacy not established. **Elderly:** No age-related precautions noted.

INTERACTIONS

DRUG: Opioids may increase levels/effect. **HERBAL:** None significant. **FOOD:** None known. **LAB VALUES:** May reduce Hgb, Hct, serum potassium.

AVAILABILITY (Rx)

Capsules: 12 mg.

ADMINISTRATION/HANDLING
PO
• First dose given 30 min to 5 hrs prior to surgery; remaining dosage given without regard to meals.

INDICATIONS/ROUTES/DOSAGE

PO: ADULTS, ELDERLY: 12 mg given 30 min to 5 hrs prior to surgery followed by 12 mg twice daily beginning the day after surgery for a maximum of 7 days or until discharge. Pts should receive no more than 15 doses.

SIDE EFFECTS

Occasional (9%–6%): Hypokalemia, constipation, flatulence, dyspepsia (epigastric distress, heartburn, indigestion). **Rare (3%):** Back pain, urinary retention.

ADVERSE EFFECTS/ TOXIC REACTIONS

None known.

NURSING CONSIDERATIONS

BASELINE ASSESSMENT

Inform pts that they must disclose long-term or intermittent opioid pain therapy, including any use of opioids in the wk prior to receiving alvimopan. Treatment should not be instituted unless pt is opioid-free for 7 days.

INTERVENTION/EVALUATION

Monitor closely for evidence of hepatotoxicity (abdominal pain lasting more than a few days, white bowel movements, dark urine, jaundice), increased AST, ALT, serum bilirubin.

PATIENT/FAMILY TEACHING

• Recent use of opioids may increase susceptibility to adverse reactions, primarily those limited to GI tract (e.g., abdominal pain, nausea, vomiting, diarrhea). • Inform pts that the most common side effects in those undergoing bowel resection are constipation, dyspepsia, flatulence. • Report abdominal pain, nausea, vomiting, diarrhea.

amantadine

a-**man**-ta-deen
(Dom-Amantadine ✽,
PMS-Amantadine ✽)

Do not confuse amantadine with ranitidine or rimantadine.

◆CLASSIFICATION

PHARMACOTHERAPEUTIC: Dopaminergic agonist. **CLINICAL:** Antiviral, antiparkinson agent (see p. 69C).

ACTION

Blocks uncoating of influenza A virus, preventing penetration into the host and inhibiting M2 protein in the assembly of progeny virions. Blocks reuptake of dopamine into presynaptic neurons and causes direct stimulation of postsynaptic receptors. **Therapeutic Effect:** Antiviral, antiparkinsonian activity.

PHARMACOKINETICS

Rapidly and completely absorbed from GI tract. Protein binding: 67%. Widely distributed. Primarily excreted in urine. Minimally removed by hemodialysis. **Half-life:** 11–15 hrs (increased in elderly, decreased in renal impairment).

USES

Prevention, treatment of respiratory tract infections due to influenza virus, Parkinson's disease, drug-induced extrapyramidal reactions.

PRECAUTIONS

Contraindications: None known. **Cautions:** History of seizures, orthostatic hypotension, CHF, peripheral edema, hepatic disease, recurrent eczematoid dermatitis, cerebrovascular disease, renal dysfunction, those receiving CNS stimulants, uncontrolled psychosis.

⌛ LIFESPAN CONSIDERATIONS

Pregnancy/Lactation: Unknown if drug crosses placenta or is distributed in breast milk. **Pregnancy Category C. Children:** No age-related precautions noted in those older than 1 yr. **Elderly:** May exhibit increased sensitivity to anticholinergic effects. Age-related renal impairment may require dosage adjustment.

✽ Canadian trade name   🔖 Non-Crushable Drug   🔲 High Alert drug

INTERACTIONS

DRUG: **Alcohol** may increase CNS effects. **Anticholinergics, antihistamines, phenothiazines, tricyclic antidepressants** may increase anticholinergic effects. **HERBAL:** None significant. **FOOD:** None known. **LAB VALUES:** None significant.

AVAILABILITY (Rx)

Capsules: 100 mg. **Solution, Oral:** 50 mg/5 ml. **Syrup:** 50 mg/5 ml. **Tablets:** 100 mg.

ADMINISTRATION/HANDLING

PO

• May give without regard to food. • Administer nighttime dose several hrs before bedtime (prevents insomnia).

INDICATIONS/ROUTES/DOSAGE

Treatment of Influenza A

PO: ADULTS: 100 mg twice a day or 200 mg once/day. Initiate within 24–48 hrs after onset of symptoms; discontinue as soon as possible based on clinical response. **ELDERLY:** 100 mg once daily. **CHILDREN 10 YRS AND OLDER, WEIGHING 40 KG OR MORE:** 100 mg twice a day. **WEIGHING LESS THAN 40 KG:** 5 mg/kg/day in 2 divided doses. **Maximum:** 150 mg/day. **CHILDREN 1–9 YRS:** 5 mg/kg/day in 2 divided doses. **Maximum:** 150 mg/day.

Prevention of Influenza A

PO: ADULTS: 100 mg twice a day or 200 mg once/day. **CHILDREN:** Refer to treatment dosing above.

Parkinson's Disease, Extrapyramidal Symptoms

PO: ADULTS, ELDERLY: 100 mg twice a day. May increase up to 400 mg/day in divided doses (300 mg/day for extrapyramidal symptoms).

Dosage in Renal Impairment

Dosage and frequency are modified based on creatinine clearance.

Creatinine Clearance	Dosage
30–50 ml/min	200 mg first day; 100 mg/day thereafter
15–29 ml/min	200 mg first day; 100 mg on alternate days
Less than 15 ml/min	200 mg every 7 days
Hemodialysis	200 mg every 7 days

SIDE EFFECTS

Frequent (10%–5%): Nausea, dizziness, poor concentration, insomnia, nervousness. **Occasional (5%–1%):** Orthostatic hypotension, anorexia, headache, livedo reticularis (reddish-blue, netlike blotching of skin), blurred vision, urinary retention, dry mouth or nose, agitation, confusion, hallucinations. **Rare:** Vomiting, depression, irritation or swelling of eyes, rash.

ADVERSE EFFECTS/ TOXIC REACTIONS

CHF, leukopenia, neutropenia occur rarely. Hyperexcitability, seizures, ventricular arrhythmias may occur. Neuroleptic malignant syndrome (NMS) occurs rarely.

NURSING CONSIDERATIONS

BASELINE ASSESSMENT

When treating infections caused by influenza A virus, obtain specimens for viral diagnostic tests before giving first dose (therapy may begin before results are known).

INTERVENTION/EVALUATION

Monitor I&O, renal function tests; check for peripheral edema. Evaluate food tolerance, vomiting. Assess skin for mottling or rash. Assess for dizziness. **Parkinson's disease:** Assess for clinical reversal of symptoms (improvement of tremor of head/hands at rest, mask-like facial expression, shuffling gait, muscular rigidity).

PATIENT/FAMILY TEACHING

• Do not take any other medications without consulting physician. • Avoid alcohol.

• Avoid tasks that require alertness, motor skills until response to drug is established (may cause dizziness, blurred vision). • Get up slowly from a sitting or lying position. • Report new symptoms, esp. blotching, rash, dizziness, blurred vision, nausea/vomiting, muscle rigidity. • Take nighttime dose several hours before bedtime to prevent insomnia.

ambrisentan

am-**bri**-sen-tan
(Letairis, Volibris ✤)
BLACK BOX ALERT Likely to produce serious birth defects if used by pregnant women.

◆CLASSIFICATION

PHARMACOTHERAPEUTIC: Endothelin receptor antagonist. **CLINICAL:** Vasodilator.

ACTION

Blocks endothelin receptor subtypes ET_A and ET_B on vascular endothelium and smooth muscle, leading to vasodilation. **Therapeutic Effect:** Improves symptoms of pulmonary arterial hypertension (e.g., improves exercise ability), decreases rate of clinical deterioration.

PHARMACOKINETICS

Rapidly absorbed. Protein binding: 99%. Not eliminated by renal pathways. **Half-life:** 9 hrs.

USES

Treatment of pulmonary arterial hypertension (PAH) to improve exercise ability, decrease rate of clinical deterioration.

PRECAUTIONS

Contraindications: Pregnancy, women who may become pregnant, idiopathic pulmonary fibrosis. **Extreme Caution:** Moderate to severe hepatic impairment. **Cautions:** Mild hepatic impairment, low hemoglobin levels, clinically significant anemia.

⏳ LIFESPAN CONSIDERATIONS

Pregnancy/Lactation: May cause serious birth defects, including malformation of heart and great vessels, facial abnormalities. Breastfeeding not recommended. **Pregnancy Category X. Children:** Safety and efficacy not established. **Elderly:** Age-related hepatic impairment requires strict monitoring.

INTERACTIONS

DRUG: Cyclosporine may increase plasma concentration. **FOOD: Grapefruit/grapefruit juice** may increase levels/effect. **HERBAL: St. John's wort** may decrease levels/effect. **LAB VALUES:** May increase serum AST, ALT to at least 3 times upper limit of normal levels (ULN). May increase serum aminotransferase more than 3 times ULN. May increase serum bilirubin more than 2 times ULN. May cause marked decrease in Hgb, Hct.

AVAILABILITY (Rx)

📋 **Tablets, Film-Coated:** 5 mg, 10 mg.

ADMINISTRATION/HANDLING

PO
• Swallow whole. Do not crush/break or chew tablets. • Give without regard to food.

INDICATIONS/ROUTES/DOSAGE

Pulmonary Arterial Hypertension (PAH)
PO: ADULTS, ELDERLY: Initially, 5 mg once a day. Dose may be increased to 10 mg once a day if 5 mg is tolerated. Dosage modification based on transaminase elevation.
Coadministration with cyclosporine: 5 mg/day maximum.

SIDE EFFECTS

Frequent (17%–15%): Peripheral edema, headache. **Occasional (6%–3%):** Nasal congestion, palpitations, constipation, flushing, nasopharyngitis, dyspnea, abdominal pain, sinusitis.

ADVERSE EFFECTS/ TOXIC REACTIONS

Potential for serious hepatic injury has been noted.

NURSING CONSIDERATIONS

BASELINE ASSESSMENT

Pregnancy must be excluded before the start of treatment and prevented thereafter. Obtain negative pregnancy test prior to initiation of treatment and monthly during treatment. Measure Hgb prior to therapy, at 1 mo, and periodically thereafter. Assess hepatic function tests prior to initiating therapy and then monthly thereafter.

INTERVENTION/EVALUATION

If elevation in hepatic enzymes noted, changes in monitoring and treatment must be initiated. If bilirubin level increases, stop treatment. Monitor Hgb, Hct levels at 1 and 3 mos of treatment, then every 3 mos. Monitor Hgb, Hct levels for decrease. Monitor for signs/symptoms of hepatotoxicity (abdominal pain, fever, jaundice).

PATIENT/FAMILY TEACHING

• Female pts should take measures to avoid pregnancy during treatment (Pregnancy Category X). • Hepatic function tests, pregnancy test must be obtained every mo during treatment. • Report clinical symptoms of hepatic injury (nausea, vomiting, fever, abdominal pain, fatigue, jaundice) immediately.

amikacin

am-i-**kay**-sin
(Amikin ✤)

BLACK BOX ALERT May cause ototoxicity, nephrotoxicity, and/or neuromuscular blockade and respiratory paralysis. Ototoxicity usually is irreversible; nephrotoxicity usually is reversible.

Do not confuse amikacin or Amikin with Amicar, or amikacin with anakinra.

◆CLASSIFICATION

PHARMACOTHERAPEUTIC: Aminoglycoside. **CLINICAL:** Antibiotic (see p. 22C).

ACTION

Irreversibly binds to protein on bacterial ribosomes. **Therapeutic Effect:** Interferes with protein synthesis of susceptible microorganisms.

PHARMACOKINETICS

Rapid, complete absorption after IM administration. Protein binding: 0%–10%. Widely distributed (penetrates blood-brain barrier when meninges are inflamed). Excreted unchanged in urine. Removed by hemodialysis. **Half-life:** 2–4 hrs (increased in renal impairment, neonates; decreased in cystic fibrosis, burn pts, febrile pts).

USES

Treatment of susceptible infections due to *Pseudomonas,* other gram-negative organisms (*Proteus, Serratia,* other gram-negative bacilli) including biliary tract, bone and joint, CNS, intra-abdominal, skin and soft tissue, urinary tract. Treatment of bacterial pneumonia, septicemia.

PRECAUTIONS

Contraindications: Hypersensitivity to amikacin, other aminoglycosides (cross-sensitivity), or their components. **Cautions:** Myasthenia gravis, neonates, pre-existing renal impairment, auditory or vestibular impairment, hypocalcemia.

🔲 LIFESPAN CONSIDERATIONS

Pregnancy/Lactation: Readily crosses placenta; small amounts distributed in breast milk. May produce fetal nephrotoxicity. **Pregnancy Category D. Children:** Neonates, premature infants may be more susceptible to toxicity due to immature renal function. **Elderly:** Higher risk of toxicity due to age-related renal impairment, increased risk of hearing loss.

INTERACTIONS

DRUG: Nephrotoxic and ototoxic medications may increase toxicity. May increase effects of **cyclosporine, neuromuscular blocking agents. HERBAL:** None significant. **FOOD:** None known. **LAB VALUES:** May increase serum creatinine, BUN, AST, ALT, bilirubin, LDH. May decrease serum calcium, magnesium, potassium, sodium concentrations. **Therapeutic levels:** Peak: life-threatening infections: 25–40 mcg/ml; serious infections: 20–25 mcg/ml; urinary tract infections: 15–20 mcg/ml. **Trough:** Less than 8 mcg/ml. **Toxic levels:** Peak: greater than 40 mcg/ml; **trough:** greater than 10 mcg/ml.

AVAILABILITY (Rx)

Injection Solution: 250 mg/ml (Amikin).

ADMINISTRATION/HANDLING

🖫 IV

Reconstitution • Dilute to concentration of 0.25–5 mg/ml in 0.9% NaCl or D₅W.
Rate of Administration • Infuse over 30–60 min.
Storage • Store vials at room temperature. • Solution appears clear but may become pale yellow (does not affect potency). • Intermittent IV infusion (piggyback) is stable for 24 hrs at room temperature, 2 days if refrigerated. • Discard if precipitate forms or dark discoloration occurs.

IM

• To minimize discomfort, give deep IM slowly. • Less painful if injected into gluteus maximus rather than in lateral aspect of thigh.

🖫 IV INCOMPATIBILITIES

Amphotericin, azithromycin (Zithromax), propofol (Diprivan).

🖫 IV COMPATIBILITIES

Amiodarone (Cordarone), aztreonam (Azactam), calcium gluconate, cefepime (Maxipime), cimetidine (Tagamet), cipro-floxacin (Cipro), clindamycin (Cleocin), dexmedetomidine (Precedex), diltiazem (Cardizem), diphenhydramine (Benadryl), enalapril (Vasotec), esmolol (BreviBloc), fluconazole (Diflucan), furosemide (Lasix), levofloxacin (Levaquin), lorazepam (Ativan), magnesium sulfate, midazolam (Versed), morphine, ondansetron (Zofran), potassium chloride, ranitidine (Zantac), vancomycin.

INDICATIONS/ROUTES/DOSAGE

Usual Parenteral Dosage
IV, IM: ADULTS, ELDERLY, CHILDREN, INFANTS: 5–7.5 mg/kg/dose q8h. **NEONATES:** 15 mg/kg/dose q12–48h (based on wgt).

Dosage in Renal Impairment
Dosage and frequency are modified based on degree of renal impairment and serum drug concentration. After a loading dose of 5–7.5 mg/kg, maintenance dose and frequency are based on serum creatinine levels and creatinine clearance.

Creatinine Clearance	Dosing Interval
60 ml/min or greater	q8h
40–59 ml/min	q12h
20–39 ml/min	q24h
Less than 20 ml/min	Loading dose, monitor levels
Hemodialysis	q48–72h (give after HD on dialysis days)
Continuous renal replacement therapy (CRRT)	Initially, 10 mg/kg, then 7.5 mg/kg q24h

SIDE EFFECTS

Frequent: Phlebitis, thrombophlebitis. **Occasional:** Hypersensitivity reactions (rash, fever, urticaria, pruritus). **Rare:** Neuromuscular blockade (difficulty breathing, drowsiness, weakness).

ADVERSE EFFECTS/TOXIC REACTIONS

Serious reactions include nephrotoxicity (as evidenced by increased thirst, decreased appetite, nausea, vomiting, increased BUN and serum creatinine levels, decreased creatinine clearance); neurotoxicity (manifested as muscle twitching, visual disturbances, seizures, paresthesia); ototoxicity (as evidenced by tinnitus, dizziness, loss of hearing).

NURSING CONSIDERATIONS

BASELINE ASSESSMENT

Dehydration must be treated prior to aminoglycoside therapy. Establish baseline hearing acuity before beginning therapy. Question for history of allergies, esp. to aminoglycosides and sulfite. Obtain specimen for culture, sensitivity before giving first dose (therapy may begin before results are known).

INTERVENTION/EVALUATION

Monitor I&O (maintain hydration), urinalysis (casts, RBC, WBC, increase in specific gravity). Monitor results of serum peak/trough levels. Be alert to ototoxic, neurotoxic, nephrotoxic symptoms (see Adverse Effects/Toxic Reactions). Check IM injection site for pain, induration. Evaluate IV site for phlebitis (heat, pain, red streaking over vein). Assess for skin rash, diarrhea, superinfection (particularly genital/anal pruritus), changes of oral mucosa. When treating pts with neuromuscular disorders, assess respiratory response carefully. **Therapeutic levels:** Peak: life-threatening infections: 25–40 mcg/ml; serious infections: 20–25 mcg/ml; urinary tract infections: 15–20 mcg/ml. **Trough:** Less than 8 mcg/ml. **Toxic levels:** Peak: greater than 40 mcg/ml; **trough:** greater than 10 mcg/ml.

PATIENT/FAMILY TEACHING

• Continue antibiotic for full length of treatment. • Space doses evenly. • IM injection may cause discomfort. • Report any hearing, visual, balance, urinary problems, even after therapy is completed. • Do not take other medications without consulting physician.

amiodarone

TOP 200 **HIGH ALERT**

a-mi-**oh**-da-rone
(Apo-Amiodarone ✦, Cordarone, Nexterone, Novo-Amiodarone ✦, Pacerone)

BLACK BOX ALERT Pts should be hospitalized when amiodarone is initiated. Alternative therapies to be tried first before using amiodarone. Only indicated for pts with life-threatening arrhythmias due to risk of toxicity. Lung damage may occur without symptoms. Hepatotoxicity is common, usually mild (rarely possible). Can exacerbate arrhythmias. **Do not confuse amiodarone with amiloride, or Cordarone with Cardura.**

◆CLASSIFICATION

PHARMACOTHERAPEUTIC: Cardiac agent. **CLINICAL:** Antiarrhythmic (see p. 18C).

ACTION

Prolongs duration of myocardial cell action potential and refractory period by acting directly on all cardiac tissue. Decreases AV and sinus node function. **Therapeutic Effect:** Suppresses arrhythmias.

PHARMACOKINETICS

Route	Onset	Peak	Duration
PO	3 days–3 wks	1 wk–5 mos	7–50 days after discontinuation

Slowly, variably absorbed from GI tract. Protein binding: 96%. Extensively metabolized in liver to active metabolite. Excreted via bile; not removed by hemodialysis. **Half-life:** 26–107 days; metabolite, 61 days.

USES

Management of life-threatening recurrent ventricular fibrillation, hemodynamically unstable ventricular tachycardia (VT) unresponsive to other therapy. **OFF-**

LABEL: Treatment of atrial fibrillation, paroxysmal supraventricular tachycardia (SVT); ventricular tachyarrhythmias.

PRECAUTIONS

Contraindications: Bradycardia-induced syncope (except in the presence of a pacemaker), second- and third-degree AV block (except in presence of a pacemaker), severe sinus node dysfunction, cardiogenic shock. Hypersensitivity to iodine. **Cautions:** May prolong QT interval. Thyroid disease, electrolyte imbalance, hepatic disease, hypotension, left ventricular dysfunction, pulmonary disease. Pts taking warfarin, surgical pts.

LIFESPAN CONSIDERATIONS

Pregnancy/Lactation: Crosses placenta; distributed in breast milk. May adversely affect fetal development. **Pregnancy Category D. Children:** Safety and efficacy not established. **Elderly:** May be more sensitive to effects on thyroid function. May experience increased incidence of ataxia, other neurotoxic effects.

INTERACTIONS

DRUG: May increase thioridazine concentration and produce additive prolongation of QT interval. May increase cardiac effects with **other antiarrhythmics.** May increase effect of **beta-blockers, oral anticoagulants (e.g., warfarin).** May increase concentration, toxicity of **aripiprazole, colchicine, digoxin, phenytoin.** May increase risk of **simvastatin** toxicity, myopathy, rhabdomyolysis. **HERBAL: St. John's wort** may decrease effect. **Ephedra** may worsen arrhythmia. **FOOD: Grapefruit, grapefruit juice** may alter effects. Avoid use during therapy. **LAB VALUES:** May increase serum AST, ALT, alkaline phosphatase, ANA titer. May cause changes in EKG, thyroid function test results. **Therapeutic serum level:** 0.5–2.5 mcg/ml; toxic serum level not established.

AVAILABILITY (Rx)

Infusion (Pre-Mix): Nexterone: 150 mg/100 ml; 360 mg/200 ml. **Injection, Solution (Cordarone IV):** 50 mg/ml. **Tablets:** 100 mg (Pacerone), 200 mg (Cordarone, Pacerone), 400 mg (Pacerone).

ADMINISTRATION/HANDLING

 IV

Reconstitution • Infusions longer than 2 hrs must be administered/diluted in glass or polyolefin bottles. • Dilute loading dose (150 mg) in 100 ml D₅W (1.5 mg/ml). • Dilute maintenance dose (900 mg) in 500 ml D₅W (1.8 mg/ml). Concentrations greater than 3 mg/ml cause peripheral vein phlebitis.
Rate of Administration • Does not need protection from light during administration. • Administer through central venous catheter (CVC) if possible, using in-line filter. • Bolus over 10 min (15 mg/min) not to exceed 30 mg/min; then 1 mg/min over 6 hrs; then 0.5 mg/min over 18 hrs. • Infusions longer than 1 hr, concentration not to exceed 2 mg/ml unless CVC used.
Storage • Store at room temperature. • Stable for 24 hrs when diluted in glass or polyolefin containers; stable for 2 hrs when diluted in PVC containers.

PO
• Give consistently with regard to meals to reduce GI distress. • Tablets may be crushed • Do not give with grapefruit juice, grapefruit.

IV INCOMPATIBILITIES

Cefazolin (Ancef), heparin, sodium bicarbonate.

IV COMPATIBILITIES

Dexmedetomidine (Precedex), dobutamine (Dobutrex), dopamine (Intropin), furosemide (Lasix), insulin (regular), labetalol (Normodyne), lidocaine, lorazepam (Ativan), midazolam (Versed), morphine, nitroglycerin, norepinephrine (Levophed), phenylephrine (Neo-Synephrine), potassium chloride, vancomycin.

✦ Canadian trade name   🍸 Non-Crushable Drug   🔲 High Alert drug

INDICATIONS/ROUTES/DOSAGE

Ventricular Arrhythmias

PO: ADULTS, ELDERLY: Initially, 800–1,600 mg/day in 1–2 divided doses for 1–3 wks. After arrhythmia is controlled or side effects occur, reduce to 600–800 mg/day for 4 wks. Maintenance: 200–600 mg/day. CHILDREN: Initially, 10–20 mg/kg/day for 4–14 days, then 5 mg/kg/day for several wks. Maintenance: 5 mg/kg/day or lowest effective maintenance dose for 5–7 days/wk. NEONATE: 10–20 mg/kg/day in 2 divided doses for 7–10 days, then 5–10 mg/kg once daily.

IV Infusion: ADULTS: Initially, 1,050 mg over 24 hrs; 150 mg over 10 min, then 360 mg over 6 hrs; then 540 mg over 18 hrs. May continue at 0.5 mg/min. After first 24 hrs, infuse 720 mg/24 hrs (0.5 mg/min) with a concentration of 1–6 mg/ml. CHILDREN, NEONATES: Loading dose: 5 mg/kg over 60 min. May repeat loading dose. Then, if needed, IV infusion of 5 mcg/kg/min. May increase up to 15 mcg/kg/min.

SIDE EFFECTS

Expected: Corneal microdeposits noted in almost all pts treated for more than 6 mos (can lead to blurry vision). Occasional (greater than 3%): PO: Constipation, headache, decreased appetite, nausea, vomiting, paresthesia, photosensitivity, muscular incoordination. Parenteral: Hypotension, nausea, fever, bradycardia. Rare (less than 3%): PO: Bitter or metallic taste, decreased libido, dizziness, facial flushing, blue-gray coloring of skin (face, arms, and neck), blurred vision, bradycardia, asymptomatic corneal deposits, rash, visual disturbances, halo vision.

ADVERSE EFFECTS/ TOXIC REACTIONS

Serious, potentially fatal pulmonary toxicity (alveolitis, pulmonary fibrosis, pneumonitis, acute respiratory distress syndrome) may begin with progressive dyspnea and cough with crackles, decreased breath sounds, pleurisy, CHF, or hepatotoxicity. May worsen existing arrhythmias or produce new arrhythmias.

NURSING CONSIDERATIONS

BASELINE ASSESSMENT

Obtain baseline pulmonary function tests, chest X-ray, serum AST, ALT, alkaline phosphatase, EKG. Assess B/P, apical pulse immediately before drug is administered (if pulse is 60/min or less or systolic B/P is less than 90 mm Hg, withhold medication, contact physician).

INTERVENTION/EVALUATION

Monitor for symptoms of pulmonary toxicity (progressively worsening dyspnea, cough). Dosage should be discontinued or reduced if toxicity occurs. Assess pulse for quality, rhythm, bradycardia. Monitor EKG for cardiac changes (e.g., widening of QRS, prolongation of PR and QT intervals). Notify physician of any significant interval changes. Assess for nausea, fatigue, paresthesia, tremor. Monitor for signs of hypothyroidism (periorbital edema, lethargy, pudgy hands/feet, cool/pale skin, vertigo, night cramps) and hyperthyroidism (hot/dry skin, bulging eyes [exophthalmos], frequent urination, eyelid edema, weight loss, difficulty breathing). Monitor serum AST, ALT, alkaline phosphatase for evidence of hepatic toxicity. Assess skin, cornea for bluish discoloration in those who have been on drug therapy longer than 2 mos. Monitor thyroid function test results. If elevated hepatic enzymes occur, dosage reduction or discontinuation is necessary. Monitor for therapeutic serum level (0.5–2.5 mcg/ml). Toxic serum level not established.

PATIENT/FAMILY TEACHING

• Protect against photosensitivity reaction on skin exposed to sunlight. • Bluish skin discoloration gradually disappears when drug is discontinued. • Report shortness of breath, cough. • Outpatients should monitor pulse before taking medication. • Do not abruptly discontinue medication. • Compliance with therapy regimen is essential to control arrhythmias. • Restrict salt, alcohol intake. • Avoid grapefruit, grapefruit juice. • Recommend ophthalmic exams q6mos. • Report any vision changes, signs/symptoms of cardiac arrhythmias.

amitriptyline

a-mi-**trip**-ti-leen
(Elavil ✤, Levate ✤, Novo-Tryptyn ✤)

BLACK BOX ALERT Increased risk of suicidal thinking and behavior in children, adolescents, young adults 18–24 yrs with major depressive disorder, other psychiatric disorders.
Do not confuse amitriptyline with aminophylline, imipramine, or nortriptyline, or Elavil with Eldepryl, enalapril, Equanil, or Mellaril.

FIXED-COMBINATION(S)

Limbitrol: amitriptyline/chlordiazepoxide (an antianxiety): 12.5 mg/5 mg, 25 mg/10 mg.

◆CLASSIFICATION

PHARMACOTHERAPEUTIC: Tricyclic. **CLINICAL:** Antidepressant, antineuralgic, antibulimic (see p. 39C).

ACTION

Blocks reuptake of neurotransmitters (norepinephrine, serotonin) at presynaptic membranes, increasing availability at postsynaptic receptor sites. Strong anticholinergic activity. **Therapeutic Effect:** Antidepressant effect.

PHARMACOKINETICS

Rapidly and well absorbed from GI tract. Protein binding: 90%. Undergoes first-pass metabolism in liver. Primarily excreted in urine. Minimal removal by hemodialysis. **Half-life:** 10–26 hrs.

USES

Treatment of various forms of depression, exhibited as persistent, prominent dysphoria (occurring nearly every day for at least 2 wks) manifested by 4 of 8 symptoms: appetite change, sleep pattern change, increased fatigue, impaired concentration, feelings of guilt or worthlessness, loss of interest in usual activities, psychomotor agitation or retardation, suicidal tendencies. **OFF-LABEL:** Relief of neuropathic pain, related to diabetic neuropathy or postherpetic neuralgia; treatment of migraine. Treatment of depression in children, post-traumatic stress disorder (PTSD).

PRECAUTIONS

Contraindications: Acute recovery period after MI, use within 14 days of MAOIs. **Cautions:** Prostatic hypertrophy, history of urinary retention or obstruction, narrow-angle glaucoma, diabetes mellitus, seizures, hyperthyroidism, cardiac/hepatic/renal disease, schizophrenia, xerostomia, visual problems, constipation or history of bowel obstruction, elderly, increased intraocular pressure (IOP), hiatal hernia.

⏳ LIFESPAN CONSIDERATIONS

Pregnancy/Lactation: Crosses placenta; minimally distributed in breast milk. **Pregnancy Category C. Children:** More sensitive to increased dosage, toxicity, increased risk of suicidal ideation, worsening of depression. **Elderly:** Increased risk of toxicity. Increased sensitivity to anticholinergic effects. Cautions in those with cardiovascular disease.

INTERACTIONS

DRUG: CNS depressants (including alcohol, anticonvulsants, barbiturates, phenothiazines, sedative-hypnotics) may increase sedation, respiratory depression, hypotensive effects. **Dronedarone, thioridazine, toremefine, ziprasidone** levels may be increased. **Quetiapine** may increase levels/effects. May increase risk of hypertensive crisis, hyperpyresis, seizures with **MAOIs**. **HERBAL**: **St. John's wort** may decrease levels. **Gotu kola, kava kava, St. John's wort, valerian** may increase CNS depression. **FOOD**: None known. **LAB VALUES**: May alter EKG readings (flattened T wave), serum glucose (increase or decrease). **Therapeutic serum level**: Peak: 120–250 ng/ml; **toxic serum level**: greater than 500 ng/ml.

AVAILABILITY (Rx)

Tablets (Elavil): 10 mg, 25 mg, 50 mg, 75 mg, 100 mg, 150 mg.

ADMINISTRATION/HANDLING

PO
• Give with food or milk if GI distress occurs.

INDICATIONS/ROUTES/DOSAGE

Depression
PO: ADULTS: 25–150 mg/day as a single dose at bedtime or in divided doses. May gradually increase up to 300 mg/day. Titrate to lowest effective dosage. **ELDERLY**: Initially, 10–25 mg at bedtime. May increase by 10–25 mg at weekly intervals. Range: 25–150 mg/day. **CHILDREN 6–12 YRS**: 1–5 mg/kg/day in divided doses.

Pain Management
PO: ADULTS, ELDERLY: 25–100 mg at bedtime. **CHILDREN**: Initially, 0.1 mg/kg. May increase over 2 wks to 0.5–2 mg/kg at bedtime.

SIDE EFFECTS

Frequent: Dizziness, drowsiness, dry mouth, orthostatic hypotension, headache, increased appetite, weight gain, nausea, unusual fatigue, unpleasant taste. **Occasional**: Blurred vision, confusion, constipation, hallucinations, delayed micturition, eye pain, arrhythmias, fine muscle tremors, parkinsonian syndrome, anxiety, diarrhea, diaphoresis, heartburn, insomnia. **Rare**: Hypersensitivity,

alopecia, tinnitus, breast enlargement, photosensitivity.

ADVERSE EFFECTS/ TOXIC REACTIONS

Overdose may produce confusion, seizures, severe drowsiness, changes in cardiac conduction, fever, hallucinations, agitation, dyspnea, vomiting, unusual fatigue, weakness. Abrupt withdrawal after prolonged therapy may produce headache, malaise, nausea, vomiting, vivid dreams. Blood dyscrasias, cholestatic jaundice occur rarely.

NURSING CONSIDERATIONS

BASELINE ASSESSMENT

Observe and record behavior. Assess psychological status, thought content, suicidal ideation, sleep patterns, appearance, interest in environment. For those on long-term therapy, hepatic/renal function tests, blood counts should be performed periodically.

INTERVENTION/EVALUATION

Supervise suicidal-risk pt closely during early therapy (as depression lessens, energy level improves, increasing suicide potential). Assess appearance, behavior, speech pattern, level of interest, mood. Monitor B/P for hypotension, pulse, arrhythmias. **Therapeutic serum level**: Peak: 120–250 ng/ml; **toxic serum level**: greater than 500 ng/ml.

PATIENT/FAMILY TEACHING

• Change positions slowly to avoid hypotensive effect. • Tolerance to postural hypotension, sedative and anticholinergic effects usually develop during early therapy. • Maximum therapeutic effect may be noted in 2–4 wks. • Sensitivity to sun may occur. • Report visual disturbances. • Do not abruptly discontinue medication. • Avoid tasks that require alertness, motor skills until response to drug is established. • Avoid alcohol. • Sips of tepid water may relieve dry mouth.

amlodipine

am-**loe**-di-peen
(Apo-Amlodipine ✢, Norvasc)
**Do not confuse amlodipine
with amiloride, or Norvasc with
Navane or Vascor.**

FIXED-COMBINATION(S)

Anturnide: amlodipine/aliskiren (a renin inhibitor)/hydrochlorothiazide (a diuretic): 5 mg/150 mg/12.5 mg, 5 mg/300 mg/12.5 mg, 5 mg/300 mg/25 mg, 10 mg/300 mg/12.5 mg, 10 mg/300 mg/25 mg. **Azor:** amlodipine/olmesartan (an angiotensin II receptor antagonist): 5 mg/20 mg, 10 mg/20 mg, 5 mg/40 mg, 10 mg/40 mg. **Caduet:** amlodipine/atorvastatin (hydroxamethylglutaryl-CoA [HMG-CoA] reductase inhibitor): 2.5 mg/10 mg, 2.5 mg/20 mg, 2.5 mg/40 mg, 5 mg/10 mg, 10 mg/10 mg, 5 mg/20 mg, 10 mg/20 mg, 5 mg/40 mg, 10 mg/40 mg, 5 mg/80 mg, 10 mg/80 mg. **Exforge:** amlodipine/valsartan (an angiotensin II receptor antagonist): 5 mg/160 mg, 10 mg/160 mg, 5 mg/320 mg, 10 mg/320 mg. **Exforge HCT:** amlodipine/valsartan/hydrochlorothiazide (a diuretic): 5 mg/160 mg/12.5 mg, 5 mg/160 mg/25 mg, 10 mg/160 mg/12.5 mg, 10 mg/160 mg/25 mg, 10 mg/320 mg/25 mg. **Lotrel:** amlodipine/benazepril (an angiotensin-converting enzyme [ACE] inhibitor): 2.5 mg/10 mg, 5 mg/10 mg, 5 mg/20 mg, 5 mg/40 mg, 10 mg/20 mg, 10 mg/40 mg. **Tekamlo:** amlodipine/aliskiren (a renin inhibitor): 5 mg/150 mg, 5 mg/300 mg, 10 mg/150 mg, 10 mg/300 mg. **Tribenzor:** amlodipine/olmesartan/hydrochlorothiazide: 5 mg/20 mg/12.5 mg, 5 mg/40 mg/12.5 mg, 5 mg/40 mg/25 mg, 10 mg/40 mg/12.5 mg, 10 mg/40 mg/25 mg. **Twynsta:** amlodipine/telmisartan (an angiotensin II receptor antagonist): 5 mg/40 mg, 5 mg/80 mg, 10 mg/40 mg, 10 mg/80 mg.

◆ CLASSIFICATION

PHARMACOTHERAPEUTIC: Calcium channel blocker. **CLINICAL:** Antihypertensive, antianginal (see p. 62C, 79C).

ACTION

Inhibits calcium movement across cardiac and vascular smooth muscle cell membranes. **Therapeutic Effect:** Dilates coronary arteries, peripheral arteries/arterioles. Decreases total peripheral vascular resistance and B/P by vasodilation.

PHARMACOKINETICS

Route	Onset	Peak	Duration
PO	0.5–1 hr	N/A	24 hrs

Slowly absorbed from GI tract. Protein binding: 95%–98%. Undergoes first-pass metabolism in liver. Excreted primarily in urine. Not removed by hemodialysis. **Half-life:** 30–50 hrs (increased in elderly, those with hepatic cirrhosis).

USES

Management of hypertension, chronic stable angina, vasospastic (Prinzmetal's or variant) angina. May be used alone or with other antihypertensives or antianginals.

PRECAUTIONS

Contraindications: None known. **Cautions:** Hepatic impairment, aortic stenosis, hypertophic cardiomyopathy.

⚕ LIFESPAN CONSIDERATIONS

Pregnancy/Lactation: Unknown if drug crosses placenta or is distributed in breast milk. **Pregnancy Category C. Children:** Safety and efficacy not established. **Elderly:** Half-life may be increased, more sensitive to hypotensive effects.

INTERACTIONS

DRUG: May increase levels of **simvastatin. Azole antifungals, cyclosporine protease inhibitors** may increase concentration. **Carbamazepine, rifampin** may decrease levels/effect. **HERBAL: St. John's wort** may decrease concentration. **Ephe-**

✢ Canadian trade name   ☒ Non-Crushable Drug   🅷🅸 High Alert drug

dra, yohimbe may worsen hypertension. **Garlic** may increase antihypertensive effect. **FOOD: Grapefruit, grapefruit juice** may increase concentration, hypotensive effects. **LAB VALUES:** May increase hepatic enzyme levels.

AVAILABILITY (Rx)

Tablets: 2.5 mg, 5 mg, 10 mg.

ADMINISTRATION/HANDLING

PO
• May give without regard to food.

INDICATIONS/ROUTES/DOSAGE

Hypertension
PO: ADULTS: Initially, 5 mg/day as a single dose. May increase by 2.5 mg/day every 7–14 days. **Maximum:** 10 mg/day. **SMALL-FRAME, FRAGILE, ELDERLY:** 2.5 mg/day as a single dose. **CHILDREN 6–17 YRS:** 2.5–5 mg/day.

Angina (Chronic Stable or Vasospastic)
PO: ADULTS: 5–10 mg/day as a single dose. **ELDERLY, PTS WITH HEPATIC INSUFFICIENCY:** 5 mg/day as a single dose.

Dosage in Hepatic Impairment
ADULTS, ELDERLY: (Hypertension) 2.5 mg/day. (Angina) 5 mg/day.

SIDE EFFECTS

Frequent (greater than 5%): Peripheral edema, headache, flushing. **Occasional (5%–1%):** Dizziness, palpitations, nausea, unusual fatigue or weakness (asthenia). **Rare (less than 1%):** Chest pain, bradycardia, orthostatic hypotension.

ADVERSE EFFECTS/ TOXIC REACTIONS

Overdose may produce excessive peripheral vasodilation, marked hypotension with reflex tachycardia, syncopy.

NURSING CONSIDERATIONS

BASELINE ASSESSMENT

Assess baseline renal/hepatic function tests, B/P, apical pulse.

INTERVENTION/EVALUATION

Assess B/P (if systolic B/P is less than 90 mm Hg, withhold medication, contact physician). Assess for peripheral edema behind medial malleolus (sacral area in bedridden pts). Assess skin for flushing. Question for headache, asthenia (loss of strength, energy).

PATIENT/FAMILY TEACHING

• Do not abruptly discontinue medication. • Compliance with therapy regimen is essential to control hypertension. • Avoid tasks that require alertness, motor skills until response to drug is established. • Do not ingest grapefruit, grapefruit juice.

---

amoxicillin

a-**mox**-i-sil-in
(Apo-Amoxi ❖, Moxatag, Novamoxin ❖)
Do not confuse amoxicillin with amoxapine or Atarax.

◆CLASSIFICATION

PHARMACOTHERAPEUTIC: Penicillin. **CLINICAL:** Antibiotic (see p. 29C).

ACTION

Inhibits bacterial cell wall synthesis. **Therapeutic Effect:** Bactericidal in susceptible microorganisms.

PHARMACOKINETICS

Well absorbed from GI tract. Protein binding: 20%. Partially metabolized in liver. Primarily excreted in urine. Removed by hemodialysis. **Half-life:** 1–1.3 hrs (increased in renal impairment).

USES

Treatment of susceptible infections due to streptococci, *E. coli, E. faecalis, P. mirabilis, H. influenzae, N. gonorrhoeae* including ear, nose, and throat; lower respiratory tract; skin and skin structure; UTIs;

acute uncomplicated gonorrhea; *H. pylori*. OFF-LABEL: Treatment of Lyme disease and typhoid fever. Postexposure prophylaxis for anthrax exposure.

PRECAUTIONS

Contraindications: Hypersensitivity to any penicillin. **Cautions:** History of allergies (esp. cephalosporins), infectious mononucleosis, renal impairment, asthma.

⧗ LIFESPAN CONSIDERATIONS

Pregnancy/Lactation: Crosses placenta, appears in cord blood, amniotic fluid. Distributed in breast milk in low concentrations. May lead to allergic sensitization, diarrhea, candidiasis, skin rash in infant. **Pregnancy Category B. Children:** Immature renal function in neonate/young infant may delay renal excretion. **Elderly:** Age-related renal impairment may require dosage adjustment.

INTERACTIONS

DRUG: Allopurinol may increase incidence of rash. **Probenecid** may increase concentration, toxicity risk. May decrease effects of **oral contraceptives.** **HERBAL:** None significant. **FOOD:** None known. **LAB VALUES:** May increase serum AST, ALT, LDH, bilirubin, creatinine, BUN. May cause positive Coombs' test.

AVAILABILITY (Rx)

Capsules: 250 mg, 500 mg. **Powder for Oral Suspension:** 125 mg/5 ml, 200 mg/5 ml, 250 mg/5 ml, 400 mg/5ml. **Tablets:** 500 mg, 875 mg. **Tablets (Chewable):** 125 mg, 200 mg, 250 mg, 400 mg. **Tablets, Extended-Release (Moxatag):** 775 mg.

ADMINISTRATION/HANDLING

PO
• Give without regard to meals. • Instruct pt to chew/crush chewable tablets thoroughly before swallowing. • Oral suspension dose may be mixed with formula, milk, fruit juice, water, cold drink. • Give immediately after mixing. • After reconstitution, oral suspension is stable for 14 days at either room temperature or refrigerated. **Moxatag:** Take within 1 hr of finishing a meal.

INDICATIONS/ROUTES/DOSAGE
Susceptible Infections
PO: ADULTS, ELDERLY, CHILDREN 12 YRS AND OLDER: 250–500 mg q8h or 500–875 mg q12h or 775 mg (Moxatag) once daily. **CHILDREN OLDER THAN 3 MOS:** 20–50 mg/kg/day in divided doses q8–12h. **CHILDREN 3 MOS AND YOUNGER:** 20–30 mg/kg/day in divided doses q12h. **NEONATE:** 20–30 mg/kg/day in divided doses q12h.

Lower Respiratory Tract Infection
PO: ADULTS, ELDERLY: 500 mg q8h or 875 mg q12h. **CHILDREN:** 45 mg/kg/day in divided doses q12h or 40 mg/kg/day in divided doses q8h.

H. Pylori Infection
PO: ADULTS, ELDERLY: 1 g twice a day in combination with at least 1 other antibiotic and an acid-suppressing agent (proton pump inhibitor or H_2 antagonist).

Otitis Media
PO: CHILDREN: 80–90 mg/kg/day in 2 divided doses.

Pharyngitis/Tonsillitis
PO *(Moxatag)*: **ADULTS, CHILDREN 12 YRS AND OLDER:** 775 mg once daily.

Endocarditis Prophylaxis
PO: ADULTS, ELDERLY: 2 g 1 hr before procedure. **CHILDREN:** 50 mg/kg 1 hr before procedure. **Maximum:** 2 g.

Dosage in Renal Impairment
◀**ALERT**▶ Immediate-release 875-mg tablet or 775-mg extended-release tablet should not be used in pts with creatinine clearance less than 30 ml/min. Dosage interval is modified based on creatinine clearance. **Creatinine clearance 10–30 ml/min:** 250–500 mg q12h. **Creatinine clearance less than 10 ml/min:** 250–500 mg q24h.

SIDE EFFECTS

Frequent: GI disturbances (mild diarrhea, nausea, vomiting), headache, oral/vaginal candidiasis. Occasional: Generalized rash, urticaria.

ADVERSE EFFECTS/ TOXIC REACTIONS

Antibiotic-associated colitis, other superinfections (abdominal cramps, severe watery diarrhea, fever) may result from altered bacterial balance of GI tract. Severe hypersensitivity reactions, including anaphylaxis, acute interstitial nephritis, occur rarely.

NURSING CONSIDERATIONS

BASELINE ASSESSMENT

Question for history of allergies, esp. penicillins, cephalosporins, renal impairment.

INTERVENTION/EVALUATION

Hold medication and promptly report rash, diarrhea (fever, abdominal pain, mucus and blood in stool may indicate antibiotic-associated colitis). Be alert for superinfection: fever, vomiting, diarrhea, anal/genital pruritus, black "hairy" tongue, oral mucosal changes (ulceration, pain, erythema). Monitor renal/hepatic function tests.

PATIENT/FAMILY TEACHING

• Continue antibiotic for full length of treatment. • Space doses evenly. • Take with meals if GI upset occurs. • Thoroughly chew the chewable tablets before swallowing. • Report rash, diarrhea, other new symptoms.

---

amoxicillin/ clavulanate

TOP 200

a-**mox**-i-sil-in/**klav**-yoo-la-nate
(<u>Amoclan</u>, Apo-Amoxi-Clav ✤, <u>Augmentin</u>, Augmentin ES 600, <u>Augmentin XR</u>, Clavulin ✤, Novo-Clavamoxin ✤)

> Do not confuse Augmentin with amoxicillin or Azulfidine.

◆CLASSIFICATION

PHARMACOTHERAPEUTIC: Penicillin.
CLINICAL: Antibiotic (see p. 29C).

ACTION

Amoxicillin inhibits bacterial cell wall synthesis. Clavulanate inhibits bacterial beta-lactamase. Therapeutic Effect: Amoxicillin is bactericidal in susceptible microorganisms. Clavulanate protects amoxicillin from enzymatic degradation.

PHARMACOKINETICS

Well absorbed from GI tract. Protein binding: 20%. Partially metabolized in liver. Primarily excreted in urine. Removed by hemodialysis. Half-life: 1–1.3 hrs (increased in renal impairment).

USES

Treatment of susceptible infections due to *streptococci, E. coli, E. faecalis, P. mirabilis,* beta-lactamase producing *H. influenzae, Klebsiella* spp., *M. catarrhalis,* and *S. aureus* (not methicillin-resistant *Staphylococcus aureus* [MRSA]) including lower respiratory, skin and skin structure, UTIs, otitis media, sinusitis. OFF-LABEL: Treatment of bronchitis, chancroid.

PRECAUTIONS

Contraindications: Hypersensitivity to any penicillins, history of cholestatic jaundice or hepatic impairment. Augmentin XR: Severe renal impairment, hemodialysis pt. Cautions: History of allergies, esp. cephalosporins; renal impairment.

⧗ LIFESPAN CONSIDERATIONS

Pregnancy/Lactation: Crosses placenta, appears in cord blood, amniotic fluid. Distributed in breast milk in low concentrations. May lead to allergic sensitization, diarrhea, candidiasis, skin rash in infant. Pregnancy Category B. Children: Immature renal function in neonate/young infant may delay renal excretion. **Elderly:** Age-related renal impairment may require dosage adjustment.

INTERACTIONS

DRUG: Allopurinol may increase incidence of rash. **Probenecid** may increase concentration, toxicity risk. May decrease effects of **oral contraceptives. HERBAL:** None significant. **FOOD:** None known. **LAB VALUES:** May increase serum AST, ALT. May cause positive Coombs' test.

AVAILABILITY (Rx)

Powder for Oral Suspension (Amoclan, Augmentin): 125 mg–31.25 mg/5 ml, 200 mg–28.5 mg/5 ml, 250 mg–62.5 mg/5 ml, 400 mg–57 mg/5 ml, 600 mg–42.9 mg/5 ml. **Tablets (Augmentin):** 250 mg–125 mg, 500 mg–125 mg, 875 mg–125 mg. **Tablets (Chewable [Augmentin]):** 200 mg–28.5 mg, 400 mg–57 mg.

🍂 **Tablets (Extended-Release [Augmentin XR]):** 1,000 mg–62.5 mg.

ADMINISTRATION/HANDLING

PO
- Store tablets at room temperature.
- After reconstitution, oral suspension is stable for 10 days but should be refrigerated. • May mix dose of suspension with milk, formula, or juice and give immediately. • Give without regard to meals.
- Give with food to increase absorption, decrease stomach upset. • Instruct pt to chew/crush chewable tablets thoroughly before swallowing. • Do not break, crush, chew, divide extended-release tablets.

INDICATIONS/ROUTES/DOSAGE

Usual Adult Dosage
PO: ADULTS: 250–500 mg q8h or 875 mg q12h.

Usual Pediatric Dosage
PO: CHILDREN OLDER THAN 3 MOS, WEIGHING 40 KG OR LESS: 20–90 mg/kg/day divided q8–12h.

Otitis Media
PO: CHILDREN: 90 mg/kg/day (600 mg/ 5 ml suspension) in divided doses q12h for 10 days.

Usual Neonate Dosage
PO: NEONATES, CHILDREN YOUNGER THAN 3 MOS: 30 mg/kg/day (125 mg/5 ml suspension) in divided doses q12h.

Dosage in Renal Impairment
◄ **ALERT** ► Do not use 875-mg tablet or extended-release tablets for creatinine clearance less than 30 ml/min.
Dosage and frequency are modified based on creatinine clearance. **Creatinine clearance 10–30 ml/min:** 250–500 mg q12h. **Creatinine clearance less than 10 ml/min:** 250–500 mg q24h. **HD:** 250–500 mg q24h, give dose during and after dialysis. **PD:** 250 mg q12h

SIDE EFFECTS

Occasional (9%–4%): Diarrhea, loose stools, nausea, skin rashes, urticaria. **Rare (less than 3%):** Vomiting, vaginitis, abdominal discomfort, flatulence, headache.

ADVERSE EFFECTS/ TOXIC REACTIONS

Antibiotic-associated colitis, other superinfections (abdominal cramps, severe watery diarrhea, fever) may result from altered bacterial balance. Severe hypersensitivity reactions, including anaphylaxis, acute interstitial nephritis, occur rarely.

NURSING CONSIDERATIONS

BASELINE ASSESSMENT

Question for history of allergies, esp. penicillins, cephalosporins, renal impairment.

INTERVENTION/EVALUATION

Hold medication and promptly report rash, diarrhea (fever, abdominal pain, mucus and blood in stool may indicate antibiotic-associated colitis). Be alert for

---

signs of superinfection including fever, vomiting, diarrhea, black "hairy" tongue, ulceration or changes of oral mucosa, anal/genital pruritus. Monitor renal/hepatic tests with prolonged therapy.

PATIENT/FAMILY TEACHING
• Continue antibiotic for full length of treatment. • Space doses evenly. • Take with meals if GI upset occurs. • Thoroughly chew the chewable tablets before swallowing. • Notify physician if rash, diarrhea, other new symptoms occur.

---

amphotericin B   **HIGH ALERT**

am-foe-**ter**-i-sin
(<u>Abelcet</u>, <u>AmBisome</u>, Amphotec, Fungizone)

BLACK BOX ALERT (Nonliposomal) To be used primarily for pts with progressive, potentially fatal fungal infection. Not to be used for noninvasive forms of fungal disease (oral thrush, vaginal candidiasis).

◆CLASSIFICATION

PHARMACOTHERAPEUTIC: Polyene antifungal. **CLINICAL:** Antifungal, antiprotozoal (see p. 47C).

ACTION

Generally fungistatic but may become fungicidal with high dosages or very susceptible microorganisms. Binds to sterols in fungal cell membrane. **Therapeutic Effect:** Increases fungal cell membrane permeability, allowing loss of potassium, other cellular components, resulting in cell death.

PHARMACOKINETICS

Protein binding: 90%. Widely distributed. Metabolic fate unknown. Cleared by nonrenal pathways. Minimal removal by hemodialysis. Amphotec and Abelcet are not dialyzable. **Half-life:** Fungizone, 24 hrs (increased in neonates and chil-

dren); Abelcet, 7.2 days; AmBisome, 100–153 hrs; Amphotec, 26–28 hrs.

USES

Abelcet: Treatment of aspergillosis or any type of invasive fungal infections refractory or intolerant to Fungizone. **AmBisome:** Empiric treatment of fungal infection in febrile neutropenic pts. *Aspergillus, Candida* species, *Cryptococcus* infections refractory to Fungizone or pt with renal impairment or toxicity with Fungizone. Treatment of cryptococcal meningitis in HIV-infected pts. Treatment of visceral leishmaniasis. **Amphotec:** Treatment of invasive aspergillosis in pts with renal impairment or toxicity or prior treatment failure with Fungizone. **Fungizone:** Treatment of severe systemic and CNS infections caused by susceptible fungi including *Candida* spp., *Histoplasma, Cryptococcus, Aspergillus, Blastomyces.* Treatment of fungal peritonitis. **OFF-LABEL: Abelcet, Amphotec:** Serious *Candida* infections. **AmBisome:** Treatment of systemic histoplasmosis infection.

PRECAUTIONS

Contraindications: Hypersensitivity to amphotericin B or sulfites. **Cautions:** Renal impairment; in combination with antineoplastic therapy. Give only for progressive, potentially fatal fungal infection.

⧗ LIFESPAN CONSIDERATIONS

Pregnancy/Lactation: Crosses placenta; unknown if distributed in breast milk. **Pregnancy Category B. Children:** Safety and efficacy not established, but use the least amount for therapeutic regimen. **Elderly:** No age-related precautions noted.

INTERACTIONS

DRUG: Antineoplastic agents may increase potential for bronchospasm, renal toxicity, hypotension. **Steroids** may cause severe hypokalemia. May increase **digoxin** toxity (due to hypokalemia). **Nephrotoxic medications** may increase nephrotoxicity. **HERBAL:** None significant. **FOOD:** None known. **LAB VALUES:** May increase serum AST, ALT, alkaline phosphatase, BUN, creatinine. May decrease serum calcium, magnesium, potassium.

AVAILABILITY (Rx)

Injection, Powder for Reconstitution: 50 mg (AmBisome, Amphotec, Fungizone), 100 mg (Amphotec). **Injection, Suspension (Abelcet):** 5 mg/ml.

ADMINISTRATION/HANDLING

 IV

• Observe strict aseptic technique; no bacteriostatic agent or preservative is present in diluent.

Reconstitution

ABELCET

• Shake 20-ml (100-mg) vial gently until contents are dissolved. Withdraw required dose using 5-micron filter needle (supplied by manufacturer). • Dilute with D_5W to 1–2 mg/ml.

AMBISOME

• Reconstitute each 50-mg vial with 12 ml Sterile Water for Injection to provide concentration of 4 mg/ml. • Shake vial vigorously for 30 sec. Withdraw required dose and empty syringe contents through a 5-micron filter into an infusion of D_5W to provide final concentration of 1–2 mg/ml (0.2–0.5 mg/ml for infants and small children).

AMPHOTEC

• Add 10 ml Sterile Water for Injection to each 50-mg vial to provide concentration of 5 mg/ml. Shake gently. • Further dilute **only** with D_5W to a concentration of 0.1–2 mg/ml.

FUNGIZONE

• Add 10 ml Sterile Water for Injection to each 50-mg vial. • Further dilute with 250–500 ml D_5W. • Final concentration should not exceed 0.1 mg/ml (0.25 mg/ml for central infusion).

Rate of Administration

• Give by slow IV infusion. Infuse conventional amphotericin over 4–6 hrs; Abelcet over 2 hrs (shake contents if infusion longer than 2 hrs); Amphotec over 2–4 hrs (avoid rate faster than 1 mg/kg/hr); AmBisome over 1–2 hrs.

Storage

ABELCET

• Refrigerate unreconstituted solution. Reconstituted solution is stable for 48 hrs if refrigerated, 6 hrs at room temperature.

AMBISOME

• Refrigerate unreconstituted solution. Reconstituted solution of 4 mg/ml is stable for 24 hrs. Concentration of 1–2 mg/ml is stable for 6 hrs.

AMPHOTEC

• Refrigerate intact vials.• Reconstituted solution is stable for 24 hrs if refrigerated.

FUNGIZONE

• Refrigerate intact vials. • Once reconstituted, vials stable for 24 hrs at room temperature, 7 days if refrigerated. • Diluted solutions stable for 24 hrs at room temperature, 2 days if refrigerated.

IV INCOMPATIBILITIES

Note: Abelcet, AmBisome, Amphotec: Do not mix with any other drug, diluent, or solution. Fungizone: Allopurinol (Aloprim), aztreonam (Azactam), calcium gluconate, cefepime (Maxipime), cimetidine (Tagamet), ciprofloxacin (Cipro), dexmedetomidine (Precedex), diphenhydramine (Benadryl), dopamine (Intropin), enalapril (Vasotec), filgrastim (Neupogen), fluconazole (Diflucan), foscarnet (Foscavir), magnesium sulfate, meropenem (Merrem IV), ondansetron (Zofran), piperacillin and tazobactam (Zosyn), potassium chloride, propofol (Diprivan).

IV COMPATIBILITY

Lorazepam (Ativan).

INDICATIONS/ROUTES/DOSAGE

Usual Abelcet Dose

IV Infusion *(Abelcet):* **ADULTS, CHILDREN:** 2.5–5 mg/kg/day at rate of 2.5 mg/kg/hr.

 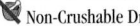

Usual AmBisome Dose
IV Infusion *(Ambisome)*: **ADULTS, CHILDREN**: 3–6 mg/kg/day over 2 hrs.

Usual Amphotec Dose
IV Infusion *(Amphotec)*: **ADULTS, CHILDREN**: 3–4 mg/kg/day at rate no faster than 1 mg/kg/hr. **Maximum:** 7.5 mg/kg/day.

Fungizone, Usual Dose
IV Infusion: ADULTS, ELDERLY: Dosage based on pt tolerance and severity of infection. Initially, 1-mg test dose is given over 20–30 min. If tolerated, usual dose is 0.3–1.5 mg/kg/day. **Maximum:** 1.5 mg/kg/day. **CHILDREN:** Test dose of 0.1 mg/kg/dose (**maximum:** 1 mg) is infused over 20–60 min. If test dose is tolerated. **NEONATES:** Initially, 0.5 mg/kg/dose once daily. May increase to maximum of 1.5 mg/kg/day. Maintenance dose: 0.25–1 mg/kg/day.

SIDE EFFECTS

Frequent (greater than 10%): Abelcet: Chills, fever, increased serum creatinine, multiple organ failure. **AmBisome:** Hypokalemia, hypomagnesemia, hyperglycemia, hypocalcemia, edema, abdominal pain, back pain, chills, chest pain, hypotension, diarrhea, nausea, vomiting, headache, fever, rigors, insomnia, dyspnea, epistaxis, increased hepatic/renal function test results. **Amphotec:** Chills, fever, hypotension, tachycardia, increased serum creatinine, hypokalemia, bilirubinemia. **Amphocin:** Fever, chills, headache, anemia, hypokalemia, hypomagnesemia, anorexia, malaise, generalized pain, nephrotoxicity.

ADVERSE EFFECTS/ TOXIC REACTIONS

Cardiovascular toxicity (hypotension, ventricular fibrillation), anaphylaxis occur rarely. Altered vision/hearing, seizures, hepatic failure, coagulation defects, multiple organ failure, sepsis may be noted. Each alternative formulation is less nephrotoxic than conventional amphotericin (Amphocin).

NURSING CONSIDERATIONS

BASELINE ASSESSMENT

Obtain baseline liver function test, chemistries, ionized calcium, renal function test. Question for history of allergies, esp. to amphotericin B, sulfite. Avoid, if possible, other nephrotoxic medications. Obtain premedication orders to reduce adverse reactions during IV therapy (antipyretics, antihistamines, antiemetics, corticosteroids).

INTERVENTION/EVALUATION

Monitor B/P, temperature, pulse, respirations; assess for adverse reactions (fever, tremors, chills, anorexia, nausea, vomiting, abdominal pain) q15min twice, then q30min for 4 hrs of initial infusion. If symptoms occur, slow infusion, administer medication for symptomatic relief. For severe reaction, stop infusion and notify physician. Evaluate IV site for phlebitis (heat, pain, red streaking over vein). Monitor I&O, renal function tests for nephrotoxicity. Monitor serum potassium and magnesium levels, hematologic and hepatic function test results.

PATIENT/FAMILY TEACHING

• Prolonged therapy (wks or mos) is usually necessary. • Fever reaction may decrease with continued therapy. • Muscle weakness may be noted during therapy (due to hypokalemia).

ampicillin

am-pi-**sil**-in
(Apo-Ampi ✦, Novo-Ampicillin ✦, Nu-Ampi ✦)
Do not confuse ampicillin with aminophylline.

◆CLASSIFICATION

PHARMACOTHERAPEUTIC: Penicillin.
CLINICAL: Antibiotic (see p. 30C).

ACTION

Inhibits cell wall synthesis in susceptible microorganisms. **Therapeutic Effect:** Bactericidal in susceptible microorganisms.

PHARMACOKINETICS

Moderately absorbed from GI tract. Protein binding: 15%–25%. Widely distributed. Partially metabolized in liver. Primarily excreted in urine. Removed by hemodialysis. **Half-life:** 1–1.5 hrs (increased in renal impairment).

USES

Treatment of susceptible infections due to streptococci, *S. pneumoniae,* staphylococci (non–penicillinase producing), meningococci, *Listeria*, some *Klebsiella, E. coli, H. influenzae, Salmonella, Shigella* including GI, GU, respiratory infections, meningitis, endocarditis prophylaxis.

PRECAUTIONS

Contraindications: Hypersensitivity to any penicillin. **Cautions:** History of allergies, esp. cephalosporins, renal impairment, asthmatic pts, infectious mononucleosis.

⧖ LIFESPAN CONSIDERATIONS

Pregnancy/Lactation: Crosses placenta; appears in cord blood, amniotic fluid. Distributed in breast milk in low concentrations. May lead to allergic sensitization, diarrhea, candidiasis, skin rash in infant. **Pregnancy Category B. Children:** Immature renal function in neonates/young infants may delay renal excretion. **Elderly:** Age-related renal impairment may require dosage adjustment.

INTERACTIONS

DRUG: **Allopurinol** may increase incidence of rash. **Probenecid** may increase concentration, toxicity risk. May decrease effects of **oral contraceptives.** May increase level/effects of **methotrexate. HERBAL:** None significant. **FOOD:** None known. **LAB VALUES:** May increase serum AST, ALT. May cause positive Coombs' test.

AVAILABILITY (Rx)

Capsules: 250 mg, 500 mg. **Injection, Powder for Reconsitution:** 125 mg, 250 mg, 500 mg, 1 g, 2 g. **Powder for Oral Suspension:** 125 mg/5 ml, 250 mg/5 ml.

ADMINISTRATION/HANDLING

 IV

Reconstitution • For IV injection, dilute each vial with 5 ml Sterile Water for Injection or 0.9% NaCl (10 ml for 1- and 2-g vials). **Maximum concentration:** 100 mg/ml for IV push. • For intermittent IV infusion (piggyback), further dilute with 50–100 ml 0.9% NaCl. **Maximum concentration:** 30 mg/ml.
Rate of Administration • For IV injection, give over 3–5 min at a rate not to exceed 100 mg/min. • For intermittent IV infusion (piggyback), infuse over 15–30 min. • Due to potential for hypersensitivity/anaphylaxis, start initial dose at few drops per min, increase slowly to ordered rate; stay with pt first 10–15 min, then check q10min.
Storage • IV solution, diluted with 0.9% NaCl, is stable for 8 hrs at room temperature or 2 days if refrigerated. • If diluted with D₅W, is stable for 2 hrs at room temperature or 3 hrs if refrigerated. • Discard if precipitate forms.

IM
• Reconstitute each vial with Sterile Water for Injection or Bacteriostatic Water for Injection (consult individual vial for specific volume of diluent). • Stable for 1 hr. • Give deeply in large muscle mass.

PO
• Oral suspension, after reconstitution, is stable for 7 days at room temperature, 14 days if refrigerated. • Give orally 1–2 hrs before meals for maximum absorption. • Shake oral suspension well before using.

▦ IV INCOMPATIBILITIES

Diltiazem (Cardizem), midazolam (Versed), ondansetron (Zofran).

 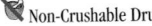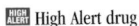

🎛 IV COMPATIBILITIES

Calcium gluconate, cefepime (Maxipime), dexmedetomidine (Precedex), dopamine (Intropin), famotidine (Pepcid), furosemide (Lasix), heparin, hydromorphone (Dilaudid), insulin (regular), levofloxacin (Levaquin), lipids, magnesium sulfate, morphine, multivitamins, potassium chloride, propofol (Diprivan).

INDICATIONS/ROUTES/DOSAGE

Usual Dosage
PO: ADULTS, ELDERLY: 250–500 mg q6h. **CHILDREN:** 50–100 mg/kg/day in divided doses q6h. **Maximum:** 2–4 g/day.
IV, IM: ADULTS, ELDERLY: 500 mg–3 g q4–6h. **Maximum:** 14 g/day. **CHILDREN:** 100–400 mg/kg/day in divided doses q6h. **Maximum:** 12 g/day. **NEONATES:** 50 mg/kg/dose q6–12h.

Dosage in Renal Impairment

Creatinine Clearance	Dosage
10–50 ml/min	Administer q6–12h
Less than 10 ml/min	Administer q12–24h
Hemodialysis	1–2 g q12–24h
Peritoneal dialysis	250 mg q12h
Continuous renal replacement therapy (CRRT)	2g, then 1–2 g q6–8h

SIDE EFFECTS

Frequent: Pain at IM injection site, GI disturbances (mild diarrhea, nausea, vomiting), oral or vaginal candidiasis. **Occasional:** Generalized rash, urticaria, phlebitis, thrombophlebitis (with IV administration), headache. **Rare:** Dizziness, seizures (esp. with IV therapy).

ADVERSE EFFECTS/ TOXIC REACTIONS

Antibiotic-associated colitis, other superinfections (abdominal cramps, severe watery diarrhea, fever) may result from altered bacterial balance in GI tract. Severe hypersensitivity reactions, including anaphylaxis, acute interstitial nephritis occur rarely.

NURSING CONSIDERATIONS

BASELINE ASSESSMENT

Question for history of allergies, esp. penicillins, cephalosporins, renal impairment.

INTERVENTION/EVALUATION

Hold medication and promptly report rash (although common with ampicillin, may indicate hypersensitivity) or diarrhea (fever, abdominal pain, mucus and blood in stool may indicate antibiotic-associated colitis). Evaluate IV site for phlebitis (heat, pain, red streaking over vein). Check IM injection site for pain, induration. Monitor I&O, urinalysis, renal function tests. Be alert for superinfection: fever, vomiting, diarrhea, anal/genital pruritus, oral mucosal changes (ulceration, pain, erythema).

PATIENT/FAMILY TEACHING

• Continue antibiotic for full length of treatment. • Space doses evenly. • More effective if taken 1 hr before or 2 hrs after food/beverages. • Discomfort may occur with IM injection. • Report rash, diarrhea, or other new symptoms.

ampicillin/ sulbactam

amp-i-**sil**-in/sul-**bak**-tam
(<u>Unasyn</u>)

◆CLASSIFICATION

PHARMACOTHERAPEUTIC: Penicillin. **CLINICAL:** Antibiotic (see p. 30C).

ACTION

Ampicillin inhibits bacterial cell wall synthesis. Sulbactam inhibits bacterial beta-lactamase. **Therapeutic Effect:** Ampicillin is bactericidal in susceptible microorganisms. Sulbactam protects ampicillin from enzymatic degradation.

PHARMACOKINETICS

Protein binding: 28%–38%. Widely distributed. Partially metabolized in liver. Primarily excreted in urine. Removed by hemodialysis. **Half-life:** 1–1.3 hrs (increased in renal impairment).

USES

Treatment of susceptible infections, including intra-abdominal, skin/skin structure, gynecologic infections, due to beta-lactamase-producing organisms including *H. influenzae, E. coli, Klebsiella, Acinetobacter, Enterobacter, S. aureus,* and *Bacteroides* spp.

PRECAUTIONS

Contraindications: Hypersensitivity to any penicillins or sulbactam. **Cautions:** History of allergies, esp. cephalosporins, renal impairment, infectious mononucleosis, asthmatic pts.

⌛ LIFESPAN CONSIDERATIONS

Pregnancy/Lactation: Crosses placenta; appears in cord blood, amniotic fluid. Distributed in breast milk in low concentrations. May lead to allergic sensitization, diarrhea, candidiasis, skin rash in infant. **Pregnancy Category B. Children:** Safety and efficacy not established in those younger than 1 yr. **Elderly:** Age-related renal impairment may require dosage adjustment.

INTERACTIONS

DRUG: Allopurinol may increase incidence of rash. **Probenecid** may increase concentration, toxicity risk. May decrease effects of **oral contraceptives.** May increase level/effects of **methotrexate.** **HERBAL:** None significant. **FOOD:** None known. **LAB VALUES:** May increase serum AST, ALT, alkaline phosphatase, LDH, creatinine. May cause positive Coombs' test.

AVAILABILITY (Rx)

Injection, Powder for Reconstitution: 1.5 g (ampicillin 1 g/sulbactam 500 g), 3 g (ampicillin 2 g/sulbactam 1 g).

ADMINISTRATION/HANDLING

 IV

Reconstitution • For IV injection, dilute with Sterile Water for Injection to provide concentration of 375 mg/ml. • For intermittent IV infusion (piggyback), further dilute with 50–100 ml 0.9% NaCl. **Rate of Administration •** For IV injection, give slowly over minimum of 10–15 min. • For intermittent IV infusion (piggyback), infuse over 15–30 min. • Due to potential for hypersensitivity/anaphylaxis, start initial dose at few drops per min, increase slowly to ordered rate; stay with pt first 10–15 min, then check q10min. **Storage •** IV solution, diluted with 0.9% NaCl, is stable for 8 hrs at room temperature, 72 hrs if refrigerated. • Discard if precipitate forms.

IM

• Reconstitute each 1.5-g vial with 3.2 ml Sterile Water for Injection or lidocaine to provide concentration of 250 mg ampicillin/125 mg sulbactam/ml. • Give deeply into large muscle mass within 1 hr after preparation.

⊞ IV INCOMPATIBILITIES

Amiodarone (Cordarone), diltiazem (Cardizem), idarubicin (Idamycin), ondansetron (Zofran).

⊞ IV COMPATIBILITIES

Famotidine (Pepcid), heparin, insulin (regular), morphine.

INDICATIONS/ROUTES/DOSAGE

Usual Dosage Range
IV, IM: ADULTS, ELDERLY, CHILDREN 13 YRS AND OLDER: 1.5 g (1 g ampicillin/500 mg sulbactam) to 3 g (2 g ampicillin/1 g sulbactam) q6h. **Maximum:** 12 g/day (Unasyn). **IV: CHILDREN 12 YRS AND YOUNGER:** 100–400 mg ampicillin/kg/day

in divided doses q6h. **Maximum:** 12 g/day (Unasyn). 8 g/day (ampicillin). **NEONATES:** 100 mg/kg/day in divided doses q8–12h.

Dosage in Renal Impairment

Dosage and frequency are modified based on creatinine clearance and severity of infection.

Creatinine Clearance	Dosage
Greater than 30 ml/min	1.5–3 g q6–8h
15–30 ml/min	1.5–3 g q12h
5–14 ml/min	1.5–3 g q24h
Hemodialysis	1.5–3 g q12–24h
Peritoneal dialysis	3 g q24h
Continuous renal replacement therapy (CRRT)	3 g, then 1.5–3 g q6–12h

SIDE EFFECTS

Frequent: Diarrhea, rash (most common), urticaria, pain at IM injection site, thrombophlebitis with IV administration, oral or vaginal candidiasis. **Occasional:** Nausea, vomiting, headache, malaise, urinary retention.

ADVERSE EFFECTS/ TOXIC REACTIONS

Antibiotic-associated colitis, other superinfections (abdominal cramps; severe, watery diarrhea; fever) may result from altered bacterial balance in GI tract. Severe hypersensitivity reactions, including anaphylaxis, acute interstitial nephritis, blood dyscrasias may occur. High dosage may produce seizures.

NURSING CONSIDERATIONS

BASELINE ASSESSMENT

Question for history of allergies, esp. penicillins, cephalosporins, renal impairment.

INTERVENTION/EVALUATION

Hold medication and promptly report rash (although common with ampicillin, may indicate hypersensitivity) or diarrhea (fever, abdominal pain, mucus and blood in stool may indicate antibiotic-associated colitis). Evaluate IV site for phlebitis (heat, pain, red streaking over vein). Check IM injection site for pain, induration. Monitor I&O, urinalysis, renal function tests. Be alert for superinfection: fever, vomiting, diarrhea, anal/genital pruritus, oral mucosal changes (ulceration, pain, erythema).

PATIENT/FAMILY TEACHING

• Take antibiotic for full length of treatment. • Space doses evenly. • Discomfort may occur with IM injection. • Report rash, diarrhea, or other new symptoms.

anakinra

an-a-**kin**-ra
(Kineret)
Do not confuse anakinra with amikacin or Ampyra.

◆CLASSIFICATION

PHARMACOTHERAPEUTIC: Interleukin-1 receptor antagonist. **CLINICAL:** Anti-inflammatory.

ACTION

Blocks the binding of interleukin-1 (IL-1), a protein that is a major mediator of joint pathology and is present in excess amounts in pts with rheumatoid arthritis. **Therapeutic Effect:** Inhibits inflammatory response.

PHARMACOKINETICS

No accumulation of anakinra in tissues or organs was observed after daily subcutaneous doses. Excreted in urine. **Half-life:** 4–6 hrs.

USES

Treatment of signs and symptoms or to slow progression of structural damage of moderate to severely active rheumatoid arthritis (RA) in pts who have failed treatment with one or more disease-modifying antirheumatic drugs. May use alone or with other disease-modifying antirheumatic drugs (other than tumor necrosis factor blocking medications).

PRECAUTIONS

Contraindications: Known hypersensitivity to *Escherichia coli*–derived proteins. **Cautions:** Renal impairment (risk of toxic reaction is increased), asthma (higher incidence of serious infection), elderly, history of significant hematologic abnormalities. Avoid use in pts with active infection.

⌛ LIFESPAN CONSIDERATIONS

Pregnancy/Lactation: Unknown if distributed in breast milk. **Pregnancy Category B. Children:** Safety and efficacy not established. **Elderly:** Age-related renal impairment may require caution.

INTERACTIONS

DRUG: Increased risk of infection with **etanercept. HERBAL: Echinacea** may decrease effect. **FOOD:** None known. **LAB VALUES:** May decrease WBC count, platelet count, absolute neutrophil count (ANC). May increase eosinophil count.

AVAILABILITY (Rx)

Injection Solution: 100-mg syringe.

ADMINISTRATION/HANDLING

Subcutaneous
• Store in refrigerator; do not freeze or shake. • Do not use if particulate or discoloration is noted. • Give by subcutaneous route (thigh, abdomen, upper arm).

INDICATIONS/ROUTES/DOSAGE

Rheumatoid Arthritis (RA)
Subcutaneous: ADULTS, ELDERLY: 100 mg/day, given at same time each day.

Dosage in Renal Impairment
Creatinine clearance less than 30 ml/min and/or end-stage renal disease: 100 mg every other day.

SIDE EFFECTS

Occasional: Injection site ecchymosis, erythema, inflammation. **Rare:** Headache, nausea, diarrhea, abdominal pain.

ADVERSE EFFECTS/ TOXIC REACTIONS

Infections, including upper respiratory tract infection, sinusitis, flu-like symptoms, cellulitis, have been noted. Neutropenia may occur, particularly when anakinra is used in combination with tumor necrosis factor blocking agents.

NURSING CONSIDERATIONS

BASELINE ASSESSMENT
Assess pt's range of motion, pain, swelling in joints.

INTERVENTION/EVALUATION
Monitor neutrophil count before therapy begins, monthly for 3 mos while receiving therapy, then quarterly for up to 1 yr. Assess for hypersensitivity reaction, esp. during first 4 wks of therapy (uncommon after first mo of therapy).

PATIENT/FAMILY TEACHING
• Follow dosage and administration procedures carefully. • Dispose of syringes and needles properly. • Avoid live/inactive virus vaccines during therapy.

---

anastrozole

an-**as**-troe-zole
(Arimidex)
Do not confuse anastrozole with letrozole, or Arimidex with Imitrex.

◆CLASSIFICATION

PHARMACOTHERAPEUTIC: Aromatase inhibitor. **CLINICAL:** Antineoplastic hormone (see p. 82C).

 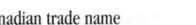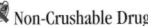

ACTION

Decreases circulating estrogen level by inhibiting aromatase, the enzyme that catalyzes the final step in estrogen production. **Therapeutic Effect:** Inhibits growth of breast cancers that are stimulated by estrogens by lowering serum estradiol concentration.

PHARMACOKINETICS

Well absorbed into systemic circulation (absorption not affected by food). Protein binding: 40%. Extensively metabolized in liver. Eliminated by biliary system and, to a lesser extent, kidneys. **Mean half-life:** 50 hrs in postmenopausal women. Steady-state plasma levels reached in about 7 days.

USES

Treatment of advanced breast cancer in postmenopausal women who have developed progressive disease while receiving tamoxifen therapy. First-line therapy in advanced or metastatic breast cancer in postmenopausal women. Adjuvant treatment in early breast cancer in postmenopausal women. **OFF-LABEL:** Treatment of recurrent or metastatic endometrial or uterine cancers; treatment of ovarian cancer.

PRECAUTIONS

Contraindications: Pregnancy, those who may become pregnant. **Cautions:** Preexisting ischemic cardiac disease or osteopenia.

⏳ LIFESPAN CONSIDERATIONS

Pregnancy/Lactation: Crosses placenta; may cause fetal harm. Unknown if distributed in breast milk. **Pregnancy Category D. Children:** Safety and efficacy not established. **Elderly:** No age-related precautions noted.

INTERACTIONS

DRUG: Estrogen therapies may reduce concentration/effects. **Tamoxifen** may reduce plasma concentration. **HERBAL:** Avoid **black cohosh, dong quai, licorice, red clover. FOOD:** None known. **LAB VALUES:** May elevate serum GGT level in pts with liver metastases. May increase serum AST, ALT, alkaline phosphate, total cholesterol, LDL.

AVAILABILITY (Rx)

Tablets: 1 mg.

ADMINISTRATION/HANDLING

PO
• Give without regard to food.

INDICATIONS/ROUTES/DOSAGE

Breast Cancer
PO: ADULTS, ELDERLY: 1 mg once a day.

SIDE EFFECTS

Frequent (16%–8%): Asthenia (loss of strength, energy), nausea, headache, hot flashes, back pain, vomiting, cough, diarrhea. **Occasional (6%–4%):** Constipation, abdominal pain, anorexia, bone pain, pharyngitis, dizziness, rash, dry mouth, peripheral edema, pelvic pain, depression, chest pain, paresthesia. **Rare (2%–1%):** Weight gain, diaphoresis.

ADVERSE EFFECTS/TOXIC REACTIONS

Thrombophlebitis, anemia, leukopenia occur rarely. Vaginal hemorrhage occurs rarely (2%).

NURSING CONSIDERATIONS

INTERVENTION/EVALUATION

Monitor for asthenia (loss of strength, energy), dizziness; assist with ambulation if needed. Assess for headache, pain. Offer antiemetic for nausea, vomiting. Monitor for onset of diarrhea; offer antidiarrheal medication.

PATIENT/FAMILY TEACHING

• Notify physician if nausea, asthenia (loss of strength, energy), hot flashes become unmanageable.

anidulafungin

a-**nid**-ue-la-**fun**-jin
(Eraxis)

◆ CLASSIFICATION

PHARMACOTHERAPEUTIC: Echinocandin. **CLINICAL:** Antifungal (see p. 48C).

ACTION

Inhibits synthesis of the enzyme glucan, (vital component of fungal cell formation), preventing fungal cell wall formation. **Therapeutic Effect:** Fungistatic.

PHARMACOKINETICS

Distributed in tissue. Moderately bound to albumin. Protein binding: 84%–99%. Slow chemical degradation; 30% excreted in feces over 9 days. Not removed by hemodialysis. **Half-life:** 40–50 hrs.

USES

Treatment of candidemia, other forms of *Candida* infections (intra-abdominal abscess, peritonitis), esophageal candidiasis. **OFF-LABEL:** Treatment of infections due to *Aspergillus*.

PRECAUTIONS

Contraindications: Hypersensitivity to anidulafungin, other echinocandins. **Cautions:** Hepatic impairment.

⌛ LIFESPAN CONSIDERATIONS

Pregnancy/Lactation: May be embryotoxic. Crosses placental barrier. Unknown if distributed in breast milk. **Pregnancy Category C. Children:** Safety and efficacy not established. **Elderly:** No age-related precautions noted.

INTERACTIONS

DRUG: None significant. **HERBAL:** None significant. **FOOD:** None known. **LAB VALUES:** May increase serum ALT, AST, bilirubin, alkaline phosphatase, LDH, transferase, amylase, lipase, CPK, creatinine, calcium. May decrease serum albumin, bicarbonate, magnesium, protein, potassium, Hgb, Hct, WBCs, neutrophils, platelet count. May prolong prothrombin time (PT).

AVAILABILITY (Rx)

Injection, Powder for Reconstitution: 50-mg vial, 100-mg vial.

ADMINISTRATION/HANDLING

 IV

Reconstitution • Reconstitute each 50-mg vial with 15 ml Sterile Water for Injection (100 mg with 30 ml). Swirl, do not shake. • Further dilute 50 mg with 50 ml D₅W or 0.9% NaCl (100 mg with 100 ml, 200 mg with 200 ml).
Rate of Administration • Do not exceed infusion rate of 1.1 mg/min. Not for IV bolus injection.
Storage • Refrigerate unreconstituted vials. • Final reconstituted infusion solution stable for 24 hrs refrigerated.

▦ IV INCOMPATIBILITIES

Amphotericin B (Abelcet, AmBisome), ertapenem (Invanz), sodium bicarbonate.

▦ IV COMPATIBILITIES

Dexamethasone (Decadron), famotidine (Pepcid), furosemide (Lasix), hydromorphone (Dilaudid), lorazepam (Ativan), methylprednisolone (Solu-Medrol), morphine. Refer to IV Compatibility Chart in front of book.

INDICATIONS/ROUTES/DOSAGE

◀ ALERT ▶ Duration of treatment based on pt's clinical response. In general, treatment is continued for at least 14 days after last positive culture.

Candidemia, Other Candida Infections
IV: ADULTS, ELDERLY: Give single 200-mg loading dose on day 1, followed by 100 mg/day thereafter for at least 14 days after last positive culture.

Esophageal Candidiasis
IV: ADULTS, ELDERLY: Give single 100-mg loading dose on day 1, followed by 50

mg/day thereafter for a minimum of 14 days and for at least 7 days following resolution of symptoms.

SIDE EFFECTS

Rare (3%–1%): Diarrhea, nausea, headache, rigors, peripheral edema.

ADVERSE EFFECTS/ TOXIC REACTIONS

Hypokalemia occurs in 4% of pts. Hypersensitivity reaction characterized by facial flushing, hypotension, pruritus, urticaria, rash occurs rarely.

NURSING CONSIDERATIONS

BASELINE ASSESSMENT

Obtain specimens for fungal culture prior to therapy. Treatment may be instituted before results are known. Obtain baseline CBC, serum chemistry, hepatic enzyme levels.

INTERVENTION/EVALUATION

Monitor serum chemistry, hepatic function results for evidence of hepatic dysfunction, hypokalemia. Monitor daily pattern of bowel activity, stool consistency. Assess for rash, urticaria.

PATIENT/FAMILY TEACHING

• For esophageal candidiasis, maintain diligent oral hygiene.

antihemophilic factor (factor VIII, AHF)

an-tee-hee-moe-**fil**-ik **fak**-tor (**Antihemophilic Factor/von Willebrand Factor Complex:** Alphanate, Humate-P, Wilate. **Human:** Hemofil M, Koate-DVI, Monarc-M, Monoclate-P. **Recombinant:** Advate, Hexilate FS, Kogenate FS, Recombinate, Refacto, Xyntha)

◆ CLASSIFICATION

PHARMACOTHERAPEUTIC: Antihemophilic agent. **CLINICAL:** Hemostatic.

ACTION

Assists in conversion of prothrombin to thrombin, essential for blood coagulation. Replaces missing clotting factor VIII. **Therapeutic Effect:** Produces hemostasis; corrects or prevents bleeding episodes.

PHARMACOKINETICS

Half-life: 8–27 hrs.

USES

Human: Prevention/treatment of hemorrhagic episodes, perioperative management of hemophilia A. **Alphanate, Humate-P, Wilate:** Prevention/treatment of hemorrhagic episodes in pts with hemophilia A. Prophylaxis with surgical/invasive procedures, treatment of bleeding in pts with von Willebrand disease (vWD) when desmopressin is known or suspected to be inadequate. **Recombinant:** Management of hemophilia A, prevention and control of bleeding episodes, perioperative management of hemophilia A, prophylaxis of joint bleeding and reduce risk of joint damage in children with hemophilia A. **OFF-LABEL:** Treatment of disseminated intravascular coagulation.

PRECAUTIONS

Contraindications: None known. **Cautions:** Hepatic disease, those with blood types A, B, AB.

⧖ LIFESPAN CONSIDERATIONS

Pregnancy/Lactation: Unknown if drug crosses placenta or is distributed in breast milk. **Pregnancy Category C. Children:** Safety and efficacy not established. **Elderly:** No age-related precautions noted.

INTERACTIONS

DRUG: None significant. **HERBAL:** None significant. **FOOD:** None known. **LAB VALUES:** None significant.

AVAILABILITY (Rx)

Human: Injection, Powder for Reconstitution (Hemofil M, Koate-DVI, Monarc-M, Monoclate-P): Actual number of units listed on each vial. **Alphanate:** 250 units, 500 units, 1,000 units, 1,500 units. **Humate-P:** 250 units, 500 units, 1,000 units. **Recombinant:** Injection, Powder for Reconsitution: **Advate:** 250 units, 500 units, 1,000 units, 1,500 units, 2,000 units, 3,000 units. **Hexilate, Kogenate, Recombinate:** 250 units, 500 units, 1,000 units. **Refacto, Xyntha:** 250 units, 500 units, 1,000 units, 2,000 units.

ADMINISTRATION/HANDLING

 IV

Reconstitution • Warm concentrate and diluent to room temperature. • Using needle supplied by the manufacturer, add diluent to powder to dissolve, gently agitate or rotate. Do not shake vigorously. Complete dissolution may take 5–10 min. • Use second filtered needle supplied by the manufacturer, and add to infusion bag.
Rate of Administration • **Advate:** Over 5 min or less. **Maximum:** 10 ml/min. • **Hexilate FS, Kogenate FS:** Over 1–15 min based on pt tolerance. • **Xyntha:** Over several min. • **Hemofil M, Koate-DVI, Monarc-M:** Over 5–10 min. **Maximum:** 10 ml/min. • **Monoclate-P:** Infuse at 2 ml/min. • **Alphanate:** 10 ml/min. **Humate-P:** 4 ml/min.
Administration Precautions • Check pulse rate prior to and following administration. If pulse rate increases, reduce or stop administration. • After administration, apply prolonged pressure on venipuncture site. • Monitor IV site for oozing q5–15min for 1–2 hrs following administration.
Storage • May refrigerate or store at room temperature. • See individual products for specific storage durations.

⚠ IV INCOMPATIBILITIES

Do not mix with other IV solutions or medications.

INDICATIONS/ROUTES/DOSAGE

Hemophilia A, Von Willebrand Disease
IV: ADULTS, ELDERLY, CHILDREN: Dosage is highly individualized and is based on pt's weight, severity of bleeding, coagulation studies.

SIDE EFFECTS

Occasional: Allergic reaction, including fever, chills, urticaria, wheezing, hypotension, nausea, feeling of chest tightness, stinging at injection site, dizziness, dry mouth, headache, altered taste.

ADVERSE EFFECTS/ TOXIC REACTIONS

Risk of transmitting viral hepatitis. Intravascular hemolysis may occur if large or frequent doses are used with blood group A, B, or AB.

NURSING CONSIDERATIONS

BASELINE ASSESSMENT

When monitoring B/P, avoid overinflation of cuff. Remove adhesive tape from any pressure dressing carefully and slowly.

INTERVENTION/EVALUATION

Following IV administration, apply prolonged pressure on venipuncture site. Monitor IV site for oozing q5–15 min for 1–2 hrs following administration. Assess for allergic reaction. Immediately report any evidence of hematuria or change in vital signs. Assess for decreases in B/P, increased pulse rate, complaint of abdominal or back pain, severe headache (may be evidence of hemorrhage). Question for increased discharge during menses. Assess skin for bruises, petechiae. Check for excessive bleeding from minor cuts, scratches. Assess gums for erythema, gingival bleeding. Assess urine for hematuria. Evaluate for therapeutic relief of pain, reduction of swelling, restricted joint movement.

PATIENT/FAMILY TEACHING

• Use electric razor, soft toothbrush to prevent bleeding. • Report any sign of bleeding, including red or dark urine, black/red stool, coffee-ground vomitus, blood-tinged mucus from cough. • Wear identification indicating a hemolytic condition. • Bring adequate supply of agent when traveling.

apixaban

a-**pix**-a-ban
(Eliquis)
Do not confuse apixaban with rivaroxaban, argatroban, or dabigatran.

BLACK BOX ALERT Discontinuation in absence of alternative anticoagulation increases risk for thrombotic events. An increased rate of stroke noted following discontinuation in pts with non-valvular atrial fibrillation. If apixaban must be discontinued based on other than pathologic bleeding, coverage with another anticoagulant should be strongly considered.

◆CLASSIFICATION

PHARMACOTHERAPEUTIC: Factor Xa inhibitor. **CLINICAL:** Anticoagulant.

ACTION

Selectively blocks active site of factor Xa, a key factor in the intrinsic and extrinsic pathway of blood coagulation cascade. Prevents new clot formation, secondary thromboembolic complications. **Therapeutic Effect:** Inhibits clot-induced platelet aggregation, fibrin clot formation.

PHARMACOKINETICS

Readily absorbed after PO administration. Peak plasma concentration: 3–4 hrs. Protein binding: 87%. Metabolized in liver. Excreted primarily in urine, feces. **Half-life:** 12 hrs.

USES

Reduces risk for stroke, systemic embolism in pts with nonvalvular atrial fibrilla-

tion. **OFF-LABEL:** Reduces risk of recurrent DVT and/or PE.

PRECAUTIONS

Contraindications: Active pathologic bleeding. **Cautions:** Mild to moderate hepatic impairment, severe renal impairment. Avoid use in those with severe hepatic impairment, prosthetic heart valve.

⏳ LIFESPAN CONSIDERATIONS

Pregnancy/Lactation: Unknown if distributed in breast milk. **Pregnancy Category B. Children:** Safety and efficacy not established. **Elderly:** No age-related precautions noted.

INTERACTIONS

DRUG: CYP3A4 inducers (e.g., carbamazepine, rifampin) may decrease levels/effects. **Aspirin, NSAIDs, warfarin, heparin, antiplatelet agents, CYP3A4 inhibitors, (e.g., ketoconazole, clarithromycin)** may increase concentration, bleeding risk. **HERBAL: St. John's wort** may decrease levels/effects. **Flaxseed, garlic, ginger, ginko biloba, ginseng, Omega-3** may increase risk of bleeding. **FOOD: Grapefruit juice** may increase levels/adverse effects. **LAB VALUES:** May decrease platelet count, Hgb, LFTs.

AVAILABILITY (Rx)

Tablets: 2.5 mg, 5 mg.

ADMINISTRATION/HANDLING

◀ALERT▶ Discontinuation in absence of alternative anticoagulation increases risk for thrombotic events.

PO
• Give without regard to meals. • If elective surgery or invasive procedures with moderate or high risk for bleeding, discontinue apixaban 24 hrs prior to procedure.

INDICATIONS/ROUTES/DOSAGE

Anticoagulant
PO: ADULTS, ELDERLY: 5 mg twice daily. In those with at least 2 of the following characteristics: age 80 yrs or older, body

weight 60 kg or less, serum creatinine 1.5 mg/dl or greater, concurrent use with CYP3A4, P-gp inhibitors (e.g., ketoconazole, ritonavir); then reduce dose to 2.5 mg twice daily.

SIDE EFFECTS

Rare (3%–1%): Nausea, ecchymosis.

ADVERSE EFFECTS/ TOXIC REACTIONS

Increased risk for bleeding/hemorrhagic events. May cause serious, potentially fatal, bleeding, accompanied by one or more of the following: a decrease in Hgb of 2 g/dl or more; a need for 2 or more units of packed RBCs; bleeding occurring at one of the following sites: intracranial, intraspinal, intraocular, pericardial, intra-articular, intramuscular with compartment syndrome, retroperitoneal. Serious reactions include jaundice, cholestasis, cytolytic hepatitis, Stevens-Johnson syndrome, hypersensitivity reaction, anaphylaxis.

NURSING CONSIDERATIONS

BASELINE ASSESSMENT

Obtain baseline CBC, PT/INR. Question history of bleeding disorders, recent surgery, spinal punctures, intracranial hemorrhage, bleeding ulcers, open wounds, anemia, hepatic impairment. Obtain full medication history including herbal products.

INTERVENTION/EVALUATION

Periodically monitor CBC, stool for occult blood. Be alert for complaints of abdominal/back pain, headache, confusion, weakness, vision change (may indicate hemorrhage). Question for increased menstrual bleeding/discharge. Assess for any sign of bleeding: bleeding at surgical site, hematuria, blood in stool, bleeding from gums, petechiae, ecchymosis.

PATIENT/FAMILY TEACHING

• Do not take/discontinue any medication except on advice from physician. • Avoid alcohol, aspirin, NSAIDs. • Consult physi-cian before surgery, dental work. • Use electric razor, soft toothbrush to prevent bleeding. • Report blood-tinged mucus from coughing, heavy menstrual bleeding, headache, vision problems, weakness, abdominal pain, frequent bruising, bloody urine or stool, joint pain or swelling.

aprepitant/ fosaprepitant

a-**prep**-i-tant/fos-a-**prep**-i-tant
(Emend, Emend for Injection)
Do not confuse fosaprepitant with aprepitant, fosamprenavir, or fospropofol.

◆CLASSIFICATION

PHARMACOTHERAPEUTIC: Selective receptor antagonist. CLINICAL: Anti-nausea, antiemetic.

ACTION

Inhibits chemotherapy-induced nausea, vomiting centrally in the chemoreceptor trigger zone. **Therapeutic Effect:** Prevents acute and delayed phases of chemotherapy-induced emesis, including vomiting caused by high-dose cisplatin.

PHARMACOKINETICS

Moderately absorbed from GI tract. Crosses blood-brain barrier. Extensively metabolized in liver. Protein binding: greater than 95%. Eliminated primarily by liver metabolism (not excreted renally). **Half-life:** 9–13 hrs.

USES

PO/IV: Prevention of nausea, vomiting associated with repeat courses of moderate to high emetogenic cancer chemotherapy, including high-dose cisplatin. PO: Prevention of postop nausea, vomiting.

PRECAUTIONS

Contraindications: None known. Cautions: Severe hepatic impairment. Concurrent use of medications metabolized through CYP3A4 **(docetaxol, etoposide, ifosfamide, imatinib, irinotecan, paclitaxel, vinbastine, vincristine, vinorelbine).**

LIFESPAN CONSIDERATIONS

Pregnancy/Lactation: Unknown if drug crosses placenta or is distributed in breast milk. **Pregnancy Category B. Children:** Safety and efficacy not established. **Elderly:** No age-related precautions noted.

INTERACTIONS

DRUG: Strong **CYP3A4 inhibitors (e.g., ketoconazole, clarithromycin)** may increase concentration. Strong **CYP3A4 inducers (e.g., carbamazepine, rifampin)** may decrease concentration. May decrease effectiveness of **hormonal contraceptives.** May decrease effectiveness of **warfarin. HERBAL: St. John's wort** may decrease plasma concentration. **FOOD: Grapefruit, grapefruit juice** may increase plasma concentration. **LAB VALUES:** May increase BUN, serum creatinine, glucose, alkaline phosphatase, AST, ALT. May produce proteinuria.

AVAILABILITY (Rx)

Capsules (Emend): 40 mg, 80 mg, 125 mg. **Emend (Combination):** 80 mg (2), 125 mg (1). **Injection, Powder for Reconstitution (Fosaprepitant):** 115 mg, 150 mg.

ADMINISTRATION/HANDLING

PO
• Give without regard to food.

 IV

Reconstitution • Reconstitute each vial with 5 ml 0.9% NaCl. • Add 0.9% NaCl to provide a final concentration of 1 mg/ml. **Rate of Administration** • Infuse 110 mg over 15 min 30 min prior to chemotherapy, 150 mg over 20–30 min 30 min prior to chemotherapy. **Storage** • Refrigerate unreconstituted vials. • After reconstitution, solution is stable at room temperature for 24 hrs.

IV INCOMPATIBILITIES

Do not infuse with any solutions containing calcium or magnesium.

INDICATIONS/ROUTES/DOSAGE

Prevention of Chemotherapy-Induced Nausea, Vomiting
PO: ADULTS, ELDERLY: 125 mg 1 hr before chemotherapy on day 1 and 80 mg once a day in the morning on days 2 and 3. **Note:** Emend for Injection 115 mg may be substituted for Emend 125 mg on day 1 only.
IV: ADULTS, ELDERLY (SINGLE-DOSE REGIMEN): 150 mg over 20–30 min 30 min prior to chemotherapy (in combination with a 5-HT$_3$ antagonist on day 1 and dexamethasone on days 1 to 4). **(3-day regimen):** 115 mg over 15 min 30 min prior to chemotherapy, followed by aprepitant 80 mg orally on days 2 and 3 (in combination with a 5-HT$_3$ antagonist and dexamethasone).

Prevention of Postop Nausea, Vomiting
PO: ADULTS, ELDERLY: 40 mg once within 3 hrs prior to induction of anesthesia.

SIDE EFFECTS

Frequent (17%–10%): Fatigue, nausea, hiccups, diarrhea, constipation, anorexia. **Occasional (8%–4%):** Headache, vomiting, dizziness, dehydration, heartburn. **Rare (3% or less):** Abdominal pain, epigastric discomfort, gastritis, tinnitus, insomnia.

ADVERSE EFFECTS/
TOXIC REACTIONS

Neutropenia, mucous membrane disorders occur rarely.

NURSING CONSIDERATIONS

BASELINE ASSESSMENT

Assess for dehydration (poor skin turgor, dry mucous membranes, longitudinal furrows in tongue).

INTERVENTION/EVALUATION

Monitor hydration, nutritional status, I&O. Assess bowel sounds for peristalsis. Assist with ambulation if dizziness occurs. Provide supportive measures. Monitor daily pattern of bowel activity, stool consistency.

PATIENT/FAMILY TEACHING
• Relief from nausea/vomiting generally occurs shortly after drug administration.
• Report persistent vomiting, headache.
• May decrease effectiveness of oral contraceptives.

---

argatroban

ar-gat-roe-ban
Do not confuse argatroban with Aggrestat.

◆CLASSIFICATION
PHARMACOTHERAPEUTIC: Thrombin inhibitor. **CLINICAL:** Anticoagulant (see p. 32C).

ACTION
Direct thrombin inhibitor that reversibly binds to thrombin-active sites. Inhibits thrombin-catalyzed or thrombin-induced reactions, including fibrin formation, activation of coagulant factors V, VIII, and XIII; inhibits protein C formation, platelet aggregation. **Therapeutic Effect:** Produces anticoagulation.

PHARMACOKINETICS
Distributed primarily in extracellular fluid. Protein binding: 54%. Metabolized in liver. Primarily excreted in the feces, presumably through biliary secretion. **Half-life:** 39–51 min.

USES
Prophylaxis or treatment of thrombosis in heparin-induced thrombocytopenia (HIT). Prevention of HIT during percutaneous coronary procedures. **OFF-LABEL:** Maintain extracorporeal circuit patency of continuous renal replacement therapy (CRRT) in pts with HIT.

PRECAUTIONS
Contraindications: Active major bleeding. **Cautions:** Severe hypertension, immediately following lumbar puncture, spinal anesthesia, major surgery, pts with congenital or acquired bleeding disorders, ulcerations, hepatic impairment, critically ill pts.

⏳ LIFESPAN CONSIDERATIONS
Pregnancy/Lactation: Unknown if excreted in breast milk. **Pregnancy Category C. Children:** Safety and efficacy not established in those younger than 18 yrs. **Elderly:** No age-related precautions noted.

INTERACTIONS
DRUG: Antiplatelet agents, other anticoagulants, thrombolytics, NSAIDs may increase the risk of bleeding. **HERBAL: Dong quai, evening primrose oil, ginkgo, policosanol, willow bark** may increase risk of bleeding. **FOOD:** None known. **LAB VALUES:** Increases prothrombin time (PT), activated partial thromboplastin time (aPTT), international normalized ratio (INR). May decrease Hgb, Hct.

AVAILABILITY (Rx)
Infusion (Pre-Mix): 125 mg/125 ml 0.9% NaCl; 50 mg/50 ml Sterile Water for Injection. **Injection Solution:** 100 mg/ml (2.5 ml).

ADMINISTRATION/HANDLING
 IV

Reconstitution • Dilute each 250-mg vial with 250 ml 0.9% NaCl, D₅W, or lactated Ringer's solution to provide a final concentration of 1 mg/ml. • The solution must be mixed by repeated inversion of the diluent bag for 1 min. • After reconstitution, solution may show a brief haziness due to formation of microprecipitates that rapidly dissolve upon mixing.
Rate of Administration • Rate of administration is based on body weight at 2 mcg/kg/min (e.g., 50-kg pt infuse at 6 ml/hr).
Storage • Discard if solution appears cloudy or an insoluble precipitate is

noted. • Following reconstitution, stable for 96 hrs at room temperature or refrigerated. • Avoid direct sunlight.

🞖 IV INCOMPATIBILITY

Amiodarone (Cardarone).

🞖 IV COMPATIBILITIES

Diphenhydramine (Benadryl), dobutamine (Dobutrex), dopamine (Intropin), furosemide (Lasix), midazolam (Versed), morphine, vasopressin (Pitressin). Refer to IV Compatibility Chart in front of book.

INDICATIONS/ROUTES/DOSAGE

Heparin-Induced Thrombocytopenia (HIT)
IV Infusion: ADULTS, ELDERLY: Initially, 2 mcg/kg/min administered as a continuous infusion. After initial infusion, dose may be adjusted until steady-state aPTT is 1.5–3 times initial baseline value, not to exceed 100 sec. Dosage should not exceed 10 mcg/kg/min.

Percutaneous Coronary Intervention
IV Infusion: ADULTS, ELDERLY: Initially, administer bolus of 350 mcg/kg over 3–5 min, then infuse at 25 mcg/kg/min. Check ACT (activated clotting time) 5–10 min following bolus. If ACT is less than 300 sec, give additional bolus 150 mcg/kg, increase infusion to 30 mcg/kg/min. If ACT is greater than 450 sec, decrease infusion to 15 mcg/kg/min. Once ACT of 300–450 sec achieved, continue dose through duration of procedure.

Dosage in Hepatic Impairment
ADULTS, ELDERLY: Initially, 0.5 mcg/kg/min. **CHILDREN:** Initially, 0.2 mcg/kg/min. Adjust dose in increments of 0.05 mcg/kg/min or less.

SIDE EFFECTS

Frequent (8%–3%): Dyspnea, hypotension, fever, diarrhea, nausea, pain, vomiting, infection, cough.

ADVERSE EFFECTS/TOXIC REACTIONS

Ventricular tachycardia, atrial fibrillation occur occasionally. Major bleeding, sepsis occur rarely.

NURSING CONSIDERATIONS

BASELINE ASSESSMENT

Check CBC, PT, PTT. Determine initial B/P. Minimize need for multiple injection sites, blood draws, catheters.

INTERVENTION/EVALUATION

Assess for any sign of bleeding: bleeding at surgical site, hematuria, blood in stool, bleeding from gums, petechiae, ecchymoses, bleeding from injection sites. Handle pt carefully and infrequently to prevent bleeding. Do not obtain B/P in lower extremities (possible deep vein thrombi). Assess for decreased B/P, increased pulse rate, complaint of abdominal/back pain, severe headache (indicates evidence of hemorrhage). Monitor ACT, PT, aPTT, platelet count, Hgb, Hct. Question for increase in discharge during menses. Assess urinary output for hematuria. Observe skin for any occurring ecchymoses, petechiae, hematoma. Use care in removing any dressing, tape.

PATIENT/FAMILY TEACHING

• Use electric razor, soft toothbrush to prevent cuts, gingival trauma. • Report any sign of bleeding, including red/dark urine, black/red stool, coffee-ground vomitus, blood-tinged mucus from cough.

---

aripiprazole

ar-i-**pip**-ra-zole
(<u>Abilify</u>, Abilify Discmelt, Abilify Maintena)

BLACK BOX ALERT Increased risk of mortality in elderly pts with dementia-related psychosis, mainly due to pneumonia, heart failure. Risk may be increased by dehydration. Increased risk of suicidal thinking and behavior in children, adolescents, young adults 18–24 yrs with major depressive disorder, other psychiatric disorders.

Do not confuse Abilify with Ambien, or aripiprazole with esomeprazole, omeprazole, pantoprazole, or rabeprazole (proton pump inhibitors).

◆ CLASSIFICATION

PHARMACOTHERAPEUTIC: Dopamine agonist. **CLINICAL:** Antipsychotic agent (see p. 66C).

ACTION

Provides partial agonist activity at dopamine and serotonin (5-HT$_{1A}$) receptors and antagonist activity at serotonin (5-HT$_{2A}$) receptors. **Therapeutic Effect:** Diminishes schizophrenic behavior.

PHARMACOKINETICS

Well absorbed through GI tract. Protein binding: 99% (primarily albumin). Reaches steady levels in 2 wks. Metabolized in liver. Eliminated primarily in feces and, to a lesser extent, in urine. Not removed by hemodialysis. **Half-life:** 75 hrs.

USES

PO: Treatment of schizophrenia. Maintains stability in pts with schizophrenia. Treatment of bipolar disorder. Maintenance treatment of bipolar disorder as an adjunct to either lithium or valproate. Adjunct treatment in major depressive disorder. Treatment of irritability associated with autistic disorder in children 6–17 yrs of age. **IM:** Agitation associated with schizophrenia/bipolar disorder. **Abilify Maintena:** Treatment of schizophrenia. **OFF-LABEL:** Schizoaffective disorder, depression with psychotic features, aggression, bipolar disorder (children), conduct disorder (children), Tourette's syndrome (children), psychosis/agitation related to Alzheimer's dementia.

PRECAUTIONS

Contraindications: None known. **Cautions:** Concurrent use of CNS depressants (including alcohol), cardiovascular or cerebrovascular diseases (may induce hypotension), Parkinson's disease (potential for exacerbation), history of seizures or conditions that may lower seizure threshold (Alzheimer's disease), diabetes mellitus. Pts at risk for pneumonia.

⧖ LIFESPAN CONSIDERATIONS

Pregnancy/Lactation: Unknown if drug crosses placenta. May be distributed in breast milk. Breast-feeding not recommended. **Pregnancy Category C. Children:** Safety and efficacy not established. **Elderly:** May increase serum glucose. May decrease neutrophils, leukocytes.

INTERACTIONS

DRUG: **Alcohol** may potentiate cognitive and motor effects. **CYP3A4 inducers (e.g., carbamazepine)** may decrease concentration. **CYP3A4 inhibitors (e.g., itraconazole, ketoconazole)** may increase concentrations. **HERBAL:** **St. John's wort** may decrease levels. **Gotu kola, kava kava, St. John's wort, valerian** may increase CNS depression. **FOOD:** None known. **LAB VALUES:** None significant.

AVAILABILITY (Rx)

Injection, Solution: 9.75 mg/1.3 ml (7.5 mg/ml). **Solution, Oral:** 1 mg/ml. **Tablets:** 2 mg, 5 mg, 10 mg, 15 mg, 20 mg, 30 mg. **Tablets, Orally Disintegrating:** 10 mg, 15 mg. **Injection, Powder for Reconstitution (Abilify Maintena):** 300 mg, 400 mg.

ADMINISTRATION/HANDLING

IM
• For IM use only (inject slowly into deep muscle mass). Do not administer IV or subcutaneous.

IM (Abilify Maintena)
• Reconstitute 400-mg vial with 1.9 ml Sterile Water for Injection (300-mg vial with 1.5 ml) to provide a concentration

of 100 mg/0.5 ml. Once reconstituted, administer in gluteal muscle.

PO
• Give without regard to food.

Orally Disintegrating Tablet
• Remove tablet, place entire tablet on tongue. • Do not break, split tablet. • May give without liquid.

INDICATIONS/ROUTES/DOSAGE

Schizophrenia
PO: ADULTS, ELDERLY: Initially, 10–15 mg once a day. May increase up to 30 mg/day. Titrate dose at minimum of 2-wk intervals. **CHILDREN 13–17 YRS:** Initially, 2 mg/day for 2 days, then 5 mg/day for 2 days. May further increase to target dose of 10 mg/day. May then increase in increments of 5 mg up to maximum of 30 mg/day. **IM:** *(Ability Maintena):* **ADULTS, ELDERLY:** Initially, 400 mg monthly.

Bipolar Disorder
PO: ADULTS, ELDERLY: (15 mg once a day with lithium/valproic acid): Initially, 10–15 mg. May increase to 30 mg/day based on pt tolerance. **CHILDREN 10–17 YRS:** Initially, 2 mg/day for 2 days, then 5 mg/day for 2 days. May further increase to a target of 10 mg/day. Give subsequent dose increases of 5 mg/day. **Maximum:** 30 mg/day.

Major Depressive Disorder (Adjunct to Antidepressants)
PO: ADULTS, ELDERLY: Initially, 2–5 mg/day. May increase up to 15 mg/day. Titrate dose in 5-mg increments of at least 1-wk intervals.

Agitation with Schizophrenia/Bipolar Disorder
IM: ADULTS, ELDERLY: 5.25–15 mg as a single dose. May repeat after 2 hrs. **Maximum:** 30 mg/day.

Irritability with Autistic Disorder
PO: CHILDREN 6–17 YRS: Initially, 2 mg/day for 7 days followed by increase to 5 mg/day. Subsequent increases made in 5-mg increments at intervals of at least 1 wk. **Maximum:** 15 mg/day.

SIDE EFFECTS

Frequent (11%–5%): Weight gain, headache, insomnia, vomiting. **Occasional (4%–3%):** Light-headedness, nausea, akathisia, drowsiness. **Rare (2% or less):** Blurred vision, constipation, asthenia (loss of strength, energy), anxiety, fever, rash, cough, rhinitis, orthostatic hypotension.

ADVERSE EFFECTS/ TOXIC REACTIONS

Extrapyramidal symptoms, neuroleptic malignant syndrome, tardive dyskinesia, hyperglycemia, ketoacidosis, hyperosmolar coma occur rarely. Prolonged QT interval occurs rarely. May cause leukopenia, neutropenia, agranulocytosis.

NURSING CONSIDERATIONS

BASELINE ASSESSMENT
Assess behavior, appearance, emotional status, response to environment, speech pattern, thought content. Correct dehydration, hypovolemia. Assess for suicidal tendencies.

INTERVENTION/EVALUATION
Periodically monitor weight. Monitor for extrapyramidal symptoms (abnormal movement), tardive dyskinesia (protrusion of tongue, puffing of cheeks, chewing/puckering of the mouth). Periodically monitor B/P, pulse (particularly in those with preexisting cardiovascular disease). Assess for therapeutic response (greater interest in surroundings, improved self-care, increased ability to concentrate, relaxed facial expression).

PATIENT/FAMILY TEACHING
• Avoid alcohol. • Avoid tasks that require alertness, motor skills until response to drug is established. • Report worsening depression, suicidal ideation, unusual changes in behavior, extrapyramidal effects.

armodafinil

ar-moe-**daf**-i-nil
(Nuvigil)

◆CLASSIFICATION

PHARMACOTHERAPEUTIC: Alpha₁ agonist. **CLINICAL:** Antinarcoleptic (stimulant).

ACTION

Binds to dopamine reuptake carrier sites in the brain, increasing alpha activity, decreasing delta, theta, and beta activity. **Therapeutic Effect:** Reduces number of sleep episodes, total daytime sleep.

PHARMACOKINETICS

Well absorbed. Widely distributed. Mainly eliminated by hepatic metabolism with less than 10% excreted by kidneys. Unknown if removed by hemodialysis. **Half-life:** 15 hrs.

USES

Treatment of excessive daytime sleepiness associated with obstructive sleep apnea–hypopnea syndrome, narcolepsy, shift-work sleep disorder.

PRECAUTIONS

Contraindications: History of sensitivity to modafinil. **Cautions:** History of mitral valve prolapse, left ventricular hypertrophy, hepatic impairment, recent history of MI, unstable angina, cardiac ischemia. History of psychosis, depression, mania, renal impairment, elderly.

⧖ LIFESPAN CONSIDERATIONS

Pregnancy/Lactation: Unknown if distributed in breast milk. Use caution if given to pregnant women. **Pregnancy Category C. Children:** Safety and efficacy not established in those younger than 17 yrs. **Elderly:** Age-related renal/hepatic impairment may require decreased dosage.

INTERACTIONS

DRUG: Carbamazine, erythromycin, ketoconazole, phenobarbital, rifampin can alter plasma levels of armodafinil. May reduce effects of **cyclosporine, oral contraceptives.** May increase concentrations of **diazepam, omeprazole, phenytoin, propranolol, tricyclic antidepressants, warfarin. HERBAL:** None significant. **FOOD: Food** slows peak concentration by 2–4 hrs; may affect time of onset, length of drug action. **LAB VALUES:** May increase alkaline phosphatase, GGT. May decrease serum uric acid.

AVAILABILITY (Rx)

Tablets: 50 mg, 150 mg, 250 mg.

ADMINISTRATION/HANDLING

PO
• May give without regard to food. • Food slows peak concentration by 2–4 hrs, may affect time of onset, length of action. • Tablets may be crushed.

INDICATIONS/ROUTES/DOSAGE

Narcolepsy, Obstructive Sleep Apnea–Hypopnea Syndrome
PO: ADULTS, ELDERLY: 150 or 250 mg/day given as a single dose in the morning.

Shift-Work Sleep Disorder
PO: ADULTS, ELDERLY: 150 mg given daily approximately 1 hr prior to the start of work shift.

SIDE EFFECTS

Frequent (17%–7%): Headache, nausea. **Occasional (5%–4%):** Dizziness, insomnia, dry mouth, diarrhea, anxiety. **Rare (2%):** Depression, fatigue, palpitations, dyspepsia, rash, upper abdominal pain.

ADVERSE EFFECTS/ TOXIC REACTIONS

Small risk of serious rash, including Stevens-Johnson syndrome.

 Canadian trade name   Non-Crushable Drug   High Alert drug

NURSING CONSIDERATIONS

BASELINE ASSESSMENT

Obtain baseline evidence of narcolepsy or other sleep disorders, including pattern, environmental situations, lengths of time of sleep episodes. Question for sudden loss of muscle tone (cataplexy) precipitated by strong emotional responses before sleep episode. Assess frequency/severity of sleep episodes prior to drug therapy.

INTERVENTION/EVALUATION

Monitor sleep pattern, evidence of restlessness during sleep, length of insomnia episodes at night. Assess for dizziness, anxiety; initiate fall precautions. Sips of tepid water may relieve dry mouth.

PATIENT/FAMILY TEACHING

• Avoid tasks that require alertness, motor skills until response to drug is established. • Avoid or limit alcohol. • Use alternative contraceptives during therapy and 1 mo after discontinuing drug (reduces effectiveness of oral contraceptives). Report rash, depression, diarrhea, insomnia.

---

arsenic trioxide `HIGH ALERT`

ar-sen-ik tri-**ox**-ide
(Trisenox)

BLACK BOX ALERT May prolong QT interval. May lead to multiform ventricular tachycardia (torsade de pointes) or complete AV block. May cause retinoic acid–acute promyelocytic leukemia (RA-APL) syndrome or acute promyelocytic leukemia.

◆CLASSIFICATION

PHARMACOTHERAPEUTIC: Antineoplastic. **CLINICAL:** Antineoplastic (see p. 82C).

ACTION

Produces morphologic changes and DNA fragmentation in promyelocytic leukemia cells. **Therapeutic Effect:** Produces cell death.

PHARMACOKINETICS

Distributed in liver, kidneys, heart, lungs, hair, and nails. Metabolized in liver. Eliminated by kidneys. **Half-life:** Not available.

USES

Induction of remission and consolidations in pts with acute promyelocytic leukemia (APL). **OFF-LABEL:** Treatment of myelodysplastic syndrome; initial treatment of APL.

PRECAUTIONS

Contraindications: None known. **Cautions:** Renal/hepatic impairment, preexisting QT-interval prolongation, concomitant medications that prolong QT interval.

⧗ LIFESPAN CONSIDERATIONS

Pregnancy/Lactation: Distributed in breast milk. May cause fetal harm. **Pregnancy Category D. Children:** Safety and efficacy not established in those younger than 5 yrs. **Elderly:** Age-related renal impairment may require dosage adjustment.

INTERACTIONS

DRUG: May prolong QT interval in those taking **antiarrhythmics, moxifloxacin, thioridazine. Amphotericin B, cyclosporine, diuretics** may produce electrolyte abnormalities. **HERBAL: Bilberry, fenugreek, garlic, ginger, ginseng** may worsen hypoglycemia. **FOOD:** None known. **LAB VALUES:** May decrease WBC count, Hgb, platelet count, serum magnesium, calcium. May increase serum AST, ALT. Higher risk of hypokalemia than hyperkalemia, hyperglycemia than hypoglycemia.

AVAILABILITY (Rx)

Injection Solution: 1 mg/ml.

ADMINISTRATION/HANDLING

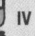 IV

◀ALERT▶ Central venous line is not required for drug administration.

Reconstitution • After withdrawing drug from ampule, dilute with 100–250 ml D₅W or 0.9% NaCl.

Rate of Administration • Infuse over 1–2 hrs. • Duration of infusion may be extended up to 4 hrs if acute vasomotor reactions occur.

Storage • Store at room temperature. • Diluted solution is stable for 24 hrs at room temperature, 48 hrs if refrigerated.

🚫 IV INCOMPATIBILITIES
Do not mix with any other medications.

INDICATIONS/ROUTES/DOSAGE

Acute Promyelocytic Leukemia
IV: ADULTS, ELDERLY, CHILDREN 5 YRS AND OLDER: Induction: 0.15 mg/kg/day until bone marrow remission. Do not exceed 60 induction doses. **Consolidation:** Beginning 3–6 wks after completion of induction therapy, 0.15 mg/kg/day for maximum 25 doses over a period of up to 5 wks.

SIDE EFFECTS

Expected (75%–50%): Nausea, cough, fatigue, fever, headache, vomiting, abdominal pain, tachycardia, diarrhea, dyspnea. **Frequent (43%–30%):** Dermatitis, insomnia, edema, rigors, prolonged QT interval, sore throat, pruritus, arthralgia, paresthesia, anxiety. **Occasional (28%–20%):** Constipation, myalgia, hypotension, epistaxis, anorexia, dizziness, sinusitis. **(15%–8%):** Ecchymosis, nonspecific pain, weight gain, herpes simplex infections, wheezing, flushing, diaphoresis, tremor, hypertension, palpitations, dyspepsia, eye irritation, blurred vision, asthenia (loss of strength, energy), adventitious or diminished breath sounds (crackles). **Rare:** Confusion, petechiae, dry mouth, oral candidiasis, incontinence, pulmonary rhonchi.

ADVERSE EFFECTS/ TOXIC REACTIONS

Seizures, GI hemorrhage, renal impairment or failure, pleural or pericardial effusion, hemoptysis, sepsis occur rarely.

Prolonged QT interval, complete AV block, unexplained fever, dyspnea, weight gain, effusion are evidence of arsenic toxicity. Treatment should be halted, steroid therapy instituted.

NURSING CONSIDERATIONS

BASELINE ASSESSMENT
Assess platelet count, Hgb, Hct, WBC, serum electrolytes, hepatic function, coagulation profiles before and frequently during treatment. Ask if pt is breastfeeding.

INTERVENTION/EVALUATION
Monitor hepatic function test results, CBC, serum values. Monitor for arsenic toxicity syndrome (fever, dyspnea, weight gain, confusion, muscle weakness, seizures).

PATIENT/FAMILY TEACHING
• Avoid crowds, those with known infection. • Avoid tasks that require alertness, motor skills until response to drug is established. • Report high fever, vomiting, difficulty breathing, or rapid heart rate.

ascorbic acid (vitamin C)

a-**skor**-bic **as**-id
(C-Gram, Proflavanol C 🍁, Revitalose C-1000 🍁, Vita-C)

◆ CLASSIFICATION
CLINICAL: Vitamin (see p. 158C).

ACTION
Assists in collagen formation, tissue repair, and is involved in oxidation reduction reactions, other metabolic reactions. **Therapeutic Effect:** Involved in carbohydrate utilization and metabolism, as well as synthesis of carnitine, lipids, proteins. Preserves blood vessel integrity.

🍁 Canadian trade name   🗲 Non-Crushable Drug   ⬛ High Alert drug

PHARMACOKINETICS

Readily absorbed from GI tract. Protein binding: 25%. Metabolized in liver. Excreted in urine. Removed by hemodialysis.

USES

Prevention and treatment of scurvy, acidification of urine, dietary supplement. **OFF-LABEL:** Prevention of common cold, urinary acidifier.

PRECAUTIONS

Contraindications: None known. **Cautions:** None significant.

⌛ LIFESPAN CONSIDERATIONS

Pregnancy/Lactation: Crosses placenta; excreted in breast milk. Large doses during pregnancy may produce scurvy in neonates. **Pregnancy Category A (C if used in doses above recommended daily allowance). Children/Elderly:** No age-related precautions noted.

INTERACTIONS

DRUG: May increase levels of **estrogen.** May decrease levels of **cyclosporine.** **HERBAL:** None significant. **FOOD:** None known. **LAB VALUES:** May decrease serum bilirubin, urinary pH. May increase serum uric acid, urinary oxalate.

AVAILABILITY

Capsules: 500 mg, 1,000 mg. **Crystals:** 4 g/tsp. **Injection, Solution:** 500 mg/ml. **Liquid, Oral:** 500 mg/5 ml. **Tablets:** 100 mg, 250 mg, 500 mg, 1,000 mg. **Tablets (Chewable):** 250 mg, 500 mg.

 Capsules (Timed-Release): 500 mg. **Tablets (Timed-Release):** 500 mg, 1,000 mg.

ADMINISTRATION/HANDLING
 IV

Rate of Administration • May give undiluted or dilute in D_5W, 0.9% NaCl, lactated Ringer's solution. • For IV push,

dilute with equal volume D_5W or 0.9% NaCl and infuse over 10 min.
Storage • Refrigerate. • Protect from freezing and light.

PO
• Give without regard to food but best given with meals. • Do not crush time-release formulations.

INDICATIONS/ROUTES/DOSAGE

Dietary Supplement
PO: ADULTS, ELDERLY: 50–200 mg/day. **CHILDREN:** 35–100 mg/day.

Acidification of Urine
PO: ADULTS, ELDERLY: 4–12 g/day in 3–4 divided doses. **CHILDREN:** 500 mg q6–8h.

Scurvy
PO: ADULTS, ELDERLY: 100–250 mg 1–2 times a day for at least 2 wks. **CHILDREN:** 100–300 mg/day in divided doses for at least 2 wks.

Prevention, Reduction of Severity of Colds
PO: ADULTS, ELDERLY: 1–3 g/day in divided doses.

SIDE EFFECTS

Rare: Abdominal cramps, nausea, vomiting, diarrhea, increased urination with doses exceeding 1 g. **Parenteral:** Flushing, headache, dizziness, sleepiness or insomnia, soreness at injection site.

ADVERSE EFFECTS/ TOXIC REACTIONS

May acidify urine, leading to crystalluria. Large doses of IV ascorbic acid may lead to deep vein thrombosis. Prolonged use of large doses may produce rebound ascorbic acid deficiency when dosage is reduced to normal range.

NURSING CONSIDERATIONS

INTERVENTION/EVALUATION

Assess for clinical improvement (improved sense of well-being and sleep patterns). Observe for reversal of deficiency symptoms (improving gingivitis, bleeding gums, poor wound healing, digestive difficulties, joint pain).

PATIENT/FAMILY TEACHING
• Larger doses may cause diarrhea, nausea, abdominal cramping. • Foods rich in vitamin C include rose hips, guava, black currant jelly, Brussels sprouts, green peppers, spinach, watercress, strawberries, citrus fruits.

---

asparaginase [HIGH ALERT]

as-par-**a**-jin-ace
(Elspar, Erwinaze, Kidrolase ✤)
Do not confuse asparaginase with pegaspargase.

◆CLASSIFICATION
PHARMACOTHERAPEUTIC: Enzyme.
CLINICAL: Antineoplastic (see p. 82C).

ACTION
Inhibits DNA, RNA, protein synthesis by breaking down asparagine, depriving tumor cells of this essential amino acid. Cell cycle–specific for G_1 phase of cell division. **Therapeutic Effect:** Toxic to leukemic cells.

PHARMACOKINETICS
Metabolized by reticuloendothelial system through slow sequestration. **Half-life: IM:** 39–49 hrs; **IV:** 8–30 hrs.

USES
Treatment of acute lymphocytic leukemia (ALL). **OFF-LABEL:** Treatment of chronic lymphocytic leukemia (CLL).

PRECAUTIONS
Contraindications: History of hypersensitivity to asparaginase. History of serious thrombosis, pancreatitis, or hemorrhagic events with prior asparaginase therapy. **Cautions:** Underlying coagulopathy, pre-existing hepatic impairment.

⧖ LIFESPAN CONSIDERATIONS
Pregnancy/Lactation: If possible, avoid use during pregnancy, esp. first trimester. Breastfeeding not recommended. **Pregnancy Category C. Children/Elderly:** No age-related precautions noted.

INTERACTIONS
DRUG: May increase levels of **dexamethasone. HERBAL:** None significant. **FOOD:** None known. **LAB VALUES:** May increase serum ammonia, BUN, uric acid, glucose, partial thromboplastin time (PTT), platelet count, prothrombin time (PT), thrombin time (TT), AST, ALT, alkaline phosphatase, bilirubin. May decrease blood clotting factors (plasma fibrinogen, antithrombin, plasminogen), serum albumin, calcium, cholesterol.

AVAILABILITY (Rx)
Injection, Powder for Reconstitution: 10,000 international units.

ADMINISTRATION/HANDLING
◀ALERT▶ May be carcinogenic, mutagenic, teratogenic. Handle with extreme care during preparation/administration. Handle voided urine as infectious waste. Powder, solution may irritate skin on contact. Wash area for 15 min if contact occurs.

 IV

◀ALERT▶ Administer intradermal test dose (2 international units) before initiating therapy or when longer than 1 wk has elapsed between doses.
• Observe pt for 1 hr for appearance of wheal or erythema.
Test Solution • Reconstitute 10,000 international units vial with 5 ml Sterile Water for Injection or 0.9% NaCl. • Shake to dissolve.
Reconstitution • Test Dose: Withdraw 0.1 ml, inject into vial containing 9.9 ml same diluent for concentration of 20 international units/ml. • **Regular dose:** Reconstitute 10,000 international units

vial with 5 ml Sterile Water for Injection or 0.9% NaCl to provide a concentration of 2,000 international units/ml. • Shake gently to ensure complete dissolution (vigorous shaking produces foam, some loss of potency). Further dilute in 50–250 ml D₅W or 0.9% NaCl.

Rate of Administration • Infuse over at least 30–60 min.

Storage • Refrigerate powder for reconstitution. • Reconstituted solution stable for 8 hrs if refrigerated. • Gelatinous fiber-like particles may develop (remove via 5-micron filter during administration).

IM

• Add 2 ml 0.9% NaCl injection to 10,000 international units vial to provide a concentration of 5,000 international units/ml. • Administer no more than 2 ml into large muscle mass.

🔲 IV COMPATIBILITIES

Methotrexate, sodium bicarbonate.

INDICATIONS/ROUTES/DOSAGE

Usual Dosage

IV: ADULTS, ELDERLY, CHILDREN: (Elspar): 6,000 units/m²/dose 3 times/wk for 6–9 doses or 1,000 units/kg/day for 10 days.
IM: ADULTS, ELDERLY, CHILDREN: (Elspar): 6,000 units/m²/dose 3 times/wk for 6–9 doses.

Erwinaze

IM: ADULTS, ELDERLY, CHILDREN: As a substitute for pegaspargase: 25,000 units/m² 3 times/wk for 6 doses. As a substitute for Elspar: 25,000 units/m² for each planned Elspar dose.

SIDE EFFECTS

Frequent: Allergic reaction (rash, urticaria, arthralgia, facial edema, hypotension, respiratory distress), pancreatitis (severe abdominal pain, nausea and vomiting). **Occasional:** CNS effects (confusion, drowsiness, depression, anxiety, fatigue), stomatitis, hypoalbuminemia

or uric acid nephropathy (manifested as pedal or lower extremity edema), hyperglycemia. **Rare:** Hyperthermia (including fever or chills), thrombosis, seizures.

ADVERSE EFFECTS/ TOXIC REACTIONS

Hepatotoxicity usually occurs within 2 wks of initial treatment. Risk of allergic reaction, including anaphylaxis, increases after repeated therapy. Myelosuppression may be severe.

NURSING CONSIDERATIONS

BASELINE ASSESSMENT

Before giving medication, agents for adequate airway and allergic reaction (antihistamine, epinephrine, O₂, IV corticosteroid) should be readily available. Assess baseline CNS functions. CBC, comprehensive serum chemistry should be performed before therapy begins and when 1 or more wks have elapsed between doses.

INTERVENTION/EVALUATION

Monitor vital signs, CBC, urinalysis, serum amylase, hepatic enzymes, coagulation profile, glucose, uric acid. Discontinue medication at first sign of renal dysfunction (oliguria, anuria), pancreatitis (abdominal pain, nausea, vomiting). Monitor for hematologic toxicity (fever, sore throat, signs of local infection, unusual bruising/bleeding), symptoms of anemia (excessive fatigue, weakness), hypersensitivity reaction.

PATIENT/FAMILY TEACHING

• Increase fluid intake (protects against renal impairment). • Nausea may decrease during therapy. • Do not have immunizations without physician's approval (drug lowers body's resistance). • Avoid contact with those who have recently received a live virus vaccine. • Notify physician if abdominal pain, rash, nausea, vomiting occurs.

aspirin (acetylsalicylic acid, ASA)

TOP 200   HIGH ALERT

as-pir-in
(Asaphen E.C. ♣, Ascriptin, Bayer, Bufferin, Ecotrin, Entrophen ♣, Halfprin, Novasen ♣)
Do not confuse aspirin or Ascriptin with Afrin, Aricept, or Asendin, Ecotrin with Epogen.

FIXED-COMBINATION(S)

Aggrenox: aspirin/dipyridamole (an antiplatelet agent): 25 mg/200 mg. **Fiorinal:** aspirin/butalbital/caffeine (a barbiturate): 325 mg/50 mg/40 mg. **Lortab/ASA:** aspirin/hydrocodone (an analgesic): 325 mg/5 mg. **Percodan:** aspirin/oxycodone (an analgesic): 325 mg/2.25 mg, 325 mg/4.5 mg. **Pravigard:** aspirin/pravastatin (a cholesterol-lowering agent): 81 mg/20 mg, 81 mg/40 mg, 81 mg/80 mg, 325 mg/20 mg, 325 mg/40 mg, 325 mg/80 mg.

◆CLASSIFICATION

PHARMACOTHERAPEUTIC: Nonsteroidal salicylate. **CLINICAL:** Antiinflammatory, antipyretic, anticoagulant (see pp. 33C, 129C).

ACTION

Inhibits prostaglandin synthesis, acts on the hypothalamus heat-regulating center, interferes with production of thromboxane A, a substance that stimulates platelet aggregation. **Therapeutic Effect:** Reduces inflammatory response, intensity of pain; decreases fever; inhibits platelet aggregation.

PHARMACOKINETICS

Route	Onset	Peak	Duration
PO	1 hr	2–4 hrs	4–6 hrs

Rapidly and completely absorbed from GI tract; enteric-coated absorption delayed; rectal absorption delayed and incomplete. Protein binding: High. Widely distributed. Rapidly hydrolyzed to salicylate. **Half-life:** 15–20 min (aspirin); 2–3 hrs (salicylate at low dose); more than 20 hrs (salicylate at high dose).

USES

Treatment of mild to moderate pain, fever. Reduces inflammation related to rheumatoid arthritis (RA), juvenile arthritis, osteoarthritis, rheumatic fever. As platelet aggregation inhibitor in the prevention of transient ischemic attacks (TIAs), cerebral thromboembolism, MI or reinfarction. Adjunctive treatment of Kawasaki's disease. **OFF-LABEL:** Prevention of preeclampsia; alternative therapy for preventing thromboembolism associated with atrial fibrillation where warfarin cannot be used; pericarditis associated with MI; prosthetic valve thromboprophylaxis.

PRECAUTIONS

Contraindications: Hypersensitivity to salicylates, NSAIDs; asthma, rhinitis, nasal polyps; inherited or acquired bleeding disorders; use in children for viral infections; pregnancy. **Cautions:** Platelet/bleeding disorders, severe renal/hepatic impairment, dehydration, erosive gastritis, peptic ulcer disease, sensitivity to tartrazine dyes.

⬛ LIFESPAN CONSIDERATIONS

Pregnancy/Lactation: Readily crosses placenta; distributed in breast milk. May prolong gestation and labor; decrease fetal birth weight; increase incidence of stillbirths, neonatal mortality, hemorrhage. Avoid use during last trimester (may adversely affect fetal cardiovascular system: premature closure of ductus arteriosus). **Pregnancy Category C (D if full dose used in third trimester of pregnancy). Children:** Caution in those with acute febrile illness (Reye's syndrome). **Elderly:** May be more susceptible to toxicity; lower dosages recommended.

♣ Canadian trade name   🗑 Non-Crushable Drug   HIGH ALERT High Alert drug

INTERACTIONS

DRUG: **Alcohol, NSAIDs** may increase risk of GI effects (e.g., ulceration). **Antacids, urinary alkalinizers** increase excretion. **Anticoagulants, heparin, thrombolytics, rivaroxaban, ticagrelor** increase risk of bleeding. **HERBAL:** Avoid **cat's claw, dong quai, evening primrose, feverfew, garlic, ginger, ginkgo, ginseng, green tea, horse chestnut, red clover** (possess antiplatelet activity). **FOOD:** None known. **LAB VALUES:** May alter serum AST, ALT, alkaline phosphatase, uric acid; prolongs prothrombin time (PT), bleeding time. May decrease serum cholesterol, potassium, T_3, T_4.

AVAILABILITY (OTC)

Caplets (Bayer): 81 mg, 325 mg, 500 mg. **Suppositories:** 300 mg, 600 mg. **Tablets:** 325 mg. **Tablets (Chewable [Bayer, St. Joseph]):** 81 mg.

⬥ **Tablets (Enteric-Coated [Bayer, Ecotrin, St. Joseph]):** 81 mg, 325 mg, 500 mg, 650 mg.

ADMINISTRATION/HANDLING

PO
• Do not break, chew, crush, or divide enteric-coated tablets. • May give with water, milk, meals if GI distress occurs.

Rectal
• Refrigerate suppositories; do not freeze. • If suppository is too soft, chill for 30 min in refrigerator or run cold water over foil wrapper. • Moisten suppository with cold water before inserting well into rectum.

INDICATIONS/ROUTES/DOSAGE

Analgesia, Fever
PO, Rectal: ADULTS, ELDERLY: 325–650 mg q4–6h. **CHILDREN:** 10–15 mg/kg/dose q4–6h. **Maximum:** 4 g/day.

Anti-Inflammatory
PO: ADULTS, ELDERLY: Initially, 2.4–3.6 g/day in divided doses, then 3.6–5.4 g/day. **CHILDREN:** Initially, 60–90 mg/kg/day in divided doses, then 80–100 mg/kg/day.

Platelet Aggregation Inhibitor
PO: ADULTS, ELDERLY: 80–325 mg/day.

Kawasaki's Disease
PO: CHILDREN: 80–100 mg/kg/day in divided doses q6h. After fever resolves, 1–5 mg/kg once a day.

SIDE EFFECTS

Occasional: GI distress (including abdominal distention, cramping, heartburn, mild nausea); allergic reaction (including bronchospasm, pruritus, urticaria).

ADVERSE EFFECTS/ TOXIC REACTIONS

High doses of aspirin may produce GI bleeding and/or gastric mucosal lesions. Dehydrated, febrile children may experience aspirin toxicity quickly. Reye's syndrome, characterized by persistent vomiting, signs of brain dysfunction, may occur in children taking aspirin with recent viral infection (chickenpox, common cold, or flu). Low-grade aspirin toxicity characterized by tinnitus, generalized pruritus (may be severe), headache, dizziness, flushing, tachycardia, hyperventilation, diaphoresis, thirst. Marked toxicity characterized by hyperthermia, restlessness, seizures, abnormal breathing patterns, respiratory failure, coma.

NURSING CONSIDERATIONS

BASELINE ASSESSMENT

Do not give to children or teenagers who have or recently had viral infections (increases risk of Reye's syndrome). Do not use if vinegar-like odor is noted (indicates chemical breakdown). Assess type, location, duration of pain, inflammation. Inspect appearance of affected joints for immobility, deformities, skin condition. **Therapeutic serum level for antiarthritic effect:** 20–30 mg/dl (toxicity occurs if level is greater than 30 mg/dl).

INTERVENTION/EVALUATION

Monitor urinary pH (sudden acidification, pH from 6.5 to 5.5, may result in toxicity). Assess skin for evidence of ecchymosis. If given as antipyretic, assess temperature directly before and 1 hr after giving medication. Evaluate for therapeutic response: relief of pain, stiffness, swelling; increased joint mobility; reduced joint tenderness; improved grip strength.

PATIENT/FAMILY TEACHING

• Do not break, chew, crush, or divide enteric-coated tablets. • Avoid alcohol. • Report tinnitus or persistent abdominal GI pain, bleeding. • Therapeutic anti-inflammatory effect noted in 1–3 wks. • Behavioral changes, persistent vomiting may be early signs of Reye's syndrome. Contact physician.

---

atazanavir
TOP 200

a-ta-**zan**-a-veer
(Reyataz)
Do not confuse Reyataz with Retavase.

◆CLASSIFICATION

PHARMACOTHERAPEUTIC: Antiretroviral. **CLINICAL:** Protease inhibitor (see p. 119C).

ACTION

Acts as an HIV-1 protease inhibitor, selectively preventing the processing of viral precursors found in cells infected with HIV-1. **Therapeutic Effect:** Prevents formation of mature HIV viral cells.

PHARMACOKINETICS

Rapidly absorbed after PO administration. Protein binding: 86%. Extensively metabolized in liver. Excreted primarily in urine and, to a lesser extent, in feces. **Half-life:** 5–8 hrs.

USES

Treatment of HIV-1 infection in combination with other antiretroviral agents.

PRECAUTIONS

Contraindications: Concurrent use with alfuzosin, ergot derivatives, indinavir, lovastatin, midazolam (oral), pimozide, rifampin, sildenafil (for pulmonary arterial hypertension), St. John's wort, simvastatin, triazolam. **Cautions:** Preexisting conduction system defects (first-, second-, or third-degree AV block), diabetes mellitus, elderly, renal impairment, hemophilia A or B, hepatitis B or C.

⌛ LIFESPAN CONSIDERATIONS

Pregnancy/Lactation: Unknown if drug crosses placenta or distributed in breast milk. Lactic acidosis syndrome, hyperbilirubinemia, kernicterus have been reported. **Pregnancy Category B. Children:** Safety and efficacy not established in those younger than 3 mos. **Elderly:** Age-related hepatic impairment may require dose reduction.

INTERACTIONS

DRUG: May increase concentration, toxicity of **amiodarone, atorvastatin, bepridil, clarithromycin, cyclosporine, diltiazem, felodipine, lidocaine, lovastatin, nicardipine, nifedipine, rosuvastatin, sildenafil, simvastatin, sirolimus, tacrolimus, tadalafil, tricyclic antidepressants, vardenafil, verapamil, warfarin. H₂-receptor antagonists, proton pump inhibitors, rifampin** may decrease concentration/effects. **Ritonavir, voriconazole** may increase concentration. **HERBAL: St. John's wort** may decrease concentration/effects. **FOOD: High-fat meals** may decrease absorption. **LAB VALUES:** May increase serum bilirubin, AST, ALT, amylase, lipase. May decrease Hgb, neutrophil count, platelets. May alter LDL, triglycerides.

AVAILABILITY (Rx)

Capsules: 100 mg, 150 mg, 200 mg, 300 mg.

 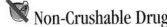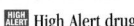

ADMINISTRATION/HANDLING

PO

• Give with food. • Swallow whole; do not open. • Administer at least 2 hrs before or 10 hrs after H$_2$ antagonist, 12 hrs after proton pump inhibitor.

INDICATIONS/ROUTES/DOSAGE

Note: Dosage adjustment may be necessary with colchicine, bosentin, H$_2$ antagonists, proton pump inhibitors, PDE5 inhibitors.

HIV-1 Infection
PO: ADULTS, ELDERLY (ANTIRETROVIRAL-NAIVE): 300 mg and ritonavir 100 mg, once a day, or 400 mg (2 capsules) once a day with food. **CHILDREN 6–17 YRS WEIGHING 39 KG OR MORE:** 300 mg and ritonavir 100 mg once daily. **WEIGHING 32–38 KG:** 250 mg and ritonavir 100 mg once daily. **WEIGHING 25–31 KG:** 200 mg and ritonavir 100 mg once daily. **WEIGHING 15–24 KG:** 150 mg and ritonavir 80 mg once daily. **ADULTS, ELDERLY (ANTIRETROVIRAL-EXPERIENCED):** 300 mg and ritonavir (Norvir) 100 mg once a day.

HIV-1 Infection (Concurrent Therapy with Efavirenz)
PO: ADULTS, ELDERLY: 400 mg atazanavir, 100 mg ritonavir (as a single dose given with food), and 600 mg efavirenz as a single daily dose on an empty stomach (preferably at bedtime).

HIV-1 Infection (Concurrent Therapy with Didanosine)
PO: ADULTS, ELDERLY: Give atazanavir with food 2 hrs before or 1 hr after didanosine.

HIV-1 Infection (Concurrent Therapy with Tenofovir)
PO: ADULTS, ELDERLY: 300 mg atazanavir, 100 mg ritonavir, and 300 mg tenofovir given as a single daily dose with food. **For treatment-experienced pregnant women during 2nd or 3rd trimester:** 400 mg with ritonavir 100 mg once daily.

HIV-1 Infection (Concurrent Therapy with Maraviroc)
PO: ADULTS, ELDERLY: 300 mg atazanavir, 100 mg ritonavir once daily, and 150 mg maraviroc twice daily.

HIV-1 Infection in Pts with Mild to Moderate Hepatic Impairment
◄ALERT► Avoid use in pts with severe hepatic impairment.
PO: ADULTS, ELDERLY: 300 mg once a day with food.

SIDE EFFECTS

Frequent (16%–14%): Nausea, headache. **Occasional (9%–4%):** Rash, vomiting, depression, diarrhea, abdominal pain, fever. **Rare (3% or less):** Dizziness, insomnia, cough, fatigue, back pain.

ADVERSE EFFECTS/ TOXIC REACTIONS

Severe hypersensitivity reaction (angioedema, chest pain), jaundice may occur.

NURSING CONSIDERATIONS

BASELINE ASSESSMENT

Obtain baseline CBC, serum chemistries, hepatic function tests before beginning therapy and at periodic intervals during therapy. Offer emotional support.

INTERVENTION/EVALUATION

Monitor lab results. Assess for nausea, vomiting; assess eating pattern. Monitor daily pattern of bowel activity, stool consistency. Assess skin for rash. Question for evidence of headache. Assess mood for evidence of depression.

PATIENT/FAMILY TEACHING

• Take with food. • Small, frequent meals may offset nausea, vomiting. • Pt must continue practices to prevent HIV transmission. • Atazanavir is not a cure for HIV infection, nor does it reduce risk of transmission to others. • Report dizziness, light-headedness, yellowing of skin or whites of eyes, pain in side or when urinating, blood in urine, skin rash.

atenolol

a-**ten**-oh-lol
(Apo-Atenol ✤, Tenormin)
BLACK BOX ALERT Do not abruptly discontinue; taper gradually to avoid acute tachycardia, hypertension, ischemia.
Do not confuse atenolol with albuterol, timolol, or Tylenol, or Tenormin with Imuran, Norpramin, or thiamine.

◆CLASSIFICATION

PHARMACOTHERAPEUTIC: Beta₁-adrenergic blocker. **CLINICAL:** Antihypertensive, antianginal, antiarrhythmic (see pp. 62C, 72C).

ACTION

Blocks beta₁-adrenergic receptors in cardiac tissue. **Therapeutic Effect:** Slows sinus node heart rate, decreasing cardiac output, B/P. Decreases myocardial oxygen demand.

PHARMACOKINETICS

Route	Onset	Peak	Duration
PO	1 hr	2–4 hrs	24 hrs

Incompletely absorbed from GI tract. Protein binding: 6%–16%. Minimal liver metabolism. Primarily excreted unchanged in urine. Removed by hemodialysis. **Half-life:** 6–9 hrs (increased in renal impairment).

USES

Treatment of hypertension, alone or in combination with other agents; management of angina; secondary prevention of post-MI. **OFF-LABEL:** Acute alcohol withdrawal, arrhythmia (esp. supraventricular and ventricular tachycardia), prevention of migraine.

PRECAUTIONS

Contraindications: Cardiogenic shock, uncompensated heart failure, second- or third-degree heart block (except with functioning pacemaker), sinus bradycardia, sinus node dysfunction, pulmonary edema, pregnancy. **Cautions:** Renal impairment, peripheral vascular disease, diabetes, thyroid disease, bronchospastic disease, compensated heart failure, concurrent use with digoxin, verapamil or diltiazem, myasthenia gravis, psychiatric disease. History of anaphylaxis to allergens.

⌛ LIFESPAN CONSIDERATIONS

Pregnancy/Lactation: Readily crosses placenta; distributed in breast milk. Avoid use during first trimester. May produce bradycardia, apnea, hypoglycemia, hypothermia during delivery; low birthweight infants. **Pregnancy Category D. Children:** No age-related precautions noted. **Elderly:** Age-related peripheral vascular disease, renal impairment require caution.

INTERACTIONS

DRUG: Diuretics, other antihypertensives may increase hypotensive effects. **Sympathomimetics, xanthines** may mutually inhibit effects. May mask symptoms of hypoglycemia, prolong hypoglycemic effect of **insulin, oral antidiabetic medications. NSAIDs** may decrease antihypertensive effect. **HERBAL: Ephedra, ginseng, yohimbe** may worsen hypertension. **Garlic** may increase antihypertensive effect. **FOOD:** None known. **LAB VALUES:** May increase serum ANA titer, BUN, serum creatinine, potassium, uric acid, lipoprotein, triglycerides.

AVAILABILITY (Rx)

Tablets: 25 mg, 50 mg, 100 mg.

ADMINISTRATION/HANDLING

PO
• Give without regard to food. • Tablets may be crushed.

 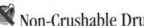

INDICATIONS/ROUTES/DOSAGE

Hypertension

PO: ADULTS: Initially, 25–50 mg once a day. May increase dose up to 100 mg once a day. **ELDERLY:** Usual initial dose, 25 mg/day. **CHILDREN:** Initially, 0.5–1 mg/kg/dose given once a day. Range: 0.5–1.5 mg/kg/day. **Maximum:** 2 mg/kg/day up to 100 mg/day.

Angina Pectoris

PO: ADULTS: Initially, 50 mg once a day. May increase dose up to 200 mg once a day. **ELDERLY:** Usual initial dose, 25 mg/day.

Post-MI

PO: ADULTS: 100 mg once a day or 50 mg twice a day for 6–9 days post-MI.

Dosage in Renal Impairment

Dosage interval is modified based on creatinine clearance.

Creatinine Clearance	Maximum Dosage
15–35 ml/min	50 mg/day
Less than 15 ml/min	25 mg/day
Hemodialysis (HD)	Give dose post-HD or give 25–50 mg supplemental dose

SIDE EFFECTS

Atenolol is generally well tolerated, with mild and transient side effects. **Frequent:** Hypotension manifested as cold extremities, constipation or diarrhea, diaphoresis, dizziness, fatigue, headache, nausea. **Occasional:** Insomnia, flatulence, urinary frequency, impotence or decreased libido, depression. **Rare:** Rash, arthralgia, myalgia, confusion (esp. in the elderly), altered taste.

ADVERSE EFFECTS/ TOXIC REACTIONS

Overdose may produce profound bradycardia, hypotension. Abrupt withdrawal may result in diaphoresis, palpitations, headache, tremors. May precipitate CHF, MI in pts with cardiac disease; thyroid storm in those with thyrotoxicosis; peripheral ischemia in those with existing peripheral vascular disease. Hypoglycemia may occur in previously controlled diabetes. Thrombocytopenia (unusual bruising, bleeding) occurs rarely. **Antidote:** Glucagon (see Appendix K for dosage).

NURSING CONSIDERATIONS

BASELINE ASSESSMENT

Assess B/P, apical pulse immediately before drug is administered (if pulse is 60/min or less, or systolic B/P is less than 90 mm Hg, withhold medication, contact physician). **Antianginal:** Record onset, quality (sharp, dull, squeezing), radiation, location, intensity, duration of anginal pain, precipitating factors (exertion, emotional stress). Assess baseline renal/hepatic function tests.

INTERVENTION/EVALUATION

Monitor B/P for hypotension, pulse for bradycardia, respiration for difficulty in breathing, EKG. Monitor daily pattern of bowel activity, stool consistency. Assess for evidence of CHF: dyspnea (particularly on exertion or lying down), nocturnal cough, peripheral edema, distended neck veins. Monitor I&O (increased weight, decreased urinary output may indicate CHF). Assess extremities for pulse quality, changes in temperature (may indicate worsening peripheral vascular disease). Assist with ambulation if dizziness occurs.

PATIENT/FAMILY TEACHING

• Do not abruptly discontinue medication. • Compliance with therapy essential to control hypertension, angina. • To reduce hypotensive effect, rise slowly from lying to sitting position and permit legs to dangle from bed momentarily before standing. • Avoid tasks that require alertness, motor skills until response to drug is established. • Advise diabetic pts to monitor blood glucose carefully (may mask signs of hypoglycemia). • Report dizziness, depression, confusion, rash, unusual bruising/bleeding. • Outpatients should monitor B/P, pulse before taking medication, following correct technique. • Restrict salt, alcohol intake. • Therapeutic antihypertensive effect noted in 1–2 wks.

atomoxetine `TOP 200`

at-oh-**mox**-e-teen
(Strattera)

BLACK BOX ALERT Increased risk of suicidal thinking and behavior in children and adolescents with attention-deficit hyperactivity disorder (ADHD).
Do not confuse atomoxetine with atorvastatin.

◆CLASSIFICATION

PHARMACOTHERAPEUTIC: Norepinephrine reuptake inhibitor. **CLINICAL:** Psychotherapeutic agent.

ACTION

Enhances noradrenergic function by selective inhibition of the presynaptic norepinephrine transporter. **Therapeutic Effect:** Improves symptoms of ADHD.

PHARMACOKINETICS

Rapidly absorbed after PO administration. Protein binding: 98% (primarily to albumin). Eliminated primarily in urine and, to a lesser extent, in feces. Not removed by hemodialysis. **Half-life:** 4–5 hrs (increased in moderate to severe hepatic insufficiency).

USES

Treatment of ADHD.

PRECAUTIONS

Contraindications: Narrow-angle glaucoma, use within 14 days of MAOIs. Pheochromocytoma or history of pheochromocytoma. Severe cardiovascular disease. **Cautions:** Hypertension, tachycardia, cardiovascular disease (e.g., structural abnormalities, cardiomyopa-

thy), urinary retention, moderate or severe hepatic impairment, suicidal ideation, emergent psychotic or manic symptoms, renal impairment, poor metabolizers of CYP2D6 metabolized drugs (e.g., fluoxetine, paroxetine).

⌛ LIFESPAN CONSIDERATIONS

Pregnancy/Lactation: Unknown if distributed in breast milk. **Pregnancy Category C. Children:** Safety and efficacy not established in those younger than 6 yrs. May produce suicidal thoughts in children and adolescents. **Elderly:** Age-related hepatic/renal impairment, cardiovascular or cerebrovascular disease may increase risk of effects.

INTERACTIONS

DRUG: MAOIs may increase concentration and toxic effects. **Fluoxetine, paroxetine** may increase concentration. Avoid concurrent use of **medications that can increase heart rate or B/P.** **HERBAL:** None significant. **FOOD:** None known. **LAB VALUES:** May increase hepatic enzymes, serum bilirubin.

AVAILABILITY (Rx)

Capsules: 10 mg, 18 mg, 25 mg, 40 mg, 60 mg, 80 mg, 100 mg.

ADMINISTRATION/HANDLING

PO
• Give without regard to food. • Swallow capsules whole, do not open (powder in capsule is ocular irritant).

INDICATIONS/ROUTES/DOSAGE

Attention-Deficit Hyperactivity Disorder (ADHD)
PO: ADULTS, CHILDREN 6 YRS AND OLDER WEIGHING 70 KG OR MORE: 40 mg once a day. May increase after at least 3 days to 80 mg as a single daily dose or in divided doses. **Maximum:** 100 mg. **CHILDREN 6 YRS AND OLDER WEIGHING LESS THAN 70 KG:** Initially, 0.5 mg/kg/day. May increase after at least 3 days to 1.2 mg/kg/day. **Maximum:** 1.4 mg/kg/day or 100 mg, whichever is less.

Dosage in Hepatic Impairment

Expect to administer 50% of normal atomoxetine dosage to pts with moderate hepatic impairment and 25% of normal dosage to those with severe hepatic impairment.

Dosage with Strong CYP2D6 Inhibitors

ADULTS: Do not exceed 80 mg/day with dosage adjustments at 4-wk intervals. **CHILDREN:** 1.2 mg/kg/day only after 4-wk interval.

SIDE EFFECTS

Frequent: Headache, dyspepsia, nausea, vomiting, fatigue, decreased appetite, dizziness, altered mood. **Occasional:** Tachycardia, hypertension, weight loss, delayed growth in children, irritability. **Rare:** Insomnia, sexual dysfunction in adults, fever.

ADVERSE EFFECTS/ TOXIC REACTIONS

Urinary retention, urinary hesitancy may occur. In overdose, gastric lavage, activated charcoal may prevent systemic absorption. Severe hepatic injury occurs rarely.

NURSING CONSIDERATIONS

BASELINE ASSESSMENT

Assess pulse, B/P before therapy, following dose increases, and periodically during therapy. Assess attention span, interactions with others.

INTERVENTION/EVALUATION

Monitor urinary output; complaints of urinary retention/hesitancy may be a related adverse reaction. Monitor B/P, pulse periodically and following dose increases. Monitor growth, attention span, hyperactivity, unusual changes in behavior, suicidal ideation. Assist with ambulation if dizziness occurs. Be alert to mood changes. Monitor fluid and electrolyte status in those with significant vomiting.

PATIENT/FAMILY TEACHING

• Avoid tasks that require alertness, motor skills until response to drug is established. • Take last dose early in evening to avoid insomnia. • Report palpitations, fever, vomiting, irritability. • Monitor growth rate, weight. • Report changes in behavior, suicidal ideation, chest pain, palpitations, dyspnea.

---

atorvastatin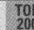

a-**tor**-va-sta-tin
(Apo-Atorvastatin ✦, <u>Lipitor</u>, Novo-Atorvastatin ✦)
Do not confuse atorvastatin with atomoxetine, lovastatin, nystatin, pitavastatin, pravastatin, or simvastatin, or Lipitor with labetalol, Levatol, lisinopril, or Zocor.

FIXED-COMBINATION(S)

Caduet: atorvastatin/amlodipine (calcium channel blocker): 10 mg/2.5 mg, 10 mg/5 mg, 10 mg/10 mg, 20 mg/2.5 mg, 20 mg/5 mg, 20 mg/10 mg, 40 mg/2.5 mg, 40 mg/5 mg, 40 mg/10 mg, 80 mg/5 mg, 80 mg/10 mg.

◆CLASSIFICATION

PHARMACOTHERAPEUTIC: Hydroxymethylglutaryl CoA (HMG-CoA) reductase inhibitor. **CLINICAL:** Antihyperlipidemic (see p. 58C).

ACTION

Inhibits HMG-CoA reductase, the enzyme that catalyzes the early step in cholesterol synthesis. **Therapeutic Effect:** Decreases LDL and VLDL, plasma triglyceride levels; increases HDL concentration.

PHARMACOKINETICS

Poorly absorbed from GI tract. Protein binding: greater than 98%. Metabolized in liver. Minimally eliminated in urine, primarily eliminated in feces (biliary). **Half-life:** 14 hrs.

USES

Primary prevention of cardiovascular disease in high-risk pts. Reduces risk of

stroke and heart attack in pts with type 2 diabetes with or without evidence of heart disease. Reduces risk of stroke in pts with or without evidence of heart disease with multiple risk factors other than diabetes. Adjunct to diet therapy in management of hyperlipidemias (reduces elevations in total cholesterol, LDL-C, apolipoprotein B triglycerides in pts with primary hypercholesterolemia), homozygous familial hypercholesterolemia, heterozygous familial hypercholesterolemia in pts 10–17 yrs of age, females more than 1 yr postmenarche. **OFF-LABEL:** Secondary prevention of myocardial ischemia in pts with CHF. Secondary prevention in pts who have experienced a noncardioembolic stroke/TIA or following an acute coronary syndrome (ACS) event.

PRECAUTIONS

Contraindications: Active hepatic disease, lactation, pregnancy, unexplained elevated hepatic function test results. **Cautions:** Anticoagulant therapy; history of hepatic disease; substantial alcohol consumption; major surgery; severe acute infection; trauma; hypotension; severe metabolic, endocrine, electrolyte disorders; uncontrolled seizures; elderly (predisposed to myopathy).

⧗ LIFESPAN CONSIDERATIONS

Pregnancy/Lactation: Distributed in breast milk. Contraindicated during pregnancy. May produce skeletal malformation. **Pregnancy Category X. Children:** Safety and efficacy not established. **Elderly:** No age-related precautions noted.

INTERACTIONS

DRUG: Strong **CYP3A4 inhibitors** (e.g., **clarithromycin, protease inhibitors, itraconazole**) may increase concentration. **Cyclosporine** may increase concentration. **Gemfibrozil, fibrates, niacin, colchicine** may increase risk of myopathy, rhabdomyolysis. Strong **CYP3A4 inducers** (e.g., **rifampin, efavirenz**)

may decrease concentration. **HERBAL: St. John's wort** may decrease levels. **FOOD: Grapefruit juice in large quantities (greater than 1 quart/day)** may increase serum concentrations. **Red yeast rice** may increase serum levels (2.4 mg lovastatin per 600 mg rice). **LAB VALUES:** May increase serum transaminase, creatinine kinase concentrations.

AVAILABILITY (Rx)

🔖 **Tablets:** 10 mg, 20 mg, 40 mg, 80 mg.

ADMINISTRATION/HANDLING

PO
• Give without regard to food or time of day. • Do not break film-coated tablets.

INDICATIONS/ROUTES/DOSAGE

Do not use in active hepatic disease.

Hyperlipidemias
PO: ADULTS, ELDERLY: Initially, 10–20 mg/day (40 mg in pts requiring greater than 45% reduction in LDL-C). Range: 10–80 mg/day.

Heterozygous Hypercholesterolemia
PO: CHILDREN 10–17 YRS: Initially, 10 mg/day. **Maximum:** 20 mg/day.

SIDE EFFECTS

Common: Atorvastatin is generally well tolerated. Side effects are usually mild and transient. **Frequent (16%):** Headache. **Occasional (5%–2%):** Myalgia, rash, pruritus, allergy. **Rare (less than 2%–1%):** Flatulence, dyspepsia, depression.

ADVERSE EFFECTS/ TOXIC REACTIONS

Potential for cataracts, photosensitivity, myalgia, rhabdomyolysis.

NURSING CONSIDERATIONS

BASELINE ASSESSMENT

Question for possibility of pregnancy before initiating therapy (Pregnancy Category X). Assess baseline lab results: cho-

lesterol, triglycerides, hepatic function tests. Obtain dietary history.

INTERVENTION/EVALUATION

Monitor for headache. Assess for rash, pruritus, malaise. Monitor cholesterol, triglyceride lab values for therapeutic response. Monitor hepatic function tests, CPK.

PATIENT/FAMILY TEACHING

• Follow special diet (important part of treatment). • Periodic lab tests are essential part of therapy. • Do not take other medications without consulting physician. • Report dark urine, muscle fatigue, bone pain. • Avoid excessive alcohol intake, large quantities of grapefruit juice.

---

atovaquone

a-**toe**-va-kwone
(Mepron)

◆CLASSIFICATION

PHARMACOTHERAPEUTIC: Systemic anti-infective. **CLINICAL:** Antiprotozoal.

ACTION

Inhibits mitochondrial electron transport system at the cytochrome bc1 complex (Complex III) interrupting nucleic acid, adenosine triphosphate synthesis. **Therapeutic Effect:** Antiprotozoal, antipneumocystic activity.

USES

Treatment or prevention of mild to moderate *Pneumocystis jiroveci* pneumonia (PCP) in those intolerant to trimethoprim-sulfamethoxazole (TMP-SMZ). **OFF-LABEL:** Treatment of babesiosis. Prophylaxis in HIV pts at high risk for developing *Toxoplasma gondii* encephalitis.

PRECAUTIONS

Contraindications: Development or history of potentially life-threatening allergic reaction to the drug. **Cautions:** Elderly, pts with severe PCP, chronic diarrhea, malabsorption syndromes, severe hepatic impairment. **Pregnancy Category C.**

INTERACTIONS

DRUG: Rifabutin, rifampin may decrease concentration. May increase **rifampin** concentration. **HERBAL: Bilberry, fenugreek, garlic, ginger, ginseng** may enhance risk of hypoglycemia. **FOOD: High-fat meals** increase absorption. **LAB VALUES:** May elevate serum AST, ALT, alkaline phosphatase, amylase. May decrease serum sodium.

AVAILABILITY (Rx)

Suspension, Oral: 750 mg/5 ml.

ADMINISTRATION/HANDLING

PO
• Must give with food or high-fat meals. Shake gently prior to using.

INDICATIONS/ROUTES/DOSAGE

Pneumocystis Jiroveci Pneumonia (PCP)
PO: ADULTS, CHILDREN OLDER THAN 12 YRS: 750 mg twice a day with food for 21 days. **CHILDREN 4–24 MOS:** 45 mg/kg/day in 2 divided doses with food. **Maximum:** 1,500 mg/day. **CHILDREN 1–3 MOS OR OLDER THAN 24 MOS:** 30–40 mg/kg/day in 2 divided doses with food. **Maximum:** 1,500 mg/day.

Prevention of PCP
PO: ADULTS, CHILDREN OLDER THAN 12 YRS: 1,500 mg once a day with food. **CHILDREN 4–24 MOS:** 45 mg/kg/day as single dose. **Maximum:** 1,500 mg/day. **CHILDREN 1–3 MOS OR OLDER THAN 24 MOS:** 30 mg/kg/day as single dose. **Maximum:** 1,500 mg/day. **NEONATES:** 30–40 mg/kg/day in 2 divided doses.

SIDE EFFECTS

Frequent (greater than 10%): Rash, nausea, diarrhea, headache, vomiting, fever, insomnia, cough. **Occasional (less than 10%):** Abdominal discomfort, thrush, asthenia (loss of strength, energy), anemia, neutropenia.

ADVERSE EFFECTS/ TOXIC REACTIONS

None known.

NURSING CONSIDERATIONS

BASELINE ASSESSMENT

Obtain baseline lab studies, esp. hepatic function tests.

INTERVENTION/EVALUATION

Assess for GI discomfort, nausea, vomiting. Monitor daily pattern of bowel activity, stool consistency. Assess skin for rash. Monitor I&O, renal function tests, CBC, hepatic enzymes, serum chemistries, amylase. Monitor elderly closely for decreased hepatic, renal, cardiac function.

PATIENT/FAMILY TEACHING

• Continue therapy for full length of treatment. • Do not take any other medications unless approved by physician. • Report rash, diarrhea, or other new symptoms. • Must be taken with high-fat meal or food.

atropine

at-roe-peen
(AtroPen Auto Injector, Atropine-Care, Isopto Atropine, Sal-Tropine)

FIXED-COMBINATION(S)

Donnatal: atropine/hyoscyamine (anticholinergic)/phenobarbital (sedative)/scopolamine (anticholinergic): 0.0194 mg/0.1037 mg/16.2 mg/0.0065 mg. **Lomotil:** atropine/diphenoxylate (peristaltic inhibitor): 0.025 mg/2.5 mg.

◆CLASSIFICATION

PHARMACOTHERAPEUTIC: Acetylcholine antagonist. **CLINICAL:** Antiarrhythmic, antispasmodic, antidote, cycloplegic, antisecretory, anticholinergic.

ACTION

Competes with acetylcholine for common binding sites on muscarinic receptors located on exocrine glands, cardiac and smooth muscle ganglia, intramural neurons. **Therapeutic Effect:** Decreases GI motility, secretory activity, GU muscle tone (ureter, bladder); produces ophthalmic cycloplegia, mydriasis; abolishes various types of reflex vagal cardiac slowing or asystole.

PHARMACOKINETICS

Rapidly and well absorbed after IM administration. Widely distributed. Metabolized in liver. Excreted in urine (30%–50% as unchanged drug). **Half-life:** 2–3 hrs.

USES

Injection: Preop to inhibit salivation/secretions; treatment of symptomatic sinus bradycardia; AV block; ventricular asystole; antidote for organophosphate pesticide poisoning. Adjuvant to decrease side effects during reversal of neuromuscular blockage. **Ophthalmic:** Produce mydriasis and cycloplegia for examination of retina and optic disc; uveitis. **OFF-LABEL:** Malignant glaucoma, pulseless electric activity, asystole, neuromuscular blockage reversal.

PRECAUTIONS

Contraindications: Narrow-angle glaucoma, pyloric stenosis, prostatic hypertrophy. **Cautions:** Autonomic neuropathy, paralytic ileus, intestinal atony, severe ulcerative colitis, toxic megacolon, renal/hepatic impairment, myocardial ischemia, hyperthyroidism, hypertension, tachyarrhythmias, CHF, coronary artery disease, esophageal reflux or hiatal hernia associated with reflux esophagitis; infants, children with spastic paralysis or brain damage; elderly; biliary tract disease, chronic pulmonary disease. **Ophthalmic:** Spastic paralysis, brain injury, Down syndrome.

⌛ LIFESPAN CONSIDERATIONS

Pregnancy/Lactation: Crosses placenta; distributed in breast milk. **Preg-**

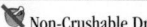

nancy Category C. **Children/Elderly:** Increased susceptibility to atropine effects.

INTERACTIONS

DRUG: Anticholinergics may increase effects. **HERBAL:** None significant. **FOOD:** None known. **LAB VALUES:** None significant.

AVAILABILITY (Rx)

Injection (AtroPen): 0.25 mg/0.3 ml, 0.5 mg/0.7 ml, 1 mg/0.7 ml, 2 mg/0.7 ml. **Injection, Solution:** 0.4 mg/ml, 1 mg/ml. **Ophthalmic Ointment:** 1%. **Ophthalmic Solution:** 1%.

ADMINISTRATION/HANDLING

 IV

• Must be given rapidly (prevents paradoxical slowing of heart rate).

IM

• May be given subcutaneously or IM.

IM, AtroPen

• Store at room temperature. • Give as soon as symptoms of organophosphate or carbamate poisoning appear. • Do not use more than three AtroPen autoinjectors for each person at risk for carbamate or organophosphate poisoning.

Ophthalmic

• Place gloved finger on lower eyelid and pull out until a pocket is formed between eye and lower lid. • Hold dropper above pocket and place prescribed number of drops or ¼–½ inch of ointment into pocket. • Instruct pt to close eye gently (so medication will not be squeezed out of the sac). • For solution, apply digital pressure to lacrimal sac at inner canthus for 1 min to minimize systemic absorption. • For ointment, instruct pt to roll eyeball to increase contact area of drug to eye.

⬛ IV INCOMPATIBILITY

None known.

⬛ IV COMPATIBILITIES

Diphenhydramine (Benadryl), droperidol (Inapsine), fentanyl (Sublimaze), glycopyrrolate (Robinul), heparin, hydromorphone (Dilaudid), midazolam (Versed), morphine, potassium chloride, propofol (Diprivan).

INDICATIONS/ROUTES/DOSAGE

Preanesthetic

IV, IM, Subcutaneous: ADULTS, ELDERLY: 0.4–0.6 mg 30–60 min preop. **CHILDREN WEIGHING 5 KG OR MORE:** 0.01–0.02 mg/kg/dose to maximum of 0.4 mg/dose. Minimum dose: 0.1 mg. **CHILDREN WEIGHING LESS THAN 5 KG:** 0.02 mg/kg/dose 30–60 min preop.

Bradycardia

IV: ADULTS, ELDERLY: 0.5–1 mg q5min, not to exceed total of 3 mg or 0.04 mg/kg. **CHILDREN:** 0.02 mg/kg with a minimum of 0.1 mg to a maximum of 0.5 mg as a single dose. May repeat in 5 min. **Maximum total dose:** 1 mg.

Cycloplegic Refraction, Postop Mydriasis, Uveitis

Ophthalmic Solution: ADULTS, ELDERLY: Instill 1 drop in affected eye(s) up to 4 times a day.
Ophthalmic Ointment: ADULTS, ELDERLY: Apply ointment several hours prior to examination when used for refraction.

Antidote for Organophosphate or Carbamate Poisoning

IM: ADULTS, CHILDREN WEIGHING MORE THAN 90 LB: AtroPen 2 mg (green). May repeat in 10 min. **Maximum:** 3 doses. **CHILDREN WEIGHING 40–90 LB:** AtroPen 1 mg (dark red). **CHILDREN WEIGHING 15–39 LB:** AtroPen 0.5 mg (blue). **INFANTS WEIGHING LESS THAN 15 LB:** 0.05 mg/kg. Do not use AtroPen.

SIDE EFFECTS

Frequent: Dry mouth, nose, throat (may be severe); decreased diaphoresis; constipation; irritation at subcutaneous or

IM injection site. **Occasional:** Dysphagia, blurred vision, bloated feeling, impotence, urinary hesitancy. **Ophthalmic:** Mydriasis, blurred vision, photophobia, decreased visual acuity, tearing, dry eyes or dry conjunctiva, eye irritation, crusting of eyelid. **Rare:** Allergic reaction, including rash, urticaria; mental confusion or excitement, particularly in children; fatigue.

ADVERSE EFFECTS/ TOXIC REACTIONS

Overdose may produce tachycardia, palpitations, hot/dry/flushed skin, absence of bowel sounds, increased respiratory rate, nausea, vomiting, confusion, drowsiness, slurred speech, dizziness, CNS stimulation. Overdose may also produce psychosis as evidenced by agitation, restlessness, rambling speech, visual hallucinations, paranoid behavior, delusions, followed by depression. Ophthalmic form may rarely produce increased IOP.

NURSING CONSIDERATIONS

BASELINE ASSESSMENT

Determine if pt is sensitive to atropine, homatropine, scopolamine. Treatment with AtroPen autoinjector may be instituted without waiting for lab results.

INTERVENTION/EVALUATION

Monitor changes in B/P, pulse, temperature. Observe for tachycardia if pt has cardiac abnormalities. Assess skin turgor, mucous membranes to evaluate hydration status (encourage adequate fluid intake unless NPO for surgery), bowel sounds for peristalsis. Be alert for fever (increased risk of hyperthermia). Monitor I&O, palpate bladder for urinary retention. Monitor daily pattern of bowel activity, stool consistency.

PATIENT/ FAMILY TEACHING

* For preop use, explain that warm, dry, flushing feeling may occur.

avanafil

a-**van**-a-fil
(Stendra)
Do not confuse with Stelara, avanafil with sildenafil, vardenafil or tadalafil.

◆CLASSIFICATION

PHARMACOTHERAPEUTIC: Phosphodiesterase inhibitor. **CLINICAL:** Erectile dysfunction adjunct.

ACTION

Inhibits PDE5, a phosphodiesterase type 5 enzyme responsible for degradation of cyclic GMP, predominant isoenzyme in human corpus cavernosum in the penis, resulting in smooth muscle relaxation, increased blood flow. **Therapeutic Effect:** Facilitates erection.

PHARMACOKINETICS

Onset: PO: 15–30 min. Rapidly absorbed. Protein binding: 99%. Extensively metabolized in liver. Primarily excreted in feces with a smaller amount eliminated in urine. **Half-life:** 5 hrs.

USES

Treatment of male erectile dysfunction.

PRECAUTIONS

Contraindications: Concurrent use of nitrates in any form. **Cautions:** Renal/hepatic dysfunction; anatomical deformation of the penis; cardiovascular disease, particularly myocardial infarction, stroke, life-threatening arrhythmia, or coronary revascularization within the last 6 months; those with resting hypotension or hypertension, unstable angina, New York Heart Association class 2 or greater CHF; pts who may be predisposed to priapism (sickle cell anemia, multiple myeloma, leukemia); left ventricular outflow obstruction (e.g., aortic stenosis); concurrent use of alpha-adrenergic blockers.

⧗ LIFESPAN CONSIDERATIONS

Pregnancy/Lactation: Not indicated for use in women, newborns. **Pregnancy Category C. Children:** Not indicated in pt population. **Elderly:** No age-related precautions noted.

INTERACTIONS

DRUG: Nitrates, **alpha-adrenergic blockers (alfuzosin, doxazosin, prazosin, tamsulosin, terazosin)** may produce severe hypotension. Strong **CYP3A4 inhibitors (erythromycin, itraconazole, indinavir, ketoconazole, nelfinavir, ritonavir, saquinavir)** may significantly increase concentration; do not use. **Antihypertensives, especially amlodipine, enalapril** may potentiate hypotension. **HERBAL:** None significant. **FOOD:** **High-fat meals** reduce rate of absorption. **LAB VALUES:** May increase serum glucose.

AVAILABILITY (Rx)

Tablets: 50 mg, 100 mg, 200 mg.

ADMINISTRATION/HANDLING

PO

• May take without regard to food. • May take approximately 30 min before sexual activity. • Use the lowest effective dose.

INDICATIONS/ROUTES/DOSAGE

Erectile Dysfunction

PO: ADULTS, ELDERLY: Initially, 100 mg 30 min prior to sexual activity. May increase to 200 mg. **Range:** 50–200 mg. **Maximum dosing frequency:** Once daily.

Dosage with Concurrent Alpha Blocker (e.g., Alfuzosin, Doxazosin, Prazosin, Terazosin)

PO: ADULTS, ELDERLY: Initially, 50 mg. **Maximum dosing frequency:** Once daily.

Dosage with Concurrent Moderate CYP3A4 Inhibitors (e.g., Amprenavir, Aprepitant, Diltiazem, Fluconazole, Fosamprenavir, Verapamil)

PO: ADULTS, ELDERLY: Initially, 50 mg. **Maximum dosing frequency:** Once daily.

SIDE EFFECTS

Occasional (6%–4%): Headache, flushing. **Rare (3%–2%):** Nasal congestion, nasopharyngitis, back pain. **Less than 2%:** Dizziness, arthralgia, diarrhea, insomnia.

ADVERSE EFFECTS/TOXIC REACTIONS

Sudden hearing decrease, sudden loss of vision in one or both eyes noted rarely.

NURSING CONSIDERATIONS

BASELINE ASSESSMENT

Assess cardiovascular status before initiating treatment for erectile dysfunction.

PATIENT/FAMILY TEACHING

• Medication has no effect in absence of sexual stimulation. • Seek treatment immediately if erection lasts longer than 4 hrs. • Avoid nitrate drugs while taking avanafil. • Report sudden decrease or loss of hearing or vision.

axitinib

aks-**it**-i-nib
(Inlyta)

◆CLASSIFICATION

PHARMACOTHERAPEUTIC: Tyrosine kinase inhibitor. **CLINICAL:** Antineoplastic (see p. 82C).

ACTION

Interferes with proliferation of tumor vasculature, preventing tumor growth. **Therapeutic Effect:** Blocks tumor growth, inhibits angiogenesis.

PHARMACOKINETICS

Undergoes extensive hepatic metabolism. Protein binding: greater than 99%. Eliminated primarily in feces with a lesser amount excreted in urine. **Half-life:** 2.5–6 hrs.

USES

Treatment of advanced renal cell carcinoma after failure of one prior systemic chemotherapy.

PRECAUTIONS

Contraindications: None significant. Do not use in those with untreated brain metastasis or recent active GI bleeding. **Cautions:** Those with increased risk or history of thrombotic events, GI perforation or fistula formation, renal/hepatic impairment, hypertension.

⧗ LIFESPAN CONSIDERATIONS

Pregnancy/Lactation: May cause fetal harm. Unknown whether distributed in breast milk. **Pregnancy Category D. Children:** Safety and efficacy not established in children younger than 18 yrs. **Elderly:** No age-related precautions noted.

INTERACTIONS

DRUG: Strong **CYP3A4/5 inhibitors (e.g., erythromycin, itraconazole, indinavir, ketoconazole, nelfinavir, ritonavir, saquinavir)** may significantly increase concentration; do not use concurrently. Coadministration with strong **CYP3A4/5 inducers (e.g., rifampin, dexamethasone, phenytoin, carbamazepine, rifabutin, rifapentine, phenobarbital)** may significantly decrease concentration; do not use concurrently. **HERBAL:** St. John's wort may decrease concentration. **FOOD:** **Grapefruit, grapefruit juice** may increase concentration. **LAB VALUES:** May decrease Hgb, WBC count, platelets, serum calcium, alkaline phosphatase, albumin, sodium. May increase serum ALT, AST, bilirubin, BUN, creatinine, serum potassium, lipase, amylase. May alter serum glucose.

AVAILABILITY (Rx)

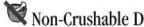 Tablets film-coated: 1 mg, 5 mg.

ADMINISTRATION/HANDLING

PO
• Give without regard to food. • Swallow tablets whole with full glass of water; do not break, crush, dissolve, or divide.

INDICATIONS/ROUTES/DOSAGE

Renal Cell Carcinoma
PO: ADULTS, ELDERLY: Initially, 5 mg twice daily, given approximately 12 hrs apart.

Moderate Hepatic Impairment
PO: ADULTS, ELDERLY: Reduce initial dose by half. May be increased or decreased based on individual safety, tolerability. Not recommended in pts with severe hepatic impairment.

SIDE EFFECTS

Frequent (55%–20%): Diarrhea, hypertension, fatigue, decreased appetite, nausea, dysphonia, palmar-plantar erythrodysesthesia (hand-foot) syndrome, weight loss, vomiting, asthenia, constipation. **Occasional (19%–11%):** Hypothyroidism, cough, stomatitis, arthralgia, dyspnea, abdominal pain, headache, peripheral pain, rash, proteinuria, dysgeusia (altered sense of taste). **Rare (10%–2%):** Dry skin, dyspepsia, dizziness, myalgia, pruritus, epistaxis, alopecia, hemorrhoids, tinnitus, erythema.

ADVERSE EFFECTS/TOXIC REACTIONS

Arterial and venous thrombotic events (MI, CVA), GI perforation, fistula have been observed and can be fatal. Hypothyroidism requiring thyroid hormone replacement has been noted. Reversible posterior leukoencephalopathy syndrome (RPLS) has been observed.

NURSING CONSIDERATIONS

BASELINE ASSESSMENT

Offer emotional support. Assess medical history, esp. hepatic function abnormali-

 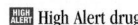

ties. Obtain baseline EKG, CBC, serum chemistries, and renal/hepatic function tests (BUN, creatinine, ALT, AST, bilirubin) before initiation of, and periodically throughout, treatment. B/P should be well controlled prior to initiating treatment. Stop medication at least 24 hrs prior to scheduled surgery. Monitor thyroid function before initiation of, and periodically throughout, treatment.

INTERVENTION/EVALUATION

Monitor CBC, serum chemistries, urinalysis, thyroid tests for changes from baseline. Monitor daily pattern of bowel activity, stool consistency. Assess for evidence of bleeding or hemorrhage. Assess for hypertension. For persistent hypertension despite use of antihypertensive medications, dose should be reduced. Permanently discontinue if signs or symptoms of RPLS occur (extreme lethargy, increased B/P from pt baseline, pyuria). Contact physician if changes in voice, redness of skin, or rash is noted.

PATIENT/FAMILY TEACHING

• Avoid crowds, those with known infection. • Avoid contact with anyone who recently received live virus vaccine; do not receive vaccinations. • Swallow tablet whole; do not chew, crush, dissolve, or divide. • Avoid grapefruit products. • Report persistent diarrhea, extreme fatigue, easy bruising, or unusual bleeding from any site.

---

azacitidine   `HIGH ALERT`

a-za-**sye**-ti-deen
(Vidaza)
Do not confuse azacitidine with azathioprine.

◆CLASSIFICATION

PHARMACOTHERAPEUTIC: DNA demethylation agent. **CLINICAL:** Antineoplastic (see p. 82C).

ACTION

Exerts cytotoxic effect on rapidly dividing cells by causing demethylation of DNA in abnormal hematopoietic cells in bone marrow. **Therapeutic Effect:** Restores normal function to tumor-suppressor genes regulating cellular differentiation, proliferation.

PHARMACOKINETICS

Rapidly absorbed after subcutaneous administration. Metabolized by liver. Eliminated in urine. **Half-life:** 4 hrs.

USES

Treatment of myelodysplastic syndromes (MDS), specifically refractory anemia, myelomonocytic leukemia. **OFF-LABEL:** Treatment of acute myelogenous leukemia.

PRECAUTIONS

Contraindications: Advanced malignant hepatic tumors, hypersensitivity to mannitol. **Cautions:** Hepatic disease, renal impairment.

LIFESPAN CONSIDERATIONS

Pregnancy/Lactation: May be embryotoxic; may cause developmental abnormalities of the fetus. Mothers should avoid breast-feeding. **Pregnancy Category D. Children:** Safety and efficacy not established. **Elderly:** Age-related renal impairment may increase risk of renal toxicity.

INTERACTIONS

DRUG: Bone marrow suppressants may increase myelosuppression. May alter effects of **live virus vaccines.** May increase levels of **clozapine, natalizumab. Pimecrolimus, tacrolimus** (topical) may increase concentration. **HERBAL: Echinacea** may decrease effect. **FOOD:** None known. **LAB VALUES:** May decrease Hgb, Hct, WBC, RBC, platelet counts. May increase serum creatinine, potassium, AST, ALT, alkaline phosphatase.

AVAILABILITY (Rx)

Injection, Powder for Reconstitution: 100 mg.

ADMINISTRATION/HANDLING

 IV

Reconstitution • Reconstitute each vial with 10 ml Sterile Water for Injection to provide a concentration of 10 mg/ml. • Vigorously shake/roll vial until all solids are dissolved. • Solution should be clear. • Further dilute desired dose with 50–100 ml 0.9% NaCl.

Rate of Administration • Administer total dose over 10–40 min. • Administer within 1 hr of reconstitution of vial.

Stability • Store unreconstituted vial at room temperature. • Solution is stable for 1 hr following reconstitution.

SUBCUTANEOUS

Reconstitution • Reconstitute with 4 ml Sterile Water for Injection. • Reconstituted solution will appear cloudy.

Rate of Administration • Doses greater than 4 ml should be divided equally into 2 syringes. • Contents of syringe must be resuspended by inverting the syringe 2–3 times and rolling the syringe between the palms for 30 sec immediately before administration. • Rotate site for each injection (thigh, upper arm, abdomen). New injections should be administered at least 1 inch from the old site.

Storage • Store vials at room temperature. • Reconstituted solution may be stored for up to 1 hr at room temperature or up to 8 hrs if refrigerated. • Solution may be allowed to return to room temperature and used within 30 min.

☒ IV INCOMPATIBILITIES

Dextrose, solutions containing sodium bicarbonate.

☒ IV COMPATIBILITIES

Lactated Ringer's, sodium chloride.

INDICATIONS/ROUTES/DOSAGE

MDS

◀ALERT▶ Dosage adjustment based on hematology testing.

IV/Subcutaneous: ADULTS, ELDERLY: 75 mg/m²/day for 7 days every 4 wks. Dosage may be increased to 100 mg/m² if initial dose is insufficient and toxicity is manageable. Treatment recommended for at least 4 cycles.

SIDE EFFECTS

Frequent (71%–29%): **IV/Subcutaneous:** Nausea, vomiting, fever, diarrhea, fatigue, injection site erythema, constipation, ecchymosis, cough, dyspnea, weakness. **IV:** Petechiae, weakness, rigors, hypokalemia. Occasional (26%–16%): **IV/Subcutaneous:** Rigors, petechiae, injection site pain, pharyngitis, arthralgia, headache, limb pain, dizziness, peripheral edema, back pain, erythema, epistaxis, weight loss, myalgia. Rare (13%–8%): **IV/Subcutaneous:** Anxiety, abdominal pain, rash, depression, tachycardia, insomnia, night sweats, stomatitis.

ADVERSE EFFECTS/ TOXIC REACTIONS

Hematologic toxicity, manifested as anemia, leukopenia, neutropenia, thrombocytopenia, occurs commonly.

NURSING CONSIDERATIONS

BASELINE ASSESSMENT

Offer emotional support. Use strict aseptic technique and protect pt from infection. Obtain CBC, electrolytes, BUN, serum creatinine, hepatic enzyme levels routinely to monitor response and toxicity but particularly before each dosing cycle.

INTERVENTION/EVALUATION

Monitor for hematologic toxicity (fever, sore throat, signs of local infections, unusual bruising/bleeding), symptoms of anemia (excessive fatigue, weakness). Assess response to medication; monitor and report nausea, vomiting, diarrhea.

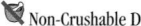

✦ Canadian trade name · Non-Crushable Drug · HIGH ALERT High Alert drug

Avoid rectal temperatures, other traumas that may induce bleeding.

PATIENT/FAMILY TEACHING

• Do not receive vaccines without physician's approval (drug lowers body's resistance). • Avoid crowds, persons with known infections. • Report signs of infection (fever, flu-like symptoms) immediately. • Contact physician if nausea/vomiting continues at home. • Men should use barrier contraception while receiving treatment.

azathioprine

a-za-**thy**-o-preen
(Apo-Azathioprine ❖, Azasan, Imuran)

BLACK BOX ALERT Chronic immunosuppression increases risk of neoplastic syndrome, serious infections.
Do not confuse azathioprine with Azulfidine, azacitidine, or azithromycin, or Imuran with Elmiron, Imdur, or Inderal.

◆CLASSIFICATION

PHARMACOTHERAPEUTIC: Immunologic agent. **CLINICAL:** Immunosuppressant.

ACTION

Antagonizes purine metabolism, inhibits DNA, protein, and RNA synthesis. **Therapeutic Effect:** Suppresses cell-mediated hypersensitivities; alters antibody production, immune response in transplant recipients. Reduces symptoms of arthritis severity.

USES

Adjunct in prevention of rejection in kidney transplantation; treatment of rheumatoid arthritis (RA) in those unresponsive to conventional therapy. **OFF-LABEL:** Treatment of dermatomyositis, polymyositis.

Adjunct in preventing rejection of solid organ (nonrenal) transplants. Maintenance, remission, or reduction of steroid use in Crohn's disease, erythema multiforme, pemphigus vulgaris, lupus nephritis, chronic refractory immune thrombocytopenic purpura, relapsing/remitting multiple sclerosis.

PRECAUTIONS

Contraindications: Pregnant women with rheumatoid arthritis (RA), those previously treated for RA with alkylating agents (cyclophosphamide, chlorambucil, melphalan). **Cautions:** Immunosuppressed pts, those with hepatic/renal impairment, active infection. Testing for genetic deficiency of thiopurine methyltransferase should be obtained. (Absence or reduced levels increase risk of myelosuppression.)

⚠ LIFESPAN CONSIDERATIONS

Pregnancy/Lactation: May depress spermatogenesis, reduction of sperm viability, count. May cause fetal harm. Do not breast-feed. **Pregnancy Category D. Children:** Safety and efficacy not established. **Elderly:** No age-related precautions noted.

INTERACTIONS

DRUG: Allopurinol, sulfamethoxazole/trimethoprim may increase activity, toxicity. **Bone marrow depressants** may increase myelosuppression. **Other immunosuppressants** may increase risk of infection or development of neoplasms. May increase effects of **live virus vaccines. HERBAL:** Avoid **cat's claw, echinacea** (immunostimulant properties). **FOOD:** None known. **LAB VALUES:** May decrease Hgb, serum albumin, uric acid, leukocytes, platelet count. May increase serum AST, ALT, alkaline phosphatase, amylase, bilirubin.

AVAILABILITY (Rx)

Injection, Powder for Reconstitution (Imuran): 100-mg vial. **Tablets:** 50 mg (Imuran), 75 mg (Azasan), 100 mg (Azasan).

ADMINISTRATION/HANDLING

IV

Reconstitution • Reconstitute 100-mg vial with 10 ml Sterile Water for Injection to provide concentration of 10 mg/ml. • Swirl vial gently to mix and dissolve solution. • May further dilute in 50 ml D₅W or 0.9% NaCl.
Rate of Administration • Give IVP over 5 min at concentration not to exceed 10 mg/ml or as intermittent infusion over 15–60 min.
Storage • Store parenteral form at room temperature. • After reconstitution, IV solution stable for 24 hrs.

PO

• Give with food or in divided doses to reduce potential for GI disturbances.
• Store oral form at room temperature.

IV INCOMPATIBILITIES

None known.

INDICATIONS/ROUTES/DOSAGE

◀ALERT▶ Reduce dose to 1/3 or 1/4 usual dose when used with allopurinol or low/absent thiopurine methyltransfurase genetic deficiency.

Prevention of Renal Allograft Rejection
PO, IV: ADULTS, ELDERLY, CHILDREN: 3–5 mg/kg/day on day of transplant (or 1–3 days prior to transplant), then 1–3 mg/kg/day as maintenance dose.

Rheumatoid Arthritis (RA)
PO: ADULTS: Initially, 1 mg/kg/day (50–100 mg) as a single dose or in 2 divided doses for 6–8 wks. May increase by 0.5 mg/kg/day after 6–8 wks at 4-wk intervals. **Maximum:** 2.5 mg/kg/day. Maintenance: Lowest effective dosage. May decrease dose by 0.5 mg/kg or 25 mg/day q4wks (while other therapies, such as rest, physiotherapy, and salicylates, are maintained). **ELDERLY:** Initially, 1 mg/kg/day (50–100 mg); may increase by 25 mg/day until response or toxicity.

Dosage in Renal Impairment
Dosage is modified based on creatinine clearance.

Creatinine Clearance	Dosage
10–50 ml/min	75% of normal
Less than 10 ml/min	50% of normal
Hemodialysis	50% of normal (Adults: additional 0.25 mg/kg)
Continuous renal replacement therapy (CRRT)	75% of normal

SIDE EFFECTS

Frequent: Nausea, vomiting, anorexia (particularly during early treatment and with large doses). **Occasional:** Rash. **Rare:** Severe nausea/vomiting with diarrhea, abdominal pain, hypersensitivity reaction.

ADVERSE EFFECTS/ TOXIC REACTIONS

Increases risk of neoplasia (new abnormal-growth tumors). Significant leukopenia and thrombocytopenia may occur, particularly in those undergoing renal transplant rejection. Hepatotoxicity occurs rarely.

NURSING CONSIDERATIONS

BASELINE ASSESSMENT

Arthritis: Assess onset, type, location, and duration of pain, fever, inflammation. Inspect appearance of affected joints for immobility, deformities, skin condition.

INTERVENTION/EVALUATION

CBC, platelet count, hepatic function studies should be performed weekly during first mo of therapy, twice monthly during second and third mos of treatment, then monthly thereafter. If WBC falls rapidly, dosage should be reduced or discontinued. Assess particularly for delayed myelosuppression. Routinely watch for any change from baseline. **Arthritis:** Assess for therapeutic response:

relief of pain, stiffness, swelling; increased joint mobility; reduced joint tenderness; improved grip strength.

PATIENT/FAMILY TEACHING

• Contact physician if unusual bleeding/ bruising, sore throat, mouth sores, abdominal pain, fever occurs. • Therapeutic response in rheumatoid arthritis may take up to 12 wks. • Women of childbearing age must avoid pregnancy.

azelastine

a-**zel**-as-teen
(<u>Astelin</u>, Astepro, Optivar)
Do not confuse Astelin with Astepro, or Optivar with Optiray.

FIXED COMBINATION(S)

Dymista: azelastine/fluticasone (a corticosteroid): 137 mcg/50 mcg per spray.

◆CLASSIFICATION

PHARMACOTHERAPEUTIC: Antihistamine. **CLINICAL:** Antiallergy (see p. 3C, 140C).

ACTION

Competes with histamine for histamine receptor sites on cells in blood vessels, GI tract, respiratory tract. **Therapeutic Effect:** Relieves symptoms associated with seasonal allergic rhinitis (increased mucus production, sneezing) and symptoms associated with allergic conjunctivitis (redness, itching, excessive tearing).

PHARMACOKINETICS

Route	Onset	Peak	Duration
Nasal spray	0.5–1 hr	2–3 hrs	12 hrs
Ophthalmic	N/A	3 min	8 hrs

Well absorbed through nasal mucosa. Primarily excreted in feces. Protein binding: 88%. Metabolized in liver. **Half-life:** 22 hrs.

USES

Nasal: Treatment of symptoms of seasonal and vasomotor rhinitis. **Ophthalmic:** Treatment of itching associated with allergic conjunctivitis.

PRECAUTIONS

Contraindications: None known. **Cautions:** None known.

⌛ LIFESPAN CONSIDERATIONS

Pregnancy/Lactation: Unknown if drug crosses placenta or is distributed in breast milk. Do not use during third trimester. **Pregnancy Category C. Children:** Safety and efficacy not established in those younger than 12 yrs. **Elderly:** No age-related precautions noted.

INTERACTIONS

DRUG: Alcohol, CNS depressants, anticholinergics may increase CNS depression. **Cimetidine** may increase plasma concentration. **HERBAL:** None significant. **FOOD:** None known. **LAB VALUES:** May suppress wheal and flare reaction to antigen skin testing unless drug is discontinued 4 days before testing. May increase serum ALT.

AVAILABILITY (Rx)

Nasal Spray (Astelin): (0.1%) 137 mcg/ spray; **(Astepro):** (0.15%) 205.5 mcg/ spray. **Ophthalmic Solution (Optivar):** 0.05%.

ADMINISTRATION/HANDLING

Nasal

• Instruct pt to clear nasal passages as much as possible before use. • Tilt pt's head slightly forward. • Insert spray tip into nostril, pointing toward nasal passage, away from nasal septum. • Spray into nostril while pt holds the other nostril closed and concurrently inhales through nose to permit medication as high into nasal passage as possible.

Ophthalmic

• Place gloved finger on lower eyelid and pull out until a pocket is formed between eye and lower lid. • Place prescribed number of drops into pocket. • Instruct pt to close eye gently for 1–2 min (so medication will not be squeezed out of the sac) and to apply digital pressure to lacrimal sac at inner canthus for 1 min to minimize systemic absorption.

INDICATIONS/ROUTES/DOSAGE

Seasonal Allergic Rhinitis
Nasal: ADULTS, ELDERLY, CHILDREN 12 YRS AND OLDER: (Astelin, Astepro): 1–2 sprays in each nostril twice a day. **CHILDREN 5–11 YRS: (Astelin):** 1 spray in each nostril twice a day.

Vasomotor Rhinitis
Nasal: ADULTS, ELDERLY, CHILDREN 12 YRS AND OLDER: 2 sprays in each nostril twice daily.

Allergic Conjunctivitis
Ophthalmic: ADULTS, ELDERLY, CHILDREN 3 YRS AND OLDER: 1 drop into affected eye twice a day.

SIDE EFFECTS

Nasal: Frequent (20%–15%): Headache, bitter taste. **Rare:** Nasal burning, paroxysmal sneezing, drowsiness. **Ophthalmic:** Transient eye burning or stinging, bitter taste, headache.

ADVERSE EFFECTS/ TOXIC REACTIONS

Epistaxis occurs rarely.

NURSING CONSIDERATIONS

BASELINE ASSESSMENT
Question for hypersensitivity to antihistamines.

INTERVENTION/EVALUATION
Assess therapeutic response to medication.

PATIENT/FAMILY TEACHING
• May cause drowsiness; avoid tasks that require alertness, motor skills until response to drug is established. • Avoid alcohol.

azilsartan

a-zil-**sar**-tan
(Edarbi)

BLACK BOX ALERT May cause fetal injury, mortality if used during second or third trimester of pregnancy.

FIXED-COMBINATION(S)

Edarbyclor: azilsartan/chlorthalidone, a diuretic: 40 mg/12.5 mg, 40 mg/25 mg.

◆CLASSIFICATION

PHARMACOTHERAPEUTIC: Angiotensin II receptor blocker (ARB). **CLINICAL:** Antihypertensive (see p. 10C, 61C).

ACTION

Potent vasodilator. Blocks vasoconstriction, aldosterone-secreting effects of angiotension II, inhibiting binding of angiotension II to AT_1 receptors. **Therapeutic Effect:** Produces vasodilation, decreases peripheral resistance, decreases B/P.

PHARMACOKINETICS

Hydrolyzed to active metabolite in GI tract. Moderately absorbed (60%). Peak plasma concentration: 1.5–3 hrs. Metabolized in liver. Protein binding: greater than 99%. Excreted primarily in feces and urine. **Half-life:** 11 hrs.

USES

Treatment of hypertension alone or in combination with other antihypertensives. Lowers risk of stroke and myocardial infarction related to hypertension.

PRECAUTIONS

Contraindications: Concomitant use with aliskiren in pts with diabetes mellitus. **Cautions:** Renal/hepatic impairment, unstented renal artery stenosis, significant aortic/mitral stenosis, severe CHF, volume depletion/salt-depleted pts.

 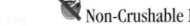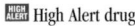

⌛ LIFESPAN CONSIDERATIONS

Pregnancy/Lactation: May cause fetal harm when administered during third trimester. Unknown if distributed in breast milk. Breast-feeding not recommended. **Pregnancy Category C (D if used in second and third trimester). Children:** Safety and efficacy not established. **Elderly:** Elevated creatinine levels may occur in pts older than 75 yrs.

INTERACTIONS

DRUG: ACE inhibitors, potassium-sparing diuretics, potassium supplements may increase risk of hyperkalemia. **NSAIDs, COX-2 inhibitors (e.g., celecoxib)** may decrease effect. **Hypotensive agents** may increase hypotensive effects. **HERBAL: Yohimbe, ephedra, licorice, ginseng** may increase B/P. **Garlic** may enhance antihypertensive effect. **FOOD:** None known. **LAB VALUES:** May increase serum creatinine. May decrease Hgb, Hct.

AVAILABILITY (Rx)

Tablets: 40 mg, 80 mg.

ADMINISTRATION/HANDLING

PO
• May give without regard to food.

INDICATIONS/ROUTES/DOSAGE

Hypertension
PO: ADULTS, ELDERLY: 80 mg once daily. Reduce to 40 mg once daily if giving high-dose diuretic concurrently.

SIDE EFFECTS

Occasional (2%–0.4%): Diarrhea, orthostatic hypotension. **Rare (0.3%):** Nausea, fatigue, muscle spasm, cough.

ADVERSE EFFECTS/ TOXIC REACTIONS

Oliguria, acute renal failure may occur in pts with history of renal artery stenosis, severe CHF, volume depletion.

NURSING CONSIDERATIONS

BASELINE ASSESSMENT

Obtain B/P, apical pulse immediately before each dose, in addition to regular monitoring (be alert to fluctuations). Question possibility of pregnancy. Assess medication history (esp. diuretics). Question history of hepatic/renal impairment, renal artery stenosis, severe CHF. Obtain baseline Hgb, Hct, serum chemistries, BUN, creatinine, AST, ALT, alkaline phosphatase, bilirubin.

INTERVENTION/EVALUATION

Maintain hydration (offer fluids frequently). Monitor serum electrolytes, B/P, pulse, hepatic/renal function. Observe for symptoms of hypotension. If excessive reduction in B/P occurs, place pt in supine position, feet slightly elevated. Correct volume or salt depletion prior to treatment.

PATIENT/FAMILY TEACHING

• Take measures to avoid pregnancy. If pregnancy occurs, inform physician immediately. • Low blood pressure is more likely to occur if pt takes diuretics or other medications to control hypertension, consumes low-salt diet, experiences vomiting or diarrhea, or becomes dehydrated. • Change positions slowly, particularly from lying to standing position. • If light-headedness or dizziness occurs, immediately lie down and call physician. • Report swollen extremities or decreased urine output despite fluid intake.

---

azithromycin   TOP 200

a-**zith**-roe-**mye**-sin
(Apo-Azithromycin ✹, AzaSite, Novo-Azithromycin ✹, <u>Zithromax</u>, Zithromax TRI-PAK, Zithromax Z-PAK, <u>Zmax</u>)
Do not confuse azithromycin with azathioprine or erythromy-

---

cin, or **Zithromax** with **Fosamax** or **Zovirax**.

◆CLASSIFICATION

PHARMACOTHERAPEUTIC: Macrolide. **CLINICAL:** Antibiotic (see p. 27C).

ACTION

Binds to ribosomal receptor sites of susceptible organisms, inhibiting RNA-dependent protein synthesis. **Therapeutic Effect:** Bacteriostatic or bactericidal, depending on drug dosage.

PHARMACOKINETICS

Rapidly absorbed from GI tract. Protein binding: 7%–50%. Widely distributed. Metabolized in liver. Eliminated primarily by biliary excretion. **Half-life:** 68 hrs.

USES

IV/PO: Treatment of susceptible infections due to *Chlamydia pneumoniae, C. trachomatis, H. influenzae, Legionella, M. catarrhalis, Mycoplasma pneumoniae, N. gonorrhoeae, S. aureus., S. pneumoniae, S. pyogenes,* including mild to moderate infections of upper respiratory tract (pharyngitis, tonsillitis), lower respiratory tract (acute bacterial exacerbations, COPD, pneumonia), uncomplicated skin and skin-structure infections, sexually transmitted diseases (nongonococcal urethritis, cervicitis due to *C. trachomatis*), chancroid. Prevents disseminated *Mycobacterium avium* complex (MAC). Treatment of mycoplasma pneumonia, community-acquired pneumonia, pelvic inflammatory disease (PID). Prevention/treatment of MAC in pts with advanced HIV infection. **Ophthalmic:** Treatment of bacterial conjunctivitis caused by susceptible infections due to *H. influenzae, S. aureus, S. mitis, S. pneumoniae.* **OFF-LABEL:** Prophylaxis of endocarditis, pertussis.

PRECAUTIONS

Contraindications: Hypersensitivity to other macrolide antibiotics. History of cholestatic jaundice/hepatic dysfunction associated with prior azithromycin therapy. **Cautions:** Hepatic/renal dysfunction. Hepatocellular and/or cholestatic hepatitis (with or without jaundice), hepatic necrosis. May prolong QT interval (rare), myasthenia gravis.

⌛ LIFESPAN CONSIDERATIONS

Pregnancy/Lactation: Unknown if distributed in breast milk. **Pregnancy Category B. Children:** Safety and efficacy not established in those younger than 16 yrs for IV use and younger than 6 mos for oral use. **Elderly:** No age-related precautions in those with normal renal function.

INTERACTIONS

DRUG: **Aluminum/magnesium-containing antacids** may decrease concentration (give 1 hr before or 2 hrs after antacid). May increase levels of **amiodarone, cyclosporine, dronedarone, QT-prolonging medications, thioridazine, toremifene, ziprasidone. Quetiapine** may increase concentration. **HERBAL:** None significant. **FOOD:** None known. **LAB VALUES:** May increase serum creatine phosphokinase (CPK), AST, ALT, bilirubin, LDH, potassium.

AVAILABILITY (Rx)

Injection, Powder for Reconstitution (Zithromax): 500 mg. **Ophthalmic Solution (AzaSite):** 1%. **Suspension, Oral (Zithromax):** 100 mg/5 ml, 200 mg/5 ml, 1-g single dose packet. **Suspension, Oral (Extended-Release [Zmax]):** 2-g single-dose packet. **Tablets:** 250 mg, 500 mg, 600 mg (Zithromax). Tri-Pak: 3 × 500 mg (Zithromax TRI-PAK). Z-PAK: 6 × 250 mg (Zithromax Z-PAK).

ADMINISTRATION/HANDLING

 IV

Reconstitution • Reconstitute each 500-mg vial with 4.8 ml Sterile Water for Injection to provide concentration of 100 mg/ml. • Shake well to ensure dissolution. • Further dilute with 250 or 500 ml

0.9% NaCl or D₅W to provide final concentration of 2 mg/ml with 250 ml diluent or 1 mg/ml with 500 ml diluent.

Rate of Administration • Infuse over 60 min (2 mg/ml). Infuse over 3 hrs (1 mg/ml).

Storage • Store vials at room temperature. • Following reconstitution, diluted solution is stable for 24 hrs at room temperature or 7 days if refrigerated.

PO (Immediate-Release Suspension)
• Give tablets without regard to food.
• May store suspension at room temperature. Stable for 10 days after reconstitution.

PO (Extended-Release Suspension)
• Do not administer oral suspension with food. Give at least 1 hr before or 2 hrs after meals. • Give Zmax within 12 hrs of reconstitution. • Give tablets with food to decrease GI effects.

PO
• Tablets: May give with food to decrease GI effects.

Ophthalmic
• Place gloved finger on lower eyelid and pull out until a pocket is formed between eye and lower lid. • Place prescribed number of drops into pocket. • Instruct pt to close eye gently for 1 to 2 min (so medication will not be squeezed out of sac) and to apply digital pressure to lacrimal sac at inner canthus for 1 min to minimize systemic absorption.

⚙ IV INCOMPATIBILITIES

Ceftriaxone (Rocephin), ciprofloxacin (Cipro), famotidine (Pepcid), furosemide (Lasix), ketorolac (Toradol), levofloxacin (Levaquin), morphine, piperacillin/tazobactam (Zosyn), potassium chloride.

⚙ IV COMPATIBILITIES

Ceftaroline (Teflaro), doripenem (Doribax), ondansetron (Zofran), tigecycline (Tygacil), diphenhydramine (Benadryl).

INDICATIONS/ROUTES/DOSAGE

Usual Dosage Range
PO: ADULTS, ELDERLY: 250–600 mg once daily or 1–2 g as single dose. **CHILDREN 6 MOS AND OLDER:** 5–12 mg/kg (**maximum:** 500 mg) once daily or 30 mg/kg (**maximum:** 1,500 mg) as single dose. **NEONATES:** 10–20 mg/kg once daily.
IV: ADULTS, ELDERLY: 250–500 mg once daily (not currently approved in children).

Acute Exacerbations of COPD
PO: ADULTS, ELDERLY, CHILDREN 16 YRS AND OLDER: 500 mg/day for 3 days or 500 mg on day 1, then 250 mg/day on days 2–5.

Acute Bacterial Sinusitis
PO (Zmax): ADULTS, ELDERLY: 2 g as a single dose.
PO: ADULTS, ELDERLY: 500 mg/day for 3 days. **CHILDREN 6 MOS AND OLDER:** 10 mg/kg for 3 days. **Maximum:** 500 mg/day.

Cervicitis
PO: ADULTS, ELDERLY: 1–2 g as single dose.

Chancroid
PO: ADULTS, ELDERLY: 1 g as single dose.

MAC Prevention
PO: ADULTS, ELDERLY: 1,200 mg once weekly. **CHILDREN:** 20 mg/kg once weekly. **Maximum:** 1,200 mg/dose.

MAC Treatment
PO: ADULTS, ELDERLY: 600 mg/day with ethambutol. **CHILDREN:** 10–12 mg/kg/day (**maximum:** 500 mg) with ethambutol.

Otitis Media
PO: CHILDREN 6 MOS AND OLDER: 30 mg/kg as single dose (**maximum:** 1,500 mg) or 10 mg/kg/day for 3 days (**maximum:** 500 mg) or 10 mg/kg on day 1 (**maximum:** 500 mg), then 5 mg/kg on days 2–5 (**maximum:** 250 mg).

---

underlined – top prescribed drug

Pharyngitis, Tonsillitis
PO: ADULTS, ELDERLY, CHILDREN 16 YRS AND OLDER: 500 mg on day 1, then 250 mg on days 2–5. **CHILDREN 2–15 YRS:** 12 mg/kg daily for 5 days (**maximum:** 500 mg).

Pneumonia, Community-Acquired
PO *(Zmax)*: **ADULTS, ELDERLY:** 2 g as single dose.
PO: ADULTS, ELDERLY, CHILDREN 16 YRS AND OLDER: 500 mg on day 1, then 250 mg on days 2–5 or 500 mg/day IV for 2 days, then 500 mg/day PO to complete course of therapy. **CHILDREN 6 MOS–15 YRS:** 10 mg/kg on day 1 (**maximum:** 500 mg), then 5 mg/kg (**maximum:** 250 mg) on days 2–5.

Skin and Skin-Structure Infections
PO: ADULTS, ELDERLY, CHILDREN 16 YRS AND OLDER: 500 mg on day 1, then 250 mg on days 2–5.

Pelvic Inflammatory Disease (PID)
IV: ADULTS, ELDERLY: 500 mg/day for at least 2 days, then 250 mg/day to complete a 7-day course of therapy.

Bacterial Conjunctivitis
Ophthalmic: ADULTS, ELDERLY: 1 drop in affected eye twice a day for 2 days, then 1 drop once a day for 5 days.

SIDE EFFECTS

Occasional: Systemic: Nausea, vomiting, diarrhea, abdominal pain. **Ophthalmic:** Eye irritation. **Rare: Systemic:** Headache, dizziness, allergic reaction.

ADVERSE EFFECTS/ TOXIC REACTIONS

Antibiotic-associated colitis, other superinfections (abdominal cramps, severe watery diarrhea, fever) may result from altered bacterial balance. Acute interstitial nephritis, hepatotoxicity occur rarely.

NURSING CONSIDERATIONS

BASELINE ASSESSMENT
Question for history of hepatitis, allergies to azithromycin, erythromycins. Assess for infection (WBC count, appearance of wound, evidence of fever).

INTERVENTION/EVALUATION
Check for GI discomfort, nausea, vomiting. Monitor daily pattern of bowel activity and stool consistency. Monitor hepatic function tests, CBC. Assess for hepatotoxicity: malaise, fever, abdominal pain, GI disturbances. Be alert for superinfection: fever, vomiting, diarrhea, anal/genital pruritus, oral mucosal changes (ulceration, pain, erythema).

PATIENT/FAMILY TEACHING
• Continue therapy for full length of treatment. • Avoid concurrent administration of aluminum- or magnesium-containing antacids. • Bacterial conjunctivitis: Do not wear contact lenses.

aztreonam

az-**tree**-o-nam
(Azactam, Cayston)

◆**CLASSIFICATION**
PHARMACOTHERAPEUTIC: Monobactam. **CLINICAL:** Antibiotic.

ACTION

Inhibits bacterial cell wall synthesis. **Therapeutic Effect:** Bactericidal.

PHARMACOKINETICS

Completely absorbed after IM administration. Protein binding: 56%–60%. Partially metabolized by hydrolysis. Primarily excreted unchanged in urine. Removed by hemodialysis. **Half-life:** 1.4–2.2 hrs (increased in renal/hepatic impairment).

USES

Treatment of infections caused by susceptible gram-negative microorganisms *P. aeruginosa, E. coli, S. marcescens, K. pneumoniae, P. mirabilis, H. influenzae, Enterobacter, Citrobacter* spp. including lower respiratory tract, skin/skin structure, intraabdominal, gynecologic, complicated/uncomplicated UTIs; septicemia; cystic fibrosis. **Cayston:** Improve respiratory symptoms in cystic fibrosis pts with *P. aeruginosa.* **OFF-LABEL:** Treatment of bone and joint infections.

PRECAUTIONS

Contraindications: None known. **Cautions:** History of allergy, esp. cephalosporins, penicillins; renal impairment.

⌛ LIFESPAN CONSIDERATIONS

Pregnancy/Lactation: Crosses placenta, distributed in amniotic fluid; low concentration in breast milk. **Pregnancy Category B. Children:** Safety and efficacy not established in those younger than 9 mos. **Elderly:** Age-related renal impairment may require dosage adjustment.

INTERACTIONS

DRUG: None significant. **HERBAL:** None significant. **FOOD:** None known. **LAB VALUES:** May increase serum alkaline phosphatase, creatinine, LDH, AST, ALT levels. Produces a positive Coombs' test. May prolong partial thromboplastin time (PTT), prothrombin time (PT).

AVAILABILITY (Rx)

Injection, Infusion Solution (Azactam): Premix 1 g/50 ml, 2 g/50 ml. **Injection, Powder for Reconstitution (Azactam):** 1 g, 2 g. **Oral Inhalation, Powder for Reconstitution (Cayston):** 75 mg.

ADMINISTRATION/HANDLING

 IV

Reconstitution • For IV push, dilute each gram with 6–10 ml Sterile Water for Injection. • For intermittent IV infusion, further dilute with 50–100 ml D₅W or 0.9% NaCl.
Rate of Administration • For IV push, give over 3–5 min. • For IV infusion, administer over 20–60 min.
Storage • Store vials at room temperature. • Solution appears colorless to light yellow. • Following reconstitution, solution is stable for 48 hrs at room temperature or 7 days if refrigerated. • Discard if precipitate forms. Discard unused portions.

IM

• Shake immediately, vigorously after adding diluent. • Inject deeply into large muscle mass. • Following reconstitution, solution is stable for 48 hrs at room temperature or 7 days if refrigerated.

Inhalation

• Administer only with an Altera nebulizer system. • Nebulize over 2–3 min. • Give bronchodilator 15 min–4 hrs (short-acting) or 30 min–12 hrs (long-acting) before administration. • Reconstituted solution must be used immediately.

🔲 IV INCOMPATIBILITIES

Acyclovir (Zovirax), amphotericin (Fungizone), lorazepam (Ativan), metronidazole (Flagyl), vancomycin (Vancocin).

🔲 IV COMPATIBILITIES

Bumetanide (Bumex), calcium gluconate, cimetidine (Tagamet), diltiazem (Cardizem), diphenhydramine (Benadryl), dobutamine (Dobutrex), dopamine (Intropin), famotidine (Pepcid), furosemide (Lasix), heparin, hydromorphone (Dilaudid), insulin (regular), magnesium sulfate, morphine, potassium chloride, propofol (Diprivan).

INDICATIONS/ROUTES/DOSAGE

Severe Infections
IV: ADULTS, ELDERLY: 2 g q6–8h. **Maximum:** 8 g/day. **CHILDREN:** 30 mg/kg q6–8h. **Maximum:** 8 g/day.

Mild–Moderate Infections
IV: ADULTS, ELDERLY: 1–2 g q8–12h. **CHILDREN:** 30 mg/kg q8h. **Maximum:** 3 g/day. **USUAL NEONATE DOSAGE:** 30 mg/kg/dose q6–12h.

Cystic Fibrosis
IV: CHILDREN: 50 mg/kg/dose q6–8h up to 200 mg/kg/day. **Maximum:** 8 g/day. **Inhalation (Nebulizer): ADULTS, CHILDREN 7 YRS OR OLDER:** 75 mg 3 times/day (at least 4 hrs apart) for 28 days, then off for 28-day cycle.

Moderate to Severe Infections in Children
IV: CHILDREN: 30 mg/kg q6–8h. **Maximum:** 120 mg/kg/day. **NEONATES:** 60–120 mg/kg/day divided q6–12h (dosage based on age and weight).

Dosage in Renal Impairment
Dosage and frequency are modified based on creatinine clearance and severity of infection:

Creatinine Clearance	Dosage
10–30 ml/min	50% usual dose at usual intervals
Less than 10 ml/min	25% usual dose at usual intervals
Hemodialysis	500 mg–2 g, then 25% of initial dose at usual interval
Continuous renal replacement therapy (CRRT)	2 g, then 1 g q8–12h or 2g q12h

SIDE EFFECTS
Frequent (greater than 5%): Cayston: Cough, nasal congestion, wheezing, pharyngolaryngeal pain, pyrexia, chest discomfort, abdominal pain, vomiting.

Occasional (less than 3%): Discomfort and swelling at IM injection site, nausea, vomiting, diarrhea, rash. **Rare (less than 1%):** Phlebitis or thrombophlebitis at IV injection site, abdominal cramps, headache, hypotension.

ADVERSE EFFECTS/ TOXIC REACTIONS
Antibiotic-associated colitis, other superinfections (abdominal cramps, severe watery diarrhea, fever) may result from altered bacterial balance. Severe hypersensitivity reactions, including anaphylaxis, occur rarely.

NURSING CONSIDERATIONS
BASELINE ASSESSMENT
Question for history of allergies, esp. to aztreonam, other antibiotics.

INTERVENTION/EVALUATION
Evaluate for phlebitis (heat, pain, red streaking over vein), pain at IM injection site. Assess for GI discomfort, nausea, vomiting. Monitor daily pattern of bowel activity, stool consistency. Assess skin for rash. Be alert for superinfection: fever, vomiting, diarrhea, anal/genital pruritus, oral mucosal changes (ulceration, pain, erythema). Monitor renal/hepatic function.

PATIENT/FAMILY TEACHING
• Report nausea, vomiting, diarrhea, rash.

baclofen

bak-loe-fen
(Apo-Baclofen ✸, Lioresal,
Novo-Baclofen ✸, Nu-Baclo ✸)

BLACK BOX ALERT Abrupt withdrawal of intrathecal form has resulted in severe hyperpyrexia, obtundation, rebound or exaggerated spasticity, muscle rigidity, leading to organ failure, death.
Do not confuse baclofen with Bactroban or Beclovent, or Lioresal with lisinopril or Lotensin.

◆CLASSIFICATION

PHARMACOTHERAPEUTIC: Skeletal muscle relaxant. **CLINICAL:** Antispastic, analgesic in trigeminal neuralgia (see p. 150C).

ACTION

Inhibits transmission of reflexes at spinal cord level. **Therapeutic Effect:** Relieves muscle spasticity.

PHARMACOKINETICS

Well absorbed from GI tract. Protein binding: 30%. Partially metabolized in liver. Primarily excreted in urine. **Half-life:** 2.5–4 hrs.

USES

Treatment of cerebral spasticity, reversible spasticity associated with multiple sclerosis, spinal cord lesions. **Intrathecal:** For those unresponsive to oral therapy or exhibiting intolerable side effects. **OFF-LABEL:** Treatment of bladder spasms, cerebral palsy, intractable hiccups or pain, Huntington's chorea, trigeminal neuralgia.

PRECAUTIONS

Contraindications: None known. **Cautions:** Renal impairment, seizure disorder.

⧗ LIFESPAN CONSIDERATIONS

Pregnancy/Lactation: Unknown if drug crosses placenta or is distributed in breast milk. **Pregnancy Category C. Children:** Safety and efficacy not established in those younger than 12 yrs. Limited published data in children. **Elderly:** Increased risk of CNS toxicity (hallucinations, sedation, confusion, mental depression); age-related renal impairment may require decreased dosage.

INTERACTIONS

DRUG: Potentiated effects when used with other **CNS depressants (including alcohol). HERBAL: Gotu kola, kava kava, St. John's wort, valerian** may increase CNS sedation. **FOOD:** None known. **LAB VALUES:** May increase serum AST, ALT, alkaline phosphatase, glucose.

AVAILABILITY (Rx)

Intrathecal Injection Solution: 50 mcg/ml, 500 mcg/ml, 2,000 mcg/ml. **Tablets:** 10 mg, 20 mg.

ADMINISTRATION/HANDLING

PO
• Give with food or milk. • Tablets may be crushed.

Intrathecal
• For screening, a 50 mcg/ml concentration should be used for injection. • For maintenance therapy, solution should be diluted for pts who require concentrations other than 500 mcg/ml or 2,000 mcg/ml.

INDICATIONS/ROUTES/DOSAGE

◀ALERT▶ Avoid abrupt withdrawal.
Spasticity
PO: ADULTS: Initially, 5 mg 3 times a day. May increase by 15 mg/day (5 mg/dose) at 3-day intervals. Range: 40–80 mg/day. **Maximum:** 80 mg/day. **ELDERLY:** Initially, 5 mg 2–3 times a day. May gradually increase dosage. **CHILDREN 8 YRS AND OLDER:** 30–40 mg/day in divided doses q8h. May increase dose by 5–15 mg/day q3days. **Maximum:** 120 mg/day. **CHILDREN 2–7 YRS:** 20–30 mg/day in divided doses q8h. May increase dose by 5–15

mg/day q3days. **Maximum:** 60 mg/day. **CHILDREN YOUNGER THAN 2 YRS:** 10–20 mg/day in divided doses q8h. May increase dose by 5–15 mg/day. **Maximum:** 40 mg/day.

Intrathecal Dose

ADULTS, ELDERLY, CHILDREN: Test dose: 50–100 mcg. Dose greater than 50 mcg given in 25-mcg increments, separated by 24 hrs. Following positive response to test dose, maintenance infusion can be given via implanted intrathecal pump. Initial dose is twice the test dose.

SIDE EFFECTS

Frequent (greater than 10%): Transient drowsiness, asthenia (loss of strength, energy), dizziness, light-headedness, nausea, vomiting. **Occasional (10%–2%):** Headache, paresthesia, constipation, anorexia, hypotension, confusion, nasal congestion. **Rare (less than 1%):** Paradoxical CNS excitement or restlessness, slurred speech, tremor, dry mouth, diarrhea, nocturia, impotence.

ADVERSE EFFECTS/ TOXIC REACTIONS

Abrupt discontinuation may produce hallucinations, seizures. Overdose results in blurred vision, seizures, myosis, mydriasis, severe muscle weakness, strabismus, respiratory depression, vomiting.

NURSING CONSIDERATIONS

BASELINE ASSESSMENT

Record onset, type, location, duration of muscular spasm. Check for immobility, stiffness, swelling.

INTERVENTION/EVALUATION

Assess for paradoxical reaction. Observe for drowsiness, dizziness, ataxia. Assist with ambulation at all times. For those on long-term therapy, hepatic/renal function tests, blood counts should be performed periodically. Evaluate for therapeutic response: decreased intensity of skeletal muscle spasm, pain.

PATIENT/FAMILY TEACHING

• Drowsiness usually diminishes with continued therapy. • Avoid tasks that require alertness, motor skills until response to drug is established. • Do not abruptly withdraw medication after long-term therapy (may result in muscle rigidity, rebound spasticity, high fever, altered mental status). • Avoid alcohol, CNS depressants.

---

basiliximab

ba-si-**lik**-si-mab
(Simulect)

BLACK BOX ALERT Must be prescribed by a physician experienced in immunosuppression therapy and organ transplant management.
Do not confuse basiliximab with daclizumab.

◆CLASSIFICATION

PHARMACOTHERAPEUTIC: Monoclonal antibody. **CLINICAL:** Immunosuppressive (see p. 123C).

ACTION

Binds to and blocks receptor of interleukin-2, a protein that stimulates proliferation of T-lymphocytes, which play a major role in organ transplant rejection. **Therapeutic Effect:** Prevents lymphocytic activity, impairs response of immune system to antigens, prevents acute renal transplant rejection.

PHARMACOKINETICS

Half-life: 4–10 days (adults); 5–17 days (children).

USES

Adjunct with cyclosporine, corticosteroids in prevention of acute organ rejection in pts receiving renal transplant. **OFF-LABEL:** Treatment of refractory graft-vs-host disease, prevention of liver or cardiac transplant rejection.

PRECAUTIONS

Contraindications: Hypersensitivity to basiliximab. **Cautions:** Anemia, HF, chronic wounds, diabetes mellitus, dehydration, electrolyte imbalance, generalized/peripheral edema, HTN.

⌛ LIFESPAN CONSIDERATIONS

Pregnancy/Lactation: Unknown if drug crosses placenta or is distributed in breast milk. Breastfeeding not recommended. **Pregnancy Category B. Children/Elderly:** No age-related precautions noted.

INTERACTIONS

DRUG: Tacrolimus (topical), **trastuzumab** may increase concentration. **HERBAL: Echinacea** may decrease therapeutic effect. **Bilberry, garlic, ginger, ginseng** may increase hypoglycemic effect. **FOOD:** None known. **LAB VALUES:** May alter serum calcium, glucose, potassium, Hgb, Hct. May increases serum cholesterol, BUN, creatinine, uric acid. May decrease serum magnesium, phosphate, platelet count.

AVAILABILITY (Rx)

Injection, Powder for Reconstitution: 10 mg, 20 mg.

ADMINISTRATION/HANDLING

 IV

Reconstitution • Reconstitute 10-mg vial with 2.5 ml or 20-mg vial with 5 ml Sterile Water for Injection. • Shake gently to dissolve. • May further dilute with 25–50 ml 0.9% NaCl or D_5W to a final concentration of 0.4 mg/ml. • Gently invert to avoid foaming. • Do not shake.
Rate of Administration • IV bolus over 10 min. • IV infusion over 20–30 min.
Storage • Refrigerate unused vials. • After reconstitution, use within 4 hrs (24 hrs if refrigerated). • Discard if precipitate forms.

🚫 IV INCOMPATIBILITIES

Specific information not available. Do not add other medications simultaneously through same IV line.

INDICATIONS/ROUTES/DOSAGE

Prophylaxis of Organ Rejection
IV: ADULTS, ELDERLY, CHILDREN WEIGHING 35 KG OR MORE: 20 mg within 2 hrs before transplant surgery and 20 mg 4 days after transplant. **CHILDREN WEIGHING LESS THAN 35 KG:** 10 mg within 2 hrs before transplant surgery and 10 mg 4 days after transplant.

SIDE EFFECTS

Frequent (greater than 10%): GI disturbances (constipation, diarrhea, dyspepsia), CNS effects (dizziness, headache, insomnia, tremor), respiratory tract infection, dysuria, acne, leg or back pain, peripheral edema, hypertension. **Occasional (10%–3%):** Angina, neuropathy, abdominal distention, tachycardia, rash, hypotension, urinary disturbances (urinary frequency, genital edema, hematuria), arthralgia, hirsutism, myalgia.

ADVERSE EFFECTS/ TOXIC REACTIONS

Severe, acute hypersensitivity reactions including anaphylaxis characterized by hypotension, tachycardia, cardiac failure, dyspnea, wheezing, bronchospasm, pulmonary edema, respiratory failure, urticaria, rash, pruritus, sneezing, as well as capillary leak syndrome and cytokine release syndrome, have been reported.

NURSING CONSIDERATIONS

BASELINE ASSESSMENT

Obtain baseline BUN, serum creatinine, potassium, uric acid, glucose, calcium, phosphatase levels and vital signs, particularly B/P, pulse rate. Breastfeeding not recommended.

INTERVENTION/EVALUATION

Diligently monitor CBC, serum chemistry results. Assess B/P for hypertension/hypotension; pulse for evidence of tachycardia.

Question for GI disturbances, CNS effects, urinary changes. Monitor for presence of wound infection, signs of infection (fever, sore throat, unusual bleeding/bruising), hypersensitivity reaction.

PATIENT/FAMILY TEACHING

• Report difficulty in breathing or swallowing, palpitations, bruising/bleeding, rash, itching, swelling of lower extremities, weakness. • Female pts should take measures to avoid pregnancy; avoid breast-feeding.

TOP 200

beclomethasone

be-kloe-**meth**-a-sone
(Apo-Beclomethasone , Beconase AQ, QNASL, QVAR, Rivanase AQ)
Do not confuse Beconase with baclofen.

◆CLASSIFICATION

PHARMACOTHERAPEUTIC: Adrenocorticosteroid. **CLINICAL:** Anti-inflammatory, immunosuppressant (see pp. 2C, 77C, 99C).

ACTION

Controls or prevents inflammation by altering rate of protein synthesis; migration of polymorphonuclear leukocytes, fibroblasts; reverses capillary permeability. **Therapeutic Effect: Inhalation:** Inhibits bronchoconstriction, produces smooth muscle relaxation, decreases mucus secretion. **Intranasal:** Decreases response to seasonal, perennial rhinitis.

PHARMACOKINETICS

Rapidly absorbed from pulmonary, nasal, GI tissue. Hydrolyzed by pulmonary esterase prior to absorption. Metabolized in liver. Protein binding: 87%. Primarily eliminated in feces. **Half-life:** 15 hrs.

USES

Inhalation: Long-term control of bronchial asthma. Reduces need for oral corticosteroid therapy for asthma. **Intranasal:** Relief of seasonal/perennial rhinitis; prevention of nasal polyp recurrence after surgical removal; treatment of nonallergic rhinitis. **QNASL:** Treatment of seasonal and perennial allergic rhinitis in adults and adolescents 12 yrs and older. **OFF-LABEL:** Prevention of seasonal rhinitis (nasal form).

PRECAUTIONS

Contraindications: Hypersensitivity to beclomethasone, acute exacerbation of asthma, status asthmaticus. **Cautions:** Thyroid disease, hepatic impairment, renal impairment, cardiovascular disease, diabetes, glaucoma, cataracts, myasthenia gravis, seizures, risk for osteoporosis, peptic ulcer, ulcerative colitis, following acute MI, elderly. Avoid use in pts with untreated viral, fungal, or bacterial systemic infections.

⌛ LIFESPAN CONSIDERATIONS

Pregnancy/Lactation: Unknown if drug crosses placenta or is distributed in breast milk. **Pregnancy Category C. Children:** Prolonged treatment/high dosages may decrease short-term growth rate, cortisol secretion. **Elderly:** No age-related precautions noted.

INTERACTIONS

DRUG: May decrease effect of **antidiabetic agents. HERBAL:** Echinacea may decrease effects. **FOOD:** None known. **LAB VALUES:** None significant.

AVAILABILITY (Rx)

Inhalation, Oral (Qvar): 40 mcg/inhalation, 80 mcg/inhalation. **QNASL:** 80 mcg/actuation. **Nasal Inhalation (Beconase AQ):** 42 mcg/inhalation.

ADMINISTRATION/HANDLING

Inhalation
• Shake container well. • Instruct pt to exhale completely, place mouthpiece be-

tween lips, inhale, hold breath as long as possible before exhaling. • Allow at least 1 min between inhalations. • Rinsing mouth after each use decreases dry mouth, hoarseness, thrush.

Intranasal
• Instruct pt to clear nasal passages as much as possible before use. • Tilt pt's head slightly forward. • Insert spray tip into nostril, pointing toward nasal passages, away from nasal septum. • Spray into one nostril while pt holds the other nostril closed, concurrently inhaling through nose to permit medication as high into nasal passages as possible.

INDICATIONS/ROUTES/DOSAGE

Long-Term Control of Bronchial Asthma
Oral Inhalation *(QVAR):* **ADULTS, ELDERLY, CHILDREN 12 YRS AND OLDER:** 40–160 mcg twice a day. **Maximum:** 320 mcg twice a day. **CHILDREN 5–11 YRS:** 40 mcg twice a day. **Maximum:** 80 mcg twice a day.

Rhinitis, Prevention of Recurrence of Nasal Polyps
Nasal Inhalation *(QVAR):* **ADULTS, ELDERLY, CHILDREN 6 YRS AND OLDER:** 1–2 sprays in each nostril twice a day.

Allergic Rhinitis
Oral Inhalation *(QNASL):* **ADULTS, ELDERLY, CHILDREN 12 YRS AND OLDER:** 2 sprays in each nostril daily.

SIDE EFFECTS

Frequent: Inhalation (14%–4%): Throat irritation, dry mouth, hoarseness, cough. **Intranasal:** Nasal burning, mucosal dryness. **Occasional: Inhalation (3%–2%):** Localized fungal infection (thrush). **Intranasal:** Nasal-crusting epistaxis, sore throat, ulceration of nasal mucosa. **Rare: Inhalation:** Transient bronchospasm, esophageal candidiasis. **Intranasal:** Nasal and pharyngeal candidiasis, eye pain.

ADVERSE EFFECTS/ TOXIC REACTIONS

Acute hypersensitivity reaction (urticaria, angioedema, severe bronchospasm) occurs rarely. Change from systemic to local steroid therapy may unmask previously suppressed bronchial asthma condition.

NURSING CONSIDERATIONS

BASELINE ASSESSMENT

Establish baseline history for asthma, rhinitis. Question for hypersensitivity to any corticosteroids.

INTERVENTION/EVALUATION

Monitor respiratory status, lung sounds; observe for signs of oral candidiasis. In those receiving bronchodilators by inhalation concomitantly with inhaled steroid therapy, advise to use bronchodilator several minutes before corticosteroid aerosol (enhances penetration of steroid into bronchial tree).

PATIENT/FAMILY TEACHING

• Do not change dose schedule or stop taking drug; must taper off gradually under medical supervision. • **Inhalation:** Maintain diligent oral hygiene. • Rinse mouth with water immediately after inhalation (prevents mouth/throat dryness, fungal infection of mouth). • Contact physician if sore throat or mouth occurs. • **Intranasal:** Contact physician if symptoms do not improve or sneezing, nasal irritation occurs. • Clear nasal passages prior to use. • Improvement noted after several days.

bedaquiline

bed-**ak**-wi-leen
(Sirturo)
Do not confuse bedaquiline with quinidine or quetiapine.
BLACK BOX ALERT QT prolongation may occur. Concurrent use with

other drugs that prolong QT interval may produce additive QT prolongation. To be used only when current treatment regimen is ineffective. Placebo-controlled trial: increased risk of death (11.4% bedaquiline vs. 2.5% placebo).

◆CLASSIFICATION

PHARMACOTHERAPEUTIC: Diaryl-quinoline antimycobacterial. **CLINICAL:** Antitubercular.

ACTION

Inhibits mycobacterial adenosine triphosphate (ATP) synthase, an enzyme essential for generation of energy in mycobacterium tuberculosum. **Therapeutic Effect:** Treatment of multidrug-resistant mycobacterium tuberculosis (TB).

PHARMACOKINETICS

Absorbed from GI tract. Peak plasma concentration: 5 hrs. Metabolized in liver. Mainly excreted in feces. Protein binding: 99.9%. **Half-life:** 5.5 mos.

USES

Treatment of pulmonary multidrug-resistant TB in adults 18 yrs and older when other alterations are not available. Not recommended for pts with extrapulmonary TB (e.g., central nervous system), latent or drug-sensitive TB.

PRECAUTIONS

Contraindications: None known. **Cautions:** Severe hepatic/renal impairment, history of or risk of QT prolongation (e.g., torsades de pointes, bradyarrhythmias, hypothyroidism).

⌛ LIFESPAN CONSIDERATIONS

Pregnancy/Lactation: Unknown if distributed in breast milk. **Pregnancy Category B. Children:** Safety and efficacy not established in those younger than 18 yrs. **Elderly:** No age-related precautions noted.

INTERACTIONS

DRUG: CYP3A4 inducers (e.g., carbamazepine, rifampin) may reduce concentration/effect. **CYP3A4 inhibitors (e.g., ketoconazole)** may increase concentration/effect. **Macrolide antibacterial (e.g., clarithromycin), fluoroquinolones (e.g., levofloxacin), clofazimine** may increase risk of prolonged QT interval. **HERBAL: St. John's wort** decreases concentration/effect. **FOOD:** Food enhances bioavailability. **LAB VALUES:** May increase serum ALT, AST, alkaline phosphatase, amylase.

AVAILABILITY (Rx)

Tablets: 100 mg.

ADMINISTRATION/HANDLING

PO
• Give with food (increases bioavailability). • Swallow tablet whole with water.

INDICATIONS/ROUTES/DOSAGE

Tuberculosis
PO: ADULTS 18 YRS AND OLDER, ELDERLY: Note: Initiate medication with at least 3 other antitubercular drugs.
Weeks 1–2: 400 mg (4 tablets of 100 mg) once daily with food. **Weeks 3–24:** 200 mg (2 tablets of 100 mg) 3 times per week with food (at least 48 hrs between doses) for a total dose of 600 mg per wk. Total duration of treatment: 24 wks.

SIDE EFFECTS

Frequent (33%–28%): Arthralgia, nausea, headache. **Occasional (9%–8%):** Anorexia, rash.

ADVERSE EFFECTS/ TOXIC REACTIONS

Hemoptysis, chest pain occur in 18% and 11%, respectively. May prolong QT interval.

NURSING CONSIDERATIONS

BASELINE ASSESSMENT

Obtain baseline laboratory results prior to initiation of treatment, particularly serum potassium, calcium, magnesium (may alter QT interval), ALT, AST, alkaline phosphatase, bilirubin and correct if abnormal. Obtain EKG and assess for prolonged QT. Test for viral hepatitis.

INTERVENTION/EVALUATION

Follow-up monitoring of electrolytes should be performed if QT prolongation is detected. If baseline EKG presents with prolonged QT interval, monitor EKG frequently to confirm QT interval has returned to baseline (monitor for syncope). Monitor serum chemistries monthly while on treatment. Aminotransferase 3 × the ULN or higher should be followed by repeat testing within 48 hrs. Diligently monitor for any signs or symptoms of bleeding, fatigue, anorexia, nausea, jaundice, melanuria, hepatic tenderness, hepatomegaly.

PATIENT/FAMILY TEACHING

• Avoid alcohol. • Report fatigue, loss of appetite, nausea, yellowing of skin or eyes, change in urine color, abdominal tenderness. • Strict compliance with drug regimen is essential.

belatacept

bel-**at**-a-sept
(Nulojix)

BLACK BOX ALERT Must be administered by personnel trained in administration/handling of therapy at appropriate medical facility. Increased risk of malignancies, tuberculosis, and opportunistic infection. Test for tuberculosis prior to and during treatment, regardless of initial result. Increased risk of posttransplant lymphoproliferative disorder (PTLD), mainly in central nervous system. JC virus-associated progressive multifocal leukoencephalopathy (PML) and polyoma virus nephropathy may lead to graft loss, deteriorated renal function, or death. Pts who are Epstein-Barr virus (EBV) antibody negative are at increased risk of developing PTLD.

Cytomegalovirus and pneumocystitis prophylaxis are recommended after transplantation. Not recommended for hepatic transplants due to increased risk of graft loss, death.

◆CLASSIFICATION

PHARMACOTHERAPEUTIC: Selective T-cell costimulation blocker. **CLINICAL:** Immunosuppressive agent.

ACTION

Inhibits T-lymphocyte proliferation and production of cytokines including interleukin-2 (IL-2), interferon-γ, interleukin-4 (IL-4), TNF-α; a critical pathway in cellular immune response involved in allograft rejection. **Therapeutic Effect:** Prevents renal transplant rejection. Decreases production of antidonor antibodies.

PHARMACOKINETICS

Half-life: 8–10 days.

USES

Prevention of acute organ rejection in pts receiving renal transplants (in combination with basiliximab induction, mycophenolate mofetil, corticosteroids). For use in Epstein-Barr virus (EBV) seropositive renal transplant recipients.

PRECAUTIONS

Contraindications: Transplant pts who are Epstein-Barr virus (EBV) seronegative or unknown sero-status. **Cautions:** History of opportunistic infections: bacterial, mycobacterial, invasive fungal, viral, protozoal, (histoplasmosis, aspergillosis, candidiasis, coccidioidomycosis, listeriosis, HIV, tuberculosis, pneumocystosis). Recent open wounds, ulcerations. Not recommended in liver transplants. Avoid use of live vaccines.

⧖ LIFESPAN CONSIDERATIONS

Pregnancy/Lactation: Unknown if drug crosses placenta or is distributed in breast milk. Must either discontinue breastfeeding or discontinue drug. **Pregnancy Category C. Children:** Safety and efficacy not established. **Elderly:** No age-related precautions noted.

INTERACTIONS

DRUG: May increase concentration/effects of **belimumab, mycophenolate. Pimecrolimus, tacrolimus** (topical) may increase belatacept concentration. **Live vaccines** not recommended. **HERBAL:** **Echinacea** may reduce belatacept effects. **FOOD:** None known. **LAB VALUES:** May increase serum potassium, cholesterol, uric acid, urine protein, glucose. May decrease serum phosphate, potassium, calcium, magnesium, WBC, Hgb, Hct.

AVAILABILITY (Rx)

Lyophilized Powder for Injection: 250 mg per vial.

ADMINISTRATION/HANDLING

◄**ALERT**► Use only silicone-free disposable syringe provided. Using different syringe may produce translucent particles. Must infuse with sterile, nonpyrogenic, low protein-binding filter (pore size 0.2–1.2 μm). Administer with dedicated line only.

IV

Reconstitution • Calculate number of vials needed for injection (solution will equal 25 mg/ml after mixing). • Reconstitute vial with 10.5 ml of suitable diluent (0.9% NaCl, D_5W, or Sterile Water for Injection) using provided syringe, 18- to 20-gauge needle. • Direct stream to glass wall (avoids foaming). • Swirl gently (do not shake). • Discard if opaque particles, discoloration, or foreign particles are present. • Infusion bag must match diluent (0.9% NaCl with 0.9% NaCl, D_5W with D_5W, Sterile Water for Injection with NaCl or D_5W). • To mix infusion bag, withdraw and discard volume equal to the volume of reconstituted solution. • Using same silicone-free disposable syringe, gently inject reconstituted solution into 100- to 250-ml bag (based on concentration). • Final concentration of infusion bag should range from 2 mg/ml to 10 mg/ml. • IV infusion stable for 24 hrs at room temperature.

Rate of Administration • Infuse over 30 min.

Storage • Solution should be clear to slightly opalescent and colorless to slightly yellow. • May refrigerate solution up to 24 hrs. • Discard if reconstituted solution remains at room temperature longer than 24 hrs.

INDICATIONS/ROUTES/DOSAGE

Prophylaxis of Acute Renal Transplant Rejection (in Combination with an Immunosuppressant)

IV: ADULTS, ELDERLY: 10 mg/kg on day 1 (day of transplantation, prior to implantation), day 5, end of wk 2, 4, 8, and 12 after transplantation. 5 mg/kg end of wk 16 and q4wks thereafter. **Dosage Modification:** Infusion is based on actual body weight at the time of transplantation; modify dose for weight changes greater than 10% during treatment. Prescribed dose must be evenly divisible by 12.5 to match closest increment (0, 12.5, 25, 37.5, 50, 62.5, 75, 87.5, 100) in mg. For example, the actual dose for a 64-kg pt is 637.5 mg, not 640 mg.

SIDE EFFECTS

Frequent (45%–20%): Anemia, diarrhea, UTI, peripheral edema, constipation, hypertension, pyrexia, nausea, cough, vomiting, headache. **Occasional (19%–5%):** Abdominal pain, hypotension, arthralgia, hematuria, upper respiratory infection, insomnia, nasopharyngitis, back pain, dyspnea, influenza, dysuria, bronchitis, stomatitis, anxiety, dizziness, abdominal pain, muscle tremor, acne, alopecia, hyperhidrosis.

ADVERSE EFFECTS/ TOXIC REACTIONS

Serious conditions including malignancies (esp. skin cancer), progressive multifocal leukoencephalopathy (caused by

JC virus), cytomegalovirus, polyoma virus nephropathy, viral reactivation (herpes zoster, hepatitis). Other opportunistic infections such as bacterial, fungal, viral, protozoal may cause tuberculosis, cryptococcal meningitis, Chagas' disease, West Nile encephalitis, Guillain-Barré syndrome, cerebral aspergillosis. Additional complications including chronic allograft nephropathy, renal tubular necrosis, renal artery necrosis, atrial fibrillation, hematoma at incision site, wound dehiscence, lymphocele, arteriovenous fistula thrombosis, hydronephrosis, urinary incontinence, anti-belatacept antibody formation have been reported.

NURSING CONSIDERATIONS

BASELINE ASSESSMENT

Evaluate pt for active tuberculosis or latent infection prior to initiating treatment and periodically during therapy. Induration of 5 mm or greater with tuberculin skin test should be considered a positive result when assessing whether treatment for latent tuberculosis is necessary. Assess baseline mental status to compare any worsening cognitive symptoms. Obtain Epstein-Barr virus (EBV) serology prior to treatment (contraindicated in pts who are EBV seronegative). Note any skin discoloration, ulcers, excoriation, lesions. Question history of hypertension/hypotension, arrhythmia, diabetes, HIV, hepatitis, home medications. Question possibility of pregnancy. Obtain baseline CBC, serum chemistries, renal function, glomerular filtration rate (GFR), magnesium, ionized calcium, phosphate, lipid panel, urinalysis, urine pregnancy if applicable.

INTERVENTION/EVALUATION

Monitor B/P, vital signs, I&O, weight. Diligently monitor CBC, renal function, serum electrolytes (hypokalemia may result in changes in muscle strength, muscle cramps, altered mental status, cardiac arrhythmias). Routinely monitor serum glucose levels for new-onset diabetes after transplantation, corticosteroid use. Monitor for fever, tenderness over transplantation site, skin lesions, changing characteristics of moles, neurologic deterioration related to PTLD or PML.

PATIENT/FAMILY TEACHING

• Inform pt that therapy may increase risk of malignancies and life-threatening infections. • Detail concomitant immunosuppressive therapy with basiliximab induction, corticosteroids. • Report history of HIV, opportunistic infections, hepatitis, coughing of blood, or close relatives with active tuberculosis. • Avoid sunlight, sunlamps. • Seek immediate attention if adverse reactions occur. • Do not receive live vaccines. • Notify physician if pregnant or plan on becoming pregnant. • Pt must adhere to strict dosing schedule. • Report any chest pain, palpitations, edema, fever, night sweats, weight loss, swollen glands, flu-like symptoms, stomach pain, vomiting, diarrhea, weakness, or urinary changes (color, frequency, odor, concentration, burning, blood).

belimumab

be-**lim**-oo-mab
(Benlysta)
Do not confuse belimumab with bevacizumab.

◆CLASSIFICATION

PHARMACOTHERAPEUTIC: Monoclonal antibody. **CLINICAL:** Immunosuppressant, Anti-Lupus agent.

ACTION

Inhibits binding of B-lymphocyte stimulator (BLYS) to B-cell receptors. Inhibits survival of B cells, including autoreactive B cells, and reduces differentiation into immunoglobulin-producing plasma cells. **Therapeutic Effect:** Limits lupus erythematosus disease activity.

PHARMACOKINETICS

Half-life: 19 days.

USES

Treatment for active, autoantibody-positive, systemic lupus erythematosus, in addition to standard therapy.

PRECAUTIONS

Contraindications: Prior anaphylaxis with belimumab. **Cautions:** Severe, active infections. Depression, pts at risk for suicide, other mood changes. Avoid live vaccines.

⏳ LIFESPAN CONSIDERATIONS

Pregnancy/Lactation: Not recommended in pregnancy unless benefits outweigh risks. Unknown if crosses placenta or distributed in breast milk. Contraception should be considered during therapy and for at least 4 wks after final treatment. **Pregnancy Category C. Children:** Safety and efficacy not established. **Elderly:** No age-related precautions noted.

INTERACTIONS

DRUG: Abatacept, belatacept, etanercept, pimecrolimus, tacrolimus (topical) may increase concentration. **Cyclophosphamide** not recommended. **HERBAL: Echinacea** may decrease effect. **FOOD:** None known. **LAB VALUES:** May decrease WBC.

AVAILABILITY (Rx)

Lyophilized Powder for Injection: 120 mg, 400 mg.

ADMINISTRATION/HANDLING

Reconstitution • Remove vials from refrigerator and let stand until room temperature (10–15 min). • Reconstitute 120-mg vial with 1.5 ml Sterile Water for Injection or 400-mg vial with 4.8 ml Sterile Water for Injection (both vials will have concentration of 80 mg/ml after reconstitution). • Direct stream toward glass wall to avoid foaming. • Gently swirl for 60 sec every 5 min until fully dissolved (usually 10–30 min). • If me-

chanical reconstitution device used, do not swirl greater than 30 min or exceed 500 rpm. • Small air bubbles expected, acceptable. • Dilute in 250 ml 0.9% NaCl only. • From infusion bag, withdraw and discard volume equal to the volume of reconstituted solution. • Invert bag and gently inject to mix. • Infuse within 8 hrs of reconstitution.
Rate of Administration • Infuse over 1 hr.
Storage • Refrigerate vials/infusion bag until time of use. • Solution should be opalescent and colorless to pale yellow with no particles present. • Discard solution if particulate matter or discoloration observed. • Protect from sunlight.

🚫 IV INCOMPATIBILITIES

Do not infuse with dextrose-based solution. Use dedicated line only.

INDICATIONS/ROUTES/DOSAGE

Active Systemic Lupus Erythematosus
IV: ADULTS: 10 mg/kg at 2-wk intervals for 3 doses, then every 4 wks thereafter.

SIDE EFFECTS

Frequent (15%–12%): Nausea, diarrhea. **Occasional (10%–5%):** Pyrexia, nasopharyngitis, bronchitis, insomnia, extremity pain, depression, migraine, pharyngitis. **Rare (less than 4%):** Cystitis, viral gastroenteritis.

ADVERSE EFFECTS/ TOXIC REACTIONS

May increase risk of mortality. Anti-belimumab antibody formation reported in less than 1%. Hypersensitivity reaction including anaphylactic reaction may include uticaria, pruritus, erythema, dyspnea, angioedema, hypotension (13% of pts). Infusion reactions such as nausea, headaches, flushing occur more frequently. Serious infections related to immunosuppression including respiratory tract infection, pneumonia, nasopharyngitis, sinusitis, influenza, UTI, cellulitis, bronchitis, viral reactivation may occur. Mental health issues including psychiatric events (16%)

♣ Canadian trade name   🚫 Non-Crushable Drug   🔺 High Alert drug

and depression (6%) have been noted. Life-threatening psychiatric events and depression (including suicide) reported in less than 1%. Those who experienced life-threatening episodes had prior psychiatric history.

NURSING CONSIDERATIONS

BASELINE ASSESSMENT

Obtain baseline vital signs, CBC with differential, serum chemistries, IgG level. Assess history of recent immunizations, malignancies, open sores, ulcerations, weight loss, HIV, chronic infection. Assess psychiatric history including insomnia, anxiety, depression, impulsiveness, suicidal ideations, mood changes. Question possibility of pregnancy, current breast-feeding.

INTERVENTION/EVALUATION

Monitor vital signs, CBC. If hypersensitivity reaction occurs, immediately notify physician. Premedication with antihistamines, antipyretics, and/or corticosteroids may prevent subsequent reactions. Discontinue treatment if anaphylactic reaction occurs; initiate appropriate medical treatment. Routinely inspect skin, paying close attention to areas that are discolored, irregular, or have ill-defined borders (may indicate malignancies). Obtain anti-belimumab antibody titer if immunogenicity suspected. Consider interrupting therapy if acute infection occurs.

PATIENT/FAMILY TEACHING

• Report any signs of hypersensitivity reaction (see Adverse Effects/Toxic Reactions). • If anaphylactic reaction occurs, pt may require rapid sequence intubation. • Hypersensitivity reactions include itching, hives, dizziness, or difficulty breathing. • Notify physician if pregnant or plan on becoming pregnant. • Contraception recommended during treatment and at least 4 mos after treatment. • Report suicidal ideation, mood changes, or worsening depression. • Do not receive live vaccines 30 days before

or during treatment. • Report any fever, cough, night sweats, flu-like symptoms, skin changes, or painful/burning urination.

benazepril   TOP 200

ben-**ay**-ze-pril
(<u>Lotensin</u>)

BLACK BOX ALERT May cause fetal injury, mortality if used during second or third trimester of pregnancy. **Do not confuse benazepril with Benadryl, or Lotensin with Lioresal.**

FIXED-COMBINATION(S)

Lotensin HCT: benazepril/hydrochlorothiazide (a diuretic): 5 mg/625 mg, 10 mg/12.5 mg, 20 mg/12.5 mg, 20 mg/25 mg. **Lotrel:** benazepril/amlodipine (a calcium blocker): 2.5 mg/10 mg, 5 mg/10 mg, 5 mg/20 mg, 5 mg/40 mg, 10 mg/20 mg, 10 mg/40 mg.

◆CLASSIFICATION

PHARMACOTHERAPEUTIC: Angiotensin-converting enzyme (ACE) inhibitor. **CLINICAL:** Antihypertensive (see p. 9C, 60C).

ACTION

Decreases rate of conversion of angiotensin I to angiotensin II, a potent vasoconstrictor. Reduces peripheral arterial resistance. **Therapeutic Effect:** Lowers B/P.

PHARMACOKINETICS

Route	Onset	Peak	Duration
PO	1 hr	2–4 hrs	24 hrs

Partially absorbed from GI tract. Protein binding: 97%. Metabolized in liver to active metabolite. Primarily excreted in urine. Minimal removal by hemodialysis. **Half-life:** 35 min; metabolite, 10–11 hrs.

USES

Treatment of hypertension. Used alone or in combination with other antihypertensives.

PRECAUTIONS

Contraindications: History of angioedema with or without previous treatment with ACE inhibitors. **Cautions:** Renal impairment; hypertophic cardiomyopathy without flow tract obstruction; severe aortic stenosis; before, during, or immediately following major surgery; unstented renal artery stenosis; diabetes mellitus.

⌛ LIFESPAN CONSIDERATIONS

Pregnancy/Lactation: Crosses placenta. Unknown if distributed in breast milk. May cause fetal, neonatal mortality or morbidity. **Pregnancy Category D. Children:** Safety and efficacy not established. **Elderly:** May be more sensitive to hypotensive effects.

INTERACTIONS

DRUG: Diuretics, hypotensive agents may increase effects. **NSAIDs, sympathomimetics** may decrease effect. **Potassium-sparing diuretics, potassium supplements** may cause hyperkalemia. May increase **cyclosporine, lithium** concentration/effect. **HERBAL: Ephedra, ginseng, licorice** may worsen hypertension. **Black cohosh, periwinkle** may have increased antihypertensive effect. **FOOD:** None known. **LAB VALUES:** May increase serum potassium, AST, ALT, alkaline phosphatase, bilirubin, BUN, creatinine, glucose. May decrease serum sodium, Hgb, Hct. May cause positive ANA titer.

AVAILABILITY (Rx)

Tablets: 5 mg, 10 mg, 20 mg, 40 mg.

ADMINISTRATION/HANDLING

• Give without regard to food.

INDICATIONS/ROUTES/DOSAGE

Hypertension (Monotherapy)
PO: ADULTS: Initially, 10 mg/day. Maintenance: 20–40 mg/day as single dose or in 2 divided doses. **Maximum:** 80 mg/day. **ELDERLY:** Initially, 5–10 mg/day. Range: 20–40 mg/day.

Hypertension (Combination Therapy)
PO: ADULTS: Discontinue diuretic 2–3 days prior to initiating benazepril, then dose as noted above. If unable to discontinue diuretic, begin benazepril at 5 mg/day.

Usual Pediatric Dosage
PO: CHILDREN 6 YRS AND OLDER: Initially, 0.2 mg/kg/day (up to 10 mg/day). Range: 0.1–0.6 mg/kg/day. **Maximum:** 40 mg/day.

Dosage in Renal Impairment
For adult pts with creatinine clearance less than 30 ml/min: Initially, 5 mg/day titrated up to maximum of 40 mg/day. **HD:** Give dose post-HD or administer 25–35% supplemental dose.

SIDE EFFECTS

Frequent (6%–3%): Cough, headache, dizziness. **Occasional (2%):** Fatigue, drowsiness, nausea. **Rare (less than 1%):** Rash, fever, myalgia, diarrhea, loss of taste.

ADVERSE EFFECTS/ TOXIC REACTIONS

Excessive hypotension ("first-dose syncope") may occur in those with CHF, severe salt or volume depletion. Angioedema (swelling of face, lips, tongue), hyperkalemia occur rarely. Agranulocytosis, neutropenia may be noted in those with renal impairment, collagen vascular disease (scleroderma, systemic lupus erythematosus). Nephrotic syndrome may be noted in pts with history of renal disease.

NURSING CONSIDERATIONS

BASELINE ASSESSMENT

Obtain B/P immediately before each dose, in addition to regular monitoring (be alert to fluctuations). If excessive reduction in B/P occurs, place pt in supine position with legs elevated. Pts with renal impairment, autoimmune disease, or taking

B

drugs that affect leukocytes or immune response. Obtain CBC before therapy begins and q2wks for 3 mos, then periodically thereafter.

INTERVENTION/EVALUATION

Assist with ambulation if dizziness occurs. Monitor B/P, renal function, urinary protein, serum potassium. Monitor CBC with differential if pt has collagen vascular disease or renal impairment.

PATIENT/FAMILY TEACHING

• To reduce hypotensive effect, rise slowly from lying to sitting position, permit legs to dangle from bed momentarily before standing. • Full therapeutic effect may take 2–4 wks. • Skipping doses or noncompliance with drug therapy may produce severe, rebound hypertension. • Report light-headedness, dizziness, persistent cough.

bendamustine

ben-da-**mus**-teen
(Treanda)
Do not confuse bendamustine with carmustine or lomustine.

◆CLASSIFICATION

PHARMACOTHERAPEUTIC: Alkylating agent. **CLINICAL:** Antineoplastic (see p. 82C).

ACTION

Alkylates and cross-links macromolecules, resulting in DNA, RNA, and protein synthesis inhibition. **Therapeutic Effect:** Inhibits tumor cell growth, causes cell death.

PHARMACOKINETICS

Metabolized via hydrolysis to metabolites. Protein binding: 64%–95%. Eliminated primarily in feces. **Half-life:** 40 min.

USES

Treatment of chronic lymphocytic leukemia (CLL). Treatment of indolent B-cell non-Hodgkin's lymphoma (NHL) that has progressed during or within 6 mos of treatment with rituximab or a rituximab-containing regimen. **OFF-LABEL:** Treatment of mantle cell lymphoma, relapsed multiple myeloma. First-line treatment for follicular lymphoma. Treatment of Waldenström's macroglobulinemia.

PRECAUTIONS

Contraindications: Known hypersensitivity to bendamustine or mannitol. **Cautions:** Myelosuppression (may increase risk of infection), renal/hepatic impairment, dehydration, HF.

⏳ LIFESPAN CONSIDERATIONS

Pregnancy/Lactation: May cause fetal harm. Unknown if distributed in breast milk. **Pregnancy Category D.** Impaired spermatogenesis, azoospermia have been reported in male pts. **Children:** Safety and efficacy not established. **Elderly:** No age-related precautions noted.

INTERACTIONS

Ciprofloxacin, fluvoxamine may increase bendamustine concentration, decrease plasma concentrations of active metabolites. **CYP1A2 inducers (e.g., omeprazole), nicotine** may decrease concentration. **HERBAL:** None known. **FOOD:** None known. **LAB VALUES:** May increase serum AST, bilirubin, creatinine, glucose, uric acid. May decrease WBCs, neutrophils, Hgb, platelets, serum potassium, sodium, calcium.

AVAILABILITY (Rx)

Injection, Powder for Reconstitution: 25 mg, 100 mg.

ADMINISTRATION/HANDLING
 IV

Reconstitution • Reconstitute each 100-mg vial with 20 ml Sterile Water for Injection (25-mg vial with 5 ml) for a concentration of 5 mg/ml. • Powder should completely dissolve in 5 min. • Discard if particulate matter is observed. • Withdraw volume needed for required dose (based on 5 mg/ml concentration) and immediately transfer to 500-ml infusion bag of 0.9% NaCl for final concentration of 0.2–0.6 mg/ml. • Reconstituted solution must be transferred to infusion bag within 30 min of reconstitution. • After transferring, thoroughly mix contents of infusion bag.

Rate of Administration • Infuse over 30 min for CLL and 60 min for NHL.

Storage • Reconstituted solution appears clear and colorless to pale yellow. • Final solution is stable for 24 hrs if refrigerated or 3 hrs at room temperature. • Administration must be completed within these stability time frames.

INDICATIONS/ROUTES/DOSAGE

◄ **ALERT** ► During first few wks of treatment, allopurinol should be given as a preventive measure in those at risk for tumor lysis syndrome.

Chronic Lymphocytic Leukemia
IV Infusion: ADULTS/ELDERLY: 100 mg/m^2 given over 30 min daily on days 1 and 2 of a 28-day cycle, up to 6 cycles.

Non-Hodgkin's Lymphoma
IV Infusion: ADULTS/ELDERLY: 120 mg/m^2 on days 1 and 2 of a 21-day cycle, up to 8 cycles.

SIDE EFFECTS

Frequent (24%–16%): Fever, nausea, vomiting. **Occasional (9%–8%):** Diarrhea, fatigue, asthenia (loss of strength, energy), rash, decreased weight, nasopharyngitis. **Rare (6%–3%):** Chills, pruritus, cough, herpes simplex infections.

ADVERSE EFFECTS/ TOXIC REACTIONS

Myelosuppression characterized as neutropenia (75%), thrombocytopenia (77%), anemia (89%), leukopenia (61%). Infection, including pneumonia, sepsis may occur. Tumor lysis syndrome may lead to acute renal failure. Worsening hypertension occurs rarely.

NURSING CONSIDERATIONS

BASELINE ASSESSMENT

Question for possibility of pregnancy. Offer emotional support. Obtain baseline CBC, serum chemistries including hepatic function tests (bilirubin, ALT, AST, alkaline phosphatase) before treatment begins and routinely thereafter.

INTERVENTION/EVALUATION

Offer antiemetics to control nausea, vomiting. Monitor daily pattern of bowel activity, stool consistency. Assess skin for evidence of rash. Monitor for signs of infection (fever, chills, cough, flu-like symptoms). Monitor for hypertension. Hematologic nadirs occur in 3rd week of therapy and may require dose delays if recovery to recommended values has not occurred by day 28.

PATIENT/FAMILY TEACHING

• Avoid crowds, those with known infection. • Avoid contact with anyone who recently received live virus vaccine. • Do not have immunizations without physician's approval (drug lowers body resistance). • Promptly report fever, chills, flu-like symptoms, sore throat, unusual bruising/bleeding from any site. • Male pts should be warned of potential risk to their reproductive capacities.

benzonatate

ben-**zoe**-na-tate
(Tessalon Perles, Zonatuss)
Do not confuse benzonatate with benazepril, benzocaine, benztropine, or Tessalon with Tussionex.

◆ CLASSIFICATION

PHARMACOTHERAPEUTIC: Non-narcotic antitussive. **CLINICAL:** Cough suppressant.

ACTION

Anesthetizes stretch or cough receptors in alveoli of lungs, bronchi, and pleura, suppressing the cough reflex. **Therapeutic Effect:** Reduces cough production.

PHARMACOKINETICS

Route	Onset	Peak	Duration
PO	15–20 min	—	3–8 hrs

Metabolized in liver. Primarily excreted in urine. **Half-life:** Unknown.

USES

Relief of nonproductive cough, including acute cough of minor throat/bronchial irritation.

PRECAUTIONS

Contraindications: Allergy to topical anesthetic medicines (tetracaine, procaine). **Cautions:** Productive cough.

⌛ LIFESPAN CONSIDERATIONS

Pregnancy/Lactation: Unknown if drug crosses placenta or is distributed in breast milk. **Pregnancy Category C. Children:** Safety and efficacy not established in those younger than 10 yrs. **Elderly:** No age-related precautions noted.

INTERACTIONS

DRUG: CNS depressants may increase effect. **HERBAL:** None significant. **FOOD:** None known. **LAB VALUES:** None significant.

AVAILABILITY (Rx)

Capsules, Liquid Filled (Tessalon Perles): 100 mg, 200 mg. **Capsules (Zonatuss):** 150 mg.

ADMINISTRATION/HANDLING

PO

• Give without regard to meals. • Administer whole; do not break, chew, crush, or allow pt to dissolve in mouth (may produce temporary local anesthesia of oral mucosa). • Give with full glass of water.

INDICATIONS/ROUTES/DOSAGE

Antitussive
PO *(Tessalon Perles)*: ADULTS, ELDERLY, CHILDREN OLDER THAN 10 YRS: 100–200 mg 3 times a day, or every 4 hrs up to 600 mg/day. *(Zouatuss):* 150 mg 3 times a day. **Maximum:** 600 mg/day.

SIDE EFFECTS

Occasional (10%–5%): Mild drowsiness, mild dizziness, constipation, nausea, skin eruptions, nasal congestion.

ADVERSE EFFECTS/TOXIC REACTIONS

Paradoxical reaction (restlessness, insomnia, euphoria, nervousness, tremors) has been noted. Chest pain or numbness, choking feeling, sense of faintness, confusion, hallucinations may result from chewing or sucking on capsule.

NURSING CONSIDERATIONS

BASELINE ASSESSMENT

Assess type, severity, frequency of cough. Monitor amount, color, consistency of sputum.

INTERVENTION/EVALUATION

Initiate deep breathing and coughing exercises, particularly in pts with impaired pulmonary function. Monitor for paradoxical reaction. Increase fluid intake and environmental humidity to lower viscosity of lung secretions. Assess for clinical improvement and record onset of cough relief.

PATIENT/FAMILY TEACHING

• Avoid tasks that require alertness, motor skills until response to drug is established. • Dry mouth, drowsiness, dizziness may be expected responses to drug. • Sucking or chewing on capsule may cause numbness of mouth or throat.

benztropine

benz-**trow**-peen
(Apo-Benztropine ✤, Cogentin)

Do not confuse benztropine with bromocriptine or benzonatate.

◆CLASSIFICATION

PHARMACOTHERAPEUTIC: Anticholinergic. **CLINICAL:** Antiparkinson agent.

ACTION

Selectively blocks central cholinergic receptors, assists in balancing cholinergic/dopaminergic activity. **Therapeutic Effect:** Reduces incidence/severity of akinesia, rigidity, tremor.

PHARMACOKINETICS

Well absorbed following PO and IM administration. Metabolized in liver. PO onset of action: 1–2 hrs, IM onset of action: minutes. Pharmacologic effects may not be apparent until 2–3 days after initiation of therapy and may persist for up to 24 hrs after discontinuation of drug. **Half-life:** Extended (no specific determination).

USES

Treatment of Parkinson's disease, drug-induced extrapyramidal reactions (except tardive dyskinesia).

PRECAUTIONS

Contraindications: Stenosing peptic ulcer, children younger than 3 yrs, pyloric or duodenal obstruction, myasthenia gravis, bladder neck obstruction, esophageal achalasia. **Cautions:** Glaucoma, heart disease, hypertension, hypotension; pts with tachycardia, arrhythmias, prostatic hypertrophy, hepatic/renal impairment, obstructive diseases of GI/GU tract, urinary retention.

⧖ LIFESPAN CONSIDERATIONS

Pregnancy/Lactation: Unknown if drug crosses placenta or is distributed in breast milk. **Pregnancy Category C. Children:** Safety and efficacy not established in pts younger than 3 yrs. **Elderly:** Increased risk for adverse reactions.

INTERACTIONS

DRUG: Alcohol, CNS depressants may increase sedation. May increase effects of **anticholinergics. HERBAL:** None significant. **FOOD:** None known. **LAB VALUES:** None significant.

AVAILABILITY (Rx)

Injection, Solution: 1 mg/ml. **Tablets:** 0.5 mg, 1 mg, 2 mg.

ADMINISTRATION/HANDLING

IM
• Inject slow, deep IM.

PO
• Give without regard to food. • Give with food if GI upset occurs.

INDICATIONS/ROUTES/DOSAGE

Parkinsonism
PO: ADULTS: 0.5–6 mg/day as a single dose or in 2 divided doses (usual dose: 1–2 mg/day). Titrate by 0.5 mg at 5–6 day intervals. **ELDERLY:** Initially, 0.5 mg once or twice a day. Titrate by 0.5 mg at 5–6 day intervals. **Maximum:** 4 mg/day.

Drug-Induced Extrapyramidal Symptoms
PO, IM, IV: ADULTS: 1–4 mg once or twice a day or 1–2 mg 2–3 times/day. **CHILDREN OLDER THAN 3 YRS:** 0.02–0.05 mg/kg/dose once or twice a day.

Acute Dystonic Reactions
IV, IM: ADULTS: Initially, 1–2 mg as a single dose.

SIDE EFFECTS

Frequent: Drowsiness, dry mouth, blurred vision, constipation, urinary retention, GI upset, photosensitivity. **Occasional:** Headache, memory loss, muscle cramps, anxiety, peripheral paresthesia, orthostatic hypotension, abdominal cramps. **Rare:** Rash, confusion, eye pain.

ADVERSE EFFECTS/ TOXIC REACTIONS

Overdose may produce severe anticholinergic effects (unsteadiness, drowsiness, tachycardia, paralytic ileus, malignant hyperthermia, urinary retention, dyspnea, skin flushing, dryness of mouth/nose/throat). Severe paradoxical reactions (hallucinations, tremor, seizures, toxic psychosis) may occur.

NURSING CONSIDERATIONS

BASELINE ASSESSMENT

Assess mental status for confusion, disorientation, agitation, psychotic-like symptoms (medication frequently produces such side effects in those older than 60 yrs). Note severity of baseline rigidity, tremors.

INTERVENTION/EVALUATION

Be alert to neurologic effects: headache, drowsiness, mental confusion, agitation. Assess for clinical reversal of symptoms (improvement of tremor of head and hands at rest, mask-like facial expression, shuffling gait, muscular rigidity). Monitor daily pattern of bowel activity, stool consistency, esp. constipation. Monitor I/O. Assess for urinary retention.

PATIENT/FAMILY TEACHING

• Avoid tasks that require alertness, motor skills until response to drug is established. • Dry mouth, drowsiness, dizziness may be an expected response to drug. • Drowsiness tends to diminish or disappear with continued therapy. • Avoid alcohol. • Report sudden muscle weakness or stiffness.

---

beractant

ber-**ak**-tant
(Survanta)
Do not confuse Survanta with Sufenta.

◆CLASSIFICATION

PHARMACOTHERAPEUTIC: Natural bovine lung extract. **CLINICAL:** Pulmonary surfactant.

ACTION

Lowers alveolar surface tension during respiration, stabilizing alveoli. **Therapeutic Effect:** Improves lung compliance, respiratory gas exchange.

PHARMACOKINETICS

Not absorbed systemically.

USES

Prevention and treatment (rescue therapy) of respiratory distress syndrome (RDS—hyaline membrane disease) in premature infants. **Prevention:** Body weight less than 1,250 g in infants at risk for developing or with evidence of surfactant deficiency (give within 15 min of birth). **Rescue Therapy:** Treatment of infants with RDS confirmed by X-ray, requiring mechanical ventilation (give within 8 hrs of birth).

PRECAUTIONS

Contraindications: None known. **Cautions:** Those at risk for circulatory overload. This drug is for use only in neonates. **Pregnancy Category:** Not indicated for use in pregnant women.

INTERACTIONS

DRUG: None significant. **HERBAL:** None significant. **FOOD:** None known. **LAB VALUES:** None significant.

AVAILABILITY (Rx)

Suspension, Intratracheal: 25 mg/ml (4 ml, 8 ml).

ADMINISTRATION/HANDLING

Intratracheal
Rate of Administration • Instill through catheter inserted into infant's endotracheal tube. Do not instill into main-stem bronchus. • Administer dose in 4-ml/kg aliquots over 2–3 sec with infant in different positions. • Monitor for bradycardia, decreased O_2 saturation during administration. Stop dosing procedure if these effects occur; begin appropriate measures before reinstituting therapy.

Storage • Refrigerate vials. • Warm by standing vial at room temperature for 20 min or warm in hand 8 min. • If settling occurs, gently swirl vial (do not shake) to redisperse. • After warming, may return to refrigerator within 8 hrs one time only. • Each vial should be injected through needle only one time; discard unused portions. • Color appears off-white to light brown.

INDICATIONS/ROUTES/DOSAGE

Prevention and Treatment (Rescue Therapy) of RDS or Hyaline Membrane Disease in Premature Infants
Intratracheal: INFANTS: 100 mg of phospholipids/kg birth weight (4 ml/kg). Give within 15 min of birth if infant weighs less than 1,250 g and has evidence of surfactant deficiency; give within 8 hrs when RDS is confirmed by X-ray and pt requires mechanical ventilation. May repeat in 6 hrs or longer after preceding dose. **Maximum:** 4 doses in the first 48 hrs of life.

SIDE EFFECTS

Frequent: Transient bradycardia, oxygen (O_2) desaturation, carbon dioxide (CO_2) retention. **Occasional:** Endotracheal tube reflux. **Rare:** Apnea, endotracheal tube blockage, hypotension or hypertension, pallor, vasoconstriction.

ADVERSE EFFECTS/ TOXIC REACTIONS

Life-threatening nosocomial sepsis may occur.

NURSING CONSIDERATIONS

BASELINE ASSESSMENT

Drug must be administered in highly supervised setting. Clinicians caring for neonate must be experienced with intubation, ventilator management. Offer emotional support to parents.

INTERVENTION/EVALUATION

Monitor infant with arterial or transcutaneous measurement of systemic O_2, CO_2. Assess for adventitious breath sounds (rales, rhonchi).

betamethasone

bay-ta-**meth**-a-sone
(Betaderm ✤, Betaject ✤, Betnesol ✤, Betnovate ✤, Celestone, Celestone Soluspan, Diprolene, Diprolene AF, Ectosone ✤, Luxiq)
Do not confuse betamethasone with dexamethasone or Luxiq with Lasix.

FIXED-COMBINATION(S)

Lotrisone: betamethasone/clotrimazole (an antifungal): 0.05%/1%. **Taclonex:** betamethasone/calcipotriene (an antipsoriatic): 0.064%/0.005%.

◆CLASSIFICATION

PHARMACOTHERAPEUTIC: Adrenocorticosteroid. **CLINICAL:** Anti-inflammatory, immunosuppressant (see pp. 99C, 101C, 102C).

ACTION

Controls rate of protein synthesis, depresses migration of polymorphonuclear leukocytes/fibroblasts, reverses capillary permeability, prevents or controls inflammation. **Therapeutic Effect:** Decreases tissue response to inflammatory process.

PHARMACOKINETICS

Rapidly absorbed following PO administration. Protein binding: 64%. After topical application, limited absorption systemically. Metabolized in liver. Excreted in urine. **Half-life:** 6.5 hrs.

USES

Systemic: Anti-inflammatory, immunosuppressant, or corticosteroid replacement therapy. **Topical:** Relief of inflammatory and pruritic dermatoses. **Foam:** Relief of inflammation, itching associated with dermatosis. **OFF-LABEL:** Accelerate fetal lung maturation in pts with preterm labor.

✤ Canadian trade name   🦌 Non-Crushable Drug   HIGH ALERT High Alert drug

PRECAUTIONS

Contraindications: Systemic fungal infections; IM administration in idiopathic thrombocytopenia purpura. **Cautions:** Hypothyroidism, hepatic/renal impairment, cardiovascular disease, diabetes, glaucoma, cataracts, myasthenia gravis, pts at risk for osteoporosis/seizures/GI disease, following acute MI, elderly.

⧗ LIFESPAN CONSIDERATIONS

Pregnancy/Lactation: Crosses placenta, distributed in breast milk. **Pregnancy Category C (D if used in first trimester).** **Children:** Prolonged treatment, high-dose therapy may decrease short-term growth rate, cortisol secretion. **Elderly:** Higher risk for developing hypertension, osteoporosis.

INTERACTIONS

DRUG: Amphotericin may increase risk of hypokalemia. May decrease effect of **insulin, oral hypoglycemics, potassium supplements.** May increase **digoxin** toxicity (due to hypokalemia). **Hepatic enzyme inducers** may decrease effect. **Live virus vaccines** may potentiate virus replication, increase vaccine side effects, decrease pt's antibody response to vaccine. **HERBAL: Cat's claw, echinacea** possess immunostimulant effects. **FOOD:** None known. **LAB VALUES:** May decrease serum calcium, potassium, thyroxine. May increase serum cholesterol, lipids, glucose, sodium, amylase.

AVAILABILITY (Rx)

Cream (Diprolene AF): 0.05%. **Foam (Luxiq):** 0.12%. **Gel:** 0.05%. **Injection, Suspension (Celestone Soluspan):** 3 mg/ml. **Lotion (Diprolene):** 0.05%. **Ointment:** 0.05%, 0.1%. **Solution, Oral:** 0.6 mg/5 ml.

ADMINISTRATION/HANDLING

IM
• Inject slowly, deep IM into large muscle mass.

PO
• Give with milk or food (decreases GI upset). • Give single doses in the morning; give multiple doses at evenly spaced intervals.

Topical
• Gently cleanse area before application. • Apply sparingly and rub into area thoroughly. • Do not apply to face, groin, axillae, or inguinal areas. Not for use on broken skin, areas of infection, or in diaper area. • Do not dispense foam directly into hands; use fingers to apply small amounts.

INDICATIONS/ROUTES/DOSAGE

Anti-Inflammation, Immunosuppression, Corticosteroid Replacement Therapy
PO: ADULTS, ELDERLY: 0.6–7.2 mg/day. **CHILDREN:** 0.0175–0.25 mg/kg/day in 3–4 divided doses.
IM: ADULTS, ELDERLY: 0.6–9 mg/day in 2 divided doses. **CHILDREN:** 0.0175–0.125 mg/kg/day in 3–4 divided doses.

Relief of Inflamed and Pruritic Dermatoses
Topical: ADULTS, ELDERLY: 1–3 times a day. **Foam:** Apply twice a day (morning and night).

SIDE EFFECTS

Frequent: Systemic: Increased appetite, abdominal distention, nervousness, insomnia, false sense of well-being. **Topical:** Burning, stinging, pruritus. **Occasional: Systemic:** Dizziness, facial flushing, diaphoresis, decreased or blurred vision, mood swings. **Topical:** Allergic contact dermatitis, purpura or blood-containing blisters, thinning of skin with easy bruising, telangiectases, raised dark red spots on skin, angiomas.

ADVERSE EFFECTS/ TOXIC REACTIONS

Overdose may cause systemic hypercorticism, adrenal suppression.

NURSING CONSIDERATIONS

BASELINE ASSESSMENT

Question for hypersensitivity to any corticosteroid, sulfite. Obtain baseline values for height, weight, B/P, serum glucose, electrolytes. Obtain baseline results of initial tests (tuberculosis [TB] skin test, X-rays, EKG).

INTERVENTION/EVALUATION

Monitor B/P, blood glucose, electrolytes. Apply topical preparation sparingly. Do not use on broken skin or in areas of infection. Do not apply to wet skin, face, inguinal areas.

PATIENT/FAMILY TEACHING

• Take with food, milk. • Take single daily dose in the morning. • Do not stop abruptly. • Apply topical preparations in a thin layer. • Do not receive smallpox vaccination during or immediately after therapy.

---

bethanechol

be-**than**-e-kole
(Duvoid ✦, Urecholine)
Do not confuse bethanechol with betaxolol.

✦CLASSIFICATION

PHARMACOTHERAPEUTIC: Parasympathomimetic choline ester. **CLINICAL:** Cholinergic.

ACTION

Acts directly at cholinergic receptors in smooth muscle of urinary bladder, GI tract. Increases detrusor muscle tone. **Therapeutic Effect:** May initiate urination, bladder emptying. Stimulates gastric, intestinal motility.

PHARMACOKINETICS

Route	Onset	Peak	Duration
PO	30–90 min	60 min	6 hrs

Poorly absorbed following PO administration. Does not cross blood-brain barrier. **Half-life:** Unknown.

USES

Treatment of acute postoperative and postpartum nonobstructive urinary retention, retention due to neurogenic bladder. **OFF-LABEL:** Treatment of gastroesophageal reflux.

PRECAUTIONS

Contraindications: Mechanical obstruction of GI/GU tract. GI or bladder wall instability, hyperthyroidism, epilepsy, bronchial asthma, coronary artery disease, hypotension, parkinsonism, peptic ulcer, pronounced bradycardia, vasomotor instability. **Cautions:** None known.

⧖ LIFESPAN CONSIDERATIONS

Pregnancy/Lactation: Unknown if drug crosses placenta or is distributed in breast milk. **Pregnancy Category C. Children/Elderly:** No age-related precautions noted.

INTERACTIONS

DRUG: Beta-blockers, anticholinesterase inhibitors may increase effects/toxicity. **HERBAL:** None significant. **FOOD:** None known. **LAB VALUES:** May increase serum amylase, lipase, AST, ALT.

AVAILABILITY (Rx)

Tablets: 5 mg, 10 mg, 25 mg, 50 mg.

ADMINISTRATION/HANDLING

PO

• Administer 1 hr before or 2 hrs after meals.

INDICATIONS/ROUTES/DOSAGE

Nonobstructive Urinary Retention, Atony of Bladder
PO: ADULTS, ELDERLY: 10–50 mg 3–4 times a day. Minimum effective dose determined by giving 5–10 mg initially, repeating same amount at 1-hr intervals until desired response is achieved. **CHILDREN:** 0.3–0.6 mg/kg/day in 3–4 divided doses.

✦ Canadian trade name   🐄 Non-Crushable Drug   🔺 High Alert drug

SIDE EFFECTS

Occasional: Belching, changes in vision, blurred vision, diarrhea, urinary urgency or frequency. **Rare:** Shortness of breath, chest tightness, bronchospasm.

ADVERSE EFFECTS/ TOXIC REACTIONS

Overdose produces CNS stimulation (insomnia, anxiety, orthostatic hypotension), cholinergic stimulation (headache, increased salivation/diaphoresis, nausea, vomiting, flushed skin, abdominal pain, seizures).

NURSING CONSIDERATIONS

BASELINE ASSESSMENT

Ensure pt has emptied bladder prior to procedure.

INTERVENTION/EVALUATION

Monitor urine output. Palpate bladder for evidence of urinary retention.

PATIENT/FAMILY TEACHING

• Report nausea, vomiting, diarrhea, diaphoresis, increased salivary secretions, irregular heartbeat, muscle weakness, severe abdominal pain, difficulty breathing.

---

bevacizumab   TOP 200 HIGH ALERT

be-va-**siz**-ue-mab
(Avastin)

 BLACK BOX ALERT May result in development of GI perforation, presented as intra-abdominal abscess, fistula, wound dehiscence, wound healing complications. Severe, sometimes fatal, hemorrhagic events including central nervous system/GI/vaginal bleeding, epistaxis, hemoptysis, pulmonary hemorrhage has occurred.

Do not confuse Avastin with Astelin, or bevacizumab with cetuximab or rituximab.

◆CLASSIFICATION

PHARMACOTHERAPEUTIC: Monoclonal antibody. **CLINICAL:** Antineoplastic (see p. 82C).

ACTION

Binds to and inhibits vascular endothelial growth factor, a protein that plays a major role in formation of new blood vessels to tumors. **Therapeutic Effect:** Inhibits metastatic disease progression.

PHARMACOKINETICS

Clearance varies by body weight, gender, tumor burden. **Half-life:** 20 days (range: 11–50 days).

USES

Combination chemotherapy with 5-fluorouracil (5-FU) for treatment of pts with colorectal cancer. Treatment with carboplatin and paclitaxel for nonsquamous, non–small-cell lung cancer (NSCLC). Treatment of renal cell carcinoma (metastatic) with interferon alfa, brain cancer (glioblastoma) that has progressed following prior therapy. **OFF-LABEL:** Adjunctive therapy in malignant mesothelioma, ovarian cancer, prostate cancer, age-related macular degeneration. Treatment of metastatic breast cancer.

PRECAUTIONS

Contraindications: None known. **Cautions:** Cardiovascular disease, acquired coagulopathy, preexisting hypertension, pts at risk of thrombocytopenia. Pts with CNS metastasis. Do not administer within 28 days of major surgery or active bleeding.

⧖ LIFESPAN CONSIDERATIONS

Pregnancy/Lactation: Teratogenic. Potential for fertility impairment. May decrease maternal and fetal body weight; increase risk of skeletal fetal abnormalities. Breast-feeding not recommended. **Pregnancy Category C. Children:** Safety and efficacy not established. **Elderly:** Higher incidence of severe adverse reactions in those older than 65 yrs.

INTERACTIONS

DRUG: Sunitinib may increase concentration/effectiveness. May increase levels of **clozapine, sorafenib, sunitinib.** **HERBAL:** None significant. **FOOD:** None known. **LAB VALUES:** May decrease serum potassium, sodium, WBC count, Hgb, Hct, platelet count. May increase urine protein.

AVAILABILITY (Rx)

Injection, Solution: 25-mg/ml vial.

ADMINISTRATION/HANDLING

IV

◄ALERT► Do not give by IV push or bolus.

Reconstitution • Dilute prescribed dose in 100 ml 0.9% NaCl. • Avoid dextrose-containing solutions. • Discard any unused portion.

Rate of Administration • Usually given following other chemotherapy. Infuse initial dose over 90 min. • If first infusion is well tolerated, second infusion may be administered over 60 min. • If 60-min infusion is well tolerated, all subsequent infusions may be administered over 30 min.

Storage • Refrigerate vials. • Diluted solution may be stored for up to 8 hrs if refrigerated.

IV INCOMPATIBILITIES

Do not mix with dextrose solutions.

INDICATIONS/ROUTES/DOSAGE

Colorectal Cancer
IV: **ADULTS, ELDERLY:** 5–10 mg/kg once every 14 days (with fluorouracil-based chemotherapy).

Non–Small-Cell Lung Cancer (NSCLC)
IV: **ADULTS, ELDERLY:** 15 mg/kg every 3 wks (in combination with carboplatin and paclitaxel).

Metastatic Renal Cell Carcinoma
IV: **ADULTS, ELDERLY:** 10 mg/kg once every 2 wks (with interferon alfa).

Brain Cancer
IV: **ADULTS, ELDERLY:** 10 mg/kg every 2 wks (as monotherapy).

Dose Adjustment for Toxicity
Temporary suspension: Mild to moderate proteinuria, severe hypertension not controlled with medical management. **Permanent discontinuation:** Wound dehiscence requiring intervention, GI perforation, hypertensive crises, serious bleeding, nephrotic syndrome.

SIDE EFFECTS

Frequent (73%–25%): Asthenia (loss of strength, energy), vomiting, anorexia, hypertension, epistaxis, stomatitis, constipation, headache, dyspnea. **Occasional (21%–15%):** Altered taste, dry skin, exfoliative dermatitis, dizziness, flatulence, excessive lacrimation, skin discoloration, weight loss, myalgia. **Rare (8%–6%):** Nail disorder, skin ulcer, alopecia, confusion, abnormal gait, dry mouth.

ADVERSE EFFECTS/ TOXIC REACTIONS

UTI, manifested as urinary frequency/urgency, proteinuria, occurs frequently. Most serious adverse effects include CHF, deep vein thrombosis, GI perforation, wound dehiscence, hypertensive crisis, nephrotic syndrome, severe hemorrhage. Anemia, neutropenia, thrombocytopenia occur occasionally. Hypersensitivity reactions occur rarely. May increase risk of tracheoesophageal fistula development.

NURSING CONSIDERATIONS

BASELINE ASSESSMENT

Assess for proteinuria with urinalysis. For those with 2+ or greater urine dipstick reading, a 24-hr urine collection is advised. Obtain baseline CBC, serum potassium, sodium levels and at regular intervals during therapy.

INTERVENTION/EVALUATION

Monitor B/P regularly for hypertension. Assess for asthenia (loss of strength, energy). Assist with ambulation if asthenia occurs. Monitor for fever, chills, abdominal pain, epistaxis. Offer antiemetic if nausea, vomiting occurs. Monitor daily pattern of bowel activity, stool consistency.

PATIENT/FAMILY TEACHING

• Report abdominal pain, vomiting, constipation, headache. • Do not receive immunizations without physician's approval (lowers body's resistance). • Avoid contact with anyone who recently received a live virus vaccine. • Avoid crowds, those with infection. • Female pts should take measures to avoid pregnancy during treatment.

---

bexarotene   HIGH ALERT

beks-**ar**-oh-teen
(Targretin)

BLACK BOX ALERT Do not administer to pregnant women (high risk of birth defects).

◆CLASSIFICATION

PHARMACOTHERAPEUTIC: Retinoid. **CLINICAL:** Antineoplastic (see p. 82C).

ACTION

Binds to and activates retinoid X receptor subtypes that regulate the genes controlling cellular differentiation and proliferation. **Therapeutic Effect:** Inhibits growth of tumor cell lines of hematopoietic and squamous cell origin, induces tumor regression.

PHARMACOKINETICS

Moderately absorbed from GI tract. Protein binding: greater than 99%. Metabolized in liver. Primarily eliminated through the hepatobiliary system. **Half-life:** 7 hrs.

USES

PO: Treatment of cutaneous T-cell lymphoma (CTCL) in those refractory to at least one prior systemic therapy. **Topical:** Treatment of cutaneous lesions in those with refractory CTCL (stage 1A and 1B) or not tolerant of other therapies.

OFF-LABEL: Treatment of diabetes mellitus; head, neck, lung, renal cell carcinomas; Kaposi's sarcoma.

PRECAUTIONS

Contraindications: Pregnancy. **Cautions:** Hepatic impairment, diabetes mellitus, lipid abnormalities, excessive alcohol consumption, biliary tract disease.

LIFESPAN CONSIDERATIONS

Pregnancy/Lactation: May cause fetal harm. Unknown if distributed in breast milk. **Pregnancy Category X. Children:** Safety and efficacy not established. **Elderly:** No age-related precautions noted.

INTERACTIONS

DRUG: **Bone marrow depressants, medications causing blood dyscrasias** may have adverse additive effects. **CYP3A4 inducers (e.g., phenobarbital, phenytoin, rifampin)** may decrease plasma concentration. **CYP3A4 inhibitors (e.g., erythromycin, gemfibrozil, itraconazole, ketoconazole)** may increase plasma concentration. Bexarotene may reduce **tamoxifen** concentration. **HERBAL: Dong quai, St. John's wort** may cause photosensitization. **St. John's wort** may decrease plasma concentration. **FOOD: Grapefruit, grapefruit juice** may increase concentration/toxicity. **LAB VALUES:** May increase serum bilirubin, AST, ALT, cholesterol, glucose, potassium, triglycerides, total cholesterol, LDL. May decrease HDL. CA-125 in ovarian cancer may be increased.

AVAILABILITY (Rx)

Capsules (Soft Gelatin [Targretin]): 75 mg.
Topical Gel (Targretin): 1%.

ADMINISTRATION/HANDLING

PO

• Give following a high-fat meal.

Topical

• Generously coat lesions with gel. • Allow to dry before covering. • Avoid applying gel to normal skin surrounding lesions or near mucosal surfaces. • Use of occlusive dressings not recommended.

INDICATIONS/ROUTES/DOSAGE

Cutaneous T-Cell Lymphoma Refractory to at Least One Prior Systemic Therapy

PO: ADULTS: 300 mg/m²/day. If no tumor response after 8 wks and initial dose is well tolerated, may be increased to 400 mg/m²/day. If not tolerated, may be decreased to 200 mg/m²/day, then to 100 mg/m²/day, or temporarily suspended to manage toxicity. **Topical: ADULTS:** Initially, apply once every other day for first wk. May increase at weekly intervals to once a day, then twice a day, then 3 times a day, up to 4 times a day based on tolerance.

SIDE EFFECTS

Frequent: Hyperlipidemia (79%), headache (30%), hypothyroidism (29%), asthenia (loss of strength, energy) (20%). **Occasional:** Rash (17%); nausea (15%); peripheral edema (13%); dry skin, abdominal pain (11%); chills, exfoliative dermatitis (10%); diarrhea (7%).

ADVERSE EFFECTS/ TOXIC REACTIONS

Pancreatitis, hepatic failure, pneumonia occur rarely.

NURSING CONSIDERATIONS

BASELINE ASSESSMENT

Assess baseline lipid profile, WBC, hepatic function, thyroid function. Question for possibility of pregnancy (Pregnancy Category X).

INTERVENTION/EVALUATION

Monitor serum cholesterol, triglycerides, CBC, hepatic, thyroid function tests.

PATIENT/FAMILY TEACHING

• Do not use medicated, drying, abrasive soaps; wash with gentle, bland soap. • Inform physician if pregnant or planning to become pregnant (Pregnancy Category X). • Warn women of childbearing age about potential fetal risk if pregnancy occurs. • Instruct on need for use of 2 reliable forms of contraceptives concurrently during therapy and for 1 mo after discontinuation of therapy, even in infertile, premenopausal women.

---

bicalutamide

bye-ka-**loo**-ta-mide
(Apo-Bicalutamide ✤, Casodex, Novo-Bicalutamide ✤)

◆CLASSIFICATION

PHARMACOTHERAPEUTIC: Antiandrogen hormone. **CLINICAL:** Antineoplastic (see p. 83C).

ACTION

Competitively inhibits androgen action by binding to androgen receptors in target tissue. **Therapeutic Effect:** Decreases growth of prostatic carcinoma.

PHARMACOKINETICS

Well absorbed from GI tract. Protein binding: 96%. Metabolized in liver to inactive metabolite. Excreted in urine and feces. Not removed by hemodialysis. **Half-life:** 5.8–7 days.

USES

Treatment of advanced metastatic prostatic carcinoma (in combination with luteinizing hormone-releasing hormone [LHRH] agonist analogues, e.g., leuprolide). Treatment with both drugs must be started at same time. **OFF-LABEL:** Monotherapy for locally advanced prostate cancer.

PRECAUTIONS

Contraindications: Women, esp. those who are or may become pregnant. **Cautions:** Moderate to severe hepatic impairment, diabetes.

⧗ LIFESPAN CONSIDERATIONS

Pregnancy/Lactation: May inhibit spermatogenesis, not used in women. **Pregnancy Category X. Children:** Safety

---

and efficacy not established. **Elderly:** No age-related precautions noted.

INTERACTIONS

DRUG: May increase effect of **aripiprazole, budesonide, colchicine, fentanyl, salmeterol, saxagliptan. HERBAL:** None significant. **FOOD:** None known. **LAB VALUES:** May increase serum AST, ALT, alkaline phosphatase, creatinine, bilirubin, BUN, glucose. May decrease WBC, Hgb.

AVAILABILITY (Rx)

Tablets: 50 mg.

ADMINISTRATION/HANDLING

PO

• Give without regard to food. • Give at same time each day.

INDICATIONS/ROUTES/DOSAGE

Prostatic Carcinoma

PO: ADULTS, ELDERLY: 50 mg once a day in morning or evening, given concurrently with an LHRH analogue or after surgical castration.

SIDE EFFECTS

Frequent: Hot flashes (49%), breast pain (38%), muscle pain (27%), constipation (17%), asthenia (loss of strength, energy) (15%), diarrhea (10%), nausea (11%). **Occasional (9%–8%):** Nocturia, abdominal pain, peripheral edema. **Rare (7%–3%):** Vomiting, weight loss, dizziness, insomnia, rash, impotence, gynecomastia.

ADVERSE EFFECTS/ TOXIC REACTIONS

Sepsis, CHF, hypertension, iron deficiency anemia, interstitial pneumonitis, pulmonary fibrosis may occur. Severe hepatotoxicity occurs rarely within the first 3–4 mos after treatment initiation.

NURSING CONSIDERATIONS

BASELINE ASSESSMENT

Obtain baseline lab tests including CBC, hepatic function, PSA, serum testosterone, leutinizing hormone (LH) levels.

INTERVENTION/EVALUATION

Monitor lab studies for changes from baseline. Perform periodic hepatic function tests. If AST, ALT increase over 2 times the upper limit of normal (ULN) or jaundice is noted, discontinue treatment. Monitor for diarrhea, nausea, vomiting.

PATIENT/FAMILY TEACHING

• Do not stop taking either medication (both drugs must be continued). • Take medications at same time each day. • Explain possible expectancy of frequent side effects. • Report persistent nausea, vomiting, diarrhea or yellowing of skin or eyes.

---

bisacodyl

bis-**ak**-oh-dil
(Alophen, Apo-Bisacodyl ✜,
Dulcolax, Fleet Bisacodyl Enema,
Veracolate)

◆CLASSIFICATION

PHARMACOTHERAPEUTIC: GI stimulant. **CLINICAL:** Laxative (see p. 126C).

ACTION

Direct effect on colonic smooth musculature by stimulating intramural nerve plexi. **Therapeutic Effect:** Promotes fluid and ion accumulation in colon, increasing peristalsis, producing laxative effect.

PHARMACOKINETICS

Route	Onset	Peak	Duration
PO	6–12 hrs	N/A	N/A
Rectal	15–60 min	N/A	N/A

Minimal absorption following PO and rectal administration. Absorbed drug is excreted in urine; remainder is eliminated in feces.

USES

Treatment of constipation, colonic evacuation before examinations or procedures.

PRECAUTIONS

Contraindications: Abdominal pain, appendicitis, intestinal obstruction, nausea, undiagnosed rectal bleeding, vomiting, pregnancy, lactation. **Cautions:** Excessive use may lead to fluid, electrolyte imbalance.

⧖ LIFESPAN CONSIDERATIONS

Pregnancy/Lactation: Unknown if drug crosses placenta or is distributed in breast milk. **Pregnancy Category C. Children:** Use with caution in those younger than 6 yrs (usually unable to describe symptoms or more severe side effects). **Elderly:** Repeated use may cause weakness, orthostatic hypotension due to fluid, electrolyte imbalance.

INTERACTIONS

DRUG: Antacids may decrease effect, cause premature dissolution of enteric coating and possible gastric irritation. **HERBAL:** None significant. **FOOD: Milk** may cause rapid dissolution of bisacodyl. **LAB VALUES:** May increase serum glucose concentration. May decrease serum potassium (due to fluid loss).

AVAILABILITY (OTC)

Rectal Enema (Fleet Bisacodyl Enema): 10 mg/30 ml. **Suppositories (Dulcolax):** 10 mg.
🥦 **Tablets (Enteric-Coated [Dulcolax]):** 5 mg.

ADMINISTRATION/HANDLING

PO
• Give on empty stomach (faster action). • Offer 6–8 glasses of water a day (aids stool softening). • Administer tablets whole; do not break, crush, or divide. • Avoid giving within 1 hr of antacids, milk, other oral medication.

Rectal, Enema
• Shake bottle, and remove orange protective shield from tip. • Position pt on left side with left knee slightly bent and right leg drawn up, or in knee-chest position. • Insert tip into rectum, aiming at pt's umbilicus.

Rectal, Suppository
• If suppository is too soft, chill for 30 min in refrigerator or run cold water over foil wrapper. • Moisten suppository with cold water before inserting well into rectum.
Storage • Store rectal enema, suppositories at room temperature.

INDICATIONS/ROUTES/DOSAGE

Treatment of Constipation
PO: ADULTS, CHILDREN OLDER THAN 12 YRS: 5–15 mg as needed. **Maximum:** 30 mg. **CHILDREN 3–12 YRS:** 5–10 mg or 0.3 mg/kg at bedtime or after breakfast. **ELDERLY:** Initially, 5 mg/day.
Rectal, Enema: ADULTS, CHILDREN OLDER THAN 12 YRS: One 1.25-oz bottle as a single daily dose.
Rectal, Suppository: ADULTS, CHILDREN OLDER THAN 12 YRS: 10 mg to induce bowel movement. **CHILDREN 2–12 YRS:** 5–10 mg as a single dose. **CHILDREN YOUNGER THAN 2 YRS:** 5 mg. **ELDERLY:** 5–10 mg/day.

SIDE EFFECTS

Frequent: Some degree of abdominal discomfort, nausea, mild cramps, faintness. **Occasional:** Rectal administration: burning of rectal mucosa, mild proctitis.

ADVERSE EFFECTS/ TOXIC REACTIONS

Long-term use may result in laxative dependence, chronic constipation, loss of normal bowel function. Overdose may result in electrolyte or metabolic disturbances (hypokalemia, hypocalcemia, metabolic acidosis, alkalosis), persistent diarrhea, vomiting, muscle weakness, malabsorption, weight loss.

NURSING CONSIDERATIONS

BASELINE ASSESSMENT
Observe for evidence of constipation. Assess pattern of bowel activity, stool consistency.

INTERVENTION/EVALUATION
Encourage adequate fluid intake. Assess bowel sounds for peristalsis. Monitor daily

pattern of bowel activity, stool consistency; record time of evacuation. Assess for abdominal disturbances. Monitor serum electrolytes in those exposed to prolonged, frequent, or excessive use of medication.

PATIENT/FAMILY TEACHING

• Institute measures to promote defecation: increase fluid intake, exercise, high-fiber diet. • Do not take antacids, milk, or other medication within 1 hr of taking medication (decreased effectiveness). • Report unrelieved constipation, rectal bleeding, muscle pain or cramps, dizziness, weakness. • Do not break, chew, crush, or divide tablets.

bismuth

bis-muth
(Diotame, Kaopectate, Pepto-Bismol)
Do not confuse Kaopectate with Kayexalate.

FIXED-COMBINATION(S)

Helidac: bismuth/metronidazole/tetracycline: 262 mg/250 mg/500 mg.

◆CLASSIFICATION

PHARMACOTHERAPEUTIC: Antisecretory, antimicrobial. **CLINICAL:** Antidiarrheal, antinausea, antiulcer (see p. 46C).

ACTION

Absorbs water, toxins in large intestine. Forms a protective coating in intestinal mucosa. Possesses antisecretory and antimicrobial effects. **Therapeutic Effect:** Prevents diarrhea.

USES

Treatment of mild, nonspecific diarrhea, indigestion, nausea. Part of multidrug regimen in treatment of *H. pylori* eradication to reduce risk of duodenal ulcer recurrence. Prevention of traveler's diarrhea.

PRECAUTIONS

Contraindications: History of severe GI bleeding or coagulopathy. **Cautions:** Elderly, diabetes. History of bleeding disorder; gastric ulcer disease; concomitant use of anticoagulants, clopidogrel, NSAIDs, or oral antidiabetic agents. **Pregnancy Category C (D if used in third trimester).**

INTERACTIONS

DRUG: May decrease absorption of **tetracyclines**. **HERBAL:** None significant. **FOOD:** None known. **LAB VALUES:** May alter serum alkaline phosphatase, AST, ALT, uric acid levels. May decrease serum potassium. May prolong prothrombin time (PT).

AVAILABILITY (OTC)

Caplets: (Pepto-Bismol): 262 mg. **Liquid:** 262 mg/15 ml (Diotame, Kaopectate, Pepto-Bismol), 525 mg/15 ml (Kaopectate Extra Strength, Maalox Total Stomach Relief, Pepto-Bismol Maximum Strength). **Suspension:** 262 mg/15 ml. **Tablets, Chewable** (Diotame, Pepto-Bismol): 262 mg.

ADMINISTRATION/HANDLING

• Shake suspension well. • Instruct pt to chew or dissolve chewable tablet before swallowing.

INDICATIONS/ROUTES/DOSAGE

Diarrhea, Gastric Distress
PO: ADULTS, ELDERLY, CHILDREN OLDER THAN 12 YRS: 2 tablets (30 ml) q30–60min. **Maximum:** 8 doses in 24 hrs. **CHILDREN 9–12 YRS:** 1 tablet or 15 ml q30–60min. **Maximum:** 8 doses in 24 hrs. **CHILDREN 6–8 YRS:** $\frac{2}{3}$ tablet or 10 ml q30–60min. **Maximum:** 8 doses in 24 hrs. **CHILDREN 3–5 YRS:** $\frac{1}{3}$ tablet or 5 ml q30–60min. **Maximum:** 8 doses in 24 hrs.

H. Pylori–Associated Duodenal Ulcer, Gastritis
PO: ADULTS, ELDERLY: 525 mg 4 times a day, requires combination therapy.

Chronic Infant Diarrhea
PO: CHILDREN 2–24 MOS: 2.5 ml q4h; **25–48 MOS:** 5 ml q4h; **49–70 MOS:** 10 ml q4h.

SIDE EFFECTS

Frequent: Grayish black stools. **Rare:** Constipation.

ADVERSE EFFECTS/ TOXIC REACTIONS

Debilitated pts and infants may develop impaction.

NURSING CONSIDERATIONS

INTERVENTION/EVALUATION

Encourage adequate fluid intake. Assess bowel sounds for peristaltic activity. Monitor daily pattern of bowel activity, stool consistency.

PATIENT/FAMILY TEACHING

• Stool may appear gray/black. • Chew chewable tablets thoroughly before swallowing. • Report diarrhea lasting more than 2 days.

---

bisoprolol `HIGH ALERT`

bi-**soe**-proe-lol
(Apo-Bisoprolol ✦, Novo-Bisoprolol ✦, Zebeta)
Do not confuse Zebeta with DiaBeta or Zetia.

FIXED-COMBINATION(S)

Ziac: bisoprolol/hydrochlorothiazide (a diuretic): 2.5 mg/6.25 mg, 5 mg/6.25 mg, 10 mg/6.25 mg.

◆CLASSIFICATION

PHARMACOTHERAPEUTIC: Beta-adrenergic blocker. **CLINICAL:** Antihypertensive (see p. 62C, 72C).

ACTION

Blocks beta₁-adrenergic receptors in cardiac tissue. **Therapeutic Effect:** Slows sinus heart rate, decreases B/P.

PHARMACOKINETICS

Well absorbed from GI tract. Protein binding: 26%–33%. Metabolized in liver.

Primarily excreted in urine. Not removed by hemodialysis. **Half-life:** 9–12 hrs (increased in renal impairment).

USES

Management of hypertension, alone or in combination with other medications. **OFF-LABEL:** Angina pectoris, premature ventricular contractions, supraventricular arrhythmias, CHF.

PRECAUTIONS

Contraindications: Cardiogenic shock, marked sinus bradycardia, overt cardiac failure, second- or third-degree heart block (except in pts with pacemaker). **Cautions:** Renal/hepatic impairment, hyperthyroidism, diabetes, bronchospastic disease, myasthenia gravis, psychiatric disease.

⌛ LIFESPAN CONSIDERATIONS

Pregnancy/Lactation: Readily crosses placenta; distributed in breast milk. Avoid use during first trimester. May produce bradycardia, apnea, hypoglycemia, hypothermia during delivery, low birth-weight infants. **Pregnancy Category C (D if used in second or third trimester). Children:** Safety and efficacy not established. **Elderly:** Age-related peripheral vascular disease may increase risk of decreased peripheral circulation.

INTERACTIONS

DRUG: Diuretics, other antihypertensives may increase hypotensive effect. May mask symptoms of hypoglycemia, prolong hypoglycemic effect of **insulin, oral hypoglycemics. NSAIDs** may decrease antihypertensive effect. **Verapamil, diltiazem, digoxin** may increase risk of bradycardia or heart block. **HERBAL: Ephedra, ginseng, yohimbe** may worsen hypertension. **Garlic** may have increased antihypertensive effect. **FOOD:** None known. **LAB VALUES:** May increase ANA titer, BUN, serum creatinine, potassium, uric acid, lipoproteins, triglycerides.

✦ Canadian trade name   ✇ Non-Crushable Drug   `HIGH` High Alert drug

AVAILABILITY (Rx)

Tablets: 5 mg, 10 mg.

ADMINISTRATION/HANDLING

PO
• Give without regard to food. • Scored tablet may be crushed.

INDICATIONS/ROUTES/DOSAGE

Hypertension
PO: ADULTS: Initially, 2.5–5 mg/day. May increase up to 20 mg/day. **ELDERLY:** Initially, 2.5 mg/day. May increase by 2.5–5 mg/day. **Maximum:** 20 mg/day.

Dosage in Renal Impairment
For adults and elderly pts whose creatinine clearance is less than 40 ml/min, initially give 2.5 mg.

SIDE EFFECTS

Frequent (11%–8%): Fatigue, headache. **Occasional (4%–2%):** Dizziness, arthralgia, peripheral edema, URI, rhinitis, pharyngitis, diarrhea, nausea, insomnia. **Rare (less than 2%):** Chest pain, asthenia (loss of strength, energy), dyspnea, vomiting, bradycardia, dry mouth, diaphoresis, decreased libido, impotence.

ADVERSE EFFECTS/TOXIC REACTIONS

Overdose may produce profound bradycardia, hypotension. Abrupt withdrawal may result in diaphoresis, palpitations, headache, tremors. May precipitate CHF, MI in pts with cardiac disease, thyroid storm in those with thyrotoxicosis, peripheral ischemia in those with existing peripheral vascular disease. Hypoglycemia may occur in previously controlled diabetes. Thrombocytopenia, unusual bruising/bleeding occur rarely.

NURSING CONSIDERATIONS

BASELINE ASSESSMENT

Assess baseline renal/hepatic function tests. Assess B/P, apical pulse immediately before drug is administered (if pulse is 60/min or less or systolic B/P is less than 90 mm Hg, withhold medication, contact physician).

INTERVENTION/EVALUATION

Monitor B/P, pulse for quality, irregular rate, bradycardia. Assist with ambulation if dizziness occurs. Assess for peripheral edema (usually, first area of lower extremity swelling is behind medial malleolus in ambulatory, sacral area in bedridden). Monitor daily pattern of bowel activity, stool consistency. Assess neurologic status.

PATIENT/FAMILY TEACHING

• Do not abruptly discontinue medication. • Compliance with therapy regimen is essential to control hypertension. • If dizziness occurs, sit or lie down immediately. • Avoid tasks that require alertness, motor skills until response to drug is established. • Teach pts how to take pulse properly before each dose and to report excessively slow pulse rate (less than 60 beats/min), peripheral numbness, dizziness. • Do not use nasal decongestants, OTC cold preparations (stimulants) without physician's approval. • Restrict salt, alcohol intake.

---

bivalirudin

bye-**val**-i-rue-din
(<u>Angiomax</u>)

◆ **CLASSIFICATION**

PHARMACOTHERAPEUTIC: Thrombin inhibitor. **CLINICAL:** Anticoagulant (see p. 32C).

ACTION

Specifically and reversibly inhibits thrombin by binding to its receptor sites. **Therapeutic Effect:** Decreases acute myocardial ischemic complications in pts with unstable angina pectoris.

PHARMACOKINETICS

Route	Onset	Peak	Duration
IV	Immediate	N/A	1 hr

Primarily eliminated by kidneys. Twenty-five percent removed by hemodialysis. **Half-life:** 25 min (increased in moderate to severe renal impairment).

USES

Anticoagulant in pts with unstable angina undergoing percutaneous transluminal coronary angioplasty (PTCA) in conjunction with aspirin. Pts with heparin-induced thrombocytopenia (HIT) and thrombosis syndrome (HITTS) while undergoing percutaneous coronary intervention (PCI) (in conjunction with aspirin). **OFF-LABEL:** HIT; ST-segment elevation MI (STEMI) undergoing PCI.

PRECAUTIONS

Contraindications: Active major bleeding. **Cautions:** Renal impairment. Conditions associated with increased risk of bleeding (e.g., bacterial endocarditis, recent major bleeding, CVA, stroke, intracerebral surgery, hemorrhagic diathesis, severe hypertension, severe renal/hepatic impairment, recent major surgery).

⌛ LIFESPAN CONSIDERATIONS

Pregnancy/Lactation: Unknown if drug crosses placenta or is distributed in breast milk. **Pregnancy Category B. Children:** Safety and efficacy not established. **Elderly:** Age-related renal impairment may require dosage adjustment.

INTERACTIONS

DRUG: Antiplatelets, NSAIDs, salicylates, thrombolytics may increase effects. **HERBAL: Ginkgo biloba,** other herbs with anticoagulant/antiplatelet properties may increase risk of bleeding. **FOOD:** None known. **LAB VALUES:** Prolongs activated partial thromboplastin time (aPTT), prothrombin time (PT).

AVAILABILITY (Rx)

Injection, Powder for Reconstitution: 250 mg.

ADMINISTRATION/HANDLING

 IV

Reconstitution • To each 250-mg vial add 5 ml Sterile Water for Injection. • Gently swirl until fully dissolved. • Dilute each vial in 50 ml D₅W or 0.9% NaCl bag to yield final concentration of 5 mg/ml (1 vial in 50 ml, 2 vials in 100 ml, 5 vials in 250 ml). • If low-rate infusion is used after initial infusion, reconstitute the 250-mg vial with added 5 ml Sterile Water for Injection. • Gently swirl until fully dissolved. • Dilute each vial in 500 ml D₅W or 0.9% NaCl bag to yield final concentration of 0.5 mg/ml. • Produces a clear, colorless solution (do not use if cloudy or contains a precipitate).
Rate of Administration • Adjust IV infusion based on aPTT or pt's body weight.
Storage • Store unreconstituted vials at room temperature. • Reconstituted solution may be refrigerated for up to 24 hrs. • Final dilution with a concentration of 0.5–5 mg/ml is stable at room temperature for up to 24 hrs.

▒ IV INCOMPATIBILITIES

Alteplase (Activase), amiodarone (Cordarone), amphotericin B (AmBisome, Abelcet), diazepam (Valium), dobutamine (Dobutrex), reteplase (Retavase), streptokinase (Streptase), vancomycin (Vancocin).

▒ IV COMPATIBILITIES

Refer to chart in front of book.

INDICATIONS/ROUTES/DOSAGE

Anticoagulant in Pts with Unstable Angina, HIT, or HITTS Undergoing PTCA
IV: **ADULTS, ELDERLY:** 0.75 mg/kg as IV bolus, followed by IV infusion at rate of 1.75 mg/kg/hr for duration of procedure and up to 4 hrs postprocedure. IV infusion may be continued beyond initial 4 hrs at rate of 0.2 mg/kg/hr for up to 20 hrs.

Dosage in Renal Impairment
◀**ALERT**▶ Initial bolus dose remains unchanged.

Creatinine Clearance	Dosage
30 ml/min or greater	1.75 mg/kg/hr
10–29 ml/min	1 mg/kg/hr
Dialysis	0.25 mg/kg/hr

SIDE EFFECTS

Frequent (42%): Back pain. **Occasional (15%–12%):** Nausea, headache, hypotension, generalized pain. **Rare (8%–4%):** Injection site pain, insomnia, hypertension, anxiety, vomiting, pelvic or abdominal pain, bradycardia, nervousness, dyspepsia, fever, urinary retention.

ADVERSE EFFECTS/ TOXIC REACTIONS

Hemorrhagic events occur rarely, characterized by significant fall in B/P or Hct.

NURSING CONSIDERATIONS

BASELINE ASSESSMENT

Assess CBC, bleeding time, renal function. Determine initial B/P.

INTERVENTION/EVALUATION

Monitor aPTT, Hct, urine and stool specimen for occult blood, renal function studies. Monitor for evidence of bleeding. Assess for decrease in B/P, increase in pulse rate. Question for increase in vaginal bleeding during menses. Assess urine for hematuria.

---

bleomycin HIGH ALERT

blee-oh-**mye**-sin
(Blenoxane)

BLACK BOX ALERT Pulmonary fibrosis (commonly presenting as pneumonitis) occurs more often in elderly, pts receiving more than 400 units total lifetime dose or single dose more than 30 units, smokers, prior radiation treatment, or receiving concurrent oxygen. Severe reactions (hypotension, mental confusion, fever, chills, wheezing) is reported rarely.

◆CLASSIFICATION

PHARMACOTHERAPEUTIC: Glycopeptide antibiotic. **CLINICAL:** Antineoplastic, sclerosing agent (see p. 83C).

ACTION

Binds to portions of DNA, producing DNA single-strand breaks. Most effective in G_2 phase of cell division. **Therapeutic Effect:** Inhibits cell replication.

PHARMACOKINETICS

Protein binding: Low (1%). Metabolism varies. Excreted in urine as unchanged drug. **Half-life:** 115 min.

USES

Treatment of Hodgkin's and non-Hodgkin's lymphoma, sclerosing agent for malignant pleural effusions, squamous cell carcinoma (e.g., head, neck, penis, cervix, vulva), testicular carcinoma. **OFF-LABEL:** Ovarian tumors.

PRECAUTIONS

Contraindications: Previous allergic reaction to bleomycin. **Cautions:** Severe renal or pulmonary impairment.

LIFESPAN CONSIDERATIONS

Pregnancy/Lactation: May cause fetal harm. Breastfeeding not recommended. **Pregnancy Category D. Children:** Safety and efficacy not established. **Elderly:** Increased risk of pulmonary toxicity.

INTERACTIONS

DRUG: May alter effects of **live vaccines. Pimecrolimus, tacrolimus** (topical) may increase concentration/effect. **HERBAL: Echinacea** may decrease effect. **FOOD:** None known. **LAB VALUES:** None significant.

AVAILABILITY (Rx)

Injection, Powder for Reconstitution (Blenoxane): 15 units, 30 units.

ADMINISTRATION/HANDLING

◀ALERT▶ May be carcinogenic, mutagenic, teratogenic. Handle with extreme care during preparation/administration.

 IV

Reconstitution • Reconstitute 15-unit vial with at least 5 ml (30-unit vial with at least 10 ml) 0.9% NaCl to provide a concentration no greater than 3 units/ml.

Rate of Administration • Administer over at least 10 min for IV injection.

Storage • Refrigerate vials. Intact vials are stable for 4 wks at room temperature. • After reconstitution with 0.9% NaCl, solution is stable for 24 hrs at room temperature.

IM, Subcutaneous

Rate of Administration • Reconstitute 15-unit vial with 1–5 ml (30-unit vial with 2–10 ml) Sterile Water for Injection, 0.9% NaCl, or Bacteriostatic Water for Injection to provide concentration of 3–15 units/ml. Do not use D_5W.

Storage • Refrigerate vials. • After reconstitution, solution is stable for 24 hrs at room temperature.

🔬 IV INCOMPATIBILITIES

Diazepam (Valium), hydrocortisone sodium succinate (Solu-Cortef).

🔬 IV COMPATIBILITIES

Furosemide (Lasix), cefepime (Maxipime), dacarbazine (DTIC), dexamethasone (Decadron), diphenhydramine (Benadryl), fludarabine (Fludara), gemcitabine (Gemzar), ondansetron (Zofran), paclitaxel (Taxol), piperacillin/tazobactam (Zosyn), vinblastine (Velban), vinorelbine (Navelbine).

INDICATIONS/ROUTES/DOSAGE

◀ALERT▶ Maximum lifetime dose = 400 units.

Usual Dosage
(Refer to individual protocols)
**IV, IM, Subcutaneous: ADULTS, EL-
DERLY:** 10–20 units/m² (0.25–0.5 units/kg) 1–2 times a wk.

Sclerosing Agent
ADULTS, ELDERLY: 60 units as a single instillation (mix with 50–100 ml 0.9% NaCl). May repeat at intervals of several days if fluid continues to accumulate.

Dosage in Renal Impairment

Creatinine Clearance	Dosage
40–50 ml/min	70% of normal
30–39 ml/min	60% of normal
20–29 ml/min	55% of normal
10–19 ml/min	45% of normal
5–9 ml/min	40% of normal

SIDE EFFECTS

Frequent: Anorexia, weight loss, erythematous skin swelling, urticaria, rash, striae, vesiculation, hyperpigmentation (particularly at areas of pressure, skin folds, cuticles, IM injection sites, scars), stomatitis (usually evident 1–3 wks after initial therapy); may be accompanied by decreased skin sensitivity followed by skin hypersensitivity, nausea, vomiting, alopecia. With parenteral form, fever, chills typically occurring a few hrs after large single dose, lasting 4–12 hrs occur frequently.

ADVERSE EFFECTS/TOXIC REACTIONS

Interstitial pneumonitis occurs in 10% of pts, occasionally progresses to pulmonary fibrosis. Appears to be dose, age related (older than 70 yrs, those receiving total dose greater than 400 units). Nephrotoxicity, hepatotoxicity occur infrequently.

NURSING CONSIDERATIONS

BASELINE ASSESSMENT

Obtain baseline pulmonary, renal function tests. Obtain baseline chest X-ray.

INTERVENTION/EVALUATION

Adventitious breath sounds may indicate pulmonary toxicity (rales, rhonchi). Observe for dyspnea. Monitor hematologic, pulmonary, hepatic, renal function tests. Assess skin daily for cutaneous toxicity (erythema, rash, vesiculation). Monitor for stomatitis (burning, erythema of oral mucosa at inner margin of lips), hematologic toxicity (fever, sore throat, signs of local infection, unusual bruising/bleeding), symptoms of anemia (excessive fatigue, weakness).

PATIENT/FAMILY TEACHING

• Report fever, chills, wheezing, difficulty breathing, prolonged nausea, vomiting, oral pain, or lesions. • Fever or chills reaction occurs less frequently with continued therapy. • Improvement of Hodgkin's disease, testicular tumors noted within 2 wks, squamous cell carcinoma within 3 wks. • Do not have immunizations without physician's approval (drug lowers body's resistance). • Avoid contact with those who have recently received live virus vaccine or had a viral infection (e.g., cold virus, herpetic infection).

---

boceprevir

boe-**sep**-re-veer
(Victrelis)

◆**CLASSIFICATION**

PHARMACOTHERAPEUTIC: Protease inhibitor. **CLINICAL:** Antiviral.

ACTION

Inhibits hepatitis C virus (HCV) protease needed for cleavage of HCV-encoded polyproteins by binding to active serine protease sites. **Therapeutic Effect:** Inhibits viral replication of hepatitis C virus.

PHARMACOKINETICS

Well absorbed after PO administration. Protein binding: 75%. Extensively metabolized in liver. Excreted primarily in feces. Minimal removal by hemodialysis. **Half-life:** 3.4 hrs.

USES

Treatment of chronic hepatitis C genotype 1 in combination with peginterferon alfa and ribavirin. Indicated for compensated liver disease, including cirrhosis, in pts who are previously untreated or who have failed previous interferon and ribavirin therapy.

PRECAUTIONS

◄**ALERT**► Safety and efficacy not established in decompensated cirrhosis, organ transplant, coinfected with HIV, hepatitis B, previous failed therapies with protease inhibitors. **Contraindications:** Pregnancy, breastfeeding, male partners of pregnant women, drugs utilizing CYP3A4/5 for clearance, CYP3A4/5 inducers (e.g., rifampin, carbamazepine), contraindications to peginterferon alfa or ribavirin. **Cautions:** Anemia, neutropenia, thrombocytopenia, HIV.

⏳ LIFESPAN CONSIDERATIONS

Pregnancy/Lactation: Strictly avoid pregnancy. May cause birth defects or fetal demise. **Pregnancy Category B (X when used in ribavirin).** Women of childbearing age must use two different forms of birth control: intrauterine device and barrier methods during treatment and at least 6 mos after treatment. Hormonal contraceptives may have decreased effectiveness. Do not initiate therapy until negative pregnancy test confirmed. Unknown if crosses placenta or into breast milk. Breastfeeding contraindicated. **Children:** Safety and efficacy not established. **Elderly:** No age-related precautions noted.

INTERACTIONS

DRUG: Contraindicated with **alfuzosin, carbamazepine, dihydroergotamine, ergonovine, ergotamine, lovastatin, methylergonovine, midazolam, phenobarbital, phenytoin, pimozide, rifampin, sildenafil, simvastatin,**

tadalafil, triazolam. May increase concentrations of **antiarrhythmics (amiodarone, bepridil, digoxin, flecanide, propafenone, quinidine), antifungals (itraconazole, ketoconazole, posaconazole, voriconazole), atorvastatin, budesonide, calcium channel blockers (dihydropyridine, felodipine, nicardipine, nifedipine), colchicine, clarithromycin, desipramine, dexamethasone, fluticasone, HIV non-nucleoside reverse transcriptase inhibitors, immunosuppressants, opioid analgesics, oral contraceptives, rifabutin, salmeterol, sildenafil, trazadone, warfarin.** May alter therapeutic levels of **buprenorphine, ethinyl estradiol, HIV protease inhibitors, methadone, warfarin. Dexamethasone, HIV non-nucleoside reverse transcriptase inhibitors, rifabutin** may decrease antiviral effectiveness. **HERBAL: St. John's wort** may decrease effectiveness (contraindicated). **FOOD:** None known. **LAB VALUES:** May decrease RBC, Hgb, Hct, neutrophils, platelets.

AVAILABILITY (Rx)

Capsules: 200 mg.

ADMINISTRATION/HANDLING

• Give with food.

INDICATIONS/ROUTES/DOSAGE

Chronic Hepatitis C with Non-Cirrhosis, Previously Untreated or Previous Partial Responders or Relapsers
PO: ADULTS, ELDERLY: 800 mg 3 times a day with food. Begin after 4 wks of peginterferon alfa, ribavirin therapy. Duration based on Response-Guided Therapy (RGT) guidelines. **Response-Guided Therapy Guidelines with HCV-RNA Level** Based on prior treatment and HCV-RNA results at wks 8, 12, 24. For previously untreated pts, if HCV-RNA undetectable at wk 8 to wk 24, complete three-medicine regimen at wk 28. If HCV-RNA detectable at wk 8 but undetectable at wk 24, continue three-medicine regimen until wk 36, then finish with peginterferon alfa, ribavirin until wk

48. For previous partial responders or relapsers, if HCV-RNA undetectable at wk 8 to wk 24, complete three-medicine regimen at wk 36. If HCV-RNA detectable at wk 8 but undetectable at wk 24, continue three-medicine regimen until wk 36, then finish with peginterferon alfa, ribavirin until wk 48. **Treatment Futility** Discontinue treatment if HCV-RNA viral load greater than or equal to 100 international units/ml at wk 12, or HCV-RNA detectable at wk 24.

Chronic Hepatitis C with Cirrhosis, or Poor Responders to Interferon
PO: ADULTS, ELDERLY: 800 mg 3 times a day with food for 44 wks. Start after 4 wks with peginterferon alfa, ribavirin therapy.

Dosage Modification
Do not reduce boceprevir during treatment. If adverse reaction or neutropenia occurs, recommend reduction/discontinuation of peginterferon alfa and/or ribavirin. If Hgb less than 10 g/dl, reduce or interrupt ribavirin. If Hgb less than 8.5 g/dl, discontinue ribavirin.

SIDE EFFECTS

Frequent (58%–25%): Fatigue, anemia, nausea, dysgeusia (altered taste), chills, insomnia, alopecia, decreased appetite, diarrhea. **Occasional (22%–8%):** Irritability, vomiting, arthralgia, dizziness, dry skin, rash, asthenia (loss of strength, energy), dry mouth, exertional dyspnea.

ADVERSE EFFECTS/ TOXIC REACTIONS

Increased risk of thromboembolic events associated with peginterferon alfa, erythropoiesis-stimulating agent. Life-threatening infections related to neutropenia. Simultaneous use of contraindicated medications use may result in hypertension/hypotension, peripheral vasospasm/ischemia (ergot toxicity), arrhythmias, rhabdomyolysis (statins), hyperkalemia (oral contraception), visual abnormalities, syncope, increased sedation or respiratory depression (sedative/hypnotics), loss of virologic response.

NURSING CONSIDERATIONS

BASELINE ASSESSMENT

Assess vital signs, O_2 saturation. Obtain CBC, HCV-RNA level, INR if on warfarin. Receive full history of home medications including vitamins, minerals, herbal products, and screen contraindications. Confirm negative pregnancy test before initiating treatment. Question history of anemia, HIV, hepatitis B, organ transplant.

INTERVENTION/EVALUATION

Assess vital signs, O_2 saturation routinely. Monitor CBC with differential (wk 4, 8, 12), and HCV-RNA levels (wk 4, 8, 12, 24), urine pregnancy every month and 6 mos after final treatment. Assess for anemia-related dizziness, exertional dyspnea, fatigue, weakness, syncope. Report decreases in Hgb, Hct, platelets, neutrophils. Monitor INR if on warfarin. Monitor for acute infection (fever, diaphoresis, lethargy, oral mucosal changes, productive cough), bloody stools, bruising, hematuria, DVT, pulmonary embolism. Encourage nutritional intake and assess anorexia, weight loss. Obtain EKG for hypokalemia, palpitations, tachycardia. Reinforce birth control compliance.

PATIENT/FAMILY TEACHING

• Must be used in combination with peginterferon alfa, ribavirin. • Inform side effects/contraindications of three-medication regimen. • Blood levels will be drawn routinely. • Immediately report any newly prescribed medications. • Women of childbearing age must use two different forms of birth control: intrauterine device and barrier methods during treatment and for at least 6 mos after treatment. • Hormonal birth control (oral, vaginal rings, injections) may be ineffective. • Immediately notify physician if partner becomes pregnant. • May alter taste of food or decrease appetite. • Report bloody stool/urine, increased bruising, difficulty breathing, weakness, dizziness, palpitations, weight loss. • Avoid alcohol. • Take with meals.

bortezomib

bor-**tez**-oh-mib
(Velcade)

◆CLASSIFICATION

PHARMACOTHERAPEUTIC: Protease inhibitor. **CLINICAL:** Antineoplastic (see p. 83C).

ACTION

Degrades conjugated proteins required for cell-cycle progression and mitosis, disrupting cell proliferation. **Therapeutic Effect:** Produces antitumor and chemosensitizing activity, cell death.

PHARMACOKINETICS

Widely distributed. Protein binding: 83%. Primarily metabolized by enzymatic action. Significant biliary excretion, with lesser amount excreted in urine. **Half-life:** 9–15 hrs.

USES

Treatment of relapsed or refractory multiple myeloma, mantle cell lymphoma. Initial treatment of multiple myeloma. **OFF-LABEL:** Treatment of Waldenström's macroglobulinemia; peripheral or cutaneous T-cell lymphoma; systemic light-chain amyloidosis.

PRECAUTIONS

Contraindications: Hypersensitivity to boron or mannitol, intrathecal administration. **Cautions:** History of syncope, pts receiving medication known to be associated with hypotension, dehydration, diabetes, hepatic impairment, preexisting cardiac disease.

⌛ LIFESPAN CONSIDERATIONS

Pregnancy/Lactation: May induce degenerative effects in ovary, degenerative changes in testes. May affect male/female fertility. Breastfeeding not recommended. **Pregnancy Category D. Children:** Safety and efficacy not established.

Elderly: Increased incidence of grades 3 or 4 thrombocytopenia.

INTERACTIONS

DRUG: CYP3A4 inhibitors (e.g., itraconazole, ketoconazole) may increase concentration/effect. **CYP3A4 inducers (e.g., rifampin)** may decrease concentration/effect. **HERBAL: Green tea, green tea extracts** may diminish effect. **St. John's wort** may decrease level/effect. **FOOD: Grapefruit juice** may increase drug level. **LAB VALUES:** May significantly decrease WBC, Hgb, Hct, platelet count, neutrophils.

AVAILABILITY (Rx)

Injection, Powder for Reconstitution: 3.5 mg.

ADMINISTRATION/HANDLING

 IV

Reconstitution • Reconstitute vial with 3.5 ml 0.9% NaCl to provide a concentration of 1 mg/ml.
Rate of Administration • Give as bolus IV injection over 3–5 sec.
Storage • Store unopened vials at room temperature. • Once reconstituted, solution may be stored at room temperature for up to 3 days or for 5 days if refrigerated.

SUBCUTANEOUS

Reconstitution • Reconstitute vial with 1.4 ml 0.9% NaCl to provide a concentration of 2.5 mg/ml.

INDICATIONS/ROUTES/DOSAGE

Relapsed or Refractory Multiple Myeloma, Mantle Cell Lymphoma
IV: Subcutaneous: ADULTS, ELDERLY: Treatment cycle consists of 1.3 mg/m² twice weekly on days 1, 4, 8, and 11 for 2 wks followed by a 10-day rest period on days 12 to 21. Consecutive doses separated by at least 72 hrs.

Multiple Myeloma (Initial Treatment)
IV: Subcutaneous: ADULTS, ELDERLY: 1.3 mg/m² (with melphalan and predni-sone) for a total of nine 6-wk treatment cycles (cycles 1–4 administer twice weekly; cycles 5–9 administer once weekly).

Dosage Adjustment Guidelines

Therapy is withheld at onset of grade 3 nonhematologic or grade 4 hematologic toxicities, excluding neuropathy. When symptoms resolve, therapy is restarted at a 25% reduced dosage.

Dosage Adjustment Guidelines with Neuropathic Pain, Peripheral Sensory Neuropathy

For grade 1 toxicity with pain or grade 2 (interfering with function but not activities of daily living [ADL]), 1 mg/m². For grade 2 toxicity with pain or grade 3 (interfering with ADL), withhold drug until toxicity is resolved, then reinitiate with 0.7 mg/m². For grade 4 toxicity (permanent sensory loss that interferes with function), discontinue bortezomib.

SIDE EFFECTS

Expected (65%–36%): Fatigue, malaise, asthenia (loss of strength, energy), nausea, diarrhea, anorexia, constipation, fever, vomiting. **Frequent (28%–21%):** Headache, insomnia, arthralgia, limb pain, edema, paresthesia, dizziness, rash. **Occasional (18%–11%):** Dehydration, cough, anxiety, bone pain, muscle cramps, myalgia, back pain, abdominal pain, taste alteration, dyspepsia, pruritus, hypotension (including orthostatic hypotension), rigors, blurred vision.

ADVERSE EFFECTS/ TOXIC REACTIONS

Thrombocytopenia occurs in 40% of pts. Platelet count peaks at day 11, returns to baseline by day 21. GI, intracerebral hemorrhage are associated with drug-induced thrombocytopenia. Anemia occurs in 32% of pts. New onset or worsening of existing neuropathy occurs in 37% of pts. Symptoms may improve in some pts upon drug discontinuation. Pneumonia occurs occasionally.

NURSING CONSIDERATIONS

BASELINE ASSESSMENT

Obtain baseline CBC. Ensure adequate hydration prior to initiation of therapy. Antiemetics, antidiarrheals may be effective in preventing, treating nausea, vomiting, diarrhea.

INTERVENTION/EVALUATION

Routinely assess B/P; monitor pt for orthostatic hypotension. Maintain strict I&O. Monitor CBC, esp. platelet count, throughout treatment. Monitor renal, hepatic, pulmonary function throughout therapy. Encourage adequate fluid intake to prevent dehydration. Monitor temperature and be alert to high potential for fever. Monitor for peripheral neuropathy (burning sensation, neuropathic pain, paresthesia, hyperesthesia). Avoid IM injections, rectal temperatures, other traumas that may induce bleeding.

PATIENT/FAMILY TEACHING

• Report new/worsening vomiting, bruising/bleeding, breathing difficulties. • Discuss importance of pregnancy testing, avoidance of pregnancy, measures to prevent pregnancy. • Increase fluid intake. • Avoid tasks that require mental alertness, motor skills until response to drug is established.

bosentan

boe-sen-tan
(Tracleer)
BLACK BOX ALERT Do not use in pregnancy (may cause birth defects) or in moderate to severe hepatic impairment.
Do not confuse Tracleer with Tricor.

◆CLASSIFICATION

PHARMACOTHERAPEUTIC: Endothelin receptor antagonist. **CLINICAL:** Vasodilator, neurohormonal blocker.

ACTION

Blocks the neurohormone that constricts pulmonary arteries. **Therapeutic Effect:** Improves exercise ability, slows clinical worsening of pulmonary arterial hypertension (PAH).

PHARMACOKINETICS

Protein binding: greater than 98%. Metabolized in liver. Eliminated by biliary excretion. **Half-life:** Approximately 5 hrs (increased in cardiac failure).

USES

Treatment of PAH World Health Organization group I to improve exercise ability and to decrease clinical worsening. **OFF-LABEL:** Pts with New York Heart Association class II, III, IV symptoms; HF, PAH-scleroderma; PAH-associated congenital heart disease with left-to-right shunts.

PRECAUTIONS

Contraindications: Administration with cyclosporine or glyburide, pregnancy. **Extreme Caution:** Moderate to severe hepatic impairment. **Cautions:** Mild hepatic impairment, anemia.

⌛ LIFESPAN CONSIDERATIONS

Pregnancy/Lactation: May induce male infertility, atrophy of seminiferous tubules of testes; reduce sperm count. Expected to cause fetal harm, teratogenic effects, including malformations of head, mouth, face, large vessels. Breastfeeding not recommended. **Pregnancy Category X. Children:** Safety and efficacy not established. **Elderly:** Use with caution. May have increased frequency of decreased hepatic, renal, cardiac function.

INTERACTIONS

DRUG: May decrease concentration of **atorvastatin, glyburide, hormonal contraceptives (oral, injectable, implantable), lovastatin, simvastatin, warfarin. Cyclosporine, ketoconazole** may increase plasma concentration. **Clarithromycin** may increase risk of hepatotoxicity. **PDE5 inhibitors**

(e.g., sildenafil) may increase concentration/effect. HERBAL: St. John's wort may decrease concentration. FOOD: Grapefruit, grapefruit juice may increase concentration/effect. LAB VALUES: May increase serum bilirubin, AST, ALT levels. May decrease Hgb, Hct levels.

AVAILABILITY (Rx)

 Tablets: 62.5 mg, 125 mg.

ADMINISTRATION/HANDLING

• Give in morning and evening, with or without food. • Instruct pt to not break, chew, crush, or divide film-coated tablets. • Avoid grapefruit, grapefruit juice.

INDICATIONS/ROUTES/DOSAGE

Pulmonary Arterial Hypertension
PO: ADULTS, ELDERLY, CHILDREN OLDER THAN 12 YRS AND WEIGHING 40 KG OR GREATER: 62.5 mg twice a day for 4 wks; then increase to maintenance dosage of 125 mg twice a day. **ADULTS, ELDERLY, CHILDREN WEIGHING LESS THAN 40 KG:** 62.5 mg twice a day.
◀ALERT▶ When discontinuing adult/elderly dosage, reduce dosage to 62.5 mg twice a day for 3–7 days to avoid clinical deterioration.

Dosage Based on Hepatic Enzyme Elevations
Any elevation accompanied by symptoms of hepatic injury or serum bilirubin 2 or more times upper limit of normal (ULN), stop treatment. AST/ALT greater than 3 or less than 6 times ULN, reduce dose or interrupt treatment. AST/ALT greater than 5 and up to 8 times ULN, confirm with additional test and, if confirmed, stop treatment. AST/ALT greater than 8 times ULN, stop treatment.

SIDE EFFECTS

Frequent (22%–11%): Headache, nasopharyngitis. **Occasional (9%–5%):** Flushing, peripheral edema, palpitations. **Rare (less than 5%):** Fatigue, dyspepsia, pruritus.

ADVERSE EFFECTS/TOXIC REACTIONS

Serious hepatic injury has been reported.

NURSING CONSIDERATIONS

BASELINE ASSESSMENT
Pregnancy must be excluded before starting treatment and prevented thereafter. A negative pregnancy test performed during the first 5 days of a normal menstrual period and at least 11 days after the last act of sexual intercourse must be obtained. Monthly follow-up pregnancy tests must be maintained. Obtain, assess baseline lab tests, esp. hepatic function.

INTERVENTION/EVALUATION
Assess hepatic enzyme levels before initiating therapy, then monthly thereafter. If elevation in hepatic enzymes is noted, changes in monitoring and treatment must be initiated. If clinical symptoms of hepatic injury (nausea, vomiting, fever, abdominal pain, fatigue, jaundice) occur or if serum bilirubin level increases to 2 or more times ULN, stop treatment. Assess for peripheral edema. Monitor Hgb levels at 1 mo and 3 mos of treatment, then q3mos for decrease.

PATIENT/FAMILY TEACHING
• Discuss importance of pregnancy testing, avoidance of pregnancy, measures to prevent pregnancy. • Report palpitations, extremity swelling, unusual weight gain, fatigue, yellowing of skin or eyes, change in color of stool, urine. • Do not break, chew, crush, or divide film-coated tablets. • Avoid grapefruit products.

---

bosutinib

boe-**sue**-ti-nib
(Bosulif)

◆CLASSIFICATION
PHARMACOTHERAPEUTIC: Tyrosine kinase inhibitor. **CLINICAL:** Antineoplastic (see p. 83C).

ACTION

Inhibits Bcr-Abl tyrosine kinase, a translocation-created enzyme, created by the Philadelphia chromosome (Ph[1]) abnormality noted in chronic myelogenous leukemia (CML). Inhibits Src-family kinase including Src, Lyn, and Hck. **Therapeutic Effect:** Inhibits tumor cell growth and proliferation in chronic, accelerated, or blast phase CML.

PHARMACOKINETICS

Well absorbed following oral administration. Protein binding: 94%. Metabolized in liver. Eliminated in feces (91%), urine (3%). **Half-life:** 22.5 hrs.

USES

Treatment of chronic, accelerated, or blast phase Ph[+] chronic myelogenous leukemia with resistance or intolerance to prior therapy.

PRECAUTIONS

Contraindications: Hypersensitivity to bosutinib. **Cautions:** Baseline anemia, thrombocytopenia, neutropenia, hepatic impairment, recent history of diarrhea, pulmonary edema, CHF, fluid retention.

⌛ LIFESPAN CONSIDERATIONS

Pregnancy/Lactation: Potential for embryo/fetal toxicity. Avoid pregnancy. Must use effective contraception during, and for at least 30 days after treatment. Unknown if distributed in breast milk. Avoid breastfeeding. **Pregnancy Category D. Children:** Safety and efficacy not established in those younger than 18 yrs. **Elderly:** No age-related precautions noted.

INTERACTIONS

DRUG: Strong CYP3A inhibitors and/ or P-glycoprotein (P-gp) inhibitors (e.g., clarithromycin, ketoconazole, ritonavir, misoprostol, nafcillin, salmeterol) and **moderate CYP3A4 inhibitors (ciprofloxacin, diltiazem, erythromycin, verapamil)** may increase concentration/effectiveness. **Strong CYP3A4 inducers (e.g., rifampin, phenytoin, phenobarbital)** and **moderate CYP3A4 inducers (bosentan, nafcillin, modafinil)** may decrease plasma concentration/effectiveness. **Proton pump inhibitors (e.g., omeprazole, lansoprazole, pantoprazole)** may reduce absorption, concentration of bosutinib. **HERBAL:** St. John's wort may decrease effectiveness. **FOOD: Grapefruit, grapefruit juice** may decrease bosutinib concentration. **LAB VALUES:** May decrease Hgb, platelets, WBCs, phosphorous. May increase ALT, AST, bilirubin, lipase.

AVAILABILITY (Rx)

▧ **Tablets:** 100 mg, 500 mg.

ADMINISTRATION/HANDLING

PO
• Give with food. Do not break, crush, divide, or dissolve tablets.

INDICATIONS/ROUTES/DOSAGE

Chronic Myelogenous Leukemia (CML)
PO: ADULTS: 500 mg once daily with food. May increase to 600 mg once daily for poor responders without high-grade adverse reactions.

CML with Baseline Hepatic Impairment
PO: ADULTS: 200 mg once daily with food.

Dosage Modification
Hepatotoxicity: Withhold treatment until AST/ALT less than or equal to 2.5× ULN. Then, resume at 400 mg once daily with food. Discontinue if recovery lasts longer than 4 wks or hepatotoxicity including elevated bilirubin levels are greater than 2× ULN. **Severe Diarrhea:** Withhold until recovery to low-grade diarrhea. Then, resume at 400 mg once daily with food. **Myelosuppression:** Withhold until neutrophil count greater than 1000 × 10^6 L and platelet count greater than 50,000 × 10^6 L. Then, resume at same dose if recovery occurs within 2 wks. May reduce dose to 400 mg for recovery lasting greater than 2 wks.

SIDE EFFECTS

Frequent (82%–35%): Diarrhea, nausea, vomiting, abdominal pain, rash. **Occasional (26%–10%):** Pyrexia, fatigue, headache, cough, peripheral edema, arthralgia, anorexia, upper respiratory infection, asthenia (loss of strength, energy), back pain, nasopharyngitis, dizziness, pruritus.

ADVERSE EFFECTS/ TOXIC REACTIONS

Severe fluid retention may result in pleural effusion, pericardial effusion, pulmonary edema, ascites. Neutropenia, thrombocytopenia, or anemia is an expected response of drug therapy. Severe diarrhea may result in fluid loss, electrolyte imbalance, hypotension. Hepatotoxicity occurred in 7%–9% of pts.

NURSING CONSIDERATIONS

BASELINE ASSESSMENT

Offer emotional support. Assess baseline weight, serum chemistries, particularly renal, hepatic function. Confirm negative pregnancy test before initiating treatment. Obtain full medication history including vitamins, minerals, herbal products. Screen for peripheral edema, signs/symptoms of CHF, anemia.

INTERVENTION/EVALUATION

Weigh daily and monitor for unexpected rapid weight gain, edema. Monitor for changes in serum chemistry tests, liver function tests during treatment. Offer antiemetics for nausea, vomiting. Monitor daily pattern of bowel activity, stool consistency. Monitor CBC for neutropenia, thrombocytopenia, anemia. Assess for bruising, hematuria, jaundice, right upper abdominal pain, weight loss, or acute infection (fever, diaphoresis, lethargy, productive cough).

PATIENT/FAMILY TEACHING

• Serum lab studies will be obtained routinely. • Take medication with meals. • Encourage fluid intake (diarrhea may result in dehydration). • Swallow whole; do not break, chew, crush, or dissolve tablets. • Strictly avoid pregnancy. • Use contraception during treatment and for at least 30 days after treatment. • Report urine changes, bloody or clay-colored stools, upper abdominal pain, nausea, vomiting, bruising, persistent diarrhea, fever, cough, difficulty breathing, chest pain. • Immediately report any newly prescribed medications. • Avoid alcohol, grapefruit products. • Discuss using antacids for indigestion, heartburn, upset stomach (omeprazole, lansoprazole, pantoprazole may reduce absorption, concentration of bosutinib). • Separate antacid dosing by more than 2 hrs before and after medication.

brentuximab vedotin

bren-**tux**-i-mab ve-**doe**-tin
(Adcetris)

BLACK BOX ALERT JC virus infection resulting in progressive multifocal leukoencephalopathy and death can occur.

◆CLASSIFICATION

PHARMACOTHERAPEUTIC: Monoclonal antibody, antimitotic. **CLINICAL:** Antineoplastic (see p. 83C).

ACTION

Binds to CD30-expressing cells, allowing the antibody to direct the drug to a target on lymphoma cells, disrupting the microtubule network within the cell. **Therapeutic Effect:** Induces cell cycle arrest, cell death.

PHARMACOKINETICS

Minimally metabolized. Protein binding: 68%–82%. Eliminated primarily in feces (72%). **Half-life:** 4–6 days.

USES

Treatment of Hodgkin's lymphoma after failure of autologous stem cell transplant or after failure of at least two prior multiagent chemotherapy regimens in pts who are not transplant candidates. Treatment of systemic anaplastic large-cell lymphoma after failure of at least one prior multiagent chemotherapy regimen.

PRECAUTIONS

Contraindications: Avoid use with bleomycin (increased risk for pulmonary toxicity). **Cautions:** Peripheral neuropathy, infusion reactions, neutropenia, tumor lysis syndrome, Stevens-Johnson syndrome, pregnancy.

⧖ LIFESPAN CONSIDERATIONS

Pregnancy/Lactation: May cause fetal harm (embryo-fetal toxicities). Unknown if distributed in breast milk. **Pregnancy Category D. Children:** Safety and efficacy not established. **Elderly:** Safety and efficacy not established.

INTERACTIONS

DRUG: Strong **CYP3A4 inhibitors (e.g., atazanavir, itraconazole, clarithromycin, ketoconazole)** increase concentration/effect. **CYP3A4 inducers (e.g., rifampin)** reduce concentration/effect. **FOOD:** None known. **HERBAL:** Echinacea may decrease effect. **LAB VALUES:** May decrease Hgb, Hct, WBC, RBC, platelets. May increase serum bicarbonate, lactate dehydrogenase, glucose, albumin, magnesium, sodium.

AVAILABILITY (Rx)

Injection, Powder for Reconstitution: 50-mg single-use vial.

ADMINISTRATION/HANDLING
 IV

Reconstitution • Reconstitute each 50-mg vial with 10.5 ml Sterile Water for Injection, directing the stream toward wall of vial and not at powder. • Gently swirl (do not shake). • This will yield a concentration of 5 mg/ml. • The dose for pts weighing over 100 kg should be calculated for 100 kg. • Reconstituted solution must be transferred to infusion bag with a minimum 100 ml diluent, yielding a final concentration range of 0.4 mg/ml to 1.8 mg/ml brentuximab. • Gently invert bag to mix solution.

Rate of Administration • Infuse over 30 min.

Storage • Discard if solution contains particulate or is discolored; solution should appear clear to slightly opalescent, colorless. • May store solution at 36°–46°F. • Use within 24 hrs after reconstitution.

▦ IV COMPATIBILITIES

0.9% NaCl, D₅W, lactated Ringer's.

INDICATIONS/ROUTES/DOSAGE

◀ALERT▶ Do not give by IV bolus or IV push.

Hodgkin's Lymphoma
IV Infusion: ADULTS/ELDERLY: 1.8 mg/kg IV infused over 30 min every 3 wks. Continue treatment until a maximum of 16 cycles, disease progression, or unacceptable toxicity occurs.

Systemic Anaplastic Large-Cell Lymphoma
IV Infusion: ADULTS/ELDERLY: 1.8 mg/kg IV infused over 30 min every 3 wks. Continue treatment until a maximum of 16 cycles, disease progression, or unacceptable toxicity occurs.

SIDE EFFECTS

◀ALERT▶ Effects present as mild, manageable.
Frequent (52%–22%): Peripheral neuropathy, fatigue, respiratory tract infection, nausea, diarrhea, fever, rash, abdominal pain, cough, vomiting. **Occasional (19%–11%):** Headache, dizziness, constipation, chills, bone/muscle pain, insomnia, peripheral edema, alopecia. **Rare (10%–5%):** Anxiety, muscle spasm, decreased appetite, dry skin.

ADVERSE EFFECTS/ TOXIC REACTIONS

Myelosuppression characterized as neutropenia (54%), peripheral neuropathy (52%), thrombocytopenia (28%), anemia (19%) was noted. Infusion reactions (including anaphylaxis), Stevens-Johnson syndrome have been reported. Tumor lysis syndrome may lead to acute renal failure. Progressive multifocal leukoencephalopathy (changes in mood, confusion, loss of memory, changes in speech, walking, and vision, decreased strength or weakness on one side of body) has been reported.

NURSING CONSIDERATIONS

BASELINE ASSESSMENT

Question for evidence of peripheral neuropathy (hypoesthesia, hyperesthesia, paresthesia, burning sensation, neuropathic pain or weakness). Those experiencing new or worsening neuropathy may require a delay, dose change, or discontinuation of treatment. Obtain baseline CBC before treatment begins and as needed to monitor response and toxicity but particularly prior to each dosing cycle. Use strict aseptic technique and protect pt from infection.

INTERVENTION/EVALUATION

Offer antiemetics to control nausea, vomiting. Monitor for hematologic toxicity (fever, sore throat, signs of local infection, easy bruising, unusual bleeding), symptoms of anemia (excessive fatigue, weakness). Assess response to medication; monitor and report nausea, vomiting, diarrhea. Monitor daily pattern of bowel activity, stool consistency. Assess skin for evidence of rash.

PATIENT/FAMILY TEACHING

• Avoid crowds, persons with known infections. • Report signs of infection at once (fever, flu-like symptoms). • Avoid contact with anyone who recently received live virus vaccine. • Do not receive immunizations without physician's approval (drug lowers body resistance).

• Promptly report fever, easy bruising or unusual bleeding from any site. • Male pts should be warned of potential risk to their reproductive capacities.

bromocriptine

broe-moe-**krip**-teen
(PMS-Bromocriptine ✤, Cycloset, Parlodel)
Do not confuse bromocriptine with benztropine, Cycloset with Glyset, or Parlodel with pindolol or Provera.

◆CLASSIFICATION

PHARMACOTHERAPEUTIC: Dopamine agonist. **CLINICAL:** Infertility therapy adjunct, antihyperprolactinemic, lactation inhibitor, antidyskinetic, growth hormone suppressant (see p. 45C, 144C, 145C).

ACTION

Directly stimulates dopamine receptors in corpus striatum, inhibits prolactin secretion. Suppresses secretion of growth hormone. **Therapeutic Effect:** Improves symptoms of parkinsonism, suppresses galactorrhea, reduces serum growth hormone concentrations in acromegaly.

PHARMACOKINETICS

Indication	Onset	Peak	Duration
Prolactin lowering	1–2 hrs	5–10 hrs	8–12 hrs

Minimally absorbed from GI tract. Protein binding: 90%–96%. Metabolized in liver. Excreted in feces by biliary secretion. **Half-life:** 15 hrs.

USES

Treatment of pituitary prolactinomas, conditions associated with hyperprolactinemia (amenorrhea, galactorrhea, hypogonadism, infertility), parkinsonism, acromegaly. **Cycloset:** Control blood glucose in type 2 diabetes. **OFF-LABEL:** Neuroleptic malignant syndrome.

PRECAUTIONS

Contraindications: Hypersensitivity to ergot alkaloids, peripheral vascular disease, pregnancy, severe ischemic heart disease, uncontrolled hypertension. Concomitant use with serotonin agonists (e.g., buspirone, sumatriptan, trazodone). **Cautions:** Impaired hepatic or cardiac function, hypertension, psychiatric disorders, peptic ulcer disease.

⧗ LIFESPAN CONSIDERATIONS

Pregnancy/Lactation: Not recommended during pregnancy or breastfeeding. **Pregnancy Category B. Children:** Safety and efficacy not established. **Elderly:** CNS effects may occur more frequently.

INTERACTIONS

DRUG: May increase concentration/side effects of **salicylates, sulfonamides, probenecid. Phenothiazines, thioxanthenes** may diminish effect. May increase **ergot-related drugs** side effects (e.g., nausea, vomiting), reduce effect of ergot drugs. **CYP3A4 inhibitors** may increase concentration; **CYP3A4 inducers** may decrease concentration/effects. **HERBAL:** St. John's wort may decrease concentration. **FOOD:** None known. **LAB VALUES:** May increase plasma concentration of growth hormone.

AVAILABILITY (Rx)

Capsules: 5 mg. **Tablets:** 2.5 mg. (Cycloset): 0.8 mg.

ADMINISTRATION/HANDLING

PO
• Give with food (decreases incidence of nausea). • **Cycloset:** Take in morning, within 2 hrs of awakening.

INDICATIONS/ROUTES/DOSAGE

Hyperprolactinemia
PO: ADULTS, ELDERLY, CHILDREN OLDER THAN 15 YRS: Initially, 1.25–2.5 mg at bedtime. May increase by 2.5 mg q3–7days up to 5–7.5 mg/day in divided doses. Maintenance: 2.5 mg 2–3 times a day. Range: 2.5–15 mg/day. **CHILDREN, 11–15 YRS:** Initially, 1.25–2.5 mg daily. May increase up to 10 mg/day. Range: 2.5–10 mg/day.

Parkinsonism
PO: ADULTS, ELDERLY: Initially, 1.25 mg 1–2 times a day. May take single doses at bedtime. May increase by 2.5 mg/day at 14- to 28-day intervals. Maintenance: 2.5–40 mg/day in divided doses. Range: 30–90 mg/day in 3 divided doses. **Maximum:** 100 mg/day.

Acromegaly
PO: ADULTS, ELDERLY: Initially, 1.25–2.5 mg at bedtime. May increase by 1.25–2.5 mg q3–7days up to 30 mg/day in divided doses. Maintenance: 20–30 mg/day in divided doses. **Maximum:** 100 mg/day.

Type 2 Diabetes (Cycloset)
PO: ADULTS, ELDERLY: Initially, 0.8 mg once daily (within 2 hrs of waking). Increase by 0.8 mg/day weekly up to maximum of 4.8 mg/day. Range: 1.6–4.8 mg/day.

SIDE EFFECTS

Cycloset: Somnolence, hypotension, syncope during initiation and dose titration. **Frequent:** Nausea (49%), headache (19%), dizziness (17%). **Occasional (7%–3%):** Fatigue, light-headedness, vomiting, abdominal cramps, diarrhea, constipation, nasal congestion, drowsiness, dry mouth. **Rare:** Muscle cramps, urinary hesitancy.

ADVERSE EFFECTS/ TOXIC REACTIONS

Visual or auditory hallucinations in pts with Parkinson's disease have been reported. Long-term, high-dose therapy may produce syncope, GI hemorrhage, peptic ulcer, severe abdominal pain, chronic rhinorrhea.

NURSING CONSIDERATIONS

BASELINE ASSESSMENT

Evaluation of pituitary gland (rule out tumor) should be done before treatment for hyperprolactinemia with amenorrhea or galactorrhea, infertility. Obtain baseline lab tests including CBC, hepatic function, prolactin level, pregnancy test.

INTERVENTION/EVALUATION

Assist with ambulation if dizziness is noted after administration. Assess for therapeutic response (decrease in engorgement, parkinsonism symptoms). Monitor daily pattern of bowel activity, stool consistency. Monitor cardiac function.

PATIENT/FAMILY TEACHING

• To diminish light-headedness, rise slowly from lying to sitting position, permit legs to dangle momentarily before standing. • Avoid sudden changes in posture. • Avoid tasks that require alertness, motor skills until response to drug is established. • Use contraceptive measures (other than oral) during treatment. • Report watery nasal discharge. • Avoid alcohol intake.

---

budesonide
TOP 200

bue-**des**-oh-nide
(Entocort EC, Pulmicort Flexhaler, Pulmicort Respules, Rhinocort Aqua, Uceris)
Do not confuse budesonide with Budeprion.

FIXED-COMBINATION(S)

Symbicort: budesonide/formoterol (bronchodilator): 80 mcg/4.5 mcg, 160 mcg/4.5 mcg.

◆CLASSIFICATION

PHARMACOTHERAPEUTIC: Glucocorticosteroid. **CLINICAL:** Anti-inflammatory, antiallergy (see pp. 2C, 77C, 99C).

ACTION

Inhibits accumulation of inflammatory cells, decreases and prevents tissues from responding to inflammatory process. **Therapeutic Effect:** Relieves symptoms of allergic rhinitis, Crohn's disease.

PHARMACOKINETICS

Form	Onset	Peak	Duration
Pulmicort Respules	2–8 days	4–6 wks	—
Rhinocort Aqua	10 hrs	2 wks	—

Minimally absorbed from nasal tissue; moderately absorbed from inhalation. Protein binding: 88%. Primarily metabolized in liver. **Half-life:** 2–3 hrs.

USES

Nasal: Management of seasonal or perennial allergic rhinitis, nonallergic rhinitis. **Nebulization:** Maintenance or prophylaxis therapy for bronchial asthma. **PO: (Entocort EC):** Treatment of mild to moderate active Crohn's disease. Maintenance of clinical remission of mild to moderate Crohn's disease. **(Uceris):** Induction of remission in active, mild to moderate ulcerative colitis. **Oral Inhalation:** Maintenance and prophylactic treatment of asthma. **OFF-LABEL:** Treatment of vasomotor rhinitis.

PRECAUTIONS

Contraindications: Hypersensitivity to any corticosteroid or its components, primary treatment of status asthmaticus, acute episodes of asthma. Not for relief of acute bronchospasms. **Cautions:** Thyroid disease, hepatic impairment, renal impairment, cardiovascular disease, diabetes, glaucoma, cataracts, myasthenia gravis, pts at risk for osteoporosis, seizures, GI disease, post acute MI, elderly.

⧗ LIFESPAN CONSIDERATIONS

Pregnancy/Lactation: Unknown if drug crosses placenta or is distributed in breast milk. **Pregnancy Category B (Inhalation); C (PO). Children:** Prolonged treatment or

---

high dosages may decrease short-term growth rate, cortisol secretion. **Elderly:** No age-related precautions noted.

INTERACTIONS

DRUG: CYP3A4 inhibitors (e.g., itraconazole, ketoconazole) may increase plasma concentration. **HERBAL: Echinacea** may decrease effects. **FOOD: Grapefruit, grapefruit juice** may increase systemic exposure of budesonide. **LAB VALUES:** May decrease serum potassium.

AVAILABILITY (Rx)

Oral Inhalation Powder (Pulmicort Flexhaler): 90 mcg per inhalation; 180 mcg per inhalation. **Inhalation Suspension for Nebulization (Pulmicort Respules):** 0.25 mg/2 ml; 0.5 mg/2 ml; 1 mg/2 ml. **Nasal Spray (Rhinocort Aqua):** 32 mcg/spray. **Capsules, Enteric-Coated (Entocort EC):** 3 mg. **Tablets, Extended-Release: (Uceris):** 9 mg.

ADMINISTRATION/HANDLING

Inhalation
• Shake container well. Instruct pt to exhale completely, place mouthpiece between lips, inhale, hold breath as long as possible before exhaling. • Allow at least 1 min between inhalations. • Rinsing mouth after each use decreases dry mouth, hoarseness.

Intranasal
• Instruct pt to clear nasal passages before use. • Tilt pt's head slightly forward. • Insert spray tip into nostril, pointing toward nasal passages, away from nasal septum. • Spray into one nostril while pt holds other nostril closed and concurrently inspires through nostril to allow medication as high into nasal passages as possible.

Nebulization
• Shake well before use. • Administer with mouthpiece or face mask. • Rinse mouth following treatment.

PO
• May take with or without food. Swallow whole. Do not crush or chew capsule or tablet.

INDICATIONS/ROUTES/DOSAGE

Rhinitis

Intranasal: ADULTS, ELDERLY, CHILDREN 6 YRS AND OLDER: 1 spray (32 mcg) in each nostril once a day. **Maximum:** 8 sprays (256 mcg)/day for adults and children 12 yrs and older; 4 sprays (128 mcg)/day for children younger than 12 yrs.

Bronchial Asthma

Nebulization: CHILDREN 12 MOS–8 YRS: *(Previous therapy with bronchodilators alone):* 0.5 mg/day as single dose or 2 divided doses. **Maximum:** 0.5 mg/day. *(Previous therapy with inhaled corticosteroids):* 0.5 mg/day as single dose or 2 divided doses. **Maximum:** 1 mg/day. *(Previous therapy of oral corticosteroids):* 1 mg/day as single dose in 2 divided doses. **Maximum:** 1 mg/day.

Oral Inhalation: *(Pulmicort Flexhaler):* **ADULTS, ELDERLY:** Initially, 360 mcg 2 times/day. **Maximum:** 720 mcg 2 times/day. **CHILDREN, 6 YRS AND OLDER:** 180 mcg 2 times/day. **Maximum:** 360 mcg 2 times/day.

Crohn's Disease
PO: ADULTS, ELDERLY: 9 mg once a day for up to 8 wks. Recurring episodes may be treated with a repeat 8-wk course of treatment. Maintenance of remission: 6 mg once daily for 3 mos.

Ulcerative Colitis
PO: ADULTS, ELDERLY: 9 mg once daily in morning for up to 8 wks.

SIDE EFFECTS

Frequent (greater than 3%): Nasal: Mild nasopharyngeal irritation, burning, stinging, dryness; headache, cough. **Inhalation:** Flu-like symptoms, headache, pharyngitis. **Occasional (3%–1%): Nasal:** Dry mouth, dyspepsia, rebound congestion, rhinorrhea, loss of taste. **Inhalation:** Back pain, vomiting, altered taste, voice changes, abdominal pain, nausea, dyspepsia.

ADVERSE EFFECTS/ TOXIC REACTIONS

Acute hypersensitivity reaction (urticaria, angioedema, severe bronchospasm) occurs rarely.

NURSING CONSIDERATIONS

BASELINE ASSESSMENT

Question for hypersensitivity to any corticosteroids, components.

INTERVENTION/EVALUATION

Monitor for relief of symptoms.

PATIENT/FAMILY TEACHING

• Improvement noted in 24 hrs, but full effect may take 3–7 days. • Contact physician if no improvement in symptoms, sneezing, nasal irritation occurs.

bumetanide

bue-**met**-a-nide
(Burinex ✤)

BLACK BOX ALERT Excess dosage can lead to profound diuresis with fluid and electrolyte loss.
Do not confuse bumetanide with Buminate.

◆ CLASSIFICATION

PHARMACOTHERAPEUTIC: Loop diuretic. **CLINICAL:** Diuretic (see p. 104C).

ACTION

Enhances excretion of sodium, chloride, and, to lesser degree, potassium, by direct action at ascending limb of loop of Henle and in proximal tubule. **Therapeutic Effect:** Produces diuresis.

PHARMACOKINETICS

Route	Onset	Peak	Duration
PO	30–60 min	60–120 min	4–6 hrs
IV	Rapid	15–30 min	2–3 hrs

Completely absorbed from GI tract (absorption decreased in CHF, nephrotic syndrome). Protein binding: 94%–96%. Partially metabolized in liver. Primarily excreted in urine. Not removed by hemodialysis. **Half-life:** 1–1.5 hrs.

USES

Treatment of edema associated with CHF, chronic renal failure (including nephrotic syndrome), hepatic cirrhosis with ascites. **OFF-LABEL:** Treatment of hypertension.

PRECAUTIONS

Contraindications: Anuria, hepatic coma, severe electrolyte depletion (until condition improves or is corrected). **Cautions:** Hypersensitivity to sulfonamides, hypotension.

⧗ LIFESPAN CONSIDERATIONS

Pregnancy/Lactation: Unknown if drug is distributed in breast milk. **Pregnancy Category C (D if used in pregnancy-induced hypertension). Children:** Safety and efficacy not established. **Elderly:** May be more sensitive to hypotension/electrolyte effects. Increased risk for circulatory collapse or thrombolytic episode. Age-related renal impairment may require reduced or extended dosage interval.

INTERACTIONS

DRUG: Agents inducing hypokalemia (e.g., metolazone, hydrochlorothiazide) may have increased hypokalemic effect. May increase risk of **lithium** toxicity. **NSAIDs** may reduce effect. **HERBAL: Ephedra, ginseng, yohimbe** may worsen hypertension. **Garlic** may have increased antihypertensive effect. **FOOD:** None known. **LAB VALUES:** May increase serum glucose, BUN, uric acid, urinary phosphate. May decrease serum calcium, chloride, magnesium, potassium, sodium.

AVAILABILITY (Rx)

Injection Solution: 0.25 mg/ml. Tablets: 0.5 mg, 1 mg, 2 mg.

ADMINISTRATION/HANDLING

 IV

Rate of Administration • May give undiluted but is compatible with D₅W, 0.9% NaCl, or lactated Ringer's solution. • Administer IV push over 1–2 min. • May give through Y tube or 3-way stopcock. • May give as continuous infusion.

Storage • Store at room temperature. • Stable for 24 hrs if diluted.

PO

• Give with food to avoid GI upset, preferably with breakfast (may prevent nocturia).

▨ IV INCOMPATIBILITY

Midazolam (Versed).

▨ IV COMPATIBILITIES

Aztreonam (Azactam), cefepime (Maxipime), dexmedetomidine (Precedex), diltiazem (Cardizem), dobutamine (Dobutrex), furosemide (Lasix), lorazepam (Ativan), milrinone (Primacor), morphine, piperacillin and tazobactam (Zosyn), propofol (Diprivan).

INDICATIONS/ROUTES/DOSAGE

Edema
PO: ADULTS: 0.5–2 mg as a single dose in the morning. May repeat q4–5h. **Maximum:** 10 mg/day. **ELDERLY:** 0.5 mg/day, increased as needed.

IV, IM: ADULTS, ELDERLY: 0.5–2 mg/dose; may repeat in 2–3 hrs (**maximum:** 10 mg/day) or 0.5–2 mg/hr by continuous IV infusion.

Hypertension
PO: ADULTS, ELDERLY: Initially, 0.5 mg/day. Range: 0.5–2 mg/day in 2 divided doses. **Maximum:** 5 mg/day. Larger doses may be given 2–3 doses/day.

Usual Pediatric Dosage
IV, IM, PO: CHILDREN: 0.015–0.1 mg/kg/dose q6–24h. **Maximum:** 10 mg/day. **NEONATES:** 0.01–0.05 mg/kg/dose q12–48h.

SIDE EFFECTS

Expected: Increased urinary frequency and urine volume. **Frequent (5%):** Muscle cramps, dizziness, hypotension, headache, nausea. **Occasional (3%–1%):** Impaired hearing, pruritus, EKG changes, weakness, hives, abdominal pain, dyspepsia, musculoskeletal pain, rash, nausea, vomiting. **Rare (less than 1%):** Chest pain, ear pain, fatigue, dry mouth, premature ejaculation, impotence, nipple tenderness.

ADVERSE EFFECTS/ TOXIC REACTIONS

Vigorous diuresis may lead to profound water and electrolyte depletion, resulting in hypokalemia, hyponatremia, dehydration, coma, circulatory collapse. Ototoxicity manifested as deafness, vertigo, tinnitus may occur, esp. in pts with severe renal impairment or those taking other ototoxic drugs. Blood dyscrasias, acute hypotensive episodes have been reported.

NURSING CONSIDERATIONS

BASELINE ASSESSMENT

Obtain baseline vital signs, esp. B/P for hypotension, before administration. Assess baseline electrolytes, particularly for hypokalemia, hyponatremia. Assess for edema. Observe skin turgor, mucous membranes for hydration status. Initiate I&O, obtain baseline weight.

INTERVENTION/EVALUATION

Continue to monitor B/P, vital signs, electrolytes, I&O, weight. Note extent of diuresis. Watch for changes from initial assessment (hypokalemia may result in muscle weakness, tremor, muscle cramps, altered mental status, cardiac arrhythmias; hyponatremia may result in confusion, thirst, cold/clammy skin).

PATIENT/FAMILY TEACHING

• Expect increased urinary frequency/volume. • Report auditory abnormalities (e.g., sense of fullness in ears, tinnitus). • Eat foods high in potassium such as whole grains (cereals), legumes, meat, bananas, apricots, orange juice, potatoes (white, sweet), raisins. • Rise slowly from sitting/lying position.

---

buprenorphine 🔲TOP 200

bue-pre-**nor**-feen
(Buprenex, Butrans, Suboxone, Subutex)

BLACK BOX ALERT Transdermal: Potential for abuse, misuse, and diversion. Do not exceed dose of one 20 mcg/hr patch due to risk of QT interval prolongation. May cause potentially life-threatening respiratory depression.

Do not confuse Buprenex with Bumex, or buprenorphine with bupropion.

FIXED-COMBINATION(S)

Suboxone: buprenorphine/naloxone (narcotic antagonist): 2 mg/0.5 mg, 8 mg/2 mg.

◆CLASSIFICATION

PHARMACOTHERAPEUTIC: Opioid agonist, antagonist injection **(Schedule V)**; tablet **(Schedule III)**. **CLINICAL:** Opioid dependence adjunct, analgesic.

ACTION

Binds to opioid receptors within CNS. **Therapeutic Effect:** Suppresses opioid withdrawal symptoms, cravings. Alters pain perception, emotional response to pain.

PHARMACOKINETICS

Route	Onset	Peak	Duration
Sublingual	15 min	1 hr	6 hrs
IV	Less than 15 min	Less than 1 hr	6 hrs
IM	15 min	1 hr	6 hrs

Excreted primarily in feces with lesser amount eliminated in urine. Protein binding: High. **Half-life: Parenteral:** 2–3 hrs; **Sublingual:** 37 hrs (increased in hepatic impairment).

USES

Tablet: Treatment of opioid dependence. **Injection:** Relief of moderate to severe pain. **Transdermal:** Moderate to severe chronic pain requiring continuous around-the-clock opioid analgesic for extended period. **OFF-LABEL:** Injection: Heroin/opioid withdrawal in hospitalized pts.

PRECAUTIONS

Contraindications: Transdermal patch: Significant respiratory depression; severe asthma; paralytic ileus. **Cautions:** Hepatic/renal impairment, elderly, debilitated, pediatric pts, head injury/increased intracranial pressure, pts at risk for respiratory depression, hyperthyroidism, myxedema, adrenal cortical insufficiency (e.g., Addison's disease), urethral stricture, CNS depression, morbid obesity, toxic psychosis, prostatic hypertrophy, delirium tremens, kyphoscoliosis, biliary tract dysfunction, acute pancreatitis, acute abdominal conditions, acute alcoholism, pts with prolonged QT syndrome, concurrent use of antiarrhythmics.

🔲 LIFESPAN CONSIDERATIONS

Pregnancy/Lactation: Crosses placenta. Distributed in breast milk. Breastfeeding not recommended. Neonatal withdrawal noted in infant if mother was treated with buprenorphine during pregnancy with onset of withdrawal symptoms generally noted on day 1, manifested as hypertonia, tremor, agitation, myoclonus. Apnea, bradycardia, seizures occur rarely. **Pregnancy Category C. Children:**

Safety and efficacy of injection form not established in those 2–12 yrs. Safety and efficacy of tablet, fixed-combination form not established in those 16 yrs or younger. **Elderly:** Age-related hepatic impairment may require dosage adjustment.

INTERACTIONS

DRUG: CNS depressants, MAOIs may increase CNS or respiratory depression, hypotension. **CYP3A4 inhibitors (e.g., azole antifungals, macrolide antibiotics, protease inhibitors)** may increase plasma concentration. **CYP3A4 inducers (e.g., carbamazepine, phenobarbital, phenytoin, rifampin)** may cause increased clearance of buprenorphine. May decrease effects of **other opioid analgesics. HERBAL: St. John's wort, kava kava, gotu kola, valerian** may increase CNS depression. **FOOD:** None known. **LAB VALUES:** May increase serum amylase, lipase.

AVAILABILITY (Rx)

Injection Solution (Buprenex): 0.3 mg/1 ml.
Tablets, Sublingual (Fixed-Combination [Suboxone]): 2 mg/0.5 mg, 8 mg/2 mg.
Transdermal (Butrans): 5 mcg/hr, 10 mcg/hr, 20 mcg/hr.

ADMINISTRATION/HANDLING

 IV

Reconstitution • May be diluted with lactated Ringer's solution, D₅W, 0.9% NaCl.
Rate of Administration • If given as IV push, administer over at least 2 min.

IM
• Give deep IM into large muscle mass.

Sublingual
• Instruct pt to dissolve tablet(s) under tongue; avoid swallowing (reduces drug bioavailability). • For doses greater than 2 tablets, either place all tablets at once or 2 tablets at a time under the tongue.
Storage • Store parenteral form at room temperature. • Protect from pro-longed exposure to light. • Store tablets at room temperature.

Transdermal
• Apply to clean, dry, intact skin of upper outer arm, upper chest, upper back, or side of chest. • Wear for 7 days. • Wait minimum of 21 days before reapplying to same site. • If patch falls off during 7-day dosing interval, apply new patch to a different skin site.

▦ IV INCOMPATIBILITIES

Diazepam (Valium), furosemide (Lasix), lorazepam (Ativan).

▦ IV COMPATIBILITIES

Allopurinol (Aloprim, Zyloprim), aztreonam (Azactam), cefepime (Maxipime), diphenhydramine (Benadryl), granisetron (Kytril), haloperidol (Haldol), heparin, linezolid (Zyvox), midazolam (Versed), piperacillin/tazobactam (Zosyn), promethazine (Phenergan), propofol (Diprivan).

INDICATIONS/ROUTES/DOSAGE

Opioid Dependence
Sublingual: **ADULTS, CHILDREN 13 YRS AND OLDER:** 8 mg on day 1, then 16 mg on day 2 and subsequent induction days. Range: 12–16 mg/day of Subutex used as induction with switch to Suboxone for maintenance.

Moderate to Severe Pain
IM/IV: **ADULTS, CHILDREN 13 YRS AND OLDER:** 0.3 mg (1 ml) q6–8h prn; may repeat once 30–60 min after initial dose. Range: 0.15–0.6 mg q4–8h prn. **CHILDREN 2–12 YRS:** 2–6 mcg/kg q4–6h prn.

Usual Elderly Dosage
IM/IV: 0.15 mg q6h prn.

Sublingual: **ADULTS, ELDERLY:** For pts taking heroin/other short-acting opioids, give at least 4 hrs after pt last used opioids or when early signs of withdrawal appear. Maintenance: 16 mg/day. Range: 4–24 mg/day.

Transdermal: **ADULTS, ELDERLY: (OPIOID NAIVE):** Initial dose always 5 mcg/hr once q7days. **THOSE ALREADY RECEIVING OPIOIDS:** Refer to conversion chart in package insert. Do not increase dose until pt exposed to previous dose for 72 hrs.

SIDE EFFECTS

Frequent: Sedation (67%), dizziness, nausea (10%). **Butrans (more than 5%):** Nausea, headache, pruritus at application site, dizziness, rash, vomiting, constipation, dry mouth. **Occasional (5%–1%):** Headache, hypotension, vomiting, miosis, diaphoresis. **Rare (less than 1%):** Dry mouth, pallor, visual abnormalities, injection site reaction.

ADVERSE EFFECTS/ TOXIC REACTIONS

Overdosage results in cold, clammy skin, weakness, confusion, severe respiratory depression, cyanosis, pinpoint pupils, seizures, extreme drowsiness progressing to stupor, coma.

NURSING CONSIDERATIONS

BASELINE ASSESSMENT

Obtain baseline B/P, pulse rate. Assess mental status, alertness. Assess type, location, intensity of pain. Obtain history of pt's last opioid use. Assess for early signs of withdrawal symptoms before initiating therapy.

INTERVENTION/EVALUATION

Monitor for change in respirations, B/P, rate/quality of pulse, mental status. Assess lab results. Initiate deep breathing, coughing exercises, particularly in those with pulmonary impairment. Assess for clinical improvement; record onset of relief of pain.

PATIENT/FAMILY TEACHING

• Change positions slowly to avoid dizziness, orthostatic hypotension. • Avoid tasks that require alertness, motor skills until response to drug is established. • Avoid alcohol, sedatives, antidepressants, tranquilizers.

*buPROPion

bue-**proe**-pee-on
(Aplenzin, Budeprion SR, Buproban, Forfivo XL, Wellbutrin, Wellbutrin SR, Wellbutrin XL, Zyban)

BLACK BOX ALERT Increased risk of suicidal thinking and behavior in children, adolescents, young adults 18–24 yrs with major depressive disorder, other psychiatric disorders. Agitation, hostility, depressed mood also reported. Use in smoking cessation may cause serious neuropsychiatric events.
Do not confuse Aplenzin with Relenza, bupropion with buspirone, Wellbutrin SR with Wellbutrin XL, or Zyban with Diovan or Zagam.

CLASSIFICATION

PHARMACOTHERAPEUTIC: Aminoketone. **CLINICAL:** Antidepressant, smoking cessation aid (see pp. 41C, 153C).

ACTION

Blocks reuptake of neurotransmitters, (serotonin, norepinephrine) at CNS presynaptic membranes, increasing availability at postsynaptic receptor sites. Reduces firing rate of noradrenergic neurons. **Therapeutic Effect:** Relieves depression. Eliminates nicotine withdrawal symptoms.

PHARMACOKINETICS

Rapidly absorbed from GI tract. Protein binding: 84%. Crosses the blood-brain barrier. Undergoes extensive first-pass metabolism in liver to active metabolite. Primarily excreted in urine. **Half-life:** 14 hrs.

USES

Treatment of depression, particularly endogenous depression, exhibited as persistent and prominent dysphoria (occurring nearly every day for at least 2 wks) manifested by 4 of 8 symptoms: appetite change, sleep pattern change, increased fatigue, impaired concentration, feelings of guilt or worthlessness, loss of interest in usual activities, psychomotor agitation or retardation, suicidal tendencies. Prevents depression in pts with seasonal affective disorder (SAD). Zyban assists in smoking cessation. **OFF-LABEL:** Treatment of ADHD in adults, children. Depression associated with bipolar disorder.

PRECAUTIONS

Contraindications: Current or prior diagnosis of anorexia nervosa or bulimia, seizure disorder, use within 14 days of MAOIs, concomitant use of other bupropion products, pts undergoing abrupt discontinuation of alcohol or sedatives. **Cautions:** History of seizure, cranial or head trauma, cardiovascular disease, history of hypertension or coronary artery disease, elderly, pts at high risk for suicide, renal/hepatic impairment.

⧗ LIFESPAN CONSIDERATIONS

Pregnancy/Lactation: Unknown if drug crosses placenta or is distributed in breast milk. **Pregnancy Category C. Children:** More sensitive to increased dosage, toxicity, increased risk of suicidal ideation, worsening of depression. Safety and efficacy not established in those younger than 18 yrs. **Elderly:** More sensitive to anticholinergic, sedative, cardiovascular effects. Age-related renal impairment may require dosage adjustment.

INTERACTIONS

DRUG: Ritonavir, efavirenz may reduce concentration. **Carbamazepine, phenobarbital, phenytoin** may decrease effectiveness. **MAOIs** may increase risk of toxicity. **Levodopa, amantadine** may increase risk of side effects. **HERBAL:** Gotu kola, kava kava, St. John's wort, valerian may increase CNS depression. **FOOD:** None known. **LAB VALUES:** May decrease WBC.

AVAILABILITY (Rx)

Tablets (Wellbutrin): 75 mg, 100 mg.

Tablets, Extended-Release: 174 mg, 348 mg, 522 mg (Aplenzin); 100 mg, 150 mg (Budeprion SR); 450 mg (Forfivo XL); 150 mg, 300 mg (Wellbutrin XL). Tablets (Sustained-Release): 100 mg, 150 mg, 200 mg (Wellbutrin SR), 150 mg (Zyban).

ADMINISTRATION/HANDLING

PO

• Give without regard to food (give with food if GI irritation occurs). • Give at least 4-hr interval for immediate onset and 8-hr interval for sustained-release tablet to avoid seizures. • Give Aplenzin once daily in the morning. • Avoid bedtime dosage (decreases risk of insomnia). • Do not crush, chew, or divide extended-release preparations.

INDICATIONS/ROUTES/DOSAGE

Depression

PO (Immediate-Release): ADULTS: Initially, 100 mg twice a day. May increase to 100 mg 3 times a day no sooner than 3 days after beginning therapy. **Maximum:** 150 mg 3 times/day. **ELDERLY:** Initially, 50–100 mg/day. May increase by 50–100 mg/day q3–4 days. Maintenance: Lowest effective dosage.

PO (Sustained-Release): ADULTS: Initially, 150 mg/day as a single dose in the morning. May increase to 150 mg twice a day as early as day 4 after beginning therapy. **Maximum:** 400 mg/day in 2 divided doses.

PO (Extended-Release): ADULTS: 150 mg once a day. May increase to 300 mg once a day. **Maximum:** 450 mg/day. **(Forfivo XL):** Use only after initial dose titration. **(Aplenzin):** Initially, 174 mg once daily in morning; may increase as soon as 4 days to 348 mg/day. **Maximum:** 522 mg/day.

Smoking Cessation

PO: ADULTS: (Zyban): Initially, 150 mg a day for 3 days, then 150 mg twice a day for 7–12 wks.

Prevention of Seasonal Affective Disorder

PO: ADULTS, ELDERLY: (Wellbutrin XL): 150 mg/day for 1 wk, then 300 mg/day.

Begin in autumn (Sept–Nov). End of treatment begins in spring (Mar–Apr) by decreasing dose to 150 mg/day for 2 wks before discontinuation. **(Aplenzin):** 174 mg once daily. May increase after 1 wk to 348 mg once daily.

Dosage in Hepatic Impairment

Mild to moderate: Use caution, reduce dosage. **Severe:** Use extreme caution. Maximum dose: Aplenzin: 174 mg every other day. Wellbutrin: 75 mg/day. Wellbutrin SR: 100 mg/day or 150 mg every other day. Wellbutrin XL: 150 mg every other day. Zyban: 150 mg every other day.

SIDE EFFECTS

Frequent (32%–18%): Constipation, weight gain or loss, nausea, vomiting, anorexia, dry mouth, headache, diaphoresis, tremor, sedation, insomnia, dizziness, agitation. **Occasional (10%–5%):** Diarrhea, akinesia, blurred vision, tachycardia, confusion, hostility, fatigue.

ADVERSE EFFECTS/ TOXIC REACTIONS

Risk of seizures increases in pts taking more than 150 mg/dose; history of bulimia, seizure disorders, discontinuing drugs that may lower seizure threshold.

NURSING CONSIDERATIONS

BASELINE ASSESSMENT

Assess psychological status, thought content, suicidal tendencies, appearance. For those on long-term therapy, hepatic/renal function tests should be performed periodically.

INTERVENTION/EVALUATION

Supervise suicidal-risk pt closely during early therapy and dose changes (as depression lessens, energy level improves, increasing suicide potential). Assess appearance, behavior, speech pattern, level of interest, mood changes.

PATIENT/FAMILY TEACHING

• Full therapeutic effect may be noted in 4 wks. • Avoid tasks that require alertness, motor skills until response to drug is established. • Report signs/symptoms of seizure, worsening depression, suicidal ideation, unusual behavioral changes. • Avoid alcohol.

*busPIRone

bue-**spye**-rone
(Apo-Buspirone ♣, BuSpar ♣, Bustab ♣, Novo-Buspirone ♣)
Do not confuse buspirone with bupropion.

◆ CLASSIFICATION

PHARMACOTHERAPEUTIC: Nonbarbiturate. **CLINICAL:** Antianxiety (see p. 15C).

ACTION

Binds to serotonin, dopamine at presynaptic neurotransmitter receptors in CNS. **Therapeutic Effect:** Produces anxiolytic effect.

PHARMACOKINETICS

Rapidly and completely absorbed from GI tract. Protein binding: 95%. Undergoes extensive first-pass metabolism. Metabolized in liver to active metabolite. Primarily excreted in urine. Not removed by hemodialysis. **Half-life:** 2–3 hrs.

USES

Short-term management (up to 4 wks) of generalized anxiety disorder (GAD). **OFF-LABEL:** Augmenting medication for antidepressants; management of aggression in mentally challenged, secondary mental disorders, major depression; premenstrual syndrome (aches, pain, fatigue, irritability).

PRECAUTIONS

Contraindications: None known. **Cautions:** Concurrent use of MAOIs, severe hepatic/renal impairment.

LIFESPAN CONSIDERATIONS

Pregnancy/Lactation: Unknown if drug crosses placenta or is distributed in breast milk. **Pregnancy Category B. Children:** Safety and efficacy not established. **Elderly:** No age-related precautions noted.

INTERACTIONS

DRUG: Alcohol, other CNS depressants potentiate effects, may increase sedation. **CYP3A4 inhibitors (e.g., erythromycin, ketoconazole)** may increase concentration/effect. **CYP3A4 inducers (e.g., rifampin)** may decrease concentration/effect. May increase effects of **MAOIs. HERBAL: Gotu kola, kava kava, St. John's wort, valerian** may increase CNS depression. **FOOD: Grapefruit, grapefruit juice** may increase concentration, risk of toxicity. **LAB VALUES:** May produce false positive for urine metanephrine/catecholamine assay test.

AVAILABILITY (Rx)

Tablets: 5 mg, 7.5 mg, 10 mg, 15 mg, 30 mg.

ADMINISTRATION/HANDLING

PO
• Give without regard to food. • Tablets may be crushed.

INDICATIONS/ROUTES/DOSAGE

Short-Term Management (up to 4 wks) of Anxiety Disorders
PO: ADULTS: 5 mg 2–3 times a day or 7.5 mg twice a day. May increase by 5 mg/day every 2–4 days. Maintenance: 15–30 mg/day in 2–3 divided doses. **Maximum:** 60 mg/day. **ELDERLY:** Initially, 5 mg twice a day. May increase by 5 mg/day every 2–3 days. **Maximum:** 60 mg/day. **CHILDREN 6 YRS AND OLDER:** Initially, 5 mg/day. May increase by 5 mg/day at weekly intervals. **Maximum:** 60 mg/day in 2–3 divided doses.

SIDE EFFECTS

Frequent (12%–6%): Dizziness, drowsiness, nausea, headache. **Occasional (5%–2%):** Nervousness, fatigue, insomnia, dry mouth, light-headedness, mood swings, blurred vision, poor concentration, diarrhea, paresthesia. **Rare:** Muscle pain/stiffness, nightmares, chest pain, involuntary movements.

ADVERSE EFFECTS/ TOXIC REACTIONS

No evidence of drug tolerance, psychological or physical dependence, withdrawal syndrome. Overdose may produce severe nausea, vomiting, dizziness, drowsiness, abdominal distention, excessive pupil constriction.

NURSING CONSIDERATIONS

BASELINE ASSESSMENT

Assess degree/manifestations of anxiety. Offer emotional support to anxious pt. Assess motor responses (agitation, trembling, tension), autonomic responses (cold, clammy hands; diaphoresis).

INTERVENTION/EVALUATION

For those on long-term therapy, CBC, hepatic/renal function tests should be performed periodically. Assist with ambulation if drowsiness, light-headedness occur. Evaluate for therapeutic response: calm facial expression, decreased restlessness, insomnia, mental status.

PATIENT/FAMILY TEACHING

• Improvement may be noted in 7–10 days, but optimum therapeutic effect generally takes 3–4 wks. • Drowsiness usually disappears during continued therapy. • If dizziness occurs, change position slowly from recumbent to sitting position before standing. • Avoid tasks that require alertness, motor skills until response to drug is established. • Avoid alcohol, grapefruit products.

---

busulfan `HIGH ALERT`

bue-**sul**-fan
(Busulfex, Myleran)

BLACK BOX ALERT Must be administered by certified chemotherapy personnel. Major effect characterized by severe bone marrow suppression. **Do not confuse Myleran with Alkeran, Leukeran, or Mylicon.**

◆CLASSIFICATION

PHARMACOTHERAPEUTIC: Alkylating agent. **CLINICAL:** Antineoplastic (see p. 83C).

ACTION

Interferes with DNA replication, RNA synthesis. Cell cycle–phase nonspecific. **Therapeutic Effect:** Disrupts nucleic acid function. Myelosuppressant.

PHARMACOKINETICS

Completely absorbed from GI tract. Protein binding: 33%. Metabolized in liver. Primarily excreted in urine. Minimally removed by hemodialysis. **Half-life:** 2.5 hrs.

USES

PO: Treatment of chronic myelogenous leukemia (CML), conditioning regimen for bone marrow transplant. **IV:** Conditioning regimen prior to allogeneic hematopoietic progenitor cell transplantation for chronic myelogenous leukemia. **OFF-LABEL:** Treatment of acute myelocytic leukemia. **PO:** Bone marrow disorders (e.g., polycythemia vera), Thrombocytosis.

PRECAUTIONS

Contraindications: PO treatment without a definitive diagnosis of CML. **Extreme Caution:** Compromised bone marrow reserve. **Cautions:** History of seizure disorder, head trauma.

⌛ LIFESPAN CONSIDERATIONS

Pregnancy/Lactation: Avoid use during pregnancy, esp. first trimester. May cause fetal harm. Unknown if distributed in breast milk. Breast-feeding not recommended. **Pregnancy Category D. Children/Elderly:** No age-related precautions noted.

INTERACTIONS

DRUG: Cytotoxic agents may increase cytotoxicity. **Bone marrow depressants** may increase risk of myelosuppression. **Live virus vaccines** may potentiate virus replication, increase vaccine side effects, decrease antibody response to vaccine. **HERBAL: St. John's wort** may decrease concentration. **Echinacea** may decrease effects. **FOOD:** None known. **LAB VALUES:** May decrease serum magnesium, potassium, phosphate, sodium. May increase serum glucose, calcium, bilirubin, AST, ALT, creatinine, alkaline phosphatase, BUN.

AVAILABILITY (Rx)

Injection Solution (Busulfex): 6 mg/ml.
Tablets (Myleran): 2 mg.

ADMINISTRATION/HANDLING

◀ALERT▶ May be carcinogenic, mutagenic, teratogenic. Handle with extreme care during administration. Use of gloves recommended. If contact occurs with skin/mucosa, wash thoroughly with water.

 IV

Reconstitution • Dilute with 0.9% NaCl or D₅W only. Diluent quantity must be 10 times the volume of busulfan (e.g., 9.3 ml busulfan must be diluted with 93 ml diluent). • Use filter to withdraw busulfan from ampule. • Add busulfan to calculated diluent. • Use infusion pump to administer busulfan.
Rate of Administration • Infuse over 2 hrs. • Before and after infusion, flush catheter line with 5 ml 0.9% NaCl or D₅W.
Storage • Refrigerate ampules. • Following dilution, stable for 8 hrs at room temperature, 12 hrs if refrigerated when diluted with 0.9% NaCl. • Infusion must be completed within 8- or 12-hr time frame.

PO
• May give without regard to meals.

🔲 IV INCOMPATIBILITIES

Do not mix busulfan with any other medications.

INDICATIONS/ROUTES/DOSAGE

Remission Induction in CML
PO: ADULTS, ELDERLY: Induction: 4–8 mg/day or 0.06 mg/kg/day. **Maintenance:** 1–4 mg/day to 2 mg/wk. Reduce dose in proportion to decrease in leukocyte count or discontinue when leukocyte count falls to ≤20,000/mm³. **CHILDREN:** 0.06–0.12 mg/kg/day. **Maintenance:** Titrate to maintain leukocyte count above 40,000/mm³, reduce dose by 50% if count is 30,000–40,000/mm³, and discontinue if the count is 20,000/mm³ or less.

Marrow Ablative Conditioning and Bone Marrow Transplantation
IV: ADULTS, ELDERLY, CHILDREN WEIGHING MORE THAN 12 KG: 0.8 mg/kg/dose q6h for total of 16 doses. (Use ideal body weight [IBW] or actual body weight [ABW], whichever is lower.) **CHILDREN WEIGHING 12 KG OR LESS:** 1.1 mg/kg/dose (IBW) q6h for 16 doses.
PO: ADULTS, ELDERLY, CHILDREN: 1 mg/kg/dose (IBW) q6h for 16 doses (in combination with cyclophosphamide).

SIDE EFFECTS

Expected (98%–72%): Nausea, stomatitis, vomiting, anorexia, insomnia, diarrhea, fever, abdominal pain, anxiety. **Frequent (69%–44%):** Headache, rash, asthenia (loss of strength, energy), infection, chills, tachycardia, dyspepsia. **Occasional (38%–16%):** Constipation, dizziness, edema, pruritus, cough, dry mouth, depression, abdominal enlargement, pharyngitis, hiccups, back pain, alopecia, myalgia. **Rare (13%–5%):** Injection site pain, arthralgia, confusion, hypotension, lethargy.

ADVERSE EFFECTS/ TOXIC REACTIONS

Major adverse effect is myelosuppression resulting in hematologic toxicity (anemia, severe leukopenia, severe thrombocytopenia). Very high dosages may produce blurred vision, muscle twitching, tonic-clonic seizures. Long-term therapy (more than 4 yrs) may produce pulmonary syndrome ("busulfan lung"), characterized by persistent cough, congestion, adventitious breath sounds (rales, crackles), dyspnea. Hyperuricemia may produce uric acid nephropathy, renal calculi, acute renal failure.

NURSING CONSIDERATIONS

BASELINE ASSESSMENT
CBC with differential, hepatic/renal function studies should be performed weekly (dosage based on hematologic values).

INTERVENTION/EVALUATION
Monitor lab values diligently for evidence of bone marrow depression. Assess oral cavity for onset of stomatitis (redness/ulceration of oral mucous membranes, gum inflammation, difficulty swallowing). Initiate antiemetics to prevent nausea/vomiting. Monitor daily pattern of bowel activity, stool consistency.

PATIENT/FAMILY TEACHING
• Educate pt/family regarding expected effects of therapy. • Maintain adequate daily fluid intake (may protect against renal impairment). • Report persistent cough, congestion, difficulty breathing. • Promptly report fever, sore throat, signs of local infection, unusual bruising/bleeding from any site. • Report signs of abrupt weakness, fatigue, weight loss, nausea, vomiting. • Do not have immunizations without physician's approval (drug lowers body's resistance). • Avoid contact with those who have recently received live virus vaccine. • Take medication at same time each day. • Contraception is recommended during therapy.

cabazitaxel

ka-**baz**-i-**tax**-el
(Jevtana)

BLACK BOX ALERT All pts should be premedicated with a corticosteroid, an antihistamine, and an H₂ antagonist prior to infusion. Severe hypersensitivity reaction has occurred. Immediately discontinue infusion and give appropriate treatment if hypersensitivity reaction occurs. Neutropenic deaths reported. CBC, particularly ANC, should be obtained prior to and during treatment. Do not administer with neutrophil count 1,500/mm³ or less.

Do not confuse cabazitaxel with paclitaxel or Paxil, or Jevtana with Januvia, Levitra, or Sentra.

◆ CLASSIFICATION

PHARMACOTHERAPEUTIC: Microtubule inhibitor. **CLINICAL:** Antineoplastic (see p. 83C).

ACTION

Disrupts microtubular cell network, essential for cellular function. Results in inhibition of mitotic and interphase cellular functions. **Therapeutic Effect:** Blocks cells in mitotic phase of cell cycle, leading to cell death.

PHARMACOKINETICS

Widely distributed. Protein binding: 89%–92%. Metabolized in liver. Excreted in feces (76%), urine (3.7%). **Half-life:** 95 hrs.

USES

Used in combination with prednisone for treatment of hormone-refractory metastatic prostate cancer previously treated with docetaxel-containing regimen.

PRECAUTIONS

Contraindications: Those with neutrophil count of 1,500/mm³ or less, history of hypersensitivity to polysorbate 80. **Caution:** Severe hepatic impairment (bilirubin equal to or greater than ULN or AST and/or ALT over 1.5 times ULN), elderly, pregnancy, renal impairment (creatinine clearance less than 50 ml/min). Avoid concurrent use of strong CYP3A4 inhibitors (e.g., atazanavir, clarithromycin, indinavir, itraconazole, ketoconazole, nelfinavir, ritonavir, saquinavir, voriconazole). Concurrent use of moderate CYP3A4 inhibitors (e.g., diltiazem, erythromycin, fluconazole, fosamprenavir, verapamil) or strong CYP3A4 inducers (e.g., carbamazepine, phenytoin, rifampin).

⌛ LIFESPAN CONSIDERATIONS

Pregnancy/Lactation: May cause fetal harm. Crosses placental barrier. Do not breastfeed. **Pregnancy Category D. Children:** Safety and effectiveness not established. **Elderly:** Those 65 yrs and older have 5% greater risk of developing neutropenia, fatigue, dizziness, fever, urinary tract infection, dehydration.

INTERACTIONS

DRUG: Concurrent use of strong **CYP3A4 inhibitors (atazanavir, clarithromycin, indinavir, itraconazole, ketoconazole, nefazodone, nelfinavir, ritonavir, saquinavir, voriconazole)** may increase concentration of cabazitaxel and is not recommended. Strong **CYP3A4 inducers (carbamazepine, phenobarbital, phenytoin, rifabutin, rifampin, rifapentine)** may decrease cabazitaxel concentration. **Live virus vaccine** may potentiate virus replication, increase vaccine's side effects, decrease response to vaccine. **HERBAL: St. John's wort, valerian** may increase CNS depression. **Echinacea** may decrease effect. **FOOD: Grapefruit, grapefruit juice** may increase concentration/effects. **LAB VALUES:** May increase serum bilirubin AST, ALT. May decrease Hgb, Hct, neutrophils, platelets.

AVAILABILITY (Rx)

Injection, Single-Use Vials, 2 per Kit: 60 mg/1.5 ml polysorbate 80 vial and one vial containing 13% ethanol (in diluent).

✚ Canadian trade name   🚫 Non-Crushable Drug   🔴 High Alert drug

ADMINISTRATION/HANDLING

◄ALERT► Wear gloves during preparation, handling. Two-step dilution process must be performed under aseptic conditions to prepare second (final) infusion solution. Medication undergoes two dilutions. After second dilution, administration should be initiated within 30 min.

Reconstitution

Step 1, First Dilution: • Each vial of cabazitaxel contains 60 mg/1.5 ml; must first be mixed with entire contents of supplied diluent. • Once reconstituted, resultant solution contains 10 mg/ml of cabazitaxel. • When transferring diluent, direct needle onto inside vial wall and inject slowly to limit foaming. • Remove syringe and needle, then gently mix initial diluted solution by repeated inversions for at least 45 sec to ensure full mixing of drug and diluent. • Do not shake. • Allow any foam to dissipate.

Step 2, Final Dilution: • Withdraw recommended dose and further dilute with 250 ml 0.9% NaCl or D$_5$W. • If dose greater than 65 mg is required, use larger volume of 0.9% NaCl or D$_5$W so that concentration of 0.26 mg/ml is not exceeded. • Concentration of final infusion should be between 0.10 and 0.26 mg/ml.

Rate of Administration • Use in-line 0.22-micron filter during administration. • Infuse over 1 hr.

Storage • Store vials at room temperature. • First dilution solution stable for 30 min. • Final dilution solution stable for 8 hrs at room temperature or 24 hrs if refrigerated.

INDICATIONS/ROUTES/DOSAGE

◄ALERT► Antihistamine (dexchlorpheniramine 5 mg, diphenhydramine 25 mg, or equivalent antihistamine), corticosteroid (dexamethasone 8 mg or equivalent steroid), and H$_2$ antagonist (ranitidine 50 mg or equivalent H$_2$ antagonist) should be given at least 30 min prior to each dose to reduce risk/severity of hypersensitivity.

Hormone-Refractory Metastatic Prostate Cancer

◄ALERT► Monitoring of CBC is essential on weekly basis during cycle 1 and before each treatment cycle thereafter so that the dose can be adjusted.

IV Infusion: ADULTS, ELDERLY: 25 mg/m^2 given as 1-hr infusion every 3 wks in combination with 10 mg prednisone daily throughout treatment. **Dose modifications: grade 3 neutropenia, febrile neutropenia, severe or persistent diarrhea:** Reduce dosage to 20 mg/m^2.

SIDE EFFECTS

Frequent (47%–16%): Diarrhea, fatigue, nausea, vomiting, constipation, esthesia (decreased sensitivity to touch), abdominal pain, anorexia, back pain. **Occasional (13%–5%):** Peripheral neuropathy, fever, dyspnea, cough, arthralgia, dysgeusia, dyspepsia, alopecia, peripheral edema, weight decrease, urinary tract infection, dizziness, headache, muscle spasm, dysuria, hematuria, mucosal inflammation, dehydration.

ADVERSE EFFECTS/ TOXIC REACTIONS

Hypersensitivity reaction may include generalized rash, erythema, hypotension, bronchospasm. 94% of pts develop grade 1–4 neutropenia and associated complications, including anemia, thrombocytopenia, sepsis. GI abnormalities, hypertension, arrhythmias, renal failure may occur.

NURSING CONSIDERATIONS

BASELINE ASSESSMENT

Offer emotional support. Obtain baseline EKG, electrolytes, CBC, liver function test, testosterone levels prior to initiation of therapy.

INTERVENTION/EVALUATION

Assess CBC, ANC prior to each infusion. Monitoring of CBC, ANC on weekly basis during cycle 1 and before each treatment cycle thereafter; do not administer if ANC less than 1,500 cells/mm³. Monitor ALT, AST. Monitor for hypersensitivity reaction (rash, erythema, dyspnea). Encourage adequate fluid intake. Monitor daily pattern of bowel activity, stool consistency. Offer antiemetics if nausea, vomiting occur. Closely monitor for signs/symptoms of neutropenia.

PATIENT/FAMILY TEACHING

• Report fever, chills, persistent sore throat, unusual bruising/bleeding, pale skin, fatigue. • Avoid tasks that require alertness, motor skills until response to drug is established. • Maintain strict oral hygiene. • Do not have immunizations without physician approval (drug lowers body's resistance). • Avoid those who have received a live virus vaccine. • Avoid crowds, those with cough, sneezing.

cabozantinib

ka-boe-**zan**-ti-nib
(Cometriq)
BLACK BOX ALERT Complications including GI perforation and fistula formation have occurred. Severe and sometimes fatal hemorrhaging including hemoptysis, GI bleeding occurred in 3% of pts. Discontinue if visceral perforation, fistula formation (GI, tracheal/esophageal), severe hemorrhaging occurs.

◆ CLASSIFICATION

PHARMACOTHERAPEUTIC: Tyrosine kinase inhibitor. **CLINICAL:** Antineoplastic.

ACTION

Inhibits tyrosine kinase activity in tumor cells. Inhibits cell migration, proliferation, survival, and angiogenesis (new blood vessel formation). **Therapeutic Effect:** Inhibits thyroid tumor cell growth and metastasis.

PHARMACOKINETICS

Well absorbed after PO administration. Metabolized in liver. Protein binding: greater than 99%. Peak plasma concentration: 2–5 hrs. Excreted in feces (54%), urine (27%). **Half-life:** 55 hrs.

USES

Treatment of progressive, metastatic medullary thyroid cancer.

PRECAUTIONS

Contraindications: None known. **Cautions:** Moderate to severe hepatic impairment, baseline thrombocytopenia, anemia, neutropenia, recent surgery or dental procedures, open wounds, chronic electrolyte imbalance, dehydration, diarrhea, hypertension, recent history of hemorrhage or hemoptysis.

⌛ LIFESPAN CONSIDERATIONS

Pregnancy/Lactation: May cause fetal harm. Not recommended in nursing mothers. Must either discontinue drug or discontinue breastfeeding. Unknown if distributed in breast milk. Contraception recommended during treatment and up to 4 mos after discontinuation. **Pregnancy Category D. Children:** Safety and efficacy not established. **Elderly:** No age-related precautions noted.

INTERACTIONS

DRUG: CYP3A4 inhibitors (e.g., **atazanavir, clarithromycin, itraconazole, ketoconazole, saquinavir, voriconazole**) may increase concentration. CYP3A4 inducers (e.g., **carbamazepine, phenobarbital, phenytoin, rifampin**) may decrease concentration. **HERBAL:** St. John's wort may decrease effect. **FOOD:** **Grapefruit, grapefruit juice** may increase concentration. **High fatty meals** may increase absorption/ exposure. **LAB VALUES:** May decrease lymphocytes, neutrophils, platelets, se-

---

rum calcium, magnesium, phosphorus, potassium, sodium. May increase serum ALT, AST, alkaline phosphatase, bilirubin, lipase, TSH, urine protein.

AVAILABILITY (Rx)

Capsules: 20 mg, 80 mg.

ADMINISTRATION/HANDLING

PO
• Give on empty stomach only; do not eat for at least 2 hrs before or 1 hr after administration. • Give with water. • Avoid grapefruit juice. • Do not break, crush, dissolve, or divide capsules.

INDICATIONS/ROUTES/DOSAGE

Metastatic Medullary Thyroid Cancer
PO: ADULTS: 140 mg once daily.

Dosage Modification
Hematologic/Nonhematologic Reaction, Drug Intolerance: Interrupt treatment and restart at 100 mg once daily (if previously taking 140 mg), or 60 mg once daily (if previously taking 100 mg). If previously taking 60 mg/day, resume 60 mg once daily once effects resolve.

SIDE EFFECTS

Frequent (63%–34%): Diarrhea, stomatitis, weight loss, decreased appetite, nausea, fatigue, oral pain, dysgeusia. **Occasional (27%–7%):** Constipation, abdominal pain, vomiting, asthenia, dysphonia, dry skin, headache, alopecia, dizziness, arthralgia, dysphagia, muscle spasms, erythema, dyspepsia, anxiety, musculoskeletal pain, paresthesia, peripheral neuropathy, hyperkeratosis.

ADVERSE EFFECTS/ TOXIC REACTIONS

May cause GI perforation (3%), GI fistula formation (1%), severe GI hemorrhaging (3%). Malignant hypertension may occur despite continued medical management. Thromboembolic events including venous/arterial thromboembolism, cerebral infarction, myocardial infarction have been reported. May cause ineffective wound healing or wound dehiscence requiring medical intervention. Osteonecrosis of the jaw may include mandibular pain, jaw bone erosion, periodontal/gingival infection or ulceration, osteomyelitis, impaired healing of the mouth after dental procedures. Palmar-plantar erythrodysesthesia syndrome (PPES), a chemotherapy-induced skin condition that presents as redness, swelling, numbness, skin sloughing of the hands and feet, has been reported. Reversible posterior leukoencephalopathy syndrome (RPLS) was reported in less than 1% of pts. Proteinuria may indicate nephrotic syndrome.

NURSING CONSIDERATIONS

BASELINE ASSESSMENT

Obtain vital signs, baseline CBC, serum chemistries, magnesium, phosphate, ionized calcium, urinalysis. Assess for recent surgeries, dental procedures. Question for possibility of pregnancy, current breastfeeding status. Obtain negative urine pregnancy before initiating treatment. Obtain full medication history including vitamins, supplements, herbal products. Question for history of hypertension, hepatic impairment.

INTERVENTION/EVALUATION

Monitor CBC, electrolytes, urinalysis. Routinely assess vital signs and report any change in blood pressure. Persistent diastolic hypertension may indicate hypertensive crisis. Reversible posterior leukoencephalopathy syndrome should be considered in pts with seizure, headache, visual disturbances, confusion, altered mental status. Assess hydration status; encourage PO intake; monitor daily pattern of bowel activity, stool consistency. Immediately report any hemorrhaging, bloody stools, abdominal pain, hemoptysis (may indicate GI perforation/ fistula formation). Obtain EKG for palpitations, chest pain, hypokalemia, hyperkalemia, hypocalcemia, bradycardia, ventricular arrhythmias.

PATIENT/FAMILY TEACHING

• Blood levels will be routinely monitored. • Strictly avoid pregnancy. • Contraception should be utilized during treatment and up to 4 mos after discontinuation. • Report any yellowing of skin or eyes, abdominal pain, bruising, black/tarry stools, dark urine, decreased urine output, skin changes. • Report neurologic changes including altered mental status, seizures, headache, blurry vision, difficulty speaking, one-sided weakness (may indicate stroke, high blood pressure crisis, or life-threatening brain swelling). • Do not take herbal supplements. • Report any jaw pain or oral lesions, skin changes including skin sloughing or rash. • Notify physician before any planned surgeries or dental procedures. • Do not ingest grapefruit products. • Do not take with food; wait at least 2 hrs before or 1 hr after.

---

caffeine citrate

kaf-een **sit**-rate
(Cafcit)

◆CLASSIFICATION

PHARMACOTHERAPEUTIC: Citrate salt of caffeine. **CLINICAL:** Bronchial smooth muscle relaxant.

ACTION

Stimulates medullary respiratory center. Appears to increase sensitivity of respiratory center to stimulatory effects of CO_2. **Therapeutic Effect:** Increases alveolar ventilation, reducing severity, frequency of apneic episodes.

USES

Short-term treatment of apnea in premature infants from 28 wks to younger than 33 wks gestational age.

PRECAUTIONS

Pregnancy Category C.

INTERACTIONS

DRUG: CNS stimulants may cause excessive CNS stimulation (e.g., nervousness, insomnia, seizures, arrhythmias). **CYP1A2 inhibitors (e.g., cimetidine, ciprofloxacin)** may increase concentration, risk of side effects. **HERBAL:** None significant. **FOOD:** None known. **LAB VALUES:** May increase or decrease serum glucose.

AVAILABILITY (Rx)

Injection Solution: 20 mg/ml. **Oral Solution:** 20 mg/ml.

ADMINISTRATION/HANDLING

PO
• May give without regard to meals. • May administer injectable solution orally.
IV
• Infuse loading dose over at least 30 min; maintenance dose over at least 10 min. • May give without further dilution.

▓ IV COMPATIBILITIES

Alprostadil, calcium gluconate, cefotoxime, dexamethasone, dobutamine, dopamine, gentamicin, heparin, vancomycin.

▓ IV INCOMPATIBILITIES

Acyclovir, furosemide.

INDICATIONS/ROUTES/DOSAGE

Apnea
PO, IV: Loading dose: 10–20 mg/kg as caffeine citrate (5–10 mg/kg as caffeine base). If theophylline given within previous 72 hrs, a modified dose (50%–75%) may be given. Maintenance: 5 mg/kg/day as caffeine citrate (2.5 mg/kg/day as caffeine base) starting 24 hrs after loading dose. Dosage adjusted based on pt response. **Maximum:** 20 mg/kg/day.

SIDE EFFECTS

Frequent (10%–5%): Feeding intolerance, rash.

ADVERSE EFFECTS/ TOXIC REACTIONS

Sepsis, necrotizing enterocolitis may occur.

NURSING CONSIDERATIONS

BASELINE ASSESSMENT

Baseline serum caffeine levels should be measured in infants previously treated with theophylline (preterm infants metabolize theophylline to caffeine).

INTERVENTION/EVALUATION

Monitor respirations diligently. Assess skin for rash. Monitor heart rate, number/severity of apnea spells, serum caffeine levels.

calcitonin

kal-si-**toe**-nin
(Apo-Calcitonin ✤, Calcimar ✤, Caltine ✤, Fortical, Miacalcin)
Do not confuse calcitonin with calcitriol, or Miacalcin with Micatin.

◆**CLASSIFICATION**

PHARMACOTHERAPEUTIC: Synthetic hormone. **CLINICAL:** Calcium regulator, bone resorption inhibitor (see p. 143C).

ACTION

Decreases osteoclast activity in bones, decreases tubular reabsorption of sodium and calcium in kidneys, increases absorption of calcium in GI tract. **Therapeutic Effect:** Regulates serum calcium concentrations.

PHARMACOKINETICS

Nasal form rapidly absorbed. Injection form rapidly metabolized primarily in kidneys; primarily excreted in urine. **Half-life: Nasal:** 43 min; **Injection:** 70–90 min.

USES

Parenteral: Treatment of Paget's disease, hypercalcemia, postmenopausal osteoporosis. **Intranasal**: Postmenopausal osteoporosis. **OFF-LABEL**: Treatment of secondary osteoporosis due to drug therapy or hormone disturbance.

PRECAUTIONS

Contraindications: Hypersensitivity to salmon protein. **Cautions:** None known.

⧖ LIFESPAN CONSIDERATIONS

Pregnancy/Lactation: Does not cross placenta; unknown if distributed in breast milk. Safe usage during lactation not established (inhibits lactation in animals). **Pregnancy Category C. Children:** Safety and efficacy not established. **Elderly:** No age-related precautions noted.

INTERACTIONS

DRUG: May decrease **lithium** concentration/effects. **HERBAL:** None significant. **FOOD:** None known. **LAB VALUES:** None significant.

AVAILABILITY (Rx)

Injection Solution (Miacalcin): 200 international units/ml (calcitonin-salmon). **Nasal Spray (Fortical, Miacalcin Nasal):** 200 international units/activation (calcitonin-salmon).

ADMINISTRATION/HANDLING

IM, Subcutaneous
• IM route preferred if injection volume greater than 2 ml. Subcutaneous injection for outpatient self-administration unless volume greater than 2 ml. • Skin test should be performed before therapy in pts suspected of sensitivity to calcitonin. • Bedtime administration may reduce nausea, flushing.

Intranasal
• Refrigerate unopened nasal spray. Store at room temperature after initial use. • Instruct pt to clear nasal passages. • Tilt head slightly forward. • Insert

spray tip into nostril, pointing toward nasal passages, away from nasal septum.
• Spray into one nostril while pt holds other nostril closed and concurrently inspires through nose to deliver medication as high into nasal passage as possible. Spray into one nostril daily.

INDICATIONS/ROUTES/DOSAGE

Skin Testing before Treatment in Pts with Suspected Sensitivity to Calcitonin-Salmon

Intracutaneous: ADULTS, ELDERLY: Prepare a 10-international units/ml dilution; withdraw 0.05 ml from a 200-international units/ml vial in a tuberculin syringe; fill up to 1 ml with 0.9% NaCl. Give 0.1 ml intradermally on inner aspect of forearm. Observe after 15 min; a positive response is the appearance of more than mild erythema or wheal.

Paget's Disease

IM, Subcutaneous: ADULTS, ELDERLY: Initially, 100 international units/day. Maintenance: 50 international units/day or 50–100 international units every 1–3 days.

Postmenopausal Osteoporosis

IM, Subcutaneous: ADULTS, ELDERLY: 100 international units every other day with adequate calcium and vitamin D intake.

Intranasal: ADULTS, ELDERLY: 200 international units/day as a single spray, alternating nostrils daily.

Hypercalcemia

IM, Subcutaneous: ADULTS, ELDERLY: Initially, 4 international units/kg q12h; may increase to 8 international units/kg q12h if no response in 2 days; may further increase to 8 international units/kg q6h if no response in another 2 days.

SIDE EFFECTS

Frequent: IM, Subcutaneous (10%): Nausea (may occur soon after injection, usually diminishes with continued ther-

apy), inflammation at injection site. **Nasal (12%–10%):** Rhinitis, nasal irritation, redness, mucosal lesions. **Occasional: IM, Subcutaneous (5%–2%):** Flushing of face, hands. **Nasal (5%–3%):** Back pain, arthralgia, epistaxis, headache. **Rare: IM, Subcutaneous:** Epigastric discomfort, dry mouth, diarrhea, flatulence. **Nasal:** Itching of earlobes, pedal edema, rash, diaphoresis.

ADVERSE EFFECTS/ TOXIC REACTIONS

Pts with a protein allergy may develop a hypersensitivity reaction (rash, dyspnea, hypotension, tachycardia).

NURSING CONSIDERATIONS

BASELINE ASSESSMENT
Establish baseline serum electrolyte levels.

INTERVENTION/EVALUATION
Ensure rotation of injection sites; check for inflammation. Assess vertebral bone mass (document stabilization/improvement). Assess for allergic response: rash, urticaria, swelling, shortness of breath, tachycardia, hypotension. Monitor serum electrolytes, calcium, alkaline phosphatase.

PATIENT/FAMILY TEACHING
• Instruct pt/family on aseptic technique, proper injection method of subcutaneous medication, including rotation of sites, proper administration of nasal medication. • Nausea is transient and usually decreases over time. • Immediately report rash, itching, shortness of breath, significant nasal irritation. • Improvement in biochemical abnormalities and bone pain usually occurs in the first few months of treatment. • Improvement of neurologic lesions may take more than a year.

calcium acetate

(Eliphos, PhosLo)

 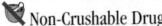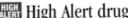

calcium carbonate

(Apo-Cal ✦, Caltrate 600 ✦, OsCal ✦, Titralac, Tums)

calcium chloride
calcium citrate

(Cal-Citrate, Citracal, Osteocit ✦)

calcium glubionate
calcium gluconate

kal-si-um
Do not confuse Citracal with Citrucel, OsCal with Asacol, or PhosLo with ProSom.

✦CLASSIFICATION

PHARMACOTHERAPEUTIC: Electrolyte replenisher. **CLINICAL:** Antacid, antihypocalcemic, antihyperkalemic, antihypermagnesemic, antihyperphosphatemic (see p. 13C).

ACTION

Essential for function, integrity of nervous, muscular, skeletal systems. Plays an important role in normal cardiac/renal function, respiration, blood coagulation, cell membrane and capillary permeability. Assists in regulating release/storage of neurotransmitters/hormones. Neutralizes/reduces gastric acid (increases pH). **Calcium acetate:** Binds with dietary phosphate, forming insoluble calcium phosphate. **Therapeutic Effect:** Replaces calcium in deficiency states; controls hyperphosphatemia in end-stage renal disease, relieves heartburn, indigestion.

PHARMACOKINETICS

Moderately absorbed from small intestine (absorption depends on presence of vitamin D metabolites, pH). Primarily eliminated in feces.

USES

Parenteral (calcium chloride, calcium gluconate): Acute hypocalcemia (e.g., neonatal hypocalcemic tetany, alkalosis), electrolyte depletion, cardiac arrest (strengthens myocardial contractions), hyperkalemia (reverses cardiac depression), hypermagnesemia (aids in reversing CNS depression). **Calcium carbonate:** Antacid, treatment/prevention of calcium deficiency, hyperphosphatemia. **Calcium citrate:** Antacid, treatment/prevention of calcium deficiency, hyperphosphatemia. **Calcium acetate:** Controls hyperphosphatemia in end-stage renal disease. **OFF-LABEL (Calcium chloride):** Calcium channel blocker overdose, severe hyperkalemia, malignant arrhythmias associated with hypermagnesemia.

PRECAUTIONS

Contraindications: All preparations: Calcium-based renal calculi, hypercalcemia, ventricular fibrillation. **Calcium chloride:** Digoxin toxicity. **Calcium gluconate: Neonates:** concurrent IV use with ceftriaxone. **Cautions:** Chronic renal impairment, hypokalemia, concurrent use with digoxin.

⌛ LIFESPAN CONSIDERATIONS

Pregnancy/Lactation: Distributed in breast milk. Unknown whether calcium chloride or gluconate is distributed in breast milk. **Pregnancy Category C. Children:** Extreme irritation, possible tissue necrosis or sloughing with IV. Restrict IV use due to small vasculature. **Elderly:** Oral absorption may be decreased.

INTERACTIONS

DRUG: Hypercalcemia may increase **digoxin** toxicity. Oral form may decrease absorption of **biphosphonates (e.g., risedronate), calcium channel blockers, tetracycline derivatives, thyroid products. HERBAL:** None significant. **FOOD:** Food may increase calcium absorption. **LAB VALUES:** May increase serum pH, calcium, gastrin. May decrease serum phosphate, potassium.

AVAILABILITY

CALCIUM ACETATE
Gelcap (PhosLo): 667 mg (equivalent to 169 mg elemental calcium). **Tablets (Eliphos):** 667 mg (equivalent to 169 mg elemental calcium).
CALCIUM CARBONATE
Tablets: 1,250 mg (equivalent to 500 mg elemental calcium); 1,500 mg (equivalent to 600 mg elemental calcium) (Caltrate 600). **Tablets (Chewable):** 500 mg (equivalent to 200 mg elemental calcium) (Tums); 1,250 mg (equivalent to 500 mg elemental calcium).
CALCIUM CHLORIDE
Injection Solution: 10% (100 mg/ml) equivalent to 27.2 mg elemental calcium per ml.
CALCIUM GLUBIONATE
Syrup: 1.8 g/5 ml (equivalent to 115 mg elemental calcium per 5 ml).
CALCIUM GLUCONATE
Injection Solution: 10% (equivalent to 9 mg elemental calcium per ml).

ADMINISTRATION/HANDLING

 IV

Dilution
Calcium Chloride • May give undiluted or may dilute with 0.9% NaCl or Sterile Water for Injection.
Calcium Gluconate • May give undiluted or may dilute with 100 ml 0.9% NaCl or D₅W.

Rate of Administration
Calcium Chloride • **Note:** Rapid administration may produce bradycardia, metallic/chalky taste, hypotension, sensation of heart, peripheral vasodilation. • **IV push:** Infuse slowly at maximum rate of 50–100 mg/min (in cardiac arrest, may administer over 10–20 sec). • **IV infusion:** Dilute to maximum final concentration of 20 mg/ml and infuse over 1 hr or no faster than 45–90 mg/kg/hr. Give via a central line. Do **NOT** use scalp, small hand or foot veins. Stop infusion if pt complains of pain or discomfort.

Calcium Gluconate • **Note:** Rapid administration may produce vasodilation, hypotension, arrhythmias, syncope, cardiac arrest. • **IV push:** Infuse slowly over 3–5 min or at maximum rate of 50–100 mg/min (in cardiac arrest, may administer over 10–20 sec). • **IV infusion:** Dilute 1–2 g in 100 ml 0.9% NaCl or D₅W and infuse over 1 hr.

Storage • Store at room temperature. • Once diluted, stable for 24 hrs at room temperature.

PO
Calcium Acetate • Administer with plenty of fluids during meals to optimize effectiveness.

Calcium Carbonate • Administer with or immediately following meals with plenty of water (give with meals if used for phosphate binding). Thoroughly chew chewable tablets before swallowing.

Calcium Citrate • Give without regard to food (give with food when used to treat hyperphosphatemia).

Calcium Glucobionate • Give with or following meals (give on empty stomach before meals when used to treat hyperphosphatemia).

▨ IV INCOMPATIBILITIES

Calcium chloride: Amphotericin B complex (Abelcet, AmBisome, Amphotec), pantoprazole (Protonix), phosphate-containing solutions, propofol (Diprivan), sodium bicarbonate. **Calcium gluconate:** Amphotericin B complex (Abelcet, AmBisome, Amphotec), fluconazole (Diflucan).

▨ IV COMPATIBILITIES

Calcium chloride: Amikacin (Amikin), dobutamine (Dobutrex), lidocaine, milrinone (Primacor), morphine, norepinephrine (Levophed). **Calcium gluconate:** Ampicillin, aztreonam (Azactam), cefazolin (Ancef), cefepime (Maxipime), ciprofloxacin (Cipro), dobutamine (Dobutrex), enalapril (Vasotec), famotidine (Pepcid), furosemide (Lasix), heparin, lidocaine, lip-

C

ids, magnesium sulfate, meropenem (Merrem IV), midazolam (Versed), milrinone (Primacor), norepinephrine (Levophed), piperacillin and tazobactam (Zosyn), potassium chloride, propofol (Diprivan).

INDICATIONS/ROUTES/DOSAGE

Hyperphosphatemia

PO *(Calcium Acetate)*: ADULTS, ELDERLY: 2 tablets 3 times a day with meals. May increase gradually up to 4 tablets 3 times a day to decrease serum phosphate level to less than 6 mg/dl as long as hypercalcemia does not develop.

PO *(Calcium Carbonate)*: ADULTS, ELDERLY, CHILDREN: 1 g with each meal. **Maximum:** 4–7 g/day.

Hypocalcemia

PO *(Calcium Carbonate)*: ADULTS, ELDERLY: 1–2 g/day in 3–4 divided doses. CHILDREN: 45–65 mg/kg/day in 3–4 divided doses. NEONATES: 50–150 mg/kg/day in 4–6 divided doses. **Maximum:** 1 g/day.

PO *(Calcium Glubionate)*: ADULTS, ELDERLY: 6–18 g/day in 4–6 divided doses. CHILDREN, INFANTS: 0.6–2 g/kg/day in 4 divided doses. NEONATES: 1.2 g/kg/day in 4–6 divided doses.

IV *(Calcium Gluconate)*: ADULTS, ELDERLY: 1–2 g over 2 hrs. May repeat q60 min until level resolved. CHILDREN: 200–500 mg/kg/day in 4 divided doses. NEONATES: 200–800 mg/kg/day in 4 divided doses.

Antacid

PO *(Calcium Carbonate)*: ADULTS, ELDERLY: 1–2 tabs (5–10 ml) q2h as needed. CHILDREN 6–11 YRS: 2 tabs (800 mg). **Maximum:** 6 tabs/day. CHILDREN 2–5 YRS: 1 tab (400 mg). **Maximum:** 3 tabs/day.

Osteoporosis

PO *(Calcium Carbonate)*: ADULTS, ELDERLY: 1,200 mg/day.

Cardiac Arrest

IV *(Calcium Chloride)*: ADULTS, ELDERLY: 500–1,000 mg over 2–5 min. May repeat as necessary. CHILDREN, NEONATES: 20 mg/kg. May repeat in 10 min as necessary.

Hypocalcemia Tetany

IV *(Calcium Chloride)*: CHILDREN, NEONATES: 10 mg/kg over 5–10 min. May repeat q6–8h. **Maximum:** 200 mg/kg/day.

IV *(Calcium Gluconate)*: ADULTS, ELDERLY: 1–3 g over 10–30 min; may repeat after 6 hrs. CHILDREN, NEONATES: 100–200 mg/kg/dose over 5–10 min. May repeat after 6 hrs. **Maximum:** 500 mg/kg/day.

Supplement

PO *(Calcium Citrate)*: ADULTS, ELDERLY: 0.5–2 g 2–4 times a day. CHILDREN: 45–65 mg/kg/day in 4 divided doses.

SIDE EFFECTS

Frequent: **PO:** Chalky taste. **Parenteral:** Pain, rash, redness, burning at injection site; flushing; nausea; vomiting; diaphoresis; hypotension. Occasional: **PO:** Mild constipation, fecal impaction, peripheral edema, metabolic alkalosis (muscle pain, restlessness, slow respirations, altered taste). **Calcium carbonate:** Milkalkali syndrome (headache, decreased appetite, nausea, vomiting, unusual fatigue). Rare: Urinary urgency, painful urination.

ADVERSE EFFECTS/ TOXIC REACTIONS

Hypercalcemia: Early signs: Constipation, headache, dry mouth, increased thirst, irritability, decreased appetite, metallic taste, fatigue, weakness, depression. **Later signs:** Confusion, drowsiness, hypertension, photosensitivity, arrhythmias, nausea, vomiting, painful urination.

NURSING CONSIDERATIONS

BASELINE ASSESSMENT

Assess B/P, EKG and cardiac rhythm, renal function, serum magnesium, phosphate, potassium.

INTERVENTION/EVALUATION

Monitor B/P, EKG, cardiac rhythm, serum magnesium, phosphate, potassium, renal function. Monitor serum, urine calcium. Monitor for signs of hypercalcemia.

PATIENT/FAMILY TEACHING

• Do not take within 1–2 hrs of other oral medications, fiber-containing foods. • Avoid excessive alcohol, tobacco, caffeine.

calfactant

cal-**fak**-tant
(Infasurf)

◆CLASSIFICATION

PHARMACOTHERAPEUTIC: Natural lung extract. **CLINICAL:** Pulmonary surfactant.

ACTION

Reduces alveolar surface tension, stabilizing the alveoli. **Therapeutic Effect:** Restores surface activity to infant lungs, improves lung compliance, respiratory gas exchange.

PHARMACOKINETICS

No studies have been performed.

USES

Prevention of respiratory distress syndrome (RDS) in premature infants younger than 29 wks of gestational age; treatment of premature infants younger than 72 hrs of age who develop RDS and require endotracheal intubation.

PRECAUTIONS

Contraindications: None known. **Cautions:** None known.

⌛ LIFESPAN CONSIDERATIONS

Pregnancy/Lactation: Not indicated in this pt population. **Pregnancy Category:** Not indicated for use in pregnant women. **Children:** Used only in neonates. No age-related precautions noted. **Elderly:** Not indicated in this pt population.

INTERACTIONS

DRUG: None significant. **HERBAL:** None significant. **FOOD:** None known. **LAB VALUES:** None significant.

AVAILABILITY (Rx)

Intratracheal Suspension: 35-mg/ml vials.

ADMINISTRATION/HANDLING

Intratracheal
• Refrigerate. • Unused vials may be returned to refrigerator within 24 hrs for future use. Avoid repeated warming to room temperature. • Do not shake. • Enter vial only once, discard unused suspension.

INDICATIONS/ROUTES/DOSAGE

Respiratory Distress Syndrome (RDS)
Intratracheal: NEONATES: 3 ml/kg of birth weight administered as soon as possible after birth in 2 doses of 1.5 ml/kg. Repeat 3-ml/kg doses, up to a total of 3 doses given 12 hrs apart.

SIDE EFFECTS

Frequent: Cyanosis (65%), airway obstruction (39%), bradycardia (34%), reflux of surfactant into endotracheal tube (21%), need for manual ventilation (16%). **Occasional:** Need for reintubation (3%).

ADVERSE EFFECTS/ TOXIC REACTIONS

Reflux of calfactant into endotracheal tube, cyanosis, bradycardia, airway obstruction have occurred.

NURSING CONSIDERATIONS

BASELINE ASSESSMENT

Drug must be administered in highly supervised setting. Clinicians must be experienced with intubation, ventilator management. Offer emotional support to parents.

INTERVENTION/EVALUATION

Monitor infant with arterial or transcutaneous measurement of systemic O_2, CO_2. Auscultate lungs for adventitious breath sounds (rales, crackles, rhonchi). Frequent ABG sampling necessary to prevent post-dosing hyperoxia and hypocarbia.

canagliflozin

kan-a-gli-**floe**-zin
(Invokana)

◆CLASSIFICATION

PHARMACOTHERAPEUTIC: Sodium-glucose co-transporter 2 (SGLT2) inhibitor. **CLINICAL:** Antidiabetic.

ACTION

Increases excretion of urinary glucose by inhibiting reabsorption of filtered glucose in kidney. Inhibits SGLT2 in proximal renal tubule. **Therapeutic Effect:** Lowers serum glucose levels.

PHARMACOKINETICS

Readily absorbed following PO administration. Metabolized in liver. Peak plasma concentration: 1–2 hrs. Protein binding: 99%. Excreted in feces (42%), urine (33%). **Half-life:** 11–13 hrs.

USES

Adjunctive treatment to diet and exercise to improve glycemic controls in pts with type 2 diabetes mellitus.

PRECAUTIONS

Contraindications: History of hypersensitivity to SGLT2 inhibitors, severe renal impairment, end-stage renal disease, dialysis. **Cautions:** Not recommended in type 1 diabetes, diabetic ketoacidosis. Concurrent use of diuretics, ACE inhibitors, angiotensin receptor blockers (ARB), other hypoglycemic or nephrotoxic medications, mild to moderate renal impairment, hypovolemia (dehydration/anemia), elderly, episode hypotension, hyperkalemia, genital mycotic infection.

⌛ LIFESPAN CONSIDERATIONS

Pregnancy/Lactation: Unknown if distributed in breast milk. Must either discontinue drug or discontinue breastfeeding. **Pregnancy Category C. Children:** Safety and efficacy not established in pts younger than 18 yrs of age. **Elderly:** May have increased risk for adverse reactions (e.g., hypotension, syncope, dehydration).

INTERACTIONS

DRUG: Rifampin, phenytoin may decrease concentration/effect. **Potassium-sparing diuretics** may increase serum potassium levels. **ACE inhibitors, angiotension receptor blockers, calcium channel blockers, diuretics** may increase risk of hypotension. **Insulin, oral hypoglycemics** may increase risk of hypoglycemia. May increase concentration/effect of **digoxin**. **HERBAL:** Herbs with hypoglycemic properties **(e.g., fenugreek, garlic, ginger, ginseng, gotu)** may increase risk of hypoglycemia. **FOOD:** None known. **LAB VALUES:** May increase low-density lipoprotein-cholesterol (LDL-C), hemoglobin, serum creatinine, magnesium, phosphate, potassium. May decrease glomerular filtration rate.

AVAILABILITY (Rx)

Tablets: 100 mg, 300 mg.

ADMINISTRATION/HANDLING

PO

• May give without regard to food. Give before first meal of the day.

INDICATIONS/ROUTES/DOSAGE

Type 2 Diabetes Mellitus

PO: ADULTS/ELDERLY: 100 mg daily before first meal. May increase to 300 mg daily if glomerular filtration rate (GFR) greater than 60 ml/min.

Renal Impairment
GFR 45–60 ml/min: 100 mg daily (maximum). **GFR less than 40 ml/min:** Discontinue.

SIDE EFFECTS

Occasional (5%): Increased urination. **Rare (3%–2%):** Thirst, nausea, constipation.

ADVERSE EFFECTS/ TOXIC REACTIONS

Symptomatic hypotension (postural dizziness, orthostatic hypotension, syncope) may occur. Genital myocotic (yeast) infections reported in 10% of pts. Hypoglycemic events reported in 1.5% of pts (5% in elderly). Concomitant use of hypoglycemic medications may increase hypoglycemic risk. Hypersensitivity reactions including angioedema (tongue/lip swelling), urticaria, rash, pruritus, erythema occurred in 3%–4% of pts. May cause hyperkalemia (muscle weakness, palpitation, EKG changes).

NURSING CONSIDERATIONS

BASELINE ASSESSMENT

Assess hydration status. Obtain serum chemistries, capillary blood glucose, hemoglobin A1C, LDL-C, digoxin level (if applicable). Assess pt's understanding of diabetes management, routine home glucose monitoring. Receive full medication history including minerals, herbal products. Question history of co-morbidities, esp. renal or hepatic impairment.

INTERVENTION/EVALUATION

Monitor digoxin levels, serum potassium, cholesterol, capillary blood glucose, hepatic/renal function tests. Assess for hypoglycemia (diaphoresis, tremors, dizziness, anxiety, headache, tachycardia, perioral numbness, hunger, diplopia, difficulty concentrating), hyperglycemia (polyuria, polyphagia, polydipsia, nausea, vomiting, fatigue, Kussmaul respirations), hypersensitivity reaction. Monitor for signs of hyperkalemia (palpitations, muscle weakness). Screen for glucose-altering conditions: fever, increased activity or stress, surgical procedures. Dietary consult for nutritional education. Encourage PO intake.

PATIENT/FAMILY TEACHING

• Diabetes mellitus requires lifelong control. • Diet and exercise are principal parts of treatment; do not skip or delay meals. • Test blood sugar regularly. • When taking combination drug therapy or when glucose demands are altered (fever, infection, trauma, stress), have low blood sugar treatment available (glucagon, oral dextrose). • Report suspected pregnancy or plans of breastfeeding. • Monitor daily calorie intake. • Go from lying to standing slowly to prevent dizziness. • Genital itching may indicate yeast infection. • Therapy may increase risk for dehydration/ low blood pressure. • Report any palpitations or muscle weakness.

candesartan

kan-de-**sar**-tan
(Apo-Candesartan ✲, Atacand)
BLACK BOX ALERT May cause fetal injury, mortality if used during second or third trimester of pregnancy.

FIXED-COMBINATION(S)

Atacand HCT: candesartan/hydrochlorothiazide (a diuretic): 16 mg/12.5 mg, 32 mg/12.5 mg.

◆CLASSIFICATION

PHARMACOTHERAPEUTIC: Angiotensin II receptor antagonist. **CLINICAL:** Antihypertensive (see p. 10C, 61C).

ACTION

Blocks vasoconstriction, aldosterone-secreting effects of angiotensin II, inhibiting binding of angiotensin II to AT_1 receptors. **Therapeutic Effect:** Produces vasodilation; decreases peripheral resistance, B/P.

✤ Canadian trade name   🔪 Non-Crushable Drug   🔲 High Alert drug

PHARMACOKINETICS

Route	Onset	Peak	Duration
PO	2–3 hrs	6–8 hrs	Greater than 24 hrs

Rapidly, completely absorbed. Protein binding: greater than 99%. Undergoes minor hepatic metabolism to inactive metabolite. Excreted unchanged in urine and in feces through biliary system. Not removed by hemodialysis. **Half-life:** 9 hrs.

USES

Treatment of hypertension alone or in combination with other antihypertensives, heart failure: NYHA class II–IV.

PRECAUTIONS

Contraindications: Severe hepatic impairment and/or cholestasis, pregnancy, breastfeeding, concomitant use with aliskiren in pts with diabetes mellitus. **Cautions:** Significant aortic/mitral stenosis, renal/hepatic impairment, unstented (unilateral/bilateral) renal artery stenosis.

⌛ LIFESPAN CONSIDERATIONS

Pregnancy/Lactation: Unknown if distributed in breast milk. May cause fetal/neonatal morbidity/mortality. **Pregnancy Category C (D if used in second or third trimester). Children:** Safety and efficacy not established in pts younger than 1 yr. **Elderly:** No age-related precautions noted.

INTERACTIONS

DRUG: May increase risk of **lithium** toxicity. **NSAIDs** may decrease effects. **HERBAL: Ephedra, ginseng, yohimbe** may worsen hypertension. **Garlic** may increase antihypertensive effect. **FOOD:** None known. **LAB VALUES:** May increase BUN, serum alkaline phosphatase, bilirubin, creatinine, AST, ALT. May decrease Hgb, Hct.

AVAILABILITY (Rx)

Tablets: 4 mg, 8 mg, 16 mg, 32 mg.

ADMINISTRATION/HANDLING

PO
• Give without regard to food.

INDICATIONS/ROUTES/DOSAGE

Hypertension
PO: ADULTS, ELDERLY, PTS WITH MILD HEPATIC OR RENAL IMPAIRMENT: Initially, 16 mg once a day in those who are not volume depleted. Can be given once or twice a day with total daily doses of 8–32 mg. Give lower dosage in those treated with diuretics or with severe renal impairment. **CHILDREN 6–16 YRS, GREATER THAN 50 KG:** Initially, 8–16 mg/day in 1–2 divided doses. **Range:** 4–32 mg. **Maximum:** 32 g/day. **50 KG OR LESS:** Initially, 4–8 mg in 1–2 divided doses. **Range:** 2–16 mg/day. **Maximum:** 32 mg/day. **CHILDREN 1–5 YRS:** Initially, 0.2 mg/kg/day in 1–2 divided doses. **Range:** 0.05–0.4 mg/kg/day.

Heart Failure
PO: ADULTS, ELDERLY: Initially, 4 mg once daily. May double dose at approximately 2-wk intervals up to a target dose of 32 mg/day.

SIDE EFFECTS

Occasional (6%–3%): Upper respiratory tract infection, dizziness, back/leg pain. **Rare (2%–1%):** Pharyngitis, rhinitis, headache, fatigue, diarrhea, nausea, dry cough, peripheral edema.

ADVERSE EFFECTS/ TOXIC REACTIONS

Overdosage may manifest as hypotension, tachycardia. Bradycardia occurs less often. May increase risk of renal failure, hyperkalemia.

NURSING CONSIDERATIONS

BASELINE ASSESSMENT

Obtain B/P, apical pulse immediately before each dose, in addition to regular monitoring (be alert to fluctuations). Question for possibility of pregnancy. Assess medication history (esp. diuretic).

Question for history of hepatic/renal impairment, renal artery stenosis. Obtain BUN, serum creatinine, AST, ALT, alkaline phosphatase, bilirubin, Hgb, Hct.

INTERVENTION/EVALUATION

Maintain hydration (offer fluids frequently). Assess for evidence of upper respiratory infection. Assist with ambulation if dizziness occurs. Monitor electrolytes, serum creatinine, BUN, urinalysis. Assess B/P for hypertension/hypotension. If excessive reduction in B/P occurs, place pt in supine position, feet slightly elevated.

PATIENT/FAMILY TEACHING

• Inform female pt regarding potential for fetal injury, mortality with second- and third-trimester exposure to candesartan. • Report suspected pregnancy. • Avoid tasks that require alertness, motor skills until response to drug is established. • Report any sign of infection (sore throat, fever). • Do not stop taking medication. • Hypertension requires lifelong control. • Caution against exercising during hot weather (risk of dehydration, hypotension).

---

capecitabine

kap-e-**sye**-ta-bine
(<u>Xeloda</u>)
BLACK BOX ALERT May increase anticoagulant effect of warfarin. **Do not confuse Xeloda with Xenical.**

◆CLASSIFICATION

PHARMACOTHERAPEUTIC: Antimetabolite. **CLINICAL:** Antineoplastic (see p. 83C).

ACTION

Enzymatically converted to 5-fluorouracil (5-FU). Inhibits enzymes necessary for synthesis of essential cellular compo-

nents. **Therapeutic Effect:** Interferes with DNA synthesis, RNA processing, protein synthesis.

PHARMACOKINETICS

Readily absorbed from GI tract. Protein binding: less than 60%. Metabolized in liver. Primarily excreted in urine. **Half-life:** 45 min.

USES

Treatment of metastatic breast cancer resistant to other therapy, colorectal cancer. Adjuvant (postsurgical) treatment of Dukes C colon cancer. **OFF-LABEL:** Gastric cancer, pancreatic cancer, esophageal cancer, ovarian cancer, metastatic renal cell cancer, metastatic CNS lesions, neuroendocrine tumors.

PRECAUTIONS

Contraindications: Severe renal impairment (creatinine clearance less than 30 ml/min), dihydropyrimidine dehydrogenase (DPD) deficiency, hypersensitivity to 5-fluorouracil (5-FU). **Cautions:** Existing bone marrow depression, hepatic impairment, moderate renal impairment, previous cytotoxic therapy/radiation therapy, elderly (80 yrs of age or older).

⚕ LIFESPAN CONSIDERATIONS

Pregnancy/Lactation: May cause fetal harm. Unknown if distributed in breast milk. **Pregnancy Category D. Children:** Safety and efficacy not established in those younger than 18 yrs. **Elderly:** May be more sensitive to GI side effects.

INTERACTIONS

DRUG: May increase concentration, toxicity of **warfarin, phenytoin.** Myelosuppression may be enhanced when given concurrently with **bone marrow depressants. Live virus vaccines** may potentiate virus replication, increase vaccine side effects, decrease pt's antibody response to vaccine. **HERBAL: Echinacea** may decrease levels/effect. **FOOD:** None known. **LAB VALUES:** May increase serum alkaline phosphatase, bilirubin,

AST, ALT. May decrease Hgb, Hct, WBC count. May increase PT/INR.

AVAILABILITY (Rx)

Tablets: 150 mg, 500 mg.

ADMINISTRATION/HANDLING

• Give within 30 min after meals with water.

INDICATIONS/ROUTES/DOSAGE

Metastatic Breast Cancer, Colorectal Cancer, Adjuvant (Postsurgery) Treatment of Dukes C Colon Cancer
PO: ADULTS, ELDERLY: Initially, 2,500 mg/m^2/day in 2 equally divided doses approximately q12h apart for 2 wks. Follow with a 1-wk rest period; given in 3-wk cycles.

Dosage in Renal Impairment
Creatinine clearance 50–80 ml/min: No adjustment. **Creatinine clearance 30–49 ml/min:** 75% of normal dose. **Creatinine clearance less than 30 ml/min:** Contraindicated.

SIDE EFFECTS

Frequent (55%–25%): Diarrhea; nausea; vomiting; stomatitis; palmar-plantar erythrodysesthesia syndrome (PPES) presenting as redness, swelling, numbness, skin sloughing of hands and feet; fatigue; anorexia; dermatitis. **Occasional (24%–10%):** Constipation, dyspepsia, headache, dizziness, insomnia, edema, myalgia, pyrexia, dehydration, dyspnea, back pain. **Rare (less than 10%):** Mood changes, depression, sore throat, epistaxis, cough, visual abnormalities.

ADVERSE EFFECTS/ TOXIC REACTIONS

Serious reactions include myelosuppression (neutropenia, thrombocytopenia, anemia), cardiovascular toxicity (angina, cardiomyopathy, deep vein thrombosis), respiratory toxicity (dyspnea, epistaxis, pneumonia), lymphedema.

NURSING CONSIDERATIONS

BASELINE ASSESSMENT

Assess sensitivity to capecitabine or 5-fluorouracil. Obtain baseline Hgb, Hct, serum chemistries, renal function.

INTERVENTION/EVALUATION

Monitor for severe diarrhea, nausea, vomiting; if dehydration occurs, fluid and electrolyte replacement therapy should be initiated. Assess hands/feet for PPES. Monitor CBC for evidence of bone marrow depression. Monitor renal/hepatic function. Monitor for blood dyscrasias (fever, sore throat, signs of local infection, unusual bruising/bleeding from any site), symptoms of anemia (excessive fatigue, weakness).

PATIENT/FAMILY TEACHING

• Report nausea, vomiting, diarrhea, hand-and-foot syndrome, stomatitis. • Do not have immunizations without physician's approval (drug lowers body's resistance). • Avoid contact with those who have recently received live virus vaccine. • Promptly report fever higher than 100.5°F, sore throat, signs of local infection, unusual bruising/bleeding from any site.

captopril

kap-toe-pril
(Apo-Capto ✺, Capoten ✺)
BLACK BOX ALERT May cause fetal injury, mortality if used during second or third trimester of pregnancy.
Do not confuse captopril with calcitriol, Capitrol, or carvedilol.

FIXED-COMBINATION(S)

Capozide: captopril/hydrochlorothiazide (a diuretic): 25 mg/15 mg, 25 mg/25 mg, 50 mg/15 mg, 50 mg/25 mg.

◆ CLASSIFICATION

PHARMACOTHERAPEUTIC: Angiotensin-converting enzyme (ACE) inhibitor. **CLINICAL:** Antihypertensive, vasodilator (see p. 9C).

ACTION

Suppresses renin-angiotensin-aldosterone system (prevents conversion of angiotensin I to angiotensin II, a potent vasoconstrictor; may inhibit angiotensin II at local vascular and renal sites). Decreases plasma angiotensin II, increases plasma renin activity, decreases aldosterone secretion. **Therapeutic Effect:** Reduces peripheral arterial resistance, pulmonary capillary wedge pressure; improves cardiac output, exercise tolerance.

PHARMACOKINETICS

Route	Onset	Peak	Duration
PO	0.25 hr	0.5–1.5 hrs	Dose-related

Rapidly, well absorbed from GI tract (absorption decreased in presence of food). Protein binding: 25%–30%. Metabolized in liver. Primarily excreted in urine. Removed by hemodialysis. **Half-life:** Less than 3 hrs (increased in renal impairment).

USES

Treatment of hypertension, HF, diabetic nephropathy, post-MI for prevention of ventricular failure. **OFF-LABEL:** Delays progression of nephropathy and reduces risk of cardiovascular events in hypertensive pts with type 1 and type 2 diabetes. Treatment of hypertensive crisis, rheumatoid arthritis; hypertension secondary to scleroderma renal crisis; diagnosis of aldosteronism; diagnosis of renal artery stenosis; idiopathic edema; Bartter's syndrome; increases circulation in Raynaud's syndrome.

PRECAUTIONS

Contraindications: History of angioedema from previous treatment with ACE inhibi-tors, concomitant use with aliskiren in pts with diabetes mellitus. **Cautions:** Renal impairment, collagen vascular disease, dehydration. Unstented unilateral/bilateral renal artery stenosis.

⌛ LIFESPAN CONSIDERATIONS

Pregnancy/Lactation: Crosses placenta; distributed in breast milk. May cause fetal/neonatal mortality/morbidity. **Pregnancy Category C (D if used in second or third trimester). Children:** Safety and efficacy not established. **Elderly:** May be more sensitive to hypotensive effects.

INTERACTIONS

DRUG: Antihypertensives, diuretics may increase hypotensive effects. May increase **lithium** concentration, toxicity. **NSAIDs** may decrease antihypertensive effect. **Potassium-sparing diuretics, potassium supplements** may cause hyperkalemia. **HERBAL: Ephedra, ginseng, yohimbe** may worsen hypertension. **Garlic** may increase antihypertensive effect. **FOOD: Licorice** may cause sodium and water retention, hypokalemia. **LAB VALUES:** May increase BUN, serum alkaline phosphatase, bilirubin, creatinine, potassium, AST, ALT. May decrease serum sodium. May cause positive ANA titer.

AVAILABILITY (Rx)

Tablets: 12.5 mg, 25 mg, 50 mg, 100 mg.

ADMINISTRATION/HANDLING

PO

• Administer 1 hr before or 2 hrs after meals for maximum absorption (food may decrease drug absorption). • Tablets may be crushed.

INDICATIONS/ROUTES/DOSAGE

Hypertension

PO: ADULTS, ELDERLY: Initially, 12.5–25 mg 2–3 times a day. May increase by 12.5–25 mg/dose at 1–2 wk intervals up to 50 mg 3 times/day. **Maximum:** 450 mg/day in 3 divided doses. **CHILDREN:**

0.3–0.5 mg 3 times a day. **Maximum:** 6 mg/kg/day in 2–4 divided doses. **INFANTS:** 0.15–0.3 mg/kg/dose. May titrate up to maximum of 6 mg/kg/day in 1–4 divided doses. Usual range: 2.5–6 mg/kg/day. **NEONATES:** 0.01–0.1 mg/kg/dose q8–24h. **Maximum:** 0.5 mg/kg/dose q6–24h.

HF
PO: **ADULTS, ELDERLY:** Initially, 6.25–25 mg 3 times a day. **Target dose:** 50 mg 3 times/day.

Post-MI
PO: **ADULTS, ELDERLY:** Initially, 6.25 mg, then 12.5 mg 3 times a day. Increase to 25 mg 3 times a day over several days, up to 50 mg 3 times a day over several wks.

Diabetic Nephropathy, Prevention of Renal Failure
PO: **ADULTS, ELDERLY:** 25 mg 3 times a day.

Dosage in Renal Impairment
Creatinine clearance 10–50 ml/min: 75% of normal dosage. **Creatinine clearance less than 10 ml/min:** 50% of normal dosage.

SIDE EFFECTS

Frequent (7%–4%): Rash. **Occasional (4%–2%):** Pruritus, dysgeusia (altered taste). **Rare (less than 2%):** Headache, cough, insomnia, dizziness, fatigue, paresthesia, malaise, nausea, diarrhea or constipation, dry mouth, tachycardia.

ADVERSE EFFECTS/ TOXIC REACTIONS

Hypotension ("first-dose syncope") may occur in pts with HF and in those who are severely sodium/volume depleted. Angioedema (swelling of face/tongue/lips), hyperkalemia occur rarely. Agranulocytosis, neutropenia noted in those with collagen vascular disease (scleroderma, systemic lupus erythematosus), renal im-

pairment. Nephrotic syndrome noted in those with history of renal disease.

NURSING CONSIDERATIONS

BASELINE ASSESSMENT
Obtain B/P immediately before each dose, in addition to regular monitoring (be alert to fluctuations). If hypotension occurs, place pt in supine position with legs elevated. In pts with prior renal disease or receiving dosages greater than 150 mg/day, test urine for protein by dipstick method with first urine of day before therapy begins and periodically thereafter. In pts with renal impairment, autoimmune disease, or taking drugs that affect leukocytes or immune response, obtain CBC before beginning therapy, q2wks for 3 mos, then periodically thereafter.

INTERVENTION/EVALUATION
Assess skin for rash, pruritus. Assist with ambulation if dizziness occurs. Monitor urinalysis for proteinuria. Monitor serum potassium levels in those on concurrent diuretic therapy. Monitor B/P, BUN, serum creatinine, CBC. Discontinue medication, contact physician if angioedema (swelling of face, lips, tongue) occurs.

PATIENT/FAMILY TEACHING
• Full therapeutic effect of B/P reduction may take several wks. • Skipping doses or voluntarily discontinuing drug may produce severe rebound hypertension. • Limit alcohol. • Immediately report if swelling of face, lips, or tongue, difficulty breathing, vomiting, diarrhea, excessive perspiration, dehydration, persistent cough, sore throat, fever occur. • Inform physician if pregnant or planning to become pregnant. • Rise slowly from sitting/lying position.

TOP
200

carbamazepine

kar-ba-**maz**-e-peen

underlined – top prescribed drug

(Apo-Carbamazepine ✦, Carbatrol, Epitol, Equetro, Tegretol, Tegretol XR)

BLACK BOX ALERT Potentially fatal aplastic anemia, agranulocytosis reported. Potentially fatal, severe dermatologic reactions (e.g., Stevens-Johnson syndrome, toxic epidermal necrolysis) may occur. Risk increased in pts of Asian descent.

Do not confuse carbamazepine with oxcarbazepine, or Tegretol with Mebaral, Toprol XL, Toradol, or Trental.

◆CLASSIFICATION

PHARMACOTHERAPEUTIC: Iminostilbene derivative. **CLINICAL:** Anticonvulsant, antineuralgic, antimanic, antipsychotic (see p. 35C).

ACTION

Decreases sodium, calcium ion influx into neuronal membranes, reducing post-tetanic potentiation at synapses. **Therapeutic Effect:** Produces anticonvulsant effect; decreases pain response.

PHARMACOKINETICS

Slowly, completely absorbed from GI tract. Protein binding: 75%–90%. Metabolized in liver. Primarily excreted in urine. Not removed by hemodialysis. **Half-life:** 25–65 hrs (decreased with chronic use).

USES

Carbatrol, Epitol, Tegretol, Tegretol XR: Treatment of partial seizures with complex symptomatology, generalized tonic-clonic seizures, mixed seizure patterns, pain relief of trigeminal neuralgia, diabetic neuropathy. **Equetro:** Acute manic and mixed episodes associated with bipolar disorder. **OFF-LABEL:** Post-traumatic stress disorder, restless legs syndrome.

PRECAUTIONS

Contraindications: Concomitant or within 14 days of use of MAOIs, myelosuppression, delavirdine or other NNRT inhibitors, hypersensitivity to tricyclic antidepressants. **Cautions:** High risk of suicide; increased IOP; concurrent use of strong CYP3A4 inhibitors or inducers; hepatic, renal impairment; history of cardiac impairment; EKG abnormalities.

⧗ LIFESPAN CONSIDERATIONS

Pregnancy/Lactation: Crosses placenta; distributed in breast milk. Accumulates in fetal tissue. **Pregnancy Category D. Children:** Behavioral changes more likely to occur. **Elderly:** More susceptible to confusion, agitation, AV block, bradycardia, syndrome of inappropriate antidiuretic hormone (SIADH).

INTERACTIONS

DRUG: CYP3A4 inhibitors (e.g., **cimetidine, clarithromycin, azole antifungals, protease inhibitors**) may increase concentration of **carbamazepine.** **CYP3A4 inducers (e.g., rifampin, phenytoin)** may decrease concentration/ effect. May decrease concentration/effect of **hormonal contraceptives, warfarin, trazodone.** **HERBAL: Evening primrose** may decrease seizure threshold. **Gotu kola, kava kava, St. John's wort, valerian** may increase CNS depression. **FOOD: Grapefruit, grapefruit juice** may increase absorption, concentration. **LAB VALUES:** May increase BUN, serum glucose, alkaline phosphatase, bilirubin, AST, ALT, protein, cholesterol, HDL, triglycerides. May decrease serum calcium, thyroid hormone (T_3, T_4 index) levels. **Therapeutic serum level:** 4–12 mcg/ml; **toxic serum level:** greater than 12 mcg/ml.

AVAILABILITY (Rx)

Suspension (Tegretol): 100 mg/5 ml. **Tablets (Epitol, Tegretol):** 200 mg. **Tablets (Chewable [Tegretol]):** 100 mg.

🔖 **Capsules (Extended-Release [Carbatrol, Equetro]):** 100 mg, 200 mg, 300 mg.

C

Tablets (Extended-Release [Tegretol XR]): 100 mg, 200 mg, 400 mg.

ADMINISTRATION/HANDLING

PO

• Store oral suspension, tablets at room temperature. • Give with meals to reduce GI distress. • May give extended-release capsules without regard to food. • Extended-release tablets should be given with meals. • Shake oral suspension well. Do not administer simultaneously with other liquid medicine. • Do not crush or open extended-release capsules or tablets. • Extended-release capsules may be opened and sprinkled over food (e.g., applesauce).

INDICATIONS/ROUTES/DOSAGE

◄**ALERT►** Suspension must be given on a 3–4 times/day schedule; tablets on a 2–4 times/day schedule; extended-release capsules 2 times/day.

Seizure Control
PO: ADULTS, CHILDREN OLDER THAN 12 YRS: Initially, 200 mg twice a day. May increase dosage by 200 mg/day at weekly intervals. Range: 400–1,200 mg/day in 2–4 divided doses. **Maximum: ADULTS:** 1.6–2.4 g/day; **CHILDREN OLDER THAN 15 YRS:** 1,200 mg/day; **CHILDREN 13–15 YRS:** 1,000 mg/day. **CHILDREN 6–12 YRS:** Initially, 100 mg twice a day (tablets) or 4 times/day (oral suspension). May increase by 100 mg/day at weekly intervals. Range: 400–800 mg/day. **Maximum:** 1,000 mg/day. **CHILDREN YOUNGER THAN 6 YRS:** Initially, 10–20 mg/kg/day in 2–3 divided doses. May increase at weekly intervals until optimal response and therapeutic levels are achieved. **Maximum:** 35 mg/kg/day. **ELDERLY:** Initially, 100 mg 1–2 times a day. May increase by 100 mg/day at weekly intervals. Usual dose 400–1,000 mg/day.

Trigeminal Neuralgia, Diabetic Neuropathy
PO: ADULTS: Initially, 100 mg twice a day (tablets) or 4 times/day (oral suspen-

sion). May increase by 100 mg twice a day up to 400–800 mg/day. **Maximum:** 1,200 mg/day. **ELDERLY:** Initially 100 mg 1–2 times/day. May increase by 100 mg/day at weekly intervals. Usual dose 400–1,000 mg/day.

Bipolar Disorder
PO: ADULTS, ELDERLY (Equetro): Initially, 400 mg/day in 2 divided doses (tablets) or 4 times/day (oral suspension). May adjust dose in 200-mg increments. **Maximum:** 1,600 mg/day in divided doses.

Dosage in Renal Impairment
CrCl less than 10 ml/min: 75% of normal dose. **HD:** 75% of normal dose. **CRRT:** 75% of normal dose.

SIDE EFFECTS

Frequent (greater than 10%): Vertigo, somnolence, ataxia, fatigue, leucopenia, rash, urticaria, nausea, vomiting. **Occasional (10%–1%):** Headache, diplopia, blurred vision, thrombocytopenia, dry mouth, edema, fluid retention, increased weight. **Rare (less than 1%):** Tremors, visual disturbances, lymphadenopathy, jaundice, involuntary muscle movements, nystagmus, dermatitis.

ADVERSE EFFECTS/ TOXIC REACTIONS

Toxic reactions appear as blood dyscrasias (aplastic anemia, agranulocytosis, thrombocytopenia, leukopenia, leukocytosis, eosinophilia), cardiovascular disturbances (HF, hypotension/hypertension, thrombophlebitis, arrhythmias), dermatologic effects (rash, urticaria, pruritus, photosensitivity). Abrupt withdrawal may precipitate status epilepticus.

NURSING CONSIDERATIONS

BASELINE ASSESSMENT
Seizures: Review history of seizure disorder (intensity, frequency, duration, level of consciousness [LOC]). Initiate seizure precautions. **Neuralgia:** Assess facial pain, stimuli that may cause facial

pain. **Bipolar:** Assess mental status, cognitive abilities. CBC, serum iron determination, urinalysis, BUN should be performed before therapy begins and periodically during therapy.

INTERVENTION/EVALUATION

Seizures: Observe frequently for recurrence of seizure activity. Monitor for therapeutic levels. Assess for clinical improvement (decrease in intensity, frequency of seizures). Assess for clinical evidence of early toxicity (fever, sore throat, mouth ulcerations, unusual bruising/bleeding, joint pain). **Neuralgia:** Avoid triggering tic douloureux (draft, talking, washing face, jarring bed, hot/warm/cold food or liquids). **Bipolar:** Monitor for suicidal ideation, behavioral changes. Observe for excessive sedation. **Therapeutic serum level:** 4–12 mcg/ml; **toxic serum level:** greater than 12 mcg/ml.

PATIENT/FAMILY TEACHING

• Do not abruptly discontinue medication after long-term use (may precipitate seizures). • Strict maintenance of therapy is essential for seizure control. • Avoid tasks that require alertness, motor skills until response to drug is established. • Report visual disturbances. • Blood tests should be repeated frequently during first 3 mos of therapy and at monthly intervals thereafter for 2–3 yrs. • Do not take oral suspension simultaneously with other liquid medicine. • Do not take with grapefruit products. • Report serious skin reactions.

carbidopa/levodopa

kar-bi-doe-pa/**lee**-voe-doe-pa
(Apo-Levocarb ✦, Parcopa, Sinemet, Sinemet CR)
Do not confuse Sinemet with Serevent.

FIXED-COMBINATION(S)

Stalevo: carbidopa/levodopa/entacapone (antiparkinson agent): 12.5 mg/50 mg/200 mg, 18.75 mg/75 mg/200 mg, 25 mg/100 mg/200 mg, 31.25 mg/125 mg/200 mg, 37.5 mg/150 mg/200 mg, 50 mg/200 mg/200 mg.

◆CLASSIFICATION

PHARMACOTHERAPEUTIC: Dopamine precursor. **CLINICAL:** Antiparkinson agent (see p. 145C).

ACTION

Converted to dopamine in basal ganglia, increasing dopamine concentration in brain, inhibiting hyperactive cholinergic activity. Carbidopa prevents peripheral breakdown of levodopa, making more levodopa available for transport into brain. **Therapeutic Effect:** Reduces tremor.

PHARMACOKINETICS

Rapidly and completely absorbed from GI tract. Widely distributed. Excreted primarily in urine. Levodopa is converted to dopamine. Excreted primarily in urine. **Half-life:** 1–2 hrs (carbidopa); 1–3 hrs (levodopa).

USES

Treatment of idiopathic Parkinson's disease (paralysis agitans), postencephalitic parkinsonism, symptomatic parkinsonism following CNS injury by CO_2 poisoning, manganese intoxication. **OFF-LABEL:** Restless legs syndrome.

PRECAUTIONS

Contraindications: Narrow-angle glaucoma, use within 14 days of MAOIs, undiagnosed skin lesions, history of melanoma. **Cautions:** History of MI, arrhythmias, bronchial asthma (tartrazine sensitivity), emphysema; severe cardiac, pulmonary, endocrine disease; severe renal/hepatic impairment; active peptic ulcer; treated open-angle glaucoma; seizure disorder; pts at risk for hypotension.

⌛ LIFESPAN CONSIDERATIONS

Pregnancy/Lactation: Unknown if drug crosses placenta or is distributed in breast milk. May inhibit lactation. Breastfeeding not recommended. **Pregnancy Category C. Children:** Safety and efficacy not established in those younger than 18 yrs. **Elderly:** More sensitive to effects of levodopa. Anxiety, confusion, nervousness more common when receiving anticholinergics.

INTERACTIONS

DRUG: Isoniazid, antipsychotics, phenytoin, pyridoxine may decrease effects. **MAOIs** may increase levels, effects of orthostatic hypotension. **Selegiline, antihypertensives** may increase risk of orthostatic hypotension. **HERBAL: Kava kava** may decrease effect. **FOOD: High-protein** diets may cause decreased or erratic response to levodopa. **LAB VALUES:** May increase BUN, serum LDH, alkaline phosphatase, bilirubin, AST, ALT. May decrease Hgb, Hct, WBC count.

AVAILABILITY (Rx)

Tablets (Immediate-Release [Sinemet]): 10 mg carbidopa/100 mg levodopa, 25 mg carbidopa/100 mg levodopa, 25 mg carbidopa/250 mg levodopa. **Tablets (Orally-Disintegrating [Parcopa], Immediate-Release):** 10 mg carbidopa/100 mg levodopa, 25 mg carbidopa/100 mg levodopa, 25 mg carbidopa/250 mg levodopa.

🍶 **Tablets (Extended-Release [Sinemet CR]):** 25 mg carbidopa/100 mg levodopa, 50 mg carbidopa/200 mg levodopa.

ADMINISTRATION/HANDLING

Note: Space doses evenly over waking hours.

PO
• Scored tablets may be crushed. • Give with meals to decrease GI upset. • Do not crush extended-release tablets; may cut in half.

PO (Parcopa)
• Place orally-disintegrating tablet on top of tongue. Tablet will dissolve in seconds, pt to swallow with saliva. Not necessary to administer with liquid.

INDICATIONS/ROUTES/DOSAGE

Parkinsonism
PO: ADULTS (IMMEDIATE-RELEASE ORALLY-DISINTEGRATING TABLET): Initially, 25/100 mg 3 times a day. May increase every other day by 1 tablet up to 200/2,000 mg daily. **ELDERLY:** Initially, 25/100 mg twice a day. May increase as necessary. **(EXTENDED-RELEASE):** 50/200 mg 2 times a day at least 6 hrs apart. Intervals between doses of Sinemet CR should be 4–8 hrs while awake, with smaller doses at end of day if doses are not equal.

SIDE EFFECTS

Frequent: Involuntary movements of face, tongue, arms, upper body; nausea/vomiting (80%); anorexia (50%). **Occasional:** Depression, anxiety, confusion, nervousness, urinary retention, palpitations, dizziness, light-headedness, decreased appetite, blurred vision, constipation, dry mouth, flushed skin, headache, insomnia, diarrhea, unusual fatigue, darkening of urine and sweat. **Rare:** Hypertension, ulcer, hemolytic anemia (marked by fatigue).

ADVERSE EFFECTS/ TOXIC REACTIONS

High incidence of involuntary choreiform, dystonic, dyskinetic movements in those on long-term therapy. Numerous mild to severe CNS and psychiatric disturbances may occur (reduced attention span, anxiety, nightmares, daytime drowsiness, euphoria, fatigue, paranoia, psychotic episodes, depression, hallucinations).

NURSING CONSIDERATIONS

BASELINE ASSESSMENT

Assess symptoms of Parkinson's disease (e.g., rigidity, pill rolling, gait).

INTERVENTION/EVALUATION

Be alert to neurologic effects (headache, lethargy, mental confusion, agitation). Monitor for evidence of dyskinesia (difficulty with movement). Assess for clinical reversal of symptoms (improvement of tremor of head and hands at rest, mask-like facial expression, shuffling gait, muscular rigidity). Monitor B/P (standing, sitting, supine).

PATIENT/FAMILY TEACHING

• Avoid tasks that require alertness, motor skills until response to drug is established. • Sugarless gum, sips of tepid water may relieve dry mouth. • Take with food to minimize GI upset. • Effects may be delayed from several wks to mos. • May cause darkening of urine or sweat (not harmful). • Report any uncontrolled movement of face, eyelids, mouth, tongue, arms, hands, legs; mental changes; palpitations; severe or persistent nausea/vomiting; difficulty urinating. • Report exacerbations of asthma, underlying depression, psychosis.

carboplatin

HIGH ALERT

kar-boe-**plat**-in
(Carboplatin Injection)

BLACK BOX ALERT Must be administered by personnel trained in administration/handling of chemotherapeutic agents (high potential for severe reactions, including anaphylaxis [may occur within minutes of administration] and sudden death). Profound myelosuppression (anemia, thrombocytopenia) has occurred.

Do not confuse carboplatin with Cisplatin or oxaliplatin, or with Platinol.

◆CLASSIFICATION

PHARMACOTHERAPEUTIC: Platinum coordination complex. **CLINICAL:** Antineoplastic (see p. 83C).

ACTION

Inhibits DNA synthesis by cross-linking with DNA strands, preventing cell division. Cell cycle–phase nonspecific. **Therapeutic Effect:** Interferes with DNA function.

PHARMACOKINETICS

Protein binding: Low. Hydrolyzed in solution to active form. Primarily excreted in urine. **Half-life:** 2.6–5.9 hrs.

USES

Treatment of ovarian carcinoma. Palliative treatment of recurrent ovarian cancer. **OFF-LABEL:** Brain tumors, Hodgkin's and non-Hodgkin's lymphomas, malignant melanoma, retinoblastoma, treatment of breast, bladder, cervical, endometrial, esophageal, small-cell lung, non–small-cell lung, head and neck, testicular carcinomas, germ cell tumors, osteogenic sarcoma.

PRECAUTIONS

Contraindications: History of severe allergic reaction to cisplatin, platinum compounds, mannitol; severe bleeding, severe myelosuppression. **Cautions:** Moderate bone marrow depression, renal impairment.

⌛ LIFESPAN CONSIDERATIONS

Pregnancy/Lactation: If possible, avoid use during pregnancy, esp. first trimester. May cause fetal harm. Unknown if distributed in breast milk. Breastfeeding not recommended. **Pregnancy Category D. Children:** Safety and efficacy not established. **Elderly:** Peripheral neurotoxicity increased, myelotoxicity may be more severe. Age-related renal impairment may require decreased dosage, careful monitoring of blood counts.

INTERACTIONS

DRUG: Bone marrow depressants may increase myelosuppression. **Live virus vaccines** may potentiate virus replication, increase vaccine side effects, decrease pt's antibody response to vaccine. **Nephrotoxic, ototoxic medications** may increase risk of toxicity. **HERBAL:** Avoid **black cohosh, dong quai** in estrogen-dependent tumors. **Echinacea** may decrease levels/effects. **FOOD:** None known. **LAB VALUES:** May decrease serum calcium, magnesium, potassium, sodium. May increase BUN, serum alkaline phosphatase, bilirubin, creatinine, AST.

AVAILABILITY (Rx)

Injection Solution: 10 mg/ml.

ADMINISTRATION/HANDLING

◄ **ALERT** ► May be carcinogenic, mutagenic, teratogenic. Handle with extreme care during preparation/administration.

 IV

Reconstitution • Dilute with D₅W or 0.9% NaCl to a final concentration of 0.5–2 mg/ml.
Rate of Administration • Infuse over 15–60 min. • Rarely, anaphylactic reaction occurs minutes after administration. Use of epinephrine, corticosteroids alleviates symptoms.
Storage • Store vials at room temperature. •After dilution, solution is stable for 8 hrs.

IV INCOMPATIBILITY

Amphotericin B complex (Abelcet, AmBisome, Amphotec).

IV COMPATIBILITIES

Etoposide (VePesid), granisetron (Kytril), ondansetron (Zofran), paclitaxel (Taxol), palonosetron (Aloxi).

INDICATIONS/ROUTES/DOSAGE

Ovarian Carcinoma (Monotherapy)
IV: ADULTS: 360 mg/m² on day 1, every 4 wks. Do not repeat dose until neutrophil and platelet counts are within acceptable levels. Adjust dosage in previously treated pts based on lowest post-treatment platelet or neutrophil count. Increase dosage only once to no more than 125% of starting dose.

Ovarian Carcinoma (Combination Therapy)
IV: ADULTS: 300 mg/m² (with cyclophosphamide) on day 1, every 4 wks. Do not repeat dose until neutrophil and platelet counts are within acceptable levels.

Dosage in Renal Impairment
Initial dosage is based on creatinine clearance; subsequent dosages are based on pt's tolerance, degree of myelosuppression.

Creatinine Clearance	Dosage Day 1
60 ml/min or greater	360 mg/m²
41–59 ml/min	250 mg/m²
16–40 ml/min	200 mg/m²

SIDE EFFECTS

Frequent: Nausea (80%–75%), vomiting (65%). **Occasional:** Generalized pain (17%), diarrhea/constipation (6%), peripheral neuropathy (4%). **Rare (3%–2%):** Alopecia, asthenia (loss of strength, energy), hypersensitivity reaction (erythema, pruritus, rash, urticaria).

ADVERSE EFFECTS/ TOXIC REACTIONS

Myelosuppression may be severe, resulting in anemia, infection (sepsis, pneumonia), major bleeding. Prolonged treatment may result in peripheral neurotoxicity.

NURSING CONSIDERATIONS

BASELINE ASSESSMENT

Obtain EKG, CBC, serum chemistries with renal function tests. Offer emotional support. Do not repeat treatment until WBC recovers from previous therapy. Transfusions may be needed in those receiving prolonged therapy (myelosuppression increased in those with previous therapy, renal impairment).

INTERVENTION/EVALUATION

Monitor hematologic status, pulmonary function studies, hepatic/renal function tests, CBC, serum electrolytes. Monitor for fever, sore throat, signs of local infection, unusual bruising/bleeding from any site, symptoms of anemia (excessive fatigue, weakness).

PATIENT/FAMILY TEACHING

• Nausea, vomiting generally abate within 24 hrs. • Do not have immunizations without physician's approval (drug lowers body's resistance). • Avoid contact with those who have recently received live virus vaccine.

carfilzomib

kar-**fil**-zoh-mib
(Kyprolis)
Do not confuse carfilzomib with crizotinib, pazopanib.

◆CLASSIFICATION

PHARMACOTHERAPEUTIC: Proteasome inhibitor. **CLINICAL:** Antineoplastic (see p. 83C).

ACTION

Blocks action of proteasomes, intracellular proteins to induce cell death in rapidly dividing cells. **Therapeutic Effect:** Inhibits activity, delays tumor growth in multiple myeloma, hematologic, and solid tumors.

PHARMACOKINETICS

Protein Binding: 97%. Rapidly, extensively metabolized. Excreted primarily extrahepatically. Minimal removal by hemodialysis. **Half-life:** Equal to or less than 1 hr on day 1 of cycle 1. Proteasome inhibition was maintained for 48 hrs or longer following first dose of carfilzomib for each week of dosing.

USES

Treatment of pts with multiple myeloma who have received at least 2 prior therapies including bortezomib and an immunomodulatory agent and have demonstrated disease progression on or within 60 days of completion of last therapy.

PRECAUTIONS

Contraindications: None known. **Cautions:** Preexisting HF, myocardial abnormalities, complications of pulmonary hypertension (e.g., dyspnea), hepatic impairment, thrombocytopenia.

⌛ LIFESPAN CONSIDERATIONS

Pregnancy/Lactation: Avoid pregnancy. May cause fetal harm. Unknown if excreted in breast milk. **Pregnancy Category D. Children:** Safety and efficacy not established. **Elderly:** No age-related precautions noted.

INTERACTIONS

DRUG: None significant. **HERBAL:** None significant. **FOOD:** None significant. **LAB VALUES:** May increase serum creatinine, glucose, creatinine, AST, ALT, bilirubin, calcium. May decrease RBC count, Hgb, Hct, absolute neutrophil count (ANC), platelet count, serum magnesium, phosphate, potassium, sodium.

AVAILABILITY (Rx)

Injection Powder for Reconstitution (Single-Use Vial): 60 mg.

ADMINISTRATION/HANDLING

◀**ALERT**▶ Dose is calculated using pts' actual body surface area at baseline. Pts with a body surface area greater than 2.2 m² should receive dose based on a body surface area of 2.2 m². No dose adjustment needed for weight changes of less than or equal to 20%.

❖ Canadian trade name   🦊 Non-Crushable Drug   🔲 High Alert drug

C

IV

Reconstitution • Slowly inject 29 ml Sterile Water for Injection, directing solution to inside wall of vial (minimizes foaming). • Swirl and invert vial slowly for 1 min or until completely dissolved. • Do not shake. • If foaming occurs, rest vial for 2–5 min until subsided. • Withdraw calculated dose from vial and dilute into 50 ml D5W. • Final concentration of reconstituted solution: 2 mg/ml.

Rate of administration • Infuse over 2–10 min. • Do not administer as a bolus.

Storage • Refrigerate undiluted vial. • Reconstituted solution may be refrigerated up to 24 hrs. • At room temperature, use diluted solution within 4 hrs.

▨ IV INCOMPATIBILITIES

Do not mix with other IV medications or additives. Infuse via dedicated line. Flush IV administration line with NaCl or D5W immediately before and after carfilzomib administration.

INDICATIONS/ROUTES/DOSAGE

◀**ALERT**▶ Prior to each dose in cycle 1, give 250 ml to 500 ml NaCl bolus. Give an additional 250 ml to 500 ml IV fluid following administration. Continue IV hydration in subsequent cycles (reduces risk of renal toxicity, tumor lysis syndrome).

Premedicate with dexamethasone 4 mg PO or IV prior to all doses during cycle 1 and prior to all doses during first cycle of dose escalation to 27 mg/m² (reduces incidence, severity of infusion reactions). Reinstate dexamethasone premedication (4 mg PO or IV) if symptoms develop or reappear during subsequent cycles.

Multiple Myeloma
IV Infusion: ADULTS, ELDERLY: 20 mg/m², given on 2 consecutive days, each wk for 3 wks (days 1, 2, 8, 9, 15, and 16), followed by a 12-day rest period (days 17 to 28). Each 28-day period is considered one treatment cycle. If tolerated in cycle 1, escalate dose to 27 mg/m² beginning in cycle 2 and continue at 27 mg/m² in subsequent cycles. Treatment may be continued until disease progression or unacceptable toxicity occurs. Dosage should be modified if hematologic, cardiac, pulmonary, renal/hepatic toxicities, peripheral neuropathy occurs.

SIDE EFFECTS

Frequent (56%–20%): Fatigue, anemia, nausea, exertional dyspnea, diarrhea, fever, headache, cough, peripheral edema, vomiting, constipation, back pain. **Occasional (18%–14%):** Insomnia, chills, arthralgia, muscle spasms, hypertension, asthenia (loss of strength, energy), extremity pain, dizziness, hypoesthesia (decreased sensitivity to touch), anorexia.

ADVERSE EFFECTS/ TOXIC REACTIONS

Pneumonia (10%), acute renal failure (4%), pyrexia (3%), and HF (3%) were reported. Adverse reactions leading to discontinuation occurred in 15% of pts. Upper respiratory tract infection was seen in 28% of pts. HF, pulmonary edema, decrease in ejection fraction were reported in 7% of pts. Infusion reaction characterized by chills, fever, wheezing, facial flushing, dyspnea, vomiting, chest tightness can occur immediately following or up to 24 hrs after administration. Tumor lysis syndrome occurs rarely.

NURSING CONSIDERATIONS

BASELINE ASSESSMENT

Obtain full history of home medications including vitamins, minerals, herbal products. Ensure hydration status and maintain throughout treatment. Obtain CBC, serum chemistries. Assess vital signs, O₂ saturation. Obtain AST, ALT, bilirubin for evidence of hepatotoxicity. Platelet nadirs occur around day 8 of each 28-day cycle and recover to baseline by start of the next 28-day cycle.

INTERVENTION/EVALUATION

Monitor for fluid overload. Monitor platelet count frequently; adjust dose according to grade of thrombocytopenia. Monitor vital signs, O_2 saturation routinely. Monitor cardiac function and manage as needed. Assess for palpitations, tachycardia. Assess for anemia-related dizziness, exertional dyspnea, fatigue, weakness, syncope. Report decreases in Hgb, Hct, platelets, neutrophils. Monitor for acute infection (fever, diaphoresis, lethargy, oral mucosal changes, productive cough), bloody stools, bruising, hematuria, DVT, pulmonary embolism. Encourage nutritional intake and assess anorexia, weight loss. Reinforce birth control compliance. Monitor daily pattern of bowel activity, stool consistency. Offer antiemetics if nausea, vomiting occur. Monitor for symptoms of neutropenia.

PATIENT/FAMILY TEACHING

• Blood levels will be drawn routinely. • Immediately report any newly prescribed medications. • May alter taste of food or decrease appetite. • Report bloody stool/ urine, increased bruising, difficulty breathing, weakness, dizziness, palpitation, weight loss. • Maintain strict oral hygiene. • Do not have immunizations without physician approval (drug lowers body's resistance). • Avoid those who have recently taken live virus vaccine. • Avoid crowds, those with symptoms of viral illness.

carisoprodol

kar-eye-soe-**proe**-dole
(Soma)
Do not confuse carisoprodol with carbamazepine, or Soma with senna.

FIXED-COMBINATION(S)

Soma Compound: carisoprodol/aspirin (a nonsteroidal salicylate): 200 mg/325 mg.

◆CLASSIFICATION

PHARMACOTHERAPEUTIC: Carbamic acid ester. **CLINICAL:** Skeletal muscle relaxant (see p. 151C).

ACTION

Skeletal muscle relaxant action may be related to its sedative properties. May produce muscle relaxation by altering interneuronal activity in the descending reticular formation of the brain and spinal cord. Does not directly affect skeletal muscle. **Therapeutic Effect:** Relieves musculoskeletal pain.

PHARMACOKINETICS

Route	Onset	Peak	Duration
PO	30 min	—	4–6 hrs

Readily absorbed from GI tract. Distributed throughout CNS. Protein binding: 60%. Metabolized in liver; excreted in urine. Removed by hemodialysis, peritoneal dialysis. **Half-life:** 2 hrs.

USES

Relief of discomfort associated with acute, painful musculoskeletal conditions. Not to be used for more than 3 wks.

PRECAUTIONS

Contraindications: Acute intermittent porphyria, hypersensitivity to meprobamate. **Cautions:** History of seizures, addiction-prone pts, elderly, debilitated pts, poor CYP2C19 metabolizers, renal/hepatic impairment.

⌛ LIFESPAN CONSIDERATIONS

Pregnancy/Lactation: Distributed in breast milk; decreases milk production. Crosses placenta. **Pregnancy Category C. Children:** Safety and efficacy not established in those younger than 16 yrs. **El-**

C

derly: No age-related precautions noted.

INTERACTIONS

DRUG: CNS depressants, including alcohol, benzodiazepines, tricyclic antidepressants, opiates may increase CNS effects. CYP2C19 inhibitors (e.g., omeprazole) may increase concentration. CYP2C19 inducers (e.g., rifampin) may decrease concentration. HERBAL: None significant. FOOD: None known. LAB VALUES: None significant.

AVAILABILITY (Rx)

Tablets: 250 mg, 350 mg.

ADMINISTRATION/HANDLING

• Give without regard to food.

INDICATIONS/ROUTES/DOSAGE

PO: ADULTS, ELDERLY, CHILDREN OLDER THAN 16 YRS: 250–350 mg 4 times daily with last dose at bedtime.

SIDE EFFECTS

Frequent (17%–13%): Drowsiness. Occasional (8%–3%): Dizziness, headache.

ADVERSE EFFECTS/ TOXIC REACTIONS

Idiosyncratic reactions and/or severe allergic reactions may occur within min or hr of first dose (severe weakness, transient quadriplesia, euphoria, temporary vision loss). Prolonged use at high dosage can lead to tolerance, dependence, withdrawal symptoms. Abrupt withdrawal following long-term use results in anxiety, abdominal cramps, insomnia, nausea, vomiting, confusion, and occasionally chills, seizures, hallucinations. Onset of withdrawal occurs 12–48 hrs following cessation and can last another 12–48 hrs. Overdose may result in tachycardia, facial flushing, ataxia, tremors, agitation, irritability. Overdose has resulted in stupor, coma, shock, respiratory depression, death.

NURSING CONSIDERATIONS

BASELINE ASSESSMENT

Record onset, type, location, duration of musculoskeletal pain, inflammation. Inspect appearance of affected joints for immobility, stiffness, swelling.

INTERVENTION/EVALUATION

Assist with ambulation. Initiate fall precautions. Evaluate for therapeutic response: relief of pain, stiffness, swelling; improved mobility; reduced joint tenderness; improved grip strength.

PATIENT/FAMILY TEACHING

• Avoid tasks that require alertness, motor skills until response to drug is established. • Avoid alcohol. • Should only be used for short periods (2–3 wks). • Report withdrawal symptoms (syncope, tachyarrhythmia or excessive fatigue, unusual mental status changes).

carmustine

kar-**mus**-teen
(BiCNU, Gliadel Wafer)
BLACK BOX ALERT Profound myelosuppression (leukopenia, thrombocytopenia) is major toxicity. High risk of pulmonary toxicity. Must be administered by personnel trained in administration/handling of chemotherapeutic agents (high potential for severe reactions, including anaphylaxis, sudden death).
Do not confuse carmustine with bendamustine or lomustine.

◆ CLASSIFICATION

PHARMACOTHERAPEUTIC: Alkylating agent, nitrosourea. CLINICAL: Antineoplastic (see p. 83C).

ACTION

Inhibits DNA, RNA synthesis by crosslinking with DNA, RNA strands, preventing cell division. Cell cycle–phase nonspecific. **Therapeutic Effect:** Interferes with DNA, RNA function.

PHARMACOKINETICS

Crosses blood-brain barrier. Metabolized in liver. Excreted in urine. **Half-life:** 15–30 min.

USES

BiCNU: Treatment of brain tumors, Hodgkin's lymphomas, non-Hodgkin's lymphomas, multiple myeloma. **Gliadel Wafer:** Adjunct to surgery to prolong survival in recurrent glioblastoma multiforme. OFF-LABEL: Treatment of mycosis fungoides (topical).

PRECAUTIONS

Contraindications: None known. **Cautions:** Thrombocytopenia leukopenia, anemia; renal/hepatic impairment.

⧖ LIFESPAN CONSIDERATIONS

Pregnancy/Lactation: Avoid pregnancy; particularly first trimester; may cause fetal harm. Unknown if distributed in breast milk. Breastfeeding not recommended. **Pregnancy Category D. Children:** Safety and efficacy not established. **Elderly:** No age-related precautions noted.

INTERACTIONS

DRUG: **Bone marrow depressants, cimetidine** may enhance myelosuppressive effect. **Hepatotoxic, nephrotoxic medications** may increase risk of hepatotoxicity, nephrotoxicity. **Live-virus vaccines** may potentiate virus replication, increase vaccine side effects, decrease pt's antibody response to vaccine. HERBAL: **Echinacea** may decrease effects. FOOD: None known. LAB VALUES: May increase BUN, serum alkaline phosphatase, bilirubin, AST, ALT.

AVAILABILITY (Rx)

Injection, Powder for Reconstitution (BiCNU): 100 mg. Implant Device (Gliadel Wafer): 7.7 mg.

ADMINISTRATION/HANDLING

◄ALERT► May be carcinogenic, mutagenic, teratogenic. Wear protective gloves during preparation of drug; may cause transient burning, brown staining of skin.

 IV

Reconstitution • Reconstitute 100-mg vial with 3 ml sterile dehydrated (absolute) alcohol, followed by 27 ml Sterile Water for Injection to provide concentration of 3.3 mg/ml. • Further dilute with 50–250 ml D_5W or 0.9% NaCl to final concentration of 0.2–1 mg/ml.
Rate of Administration • Infuse over 1–2 hrs (shorter duration may produce intense burning pain at injection site, intense flushing of skin, conjunctiva). • Flush IV line with 5–10 ml 0.9% NaCl or D_5W before and after administration to prevent irritation at injection site.
Storage • Refrigerate unused vials. • Reconstituted vials are stable for 8 hrs at room temperature or 24 hrs if refrigerated. • Solutions further diluted with D_5W or 0.9% NaCl are stable for 48 hrs if refrigerated or an additional 8 hrs at room temperature. • Solutions appear clear, colorless to yellow. • Discard if precipitate forms, color change occurs, or oily film develops on bottom of vial. **Gliadel Wafers:** Store at or below −20°C (−4°F). Unopened pouches may be kept at room temperature for maximum of 6 hrs.

▩ IV INCOMPATIBILITY

Allopurinol (Aloprim), sodium bicarbonate.

▩ IV COMPATIBILITY

Granisetron (Kytril), ondansetron (Zofran).

INDICATIONS/ROUTES/DOSAGE

◄ALERT► Refer to individual oncology protocols.
Usual Dosage (Refer to Individual Protocols)
IV *(BiCNU)*: ADULTS, ELDERLY: 150–200 mg/m² as a single dose q6wks or 75–100

C

mg/m^2 on 2 successive days q6wks. **CHILDREN:** 200–250 mg/m^2 q4–6wks as a single dose.
◄**ALERT**► Next dosage is based on clinical and hematologic response to previous dose (platelets greater than 100,000/mm^3 and leukocytes greater than 4,000/mm^3).

Implantation *(Gliadel Wafer):* **ADULTS, ELDERLY, CHILDREN:** Up to 8 wafers (62.6 mg) may be placed in resection cavity.

Dosage in Renal Impairment

Creatinine Clearance (ml/min)	Dosage
46–60	80% of dose
31–45	75% of dose
Less than 31	Not recommended

SIDE EFFECTS

Frequent: Nausea/vomiting (may last up to 6 hrs). **Occasional:** Diarrhea, esophagitis, anorexia, dysphagia, hyperpigmentation. **Rare:** Thrombophlebitis, burning sensation, pain at injection site.

ADVERSE EFFECTS/ TOXIC REACTIONS

Hematologic toxicity due to myelosuppression occurs frequently. Thrombocytopenia occurs approximately 4 wks after treatment begins and lasts 1–2 wks. Leukopenia is evident 5–6 wks after treatment begins and lasts 1–2 wks. Anemia occurs less frequently. Mild, reversible hepatotoxicity occurs frequently. Prolonged, high-dose therapy may produce impaired renal function, pulmonary toxicity (pulmonary infiltrate/fibrosis).

NURSING CONSIDERATIONS

BASELINE ASSESSMENT

Obtain CBC, renal/hepatic function studies before initiation and periodically thereafter.

INTERVENTION/EVALUATION

Monitor renal/hepatic function tests. Obtain CBC weekly during and for at least 6 wks after therapy ends. Monitor for hematologic toxicity (fever, sore throat, signs of local infection, unusual bruising/bleeding from any site), symptoms of anemia (excessive fatigue, weakness). Monitor for pulmonary toxicity; observe for dyspnea, adventitious breath sounds (rales, rhonchi, crackles).

PATIENT/FAMILY TEACHING

• Maintain adequate hydration (may protect against renal impairment). • Do not have immunizations without physician's approval (drug lowers body's resistance). • Avoid contact with those who have recently received live virus vaccine. • Report nausea/vomiting, fever, sore throat, chills, unusual bleeding/bruising.

---

carvedilol   TOP 200   HIGH ALERT

kar-**ve**-dil-ole
(Apo-Carvedilol , <u>Coreg</u>, Coreg CR, Novo-Carvedilol)
Do not confuse carvedilol with atenolol or carteolol, or Coreg with Corgard, Cortef, or Cozaar.

◆CLASSIFICATION

PHARMACOTHERAPEUTIC: Beta-adrenergic blocker. **CLINICAL:** Antihypertensive (see p. 73C).

ACTION

Possesses nonselective beta-blocking and alpha-adrenergic blocking activity. Causes vasodilation. **Therapeutic Effect:** Reduces cardiac output, exercise-induced tachycardia, reflex orthostatic tachycardia; reduces peripheral vascular resistance.

PHARMACOKINETICS

Route	Onset	Peak	Duration
PO	30 min	1–2 hrs	24 hrs

Rapidly, extensively absorbed from GI tract. Protein binding: 98%. Metabolized in liver. Excreted primarily via bile into feces. Minimally removed by hemodialysis. **Half-life:** 7–10 hrs. Food delays rate of absorption.

USES

Treatment of mild to severe heart failure, left ventricular dysfunction following MI, hypertension. **OFF-LABEL:** Treatment of angina pectoris, idiopathic cardiomyopathy.

PRECAUTIONS

Contraindications: Bronchial asthma or related bronchospastic conditions, cardiogenic shock, decompensated HF requiring intravenous inotropic therapy, severe hepatic impairment, second- or third-degree AV block, severe bradycardia, or sick sinus syndrome (except in pts with pacemaker). **Cautions:** Concurrent use of digoxin, diltiazem, or verapamil; diabetes, myasthenia gravis; psychiatric disease; mild to moderate hepatic impairment. Withdraw gradually to avoid acute tachycardia, hypertension, and/or ischemia.

⧗ LIFESPAN CONSIDERATIONS

Pregnancy/Lactation: Unknown if drug crosses placenta or is distributed in breast milk. May produce bradycardia, apnea, hypoglycemia, hypothermia during delivery; may contribute to low birthweight infants. **Pregnancy Category C (D if used in the second or third trimester). Children:** Safety and efficacy not established. **Elderly:** Incidence of dizziness may be increased.

INTERACTIONS

DRUG: Calcium channel blockers, digoxin, beta-blockers, CYP2C9 inhibitors (e.g., amiodarone, fluconazole) increase risk of cardiac conduction disturbances. **Diuretics, other antihypertensives** may potentiate hypotensive effects. **Cimetidine** may increase concentration. May increase concentration of **cyclosporine, digoxin. CYP2D6 inhibitors (e.g., fluoxetine, paroxetine);** may increase concentration/side effects; may enhance slowing of HR or cardiac conduction. May increase effect of **insulin, oral hypoglycemics. Rifampin** decreases concentration. **HERBAL: Ephedra, ginseng, yohimbe** may worsen hypertension. **Garlic** may increase antihypertensive effect. **FOOD:** None known. **LAB VALUE:** May increase serum creatinine, bilirubin, AST, ALT, PT.

AVAILABILITY (Rx)

Tablets (Immediate-Release): 3.125 mg, 6.25 mg, 12.5 mg, 25 mg.

▥ **Capsules (Extended-Release [Coreg CR]):** 10 mg, 20 mg, 40 mg, 80 mg.

ADMINISTRATION/HANDLING

PO
• Give with food (slows rate of absorption, reduces risk of orthostatic effects).
• Do not crush or cut extended-release capsules. • Capsules may be opened and sprinkled on applesauce for immediate use.

INDICATIONS/ROUTES/DOSAGE

Hypertension
PO *(Immediate-Release):* ADULTS, ELDERLY: Initially, 6.25 mg twice a day. May double at 1–2 wk intervals to highest tolerated dosage. **Maximum:** 50 mg/day. *(Extended-Release):* Initially, 20 mg once daily. May increase to 40 mg once daily after 1–2 wks. **Maximum:** 80 mg once daily.

HF
PO *(Immediate-Release):* ADULTS, ELDERLY: Initially, 3.125 mg twice a day. May double at 2-wk intervals to highest tolerated dosage. **Maximum: Greater than 85 kg:** 50 mg twice a day; **Less than 85 kg:** 25 mg twice a day. *(Extended-Release):* Initially, 10 mg once daily for 2 wks. May increase to 20 mg, 40 mg, and 80 mg over successive intervals of at least 2 wks.

Left Ventricular Dysfunction Following MI
PO *(Immediate-Release)*: **ADULTS, ELDERLY**: Initially, 3.125–6.25 mg twice a day. May increase at intervals of 3–10 days up to 25 mg twice a day. *(Extended-Release)*: Initially, 10–20 mg once daily. May increase to 40 mg and 80 mg once daily in intervals of 3–10 days.

SIDE EFFECTS

Frequent (6%–4%): Fatigue, dizziness. **Occasional (2%):** Diarrhea, bradycardia, rhinitis, back pain. **Rare (less than 2%):** Orthostatic hypotension, drowsiness, UTI, viral infection.

ADVERSE EFFECTS/ TOXIC REACTIONS

Overdose may produce profound bradycardia, hypotension, bronchospasm, cardiac insufficiency, cardiogenic shock, cardiac arrest. Abrupt withdrawal may result in diaphoresis, palpitations, headache, tremors. May precipitate HF, MI in pts with cardiac disease; thyroid storm in those with thyrotoxicosis; peripheral ischemia in those with existing peripheral vascular disease. Hypoglycemia may occur in pts with previously controlled diabetes.

NURSING CONSIDERATIONS

BASELINE ASSESSMENT

Assess B/P, apical pulse immediately before drug is administered (if pulse is 60 beats/min or less or systolic B/P is less than 90 mm Hg, withhold medication, contact physician).

INTERVENTION/EVALUATION

Monitor B/P for hypotension, respirations for dyspnea. Take standing systolic B/P 1 hr after dosing as guide for tolerance. Assess pulse for quality, regularity, rate; monitor for bradycardia. Monitor EKG for cardiac arrhythmias. Assist with ambulation if dizziness occurs. Assess for evidence of HF: dyspnea (particularly on exertion or lying down), night cough, peripheral edema, distended neck veins. Monitor I&O (increase in weight, decrease in urine output may indicate HF). Monitor renal/hepatic function tests.

PATIENT/FAMILY TEACHING

• Full antihypertensive effect noted in 1–2 wks. • Contact lens wearers may experience decreased lacrimation. • Take with food. • Do not abruptly discontinue medication. • Compliance with therapy regimen is essential to control hypertension. • Avoid tasks that require alertness, motor skills until response to drug is established. • Report excessive fatigue, prolonged dizziness. • Do not use nasal decongestants, OTC cold preparations (stimulants) without physician's approval. • Monitor B/P, pulse before taking medication. • Restrict salt, alcohol intake.

caspofungin

kas-poe-**fun**-jin
(<u>Cancidas</u>)

◆CLASSIFICATION

PHARMACOTHERAPEUTIC: Echinocandin antifungal. **CLINICAL:** Antifungal (see p. 48C).

ACTION

Inhibits synthesis of glucan, a vital component of fungal cell wall formation, damaging fungal cell membrane. **Therapeutic Effect:** Fungistatic.

PHARMACOKINETICS

Distributed in tissue. Protein binding: 97%. Metabolized in liver to active metabolite. Excreted primarily in urine and, to a lesser extent, in feces. Not removed by hemodialysis. **Half-life:** 40–50 hrs.

USES

Treatment of invasive aspergillosis, candidemia, *Candida* infection (intra-abdominal abscess, peritonitis, esophageal, pleural space). Empiric therapy for presumed fungal infections in febrile neutropenia.

PRECAUTIONS

Contraindications: None known. **Cautions:** Concurrent use of cyclosporine, hepatic impairment.

⌛ LIFESPAN CONSIDERATIONS

Pregnancy/Lactation: May be embryotoxic. Crosses placental barrier. Distributed in breast milk. **Pregnancy Category C. Children:** Safety and efficacy not established. **Elderly:** Age-related moderate renal impairment may require dosage adjustment.

INTERACTIONS

DRUG: Cyclosporine may increase concentration. **Rifampin** may decrease concentration. May decrease concentration/effects of **tacrolimus**. **HERBAL:** None significant. **FOOD:** None known. **LAB VALUES:** May increase serum alkaline phosphatase, bilirubin, creatinine, AST, ALT, urine protein, RBCs. May decrease serum albumin, bicarbonate, potassium, magnesium, Hgb, Hct.

AVAILABILITY (Rx)

Injection, Powder for Reconstitution: 50-mg, 70-mg vials.

ADMINISTRATION/HANDLING

 IV

Reconstitution • Reconstitute 50-mg or 70-mg vial with 0.9% NaCl, Sterile Water for Injection, or Bacteriostatic Water for Injection. Further dilute in 0.9% NaCl or D_5W to maximum concentration of 0.5 mg/ml.
Rate of Administration • Infuse over 60 min.
Storage • Refrigerate vials but warm to room temperature before preparing with diluent. • Reconstituted solution, prior to preparation of pt infusion solution, may be stored at room temperature for 1 hr before infusion. • Final infusion solution can be stored at room temperature for 24 hrs or 48 hrs if refrigerated. • Discard if solution contains particulate or is discolored.

🔃 IV COMPATIBILITIES

Aztreonam (Azactam), daptomycin (Cubicin), fluconazole (Diflucan), linezolid (Zyvox), meropenem (Merrem IV), piperacillin/tazobactam (Zosyn), vancomycin.

🔃 IV INCOMPATIBILITIES

Cefepime (Maxipime), ceftaroline (Teflaro), ceftazidime (Fortaz), ceftriaxone (Rocephin), furosemide (Lasix).

INDICATIONS/ROUTES/DOSAGE

Aspergillosis
IV: ADULTS, ELDERLY: Give single 70-mg loading dose on day 1, followed by 50 mg/day thereafter. For pts with moderate hepatic insufficiency, reduce daily dose to 35 mg. **CHILDREN 3 MOS–17 YRS:** 70 mg/m^2 on day 1, then 50 mg/m^2 daily. **Maximum:** 70-mg loading dose, 50-mg daily dose.

Invasive Candidiasis
IV: ADULTS, ELDERLY: Initially, 70 mg followed by 50 mg daily. **CHILDREN 3 MOS–17 YRS:** 70 mg/m^2 on day 1, then 50 mg/m^2 daily. **Maximum:** 70-mg loading dose, 50-mg daily dose.

Esophageal Candidiasis
IV: ADULTS, ELDERLY: 50 mg a day. **CHILDREN 3 MOS–17 YRS:** 50 mg/m^2 daily. **Maximum:** 50 mg.

Empiric Therapy
IV: ADULTS, ELDERLY: Initially, 70 mg then 50 mg/day. May increase to 70 mg/day. **CHILDREN 3 MOS–17 YRS:** 70 mg/m^2 on day 1, then 50 mg/m^2 daily. **Maximum:** 70 mg.

C

**Usual Dosage Neonatal—
Less Than 3 mos
IV:** 25 mg/mm²/dose once daily.

Dosage in Hepatic Impairment

Mild	No adjustment
Moderate	(Child-Pugh score 7–9): 35 mg/day
Severe	No clinical experience

SIDE EFFECTS

Frequent (26%): Fever. **Occasional (11%–4%):** Headache, nausea, phlebitis. **Rare (3% or less):** Paresthesia, vomiting, diarrhea, abdominal pain, myalgia, chills, tremor, insomnia.

ADVERSE EFFECTS/ TOXIC REACTIONS

Hypersensitivity reaction (rash, facial edema, pruritus, sensation of warmth) including anaphylaxis may occur. May cause hepatic disfunction, hepatitis (drug-induced), or hepatic failure.

NURSING CONSIDERATIONS

BASELINE ASSESSMENT

Obtain baseline CBC, serum chemistries, hepatic function test, magnesium. Determine baseline temperature, hepatic function tests. Assess for allergic or hypersensitivity reactions.

INTERVENTION/EVALUATION

Assess for signs/symptoms of hepatic dysfunction. Monitor hepatic enzyme tests in pts with preexisting hepatic dysfunction. Monitor CBC, serum potassium, Hgb. Monitor for fever, chills.

PATIENT/FAMILY TEACHING

• Report rash, facial swelling, itching, difficulty breathing, abdominal pain, yellowing of skin or eyes, dark colored urine, nausea.

cefaclor

sef-a-klor
(Apo-Cefaclor ✦, Ceclor ✦, Novo-Cefaclor ✦)
Do not confuse Cefaclor with cephalexin.

◆CLASSIFICATION

PHARMACOTHERAPEUTIC: Second-generation cephalosporin. **CLINICAL:** Antibiotic (see p. 24C).

ACTION

Binds to bacterial cell membranes, inhibits cell wall synthesis. **Therapeutic Effect:** Bactericidal.

PHARMACOKINETICS

Well absorbed from GI tract. Protein binding: 25%. Widely distributed. Partially metabolized in liver. Primarily excreted in urine. Moderately removed by hemodialysis. **Half-life:** 0.6–0.9 hr (increased in renal impairment).

USES

Treatment of susceptible infections due to *S. pneumoniae, S. pyogenes, S. aureus, H. influenzae, E. coli, M. catarrhalis, Klebsiella* spp., *P. mirabilis,* including acute otitis media, bronchitis, pharyngitis/tonsillitis, respiratory tract, skin/skin structure, UTIs.

PRECAUTIONS

Contraindications: History of hypersensitivity/anaphylactic reaction to cephalosporins. **Cautions:** Severe renal impairment, history of penicillin allergy.

⌛ LIFESPAN CONSIDERATIONS

Pregnancy/Lactation: Readily crosses placenta. Distributed in breast milk. **Pregnancy Category B. Children:** No age-related precautions noted in pts older than 1 mo. **Elderly:** Age-related renal impairment may require dosage adjustment.

INTERACTIONS

DRUG: Probenecid may increase concentration. **HERBAL:** None significant. **FOOD:** None known. **LAB VALUES:** May increase BUN, serum alkaline phosphatase, bilirubin, creatinine, LDH, AST, ALT. May cause positive direct/indirect Coombs' test.

AVAILABILITY (Rx)

Capsules: 250 mg, 500 mg. **Powder for Oral Suspension:** 125 mg/5 ml, 250 mg/5 ml, 375 mg/5 ml.

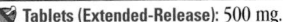 **Tablets (Extended-Release):** 500 mg.

ADMINISTRATION/HANDLING

PO

• After reconstitution, oral solution is stable for 14 days if refrigerated. • Shake oral suspension well before using. • Chewable tablet must be chewed before swallowing; do not swallow whole. • Give without regard to food; if GI upset occurs, give with food, milk.

INDICATIONS/ROUTES/DOSAGE

Usual Dosage
PO: ADULTS, ELDERLY: 250–500 mg q8h. **CHILDREN:** 20–40 mg/kg/day divided q8–12h. **Maximum:** 1 g/day.

Otitis Media
PO: CHILDREN: 40 mg/kg/day divided q12h. **Maximum:** 1 g/day.

Pharyngitis
CHILDREN: 20 mg/kg/day divided q12h. **Maximum:** 1 g/day.

Dosage in Renal Impairment

Creatinine Clearance	Dosage
10–50 ml/min	50%–100% of normal
Less than 10 ml/min	50% of normal

SIDE EFFECTS

Frequent: Oral candidiasis, mild diarrhea, mild abdominal cramping, vaginal candidiasis. **Occasional:** Nausea, serum sickness-like reaction (fever, joint pain; usually occurs after second course of therapy and resolves after drug is discontinued). **Rare:** Allergic reaction (pruritus, rash, urticaria).

ADVERSE EFFECTS/ TOXIC REACTIONS

Antibiotic-associated colitis, other (abdominal cramps, severe watery diarrhea, fever) superinfections may result from altered bacterial balance. Nephrotoxicity may occur, esp. in pts with pre-existing renal disease. Pts with history of penicillin allergy are at increased risk for developing a severe hypersensitivity reaction (severe pruritus, angioedema, bronchospasm, anaphylaxis).

NURSING CONSIDERATIONS

BASELINE ASSESSMENT

Obtain baseline CBC, renal function tests. Question for history of allergies, particularly cephalosporins, penicillins.

INTERVENTION/EVALUATION

Assess oral cavity for white patches on mucous membranes, tongue (thrush). Monitor daily pattern of bowel activity, stool consistency. Mild GI effects may be tolerable (increasing severity may indicate onset of antibiotic-associated colitis). Monitor I&O, renal function tests for nephrotoxicity. Be alert for superinfection: fever, vomiting, diarrhea, anal/genital pruritus, oral mucosal changes (ulceration, pain, erythema).

PATIENT/FAMILY TEACHING

• Continue therapy for full length of treatment. • Doses should be evenly spaced. • May cause GI upset (may take with food, milk). • Refrigerate oral suspension. • Report persistent diarrhea.

cefadroxil

sef-a-**drox**-il
(Apo-Cefadroxil ✤)

✤ Canadian trade name   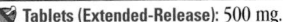 Non-Crushable Drug   ⬛ High Alert drug

◆CLASSIFICATION

PHARMACOTHERAPEUTIC: First-generation cephalosporin. **CLINICAL:** Antibiotic (see p. 23C).

ACTION

Binds to bacterial cell membranes, inhibits cell wall synthesis. **Therapeutic Effect:** Bactericidal.

PHARMACOKINETICS

Well absorbed from GI tract. Protein binding: 15%–20%. Widely distributed. Primarily excreted unchanged in urine. Removed by hemodialysis. **Half-life:** 1.2–1.5 hrs (increased in renal impairment).

USES

Treatment of susceptible infections due to group A streptococci, staphylococci, *S. pneumoniae, H. influenzae, Klebsiella* spp., *E. coli, P. mirabilis*, including impetigo, pharyngitis/tonsillitis, skin/skin structure, UTIs.

PRECAUTIONS

Contraindications: History of hypersensitivity/anaphylactic reaction to cephalosporins. **Cautions:** Severe renal impairment, history of penicillin allergy.

⌛ LIFESPAN CONSIDERATIONS

Pregnancy/Lactation: Readily crosses placenta. Distributed in breast milk. **Pregnancy Category B. Children:** No age-related precautions noted. **Elderly:** Age-related renal impairment may require dosage adjustment.

INTERACTIONS

DRUG: Probenecid may increase concentration. **HERBAL:** None significant. **FOOD:** None known. **LAB VALUES:** May increase BUN, serum alkaline phosphatase, bilirubin, creatinine, LDH, AST, ALT. May cause positive direct/indirect Coombs' test.

AVAILABILITY (Rx)

Capsules: 500 mg. Powder for Oral Suspension: 250 mg/5 ml, 500 mg/5 ml. Tablets: 1 g.

ADMINISTRATION/HANDLING

PO

• After reconstitution, oral solution is stable for 14 days if refrigerated. • Shake oral suspension well before using. • Give without regard to meals; if GI upset occurs, give with food, milk.

INDICATIONS/ROUTES/DOSAGE

Usual Dosage

PO: ADULTS, ELDERLY: 1–2 g/day in 2 divided doses. **CHILDREN:** 30 mg/kg/day in 2 divided doses. **Maximum:** 2 g/day.

Dosage in Renal Impairment

After initial 1-g dose, dosage and frequency are modified based on creatinine clearance and severity of infection.

Creatinine Clearance	Dosage
10–25 ml/min	q24h
Less than 10 ml/min	q36h

SIDE EFFECTS

Frequent: Oral candidiasis, mild diarrhea, mild abdominal cramping, vaginal candidiasis. **Occasional:** Nausea, unusual bruising/bleeding, serum sickness-like reaction (fever, joint pain; usually occurs after second course of therapy and resolves after drug is discontinued). **Rare:** Allergic reaction (rash, pruritus, urticaria), thrombophlebitis (pain, redness, swelling at injection site).

ADVERSE EFFECTS/ TOXIC REACTIONS

Antibiotic-associated colitis, other superinfections (abdominal cramps, severe watery diarrhea, fever) may result from altered bacterial balance. Nephrotoxicity may occur, esp. in pts with preexisting renal disease. Pts with history of penicillin allergy are at increased risk for developing a severe hypersensitivity reaction (severe pruritus, angioedema, broncho-spasm, anaphylaxis).

NURSING CONSIDERATIONS

BASELINE ASSESSMENT
Obtain CBC, renal function tests. Question for history of allergies, particularly cephalosporins, penicillins.

INTERVENTION/EVALUATION
Assess oral cavity for white patches on mucous membranes, tongue (thrush). Monitor daily pattern of bowel activity, stool consistency. Mild GI effects may be tolerable (increasing severity may indicate onset of antibiotic-associated colitis). Monitor I&O, renal function tests for nephrotoxicity. Be alert for superinfection: fever, vomiting, diarrhea, anal/genital pruritus, oral mucosal changes (ulceration, pain, erythema).

PATIENT/FAMILY TEACHING
• Continue therapy for full length of treatment. • Doses should be evenly spaced. • May cause GI upset (may take with food, milk). • Refrigerate oral suspension. • Report persistent diarrhea.

---

cefazolin

sef-a-**zoe**-lin
(Ancef)
Do not confuse cefazolin with cefoxitin, cefprozil, ceftriaxone, or cephalexin.

◆ CLASSIFICATION
PHARMACOTHERAPEUTIC: First-generation cephalosporin. **CLINICAL:** Antibiotic (see p. 24C).

ACTION
Binds to bacterial cell membranes, inhibits cell wall synthesis. **Therapeutic Effect:** Bactericidal.

PHARMACOKINETICS
Widely distributed. Protein binding: 85%. Primarily excreted unchanged in urine. Moderately removed by hemodialysis. **Half-life:** 1.4–1.8 hrs (increased in renal impairment).

USES
Treatment of susceptible infections due to *S. aureus, S. epidermidis,* group A beta-hemolytic streptococci, *S. pneumoniae, E. coli, P. mirabilis, Klebsiella* spp., *H. influenzae* including biliary tract, bone and joint, genital, respiratory tract, skin/skin structure, UTIs, endocarditis, perioperative prophylaxis, septicemia. **OFF-LABEL:** Prophylaxis against infective endocarditis.

PRECAUTIONS
Contraindications: History of hypersensitivity/anaphylactic reaction to cephalosporins. **Cautions:** Severe renal impairment, history of penicillin allergy, history of seizures.

⌛ LIFESPAN CONSIDERATIONS
Pregnancy/Lactation: Readily crosses placenta; distributed in breast milk. **Pregnancy Category B. Children:** No age-related precautions noted. **Elderly:** Age-related renal impairment may require reduced dosage.

INTERACTIONS
DRUG: Probenecid may increase concentration. **HERBAL:** None significant. **FOOD:** None known. **LAB VALUES:** May increase BUN, serum alkaline phosphatase, bilirubin, creatinine, LDH, AST, ALT. May cause positive direct/indirect Coombs' test.

AVAILABILITY (Rx)
Injection, Powder for Reconstitution (Ancef): 500 mg, 1 g. Ready-to-Hang Infusion (Ancef): 1 g/50 ml, 2 g/100 ml.

ADMINISTRATION/HANDLING
 IV

Reconstitution • Reconstitute each 1 g with at least 10 ml Sterile Water for Injection or 0.9% NaCl. • May further dilute in 50–100 ml D$_5$W or 0.9% NaCl (decreases incidence of thrombophlebitis).

Rate of Administration • For IV push, administer over 3–5 min (**maximum concentration: 100 mg/ml**). • For intermittent IV infusion (piggyback), infuse over 10–60 min (**maximum concentration: 20 mg/ml**).

Storage • Solution appears light yellow to yellow. • Reconstituted solution stable for 24 hrs at room temperature or for 10 days if refrigerated. • IV infusion (piggyback) stable for 48 hrs at room temperature or for 14 days if refrigerated.

IM
• To minimize discomfort, inject deep IM slowly. • Less painful if injected into gluteus maximus rather than lateral aspect of thigh.

▦ IV INCOMPATIBILITIES

Amikacin (Amikin), amiodarone (Cordarone), hydromorphone (Dilaudid).

▦ IV COMPATIBILITIES

Calcium gluconate, dexamethasone (Decadron), diltiazem (Cardizem), famotidine (Pepcid), heparin, insulin (regular), lidocaine, lorazepam (Ativan), magnesium sulfate, meperidine (Demerol), metoclopramide (Reglan), midazolam (Versed), morphine, multivitamins, ondansetron (Zofran), potassium chloride, propofol (Diprivan).

INDICATIONS/ROUTES/DOSAGE

Usual Dosage Range
IV, IM: ADULTS: 250 mg to 1.5 g q6–12h (usually q8h). **Maximum:** 12 g/day. **CHILDREN OLDER THAN 1 MO:** 25–100 mg/kg/day divided q6–8h. **Maximum:** 6 g/day. **NEONATES OLDER THAN 7 DAYS:** 25 mg/kg/dose q8h. **NEONATES 7 DAYS AND YOUNGER:** 25 mg/kg/dose q12h.

Uncomplicated UTI
IV, IM: ADULTS, ELDERLY: 1 g q12h.

Mild to Moderate Infections
IV, IM: ADULTS, ELDERLY: 500 mg–1 g q6–8h.

Severe Infections
IV, IM: ADULTS, ELDERLY: 1–1.5 g q6–8h.

Perioperative Prophylaxis
IV, IM: ADULTS, ELDERLY: 1–2 g 30–60 min before surgery, 0.5–1 g during surgery, and q6–8h for up to 24 hrs postoperatively.

Dosage in Renal Impairment
Dosing frequency is modified based on creatinine clearance.

Creatinine Clearance	Dosage
11–34 ml/min	50% usual dose q12h
10 ml/min or less	50% usual dose q18–24h

SIDE EFFECTS

Frequent: Discomfort with IM administration, oral candidiasis (thrush), mild diarrhea, mild abdominal cramping, vaginal candidiasis. **Occasional:** Nausea, serum sickness-like reaction (fever, joint pain; usually occurs after second course of therapy and resolves after drug is discontinued). **Rare:** Allergic reaction (rash, pruritus, urticaria), thrombophlebitis (pain, redness, swelling at injection site).

ADVERSE EFFECTS/ TOXIC REACTIONS

Antibiotic-associated colitis, other superinfections (abdominal cramps, severe watery diarrhea, fever) may result from altered bacterial balance. Nephrotoxicity may occur, esp. in pts with preexisting renal disease. Pts with history of penicillin allergy are at increased risk for developing severe hypersensitivity reaction (severe pruritus, angioedema, bronchospasm, anaphylaxis).

NURSING CONSIDERATIONS

BASELINE ASSESSMENT

Obtain CBC, renal function tests. Question for history of allergies, particularly cephalosporins, penicillins.

INTERVENTION/EVALUATION

Evaluate IM site for induration and tenderness. Assess oral cavity for white patches on mucous membranes, tongue (thrush). Monitor daily pattern of bowel activity, stool consistency. Mild GI effects may be tolerable (increasing severity may indicate onset of antibiotic-associated colitis). Monitor I&O, renal function tests for nephrotoxicity. Be alert for superinfection: fever, vomiting, diarrhea, anal/genital pruritus, oral mucosal changes (ulceration, pain, erythema).

PATIENT/FAMILY TEACHING

• Discomfort may occur with IM injection.

---

cefdinir

sef-di-neer

◆ CLASSIFICATION

PHARMACOTHERAPEUTIC: Third-generation cephalosporin. **CLINICAL:** Antibiotic (see p. 25C).

ACTION

Binds to bacterial cell membranes, inhibits cell wall synthesis. **Therapeutic Effect:** Bactericidal.

PHARMACOKINETICS

Moderately absorbed from GI tract. Protein binding: 60%–70%. Widely distributed. Not appreciably metabolized. Primarily excreted unchanged in urine. Minimally removed by hemodialysis. **Half-life:** 1–2 hrs (increased in renal impairment).

USES

Treatment of susceptible infections due to *S. pyogenes, S. pneumoniae, H. influenzae, H. parainfluenzae, M. catarrhalis* including community-acquired pneumonia, acute exacerbation of chronic bronchitis, acute maxillary sinusitis, pharyngitis, tonsillitis, uncomplicated skin/skin structure infections, otitis media.

PRECAUTIONS

Contraindications: History of anaphylactic reaction to cephalosporins. **Cautions:** Hypersensitivity to penicillins; renal impairment.

⌛ LIFESPAN CONSIDERATIONS

Pregnancy/Lactation: Crosses placenta. Not detected in breast milk. **Pregnancy Category B. Children:** Newborns, infants may have lower renal clearance. **Elderly:** Age-related renal impairment may require decreased dosage or increased dosing interval.

INTERACTIONS

DRUG: Antacids, iron preparations may interfere with absorption. **Probenecid** increases concentration. **HERBAL:** None significant. **FOOD:** None known. **LAB VALUES:** May produce false-positive reaction for urine ketones. May increase serum alkaline phosphatase, bilirubin, LDH, AST, ALT.

AVAILABILITY (Rx)

Capsules: 300 mg. **Powder for Oral Suspension:** 125 mg/5 ml, 250 mg/5 ml.

ADMINISTRATION/HANDLING

PO
• Give without regard to food. • Twice daily doses should be given 12 hrs apart. • Shake oral suspension well before administering. • Store mixed suspension at room temperature. Discard unused portion after 10 days.

INDICATIONS/ROUTES/DOSAGE

Usual Dosage Range
PO: ADULTS, ELDERLY: 300 mg q12h or 600 mg once daily. **CHILDREN 6 MOS–12**

YRS: 7 mg/kg q12h or 14 mg/kg once daily. **Maximum:** 600 mg/day.

Community-Acquired Pneumonia
PO: ADULTS, ELDERLY, CHILDREN 13 YRS AND OLDER: 300 mg q12h for 10 days.

Acute Exacerbation of Chronic Bronchitis
PO: ADULTS, ELDERLY: 300 mg q12h for 5–10 days or 600 mg once daily for 10 days.

Acute Maxillary Sinusitis
PO: ADULTS, ELDERLY, CHILDREN 13 YRS AND OLDER: 300 mg q12h or 600 mg q24h for 10 days. **CHILDREN 6 MOS–12 YRS:** 7 mg/kg q12h or 14 mg/kg q24h for 10 days. **Maximum:** 600 mg/day.

Pharyngitis, Tonsillitis
PO: ADULTS, ELDERLY, CHILDREN 13 YRS AND OLDER: 300 mg q12h for 5–10 days or 600 mg q24h for 10 days. **CHILDREN 6 MOS–12 YRS:** 7 mg/kg q12h for 5–10 days or 14 mg/kg q24h for 10 days. **Maximum:** 600 mg/day.

Uncomplicated Skin/Skin Structure Infections
PO: ADULTS, ELDERLY, CHILDREN 13 YRS AND OLDER: 300 mg q12h for 10 days. **CHILDREN 6 MOS–12 YRS:** 7 mg/kg q12h for 10 days. **Maximum:** 600 mg/day.

Acute Bacterial Otitis Media
PO *(Capsules)*: **CHILDREN: 6 MOS–12 YRS:** 7 mg/kg q12h or 14 mg/kg q24h for 10 days. **Maximum:** 600 mg/day.

Dosage in Renal Impairment
Creatinine clearance less than 30 ml/min: 300 mg/day or 7 mg/kg as single daily dose. **Hemodialysis pts:** 300 mg or 7 mg/kg/dose every other day.

SIDE EFFECTS

Frequent: Oral candidiasis, mild diarrhea, mild abdominal cramping, vaginal candidiasis. **Occasional:** Nausea, serum sickness-like reaction (fever, joint pain; usually occurs after second course of therapy and resolves after drug is discontinued). **Rare:** Allergic reaction (rash, pruritus, urticaria).

ADVERSE EFFECTS/ TOXIC REACTIONS

Antibiotic-associated colitis, other superinfections (abdominal cramps, severe watery diarrhea, fever) may result from altered bacterial balance. Nephrotoxicity may occur, esp. in pts with pre-existing renal disease. Pts with history of penicillin allergy are at increased risk for developing a severe hypersensitivity reaction (severe pruritus, angioedema, bronchospasm, anaphylaxis).

NURSING CONSIDERATIONS

BASELINE ASSESSMENT
Obtain CBC, renal function tests. Question for hypersensitivity to cefdinir or other cephalosporins, penicillins.

INTERVENTION/EVALUATION
Observe for rash. Monitor daily pattern of bowel activity, stool consistency. Mild GI effects may be tolerable (increasing severity may indicate onset of antibiotic-associated colitis). Be alert for superinfection: fever, vomiting, diarrhea, anal/genital pruritus, oral mucosal changes (ulceration, pain, erythema). Monitor hematology reports.

PATIENT/FAMILY TEACHING
• Take antacids 2 hrs before or following medication. • Continue medication for full length of treatment; do not skip doses. • Doses should be evenly spaced. • Report persistent severe diarrhea, rash, muscle aches, fever, enlarged lymph nodes, joint pain.

cefepime

sef-e-**peem**
(Maxipime ✦)

C

Do not confuse cefepime with cefixime or ceftazidime.

◆CLASSIFICATION

PHARMACOTHERAPEUTIC: Fourth-generation cephalosporin. **CLINICAL:** Antibiotic (see p. 25C).

ACTION

Binds to bacterial cell wall membranes, inhibits cell wall synthesis. **Therapeutic Effect:** Bactericidal.

PHARMACOKINETICS

Well absorbed after IM administration. Protein binding: 20%. Widely distributed. Primarily excreted unchanged in urine. Removed by hemodialysis. **Half-life:** 2–2.3 hrs (increased in renal impairment, elderly pts).

USES

Susceptible infections due to aerobic gram-negative organisms including *P. aeruginosa,* gram-positive organisms including *S. aureus.* Treatment of empiric febrile neutropenia, intra-abdominal infections, skin/skin structure infections, UTIs, pneumonia. **OFF-LABEL:** Brain abscess, malignant otitis externa, septic lateral/cavernous sinus thrombus.

PRECAUTIONS

Contraindications: History of anaphylactic reaction to penicillins, hypersensitivity to cephalosporins. **Cautions:** Renal impairment, history of seizure disorder.

⏳ LIFESPAN CONSIDERATIONS

Pregnancy/Lactation: Unknown if distributed in breast milk. **Pregnancy Category B. Children:** No age-related precautions noted in those older than 2 mos. **Elderly:** Age-related renal impairment may require reduced dosage or increased dosing interval.

INTERACTIONS

DRUG: Probenecid may increase concentration. May increase **aminoglyco**-side concentration. **HERBAL:** None significant. **FOOD:** None known. **LAB VALUES:** May increase BUN, serum alkaline phosphatase, bilirubin, LDH, AST, ALT. May cause positive direct/indirect Coombs' test.

AVAILABILITY (Rx)

Injection, Powder for Reconstitution: 500 mg, 1 g, 2 g. **Injection, Premix:** 1 g (50 ml), 2 g (100 ml).

ADMINISTRATION/HANDLING

 IV

Reconstitution • Add 5 ml to 500-mg vial (10 ml for 1-g and 2-g vials). • Further dilute with 50–100 ml 0.9% NaCl or D$_5$W (final concentration not to exceed 40 mg/ml).

Rate of Administration • For intermittent IV infusion (piggyback), infuse over 20–30 min. For direct IV, administer over 5 min.

Storage • Solution is stable for 24 hrs at room temperature, 7 days if refrigerated.

IM

• Add 1.3 ml Sterile Water for Injection, 0.9% NaCl, or D$_5$W to 500-mg vial (2.4 ml for 1-g and 2-g vials). • Inject into a large muscle mass (e.g., upper gluteus maximus).

🔲 IV INCOMPATIBILITIES

Acyclovir (Zovirax), amphotericin (Fungizone), cimetidine (Tagamet), ciprofloxacin (Cipro), cisplatin (Platinol), dacarbazine (DTIC), daunorubicin (Cerubidine), diazepam (Valium), diphenhydramine (Benadryl), dobutamine (Dobutrex), dopamine (Intropin), doxorubicin (Adriamycin), droperidol (Inapsine), famotidine (Pepcid), ganciclovir (Cytovene), haloperidol (Haldol), magnesium, magnesium sulfate, mannitol, metoclopramide (Reglan), morphine, ofloxacin (Floxin), ondansetron (Zofran), vancomycin (Vancocin).

🏵 IV COMPATIBILITIES

Bumetanide (Bumex), calcium gluconate, furosemide (Lasix), hydromorphone (Dilaudid), lorazepam (Ativan), propofol (Diprivan).

INDICATIONS/ROUTES/DOSAGE

Usual Dosage Range

IV: ADULTS, ELDERLY: 1–2 g q8–12h. **CHILDREN:** 50 mg/kg q8–12h not to exceed adult dosing. **NEONATES:** 30 mg/kg/dose q12h.

IM: ADULTS, ELDERLY: 0.5–1 g q12h. **CHILDREN:** 50 mg/kg/dose q8–12h not to exceed adult dosing.

Pneumonia

IV: ADULTS, ELDERLY: 1–2 g q12h for 10 days. **CHILDREN 2 MOS AND OLDER:** 50 mg/kg q12h for 10 days. **Maximum:** 2 g/dose.

Intra-Abdominal Infections

IV: ADULTS, ELDERLY: 2 g q12h for 7–10 days.

Skin/Skin Structure Infections

IV: ADULTS, ELDERLY: 2 g q12h for 10 days. **CHILDREN 2 MOS AND OLDER:** 50 mg/kg q12h for 10 days. **Maximum:** 2 g/dose.

UTI

IV: ADULTS, ELDERLY: 0.5–2 g q12h for 7–10 days. **CHILDREN 2 MOS AND OLDER:** 50 mg/kg q12h for 7–10 days. **Maximum:** 2 g/dose.

Febrile Neutropenia

IV: ADULTS, ELDERLY: 2 g q8h for 7 days or until neutropenia resolves. **CHILDREN 2 MOS AND OLDER:** 50 mg/kg q8h for 7 days or until neutropenia resolves. **Maximum:** 2 g/dose.

Dosage in Renal Impairment

Dosage and frequency are modified based on creatinine clearance and severity of infection.

Creatinine Clearance	Dosage
30–60 ml/min	500 mg q24h–2 g q12h
11–29 ml/min	500 mg–2 g q24h
10 ml/min or less	250 mg–1 g q24h
Hemodialysis	Initially, 1 g, then 0.5–1 g q24h or 1–2 g q48–72h
Peritoneal dialysis	Normal dose q48h
Continuous renal replacement therapy	Initially, 2 g, then 1 g q8h or 2 g q12h

SIDE EFFECTS

Frequent: Discomfort with IM administration, oral candidiasis (thrush), mild diarrhea, mild abdominal cramping, vaginal candidiasis. **Occasional:** Nausea, serum sickness-like reaction (fever, joint pain; usually occurs after second course of therapy and resolves after drug is discontinued). **Rare:** Allergic reaction (rash, pruritus, urticaria), thrombophlebitis (pain, redness, swelling at injection site).

ADVERSE EFFECTS/ TOXIC REACTIONS

Antibiotic-associated colitis, other superinfections (abdominal cramps, severe watery diarrhea, fever) may result from altered bacterial balance. Nephrotoxicity may occur, esp. in pts with preexisting renal disease. Pts with history of penicillin allergy are at increased risk for developing a severe hypersensitivity reaction (severe pruritus, angioedema, bronchospasm, anaphylaxis).

NURSING CONSIDERATIONS

BASELINE ASSESSMENT

Obtain CBC, renal function tests. Question for history of allergies, particularly cephalosporins, penicillins.

INTERVENTION/EVALUATION

Evaluate IM site for induration and tenderness. Assess oral cavity for white patches on mucous membranes, tongue (thrush). Monitor daily pattern of bowel activity, stool consistency. Mild GI effects may be tolerable (increasing severity may indicate onset of antibiotic-associated colitis). Monitor I&O, CBC, renal function tests for nephrotoxicity. Be alert for superinfection: fever, vomiting, diarrhea, anal/genital pruritus, oral mucosal changes (ulceration, pain, erythema).

PATIENT/FAMILY TEACHING

• Discomfort may occur with IM injection. • Continue therapy for full length of treatment. • Doses should be evenly spaced. • Report persistent diarrhea.

---

cefixime

sef-**ix**-eem
(Suprax)
Do not confuse cefixime with cefepime, or Suprax with Sporanox or Surbex.

◆ CLASSIFICATION

PHARMACOTHERAPEUTIC: Third-generation cephalosporin. **CLINICAL:** Antibiotic.

ACTION

Binds to bacterial cell membranes, inhibits cell wall synthesis. **Therapeutic Effect:** Bactericidal.

PHARMACOKINETICS

Moderately absorbed from GI tract. Protein binding: 65%–70%. Widely distributed. Primarily excreted unchanged in urine. Minimally removed by hemodialysis. **Half-life:** 3–4 hrs (increased in renal impairment).

USES

Treatment of susceptible infections due to *S. pneumoniae, S. pyogenes, M. catarrhalis, H. influenzae, E. coli, P. mirabilis* including otitis media, acute bronchitis, acute exacerbations of chronic bronchitis, pharyngitis, tonsillitis, uncomplicated UTI, uncomplicated gonorrhea.

PRECAUTIONS

Contraindications: History of hypersensitivity/anaphylactic reaction to cephalosporins. **Cautions:** History of penicillin allergy, renal impairment.

⌛ LIFESPAN CONSIDERATIONS

Pregnancy/Lactation: Not recommended during labor and delivery. Unknown if distributed in breast milk. **Pregnancy Category B. Children:** Safety and efficacy not established in those younger than 6 mos. **Elderly:** Age-related renal impairment may require dosage adjustment.

INTERACTIONS

DRUG: Probenecid may increase concentration. May increase **aminoglycoside** levels. **HERBAL:** None significant. **FOOD:** None known. **LAB VALUES:** May increase BUN, serum alkaline phosphatase, bilirubin, creatinine, LDH, AST, ALT. May cause a positive direct/indirect Coombs' test.

AVAILABILITY (Rx)

Oral Suspension: 100 mg/5 ml, 200 mg/5 ml. **Tablets:** 400 mg.

ADMINISTRATION/HANDLING

PO

• Give without regard to food. • After reconstitution, oral suspension is stable for 14 days at room temperature. • Do not refrigerate. • Shake oral suspension well before administering.

INDICATIONS/ROUTES/DOSAGE

Usual Dosage
PO: ADULTS, ELDERLY, CHILDREN 12 YRS AND OLDER WEIGHING MORE THAN 50 KG: 400 mg/day as a single dose or in 2 divided doses. **CHILDREN 6 MOS–12 YRS WEIGHING LESS THAN 50 KG:** 8 mg/kg/day as a single dose or in 2 divided doses. **Maximum:** 400 mg.

C

Dosage in Renal Impairment
Dosage is modified based on creatinine clearance.

Creatinine Clearance	Dosage
21–60 ml/min	75% of usual dose
20 ml/min or less	50% of usual dose

SIDE EFFECTS

Frequent: Oral candidiasis (thrush), mild diarrhea, mild abdominal cramping, vaginal candidiasis. **Occasional:** Nausea, serum sickness-like reaction (arthralgia, fever; usually occurs after second course of therapy and resolves after drug is discontinued). **Rare:** Allergic reaction (rash, pruritus, urticaria).

ADVERSE EFFECTS/ TOXIC REACTIONS

Antibiotic-associated colitis, other superinfections (abdominal cramps, severe watery diarrhea, fever) may result from altered bacterial balance. Nephrotoxicity may occur, esp. in pts with preexisting renal disease. Pts with history of penicillin allergy are at increased risk for developing a severe hypersensitivity reaction (severe pruritus, angioedema, bronchospasm, anaphylaxis).

NURSING CONSIDERATIONS

BASELINE ASSESSMENT

Obtain CBC, renal function tests. Question for hypersensitivity to cefixime or other cephalosporins, penicillins.

INTERVENTION/EVALUATION

Assess oral cavity for white patches on mucous membranes, tongue (thrush). Monitor daily pattern of bowel activity, stool consistency. Mild GI effects may be tolerable (increasing severity may indicate onset of antibiotic-associated colitis). Monitor renal function tests for evidence of nephrotoxicity. Be alert for superinfection: fever, vomiting, diarrhea, anal/genital pruritus, oral mucosal changes (ulceration, pain, erythema).

PATIENT/FAMILY TEACHING

• Continue medication for full length of treatment; do not skip doses. • Doses should be evenly spaced. • May cause GI upset (may take with food or milk). • Report persistent diarrhea.

cefotaxime

sef-oh-**tax**-eem
(Claforan)
Do not confuse cefotaxime with cefoxitin, ceftizoxime, or cefuroxime, or Claforan with Claritin.

◆CLASSIFICATION

PHARMACOTHERAPEUTIC: Third-generation cephalosporin. **CLINICAL:** Antibiotic (see p. 25C).

ACTION

Binds to bacterial cell membranes, inhibits cell wall synthesis. **Therapeutic Effect:** Bactericidal.

PHARMACOKINETICS

Widely distributed to CSF. Protein binding: 30%–50%. Partially metabolized in liver to active metabolite. Primarily excreted in urine. Moderately removed by hemodialysis. **Half-life:** 1 hr (increased in renal impairment).

USES

Treatment of susceptible infections (active vs. most gram-negative [not *Pseudomonas*] and gram-positive cocci [not *Enterococcus*]) including bone, joint, GU, gynecologic, intra-abdominal, lower respiratory tract, skin/skin structure infections, septicemia, meningitis, perioperative prophylaxis. **OFF-LABEL:** Treatment of Lyme disease.

PRECAUTIONS

Contraindications: History of hypersensitivity/anaphylactic reaction to cephalosporins. **Cautions:** History of penicillin allergy, renal impairment with creatinine clearance less than 30 ml/min.

⧗ LIFESPAN CONSIDERATIONS

Pregnancy/Lactation: Readily crosses placenta. Distributed in breast milk. **Pregnancy Category B. Children:** No age-related precautions noted. **Elderly:** Age-related renal impairment may require dosage adjustment.

INTERACTIONS

DRUG: Probenecid may increase concentration. May increase **aminoglycoside** concentration. **HERBAL:** None significant. **FOOD:** None known. **LAB VALUES:** May cause positive direct/indirect Coombs' test. May increase BUN, serum creatinine, AST, ALT, alkaline phosphatase.

AVAILABILITY (Rx)

Injection, Powder for Reconstitution: 500 mg, 1 g, 2 g. **Intravenous Solution (Premix):** 1 g/50 ml, 2 g/50 ml.

ADMINISTRATION/HANDLING

IV

Reconstitution • Reconstitute with 10 ml Sterile Water for Injection or 0.9% NaCl to provide a maximum concentration of 100 mg/ml. • May further dilute with 50–100 ml 0.9% NaCl or D_5W.
Rate of Administration • For IV push, administer over 3–5 min. • For intermittent IV infusion (piggyback), infuse over 15–30 min.
Storage • Solution appears light yellow to amber. • IV infusion (piggyback) is stable for 24 hrs at room temperature, 5 days if refrigerated. • Discard if precipitate forms.

IM

• Reconstitute with Sterile Water for Injection or Bacteriostatic Water for Injection to provide a concentration of 230–330 mg/ml. • To minimize discomfort, inject deep IM slowly. Less painful if injected into gluteus maximus than lateral aspect of thigh. For 2-g IM dose, give at 2 separate sites.

▦ IV INCOMPATIBILITIES

Allopurinol (Aloprim), filgrastim (Neupogen), fluconazole (Diflucan), vancomycin (Vancocin).

▦ IV COMPATIBILITIES

Diltiazem (Cardizem), famotidine (Pepcid), hydromorphone (Dilaudid), lorazepam (Ativan), magnesium sulfate, midazolam (Versed), morphine, propofol (Diprivan).

INDICATIONS/ROUTES/DOSAGE

Usual Dosage Range
IV, IM: ADULTS, ELDERLY, CHILDREN WEIGHING 50 KG OR MORE: 1–2 g q4–12h. **CHILDREN 1 MO–12 YRS WEIGHING LESS THAN 50 KG:** 50–200 mg/kg/day in divided doses q6–8h. **NEONATES:** 50 mg/kg/dose q8–12h.

Uncomplicated Infections
IV, IM: ADULTS, ELDERLY: 1 g q12h.

Mild to Moderate Infections
IV, IM: ADULTS, ELDERLY: 1–2 g q8h.

Severe Infections
IV, IM: ADULTS, ELDERLY: 2 g q6–8h.

Life-Threatening Infections
IV, IM: ADULTS, ELDERLY: 2 g q4h. **CHILDREN:** 2 g q4h. **Maximum:** 12 g/day.

Gonorrhea
IM: ADULTS: (Male): 1 g as a single dose. **(Female):** 0.5 g as a single dose.

Perioperative Prophylaxis
IV, IM: ADULTS, ELDERLY: 1 g as a single dose 30–90 min before surgery.

Cesarean Section
IV: ADULTS: 1 g as soon as umbilical cord is clamped, then 1 g 6 and 12 hrs after first dose.

Dosage in Renal Impairment

Creatinine Clearance	Dosage Interval
10–50 ml/min	8–12 hrs
Less than 10 ml/min	24 hrs
Hemodialysis	q24h
Peritoneal dialysis	q24h
Continuous renal replacement therapy	q12h

SIDE EFFECTS

Frequent: Discomfort with IM administration, oral candidiasis (thrush), mild diarrhea, mild abdominal cramping, vaginal candidiasis. **Occasional:** Nausea, serum sickness-like reaction (fever, joint pain; usually occurs after second course of therapy and resolves after drug is discontinued). **Rare:** Allergic reaction (rash, pruritus, urticaria), thrombophlebitis (pain, redness, swelling at injection site).

ADVERSE EFFECTS/ TOXIC REACTIONS

Antibiotic-associated colitis, other superinfections (abdominal cramps, severe watery diarrhea, fever) may result from altered bacterial balance. Nephrotoxicity may occur, esp. in pts with preexisting renal disease. Pts with history of penicillin allergy are at increased risk for developing a severe hypersensitivity reaction (severe pruritus, angioedema, bronchospasm, anaphylaxis).

NURSING CONSIDERATIONS

BASELINE ASSESSMENT

Question for history of allergies, particularly cephalosporins, penicillins.

INTERVENTION/EVALUATION

Check IM injection sites for induration, tenderness. Assess oral cavity for white patches on mucous membranes, tongue (thrush). Monitor daily pattern of bowel activity, stool consistency. Mild GI effects may be tolerable (increasing severity may indicate onset of antibiotic-associated colitis). Monitor I&O, renal function tests for nephrotoxicity. Be alert for superinfection: fever, vomiting, diarrhea, anal/genital pruritus, oral mucosal changes (ulceration, pain, erythema).

PATIENT/FAMILY TEACHING

• Discomfort may occur with IM injection. • Doses should be evenly spaced. • Continue antibiotic therapy for full length of treatment.

cefoxitin

sef-**ox**-i-tin
(Mefoxin)
Do not confuse cefoxitin with cefazolin, cefotaxime, ceftazidime, ceftriaxone, or Cytoxan, or Mefoxin with Lanoxin.

◆CLASSIFICATION

PHARMACOTHERAPEUTIC: Second-generation cephalosporin. **CLINICAL:** Antibiotic (see p. 24C).

ACTION

Binds to bacterial cell membranes, inhibits cell wall synthesis. **Therapeutic Effect:** Bactericidal.

PHARMACOKINETICS

Well distributed. Protein binding: 65%–79%. Primarily excreted unchanged in urine. Removed by hemodialysis. **Half-life:** 0.8–1 hr.

USES

Treatment of susceptible infections due to *S. pneumoniae, S. aureus,* gram-negative enteric bacilli, anaerobes (e.g., *Bacteroides* spp.) including bone, joint, gynecologic, intra-abdominal, lower respiratory, skin/skin structure, UTIs, perioperative prophylaxis.

PRECAUTIONS

Contraindications: History of hypersensitivity/anaphylactic reaction to cephalosporins. **Cautions:** Renal impairment, history of penicillin allergy.

⧗ LIFESPAN CONSIDERATIONS

Pregnancy/Lactation: Readily crosses placenta; distributed in breast milk. **Pregnancy Category B. Children:** No age-related precautions noted. **Elderly:** Age-related renal impairment may require dosage adjustment.

INTERACTIONS

DRUG: Probenecid may increase concentration. **HERBAL:** None significant. **FOOD:** None known. **LAB VALUES:** May increase BUN, serum alkaline phosphatase, creatinine, AST, ALT. May cause positive direct/indirect Coombs' test.

AVAILABILITY (Rx)

Injection, Powder for Reconstitution: 1 g, 2 g. **Intravenous Solution:** 1 g/50 ml, 2 g/50 ml.

ADMINISTRATION/HANDLING

◀**ALERT**▶ Give IM, IV push, intermittent IV infusion (piggyback).

 IV

Reconstitution • Reconstitute with 10 ml Sterile Water for Injection, Bacteriostatic Water for Injection, 0.9% NaCl, or D_5W to provide a maximum concentration of 100 mg/ml. • May further dilute with 50–100 ml 0.9% Sterile Water for Injection, NaCl, or D_5W.
Rate of Administration • For IV push, administer over 3–5 min. • For intermittent IV infusion (piggyback), infuse over 10–60 min.
Storage • Solution appears colorless to light amber but may darken (does not indicate loss of potency). • IV infusion (piggyback) is stable for 24 hrs at room temperature, 48 hrs if refrigerated. • Discard if precipitate forms.

IM
• Reconstitute each 1 g with 2 ml Sterile Water for Injection or lidocaine to pro-

vide concentration of 400 mg/ml. • To minimize discomfort, inject deep IM slowly. Less painful if injected into gluteus maximus than lateral aspect of thigh.

▥ IV INCOMPATIBILITIES

Vancomycin (Vancocin).

▥ IV COMPATIBILITIES

Diltiazem (Cardizem), famotidine (Pepcid), heparin, hydromorphone (Dilaudid), magnesium sulfate, morphine, multivitamins, propofol (Diprivan).

INDICATIONS/ROUTES/DOSAGE

Usual Dosage Range
IM, IV: ADULTS, ELDERLY: 1–2 g q6–8h. **Maximum:** 12 g/day. **CHILDREN OLDER THAN 3 MOS:** 80–160 mg/kg/day in 3–6 divided doses. **Maximum:** 12 g/day. **NEONATES:** 90–100 mg/kg/day in divided doses q8h.

Mild to Moderate Infections
IV, IM: ADULTS, ELDERLY: 1–2 g q6–8h. **CHILDREN:** 80 mg/kg/day divided q6–8h.

Severe Infections
IV, IM: ADULTS, ELDERLY: 1 g q4h or 2 g q6–8h up to 2 g q4h. **CHILDREN:** 160 mg/kg/day divided q6h.

Perioperative Prophylaxis
IV, IM: ADULTS, ELDERLY: 1–2 g 30–60 min before surgery, then q6h for up to 24 hrs after surgery. **CHILDREN OLDER THAN 3 MOS:** 30–40 mg/kg 30–60 min before surgery, then q6h for up to 24 hrs after surgery.

Dosage in Renal Impairment
After a loading dose of 1–2 g, dosage and frequency are modified based on creatinine clearance and severity of infection.

Creatinine Clearance	Dosage
30–50 ml/min	1–2 g q8–12h
10–29 ml/min	1–2 g q12–24h
5–9 ml/min	500 mg–1 g q12–24h
Less than 5 ml/min	500 mg–1 g q24–48h
Hemodialysis	Loading dose of 1–2 g after each HD. Maintenance dose based on creatinine clearance.
Continuous renal replacement therapy	1–2 g q8–24h.

SIDE EFFECTS

Frequent: Discomfort with IM administration, oral candidiasis (thrush), mild diarrhea, mild abdominal cramping, vaginal candidiasis. **Occasional:** Nausea, serum sickness-like reaction (fever, joint pain; usually occurs after second course of therapy and resolves after drug is discontinued). **Rare:** Allergic reaction (pruritus, rash, urticaria), thrombophlebitis (pain, redness, swelling at injection site).

ADVERSE EFFECTS/ TOXIC REACTIONS

Antibiotic-associated colitis, other superinfections (abdominal cramps, severe watery diarrhea, fever) may result from altered bacterial balance. Nephrotoxicity may occur, esp. in pts with preexisting renal disease. Pts with history of penicillin allergy are at increased risk for developing a severe hypersensitivity reaction (severe pruritus, angioedema, bronchospasm, anaphylaxis).

NURSING CONSIDERATIONS

BASELINE ASSESSMENT

Obtain CBC, renal function tests. Question for history of allergies, particularly cephalosporins, penicillins.

INTERVENTION/EVALUATION

Evaluate IV site for phlebitis (heat, pain, red streaking over vein). Assess IM injection sites for induration, tenderness. Assess oral cavity for white patches on mucous membranes, tongue (thrush). Monitor daily pattern of bowel activity, stool consistency. Mild GI effects may be tolerable (increasing severity may indicate onset of antibiotic-associated colitis). Monitor I&O, renal function tests for nephrotoxicity. Be alert for superinfection: fever, vomiting, diarrhea, anal/genital pruritus, oral mucosal changes (ulceration, pain, erythema).

PATIENT/FAMILY TEACHING

• Discomfort may occur with IM injection. • Doses should be evenly spaced. • Continue antibiotic therapy for full length of treatment.

cefpodoxime

sef-poe-**dox**-eem

◆ CLASSIFICATION

PHARMACOTHERAPEUTIC: Third-generation cephalosporin. **CLINICAL:** Antibiotic (see p. 25C).

ACTION

Binds to bacterial cell membranes, inhibits cell wall synthesis. **Therapeutic Effect:** Bactericidal.

PHARMACOKINETICS

Well absorbed from GI tract (food increases absorption). Protein binding: 18%–23%. Widely distributed. Primarily excreted unchanged in urine. Partially removed by hemodialysis. **Half-life:** 2.3 hrs (increased in renal impairment, elderly pts).

USES

Treatment of susceptible infections due to *S. pneumoniae, S. pyogenes, S. aureus, H. influenzae, M. catarrhalis, E. coli, Proteus, Klebsiella* spp., including acute maxillary sinusitis, chronic bronchitis, community-acquired pneumonia, gonorrhea, otitis media, pharyngitis, tonsillitis, skin/skin structure infections, UTIs.

PRECAUTIONS

Contraindications: History of hypersensitivity/anaphylactic reaction to cephalosporins. **Cautions:** Renal impairment, history of penicillin allergy.

⧗ LIFESPAN CONSIDERATIONS

Pregnancy/Lactation: Readily crosses placenta. Distributed in breast milk. **Pregnancy Category B. Children:** Safety and efficacy not established in those younger than 6 mos. **Elderly:** Age-related renal impairment may require dosage adjustment.

INTERACTIONS

DRUG: High doses of **antacids containing aluminum, H₂ antagonists** may decrease absorption. **Probenecid** may increase concentration. **HERBAL:** None significant. **FOOD: Food** enhances absorption. **LAB VALUES:** May increase BUN, serum alkaline phosphatase, bilirubin, creatinine, LDH, AST, ALT. May cause positive direct/indirect Coombs' test.

AVAILABILITY (Rx)

Oral Suspension: 50 mg/5 ml, 100 mg/5 ml. **Tablets:** 100 mg, 200 mg.

ADMINISTRATION/HANDLING

PO
• Administer tablet with food (enhances absorption). • Administer suspension without regard to food. • After reconstitution, oral suspension is stable for 14 days if refrigerated.

INDICATIONS/ROUTES/DOSAGE

Usual Dosage Range
PO: ADULTS, ELDERLY, CHILDREN OLDER THAN 12 YRS: 100–400 mg q12h. **CHILDREN 2 MOS–12 YRS:** 10 mg/kg/day in 2 divided doses. **Maximum:** 400 mg/day.

Chronic Bronchitis, Pneumonia
PO: ADULTS, ELDERLY, CHILDREN OLDER THAN 12 YRS: 200 mg q12h for 10–14 days.

Gonorrhea, Rectal Gonococcal Infection (Female Pts Only)
PO: ADULTS, CHILDREN OLDER THAN 12 YRS: 200 mg as a single dose.

Skin/Skin Structure Infections
PO: ADULTS, ELDERLY, CHILDREN OLDER THAN 13 YRS: 400 mg q12h for 7–14 days.

Pharyngitis, Tonsillitis
PO: ADULTS, ELDERLY, CHILDREN OLDER THAN 13 YRS: 100 mg q12h for 5–10 days. **CHILDREN 6 MOS–13 YRS:** 5 mg/kg q12h for 5–10 days. **Maximum:** 100 mg/dose.

Acute Maxillary Sinusitis
PO: ADULTS, CHILDREN OLDER THAN 13 YRS: 200 mg q12h for 10 days. **CHILDREN 2 MOS–13 YRS:** 5 mg/kg q12h for 10 days. **Maximum:** 200 mg/dose.

UTI
PO: ADULTS, ELDERLY, CHILDREN OLDER THAN 13 YRS: 100 mg q12h for 7 days.

Acute Otitis Media
PO: CHILDREN 6 MOS–13 YRS: 5 mg/kg q12h for 5 days. **Maximum:** 400 mg/dose.

Dosage in Renal Impairment
For pts with creatinine clearance less than 30 ml/min, usual dose is given q24h. For pts on hemodialysis, usual dose is given 3 times a wk after dialysis.

SIDE EFFECTS

Frequent: Oral candidiasis (thrush), mild diarrhea, mild abdominal cramping, vaginal candidiasis. **Occasional:** Nausea, serum sickness-like reaction (fever, joint pain; usually occurs after second course of therapy and resolves after drug is discontinued). **Rare:** Allergic reaction (pruritus, rash, urticaria).

ADVERSE EFFECTS/ TOXIC REACTIONS

Antibiotic-associated colitis, other superinfections (abdominal cramps, severe watery diarrhea, fever) may result from altered bacterial balance. Nephrotoxicity may occur, esp. in pts with preexisting renal disease. Pts with history of penicillin allergy are at increased risk for developing a severe hypersensitivity reaction (severe pruritus, angioedema, bronchospasm, anaphylaxis).

NURSING CONSIDERATIONS

BASELINE ASSESSMENT
Obtain CBC, renal function tests. Question for history of allergies, particularly cephalosporins, penicillins.

INTERVENTION/EVALUATION
Assess oral cavity for white patches on mucous membranes, tongue (thrush). Monitor daily pattern of bowel activity, stool consistency. Mild GI effects may be tolerable (increasing severity may indicate onset of antibiotic-associated colitis). Monitor I&O, renal function tests for nephrotoxicity. Be alert for superinfection: fever, vomiting, diarrhea, anal/genital pruritus, oral mucosal changes (ulceration, pain, erythema).

PATIENT/FAMILY TEACHING
• Doses should be evenly spaced.
• Shake oral suspension well before using. • Continue antibiotic therapy for full length of treatment. • Refrigerate oral suspension. • Report persistent diarrhea.

cefprozil

sef-proe-zil
(Apo-Cefprozil ✦, Cefzil ✦)
Do not confuse cefprozil with cefazolin, or Cefzil with Cefol, Ceftin, or Kefzol.

◆CLASSIFICATION

PHARMACOTHERAPEUTIC: Second-generation cephalosporin. **CLINICAL:** Antibiotic (see p. 24C).

ACTION
Binds to bacterial cell membranes, inhibits cell wall synthesis. **Therapeutic Effect:** Bactericidal.

PHARMACOKINETICS
Well absorbed from GI tract. Protein binding: 36%–45%. Widely distributed. Primarily excreted unchanged in urine. Moderately removed by hemodialysis. **Half-life:** 1.3 hrs (increased in renal impairment).

USES
Treatment of susceptible infections due to *S. pneumoniae, S. pyogenes, S. aureus, H. influenzae, M. catarrhalis* including pharyngitis, tonsillitis, otitis media, secondary bacterial infection of acute bronchitis, acute bacterial exacerbation of chronic bronchitis, uncomplicated skin/skin structure infections, acute sinusitis.

PRECAUTIONS
Contraindications: History of hypersensitivity/anaphylactic reaction to cephalosporins. **Cautions:** Severe renal impairment, history of penicillin allergy.

⏳ LIFESPAN CONSIDERATIONS
Pregnancy/Lactation: Readily crosses placenta. Distributed in breast milk. **Pregnancy Category B. Children:** Safety and efficacy not established in those younger than 6 mos. **Elderly:** Age-related renal impairment may require dosage adjustment.

INTERACTIONS
DRUG: Probenecid may increase concentration. May increase **aminoglycoside** concentration. **HERBAL:** None significant. **FOOD:** None known. **LAB VALUES:** May cause positive direct/indirect Coombs' test. May increase BUN, serum creatinine, alkaline phosphatase, AST, ALT.

AVAILABILITY (Rx)
Oral Suspension: 125 mg/5 ml, 250 mg/5 ml. **Tablets:** 250 mg, 500 mg.

ADMINISTRATION/HANDLING

PO

• Give without regard to food; if GI upset occurs, give with food, milk. • After reconstitution, oral suspension is stable for 14 days if refrigerated. • Shake oral suspension well before using.

INDICATIONS/ROUTES/DOSAGE

Usual Dosage Range

PO: ADULTS, ELDERLY, CHILDREN OLDER THAN 12 YRS: 250–500 mg q12h or 500 mg q24h. **CHILDREN OLDER THAN 6 MOS–12 YRS:** 7.5–15 mg/kg/day in 2 divided doses.

Pharyngitis, Tonsillitis

PO: ADULTS, ELDERLY: 500 mg q24h for 10 days. **CHILDREN 2–12 YRS:** 7.5 mg/kg q12h for 10 days. **Maximum:** 1 g/day.

Acute Bacterial Exacerbation of Chronic Bronchitis, Secondary Bacterial Infection of Acute Bronchitis

PO: ADULTS, ELDERLY: 500 mg q12h for 10 days.

Skin/Skin Structure Infections

PO: ADULTS, ELDERLY, CHILDREN OLDER THAN 12 YRS: 250–500 mg q12h for 10 days. **CHILDREN 2–12 YRS:** 20 mg/kg q24h for 10 days. **Maximum:** 1 g/day.

Acute Sinusitis

PO: ADULTS, ELDERLY: 250–500 mg q12h for 10 days. **CHILDREN 6 MOS–12 YRS:** 7.5–15 mg/kg q12h for 10 days.

Otitis Media

PO: CHILDREN 6 MOS–12 YRS: 15 mg/kg q12h for 10 days. **Maximum:** 1 g/day.

Dosage in Renal Impairment

Creatinine clearance less than 30 ml/min: 50% of usual dose at usual interval. **Hemodialysis:** Administer dose after completion of dialysis.

SIDE EFFECTS

Frequent: Oral candidiasis (thrush), mild diarrhea, mild abdominal cramping, vaginal candidiasis. **Occasional:** Nausea, serum sickness reaction (fever, joint pain; usually occurs after second course of therapy and resolves after drug is discontinued). **Rare:** Allergic reaction (pruritus, rash, urticaria).

ADVERSE EFFECTS/ TOXIC REACTIONS

Antibiotic-associated colitis, other superinfections (abdominal cramps, severe watery diarrhea, fever) may result from altered bacterial balance. Nephrotoxicity may occur, esp. in pts with preexisting renal disease. Pts with history of penicillin allergy are at increased risk for developing a severe hypersensitivity reaction (severe pruritus, angioedema, bronchospasm, anaphylaxis).

NURSING CONSIDERATIONS

BASELINE ASSESSMENT

Obtain CBC, renal function tests. Question for history of allergies, particularly cephalosporins, penicillins.

INTERVENTION/EVALUATION

Assess oral cavity for evidence of stomatitis. Monitor daily pattern of bowel activity, stool consistency. Mild GI effects may be tolerable (but increasing severity may indicate onset of antibiotic-associated colitis). Monitor I&O, renal function tests for nephrotoxicity. Be alert for superinfection: fever, vomiting, diarrhea, anal/genital pruritus, oral mucosal changes (ulceration, pain, erythema).

PATIENT/FAMILY TEACHING

• Doses should be evenly spaced. • Continue antibiotic therapy for full length of treatment. • May cause GI upset (may take with food or milk). • Report persistent diarrhea.

ceftaroline

sef-**tar**-o-leen
(Teflaro)

 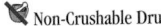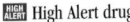

◆CLASSIFICATION

PHARMACOTHERAPEUTIC: Fifth-generation cephalosporin. **CLINICAL:** Antibiotic (see p. 25C).

ACTION

Binds to bacterial cell membranes, inhibits cell wall synthesis. **Therapeutic Effect:** Bactericidal.

PHARMACOKINETICS

Protein binding: 20%. Widely distributed in plasma. Not metabolized. Primarily excreted unchanged in urine. Hemodialyzable. **Half-life:** 1.6 hrs (increased in renal impairment).

USES

Treatment of susceptible infections due to gram-positive and gram-negative organisms including *S. pneumoniae, S. aureus* (methicillin susceptible only), *H. influenzae, Klebsiella pneumoniae, E. coli* including acute bacterial skin and skin structure infections, community-acquired bacterial pneumonia.

PRECAUTIONS

Contraindications: History of hypersensitivity/anaphylactic reaction to cephalosporins. **Cautions:** History of allergy to penicillin, severe renal impairment with creatinine clearance less than 50 ml/min.

☒ LIFESPAN CONSIDERATIONS

Pregnancy/Lactation: Unknown if distributed in breast milk. **Pregnancy Category B. Children:** Safety and efficacy not established in those younger than 18 yrs. **Elderly:** Age-related renal impairment may require dose adjustment.

INTERACTIONS

DRUG: Probenecid may increase concentration. **HERBAL:** None significant. **FOOD:** None known. **LAB VALUES:** May cause positive direct/indirect Coombs' test. May increase BUN, serum creatinine. May decrease serum potassium.

AVAILABILITY (Rx)

Injection, Powder for Reconstitution: 400-mg, 600-mg single-use vial.

ADMINISTRATION/HANDLING

◀**ALERT**▶ Give by intermittent IV infusion (piggyback). Do not give IV push.
Reconstitution • Reconstitute either 400-mg or 600-mg vial with 20 ml Sterile Water for Injection. • Mix gently to dissolve powder. • Further dilute with 250 ml D₅W, 0.9% NaCl, or 0.45% NaCl to provide concentration of 20 mg/ml for 400-mg dose or 30 mg/ml for 600-mg dose.
Rate of Administration • Infuse over 60 min.
Storage • Discard if particulate is present. • Following reconstitution, solution should appear clear, light to dark yellow. • Solution is stable for 6 hrs at room temperature or 24 hrs if refrigerated.

▦ IV INCOMPATIBILITIES

Fluconazole (Diflucan), vancomycin (Vancocin).

▦ IV COMPATIBILITIES

Famotidine (Pepcid), hydromorphone (Dilaudid), lorazepam (Ativan), magnesium sulfate, midazolam (Versed), morphine, propofol (Diprivan).

INDICATIONS/ROUTES/DOSAGE

Acute Bacterial Skin/Skin Structure Infections
IV Infusion: ADULTS, ELDERLY: 600 mg every 12 hrs for 5–14 days.

Community-Acquired Bacterial Pneumonia
IV Infusion: ADULTS, ELDERLY: 600 mg every 12 hrs for 5–7 days.

Dosage in Renal Impairment

Creatinine Clearance	Dosage
30–50 ml/min	400 mg q12h
15–29 ml/min	300 mg q12h
End-stage renal disease, hemodialysis	200 mg every 12 hrs (give after dialysis)

SIDE EFFECTS

Occasional (5%–4%): Diarrhea, nausea. **Rare (3%–2%):** Allergic reaction (rash, pruritus, urticaria), phlebitis.

ADVERSE EFFECTS/ TOXIC REACTIONS

Antibiotic-associated colitis, other super infections (abdominal cramps, severe watery diarrhea, fever) may result from altered bacterial balance. Nephrotoxicity may occur, esp. with preexisting renal disease. Pts with history of penicillin allergy are at increased risk for developing a severe hypersensitivity reaction (severe pruritus, angioedema, bronchospasm, anaphylaxis).

NURSING CONSIDERATIONS

BASELINE ASSESSMENT

Obtain CBC, renal function tests. Question for hypersensitivity to other cephalosporins, penicillins. For those on hemodialysis, administer medication after dialysis.

INTERVENTION/EVALUATION

Assess oral cavity for white patches on mucous membranes, tongue. Monitor daily pattern of bowel activity, stool consistency. Mild GI effects may be tolerable, but increasing severity may indicate onset of antibiotic-associated colitis. Monitor I&O, renal function tests for evidence of nephrotoxicity. Be alert for superinfection: fever, vomiting, severe genital/anal pruritus, moderate to severe diarrhea, oral mucosal changes (ulceration, pain, erythema).

PATIENT/FAMILY TEACHING

• Continue medication for full length of treatment. • Doses should be evenly spaced.

ceftazidime

sef-**taz**-i-deem
(Fortaz, Tazicef)

Do not confuse ceftazidime with cefazolin, cefepime, or ceftriaxone.

◆**CLASSIFICATION**

PHARMACOTHERAPEUTIC: Third-generation cephalosporin. **CLINICAL:** Antibiotic (see p. 25C).

ACTION

Binds to bacterial cell membranes, inhibits cell wall synthesis. **Therapeutic Effect:** Bactericidal.

PHARMACOKINETICS

Widely distributed including to CSF. Protein binding: 5%–17%. Primarily excreted unchanged in urine. Removed by hemodialysis. **Half-life:** 2 hrs (increased in renal impairment).

USES

Treatment of susceptible infections due to gram-negative organisms (including *Pseudomonas* and *Enterobacteriaceae*) including bone, joint, CNS (including meningitis), gynecologic, intra-abdominal, lower respiratory tract, skin/skin structure, UTI, septicemia. Treatment of CNS infections due to *H. influenzae, N. meningitidis,* including meningitis. **OFF-LABEL:** Bacterial endophthalmitis.

PRECAUTIONS

Contraindications: History of hypersensitivity/anaphylactic reaction to cephalosporins. **Cautions:** Severe renal impairment, history of penicillin allergy, seizure disorder.

⌛ LIFESPAN CONSIDERATIONS

Pregnancy/Lactation: Readily crosses placenta. Distributed in breast milk. **Pregnancy Category B. Children:** No age-related precautions noted. **Elderly:** Age-related renal impairment may require dosage adjustment.

INTERACTIONS

DRUG: Probenecid may increase concentration. May increase **aminoglyco-**

side levels. **HERBAL:** None significant. **FOOD:** None known. **LAB VALUES:** May increase BUN, serum alkaline phosphatase, creatinine, LDH, AST, ALT. May cause positive direct/indirect Coombs' test.

AVAILABILITY (Rx)

Injection, Powder for Reconstitution (Fortaz, Tazicef): 500 mg, 1 g, 2 g. **Injection, Premix:** 1 g/50 ml, 2 g/50 ml.

ADMINISTRATION/HANDLING

◄**ALERT**► Give by IM injection, direct IV injection (IV push), or intermittent IV infusion (piggyback).

 IV

Reconstitution • Add 10 ml Sterile Water for Injection to each 1 g to provide concentration of 90 mg/ml. • May further dilute with 50–100 ml 0.9% NaCl, D_5W, or other compatible diluent.
Rate of Administration • For IV push, administer over 3–5 min (**maximum concentration:** 180 mg/ml). • For intermittent IV infusion (piggyback), infuse over 15–30 min.
Storage • Solution appears light yellow to amber, tends to darken (color change does not indicate loss of potency). • IV infusion (piggyback) stable for 12 hrs at room temperature or 3 days if refrigerated. • Discard if precipitate forms.

IM
• For reconstitution, add 1.5 ml Sterile Water for Injection or lidocaine 1% to 500-mg vial or 3 ml to 1-g vial to provide a concentration of 280 mg/ml. • To minimize discomfort, inject deep IM slowly. Less painful if injected into gluteus maximus than lateral aspect of thigh.

▦ IV INCOMPATIBILITIES

Amphotericin B complex (Abelcet, AmBisome, Amphotec), fluconazole (Diflucan), idarubicin, midazolam (Versed), <u>vancomycin</u> (Vancocin).

▦ IV COMPATIBILITIES

Diltiazem (Cardizem), famotidine (Pepcid), heparin, hydromorphone (Dilaudid), lipids, morphine, propofol (Diprivan).

INDICATIONS/ROUTES/DOSAGE

Usual Dosage Range
IV, IM: ADULTS, ELDERLY: 500 mg–2 g q8–12h.
IV: CHILDREN 1 MO–12 YRS: 90–150 mg/kg/day in divided doses q8h. **Maximum:** 6 g/day. **NEONATES 0–4 WKS:** 50 mg/kg/dose q8–12h.

Usual Elderly Dosage
ELDERLY (NORMAL RENAL FUNCTION): 500 mg–1 g q12h.

Dosage in Renal Impairment
Dosage and frequency are modified based on creatinine clearance and severity of infection.

Creatinine Clearance	Dosage
31–50 ml/min	q12h
10–30 ml/min	q24h
Less than 10 ml/min	q48–72h
Hemodialysis	0.5–1 g q24h or 1–2 g q48–72h (give post hemodialysis on dialysis days)
Peritoneal dialysis	Initially, 1 g, then 0.5 g q24h
Continuous renal replacement therapy	Initially, 2 g, then 1 g q8h or 2 g q12h

SIDE EFFECTS

Frequent: Discomfort with IM administration, oral candidiasis (thrush), mild diarrhea, mild abdominal cramping, vaginal candidiasis. **Occasional:** Nausea, serum sickness-like reaction (fever, joint pain; usually occurs after second course of therapy and resolves after drug is discontinued). **Rare:** Allergic reaction (pruritus, rash, urticaria), thrombophlebitis (pain, redness, swelling at injection site).

<u>underlined</u> – top prescribed drug

ADVERSE EFFECTS/ TOXIC REACTIONS

Antibiotic-associated colitis, other super-infections (abdominal cramps, severe watery diarrhea, fever) may result from altered bacterial balance. Nephrotoxicity may occur, esp. in pts with preexisting renal disease. Pts with history of penicillin allergy are at increased risk for developing a severe hypersensitivity reaction (severe pruritus, angioedema, bronchospasm, anaphylaxis).

NURSING CONSIDERATIONS

BASELINE ASSESSMENT

Obtain CBC, renal function tests. Question for history of allergies, particularly cephalosporins, penicillins.

INTERVENTION/EVALUATION

Evaluate IV site for phlebitis (heat, pain, red streaking over vein). Assess IM injection sites for induration, tenderness. Check oral cavity for white patches on mucous membranes, tongue (thrush). Monitor daily pattern of bowel activity, stool consistency. Mild GI effects may be tolerable (increasing severity may indicate onset of antibiotic-associated colitis). Monitor I&O, renal function tests for nephrotoxicity. Be alert for superinfection: fever, vomiting, diarrhea, anal/genital pruritus, oral mucosal changes (ulceration, pain, erythema).

PATIENT/FAMILY TEACHING

• Discomfort may occur with IM injection. • Doses should be evenly spaced. • Continue antibiotic therapy for full length of treatment.

ceftibuten

sef-tye-**bue**-ten
(Cedax)
Do not confuse Cedax with Cidex.

◆**CLASSIFICATION**

PHARMACOTHERAPEUTIC: Third-generation cephalosporin. **CLINICAL:** Antibiotic (see p. 25C).

ACTION

Binds to bacterial cell membranes, inhibits cell wall synthesis. **Therapeutic Effect:** Bactericidal.

PHARMACOKINETICS

Rapidly absorbed from GI tract. Protein binding: 65%–77%. Excreted primarily unchanged in urine. **Half-life:** 2–3 hrs.

USES

Treatment of susceptible infections due to *S. pneumoniae, S. pyogenes, H. influenzae, M. catarrhalis* including chronic bronchitis, acute bacterial otitis media, pharyngitis, tonsillitis.

PRECAUTIONS

Contraindications: History of hypersensitivity/anaphylactic reaction to cephalosporins. **Cautions:** History of penicillin allergy, moderate to severe renal impairment.

⧗ LIFESPAN CONSIDERATIONS

Pregnancy/Lactation: Unknown if drug crosses placenta or is distributed in breast milk. **Pregnancy Category B. Children:** Safety and efficacy not established in those younger than 6 mos. **Elderly:** Age-related renal impairment may require dosage adjustment.

INTERACTIONS

DRUG: Probenecid may increase concentration. May increase **aminoglycoside** concentration. **HERBAL:** None significant. **FOOD:** None known. **LAB VALUES:** May increase BUN, serum alkaline phosphatase, bilirubin, creatinine, LDH, AST, ALT. May cause positive direct/indirect Coombs' test.

AVAILABILITY (Rx)

Capsules: 400 mg. **Oral Suspension:** 90 mg/5 ml, 180 mg/5 ml.

 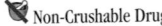

C

ADMINISTRATION/HANDLING

Capsules: Administer without regard to food. **Suspension:** Shake well, give 2 hrs before or 1 hr after meals.

INDICATIONS/ROUTES/DOSAGE

Usual Dosage
PO: ADULTS, ELDERLY: 400 mg once daily for 10 days. **CHILDREN 6 MOS–11 YRS:** 9 mg/kg/day for 10 days. **Maximum:** 400 mg/day.

Chronic Bronchitis
PO: ADULTS, ELDERLY: 400 mg/day once a day for 10 days.

Pharyngitis, Tonsillitis
PO: ADULTS, ELDERLY: 400 mg once a day for 10 days. **CHILDREN OLDER THAN 6 MOS:** 9 mg/kg once a day for 10 days. **Maximum:** 400 mg/day.

Otitis Media
PO: CHILDREN OLDER THAN 6 MOS: 9 mg/kg once a day for 10 days. **Maximum:** 400 mg/day.

Dosage in Renal Impairment
Dosage is modified based on creatinine clearance.

Creatinine Clearance	Dosage
50 ml/min and higher	400 mg or 9 mg/kg q24h
30–49 ml/min	200 mg or 4.5 mg/kg q24h
Less than 30 ml/min	100 mg or 2.25 mg/kg q24h
Hemodialysis	400 mg or 9 mg/kg (**maximum:** 400 mg) after each dialysis session.

SIDE EFFECTS

Frequent: Oral candidiasis (thrush), mild diarrhea (discharge, itching). **Occasional:** Nausea, serum sickness-like reaction (fever, joint pain; usually occurs after second course of therapy and resolves after drug is discontinued).

Rare: Allergic reaction (rash, pruritus, urticaria).

ADVERSE EFFECTS/ TOXIC REACTIONS

Antibiotic-associated colitis, other superinfections (abdominal cramps, severe watery diarrhea, fever) may result from altered bacterial balance. Nephrotoxicity may occur, esp. in pts with preexisting renal disease. Pts with history of penicillin allergy are at increased risk for developing a severe hypersensitivity reaction (severe pruritus, angioedema, bronchospasm, anaphylaxis).

NURSING CONSIDERATIONS

BASELINE ASSESSMENT
Obtain CBC, renal function tests. Question for history of allergies, particularly cephalosporins, penicillins.

INTERVENTION/EVALUATION
Assess oral cavity for white patches on mucous membranes, tongue (thrush). Monitor daily pattern of bowel activity, stool consistency. Mild GI effects may be tolerable (increasing severity may indicate onset of antibiotic-associated colitis). Monitor I&O, serum renal function tests for nephrotoxicity. Be alert for superinfection: fever, vomiting, diarrhea, anal/genital pruritus, oral mucosal changes (ulceration, pain, erythema).

PATIENT/FAMILY TEACHING
• Continue medication for full length of treatment; do not skip doses. • May cause GI upset (may take with food or milk). • Report persistent diarrhea.

ceftriaxone

sef-trye-**ax**-own
(Rocephin)
Do not confuse ceftriaxone with cefazolin, cefoxitin, or ceftazidine.

◆CLASSIFICATION

PHARMACOTHERAPEUTIC: Third-generation cephalosporin. **CLINICAL:** Antibiotic (see p. 25C).

ACTION

Binds to bacterial cell membranes, inhibits cell wall synthesis. **Therapeutic Effect:** Bactericidal.

PHARMACOKINETICS

Widely distributed including to CSF. Protein binding: 83%–96%. Primarily excreted unchanged in urine. Not removed by hemodialysis. **Half-life: IV:** 4.3–4.6 hrs; **IM:** 5.8–8.7 hrs (increased in renal impairment).

USES

Treatment of susceptible infections due to gram-negative aerobic organisms, some gram-positive organisms including respiratory tract, GU tract, skin and skin structure, bone and joint, intra-abdominal, pelvic inflammatory disease (PID), biliary tract/urinary tract infections, bacterial septicemia, meningitis, perioperative prophylaxis, acute bacterial otitis media. **OFF-LABEL:** Complicated gonococcal infections, STDs, Lyme disease, salmonellosis, shigellosis, atypical community-acquired pneumonia.

PRECAUTIONS

Contraindications: History of hypersensitivity/anaphylactic reaction to cephalosporins. Hyperbilirubinemic neonates, esp. premature infants, should not be treated with ceftriaxone (can displace bilirubin from its binding to serum albumin, causing bilirubin encephalopathy). Do not administer with calcium-containing IV solutions, including continuous calcium-containing infusion such as parenteral nutrition (in neonates) due to the risk of precipitation of ceftriaxone-calcium salt. **Cautions:** Hepatic impairment, history of GI disease (esp. ulcerative colitis, antibiotic-associated colitis). Severe renal impairment, history of penicillin allergy.

⧗ LIFESPAN CONSIDERATIONS

Pregnancy/Lactation: Readily crosses placenta. Distributed in breast milk. **Pregnancy Category B. Children:** May displace bilirubin from serum albumin. Contraindicated in hyperbilirubinemic neonates. **Elderly:** Age-related renal impairment may require dosage adjustment.

INTERACTIONS

DRUG: Probenecid may increase excretion. May increase **aminoglycoside** concentration. **HERBAL:** None significant. **FOOD:** None known. **LAB VALUES:** May increase BUN, serum alkaline phosphatase, bilirubin, creatinine, LDH, AST, ALT. May cause positive direct/indirect Coombs' test.

AVAILABILITY (Rx)

Injection, Powder for Reconstitution (Rocephin): 250 mg, 500 mg, 1 g, 2 g. **Intravenous Solution (Rocephin):** 1 g/50 ml, 2 g/50 ml.

ADMINISTRATION/HANDLING

IV

Reconstitution • Add 2.4 ml Sterile Water for Injection to each 250 mg to provide concentration of 100 mg/ml. • May further dilute with 50–100 ml 0.9% NaCl, D$_5$W.

Rate of Administration • For IV push, administer over 2–4 min (**maximum concentration:** 40 mg/ml). • For intermittent IV infusion (piggyback), infuse over 15–30 min for adults, 10–30 min in children, neonates. • Alternating IV sites, use large veins to reduce potential for phlebitis.

Storage • Solution appears light yellow to amber. • IV infusion (piggyback) is stable for 2 days at room temperature, 10 days if refrigerated. • Discard if precipitate forms.

IM

• Add 0.9 ml Sterile Water for Injection, 0.9% NaCl, D$_5$W, or lidocaine to each 250 mg to provide concentration of 250 mg/ml. • To minimize discomfort, inject deep IM slowly. Less painful if injected into gluteus maximus than lateral aspect of thigh.

🔲 IV INCOMPATIBILITIES

Amphotericin B complex (Abelcet, AmBisome, Amphotec), famotidine (Pepcid), fluconazole (Diflucan), labetalol (Normodyne), vancomycin (Vancocin).

🔲 IV COMPATIBILITIES

Diltiazem (Cardizem), heparin, lidocaine, metronidazole (Flagyl), morphine, propofol (Diprivan).

INDICATIONS/ROUTES/DOSAGE

Usual Dosage Range
IM/IV: ADULTS, ELDERLY: 1–2 g q12–24h. **CHILDREN:** 50–100 mg/kg/day in 1–2 divided doses. **Maximum:** 4 g/day (meningitis), 2 g/day (other). **NEONATES:** 50 mg/kg/dose given once daily.

Mild to Moderate Infections
IV, IM: ADULTS, ELDERLY: 1–2 g as a single dose or in 2 divided doses. **CHILDREN:** 50–75 mg/kg/day in 1–2 divided doses q12–24h. **Maximum:** 2 g/day.

Serious Infections
IV, IM: ADULTS, ELDERLY: Up to 4 g/day in 2 divided doses. **CHILDREN:** 80–100 mg/kg/day in divided doses q12h. **Maximum:** 4 g/day.

Meningitis
IV: CHILDREN: Initially, 75–100 mg/kg, then 100 mg/kg/day as a single dose or in divided doses q12h. **Maximum:** 4 g/day.

Lyme Disease
IV: ADULTS, ELDERLY: 2 g/day for 14–28 days.

Acute Bacterial Otitis Media
IM: CHILDREN: 50 mg/kg once. **Maximum:** 1 g/day.

Perioperative Prophylaxis
IV, IM: ADULTS, ELDERLY: 1 g 0.5–2 hrs before surgery.

Dosage in Renal Impairment
Dosage modification is usually unnecessary but hepatic/renal function test results should be monitored in those with renal and hepatic impairment or severe renal impairment.

SIDE EFFECTS

Frequent: Discomfort with IM administration, oral candidiasis (thrush), mild diarrhea, mild abdominal cramping, vaginal candidiasis. **Occasional:** Nausea, serum sickness-like reaction (fever, joint pain; usually occurs after second course of therapy and resolves after drug is discontinued). **Rare:** Allergic reaction (rash, pruritus, urticaria), thrombophlebitis (pain, redness, swelling at injection site).

ADVERSE EFFECTS/ TOXIC REACTIONS

Antibiotic-associated colitis, other superinfections (abdominal cramps, severe watery diarrhea, fever) may result from altered bacterial balance. Nephrotoxicity may occur, esp. in pts with preexisting renal disease. Pts with history of penicillin allergy are at increased risk for developing a severe hypersensitivity reaction (severe pruritus, angioedema, bronchospasm, anaphylaxis).

NURSING CONSIDERATIONS

BASELINE ASSESSMENT
Obtain CBC, renal function tests. Question for history of allergies, particularly cephalosporins, penicillins.

INTERVENTION/EVALUATION
Assess oral cavity for white patches on mucous membranes, tongue (thrush). Monitor daily pattern of bowel activity, stool consistency. Mild GI effects may be tolerable (increasing severity may indicate onset of antibiotic-associated colitis). Monitor I&O, renal function tests for nephrotoxicity, CBC. Be alert for superinfection: fever, vomiting, diarrhea, anal/genital pruritus, oral mucosal changes (ulceration, pain, erythema).

PATIENT/FAMILY TEACHING
• Discomfort may occur with IM injection. • Doses should be evenly spaced. • Continue antibiotic therapy for full length of treatment.

cefuroxime

sef-ue-**rox**-eem
(Apo-Cefuroxime ❧, Ceftin, Zinacef)
Do not confuse Ceftin with Cefzil or Cipro, cefuroxime with cefotaxime, cefprozil, or deferoxamine, or Zinacef with Zithromax.

◆ CLASSIFICATION

PHARMACOTHERAPEUTIC: Second-generation cephalosporin. **CLINICAL:** Antibiotic (see p. 24C).

ACTION

Binds to bacterial cell membranes, inhibits cell wall synthesis. **Therapeutic Effect:** Bactericidal.

PHARMACOKINETICS

Rapidly absorbed from GI tract. Protein binding: 33%–50%. Widely distributed including to CSF. Primarily excreted unchanged in urine. Moderately removed by hemodialysis. **Half-life:** 1.3 hrs (increased in renal impairment).

USES

Treatment of susceptible infections due to group B streptococci, pneumococci, staphylococci, *H. influenzae, E. coli, Enterobacter, Klebsiella* including acute/chronic bronchitis, gonorrhea, impetigo, early Lyme disease, otitis media, pharyngitis/tonsillitis, sinusitis, skin/skin structure, UTI, perioperative prophylaxis.

PRECAUTIONS

Contraindications: History of hypersensitivity/anaphylactic reaction to cepha-losporins. **Cautions:** Severe renal impairment, history of penicillin allergy.

⏳ LIFESPAN CONSIDERATIONS

Pregnancy/Lactation: Readily crosses placenta. Distributed in breast milk. **Pregnancy Category B. Children:** No age-related precautions noted. **Elderly:** Age-related renal impairment may require dosage adjustment.

INTERACTIONS

DRUG: Probenecid may increase concentration. **Antacids, H₂-receptor antagonists (e.g, cimetidine, famotidine)** may decrease absorption. **HERBAL:** None significant. **FOOD:** None known. **LAB VALUES:** May increase BUN, serum creatinine, alkaline phosphatase, bilirubin, LDH, AST, ALT. May cause positive direct/indirect Coombs' test.

AVAILABILITY (Rx)

Injection, Powder for Reconstitution: 750 mg, 1.5 g. **Injection, Solution:** 750 mg/50 ml, 1.5 g/50 ml. **Oral Suspension (Ceftin):** 125 mg/5 ml, 250 mg/5 ml. **Tablets (Ceftin):** 250 mg, 500 mg.

ADMINISTRATION/HANDLING

 IV

Reconstitution • Reconstitute 750 mg in 8 ml (1.5 g in 14 ml) Sterile Water for Injection to provide a concentration of 100 mg/ml. • For intermittent IV infusion (piggyback), further dilute with 50–100 ml 0.9% NaCl or D₅W.
Rate of Administration • For IV push, administer over 3–5 min. • For intermittent IV infusion (piggyback), infuse over 15–30 min.
Storage • Solution appears light yellow to amber (may darken, but color change does not indicate loss of potency). • IV infusion (piggyback) is stable for 24 hrs at room temperature, 48 hrs if refrigerated. • Discard if precipitate forms.

C

IM

• To minimize discomfort, inject deep IM slowly. Less painful if injected into gluteus maximus than lateral aspect of thigh.

PO

• Give tablets without regard to food (give 400-mg dose with food). • If GI upset occurs, give with food, milk. • Avoid crushing tablets due to bitter taste. • Suspension must be given with food. • Suspension stable at room temperature or refrigerated for 10 days.

🔲 IV INCOMPATIBILITIES

Fluconazole (Diflucan), midazolam (Versed), vancomycin (Vancocin).

🔲 IV COMPATIBILITIES

Diltiazem (Cardizem), hydromorphone (Dilaudid), morphine, propofol (Diprivan).

INDICATIONS/ROUTES/DOSAGE

Usual Dosage
IV, IM: ADULTS, ELDERLY: 750 mg–1.5 g q8h. **CHILDREN:** 75–150 mg/kg/day divided q8h. **Maximum:** 6 g/day. **NEONATES:** 50 mg/kg/dose q8–12h.
PO: ADULTS, ELDERLY: 250–500 mg twice a day. **CHILDREN:** 20–30 mg/kg/day in 2 divided doses. **Maximum:** 1 g/day.

Pharyngitis, Tonsillitis
PO: CHILDREN 3 MOS–12 YRS: 125 mg (tablets) q12h or 20 mg/kg/day (suspension) in 2 divided doses for 10 days. **Maximum:** 500 mg/day.

Acute Otitis Media, Acute Bacterial Maxillary Sinusitis, Impetigo
PO: CHILDREN 3 MOS–12 YRS: 250 mg (tablets) q12h or 30 mg/kg/day (suspension) in 2 divided doses for 10 days. **Maximum:** 1 g/day.

Gonorrhea
PO: ADULTS, ELDERLY: 1 g as single dose.
IM: 1.5 g as single dose.

UTI
PO: ADULTS, ELDERLY: 125–250 mg q12h for 7–10 days.

Perioperative Prophylaxis
IV: ADULTS, ELDERLY: 1.5 g 30–60 min before surgery.

Dosage in Renal Impairment
Adult dosage frequency is modified based on creatinine clearance and severity of infection.

Creatinine Clearance	Dosage
Greater than 20 ml/min	q8h
10–20 ml/min	q12h
Less than 10 ml/min	q24h
Peritoneal dialysis	Dose q24h
Continuous renal replacement therapy	1 g q12h

SIDE EFFECTS

Frequent: Discomfort with IM administration, oral candidiasis (thrush), mild diarrhea, mild abdominal cramping, vaginal candidiasis. **Occasional:** Nausea, serum sickness–like reaction (fever, joint pain; usually occurs after second course of therapy and resolves after drug is discontinued). **Rare:** Allergic reaction (rash, pruritus, urticaria), thrombophlebitis (pain, redness, swelling at injection site).

ADVERSE EFFECTS/ TOXIC REACTIONS

Antibiotic-associated colitis, other superinfections (abdominal cramps, severe watery diarrhea, fever) may result from altered bacterial balance. Nephrotoxicity may occur, esp. in pts with pre-existing renal disease. Pts with history of penicillin allergy are at increased risk for developing a severe hypersensitivity reaction (severe pruritus, angioedema, bronchospasm anaphylaxis).

NURSING CONSIDERATIONS

BASELINE ASSESSMENT

Obtain CBC, renal function tests. Question for history of allergies, particularly cephalosporins, penicillins.

INTERVENTION/EVALUATION

Assess oral cavity for white patches on mucous membranes, tongue (thrush). Monitor daily pattern of bowel activity, stool consistency. Mild GI effects may be tolerable (increasing severity may indicate onset of antibiotic-associated colitis). Monitor I&O, renal function tests for nephrotoxicity. Be alert for superinfection: fever, vomiting, diarrhea, anal/genital pruritus, oral mucosal changes (ulceration, pain, erythema).

PATIENT/FAMILY TEACHING

• Discomfort may occur with IM injection. • Doses should be evenly spaced. • Continue antibiotic therapy for full length of treatment. • May cause GI upset (may take with food, milk).

---

celecoxib

TOP 200

sel-e-**kox**-ib
(Celebrex)

BLACK BOX ALERT Increased risk of serious cardiovascular thrombotic events, including MI, CVA. Increased risk of severe GI reactions, including ulceration, bleeding, perforation of stomach, intestines.
Do not confuse Celebrex with Celexa, Cerebyx, or Clarinex.

◆CLASSIFICATION

PHARMACOTHERAPEUTIC: NSAID. **CLINICAL:** Anti-inflammatory (see p. 129C).

ACTION

Inhibits cyclooxygenase-2, the enzyme responsible for prostaglandin synthesis.

Therapeutic Effect: Reduces inflammation, relieves pain.

PHARMACOKINETICS

Rapidly absorbed from GI tract. Widely distributed. Protein binding: 97%. Metabolized in liver. Primarily eliminated in feces. **Half-life:** 11.2 hrs.

USES

Relief of signs/symptoms of osteoarthritis, rheumatoid arthritis (RA) in adults. Treatment of acute pain, primary dysmenorrhea. Relief of signs/symptoms associated with ankylosing spondylitis. Treatment of juvenile rheumatoid arthritis (JRA).

PRECAUTIONS

◄ALERT► May increase cardiovascular risk when high doses given to prevent colon cancer.
Contraindications: Hypersensitivity to aspirin, NSAIDs, sulfonamides. Treatment of perioperative pain in coronary artery bypass graft (CABG) surgery. **Cautions:** History of GI disease (bleeding/ulcers); concurrent use with aspirin, anticoagulants; smoking; alcohol; elderly; debilitated pts; asthma; renal/hepatic impairment. Pts with edema, cerebrovascular disease, ischemic heart disease, heart failure, known or suspected deficiency of cytochrome P450 isoenzyme 2C9.

⌛ LIFESPAN CONSIDERATIONS

Pregnancy/Lactation: Unknown if drug crosses placenta or is distributed in breast milk. Avoid use during third trimester (may adversely affect fetal cardiovascular system: premature closure of ductus arteriosus). **Pregnancy Category C (D if used in third trimester or near delivery). Children:** Safety and efficacy not established in those younger than 18 yrs. **Elderly:** No age-related precautions noted.

INTERACTIONS

DRUG: May decrease antihypertensive effect of **ACE inhibitors and angiotensin II antagonists. Fluconazole** may significantly increase concentration. May increase **lithium** concentration. **Warfarin** may increase risk of bleeding. **Aspirin** may increase risk of celecoxib-induced GI ulceration, other GI complications. **HERBAL:** Avoid herbs with anticoagulant or antiplatelet activity **(e.g., evening primrose, garlic, ginger, ginseng). FOOD:** None known. **LAB VALUES:** May increase serum AST, ALT, alkaline phosphatase, creatinine, BUN. May decrease serum phosphate.

AVAILABILITY (Rx)

 Capsules: 50 mg, 100 mg, 200 mg, 400 mg.

ADMINISTRATION/HANDLING

PO

• Lower doses (200 mg): Give without regard to food; higher doses (400 mg): Give with food. • Do not give with antacids. • Capsules may be swallowed whole or opened and mixed with applesauce.

INDICATIONS/ROUTES/DOSAGE

Osteoarthritis
PO: ADULTS, ELDERLY: 200 mg/day as a single dose or 100 mg twice a day.

Rheumatoid Arthritis (RA)
PO: ADULTS, ELDERLY: 100–200 mg twice a day.

Juvenile Rheumatoid Arthritis (JRA)
PO: CHILDREN 2 YRS AND OLDER, WEIGHING MORE THAN 25 KG: 100 mg twice a day. **WEIGHING 10–25 KG:** 50 mg twice a day.

Acute Pain
PO: ADULTS, ELDERLY: Initially, 400 mg with additional 200 mg on day 1, if needed. Maintenance: 200 mg twice a day as needed.

Ankylosing Spondylitis
PO: ADULTS, ELDERLY: 200 mg/day as a single dose or in 2 divided doses. May increase to 400 mg/day if no effect is seen after 6 wks.

Dosage in Hepatic Impairment
Decrease dose by 50% in pts with moderate hepatic impairment. Not recommended in severe hepatic impairment.

SIDE EFFECTS

Frequent (16%–5%): Diarrhea, dyspepsia, headache, upper respiratory tract infection. **Occasional (less than 5%):** Abdominal pain, flatulence, nausea, back pain, peripheral edema, dizziness, insomnia, rash.

ADVERSE EFFECTS/ TOXIC REACTIONS

Increased risk of cardiovascular events, (MI, CVA), serious, potentially life-threatening GI bleeding.

NURSING CONSIDERATIONS

BASELINE ASSESSMENT

Assess onset, type, location, duration of pain/inflammation. Inspect appearance of affected joints for immobility, deformity, skin condition. Assess for allergy to sulfa, aspirin, or NSAIDs (contraindicated).

INTERVENTION/EVALUATION

Assess for therapeutic response: pain relief; decreased stiffness, swelling; increased joint mobility; reduced joint tenderness; improved grip strength. Observe for bleeding, bruising, weight gain.

PATIENT/FAMILY TEACHING

• If GI upset occurs, take with food. • Avoid aspirin, alcohol (increases risk of GI bleeding). • Immediately report chest pain, jaw pain, sweating; or confusion, difficulty speaking, one sided weakness (may indicate heart attack or stroke).

cephalexin   TOP 200

sef-a-**lex**-in
(Apo-Cephalex ✤, Keflex, Novo-Lexin ✤)
Do not confuse cephalexin with cefaclor, cefazolin, or ciprofloxacin.

C

◆**CLASSIFICATION**

PHARMACOTHERAPEUTIC: First-generation cephalosporin. **CLINICAL:** Antibiotic (see p. 24C).

ACTION

Binds to bacterial cell membranes, inhibits cell wall synthesis. **Therapeutic Effect:** Bactericidal.

PHARMACOKINETICS

Rapidly absorbed from GI tract (delayed in young children). Protein binding: 10%–15%. Widely distributed. Primarily excreted unchanged in urine. Moderately removed by hemodialysis. **Half-life:** 0.9–1.2 hrs (increased in renal impairment).

USES

Treatment of susceptible infections due to staphylococci, group A *streptococcus, K. pneumoniae, E. coli, P. mirabilis, H. influenzae, M. catarrhalis* including respiratory tract, genitourinary tract, skin, soft tissue, bone infections; otitis media; rheumatic fever prophylaxis; follow-up to parenteral therapy.

PRECAUTIONS

Contraindications: History of hypersensitivity/anaphylactic reaction to cephalosporins. **Cautions:** Renal/hepatic impairment, history of GI disease (esp. ulcerative colitis, antibiotic-associated colitis).

⧖ LIFESPAN CONSIDERATIONS

Pregnancy/Lactation: Readily crosses placenta. Distributed in breast milk. **Pregnancy Category B. Children:** No age-related precautions noted. **Elderly:** Age-related renal impairment may require dosage adjustment.

INTERACTIONS

DRUG: Probenecid may increase concentration. **HERBAL:** None significant. **FOOD:** None known. **LAB VALUES:** May increase BUN, serum creatinine, alkaline phosphatase, bilirubin, LDH, AST, ALT. May cause positive direct/indirect Coombs' test.

AVAILABILITY (Rx)

Capsules: 250 mg, 500 mg, 750 mg. **Powder for Oral Suspension:** 125 mg/5 ml, 250 mg/5 ml. **Tablets:** 250 mg, 500 mg.

ADMINISTRATION/HANDLING

PO

• After reconstitution, oral suspension is stable for 14 days if refrigerated. • Shake oral suspension well before using. • Give without regard to food. If GI upset occurs, give with food, milk.

INDICATIONS/ROUTES/DOSAGE

Usual Dosage Range
PO: ADULTS, ELDERLY: 250–1,000 mg q6h. **Maximum:** 4 g/day. **CHILDREN:** 25–100 mg/kg/day in 3–4 divided doses. **Maximum:** 4 g/day.

Streptococcal Pharyngitis, Skin/Skin Structure Infections
PO: ADULTS, ELDERLY: 500 mg q12h. **CHILDREN:** 25–50 mg/kg/day in 2 divided doses.

Uncomplicated Cystitis
PO: ADULTS, ELDERLY, CHILDREN OLDER THAN 15 YRS: 500 mg q12h for 7–14 days.

Otitis Media
PO: CHILDREN: 75–100 mg/kg/day in 4 divided doses.

Dosage in Renal Impairment
After usual initial dose, dosing frequency is modified based on creatinine clearance and severity of infection.

Creatinine Clearance	Dosage
10–50 ml/min	500 mg q8–12h
Less than 10 ml/min	250–500 mg q12–24h
Hemodialysis	250 mg q12–24h

SIDE EFFECTS

Frequent: Oral candidiasis, mild diarrhea, mild abdominal cramping, vaginal candidiasis. **Occasional:** Nausea, serum sickness–like reaction (fever, joint pain; usually occurs after second course of therapy and resolves after drug is discontinued). **Rare:** Allergic reaction (rash, pruritus, urticaria).

ADVERSE EFFECTS/ TOXIC REACTIONS

Antibiotic-associated colitis, other superinfections (abdominal cramps, severe watery diarrhea, fever) may result from altered bacterial balance. Nephrotoxicity may occur, esp. in pts with preexisting renal disease. Pts with history of penicillin allergy are at increased risk for developing a severe hypersensitivity reaction (severe pruritus, angioedema, bronchospasm, anaphylaxis).

NURSING CONSIDERATIONS

BASELINE ASSESSMENT

Obtain CBC, renal function tests. Question for history of allergies, particularly cephalosporins, penicillins.

INTERVENTION/EVALUATION

Assess oral cavity for white patches on mucous membranes, tongue (thrush). Monitor daily pattern of bowel activity, stool consistency. Mild GI effects may be tolerable (increasing severity may indicate onset of antibiotic-associated colitis). Monitor I&O, renal function tests for nephrotoxicity. Be alert for superinfection: fever, vomiting, diarrhea, anal/genital pruritus, oral mucosal changes (ulceration, pain, erythema). With prolonged therapy, monitor renal/hepatic function tests.

PATIENT/FAMILY TEACHING

• Doses should be evenly spaced. • Continue therapy for full length of treatment. • May cause GI upset (may take with food, milk). • Refrigerate oral suspension. • Report persistent diarrhea.

certolizumab

ser-toe-**liz**-ue-mab
(Cimzia)

BLACK BOX ALERT Serious, sometimes fatal, cases of tuberculosis, other fungal infections, or other opportunistic infections including viral and bacterial events have been reported. Lymphoma reported in children/adolescents receiving other TNF-blocking medications.

◆ CLASSIFICATION

PHARMACOTHERAPEUTIC: Tumor necrosis factor (TNF) blocker. **CLINICAL:** Crohn's disease agent.

ACTION

Binds specifically to TNF-alpha cell, a protein in the immune system that causes inflammation. **Therapeutic Effect:** Reduces signs and symptoms of Crohn's disease in those with inadequate response to conventional therapy.

PHARMACOKINETICS

Higher clearance with increasing body weight. Peak plasma concentrations: 54–171 hrs. **Half-life:** 14 days.

USES

Reduction of signs and symptoms of Crohn's disease, maintenance of clinical response in pts with moderate to severely active disease. Treatment of moderately to severely active rheumatoid arthritis.

PRECAUTIONS

Contraindications: None known. **Cautions:** Chronic, latent, or localized infection, preexisting or recent-onset CNS demyelinating disorders, heart failure, underlying hematologic disorders, elderly. May increase risk of malignancies (e.g., lymphoma). Pts who have resided in regions where TB is endemic, pts who are hepatitis B virus carriers. Use of live vaccines.

⌛ LIFESPAN CONSIDERATIONS

Pregnancy/Lactation: Unknown if distributed in breast milk. **Pregnancy Category B. Children:** Safety and efficacy not established. **Elderly:** Use cautiously due to higher rate of infection.

INTERACTIONS

DRUG: Anakinra, other TNF antagonists (adalimumab, etanercept, infliximab) may increase risk of infection. **Live virus vaccines** may decrease immune response. **HERBAL: Echinacea** may decrease effect. **FOOD:** None known. **LAB VALUES:** May increase serum alkaline phosphatase, AST, ALT, bilirubin, aPTT.

AVAILABILITY (Rx)

Injection, Powder for Reconstitution: 200 mg. **Injection, Solution:** 200 mg/ml in a single-use prefilled syringe.

ADMINISTRATION/HANDLING

Subcutaneous

Reconstitution • Bring to room temperature before reconstitution. • Reconstitute with 1 ml Sterile Water for Injection. • Gently swirl without shaking, using syringe with 20-gauge needle. • Leave undisturbed to fully reconstitute (may take as long as 30 min). • Using a new 20-gauge needle, withdraw reconstituted solution into syringe for final concentration of 1 ml (200 mg). Use separate syringes for multiple vials. • Switch each 20-gauge needle to a 23-gauge needle and inject full contents of each syringe subcutaneously into separate sites on the abdomen or thigh.

Storage • Store vial in refrigerator. • Once powder reconstituted, solution should appear clear to opalescent, colorless to pale yellow. • Discard if solution is discolored or contains precipitate. • Reconstituted solution is stable for up to 2 hrs at room temperature or 24 hrs if refrigerated.

INDICATIONS/ROUTES/DOSAGE

Crohn's Disease

Subcutaneous: Initially, 400 mg (given as 2 subcutaneous injections of 200 mg) and at weeks 2 and 4. Maintenance: In pts who obtain a therapeutic response, 400 mg every 4 wks.

Rheumatoid Arthritis

Subcutaneous: ADULTS, ELDERLY: Initially, 400 mg and at weeks 2 and 4. Maintenance: 200 mg q2wks or 400 mg q4wks.

SIDE EFFECTS

Occasional (6%): Arthralgia. **Rare (less than 1%):** Abdominal pain, diarrhea.

ADVERSE EFFECTS/TOXIC REACTIONS

Upper respiratory tract infection occurs in 20% of pts. UTI occurs in 7% of pts. Serious infections such as pneumonia, pyelonephritis occur in 3% of pts. Hypersensitivity reaction (rash, urticaria, hypotension, dyspnea) occurs rarely.

NURSING CONSIDERATIONS

BASELINE ASSESSMENT

Do not initiate treatment in pts with active infections, including chronic or localized infection. TB test should be obtained before initiation. Obtain baseline WBC count, urinalysis, C-reactive protein.

INTERVENTION/EVALUATION

Monitor pts for infection during and after treatment. Monitor temperature. If pt develops an infection, treatment should be discontinued. Monitor lab results, especially WBC count, urinalysis, C-reactive protein for evidence of infection.

PATIENT/FAMILY TEACHING

• Report cough, fever, flu-like symptoms. • Do not receive live virus vaccine during treatment or within 3 months of its discontinuation.

C

cetirizine

se-**teer**-i-zeen
(Apo-Cetirizine ♥, Reactine ♥, Zyrtec)
Do not confuse cetirizine with levocetirizine, or Zyrtec with Xanax, Zantac, Zocor, or Zyprexa.

FIXED-COMBINATION(S)

Zyrtec D 12 Hour Tablets: cetirizine/pseudoephedrine: 5 mg/120 mg.

◆CLASSIFICATION

PHARMACOTHERAPEUTIC: Second-generation piperazine. **CLINICAL:** Antihistamine (see p. 54C).

ACTION

Competes with histamine for H_1-receptor sites on effector cells in GI tract, blood vessels, respiratory tract. **Therapeutic Effect:** Prevents allergic response, produces mild bronchodilation, blocks histamine-induced bronchitis.

PHARMACOKINETICS

Route	Onset	Peak	Duration
PO	Less than 1 hr	4–8 hrs	Less than 24 hrs

Well absorbed from GI tract. Protein binding: 93%. Undergoes low first-pass metabolism; not extensively metabolized. Primarily excreted in urine (more than 80% as unchanged drug). **Half-life:** 6.5–10 hrs.

USES

Relief of symptoms (sneezing, rhinorrhea, postnasal discharge, nasal pruritus, ocular pruritus, tearing) of seasonal and perennial allergic rhinitis (hay fever). Treatment of chronic urticaria (hives).

PRECAUTIONS

Contraindications: Hypersensitivity to cetirizine, hydroxyzine. **Cautions:** Hepatic/renal impairment.

⧖ LIFESPAN CONSIDERATIONS

Pregnancy/Lactation: Not recommended during first trimester of pregnancy. Distributed in breast milk. Breastfeeding not recommended. **Pregnancy Category B. Children:** Less likely to cause anticholinergic effects. **Elderly:** More sensitive to anticholinergic effects (e.g., dry mouth, urinary retention). Dizziness, sedation, confusion may occur.

INTERACTIONS

DRUG: Alcohol, other CNS depressants may increase CNS depression. **Anticholinergics** may increase anticholinergic effects. **HERBAL:** None significant. **FOOD:** None known. **LAB VALUES:** May suppress wheal and flare reactions to antigen skin testing unless drug is discontinued 4 days before testing.

AVAILABILITY (Rx)

Capsule: 10 mg. **Syrup:** 5 mg/5 ml. **Tablets:** 5 mg, 10 mg. **Tablets (Chewable):** 5 mg, 10 mg.

ADMINISTRATION/HANDLING

PO
• Give without regard to food.

INDICATIONS/ROUTES/DOSAGE

◀**ALERT**▶ May cause drowsiness at dosage greater than 10 mg/day.

Allergic Rhinitis, Urticaria
PO: ADULTS, ELDERLY, CHILDREN OLDER THAN 5 YRS: Initially, 5–10 mg/day as single dose. **CHILDREN 2–5 YRS:** 2.5 mg/day. May increase up to 5 mg/day as a single dose or in 2 divided doses. **CHILDREN 12–23 MOS:** Initially, 2.5 mg/day. May increase up to 5 mg/day in 2 divided doses. **CHILDREN 6–11 MOS:** 2.5 mg once a day.

Dosage in Renal/Hepatic Impairment
Adult/elderly pts with renal impairment (creatinine clearance 11–31 ml/min), pts receiving hemodialysis (creatinine clearance less than 7 ml/min), pts with hepatic impairment:

Dosage is decreased to 5 mg once a day. **CHILDREN 6–11 YRS:** Less than 2.5 mg once daily.

SIDE EFFECTS

Occasional (10%–2%): Pharyngitis, dry mucous membranes, nausea/vomiting, abdominal pain, headache, dizziness, fatigue, thickening of mucus, drowsiness, photosensitivity, urinary retention.

ADVERSE EFFECTS/ TOXIC REACTIONS

Children may experience paradoxical reaction (restlessness, insomnia, euphoria, nervousness, tremor). Dizziness, sedation, confusion more likely to occur in elderly.

NURSING CONSIDERATIONS

BASELINE ASSESSMENT

Assess lung sounds. Assess severity of rhinitis, urticaria, other symptoms. Obtain baseline renal/hepatic function tests.

INTERVENTION/EVALUATION

For upper respiratory allergies, increase fluids to maintain thin secretions and offset thirst. Monitor symptoms for therapeutic response.

PATIENT/FAMILY TEACHING

• Avoid tasks that require alertness, motor skills until response to drug is established. • Avoid alcohol.

---

cetuximab TOP 200 HIGH ALERT

se-**tux**-ih-mab
(Erbitux)

BLACK BOX ALERT Severe infusion reactions (bronchospasm, stridor, urticaria, hypotension, cardiac arrest) have occurred, especially with first infusion. Cardiopulmonary arrest reported in pts receiving radiation in combination with cetuximab.

Do not confuse cetuximab with bevacizumab.

◆CLASSIFICATION

PHARMACOTHERAPEUTIC: Monoclonal antibody. **CLINICAL:** Antineoplastic (see p. 83C).

ACTION

Binds to the epidermal growth factor receptor (EGFR), a glycoprotein on normal and tumor cells. **Therapeutic Effect:** Inhibits tumor cell growth, inducing apoptosis (cell death).

PHARMACOKINETICS

Reaches steady-state levels by the third weekly infusion. Clearance decreases as dose increases. **Half-life:** 114 hrs (range: 75–188 hrs).

USES

As a single agent or in combination with irinotecan for treatment of EGFR-expressing, metastatic colorectal carcinoma in pts who are refractory or intolerant to irinotecan-based chemotherapy. Treatment of advanced squamous cell cancer of head/neck (with radiation). Treatment of recurrent or metastasized squamous cell carcinoma of head/neck progressing after platinum-based therapy. First-line treatment of squamous cell carcinoma of head and neck in combination with platinum-based therapy with 5-FU. **OFF-LABEL:** EGFR-expressing advanced non–small-cell lung cancer (NSCLC). Treatment of unresectable squamous cell skin cancer.

PRECAUTIONS

Contraindications: None known. **Cautions:** Preexisting IgE antibodies to cetuximab, coronary artery disease, heart failure, arrythmias, pulmonary disease.

⌛ LIFESPAN CONSIDERATIONS

Pregnancy/Lactation: Crosses placental barrier; may cause fetal harm, abortifactant. Breast-feeding not recom-

---

C

mended. **Pregnancy Category C. Children:** Safety and efficacy not established. **Elderly:** No age-related precautions noted.

INTERACTIONS

DRUG: None significant. **HERBAL:** None significant. **FOOD:** None known. **LAB VALUES:** May decrease WBCs, calcium, magnesium, potassium.

AVAILABILITY (Rx)

Injection Solution: 2 mg/ml (50 ml, 100 ml).

ADMINISTRATION/HANDLING

 IV

◀**ALERT**▶ Do not give by IV push or bolus.

Reconstitution • Does not require reconstitution. • Solution should appear clear, colorless; may contain a small amount of visible, white particulates. • Do not shake or dilute. • Infuse with a low protein-binding 0.22-micron in-line filter. **Rate of Administration •** First dose should be given as a 120-min infusion. • Maintenance infusion should be infused over 60 min. • Maximum infusion rate should not exceed 5 ml/min. **Storage •** Refrigerate vials. • Infusion containers are stable for up to 12 hrs if refrigerated, up to 8 hrs at room temperature. • Discard unused portions.

IV COMPATIBILITY

Irinotecan (Camptosar).

INDICATIONS/ROUTES/DOSAGE

Head/Neck Cancer, Metastatic Colorectal Carcinoma
IV: ADULTS, ELDERLY: Initially, 400 mg/m^2 as a loading dose. Maintenance: 250 mg/m^2 infused over 60 min weekly.

SIDE EFFECTS

Frequent (90%–25%): Acneiform rash, malaise, fever, nausea, diarrhea, constipation, headache, abdominal pain, anorexia, vomiting. **Occasional (16%–10%):** Nail disorder, back pain, stomatitis, peripheral edema, pruritus, cough, insomnia. **Rare (9%–5%):** Weight loss, depression, dyspepsia, conjunctivitis, alopecia.

ADVERSE EFFECTS/ TOXIC REACTIONS

Anemia occurs in 10% of pts. Severe infusion reaction (rapid onset of airway obstruction, hypotension, severe urticaria) occurs rarely. Dermatologic toxicity, pulmonary embolus, leukopenia, renal failure occur rarely.

NURSING CONSIDERATIONS

BASELINE ASSESSMENT

Monitor Hgb, Hct, serum potassium, magnesium. Assess for evidence of anemia. Question possibility of pregnancy.

INTERVENTION/EVALUATION

Monitor for evidence of infusion reaction (rapid onset of bronchospasm, stridor, hoarseness, urticaria, hypotension) during infusion and for at least 1 hr postinfusion. Pt may experience first severe infusion reaction during later infusions. Assess skin for evidence of dermatologic toxicity (development of inflammatory sequelae, dry skin, exfoliative dermatitis, rash). Monitor serum electrolytes, acute onset or worsening pulmonary symptoms.

PATIENT/FAMILY TEACHING

• Do not have immunizations without physician's approval (drug lowers resistance). • Avoid contact with anyone who recently received a live virus vaccine. • Avoid crowds, those with infection. • Wear sunscreen, limit sun exposure (sunlight can exacerbate skin reactions). • Avoid pregnancy. • Report cardiac or pulmonary symptoms, severe rash.

chlorambucil

klor-**am**-bue-sil
(Leukeran)

BLACK BOX ALERT May cause myelosuppression. Affects fertility; potential for carcinogenic, mutagenic, teratogenic effects. May cause azoospermia.

Do not confuse Leukeran with Alkeran, Leukine, or Myleran.

◆CLASSIFICATION

PHARMACOTHERAPEUTIC: Alkylating agent, nitrogen mustard. **CLINICAL:** Antineoplastic (see p. 84C).

ACTION

Inhibits DNA, RNA synthesis by cross-linking with DNA, RNA strands. Cell cycle–phase nonspecific. **Therapeutic Effect:** Interferes with nucleic acid function.

PHARMACOKINETICS

Rapidly, completely absorbed from GI tract. Protein binding: 99%. Metabolized in liver to active metabolite. Not removed by hemodialysis. **Half-life:** 1.5 hrs; metabolite, 2.5 hrs.

USES

Treatment of chronic lymphocytic leukemia (CLL), Hodgkin's and non-Hodgkin's lymphomas (NHL). **OFF-LABEL:** Nephrotic syndrome in children, Waldenström's macroglobulinemia.

PRECAUTIONS

Contraindications: Previous allergic reaction to other alkylating agents, prior resistance to chlorambucil, pregnancy. **Extreme Cautions:** Treatment within 4 wks after full-course radiation therapy or myelosuppressive drug regimen. **Cautions:** Seizure disorder, head trauma, bone marrow suppression.

⚖ LIFESPAN CONSIDERATIONS

Pregnancy/Lactation: If possible, avoid use during pregnancy, esp. first trimester. Breastfeeding not recommended. **Pregnancy Category D. Children:** No age-related precautions noted. When taken for nephrotic syndrome, may increase seizures. **Elderly:** No age-related precautions noted.

INTERACTIONS

DRUG: Bone marrow depressants may increase myelosuppression. **Other immunosuppressants (e.g., steroids)** may increase risk of infection or development of neoplasms. **Live virus vaccines** may potentiate virus replication, decrease antibody response to vaccine. **HERBAL: Echinacea** may decrease effects. **FOOD: Acidic foods, hot foods, spices** may delay absorption. **LAB VALUES:** May increase serum alkaline phosphatase, AST, uric acid.

AVAILABILITY (Rx)

Tablets: 2 mg.

ADMINISTRATION/HANDLING

PO
• Give 30–60 min before food. • Do not give with acidic foods, hot foods, spices.

INDICATIONS/ROUTES/DOSAGE

Chronic Lymphocytic Leukemia (CLL)
PO: ADULTS, ELDERLY: 0.1 mg/kg/day for 3–6 wks or 0.4 mg/kg pulsed doses administered intermittently, biweekly or monthly.

Hodgkin's Lymphoma (HL)
PO: ADULTS, ELDERLY: 0.2 mg/kg/day for 3–6 wks.

Non-Hodgkin's Lymphoma (NHL)
PO: ADULTS, ELDERLY: 0.1 mg/kg/day for 3–6 wks.

SIDE EFFECTS

Expected: GI effects (nausea, vomiting, anorexia, diarrhea, abdominal distress) generally mild, last less than 24 hrs, occur only if single dose exceeds 20 mg. **Occasional:** Rash, dermatitis, pruritus, cold sores. **Rare:** Alopecia, urticaria, erythema, hyperuricemia.

ADVERSE EFFECTS/ TOXIC REACTIONS

Hematologic toxicity due to severe myelosuppression occurs frequently, manifested as neutropenia, anemia, thrombocytopenia. After discontinuation of therapy, thrombocytopenia, neutropenia usually last for 1–2 wks, but may persist for 3–4 wks. Neutrophil count may continue to decrease for up to 10 days after last dose. Toxicity appears to be less severe with intermittent drug administration. Overdosage may produce seizures in children. Excessive serum uric acid level, hepatotoxicity occur rarely.

NURSING CONSIDERATIONS

BASELINE ASSESSMENT

Obtain CBC before therapy and each wk during therapy, WBC count 3–4 days following each weekly CBC during first 3–6 wks of therapy (4–6 wks if pt on intermittent dosing schedule).

INTERVENTION/EVALUATION

Monitor CBC, platelet count, serum uric acid, hepatic function tests. Monitor for hematologic toxicity (fever, sore throat, signs of local infection, unusual bruising/bleeding from any site), symptoms of anemia (excessive fatigue, weakness). Assess skin for rash, pruritus, urticaria.

PATIENT/FAMILY TEACHING

• Increase fluid intake (may protect against hyperuricemia). • Do not have immunizations without physician's approval (drug lowers resistance). • Avoid contact with those who have recently received live virus vaccine. • Promptly report fever, sore throat, signs of local infection, unusual bruising/bleeding from any site, nausea, vomiting, rash.

chlordiazepoxide

klor-dye-az-e-**pox**-ide
(Apo-Chlordiazepoxide ✦, Librium)
Do not confuse Librium with Librax.

FIXED-COMBINATION(S)

Limbitrol: amitriptyline/chlordiazepoxide: 5 mg/12.5 mg, 10 mg/25 mg. **Librax:** chlordiazepoxide-clidinium: 5 mg/2.5 mg.

◆ CLASSIFICATION

PHARMACOTHERAPEUTIC: Benzodiazepine **(Schedule IV). CLINICAL:** Antianxiety (see p. 14C).

ACTION

Enhances action of inhibitory neurotransmitter gamma-aminobutyric acid in CNS. **Therapeutic Effect:** Produces anxiolytic effect.

PHARMACOKINETICS

Widely distributed. Protein binding: 90%–98%. Metabolized in liver. Primarily excreted in urine. **Half-life:** 6.6–25 hrs.

USES

Management of anxiety disorders, acute alcohol withdrawal symptoms; short-term relief of symptoms of anxiety, pre-op anxiety.

PRECAUTIONS

Contraindications: None known. **Cautions:** Renal/hepatic impairment, elderly, debilitated pts, respiratory disease, impaired gag reflex, porphyria, other CNS depressants, pts at risk for falls/traumatic injury, history of drug dependence, high risk of suicidal ideation.

⧖ LIFESPAN CONSIDERATIONS

Pregnancy/Lactation: Crosses placenta; distributed in breast milk. **Pregnancy Category D. Children/Elderly:**

Reduce initial dose, increase dosage gradually (prevents excessive sedation).

INTERACTIONS

DRUG: Alcohol, other CNS depressants may increase CNS depression. **Azole antifungals (e.g., ketoconazole), CYP3A4 inhibitors (e.g., fluconazole, diltiazem)** may increase serum concentration, increase risk of toxicity. **CYP3A4 inducers (e.g., rifampin)** may decrease concentration/effects. **HERBAL: Gotu kola, kava kava, St. John's wort, valerian** may increase CNS depression. **St. John's wort** may decrease effectiveness. **FOOD:** None known. **LAB VALUES: Therapeutic serum level:** 0.1–3 mcg/ml; **toxic serum level:** greater than 23 mcg/ml.

AVAILABILITY (Rx)

Capsules (Librium): 5 mg, 10 mg, 25 mg.

ADMINISTRATION/HANDLING

PO
• May take without regard to food.

INDICATIONS/ROUTES/DOSAGE

Alcohol Withdrawal Symptoms
PO: ADULTS, ELDERLY: 50–100 mg. May repeat q2–4h as necessary. **Maximum:** 300 mg/24 hrs.

Anxiety
PO: ADULTS: 15–100 mg/day in 3–4 divided doses. **ELDERLY:** 5 mg 2–4 times a day. **CHILDREN 6 YRS AND OLDER:** 5 mg 2–4 times/day or 10 mg 2–3 times/day.

SIDE EFFECTS

Frequent: Drowsiness, ataxia, dizziness, confusion (particularly in elderly or debilitated pts). **Occasional:** Rash, peripheral edema, GI disturbances. **Rare:** Paradoxical CNS reactions (hyperactivity, nervousness in children; excitement, restlessness in the elderly, generally noted during first 2 wks of therapy, particularly in presence of uncontrolled pain).

ADVERSE EFFECTS/ TOXIC REACTIONS

Abrupt or rapid withdrawal may result in pronounced restlessness, irritability, insomnia, tremors, abdominal/muscle cramps, diaphoresis, vomiting, seizures. Overdose results in drowsiness, confusion, diminished reflexes, coma.

NURSING CONSIDERATIONS

BASELINE ASSESSMENT

Assess B/P, pulse, respirations immediately before administration. Note severity of alcohol withdrawal symptoms before each dose.

INTERVENTION/EVALUATION

Monitor vital signs, esp. B/P, for changes. Assess motor responses (agitation, tremors, tension), autonomic responses (cold/clammy hands, diaphoresis). Assess children, elderly for paradoxical reaction, particularly during early therapy. Assist with ambulation if drowsiness, ataxia occur. **Therapeutic serum level:** 0.1–3 mcg/ml; **toxic serum level:** greater than 23 mcg/ml.

PATIENT/FAMILY TEACHING

• Avoid tasks that require alertness, motor skills until response to drug is established or drowsiness has diminished. • Drowsiness usually disappears during continued therapy. • If dizziness occurs, change positions slowly from lying to sitting before standing. • Smoking reduces drug effectiveness. • Do not abruptly discontinue medication after long-term therapy. • Avoid alcohol.

---

*chlorproMAZINE

klor-**pro**-ma-zeen
(Largactil ♣, Novo-Chlorpromazine ♣)
BLACK BOX ALERT Increased risk of mortality in elderly pts with dementia-related psychosis.
Do not confuse chlorpromazine with clomipramine, prochlorperazine, or promethazine.

◆CLASSIFICATION

PHARMACOTHERAPEUTIC: Phenothiazine. **CLINICAL:** Antipsychotic, antiemetic, antianxiety, antineuralgia adjunct (see p. 66C).

ACTION

Blocks dopamine neurotransmission at postsynaptic receptor sites. Possesses strong anticholinergic, sedative, antiemetic effects; moderate extrapyramidal effects; slight antihistamine action. **Therapeutic Effect:** Improves psychotic conditions; relieves nausea/vomiting; controls intractable hiccups, porphyria.

PHARMACOKINETICS

Rapidly absorbed from GI tract. Protein binding: 92%–97%. Metabolized in liver. Excreted in urine. **Half-life:** Initial 2 hrs; **terminal:** 30 hrs.

USES

Management of psychotic disorders (control of mania, treatment of schizophrenia), severe nausea/vomiting, severe behavioral disturbances in children. Relief of intractable hiccups, acute intermittent porphyria. **OFF-LABEL:** Management of psychotic disorders, behavioral symptoms associated with dementia, agitation related to Alzheimer's dementia.

PRECAUTIONS

Contraindications: Comatose states, severe CNS depression, phenothiazine hypersensitivity. **Cautions:** Respiratory/hepatic/renal/cardiac impairment, alcohol withdrawal, subcortical brain damage, history of seizures, urinary retention, prostatic hypertrophy, hypocalcemia (increases susceptibility to dystonias), myasthenia gravis, cerebrovascular disease, pts with prolonged QT interval. Pts with hemodynamic instability, risk for aspiration pneumonia, decreased GI motility, visual problems (e.g., narrow-angle glaucoma).

⧖ LIFESPAN CONSIDERATIONS

Pregnancy/Lactation: Crosses placenta; distributed in breast milk. **Pregnancy Category C. Children:** Pts with acute illnesses (chickenpox, measles, gastroenteritis, CNS infection) are at risk for developing neuromuscular, extrapyramidal symptoms (EPS), particularly dystonias. **Elderly:** Susceptible to anticholinergic, neuromuscular effects; EPS.

INTERACTIONS

DRUG: Rifampin may decrease effect. **Alcohol, CNS depressants** may increase respiratory depression, hypotensive effects. **MAOIs, tricyclic antidepressants** may increase sedative, anticholinergic effects. **HERBAL: St. John's wort** may decrease concentration; increase photosensitization, sedative effect. **Dong quai** may increase photosensitization. **Gotu kola, kava kava, valerian** may increase sedative effect. **FOOD:** None known. **LAB VALUES:** May produce false-positive pregnancy test, phenylketonuria (PKU) test. EKG changes may occur, including QT-interval and T-wave disturbances.

AVAILABILITY (Rx)

Injection Solution: 25 mg/ml. **Tablets:** 10 mg, 25 mg, 50 mg, 100 mg, 200 mg.

ADMINISTRATION/HANDLING

IM
◄ALERT► Do not give chlorpromazine by SQ route (risk for severe tissue necrosis).
• Dilute solution as prescribed with Sodium Chloride for Injection. • Slowly inject drug deep into large muscle, such as gluteus maximus rather than lateral aspect of the thigh, to minimize discomfort.

IV
• For direct IV injection, dilute with 0.9% NaCl to maximum concentration of 1 mg/ml. • Administer slowly: 0.5 mg/min in

children, 1 mg/min in adults. • Protect from light. • A slightly yellow solution does not indicate potency loss. • Discard markedly discolored solutions.

PO

Administer with food or milk to decrease GI effects.

INDICATIONS/ROUTES/DOSAGE

Severe Nausea/Vomiting
PO: ADULTS, ELDERLY: 10–25 mg q4–6h. **CHILDREN:** 0.5–1 mg/kg q4–6h.
IV, IM: ADULTS, ELDERLY: 25–50 mg q4–6h. **CHILDREN:** 0.5–1 mg/kg q6–8h. **Maximum:** 40 mg/day for children less than 5 yrs; 75 mg/day for children 5–12 yrs.

Psychotic Disorders
PO: ADULTS, ELDERLY: 30–800 mg/day in 1–4 divided doses (usual dose: 200–600 mg/day). **CHILDREN OLDER THAN 6 MOS:** 0.5–1 mg/kg q4–6h.
IV, IM: ADULTS, ELDERLY: Initially, 25 mg; may repeat in 1–4 hrs. May gradually increase to 400 mg/dose. Usual dose: 300–800 mg/day. **CHILDREN OLDER THAN 6 MOS:** 0.5–1 mg/kg q6–8h. **Maximum:** 75 mg/day for children 5–12 yrs; 40 mg/day for children younger than 5 yrs.

Intractable Hiccups
PO, IM: ADULTS: 25–50 mg 3–4 times a day. **IV:** 25–50 mg by slow IV infusion.

Porphyria
PO: ADULTS: 25–50 mg 3–4 times a day. **IM: ADULTS, ELDERLY:** 25 mg 3–4 times a day.

SIDE EFFECTS

Frequent: Drowsiness, blurred vision, hypotension, color vision or night vision disturbances, dizziness, decreased diaphoresis, constipation, dry mouth, nasal congestion. **Occasional:** Urinary retention, photosensitivity, rash, decreased sexual function, swelling/pain in breasts, weight gain, nausea, vomiting, abdominal pain, tremors.

ADVERSE EFFECTS/ TOXIC REACTIONS

Extrapyramidal symptoms appear to be dose related (particularly high dosage) and may include: akathisia (inability to sit still, tapping of feet), parkinsonian symptoms (mask-like face, tremors, shuffling gait, hypersalivation), acute dystonias (torticollis [neck muscle spasm], opisthotonos [rigidity of back muscles], and oculogyric crisis [rolling back of eyes]). Dystonic reaction may produce diaphoresis, pallor. Tardive dyskinesia (tongue protrusion, puffing of cheeks, puckering of the mouth) occurs rarely (may be irreversible). Abrupt discontinuation after long-term therapy may precipitate nausea, vomiting, gastritis, dizziness, tremors. Blood dyscrasias, particularly agranulocytosis, mild leukopenia, may occur. May decrease seizure threshold.

NURSING CONSIDERATIONS

BASELINE ASSESSMENT
Avoid skin contact with solution (contact dermatitis). **Antiemetic:** Assess for dehydration (poor skin turgor, dry mucous membranes, longitudinal furrows in tongue). **Antipsychotic:** Assess behavior, appearance, emotional status, response to environment, speech pattern, thought content.

INTERVENTION/EVALUATION
Monitor B/P for hypotension. Assess for EPS. Monitor WBC, differential count for blood dyscrasias, fine tongue movement (may be early sign of tardive dyskinesia). Supervise suicidal-risk pt closely during early therapy (as depression lessens, energy level improves, increasing suicide potential). Assess for therapeutic response (interest in surroundings, improvement in self-care, increased ability to concentrate, relaxed facial expression). **Therapeutic serum level:** 50–300 ng/ml; **toxic serum level:** greater than 750 ng/ml.

PATIENT/FAMILY TEACHING

• Full therapeutic response may take up to 6 wks. • Urine may darken. • Do not abruptly withdraw from long-term drug therapy. • Report visual disturbances. • Drowsiness generally subsides with continued therapy. • Avoid tasks that require alertness, motor skills until response to drug is established. • Avoid alcohol, exposure to sunlight.

cholestyramine

koe-lee-**stye**-ra-meen
(Novo-Cholamine ✤, Prevalite, Questran, Questran Lite)

◆ CLASSIFICATION

PHARMACOTHERAPEUTIC: Bile acid sequestrant. **CLINICAL:** Antihyperlipoproteinemic (see p. 56C).

ACTION

Binds with bile acids in intestine, forming insoluble complex. Binding results in partial removal of bile acid from enterohepatic circulation. **Therapeutic Effect:** Removes LDL cholesterol from plasma.

PHARMACOKINETICS

Not absorbed from GI tract. Decreases in serum LDL apparent in 5–7 days and in serum cholesterol in 1 mo. Serum cholesterol returns to baseline about 1 mo after drug discontinuation.

USES

Adjunct to diet to decrease elevated serum cholesterol levels in pts with primary hypercholesterolemia. Relief of pruritus associated with elevated levels of bile acids. Regression of arteriosclerosis. **OFF-LABEL:** Treatment of diarrhea (due to bile acids), binding toxicologic agents.

PRECAUTIONS

Contraindications: Complete biliary obstruction. **Cautions:** GI dysfunction (esp. constipation), recent abdominal surgery, renal impairment, dehydration, concurrent spironolactone therapy.

⌛ LIFESPAN CONSIDERATIONS

Pregnancy/Lactation: Not systemically absorbed. May interfere with maternal absorption of fat-soluble vitamins. **Pregnancy Category B. Children:** No age-related precautions noted. Limited experience in those younger than 10 yrs. **Elderly:** Increased risk of GI side effects, adverse nutritional effects.

INTERACTIONS

DRUG: May increase effects of **anticoagulants** by decreasing vitamin K level. May decrease **warfarin** absorption. May bind with, decrease absorption of **digoxin, folic acid, penicillins, propranolol, tetracyclines, thiazides, thyroid hormones, oral vancomycin.** **HERBAL:** None significant. **FOOD:** None known. **LAB VALUES:** May increase serum alkaline phosphatase, magnesium, AST, ALT. May decrease serum calcium, potassium, sodium. May prolong PT.

AVAILABILITY (Rx)

Powder for Oral Suspension: 4 g.

ADMINISTRATION/HANDLING

PO

• Give other drugs at least 1 hr before or 4–6 hrs following cholestyramine (capable of binding drugs in GI tract). • Do not give in dry form (highly irritating). Mix with 3–6 oz water, milk, fruit juice, soup. • Place powder on surface for 1–2 min (prevents lumping), then mix thoroughly. • Excessive foaming with carbonated beverages reported; use extra large glass, stir slowly. • Administer with meals.

INDICATIONS/ROUTES/DOSAGE

Hypercholesterolemia
PO: ADULTS, ELDERLY: Initially, 4 g 1–2 times a day. Gradually increase over at

least 1-mo intervals. Maintenance: 4–16 g/day in divided doses. **Maximum:** 24 g/day, 6 doses/day. **CHILDREN:** 80 mg/kg 3 times a day. **Maximum:** 8 g/day.

Pruritis
PO: **ADULTS, ELDERLY:** Initially, 4 g 1–2 times a day. Maintenance: 4–16 g/day in divided doses. **Maximum:** 24 g/day.

SIDE EFFECTS

Frequent: Constipation (may lead to fecal impaction), nausea, vomiting, abdominal pain, indigestion. **Occasional:** Diarrhea, belching, bloating, headache, dizziness. **Rare:** Gallstones, peptic ulcer disease, malabsorption syndrome.

ADVERSE EFFECTS/ TOXIC REACTIONS

GI tract obstruction, hyperchloremic acidosis, or osteoporosis secondary to calcium excretion may occur. High dosage may interfere with fat absorption, resulting in steatorrhea.

NURSING CONSIDERATIONS

BASELINE ASSESSMENT

Question for history of hypersensitivity to cholestyramine, tartrazine, aspirin. Obtain baseline serum cholesterol, triglycerides, electrolytes, hepatic enzyme levels.

INTERVENTION/EVALUATION

Monitor daily pattern of bowel activity, stool consistency. Evaluate food tolerance, abdominal discomfort, flatulence. Monitor cholesterol, triglycerides, PT, hepatic enzymes, CBC, serum electrolytes. Encourage several glasses of water between meals.

PATIENT/FAMILY TEACHING

• Complete full course of therapy; do not stop or change doses. • Take other drugs at least 1 hr before or 4–6 hrs after cholestyramine. • Never take in dry form; mix with 3–6 oz water, milk, fruit juice, soup (place powder on surface for 1–2 min to prevent lumping, then mix well). • Use extra-large glass, stir slowly when mixing with carbonated beverages due to foaming. • Take with meals, drink several glasses of water between meals. • Eat high-fiber foods (whole-grain cereals, fruits, vegetables) to reduce potential for constipation.

ciclesonide

sye-**kles**-oh-nide
(Alvesco HFA, Omnaris, Zetonna)

◆CLASSIFICATION

PHARMACOTHERAPEUTIC: Glucocorticoid. **CLINICAL:** Anti-inflammatory (see p. 2C, 77C).

ACTION

Inhibits accumulation of inflammatory cells, decreases and prevents tissues from responding to inflammatory process. **Therapeutic Effect:** Relieves symptoms of allergic rhinitis, asthma.

PHARMACOKINETICS

Minimally absorbed from nasal tissue, moderately absorbed from inhalation. Protein binding: 99%. Metabolized in liver. Excreted in feces (66%), urine (20% or less). **Half-life:** 2–3 hrs.

USES

Intranasal: Management of seasonal or perennial allergic rhinitis. **Oral Inhalation:** Prophylactic management of bronchial asthma. **OFF-LABEL:** Adjunct to antibiotics in empiric treatment of acute bacterial rhinosinusitis.

PRECAUTIONS

Contraindications: Acute asthma or status asthmaticus; moderate to severe bronchiectasis. **Cautions:** Cataracts, severe hepatic impairment, seizures, osteoporosis, glaucoma, thyroid disease, psychiatric disturbance, cardiovascular disease, myasthenia gravis, elderly, chronic wounds.

⧗ LIFESPAN CONSIDERATIONS

Pregnancy/Lactation: Unknown if drug crosses placenta or distributed in breast milk. **Pregnancy Category C. Children:** Safety and efficacy not established in pts younger than 12 yrs. **Elderly:** No age-related precautions noted.

INTERACTIONS

DRUG: Ketoconazole may increase concentration/effects. **HERBAL:** None significant. **FOOD:** None known. **LAB VALUES:** None significant.

AVAILABILITY (Rx)

Inhalation (Alvesco HFA): 80 mcg/spray, 160 mcg/spray. **Nasal Spray (Omnaris):** 50 mcg/spray. **(Zetonna):** 37 mcg/spray.

ADMINISTRATION/HANDLING

Inhalation
• Shaking not necessary. • Wait 2 min before inhaling second dose (allows for deeper bronchial penetration). • Rinse mouth with water immediately after inhalation (prevents mouth/throat dryness).

Intranasal
• Instruct pt to clear nasal passages before use. • Tilt head slightly forward. • Insert spray tip into nostril, pointing toward nasal passages, away from nasal septum. • Spray into one nostril while pt holds other nostril closed, concurrently inspires through nose to permit medication as high into nasal passages as possible.

INDICATIONS/ROUTES/DOSAGE

Perennial Allergic Rhinitis
Intranasal: ADULTS, ELDERLY, CHILDREN 12 YRS AND OLDER: (Omnaris): 2 sprays (100 mcg) in each nostril once a day. **Maximum:** 200 mcg/day. **(Zetonna):** 1 spray (37 mcg) in each nostril daily. **Maximum:** 74 mcg/day.

Seasonal Allergic Rhinitis
Intranasal: ADULTS, ELDERLY, CHILDREN 6 YRS AND OLDER: (Omnaris): 2 sprays (100 mcg) in each nostril once a day. **Maximum:** 200 mcg/day. **(Zetonna):** 1 spray (37 mcg) in each nostril daily.. **Maximum:** 74 mcg/day.

Asthma
Inhalation: ADULTS, ELDERLY, CHILDREN 12 YRS AND OLDER (PREVIOUS THERAPY WITH BRONCHODILATORS ALONE): Initially, 80 mcg 2 times daily. **Maximum:** 320 mcg 2 times daily. **(PREVIOUS THERAPY WITH INHALED STEROIDS):** Initially, 80 mcg twice daily. **Maximum:** 640 mcg/day. **(PREVIOUS THERAPY WITH ORAL STEROIDS):** Initially, 320 mcg twice daily. **Maximum:** 640 mcg/day.

SIDE EFFECTS

Occasional (6%–4%): Headache, epistaxis, nasopharyngitis. **Rare (2%):** Ear pain.

ADVERSE EFFECTS/ TOXIC REACTIONS

Excessive doses over prolonged periods may result in systemic hypercortisolism.

NURSING CONSIDERATIONS

BASELINE ASSESSMENT

Question for hypersensitivity to any corticosteroids. Establish baseline history of asthma, rhinitis.

INTERVENTION/EVALUATION

Monitor for relief of symptoms. Monitor rate, depth, rhythm, type of respiration. Assess lung sounds for rhonchi, wheezing, rales. Assess oral mucous membranes for candidiasis.

PATIENT/FAMILY TEACHING

• Improvement noted in 24–48 hrs, but full effect may take 1–2 wks for seasonal allergic rhinitis, 5 wks for perennial allergic rhinitis. • Improvement in asthma may take 4 wks or longer. • Oral inhalation not indicated for acute asthma attacks. • Report if no improvement in symptoms, sneezing or nasal irritation occurs.

cidofovir

sye-**dof**-o-veer
(Vistide)

BLACK BOX ALERT Dose-dependent nephrotoxicity requires dose adjustment, discontinuation if changes in renal function occur (renal lab tests, urinalysis). May cause hypospermia. May be embryotoxic, teratogenic. Neutropenia reported: monitor neutrophil count.

◆ CLASSIFICATION

PHARMACOTHERAPEUTIC: Anti-infective. **CLINICAL:** Antiviral (see p. 69C).

ACTION

Inhibits viral DNA synthesis by incorporating itself into viral DNA chain. **Therapeutic Effect:** Suppresses replication of cytomegalovirus (CMV).

PHARMACOKINETICS

Protein binding: less than 6%. Excreted primarily unchanged in urine. Effect of hemodialysis unknown. **Elimination Half-life:** 1.4–3.8 hrs.

USES

Treatment of CMV retinitis in those with HIV. Should be given with probenecid.

PRECAUTIONS

Contraindications: Direct intraocular injection, history of clinically severe hypersensitivity to probenecid or other sulfa-containing drugs, renal impairment (serum creatinine level greater than 1.5 mg/dl, creatinine clearance 55 ml/min or less, or urine protein level greater than 100 mg/dl). Use with or within 7 days of nephrotoxic agent. **Caution:** History of hepatic impairment, metabolic acidosis, pancreatitis, dehydration.

⌛ LIFESPAN CONSIDERATIONS

Pregnancy/Lactation: May cause fetal harm. Unknown if distributed in breast milk. Breast-feeding not recommended.

Pregnancy Category C. Children: Safety and efficacy not established. **Elderly:** Age-related renal impairment may require dosage adjustment.

INTERACTIONS

DRUG: Nephrotoxic medications (e.g., aminoglycosides, amphotericin B, foscarnet, IV pentamidine) increase risk of nephrotoxicity. **HERBAL:** None significant. **FOOD:** None known. **LAB VALUES:** May decrease neutrophil count, serum bicarbonate, phosphate, uric acid. May elevate serum creatinine.

AVAILABILITY (Rx)

Injection Solution: 75 mg/ml (5-ml ampule).

ADMINISTRATION/HANDLING

◀ALERT▶ Do not exceed recommended dosage, frequency, infusion rate.

 IV

Reconstitution • Dilute in 100 ml 0.9% NaCl or D₅W; do not exceed concentration of 8 mg/ml.
Rate of Administration • Infuse over 1 hr. • IV hydration with 0.9% NaCl (1,000 ml prior to and after infusion). Probenecid therapy **must** be used with each cidofovir infusion (minimizes risk of nephrotoxicity). • Ingestion of food before each dose of probenecid may reduce nausea/vomiting.
Storage • Store at room temperature. • Admixtures may be refrigerated for no more than 24 hrs. • Allow refrigerated admixtures to warm to room temperature before use.

▓ IV INCOMPATIBILITIES

None known.

INDICATIONS/ROUTES/DOSAGE

Cytomegalovirus (CMV) Retinitis in Pts with HIV (in Combination with Probenecid)
IV Infusion: ADULTS: Induction: Usual dosage, 5 mg/kg at constant rate over 1 hr once weekly for 2 consecutive wks. Give 2 g of PO probenecid 3 hrs before

cidofovir dose, then give 1 g 2 hrs and 8 hrs after completion of the 1-hr cidofovir infusion (total of 4 g). In addition, give 1 L of 0.9% NaCl over 1–2 hrs immediately before cidofovir infusion. If tolerated, a second liter may be infused over 1–3 hrs at start of infusion or immediately afterward. **CHILDREN:** 5 mg/kg once with probenecid and hydration. **Maintenance: ADULTS, ELDERLY:** 5 mg/kg once every 2 wks. **CHILDREN:** 3–5 mg/kg/dose once q2wks for 2–4 doses.

Dosage in Renal Impairment

Changes during Therapy: If creatinine increases by 0.3–0.4 mg/dl, reduce dose to 3 mg/kg; if creatinine increases by 0.5 mg/dl or greater or proteinuria 3+ or greater develops, discontinue therapy.
Preexisting Renal Impairment: (See contraindications.)

SIDE EFFECTS

Frequent: Nausea, vomiting (65%), fever (57%), asthenia (loss of strength, energy) (46%), rash (30%), diarrhea (27%), headache (27%), alopecia (25%), chills (24%), anorexia (22%), dyspnea (22%), abdominal pain (17%).

ADVERSE EFFECTS/ TOXIC REACTIONS

Serious adverse effects include proteinuria (80%), nephrotoxicity (53%), neutropenia (31%), elevated serum creatinine (29%), infection (24%), anemia (20%), decrease in intraocular pressure (IOP) (12%), pneumonia (9%). Concurrent use of probenecid may produce a hypersensitivity reaction characterized by rash, fever, chills, anaphylaxis. Acute renal failure occurs rarely.

NURSING CONSIDERATIONS

BASELINE ASSESSMENT

Obtain baseline WBC, renal function tests prior to beginning therapy. For those taking zidovudine, temporarily discontinue zidovudine administration or decrease zidovudine dose by 50% on days of infusion (probenecid reduces metabolic clearance of zidovudine). Assess hydration status.

INTERVENTION/EVALUATION

Monitor WBC count, BUN, serum creatinine, electrolytes, hepatic function tests, urine protein before each dose. Proteinuria may be early indicator of dose-dependent nephrotoxicity. Periodically monitor visual acuity, ocular symptoms.

PATIENT/FAMILY TEACHING

• Obtain regular follow-up ophthalmologic exams. • Those of childbearing age should use effective contraception during and for 1 mo after treatment. • Men should wear condoms during and for 3 mos after treatment. • Breast-feeding not recommended. • Must complete full course of probenecid with each cidofovir dose. • Report rash immediately.

cilostazol

sil-o-sta-zol
(Pletal)
BLACK BOX ALERT Contraindicated in pts with HF of any severity, active bleeding.
Do not confuse Pletal with Plendil.

◆CLASSIFICATION

PHARMACOTHERAPEUTIC: Phosphodiesterase enzyme inhibitor. **CLINICAL:** Antiplatelet.

ACTION

Inhibits platelet aggregation. Dilates vascular beds with greatest dilation in femoral beds. **Therapeutic Effect:** Improves walking distance in those with intermittent claudication; usually noted in 2–4 wks but may take as long as 12 wks.

PHARMACOKINETICS

Moderately absorbed from GI tract. Protein binding: 95%–98%. Metabolized in liver. Excreted in urine (74%), feces

(20%). Not removed by hemodialysis. **Half-life:** 11–13 hrs.

USES

Management of peripheral vascular disease, primarily intermittent claudication. **OFF-LABEL:** Adjunct with aspirin and clopidogrel for prevention of stent thrombosis and restenosis after coronary stent placement.

PRECAUTIONS

Contraindications: HF of any severity, hemostatic disorders or active bleeding (bleeding peptic ulcer, intracranial bleeding). **Cautions:** Severe underlying heart disease, thrombocytopenia, pts receiving other platelet aggregation inhibitors, moderate to severe hepatic impairment, severe renal impairment.

⌛ LIFESPAN CONSIDERATIONS

Pregnancy/Lactation: Unknown if drug crosses placenta or is distributed in breast milk. **Pregnancy Category C. Children:** Safety and efficacy not established. **Elderly:** No age-related precautions noted.

INTERACTIONS

DRUG: Aspirin may potentiate inhibition of platelet aggregation. **CYP3A4 inhibitors (e.g., clarithromycin, diltiazem, erythromycin, fluconazole), CYP2C19 inhibitors (e.g., omeprazole)** may increase concentration/effects. **HERBAL: St. John's wort** may decrease effect. Avoid herbs with antiplatelet activity **(e.g., garlic, ginger, ginkgo). FOOD: Grapefruit, grapefruit juice** may increase concentration, toxicity. **LAB VALUES:** May increase BUN, serum glucose, uric acid. May decrease platelet count, WBC.

AVAILABILITY (Rx)

Tablets: 50 mg, 100 mg.

ADMINISTRATION/HANDLING

PO

• Give at least 30 min before or 2 hrs after meals. • Do not give with grapefruit products.

INDICATIONS/ROUTES/DOSAGE

Peripheral Vascular Disease
PO: ADULTS, ELDERLY: 100 mg twice a day at least 30 min before or 2 hrs after meals. Decrease to 50 mg twice a day during concurrent therapy with CYP3A4 or CYP2C19 inhibitors (e.g., clarithromycin, diltiazem, erythromycin, fluconazole, fluoxetine, omeprazole, sertraline).

SIDE EFFECTS

Frequent (34%–10%): Headache, diarrhea, palpitations, dizziness, pharyngitis. **Occasional (7%–3%):** Nausea, rhinitis, back pain, peripheral edema, dyspepsia, abdominal pain, tachycardia, cough, flatulence, myalgia. **Rare (2%–1%):** Leg cramps, paresthesia, rash, vomiting.

ADVERSE EFFECTS/ TOXIC REACTIONS

Overdose noted as severe headache, diarrhea, hypotension, cardiac arrhythmias. May increase risk of endocardial hemorrhage, fibrosis of left ventricle, intimal thickening of coronary artery.

NURSING CONSIDERATIONS

BASELINE ASSESSMENT

Assess platelet count, CBC, serum chemistries, esp. renal/hepatic function tests before treatment and periodically during treatment.

INTERVENTION/EVALUATION

Monitor for improvement of symptoms (e.g., improved walking distance). Monitor lab tests periodically. Monitor for bleeding events, cardiovascular toxicity or lesions.

PATIENT/FAMILY TEACHING

• Take on an empty stomach (at least 30 min before or 2 hrs after meals). • Do not take with grapefruit products.

cimetidine

sye-**met**-i-deen

C

(Apo-Cimetidine ✷, Novo-Cimetidine ✷, Tagamet, Tagamet HB 200)
Do not confuse cimetidine with simethicone.

◆ CLASSIFICATION

PHARMACOTHERAPEUTIC: H_2-receptor antagonist. **CLINICAL:** Antiulcer, gastric acid secretion inhibitor (see p. 110C).

ACTION

Inhibits histamine action at histamine-2 (H_2)-receptor sites of parietal cells. **Therapeutic Effect:** Inhibits gastric acid secretion.

PHARMACOKINETICS

Well absorbed from GI tract. Protein binding: 15%–20%. Widely distributed. Metabolized in liver. Primarily excreted in urine. Not removed by hemodialysis. **Half-life:** 2 hrs (increased in renal impairment).

USES

Short-term treatment of active duodenal ulcer. Prevention of duodenal ulcer recurrence. Treatment of benign gastric ulcer, pathologic GI hypersecretory conditions, gastroesophageal reflux disease (GERD). **OTC** use: Heartburn, acid indigestion. **OFF-LABEL:** *H. pylori* eradication to reduce risk of duodenal ulcer recurrence.

PRECAUTIONS

Contraindications: Hypersensitivity to other H_2 antagonists. **Cautions:** Renal/hepatic impairment, elderly. Concurrent administration of medications utilizing P450 system.

⧗ LIFESPAN CONSIDERATIONS

Pregnancy/Lactation: Distributed in breast milk. Possible adverse effects on fetal development. **Pregnancy Category B. Children:** Long-term use may induce cerebral toxicity, affect hormonal system. **Elderly:** More likely to experience confusion, esp. pt with renal impairment.

INTERACTIONS

DRUG: May increase concentration, decrease metabolism of **warfarin, phenytoin, propranolol, tricyclic antidepressants.** May decrease absorption of **itraconazole, ketoconazole. HERBAL: St. John's wort** may decrease concentration. **FOOD:** None known. **LAB VALUES:** Interferes with skin tests using allergen extracts. May increase serum prolactin, creatinine, ALT, AST. May decrease parathyroid hormone concentration.

AVAILABILITY (Rx)

Liquid, Oral: 300 mg/5 ml. **Tablets:** 200 mg (OTC), 300 mg, 400 mg, 800 mg.

ADMINISTRATION/HANDLING
PO
• Give without regard to food. • Best given with meals and at bedtime. • Do not administer within 1 hr of antacids.

INDICATIONS/ROUTES/DOSAGE

Active Duodenal Ulcer
PO: ADULTS, ELDERLY: 300 mg 4 times a day or 400 mg twice a day or 800 mg at bedtime for up to 8 wks.

Prevention of Duodenal Ulcer
PO: ADULTS, ELDERLY: 400 mg at bedtime.

Gastric Hypersecretory Secretions
PO: ADULTS, ELDERLY: 300–600 mg q6h. **Maximum:** 2,400 mg/day.

Gastroesophageal Reflux Disease (GERD)
PO: ADULTS, ELDERLY: 800 mg twice a day or 400 mg 4 times a day for 12 wks.

OTC Use
PO: ADULTS, ELDERLY: 200 mg up to 30 min before meals. **Maximum:** 2 doses/day.

Usual Pediatric/Neonatal Dosage
CHILDREN: 20–40 mg/kg/day in divided doses q6h. **INFANTS:** 10–20 mg/kg/day in divided doses q6–12h. **NEONATES:** 5–10 mg/kg/day in divided doses q8–12h.

Dosage in Renal Impairment
Dosage is modified based on creatinine clearance.

Creatinine Clearance	Dosage
Greater than 50 ml/min	No change
10–50 ml/min	50% of normal dose
Less than 10 ml/min	25% of normal dose

Give after hemodialysis and q12h between dialysis sessions.

SIDE EFFECTS

Occasional (4%–2%): Headache. **Elderly, pts with renal impairment, severely ill pts:** Confusion, agitation, psychosis, depression, anxiety, disorientation, hallucinations. Effects reverse 3–4 days after discontinuance. **Rare (less than 2%):** Diarrhea, dizziness, drowsiness, nausea, vomiting, gynecomastia, rash, impotence.

ADVERSE EFFECTS/ TOXIC REACTIONS

None known.

NURSING CONSIDERATIONS

BASELINE ASSESSMENT

Obtain baseline CBC, PT, aPTT, BUN, creatinine.

INTERVENTION/EVALUATION

Assess for GI bleeding: hematemesis, blood in stool. Monitor for changes in mental status in elderly, severely ill, those with renal impairment.

PATIENT/FAMILY TEACHING

• Do not take antacids within 1 hr of cimetidine administration. • Avoid tasks that require alertness, motor skills until response to drug is established. • Avoid smoking, excessive amounts of caffeine. • Report any blood in vomitus/stool, or dark, tarry stool.

cinacalcet   TOP 200

sin-a-**kal**-set
(Sensipar)

◆CLASSIFICATION

PHARMACOTHERAPEUTIC: Calcium receptor agonist. **CLINICAL:** Calcimimetic.

ACTION

Increases sensitivity of calcium-sensing receptor on parathyroid gland to activation by extracellular calcium, thus lowering parathyroid hormone (PTH) levels. **Therapeutic Effect:** Decreases serum calcium, PTH levels.

PHARMACOKINETICS

Extensively distributed after PO administration. Protein binding: 93%–97%. Metabolized in liver. Excreted in urine (80%), feces (15%). **Half-life:** 30–40 hrs.

USES

Treatment of hypercalcemia in pts with parathyroid carcinoma. Treatment of secondary hyperparathyroidism in pts with chronic renal disease on dialysis. Treatment of severe hypercalcemia in pts with hyperparathyroidism unable to undergo parathyroidectomy. **OFF-LABEL:** Primary hyperparathyroidism.

PRECAUTIONS

Contraindications: Hypocalcemia. **Cautions:** Moderate to severe hepatic impairment. Seizure disorder, cardiovascular disease.

⌛ LIFESPAN CONSIDERATIONS

Pregnancy/Lactation: May cross placental barrier; unknown if distributed in breast milk. Safe usage during lactation not established (potential adverse reaction in infants). **Pregnancy Category C. Children:** Safety and efficacy not established. **Elderly:** No age-related precautions noted.

✤ Canadian trade name   🔪 Non-Crushable Drug   🔺 High Alert drug

INTERACTIONS

DRUG: Strong **CYP3A4 inhibitors (e.g., erythromycin, itraconazole, ketoconazole)** increase concentration/effects. Concurrent administration of drugs metabolized by **CYP2D6 enzyme (e.g., flecainide, tricyclic antidepressants, metoprolol, carvedilol)**, may require dosage adjustment. **HERBAL:** None significant. **FOOD: High-fat meals** increase plasma concentration. **LAB VALUES:** May decrease serum calcium, phosphorus.

AVAILABILITY (Rx)

Tablets: 30 mg, 60 mg, 90 mg.

ADMINISTRATION/HANDLING

PO

• Store at room temperature. • Do not break, cut, crush, or divide film-coated tablets. • Administer with food or shortly after a meal.

INDICATIONS/ROUTES/DOSAGE

Hypercalcemia in Parathyroid Carcinoma; Primary Hyperparathyroidism

PO: ADULTS, ELDERLY: Initially, 30 mg twice a day. Titrate dosage sequentially (60 mg twice a day, 90 mg twice a day, and 90 mg 3–4 times a day) every 2–4 wks as needed to normalize serum calcium level. **Maximum:** 360 mg/day (as 90 mg 4 times/day).

Secondary Hyperparathyroidism in Pts on Dialysis

PO: ADULTS, ELDERLY: Initially, 30 mg once a day. Titrate dosage sequentially (60, 90, 120, and 180 mg once a day) every 2–4 wks to maintain iPTH level between 150 and 300 pg/ml. **Maximum:** 180 mg/day.

SIDE EFFECTS

Frequent (31%–21%): Nausea, vomiting, diarrhea. **Occasional (15%–10%):** Myalgia, dizziness. **Rare (7%–5%):** Asthenia (loss of strength, energy), hypertension, anorexia, noncardiac chest pain.

ADVERSE EFFECTS/ TOXIC REACTIONS

Overdose may lead to hypocalcemia, seizures, worsening of HF.

NURSING CONSIDERATIONS

BASELINE ASSESSMENT

Establish baseline serum electrolyte levels (esp. serum calcium, phosphorus, ionized calcium).

INTERVENTION/EVALUATION

Monitor serum calcium, phosphorus, ionized calcium for hyperparathyroidism. Monitor daily pattern of bowel activity, stool consistency. Obtain order for antidiarrhea, antiemetic medication to prevent serum electrolyte imbalance. Assess for evidence of dizziness, institute fall risk precautions.

PATIENT/FAMILY TEACHING

• Take with food or shortly after a meal. • Do not break, chew, crush, or divide film-coated tablets. • Notify physician immediately if vomiting, diarrhea, cramping, muscle pain, numbness occurs.

ciprofloxacin
TOP 200

sip-roe-**flox**-a-sin
(Apo-Ciproflox ✤, Cetraxal, Ciloxan, Cipro, Cipro IV, Novo-Ciprofloxacin ✤)
BLACK BOX ALERT May increase risk of tendonitis, tendon rupture. **Do not confuse Ciloxan with Cytoxan, or Cipro with Ceftin, or ciprofloxacin with cephalexin.**

FIXED-COMBINATION(S)

Cipro HC Otic: ciprofloxacin/hydrocortisone (a steroid): 0.2%/1%. **CiproDex Otic:** ciprofloxacin/dexamethasone (a corticosteroid): 0.3%/0.1%.

◆CLASSIFICATION

PHARMACOTHERAPEUTIC: Fluoroquinolone. **CLINICAL:** Antibiotic (see p. 26C).

ACTION

Inhibits enzyme, DNA gyrase, in susceptible bacteria, interfering with bacterial cell replication. **Therapeutic Effect:** Bactericidal.

PHARMACOKINETICS

Well absorbed from GI tract. Protein binding: 20%–40%. Widely distributed including to CSF. Metabolized in liver. Primarily excreted in urine. Minimal removal by hemodialysis. **Half-life:** 3–5 hrs (increased in renal impairment, elderly).

USES

Treatment of susceptible infections due to *E. coli, K. pneumoniae, E. cloacae, P. mirabilis, P. vulgaris, P. aeruginosa, H. influenzae, M. catarrhalis, S. pneumoniae, S. aureus* (methicillin susceptible), *S. epidermidis, S. pyogenes, C. jejuni, Shigella* spp., *S. typhi* including intra-abdominal, bone, joint, lower respiratory tract, skin/skin structure, UTIs, infectious diarrhea, prostatitis, sinusitis, typhoid fever, febrile neutropenia. **Ophthalmic:** Treatment of superficial ocular infections. **OTIC:** Treatment of acute otitis externa due to susceptible strains of *P. aeruginosa* or *S. aureus*. **OFF-LABEL:** Treatment of chancroid. Acute pulmonary exacerbations in cystic fibrosis, disseminated gonococcal infections, prophylaxis to *Neisseria meninigitidis* following close contact with infected person. Infectious diarrhea (children); periodontitis.

PRECAUTIONS

Contraindications: Hypersensitivity to any fluoroquinolones, other quinolones. Concurrent use of tizanidine. **Cautions:** Renal impairment, CNS disorders, seizures, rheumatoid arthritis, history of QT prolongation, uncorrected hypokalemia, hypomagnesemia, myasthenia gravis. Suspension not for use in NG tube.

⌛ LIFESPAN CONSIDERATIONS

Pregnancy/Lactation: Unknown if distributed in breast milk. If possible, do not use during pregnancy/lactation (risk of arthropathy to fetus/infant). **Pregnancy Category C. Children:** Arthropathy may occur if given to children younger than 18 yrs. **Elderly:** Age-related renal impairment may require dosage adjustment.

INTERACTIONS

DRUG: **Antacids, iron preparations, sucralfate** may decrease absorption. May increase effects of **caffeine, oral anticoagulants (e.g., warfarin).** May decrease concentration of **fosphenytoin, phenytoin.** May increase concentration, toxicity of **theophylline.** Decreases **theophylline** clearance. **HERBAL:** **Dong quai, St. John's wort** may increase photosensitization. **FOOD:** None known. **LAB VALUES:** May increase serum alkaline phosphatase, creatine kinase (CK), LDH, AST, ALT.

AVAILABILITY (Rx)

Infusion Solution: 200 mg/100 ml, 400 mg/200 ml. **Injection, Solution (Cipro):** 10 mg/ml. **Ophthalmic Ointment (Ciloxan):** 0.3%. **Ophthalmic Solution (Ciloxan):** 0.3%. **Otic Solution (Cetraxal):** 0.2%. **Suspension, Oral:** 250 mg/5 ml, 500 mg/5 ml. **Tablets (Cipro):** 100 mg, 250 mg, 500 mg, 750 mg.

 Tablets (Extended-Release): 500 mg, 1,000 mg.

ADMINISTRATION/HANDLING

📟 **IV**

Reconstitution • Available prediluted in infusion container ready for use. Final concentration not to exceed 2 mg/ml.
Rate of Administration • Infuse over 60 min (reduces risk of venous irritation).
Storage • Store at room temperature. • Solution appears clear, colorless to slightly yellow.

C

PO

• May be given without regard to food (preferred dosing time: 2 hrs after meals). • Do not give with dairy products. • Do not administer antacids (aluminum, magnesium) within 2 hrs of ciprofloxacin. • Do not administer suspension through feeding tubes.

Ophthalmic

• Place gloved finger on lower eyelid and pull out until a pocket is formed between eye and lower lid. • Place ointment or drops into pocket. • Instruct pt to close eye gently for 1–2 min (so medication will not be squeezed out of the sac). • Instruct pt using ointment to roll eyeball to increase contact area of drug to eye. • Instruct pt using solution to apply digital pressure to lacrimal sac at inner canthus for 1 min to minimize systemic absorption. • Do not use ophthalmic solution for injection.

▦ IV INCOMPATIBILITIES

Ampicillin and sulbactam (Unasyn), cefepime (Maxipime), dexamethasone (Decadron), furosemide (Lasix), heparin, hydrocortisone (Solu-Cortef), methylprednisolone (Solu-Medrol), phenytoin (Dilantin), sodium bicarbonate.

▦ IV COMPATIBILITIES

Calcium gluconate, diltiazem (Cardizem), dobutamine (Dobutrex), dopamine (Intropin), lidocaine, lorazepam (Ativan), magnesium, midazolam (Versed), potassium chloride.

INDICATIONS/ROUTES/DOSAGE

Note: Not recommended as first choice due to adverse events related to joints/surrounding tissue.

Usual Dosage Range
PO: ADULTS, ELDERLY: 250–750 mg q12h.
CHILDREN: 20–30 mg/kg/day in 2 divided doses. **Maximum:** 1.5 g/day.
IV: ADULTS, ELDERLY: 200–400 mg q12h.
CHILDREN: 20–30 mg/kg/day in divided doses q12h. **Maximum:** 800 mg/day.

Bone, Joint Infections
IV: ADULTS, ELDERLY: 400 mg q8–12h for 4–6 wks.
PO: ADULTS, ELDERLY: 500–750 mg q12h for 4–6 wks.

Conjunctivitis
Ophthalmic: ADULTS, ELDERLY: (Solution): 1–2 drops q2h for 2 days, then 2 drops q4h for 5 days. **(Ointment):** ½ inch 3 times a day for 2 days, then ½ inch daily for 5 days.

Corneal Ulcer
Ophthalmic: ADULTS, ELDERLY: 2 drops q15min for 6 hrs, then 2 drops q30min for the remainder of first day, 2 drops q1h on second day, and 2 drops q4h on days 3–14.

Cystic Fibrosis
IV: CHILDREN: 40 mg/kg/day in 2–3 divided doses. **Maximum:** 1.2 g/day.
PO: CHILDREN: 40 mg/kg/day. **Maximum:** 2 g/day.

Febrile Neutropenia
IV: ADULTS, ELDERLY: 400 mg q8h for 7–14 days (in combination).

Gonorrhea
PO: ADULTS, ELDERLY: 250–500 mg as a single dose.

Infectious Diarrhea
PO: ADULTS, ELDERLY: 500 mg q12h for 3–7 days.

Intra-Abdominal Infections (with Metronidazole)
IV: ADULTS, ELDERLY: 400 mg q12h for 7–14 days.
PO: ADULTS, ELDERLY: 500 mg q12h for 7–14 days.

Lower Respiratory Tract Infections
IV: ADULTS, ELDERLY: 400 mg q8–12h for 7–14 days.
PO: ADULTS, ELDERLY: 500–750 mg q12h for 7–14 days.

Nosocomial Pneumonia
IV: ADULTS, ELDERLY: 400 mg q8h for 10–14 days.

Prostatitis
IV: ADULTS, ELDERLY: 400 mg q12h for 28 days.
PO: ADULTS, ELDERLY: 500 mg q12h for 28 days.

Sinusitis
IV: ADULTS, ELDERLY: 400 mg q12h for 10 days.
PO: ADULTS, ELDERLY: 500 mg q12h for 10 days.

Skin/Skin Structure Infections
IV: ADULTS, ELDERLY: 400 mg q12h for 7–14 days.
PO: ADULTS, ELDERLY: 500–750 mg q12h for 7–14 days.

Susceptible Infections
IV: ADULTS, ELDERLY: 400 mg q8–12h.
PO: ADULTS, ELDERLY: 500–750 mg q12h.

Typhoid Fever
PO: ADULTS, ELDERLY: 500 mg q12h for 10 days.

UTI
IV: ADULTS, ELDERLY: 200–400 mg q12h for 7–14 days.
PO: ADULTS, ELDERLY: Immediate-release: 250 mg q12h for 3 days for acute uncomplicated infections; 250 mg q12h for 7–14 days for mild to moderate infections; 500 mg q12h for 7–14 days for severe or complicated infections. **Extended-release: Complicated infection:** 1,000 mg q24h for 7–14 days. **Uncomplicated infection:** 500 mg q24h for 3 days.

Otitis Externa
Otic: ADULTS, ELDERLY, CHILDREN: Contents of one single-use container twice daily for 7 days.

Dosage in Renal Impairment
Dosage and frequency are modified based on creatinine clearance and the severity of the infection.

Creatinine Clearance	Dosage
30–50 ml/min	PO: 250–500 mg q12h
Less than 30 ml/min	PO (extended-release): 500 mg q24h PO (immediate-release): 250–500 mg q18h IV: 200–400 mg q18–24h

Hemodialysis
PO: ADULTS, ELDERLY: 250–500 mg q24h (after dialysis). **IV:** 200–400 mg q24h.

Peritoneal Dialysis
PO: ADULTS, ELDERLY: 250–500 mg q24h (after dialysis).

Continuous Renal Replacement Therapy
IV: ADULTS, ELDERLY: 200–400 mg q12–24h.

SIDE EFFECTS

Frequent (5%–2%): Nausea, diarrhea, dyspepsia, vomiting, constipation, flatulence, confusion, crystalluria. **Ophthalmic:** Burning, crusting in corner of eye. **Occasional (less than 2%):** Abdominal pain/discomfort, headache, rash. **Ophthalmic:** Bad taste, sensation of foreign body in eye, eyelid redness, itching. **Rare (less than 1%):** Dizziness, confusion, tremors, hallucinations, hypersensitivity reaction, insomnia, dry mouth, paresthesia.

ADVERSE EFFECTS/ TOXIC REACTIONS

Superinfection (esp. enterococcal, fungal), nephropathy, cardiopulmonary arrest, cerebral thrombosis may occur. Hypersensitivity reaction (rash, pruritus, blisters, edema, burning skin), photosensitivity have occurred. Sensitization to ophthalmic form may contraindicate later systemic use of ciprofloxacin.

✦ Canadian trade name   � Non-Crushable Drug   🅷🅸 High Alert drug

NURSING CONSIDERATIONS

BASELINE ASSESSMENT
Question for history of hypersensitivity to ciprofloxacin, quinolones.

INTERVENTION/EVALUATION
Obtain urinalysis for microscopic analysis for crystalluria prior to and during treatment. Evaluate food tolerance. Monitor daily pattern of bowel activity, stool consistency. Encourage hydration (reduces risk of crystalluria). Monitor for dizziness, headache, visual changes, tremors. Assess for chest, joint pain. **Ophthalmic:** Observe therapeutic response.

PATIENT/FAMILY TEACHING
• Do not skip doses; take full course of therapy. • Maintain adequate hydration to prevent crystalluria. • Do not take antacids within 2 hrs of ciprofloxacin (reduces/destroys effectiveness). • Shake suspension well before using; do not chew microcapsules in suspension. • Sugarless gum, hard candy may relieve bad taste. • Avoid caffeine. • Report tendon pain or swelling. • Avoid exposure to sunlight/artificial light (may cause photosensitivity reaction). • Report persistent diarrhea. • **Ophthalmic:** Crystal precipitate may form, usual resolution in 1–7 days.

---

cisplatin

sis-**pla**-tin
(Platinol-AQ)

BLACK BOX ALERT Cumulative renal toxicity may be severe. Dose-related toxicities include myelosuppression, nausea, vomiting. Ototoxicity, especially pronounced in children, noted by tinnitus, loss of high-frequency hearing, deafness. Must be administered by personnel trained in administration/handling of chemotherapeutic agents. Anaphylactic reaction can occur within minutes of administration.

Do not confuse cisplatin with carboplatin or oxaliplatin.

◆CLASSIFICATION
PHARMACOTHERAPEUTIC: Platinum coordination complex. **CLINICAL:** Antineoplastic (see p. 84C).

ACTION
Inhibits DNA and, to a lesser extent, RNA protein synthesis by cross-linking with DNA strands. Cell cycle–phase nonspecific. **Therapeutic Effect:** Prevents cellular division.

PHARMACOKINETICS
Widely distributed. Protein binding: greater than 90%. Undergoes rapid non-enzymatic conversion to inactive metabolite. Excreted in urine. Removed by hemodialysis. **Half-life:** 58–73 hrs (increased in renal impairment).

USES
Treatment of metastatic testicular tumors, metastatic ovarian tumors, advanced bladder carcinoma. **OFF-LABEL:** Breast, cervical, endometrial, esophageal, gastric, head and neck, lung (small-cell, non–small-cell) carcinomas; Hodgkin's and non-Hodgkin's lymphomas; malignant melanoma, neuroblastoma, osteosarcoma, soft tissue sarcoma, Wilms tumor.

PRECAUTIONS
Contraindications: Hearing impairment, myelosuppression, preexisting renal impairment. **Cautions:** Elderly, renal impairment.

⧗ LIFESPAN CONSIDERATIONS
Pregnancy/Lactation: If possible, avoid use during pregnancy, esp. first trimester. Breastfeeding not recommended. **Pregnancy Category D. Children:** Ototoxic effects may be more severe. **Elderly:** Age-related renal impairment may require dosage adjustment.

INTERACTIONS
DRUG: May decrease effects of **anticonvulsant medications. Bone marrow depressants** (e.g., **paclitaxel**) may in-

crease myelosuppression. **Live virus vaccines** may potentiate virus replication, increase vaccine side effects, decrease pt's antibody response to vaccine. **Nephrotoxic, ototoxic agents (e.g., aminoglycosides)** may increase risk of toxicity. HERBAL: Avoid **black cohosh, dong quai** with estrogen-dependent tumors. **Echinacea** may decrease effects. FOOD: None known. LAB VALUES: May increase BUN, serum creatinine, uric acid, AST. May decrease creatinine clearance, serum calcium, magnesium, phosphate, potassium, sodium. May cause positive Coombs' test.

AVAILABILITY (Rx)

Injection Solution: 1 mg/ml (50 ml, 100 ml, 200 ml).

ADMINISTRATION/HANDLING

◄ALERT► Wear protective gloves during handling. May be carcinogenic, mutagenic, teratogenic. Handle with extreme care during preparation/administration.

 IV

Dilution • Dilute desired dose in 250–1,000 ml 0.9% NaCl, D$_5$/0.45% NaCl, or D$_5$/0.9% NaCl to concentration of 0.05–2 mg/ml. Solution should have final NaCl concentration of 0.2% or greater.
Rate of Administration • Infuse over 2–24 hrs (per protocol). • Avoid rapid infusion (increases risk of nephrotoxicity, ototoxicity). • Monitor for anaphylactic reaction during first few minutes of infusion.
Storage • Protect from sunlight. • Do not refrigerate (may precipitate). Discard if precipitate forms. IV infusion: Stable for 72 hrs at 39°F–77°F.

▨ IV INCOMPATIBILITIES

Amphotericin B complex (Abelcet, AmBisome, Amphotec), cefepime (Maxipime), piperacillin and tazobactam (Zosyn), sodium bicarbonate.

▨ IV COMPATIBILITIES

Etoposide (VePesid), granisetron (Kytril), heparin, hydromorphone (Dilaudid), lipids, lorazepam (Ativan), magnesium sulfate, mannitol, morphine, ondansetron (Zofran), palonosetron (Aloxi).

INDICATIONS/ROUTES/DOSAGE

Note: Pretreatment hydration with 1–2 liters of fluid recommended. Adequate hydration, urine output greater than 100 ml/hr should be maintained for 24 hrs after administration.

Bladder Carcinoma
IV: ADULTS, ELDERLY: (Single agent): 50–70 mg/m² q3–4wks.

Ovarian Tumors
IV: ADULTS, ELDERLY: 75–100 mg/m² q3–4wks (combination therapy) or 100 mg/m² q4wks (single agent).

Testicular Tumors
IV: ADULTS, ELDERLY: 20 mg/m² daily for 5 days repeated q3wks.

Dosage in Renal Impairment
Dosage is modified based on creatinine clearance, BUN.
◄ALERT► Repeated courses of cisplatin should not be given until serum creatinine is less than 1.5 mg/100 ml and/or BUN is less than 25 mg/100 ml.

Creatinine Clearance	Dosage
10–50 ml/min	75% of normal dose
Less than 10 ml/min	50% of normal dose
Hemodialysis	50% of dose post dialysis
Peritoneal dialysis	50% of dose
Continuous renal replacement therapy	75% of dose

SIDE EFFECTS

Frequent: Nausea, vomiting (occurs in more than 90% of pts, generally beginning 1–4 hrs after administration and lasting up to 24 hrs); myelosuppression (affecting 25%–30% of pts, with recovery generally occurring in 18–23 days). **Occasional:** Peripheral neuropathy (with prolonged therapy [4–7 mos]).

Pain/redness at injection site, loss of taste, appetite. **Rare:** Hemolytic anemia, blurred vision, stomatitis.

ADVERSE EFFECTS/ TOXIC REACTIONS

Anaphylactic reaction (angioedema, wheezing, tachycardia, hypotension) may occur in first few minutes of administration in pt previously exposed to cisplatin. Nephrotoxicity occurs in 28%–36% of pts treated with a single dose, usually during second wk of therapy. Ototoxicity (tinnitus, hearing loss) occurs in 31% of pts treated with a single dose (more severe in children). Symptoms may become more frequent, severe with repeated doses.

NURSING CONSIDERATIONS

BASELINE ASSESSMENT

Obtain baseline CBC, serum chemistry tests, urinalysis prior to initiation. Pts should be well hydrated before and 24 hrs after medication to ensure adequate urinary output (100 ml/hr), decrease risk of nephrotoxicity.

INTERVENTION/EVALUATION

Measure all emesis, urine output (general guideline requiring immediate notification of physician: 750 ml/8 hrs, urinary output less than 100 ml/hr). Monitor I&O q1–2h beginning with pretreatment hydration, continue for 48 hrs after dose. Assess vital signs q1–2h during infusion. Monitor urinalysis, serum electrolytes, hepatic/renal function tests, CBC, platelet count for changes from baseline.

PATIENT/FAMILY TEACHING

• Report signs of ototoxicity (tinnitus, hearing loss). • Do not have immunizations without physician's approval (lowers body's resistance). • Avoid contact with those who have recently taken oral polio vaccine. • Report if nausea/vomiting continues at home. • Report signs of peripheral neuropathy.

citalopram

sye-**tal**-o-pram
(Apo-Citalopram ✦, Celexa)

BLACK BOX ALERT Increased risk of suicidal thinking and behavior in children, adolescents, young adults 18–24 yrs with major depressive disorder, other psychiatric disorders.

Do not confuse Celexa with Celebrex, Cerebyx, Ranexa, or Zyprexa.

◆CLASSIFICATION

PHARMACOTHERAPEUTIC: Serotonin reuptake inhibitor. **CLINICAL:** Antidepressant (see p. 40C).

ACTION

Blocks uptake of the neurotransmitter serotonin at CNS presynaptic neuronal membranes, increasing its availability at postsynaptic receptor sites. **Therapeutic Effect:** Relieves depression.

PHARMACOKINETICS

Well absorbed after PO administration. Protein binding: 80%. Extensively metabolized in liver. Excreted in urine. **Half-life:** 35 hrs.

USES

Treatment of depression. **OFF-LABEL:** Treatment of alcohol abuse, diabetic neuropathy, obsessive-compulsive disorder, smoking cessation.

PRECAUTIONS

Contraindications: Sensitivity to citalopram, use within 14 days of MAOIs. **Cautions:** Hepatic/renal impairment; history of seizures; during third trimester of pregnancy; elderly; concomitant CNS depression; concomitant use of aspirin, NSAIDs, or warfarin. Not recommended in pts with congenital long QT syndrome, bradycardia, recent MI, uncompensated HF, hypokalemia, or hypomagnesemia.

⌛ LIFESPAN CONSIDERATIONS

Pregnancy/Lactation: Distributed in breast milk. **Pregnancy Category C. Children:** May cause increased anticholinergic effects, hyperexcitability. **Elderly:** More sensitive to anticholinergic effects (e.g., dry mouth), more likely to experience dizziness, sedation, confusion, hypotension, hyperexcitability.

INTERACTIONS

DRUG: **CYP2C19 inhibitors (e.g., fluconazole), other medications prolonging QT** interval may increase risk of QT prolongation. **Linezolid, MAOIs, triptans** may cause serotonin syndrome (excitement, diaphoresis, rigidity, hyperthermia, autonomic hyperactivity, coma). **HERBAL: Gotu kola, kava kava, SAMe, St. John's wort, valerian** may increase CNS depression. **St. John's wort** may increase risk of serotonin syndrome. **FOOD:** None known. **LAB VALUES:** May decrease serum sodium.

AVAILABILITY (Rx)

Oral Solution: 10 mg/5 ml. **Tablets:** 10 mg, 20 mg, 40 mg.

ADMINISTRATION/HANDLING

PO
• Give without regard to food. • Scored tablets may be crushed.

INDICATIONS/ROUTES/DOSAGE

Depression
PO: ADULTS: Initially, 20 mg once a day in the morning or evening. May increase in 20-mg increments at intervals of no less than 1 wk. **Maximum:** 40 mg/day. **ELDERLY, PTS WITH HEPATIC IMPAIRMENT: Poor Metabolizers of CYP2C19, Concurrent CYP2C19 Inhibitors:** 20 mg/day. **Maximum:** 20 mg/day.

SIDE EFFECTS

Frequent (21%–11%): Nausea, dry mouth, drowsiness, insomnia, diaphoresis. **Occasional (8%–4%):** Tremor, diarrhea, abnormal ejaculation, dyspepsia, fatigue, anxiety, vomiting, anorexia. **Rare (3%–2%):** Sinusitis, sexual dysfunction, menstrual disorder, abdominal pain, agitation, decreased libido.

ADVERSE EFFECTS/ TOXIC REACTIONS

Overdose manifested as dizziness, drowsiness, tachycardia, confusion, seizures, Torsades de Pointes, V-tach, sudden death.

NURSING CONSIDERATIONS

BASELINE ASSESSMENT

Hepatic/renal function tests, blood counts should be performed periodically for pts on long-term therapy. Observe, record behavior. Assess psychological status, thought content, sleep pattern, appearance, interest in environment. Screen for bipolar disorder.

INTERVENTION/EVALUATION

Supervise suicidal-risk pt closely during early therapy (as depression lessens, energy level improves, increasing suicide potential). Assess appearance, behavior, speech pattern, level of interest, mood. Screen for bipolar disorder.

PATIENT/FAMILY TEACHING

• Do not stop taking medication or increase dosage. • Avoid alcohol. • Avoid tasks that require alertness, motor skills until response to drug is established. • Report worsening depression, suicidal ideation, unusual changes in behavior.

---

cladribine

klad-ree-bine

BLACK BOX ALERT Must be administered by personnel trained in administration/handling of chemotherapeutic agents. Myelosuppression, neurologic toxicity, acute nephrotoxicity have been reported.
Do not confuse cladribine with clevidipine, clofarabine, or fludarabine, or Leustatin with lovastatin.

◆CLASSIFICATION

PHARMACOTHERAPEUTIC: Antimetabolite. **CLINICAL:** Antineoplastic (see p. 84C).

ACTION

Disrupts cellular metabolism by incorporating into DNA of dividing cells. Cytotoxic to both actively dividing and quiescent lymphocytes, monocytes. **Therapeutic Effect:** Prevents DNA synthesis.

PHARMACOKINETICS

Protein binding: 20%. Metabolized in liver. Primarily excreted in urine. **Half-life:** 5.4 hrs.

USES

Treatment of active hairy cell leukemia defined by clinically significant anemia, neutropenia, thrombocytopenia. **OFF-LABEL:** Treatment of chronic lymphocytic leukemia, non-Hodgkin's lymphoma, acute myeloid leukemia.

PRECAUTIONS

Contraindications: None known. **Cautions:** Renal/hepatic impairment. Preexisting hematologic or immunologic abnormalities; those with high tumor burden.

⧗ LIFESPAN CONSIDERATIONS

Pregnancy/Lactation: May produce fetal harm; may be embryotoxic, fetotoxic; potential for serious reactions in breast-fed infants. **Pregnancy Category D. Children:** Safety and efficacy not established. **Elderly:** No age-related precautions noted.

INTERACTIONS

DRUG: Bone marrow depressants may increase myelosuppression. **Live virus vaccines** may potentiate virus replication, increase vaccine side effects, decrease pt's antibody response to vaccine. **HERBAL: Echinacea** may decrease effects. **FOOD:** None known. **LAB VALUES:** May decrease platelets, Hgb, Hct, neutrophils during initial dose of

therapy. Resolution of anemia, thrombocytopenia, neutropenia indicates disease progression.

AVAILABILITY (Rx)

Injection Solution: 1 mg/ml (10 ml).

ADMINISTRATION/HANDLING

 IV

Reconstitution • Must dilute before administration. • Wear gloves, protective clothing during handling; if contact with skin, rinse with copious amounts of water. • Add calculated dose (0.09 mg/kg) to 500 ml 0.9% NaCl. Avoid D_5W (increases degradation of medication).
Rate of Administration • Infuse over 1–2 hrs.
Storage • Refrigerate unopened vials. • May refrigerate diluted solution for no more than 8 hrs. • Diluted solution is stable for at least 24 hrs at room temperature. • Discard unused portion.

▦ IV INCOMPATIBILITIES

None known.

▦ IV COMPATIBILITIES

Dexamethasone (Decadron), granisetron (Kytril), ondansetron (Zofran).

INDICATIONS/ROUTES/DOSAGE

Hairy Cell Leukemia
IV Infusion: ADULTS, CHILDREN: 0.09–0.1 mg/kg/day as continuous infusion for 7 days. May repeat every 28–35 days.

Dosage in Renal Impairment

	Children	Adults
CrCl 10–50	50% of dose	75% of dose
CrCl less than 10	30% of dose	50% of dose
Hemodialysis	30% of dose	—
Peritoneal dialysis	—	50% of dose
Continuous renal replacement therapy	50% of dose	—

SIDE EFFECTS

Frequent: Fever (69%), fatigue (45%), nausea (28%), rash (27%), headache (22%), injection site reactions (19%), anorexia (17%), vomiting (13%). **Occasional (10%–5%):** Diarrhea, cough, purpura, chills, diaphoresis, constipation, dizziness, petechiae, myalgia, shortness of breath, malaise, pruritus, erythema, insomnia, edema, tachycardia, abdominal/trunk pain, epistaxis, arthralgia.

ADVERSE EFFECTS/ TOXIC REACTIONS

Myelosuppression characterized as severe neutropenia (less than 500 cells/mm^3), severe anemia (Hgb less than 8.5 g/dl), thrombocytopenia occur commonly. High-dose treatment may produce acute nephrotoxicity (increased BUN, serum creatinine levels), neurotoxicity (irreversible motor weakness of upper/lower extremities).

NURSING CONSIDERATIONS

BASELINE ASSESSMENT

Offer emotional support. Perform neurologic exam before chemotherapy. Use strict asepsis; protect pt from infection. Obtain baseline CBC, serum chemistries.

INTERVENTION/EVALUATION

Monitor vital signs during infusion, esp. during first hour. Observe for hypotension, bradycardia (both do not usually occur during same course). Immediately discontinue if severe hypersensitivity reaction occurs. Monitor for and report fever promptly. Assess for signs of infection. Assess skin for evidence of rash, purpura, petechiae. Monitor CBC, serum creatinine, potassium, sodium.

PATIENT/FAMILY TEACHING

• There is a narrow margin between therapeutic and toxic response. • Avoid crowds, persons with known infections; report signs of infection at once (fever, flu-like symptoms). • Do not have immunizations without physician's approval (drug lowers resistance). • Avoid contact with those who have recently received live virus vaccine. • Avoid pregnancy.

---

clarithromycin

kla-**rith**-roe-**mye**-sin
(Apo-Clarithromycin ✦, Biaxin, Biaxin XL, PMS-Clarithromycin ✦)
Do not confuse clarithromycin with Claritin, clindamycin, or erythromycin.

◆ CLASSIFICATION

PHARMACOTHERAPEUTIC: Macrolide.
CLINICAL: Antibiotic (see p. 27C).

ACTION

Binds to ribosomal receptor sites of susceptible organisms, inhibiting protein synthesis of bacterial cell wall. **Therapeutic Effect:** Bacteriostatic; may be bactericidal with high dosages or very susceptible microorganisms.

PHARMACOKINETICS

Well absorbed from GI tract. Protein binding: 65%–75%. Widely distributed (except CNS). Metabolized in liver. Primarily excreted in urine. Not removed by hemodialysis. **Half-life:** 3–7 hrs; metabolite, 5–9 hrs (increased in renal impairment).

USES

Treatment of susceptible infections due to *C. pneumoniae, H. influenzae, H. parainfluenzae, H. pylori, M. catarrhalis, M. avium, M. pneumoniae, S. aureus, S. pneumoniae, S. pyogenes,* including bacterial exacerbation of bronchitis, otitis media, acute maxillary sinusitis, *Mycobacterium avium* complex (MAC), pharyngitis, tonsillitis, *H. pylori* duodenal ulcer, community acquired pneumonia, skin and soft tissue infections. Prevention of MAC disease. **OFF-**

LABEL: Prophylaxis of infective endocarditis, pertussis.

PRECAUTIONS

Contraindications: Hypersensitivity to other macrolide antibiotics. History of QT prolongation or ventricular arrhythmias including torsades de pointes. History of cholestatic jaundice or hepatic impairment with prior clarithromycin use. Concomitant use with colchicine, lovastatin, simvastatin. **Cautions:** Hepatic/renal dysfunction, elderly with severe renal impairment, myasthenia gravis, coronary artery disease. May prolong QT interval (rare).

⧗ LIFESPAN CONSIDERATIONS

Pregnancy/Lactation: Unknown if distributed in breast milk. **Pregnancy Category C. Children:** Safety and efficacy not established in those younger than 6 mos. **Elderly:** Age-related renal impairment may require dosage adjustment.

INTERACTIONS

DRUG: May increase concentration, toxicity of **carbamazepine, colchicine, digoxin, ergotamine, theophylline, sildenafil, tadalafil, vardenafil. Rifabutin, rifampin, atorvastatin, efavirenz** may decrease plasma concentration. May increase **warfarin** effects. May decrease concentration of **zidovudine. Atazanavir, ritonavir** may increase concentration of clarithromycin. **HERBAL: St. John's wort** may decrease plasma concentration. **FOOD:** None known. **LAB VALUES:** May increase BUN, serum AST, ALT, alkaline phosphatase, LDH, serum creatinine, PT. May decrease WBC.

AVAILABILITY (Rx)

Oral Suspension (Biaxin): 125 mg/5 ml, 250 mg/5 ml. **Tablets (Biaxin):** 250 mg, 500 mg.

🔖 Tablets (Extended-Release [Biaxin XL]): 500 mg.

ADMINISTRATION/HANDLING

PO
• Give immediate-release tablets, oral suspension without regard to food. • Extended-release tablets should be given with food. • Do not crush, cut, or divide extended-release tablets. • Give q12h (rather than twice daily). • Shake suspension well before each use.

INDICATIONS/ROUTES/DOSAGE

Usual Dosage Range
PO: ADULTS, ELDERLY: 250–500 mg q12h or 500–1,000 mg once daily (extended-release tablets). **CHILDREN 6 MOS AND OLDER:** 7.5 mg/kg q12h. **Maximum:** 500 mg.

Bronchitis
PO: ADULTS, ELDERLY: 250–500 mg q12h for 7–14 days.
PO *(Extended-Release)*: **ADULTS, ELDERLY:** 1 g once daily for 7 days.

Skin, Soft Tissue Infections
PO: ADULTS, ELDERLY: 250 mg q12h for 7–14 days. **CHILDREN:** 7.5 mg/kg q12h for 10 days. **Maximum:** 1 g/day.

Mycobacterium Avium **Complex (MAC) Prophylaxis**
PO: ADULTS, ELDERLY: 500 mg twice a day. **CHILDREN:** 7.5 mg/kg q12h. **Maximum:** 500 mg twice a day.

Mycobacterium Avium **Complex (MAC) Treatment**
PO: ADULTS, ELDERLY: 500 mg twice a day in combination. **CHILDREN:** 7.5 mg/kg q12h in combination. **Maximum:** 500 mg twice a day.

Pharyngitis, Tonsillitis
PO: ADULTS, ELDERLY: 250 mg q12h for 10 days. **CHILDREN:** 7.5 mg/kg q12h for 10 days. **Maximum:** 1 g/day.

Pneumonia
PO: ADULTS, ELDERLY: 250 mg q12h for 7–14 days. **CHILDREN:** 7.5 mg/kg q12h.
PO *(Extended-Release)*: **ADULTS, ELDERLY:** 1 g/day.

Maxillary Sinusitis
PO: ADULTS, ELDERLY: 500 mg q12h or 1,000 mg (2×500 mg extended-release) once daily for 14 days. **CHILDREN:** 7.5 mg/kg q12h. **Maximum:** 500 mg twice a day.

H. Pylori
PO: ADULTS, ELDERLY: 500 mg q8–12h for 10–14 days in combination.

Acute Otitis Media
PO: CHILDREN: 7.5 mg/kg q12h for 10 days. **Maximum:** 500 mg q12h.

Dosage in Renal Impairment
Creatinine clearance less than 30 ml/min: Reduce dose by 50% and administer once or twice a day. **HD:** Administer dose after dialysis complete.

Combination with atazanavir

CrCl 30–60 ml/min	Decrease dose by 50%
CrCl <30 ml/min	Decrease dose by 75%

SIDE EFFECTS

Occasional (6%–3%): Diarrhea, nausea, altered taste, abdominal pain. **Rare (2%–1%):** Headache, dyspepsia.

ADVERSE EFFECTS/ TOXIC REACTIONS

Antibiotic-associated colitis, other superinfections (abdominal cramps, severe watery diarrhea, fever) may result from altered bacterial balance in GI tract. Hepatotoxicity, thrombocytopenia occur rarely.

NURSING CONSIDERATIONS

BASELINE ASSESSMENT

Question pt for allergies to clarithromycin, erythromycins.

INTERVENTION/EVALUATION

Monitor daily pattern of bowel activity, stool consistency. Mild GI effects may be tolerable, but increasing severity may indicate onset of antibiotic-associated colitis. Be alert for superinfection: fever, vomiting, diarrhea, anal/genital pruritus, oral mucosal changes (ulceration, pain, erythema). Monitor CBC, BUN, serum creatinine.

PATIENT/FAMILY TEACHING

• Continue therapy for full length of treatment. • Doses should be evenly spaced. • Biaxin may be taken without regard to food. Take Biaxin XL with food. • Report severe diarrhea.

C

---

clevidipine

kle-**vid**-i-peen
(Cleviprex)
Do not confuse clevidipine with cladribine or clafarabine, or Cleviprex with Claravis.

◆CLASSIFICATION

PHARMACOTHERAPEUTIC: Short-acting calcium channel blocker. **CLINICAL:** Antihypertensive.

ACTION

Inhibits calcium ion movement across cell membranes, depressing contraction of cardiac, vascular smooth muscle. **Therapeutic Effect:** Decreases systemic vascular resistance, B/P.

PHARMACOKINETICS

Route	Onset	Peak	Duration
IV	2–4 min	—	—

Full recovery to therapeutic B/P reading occurs 5–15 min following termination of infusion. Rapidly distributed and metabolized. Protein binding: 99.5%. Eliminated in urine (74%), feces (22%). **Half-life:** 30 sec–1 min.

USES

Management of hypertension.

PRECAUTIONS

Contraindications: Allergy to soy or eggs, abnormal lipid metabolism, severe aortic stenosis, hypertriglyceremia. **Cautions:**

Heart failure, pts with disorders of lipid metabolism.

⌛ LIFESPAN CONSIDERATIONS

Pregnancy/Lactation: Unknown if distributed in breast milk. **Pregnancy Category C. Children:** Safety and efficacy not established in those younger than 18 yrs. **Elderly:** No age-related precautions noted.

INTERACTIONS

DRUG: Diuretics, other antihypertensives may increase hypotensive effect. **NSAIDs** may decrease antihypertensive effect. **HERBAL: Ephedra, ginger, licorice, ginseng, yohimbe** may worsen hypertension. **Garlic** may increase antihypertensive effect. **FOOD:** None known. **LAB VALUES:** May increase BUN, serum uric acid, potassium, triglycerides.

AVAILABILITY (Rx)

Injection, Emulsion: 0.5 mg/ml as 50-ml vial, 100-ml vial.

ADMINISTRATION/HANDLING
 IV

Reconstitution • Do not dilute.• Both 50-ml and 100-ml vials supplied as concentration of 0.5 mg/ml. • Invert vial gently several times before use to ensure uniformity of emulsion.
Storage • Refrigerate vials but may be held at controlled room temperature (77°F) for 2 mos. • Vial cannot be returned to refrigerator once warmed to room temperature. • Once stopper is punctured, use within 12 hrs; discard unused portion, including that currently being infused. • Discard if discoloration or particulate matter is present.

▓ IV INCOMPATIBILITIES

Do not administer in same IV line as other medications.

▓ IV COMPATIBILITIES

Sterile Water for Injection, 0.9% NaCl, D_5W, lactated Ringer's, 10% amino acid.

INDICATIONS/ROUTES/DOSAGE

◀ALERT▶ Titrate drug to achieve desired B/P reduction. Individualize dosage depending on desired B/P and pt response.

Hypertension
IV: ADULTS, ELDERLY: Initiate IV infusion at 1–2 mg/hr. Dose may be doubled at short (90-sec) intervals initially. As B/P approaches goal, an increase in doses should be less than double, and time between dose adjustments lengthened to every 5–10 min. Maintenance: Desired therapeutic response generally occurs at doses of 4–6 mg/hr. (Pts with severe hypertension may require doses up to 32 mg/hr.) **Maximum:** 16 mg/hr; no more than 21 mg/hr is recommended per 24-hr period.

SIDE EFFECTS

Generally well tolerated. **Occasional (6%–3%):** Headache, nausea, vomiting. **Rare (less than 1%):** Syncope, dyspnea.

ADVERSE EFFECTS/ TOXIC REACTIONS

Hypotension, atrial fibrillation, reflex tachycardia may occur with large doses. May exacerbate heart failure. Acute renal failure has occurred rarely.

NURSING CONSIDERATIONS

BASELINE ASSESSMENT
Assess baseline renal/hepatic function tests. Assess B/P, apical pulse immediately before drug administration.

INTERVENTION/EVALUATION
Monitor B/P, pulse rate continuously during IV infusion. Monitor cardiac pts diligently. Pts who receive prolonged IV infusion and are not changed to other antihypertensive therapy should be monitored for rebound hypertension for at least 8 hrs after infusion is stopped.

clindamycin

klin-da-**mye**-sin
(Apo-Clindamycin ✤, Cleocin,
Cleocin Pediatric, Cleocin T, Cleocin
Vaginal, Clindagel, Clindamax,
Clindesse, Novo-Clindamycin ✤)

BLACK BOX ALERT May cause severe, potentially fatal colitis characterized by severe, persistent diarrhea, severe abdominal cramps, passage of blood and mucus.

Do not confuse Cleocin with Clinoril or Cubicin, or clindamycin with clarithromycin, Claritin, or vancomycin.

◆ CLASSIFICATION

PHARMACOTHERAPEUTIC: Lincosamide. **CLINICAL:** Antibiotic.

ACTION

Inhibits protein synthesis of bacterial cell wall by binding to bacterial ribosomal receptor sites. Topically, decreases fatty acid concentration on skin. **Therapeutic Effect:** Bacteriostatic. Prevents outbreaks of acne vulgaris.

PHARMACOKINETICS

Rapidly absorbed from GI tract. Protein binding: 92%–94%. Widely distributed. Metabolized in liver. Primarily excreted in urine. Not removed by hemodialysis. **Half-life:** 1.6–5.3 hrs (increased in renal impairment, premature infants).

USES

Systemic: Treatment of aerobic gram-positive staphylococci and streptococci (not enterococci), *Fusobacterium, Bacteroides* spp., and *Actinomyces* for treatment of respiratory tract infections, skin/soft tissue infections, sepsis, intra-abdominal infections, infections of female pelvis and genital tract, bacterial endocarditis prophylaxis for dental and upper respiratory procedures in penicillin-allergic pts, perioperative prophylaxis. **Topical:** Treatment of acne vulgaris. **Intravaginal:** Treatment of bacterial vaginosis. **OFF-LABEL:** Treatment of actinomycosis, babesiosis, erysipelas, malaria, otitis media, *Pneumocystis jiroveci* pneumonia (PCP), sinusitis, toxoplasmosis. **PO:** Bacterial vaginosis.

PRECAUTIONS

Contraindications: None known. **Cautions:** Severe hepatic dysfunction; history of GI disease.

⌛ LIFESPAN CONSIDERATIONS

Pregnancy/Lactation: Readily crosses placenta. Distributed in breast milk. **Topical/vaginal:** Unknown if distributed in breast milk. **Pregnancy Category B. Children:** Caution in pt younger than 1 mo. **Elderly:** No age-related precautions noted.

INTERACTIONS

DRUG: Adsorbent antidiarrheals may delay absorption. **Erythromycin** may increase effects. May increase effects of **neuromuscular blockers. HERBAL: St. John's wort** may decrease concentration/effects. **FOOD:** None known. **LAB VALUES:** May increase serum alkaline phosphatase, AST, ALT.

AVAILABILITY (Rx)

Capsules: 75 mg, 150 mg, 300 mg. **Cream, Vaginal (Cleocin, Clindesse):** 2%. **Gel, Topical (Cleocin T, Clindagel, Clindamax):** 1%. **Infusion, Premix (Cleocin):** 300 mg/50 ml, 600 mg/50 ml, 900 mg/50 ml. **Injection Solution (Cleocin):** 150 mg/ml. **Lotion (Cleocin T, Clindamax):** 1%. **Oral Solution (Cleocin Pediatric):** 75 mg/5 ml. **Suppositories, Vaginal (Cleocin):** 100 mg. **Swabs, Topical (Cleocin T):** 1%.

ADMINISTRATION/HANDLING

🖱 IV

Reconstitution • Dilute 300–600 mg with 50 ml D₅W or 0.9% NaCl (900–1,200 mg with 100 ml). • Never exceed concentration of 18 mg/ml.

Rate of Administration • Infuse over at least 10–60 min at rate not exceeding 30 mg/min. Severe hypotension, cardiac arrest can occur with rapid administration. • No more than 1.2 g should be given in a single infusion.

Storage • Reconstituted IV infusion (piggyback) is stable for 16 days at room temperature, 32 days if refrigerated.

IM

• Do not exceed 600 mg/dose. • Administer deep IM.

PO

• Store capsules at room temperature. • After reconstitution, oral solution is stable for 2 wks at room temperature. • Do not refrigerate oral solution (avoids thickening). • Give with at least 8 oz water (minimizes esophageal ulceration). • Give without regard to food.

Topical

• Wash skin, allow to completely dry before application. • Shake topical lotion well before each use. • Apply liquid, solution, or gel in thin film to affected area. • Avoid contact with eyes or abraded areas.

Vaginal, Cream or Suppository

• Use one applicatorful or suppository at bedtime. • Fill applicator that comes with cream or suppository to indicated level. • Instruct pt to lie on back with knees drawn upward and spread apart. • Insert applicator into vagina and push plunger to release medication. • Withdraw, wash applicator with soap and warm water. • Wash hands promptly to avoid spreading infection.

▨ IV INCOMPATIBILITIES

Allopurinol (Aloprim), fluconazole (Diflucan).

▨ IV COMPATIBILITIES

Amiodarone (Cordarone), diltiazem (Cardizem), heparin, hydromorphone (Dilaudid), magnesium sulfate, mid-azolam (Versed), morphine, multivitamins, propofol (Diprivan).

INDICATIONS/ROUTES/DOSAGE

Usual Dosage

IV, IM: ADULTS, ELDERLY: 1.2–2.7 g/day in 2–4 divided doses. **Maximum:** 4.8 g/day. **CHILDREN 1 MO–16 YRS:** 20–40 mg/kg/day in 3–4 divided doses. **Maximum:** 2,700 mg. **CHILDREN YOUNGER THAN 1 MO:** 5 mg/kg/dose q6–12h.

PO: ADULTS, ELDERLY: 150–450 mg q6h. **Maximum:** 1.8 g/day. **CHILDREN 1 MO–16 YRS:** 10–40 mg/kg/day in divided doses q6–8h. **CHILDREN YOUNGER THAN 1 MO:** 5 mg/kg/dose q6–12h.

Bacterial Vaginosis

Intravaginal *(Cream)*: **ADULTS:** One applicatorful at bedtime for 3–7 days or 1 suppository at bedtime for 3 days. *(Clindesse)*: **ADULTS:** One applicatorful once daily.

Acne Vulgaris

Topical: ADULTS: Apply thin layer to affected area twice a day.

SIDE EFFECTS

Frequent: Systemic: Abdominal pain, nausea, vomiting, diarrhea. **Topical:** Dry, scaly skin. **Vaginal:** Vaginitis, pruritus. **Occasional: Systemic:** Phlebitis, pain, induration at IM injection site, allergic reaction, urticaria, pruritus. **Topical:** Contact dermatitis, abdominal pain, mild diarrhea, burning, stinging. **Vaginal:** Headache, dizziness, nausea, vomiting, abdominal pain. **Rare: Vaginal:** Hypersensitivity reaction.

ADVERSE EFFECTS/ TOXIC REACTIONS

Antibiotic-associated colitis, other superinfections (abdominal cramps, severe watery diarrhea, fever) may occur during and several wks after clindamycin therapy (including topical form). Blood dyscrasias (leukopenia, thrombocytopenia), nephrotoxicity (proteinuria, azotemia, oliguria) occur rarely. Thrombophlebitis with IV administration.

NURSING CONSIDERATIONS

BASELINE ASSESSMENT

Question pt for history of allergies. Avoid, if possible, concurrent use of neuromuscular blocking agents. Obtain baseline WBC.

INTERVENTION/EVALUATION

Monitor daily pattern of bowel activity, stool consistency. Report diarrhea promptly due to potential for serious colitis (even with topical or vaginal administration). Assess skin for rash (dryness, irritation) with topical application. With all routes of administration, be alert for superinfection: fever, vomiting, diarrhea, anal/genital pruritus, oral mucosal changes (ulceration, pain, erythema).

PATIENT/FAMILY TEACHING

• Continue therapy for full length of treatment. • Doses should be evenly spaced. • Take oral doses with at least 8 oz water. • Use caution when applying topical clindamycin concurrently with peeling or abrasive acne agents, soaps, alcohol-containing cosmetics to avoid cumulative effect. • Do not apply topical preparations near eyes, abraded areas. • Report severe persistent diarrhea, cramps, bloody stool. • **Vaginal:** In event of accidental contact with eyes, rinse with large amounts of cool tap water. • Do not engage in sexual intercourse during treatment. • Wear sanitary napkin to protect clothes against stains. Tampons should not be used.

clobazam

kloe-**ba**-zam
(Onfi)
Do not confuse clobazam with clonazepam or clozapine.

◆CLASSIFICATION

PHARMACOTHERAPEUTIC: Benzodiazepine **(Schedule IV). CLINICAL:** Anticonvulsant.

ACTION

Potentiates neurotransmission of gamma-aminobutyric acid (GABA) by binding to GABA receptor. Depresses nerve impulse transmission in motor cortex. **Therapeutic Effect:** Decreases seizure activity.

PHARMOCOKINETICS

Rapidly absorbed after PO administration. Peak plasma concentration: 0.5–4 hrs. Protein binding: 80–90%. Metabolized in liver. Primarily excreted in urine. Unknown if removed by dialysis. **Half-life:** 36–42 hrs.

USES

Adjunctive treatment of seizures associated with Lennox-Gastaut syndrome in pts 2 yrs of age and older. **OFF-LABEL:** Catamenial epilepsy; epilepsy (monotherapy).

PRECAUTIONS

Contraindications: None known. **Cautions:** Elderly, debilitated, mild to moderate hepatic impairment, preexisting muscle weakness or ataxia, concomitant CNS depressants, impaired gag reflex, respiratory disease, sleep apnea, CYP2C19 poor metabolizers, pts at risk for falls, myasthenia gravis, narrow-angle glaucoma.

⊠ LIFESPAN CONSIDERATIONS

Pregnancy/Lactation: Excreted in breast milk. **Hormonal contraceptives** may have decreased effectiveness. Nonhormonal contraception recommended. **Pregnancy Category C. Children:** Safety and efficacy not established in pts younger than 2 yrs. **Elderly:** May have decreased clearance levels (initial dose 5 mg/day).

INTERACTIONS

DRUG: CYP2C19 inhibitors (e.g., fluconazole, fluvoxamine, omeprazole, ticlopidine) may increase concentration/effects. **Alcohol, other CNS depressants** may increase CNS depression. May decrease effect of **hormonal contraceptives.** HERBAL: Gotu kola, kava kava, St. John's wort, valerian may increase CNS depression. **St. John's wort** may decrease effects. **FOOD:** None known. **LAB VALUES:** None significant.

AVAILABILITY (Rx)

Tablets: 5 mg, 10 mg, 20 mg.

ADMINISTRATION/HANDLING

- May give without regard to food.
- Tablets may be crushed and mixed with applesauce.

INDICATIONS/ROUTES/DOSAGE

Seizure Control (Lennox-Gastaut Syndrome)
PO: ADULTS, CHILDREN WEIGHING 30 KG OR LESS: Initially, 5 mg once daily. Increase to 5 mg twice daily on day 7, then increase to 10 mg twice daily on day 14. **Maximum:** 20 mg/day. **ADULTS, CHILDREN WEIGHING MORE THAN 30 KG:** Initially, 10 mg once daily. Increase to 10 mg twice daily on day 7, then increase to 20 mg twice daily on day 14. **Maximum:** 40 mg/day.
PO: ELDERLY/HEPATIC IMPAIRMENT: Initially, 5 mg once daily. Increase at weekly increments by 5–10 mg/day based on tolerability. **Maximum:** 20 mg/day or 40 mg/day based on weight group. **Discontinuation:** Gradually taper by 5–10 mg/day on weekly basis.

SIDE EFFECTS

Frequent (26%–10%): Sleepiness, URI, lethargy. **Occasional (9%–5%):** Drooling, nausea, vomiting, constipation, irritability, ataxia, insomnia, cough, fatigue. **Rare (4%–2%):** Psychomotor hyperactivity, UTI, decreased/increased appetite, dysarthria, pyrexia, dysphagia, bronchitis.

ADVERSE EFFECTS/ TOXIC REACTIONS

May increase risk of suicidal behavior/ ideation (less than 1%). Physical dependence can increase with higher doses or concomitant alcohol/drug abuse. Abrupt benzodiazepine withdrawal may present as profuse sweating, cramping, nausea, vomiting, muscle pain, convulsions, psychosis, hallucinations, aggression, tremor, anxiety, insomnia. Overdose may result in confusion, lethargy, diminished reflexes, respiratory depression, coma. **Antidote:** Flumazenil (see Appendix K for dosage). Decreased mobility may potentiate higher risk of pneumonia.

NURSING CONSIDERATIONS

BASELINE ASSESSMENT

Offer emotional support. Review history of seizure disorder (frequency, duration, intensity, level of consciousness [LOC]). Question history of alcohol use. Obtain baseline vital signs. Assess history of depression/suicidal ideation.

INTERVENTION/EVALUATION

Observe for excess sedation, respiratory depression, suicidal ideation. Implement seizure precautions, observe frequently for seizure activity. Assist with ambulation if drowsiness, dizziness occurs. Evaluate for therapeutic response. Encourage turning, coughing, deep breathing for pts with decreased mobility or who are bedridden.

PATIENT/FAMILY TEACHING

- Avoid tasks that require alertness, motor skills until response to drug is established. • Do not abruptly discontinue medication. • If tapering, monitor for drug withdrawal symptoms. • Avoid alcohol. • Report depression, aggression, thoughts of suicide/self-harm, excessive drowsiness.

clofarabine

kloe-**far**-a-been
(Clolar)
Do not confuse clofarabine with cladribine or clevidipine.

◆CLASSIFICATION

PHARMACOTHERAPEUTIC: Antimetabolite. **CLINICAL:** Antineoplastic.

ACTION

Metabolized intracellularly to ribonucleotide reductase. Alters mitochondrial membrane necessary in DNA synthesis. **Therapeutic Effect:** Decreases cell replication, inhibits cell repair. Produces cell death.

PHARMACOKINETICS

Protein binding: 47%. Metabolized intracellularly. Primarily excreted in urine (40%–60% unchanged). **Half-life:** 5.2 hrs.

USES

Treatment of pediatric pts (1–21 yrs) with relapsed or refractory acute lymphoblastic leukemia (ALL) after at least 2 prior regimens. **OFF-LABEL:** Acute myeloid leukemia (AML) in adults 60 yrs or older.

PRECAUTIONS

Contraindications: None known. **Cautions:** Dehydration, hypotension, concomitant nephrotoxic or hepatotoxic medications, renal/hepatic impairment.

⏳ LIFESPAN CONSIDERATIONS

Pregnancy/Lactation: May cause fetal harm. Breastfeeding not recommended. **Pregnancy Category D. Children:** Safety and efficacy not established in pts younger than 1 yr. **Elderly:** No age-related precautions noted.

INTERACTIONS

DRUG: Hepatotoxic, nephrotoxic medications may increase risk of hepatic/renal toxicity. **HERBAL: Echinacea** may decrease effects. **FOOD:** None known. **LAB VALUES:** May increase serum creatinine, uric acid, AST, ALT, bilirubin.

AVAILABILITY (Rx)

Injection, Solution: 1 mg/ml (20-ml vial).

ADMINISTRATION/HANDLING

 IV

Reconstitution • Filter clofarabine through sterile, 0.2-micrometer syringe filter prior to dilution with D_5W or 0.9% NaCl to final concentration of 0.15–0.4 mg/ml.
Rate of Administration • Administer over 2 hrs. • Continuously infuse IV fluids to decrease risk of tumor lysis syndrome, other adverse events.
Storage • Store undiluted or diluted solution at room temperature. • Use diluted solution within 24 hrs.

🖳 IV INCOMPATIBILITIES

Do not administer any other medication through same IV line.

INDICATIONS/ROUTES/DOSAGE

Acute Lymphoblastic Leukemia (ALL)
IV: CHILDREN 1–21 YRS: 52 mg/m² over 2 hrs once daily for 5 consecutive days; repeat q2–6wks following recovery or return to baseline organ function. (Subsequent cycles should begin no sooner than 14 days from day 1 of previous cycle.)

SIDE EFFECTS

Frequent: Vomiting (83%); nausea (75%); diarrhea (53%); pruritus (47%); headache (46%); fever, dermatitis (41%); rigors (38%); abdominal pain, fatigue (36%); tachycardia (34%); epistaxis (31%); anorexia (30%); petechiae, limb pain, hypotension (29%); anxiety (22%); constipation (21%); edema (20%). **Occasional:** Cough (19%); mucosal inflammation, erythema, flushing (18%); hematuria (17%); dizziness (16%); gingival bleeding (15%); injection site pain, respiratory distress, pharyngitis (14%); back pain, palmar-plantar erythrodysesthesia syndrome, myalgia, oral candidiasis (13%); hypertension, depression, irritability, arthralgia, anorexia (11%). **Rare (10%):** Tremor, weight gain, drowsiness.

ADVERSE EFFECTS/ TOXIC REACTIONS

Neutropenia occurs in 57% of pts; pericardial effusion in 35%; left ventricular systolic dysfunction in 27%; hepatomegaly, jaundice in 15%; pleural effusion, pneumonia, bacteremia in 10%; capillary leak syndrome in less than 10%.

NURSING CONSIDERATIONS

BASELINE ASSESSMENT

Question possibility of pregnancy. Obtain CBC, BUN, serum creatinine, AST, ALT, bilirubin, creatinine clearance levels prior to therapy.

INTERVENTION/EVALUATION

Monitor B/P, hepatic/renal function tests, cardiac function, respiratory status, CBC, platelets, uric acid. Monitor daily pattern of bowel activity, stool consistency. Assess for GI disturbances. Assess skin for pruritus, dermatitis, petechiae, erythema on palms of hands and soles of feet. Assess for fever, sore throat; obtain blood cultures to detect evidence of infection. Ensure adequate hydration.

PATIENT/FAMILY TEACHING

• Do not have immunizations without physician's approval (drug lowers resistance). • Avoid contact with anyone who recently received a live virus vaccine. • Avoid crowds, those with infection. • Avoid pregnancy; pts of childbearing potential should use effective contraception. • Maintain strict oral hygiene and frequent handwashing. • Report fever, respiratory distress, prolonged nausea, vomiting, diarrhea, easy bruising.

---

*clomiPRAMINE

kloe-**mip**-rah-meen
(Anafranil, Apo-Clomipramine ✦, Novo-Clomipramine ✦)

BLACK BOX ALERT Increased risk of suicidal ideation and behavior in children, adolescents, young adults 18–24 yrs with major depressive disorder, other psychiatric disorders.

Do not confuse Anafranil with enalapril, or clomipramine with chlorpromazine, clevidipine, clomiphene, or desipramine.

◆CLASSIFICATION

PHARMACOTHERAPEUTIC: Tricyclic. **CLINICAL:** Antidepressant (see p. 39C).

ACTION

Blocks reuptake of neurotransmitters (norepinephrine, serotonin) at CNS presynaptic membranes, increasing availability at postsynaptic receptor sites. **Therapeutic Effect:** Reduces obsessive-compulsive behavior.

PHARMACOKINETICS

Rapidly absorbed. Metabolized in liver. Eliminated in urine (51%–60%), feces (24%–32%). **Half-life:** 20–30 hrs.

USES

Treatment of obsessive-compulsive disorder manifested as repetitive tasks producing marked distress, time-consuming, or significant interference with social or occupational behavior. **OFF-LABEL:** Chronic pain, depression, panic attacks.

PRECAUTIONS

Contraindications: Acute recovery period after MI, use within 14 days of MAOIs. **Cautions:** Pts at high risk for suicide, prostatic hypertrophy, history of urinary retention/obstruction, narrow-angle glaucoma, seizures, hepatic/renal disease, alcoholism, xerostomia, visual problems, elderly, constipation, history of bowel obstruction.

⊠ LIFESPAN CONSIDERATIONS

Pregnancy/Lactation: Distributed in breast milk. **Pregnancy Category D. Children:** Increased risk of suicidal ideation, behavior noted in children, adolescents. Safety and effectiveness in those younger than 10 yrs not established. **Elderly:** No age-related precautions noted.

---

* "Tall Man" lettering   underlined – top prescribed drug

INTERACTIONS

DRUG: Alcohol, other CNS depressants may increase CNS, respiratory depression, hypotensive effects. **Cimetidine, haloperidol** may increase concentration, risk of toxicity. May decrease effects of **clonidine. Phenobarbital** may decrease concentration, antidepressant effects. **MAOIs** may increase risk of neuroleptic malignant syndrome, seizures, hyperpyresis, hypertensive crisis. **Phenothiazines** may increase anticholinergic, sedative effects. **Sympathomimetics** may increase the risk of cardiac effects. **HERBAL: Gota kola, kava kava, SAMe, St. John's wort, valerian** may increase CNS depression. **FOOD: Grapefruit, grapefruit juice** may increase concentration, toxicity. **LAB VALUES:** May alter serum glucose, ECG readings.

AVAILABILITY (Rx)

Capsules: 25 mg, 50 mg, 75 mg.

ADMINISTRATION/HANDLING

PO
• May give with food to decrease risk of GI disturbance. • Recommend bedtime administration.

INDICATIONS/ROUTES/DOSAGE

Obsessive-Compulsive Disorder (OCD)
PO: ADULTS, ELDERLY: Initially, 25 mg/day. May gradually increase to 100 mg/day in the first 2 wks. **Maximum:** 250 mg/day. **CHILDREN 10 YRS AND OLDER:** Initially, 25 mg/day. May gradually increase up to maximum of 3 mg/kg/day or 200 mg, whichever is lowest.

SIDE EFFECTS

Frequent (30%–15%): Ejaculatory failure, dry mouth, somnolence, tremors, dizziness, headache, constipation, fatigue, nausea. **Occasional (14%–5%):** Impotence, diaphoresis, dyspepsia, sexual dysfunction, dysmenorrhea, nervousness, weight gain, pharyngitis. **Rare (less than 5%):** Diarrhea, myalgia, rhinitis, increased appetite, paresthesia, memory impairment, anxiety, rash, pruritus, anorexia, abdominal pain, vomiting, flatulence, flushing, UTI, back pain.

ADVERSE EFFECTS/TOXIC REACTIONS

Overdose may produce seizures, cardiovascular effects (severe orthostatic hypotension, dizziness, tachycardia, palpitations, arrhythmias), altered temperature regulation (hyperpyrexia, hypothermia). Abrupt discontinuation after prolonged therapy may produce headache, malaise, nausea, vomiting, vivid dreams. Anemia, agranulocytosis have been noted.

NURSING CONSIDERATIONS

BASELINE ASSESSMENT

Assess psychological status, thought content, level of interest, mood, behavior, suicidal ideation.

INTERVENTION/EVALUATION

Supervise suicidal-risk pt closely during early therapy (as depression lessens, energy level improves, increasing suicide potential). Assess appearance, behavior, speech pattern, level of interest, mood.

PATIENT/FAMILY TEACHING

• May cause dry mouth, constipation, blurred vision. • Tolerance to postural hypotension, sedative, anticholinergic effects usually develop during early therapy. • Maximum therapeutic effect may be noted in 2–4 wks. • Do not abruptly discontinue medication. • Avoid tasks that require alertness, motor skills until response to drug is established. • Daily dose may be given at bedtime to minimize daytime sedation. • Avoid alcohol. • Report worsening depression, suicidal ideation, change in behavior.

---

clonazepam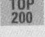

kloe-**naz**-e-pam

 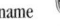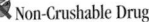 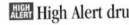

C

(Apo-Clonazepam ✤, Clonapam ✤, Klonopin, Novo-Clonazepam ✤, Rivotril ✤)

Do not confuse clonazepam or Klonopin with clobazam, clonidine, clozapine, or lorazepam.

◆CLASSIFICATION

PHARMACOTHERAPEUTIC: Benzodiazepine **(Schedule IV). CLINICAL:** Anticonvulsant, antianxiety (see p. 35C).

ACTION

Depresses all levels of CNS; depresses nerve impulse transmission in motor cortex. Suppresses abnormal discharge in petit mal seizures. **Therapeutic Effect:** Produces anxiolytic, anticonvulsant effects.

PHARMACOKINETICS

Route	Onset	Peak	Duration
PO	20–60 min	—	12 hrs or less

Well absorbed from GI tract. Protein binding: 85%. Metabolized in liver. Excreted in urine. Not removed by hemodialysis. **Half-life:** 18–50 hrs.

USES

Adjunct in treatment of Lennox-Gastaut syndrome (petit mal variant epilepsy); akinetic, myoclonic seizures; absence seizures (petit mal). Treatment of panic disorder. **OFF-LABEL:** Restless legs syndrome, neuralgia, multifocal tic disorder, parkinsonian dysarthria, bipolar disorder, adjunct therapy for schizophrenia, stomatitis.

PRECAUTIONS

Contraindications: Narrow-angle glaucoma, severe hepatic disease, pregnancy. **Cautions:** Renal/hepatic impairment, impaired gag reflex, chronic respiratory disease, elderly, debilitated pts, depres-

sion, those at suicidal risk, or drug dependence.

⌛ LIFESPAN CONSIDERATIONS

Pregnancy/Lactation: Crosses placenta. May be distributed in breast milk. Chronic ingestion during pregnancy may produce withdrawal symptoms, CNS depression in neonates. **Pregnancy Category D. Children:** Long-term use may adversely affect physical/mental development. **Elderly:** Usually more sensitive to CNS effects (e.g., ataxia, dizziness, oversedation). Use low dosage, increase gradually.

INTERACTIONS

DRUG: Alcohol, other CNS depressants may increase CNS depressant effect. **CYP3A4 inhibitors (e.g., azole antifungals)** may increase concentration, toxicity. **HERBAL: Gotu kola, kava kava, SAMe, St. John's wort, valerian** may increase CNS depression. **St. John's wort** may decrease concentration/effects. **FOOD:** None known. **LAB VALUES:** None significant.

AVAILABILITY (Rx)

Tablets (Klonopin): 0.5 mg, 1 mg, 2 mg. **Tablets (Orally Disintegrating):** 0.125 mg, 0.25 mg, 0.5 mg, 1 mg, 2 mg.

ADMINISTRATION/HANDLING

PO
• Give without regard to food. • Tablets may be crushed.

Orally Disintegrating Tablet
• Open pouch, peel back foil; do not push tablet through foil. • Remove tablet with dry hands, place in mouth. • Swallow with or without water. • Use immediately after removing from package.

INDICATIONS/ROUTES/DOSAGE

Seizures
PO: ADULTS, ELDERLY, CHILDREN 10 YRS AND OLDER: Initial dose not to exceed 1.5 mg/day in 3 divided doses; may be in-

creased in 0.5- to 1-mg increments every 3 days until seizures are controlled or adverse effects occur. **Maintenance:** 0.05–0.2 mg/kg/day. **Maximum:** 20 mg/day. **INFANTS, CHILDREN YOUNGER THAN 10 YRS OR WEIGHING LESS THAN 30 KG:** 0.01–0.03 mg/kg/day in 2–3 divided doses; may be increased by no more than 0.5 mg every 3 days until seizures are controlled or adverse effects occur. Do not exceed maintenance dosage of 0.2 mg/kg/day in 3 divided doses.

Panic Disorder
PO: **ADULTS, ELDERLY:** Initially, 0.25 mg twice a day. Increase in increments of 0.125–0.25 mg twice a day every 3 days. **Target dose:** 1 mg/day. **Maximum:** 4 mg/day.

SIDE EFFECTS

Frequent (37%–11%): Mild, transient drowsiness; ataxia; behavioral disturbances (aggression, irritability, agitation), esp. in children. **Occasional (10%–5%):** Dizziness, ataxia, URI, fatigue. **Rare (4% or less):** Impaired memory, dysarthria, nervousness, sinusitis, rhinitis, constipation, allergic reaction.

ADVERSE EFFECTS/ TOXIC REACTIONS

Abrupt withdrawal may result in pronounced restlessness, irritability, insomnia, hand tremors, abdominal/muscle cramps, diaphoresis, vomiting, status epilepticus. Overdose results in drowsiness, confusion, diminished reflexes, coma. **Antidote:** Flumazenil (see Appendix K for dosage).

NURSING CONSIDERATIONS

BASELINE ASSESSMENT
Review history of seizure disorder (frequency, duration, intensity, level of consciousness [LOC]). For panic attack, assess motor responses (agitation, trembling, tension), autonomic responses (cold/clammy hands, diaphoresis).

INTERVENTION/EVALUATION
Observe for excess sedation, respiratory depression, suicidal ideation. Assess children, elderly for paradoxical reaction, particularly during early therapy. Initiate seizure precautions, observe frequently for recurrence of seizure activity. Assist with ambulation if drowsiness, ataxia occur. For pts on long-term therapy, hepatic/renal function tests, blood counts should be performed periodically. Evaluate for therapeutic response: decreased intensity and frequency of seizures or, if used in panic attack, calm facial expression, decreased restlessness.

PATIENT/FAMILY TEACHING
• Avoid tasks that require alertness, motor skills until response to drug is established. • Do not abruptly discontinue medication after long-term therapy. • Strict maintenance of drug therapy is essential for seizure control. • Avoid alcohol. • Report depression, thoughts of suicide/self-harm, excessive drowsiness, GI symptoms, worsening or loss of seizure control.

clonidine

klon-i-deen
(Apo-Clonidine ✤, Catapres, Catapres-TTS, Dixarit ✤, Duraclon, Kapvay, Nexiclon XR, Novo-Clonidine ✤)
BLACK BOX ALERT Epidural: Not to be used for perioperative, obstetric, or postpartum pain.
Do not confuse Catapres with Cataflam, or clonidine with clomiphene, clorazepam, Klonopin, or quinidine.

◆CLASSIFICATION
PHARMACOTHERAPEUTIC: Antiadrenergic, sympatholytic. **CLINICAL:** Antihypertensive (see pp. 61C, 153C).

ACTION

Stimulates alpha-adrenergic receptors, reducing sympathetic CNS response. **Epidural:** Prevents pain signal transmission to brain and produces analgesia at pre- and post-alpha-adrenergic receptors in spinal cord. **Therapeutic Effect:** Reduces peripheral resistance; decreases B/P, heart rate. Produces analgesia.

PHARMACOKINETICS

Route	Onset	Peak	Duration
PO	0.5–1 hr	2–4 hrs	6–10 hrs

Well absorbed from GI tract. Transdermal best absorbed from chest and upper arm; least absorbed from thigh. Protein binding: 20%–40%. Metabolized in liver. Primarily excreted in urine. Minimally removed by hemodialysis. **Half-life:** 6–20 hrs (increased in renal impairment).

USES

Immediate Release: Nexiclon XR: Treatment of hypertension alone or in combination with other antihypertensive agents. **Kapvay:** Treatment of attention-deficit hyperactivity disorder (ADHD). **Epidural:** Combined with opiates for relief of severe pain. **OFF-LABEL:** Opioid or nicotine withdrawal, prevention of migraine headaches, treatment of diarrhea in diabetes mellitus, treatment of dysmenorrhea, menopausal flushing, alcohol dependence, glaucoma, clozapine-induced sialorrhea, Tourette's syndrome, insomnia in children.

PRECAUTIONS

Contraindications: Epidural: Contraindicated in pts with bleeding diathesis or infection at the injection site, those receiving anticoagulation therapy. **Cautions:** Severe coronary insufficiency; recent MI; cerebrovascular disease; chronic renal failure; pre-existing bradycardia; sinus node dysfunction; conduction disturbances; concurrent use with digoxin, diltiazem, metoprolol, verapamil; depression.

⧖ LIFESPAN CONSIDERATIONS

Pregnancy/Lactation: Crosses placenta. Distributed in breast milk. **Pregnancy Category C. Children:** More sensitive to effects; use caution. **Elderly:** May be more sensitive to hypotensive effect. Age-related renal impairment may require dosage adjustment.

INTERACTIONS

DRUG: Discontinuation of concurrent **beta-blocker** therapy may increase risk of clonidine-withdrawal hypertensive crisis. **Tricyclic antidepressants** may decrease effect (may require increased dose of clonidine). **Digoxin, diltiazem, metoprolol, verapamil** may increase risk of serious bradycardia. **HERBAL: Gotu kola, kava kava, SAMe, St. John's wort, valerian** may increase CNS depression. **Ephedra, ginseng, yohimbe** may decrease antihypertensive effects. **FOOD:** None known. **LAB VALUES:** None significant.

AVAILABILITY (Rx)

Injection Solution (Duraclon): 100 mcg/ml, 500 mcg/ml. **Tablets (Catapres):** 0.1 mg, 0.2 mg, 0.3 mg. **Transdermal Patch (Catapres-TTS):** 2.5 mg (release at 0.1 mg/24 hrs), 5 mg (release at 0.2 mg/24 hrs), 7.5 mg (release at 0.3 mg/24 hrs).

🍃 **Extended-Release Oral Suspension (Nexiclon XR):** 0.09 mg/ml. 🍃 **Extended-Release Tablets: (Kapvay):** 0.1 mg. **(Nexiclon XR):** 0.17 mg.

ADMINISTRATION/HANDLING

PO

• Give without regard to food. • Tablets may be crushed. • Give last oral dose just before bedtime. • Swallow extended-release tablets whole; do not crush, cut, or break.

Transdermal

• Apply transdermal system to dry, hairless area of intact skin on upper arm or chest. • Rotate sites (prevents skin irritation). • Do not trim patch to adjust dose.

Epidural
• Must be administered only by medical personnel trained in epidural management.

⚅ IV INCOMPATIBILITIES
None known.

⚅ IV COMPATIBILITIES
Bupivacaine (Marcaine, Sensorcaine), fentanyl (Sublimaze), heparin, ketamine (Ketalar), lidocaine, lorazepam (Ativan).

INDICATIONS/ROUTES/DOSAGE
Hypertension
PO: ADULTS: Initially, 0.1 mg twice a day. Increase by 0.1–0.2 mg q2–4days. Maintenance: 0.2–1.2 mg/day in 2–4 divided doses up to maximum of 2.4 mg/day. **ELDERLY:** Initially, 0.1 mg at bedtime. May increase gradually. **CHILDREN 12 YRS AND OLDER:** Initially, 0.2 mg/day in 2 divided doses. May increase gradually at 5- to 7-day intervals in 0.1 mg/day increments. **Maximum:** 2.4 mg/day.
Extended-Release Tablet/Suspension *(Nexiclon XR)*: **ADULTS, ELDERLY:** Initially, 0.17 mg once daily at bedtime. May increase dose by 0.09 mg/day at weekly intervals. **Range:** 0.17–0.52 mg once daily.
Transdermal: ADULTS, ELDERLY: System delivering 0.1 mg/24 hrs up to 0.6 mg/24 hrs q7days. **Usual dosage range:** 0.1–0.3 mg once weekly.

Acute Hypertension
PO: ADULTS: Initially, 0.1–0.2 mg followed by 0.1 mg every hr if necessary, up to maximum total dose of 0.7 mg.

Attention-Deficit Hyperactivity Disorder (ADHD)
PO: CHILDREN 45 KG OR LESS: Initially 0.05 mg/day at bedtime. May increase in increments of 0.05 mg/day q3–7days up to 0.2 mg/day (27–40.5 kg), 0.3 mg/day (40.5–45 kg). **GREATER THAN 45 KG:** 0.1

mg at bedtime. May increase 0.1 mg/day q3–7 days. **Maximum:** 0.4 mg/day.
Extended-Release Tablet *(Kapvay)*: **CHILDREN 6 YRS AND OLDER:** Initially, 0.1 mg daily at bedtime. May increase in increments of 0.1 mg/day at weekly intervals (**Maximum:** 0.4 mg/day). Doses should be taken twice daily with higher split dose given at bedtime.

Severe Pain
Epidural: ADULTS, ELDERLY: 30–40 mcg/hr. **CHILDREN:** Range: 0.5–2 mcg/kg/hr, not to exceed adult dose.

SIDE EFFECTS
Frequent (40%–10%): Dry mouth, drowsiness, dizziness, sedation, constipation. **Occasional (5%–1%): Tablets, Injection:** Depression, pedal edema, loss of appetite, decreased sexual function, itching eyes, dizziness, nausea, vomiting, nervousness. **Transdermal:** Pruritus, redness or darkening of skin. **Rare (less than 1%):** Nightmares, vivid dreams, feeling of coldness in distal extremities (esp. the digits).

ADVERSE EFFECTS/ TOXIC REACTIONS
Overdose produces profound hypotension, irritability, bradycardia, respiratory depression, hypothermia, miosis (pupillary constriction), arrhythmias, apnea. Abrupt withdrawal may result in rebound hypertension associated with nervousness, agitation, anxiety, insomnia, paresthesia, tremor, flushing, diaphoresis. May produce sedation in pts with acute CVA.

NURSING CONSIDERATIONS
BASELINE ASSESSMENT
Obtain B/P immediately before each dose is administered, in addition to regular monitoring (be alert to B/P fluctuations).

INTERVENTION/EVALUATION
Monitor B/P, pulse, mental status. Monitor daily pattern of bowel activity, stool consistency. If clonidine is to be with-

drawn, discontinue concurrent beta-blocker therapy several days before discontinuing clonidine (prevents clonidine withdrawal hypertensive crisis). Slowly reduce clonidine dosage over 2–4 days.

PATIENT/FAMILY TEACHING

• Sugarless gum, sips of tepid water may relieve dry mouth. • Avoid tasks that require alertness, motor skills until response to drug is established. • To reduce hypotensive effect, rise slowly from lying to sitting position. • Skipping doses or voluntarily discontinuing drug may produce severe, rebound hypertension. • Avoid alcohol. • If patch loosens during 7-day application period, secure with adhesive cover.

---

clopidogrel   TOP 200 HIGH ALERT

kloe-**pid**-oh-grel
(Apo-Clopidogrel , Plavix)
BLACK BOX ALERT Diminished effectiveness in CYP2C19 metabolizers increases risk for cardiovascular events.
Do not confuse Plavix with Elavil or Paxil.

◆CLASSIFICATION

PHARMACOTHERAPEUTIC: Thienopyridine derivative. **CLINICAL:** Antiplatelet (see p. 33C).

ACTION

Inhibits binding of enzyme adenosine phosphate (ADP) to its platelet receptor and subsequent ADP-mediated activation of a glycoprotein complex. **Therapeutic Effect:** Inhibits platelet aggregation.

PHARMACOKINETICS

Route	Onset	Peak	Duration
PO	2 hrs	5–7 days (with repeated doses of 75 mg/day)	5 days after last dose

Rapidly absorbed. Protein binding: 98%. Extensively metabolized by liver. Eliminated equally in the urine and feces. **Half-life:** 8 hrs.

USES

Reduction of atherosclerotic events (e.g., MI, stroke, vascular death) in pts with recent MI or stroke, or established peripheral artery disease (PAD). Treatment of acute coronary syndrome (ACS). Reduces rate of atherothrombotic events in pts with unstable angina (UA), non-ST segment elevation MI (non-STEMI), ST-segment elevation MI (STEMI), or with percutaneous coronary intervention (PCI) or CABG. **OFF-LABEL:** Graft patency (saphenous vein), stable coronary artery disease (in combination with aspirin). Initial treatment of acute coronary syndrome in pts allergic to aspirin.

PRECAUTIONS

Contraindications: Active bleeding (e.g., peptic ulcer, intracranial hemorrhage). **Cautions:** Severe hepatic/renal impairment, pts at risk of increased bleeding (e.g., trauma), concurrent use of anticoagulants.

⌛ LIFESPAN CONSIDERATIONS

Pregnancy/Lactation: Unknown if drug crosses placenta or is distributed in breast milk. **Pregnancy Category B. Children:** Safety and efficacy not established. **Elderly:** No age-related precautions noted.

INTERACTIONS

DRUG: Aspirin, NSAIDs, warfarin may increase risk of bleeding. **Proton pump inhibitors (e.g., omeprazole)** may decrease efficacy, increase risk of cardiovascular events. **HERBAL: Cat's claw, dong quai, evening primrose, feverfew, garlic, ginger, ginkgo, ginseng, green tea, red clover** may have additive antiplatelet effects. **FOOD: Grapefruit, grapefruit juice** may decrease effects. **LAB VALUES:** May increase bilirubin, AST, ALT, serum cholesterol, uric acid. May decrease neutrophil count, platelet count.

AVAILABILITY (Rx)
Tablets: 75 mg, 300 mg.

ADMINISTRATION/HANDLING
PO
• Give without regard to food.

INDICATIONS/ROUTES/DOSAGE
Reduction of Atherosclerotic Events (Pts with Recent MI, Stroke, PAD)
PO: ADULTS, ELDERLY: 75 mg once a day.

Acute Coronary Syndrome (ACS), Unstable Angina/NSTEMI
PO: ADULTS, ELDERLY: Initially, 300 mg loading dose, then 75 mg once a day (in combination with aspirin).

ACS (STEMI)
PO: ADULTS, ELDERLY: 75 mg once a day (in combination with aspirin).

ACS (PCI)
PO: ADULTS, ELDERLY: Initially, 600 mg, then 75 mg once daily.

SIDE EFFECTS
Frequent (15%): Skin disorders. **Occasional (8%–6%):** Upper respiratory tract infection, chest pain, flu-like symptoms, headache, dizziness, arthralgia. **Rare (5%–3%):** Fatigue, edema, hypertension, abdominal pain, dyspepsia, diarrhea, nausea, epistaxis, dyspnea, rhinitis.

ADVERSE EFFECTS/ TOXIC REACTIONS
Agranulocytosis, aplastic anemia/pancytopenia, thrombotic thrombocytopenic purpura (TTP) occur rarely. Hepatitis, hypersensitivity reaction, anaphylactoid reaction have been reported.

NURSING CONSIDERATIONS
BASELINE ASSESSMENT
Obtain baseline chemistries, platelet count, PFA level. Perform platelet counts before drug therapy, q2days during first wk of treatment, and weekly thereafter until therapeutic maintenance dose is reached. Abrupt discontinuation of drug therapy produces elevated platelet count within 5 days.

INTERVENTION/EVALUATION
Monitor platelet count for evidence of thrombocytopenia. Assess BUN, serum creatinine, bilirubin, AST, ALT, WBC, Hgb, Hct, signs/symptoms of hepatic insufficiency during therapy.

PATIENT/FAMILY TEACHING
• It may take longer to stop bleeding during drug therapy. • Report any unusual bleeding. • Inform physicians, dentists if clopidogrel is being taken, esp. before surgery is scheduled or before taking any new drug.

clorazepate

klor-**az**-e-pate
(Apo-Clorazepate ✤, Novo-Clopate ✤, Tranxene T-Tab)
Do not confuse clorazepate with clofibrate or clonazepam.

◆CLASSIFICATION
PHARMACOTHERAPEUTIC: Benzodiazepine **(Schedule IV). CLINICAL:** Antianxiety, anticonvulsant (see p. 15C).

ACTION
Depresses all levels of CNS, including limbic and reticular formation, by binding to benzodiazepine receptor sites on gamma-aminobutyric acid (GABA) receptor complex. Modulates GABA, a major inhibitory neurotransmitter in the brain. **Therapeutic Effect:** Produces anxiolytic effect, suppresses seizure activity.

PHARMACOKINETICS
Readily absorbed from GI tract. Metabolized in liver. (**Half-life:** 48–96 hrs) and oxazepam (**Half-life:** 6–8 hrs). Excreted primarily in urine.

USES

Management of generalized anxiety disorders, short-term relief of anxiety symptoms, partial seizures, acute alcohol withdrawal symptoms.

PRECAUTIONS

Contraindications: Narrow-angle glaucoma. **Cautions:** Renal/hepatic impairment, depression, high risk of suicidal ideation, history of drug dependence, elderly, debilitated pts, those with respiratory disease, sleep apnea.

⏳ LIFESPAN CONSIDERATIONS

Pregnancy/Lactation: Crosses placenta; distributed in breast milk. **Pregnancy Category D. Children:** May experience paradoxical excitement. **Elderly:** Increased risk of dizziness, sedation, confusion, hypotension, hyperexcitability.

INTERACTIONS

DRUG: Alcohol, other CNS depressants may increase CNS depressant effects. **CYP3A4 inhibitors (e.g., azole antifungals)** may increase concentration, toxicity. **HERBAL: Gotu kola, kava kava, SAMe, St. John's wort, valerian** may increase CNS depression. **FOOD:** None known. **LAB VALUES:** May increase BUN, serum creatinine, ALT, AST, alkaline phosphatase. May decrease Hct. **Therapeutic serum level:** 0.12–1 mcg/ml; **toxic serum level:** greater than 5 mcg/ml.

AVAILABILITY (Rx)

💊 **Tablets (Tranxene T-Tab):** 3.75 mg, 7.5 mg, 15 mg.

ADMINISTRATION/HANDLING

◀ **ALERT** ▶ If pt requires change to another anticonvulsant, decrease dosage gradually as low-dose therapy begins with replacement drug.

PO
• May administer with food/water to decrease risk of GI disturbance.

INDICATIONS/ROUTES/DOSAGE

Anxiety
PO: ADULTS, ELDERLY: 7.5–15 mg 2–4 times a day.

Partial Seizures
PO: ADULTS, ELDERLY, CHILDREN OLDER THAN 12 YRS: Initially, up to 7.5 mg 2–3 times a day. May increase by 7.5 mg at weekly intervals. **Maximum:** 90 mg/day. **CHILDREN 9–12 YRS:** Initially, 3.75–7.5 mg twice a day. May increase by 3.75 mg at weekly intervals. **Maximum:** 60 mg/day in 2–3 divided doses.

Alcohol Withdrawal
PO: ADULTS, ELDERLY: Initially, 30 mg, then 15 mg 2–4 times a day on first day. Gradually decrease dosage over subsequent days. **Maximum:** 90 mg/day.

SIDE EFFECTS

Frequent: Drowsiness. **Occasional:** Dizziness, GI disturbances, anxiety, blurred vision, dry mouth, headache, confusion, ataxia, rash, irritability, slurred speech. **Rare:** Paradoxical CNS reactions (hyperactivity, nervousness in children; excitement, restlessness in elderly, debilitated, generally noted during first 2 wks of therapy, particularly in presence of uncontrolled pain).

ADVERSE EFFECTS/ TOXIC REACTIONS

Abrupt or rapid withdrawal may result in pronounced restlessness, irritability, insomnia, hand tremors, abdominal/muscle cramps, diaphoresis, vomiting, seizures. Overdose results in drowsiness, confusion, diminished reflexes, coma. May increase risk of suicidal ideation or behavior.

NURSING CONSIDERATIONS

BASELINE ASSESSMENT

Anxiety: Assess autonomic response (cold/clammy hands, diaphoresis), motor response (agitation, trembling, tension). Offer emotional support. **Seizures:** Review history of seizure disorder (intensity, frequency, duration, level of consciousness [LOC]). Initiate seizure precautions.

INTERVENTION/EVALUATION

Assess for paradoxical reaction, particularly during early therapy. Assist with ambulation if drowsiness, dizziness occur. Observe for seizure activity. Evaluate for therapeutic response: **Anxiety:** Assess for calm facial expression; decreased restlessness. Monitor for signs/symptoms of depression, anxiety (loss of interest, mood swings, suicidal ideation or behavior). **Seizures:** Assess for decrease in intensity/frequency of seizures. **Therapeutic serum level:** 0.12–1 mcg/ml; **toxic serum level:** greater than 5 mcg/ml.

PATIENT/FAMILY TEACHING

• Do not abruptly discontinue medication after long-term use (may precipitate seizures). • Strict maintenance of drug therapy is essential for seizure control. • Drowsiness usually disappears during continued therapy. • Avoid tasks that require alertness, motor skills until response to drug is established. • Go from lying to standing slowly. • Smoking reduces drug effectiveness. • Avoid alcohol. • Report thoughts of suicide, worsening depression, or loss of seizure control.

---

clozapine

kloe-za-peen
(Apo-Clozapine ✤, Clozaril, FazaClo, Versacloz)

BLACK BOX ALERT Significant risk of life-threatening agranulocytosis, increased risk of potentially fatal cardiovascular events, particularly myocarditis, in elderly pts with dementia-related psychosis. May cause severe orthostatic hypotension, dose-dependent seizures.

Do not confuse clozapine with clonazepam, clonidine, or Klonopin, or Clozaril with Clinoril or Colazal.

◆CLASSIFICATION

PHARMACOTHERAPEUTIC: Dibenzodiazepine derivative. **CLINICAL:** Antipsychotic (see p. 66C).

ACTION

Interferes with binding of dopamine at dopamine receptor sites; binds primarily at nondopamine receptor sites. **Therapeutic Effect:** Diminishes schizophrenic behavior.

PHARMACOKINETICS

Readily absorbed from GI tract. Protein binding: 97%. Metabolized in liver. Excreted in urine. **Half-life:** 12 hrs.

USES

Management of severely ill schizophrenic pts who have failed to respond to other antipsychotic therapy. Treatment of recurrent suicidal behavior. **OFF-LABEL:** Schizoaffective disorder, bipolar disorder, childhood psychosis, obsessive-compulsive disorder, agitation related to Alzheimer's dementia.

PRECAUTIONS

Contraindications: Concurrent use of other drugs that may suppress bone marrow function, history of clozapine-induced agranulocytosis or severe granulocytopenia, myeloproliferative disorders, paralytic ileus, uncontrolled seizures, severe CNS depression, coma. **Cautions:** History of seizures, cardiovascular disease, myocarditis; respiratory/hepatic/renal impairment; alcohol withdrawal; high risk of suicide; paralytic ileus; myasthenia gravis; pts at risk for aspiration pneumonia; urinary retention; narrow-angle glaucoma; prostatic hypertrophy; xerostomia; visual disturbances; constipation; history of bowel obstruction; diabetes mellitus. **Pregnancy Category B.**

INTERACTIONS

DRUG: **Antihypertensive medications** may increase risk of hypotension. **Alco-**

C

hol, other **CNS depressants** may increase CNS depressant effects. **Bone marrow depressants** may increase myelosuppression. **Cimetidine, citalopram, ciprofloxacin, erythromycin** may increase concentration, risk of adverse effects. **SSRIs (e.g., paroxetine)** may increase concentration. **Lithium** may increase risk of confusion, dyskinesia, seizures. **Medications prolonging QT interval** may increase risk of QT prolongation. **CYP3A4 inducers (e.g., phenytoin, carbamazepine, rifampin)** may decrease concentration/effects. HERBAL: **St. John's wort** may decrease concentration/therapeutic effects. **Kava kava, gotu kola, valerian, St. John's wort** may increase risk of CNS depression. FOOD: None known. LAB VALUES: May increase serum glucose, cholesterol (rare), triglycerides (rare).

AVAILABILITY (Rx)

Suspension, Oral (Versacloz): 50 mg/ml (100 ml). Tablets (Clozaril): 25 mg, 50 mg, 100 mg, 200 mg. Tablets (Orally Disintegrating [FazaClo]): 12.5 mg, 25 mg, 100 mg, 150 mg, 200 mg.

ADMINISTRATION/HANDLING

PO

• Give without regard to food. • **Suspension:** Use oral syringes (provided). Shake well, administer dose immediately after preparing. Suspension stable for 100 days after initial bottle opening.

Orally Disintegrating Tablets

• Remove from foil blister; do not push tablet through foil. • Remove tablet with dry hands, place in mouth. • Allow to dissolve in mouth, swallow with saliva. • If dose requires splitting tablet, discard unused portion.

INDICATIONS/ROUTES/DOSAGE

Schizophrenic Disorders

◀ALERT▶ For initiation of therapy, must have WBC equal to or greater than 3,500 mm^3 and ANC equal to or greater than 2,000 mm^3.

PO: ADULTS: Initially, 12.5 mg once or twice a day. May increase by 25–50 mg/day over 2 wks until dosage of 300–450 mg/day is achieved. May further increase by 50–100 mg/day no more than once or twice a week. Range: 200–600 mg/day. **Maximum:** 900 mg/day. ELDERLY: Initially, 25 mg/day. May increase by 25 mg/day. **Maximum:** 450 mg/day.

Suicidal Behavior in Schizophrenia

PO: ADULTS: Initially, 12.5 mg 1–2 times/day. May increase in increments of 25–50 mg/day to a target dose of 300–450 mg/day after 2 wks. Range: 12.5–900 mg/day.

SIDE EFFECTS

Frequent (39%–14%): Drowsiness, salivation, tachycardia, dizziness, constipation. Occasional (9%–4%): Hypotension; headache; tremor, syncope, diaphoresis, dry mouth; nausea, visual disturbances; nightmares, restlessness, akinesia, agitation, hypertension, abdominal discomfort, heartburn, weight gain. Rare: Rigidity, confusion, fatigue, insomnia, diarrhea, rash.

ADVERSE EFFECTS/ TOXIC REACTIONS

Seizures occur occasionally (3%). Overdose produces CNS depression (sedation, delirium, coma), respiratory depression, hypersalivation. Blood dyscrasias, particularly agranulocytosis, mild leukopenia, may occur.

NURSING CONSIDERATIONS

BASELINE ASSESSMENT

Obtain baseline weight, glucose, Hgb A1C, WBC, absolute neutrophil count (ANC) before initiating treatment. Assess behavior, appearance, emotional status, response to environment, speech pattern, thought content.

INTERVENTION/EVALUATION

Monitor B/P for hypertension/hypotension. Assess pulse for tachycardia (common side effect). Monitor CBC for blood dyscrasias. Monitor WBC, ANC count every wk for first 6 mos, then biweekly for 6 mos. If CBC and ANC are normal after 12 mos, then monthly monitoring of CBC and ANC is recommended.Supervise suicidal-risk pt closely during early therapy (as depression lessens, energy level improves, increasing suicide potential). Assess for therapeutic response (interest in surroundings, improvement in self-care, increased ability to concentrate, relaxed facial expression).

PATIENT/FAMILY TEACHING

• Do not abruptly discontinue long-term drug therapy. • Drowsiness generally subsides during continued therapy. • Avoid tasks that require alertness, motor skills until response to drug is established. • Avoid alcohol, caffeine. • Report fever, sore throat, flu-like symptoms.

---

codeine HIGH ALERT

koe-deen
(Codeine Contin)
Do not confuse codeine with Cardene or Lodine.

FIXED-COMBINATION(S)

Capital with Codeine, Tylenol with Codeine: acetaminophen/codeine: 120 mg/12 mg per 5 ml. **Tylenol with Codeine:** acetaminophen/codeine: 300 mg/15 mg, 300 mg/30 mg, 300 mg/60 mg.

◆CLASSIFICATION

PHARMACOTHERAPEUTIC: Opioid agonist. **CLINICAL:** Analgesic: Single entity: **Schedule II:** Fixed-combination form: **Schedule III:** Less than 90 mg, fixed combinations.

ACTION

Binds to opioid receptors in CNS, particularly in medulla. Inhibits ascending pain pathways. **Therapeutic Effect:** Alters perception, emotional response to pain; suppresses cough reflex.

PHARMACOKINETICS

Route	Onset	Peak	Duration
PO	30–60 min	1–1.5 hrs	4–6 hrs
IM	10–30 min	0.5–1 hr	4–6 hrs

Well absorbed following PO administration. Protein binding: (7–25%.) Metabolized in liver. Excreted in urine. **Half-life:** 2.5–3.5 hrs.

USES

Relief of mild to moderate pain. **OFF-LABEL:** Short-term relief of cough.

PRECAUTIONS

Contraindications: Respiratory depression in absence of resuscitative equipment, acute or severe bronchial asthma or hypercarbia, paralytic ileus. **Cautions:** Adrenal insufficiency, biliary tract impairment, CNS depression/coma, morbid obesity, prostatic hyperplasia, urinary stricture, thyroid dysfunction, severe renal/hepatic impairment, COPD, respiratory disease, cardiovascular disease, hypovolemia, GI obstruction, head injury, elevated intracranial pressure, history of drug abuse, patients with 2 or more copies of variant CYP2D6*2 allele (may have extensive conversion to morphine).

⧖ LIFESPAN CONSIDERATIONS

Pregnancy Category C (D if used for prolonged periods or at high dosages at term). Children: Efficacy not established in those younger than 2 years. **Elderly:** May cause confusion, oversedation; use lower dosing range.

INTERACTIONS

DRUG: Alcohol, other CNS depressants may increase CNS, respiratory depression, hypotension. **Anticholinergics** may increase risk of urinary retention, severe constipation. **MAOIs** may produce a severe, sometimes fatal reaction (reduce dosage to ¼ usual

---

dose). **HERBAL:** **St. John's wort** may decrease concentration. **Gotu kola, kava kava, SAMe, St. John's wort, valerian** may increase CNS depression. **FOOD:** None known. **LAB VALUES:** May increase serum amylase, lipase.

AVAILABILITY (Rx)

Tablets: 15 mg, 30 mg, 60 mg.

ADMINISTRATION/HANDLING

PO
• Give with food or milk (minimizes adverse GI effects).

INDICATIONS/ROUTES/DOSAGE

◄ALERT► Reduce initial dosage in those with hypothyroidism, Addison's disease, renal insufficiency, those using other CNS depressants concurrently. Respiratory depression and death have occurred in children receiving codeine following tonsillectomy and/or adenoidectomy and found to have evidence of being ultrarapid metabolizers of codeine due to a CYP2D6 polymorphism.

Analgesia
PO: ADULTS, ELDERLY: 15–60 mg q4h as needed. **Maximum total daily dose:** 360 mg. CHILDREN: 0.5–1 mg/kg q4–6h. **Maximum:** 60 mg/dose.

Dosage in Renal Impairment
Dosage is modified based on creatinine clearance.

Creatinine Clearance	Dosage
10–50 ml/min	75% of usual dose
Less than 10 ml/min	50% of usual dose

SIDE EFFECTS

◄ALERT► Ambulatory pts, those not in severe pain may experience dizziness, nausea, vomiting, hypotension more frequently than those in supine position or with severe pain. Frequent: Constipation, drowsiness, nausea, vomiting. Occasional: Paradoxical excitement, confusion, palpitations, facial flushing, decreased urina-

tion, blurred vision, dizziness, dry mouth, headache, hypotension (including orthostatic hypotension), decreased appetite, injection site redness, burning, or pain. Rare: Hallucinations, depression, abdominal pain, insomnia.

ADVERSE EFFECTS/ TOXIC REACTIONS

Chronic use may result in paralytic ileus. Overdose may produce cold/clammy skin, confusion, seizures, decreased B/P, restlessness, pinpoint pupils, bradycardia, respiratory depression, decreased LOC, severe weakness. Tolerance to drug's analgesic effect, physical dependence may occur with chronic use.

NURSING CONSIDERATIONS

BASELINE ASSESSMENT

Analgesic: Assess onset, type, location, duration of pain. Effect of medication is reduced if full pain response recurs before next dose. **Antitussive:** Assess type, severity, frequency of cough, sputum production.

INTERVENTION/EVALUATION

Monitor daily pattern of bowel activity, stool consistency. Increase fluid intake, environmental humidity to improve viscosity of lung secretions. Initiate deep breathing, coughing exercises. Assess for clinical improvement; record onset of relief of pain, cough.

PATIENT/FAMILY TEACHING

• Change positions slowly to avoid orthostatic hypotension. • Avoid tasks that require alertness, motor skills until response to drug is established. • Tolerance, dependence may occur with prolonged use of high dosages. • Avoid alcohol.

colchicine   TOP 200   HIGH ALERT

kol-chi-seen
(Colcrys)

Do not confuse colchicine with Cortrosyn.

◆ CLASSIFICATION

PHARMACOTHERAPEUTIC: Alkaloid. **CLINICAL:** Antigout.

ACTION

Decreases leukocyte motility, phagocytosis, lactic acid production. **Therapeutic Effect:** Decreases urate crystal deposits, reduces inflammatory process.

PHARMACOKINETICS

Rapidly absorbed from GI tract. Highest concentration is in liver, spleen, kidney. Protein binding: 30%–50%. Reenters intestinal tract by biliary secretion and is reabsorbed from intestines. Partially metabolized in liver. Eliminated primarily in feces. **Half-life:** 12–30 min.

USES

Prevention, treatment of acute gouty arthritis. Used to reduce frequency of recurrence of familial Mediterranean fever (FMF). **OFF-LABEL:** Treatment of biliary cirrhosis, recurrent pericarditis.

PRECAUTIONS

Contraindications: Concomitant use of a P-glycoprotein (e.g., cyclosporine) or strong CYP3A4 inhibitor (e.g., clarithromycin) in presence of renal or hepatic impairment. **Cautions:** Hepatic impairment, elderly, debilitated, renal impairment.

⧗ LIFESPAN CONSIDERATIONS

Pregnancy/Lactation: Unknown if drug crosses placenta or is distributed in breast milk. **Pregnancy Category C. Children:** Safety and efficacy not established. **Elderly:** May be more susceptible to cumulative toxicity. Age-related renal impairment may increase risk of myopathy.

INTERACTIONS

DRUG: May increase concentration of **statins** and increase risk of rhabdomyolysis. **Atazanavir, clarithromycin, cyclo-** sporine, **diltiazem, erythromycin, fluconazole, fosamprenavir, indinavir, itraconazole, ketoconazole, nelfinavir, ranolazine, ritonavir, saquinavir, verapamil** may increase colchicine concentration, toxicity. **HERBAL:** None significant. **FOOD: Grapefruit juice, grapefruit** may increase concentration/toxicity. **LAB VALUES:** May increase serum alkaline phosphatase, AST. May decrease platelet count.

AVAILABILITY (Rx)

Tablets: 0.6 mg.

ADMINISTRATION/HANDLING

PO

• Give without regard to food. • For FMF, give in 1 or 2 divided doses. • Give with adequate water and maintain fluid intake.

INDICATIONS/ROUTES/DOSAGE

Acute Gouty Arthritis

PO: ADULTS, ELDERLY: Initially, 1.2 mg at first sign of gout flare, then 0.6 mg 1 hr later. **Coadministration with Strong CYP3A4 Inhibitors:** Initially, 0.6 mg, then 0.3 mg dose 1 hr later. Do not repeat for at least 3 days. **Coadministration with Moderate CYP3A4 Inhibitors:** 1.2 mg once. Do not repeat for at least 3 days. **Coadministration with P-Glycoprotein Inhibitors:** 0.6 mg once. Do not repeat for at least 3 days.

Gout Prophylaxis

PO: ADULTS, ELDERLY: 0.6 mg 1–2 times/day. **Maximum:** 1.2 mg/day. **Coadministration with Strong CYP3A4 Inhibitors:** If dose is 0.6 mg 2 times/day, adjust dose to 0.3 mg once daily; if dose is 0.6 mg once daily, adjust dose to 0.3 mg every other day. **Coadministration with Moderate CYP3A4 Inhibitors:** If dose is 0.6 mg 2 times/day, adjust dose to 0.3 mg twice daily or 0.6 mg once daily; if dose is 0.6 mg once daily, adjust dose to 0.3 mg once daily. **Coadministration with P-Glycoprotein Inhibitors:** If dose is 0.6 mg 2 times/day, adjust dose to 0.3 mg once daily; if dose is 0.6 mg once daily, adjust dose to 0.3 mg every other day.

FMF

PO: ADULTS, ELDERLY, CHILDREN OLDER THAN 12 YRS: 1.2–2.4 mg/day. **Coadministration with strong CYP3A4 inhibitors: Maximum:** 0.6 mg once daily (or 0.3 mg twice daily). **Coadministration with moderate CYP3A4 inhibitors:** 1.2 mg/day (0.6 mg twice daily). **Coadministration with P-glycoprotein inhibitors:** 0.6 mg once daily (or 0.3 mg twice daily). **CHILDREN 6–12 YRS:** 0.9–1.8 mg/day in 1–2 divided doses. **CHILDREN 4–5 YRS:** 0.3–1.8 mg/day in 1–2 divided doses. **Note:** Increase or decrease dose by 0.3 mg/day, not to exceed maximum dose.

Pericarditis

PO: ADULTS, ELDERLY: 0.6 mg 2 times/day.

Dosage in Renal Impairment

Creatinine Clearance	Dosage
Less than 30 ml/min	
FMF	0.3 mg initially
Gout prophylaxis	0.3 mg/day
Gout flare	No reduction
HD	
FMF	0.3 mg as single dose
Gout prophylaxis	0.3 mg 2–4 times/wk

SIDE EFFECTS

Frequent: Nausea, vomiting, abdominal discomfort. **Occasional:** Anorexia. **Rare:** Hypersensitivity reaction, including angioedema.

ADVERSE EFFECTS/ TOXIC REACTIONS

Bone marrow depression (aplastic anemia, agranulocytosis, thrombocytopenia) may occur with long-term therapy. Overdose initially causes burning feeling in skin/throat, severe diarrhea, abdominal pain. Second stage manifests as fever, seizures, delirium, renal impairment (hematuria, oliguria). Third stage causes hair loss, leukocytosis, stomatitis.

NURSING CONSIDERATIONS

BASELINE ASSESSMENT

Obtain baseline laboratory studies. **Gout:** Assess involved joints for pain, mobility, edema. **Mediterranean fever:** Assess abdominal pain, fever, chills, erythema, swollen skin lesions.

INTERVENTION/EVALUATION

Discontinue medication immediately if GI symptoms occur. Encourage high fluid intake (3,000 ml/day). Monitor I&O (output should be at least 2,000 ml/day), CBC, hepatic/renal function tests. Monitor serum uric acid. Assess for therapeutic response: relief of pain, stiffness, swelling; increased joint mobility; reduced joint tenderness; improved grip strength.

PATIENT/FAMILY TEACHING

• Drink 8–10 glasses (8 oz) of fluid daily while taking medication. • Report skin rash, sore throat, fever, unusual bruising/bleeding, weakness, fatigue, numbness. • Stop medication as soon as gout pain is relieved or at first sign of nausea, vomiting, diarrhea. • Avoid grapefruit products.

colesevelam TOP 200

(**koe**-le-**sev**-e-lam)
(Lodalis ✦, Welchol)

◆ CLASSIFICATION

PHARMACOTHERAPEUTIC: Bile acid sequestrant. **CLINICAL:** Antihyperlipidemic agent, hypoglycemic agent (see p. 45C, 56C).

ACTION

Binds with bile acids in the intestine, preventing reabsorption. Increases clearance of low-density lipoprotein cholesterol (LDL-C). Glycemic control mechanism unknown. **Therapeutic Effect:** Decreases serum LDL-C levels, Hgb A1C levels.

PHARMACOKINETICS

Not absorbed after PO administration. Strictly limited to intestines. Primarily excreted in feces.

USES

Adjunctive therapy to diet and exercise to reduce elevated LDL-C. Improves glycemic control in pts with type 2 diabetes mellitus when used with other antidiabetic agents. Used as monotherapy or in combination with other cholesterol-lowering drugs (statins). Indicated for children (10–17 yrs of age) with heterozygous familial hypercholesterolemia with LDL-C greater than 190 mg/dL or LDL-C greater than 160 mg/dL (after adequate trial of diet therapy) with positive family history of premature cardiovascular history, or two or more other cardiovascular risk factors.

PRECAUTIONS

Contraindications: Bowel obstruction, hypertriglyceridemia-induced pancreatitis, serum triglycerides greater than 500 mg/dL. **Cautions:** Chronic constipation, major GI surgery, gastroparesis, serum triglycerides 300–500 mg/dL, fat-soluble vitamin deficiency.

⧗ LIFESPAN CONSIDERATIONS

Pregnancy/Lactation: Breast milk distribution unlikely due to nonsystemic absorption. **Pregnancy Category B. Children:** Safety and efficacy not established in pts under 10 yrs of age. Oral suspension recommended. **Elderly:** No age-related precautions noted.

INTERACTIONS

DRUG: May decrease concentration/effects of **oral contraceptives** containing **ethinyl estradiol** and **norethindrone; cyclosporine, glipizide, glyburide, levothyroxine, olmesartan, phenytoin. HERBAL:** Gotu kola may decrease effectiveness. **FOOD:** None significant. **LAB VALUES:** May increase serum triglycerides, CPK, AST/ALT. Decreases glucose, Hgb A1C.

AVAILABILITY (RX)

Tablets: 625 mg. **Suspension, Oral (Packet):** 3.75 grams.

ADMINISTRATION/HANDLING

PO
• Give with meal.

Oral Suspension
• Empty packet into 4–8 ounces of water, fruit juice, soft drink.

INDICATIONS/ROUTES/DOSAGE

Hyperlipidemia
PO: ADULTS, CHILDREN (10–17 YRS): 3 tablets (1,875 mg) twice/day with meal or 6 tablets (3,750 mg) once daily with meal. **Oral Suspension:** 3.75 grams once daily with meal.
◄**ALERT**► Not indicated for treatment of type 1 diabetes, diabetic ketoacidosis.

Type 2 Diabetes
PO: ADULTS: 1,875 mg twice daily or 3,750 mg once daily.

SIDE EFFECTS

Frequent (11%–8%): Constipation, dyspepsia. **Occasional (6%–3%):** Nasopharyngitis, nausea, headache, fatigue, asthenia (loss of strength, energy), pharyngitis, flu-like symptoms. **Rare (2%):** Rhinitis, vomiting, myalgia.

ADVERSE EFFECTS/TOXIC REACTIONS

Elevated serum triglycerides may increase cardiovascular risk. Hypoglycemia reported in 3% of pts.

NURSING CONSIDERATIONS

BASELINE ASSESSMENT

Obtain enhanced lipid panel, liver function, Hgb A1C, blood glucose. Baseline therapeutic levels if applicable: TSH (hormone replacement therapy), PT/INR (warfarin), phenytoin free/total (phenytoin, fosphenytoin).

INTERVENTION/EVALUATION

Monitor lipid panel, Hgb A1C, blood glucose for therapeutic response. Monitor daily pattern of bowel activity, stool consistency. Notify physician if abdominal pain, distention occurs.

PATIENT/FAMILY TEACHING

• Instruct importance of diet, exercise. • Do not take medications within 4 hrs of dose. • Blood levels will be drawn routinely. • Sweating, confusion, dizziness, tremors may indicate low blood sugar. • Report any newly prescribed medications. • Take with meal. • Report persistent GI upset, severe abdominal pain, respiratory difficulties.

conivaptan

koe-nye-**vap**-tan
(Vaprisol)

◆CLASSIFICATION

PHARMACOTHERAPEUTIC: Vasopressin antagonist. **CLINICAL:** Hyponatremia adjunct.

ACTION

Promotes excretion of free water (without loss of serum electrolytes) resulting in net fluid loss, increased urine output, decreased urine osmolarity. **Therapeutic Effect:** Restores normal serum sodium level.

PHARMACOKINETICS

Metabolized in liver. Protein binding: 99%. Eliminated in feces (83%), urine (12%). **Half-life:** 6.7–8.6 hrs.

USES

Treatment of euvolemic and hypervolemic hyponatremia (syndrome of inappropriate secretion of antidiuretic hormone, in setting of hypothyroidism, adrenal insufficiency, pulmonary disorders) in hospitalized pts.

PRECAUTIONS

Contraindications: Hypovolemic hyponatremia; concurrent use with strong CYP3A4 inhibitors (clarithromycin, ketoconazole, ritonavir); anuria. **Cautions:** Hepatic/renal impairment, underlying congestive heart failure.

⧗ LIFESPAN CONSIDERATIONS

Pregnancy/Lactation: Accumulates in placenta; systemic exposure to fetus likely. Potential for decreased neonatal viability, delayed growth/development at doses lower than those required for therapeutic efficacy. Unknown if distributed in breast milk. **Pregnancy Category C. Children:** Safety and efficacy not established. **Elderly:** No age-related precautions noted.

INTERACTIONS

DRUG: CYP3A4 inhibitors (e.g., ketoconazole, itraconazole) may increase concentration. **CYP3A4 inducers (e.g., rifampin, carbamazepine)** may decrease concentration. May increase level/toxicity of **digoxin**. **HERBAL: St. John's wort** may decrease effects. **FOOD:** None known. **LAB VALUES:** May decrease Hgb, Hct, serum potassium, magnesium. May alter serum glucose.

AVAILABILITY (Rx)

Injection, Premix Solutions: 20 mg/100 ml D$_5$W.

ADMINISTRATION/HANDLING

◄ALERT► Administer through large veins; change peripheral IV site every 24 hrs (minimizes risk of vascular irritation).

 IV

Reconstitution • No reconstitution needed.

Rate of Administration • For loading dose, 20 mg/100 ml bag over 30 min. Follow with infusion (20 mg/100 ml) over 24 hrs.

Storage • Store infusions at room temperature. • Do not remove protective overwrap until ready for use.

🢒 IV INCOMPATIBILITIES

Do not infuse concurrently with any other medication or solution.

INDICATIONS/ROUTES/DOSAGE

Euvolemic/Hypervolemic Hyponatremia
IV: ADULTS, ELDERLY: Loading dose: 20 mg given over 30 min. Follow with 20 mg in a continuous IV infusion over 24 hrs. Administer for an additional 1–3 days as a continuous infusion of 20 mg/day. May be titrated upward to 40 mg/day as a continuous infusion if serum sodium is not rising at desired rate. Duration of infusion after loading dose should not exceed 4 days.

SIDE EFFECTS

Frequent: Peripheral injection site reactions (pain, erythema, phlebitis, swelling) (53%), headache (12%). **Occasional (10%–4%):** Thirst, vomiting, hypertension, polyuria, orthostatic hypotension, diarrhea, constipation, fever, confusion, dry mouth, nausea. **Rare (3%–2%):** Atrial fibrillation, hypotension, insomnia, dehydration, oral candidiasis.

ADVERSE EFFECTS/ TOXIC REACTIONS

Overly rapid increase in serum sodium may produce temporary neurologic symptoms. UTI, anemia, hematuria, pneumonia occur occasionally.

NURSING CONSIDERATIONS

BASELINE ASSESSMENT

Obtain baseline CBC, BUN, serum creatinine, sodium, hepatic enzyme levels. Start peripheral IV in large vein. Assess for increased pulse rate, poor skin turgor, nausea, diarrhea (signs of hyponatremia).

INTERVENTION/EVALUATION

Obtain, monitor frequent serum sodium levels. Assess peripheral IV site for pain, erythema, phlebitis, swelling; if vein irritation occurs, change IV site. New IV site should be obtained every 24 hrs (minimizes vein irritation). Monitor urine output. Observe for improvement in signs/symptoms of hyponatremia, impending signs/symptoms of hypernatremia (flushing, edema, restlessness, dry mucous membranes, fever).

PATIENT/FAMILY TEACHING

Change positions slowly to avoid orthostatic hypotension.

conjugated estrogens

TOP 200

kon-joo-gate-ed **ess**-troe-jenz
(Cenestin, Enjuvia, Premarin)

BLACK BOX ALERT Risk of dementia may be increased in postmenopausal women. Do not use to prevent cardiovascular disease. May increase risk of endometrial carcinoma in postmenopausal women.
Do not confuse Enjuvia with Januvia, or Premarin with Primaxin, Provera, or Remeron.

FIXED-COMBINATION(S)

Duavee: conjugated estrogen/bazedoxifene (estrogen agonist/antagonist): 0.45 mg/20 mg.

◆ CLASSIFICATION

PHARMACOTHERAPEUTIC: Estrogen.
CLINICAL: Hormone.

ACTION

Increases synthesis of DNA, RNA, various proteins in target tissues; reduces release of gonadotropin-releasing hormone, reduces follicle-stimulating hormone

---

(FSH), luteinizing hormone (LH). **Therapeutic Effect:** Promotes normal growth, development of female sex organs; maintains GU function, vasomotor stability. Prevents accelerated bone loss by inhibiting bone resorption, restoring balance of bone resorption/formation. Inhibits LH, decreases serum concentration of testosterone.

PHARMACOKINETICS

Well absorbed from GI tract. Widely distributed. Protein binding: 50%–80%. Metabolized in liver. Primarily excreted in urine. **Half-life (total estrone):** 27 hrs.

USES

Premarin: Management of moderate to severe vasomotor symptoms associated with menopause. Treatment of atrophic vaginitis, kraurosis vulvae, female hypogonadism and castration, primary ovarian failure. Retardation of osteoporosis in postmenopausal women. Palliative treatment of inoperable, progressive cancer of the prostate in men and of the breast in postmenopausal women. Treatment of moderate to severe postmenopausal dyspareunia (painful sexual intercourse). **Cenestin:** Treatment of moderate to severe vasomotor symptoms of menopause, treatment of vulvar/vaginal atrophy. **Enjuvia:** Treatment of moderate to severe vasomotor symptoms, moderate to severe vaginal dryness and pain with intercourse, symptoms of vulvar/vaginal atrophy associated with menopause. **OFF-LABEL:** Prevention of estrogen deficiency–induced premenopausal osteoporosis. **Cream:** Prevention of nosebleeds.

PRECAUTIONS

Contraindications: Breast cancer (except in pts being treated for metastatic disease), hepatic disease, history or current thrombophlebitis, undiagnosed abnormal vaginal bleeding, pregnancy. **Cautions:** Asthma, epilepsy, migraine headaches, diabetes, cardiac/renal dysfunction, history of severe hypocalce-mia, lupus erythematosis, porphyria, endometriosis, gallbladder disease, familial defects of lipoprotein metabolism.

⏳ LIFESPAN CONSIDERATIONS

Pregnancy/Lactation: Distributed in breast milk. May be harmful to fetus. Not for use during lactation. **Pregnancy Category X. Children:** Safety and efficacy not established. **Elderly:** No age-related precautions noted.

INTERACTIONS

DRUG: None significant. **HERBAL: Black cohosh, dong quai** may increase estrogenic activity. **Ginseng, red clover, saw palmetto** may increase hormonal effects. **St. John's wort** may decrease concentration. **FOOD: Grapefruit juice** may increase concentration/toxicity. **LAB VALUES:** May increase glucose, HDL, serum calcium, triglycerides. May decrease serum cholesterol, LDH. May affect serum metapyrone testing, thyroid function tests.

AVAILABILITY (Rx)

Cream, Vaginal (Premarin): 0.625 mg/g. **Injection, Powder for Reconstitution:** 25 mg. **Tablet (Cenestin, Enjuvia, Premarin):** 0.3 mg, 0.45 mg, 0.625 mg, 0.9 mg, 1.25 mg.

ADMINISTRATION/HANDLING

 IV

Reconstitution • Reconstitute with Sterile Water for Injection. • Slowly add diluent, shaking gently. • Avoid vigorous shaking.
Rate of Administration • Give slowly to prevent flushing reaction.
Storage • Refrigerate vials for IV use. • Use immediately following reconstitution.

PO

• Administer at same time each day.
• Give with milk, food if nausea occurs.

🖼 IV INCOMPATIBILITIES

No information available on Y-site administration.

INDICATIONS/ROUTES/DOSAGE

Vasomotor Symptoms Associated with Menopause
PO: ADULTS, ELDERLY: (Premarin): 0.3 mg/day cyclically (21 days on, 7 days off) or continuously. (Enjuvia): 0.3 mg/day. May titrate up to 1.25 mg/day. (Cenestin): 0.45 mg/day. May titrate up to 1.25 mg/day.

Vulvar and Vaginal Atrophy
PO: ADULTS, ELDERLY: (Cenestin, Enjuvia, Premarin): 0.3 mg/day.
Intravaginal: ADULTS, ELDERLY: 0.5–2 g/day cyclically, such as 21 days on and 7 days off.

Female Hypogonadism
PO: ADULTS: (Premarin): 0.3–0.625 mg/day given either as 3 wks on/1 wk off or 25 days on/5 days off.

Female Castration, Primary Ovarian Failure
PO: ADULTS: (Premarin): Initially, 1.25 mg/day cyclically given either as 3 wks on/1 wk off or 25 days on/5 days off. Adjust dosage, upward or downward, according to severity of symptoms and pt response. For maintenance, adjust dosage to lowest level that will provide effective control.

Postmenopausal Osteoporosis Prevention
PO: ADULTS, ELDERLY: (Premarin): 0.3 daily or cyclically, such as 25 days on and 5 days off or 3 wks on and 1 wk off.

Breast Cancer
PO: ADULTS, ELDERLY: (Premarin): 10 mg 3 times a day for at least 3 mos.

Prostate Cancer
PO: ADULTS, ELDERLY: (Premarin): 1.25–2.5 mg 3 times a day.

Abnormal Uterine Bleeding
IV, IM: ADULTS: 25 mg; may repeat once in 6–12 hrs.

Dyspareunia
Intravaginal: ADULTS, ELDERLY: 0.5 g daily (21 days on, 7 days off).

SIDE EFFECTS

Frequent: Vaginal bleeding (spotting, breakthrough bleeding); breast pain/tenderness; gynecomastia. **Occasional:** Headache, hypertension, intolerance to contact lenses. **High doses:** Anorexia, nausea. **Rare:** Loss of scalp hair, depression.

ADVERSE EFFECTS/TOXIC REACTIONS

Prolonged administration may increase risk of breast, cervical, endometrial, hepatic, vaginal carcinoma; cerebrovascular disease, coronary heart disease, gallbladder disease, hypercalcemia.

NURSING CONSIDERATIONS

BASELINE ASSESSMENT

Question for hypersensitivity to estrogen, hepatic dysfunction, thromboembolic disorders associated with pregnancy, estrogen therapy. Assess frequency/severity of vasomotor symptoms.

INTERVENTION/EVALUATION

Assess B/P periodically. Assess for edema; weigh daily. Monitor for loss of vision, diplopia, migraine, thromboembolic disorder, sudden onset of proptosis.

PATIENT/FAMILY TEACHING

• Avoid smoking due to increased risk of heart attack, blood clots. • Avoid grapefruit products. • Diet, exercise important part of therapy when used to retard osteoporosis. • Teach how to perform Homans' test, signs/symptoms of blood clots (report these immediately). • Promptly report signs/symptoms of thromboembolic, thrombotic disorders: sudden severe headache, shortness of breath, vision/speech disturbance, weakness/numbness of an extremity, loss of coordination, pain in chest, groin, leg. • Report abnormal vaginal bleeding, depression. • Teach fe-

C

male pts to perform breast self-exam. • Report weight gain of more than 5 lbs a wk. • Stop taking medication, contact physician if pregnancy is suspected.

cortisone

kor-ti-sone
Do not confuse cortisone with Cardizem.

◆CLASSIFICATION

PHARMACOTHERAPEUTIC: Adrenocortical steroid. **CLINICAL:** Glucocorticoid (see p. 99C).

ACTION

Inhibits accumulation of inflammatory cells at inflammation sites, phagocytosis, synthesis and release of mediators of inflammation. **Therapeutic Effect:** Prevents/suppresses cell-mediated immune reactions. Decreases/prevents tissue response to inflammatory process.

PHARMACOKINETICS

Slowly absorbed from GI tract. Widely distributed. Metabolized in liver. Excreted in urine/feces. **Half-life:** 0.5–2 hrs.

USES

Treatment of adrenocortical insufficiency, conditions treated by immunosuppression, inflammatory conditions.

PRECAUTIONS

Contraindications: Hypersensitivity to corticosteroids, administration of live virus vaccine, systemic viral or fungal infection, serious infections (except septic shock or tuberculosis meningitis). **Cautions:** Thromboembolic disorders, history of tuberculosis (may reactivate disease), hypothyroidism, cirrhosis, HF, psychosis, renal insufficiency, seizure disorders, GI disease, cardiovascular disease, peptic ulcer, myasthenia gravis, hepatic impairment, diabetes, cataracts,

or glaucoma. Prolonged therapy should be discontinued slowly.

⧗ LIFESPAN CONSIDERATIONS

Pregnancy/Lactation: Crosses placenta; distributed in breast milk. **Pregnancy Category C (D if used in the first trimester). Children:** Monitor growth, development of children, infants on prolonged steroid therapy. **Elderly:** Higher risk for hypertension, osteoporosis.

INTERACTIONS

DRUG: CYP3A4 inducers (e.g., phenobarbital, phenytoin, rifampin) may decrease concentration/effects. **CYP3A4 inhibitors (e.g., itraconazole, ketoconazole)** may increase concentration. May alter effects of **anticoagulants.** **HERBAL: Echinacea** may decrease corticosteroid effectiveness. **FOOD:** None known. **LAB VALUES:** May increase blood glucose, serum cholesterol, amylase, sodium. May decrease serum calcium, potassium, thyroxine.

AVAILABILITY (Rx)

Tablets: 25 mg.

ADMINISTRATION/HANDLING

• Administer with meals, food, or milk to decrease risk of GI disturbance.

INDICATIONS/ROUTES/DOSAGE

Dosage is dependent on condition being treated and pt response.

Physiologic Replacement
PO: ADULTS, ELDERLY: 25–35 mg/day. **CHILDREN:** 0.5–0.75 mg/kg/day in 3 divided doses.

Inflammatory Conditions
PO: ADULTS, ELDERLY: 25–300 mg/day. **CHILDREN:** 2.5–10 mg/kg/day in 3–4 divided doses.

SIDE EFFECTS

Frequent: Insomnia, heartburn, anxiety, abdominal distention, increased diaphoresis, acne, mood swings, increased appetite, facial flushing, delayed wound healing, increased susceptibility to infection, diarrhea, constipation. **Occasional:** Headache, edema, change in skin color, frequent urination. **Rare:** Tachycardia, allergic reaction (rash, urticaria), psychological changes, hallucinations, depression.

ADVERSE EFFECTS/ TOXIC REACTIONS

Long-term therapy: Hypocalcemia, hypokalemia, muscle wasting (esp. arms, legs), osteoporosis, spontaneous fractures, amenorrhea, cataracts, glaucoma, peptic ulcer, HF. **Abrupt withdrawal following long-term therapy:** Anorexia, nausea, fever, headache, joint pain, rebound inflammation, fatigue, weakness, lethargy, dizziness, orthostatic hypotension.

NURSING CONSIDERATIONS

BASELINE ASSESSMENT

Question for hypersensitivity to any corticosteroids. Obtain baseline values for weight, B/P, serum glucose, cholesterol, electrolytes.

INTERVENTION/EVALUATION

Be alert for infection (reduced immune response): sore throat, fever, vague symptoms. For pts on long-term therapy, monitor for hypocalcemia (muscle twitching, cramps, positive Trousseau's or Chvostek's signs), hypokalemia (weakness, muscle cramps, numbness/tingling [esp. lower extremities], nausea/vomiting, irritability, EKG changes). Assess emotional status, ability to sleep.

PATIENT/FAMILY TEACHING

• Do not change dose or schedule or stop taking drug; **must** taper off under medical supervision. • Notify physician of fever, sore throat, muscle aches, sudden weight gain/swelling. • Inform dentist, other physicians of cortisone therapy now or within past 12 mos.

cosyntropin

koe-sin-**troe**-pin
(Cortrosyn)
Do not confuse Cortrosyn with colchicine, cortisone, or Cotazym.

◆CLASSIFICATION

PHARMACOTHERAPEUTIC: Adrenocortical steroid. **CLINICAL:** Glucocorticoid.

ACTION

Stimulates initial reaction in synthesis of adrenal steroids from cholesterol. **Therapeutic Effect:** Increases endogenous corticoid synthesis.

USES

Diagnostic testing of adrenocortical function.

PRECAUTIONS

Contraindications: Hypersensitivity to cosyntropin, corticotropin. **Cautions:** Preexisting allergies, history of allergic reaction to corticotropin.

⧖ LIFESPAN CONSIDERATIONS

Pregnancy/Lactation: Unknown if distributed in breast milk. **Pregnancy Category C. Children/Elderly:** No age-related precautions noted.

INTERACTIONS

DRUG: None significant. **HERBAL:** None significant. **FOOD:** None known. **LAB VALUES:** None significant.

AVAILABILITY (Rx)

Powder for Injection: 0.25 mg. **Injection, Solution:** 0.25 mg/ml.

ADMINISTRATION/HANDLING

Reconstitution
IM: • Reconstitute with 1 ml 0.9% NaCl. • Give as 0.25 mg/ml concentration.

IV Push: • Dilute with 2–5 ml 0.9% NaCl over 2 min.

Storage
Powder: • Room temperature. **Solution:** • Refrigerate.

INDICATIONS/ROUTES/DOSAGE
Adrenocortical Insufficiency
IM, IV: ADULTS, ELDERLY, CHILDREN OLDER THAN 2 YRS: 0.25–0.75 mg. **CHILDREN 2 YRS AND YOUNGER:** 0.125 mg. **NEONATES:** 0.015 mg/kg/dose.
IV Infusion: ADULTS, ELDERLY, CHILDREN OLDER THAN 2 YRS: 0.25 mg over 6 hrs at 0.04 mg/hr.

SIDE EFFECTS
Occasional: Nausea, vomiting. **Rare:** Hypersensitivity reaction (fever, pruritus).

ADVERSE EFFECTS/ TOXIC REACTIONS
None known.

NURSING CONSIDERATIONS

BASELINE ASSESSMENT
Hold cortisone, hydrocortisone, spironolactone the day prior to and the day of the test. Ensure that baseline plasma cortisol concentration has been drawn before start of test or 24-hr urine for 17-KS or 17-OHCS is initiated.

INTERVENTION/EVALUATION
Adhere to time frame for blood draws; monitor urine collection if indicated.

PATIENT/FAMILY TEACHING
• Explain procedure, purpose of test.

crizotinib

kriz-**oh**-ti-nib
(Xalkori)

◆**CLASSIFICATION**

PHARMACOTHERAPEUTIC: Tyrosine kinase inhibitor. **CLINICAL:** Antineoplastic (see p. 84C).

ACTION
Inhibits receptor tyrosine kinases including anaplastic lymphoma kinase (ALK), hepatocyte growth factor receptors (HGFR, c-Met), receptor d'origine nantais (RON). **Therapeutic Effect:** Inhibits tumor cell proliferation and survival.

PHARMACOKINETICS
Well absorbed after PO administration. Peak plasma concentration: 4–6 hrs. Protein binding: 91%. Metabolized in liver. Excreted in feces (63%) and urine (22%). **Half-life:** 42 hrs.

USES
Treatment of locally advanced or metastatic non–small-cell lung cancer (NSCLC) that is anaplastic lymphoma kinase (ALK) positive.

PRECAUTIONS
Contraindications: None known. **Cautions:** Baseline hepatic impairment, congenital long QT interval syndrome. Pregnancy (avoid use).

⧖ LIFESPAN CONSIDERATIONS
Pregnancy/Lactation: Avoid pregnancy. May cause fetal harm. Contraception should be considered during therapy and for at least 12 wks after discontinuation. Do not initiate therapy until pregnancy status confirmed. Unknown if crosses placenta or distributed in breast milk. Nursing mothers must discontinue either nursing or drug therapy. **Pregnancy Category D. Children:** Safety and efficacy not established. **Elderly:** No age-related precautions noted.

INTERACTIONS
DRUG: Strong **CYP3A inhibitors** including **atazanavir, clarithromycin, itra-**

conazole, **ketoconazole**, **ritonavir**, **saquinavir**, **voriconazole** may increase concentration. Strong **CYP3A inducers** including **carbamazepine**, **phenytoin**, **rifabutin**, **rifampin** may decrease concentration. May alter plasma levels of **alfentanil**, **cyclosporine**, **dihydroergotamine**, **ergotamine**, **fentanyl**, **pimozide**, **sirolimus**. **Proton pump inhibitors**, **H_2 blockers**, **antacids** may decrease solubility. May increase plasma levels of **colchicine**, **dexamethasone**, **doxorubicin**, **etoposide**, **non-nucleoside reverse transcriptase inhibitors**, **protease inhibitors**, **quinidine**, **tacrolimus**, **vinblastine**. HERBAL: **St. John's wort** may decrease effectiveness. FOOD: **Grapefruit** or **grapefruit juice** may increase concentration/toxicity (potential for torsades, myelotoxicity). LAB VALUES: May increase serum ALT, AST, alkaline phosphatase, bilirubin. May decrease neutrophils, platelets, lymphocytes.

AVAILABILITY (Rx)

Capsules: 200 mg, 250 mg.

ADMINISTRATION/HANDLING

• May give without regard to meals.
• Avoid grapefruit or grapefruit products. • Do not crush or cut.

INDICATIONS/ROUTES/DOSAGE

Non–Small-Cell Lung Cancer (ALK-Positive)
PO: ADULTS: 250 mg twice daily. Dosage Modification: Interrupt and/or reduce to 200 mg twice daily based on graded protocol, including hematologic toxicity (grade 4), elevated LFTs with bilirubin elevation (grade 1), QT prolongation (grade 3). May reduce to 250 mg once daily if indicated. Discontinue treatment for QT prolongation (grade 4), elevated LFTs with bilirubin elevation (grade 2, 3, 4), any pneumonitis grade.

SIDE EFFECTS

Frequent (62%–27%): Diplopia, photopsia, photophobia, blurry vision, visual field defect, vitreous floaters, reduced visual acuity, nausea, diarrhea, vomiting, peripheral/localized edema, constipation. Occasional (20%–4%): Fatigue, decreased appetite, dizziness, neuropathy, paresthesia, dysgeusia, dyspepsia, dysphagia, esophageal obstruction/pain/spasm/ulcer, odynophagia, reflux esophagitis, rash, abdominal pain/tenderness, stomatitis, glossodynia, glossitis, cheilitis, mucosal inflammation, oropharyngeal pain/discomfort, bradycardia, headache, cough. Rare (3%–1%): Musculoskeletal chest pain, insomnia, dyspnea, arthralgia, nasopharyngitis, rhinitis, pharyngitis, URI, back pain, complex renal cysts, chest pain/tightness.

ADVERSE EFFECTS/ TOXIC REACTIONS

Severe, sometimes fatal treatment-related pneumonitis, pneumonia, dyspnea, pulmonary embolism in less than 2% of pts was noted. Grade 3–4 elevation of hepatic enzymes, increased QT prolongation may require discontinuation. May cause thrombocytopenia, neutropenia, lymphopenia. Severe/worsening vitreous floaters, photopsia may indicate retinal hole, retinal detachment.

NURSING CONSIDERATIONS

BASELINE ASSESSMENT

Assess vital signs, O_2 saturation. Obtain baseline CBC with differential, serum chemistries, hepatic function test, PT/INR, EKG. Question possibility of pregnancy or plans for breastfeeding. Obtain full medication history including vitamins, minerals, herbal products. Detection of ALK-positive NSCLC test needed prior to treatment. Assess history of tuberculosis, HIV, HF, bradyarrhythmias, electrolyte imbalance, medications that prolong QT interval. Assess visual acuity, history of vitreous floaters.

INTERVENTION/EVALUATION

Assess vital signs, O_2 saturation routinely. Monitor CBC with differential monthly, hepatic function tests monthly; increase testing for grades 2, 3, 4 adverse effects. Obtain EKG for bradycardia, electrolyte imbalance, chest pain, difficulty breathing. Monitor for bruising, hematuria, jaundice, right upper abdominal pain, weight loss, or acute infection (fever, diaphoresis, lethargy, oral mucosal changes, productive cough). Report decrease in RBC, Hgb, Hct, platelets, neutrophils, lymphocytes. Worsening cough, fever, or shortness of breath may indicate pneumonitis. Consider ophthalmological evaluation for vision changes. Reinforce birth control compliance.

PATIENT/FAMILY TEACHING

• Blood levels will be drawn routinely. • Report urine changes, bloody or clay-colored stools, upper abdominal pain, nausea, vomiting, bruising, fever, cough, difficulty breathing. • Report history of liver abnormalities or heart problems including long QT syndrome, syncope, palpitations, extremity swelling. • Immediately report any newly prescribed medications, suspected pregnancy, or vision changes including light flashes, blurred vision, increased floaters, photophobia, or new or increased floaters. • Contraception recommended during treatment and for at least 3 mos after treatment. • Avoid alcohol. • Do not ingest grapefruit products.

---

cyanocobalamin (vitamin B₁₂)

sye-an-oh-koe-**bal**-a-min
(Nascobal)

◆CLASSIFICATION

PHARMACOTHERAPEUTIC: Coenzyme.
CLINICAL: Vitamin, antianemic (see p. 158C).

ACTION

Coenzyme for metabolic functions (fat, carbohydrate metabolism, protein synthesis). **Therapeutic Effect:** Necessary for cell growth and replication, hematopoiesis, myelin synthesis.

PHARMACOKINETICS

In presence of calcium, absorbed systemically in lower half of ileum. Initially, bound to intrinsic factor; this complex passes down intestine, binding to receptor sites on ileal mucosa. Protein binding: High. Metabolized in liver. Primarily eliminated unchanged in urine. **Half-life:** 6 days.

USES

Treatment of pernicious anemia, vitamin B₁₂ deficiency due to malabsorption diseases, increased B₁₂ requirement due to pregnancy, thyrotoxicosis, hemorrhage, malignancy, hepatic/renal disease. **Calo-Mist:** Maintenance of vitamin B₁₂ concentrations.

PRECAUTIONS

Contraindications: Hereditary optic nerve atrophy. **Cautions:** Folic acid deficiency, anemia, premature neonates.

⧗ LIFESPAN CONSIDERATIONS

Pregnancy/Lactation: Crosses placenta. Distributed in breast milk. **Pregnancy Category A (C if used in doses above recommended daily allowance; C for intranasal). Children/Elderly:** No age-related precautions noted.

INTERACTIONS

DRUG: None significant. **HERBAL:** None significant. **FOOD:** None known. **LAB VALUES:** None significant.

AVAILABILITY (Rx)

Injection Solution: 1,000 mcg/ml. **Nasal Spray (Nascobal):** 500 mcg/spray. **Tablets:** 50 mcg, 100 mcg, 250 mcg, 500 mcg, 1,000 mcg. **Tablets (Extended-Release):** 1,000 mcg, 1,500 mcg.

ADMINISTRATION/HANDLING

IM, Subcutaneous
• Avoid IV route.

PO
• May give without regard to food.

Intranasal
• Clear both nostrils. • Pull clear cover off top of pump. • Press down firmly and quickly on pump's finger grips until a droplet of gel appears at top. Then press down on finger grips two more times. • Place the tip halfway into nostril, pointing tip toward back of nose. • Press down firmly and quickly on finger grips to release medication into one nostril while pressing other nostril closed. • Massage medicated nostril for a few seconds. • Administer nasal preparation at least 1 hr before or 1 hr after hot foods or liquids are consumed (hot foods can cause nasal secretion, resulting in loss of medication).

INDICATIONS/ROUTES/DOSAGE

Pernicious Anemia
IM, Subcutaneous: ADULTS, ELDERLY: 100 mcg/day for 7 days, then every other day for 7 days, then every 3–4 days for 2–3 wks. Maintenance: 100 mcg/mo (PO 1,000–2,000 mcg/day). **CHILDREN:** 30–50 mcg/day for 2 or more wks. Maintenance: 100 mcg/mo. **NEONATES:** 0.2 mcg/kg for 2 days, then 1,000 mcg/day for 2–7 days. Maintenance: 100 mcg/mo.

Vitamin Deficiency
IM, Subcutaneous: ADULTS, ELDERLY: 30 mcg/day for 5–10 days, then 100–200 mcg/mo.
PO: ADULTS, ELDERLY: 250 mcg/day.
Intranasal: ADULTS, ELDERLY: (NASCOBAL): 500 mcg in one nostril once weekly.

SIDE EFFECTS

Occasional: Diarrhea, pruritus.

ADVERSE EFFECTS/ TOXIC REACTIONS

Impurities in preparation may cause rare allergic reaction. Peripheral vascular thrombosis, pulmonary edema, hypokalemia, HF occur rarely.

C

NURSING CONSIDERATIONS

BASELINE ASSESSMENT
Assess for signs, symptoms of vitamin B_{12} deficiency (anorexia, ataxia, fatigue, hyporeflexia, insomnia, irritability, loss of positional sense, pallor, palpitations on exertion).

INTERVENTION/EVALUATION
Assess for HF, pulmonary edema, hypokalemia in cardiac pts receiving subcutaneous/IM therapy. Monitor serum potassium, serum B_{12}, rise in reticulocyte count (peaks in 5–8 days). Assess for reversal of deficiency symptoms (hyporeflexia, loss of positional sense, ataxia, fatigue, irritability, insomnia, anorexia, pallor, palpitations on exertion). Therapeutic response usually dramatic within 48 hrs.

PATIENT/FAMILY TEACHING
• Lifetime treatment may be necessary with pernicious anemia. • Report symptoms of infection. • Foods rich in vitamin B_{12} include clams, oysters, herring, red snapper, muscle meats, fermented cheese, dairy products, egg yolks. • Use nasal preparation at least 1 hr before or 1 hr after consuming hot foods, liquids.

TOP 200

cyclobenzaprine

sye-kloe-**ben**-za-preen
(Amrix, Apo-Cyclobenzaprine ❦,
Flexeril, Fexmid,
Novo-Cycloprine ❦)

❦ Canadian trade name   🦬 Non-Crushable Drug   🟥 High Alert drug

Do not confuse cyclobenzaprine with cycloserine or cyproheptadine, or Flexeril with Floxin.

◆**CLASSIFICATION**

CLINICAL: Skeletal muscle relaxant (see p. 151C).

ACTION

Centrally acting skeletal muscle relaxant that reduces tonic somatic muscle activity at level of brainstem. **Therapeutic Effect:** Relieves local skeletal muscle spasm.

PHARMACOKINETICS

Route	Onset	Peak	Duration
PO	1 hr	3–4 hrs	12–24 hrs

Well but slowly absorbed from GI tract. Protein binding: 93%. Metabolized in GI tract and liver. Primarily excreted in urine. **Half-life:** 8–37 hrs.

USES

Treatment of muscle spasm associated with acute, painful musculoskeletal conditions. **OFF-LABEL:** Treatment of muscle spasms associated with temporomandibular joint pain (TMJ).

PRECAUTIONS

Contraindications: Acute recovery phase of MI, arrhythmias, HF, heart block, conduction disturbances, hyperthyroidism, use within 14 days of MAOIs. **Cautions:** Hepatic impairment, history of urinary hesitancy or retention, angle-closure glaucoma, increased intraocular pressure (IOP), elderly.

⧗ LIFESPAN CONSIDERATIONS

Pregnancy/Lactation: Unknown if drug crosses placenta or is distributed in breast milk. **Pregnancy Category B. Children:** Safety and efficacy not established. **Elderly:** Increased sensitivity to anticholinergic effects (e.g., confusion, urinary retention).

INTERACTIONS

DRUG: Alcohol, other CNS depressant medications may increase CNS depression. **MAOIs** may increase risk of hypertensive crisis, seizures. **Tramadol** may increase risk of seizures. **HERBAL: Gotu kola, kava kava, SAMe, St. John's wort, valerian** may increase CNS depression. **FOOD:** None known. **LAB VALUES:** None significant.

AVAILABILITY (Rx)

Tablets: (Flexeril): 5 mg, 10 mg. (Flexmid): 7.5 mg.

▧ Capsules (Extended-Release [Amrix]): 15 mg, 30 mg.

ADMINISTRATION/HANDLING

PO

• Give without regard to food. • Do not break, chew, crush, or divide extended-release capsule. • Give extended-release capsule at same time each day.

INDICATIONS/ROUTES/DOSAGE

◄**ALERT**► Do not use longer than 2–3 wks.

Acute, Painful Musculoskeletal Conditions
PO: ADULTS, ELDERLY, CHILDREN 15 YRS AND OLDER: Initially, 5 mg 3 times a day. May increase to 7.5–10 mg 3 times a day.
PO (Extended-Release): ADULTS, ELDERLY: 15–30 mg once daily.

Dosage in Hepatic Impairment
Note: Extended-release capsule not recommended in hepatic impairment. **MILD:** 5 mg 3 times a day. **MODERATE AND SEVERE:** Not recommended.

SIDE EFFECTS

Frequent (39%–11%): Drowsiness, dry mouth, dizziness. Rare (3%–1%): Fatigue, asthenia (loss of strength, energy), blurred vision, headache, anxiety, confusion, nausea, constipation, dyspepsia, unpleasant taste.

ADVERSE EFFECTS/ TOXIC REACTIONS

Overdose may result in visual hallucinations, hyperactive reflexes, muscle rigidity, vomiting, hyperpyrexia.

NURSING CONSIDERATIONS

BASELINE ASSESSMENT

Record onset, type, location, duration of muscular spasm. Check for immobility, stiffness, swelling.

INTERVENTION/EVALUATION

Assist with ambulation. Assess for therapeutic response: relief of pain; decreased stiffness, swelling; increased joint mobility; reduced joint tenderness; improved grip strength.

PATIENT/FAMILY TEACHING

• Drowsiness usually diminishes with continued therapy. • Avoid tasks that require alertness, motor skills until response to drug is established. • Avoid alcohol, other depressants while taking medication. • Avoid sudden changes in posture. • Sugarless gum, sips of water may relieve dry mouth.

---

cyclophosphamide

sye-kloe-**foss**-fa-mide
(Procytox ✦)
Do not confuse cyclophosphamide with cyclosporine or ifosfamide.

◆CLASSIFICATION

PHARMACOTHERAPEUTIC: Alkylating agent. **CLINICAL:** Antineoplastic (see p. 84C).

ACTION

Inhibits DNA, RNA protein synthesis by cross-linking with DNA, RNA strands. Cell cycle–phase nonspecific. **Therapeutic Effect:** Prevents cell growth. Potent immunosuppressant.

PHARMACOKINETICS

Well absorbed from GI tract. Protein binding: 10%–60%. Crosses blood-brain barrier. Metabolized in liver. Primarily excreted in urine. Removed by hemodialysis. **Half-life:** 3–12 hrs.

USES

Treatment of acute lymphocytic, acute nonlymphocytic, chronic myelocytic, chronic lymphocytic leukemias; ovarian, breast carcinomas; neuroblastoma; retinoblastoma; Hodgkin's, non-Hodgkin's lymphomas; multiple myeloma; mycosis fungoides; nephrotic syndrome in children. **OFF-LABEL:** Treatment of adrenocortical, bladder, cervical, endometrial, prostatic, testicular carcinomas; Ewing's sarcoma; multiple sclerosis; non–small-cell, small-cell lung cancer; organ transplant rejection; osteosarcoma; ovarian germ cell, primary brain, trophoblastic tumors; rheumatoid arthritis; soft-tissue sarcomas; systemic dermatomyositis; systemic lupus erythematosus; Wilms' tumor.

PRECAUTIONS

Contraindications: Severe myelosuppression. **Cautions:** Severe leukopenia, thrombocytopenia, tumor infiltration of bone marrow, previous therapy with other antineoplastic agents, radiation, renal/hepatic impairment.

⌛ LIFESPAN CONSIDERATIONS

Pregnancy/Lactation: If possible, avoid use during pregnancy. May cause fetal malformations (limb abnormalities, cardiac anomalies, hernias). Distributed in breast milk. Breast-feeding not recommended. **Pregnancy Category D. Children:** No age-related precautions noted.

Elderly: Age-related renal impairment may require dosage adjustment.

INTERACTIONS

DRUG: CYP2D6 inducers (e.g., carbamazepine, phenobarbital) may decrease concentration; **CYP2D6 inhibitors (e.g., paroxetine, amiodarone)** may increase concentration. **Anthracycline agents (e.g., doxorubicin, epirubicin)** may increase risk of cardiomyopathy. **CYP3A4 inhibitors (e.g., ketoconazole)** may increase concentrations, risk of adverse effects. **Live virus vaccines** may potentiate virus replication, increase vaccine side effects, decrease pt's antibody response to vaccine. **HERBAL:** Pts with an estrogen-dependent tumor should avoid **black cohosh, dong quai. FOOD:** None known. **LAB VALUES:** May increase serum uric acid.

AVAILABILITY (Rx)

Injection, Powder for Reconstitution: 500 mg, 1 g, 2 g.

Tablets: 25 mg, 50 mg.

ADMINISTRATION/HANDLING

◄ALERT► May be carcinogenic, mutagenic, teratogenic. Handle with extreme care during preparation/administration.

 IV

Reconstitution • Reconstitute each 100 mg with 5 ml Sterile Water for Injection, 0.9% NaCl, or D₅W to provide concentration of 20 mg/ml. • Shake to dissolve. • Allow to stand until clear.
Rate of Administration • May give by IV push or further dilute with 250 ml D₅W, 0.9% NaCl. • IV infusions may be given over 1–24 hrs. • Doses of 500 mg to 2g may be given over 20–30 min. • IV route may produce faintness, facial flushing, diaphoresis, oropharyngeal sensation.
Storage • Reconstituted solution is stable for 24 hrs at room temperature or up to 6 days if refrigerated.

PO
• Give on an empty stomach. If GI upset occurs, give with food. • Do not cut or crush. • To minimize risk of bladder irritation, do not give at bedtime.

IV INCOMPATIBILITY

Amphotericin B complex (Abelcet, AmBisome, Amphotec).

IV COMPATIBILITIES

Granisetron (Kytril), heparin, hydromorphone (Dilaudid), lorazepam (Ativan), morphine, ondansetron (Zofran), propofol (Diprivan).

INDICATIONS/ROUTES/DOSAGE

Usual Dosage (Refer to Individual Protocols)
IV: ADULTS, ELDERLY, CHILDREN: (Single agent): 40–50 mg/kg in divided doses over 2–5 days or 10–15 mg/kg q7–10 days or 3–5 mg/kg twice weekly.
PO: ADULTS, ELDERLY, CHILDREN: 1–5 mg/kg/day.

Nephrotic Syndrome
PO: ADULTS, CHILDREN: 2.5–3 mg/kg/day for 60–90 days.

SIDE EFFECTS

Expected: Marked leukopenia 8–15 days after initiation. **Frequent:** Nausea, vomiting (beginning about 6 hrs after administration and lasting about 4 hrs); alopecia (33%). **Occasional:** Diarrhea, darkening of skin/fingernails, stomatitis, headache, diaphoresis. **Rare:** Pain/redness at injection site.

ADVERSE EFFECTS/ TOXIC REACTIONS

Myelosuppression resulting in blood dyscrasias (leukopenia, anemia, thrombocytopenia, hypoprothrombinemia) was noted. Expect leukopenia to resolve in 17–28 days. Anemia generally occurs after large doses or prolonged therapy. Thrombocytopenia may occur 10–15 days after drug initiation. Hemorrhagic cystitis occurs commonly in long-term therapy (esp. in children). Pulmonary fibrosis, cardiotoxicity noted with high doses. Amenorrhea, azoospermia, hyperkalemia may occur.

NURSING CONSIDERATIONS

BASELINE ASSESSMENT

Obtain CBC weekly during therapy or until maintenance dose is established, then at 2- to 3-wk intervals.

INTERVENTION/EVALUATION

Monitor CBC, serum creatinine, BUN, urine output, serum uric acid, electrolytes. Monitor WBC counts closely during initial therapy. Monitor for hematologic toxicity (fever, sore throat, signs of local infection, unusual bruising/bleeding from any site), symptoms of anemia (excessive fatigue, weakness). Recovery from marked leukopenia due to myelosuppression can be expected in 17–28 days.

PATIENT/FAMILY TEACHING

• Encourage copious fluid intake, frequent voiding (assists in preventing cystitis) at least 24 hrs before, during, after therapy. • Do not have immunizations without physician's approval (drug lowers resistance). • Avoid contact with those who have recently received live virus vaccine. • Promptly report fever, sore throat, signs of local infection, difficulty or pain with urination, unusual bruising/ bleeding from any site. • Hair loss is reversible, but new hair growth may have different color, texture.

*cycloSPORINE

sye-kloe-**spor**-in
(Gengraf, Neoral, <u>Restasis</u>, Sandimmune)

BLACK BOX ALERT Only physicians experienced in management of immunosuppressive therapy and organ transplant pts should prescribe. Renal impairment may occur with high dosage. Increased risk of neoplasia, susceptibility to infections. May cause hypertension, nephrotoxicity. Psoriasis pts: Increased risk of developing skin malignancies.

Do not confuse cyclosporine with cycloserine or cyclophosphamide, Gengraf with ProGraf, Neoral with Neurontin or Nizoral, or Sandimmune with Sandostatin.

◆CLASSIFICATION

PHARMACOTHERAPEUTIC: Cyclic polypeptide. **CLINICAL:** Immunosuppressant (see p. 123C).

ACTION

Inhibits cellular, humoral immune responses by inhibiting interleukin-2, a proliferative factor needed for T-cell activity. **Therapeutic Effect:** Prevents organ rejection, relieves symptoms of psoriasis, arthritis.

PHARMACOKINETICS

Variably absorbed from GI tract. Protein binding: 90%. Metabolized in liver. Eliminated primarily by biliary or fecal excretion. Not removed by hemodialysis. **Half-life:** Adults, 10–27 hrs; children, 7–19 hrs.

USES

Prevents organ rejection of kidney, liver, heart in combination with steroid therapy and/or azathioprine. Treatment of chronic allograft rejection in those previously treated with other immunosuppressives. **Capsules/solution:** Treatment of severe, active rheumatoid arthritis, severe recalcitrant plaque psoriasis in nonimmunocompromised adults. **Ophthalmic:** Chronic dry eyes. OFF-LABEL: Allogenic stem cell transplants for prevention/treatment of graft-vs-host disease; focal segmental glomerulosclerosis, severe ulcerative colitis.

PRECAUTIONS

Contraindications: History of hypersensitivity to cyclosporine, polyoxyethylated castor oil; uncontrolled hypertension, renal impairment, or malignancies in treatment of psoriasis or rheumatoid arthritis. **Cautions:** Hepatic/renal, impairment. **Ophthalmic:** Active eye infection.

⌛ LIFESPAN CONSIDERATIONS

Pregnancy/Lactation: Readily crosses placenta. Distributed in breast milk. Breastfeeding not recommended. **Pregnancy Category C. Children:** No age-related precautions noted in transplant pts. **Elderly:** Increased risk of hypertension, increased serum creatinine.

INTERACTIONS

DRUG: Allopurinol, bromocriptine, cimetidine, clarithromycin, danazol, diltiazem, oral contraceptives, erythromycin, fluconazole, itraconazole, ketoconazole may increase concentration, risk of hepatic/renal toxicity. **Rifampin, carbamazepine, phenytoin** may decrease **cyclosporine** concentration. **ACE inhibitors, potassium-sparing diuretics, potassium supplements** may cause hyperkalemia. **Immunosuppressants** may increase risk of infection, lymphoproliferative disorders. **Lovastatin, simvastatin, atorvastatin, pravastatin** may increase risk of rhabdomyolysis. **Live virus vaccines** may potentiate virus replication, increase vaccine side effects, decrease pt's response to vaccine. May increase concentration/toxicity of **digoxin, colchicine. HERBAL:** Avoid **cat's claw, echinacea** (possess immunostimulant properties). **St. John's wort** may decrease plasma concentration. **FOOD: Grapefruit, grapefruit products** may increase absorption/immunosupression, risk of toxicity. **LAB VALUES:** May increase BUN, serum alkaline phosphatase, amylase, bilirubin, creatinine, potassium, uric acid, AST, ALT. May decrease serum magnesium. **Therapeutic peak serum level:** 50–400 ng/ml; **toxic serum level:** greater than 400 ng/ml.

AVAILABILITY (Rx)

Capsules (Gengraf, Neoral [Modified], Sandimmune [Nonmodified]): 25 mg, 100 mg. **Injection, Solution (Sandimmune):** 50 mg/ml. **Ophthalmic Emulsion (Restasis):** 0.05%. **Oral Solution (Gengraf, Neoral [Modified], Sandimmune [Nonmodified]):** 100 mg/ml.

ADMINISTRATION/HANDLING

◀**ALERT**▶ Oral solution available in bottle form with calibrated liquid measuring device. Oral form should replace IV administration as soon as possible.

 IV

Reconstitution • Dilute each ml (50 mg) concentrate with 20–100 ml 0.9% NaCl or D_5W (**maximum concentration:** 2.5 mg/ml).
Rate of Administration • Infuse over 2–6 hrs. • Monitor pt continuously for hypersensitivity reaction (facial flushing, dyspnea).
Storage • Store parenteral form at room temperature. • Protect IV solution from light. • After diluted, stable for 6 hrs in PVC; 24 hrs in Excel or glass.

PO

• Administer consistently with relation to time of day and meals. • Oral solution may be mixed in glass container with milk, chocolate milk, orange juice, or apple juice (preferably at room temperature). Stir well. • Drink immediately. • Add more diluent to glass container. Mix with remaining solution to ensure total amount is given. • Dry outside of calibrated liquid measuring device before replacing cover. • Do not rinse with water. • Avoid refrigeration of oral solution (solution may separate). • Discard oral solution after 2 mos once bottle is opened.

Ophthalmic

• Invert vial several times to obtain uniform suspension. • Instruct pt to remove contact lenses before administration

---

(may reinsert 15 min after administration). • May use with artificial tears.

🔲 IV INCOMPATIBILITIES

Acyclovir (Zovirax), amphotericin B complex (Abelcet, AmBisome, Amphotec), magnesium.

🔲 IV COMPATIBILITIES

Propofol (Diprivan).

INDICATIONS/ROUTES/DOSAGE

Transplantation, Prevention of Organ Rejection
PO: ADULTS, ELDERLY, CHILDREN: NOT MODIFIED: 10–18 mg/kg/dose given 4–12 hrs prior to organ transplantation. Maintenance: 5–15 mg/kg/day in divided doses then tapered to 3–10 mg/kg/day. **MODIFIED:** (dose dependent upon type of transplant): Renal: 6–12 mg/kg/day in 2 divided doses. Hepatic: 4–12 mg/kg/day in 2 divided doses. Heart: 4–10 mg/kg/day in 2 divided doses.
IV: ADULTS, ELDERLY, CHILDREN: Initially, 5–6 mg/kg/dose given 4–12 hrs prior to organ transplantation. Maintenance: 2–10 mg/kg/day in divided doses.

Rheumatoid Arthritis
PO: ADULTS, ELDERLY: Initially, 2.5 mg/kg a day in 2 divided doses. May increase by 0.5–0.75 mg/kg/day. **Maximum:** 4 mg/kg/day.

Psoriasis
PO: ADULTS, ELDERLY: Initially, 2.5 mg/kg/day in 2 divided doses. May increase by 0.5 mg/kg/day after 4 wks; additional increases may be made q2wks. **Maximum:** 4 mg/kg/day.

Dry Eye
Ophthalmic: ADULTS, ELDERLY: Instill 1 drop in each affected eye q12h.

SIDE EFFECTS

Frequent (26%–12%): Mild to moderate hypertension, hirsutism, tremor. **Occasional (4%–2%):** Acne, leg cramps, gingi-

val hyperplasia (red, bleeding, tender gums), paresthesia, diarrhea, nausea, vomiting, headache. **Rare (less than 1%):** Hypersensitivity reaction, abdominal discomfort, gynecomastia, sinusitis.

ADVERSE EFFECTS/TOXIC REACTIONS

Mild nephrotoxicity occurs in 25% of renal transplants, 38% of cardiac transplants, 37% of liver transplants, generally 2–3 mos after transplantation (more severe toxicity may occur soon after transplantation). Hepatotoxicity occurs in 4% of renal, 7% of cardiac, and 4% of liver transplants, generally within first mo after transplantation. Both toxicities usually respond to dosage reduction. Severe hyperkalemia, hyperuricemia occur occasionally.

NURSING CONSIDERATIONS

BASELINE ASSESSMENT
Obtain baseline serum chemistries, esp. renal/hepatic function tests. If nephrotoxicity occurs, mild toxicity is generally noted 2–3 mos after transplantation; more severe toxicity noted early after transplantation; hepatotoxicity may be noted during first mo after transplantation.

INTERVENTION/EVALUATION
Diligently monitor BUN, serum creatinine, bilirubin, AST, ALT, LDH levels for evidence of hepatotoxicity, nephrotoxicity (mild toxicity noted by slow rise in serum levels; more overt toxicity noted by rapid rise in levels; hematuria also noted in nephrotoxicity). Monitor serum potassium for evidence of hyperkalemia. Encourage diligent oral hygiene (gingival hyperplasia). Monitor B/P for evidence of hypertension. **Note:** Reference ranges dependent on organ transplanted, organ function, cyclosporine toxicity. Trough levels should be obtained immediately prior to next dose. **Therapeutic serum level:** 50–400 ng/ml; **toxic serum level:** greater than 400 ng/ml.

PATIENT/FAMILY TEACHING

• Blood levels will be drawn routinely. • Report severe headache, persistent nausea/vomiting, unusual swelling of extremities, chest pain. • Avoid grapefruit products (increases concentration/effects), St. John's wort (decreases concentration).

---

cytarabine

sye-**tar**-ah-bine
(Ara-C, Cytosar-U ✤, Depo-Cyt)

BLACK BOX ALERT Must be administered by personnel trained in administration/handling of chemotherapeutic agents. **Conventional:** Potent myelosuppressant. High risk of multiple toxicities (GI, CNS, pulmonary, cardiac). **Liposomal:** Chemical arachnoiditis, manifested by profound nausea, vomiting, fever, may be fatal if untreated.
Do not confuse cytarabine with Cytoxan or vidarabine, or Cytosar with Cytoxan or Neosar.

◆CLASSIFICATION

PHARMACOTHERAPEUTIC: Antimetabolite. **CLINICAL:** Antineoplastic (see p. 84C).

ACTION

Converted intracellularly to nucleotide. Cell cycle–specific for S phase of cell division. **Therapeutic Effect:** Appears to inhibit DNA synthesis. Potent immunosuppressive activity.

PHARMACOKINETICS

Widely distributed; moderate amount crosses blood-brain barrier. Protein binding: 15%. Primarily excreted in urine. Half-life: 1–3 hrs.

USES

Ara-C: Treatment of acute lymphocytic, acute nonlymphocytic, chronic myelocytic, meningeal leukemias. **Depo-Cyt:** Treatment of lymphomatous meningitis. **OFF-LABEL: Ara-C:** Carcinomatous meningitis, Hodgkin's and non-Hodgkin's lymphomas, myelodysplastic syndrome.

PRECAUTIONS

Contraindications: (Liposomal): Active meningeal infection. **Cautions:** Renal/hepatic impairment, prior bone marrow suppression.

⌛ LIFESPAN CONSIDERATIONS

Pregnancy/Lactation: If possible, avoid use during pregnancy. May cause fetal malformations. Unknown if distributed in breast milk. Breastfeeding not recommended. **Pregnancy Category D. Children:** No age-related precautions noted. **Elderly:** Age-related renal impairment may require dosage adjustment.

INTERACTIONS

DRUG: May decrease concentration of **digoxin, flucytosine. Live virus vaccines** may potentiate virus replication, increase vaccine side effects, decrease pt's response to vaccine. **HERBAL: Echinacea** may decrease therapeutic effect. **FOOD:** None known. **LAB VALUES:** May increase serum alkaline phosphatase, bilirubin, uric acid, AST.

AVAILABILITY (Rx)

Injection, Powder for Reconstitution (Ara-C): 100 mg, 500 mg, 1 g, 2 g. Injection, Solution (Ara-C): 20 mg/ml, 100 mg/ml. Injection, Suspension (Depo-Cyt): 10 mg/ml.

ADMINISTRATION/HANDLING

◄**ALERT**► May give by subcutaneous, IV push, IV infusion, intrathecal routes at concentration not to exceed 100 mg/ml. May be carcinogenic, mutagenic, teratogenic (embryonic deformity). Handle with extreme care during preparation/administration. Depo-Cyt for intrathecal use only.

C

IV, Subcutaneous, Intrathecal

 IV

Reconstitution • Ara-C: Reconstitute with Bacteriostatic Water for Injection. • Dose may be further diluted with 250–1,000 ml D₅W or 0.9% NaCl for IV infusion. • For intrathecal use, reconstitute vial with preservative-free 0.9% NaCl or pt's spinal fluid. Dose usually administered in 5–15 ml of solution, after equivalent volume of CSF removed. • Depo-Cyt: No reconstitution required.

Rate of Administration • Ara-C: For IV infusion, give over 1–3 hrs or as continuous infusion.

Storage • Ara-C: Store at room temperature. • Reconstituted solution is stable for 48 hrs at room temperature. • Use diluted solution within 24 hrs. • Discard if slight haze develops. • Depo-Cyt: Refrigerate; use within 4 hrs following withdrawal from vial.

🔷 IV INCOMPATIBILITIES

Amphotericin B complex (Abelcet, AmBisome, Amphotec), ganciclovir (Cytovene), heparin, insulin (regular).

🔷 IV COMPATIBILITIES

Dexamethasone (Decadron), diphenhydramine (Benadryl), filgrastim (Neupogen), granisetron (Kytril), hydromorphone (Dilaudid), lorazepam (Ativan), morphine, ondansetron (Zofran), potassium chloride, propofol (Diprivan).

INDICATIONS/ROUTES/DOSAGE

Usual Dosage for Induction
(Refer to Individual Protocols)
IV: ADULTS, ELDERLY, CHILDREN: (Induction): 100 mg/m²/day continuous infusion for 7 days.
Intrathecal: ADULTS, ELDERLY, CHILDREN: 5–75 mg/m² daily × 4 days or once q4days.

Usual Maintenance Dosage
IV: ADULTS, ELDERLY, CHILDREN: 70–200 mg/m²/day for 2–5 days q mo.

Subcutaneous: ADULTS, ELDERLY, CHILDREN: 1–1.5 mg/m² as single dose q1–4wks.

Usual Dosage for Depo-Cyt
Intrathecal: ADULTS, ELDERLY: (Induction): 50 mg q14 days for 2 doses (wks 1, 3). **(Consolidation):** 50 mg q14 days for 3 doses (wks 5, 7, 9) followed by additional dose at wk 13. **(Maintenance):** 50 mg q28days for 4 doses (wks 17, 21, 25, 29).

SIDE EFFECTS

Frequent: **IV, Subcutaneous (33%–16%):** Asthenia (loss of strength, energy), fever, pain, altered taste/smell, nausea, vomiting (risk greater with IV push than with continuous IV infusion). **Intrathecal (28%–11%):** Headache, asthenia (loss of strength, energy), altered taste/smell, confusion, drowsiness, nausea, vomiting. **Occasional: IV, Subcutaneous (11%–7%):** Abnormal gait, drowsiness, constipation, back pain, urinary incontinence, peripheral edema, headache, confusion. **Intrathecal (7%–3%):** Peripheral edema, back pain, constipation, abnormal gait, urinary incontinence.

ADVERSE EFFECTS/ TOXIC REACTIONS

Myelosuppression resulting in blood dyscrasias (leukopenia, anemia, thrombocytopenia, megaloblastosis, reticulocytopenia) occurring minimally after single IV dose. Leukopenia, anemia, thrombocytopenia should be expected with daily or continuous IV therapy. Cytarabine syndrome (fever, myalgia, rash, conjunctivitis, malaise, chest pain), hyperuricemia may occur. High-dose therapy may produce severe CNS, GI, pulmonary toxicity.

NURSING CONSIDERATIONS

BASELINE ASSESSMENT

Obtain baseline CBC, renal/hepatic function tests. Leukocyte count decreases

---

C

within 24 hrs after initial dose, continues to decrease for 7–9 days followed by brief rise at 12 days, decreases again at 15–24 days, then rises rapidly for next 10 days. Platelet count decreases 5 days after drug initiation to its lowest count at 12–15 days, then rises rapidly for next 10 days.

INTERVENTION/EVALUATION

Monitor BUN, serum creatinine, uric acid, AST, ALT, bilirubin, alkaline phosphatase. Monitor CBC for evidence of myelosuppression. Monitor for blood dyscrasias (fever, sore throat, signs of local infection, unusual bruising/bleeding from any site), symptoms of anemia (excessive fatigue, weakness). Monitor for signs of neuropathy (gait disturbances, handwriting difficulties, paresthesia).

PATIENT/FAMILY TEACHING

• Increase fluid intake (may protect against hyperuricemia). • Do not have immunizations without physician's approval (drug lowers resistance). • Avoid contact with those who have recently received live virus vaccine. • Promptly report fever, sore throat, signs of local infection, unusual bruising/bleeding from any site.

dabigatran

dab-ih-**gah**-tran
(Pradaxa, Pradax ♣)

◆CLASSIFICATION

PHARMACOTHERAPEUTIC: Thrombin inhibitor. **CLINICAL:** Anticoagulant (see p. 32C).

ACTION

Direct thrombin inhibitor, preventing the conversion of fibrinogen into fibrin during coagulation cascade. **Therapeutic Effect:** Produces anticoagulation, preventing development of thrombus.

PHARMACOKINETICS

Metabolized in liver. Protein binding: 35%. Eliminated primarily in urine. **Half-life:** 12–17 hrs.

USES

Indicated to reduce risk of stroke, systemic embolism in pts with nonvalvular atrial fibrillation.

PRECAUTIONS

Contraindications: Active major bleeding, pts with mechanical prosthetic heart valves. **Cautions:** Renal impairment (creatinine clearance 15–30 ml/min), moderate hepatic impairment, invasive procedures, spinal anesthesia, major surgery, those with congenital or acquired bleeding disorders.

⌛ LIFESPAN CONSIDERATIONS

Pregnancy/Lactation: Unknown if distributed in breast milk. **Pregnancy Category C. Children:** Safety and efficacy not established in those younger than 18 yrs. **Elderly:** Severe renal impairment may require dosage adjustment.

INTERACTIONS

DRUG: Rifampin may decrease concentration. **Antacids, proton pump in-**hibitors may decrease levels, effect. **Antiplatelet agents, NSAIDs, other anticoagulants, thrombolytics** may increase risk of bleeding. **HERBAL: Feverfew, ginkgo biloba, green tea, red clover** may increase risk of bleeding. **St. John's wort** may decrease concentration/effect. **FOOD: High-fat meal** delays absorption approximately 2 hrs. **LAB VALUES:** May increase aPTT, PT, INR.

AVAILABILITY (Rx)

Capsules: 75 mg, 150 mg.

ADMINISTRATION/HANDLING

PO
• May be given without regard to food. Administer with water. • Do not break, cut, open capsules.

INDICATIONS/ROUTES/DOSAGE

◀**ALERT**▶ Medication should be discontinued prior to invasive or surgical procedures.

Nonvalvular Atrial Fibrillation
PO: ADULTS, ELDERLY: 150 mg twice daily.

Renal Impairment
Creatinine Clearance 15–30 ml/min: 75 mg twice daily. Creatinine clearance less than 15, or **HD:** Use not recommended (removes ~60% over 2–3 hrs).

SIDE EFFECTS

Frequent (less than 16%): Dyspepsia (heartburn, nausea, indigestion), diarrhea, upper abdominal pain.

ADVERSE EFFECTS/TOXIC REACTIONS

Gastrointestinal bleeding occurs rarely.

NURSING CONSIDERATIONS

BASELINE ASSESSMENT

Assess CBC, including platelet count. Check PT, PTT. Determine initial B/P.

INTERVENTION/EVALUATION

Assess for any sign of bleeding (hematuria, melena, bleeding from gums, petechiae, bruising). Do not obtain B/P in lower extremities (possible deep vein thrombosis). Assess for decrease in B/P, increase in pulse rate, complaint of abdominal pain, diarrhea. Obtain aPTT, PT, platelet count. Question for increase in discharge during menses. Monitor for hematoma. Use care in removing any dressing, tape.

PATIENT/FAMILY TEACHING

• Do not break, open, chew capsules. • Use electric razor, soft toothbrush to prevent bleeding. • Report any sign of red or dark urine, black or red stool, coffee-ground vomitus, red-speckled mucus from cough. • Keep in original container. Do not transfer to pill box/organizer. • Once bottle is opened, must be used within 60 days. • Open blister pack at time of use.

---

dabrafenib

da-**braf**-e-nib
(Tafinlar)
Do not confuse dabrafenib with dasatinib.

◆CLASSIFICATION

PHARMACOTHERAPEUTIC: Kinase inhibitor. **CLINICAL:** Antineoplastic.

ACTION

Inhibits BRAF kinase gene mutation, a main cause of tumor cell growth, in the absence of growth factors that are normally required for proliferation. **Therapeutic Effect:** Inhibits tumor cell growth and metastasis.

PHARMACOKINETICS

Readily absorbed after PO administration. Protein binding: 99.7%. Peak plasma concentration: 2 hrs. Metabolized in liver. Excreted in feces (71%), urine (23%). **Half-life:** 8 hrs.

USES

Treatment of unresectable or metastatic melanoma with BRAF V600E mutation as detected by FDA-approved test. **◄ALERT►** Not indicated for treatment of wild-type BRAF melanomas.

PRECAUTIONS

Contraindications: None known. **Cautions:** Diabetes mellitus, hepatic/renal impairment, dehydration, glucose-6-phosphate dehydrogenase (G6PD) deficiency.

⌛ LIFESPAN CONSIDERATIONS

Pregnancy/Lactation: Avoid pregnancy. May cause fetal harm. Must use effective nonhormonal contraception during treatment and for at least 4 wks after treatment (intrauterine device, barrier methods). Unknown if distributed in breast milk. Must either discontinue breastfeeding or discontinue therapy. **Pregnancy Category D. Children:** Safety and efficacy not established. **Elderly:** May have increased risk of adverse effects, skin lesions.

INTERACTIONS

DRUG: Antacids, **H₂-receptors blockers, proton pump inhibitors** may decrease concentration/effect. **CYP3A4 inducers (e.g., carbamazepine, phenytoin, rifampin)** may decrease concentration/effect. **CYP3A4 inhibitors (e.g., clarithromycin, gemfibrozil, ketoconazole)** may increase concentration. May decrease effectiveness of **hormonal contraceptives, warfarin.** **HERBAL: St John's wort** may decrease concentration/effect. **FOOD: High-fat meals** may decrease absorption/effect. **LAB VALUES:** May increase serum glucose, alkaline phosphatase. May decrease serum phosphate, sodium.

AVAILABILITY (Rx)

🎗 **Capsules:** 50 mg, 75 mg.

ADMINISTRATION/HANDLING

PO
• Give at least 1 hr before or at least 2 hrs after meal. Do not crush, cut, or open capsule.

INDICATIONS/ROUTES/DOSAGE

Metastatic Melanoma
PO: ADULTS/ELDERLY: 150 mg twice daily (about 12 hrs apart).

Dose Modification
Based on Common Terminology Criteria for Adverse Events (CTCAE) grading 1–4.

Reduction Levels	Dose
1st dose reduction	100 mg twice daily
2nd dose reduction	75 mg twice daily
3rd dose reduction	50 mg twice daily

Fever greater than 101.3°F or Any Grade 2 or Grade 3 Adverse Event
Withhold until fever or adverse event resolves to grade 1 or less, then reduce dose by one level. May further decrease each dose level based on tolerability.

Recurrent Grade 4 Adverse Event or 50-mg Dose Intolerability or Hemodynamic Instability
Permanently discontinue.

SIDE EFFECTS

Frequent (37%–17%): Hyperkeratosis, headache, pyrexia, arthralgia, alopecia, rash. **Occasional (12%–10%):** Back pain, cough, myalgia, constipation, nasopharyngitis, fatigue.

ADVERSE EFFECTS/ TOXIC REACTIONS

Cutaneous squamous cell carcinoma (cuSCC) and keratocanthomas reported in 11% of pts (esp. elderly, prior skin cancer, chronic sun exposure). Skin reactions including palmar-plantar erythrodysesthesia syndrome (PPES), papilloma have occurred. May increase cell proliferation of wild-type BRAF melanoma or new malignant melanomas. Eye conditions including uveitis, iritis reported. Hyperglycemia reported in 6% of pts. Serious febrile drug reactions including hypotension, rigors, dehydration reported in 4% of pts. Pts with G6PD deficiency have increased risk of hemolytic anemia. Pancreatitis, interstitial nephritis, bullous rash reported in less than 10% of pts.

NURSING CONSIDERATIONS

BASELINE ASSESSMENT
Obtain baseline serum CMP, magnesium, phosphate, capillary glucose level. Confirm presence of BRAF V600E mutation, negative urine pregnancy before initiating treatment. Assess skin for moles, lesions, papillomas. Baseline ophthalmologic exam, visual acuity. Question current breastfeeding status. Receive full medication history including herbal products.

INTERVENTION/EVALUATION
Offer emotional support. Monitor serum electrolytes, capillary blood glucose routinely. Obtain CBC if hemolytic anemia suspected. Monitor for signs of hyperglycemia (thirst, polyuria, confusion, dehydration). Assess for skin lesions every 2 mos during treatment and at least 6 mos after treatment. Immediately report any vision changes, eye pain/swelling, febrile events, renal impairment.

PATIENT/FAMILY TEACHING
• Treatment may cause hair loss. • Do not breastfeed. • Avoid pregnancy; nonhormonal contraception should be used during treatment and up to 4 wks after treatment. • Take capsule at least 1 hr before or at least 2 hrs after meal. Swallow whole; do not crush or chew. • Report any increased urination, thirst, confusion, vision changes, eye pain, fever, skin changes including moles or lesions. • Minimize exposure to sunlight. • Males may experience a decreased sperm count. • Report any newly prescribed medications.

dacarbazine

HIGH ALERT

da-**kar**-bah-zeen
(DTIC ✹)

BLACK BOX ALERT Myelosuppression is most common toxicity. May cause hepatic necrosis, hepatic vein thrombosis. May be carcinogenic or teratogenic. Administer only under supervision of an experienced cancer chemotherapy physician.
Do not confuse dacarbazine with Dicarbosil or procarbazine.

◆CLASSIFICATION

PHARMACOTHERAPEUTIC: Alkylating agent. **CLINICAL:** Antineoplastic (see p. 84C).

ACTION

Forms methyldiazonium ions, which attack nucleophilic groups in DNA. Crosslinks DNA strands. **Therapeutic Effect:** Inhibits DNA, RNA, protein synthesis.

PHARMACOKINETICS

Minimally crosses blood-brain barrier. Protein binding: 5%. Metabolized in liver. Excreted in urine. **Half-life:** 5 hrs (increased in renal impairment).

USES

Treatment of metastatic malignant melanoma, second-line therapy of Hodgkin's disease. **OFF-LABEL:** Treatment of islet cell carcinoma, soft-tissue sarcoma, pheochromocytoma, medullary carcinoma of thyroid.

PRECAUTIONS

Contraindications: Hypersensitivity to dacarbazine. **Cautions:** Renal/hepatic impairment, bone marrow suppression.

⌛ LIFESPAN CONSIDERATIONS

Pregnancy/Lactation: If possible, avoid use during pregnancy, esp. first trimester. Breastfeeding not recommended. **Pregnancy Category C. Children:** Safety and efficacy not established. **Elderly:** Age-related renal impairment may require dosage adjustment.

INTERACTIONS

DRUG: **Bone marrow depressants** may enhance myelosuppression. **CYP1A2 inducers (e.g., rifampin)** may decrease effects. **CYP1A2 inhibitors (e.g., fluoxetine, amlodipine)** may increase levels/effects. **Live virus vaccines** may potentiate virus replication, increase vaccine side effects, decrease pt's antibody response to the vaccine. **HERBAL: Dong quai, St. John's wort** may increase photosensitization. **Echinacea** may decrease effects. **FOOD:** None known. **LAB VALUES:** May increase BUN, serum alkaline phosphatase, AST, ALT.

AVAILABILITY (Rx)

Injection, Powder for Reconstitution: 100-mg vial, 200-mg vial.

ADMINISTRATION/HANDLING

◀**ALERT**▶ Give by IV push or IV infusion. May be carcinogenic, mutagenic, teratogenic. Handle with extreme care during preparation/administration.

 IV

Reconstitution • Reconstitute 100-mg vial with 9.9 ml Sterile Water for Injection (19.7 ml for 200-mg vial) to provide concentration of 10 mg/ml.
Rate of Administration • Give IV push over 2–3 min. • For IV infusion, further dilute with 250–1,000 ml D_5W or 0.9% NaCl at a concentration not to exceed 10 mg/ml. Infuse over 15–120 min. • Apply hot packs if local pain, burning sensation, irritation at injection site occur. • Avoid extravasation (stinging, swelling, coolness, slight or no blood return at injection site).
Storage • Protect from light; refrigerate vials. • Color change from ivory to pink indicates decomposition; discard. • Solution containing 10 mg/ml is stable for 8 hrs at room temperature or 72 hrs if refrigerated. • Solution diluted with D_5W or 0.9% NaCl is stable for at least 24 hrs at room temperature.

D

🔲 IV INCOMPATIBILITIES

Allopurinol (Aloprim), hydrocortisone (Solu-Cortef), heparin, piperacillin and tazobactam (Zosyn).

🔲 IV COMPATIBILITIES

Granisetron (Kytril), ondansetron (Zofran), palonosetron (Aloxi).

INDICATIONS/ROUTES/DOSAGE

Refer to individual protocols.

Metastatic Melanoma
IV: ADULTS, ELDERLY: 250 mg/m²/day for 5 days, repeat q3wks.

Hodgkin's Disease
IV: ADULTS, ELDERLY, CHILDREN: 375 mg/m² once, repeat in 15 days (as combination therapy) of every 28-day cycle.

Dosage in Renal Impairment

Creatinine Clearance	Dose
46–60 ml/min	80% of dose
31–45 ml/min	75% of dose
30 or less ml/min	70% of dose

SIDE EFFECTS

Frequent (90%): Nausea, vomiting, anorexia (occurs within 1 hr of initial dose, may last up to 12 hrs). **Occasional:** Facial flushing, paresthesia, alopecia, flu-like symptoms (fever, myalgia, malaise), dermatologic reactions, confusion, blurred vision, headache, lethargy. **Rare:** Diarrhea, stomatitis, photosensitivity.

ADVERSE EFFECTS/ TOXIC REACTIONS

Myelosuppression resulting in blood dyscrasias (leukopenia, thrombocytopenia) generally appears 2–4 wks after last dacarbazine dose. Hepatotoxicity occurs rarely.

NURSING CONSIDERATIONS

BASELINE ASSESSMENT

Obtain baseline CBC, serum chemistries, esp. hepatic function tests. Conflicting reports of antiemetic effectiveness for nausea, vomiting. Some clinicians recommend food, fluid restriction 4–6 hrs before treatment; other clinicians believe good hydration to within 1 hr of treatment will prevent dehydration due to vomiting.

INTERVENTION/EVALUATION

Monitor CBC for evidence of myelosuppression. Monitor for hematologic toxicity (fever, sore throat, signs of local infection, unusual bruising/bleeding from any site).

PATIENT/FAMILY TEACHING

• Tolerance to GI effects occurs rapidly (generally after 1–2 days of treatment). • Do not have immunizations without physician's approval (drug lowers resistance). • Avoid contact with those who have recently received live virus vaccine. • Promptly report fever, sore throat, signs of local infection, unusual bruising/bleeding from any site. • Notify physician of persistent nausea, vomiting.

---

dalfampridine

dal-**fam**-pri-deen
(Ampyra)
Do not confuse Ampyra with anakinra, or dalfampridine with desipramine.

◆CLASSIFICATION

PHARMACOTHERAPEUTIC: Potassium channel blocker. **CLINICAL:** Multiple sclerosis agent.

ACTION

Increases conduction of action potentials in demyelinated axons, inhibiting potassium channels. **Therapeutic Effect:** Improves ambulation in those with multiple sclerosis (MS).

🍁 Canadian trade name   🔲 Non-Crushable Drug   🔲 High Alert drug

PHARMACOKINETICS

Rapidly absorbed from GI tract. Minimally metabolized in liver. Primarily excreted in urine. **Half-life:** 5.2–6.5 hrs.

USES

Indicated to improve ambulation in pts with MS, as demonstrated by increase in walking speed.

PRECAUTIONS

Contraindications: History of seizures, moderate to severe renal impairment (creatinine clearance [CrCl] equal to or less than 50 ml/min). **Cautions:** Mild renal impairment (CrCl equal to 51–80 ml/min).

⌛ LIFESPAN CONSIDERATIONS

Pregnancy/Lactation: Unknown if drug crosses placenta or is distributed in breast milk. **Pregnancy Category C. Children:** Safety and efficacy not established in those younger than 18 years. **Elderly:** Age-related renal impairment may require dosage adjustment.

INTERACTIONS

DRUG: None significant. **HERBAL:** None significant. **FOOD:** None known. **LAB VALUES:** May increase creatinine clearance.

AVAILABILITY (Rx)

🔖 **Tablet, Film-Coated, Extended-Release:** 10 mg.

ADMINISTRATION/HANDLING

PO
• May give without regard to food. • Do not break, cut, crush, or divide tablets.

INDICATIONS/ROUTES/DOSAGE

Multiple Sclerosis
PO: ADULTS 18 YEARS AND OLDER, ELDERLY: 10 mg twice daily.

Dosage in Renal Impairment
Creatinine Clearance 50 ml/min or Less: Contraindicated.

SIDE EFFECTS

Frequent (9%–5%): Insomnia, dizziness, headache, nausea, asthenia (loss of strength, energy), back pain.
Rare (4%–2%): Paresthesia, nasopharyngitis, constipation, dyspepsia, pharyngolaryngeal pain.

ADVERSE EFFECTS/ TOXIC REACTIONS

Urinary tract infection occurs in 12% of pts.

NURSING CONSIDERATIONS

BASELINE ASSESSMENT

Obtain CBC, BUN, creatinine clearance, serum chemistries prior to treatment and routinely thereafter. Offer emotional support.

INTERVENTION/EVALUATION

Monitor CBC, serum chemistries, renal function tests, particularly creatinine clearance. Monitor for urinary, respiratory infection. Assess for therapeutic response (improvement in walking as demonstrated by increase in walking speed).

PATIENT/FAMILY TEACHING

• Avoid tasks that require alertness, motor skills until response to drug is established. • Report difficulty in sleeping, dizziness, headache, nausea, back pain, loss of strength or energy. • Do not break, chew, crush, or divide tablets.

dalteparin   HIGH ALERT

dal-te-par-in
(Fragmin)
BLACK BOX ALERT Epidural or spinal anesthesia greatly increases potential for spinal or epidural hematoma, subsequent long-term or permanent paralysis.

CLASSIFICATION

PHARMACOTHERAPEUTIC: Low molecular weight heparin. **CLINICAL:** Anticoagulant (see p. 32C).

ACTION

Antithrombin in presence of low molecular weight heparin inhibits factor Xa, thrombin. Only slightly influences platelet aggregation, PT, aPTT. **Therapeutic Effect:** Produces anticoagulation.

PHARMACOKINETICS

Route	Onset	Peak	Duration
Subcutaneous	N/A	4 hrs	N/A

Protein binding: less than 10%. **Half-life:** 3–5 hrs.

USES

Treatment of unstable angina, non–Q-wave MI to prevent ischemic events. Prevention of deep vein thrombosis (DVT) in pts undergoing hip replacement or abdominal surgery who are at risk for thromboembolic complications. Extended treatment of symptomatic venous thromboembolism (VTE) to reduce recurrence of VTE in cancer pts. Prevention of DVT or pulmonary embolism in acutely ill pts with severely restricted mobility. Those at risk are 40 yrs and older, obese, undergoing surgery under general anesthesia lasting longer than 30 min, malignancy, history of DVT, pulmonary embolism. **OFF-LABEL:** Treatment of DVT in noncancer pts.

PRECAUTIONS

Contraindications: Active major bleeding; concurrent heparin therapy; hypersensitivity to dalteparin, heparin, pork products; unstable angina; history of heparin-induced thrombocytopenia; non–Q-wave MI; prolonged venous thromboembolism undergoing epidural/neuraxial anesthesia. **Cautions:** Conditions with increased risk for hemorrhage, bacterial endocarditis, renal/hepatic impairment, uncontrolled hypertension, history of recent GI ulceration/hemorrhage, peptic ulcer disease, pericarditis, preexisting thrombocytopenia, recent childbirth, concurrent use of aspirin.

⧗ LIFESPAN CONSIDERATIONS

Pregnancy/Lactation: Use with caution, particularly during last trimester, immediate postpartum period (increased risk of maternal hemorrhage). Unknown if distributed in breast milk. **Pregnancy Category B. Children:** Safety and efficacy not established. **Elderly:** No age-related precautions noted.

INTERACTIONS

DRUG: Anticoagulants, NSAIDs, platelet inhibitors, thrombolytic agents may increase risk of bleeding. **HERBAL: Cat's claw, dong quai, evening primrose, garlic, ginseng, other herbs with anticoagulant/antiplatelet activity** may increase antiplatelet activity. **FOOD:** None known. **LAB VALUES:** May increase serum AST, ALT. May decrease serum triglycerides.

AVAILABILITY (Rx)

Injection, Solution: 2,500 international units/0.2 ml, 5,000 international units/0.2 ml, 7,500 international units/0.3 ml, 10,000 international units/ml, 25,000 international units/ml, 12,500 international units/0.5 ml, 15,000 international units/0.6 ml, 18,000 international units/0.72 ml.

ADMINISTRATION/HANDLING

Subcutaneous

• Store at room temperature. • Inject in U-shaped area around the navel, upper outer side of thigh, upper outer quadrangle of buttock. • Use fine needle (25–26 gauge) to minimize tissue trauma. • Introduce entire length of needle (½ inch) into skin fold held between thumb and forefinger, holding needle during injection at 45°–90° angle. • Do not rub injection site after administration (prevents bruising). • Alternate administration site with each injection. • New injections should be administered at least 1 inch from the old site.

Never inject into an area where skin is tender, bruised, red, or hard.

INDICATIONS/ROUTES/DOSAGE

Abdominal Surgery, Low to Moderate DVT Risk
Subcutaneous: ADULTS, ELDERLY: 2,500 international units 1–2 hrs before surgery, then daily for 5–10 days.

Abdominal Surgery, High DVT Risk
Subcutaneous: ADULTS, ELDERLY: 5,000 international units 1–2 hrs before surgery, then daily for 5–10 days.

Total Hip Surgery
Subcutaneous: ADULTS, ELDERLY: 2,500 international units 1–2 hrs before surgery, then 2,500 units 4–8 hrs after surgery, then 5,000 units/day (starting at least 6 hrs after postsurgical dose) for 7–10 days.

Unstable Angina, Non–Q-Wave MI
Subcutaneous: ADULTS, ELDERLY: 120 international units/kg q12h (**maximum: 10,000** international units/dose) given with aspirin until clinically stable.

Venous Thromboembolism (Cancer Pts)
Subcutaneous: ADULTS, ELDERLY: Initially (1 mo), 200 international units/kg (**maximum: 18,000** international units) daily for 30 days. Maintenance (2–6 mos): 150 international units/kg once daily (**maximum: 18,000** international units). If platelet count 50,000–100,000/mm^3, reduce dose by 2,500 units until platelet count recovers to 100,000/mm^3 or more. If platelet count less than 50,000/mm^3, discontinue until platelet count recovers to more than 50,000/mm^3.

Prevention of Deep Vein Thrombosis (DVT), Acutely Ill Pt, Immobile Pt
Subcutaneous: ADULTS, ELDERLY: 5,000 international units once a day.

Dosage in Renal Impairment
For creatinine clearance less than 30 ml/min, monitor anti-Xa levels to determine appropriate dose.

SIDE EFFECTS

Occasional (7%–3%): Hematoma at injection site. **Rare (less than 1%):** Hypersensitivity reaction (chills, fever, pruritus, urticaria, asthma, rhinitis, lacrimation, headache); mild, local skin irritation.

ADVERSE EFFECTS/ TOXIC REACTIONS

Overdose may lead to bleeding complications ranging from local ecchymoses to major hemorrhage. Thrombocytopenia occurs rarely.

NURSING CONSIDERATIONS

BASELINE ASSESSMENT

Obtain baseline coagulation studies, CBC, esp. platelet count. Determine baseline B/P.

INTERVENTION/EVALUATION

Periodically monitor CBC, platelet count, stool for occult blood (no need for daily monitoring in pts with normal presurgical coagulation parameters). Assess for any sign of bleeding (bleeding at surgical site, hematuria, blood in stool, bleeding from gums, petechiae, bruising/bleeding at injection sites).

PATIENT/FAMILY TEACHING

• Usual length of therapy is 5–10 days. • Do not take any OTC medication (esp. aspirin) without consulting physician. • Report bleeding, bruising, dizziness, light-headedness, rash, itching, fever, swelling, breathing difficulty. • Rotate injection sites daily. • Teach proper injection technique. • Excessive bruising at injection site may be lessened by ice massage before injection.

dantrolene

dan-troe-leen
(Dantrium, Revonto)
BLACK BOX ALERT Potential for hepatotoxicity.

Do not confuse Dantrium with danazol or Daraprim, Revontro with Revatio.

◆ CLASSIFICATION

CLINICAL: Skeletal muscle relaxant (see p. 151C).

ACTION

Reduces muscle contraction by interfering with release of calcium ion. Reduces calcium ion concentration. **Therapeutic Effect:** Dissociates excitation-contraction coupling. Interferes with catabolic process associated with malignant hyperthermia.

PHARMACOKINETICS

Poorly absorbed from GI tract. Protein binding: High. Metabolized in liver. Primarily excreted in urine. **Half-life: IV:** 4–8 hrs; **PO:** 8.7 hrs.

USES

PO: Relief of symptoms of spasticity due to spinal cord injuries, stroke, cerebral palsy, multiple sclerosis, esp. flexor spasms, concomitant pain, clonus, muscular rigidity. **Parenteral:** Management of fulminant hypermetabolism of skeletal muscle due to malignant hyperthermia crisis. Prevention of malignant hyperthermia (pre- or postoperative administration). **OFF-LABEL:** Neuroleptic malignant syndrome.

PRECAUTIONS

Contraindications: IV: None known. **PO:** When spasticity used to maintain posture/balance during locomotion or to obtain increased motor function. Active hepatic disease. **Cautions:** Cardiac/pulmonary impairment, history of previous hepatic disease.

⌛ LIFESPAN CONSIDERATIONS

Pregnancy/Lactation: Readily crosses placenta. Breastfeeding not recommended. **Pregnancy Category C. Children:** No age-related precautions noted

in those 5 yrs and older. **Elderly:** No precautions specified.

INTERACTIONS

DRUG: CNS depressants may increase CNS depression with short-term use. **Hepatotoxic medications** may increase risk of hepatic toxicity with chronic use. **CYP3A4 inhibitors (e.g., clarithromycin)** may increase concentration. **HERBAL: Gotu kola, kava kava, St. John's wort, valerian** may increase CNS depression. **FOOD:** None known. **LAB VALUES:** May alter serum hepatic function test.

AVAILABILITY (Rx)

Capsules (Dantrium): 25 mg, 50 mg, 100 mg. **Injection, Powder for Reconstitution (Dantrium, Revontro):** 20-mg vial.

ADMINISTRATION/HANDLING

 IV

Reconstitution • Reconstitute 20-mg vial with 60 ml Sterile Water for Injection (**not** Bacteriostatic Water for Injection). **Rate of Administration** • For therapeutic or emergency dose, give IV over 2–3 min. • For IV infusion, administer over 1 hr. • Diligently monitor for extravasation (high pH of IV preparation). May produce severe complications. **Storage** • Store at room temperature. • Use within 6 hrs after reconstitution. • Solution is clear, colorless. Discard if cloudy, precipitate forms.

PO

• Give without regard to food.

▦ IV INCOMPATIBILITY

D_5W, 0.9% NaCl.

INDICATIONS/ROUTES/DOSAGE

Spasticity

PO: ADULTS, ELDERLY: Initially, 25 mg once daily for 7 days; then 25 mg 3 times/day for 7 days; then 50 mg 3 times/day for 7 days; then 100 mg 3 times/day. **Maximum:** 400 mg/day. **CHILDREN:** Initially, 0.5 mg/kg/dose once daily for 7 days; then 0.5 mg/kg/dose 3 times/day for 7 days; then 1 mg/kg/dose 3 times/day for 7 days; then 2 mg/kg/dose 3 times/day. **Maximum:** 400 mg/day.

Perioperative Prophylaxis for Malignant Hyperthermic Crisis
PO: ADULTS, ELDERLY, CHILDREN: 4–8 mg/kg/day in 3–4 divided doses beginning 1–2 days before surgery; give last dose 3–4 hrs before surgery.
IV: ADULTS, ELDERLY, CHILDREN: 2.5 mg/kg about 1.25 hrs before surgery with additional doses as needed.

Management of Malignant Hyperthermic Crisis
IV: ADULTS, ELDERLY, CHILDREN: Initially, a minimum of 2.5 mg/kg rapid IV; may repeat up to total cumulative dose of 10 mg/kg. May follow with 4–8 mg/kg/day PO in 4 divided doses up to 3 days after crisis.

SIDE EFFECTS

Frequent: Drowsiness, dizziness, weakness, general malaise, diarrhea (mild). **Occasional:** Confusion, diarrhea (severe), headache, insomnia, constipation, urinary frequency. **Rare:** Paradoxical CNS excitement or restlessness, paresthesia, tinnitus, slurred speech, tremor, blurred vision, dry mouth, nocturia, impotence, rash, pruritus.

ADVERSE EFFECTS/ TOXIC REACTIONS

Risk of hepatotoxicity, most notably in females, pts 35 yrs and older, those taking other hepatotoxic medications concurrently. Overt hepatitis noted most frequently between 3rd and 12th mo of therapy. Overdose results in vomiting, muscular hypotonia, muscle twitching, respiratory depression, seizures.

NURSING CONSIDERATIONS

BASELINE ASSESSMENT

Obtain baseline hepatic function tests (AST, ALT, alkaline phosphatase, total bilirubin). Record onset, type, location, duration of muscular spasm. Check for immobility, stiffness, swelling.

INTERVENTION/EVALUATION

Assist with ambulation. For pts on long-term therapy, hepatic/renal function tests, CBC should be performed periodically. Assess for therapeutic response: relief of pain, stiffness, spasm.

PATIENT/FAMILY TEACHING

• Drowsiness usually diminishes with continued therapy. • Avoid tasks that require alertness, motor skills until response to drug is established. • Avoid alcohol/other depressants. • Report continued weakness, fatigue, nausea, diarrhea, skin rash, itching, bloody/tarry stools.

daptomycin TOP 200

dap-toe-mye-sin
(Cubicin)
Do not confuse Cubicin with Cleocin, or daptomycin with dactinomycin.

◆CLASSIFICATION

PHARMACOTHERAPEUTIC: Lipopeptide antibacterial agent. **CLINICAL:** Antibiotic.

ACTION

Binds to bacterial membranes and causes rapid depolarization of membrane potential. Inhibits protein, DNA, RNA synthesis. **Therapeutic Effect:** Bactericidal.

PHARMACOKINETICS

Widely distributed. Protein binding: 90%. Primarily excreted unchanged in urine. Moderately removed by hemodialysis. **Half-life:** 7–8 hrs (increased in renal impairment).

underlined – top prescribed drug

USES

Treatment of complicated skin/skin structure infections caused by susceptible strains of gram-positive pathogens, including *Staphyloccus aureus* (methicillin susceptible and methicillin resistant), *Streptococcus pyogenes, Streptococcus agalactiae.* Treatment of *S. aureus* systemic infections caused by methicillin susceptible and resistant *S. aureus.*

PRECAUTIONS

Contraindications: None known. **Cautions:** Severe renal impairment (creatinine clearance less than 30 ml/min), concurrent use of other medications associated with myopathy (e.g., statins).

⌛ LIFESPAN CONSIDERATIONS

Pregnancy/Lactation: Unknown if drug is distributed in breast milk. **Pregnancy Category B. Children:** Safety and efficacy not established in those younger than 18 yrs. **Elderly:** No age-related precautions noted.

INTERACTIONS

DRUG: Concurrent use with **HMG-CoA reductase inhibitors (statins)** may cause myopathy (discontinue use). **HERBAL:** None significant. **FOOD:** None known. **LAB VALUES:** May increase serum CPK, potassium. May alter serum hepatic function test results.

AVAILABILITY (Rx)

Injection, Powder for Reconstitution: 500 mg/vial.

ADMINISTRATION/HANDLING

 IV

Reconstitution • Reconstitute 500-mg vial with 10 ml 0.9% NaCl to provide a concentration of 50 mg/ml. May further dilute in 0.9% NaCl. • Do not shake or agitate vial.
Rate of Administration • For IV injection, give over 2 min (concentration: 50 mg/ml). • For intermittent IV infusion (piggyback), infuse over 30 min.

Storage • Refrigerate. • Appears as pale yellow to light brown lyophilized cake. • Reconstituted solution is stable for 12 hrs at room temperature or up to 48 hrs if refrigerated. • Discard if particulate forms.

🔲 IV INCOMPATIBILITIES

Diluents containing dextrose. If same IV line is used to administer different drugs, flush line with 0.9% NaCl.

🔲 IV COMPATIBILITIES

0.9% NaCl, Lactated Ringer's, aztreonam (Azactam), dopamine, fluconazole (Diflucan), gentamicin, heparin, levofloxacin (Levaquin).

INDICATIONS/ROUTES/DOSAGE

Complicated Skin/Skin Structure Infections
IV: ADULTS, ELDERLY: 4 mg/kg every 24 hrs for 7–14 days.

Systemic Infections
IV: ADULTS, ELDERLY: 6 mg/kg once daily for 2–6 wks.

Dosage in Renal Impairment
Creatinine clearance less than 30 ml/min, (HD) hemodialysis, (PD) peritoneal dialysis: Dosage is 4 mg/kg q48h for skin and soft tissue infections, 6 mg/kg q48h for staphylococcal bacteremia. **(HD) hemodialysis:** Give dose after dialysis. **(CRRT) continuous renal replacement therapy (CVVHD):** 8 mg/kg q48h, **(CVVH or CVVHDF):** 8 mg/kg q48h or 4–6 mg/kg q24h.

SIDE EFFECTS

Frequent (6%–5%): Constipation, nausea, peripheral injection site reactions, headache, diarrhea. **Occasional (4%–3%):** Insomnia, rash, vomiting. **Rare (less than 3%):** Pruritus, dizziness, hypotension.

ADVERSE EFFECTS/ TOXIC REACTIONS

Skeletal muscle myopathy (muscle pain/weakness, particularly of distal extremities) occurs rarely. Antibiotic-associated colitis, other superinfections (abdominal cramps, severe diarrhea, fever) may result from altered bacterial balance in GI tract.

NURSING CONSIDERATIONS

BASELINE ASSESSMENT

Obtain CPK, blood culture, sensitivity test before first dose (therapy may begin before results are known).

INTERVENTION/EVALUATION

Assess oral cavity for white patches on mucous membranes, tongue (thrush). Monitor for myopathy (muscle pain, weakness), CPK levels, renal function tests. Monitor daily pattern of bowel activity, stool consistency. Mild GI effects may be tolerable, but increasing severity may indicate onset of antibiotic-associated colitis. Be alert for superinfection: fever, vomiting, diarrhea, anal/genital pruritus, oral mucosal changes (ulceration, pain, erythema). Monitor for dizziness, institute appropriate measures.

PATIENT/FAMILY TEACHING

• Report rash, headache, nausea, dizziness, constipation, diarrhea, muscle pain, or any other new symptom.

darbepoetin alfa

TOP 200

dar-be-poe-**e**-tin **al**-fa
(Aranesp)

BLACK BOX ALERT Increased risk of serious cardiovascular events, thromboembolic events, mortality, time-to-tumor progression when administered to a target hemoglobin greater than 11 g/dl. Shortened overall survival and/or increased risk of tumor progression has been reported with breast, cervical, head/neck, NSCL cancers.

Do not confuse Aranesp with Aricept, or darbepoetin with dalteparin or epoetin.

◆CLASSIFICATION

PHARMACOTHERAPEUTIC: Glycoprotein. **CLINICAL:** Hematopoietic agent.

ACTION

Stimulates formation of RBCs in bone marrow; increases serum half-life of epoetin. **Therapeutic Effect:** Induces erythropoiesis, release of reticulocytes from bone marrow.

PHARMACOKINETICS

Well absorbed after subcutaneous administration. **Half-life:** 48.5 hrs.

USES

Treatment of anemia associated with chronic renal failure (including pts on dialysis and pts not on dialysis), treatment of anemia caused by concurrent myelosuppressive chemotherapy in pts planned to receive chemotherapy for minimum of 2 additional months. **OFF-LABEL:** Treatment of symptomatic anemia in myelodysplastic syndrome (MDS).

PRECAUTIONS

Contraindications: Pure red cell aplasia, uncontrolled hypertension. **Cautions:** History of seizures, hypertension.

⌛ LIFESPAN CONSIDERATIONS

Pregnancy/Lactation: Unknown if drug crosses placenta or is distributed in breast milk. **Pregnancy Category C. Children:** Safety and efficacy not established. **Elderly:** Age-related renal impairment may require dosage adjustment.

INTERACTIONS

DRUG: None significant. **HERBAL:** None significant. **FOOD:** None known. **LAB VALUES:** May decrease serum ferritin, serum transferrin saturation.

AVAILABILITY (Rx)

Injection Solution: 25 mcg/ml, 40 mcg/ml, 60 mcg/ml, 100 mcg/ml, 150 mcg/0.75 ml, 200 mcg/ml, 300 mcg/ml. **Prefilled**

Syringe: 25 mcg/0.42 ml, 40 mcg/0.4 ml, 60 mcg/0.3 ml, 100 mcg/0.5 ml, 150 mcg/0.3 ml, 200 mcg/0.4 ml, 300 mcg/0.6 ml, 500 mcg/ml.

ADMINISTRATION/HANDLING

◀ALERT▶ Avoid excessive agitation of vial; do not shake (will cause foaming).

 IV

Reconstitution • No reconstitution necessary. Do not dilute.
Rate of Administration • May be given as IV bolus.
Storage • Refrigerate vials. • Do not shake. Vigorous shaking may denature medication, rendering it inactive.

Subcutaneous
• Use 1 dose per vial; do not reenter vial. Discard unused portion.

IV INCOMPATIBILITIES

Do not mix with other medications.

INDICATIONS/ROUTES/DOSAGE

Anemia in Chronic Renal Failure
◀ALERT▶ Individualize dosing and use lowest dose to reduce need for RBC transfusions. **ON DIALYSIS:** Initiate when Hgb less than 10 g/dl; reduce or stop dose when Hgb approaches or exceeds 11 g/dl. **NOT ON DIALYSIS:** Initiate when Hgb less than 10 g/dl and Hgb decline would likely result in RBC transfusion; reduce dose or stop if Hgb exceeds 10 g/dl.
IV, Subcutaneous: ADULTS, ELDERLY: ON DIALYSIS: Initially, 0.45 mcg/kg once weekly. Alternate for nondialysis pts: 0.75 mcg/kg once q2wks. **NOT ON DIALYSIS:** 0.45 mcg/kg q4wks.
Decrease dose by 25%: If Hgb approaches 12 g/dl or increases greater than 1 g/dl in any 2-wk period.
Increase dose by 25%: If Hgb does not increase by 1 g/dl after 4 wks of therapy and Hgb is below target range (with adequate iron stores), do not increase dose more frequently than every 4 wks.

Note: If pt does not attain Hgb range of 10–12 g/dl after appropriate dosing over 12 wks, do not increase dose and use minimum effective dose to maintain Hgb level that will avoid red blood cell transfusions.

Anemia Associated with Chemotherapy
◀ALERT▶ Initiate only if Hgb less than 10 g/dl and anticipated duration of myelosuppression is 2 months or longer. Titrate dose to maintain Hgb level and avoid RBC transfusions. Discontinue upon completion of chemotherapy.
Subcutaneous: ADULTS, ELDERLY: 2.25 mcg/kg once weekly or 500 mcg every 3 wks.
Increase dose: If Hgb does not increase by 1 g/dl after 6 wks and Hgb is below target range, increase dose to 4.5 mcg/kg once weekly.
Decrease dose: Decrease dose by 40% if Hgb increases greater than 1 g/dl in any 2-wk period or Hgb reaches level that will avoid red blood cell transfusions. Note: Withhold dose when Hgb exceeds a level needed to avoid RBC transfusions, resume at dose 40% lower when Hgb approaches a level where transfusions may be required.

SIDE EFFECTS

Frequent: Myalgia, hypertension/hypotension, headache, diarrhea. **Occasional:** Fatigue, edema, vomiting, reaction at injection site, asthenia (loss of strength, energy), dizziness.

ADVERSE EFFECTS/ TOXIC REACTIONS

Vascular access thrombosis, HF, sepsis, arrhythmias, anaphylactic reaction occur rarely.

NURSING CONSIDERATIONS

BASELINE ASSESSMENT

Assess B/P before drug administration. B/P often rises during early therapy in pts with history of hypertension. Assess serum iron (transferrin saturation should

 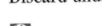

be greater than 20%), serum ferritin (greater than 100 ng/ml) before and during therapy. Consider supplemental iron therapy. Establish baseline CBC (esp. note Hct).

INTERVENTION/EVALUATION

Monitor serum ferritin, CBC with differential, serum creatinine, BUN, potassium, phosphorus, reticulocyte count. Monitor B/P aggressively for increase (25% of pts taking medication require antihypertension therapy, dietary restrictions).

PATIENT/FAMILY TEACHING

• Frequent blood tests needed to determine correct dose. • Report swollen extremities, breathing difficulty, extreme fatigue, or severe headache. • Avoid tasks requiring alertness, motor skills until response to drug is established.

darifenacin

dare-i-**fen**-a-sin
(Enablex)

◆**CLASSIFICATION**

PHARMACOTHERAPEUTIC: Muscarinic receptor antagonist. **CLINICAL:** Urinary antispasmodic.

ACTION

Acts as a direct antagonist at muscarinic receptor sites in cholinergically innervated organs; limits bladder contractions. **Therapeutic Effect:** Reduces symptoms of bladder irritability/overactivity (urge incontinence, urinary urgency/frequency), improves bladder capacity.

PHARMACOKINETICS

Well absorbed following PO administration. Protein binding: 98%. Metabolized in liver. Excreted in urine (60%), feces (40%). **Half-life:** 13–19 hrs.

USES

Management of symptoms of bladder overactivity (urge incontinence, urinary urgency/frequency).

PRECAUTIONS

Contraindications: Uncontrolled narrow-angle glaucoma, paralytic ileus, GI/GU obstruction, urine retention. **Cautions:** Bladder outflow obstruction, hepatic impairment, nonobstructive prostatic hyperplasia, decreased GI motility, constipation, hiatal hernia, reflux esophagitis, ulcerative colitis, controlled narrow-angle glaucoma, myasthenia gravis, concurrent use of CYP3A4 inhibitors.

⧖ LIFESPAN CONSIDERATIONS

Pregnancy/Lactation: Unknown if drug crosses placenta or is distributed in breast milk. **Pregnancy Category C. Children:** Safety and efficacy not established. **Elderly:** No age-related precautions noted.

INTERACTIONS

DRUG: CYP3A4 inhibitors (clarithromycin, erythromycin, isoniazid, protease inhibitors) may increase concentration/effects. **Anticholinergics** may increase side effects (e.g., dry mouth, constipation). **HERBAL: St. John's wort** may decrease concentration/effects. **FOOD:** None known. **LAB VALUES: Grapefruit** may increase potential for urinary retention; constipation.

AVAILABILITY (Rx)

Tablets (Extended-Release): 7.5 mg, 15 mg.

ADMINISTRATION/HANDLING

PO

• Give without regard to food. • Administer extended-release tablets whole; do not break, crush, or divide tablet.

INDICATIONS/ROUTES/DOSAGE

Overactive Bladder
PO: ADULTS, ELDERLY: Initially, 7.5 mg once daily. If response is not adequate after at least 2 wks, may increase to 15 mg once daily. Do not exceed 7.5 mg once daily in moderate hepatic impairment or concurrent use with CYP3A4 inhibitors (clarithromycin, fluconazole, protease inhibitors, isoniazid).

Dosage Hepatic Impairment

Moderate impairment	**Maximum dose:** 7.5 mg
Severe impairment	Not recommended

SIDE EFFECTS

Frequent (35%–21%): Dry mouth, constipation. **Occasional (8%–4%):** Dyspepsia, headache, nausea, abdominal pain. **Rare (3%–2%):** Asthenia (loss of strength, energy), diarrhea, dizziness, ocular dryness.

ADVERSE EFFECTS/ TOXIC REACTIONS

UTI occurs occasionally.

NURSING CONSIDERATIONS

BASELINE ASSESSMENT

Monitor voiding pattern, assess signs/ symptoms of overactive bladder prior to therapy as baseline.

INTERVENTION/EVALUATION

Monitor I&O. Palpate bladder for urine retention. Monitor daily pattern of bowel activity, stool consistency for evidence of constipation. Dry mouth may be relieved with sips of tepid water. Assess for relief of symptoms of overactive bladder (urge incontinence, urinary frequency/urgency).

PATIENT/FAMILY TEACHING

• Swallow tablet whole; do not break, chew, crush, or divide. • Increase fluid intake to reduce risk of constipation. • Avoid tasks that require alertness, motor skills until response to drug is established.

darunavir
TOP 200

dar-**ue**-na-veer
(Prezista)

◆ **CLASSIFICATION**

PHARMACOTHERAPEUTIC: Protease inhibitor. **CLINICAL:** Antiretroviral (see pp. 69C, 119C).

ACTION

Prevents virus-specific processing of polyproteins, HIV-1 protease infected cells. **Therapeutic Effect:** Prevents formation of mature viral cells.

PHARMACOKINETICS

Readily absorbed following PO administration. Protein binding: 95%. Metabolized in liver. Eliminated in feces (79.5%), urine (13.9%). Not significantly removed by hemodialysis. **Half-life:** 15 hrs.

USES

Treatment of HIV infection in combination with ritonavir and other antiretroviral agents in adults and children 3 yrs and older.

PRECAUTIONS

Contraindications: Concurrent therapy with alfuzosin, dihydroergotamine, ergonovine, ergotamine, lovastatin, methylergonovine, oral midazolam, pimozide, rifampin, sildenafil (for treatment of PAH), simvastatin, St. John's wort, triazolam. **Cautions:** Diabetes mellitus, hemophilia, known sulfonamide allergy, hepatic impairment.

⧗ LIFESPAN CONSIDERATIONS

Pregnancy/Lactation: Unknown if drug crosses placenta or is distributed in breast milk. Breastfeeding not recommended. **Pregnancy Category B. Children:** Safety and efficacy not established. **Elderly:** No age-related precautions noted.

INTERACTIONS

DRUG: May increase concentration/effects of **amiodarone, bepredil, lidocaine, desipramine, colchicine, beta blockers, midazolam, paroxetine, sertraline, atorvastatin, clarithromycin, cyclosporine, felodipine, inhaled fluticasone, lovastatin, nicardipine, nifedipine, pravastatin, simvastatin, sirolimus, tacrolimus, trazodone, sildenafil, tadalafil, vardenafil. CYP3A4 inhibitors (e.g., itraconazole, ketoconazole, voriconazole)** may increase concentration. May decrease effect of **methadone, oral contraceptives. HERBAL: St. John's wort** may lead to loss of virologic response, potential resistance to darunavir. **FOOD: Food** increases plasma concentration. **LAB VALUES:** May increase aPTT, PT, serum alkaline phosphatase, bilirubin, amylase, lipase, cholesterol, triglycerides, uric acid. May decrease lymphocytes/neutrophil count, platelets, WBC count, serum bicarbonate, albumin, calcium. May alter serum glucose, sodium.

AVAILABILITY (Rx)

⬥ Tablets (Prezista): 75 mg, 150 mg, 400 mg, 600 mg, 800 mg.

ADMINISTRATION/HANDLING

PO
• Give with food (increases plasma concentration). • Coadministration with ritonavir required. • Do not crush or cut film-coated tablets.

INDICATIONS/ROUTES/DOSAGE

HIV Infection, Treatment Experienced
PO: ADULTS, ELDERLY: 600 mg administered with 100 mg ritonavir with food twice daily or 800 mg (two 400-mg tablets) with 100 mg ritonavir with food once daily.

HIV Infection, Treatment Naive
PO: ADULTS, ELDERLY: 800 mg (two 400-mg tablets) administered with 100 mg ritonavir with food once daily.

Usual Pediatric Dose
◀ALERT▶ Do not use once-daily dosing in pediaric pts.

PO: CHILDREN 3 YRS OF AGE OR OLDER: 20 mg/kg twice daily.

Use Tablet or Solution
PO: CHILDREN WEIGHING 40 KG OR MORE: 600 mg twice daily with 100 mg ritonavir. **WEIGHING 30–39 KG:** 450 mg twice daily with 60 mg ritonavir. **WEIGHING 15–29 KG:** 375 mg twice daily with 50 mg ritonavir.

Use Oral Solution Only
14 KG TO < 15 KG: 280 mg (48 mg ritonavir) twice daily. **13 KG TO < 14 KG:** 250 mg (40 mg ritonavir) twice daily. **12 KG TO < 13 KG:** 240 mg (40 mg ritonavir) twice daily. **11 KG TO < 12 KG:** 220 mg (32 mg ritonavir) twice daily. **10 KG TO < 11 KG:** 200 mg (32 mg ritonavir) twice daily.

SIDE EFFECTS

Frequent (19%–13%): Diarrhea, nausea, headache, nasopharyngitis. **Occasional (3%–2%):** Constipation, abdominal pain, vomiting. **Rare (less than 2%):** Allergic dermatitis, dyspepsia, flatulence, abdominal distention, anorexia, arthralgia, myalgia, paresthesia, memory impairment.

ADVERSE EFFECTS/ TOXIC REACTIONS

Hypertension, MI, transient ischemic attack occur in less than 2% of pts. Acute renal failure, diabetes mellitus, dyspnea, worsening of hepatic impairment, skin reactions including Stevens-Johnson syndrome, toxic epidermal necrolysis occur rarely.

NURSING CONSIDERATIONS

BASELINE ASSESSMENT

Obtain baseline hepatic function tests before beginning therapy and at periodic intervals during therapy. Offer emotional support. Obtain full medication history.

D

INTERVENTION/EVALUATION

Closely monitor for GI discomfort. Monitor daily pattern of bowel activity, stool consistency. Assess skin for rash, other skin reactions, chemistries, laboratory abnormalities, particularly hepatic profile, glucose, cholesterol, triglycerides. Assess for opportunistic infections (onset of fever, oral mucosa changes, cough, other respiratory symptoms).

PATIENT/FAMILY TEACHING

• Take medication with food. • Continue therapy for full length of treatment. • Doses should be evenly spaced. • Darunavir is not a cure for HIV infection, nor does it reduce risk of transmission to others. • Pt may continue to experience illnesses, including opportunistic infections. • Diarrhea can be controlled with OTC medication. • Report any skin reactions.

---

dasatinib HIGH ALERT

da-**sa**-ti-nib
(Sprycel)
Do not confuse dasatinib with erlotinib, imatinib, or lapatinib.

◆CLASSIFICATION

PHARMACOTHERAPEUTIC: Protein-tyrosine kinase inhibitor. **CLINICAL:** Antineoplastic (see p. 84C).

ACTION

Reduces activity of proteins responsible for uncontrolled growth of leukemia cells by binding to most imatinib-resistant BCR-ABL mutations of pts with chronic myelogenous leukemia (CML) or acute lymphoblastic leukemia (ALL). **Therapeutic Effect:** Inhibits proliferation, tumor growth of CML and ALL cancer cell lines.

PHARMACOKINETICS

Extensively distributed in extravascular space. Protein binding: 96%. Metabo-lized in liver. Eliminated primarily in feces. **Half-life:** 3–5 hrs.

USES

Treatment of adults with chronic, accelerated, myeloid or lymphoid blast phase of chronic myelogenous leukemia (CML) with resistance, intolerance to prior therapy, including imatinib. Treatment of adults with Philadelphia chromosome-positive (Ph+) acute lymphoblastic leukemia (ALL) with resistance or intolerance to prior therapy. Treatment of Philadelphia chromosome-positive (Ph+) chronic myeloid leukemia (CML) in chronic phase of newly diagnosed pts. **OFF-LABEL:** Post stem cell transplant follow-up treatment of CML. Treatment of GI stromal tumor.

PRECAUTIONS

Contraindications: None known. **Cautions:** Hepatic impairment, myelosuppression (particularly thrombocytopenia), pts prone to fluid retention, those with prolonged QT interval, cardiovascular/pulmonary disease. Concomitant use of anticoagulants, CYP3A4 inducers/inhibitors may increase risk of pulmonary arterial hypertension.

⧖ LIFESPAN CONSIDERATIONS

Pregnancy/Lactation: Has potential for severe teratogenic effects, fertility impairment. Breastfeeding not recommended. **Pregnancy Category D. Children:** Safety and efficacy not established in those younger than 18 yrs. **Elderly:** No age-related precautions noted.

INTERACTIONS

DRUG: CYP3A4 inhibitors (e.g., ata-zanavir, clarithromycin, erythromycin, indinavir, ketoconazole, nefazodone, nelfinavir, ritonavir, saquinavir) may increase concentration. CYP3A4 inducers (e.g., carbamazepine, phenobarbital, phenytoin, rifampin) may decrease concentration. Antacids alter pH-dependent solubility of dasatinib. Famotidine, omeprazole may reduce dasatinib absorption. HERBAL: St. John's

---

wort, **echinacea** may decrease concentration. **FOOD: Grapefruit products** may increase concentration/toxicity (increased risk of torsades, myelotoxicity). **LAB VALUES:** May decrease WBC, platelets, Hgb, Hct, RBC, serum calcium, phosphates. May increase serum bilirubin, ALT, AST, creatinine.

AVAILABILITY (Rx)

Tablets (Film-Coated): 20 mg, 50 mg, 70 mg, 80 mg, 100 mg, 140 mg.

ADMINISTRATION/HANDLING

PO

• Give without regard to food. • Take with food or large glass of water if GI upset occurs. • Avoid grapefruit products. • Do not chew/crush/cut film-coated tablets. • Store at room temperature. • Do not give antacids either 2 hrs prior to or within 2 hrs after dasatinib administration.

INDICATIONS/ROUTES/DOSAGE

Chronic Myelogenous Leukemia (CML)
PO: ADULTS, ELDERLY: (Chronic phase): 100 mg once daily. May increase to 140 mg once daily in pts not achieving cytogenetic response. **(Accelerated or blast phase):** 140 mg once daily. May increase to 180 mg once daily in pts not achieving cytogenetic response.

CML (Newly Diagnosed)
PO: ADULTS, ELDERLY: 100 mg once daily. May increase to 140 mg/day in pts not achieving cytogenetic response.

Ph+ ALL
PO: ADULTS, ELDERLY: 140 mg once daily. May increase to 180 mg once daily in pts not achieving cytogenetic response.

SIDE EFFECTS

Frequent (50%–32%): Fluid retention, diarrhea, headache, fatigue, musculoskeletal pain, fever, rash, nausea, dyspnea. **Occasional (28%–12%):** Cough, abdominal pain, vomiting, anorexia, asthenia (loss of strength, energy), arthralgia, stomatitis, dizziness, constipation, peripheral neuropathy, myalgia. **Rare (less than 12%):** Abdominal distention, chills, weight increase, pruritus.

ADVERSE EFFECTS/ TOXIC REACTIONS

Pleural effusion occurs in 8% of pts, febrile neutropenia in 7%, GI bleeding, pneumonia in 6%, thrombocytopenia in 5%, dyspnea in 4%, anemia, cardiac failure in 3%.

NURSING CONSIDERATIONS

BASELINE ASSESSMENT

Obtain CBC weekly for first mo, biweekly for second mo, and periodically thereafter. Monitor hepatic function tests before treatment begins and monthly thereafter.

INTERVENTION/EVALUATION

Assess lower extremities for pedal edema, early evidence of fluid retention. Weigh daily, monitor for unexpected rapid weight gain. Offer antiemetics to control nausea, vomiting. Monitor daily pattern of bowel activity, stool consistency. Assess oral mucous membranes for evidence of stomatitis. Monitor CBC for neutropenia, thrombocytopenia; monitor hepatic function tests for hepatotoxicity.

PATIENT/FAMILY TEACHING

• Avoid crowds, those with known infection. • Avoid contact with anyone who recently received live virus vaccine; do not receive vaccinations. • Antacids may be taken up to 2 hrs before or 2 hrs after taking dasatinib. • Avoid grapefruit juice.

---

*DAUNOrubicin

daw-noe-**roo**-bi-sin
(Cerubidine, DaunoXome)

BLACK BOX ALERT Irreversible cardiotoxicity may occur. Myelosuppresant. Lipid component may cause infusion-related effects (back pain, flushing, chest tightness) within first 5 min of infusion. Must be administered by personnel trained in administration/handling of chemotherapeutic agents. Caution in renal impairment or hepatic dysfunction. Potent vesicant.

Do not confuse daunorubicin with dactinomycin, doxorubicin, epirubicin, idarubicin, or valrubicin.

◆CLASSIFICATION

PHARMACOTHERAPEUTIC: Anthracycline antibiotic. **CLINICAL:** Antineoplastic (see p. 84C).

ACTION

Inhibits DNA, DNA-dependent RNA synthesis by binding with DNA strands. Cell cycle–phase nonspecific. **Therapeutic Effect:** Prevents cell division.

PHARMACOKINETICS

Widely distributed. Protein binding: High. Does not cross blood-brain barrier. Metabolized in liver to active metabolite. Excreted in urine (40%); biliary excretion (40%). **Half-life:** 18.5 hrs; metabolite: 26.7 hrs.

USES

Cerubidine: Treatment of leukemias (acute lymphocytic [ALL], acute myeloid [AML]) in combination with other agents. **DaunoXome:** Advanced HIV-related Kaposi's sarcoma.

PRECAUTIONS

Contraindications: None known. **Cautions:** Renal, biliary, hepatic impairment.

⧖ LIFESPAN CONSIDERATIONS

Pregnancy/Lactation: If possible, avoid use during pregnancy, esp. first trimester. May cause fetal harm. Breastfeeding not recommended. **Pregnancy Category D. Children:** Safety and efficacy not established. **Elderly:** Cardiotoxicity may be more frequent; reduced bone marrow reserves require caution. Age-related renal impairment may require dosage adjustment.

INTERACTIONS

DRUG: Previous use of **doxorubicin**, concurrent use of **cyclophosphamide** increases risk of cardiotoxicity. **Hepatotoxic medications** increase risk of hepatotoxicity. **Bone marrow depressants** may enhance myelosuppression. **Live virus vaccines** may potentiate virus replication, increase vaccine side effects, decrease pt's antibody response to vaccine. **HERBAL:** Echinacea may decrease levels/effects. **FOOD:** None known. **LAB VALUES:** May increase serum alkaline phosphatase, bilirubin, uric acid, AST.

AVAILABILITY (Rx)

Injection, Powder for Reconstitution (Cerubidine): 20 mg. Injection Solution (Cerubidine): 5 mg/ml. Injection Solution (DaunoXome): 2 mg/ml.

ADMINISTRATION/HANDLING

 IV

◄ALERT► Cerubidine: Give by IV push or IV infusion. **DaunoXome:** Give by IV infusion. May be carcinogenic, mutagenic, teratogenic. Handle with extreme care during preparation/administration.

Reconstitution

Cerubidine • Reconstitute each 20-mg vial with 4 ml Sterile Water for Injection to provide concentration of 5 mg/ml. • Gently agitate vial until completely dissolved. • May further dilute with 100 ml D_5W or 0.9% NaCl.

DaunoXome • Must dilute with equal part D_5W to provide concentration of 1 mg/ml. • Do not use any other diluent.

Rate of Administration

Cerubidine • For IV push, withdraw desired dose into syringe containing 10–15

ml 0.9% NaCl. Inject over 1–5 min into tubing of rapidly infusing IV solution of D5W or 0.9% NaCl. • For IV infusion, further dilute with 100 ml D5W or 0.9% NaCl. Infuse over 15–30 min. • Extravasation produces immediate pain, severe local tissue damage. Aspirate as much infiltrated drug as possible, then infiltrate area with hydrocortisone sodium succinate injection (50–100 mg hydrocortisone) and/or isotonic sodium thiosulfate injection or ascorbic acid injection (1 ml of 5% injection). Apply cold compresses.
DaunoXome • Infuse over 60 min. • Do not use in-line filter.

Storage
Cerubidine • Reconstituted solution is stable for 4 days at room temperature. Diluted solution in D5W or 0.9% NaCl is stable for 4 wks at room temperature if protected from light. • Color change from red to blue-purple indicates decomposition; discard.
DaunoXome • Refrigerate unopened vials • Reconstituted solution is stable for 6 hrs if refrigerated. • Do not use if opaque.

🟦 IV INCOMPATIBILITIES

Allopurinol (Aloprim), aztreonam (Azactam), cefepime (Maxipime), dexamethasone (Decadron), heparin, piperacillin and tazobactam (Zosyn). **DaunoXome:** Do not mix with any other solution, esp. NaCl or bacteriostatic agents (e.g., benzyl alcohol).

🟦 IV COMPATIBILITIES

Granisetron (Kytril), ondansetron (Zofran).

INDICATIONS/ROUTES/DOSAGE

◀ALERT▶ Refer to individual protocols. **Cerubidine:** Cumulative dose should not exceed 550 mg/m² in adults (increased risk of cardiotoxicity) or 400 mg/m² in those receiving chest irradiation.

Acute Lymphoblastic Leukemia (ALL)
IV *(Cerubidine):* **ADULTS, ELDERLY:** 45 mg/m² on days 1, 2, and 3 of induction course. **CHILDREN 2 YRS AND OLDER, BODY SURFACE AREA 0.5 m² OR GREATER:** 25 mg/m² on day 1 of every wk for up to 4–6 cycles. Cumulative dose not to exceed 300 mg/m². **CHILDREN YOUNGER THAN 2 YRS, BODY SURFACE AREA LESS THAN 0.5 m²:** 1 mg/kg/dose per protocol. Cumulative dose not to exceed 10 mg/kg.

Acute Myeloid Leukemia (AML)
IV *(Cerubidine):* **ADULTS YOUNGER THAN 60 YRS:** 45 mg/m² on days 1, 2, and 3 of induction course, then on days 1 and 2 of subsequent courses. **ADULTS 60 YRS AND OLDER:** 30 mg/m² on days 1, 2, and 3 of induction course, then on days 1 and 2 of subsequent courses. **CHILDREN 2 YRS AND OLDER, BSA 0.5 m² OR GREATER:** 30–60 mg/m²/day on days 1–3 of cycle.

Kaposi's Sarcoma
IV *(Daunoxome):* **ADULTS:** 40 mg/m² over 1 hr repeated q2wks.

Dosage in Renal Impairment
Cerubidine: **SERUM CREATININE GREATER THAN 3 MG/DL:** 50% of normal dose.
Daunoxome: **SERUM CREATININE GREATER THAN 3 MG/DL:** 50% of normal dose.

Dosage in Hepatic Impairment
Cerubidine: **BILIRUBIN 1.2–3 MG/DL:** 75% of normal dose. **BILIRUBIN 3.1–5 MG/DL:** 50% of normal dose. **BILIRUBIN GREATER THAN 5 MG/DL:** Daunorubicin is not recommended for use in this pt population.
Daunoxome: **BILIRUBIN 1.2–3 MG/DL:** 75% of normal dose. **BILIRUBIN GREATER THAN 3 MG/DL:** 50% of normal dose.

SIDE EFFECTS

Frequent: Complete alopecia (scalp, axillary, pubic), nausea, vomiting (beginning a few hrs after administration and lasting 24–48 hrs). **DaunoXome:** Mild to moderate nausea, fatigue, fever. **Occasional:** Diarrhea, abdominal pain, esophagitis, stomatitis, transverse pigmentation of fingernails, toenails. **Rare:** Transient fever, chills.

ADVERSE EFFECTS/ TOXIC REACTIONS

Myelosuppression manifested as hematologic toxicity (severe leukopenia, anemia, thrombocytopenia). Decrease in platelet count, WBC count occurs in 10–14 days, returns to normal level by third week. Cardiotoxicity noted as either acute, transient, abnormal. EKG findings and/or cardiomyopathy manifested as HF (risk increases when cumulative dose exceeds 550 mg/m^2 in adults, 300 mg/m^2 in children 2 yrs and older, or total dosage greater than 10 mg/kg in children younger than 2 yrs).

NURSING CONSIDERATIONS

BASELINE ASSESSMENT

Obtain WBC, platelet, erythrocyte counts before and at frequent intervals during therapy. EKG should be obtained before therapy. Antiemetics may be effective in preventing, treating nausea.

INTERVENTION/EVALUATION

Monitor for stomatitis (burning, erythema of oral mucosa). May lead to ulceration within 2–3 days. Assess skin, nailbeds for hyperpigmentation. Monitor hematologic status, renal/hepatic function studies, serum uric acid. Monitor daily pattern of bowel activity, stool consistency. Monitor for hematologic toxicity (fever, sore throat, signs of local infection, unusual bruising/bleeding from any site), symptoms of anemia (excessive fatigue, weakness).

PATIENT/FAMILY TEACHING

• Urine may turn reddish color for 1–2 days after beginning therapy. • Hair loss is reversible, but new hair growth may have different color, texture. • New hair growth resumes about 5 wks after last therapy dose. • Maintain strict oral hygiene. • Do not have immunizations without physician's approval (drug lowers resistance). • Avoid contact with those who have recently received live virus vaccine. • Promptly report fever, sore throat, signs of local infection, unusual bruising/ bleeding from any site, yellowing of whites of eyes/skin, difficulty breathing. • Increase fluid intake (may protect against hyperuricemia). • Contact physician for persistent nausea, vomiting.

---

decitabine

de-**sye**-ta-bine
(Dacogen)

◆ CLASSIFICATION

PHARMACOTHERAPEUTIC: DNA demethylation agent. **CLINICAL:** Antineoplastic.

ACTION

Exerts cytotoxic effect on rapidly dividing cells by causing demethylation of DNA in abnormal hematopoietic cells in bone marrow. **Therapeutic Effect:** Restores normal function to tumor suppressor genes regulating cellular differentiation, proliferation.

PHARMACOKINETICS

Protein binding: less than 1%. Elimination appears to occur by removal of an amino group from the enzyme cytidine deaminase, found principally in liver, but also in granulocytes, intestinal epithelium, whole blood. **Half-life:** 30 min.

USES

Treatment of myelodysplastic syndromes, specifically refractory anemia, myelomonocytic leukemia. **OFF-LABEL:** Treatment of acute and chronic myelogenous leukemia, sickle cell anemia.

PRECAUTIONS

Contraindications: None known. **Cautions:** Baseline thrombocytopenia, anemia, neutrapenia, diabetes mellitus, fluid retention, hepatic/renal impairment.

⧗ LIFESPAN CONSIDERATIONS

Pregnancy/Lactation: May be embryotoxic; may cause developmental abnormalities of fetus. Breastfeeding not recommended. Men should not father a child while receiving treatment and for 2 mos after treatment. **Pregnancy Category D. Children:** Safety and efficacy not established. **Elderly:** No age-related precautions noted.

INTERACTIONS

DRUG: May increase levels/effects of **clozapine. HERBAL:** None significant. **FOOD:** None known. **LAB VALUES:** May decrease Hgb, Hct, WBC, RBC, platelets. May increase serum creatinine, AST, ACT, alkaline phosphatase, bicarbonate, lactate dehydrogenase, BUN, bilirubin, glucose, albumin, magnesium, sodium.

AVAILABILITY (Rx)

Injection, Powder for Reconstitution: 50 mg.

ADMINISTRATION/HANDLING

 IV

Reconstitution • Reconstitute with 10 ml Sterile Water for Injection. • Further dilute with 50–250 ml 0.9% NaCl, D₅W, or lactated Ringer's to a final concentration of 0.1–1 mg/ml.
Rate of Administration • Give by continuous IV infusion over 1–3 hrs.
Storage • Store vials at room temperature. • Unless used within 15 min of reconstitution, diluted solution must be prepared using cold infusion fluids and stored in refrigerator up to maximum of 7 hrs until administration.

INDICATIONS/ROUTES/DOSAGE

◀ALERT▶ Premedicate with antiemetics prior to therapy.

Myelodysplastic Syndrome
IV Infusion: ADULTS, ELDERLY: **(Option 1):** 15 mg/m² over 3 hrs q8h (45 mg/m²/day) for 3 days. Subsequent treatment cycles should be repeated every 6 wks for a minimum of 4 cycles. **(Option 2):** 20 mg/m² over 1 hr daily for 5 days. Repeat cycle q4wks. Adjust dose for delayed hematologic recovery. Hold treatment until resolution of serum creatinine 2 mg/dl or greater; ALT or bilirubin 2 times upper limit of normal; active or uncontrolled infection.

SIDE EFFECTS

Frequent (53%–20%): Fever, nausea, cough, petechiae, constipation, diarrhea, insomnia, headache, vomiting, peripheral edema, pallor, ecchymosis, rigors, arthralgia. Occasional (19%–11%): Rash, limb pain, dizziness, back pain, anorexia, pharyngitis, abdominal pain, erythema, oral mucosal, petechiae, stomatitis, confusion, lethargy, dyspepsia, anxiety, pruritus, hypoesthesia. Rare (10%–5%): Candidiasis, ascites, alopecia, chest wall pain, rales, catheter site infection, facial edema, hypotension, urticaria, dehydration, blurred vision, musculoskeletal discomfort, malaise, sinusitis, gastroesophageal reflux.

ADVERSE EFFECTS/TOXIC REACTIONS

Pneumonia occurs in 22% of pts, cellulitis in 12%. Hematologic toxicity manifested most commonly as neutropenia (90%; recovery 28–50 days), thrombocytopenia (89%), anemia (82%), febrile neutropenia (29%), leukopenia (28%), lymphadenopathy (12%). UTI occurs in 7%.

NURSING CONSIDERATIONS

BASELINE ASSESSMENT

Offer emotional support. Use strict asepsis, protect pt from infection. Perform CBC, renal/hepatic function tests as needed to monitor response, toxicity but esp. prior to each dosing cycle.

INTERVENTION/EVALUATION

Monitor for hematologic toxicity (fever, sore throat, signs of local infections, unusual bleeding/bruising), symptoms of anemia (excessive fatigue, weakness). Assess response to medication. Monitor, report nausea, vomiting, diarrhea. Avoid rectal temperatures, other traumas that may induce bleeding. Monitor CBC, platelets, serum creatinine, hepatic function tests. If serum creatinine increases to 2 mg/dl, ALT, total bilirubin at least 2 times upper limit of normal, and pt has active or uncontrolled infection, stop treatment; do not restart until toxicity is resolved.

PATIENT/FAMILY TEACHING

• Do not have immunizations without physician's approval (drug lowers resistance). • Avoid crowds, persons with known infections. • Report signs of infection (fever, flu-like symptoms) immediately. • Report persistent nausea or vomiting. • Men should use barrier contraception during therapy.

deferasirox

dee-**fur**-a-sir-ox
(Exjade)

BLACK BOX ALERT May cause renal/hepatic failure, hepatotoxicity, gastrointestinal hemorrhage.
Do not confuse deferasirox with deferoxamine.

◆CLASSIFICATION

PHARMACOTHERAPEUTIC: Iron-chelating agent. **CLINICAL:** Iron reduction agent.

ACTION

Selective for iron. Binds iron with high affinity in a 2:1 ratio. **Therapeutic Effect:** Induces iron excretion.

PHARMACOKINETICS

Well absorbed following PO administration. Protein binding: 99%. Metabolized in liver. Excreted in feces (84%), urine (8%). Half-life: 8–16 hrs.

USES

Treatment of chronic iron overload due to blood transfusions (transfusional hemosiderosis) in pts 2 yrs and older. Treatment of iron overload in pts 10 yrs and older with non–transfusion-dependent thalassemia syndrome.

PRECAUTIONS

Contraindications: Platelet counts less than 50,000/mm^3; poor performance status and high-risk myelodysplastic syndromes or advanced malignancies; creatinine clearance less than 40 ml/min or serum creatinine greater than 2 times the upper limit of normal. **Cautions:** Renal/hepatic impairment, cardiac dysfunction, elderly, concurrent medications that may increase GI effects (e.g., NSAIDs).

⌛ LIFESPAN CONSIDERATIONS

Pregnancy/Lactation: Unknown if drug crosses placenta or is distributed in breast milk. **Pregnancy Category B. Children:** Not recommended for those younger than 2 yrs. **Elderly:** No age-related precautions noted.

INTERACTIONS

DRUG: Antacids containing aluminium, cholestyramine, phenobarbital, phenytoin, rifampin, ritonavir decrease concentration/effects. May decrease effect of **cyclosporine, simvastatin, oral contraceptives.** May increase concentration of **cyclobenzapine, olanzapine, tizanidine.** HERBAL: None significant. **FOOD:** Bioavailability is variably increased when given with **food.** LAB VALUES: Decreases serum ferritin. May increase serum creatinine, AST, ALT, urine protein.

AVAILABILITY (Rx)

Tablets for Oral Suspension (Exjade): 125 mg, 250 mg, 500 mg.

ADMINISTRATION/HANDLING

PO

• Give on empty stomach 30 min before food. • Do not give simultaneously with

---

✢ Canadian trade name   🦫 Non-Crushable Drug   **HIGH ALERT** High Alert drug

aluminum-containing antacids, cholestyramine. • Tablets should not be chewed or swallowed whole. • Disperse tablet by stirring in water, apple juice, orange juice until fine suspension is achieved. • Dosage less than 1 g should be dispersed in 3.5 oz of liquid, dosage more than 1 g should be dispersed in 7 oz of liquid. If any residue remains in glass, resuspend with a small amount of liquid.

INDICATIONS/ROUTES/DOSAGE

Iron Overload
PO: ADULTS, ELDERLY, CHILDREN 2 YRS AND OLDER: Initially, 20 mg/kg once daily. Adjust dosage of 5 or 10 mg/kg/day every 3–6 mos based on serum ferritin levels. Hold dose for serum ferritin less than 500 mcg/L. **Maximum:** 40 mg/kg once daily.

Thalassemia Syndromes
PO: ADULTS, ELDERLY, CHILDREN 10 YRS AND OLDER: 10 mg/kg once daily.

Dosage in Renal Impairment
Note: See Contraindications.
ADULTS: For increase in serum creatinine greater than 33% on 2 consecutive measures, reduce daily dose by 10 mg/kg. **CHILDREN:** For increase in serum creatinine above age-appropriate upper limit of normal on 2 consecutive measures, reduce daily dose by 10 mg/kg.

Dosage in Liver Impairment
For severe or persistent elevations in hepatic function tests, consider dose reduction or discontinuation.

SIDE EFFECTS

Frequent (19%–10%): Fever, headache, abdominal pain, cough, nasopharyngitis, diarrhea, nausea, vomiting. **Occasional (9%–4%):** Rash, arthralgia, fatigue, back pain, urticaria. **Rare (1%):** Edema, sleep disorder, dizziness, anxiety.

ADVERSE EFFECTS/ TOXIC REACTIONS

Bronchitis, pharyngitis, acute tonsillitis, ear infection occur occasionally. Hepatitis, auditory disturbances, ocular abnormalities occur rarely. Acute renal failure, cytopenias (e.g., agranulocytosis, neutropenia, thrombocytopenia) may occur.

NURSING CONSIDERATIONS

BASELINE ASSESSMENT
Obtain baseline serum CBC, ferritin, iron, creatinine, ALT, AST, urine protein, then monthly thereafter. Auditory, ophthalmic testing should be obtained before therapy and annually thereafter.

INTERVENTION/EVALUATION
Treatment should be interrupted if serum ferritin levels are consistently less than 500 mcg/L. Suspend treatment if severe rash occurs.

PATIENT/FAMILY TEACHING
• Take on empty stomach 30 min before food. • Do not chew or swallow tablet whole; disperse tablet completely in water, apple juice, orange juice; drink resulting suspension immediately. • Do not take aluminum-containing antacids concurrently. • Inform physician if severe skin rash, changes in vision/hearing, or yellowing of skin/eyes occurs.

deferiprone

de-**fair**-i-prone
(Ferriprox)
BLACK BOX ALERT May cause agranulocytosis that can lead to serious infection, death. Neutropenia may precede development of agranulocytosis.

◆CLASSIFICATION

PHARMACOTHERAPEUTIC: Iron-chelating agent. **CLINICAL:** Iron reduction.

ACTION

Selective for ferric ion. Attaches to iron to form a compound that can be excreted by the body. **Therapeutic Effect:** Induces iron excretion.

PHARMACOKINETICS

Rapidly absorbed following oral administration. Peak plasma concentration: 1 hr. Protein binding: 10%. Primarily excreted in urine. **Half-life:** 1.9 hrs.

USES

Treatment of transfusional iron overload due to thalassemia syndrome (a generic blood disorder that causes anemia) when current chelation therapy is inadequate.

PRECAUTIONS

Contraindications: None known. **Cautions:** Renal/hepatic impairment, pts at increased risk of prolongation of QT interval (HF, bradycardia, diuretic use, cardiac hypertrophy, hypokalemia, hypomagnesemia).

⌛ LIFESPAN CONSIDERATIONS

Pregnancy/Lactation: May cause fetal harm. Unknown if excreted in breast milk. Do not breastfeed. **Pregnancy Category D. Children:** Safety and efficacy not established. **Elderly:** No age-related precautions noted.

INTERACTIONS

DRUG: Aluminum-containing antacids, supplements containing **iron or zinc** may decrease effects. Separate by 4 hrs. Other **iron-chelating agents** increase risk of toxic effects. **HERBAL: Milk thistle** may increase risk of side effects. **FOOD:** None known. **LAB VALUES:** Decreases serum ferritin, zinc concentration. May increase serum ALT, AST.

AVAILABILITY (Rx)

Tablets, Film-Coated, Scored: 500 mg.

ADMINISTRATION/HANDLING

PO
• Give without regard to food. • Do not give simultaneously with aluminum-con-

taining antacids or supplements containing iron or zinc; separate by 4 hrs.

INDICATIONS/ROUTES/DOSAGE

Iron Overload
PO: ADULTS, ELDERLY: Initially, 25 mg/kg 3 times daily (morning, midday, evening) for a total of 75 mg/kg per day. Adjust dosage up to 33 mg/kg 3 times daily. **Maximum:** 99 mg/kg per day. Dose should be rounded to nearest 250 mg (half-tablet).

SIDE EFFECTS

Occasional (15%–10%): Chromaturia (reddish/brown discoloration of urine), nausea, abdominal pain/discomfort, vomiting, arthralgia. **Rare (4%–2%):** Increased weight, diarrhea, headache, dyspepsia (heartburn, bloating, eructation), back pain, pain in extremity.

ADVERSE EFFECTS/ TOXIC REACTIONS

Agranulocytosis, generally preceded by neutropenia may be noted.

NURSING CONSIDERATIONS

BASELINE ASSESSMENT

Obtain baseline serum creatinine, ferritin, ALT, AST, and monthly thereafter. Measure absolute neutrophil count (ANC) prior to therapy and monitor ANC weekly during therapy. If deferiprone is used during pregnancy or if pt becomes pregnant while taking medication, pt should be apprised of potential hazard to fetus.

INTERVENTION/EVALUATION

Monitor serum ferritin concentration every 2–3 mos to assess the effects of medication on body iron stores. If serum ferritin falls consistently below 500 mcg/L, consider temporarily interrupting therapy. Interrupt treatment if infection develops or if neutropenia occurs, based on ANC. Monitor serum ALT, AST values monthly during therapy. Interruption of therapy should be considered if there is a persistent increase in serum transaminase levels.

PATIENT/FAMILY TEACHING
• Urine may show a reddish-brown discoloration. • Report any symptoms that may indicate infection (fever, sore throat, flu-like symptoms). • Avoid pregnancy. • Do not breastfeed during treatment. • Do not simultaneously take aluminum-containing antacids or supplements containing zinc or iron (separate by 4 hrs).

deferoxamine

de-fur-**ox**-a-meen
(Desferal)
Do not confuse deferoxamine with cefuroxime or deferasirox, or Desferal with Desyrel.

♦ CLASSIFICATION
CLINICAL: Antidote.

ACTION

Binds with iron to form complex. **Therapeutic Effect:** Promotes urinary excretion of iron.

PHARMACOKINETICS

Erratic absorption following IM administration. Widely distributed. Excreted in urine, eliminated in feces via biliary excretion. Removed by hemodialysis. **Half-life:** 6 hrs.

USES

Treatment of acute iron toxicity, chronic iron toxicity secondary to multiple transfusions associated with some chronic anemias (e.g., thalassemia). **OFF-LABEL:** Treatment/diagnosis of aluminum toxicity associated with chronic kidney disease.

PRECAUTIONS

Contraindications: Severe renal disease, anuria, primary hemochromatosis. **Cautions:** Renal impairment, elderly. **Pregnancy Category C.**

INTERACTIONS

DRUG: Vitamin C may increase effect. **HERBAL:** None significant. **FOOD:** None known. **LAB VALUES:** May cause falsely elevated total iron-binding capacity (TIBC).

AVAILABILITY (Rx)

Injection, Powder for Reconstitution: 500 mg, 2 g.

ADMINISTRATION/HANDLING

◀ **ALERT** ▶ **IM:** Reconstitute each 500-mg vial with 2 ml Sterile Water for Injection to provide a concentration of 210 mg/ml or 8 ml to each 2-g vial to provide a concentration of 213 mg/ml. **IV:** Reconstitute with SWFI to provide concentration of 100 mg/ml. **Subcutaneous:** Reconstitute 500 mg with 5 ml; 2 g with 20 ml SWFI to provide a concentration of 95 mg/ml.

 IV

• For IV infusion, further dilute with 0.9% NaCl, D_5W, and administer at no more than 15 mg/kg/hr for first 1,000 mg, followed by 500 mg over 4 hrs.
• Rapid IV administration may produce skin flushing, urticaria, hypotension, shock.

IM
• Inject deeply into upper outer quadrant of buttock. No further dilution necessary.

Subcutaneous
• Administer subcutaneous slowly. No further dilution necessary. Following reconstitution, stable for 7 days at room temperature.

🖳 IV INCOMPATIBILITY

Do not mix with any other IV medications.

INDICATIONS/ROUTES/DOSAGE

Acute Iron Intoxication
IV, IM: ADULTS: Initially, 1 g, then 0.5 g q4h for 2 doses; may give additional

doses of 0.5 g q4–12h. **IM: CHILDREN 3 YRS AND OLDER:** 90 mg/kg/dose q8h. **Maximum:** 6 g/day.
IV: CHILDREN: 15 mg/kg/hr. **Maximum:** 6 g/day.

Chronic Iron Overload

Subcutaneous: ADULTS: 1–2 g/day or 20–40 mg/kg/day over 8–24 hrs. **CHILDREN 3 YRS AND OLDER:** 20–40 mg/kg/day over 8–12 hrs. **Maximum:** 2 g/day.
IM: ADULTS: 0.5–1 g/day. Also, 2 g with each unit of blood.
IV: CHILDREN 3 YRS AND OLDER: 15 mg/kg/hr. **Maximum:** 6 g/24h.

SIDE EFFECTS

Frequent: Pain, induration at injection site, urine color change (to orange-rose). **Occasional:** Abdominal discomfort, diarrhea, leg cramps, impaired vision.

ADVERSE EFFECTS/ TOXIC REACTIONS

High-frequency hearing loss, tinnitus have been noted.

NURSING CONSIDERATIONS

BASELINE ASSESSMENT

Assess serum iron levels, total iron-binding capacity (TIBC) before and during therapy.

INTERVENTION/EVALUATION

Question for evidence of hearing loss (neurotoxicity). Periodic ophthalmic exams should be obtained in those treated for chronic iron overload. For IV administration, monitor serum ferritin, iron, TIBC, body weight, growth, B/P. If using subcutaneous technique, monitor for pruritus, erythema, skin irritation, edema.

PATIENT/FAMILY TEACHING

• Medication may produce discomfort at IM or subcutaneous injection site. • Urine will appear reddish. • Report hearing or vision changes.

degarelix

deg-a-**re**-lix
(Firmagon)
Do not confuse degarelix with cetrorelix or ganirelix.

◆**CLASSIFICATION**

PHARMACOTHERAPEUTIC: Gonadotropin-releasing hormone antagonist. **CLINICAL:** Antineoplastic.

ACTION

Antagonizes pituitary gonadotropin-releasing hormone (GnRH) receptors (binds immediately and reversibly), suppressing release of luteinizing hormone (LH) from pituitary gland, leading to rapid and sustained suppression of testosterone release from testes. **Therapeutic Effect:** Reduces size and growth of prostate cancer.

PHARMACOKINETICS

Distributed throughout total body water. Protein binding: 90%. Metabolized due to peptide hydrolysis during hepatobiliary system passage. Excreted in feces (70%–80%), urine (20%–30%). **Half-life:** 53 days.

USES

Treatment of advanced prostate cancer.

PRECAUTIONS

Contraindications: Pregnancy (Pregnancy Category X), potential to become pregnant. **Cautions:** History of QT prolongation, those with risk factors for QT prolongation (e.g., hypokalemia, HF), severe hepatic impairment, renal impairment (creatinine clearance less than 50 ml/min).

⧗ LIFESPAN CONSIDERATIONS

Pregnancy/Lactation: Not indicated for use in this pt population. **Pregnancy Category X. Children:** Not indicated for use in this pt population. **Elderly:** No age-related precautions noted.

INTERACTIONS

DRUG: Dronedarone, amiodarone, macrolide antibiotics other QT prolonging medications increase risk of QT prolongation. **HERBAL:** None significant. **FOOD:** None known. **LAB VALUES:** Expected to decrease serum testosterone levels. May increase serum AST, ALT levels.

AVAILABILITY (Rx)

Injection, Powder for Solution: 80 mg, 120 mg.

ADMINISTRATION/HANDLING

Subcutaneous
• Reconstitute 80-mg vial with 4.2 ml Sterile Water for Injection to provide 20 mg/ml concentration (120 mg with 3 ml SWI to provide 40 mg/ml concentration). • Administer within 1 hr following reconstitution. • Wear gloves during preparation and administration. • Vial must be kept vertical at all times; do not shake. • Administer in abdominal region in areas that will not be exposed to pressure (on or close to waistband area).

INDICATIONS/ROUTES/DOSAGE

Prostate Cancer
Subcutaneous: ADULTS, ELDERLY: Loading dose: 240 mg given as 2 injections of 120 mg (40 mg/ml). **Maintenance:** 80 mg q28days beginning 28 days after loading dose.

SIDE EFFECTS

Frequent: (27%–11%): Hot flashes, injection site pain, erythema, increased weight. **Occasional (7%–5%):** Hypertension, local edema, fatigue, back pain, constipation, urinary tract infection, asthenia (lack of strength, energy), arthralgia, chills. **Rare: (1%):** Insomnia, headache, nausea, dizziness, erectile dysfunction, gynecomastia, testicular atrophy, night sweats.

ADVERSE EFFECTS/ TOXIC REACTIONS

Long-term androgen deprivation therapy may prolong QT interval. Loss of bone density may occur.

NURSING CONSIDERATIONS

BASELINE ASSESSMENT
Obtain baseline EKG, electrolyte parameters, liver function test, prostate-specific antigen (PSA), testosterone levels prior to initiation of therapy.

INTERVENTION/EVALUATION
Monitor serum electrolytes, prostate-specific antigen (PSA) periodically. If PSA increases, measure testosterone serum concentrations. Monitor routine EKG for QT prolongation. Assess for decrease in testosterone levels throughout therapy. Monitor daily pattern of bowel activity, stool consistency.

PATIENT/FAMILY TEACHING
• Advise pt that swelling, itching, redness may occur at injection site. • Avoid tasks that require alertness, motor skills until response to drug is established.

---

delavirdine

de-la-**veer**-deen
(Rescriptor)
Do not confuse delavirdine with dalfampridine, or Rescriptor with ritonavir.

◆CLASSIFICATION

PHARMACOTHERAPEUTIC: Nonnucleoside reverse transcriptase inhibitor. **CLINICAL:** Antiretroviral (see pp. 69C, 119C).

ACTION

Binds directly to HIV-1 reverse transcriptase, blocks RNA- and DNA-dependent

DNA polymerase activities. **Therapeutic Effect:** Interrupts HIV replication, slowing progression of HIV infection.

PHARMACOKINETICS

Rapidly absorbed after PO administration. Protein binding: 98%. Primarily distributed in plasma. Metabolized in liver. Eliminated in urine (51%), feces (44%). **Half-life:** 2–11 hrs.

USES

Treatment of HIV infection (in combination with other antiretrovirals). Not recommended in initial antiretroviral regimens.

PRECAUTIONS

Contraindications: Concurrent use of alprazolam, ergot alkaloids, midazolam, rifampin, triazolam. **Cautions:** Renal/hepatic impairment. Concurrent use of CYP3A4 inhibitors/inducers (e.g., clarithromycin, fluoxetine, verapamil, phenobarbital, carbamazepine).

⌛ LIFESPAN CONSIDERATIONS

Pregnancy/Lactation: Unknown if drug crosses placenta or is distributed in breast milk. **Pregnancy Category C. Children:** Safety and efficacy not established in those younger than 16 yrs. **Elderly:** Safety and efficacy not established.

INTERACTIONS

DRUG: CYP3A4 inducers (e.g., carbamazepine, phenobarbital, phenytoin, rifabutin, rifampin) may decrease concentration/effects. May increase concentration/adverse effects of **statins, ergot derivatives, alprazolam, midazolam, triazolam. HERBAL: St. John's wort** may decrease concentration/effects. **FOOD:** None known. **LAB VALUES:** May increase serum AST, ALT. May decrease neutrophil count.

AVAILABILITY (Rx)

Tablets: 100 mg, 200 mg.

ADMINISTRATION/HANDLING

PO
• May disperse 100-mg tablets in water before consumption. 200-mg tablets should remain intact. • Give without regard to food. • Pts with achlorhydria should take with orange juice, cranberry juice.

INDICATIONS/ROUTES/DOSAGE

HIV Infection (in Combination with Other Antiretrovirals)
PO: ADULTS: 400 mg 3 times a day.

SIDE EFFECTS

Frequent (18%): Rash, pruritus. **Occasional (greater than 2%):** Headache, nausea, diarrhea, fatigue, anorexia.

ADVERSE EFFECTS/ TOXIC REACTIONS

Hepatic failure, severe rash, hemolytic anemia, rhabdomyolysis, erythema multiforme, Stevens-Johnson syndrome, acute renal failure have been reported.

NURSING CONSIDERATIONS

BASELINE ASSESSMENT

Obtain baseline lab tests, esp. hepatic function tests, before initiation of therapy and at periodic intervals during therapy. Offer emotional support.

INTERVENTION/EVALUATION

Assess skin for rash. Question for nausea, fatigue. Monitor daily pattern of bowel activity, stool consistency. Assess eating pattern; monitor for weight loss. Monitor lab values carefully, particularly hepatic function, especially if taken with saquinavir.

PATIENT/FAMILY TEACHING

• Do not take any medications, including OTC drugs, without consulting physician. • Small, frequent meals may offset anorexia, nausea. • Delavirdine is not a cure for HIV infection, nor does it reduce risk of transmission to others.

denileukin `HIGH ALERT`

de-ni-**loo**-kin
(Ontak)

BLACK BOX ALERT Must be administered by personnel trained in administration/handling of chemotherapeutic agents. Has been associated with severe capillary leak syndrome; severe and fatal infusion reactions; loss of visual acuity, usually with loss of color vision.

◆ CLASSIFICATION

PHARMACOTHERAPEUTIC: Biologic response modifier. **CLINICAL:** Antineoplastic (see p. 84C).

ACTION

Cytotoxic fusion protein that targets cells expressing interleukin-2 (IL-2) receptors. After binding to IL-2 receptor, directs cytocidal action to malignant cutaneous T-cell lymphoma (CTCL) cells. **Therapeutic Effect:** Causes inhibition of protein synthesis, cell death.

PHARMACOKINETICS

Metabolized in liver. **Half-life:** 70–80 min.

USES

Treatment of persistent/recurrent cutaneous T-cell lymphoma (CTCL) whose malignant cells express CD25 component of IL-2 receptor. **OFF-LABEL:** Treatment of relapsed/recurrent peripheral T-cell lymphoma.

PRECAUTIONS

Contraindications: None known. **Cautions:** Pts older than 65 yrs of age, hypoalbuminemia. **Pregnancy Category C.**

INTERACTIONS

DRUG: None significant. **HERBAL: Echinacea** may decrease concentration/effects. **FOOD:** None known. **LAB VALUES:** May decrease serum albumin, calcium, potassium, WBC, Hgb, Hct. May increase serum transaminase.

AVAILABILITY (Rx)

Injection Solution: 150 mcg/ml.

ADMINISTRATION/HANDLING

 IV

Reconstitution • Thaw in refrigerator for up to 24 hrs or at room temperature for 1–2 hrs. • Inject calculated dose into empty infusion bag. Dilute with 0.9% NaCl to a concentration of 15 mcg/ml or greater.
Rate of Administration • Infuse over 30–60 min.
Storage • Store frozen. • Solutions for IV infusion stable for 6 hrs.

🔀 IV INCOMPATIBILITIES

Do not mix with any other IV medications.

INDICATIONS/ROUTES/DOSAGE

Cutaneous T-Cell Lymphoma (CTCL)
IV Infusion: ADULTS: 9 or 18 mcg/kg/day for 5 consecutive days q21days for 8 cycles. Infuse over at least 30 min. Hold if serum albumin less than 3 g/dl.

SIDE EFFECTS

Frequent: Two distinct syndromes occur commonly: a hypersensitivity reaction (69%), consisting of 2 or more of the following: hypotension, back pain, dyspnea, vasodilation, vascular leak syndrome characterized by hypotension, edema, hypoalbuminemia, rash, chest tightness, tachycardia, dysphagia, syncope; and a flu-like symptom complex (91%), consisting of 2 or more of the following: fever, chills, nausea, vomiting, diarrhea, myalgia, arthralgia. **Occasional (25%–10%):** Dizziness, peripheral edema, chest pain, weight loss, rhinitis, pruritus.

ADVERSE EFFECTS/ TOXIC REACTIONS

Pancreatitis, acute renal insufficiency, hematuria, hypothyroidism/hyperthyroidism occur rarely.

NURSING CONSIDERATIONS

BASELINE ASSESSMENT

Obtain CBC, serum chemistries (including renal/hepatic function tests), chest X-ray before therapy and weekly thereafter. Assess serum albumin level before initiation of each treatment (should be equal to or greater than 3 g/dl).

INTERVENTION/EVALUATION

Monitor serum albumin for hypoalbuminemia (generally occurs 1–2 wks after administration). Monitor for evidence of infection (lowered immune response: sore throat, fever, other vague symptoms). Monitor weight, B/P, or for hypersensitivity reaction. Assess for peripheral edema.

PATIENT/FAMILY TEACHING

• Drink plenty of fluids (protects against renal impairment). • Do not have immunizations without physician's approval (drug lowers resistance); avoid contact with those who have recently taken live virus vaccine.

---

denosumab

TOP 200

den-**oh**-sue-mab
(Prolia, Xgeva)

Do not confuse denosumab with daclizumab, or Prolia with Avandia or Zebeta.

◆ CLASSIFICATION

PHARMACOTHERAPEUTIC: Monoclonal antibody. **CLINICAL:** Bone resorption inhibitor (see p. 143C).

ACTION

Binds to RANK ligand (transmembrane protein). Essential for formation, function, survival of osteoclasts. **Therapeutic Effect:** Decreases bone resorption; increases bone mass, strength.

PHARMACOKINETICS

Serum level detected 1 hr after administration. **Half-life:** 32 days.

USES

Prolia: Treatment of postmenopausal women with osteoporosis at high risk for fracture. Treatment to increase bone mass in men at high risk for fractures receiving androgen deprivation therapy for nonmetastatic prostate cancer and in women at high risk for fractures receiving adjuvant aromatase inhibitor therapy for breast cancer. Treatment to increase bone mass in men with osteoporosis at high risk for fracture. **Xgeva:** Prevention of skeletal-related events (e.g., fracture, spinal cord compression) in pts with bone metastases from solid tumor. Treatment of giant cell tumor of bone. **OFF-LABEL:** Treatment of bone destruction caused by rheumatoid arthritis.

PRECAUTIONS

Contraindications: Prolia: Preexisting hypocalcemia (must be corrected prior to surgery). **Pregnancy Cautions:** History of hypoparathyroidism, thyroid/parathyroid surgery, malabsorption syndromes, excision of small intestine, immunocompromised pts. Pts with severe renal impairment (creatinine clearance less than 30 ml/min) or receiving dialysis are at greater risk for developing hypocalcemia.

⌛ LIFESPAN CONSIDERATIONS

Pregnancy/Lactation: Approved for use only in postmenopausal women. **Pregnancy Category C. Children:** Approved for use only in postmenopausal women. **Elderly:** No age-related precautions noted.

INTERACTIONS

DRUG: None significant. **HERBAL:** None significant. **FOOD:** None known. **LAB VALUES:** May decrease serum calcium. May increase serum cholesterol.

AVAILABILITY (Rx)

Injection, Solution (Prolia): 60 mg/ml. **(Xgeva):** 70 mg/ml (1.7 ml).

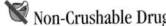

♣ Canadian trade name   🦺 Non-Crushable Drug   🔲 High Alert drug

ADMINISTRATION/HANDLING

Subcutaneous
• Administer in upper arm, upper thigh, or abdomen.
Storage • Refrigerate. • Solution appears as clear, colorless to pale yellow.

INDICATIONS/ROUTES/DOSAGE

Prolia
Osteoporosis; Increase Bone Mass
Subcutaneous: ADULTS, ELDERLY: 60 mg every 6 mos.

Xgeva
Prevention of Skeletal-Related Events
Subcutaneous: ADULTS, ELDERLY: 120 mg q4wks.

Xgeva
Giant Cell Tumor
Subcutaneous: ADULTS, ELDERLY, MATURE ADOLESCENTS: 120 mg q4wks with additional doses on days 8 and 15 of first mo of therapy.

SIDE EFFECTS

Frequent (35%–12%): Back pain, extremity pain. **Occasional (8%–5%):** Musculoskeletal pain, vertigo, peripheral edema, sciatica. **Rare (4%–2%):** Bone pain, upper abdominal pain, rash, insomnia, flatulence, pruritus, myalgia, asthenia (loss of strength, energy), GI reflux.

ADVERSE EFFECTS/ TOXIC REACTIONS

Increases risk of infection, specifically cystitis, upper respiratory tract infection, pneumonia, pharyngitis, herpes zoster (shingles) occur in 2%–6% of pts. Osteonecrosis of the jaw (OJN) was reported. Suppression of bone turnover, pancreatitis have been reported.

NURSING CONSIDERATIONS

BASELINE ASSESSMENT

Hypocalcemia must be corrected prior to treatment. Calcium 1,000 mg/day and vitamin D at least 400 international units/day should be given. Dental exam should be provided prior to treatment.

INTERVENTION/EVALUATION

Monitor serum magnesium, calcium, ionized calcium, phosphate. In pts predisposed with hypocalcemia and disturbances of mineral metabolism, clinical monitoring of calcium, mineral levels is highly recommended. Adequately supplement all pts with calcium and vitamin D. Monitor for delayed fracture healing.

PATIENT/FAMILY TEACHING

• Report rash, new-onset eczema. • Seek prompt medical attention if signs, symptoms of severe infection (rash, itching, reddened skin, cellulitis) occur. • Report muscle stiffness, numbness, cramps, spasms (signs of hypocalcemia); swelling or drainage from jaw, mouth, or teeth.

desipramine

de-**sip**-ra-meen
(Novo-Desipramine ❦, Norpramin)
BLACK BOX ALERT Increased risk of suicidal ideation and behavior in children, adolescents, young adults 18–24 yrs with major depressive disorder, other psychiatric disorders.
Do not confuse desipramine with clomipramine, dalfampridine, diphenhydramine, disopyramide, or imipramine, or Norpramin with nortriptyline.

◆ CLASSIFICATION

PHARMACOTHERAPEUTIC: Tricyclic.
CLINICAL: Antidepressant (see p. 39C).

ACTION

Blocks reuptake of neurotransmitters, (norepinephrine, serotonin) at presynaptic membranes, increasing their availability at postsynaptic receptor sites. Strong anticholinergic activity. **Therapeutic Effect:** Relieves depression.

PHARMACOKINETICS

Rapidly, well absorbed from GI tract. Protein binding: 90%. Metabolized in liver. Primarily excreted in urine. Minimally removed by hemodialysis. **Half-life:** 7–60 hrs.

USES

Treatment of depression, often in conjunction with psychotherapy. **OFF-LABEL:** Treatment of ADHD, adjunct in chronic pain treatment, neurogenic pain, depression in children 6–12 yrs.

PRECAUTIONS

Contraindications: Use within 14 days of MAOIs, acute recovery phase of MI. **Cautions:** Cardiovascular disease, cardiac conduction disturbances, urinary retention, diabetes, BPH, glaucoma, narrow-angle glaucoma, xerostomia, visual problems, constipation, history of bowel obstruction, seizure disorders, hyperthyroidism, pts taking thyroid replacement therapy, high risk of suicide, renal/hepatic impairment.

⌛ LIFESPAN CONSIDERATIONS

Pregnancy/Lactation: Crosses placenta. Minimally distributed in breast milk. **Pregnancy Category C. Children:** Not recommended in pts 6 yrs and younger. Children and adolescents with major depressive disorder (MDD), other psychiatric disorders, at increased risk for suicidal ideation, behavior, esp. during first few mos of treatment. **Elderly:** Use lower dosages (higher dosages not tolerated, increases risk of toxicity).

INTERACTIONS

DRUG: **Alcohol, other CNS depressants** may increase CNS, respiratory depression; hypotensive effects. **Cimetidine** may increase desipramine concentration, risk of toxicity. **Fluoxetine, paroxetine, phenothiazines, propafenone, flecainide** may increase concentration. **HERBAL:** **Kava kava, SAMe, St. John's wort, valerian** may increase sedation, risk of se-

rotonin syndrome. **St. John's wort** may decrease concentration. **FOOD:** **Grapefruit products** may increase concentration/toxicity. **LAB VALUES:** May alter serum glucose, EKG readings. **Therapeutic serum level:** 115–300 ng/ml; **toxic serum level:** greater than 400 ng/ml.

AVAILABILITY (Rx)

Tablets: 10 mg, 25 mg, 50 mg, 75 mg, 100 mg, 150 mg.

ADMINISTRATION/HANDLING

PO
◀ **ALERT** ▶ Fourteen days must elapse between use of MAOIs and desipramine.
• Give with food, milk if GI distress occurs.

INDICATIONS/ROUTES/DOSAGE

Depression
PO: ADULTS: 75 mg/day. May gradually increase to 150–200 mg/day. **Maximum:** 300 mg/day. **ELDERLY:** Initially, 10–25 mg/day. May gradually increase to 75–100 mg/day. **Maximum:** 150 mg/day. **CHILDREN OLDER THAN 12 YRS:** Initially, 25–50 mg/day. May gradually increase to 100 mg/day. **Maximum:** 150 mg/day. **CHILDREN 6–12 YRS (OFF-LABEL):** 1–3 mg/kg/day. **Maximum:** 5 mg/kg/day.

SIDE EFFECTS

Frequent: Drowsiness, fatigue, dry mouth, blurred vision, constipation, delayed urination, orthostatic hypotension, diaphoresis, impaired concentration, increased appetite, urinary retention. **Occasional:** GI disturbances (nausea, GI distress, metallic taste). **Rare:** Paradoxical reactions (agitation, restlessness, nightmares, insomnia), extrapyramidal symptoms (particularly fine hand tremor).

ADVERSE EFFECTS/ TOXIC REACTIONS

Overdose may produce confusion, seizures, drowsiness, arrhythmias, fever, hallucinations, dyspnea, vomiting, unusual fatigue, weakness. Abrupt discontinuation after prolonged therapy may produce severe headache, malaise, nausea, vomiting, vivid dreams.

NURSING CONSIDERATIONS

BASELINE ASSESSMENT

For pts on long-term therapy, hepatic/renal function tests, blood counts should be performed periodically. For those at risk for arrhythmias, perform baseline EKG.

INTERVENTION/EVALUATION

Monitor for worsening of depression, suicidal ideation. Assess appearance, behavior, speech pattern, level of interest, mood. **Therapeutic serum level:** 115–300 ng/ml; **toxic serum level:** greater than 400 ng/ml. Monitor EKG if pt has history of arrhythmias.

PATIENT/FAMILY TEACHING

• Go from lying to standing slowly. • Tolerance to postural hypotension, sedative, anticholinergic effects usually develops during early therapy. • Maximum therapeutic effect may be noted in 2–4 wks. • Do not abruptly discontinue medication. • Avoid alcohol, grapefruit products. • Report worsening depression, suicidal ideation, unusual changes in behavior (esp. at initiation of therapy or with changes in dosage).

desloratadine

des-lor-a-ta-deen
(Aerius ✤, Clarinex, Clarinex Redi-Tabs)
Do not confuse Clarinex with Celebrex or Claritin.

FIXED-COMBINATION(S)

Clarinex-D 24 Hour: desloratadine/pseudoephedrine (a sympathomimetic): 5 mg/240 mg. **Clarinex-D 12 Hour:** desloratadine/pseudoephedrine: 2.5 mg/120 mg.

◆CLASSIFICATION

PHARMACOTHERAPEUTIC: H_1 antagonist. **CLINICAL:** Nonsedating antihistamine (see p. 54C).

ACTION

Exhibits selective peripheral histamine H_1 receptor blocking action. Competes with histamine at receptor sites. **Therapeutic Effect:** Prevents allergic response mediated by histamine (rhinitis, urticaria).

PHARMACOKINETICS

Rapidly absorbed from GI tract. Distributed mainly in liver, lungs, GI tract, bile. Protein binding: 82%. Metabolized in liver. Eliminated in urine, feces. **Half-life:** 27 hrs (increased in elderly, renal/hepatic impairment).

USES

Relief of nasal/non-nasal symptoms of seasonal and perennial rhinitis (sneezing, rhinorrhea, itching/tearing of eyes, stuffiness), chronic idiopathic urticaria (hives).

PRECAUTIONS

Contraindications: None known. **Cautions:** Renal/hepatic impairment, breastfeeding.

⊠ LIFESPAN CONSIDERATIONS

Pregnancy/Lactation: Excreted in breast milk. **Pregnancy Category C. Children/Elderly:** More sensitive to anticholinergic effects (e.g., dry mouth, nose, throat).

INTERACTIONS

DRUG: Erythromycin, ketoconazole, fluoxetine, cimetidine may increase concentration. **HERBAL:** None significant. **FOOD:** None known. **LAB VALUES:** May suppress wheal, flare reactions to antigen skin testing unless antihistamines are discontinued 4 days before testing.

AVAILABILITY (Rx)
Syrup (Clarinex): 2.5 mg/5 ml. **Tablets** (Clarinex): 5 mg.

ADMINISTRATION/HANDLING
PO
• May give with or without food.

INDICATIONS/ROUTES/DOSAGE
Allergic Rhinitis, Urticaria
PO: ADULTS, ELDERLY, CHILDREN OLDER THAN 12 YRS: 5 mg once a day. **CHILDREN 6–12 YRS:** 2.5 mg once a day. **CHILDREN 1–5 YRS:** 1.25 mg once a day. **CHILDREN 6–11 MOS:** 1 mg once a day.

Dosage in Hepatic/Renal Impairment
Dosage is decreased to 5 mg every other day.

SIDE EFFECTS
Frequent (12%): Headache. **Occasional (3%):** Dry mouth, drowsiness. **Rare (less than 3%):** Fatigue, dizziness, diarrhea, nausea.

ADVERSE EFFECTS/ TOXIC REACTIONS
None known.

NURSING CONSIDERATIONS

BASELINE ASSESSMENT
Assess lung sounds for wheezing; skin for urticaria, hives.

INTERVENTION/EVALUATION
For upper respiratory allergies, increase fluids to decrease viscosity of secretions, offset thirst, replace loss of fluids from diaphoresis. Monitor symptoms for therapeutic response.

PATIENT/FAMILY TEACHING
• Drink plenty of water (may cause dry mouth). • Avoid tasks that require alertness, motor skills until response to drug is established (may cause drowsiness). • Avoid alcohol.

desmopressin

des-moe-**press**-in
(Apo-Desmopressin ✦, DDAVP, DDAVP Nasal, DDAVP Rhinal Tube, Minirin ✦, Novo-Desmopressin ✦, Octostim ✦, Stimate)

◆ **CLASSIFICATION**
PHARMACOTHERAPEUTIC: Synthetic pituitary hormone. **CLINICAL:** Antidiuretic.

ACTION
Increases reabsorption of water by increasing permeability of collecting ducts of kidneys. Plasminogen activator. **Therapeutic Effect:** Increases plasma factor VIII (antihemophilic factor). Decreases urinary output.

PHARMACOKINETICS

Route	Onset	Peak	Duration
PO	1 hr	2–7 hrs	8–12 hrs
IV	15–30 min	1.5–3 hrs	8–12 hrs
Intranasal	15 min–1 hr	1–5 hrs	8–12 hrs

Poorly absorbed after PO, nasal administration. Metabolism: Unknown. **Half-life: PO:** 1.5–2.5 hrs. **Intranasal:** 3.3–3.5 hrs. **IV:** 0.4–4 hrs.

USES
DDAVP Nasal: Central cranial diabetes insipidus. **Parenteral:** Central cranial diabetes insipidus. Maintain hemostasis and control bleeding in hemophilia A, von Willebrand's disease (type I). **Stimate intranasal:** Maintain hemostasis and control bleeding in hemophilia A, von Willebrand's disease (type I). **PO:** Central cranial diabetes insipidus, primary nocturnal enuresis, temporary polyuria, polydipsia following pituitary surgery or head trauma. **OFF-LABEL:** Uremic bleeding occurring with acute/chronic renal failure; prevent surgical bleeding in pts with uremia.

✦ Canadian trade name   ✔ Non-Crushable Drug   ▦ High Alert drug

PRECAUTIONS

Contraindications: Hyponatremia; history of hyponatremia; moderate to severe renal impairment. **Cautions:** Predisposition to thrombus formation; conditions with fluid, electrolyte imbalance; coronary artery disease; hypertensive cardiovascular disease. Avoid use in hemophilia A with factor VIII levels less than 5%; hemophilia B; severe type I, type IIB, platelet-type von Willebrand's disease.

⌛ LIFESPAN CONSIDERATIONS

Pregnancy/Lactation: Pregnancy Category B. Children: Caution in neonates, those younger than 3 mos (increased risk of fluid balance problems). Careful fluid restrictions recommended in infants. **Elderly:** Increased risk of hyponatremia, water intoxication.

INTERACTIONS

DRUG: Carbamazepine, lamotrigine, NSAIDs, SSRIs, tricyclic antidepressants may increase effect. **Demeclocycline, lithium** may decrease effect. **HERBAL:** None significant. **FOOD:** None known. **LAB VALUES:** May decrease serum sodium.

AVAILABILITY (Rx)

Injection Solution (DDAVP): 4 mcg/ml. **Nasal Solution (DDAVP):** 100 mcg/ml. **Nasal Spray (Stimate):** 1.5 mg/ml (150 mcg/spray). **(DDAVP):** 100 mcg/ml (10 mcg/spray). **Tablets (DDAVP):** 0.1 mg, 0.2 mg.

ADMINISTRATION/HANDLING

 IV

Reconstitution • For IV infusion, dilute in 10–50 ml 0.9% NaCl (10 ml for children 10 kg or less; 50 ml for adults, children greater than 10 kg).
Rate of Administration • Infuse over 15–30 min. • For preop use, administer 30 min before procedure.
Storage • Refrigerate. • Stable for 2 wks at room temperature.

Subcutaneous
• Withdraw dose from vial. Further dilution not required.

Intranasal
• Refrigerate DDAVP Rhinal Tube solution, Stimate nasal spray. • Rhinal Tube solution, Stimate nasal spray are stable for 3 wks at room temperature. • DDAVP nasal spray is stable at room temperature. • Calibrated catheter (rhinyle) is used to draw up measured quantity of desmopressin; with one end inserted in nose, pt blows on other end to deposit solution deep in nasal cavity. • For infants, young children, obtunded pts, air-filled syringe may be attached to catheter to deposit solution.

INDICATIONS/ROUTES/DOSAGE

Primary Nocturnal Enuresis
PO: CHILDREN 6 YRS AND OLDER: 0.2–0.6 mg once before bedtime. Limit fluid intake 1 hr prior and at least 8 hrs after dose.

Central Cranial Diabetes Insipidus
◀ALERT▶ Fluid restriction should be observed.
PO: ADULTS, ELDERLY, CHILDREN 12 YRS AND OLDER: Initially, 0.05 mg twice a day. Titrate to desired response. Range: 0.1–1.2 mg/day in 2–3 divided doses. **CHILDREN YOUNGER THAN 12 YRS:** Initially, 0.05 mg, twice a day. Titrate to desired response. Range: 0.1–1.2 mg daily.
IV, Subcutaneous: ADULTS, ELDERLY, CHILDREN 12 YRS AND OLDER: 2–4 mcg/day in 2 divided doses or $\frac{1}{10}$ of maintenance intranasal dose.
Intranasal (Use 100 mcg/ml Concentration): ADULTS, ELDERLY, CHILDREN OLDER THAN 12 YRS: 10–40 mcg (0.1–0.4 ml) in 1–3 doses/day. **CHILDREN 3 MOS–12 YRS:** Initially, 5 mcg (0.05 ml)/day. Range: 5–30 mcg (0.05–0.3 ml)/day.

Hemophilia A, von Willebrand's Disease (Type I)
IV Infusion: ADULTS, ELDERLY, CHILDREN WEIGHING MORE THAN 10 KG: 0.3 mcg/kg diluted in 50 ml 0.9% NaCl. **CHILDREN**

WEIGHING 10 KG AND LESS: 0.3 mcg/kg diluted in 10 ml 0.9% NaCl.
Intranasal *(Use 1.5 mg/ml Concentration Providing 150 mcg/Spray):* **ADULTS, ELDERLY, CHILDREN 12 YRS AND OLDER WEIGHING MORE THAN 50 KG:** 300 mcg; use 1 spray in each nostril. **ADULTS, ELDERLY, CHILDREN 12 YRS AND OLDER WEIGHING 50 KG OR LESS:** 150 mcg as a single spray.

Dosage in Renal Impairment
Creatinine clearance less than 50 ml/min: Not recommended.

SIDE EFFECTS

Occasional: IV: Pain, redness, swelling at injection site; headache; abdominal cramps; vulvular pain; flushed skin; mild B/P elevation; nausea with high dosages. **Nasal:** Rhinorrhea, nasal congestion, slight B/P elevation.

ADVERSE EFFECTS/ TOXIC REACTIONS

Water intoxication, hyponatremia (headache, drowsiness, confusion, decreased urination, rapid weight gain, seizures, coma) may occur in overhydration. Children, elderly pts, infants are esp. at risk.

NURSING CONSIDERATIONS

BASELINE ASSESSMENT

Establish baselines for B/P, pulse, weight, serum electrolytes, urine specific gravity. Check lab values for factor VIII coagulant concentration for hemophilia A, von Willebrand's disease; bleeding times.

INTERVENTION/EVALUATION

Check B/P, pulse with IV infusion. Monitor pt weight, fluid intake, urine volume, urine specific gravity, osmolality, serum electrolytes for diabetes insipidus. Assess factor VIII antigen levels, aPTT, factor VIII activity level for hemophilia.

PATIENT/FAMILY TEACHING

• Avoid overhydration. • Follow guidelines for proper intranasal administration.

• Report headache, shortness of breath, heartburn, nausea, abdominal cramps.

TOP 200

D

desvenlafaxine

des-ven-la-**fax**-een
(Pristiq)
BLACK BOX ALERT Increased risk of suicidal thinking and behavior in children, adolescents, young adults 18–24 yrs with major depressive disorder, other psychiatric disorders.

◆CLASSIFICATION

PHARMACOTHERAPEUTIC: Phenethylamine derivative. **CLINICAL:** Antidepressant (see p. 41C).

ACTION

Appears to inhibit serotonin and norepinephrine reuptake at CNS neuronal presynaptic membranes (weakly inhibits dopamine reuptake). **Therapeutic Effect:** Produces antidepressant effect.

PHARMACOKINETICS

Well absorbed from GI tract. Protein binding: 30%. Excreted primarily in urine. Steady-state plasma levels occur in 4–5 days. **Half-life:** 9–11 hrs.

USES

Treatment of major depression exhibited as persistent, prominent dysphoria (occurring nearly every day for at least 2 wks) manifested by 4 of 8 symptoms: change in appetite, change in sleep pattern, increased fatigue, impaired concentration, feelings of guilt or worthlessness, loss of interest in usual activities, psychomotor agitation or retardation, or suicidal tendencies.

PRECAUTIONS

Contraindications: Use of MAOIs within 14 days or in those currently taking

---

♣ Canadian trade name   🐢 Non-Crushable Drug   🔺HIGH ALERT High Alert drug

MAOIs (may cause neuroleptic malignant syndrome). Allow at least 7 days after discontinuation before starting an MAOI. **Cautions:** Renal impairment, history of seizures, bipolar disorder, those with suicidal ideation and behavior, increased intraocular pressure, narrow-angle glaucoma, cardiovascular or cerebrovascular disease.

⌛ LIFESPAN CONSIDERATIONS

Pregnancy/Lactation: Distributed in breast milk. **Pregnancy Category C. Children:** Safety and efficacy not established. **Elderly:** No age-related precautions noted.

INTERACTIONS

DRUG: Concurrent use of **MAOIs** may cause neuroleptic malignant syndrome: hyperthermia, rigidity, myoclonus, autonomic instability (including rapid fluctuations of vital signs), mental status changes, coma, extreme agitation. **Alcohol** increases CNS depressant effects. Decreases **midazolam** concentration. Increases **desipramine** concentration. **Aspirin, NSAIDs, warfarin** increase risk of bleeding. **Ketoconazole** may increase concentration/effect. **HERBAL: Gotu kola, kava kava, St. John's wort, valerian** may increase CNS depressant effects. **FOOD:** None known. **LAB VALUES:** May increase total serum cholesterol, LDL cholesterol, triglycerides, AST, ALT, prolactin level.

AVAILABILITY (Rx)

🐾 Tablets (Extended-Release): 50 mg, 100 mg.

ADMINISTRATION/HANDLING

PO
• Give without regard to food. • Give with food or milk if GI distress occurs. • Do not divide, crush, dissolve tablets. • Must be swallowed whole, with fluid.

INDICATIONS/ROUTES/DOSAGE

Major Depressive Disorder
PO: ADULTS: 50 mg once daily.

Dosage in Renal Impairment
Creatinine clearance less than 30 ml/min: 50 mg every other day. **HD:** 50 mg every other day.

SIDE EFFECTS

Frequent (22%–20%): Nausea, headache. **Occasional (13%–7%):** Dizziness, dry mouth, diarrhea, sweating, constipation, insomnia, fatigue. **Rare (5%–2%):** Anorexia, drowsiness, decreased libido, erectile dysfunction in men, anxiety, blurred vision, vomiting, decreased weight, tremor, paresthesia, irritability, abnormal dreams, blurred vision, tinnitus.

ADVERSE EFFECTS/ TOXIC REACTIONS

Seizures, syncope, extrapyramidal disorder, depersonalization, hypomania, epistaxis occur rarely. Ischemic cardiac events, including myocardial ischemia, MI, coronary occlusion requiring revascularization, may occur. Sustained increase in diastolic B/P (10–15 mm Hg) occurs occasionally.

NURSING CONSIDERATIONS

BASELINE ASSESSMENT
Obtain initial weight, B/P. Assess appearance, behavior, speech pattern, level of interest, mood, sleep pattern.

INTERVENTION/EVALUATION
Assess sleep pattern for evidence of insomnia. Monitor for suicidal ideation (esp. at initiation of therapy or changes in dosage). Assess appearance, behavior, speech pattern, level of interest, mood for therapeutic response. For pts on long-term therapy, serum chemistry profile to assess hepatic function should be performed periodically.

PATIENT/FAMILY TEACHING
• Take with food to minimize GI distress. • Do not increase, decrease, or suddenly discontinue medication. • Therapeutic effect may be noted within 1–4 wks. • Avoid tasks that require alertness, mo-

tor skills until response to drug is established. • Avoid alcohol. • Report worsening depression, suicidal ideation, unusual changes in behavior.

dexamethasone

dex-a-**meth**-a-sone
(Apo-Dexamethasone ✤, Baycodron, Dexamethasone Intensol, Dex-Pak TaperPak, Diodex ✤, Maxidex)
Do not confuse Decadron with Percodan, dexamethasone with dextroamphetamine, or Maxidex with Maxzide.

FIXED-COMBINATION(S)

Ciprodex Otic: dexamethasone/ciprofloxacin (antibiotic): 0.1%/0.3%.
Dexacidin, Maxitrol: dexamethasone/neomycin/polymyxin (anti-infectives): 0.1%/3.5 mg/10,000 units per g or ml.

◆CLASSIFICATION

PHARMACOTHERAPEUTIC: Long-acting glucocorticoid. **CLINICAL:** Corticosteroid (see pp. 100C, 102C).

ACTION

Inhibits accumulation of inflammatory cells at inflammation sites, phagocytosis, lysosomal enzyme release and synthesis, and/or release of mediators of inflammation. **Therapeutic Effect:** Prevents/suppresses cell/tissue immune reactions, inflammatory process.

PHARMACOKINETICS

Rapidly absorbed from GI tract after PO administration. Widely distributed. Protein binding: High. Metabolized in liver. Primarily excreted in urine. Minimally removed by hemodialysis. **Half-life:** 3–4.5 hrs.

USES

Acute exacerbations of chronic allergic disorders, cerebral edema, conditions treated by immunosuppression, inflammatory conditions, otitis externa, ophthalmic conditions (corneal injury, inflammatory conditions, allergic conjunctivitis). **OFF-LABEL:** Antiemetic, treatment of croup, dexamethasone suppression test (indicator consistent with suicide and/or depression), accelerate fetal lung maturation. Treatment of acute mountain sickness, high altitude cerebral edema.

PRECAUTIONS

Contraindications: Systemic fungal infections, cerebral malaria. **Cautions:** Thyroid disease, renal/hepatic impairment, cardiovascular disease, diabetes, glaucoma, cataracts, myasthenia gravis, pts at risk for seizures, osteoporosis, post MI.

⧗ LIFESPAN CONSIDERATIONS

Pregnancy/Lactation: Crosses placenta. Distributed in breast milk. **Pregnancy Category C (D if used in the first trimester). Children:** Prolonged treatment with high-dose therapy may decrease short-term growth rate, cortisol secretion. **Elderly:** Higher risk for developing hypertension, osteoporosis.

INTERACTIONS

DRUG: Amphotericin may increase hypokalemia. May increase **digoxin** toxicity caused by hypokalemia. **CYP3A4 inducers (e.g., carbamazepine, phenytoin, rifampin)** may decrease concentration. **CYP3A4 inhibitors (e.g., ketoconazole), macrolide antibiotics** may increase concentration. May decrease effects of **oral antidiabetic agents. Live virus vaccines** may decrease pt's antibody response to vaccine, increase vaccine side effects, potentiate virus replication. **HERBAL: Cat's claw, echinacea** may increase immunosuppressant effect. **FOOD:** Interferes with **calcium** absorption. **LAB VALUES:** May increase serum glucose, lipids, sodium levels. May decrease serum calcium, potassium, thyroxine, WBC.

AVAILABILITY (Rx)

Elixir: 0.5 mg/5 ml. Injection, Solution: 4 mg/ml, 10 mg/ml. Ophthalmic Solution: 0.1%. Ophthalmic Suspension (Maxidex): 0.1%. Solution, Oral: 0.5 mg/5 ml. Solution, Oral Concentrate (Dexamethasone Intensol): 1 mg/ml. Tablets: 0.5 mg, 0.75 mg, 1 mg, 1.5 mg, 2 mg, 4 mg, 6 mg. Tablets (TaperPak [DexPak]): 1.5 mg (35 or 51 tablets on taper dose card).

ADMINISTRATION/HANDLING

 IV

◀ALERT▶ Dexamethasone sodium phosphate may be given by IV push or IV infusion. Rapid injection may cause genital burning sensation in females.
• For IV push, give over 1–4 min if dose is less than 10 mg. • For IV infusion, mix with 50–100 ml 0.9% NaCl or D₅W and infuse over 15–30 min. • For neonates, solution must be preservative free. • IV solution must be used within 24 hrs.

IM
• Give deep IM, preferably in gluteus maximus.

PO
• Give with milk, food (to decrease GI effect).

Ophthalmic Solution, Suspension
• Place gloved finger on lower eyelid and pull out until a pocket is formed between eye and lower lid. • Place prescribed number of drops or ¼–½ inch ointment into pocket. • Instruct pt to close eye gently for 1–2 min (so medication will not be squeezed out of the sac). • Instruct pt to apply digital pressure to lacrimal sac at inner canthus for 1–2 min to minimize systemic absorption.

⊞ IV INCOMPATIBILITIES

Ciprofloxacin (Cipro), daunorubicin (Cerubidine), idarubicin (Idamycin), midazolam (Versed).

⊞ IV COMPATIBILITIES

Cimetidine (Tagamet), cisplatin (Platinol), cyclophosphamide (Cytoxan), cytarabine (Cytosar), docetaxel (Taxotere), doxorubicin (Adriamycin), etoposide (VePesid), furosemide (Lasix), granisetron (Kytril), heparin, hydromorphone (Dilaudid), lorazepam (Ativan), morphine, ondansetron (Zofran), paclitaxel (Taxol), palonosetron (Aloxi), potassium chloride, propofol (Diprivan).

INDICATIONS/ROUTES/DOSAGE

Anti-Inflammatory
PO, IV, IM: ADULTS, ELDERLY: 0.75–9 mg/day in divided doses q6–12h. CHILDREN: 0.08–0.3 mg/kg/day in divided doses q6–12h.

Cerebral Edema
IV: ADULTS, ELDERLY: Initially, 10 mg, then 4 mg (IV or IM) q6h.
PO, IV, IM: CHILDREN: Loading dose of 1–2 mg/kg, then 1–1.5 mg/kg/day in divided doses q4–6h.

Nausea/Vomiting in Chemotherapy Pts
IV: ADULTS, ELDERLY: 10–20 mg 15–30 min before treatment. CHILDREN: 10 mg/m²/dose on days of chemotherapy.

Physiologic Replacement
PO, IV, IM: ADULTS, ELDERLY, CHILDREN: 0.03–0.15 mg/kg/day in divided doses q6–12h.

Usual Ophthalmic Dosage, Ocular Inflammatory Conditions
Suspension: ADULTS, ELDERLY, CHILDREN: Initially, 2 drops q1h while awake and q2h at night for 1 day, then reduce to 3–4 times a day.

SIDE EFFECTS

Frequent: Inhalation: Cough, dry mouth, hoarseness, throat irritation. Intranasal: Burning, mucosal dryness. Ophthalmic: Blurred vision. Systemic: Insomnia, facial edema (cushingoid appearance ["moon face"]), moderate abdominal distention, indigestion, increased appetite, nervousness, facial flushing, diaphoresis. **Occasional: Inhalation:** Localized fungal infection (thrush). **Intranasal:** Crusting inside nose, epistaxis, sore throat, ulceration of nasal mucosa. **Ophthalmic:** Decreased vision; watering of eyes; eye pain; burning, stinging, redness of eyes; nausea; vomiting. **Systemic:** Dizziness, decreased/blurred vision. **Rare: Inhalation:** Increased bronchospasm, esophageal candidiasis. **Intranasal:** Nasal/pharyngeal candidiasis, eye pain. **Systemic:** Generalized allergic reaction (rash, urticaria); pain, redness, swelling at injection site; psychological changes; false sense of well-being; hallucinations; depression.

ADVERSE EFFECTS/ TOXIC REACTIONS

Long-term therapy: Muscle wasting (esp. arms, legs), osteoporosis, spontaneous fractures, amenorrhea, cataracts, glaucoma, peptic ulcer disease, HF. **Ophthalmic:** Glaucoma, ocular hypertension, cataracts. **Abrupt withdrawal following long-term therapy:** Severe joint pain, severe headache, anorexia, nausea, fever, rebound inflammation, fatigue, weakness, lethargy, dizziness, orthostatic hypotension.

NURSING CONSIDERATIONS

BASELINE ASSESSMENT

Question for hypersensitivity to any corticosteroids. Obtain baselines for height, weight, B/P, serum glucose, electrolytes.

INTERVENTION/EVALUATION

Monitor I&O, daily weight, serum glucose. Assess for edema. Evaluate food tolerance. Monitor daily pattern of bowel activity, stool consistency. Report hyperacidity promptly. Check vital signs at least twice a day. Be alert to infection (sore throat, fever, vague symptoms). Monitor serum electrolytes, esp. for hypercalcemia (muscle twitching, cramps), hypokalemia (weakness, muscle cramps, paresthesia [esp. lower extremities], nausea/vomiting,

irritability), Hgb, occult blood loss. Assess emotional status, ability to sleep.

PATIENT/FAMILY TEACHING

• Do not change dose/schedule or stop taking drug. • **Must** taper off gradually under medical supervision. • Notify physician if fever, sore throat, muscle aches, sudden weight gain, edema, exposure to measles/chickenpox occurs. • Severe stress (serious infection, surgery, trauma) may require increased dosage. • Inform dentist, other physicians of dexamethasone therapy within past 12 mos. • Avoid alcohol, limit caffeine.

TOP 200

dexlansoprazole

dex-lan-soe-**pra**-zol
(Dexilant)
Do not confuse dexlansoprazole with aripiprazole, lansoprazole, omeprazole, pantoprazole, or rabeprazole.

◆CLASSIFICATION

PHARMACOTHERAPEUTIC: Benzimidazole.
CLINICAL: Proton pump inhibitor (see p. 147C).

ACTION

Binds to and inhibits hydrogen-potassium adenosine triphosphatase, an enzyme on surface of gastric parietal cells, blocking the final step of acid production. **Therapeutic Effect:** Reduces gastric acid production.

PHARMACOKINETICS

Extensively metabolized in liver. Excreted in urine (51%), feces (48%). Protein binding: 97%. **Half-life:** 1–2 hrs.

USES

Healing of all grades of erosive esophagitis; maintenance healing of erosive esophagitis. Treatment of heartburn associated with nonerosive gastroesophageal reflux disease (GERD).

PRECAUTIONS

Contraindications: None known. **Cautions:** Hepatic impairment.

⧗ LIFESPAN CONSIDERATIONS

Pregnancy/Lactation: Unknown if distributed in breast milk. **Pregnancy Category B. Children:** Safety and efficacy not established. **Elderly:** No age-related precautions noted.

INTERACTIONS

Drug: May decrease concentration/effect of **atazanavir.** May interfere with **ampicillin, digoxin, iron salts, ketoconazole** absorption. May increase effect of **warfarin. Sucralfate** may delay dexlansoprazole absorption (give dexlansoprazole 30 min before sucralfate). **HERBAL:** None significant. **FOOD:** None known. **LAB VALUES:** May increase serum glucose, potassium, creatinine. May decrease platelets.

AVAILABILITY (Rx)

▧**Capsules (Delayed-Release):** 30 mg, 60 mg.

ADMINISTRATION/HANDLING

PO

• Do not crush or cut delayed-release capsules. • Administer whole. May take with or without regard to food. • If pt has difficulty swallowing capsules, open capsules, sprinkle granules on 1 tbsp of applesauce, and have pt swallow immediately.

INDICATIONS/ROUTES/DOSAGE

Erosive Esophagitis

PO: ADULTS, ELDERLY: 60 mg once daily for up to 8 wks. Maintenance of healed erosive esophagitis: 30 mg once daily for up to 6 mos.

GERD

PO: ADULTS, ELDERLY: 30 mg once daily for 4 wks.

Moderate Hepatic Impairment

PO: ADULTS, ELDERLY: Consider 30 mg maximum daily dose.

SIDE EFFECTS

Occasional (5%–4%): Diarrhea, abdominal pain. **Rare (3%–1%):** Nausea, vomiting, flatulence.

ADVERSE EFFECTS/TOXIC REACTIONS

Upper respiratory tract infection occurs rarely.

NURSING CONSIDERATIONS

BASELINE ASSESSMENT

Obtain baseline lab values. Assess for epigastric or abdominal pain, occult blood.

INTERVENTION/EVALUATION

Assess for therapeutic response (relief of GI symptoms). Question for occurrence of diarrhea, GI discomfort, nausea. Monitor CBC, renal/hepatic function tests.

PATIENT/FAMILY TEACHING

• Do not chew/crush delayed-release capsules. • For pts who have difficulty swallowing capsules, open capsules, sprinkle granules on 1 tbsp of applesauce, and have pt swallow immediately.

dexmedetomidine

dex-med-e-**toe**-mye-deen
(Precedex)
Do not confuse Precedex with Percocet or Peridex.

◆**CLASSIFICATION**

PHARMACOTHERAPEUTIC: Alpha₂ agonist. **CLINICAL:** Nonbarbiturate sedative, hypnotic.

ACTION

Selective alpha$_2$-adrenergic agonist. **Therapeutic Effect:** Produces analgesic, hypnotic, sedative effects.

PHARMACOKINETICS

Protein binding: 94%. Metabolized in liver. Excreted in urine. **Half-life: 2 hrs.**

USES

Sedation of initially intubated, mechanically ventilated adults in intensive care setting. Use in nonintubated pts requiring sedation before and/or during surgical and other procedures. **OFF-LABEL:** Treatment of shivering, use in children.

PRECAUTIONS

Contraindications: None known. **Cautions:** Heart block, hepatic impairment, hypovolemia, diabetes, hypotension, chronic hypertension, severe ventricular dysfunction, elderly, use of vasodilators or drugs decreasing heart rate. **Pregnancy Category C.**

INTERACTIONS

DRUG: Sedatives, opioids, hypnotics may enhance effects. **HERBAL:** None significant. **FOOD:** None known. **LAB VALUES:** May increase serum alkaline phosphatase, potassium, AST, ALT.

AVAILABILITY (Rx)

Injection Solution: 4 mcg/ml (50 ml, 100 ml), 100 mcg/ml.

ADMINISTRATION/HANDLING

 IV

Reconstitution • Dilute 2 ml of dexmedetomidine with 48 ml 0.9% NaCl.
Rate of Administration • Individualized, titrated to desired effect.
Storage • Store at room temperature.

IV INCOMPATIBILITIES

Do not mix dexmedetomidine with any other medications.

IV COMPATIBILITIES

Amiodarone (Cordarone), bumetanide (Bumex), calcium gluconate, cisatracurium (Nimbex), dexamethasone, dobutamine, dopamine, magnesium sulfate, norepinephrine (Levophed), propofol (Diprivan).

INDICATIONS/ROUTES/DOSAGE

Sedation
IV: ADULTS: Loading dose of 1 mcg/kg over 10 min followed by maintenance infusion of 0.2–0.7 mcg/kg/hr. **ELDERLY:** May require decreased dosage. No guidelines available.

SIDE EFFECTS

Frequent: Hypotension (30%), nausea (11%). **Occasional (3%–2%):** Pain, fever, oliguria, thirst.

ADVERSE EFFECTS/ TOXIC REACTIONS

Bradycardia, atrial fibrillation, hypoxia, anemia, pain, pleural effusion may occur with too-rapid IV infusion.

NURSING CONSIDERATIONS

BASELINE ASSESSMENT
Obtain baseline B/P, heart rate, LOC prior to initiation.

INTERVENTION/EVALUATION
Monitor EKG for atrial fibrillation, pulse for bradycardia, B/P for hypotension, level of sedation. Assess respiratory rate, rhythm. Monitor ventilator settings. Discontinue once pt weaned off ventilator.

TOP 200

dexmethylphenidate

dex-**meth**-il-**fen**-i-date
(Focalin, Focalin XR)

BLACK BOX ALERT Chronic use can lead to marked tolerance, psychological dependence. Severe depression may occur during drug withdrawal.
Do not confuse dexmethylphenidate with methadone.

♦CLASSIFICATION

PHARMACOTHERAPEUTIC: Cerebral cortex stimulator **(Schedule II).** **CLINICAL:** CNS stimulant.

ACTION

Blocks reuptake of norepinephrine, dopamine into presynaptic neurons, increasing release of these neurotransmitters into synaptic cleft. **Therapeutic Effect:** Decreases motor restlessness, fatigue; increases motor activity, mental alertness, attention span; elevates mood.

PHARMACOKINETICS

Readily absorbed from GI tract. Metabolized in liver. Excreted in urine. **Half-life:** 2.2 hrs.

USES

Adjunct in treatment of ADHD with moderate to severe distractability, short attention spans, hyperactivity, emotional impulsivity in children 6 yrs and older. Focalin XR extended-release capsule approved for 30-min onset of action for treatment of ADHD.

PRECAUTIONS

Contraindications: Diagnosis or family history of Tourette's syndrome, glaucoma, history of marked agitation, anxiety, tension, motor tics, use of MAOIs within 14 days. **Cautions:** Cardiovascular disease (heart failure, recent MI), seizure disorder, psychosis, emotional instability, acute stress reactions, hyperthyroidism. Avoid use in pts with history of substance abuse.

⌛ LIFESPAN CONSIDERATIONS

Pregnancy/Lactation: Unknown if excreted in breast milk. **Pregnancy Category C. Children:** May be more susceptible to developing anorexia, insomnia, abdominal pain, weight loss. Chronic use may inhibit growth. In psychotic children, may exacerbate symptoms of behavior disturbance, thought disorder. **Elderly:** No age-related precautions noted.

INTERACTIONS

DRUG: May enhance effects of **antihypertensives.** May inhibit metabolism of **phenobarbital, phenytoin, primidone, tricyclic antidepressants;** decreased dosages may be necessary. May alter effects of **warfarin. HERBAL: Ephedra** may cause hypertension, arrhythmias. **Yohimbe** may increase CNS stimulation. **FOOD:** None known. **LAB VALUES:** None known.

AVAILABILITY (Rx)

Tablets (Focalin): 2.5 mg, 5 mg, 10 mg.

🗒 Capsules (Extended-Release [Focalin XR]): 5 mg, 10 mg, 15 mg, 20 mg, 30 mg, 40 mg.

ADMINISTRATION/HANDLING

PO

• Do not give drug in afternoon or evening (causes insomnia). • Tablets may be crushed. • Give without regard to food. • Administer extended-release capsules whole; do not cut or crush. • May sprinkle contents of extended-release capsules on small amount of applesauce. • Give extended-release capsules once each day in the morning, before breakfast.

INDICATIONS/ROUTES/DOSAGE

ADHD

Pts not currently taking methylphenidate:

Capsules (Extended-Release)

PO: ADULTS, ELDERLY: Initially, 10 mg/day. May increase in increments of 10 mg/day at weekly intervals. **Maximum:** 40 mg/day. **CHILDREN 6 YRS AND OLDER:** Initially, 5 mg/day. May increase in increments of 5 mg/day at weekly intervals. **Maximum:** 30 mg/day.

Tablets (Immediate-Release)

PO: ADULTS, ELDERLY, CHILDREN 6 YRS AND OLDER: Initially, 2.5 mg 2 times a day. Doses should be given at least 4 hrs apart. May increase in increments of 2.5–5 mg at weekly intervals. **Maximum:** 20 mg/day.

SIDE EFFECTS

Frequent: Abdominal pain, nausea, anorexia, fever. **Occasional:** Tachycardia, arrhythmias, palpitations, insomnia, twitching. **Rare:** Blurred vision, rash, arthralgia.

ADVERSE EFFECTS/ TOXIC REACTIONS

Withdrawal after prolonged therapy may unmask symptoms of underlying disorder. May lower seizure threshold in pts with history of seizures. Overdose produces excessive sympathomimetic effects (vomiting, tremor, hyperreflexia, seizures, confusion, hallucinations, diaphoresis). Prolonged administration to children may delay growth. Neuroleptic malignant syndrome occurs rarely.

NURSING CONSIDERATIONS

BASELINE ASSESSMENT

Evaluate pt for cardiac disease, psychiatric conditions. Obtain baseline vital signs, CBC count.

INTERVENTION/EVALUATION

CBC, B/P, heart rate should be performed routinely during therapy. If paradoxical return of ADHD occurs, dosage should be reduced or discontinued. Weigh, measure pediatric pt regularly to detect delayed growth.

PATIENT/FAMILY TEACHING

• Report any increase in seizures, chest pain, unexplained syncope. • Avoid caffeine. • Last dose should be given in morning to prevent insomnia. • Report anxiety, fever.

dexrazoxane

dex-ra-**zox**-ane
(Tolect, Zinecard)
Do not confuse Zinecard with Gemzar.

◆CLASSIFICATION

PHARMACOTHERAPEUTIC: Cytoprotective agent. **CLINICAL:** Antineoplastic.

ACTION

Rapidly penetrates myocardial cell membrane. Binds intracellular iron, prevents generation of free radicals by anthracyclines. **Therapeutic Effect:** Protects against anthracycline-induced cardiomyopathy.

PHARMACOKINETICS

Rapidly distributed after administration. Not bound to plasma proteins. Primarily excreted in urine. Removed by peritoneal dialysis. **Half-life:** 2.1–2.5 hrs.

USES

Tolect: Treatment of anthracycline-induced extravasation. **Zinecard:** Reduction of incidence, severity of cardiomyopathy–associated with doxorubicin therapy in women with metastatic breast cancer having received a cumulative dose of 300 mg/m^2 and would benefit from continued doxorubicin therapy. Not recommended with initiation of doxorubicin therapy.

PRECAUTIONS

Contraindications: Use in nonanthracycline chemotherapy regimens. **Cautions:** Hepatic/renal impairment.

⌛ LIFESPAN CONSIDERATIONS

Pregnancy/Lactation: May be embryotoxic, teratogenic. Unknown if distributed in breast milk. Breastfeeding not recommended. **Pregnancy Category C. Children:** Safety and efficacy not established. **Elderly:** Information not available.

INTERACTIONS

DRUG: **Other myelosuppressive agents** may increase risk of myelosuppression, infection. **HERBAL:** None significant. **FOOD:** None known. **LAB VALUES:** None significant.

D

AVAILABILITY (Rx)

Injection, Powder for Reconstitution: (Zinecard): 250 mg (10 mg/ml reconstituted in 25-ml single-use vial). (Tolect, Zinecard): 500 mg (10 mg/ml reconstituted in 50-ml single-use vial).

ADMINISTRATION/HANDLING

◄ALERT► Do not mix with other drugs. Use caution in handling/preparation of reconstituted solution (glove use recommended).

 IV

Reconstitution • Reconstitute with 0.167 molar (M/6) sodium lactate injection to give concentration of 10 mg dexrazoxane for each ml of sodium lactate. • May further dilute with 0.9% NaCl or D₅W. Concentration should range from 1.3–5 mg/ml. Treatment of extravasation: Further dilute reconstituted vial in 1,000 ml 0.9% NaCl.

Rate of Administration • Give reconstituted solution by slow IV push or IV infusion over 5–15 min. • After infusion is complete and before total elapsed time of 30 min from beginning of dexrazoxane infusion, give IV injection of doxorubicin. Treatment of extravasation: Infuse over 1–2 hrs in large vein other than in area of extravasation.

Storage • Store vials at room temperature. • **Zinecard:** Reconstituted solution is stable for 6 hrs at room temperature or if refrigerated. Discard unused solution. **Tolect:** Stable for 4 hrs in 0.9% NaCl.

⚙ IV INCOMPATIBILITIES

Do not mix dexrazoxane with other medications.

INDICATIONS/ROUTES/DOSAGE

Cardioprotective

IV *(Zinecard)*: ADULTS, CHILDREN: Recommended dosage ratio is 10 parts dexrazoxane to 1 part doxorubicin (e.g., 500 mg/m² dexrazoxane for every 50 mg/m² doxorubicin).

Anthracycline Extravasation

IV *(Tolect)*: ADULTS, ELDERLY: 1,000 mg/m² on days 1 and 2 (**maximum: 2,000 mg**), then 500 mg/m² on day 3 (**maximum: 1,000 mg**). Begin treatment within 6 hrs of extravasation.

Dosage in Renal Impairment

IV: ADULTS, ELDERLY: Moderate to severe (creatinine clearance less than 40 ml/min): Reduce dose by 50%.

SIDE EFFECTS

Frequent: Alopecia (94%), nausea (82%), vomiting (63%), fatigue/malaise (62%), anorexia (50%), stomatitis (36%), fever (35%), infection (31%), diarrhea (22%). **Occasional:** Pain at injection site (11%), neurotoxicity (16%), streaking/erythema at injection site (7%), dysphagia (6%). **Rare:** Esophagitis (5%), phlebitis (5%), urticaria (4%).

ADVERSE EFFECTS/TOXIC REACTIONS

Fluorouracil, adriamycin, cyclophosphamide (FAC) therapy with dexrazoxane increases risk for severe leukopenia, granulocytopenia, thrombocytopenia compared with those receiving FAC without dexrazoxane. Overdose can be removed with peritoneal dialysis or hemodialysis.

NURSING CONSIDERATIONS

BASELINE ASSESSMENT

Obtain baseline CBC with differential, electrolytes, BUN, creatinine, liver function test, cardiac function. Use gloves when preparing solution. If powder/solution comes in contact with skin, wash immediately with soap and water. Antiemetics may be effective in preventing, treating nausea.

INTERVENTION/EVALUATION

Frequently monitor platelets, CBC with differential for evidence of blood dyscrasias. Assess for stomatitis (burning/erythema of oral mucosa at inner margin of lips, sore throat, difficulty swallowing). Monitor hematologic status, renal/hepatic function studies, cardiac function. Monitor for hematologic toxicity (fever, signs of local infection, unusual bruising/bleeding from any site).

PATIENT/FAMILY TEACHING

• Hair loss is reversible, but new hair growth may have different color/texture. • New hair growth resumes 2–3 mos after last therapy dose. • Maintain strict oral hygiene. • Promptly report fever, sore throat, signs of local infection, bleeding, bruising. • Report persistent nausea, vomiting.

TOP
200

dextroamphetamine and amphetamine

dex-troe-am-**fet**-ah-meen/am-**fet**-ah-meen
(Adderall, <u>Adderall-XR</u>)

BLACK BOX ALERT High potential for abuse. Prolonged administration may lead to drug dependence.
Do not confuse Adderall with Inderal.

◆CLASSIFICATION

PHARMACOTHERAPEUTIC: Amphetamine **(Schedule II). CLINICAL:** CNS stimulant.

ACTION

Enhances action of dopamine, norepinephrine by blocking reuptake from synapses. Inhibits monoamine oxidase, facilitates release of catecholamines. **Therapeutic Effect:** Increases motor activity, mental alertness; decreases drowsiness, fatigue; suppresses appetite.

PHARMACOKINETICS

Well absorbed following PO administration. Widely distributed including CNS. Metabolized in liver. Excreted in urine. Removed by hemodialysis. **Half-life:** 10–13 hrs.

USES

Treatment of narcolepsy; treatment of ADHD in hyperactive children.

PRECAUTIONS

Contraindications: Advanced arteriosclerosis, agitated mental states, glaucoma, history of drug abuse, hypersensitivity to sympathomimetic amines, hyperthyroidism, moderate to severe hypertension, symptomatic cardiovascular disease, use of MAOIs within 14 days. **Cautions:** Elderly, debilitated pts, history of seizures, mild hypertension.

⌛ LIFESPAN CONSIDERATIONS

Pregnancy/Lactation: Distributed in breast milk. **Pregnancy Category C. Children:** Safety and efficacy not established in those younger than 3 yrs. **Elderly:** Age-related cardiovascular, cerebrovascular disease, hepatic/renal impairment may increase risk of side effects.

INTERACTIONS

DRUG: May enhance effects of **tricyclic antidepressants, sympathomimetics. MAOIs** may prolong, intensify effects. May antagonize effects of **hypotensive agents. HERBAL:** None significant. **FOOD:** None known. **LAB VALUES:** May increase plasma corticosteroid.

AVAILABILITY (Rx)

Tablets (Adderall): 5 mg, 7.5 mg, 10 mg, 12.5 mg, 15 mg, 20 mg, 30 mg.

🔪 **Capsules (Extended-Release [Adderall-XR]):** 5 mg, 10 mg, 15 mg, 20 mg, 25 mg, 30 mg.

ADMINISTRATION/HANDLING

PO

• Give tablets at least 6 hrs before bedtime. • Extended-release capsules should be swallowed whole; do not break, crush, or cut. • Avoid afternoon doses to prevent insomnia. • May open capsules and sprin-

---

◆ Canadian trade name 　　🔪 Non-Crushable Drug 　　🔲 High Alert drug

kle on applesauce. Instruct pt not to chew sprinkled beads; take immediately.

INDICATIONS/ROUTES/DOSAGE

Narcolepsy

PO: ADULTS, CHILDREN OLDER THAN 12 YRS: Initially, 10 mg/day. Increase by 10 mg/day at weekly intervals until therapeutic response is achieved. **Maximum:** 60 mg/day given in 1–3 divided doses with interval of 4–6 hrs between doses. **CHILDREN 6–12 YRS:** Initially, 5 mg/day. Increase by 5 mg/day at weekly intervals until therapeutic response is achieved. **Maximum:** 60 mg/day given in 1–3 divided doses with interval of 4–6 hrs between doses.

ADHD

ADULTS, ELDERLY: (ADDERALL-XR): Initially, 20 mg once daily in the morning. May increase up to 60 mg/day. **CHILDREN 13–17 YRS: (ADDERALL-XR):** Initially, 10 mg once daily in the morning. May increase to 20 mg/day after 1 wk if symptoms are not controlled. May increase up to 60 mg/day. **CHILDREN 6–12 YRS: (ADDERALL):** Initially, 5 mg 1–2 times a day. May increase in 5-mg increments at weekly intervals until optimal response is obtained. **Maximum:** 40 mg/day given in 1–3 divided doses (use intervals of 4–6 hrs between additional doses). **(ADDERALL-XR):** Initially, 5–10 mg once daily in the morning. May increase daily dose in 5- to 10-mg increments at weekly intervals. **Maximum:** 30 mg/day. **CHILDREN 3–5 YRS: (ADDERALL):** Initially, 2.5 mg/day given every morning. May increase daily dose in 2.5-mg increments at weekly intervals until optimal response is obtained. **Maximum:** 40 mg/day given in 1–3 divided doses (use intervals of 4–6 hrs between additional doses). Not recommended in children younger than 3 yrs.

SIDE EFFECTS

Frequent: Increased motor activity, talkativeness, nervousness, mild euphoria, insomnia. **Occasional:** Headache, chills, dry mouth, GI distress, worsening depression in pts who are clinically de-

pressed, tachycardia, palpitations, chest pain, dizziness, decreased appetite.

ADVERSE EFFECTS/ TOXIC REACTIONS

Overdose may produce skin pallor/flushing, arrhythmias, psychosis. Abrupt withdrawal after prolonged use of high doses may produce lethargy (may last for wks). Prolonged administration to children with ADHD may temporarily suppress normal weight/height pattern.

NURSING CONSIDERATIONS

BASELINE ASSESSMENT

Assess child's attention span, impulse control, interaction with others. Screen for drug–seeking behavior, past drug abuse. Obtain baseline B/P.

INTERVENTION/EVALUATION

Monitor for CNS overstimulation, increase in B/P, growth rate, change in pulse rate, respirations, weight loss. **Narcolepsy:** Observe/document frequency of narcoleptic episodes. **ADHD:** Observe for improved attention span.

PATIENT/FAMILY TEACHING

• Normal dosage levels may produce tolerance to drug's anorexic mood-elevating effects within a few wks. • Dry mouth may be relieved with sugarless gum, sips of water. • Take early in day. • Do not break, crush, chew extended-release capsules. • May mask extreme fatigue. • Report pronounced anxiety, dizziness, decreased appetite, dry mouth, new or worsening behavior, chest pain, palpitations. • Avoid alcohol, caffeine.

---

diazepam   TOP 200

dye-**az**-e-pam
(Apo-Diazepam ✦, Diastat, Diazemuls ✦, Diazepam Intensol, Novo-Dipam ✦, Valium)
Do not confuse diazepam with diazoxide, diltiazem, Ditropan,

or lorazepam, or Valium with Valcyte.

◆ CLASSIFICATION

PHARMACOTHERAPEUTIC: Benzodiazepine **(Schedule IV). CLINICAL:** Antianxiety, skeletal muscle relaxant, anticonvulsant (see pp. 15C, 151C).

ACTION

Depresses all levels of CNS by enhancing action of gamma-aminobutyric acid, a major inhibitory neurotransmitter in the brain. **Therapeutic Effect:** Produces anxiolytic effect, elevates seizure threshold, produces skeletal muscle relaxation.

PHARMACOKINETICS

Well absorbed from GI tract. Widely distributed. Protein binding: 98%. Excreted in urine. Minimally removed by hemodialysis. **Half-life:** 20–70 hrs (increased in hepatic dysfunction, elderly).

USES

Short-term relief of anxiety symptoms, relief of acute alcohol withdrawal. Adjunct for relief of acute musculoskeletal conditions, treatment of seizures (IV route used for termination of status epilepticus). **Gel:** Control of increased seizure activity in refractory epilepsy in those on stable regimens. **OFF-LABEL:** Treatment of panic disorder. Short-term treatment of spasticity in children with cerebral palsy. Sedation for mechanically vented pts in ICU.

PRECAUTIONS

Contraindications: Acute narrow-angle glaucoma, severe respiratory depression, severe, uncontrolled pain, severe hepatic insufficiency, sleep apnea syndrome, myasthenia gravis. Children less than 6 months of age. **Cautions:** Pts receiving other CNS depressants or psychoactive agents, depression, history of drug and alcohol abuse, renal/hepatic impairment, hypoalbuminemia, respiratory disease, impaired gag reflex, concurrent use of strong CYP3A4 inhibitors or inducers.

⏳ LIFESPAN CONSIDERATIONS

Pregnancy/Lactation: Crosses placenta. Distributed in breast milk. May increase risk of fetal abnormalities if administered during first trimester of pregnancy. Chronic ingestion during pregnancy may produce withdrawal symptoms, CNS depression in neonates. **Pregnancy Category D. Children/Elderly:** Use small initial doses with gradual increases to avoid ataxia, excessive sedation.

INTERACTIONS

DRUG: Alcohol, CNS depressants may increase CNS depression. **CYP3A4 inducers (e.g., carbamazepine, rifampin)** may decrease concentration. **CYP3A4 inhibitors (e.g., itraconazole, ketoconazole)** may increase concentration. **HERBAL: Gotu kola, kava kava, St. John's wort, valerian** may increase CNS depression. **St. John's wort** may decrease concentration/effects. **FOOD: Grapefruit products** increases concentration/effects. **LAB VALUES:** None significant. **Therapeutic serum level:** 0.5–2 mcg/ml; **toxic serum level:** greater than 3 mcg/ml.

AVAILABILITY (Rx)

Injection, Solution: 5 mg/ml. **Oral Concentrate (Diazepam Intensol):** 5 mg/ml. **Oral Solution:** 5 mg/5 ml. **Rectal Gel (Diastat)** (adult rectal tip): Delivers set doses of 12.5 mg, 15 mg, 17.5 mg, 20 mg. (pediatric rectal tip): Delivers set dose of 2.5 mg. (adult/pediatric tip): Delivers set doses of 5 mg, 7.5 mg, 10 mg. **Tablet (Valium):** 2 mg, 5 mg, 10 mg.

ADMINISTRATION/HANDLING
💉 IV

Rate of Administration • Give by IV push into tubing of flowing IV solution as close as possible to vein insertion point. • Administer directly into large vein (reduces risk of thrombosis/phlebitis). Do not use small veins (e.g., wrist/dorsum of hand). • Administer IV at rate not exceeding 5 mg/min for adults. For children, give

1–2 mg/min (too-rapid IV may result in hypotension, respiratory depression). • Monitor respirations q5–15min for 2 hrs. **Storage** • Store at room temperature.

IM

• Injection may be painful. Inject deeply into large muscle mass.

PO

• Give without regard to meals. • Dilute oral concentrate with water, juice, carbonated beverages; may be mixed in semisolid food (applesauce, pudding). • Tablets may be crushed.

📋 IV INCOMPATIBILITIES

Amphotericin B complex (Abelcet, AmBisome, Amphotec), cefepime (Maxipime), diltiazem (Cardizem), fluconazole (Diflucan), foscarnet (Foscavir), furosemide (Lasix), heparin, hydrocortisone (Solu-Cortef), hydromorphone (Dilaudid), meropenem (Merrem IV), potassium chloride, propofol (Diprivan), vitamins.

📋 IV COMPATIBILITIES

Dobutamine (Dobutrex), fentanyl, morphine.

INDICATIONS/ROUTES/DOSAGE

Anxiety

PO: ADULTS: 2–10 mg 2–4 times a day. **ELDERLY:** Initially, 1–2 mg 1–2 times a day. **CHILDREN:** 0.12–0.8 mg/kg/day in divided doses q6–8h.

IV, IM: ADULTS: 2–10 mg; may repeat in 3–4 hrs if needed. **CHILDREN:** 0.04–0.3 mg/kg/dose q2–4h. **Maximum:** 0.6 mg/kg within 8-hr period.

Skeletal Muscle Relaxation

PO: ADULTS: 2–10 mg 2–4 times a day. **ELDERLY:** Initially, 1–2 mg 1–2 times a day. **CHILDREN:** 0.12–0.8 mg/kg/day in divided doses q6–8h.

Alcohol Withdrawal

PO: ADULTS, ELDERLY: 10 mg 3–4 times during first 24 hrs, then reduced to 5 mg 3–4 times a day as needed.

Status Epilepticus

IV: ADULTS, ELDERLY: 5–10 mg q5–10min. **Maximum:** 30 mg. **INFANTS, CHILDREN:** 0.1–0.3 mg/kg over 5 min or less; may repeat after 5–10 min. **Maximum:** 10 mg/dose.

Control of Increased Seizure Activity (Breakthrough Seizures) in Pts with Refractory Epilepsy Who Are on Stable Regimens of Anticonvulsants

Rectal Gel: ADULTS, CHILDREN 12 YRS AND OLDER: 0.2 mg/kg; may be repeated in 4–12 hrs. **CHILDREN 6–11 YRS:** 0.3 mg/kg; may be repeated in 4–12 hrs. **CHILDREN 2–5 YRS:** 0.5 mg/kg; may be repeated in 4–12 hrs.

SIDE EFFECTS

Frequent: Pain with IM injection, drowsiness, fatigue, ataxia. **Occasional:** Slurred speech, orthostatic hypotension, headache, hypoactivity, constipation, nausea, blurred vision. **Rare:** Paradoxical CNS reactions (hyperactivity/nervousness in children, excitement/restlessness in elderly/debilitated) generally noted during first 2 wks of therapy, particularly in presence of uncontrolled pain.

ADVERSE EFFECTS/ TOXIC REACTIONS

IV route may produce pain, swelling, thrombophlebitis, carpal tunnel syndrome. Abrupt or too-rapid withdrawal may result in pronounced restlessness, irritability, insomnia, hand tremor, abdominal/muscle cramps, diaphoresis, vomiting, seizures. Abrupt withdrawal in pts with epilepsy may produce increase in frequency/severity of seizures. Overdose results in drowsiness, confusion, diminished reflexes, CNS depression, coma. **Antidote:** Flumazenil (see Appendix K for dosage).

NURSING CONSIDERATIONS

BASELINE ASSESSMENT

Assess B/P, pulse, respirations immediately before administration. **Anxiety:** Assess autonomic response (cold, clammy hands, diaphoresis), motor response (agitation, trembling, tension). **Musculoskeletal spasm:** Record onset, type, location, duration of pain. Check for immobility, stiffness, swelling. **Seizures:** Review history of seizure disorder (length, intensity, frequency, duration, LOC). Observe frequently for recurrence of seizure activity. Initiate seizure precautions.

INTERVENTION/EVALUATION

Monitor heart rate, respiratory rate, B/P, mental status. Assess children, elderly for paradoxical reaction, particularly during early therapy. Evaluate for therapeutic response (decrease in intensity/frequency of seizures; calm facial expression, decreased restlessness; decreased intensity of skeletal muscle pain). **Therapeutic serum level:** 0.5–2 mcg/ml; **toxic serum level:** greater than 3 mcg/ml.

PATIENT/FAMILY TEACHING

• Avoid alcohol. • Limit caffeine. • May cause drowsiness. • Avoid tasks that require alertness, motor skills until response to drug is established. • May be habit forming. • Avoid abrupt discontinuation after prolonged use.

---

diclofenac

dye-**kloe**-fen-ak
(Apo-Diclo ✤, Cambia, Cataflam, Flector, Novo-Difenac ✤, Pennsaid, Solaraze, Voltaren, Voltaren Gel, Voltaren Ophthalmic, Voltaren XR, Zipsor, Zorvolex)

BLACK BOX ALERT Increased risk of serious cardiovascular thrombotic events, including myocardial infarction, CVA. Increased risk of severe GI reactions, including ulceration, bleeding, perforation of stomach, intestines. Contraindicated for treatment of perioperative pain in setting of CABG surgery.

Do not confuse Cataflam with Catapres, diclofenac with Diflucan or Duphalac, or Voltaren with tramadol, Ultram, or Verelan.

FIXED-COMBINATION(S)

Arthrotec: diclofenac/misoprostol (an antisecretory gastric protectant): 50 mg/200 mcg, 75 mg/200 mcg.

◆CLASSIFICATION

PHARMACOTHERAPEUTIC: NSAID. **CLINICAL:** Analgesic, anti-inflammatory (see p. 129C).

ACTION

Inhibits prostaglandin synthesis, intensity of pain stimulus reaching sensory nerve endings. Constricts iris sphincter. **Therapeutic Effect:** Produces analgesic, anti-inflammatory effects. Prevents miosis during cataract surgery.

PHARMACOKINETICS

Route	Onset	Peak	Duration
PO	30 min	2–3 hrs	Up to 8 hrs

Completely absorbed from GI tract; penetrates cornea after ophthalmic administration (may be systemically absorbed). Protein binding: greater than 99%. Widely distributed. Metabolized in liver. Primarily excreted in urine. Minimally removed by hemodialysis. **Half-life:** 1.2–2 hrs.

USES

PO: (Immediate-release): Treatment of rheumatoid arthritis, osteoarthritis, ankylosing spondylitis, primary dysmenorrhea. **(Zipsor, Zorvolex):** Mild to moderate pain. **(Delayed-release):** Treatment of rheumatoid arthritis, osteoarthritis, ankylosing spondylitis. **(Extended-release):** Treatment of rheumatoid arthritis, osteoarthritis. **Oral Solution (Cambia):** Treatment of migraine. **Topical Patch:** Treatment of acute pain due to minor strains, sprains, contusions. **Ophthalmic:** Treatment of photophobia, pain in pts undergoing corneal refractive surgery. **Topical Gel (3%):** Treatment of actinic keratoses. **(1%):** Treatment of osteoarthritis, joint pain (e.g., ankle, elbow, wrist). **Topical Solution:** Treatment of pain associated with osteoarthritis of knee. **OFF-**

D

LABEL: Treatment of juvenile idiopathic arthritis.

PRECAUTIONS

Contraindications: Asthmatic pts, hypersensitivity to aspirin, diclofenac, other NSAIDs; perioperative pain in setting of CABG surgery. **Cautions:** HF, hypertension, renal/hepatic impairment, history of GI disease. Avoid topical gel in open skin wounds, infections, exfoliative dermatitis, eyes, neonates, infants, children.

⧗ LIFESPAN CONSIDERATIONS

Pregnancy/Lactation: Crosses placenta. Unknown if distributed in breast milk. Avoid use during third trimester (may adversely affect fetal cardiovascular system: premature closure of ductus arteriosus). **Pregnancy Category B (D if used in third trimester or near delivery; C for ophthalmic solution). Children:** Safety and efficacy not established. **Elderly:** GI bleeding, ulceration more likely to cause serious adverse effects. Age-related renal impairment may increase risk of hepatic/renal toxicity; reduced dosage recommended.

INTERACTIONS

DRUG: May decrease effects of **acetylcholine, antihypertensives, carbachol, diuretics. Aspirin, other salicylates, warfarin** may increase risk of GI side effects/bleeding. **CYP2C9 inhibitors (e.g., voriconazole)** may increase concentration/risk of toxicity. **CYP2C9 inducers (e.g., rifampin)** may decrease effect. May increase serum **cyclosporine** concentration/toxicity. **Ophthalmic:** May decrease antiglaucoma effects of **antiglaucoma agents, epinephrine. HERBAL: Cat's claw, dong quai, evening primrose, garlic, ginseng** may increase antiplatelet activity. **FOOD:** None known. **LAB VALUES:** May increase urine protein, BUN, serum alkaline phosphatase, creatinine, LDH, potassium, AST, ALT. May decrease serum uric acid.

AVAILABILITY (Rx)

Adhesive Patch (Flector): 10×14 cm patch containing 180 mg diclofenac. **Capsules (Zipsor):** 25 mg. **(Zorvolex):** 18 mg, 35 mg. **Ophthalmic Solution (Voltaren Ophthalmic):** 0.1%. **Oral Solution (Cambia):** 25-mg, 50-mg packets. **Tablets (Cataflam):** 50 mg. **Topical Gel (Solaraze):** 3%. **(Voltaren Gel):** 1%. **Topical Solution (Pennsaid):** 1.5%.

◪ **Tablets (Delayed-Release [Voltaren]):** 25 mg, 50 mg, 75 mg. ◪ **Tablets (Extended-Release [Voltaren XR]):** 100 mg.

ADMINISTRATION/HANDLING

PO
• Do not crush, break enteric-coated tablets. • May give with food, milk, antacids if GI distress occurs. • **Cambia:** Mix one packet in 1–2 oz water, stir well, and instruct pt to drink immediately.

Ophthalmic
• Place finger on lower eyelid and pull out until pocket is formed between eye and lower lid. • Place prescribed number of drops in pocket. • Instruct pt to close eye gently for 1–2 min (so medication will not be squeezed out of the sac) and to apply digital pressure to lacrimal sac for 1 min to minimize system absorption. • Remove excess solution with tissue.

Topical Solution
• Apply only to clean, dry skin. • Squeeze 10 drops into hand or directly onto knee. • Spread evenly onto knee (front, back, sides). • Repeat until 40 drops applied and knee completely covered.

Topical Gel
• Do not apply to eyes, mucous membranes, open wounds. • Avoid sunlight exposure to treated areas.

Transdermal Patch
• Apply to intact skin; avoid contact with eyes. • Do not wear when bathing/showering. • Wash hands after handling.

D

INDICATIONS/ROUTES/DOSAGE

Osteoarthritis
PO *(Cataflam, Voltaren)*: **ADULTS, ELDERLY:** 50 mg 2–3 times a day.
PO *(Voltaren XR)*: **ADULTS, ELDERLY:** 100 mg/day as a single dose.
Topical *(Voltaren Gel)*: 2–4 g 4 times a day. **Maximum:** (upper extremities): 8g per joint per day. (lower extremities): 16 g per joint per day.
Topical *(Pennsaid)*: 40 drops to knee 4 times/day.

Rheumatoid Arthritis (RA)
PO *(Cataflam, Voltaren)*: **ADULTS, ELDERLY:** 50 mg 2–4 times a day.
PO *(Voltaren XR)*: **ADULTS, ELDERLY:** 100 mg once a day. **Maximum:** 100 mg twice a day.

Ankylosing Spondylitis
PO *(Voltaren)*: **ADULTS, ELDERLY:** 100–125 mg/day in 4–5 divided doses.

Analgesia, Primary Dysmenorrhea
PO *(Cataflam)*: **ADULTS, ELDERLY:** 50 mg 3 times a day.

Acute Pain
Topical Patch *(Flector)*: **ADULTS, ELDERLY:** Apply 2 times a day.

Mild–Moderate Pain
PO *(Zipsor)*: **ADULTS, ELDERLY:** 25 mg 4 times a day. *(Zorvolex)*: 18 mg or 35 mg 3 times a day.

Migraine (Oral Solution)
PO: ADULTS, ELDERLY: 50 mg once.

Usual Pediatric Dosage
CHILDREN: 2–3 mg/kg/day in 2–4 divided doses. **Maximum:** 200 mg/day.

Actinic Keratoses
Topical *(Solaraze)*: **ADULTS, ADOLESCENTS:** Apply twice a day to lesion for 60–90 days.

Cataract Surgery
Ophthalmic: ADULTS, ELDERLY: Apply 1 drop to eye 4 times a day commencing 24 hrs after cataract surgery. Continue for 2 wks afterward.

Pain, Relief of Photophobia in Pts Undergoing Corneal Refractive Surgery
Ophthalmic: ADULTS, ELDERLY: Apply 1–2 drops to affected eye 1 hr before surgery, within 15 min after surgery, then 4 times a day for up to 3 days.

SIDE EFFECTS

Frequent (9%–4%): PO: Headache, abdominal cramps, constipation, diarrhea, nausea, dyspepsia. **Ophthalmic:** Burning, stinging on instillation, ocular discomfort. **Occasional (3%–1%): PO:** Flatulence, dizziness, epigastric pain. **Ophthalmic:** Ocular itching, tearing. **Rare (less than 1%): PO:** Rash, peripheral edema, fluid retention, visual disturbances, vomiting, drowsiness.

ADVERSE EFFECTS/ TOXIC REACTIONS

Overdose may result in acute renal failure. In pts treated chronically, peptic ulcer, GI bleeding, gastritis, severe hepatic reaction (jaundice), nephrotoxicity (hematuria, dysuria, proteinuria), severe hypersensitivity reaction (bronchospasm, angioedema) occur rarely.

NURSING CONSIDERATIONS

BASELINE ASSESSMENT
Anti-inflammatory: Assess onset, type, location, duration of pain, inflammation. Inspect appearance of affected joints for immobility, deformities, skin condition.

INTERVENTION/EVALUATION
Monitor CBC, hepatic/renal function tests, urine output, occult blood test. Monitor for headache, dyspepsia. Monitor daily pattern of bowel activity, stool consistency. Assess for therapeutic response: relief of pain, stiffness, swelling;

✦ Canadian trade name 🦺 Non-Crushable Drug 🔺 High Alert drug

increased joint mobility; reduced joint tenderness; improved grip strength.

PATIENT/FAMILY TEACHING

• Swallow tablet whole; do not crush, chew. • Avoid aspirin, alcohol during therapy (increases risk of GI bleeding). • If GI upset occurs, take with food, milk. • Report skin rash, itching, weight gain, changes in vision, black stools, bleeding, jaundice, upper quadrant pain, persistent headache. • **Ophthalmic:** Do not use hydrogel soft contact lenses. • **Topical:** Avoid exposure to sunlight, sunlamps. • Report rash.

dicyclomine

dye-**sye**-kloe-meen
(Bentyl, Bentylol ❀, Formulex ❀, Lomine ❀)
Do not confuse Bentyl with Aventyl, Benadryl, Proventil, or Trental, or dicyclomine with diphenhydramine or doxycycline.

◆CLASSIFICATION

CLINICAL: GI antispasmodic, anticholinergic. **PHARMACOTHERAPEUTIC:** Anticholinergic, antimuscarinic agent.

ACTION

Directly acts as smooth muscle relaxant. **Therapeutic Effect:** Reduces tone, motility of GI tract.

PHARMACOKINETICS

Readily absorbed from GI tract. Widely distributed. Metabolized in liver. **Half-life:** 9–10 hrs.

USES

Treatment of functional disturbances of GI motility (e.g., irritable bowel syndrome). **OFF-LABEL:** Urinary incontinence.

PRECAUTIONS

Contraindications: Bladder neck obstruction, myasthenia gravis, narrow-angle glaucoma, obstructive disease of GI tract, severe ulcerative colitis, tachycardia, infants younger than 6 mos of age, nursing mothers. **Extreme Caution:** Autonomic neuropathy, mild to moderate ulcerative colitis. **Cautions:** Hyperthyroidism, hepatic/renal disease, hypertension, tachyarrhythmias, HF, coronary artery disease, hiatal hernia.

⌛ LIFESPAN CONSIDERATIONS

Pregnancy/Lactation: Unknown if drug crosses placenta or is distributed in breast milk. **Pregnancy Category B. Children:** Infants, young children more susceptible to toxic effects. **Elderly:** May cause excitement, agitation, drowsiness, confusion.

INTERACTIONS

DRUG: Antacids may decrease absorption. May decrease absorption of **ketoconazole.** Other **anticholinergics (e.g., tricyclic antidepressants)** may increase effects. May antagonize effects of **antiglaucoma agents. HERBAL:** None significant. **FOOD:** None known. **LAB VALUES:** None significant.

AVAILABILITY (Rx)

Capsules (Bentyl): 10 mg. **Injection Solution (Bentyl):** 10 mg/ml. **Syrup (Bentyl):** 10 mg/5 ml. **Tablets (Bentyl):** 20 mg.

ADMINISTRATION/HANDLING

IM
• Injection should appear colorless.
• Do not administer IV or subcutaneous.
• Inject deep into large muscle mass.
• Do not give for longer than 2 days.

PO
• Dilute oral solution with equal volume of water just before administration.
• Administer 30 min before food.

INDICATIONS/ROUTES/DOSAGE

Functional Disturbances of GI Motility
PO: ADULTS: 20 mg 3–4 times a day for 1 week. May increase up to 40 mg 4 times

a day. **ELDERLY:** 10–20 mg 4 times a day. May increase up to 160 mg/day. **CHILDREN OLDER THAN 2 YRS:** 10 mg 3–4 times a day. **CHILDREN 6 MOS–2 YRS:** 5 mg 3–4 times a day.

IM: ADULTS: 20 mg q4–6h.

SIDE EFFECTS

Frequent: Dry mouth (sometimes severe), constipation, diminished sweating ability. **Occasional:** Blurred vision; photophobia; urinary hesitancy; drowsiness (with high dosage); agitation, excitement, confusion, drowsiness noted in elderly (even with low dosages); transient dizziness (with IM route), irritation at injection site (with IM route). **Rare:** Confusion, hypersensitivity reaction, increased intraocular pressure, nausea, vomiting, unusual fatigue.

ADVERSE EFFECTS/ TOXIC REACTIONS

Overdose may produce temporary paralysis of ciliary muscle, pupillary dilation, tachycardia, palpitations, hot/dry/flushed skin, absence of bowel sounds, hyperthermia, increased respiratory rate, EKG abnormalities, nausea, vomiting, rash over face/upper trunk, CNS stimulation, psychosis (agitation, restlessness, rambling speech, visual hallucinations, paranoid behavior, delusions) followed by depression.

NURSING CONSIDERATIONS

BASELINE ASSESSMENT

Assess symptoms of irritable bowel syndrome (abdominal cramping, bloating, excessive flatus).

INTERVENTION/EVALUATION

Monitor daily pattern of bowel activity, stool consistency. Monitor I/O. Assess for urinary retention. Monitor changes in B/P, temperature. Be alert for fever (increased risk of hyperthermia). Assess skin turgor, mucous membranes to evaluate hydration status (encourage adequate fluid intake), bowel sounds for peristalsis.

PATIENT/FAMILY TEACHING

• Do not become overheated during exercise in hot weather (may result in heatstroke). • Avoid hot baths, saunas. • Avoid tasks that require alertness, motor skills until response to drug is established. • Do not take antacids or antidiarrheals within 1 hr of taking dicyclomine (decreased effectiveness).

didanosine

dye-**dan**-o-seen
(Videx, Videx EC)

BLACK BOX ALERT Pancreatitis, sometimes fatal, has been reported. Serious, sometimes fatal, hypersensitivity reactions, lactic acidosis, severe hepatomegaly with steatosis (fatty liver) have occurred.

Do not confuse Videx with Lidex.

◆CLASSIFICATION

PHARMACOTHERAPEUTIC: Purine nucleoside analogue. **CLINICAL:** Antiviral (see pp. 69C, 117C).

ACTION

Intracellularly converted into triphosphate, which interferes with RNA-directed DNA polymerase (reverse transcriptase). **Therapeutic Effect:** Inhibits replication of retroviruses, including HIV.

PHARMACOKINETICS

Variably absorbed from GI tract. Protein binding: less than 5%. Primarily excreted in urine. Partially (20%) removed by hemodialysis. **Half-life:** 1.5 hrs; metabolite, 8–24 hrs.

USES

Treatment of HIV infection in combination with at least two other antiretroviral agents.

PRECAUTIONS

Contraindications: Hypersensitivity to didanosine or any of its components. Concurrent therapy with allopurinol or ribavirin. **Cautions:** Renal/hepatic impairment, alcoholism, elevated triglycerides, T-cell counts less than 100 cells/mm³; extreme caution with history of pancreatitis.

⌛ LIFESPAN CONSIDERATIONS

Pregnancy/Lactation: Use during pregnancy only if clearly needed. Breast-feeding not recommended. **Pregnancy Category B. Children:** Well tolerated in those older than 3 mos. **Elderly:** Age-related renal impairment may require dosage adjustment.

INTERACTIONS

DRUG: May decrease absorption of **fluoroquinolones, itraconazole, ketoconazole, tetracyclines.** **HERBAL:** None significant. **FOOD: All foods** decrease absorption. **LAB VALUES:** May increase serum alkaline phosphatase, amylase, bilirubin, lipase, triglycerides, AST, ALT, uric acid. May decrease serum potassium, WBC, CBC.

AVAILABILITY (Rx)

◄**ALERT**► Chewable/dispersible buffered tablets not available in United States.
Pediatric Powder for Oral Solution (Videx): 2 g, 4 g (makes 10 mg/ml after final mixing).

🐾 **Capsules (Delayed-Release [Videx EC]):** 125 mg, 200 mg, 250 mg, 400 mg.

ADMINISTRATION/HANDLING

PO

• Store at room temperature. • Administer oral solution or tablets 30 min before or 2 hrs after a meal. • Pediatric powder for oral solution, following reconstitution as directed, is stable for 30 days if refrigerated. • **Powder for oral solution:** Add 100–200 ml water to 2 or 4 g, respectively, to provide concentration of 20 mg/ml. Immediately mix with equal amount of antacid to provide concentration of 10 mg/ml. Shake thoroughly before removing each dose. • **Enteric-coated capsules:** Swallow whole; do not break, open, chew capsules.

INDICATIONS/ROUTES/DOSAGE

HIV Infection

PO *(Delayed-Release Capsules)*: **ADULTS, CHILDREN 6 YRS AND OLDER, WEIGHING 60 KG OR MORE:** 400 mg once a day. **ADULTS, CHILDREN 13 YRS AND OLDER, WEIGHING 25 KG TO LESS THAN 60 KG:** 250 mg once a day. **WEIGHING 20 KG TO LESS THAN 25 KG:** 200 mg once a day.

PO *(Oral Solution)*: **ADULTS, CHILDREN 13 YRS AND OLDER, WEIGHING 60 KG OR MORE:** 200 mg q12h or 400 mg once a day. **ADULTS, CHILDREN 13 YRS AND OLDER, WEIGHING LESS THAN 60 KG:** 125 mg q12h or 250 mg once a day. **CHILDREN 8 MOS–12 YRS:** 90–150 mg/m² 2 times a day. **CHILDREN 2 WKS TO 8 MOS:** 100 mg/m² 2 times a day.

Dosage in Renal Impairment
Pts weighing less than 60 kg:

Creatinine Clearance	Oral Solution	Delayed-Release Capsules
30–59 ml/min	75 mg twice a day (or 150 mg once a day)	125 mg once a day
10–29 ml/min	100 mg once a day	125 mg once a day
Less than 10 ml/min	75 mg once a day	N/A

Pts weighing 60 kg or more:

Creatinine Clearance	Oral Solution	Delayed-Release Capsules
30–59 ml/min	100 mg twice a day (or 200 mg once a day)	200 mg once a day
10–29 ml/min	150 mg once a day	125 mg once a day
Less than 10 ml/min	100 mg once a day	125 mg once a day

SIDE EFFECTS

Frequent: Adults (greater than 10%): Diarrhea, neuropathy, chills, fever. **Children (greater than 25%):** Chills, fever, decreased appetite, pain, malaise, nausea, vomiting, diarrhea, abdominal pain, headache, nervousness, cough, rhinitis, dyspnea, asthenia (loss of strength, energy), rash, pruritus. **Occasional: Adults (9%–2%):** Rash, pruritus, headache, abdominal pain, nausea, vomiting, pneumonia, myopathy, decreased appetite, dry mouth, dyspnea. **Children (25%–10%):** Failure to thrive, weight loss, stomatitis, oral thrush, ecchymosis, arthritis, myalgia, insomnia, epistaxis, pharyngitis.

ADVERSE EFFECTS/ TOXIC REACTIONS

Pneumonia, opportunistic infections occur occasionally. Peripheral neuropathy, potentially fatal pancreatitis are major toxic effects.

NURSING CONSIDERATIONS

BASELINE ASSESSMENT

Obtain baseline values for CBC, serum renal/hepatic function tests, T-cell count, vital signs, weight.

INTERVENTION/EVALUATION

In event of abdominal pain, nausea, vomiting, elevated serum amylase, triglycerides, contact physician before administering medication (potential for pancreatitis). Monitor for burning feet, restless legs syndrome (unable to find comfortable position for legs or feet), lack of coordination, other signs of peripheral neuropathy. Monitor daily pattern of bowel activity, stool consistency. Check skin for rash, eruptions. Monitor serum electrolytes, CBC, glucose, renal/hepatic function tests, Hgb, platelet count. Assess for opportunistic infections (onset of fever, oral mucosa changes, cough, other respiratory symptoms). Check weight at least twice per wk. Assess for visual, auditory difficulty; provide protection from light if photophobia develops.

PATIENT/FAMILY TEACHING

• Avoid alcohol. • Report numbness, tingling, persistent severe abdominal pain, leg pain, nausea, vomiting, change in vision occur. • Shake oral suspension well before use, keep refrigerated. • Discard solution after 30 days, obtain new supply.

digoxin

di-**jox**-in
(Apo-Digoxin ✤, Lanoxin)
Do not confuse digoxin with Desoxyn or doxepin, or Lanoxin with Lasix, Levoxyl, Levsinex, Lonox, or Mefoxin.

◆CLASSIFICATION

PHARMACOTHERAPEUTIC: Cardiac glycoside. **CLINICAL:** Antiarrhythmic, cardiotonic.

ACTION

Increases influx of calcium from extracellular to intracellular cytoplasm. **Therapeutic Effect:** Potentiates activity of contractile cardiac muscle fibers, increases force of myocardial contraction. Slows the heart rate by decreasing conduction through SA, AV nodes.

PHARMACOKINETICS

Route	Onset	Peak	Duration
PO	0.5–2 hrs	2–8 hrs	3–4 days
IV	5–30 min	1–4 hrs	3–4 days

Readily absorbed from GI tract. Widely distributed. Protein binding: 30%. Partially metabolized in liver. Primarily excreted in urine. Minimally removed by hemodialysis. **Half-life:** 36–48 hrs (increased in renal impairment, elderly).

USES

Treatment of mild to moderate HF, atrial fibrillation (rate-controlled). **OFF-LABEL:** Fetal tachycardia with or without hydrops;

decrease ventricular rate in supraventricular tachyarrhythmias.

PRECAUTIONS

Contraindications: Ventricular fibrillation. **Cautions:** Renal impairment, sinus nodal disease, acute MI (within 6 mos), second- or third-degree heart block (unless functioning pacemaker), concurrent use of strong inducers or inhibitors of P-glycoprotein (cyclosporine), hyperthyroidism, hypothyroidism, hypokalemia, hypocalcemia.

LIFESPAN CONSIDERATIONS

Pregnancy/Lactation: Crosses placenta. Distributed in breast milk. **Pregnancy Category C. Children:** Premature infants more susceptible to toxicity. **Elderly:** Age-related hepatic/renal impairment may require dosage adjustment. Increased risk of loss of appetite.

INTERACTIONS

DRUG: Amiodarone may increase concentration/toxicity. **Beta-blockers, calcium channel blockers** may have additive effect on slowing AV nodal conduction. **Potassium-depleting diuretics** may increase toxicity due to hypokalemia. **Sympathomimetics** may increase risk of arrhythmias. **HERBAL: Ephedra** may increase risk of arrhythmias. **Licorice** may cause sodium and water retention, loss of potassium. **FOOD: Meals with increased fiber (bran) or high in pectin** may decrease absorption. **LAB VALUES:** None known.

AVAILABILITY (Rx)

Oral Solution (Lanoxin): 50 mcg/ml. **Injection Solution (Lanoxin):** 100 mcg/ml, 250 mcg/ml. **Tablets (Lanoxin):** 125 mcg, 250 mcg.

ADMINISTRATION/HANDLING

◀**ALERT**▶ IM rarely used (produces severe local irritation, erratic absorption). If no other route possible, give deep into muscle followed by massage. Give no more than 2 ml at any one site.

IV

• May give undiluted or dilute with at least a 4-fold volume of Sterile Water for Injection or D₅W (less may cause precipitate). • Use immediately. • Give IV slowly over at least 5 min.

PO

• May give without regard to meals. • Tablets may be crushed.

▦ IV INCOMPATIBILITIES

Amphotericin B complex (Abelcet, AmBisome, Amphotec), fluconazole (Diflucan), foscarnet (Foscavir), propofol (Diprivan).

▦ IV COMPATIBILITIES

Diltiazem (Cardizem), furosemide (Lasix), heparin, insulin regular, lidocaine, midazolam (Versed), milrinone (Primacor), morphine, potassium chloride.

INDICATIONS/ROUTES/DOSAGE

Loading Dose

PO: ADULTS, ELDERLY: Initially, 0.5–0.75 mg, 2 additional doses of 0.125–0.375 mg at 6- to 8-hr intervals. Range: 0.75–1.5 mg. **CHILDREN 10 YRS AND OLDER:** 10–15 mcg/kg. **CHILDREN 5–9 YRS:** 20–35 mcg/kg. **CHILDREN 2–4 YRS:** 30–40 mcg/kg. **CHILDREN 1–23 MOS:** 35–60 mcg/kg. **NEONATE, FULL-TERM:** 25–35 mcg/kg. **NEONATE, PREMATURE:** 20–30 mcg/kg.

IV: ADULTS, ELDERLY: (Atrial fibrillation in pts with HF): 0.25 mg q2h up to 1.5 mg in 24 hrs. **(Supraventricular tachyarrhythmias):** 0.5–1 mg. **CHILDREN 10 YRS AND OLDER:** 8–12 mcg/kg. **CHILDREN 5–9 YRS:** 15–30 mcg/kg. **CHILDREN 2–4 YRS:** 25–35 mcg/kg. **CHILDREN 1–23 MOS:** 30–50 mcg/kg. **NEONATES, FULL-TERM:** 20–30 mcg/kg. **NEONATES, PREMATURE:** 15–25 mcg/kg.

Maintenance Dosage

	PO	IV/IM
Preterm infant	5–7.5 mcg/kg	4–6 mcg/kg
Full-term infant	6–10 mcg/kg	5–8 mcg/kg
1 mo–2 yrs	10–15 mcg/kg	7.5–12 mcg/kg
2–5 yrs	7.5–10 mcg/kg	6–9 mcg/kg
5–10 yrs	5–10 mcg/kg	4–8 mcg/kg
11–18 yrs	2.5–5 mcg/kg	2–3 mcg/kg
Adults	0.125–0.5 mg	0.1–0.4 mg

Dosage in Renal Impairment

Dosage adjustment is based on creatinine clearance. Total digitalizing dose: decrease by 50% in end-stage renal disease.

Creatinine Clearance	Dosage
10–50 ml/min	25%–75% of usual dose or q36h
Less than 10 ml/min	10%–25% of usual dose or q48h

SIDE EFFECTS

Dizziness, headache, diarrhea, rash, visual disturbances.

ADVERSE EFFECTS/ TOXIC REACTIONS

Most common early manifestations of digoxin toxicity are GI disturbances (anorexia, nausea, vomiting), neurologic abnormalities (fatigue, headache, depression, weakness, drowsiness, confusion, nightmares). Facial pain, personality change, ocular disturbances (photophobia, light flashes, halos around bright objects, yellow or green color perception) may occur. Sinus bradycardia, AV block, ventricular arrhythmias noted. **Antidote:** Digoxin immune FAB (see Appendix K for dosage).

NURSING CONSIDERATIONS

BASELINE ASSESSMENT

Assess apical pulse. If pulse is 60 or less/min (70 or less/min for children), withhold drug, contact physician. Blood samples are best taken 6–8 hrs after dose or just before next dose.

INTERVENTION/EVALUATION

Monitor pulse for bradycardia, EKG for arrhythmias for 1–2 hrs after administration (excessive slowing of pulse may be first clinical sign of toxicity). Assess for GI disturbances, neurologic abnormalities (signs of toxicity) q2–4h during loading dose (daily during maintenance). Monitor serum potassium, magnesium, calcium, renal function. **Therapeutic serum level:** 0.8–2 ng/ml; **toxic serum level:** greater than 2 ng/ml.

PATIENT/FAMILY TEACHING

• Follow-up visits, blood tests are an important part of therapy. • Follow guidelines to take apical pulse and report pulse 60 or less/min (or as indicated by physician). • Wear/carry identification of digoxin therapy and inform dentist, other physician of taking digoxin. • Do not increase or skip doses. • Do not take OTC medications without consulting physician. • Report decreased appetite, nausea/vomiting, diarrhea, visual changes.

digoxin immune FAB

di-**jox**-in
(DigiFab)
Do not confuse digoxin immune FAB with Desoxyn or doxepin.

◆ CLASSIFICATION

CLINICAL: Antidote.

ACTION

Binds molecularly to digoxin in extracellular space. **Therapeutic Effect:** Makes digoxin unavailable for binding at site of action on cells in the body.

PHARMACOKINETICS

Route	Onset	Peak	Duration
IV	2–30 min	N/A	3–4 days

Widely distributed into extracellular space. Excreted in urine. **Half-life:** 15–20 hrs.

USES

Treatment of life-threatening or potentially life-threatening digoxin toxicity.

PRECAUTIONS

Contraindications: None known. **Cautions:** Cardiac failure, renal impairment.

⌛ LIFESPAN CONSIDERATIONS

Pregnancy/Lactation: Unknown if drug crosses placenta or is distributed in breast milk. **Pregnancy Category C. Children:** No age-related precautions noted. **Elderly:** Age-related renal impairment may require dosage adjustment.

INTERACTIONS

DRUG: None significant. **HERBAL:** None significant. **FOOD:** None known. **LAB VALUES:** May alter serum potassium. Serum digoxin may increase precipitously and persist for up to 1 wk until FAB/digoxin complex is eliminated from body.

AVAILABILITY (Rx)

Injection, Powder for Reconstitution: 40-mg vial (DigiFab).

ADMINISTRATION/HANDLING

 IV

Reconstitution • Reconstitute each 40-mg vial with 4 ml Sterile Water for Injection to provide concentration of 10 mg/ml. • Further dilute with 36 ml 0.9% NaCl to provide a concentration of 1 mg/ml. **Rate of Administration** • Infuse over 30 min (recommended that solution be infused through a 0.22-micron filter). • If cardiac arrest is imminent, may give IV push. **Storage** • Refrigerate vials. • After reconstitution, stable for 4 hrs if refrigerated. • Use immediately after reconstitution.

🔲 IV INCOMPATIBILITY

None known.

INDICATIONS/ROUTES/DOSAGE

Potentially Life-Threatening Digoxin Overdose
IV: ADULTS, ELDERLY, CHILDREN: Dosage varies according to amount of digoxin to be neutralized. Refer to manufacturer's dosing guidelines.

SIDE EFFECTS

Rare: Allergic reaction.

ADVERSE EFFECTS/TOXIC REACTIONS

Digoxin toxicity may result in hyperkalemia (diarrhea, paresthesia, heaviness of legs, decreased B/P, cold skin, grayish pallor, hypotension, mental confusion, irritability, flaccid paralysis, tented T waves, widening QRS, ST depression). When effect of digitalis is reversed, hypokalemia may develop rapidly (muscle cramping, nausea, vomiting, hypoactive bowel sounds, abdominal distention, difficulty breathing, postural hypotension). Low cardiac output conditions, HF occur rarely.

NURSING CONSIDERATIONS

BASELINE ASSESSMENT

Obtain serum digoxin level before administering drug. If drawn less than 6 hrs before last digoxin dose, test result may be unreliable. Those with renal impairment may require more than 1 wk before serum digoxin assay is reliable. Assess muscle strength, mental status.

INTERVENTION/EVALUATION

Closely monitor temperature, B/P, EKG, serum potassium during and after drug is administered. Watch for changes from initial assessment (hypokalemia may result in muscle strength changes, tremor, muscle cramps, altered mental status, cardiac arrhythmias; hyponatremia may result in confusion, thirst, cold/clammy skin).

dihydroergotamine

dye-**hye**-droe-er-**got**-a-meen
(D.H.E. 45, Migranal)

BLACK BOX ALERT Concurrent use with CYP3A4 inhibitors (macrolide antibiotics, azole antifungals, protease inhibitors) increases risk of vasospasm, producing ischemia of brain and peripheral extremities.

FIXED-COMBINATION(S)

Bellergal-S: ergotamine/belladonna (anticholinergic)/phenobarbital (sedative-hypnotic): 0.6 mg/0.2 mg/ 40 mg. **Cafergot, Wigraine:** ergotamine/caffeine (stimulant): 1 mg/100 mg, 2 mg/100 mg.
Do not confuse Cafergot with Carafate.

◆CLASSIFICATION

PHARMACOTHERAPEUTIC: Ergotamine derivative. **CLINICAL:** Antimigraine.

ACTION

Directly stimulates vascular smooth muscle, resulting in peripheral and cerebral vasoconstriction. May have antagonist effects on serotonin. **Therapeutic Effect:** Suppresses vascular headaches, migraine headaches.

PHARMACOKINETICS

Slowly, incompletely absorbed from GI tract; rapidly and extensively absorbed after rectal administration. Protein binding: greater than 90%. Eliminated in feces by the biliary system. **Half-life:** 21 hrs.

USES

Treatment of migraine headache with or without aura. Injection used to treat cluster headache. **OFF-LABEL:** Prevention of deep venous thrombosis (DVT), prevention and treatment of orthostatic hypotension, xerostomia secondary to antidepressants, pelvic congestion with pain.

PRECAUTIONS

Contraindications: Uncontrolled hypertension, ischemic heart disease, coronary artery vasospasm, hemiplegic or basilar migraine, peripheral vascular disease, sepsis, severe renal/hepatic impairment, use of MAOIs within 14 days, use of 5-HT$_B$ agonists within 24 hrs, CYP3A4 inhibitors (e.g., azole antifungals, macrolide antibiotics, protease inhibitors), pregnancy, breast-feeding. **Cautions:** Elderly.

⧗ LIFESPAN CONSIDERATIONS

Pregnancy/Lactation: Contraindicated in pregnancy (produces uterine stimulant action, resulting in possible fetal death or retarded fetal growth); increases vasoconstriction of placental vascular bed. Drug distributed in breast milk. May produce diarrhea, vomiting in neonate. May prohibit lactation. **Pregnancy Category X. Children:** No precautions in those 6 yrs and older, but use only when unresponsive to other medication. **Elderly:** Age-related occlusive peripheral vascular disease increases risk of peripheral vasoconstriction. Age-related renal impairment may require dosage adjustment.

INTERACTIONS

DRUG: **Beta-blockers, erythromycin** may increase risk of peripheral vasoconstriction. **Ergot alkaloids, 5-HT$_B$ agonists (e.g., sumatriptan), systemic vasoconstrictors** may increase pressor effect. **HERBAL:** None significant. **FOOD:** **Coffee, cola, tea** may increase absorption. **Grapefruit products** may increase concentration/toxicity. **LAB VALUES:** None significant.

AVAILABILITY (Rx)

Dihydroergotamine Injection, Solution: 1 mg/ml. **Intranasal Spray, Solution (Migranal):** 4 mg/ml (0.5 mg/spray).

INDICATIONS/ROUTES/DOSAGE

Vascular Headaches

IM/Subcutaneous: ADULTS, ELDERLY: 1 mg at onset of headache; repeat hourly. **Maximum:** 3 mg/day; 6 mg/wk.

IV: ADULTS, ELDERLY: 1 mg at onset of headache; repeat hourly. **Maximum:** 2 mg/day; 6 mg/wk.

Intranasal: ADULTS, ELDERLY: 1 spray (0.5 mg) into each nostril; repeat in 15 min. **Maximum:** 6 sprays/day; 8 sprays/wk.

SIDE EFFECTS

Occasional (5%–2%): Cough, dizziness. **Rare (less than 2%):** Myalgia, fatigue, diarrhea, upper respiratory tract infection, dyspepsia.

ADVERSE EFFECTS/TOXIC REACTIONS

Prolonged administration, excessive dosage may produce ergotamine poisoning, manifested as nausea, vomiting, paresthesia of extremities, muscle pain/weakness, precordial pain, significant changes in pulse rate and blood pressure. Vasoconstriction of peripheral arteries/arterioles may result in localized edema, pruritus. Feet, hands will become cold, pale. Muscle pain will occur when walking and later, even at rest. Other rare effects include confusion, depression, drowsiness, seizures, gangrene.

NURSING CONSIDERATIONS

BASELINE ASSESSMENT

Question for history of peripheral vascular disease, renal/hepatic impairment, possibility of pregnancy. Question onset, location, duration of migraine, possible precipitating symptoms.

INTERVENTION/EVALUATION

Monitor closely for evidence of ergotamine overdosage as result of prolonged administration or excessive dosage.

PATIENT/FAMILY TEACHING

• Initiate therapy at first sign of migraine headache. • Report if there is need to progressively increase dose to relieve vascular headaches or if palpitations, nausea, vomiting, paresthesia, pain or weakness of extremities, chest pain. Avoid grapefruit products. • Female pts should avoid pregnancy; if suspected, immediately report. (Pregnancy Category X).

---

diltiazem

dil-**tye**-a-zem
(Apo-Diltiaz ❖, <u>Cardizem</u>, Cardizem CD, Cardizem LA, Cartia XT, Dilacor XR, Dilt-CD, Dilt-XR, Diltia XT, Matzim LA, Taztia XT, Tiazac)
Do not confuse Cardizem with Cardene or Cardene SR, Cartia XT with Procardia XL, diltiazem with Calan, diazepam, or Dilantin, or Tiazac with Ziac.

FIXED-COMBINATION(S)

Teczem: diltiazem/enalapril (ACE inhibitor): 180 mg/5 mg.

◆CLASSIFICATION

PHARMACOTHERAPEUTIC: Calcium channel blocker. **CLINICAL:** Antianginal, antihypertensive, antiarrhythmic (see pp. 19C, 62C, 79C).

ACTION

Inhibits calcium movement across cardiac, vascular smooth-muscle cell membranes (causes dilation of coronary arteries, peripheral arteries, arterioles). **Therapeutic Effect:** Decreases heart rate, myocardial contractility; slows SA, AV conduction; decreases total peripheral vascular resistance by vasodilation.

PHARMACOKINETICS

Route	Onset	Peak	Duration
PO	0.5–1 hr	N/A	N/A
PO (extended-release)	2–3 hrs	N/A	N/A
IV	3 min	N/A	N/A

Well absorbed from GI tract. Protein binding: 70%–80%. Primarily excreted in urine. Not removed by hemodialysis. **Half-life:** 3–8 hrs.

USES

PO: Treatment of angina due to coronary artery spasm (Prinzmetal's variant angina), chronic stable angina (effort-associated angina). **Extended-release:** Treatment of essential hypertension, angina. **Cardizem LA:** Treatment of chronic stable angina. **Parenteral:** Temporary control of rapid ventricular rate in atrial fibrillation/flutter. Rapid conversion of paroxysmal supraventricular tachycardia (PSVT) to normal sinus rhythm. **OFF-LABEL:** Stable narrow complex tachycardia, recurrent SVT, pediatric hypertension, hypertrophic cardiomyopathy.

PRECAUTIONS

Contraindications: PO: Acute MI, pulmonary congestion, hypersensitivity to diltiazem or other calcium channel blockers, second- or third-degree AV block (except in presence of pacemaker), severe hypotension (less than 90 mm Hg, systolic), sick sinus syndrome. **IV:** Sick sinus syndrome or second- or third-degree block (except with functioning pacemaker), cardiogenic shock, administration of IV beta blocker within several hours; atrial fibrillation/flutter associated with accessory bypass tract. **Cautions:** Renal/hepatic impairment, HF, concurrent use with beta-blocker, hypertrophic obstructive cardiomyopathy.

⌛ LIFESPAN CONSIDERATIONS

Pregnancy/Lactation: Distributed in breast milk. **Pregnancy Category C. Children:** No age-related precautions noted. **Elderly:** Age-related renal impairment may require dosage adjustment.

INTERACTIONS

DRUG: Beta-blockers, digoxin may have additive effect on prolonging A-V conduction. May increase concentration, risk of toxicity with **carbamazepine, benzodiazepines.** May increase serum **digoxin**

concentration. **Rifampin** may decrease concentration/effects. May increase concentration of **statins** and risk of myopathy/rhabdomyolysis. **HERBAL: Ephedra** may worsen arrhythmias, hypertension. **Garlic** may increase antihypertensive effect. **Ginseng, yohimbe** may worsen hypertension. **St. John's wort** may decrease concentration. **FOOD:** None known. **LAB VALUES:** May increase PR interval.

AVAILABILITY (Rx)

Injection, Infusion (Ready to Hang): 1 mg/ml. **Injection, Solution:** 5 mg/ml (5 ml, 10 ml, 25 ml). **Tablets, Immediate-Release:** 30 mg, 60 mg, 90 mg, 120 mg.

🔲 **Capsules, Extended-Release: (Cardizem CD):** 120 mg, 180 mg, 240 mg, 300 mg, 360 mg. **(Cartia XT):** 120 mg, 180 mg, 240 mg, 300 mg. **(Dilacor XR, Dilt-XR, Diltia XT):** 120 mg, 180 mg, 240 mg. **(Taztia XT):** 120 mg, 180 mg, 240 mg, 300 mg, 360 mg. **(Tiazac):** 120 mg, 180 mg, 240 mg, 300 mg, 360 mg, 420 mg. 🔲 **Capsules, Sustained-Release:** 60 mg, 90 mg, 120 mg. 🔲 **Tablets, Extended-Release: (Cardizem LA):** 120 mg, 180 mg, 240 mg, 300 mg, 360 mg, 420 mg. **(Matzim LA):** 120 mg, 180 mg, 240 mg, 300 mg, 360 mg, 420 mg.

ADMINISTRATION/HANDLING

 IV

Reconstitution • Add 125 mg to 100 ml D₅W, 0.9% NaCl to provide concentration of 1 mg/ml.
Rate of Administration • Infuse per dilution/rate chart provided by manufacturer.
Storage • Refrigerate vials. • After dilution, stable for 24 hrs.

PO

• Give immediate-release tablets before meals and at bedtime. • Tablets may be crushed. • Do not open, cut, or crush sustained-release capsules or extended-release capsules or tablets. • Taztia XT capsules may be opened and mixed with applesauce; follow with glass of water.

D

• Cardizem CD, Cardizem LA, Cartia XT, Dilt-CD, Matzim LA may be given without regard to meals. • Dilacor XR, Dilt-XR, Diltia XT to be given on empty stomach.

🔳 IV INCOMPATIBILITIES

Acetazolamide (Diamox), acyclovir (Zovirax), ampicillin, ampicillin/sulbactam (Unasyn), diazepam (Valium), furosemide (Lasix), heparin, insulin, nafcillin, phenytoin (Dilantin), rifampin (Rifadin), sodium bicarbonate.

🔳 IV COMPATIBILITIES

Albumin, aztreonam (Azactam), bumetanide (Bumex), cefazolin (Ancef), cefotaxime (Claforan), ceftazidime (Fortaz), ceftriaxone (Rocephin), cefuroxime (Zinacef), ciprofloxacin (Cipro), clindamycin (Cleocin), dexmedetomidine (Precedex), digoxin (Lanoxin), dobutamine (Dobutrex), dopamine (Intropin), gentamicin, hydromorphone (Dilaudid), lidocaine, lorazepam (Ativan), metoclopramide (Reglan), metronidazole (Flagyl), midazolam (Versed), morphine, multivitamins, nitroglycerin, norepinephrine (Levophed), potassium chloride, potassium phosphate, tobramycin (Nebcin), vancomycin (Vancocin).

INDICATIONS/ROUTES/DOSAGE

Angina
PO *(Immediate-Release) (Cardizem)*: **ADULTS, ELDERLY:** Initially, 30 mg 4 times a day. Range: 120–320 mg/day.
PO *(Extended-Release) (Cardizem CD, Cartia XT, Dilacor XR, DILT-CD, DILT XR, DILT XT)*: **ADULTS, ELDERLY:** Initially, 120–180 mg once daily. Range: 120–320 mg. **Maximum:** 480 mg/day.
(Extended-Release) (Tiazac, Taztia XT): **ADULTS, ELDERLY:** Initially, 120–180 mg once daily. Range: 120–320 mg/day. **Maximum:** 540 mg/day.
(Extended-Release) (Cardizem LA, Matzim LA): Initially, 180 mg/day. Range: 120–320 mg. **Maximum:** 360 mg daily.

Hypertension
PO *(Cardizem CD, Cartia XT, Dilacor XR, DILT CD, Diltia XT, Tiazac)*: **ADULTS, ELDERLY:** Initially, 180–240 mg/day. Range: 180–420 mg/day. **Tiazac:** 120–540 mg/day.
PO *(Sustained-Release)*: **ADULTS, ELDERLY:** Initially, 60–120 mg twice a day. May increase at 14-day intervals. Maintenance: 240–360 mg/day.
PO *(Cardizem LA, Matzim LA)*: **ADULTS, ELDERLY:** Initially, 180–240 mg/day. May increase at 14-day intervals. Range: 120–540 mg/day.

Temporary Control of Rapid Ventricular Rate in Atrial Fibrillation/Flutter; Rapid Conversion of Paroxysmal Supraventricular Tachycardia to Normal Sinus Rhythm
IV Push: ADULTS, ELDERLY: Initially, 0.25 mg/kg (average dose: 20 mg) actual body weight over 2 min. May repeat in 15 min at dose of 0.35 mg/kg (average dose: 25 mg) actual body weight. Subsequent doses individualized.
IV Infusion: ADULTS, ELDERLY: After initial bolus injection, may begin infusion at 5–10 mg/hr; may increase by 5 mg/hr up to a maximum of 15 mg/hr. Infusion duration should not exceed 24 hrs. Attempt conversion to PO therapy as soon as possible.

SIDE EFFECTS

Frequent (10%–5%): Peripheral edema, dizziness, light-headedness, headache, bradycardia, asthenia (loss of strength, energy). **Occasional (5%–2%):** Nausea, constipation, flushing, EKG changes. **Rare (less than 2%):** Rash, micturition disorder (polyuria, nocturia, dysuria, frequency of urination), abdominal discomfort, drowsiness.

ADVERSE EFFECTS/ TOXIC REACTIONS

Abrupt withdrawal may increase frequency, duration of angina, HF; second- and third-degree AV block occur rarely. Overdose produces nausea, drowsiness, confusion, slurred speech, profound bradycardia. **Antidote:** Glucagon, insu-

---

lin drip with continuous calcium infusion (see Appendix K for dosage).

NURSING CONSIDERATIONS

BASELINE ASSESSMENT

Record onset, type (sharp, dull, squeezing), radiation, location, intensity, duration of anginal pain, precipitating factors (exertion, emotional stress). Assess baseline renal/hepatic function tests. Assess B/P, apical pulse immediately before drug is administered.

INTERVENTION/EVALUATION

Assist with ambulation if dizziness occurs. Assess for peripheral edema behind medial malleolus (sacral area in bedridden pts). Monitor pulse rate for bradycardia. Assess B/P, renal/hepatic function tests, EKG with IV therapy. Question for asthenia (loss of strength, energy), headache.

PATIENT/FAMILY TEACHING

• Do not abruptly discontinue medication. • Compliance with therapy regimen is essential to control anginal pain. • To avoid hypotensive effect, go from lying to standing slowly. • Avoid tasks that require alertness, motor skills until response to drug is established. • Report palpitations, shortness of breath, pronounced dizziness, nausea, constipation. • Avoid alcohol (may increase risk of hypotension or vasodilation).

dimenhydrinate

dye-men-**hye**-dra-nate
(Apo-Dimenhydrinate ✤, Dramamine, Driminate)
Do not confuse dimenhydrinate with diphenhydramine.

◆CLASSIFICATION

PHARMACOTHERAPEUTIC: Anticholinergic, antihistamine. **CLINICAL:** Antiemetic, antivertigo (see p. 55C).

ACTION

Depressant action on labyrinthine function. **Therapeutic Effect:** Prevents, treats nausea, vomiting, vertigo associated with motion sickness.

PHARMACOKINETICS

	Onset	Peak	Duration
PO	15-60 min	1–2 hrs	4–6 hrs

Well absorbed following PO administration. Metabolized in liver. Primarily excreted in urine. **Half-life:** 1.5 hrs.

USES

Prevention and treatment of nausea, vomiting, dizziness, vertigo associated with motion sickness. **OFF-LABEL:** Nausea and vomiting of pregnancy.

PRECAUTIONS

Contraindications: None known. **Cautions:** Narrow-angle glaucoma, peptic ulcer, prostatic hyperplasia, pyloroduodenal or bladder neck obstruction, asthma, COPD, increased IOP, cardiovascular disease, hyperthyroidism, hypertension, seizure disorders.

⌛ LIFESPAN CONSIDERATIONS

Pregnancy/Lactation: Small amount detected in breast milk. **Pregnancy Category B. Children/Elderly:** Paradoxical excitement may occur. **Elderly:** Increased risk for dizziness, sedation, confusion, hyperexcitability.

INTERACTIONS

DRUG: Alcohol, other CNS depressants may increase CNS depressant effects. **Anticholinergics** may increase anticholinergic, CNS depressant effects. **HERBAL: Gotu kola, kava kava, St. John's wort, valerian** may increase CNS depression. **FOOD:** None known. **LAB VALUES:** May suppress wheal/flare reactions to antigen skin testing unless antihistamines are discontinued 4 days before testing.

AVAILABILITY (OTC)

Injection, solution: 50 mg/ml. **Tablets:** 50 mg. **Tablets, Chewable:** 25 mg, 50 mg.

ADMINISTRATION/HANDLING

PO
• Give with food or water. • Scored tablets may be crushed.

IV
Must dilute with 10 ml 0.9% NaCl.

INDICATIONS/ROUTES/DOSAGE

Nausea, Vomiting, Motion Sickness
PO: ADULTS, ELDERLY: 50–100 mg q4–6h. **Maximum:** 400 mg in 24 hrs. **CHILDREN 6–12 YRS:** 25–50 mg q6–8h. **Maximum:** 150 mg in 24 hrs. **CHILDREN 2–5 YRS:** 12.5–25 mg q6–8h. **Maximum:** 75 mg in 24 hrs.
IV: ADULTS: 50 mg q4h. **Maximum:** 100 mg q4h.
IM: ADULTS: 50–100 mg q4h. **CHILDREN:** 1.25 mg/kg 4 times/day. **Maximum:** 300 mg/day.

SIDE EFFECTS

Occasional: Drowsiness, restlessness, dry mouth, hypotension, insomnia (esp. in children), excitation, lassitude. Sedation, dizziness, hypotension more likely noted in elderly. **Rare:** Visual disturbances, hearing disturbances, paresthesia.

ADVERSE EFFECTS/ TOXIC REACTIONS

Children may experience dominant paradoxical reactions (restlessness, insomnia). Overdosage may result in seizures, respiratory depression.

NURSING CONSIDERATIONS

BASELINE ASSESSMENT

Obtain baseline B/P, pulse rate. Assess for dehydration if excessive vomiting has occurred (poor skin turgor, dry mucous membranes, longitudinal furrows in tongue).

INTERVENTION/EVALUATION

Monitor B/P, esp. in elderly (increased risk of hypotension). Monitor children closely for paradoxical reaction. Monitor serum electrolytes in those with severe vomiting. Assess hydration status.

PATIENT/FAMILY TEACHING

• Avoid tasks that require alertness, motor skills until response to drug is established. • Avoid alcohol. • Sugarless gum, sips of water may relieve dry mouth. • Coffee, tea may help reduce drowsiness.

dimethyl fumarate

dye-**meth**-il-**fue**-ma-rate
(Tecfidera)

◆CLASSIFICATION

PHARMACOTHERAPEUTIC: Fumaric acid ester. **CLINICAL:** Multiple sclerosis agent.

ACTION

Exact mechanism of action unknown. May include antiinflammatory action and modulation of cellular oxidative. **Therapeutic Effect:** Modify disease progression.

PHARMACOKINETICS

Undergoes rapid hydrolysis into active metabolite, monomethyl fumarate. Peak concentration: 2–2½ hrs. Protein binding: 27%–45%. Extensively metabolized by esterases. Primarily eliminated as exhaled carbon dioxide (60%). **Half-life:** 1 hr.

USES

Treatment of relapsing-remitting multiple sclerosis.

PRECAUTIONS

Contraindications: None known. **Cautions:** Hepatic impairment (may increase hepatic transaminases, lymphopenia (may decrease lymphocyte count).

⌛ LIFESPAN CONSIDERATIONS

Pregnancy/Lactation: Unknown if distributed in breast milk. **Pregnancy Category C. Children:** Safety and efficacy not established in pts younger than 18 yrs. **Elderly:** No age-related precautions noted.

INTERACTIONS

DRUG: None known. **HERBAL:** None known. **FOOD:** None significant. **LAB VALUES:** May decrease lymphocytes. May increase serum AST, ALT, eosinophils, urine albumin.

AVAILABILITY (Rx)

Capsules, Delayed-Release: 120 mg, 240 mg.

ADMINISTRATION/HANDLING

PO
• Give capsule whole; do not crush, cut, or sprinkle capsule contents on food. May give without regard to meal. May give with food to decrease flushing reaction and GI effects. Protect from light.

INDICATIONS/ROUTES/DOSAGE

Relapsing-Remitting Multiple Sclerosis
PO: **ADULTS/ELDERLY:** Initially, 120 mg twice daily for 7 days. Then increase to 240 mg twice daily.

SIDE EFFECTS

Frequent (40%): Flushing. **Occasional (18%–5%):** Abdominal pain, diarrhea, nausea, vomiting, dyspepsia, pruritus, rash, erythema.

ADVERSE EFFECTS/ TOXIC REACTIONS

Lymphopenia may increase risk for infection. Severe flushing may lead to noncompliance of therapy.

NURSING CONSIDERATIONS

BASELINE ASSESSMENT

Obtain baseline CBC, CMP, urine pregnancy if applicable. Question any plans of breastfeeding. Assess hydration status (urine output, skin turgor). Question

history of hepatic impairment, lymphopenia.

INTERVENTION/EVALUATION

Monitor CBC annually, hepatic function test. Encourage PO intake. Offer antiemetics for nausea, vomiting. Question any episodes of noncompliance due to flushing, GI symptoms. Monitor for infectious process (fever, malaise, chills, body aches, cough).

PATIENT/FAMILY TEACHING

• Pts will most likely experience abdominal pain, diarrhea, nausea, and flushing. Side effects may decrease over time. • Take with meals to decrease flushing reaction. • Swallow capsule whole; do not crush, cut, or chew. • Two dosage strengths will be provided for starting dose and maintenance dose. • Report any yellowing of skin or eyes, upper abdominal pain, bruising, dark-colored urine, fever, body aches, cough, dehydration.

dinoprostone

dye-noe-**pros**-tone
(Cervidil, Prepidil, Prostin E₂)
BLACK BOX ALERT To be used only by personnel medically trained in dinoprostone-specific drug effects in a hospital setting.
Do not confuse Cervidil or Prepidil with bepridil.

◆CLASSIFICATION

PHARMACOTHERAPEUTIC: Prostaglandin. **CLINICAL:** Oxytocic, abortifacient.

ACTION

Directly acts on myometrium, causing softening, dilation effect of cervix. **Therapeutic Effect:** Stimulates myometrial contractions in gravid uterus.

PHARMACOKINETICS

	Onset	Peak	Duration
Uterine stimulation	10 min (contractions begin)	1–2 hrs (abortion time)	2–6 hrs (contractions persist)

Undergoes rapid enzymatic deactivation primarily in maternal lungs. Protein binding: 73%. Primarily excreted in urine. **Half-life:** Less than 5 min.

USES

Vaginal suppository: To induce abortion from wk 12 through wk 20 of pregnancy to evacuate uterine contents in missed abortion or intrauterine fetal death up to 28 wks gestational age (as calculated from first day of last normal menstrual period), benign hydatidiform mole. **Gel:** Ripening of unfavorable cervix in pregnant women at or near term with medical/obstetric need for labor induction. Induction of labor at or near term. **Vaginal insert:** Initiation and/or cervical ripening in pts with medical indication for induction of labor.

PRECAUTIONS

Contraindications: Gel: Active cardiac, hepatic, pulmonary, renal disease; acute pelvic inflammatory disease (PID); fetal malpresentation; grand multiparae with 6 or more previous term pregnancy cases with nonvertex presentation; history of cesarean section, major uterine surgery; history of difficult labor, traumatic delivery; hypersensitivity to other prostaglandins; placenta previa, unexplained vaginal bleeding during this pregnancy; pts for whom vaginal delivery is not indicated (vasa previa, active herpes genitalia); significant cephalopelvic disproportion. **Vaginal Suppository:** Active cardiac, hepatic, pulmonary, renal disease; acute PID. **Cautions:** Cervicitis, infected endocervical lesions, acute vaginitis, history of asthma, hypotension/hypertension, anemia, jaundice, diabetes, epilepsy, uterine fibroids, compromised (scarred) uterus, history of cardiovascular, renal/hepatic disease.

⏳ LIFESPAN CONSIDERATIONS

Pregnancy/Lactation: Suppository: Teratogenic, therefore abortion must be complete. **Gel:** Sustained uterine hyperstimulation may affect fetus (e.g., abnormal heart rate). **Pregnancy Category C. Children/Elderly:** Not used in these pt populations.

INTERACTIONS

DRUG: Oxytocics may cause uterine contractions, possibly resulting in uterine rupture, cervical laceration. **HERBAL:** None significant. **FOOD:** None known. **LAB VALUES:** May alter B/P, heart rate. May increase body temperature.

AVAILABILITY (Rx)

Endocervical Gel (Prepidil): 0.5 mg/3 g syringe. **Vaginal Inserts (Cervidil):** 10 mg. **Vaginal Suppositories (Prostin E₂):** 20 mg.

ADMINISTRATION/HANDLING

Gel
• Refrigerate. • Use caution in handling; prevent skin contact. Wash hands thoroughly with soap and water following administration. • Bring to room temperature just before use (avoid forcing the warming process). • Assemble dosing apparatus as described in manufacturer's insert. • Place pt in dorsal position with cervix visualized using a speculum. • Introduce gel into cervical canal just below level of internal os. • Have pt remain in supine position at least 15–30 min (minimizes leakage from cervical canal). • Wait 6–12h after gel administration before initiating oxytocin therapy.

Suppository, Vaginal Inserts
• Keep frozen (−4°F); bring to room temperature just before use. • Administer only in hospital setting with emergency equipment available. • Warm suppository to room temperature before removing foil wrapper. • Avoid skin contact (risk of absorption). • Insert high into vagina. • Pt should remain supine for 10 min after administration of suppository, 2 hrs after vaginal insert. • Wait

at least 30 min after removing insert before initiating oxytocin therapy.

INDICATIONS/ROUTES/DOSAGE

Abortifacient
Intravaginal: ADULTS (VAGINAL SUPPOSITORY): 20 mg (one suppository) high into vagina. May repeat at 3- to 5-hr intervals until abortion occurs. Do not administer for longer than 2 days.

Ripening of Unfavorable Cervix
Intracervical *(Prepidil):* **ADULTS (ENDOCERVICAL GEL):** Initially, 0.5 mg (2.5 ml); if no cervical or uterine response, may repeat 0.5-mg dose in 6 hrs. **Maximum:** 1.5 mg (7.5 ml) for a 24-hr period.
Intracervical *(Cervidil):* **ADULTS (VAGINAL INSERT):** 10 mg transversely into posterior formix of the vagina (remove upon onset of active labor or 12 hrs after insertion).

SIDE EFFECTS

Frequent: Vomiting (66%), diarrhea (40%), nausea (33%). **Occasional:** Headache (10%), chills/shivering (10%), urticaria, bradycardia, increased uterine pain accompanying abortion, peripheral vasoconstriction. **Rare:** Flushing of skin, vulvar edema.

ADVERSE EFFECTS/
TOXIC REACTIONS

Overdose may cause uterine contractions with spasm and tetanic contraction, leading to cervical laceration/perforation, uterine rupture/hemorrhage.

NURSING CONSIDERATIONS

BASELINE ASSESSMENT

Offer emotional support. **Suppository:** Obtain orders for antiemetics, antidiarrheals, meperidine, other pain medication for abdominal cramps. Assess any uterine activity, vaginal bleeding. **Gel:** Assess Bishop score. Assess degree of effacement (determines size of shielded endocervical catheter).

INTERVENTION/EVALUATION

Suppository: Check strength, duration, frequency of contractions. Monitor vital signs q15min until stable, then hourly until abortion complete. Check resting uterine tone. Administer medications for relief of GI effects if indicated or for abdominal cramps. **Gel:** Monitor uterine activity (onset of uterine contractions), fetal status (heart rate), character of cervix (dilation, effacement). Have pt remain recumbent 12 hrs after application with continuous electronic monitoring of fetal heart rate, uterine activity. Record maternal vital signs at least hourly in presence of uterine activity. Reassess Bishop score.

PATIENT/FAMILY TEACHING

• **Suppository:** Report promptly fever, chills, foul-smelling/increased vaginal discharge, uterine cramps, pain.

---

*diphenhydrAMINE

dye-fen-**hye**-dra-meen
(Allerdryl ✤, Banophen, Benadryl, Benadryl Children's Allergy, Diphen, Diphenhist, Dytan, Genahist, Nytol ✤)
Do not confuse Benadryl with benazepril, Bentyl, or Benylin, or diphenhydramine with desipramine, dicyclomine, or dimenhydrinate.

FIXED-COMBINATION(S)

Advil PM: diphenhydramine/ibuprofen (NSAID): 38 mg/200 mg. With calamine, an astringent, and camphor, a counterirritant **(Caladryl).**

✦CLASSIFICATION

PHARMACOTHERAPEUTIC: Ethanolamine. **CLINICAL:** Antihistamine, anticholinergic, antipruritic, antitussive, antiemetic, antidyskinetic (see p. 55C).

ACTION

Competitively blocks effects of histamine at peripheral H$_1$ receptor sites. **Therapeutic Effect:** Produces anticholinergic, antipruritic, antitussive, antiemetic, antidyskinetic, sedative effects.

PHARMACOKINETICS

Route	Onset	Peak	Duration
PO	15–30 min	1–4 hrs	4–6 hrs
IV, IM	Less than 15 min	1–4 hrs	4–6 hrs

Well absorbed after PO, parenteral administration. Protein binding: 98%–99%. Widely distributed. Metabolized in liver. Primarily excreted in urine. **Half-life:** 1–4 hrs.

USES

Treatment of allergic reactions including nasal allergies; parkinsonism, including drug-induced extrapyramidal symptoms; prevention/treatment of nausea, vomiting, or vertigo due to motion sickness; antitussive; short-term management of insomnia; adjunct to epinephrine in treatment of anaphylaxis. Topical form used for relief of pruritus from insect bites, skin irritations.

PRECAUTIONS

Contraindications: Acute exacerbation of asthma, neonates or premature infants, breast-feeding. **Cautions:** Narrow-angle glaucoma, stenotic peptic ulcer, prostatic hypertrophy, pyloroduodenal/bladder neck obstruction, asthma, COPD, increased IOP, cardiovascular disease, hyperthyroidism.

⧗ LIFESPAN CONSIDERATIONS

Pregnancy/Lactation: Crosses placenta. Detected in breast milk (may produce irritability in breast-fed infants). Increased risk of seizures in neonates, premature infants if used during third trimester of pregnancy. May prohibit lactation. **Pregnancy Category B. Children:** Not recommended in newborns, premature infants (increased risk of paradoxical reaction, seizures). **Elderly:** Increased risk

for dizziness, sedation, confusion, hypotension, hyperexcitability.

INTERACTIONS

DRUG: Alcohol, other CNS depressants may increase CNS depressant effects. **Anticholinergics** may increase anticholinergic effects. **HERBAL: Gotu kola, kava kava, St. John's wort, valerian** may increase CNS depression. **FOOD:** None known. **LAB VALUES:** May suppress wheal/flare reactions to antigen skin testing unless drug is discontinued 4 days before testing.

AVAILABILITY (OTC)

Capsules: 25 mg (Banophen, Diphen, Genahist), 50 mg. **Cream (Benadryl):** 1%, 2%. **Injection Solution (Benadryl):** 50 mg/ml. **Syrup (Diphen, Diphenhist):** 12.5 mg/5 ml. **Tablets (Banophen, Benadryl, Genahist):** 25 mg, 50 mg. **Tablets, Orally-Disintegrating (Benadryl Children's Allergy):** 12.5 mg, 25 mg.

ADMINISTRATION/HANDLING

 IV

• May be given undiluted. • Give IV injection over at least 1 min. **Maximum rate:** 25 mg/min.

IM

• Give deep IM into large muscle mass.

PO

• Give with food to decrease GI distress.
• Scored tablets may be crushed.

▦ IV INCOMPATIBILITIES

Allopurinol (Aloprim), cefepime (Maxipime), dexamethasone (Decadron), foscarnet (Foscavir).

▦ IV COMPATIBILITIES

Atropine, cisplatin (Platinol), cyclophosphamide (Cytoxan), cytarabine (Ara-C), fentanyl, glycopyrrolate (Robinul), heparin, hydrocortisone (Solu-Cortef), hydromorphone (Dilaudid), hydroxyzine (Vistaril), lidocaine, metoclopramide (Reglan), ondansetron (Zofran), potassium chloride, promethazine (Phenergan), propofol (Diprivan).

INDICATIONS/ROUTES/DOSAGE

Moderate to Severe Allergic Reaction
PO: ADULTS, ELDERLY: 25–50 mg q6–8h. **Maximum:** 400 mg/day. **IM, IV:** 10–50 mg/dose. **PO, IV, IM: CHILDREN:** 5 mg/kg/day in divided doses q6–8h. **Maximum:** 300 mg/day.

Motion Sickness
PO: ADULTS, ELDERLY, CHILDREN 12 YRS AND OLDER: 25–50 mg q4–6h. **Maximum:** 300 mg/day. **CHILDREN 6–11 YRS:** 12.5–25 mg q4–6h. **Maximum:** 150 mg/day. **CHILDREN 2–5 YRS:** 6.25 mg q4–6h. **Maximum:** 37.5 mg/day.

Parkinson's Disease
IM, IV *(Dystonic Reaction)*: 50 mg; may repeat in 20–30 min.

Antitussive
PO: ADULTS, ELDERLY, CHILDREN 12 YRS AND OLDER: 25 mg q4h. **Maximum:** 150 mg/day. **CHILDREN 6–11 YRS:** 12.5 mg q4h. **Maximum:** 75 mg/day. **CHILDREN 2–5 YRS:** 6.25 mg q4h. **Maximum:** 37.5 mg/day.

Nighttime Sleep Aid
PO: ADULTS, ELDERLY, CHILDREN 12 YRS AND OLDER: 25–50 mg at bedtime. **CHILDREN 2–11 YRS:** 1 mg/kg/dose. **Maximum:** 50 mg.

Pruritus
Topical: ADULTS, ELDERLY, CHILDREN 12 YRS AND OLDER: Apply 1% or 2% cream or spray 3–4 times a day. **CHILDREN 2–11 YRS:** Apply 1% cream or spray 3–4 times a day.

SIDE EFFECTS

Frequent: Drowsiness, dizziness, muscle weakness, hypotension, urinary retention, thickening of bronchial secretions, dry mouth, nose, throat, lips; in elderly: sedation, dizziness, hypotension. **Occasional:** Epigastric distress, flushing, visual/hearing disturbances, paresthesia, diaphoresis, chills.

ADVERSE EFFECTS/ TOXIC REACTIONS

Hypersensitivity reactions (eczema, pruritus, rash, cardiac disturbances, photosensitivity) may occur. Overdose symptoms may vary from CNS depression (sedation, apnea, hypotension, cardiovascular collapse, death) to severe paradoxical reactions (hallucinations, tremors, seizures). Children, infants, neonates may experience paradoxical reactions (restlessness, insomnia, euphoria, nervousness, tremors). Overdosage in children may result in hallucinations, seizures, death.

NURSING CONSIDERATIONS

BASELINE ASSESSMENT

If pt is having acute allergic reaction, obtain history of recently ingested foods, drugs, environmental exposure, emotional stress. Monitor B/P rate, depth, rhythm, type of respiration; quality, rate of pulse. Assess lung sounds for rhonchi, wheezing, rales.

INTERVENTION/EVALUATION

Monitor B/P, esp. in elderly (increased risk of hypotension). Monitor children closely for paradoxical reaction.

PATIENT/FAMILY TEACHING

• Tolerance to antihistaminic effect generally does not occur; tolerance to sedative effect may occur. • Avoid tasks that require alertness, motor skills until response to drug is established. • Dry mouth, drowsiness, dizziness may be an expected response to drug. • Avoid alcohol.

diphenoxylate with atropine

dye-fen-**ox**-i-late **at**-roe-peen
(Lomotil)
Do not confuse Lomotil with Lamictal, Lamisil, or Lasix, or

Lonox with Lanoxin, Loprox, or Lovenox.

FIXED-COMBINATION(S)

Lomotil: diphenoxylate/atropine (anticholinergic, antispasmodic): 2.5 mg/0.025 mg.

◆CLASSIFICATION

PHARMACOTHERAPEUTIC: Meperidine derivative. **CLINICAL:** Antidiarrheal (see p. 46C).

ACTION

Acts locally and centrally on gastric mucosa. **Therapeutic Effect:** Reduces intestinal motility.

PHARMACOKINETICS

	Onset	Peak	Duration
Antidiarrheal	45–60 min	—	3–4 hrs

Well absorbed from GI tract. Metabolized in liver. Primarily eliminated in feces. **Half-life:** 2.5 hrs; metabolite, 12–24 hrs.

USES

Adjunctive treatment of acute, chronic diarrhea.

PRECAUTIONS

Contraindications: Children younger than 2 yrs, dehydration, obstructive jaundice, narrow-angle glaucoma, severe hepatic disease, diarrhea associated with pseudomembranous colitis or enterotoxin-producing bacteria. **Cautions:** Cirrhosis, renal/hepatic disease, renal impairment, acute ulcerative colitis, dehydration.

⧗ LIFESPAN CONSIDERATIONS

Pregnancy/Lactation: Unknown if drug crosses placenta or is distributed in breast milk. **Pregnancy Category C. Children:** Not recommended (increased susceptibility to toxicity, including respiratory depression). **Elderly:** More susceptible to anticholinergic effects, confusion, respiratory depression.

INTERACTIONS

DRUG: Alcohol, other CNS depressants may increase CNS depressant effects. **Anticholinergics** may increase effects of atropine. **MAOIs** may precipitate hypertensive crisis. **HERBAL:** None significant. **FOOD:** None known. **LAB VALUES:** May increase serum amylase.

AVAILABILITY (Rx)

Liquid (Lomotil): 2.5 mg/5 ml. **Tablets (Lomotil):** 2.5 mg diphenoxylate/0.025 mg atropine.

ADMINISTRATION/HANDLING

PO
• Give without regard to meals. If GI irritation occurs, give with food. • Use liquid for children 2–12 yrs (use graduated dropper for administration of liquid medication).

INDICATIONS/ROUTES/DOSAGE

Diarrhea
PO: ADULTS, ELDERLY: Initially, 5 mg (2 tabs or 10 ml) 4 times/day. **Maximum:** 20 mg/day. Then reduce dose as needed. **CHILDREN:** 0.3–0.4 mg/kg/day in 4 divided doses (**maximum:** 10 mg/day); then reduce dose as needed.

SIDE EFFECTS

Frequent: Drowsiness, light-headedness, dizziness, nausea. **Occasional:** Headache, dry mouth. **Rare:** Flushing, tachycardia, urinary retention, constipation, paradoxical reaction (marked by restlessness, agitation), blurred vision.

ADVERSE EFFECTS/ TOXIC REACTIONS

Dehydration may predispose pt to diphenoxylate toxicity. Paralytic ileus, toxic megacolon (constipation, decreased appetite, abdominal pain with nausea/vomiting) occur rarely. Severe anticholinergic reaction (severe lethargy, hypotonic reflexes, hyperthermia) may result in severe respiratory depression, coma.

NURSING CONSIDERATIONS

BASELINE ASSESSMENT

Check baseline hydration status: skin turgor, mucous membranes for dryness, urinary status.

INTERVENTION/EVALUATION

Encourage adequate fluid intake. Assess bowel sounds for peristalsis. Monitor daily pattern of bowel activity, stool consistency. Record time of evacuation. Assess for abdominal disturbances. Discontinue medication if abdominal distention occurs.

PATIENT/FAMILY TEACHING

• Avoid tasks that require alertness, motor skills until response to drug is established. • Avoid alcohol. • Report persistent fever, palpitations, diarrhea. • Report abdominal distention.

---

dipyridamole [HIGH ALERT]

dye-peer-**id**-a-mole
(Apo-Dipyridamole FC ❦,
Persantine)
Do not confuse Aggrenox with Aggrastat, dipyridamole with disopyramide, or Persantine with Periactin.

FIXED-COMBINATION(S)

Aggrenox: dipyridamole/aspirin (antiplatelet): 200 mg/25 mg.

◆CLASSIFICATION

PHARMACOTHERAPEUTIC: Blood modifier, platelet aggregation inhibitor, coronary vasodilator. **CLINICAL:** Antiplatelet, antianginal, diagnostic agent (see p. 34C).

ACTION

Inhibits activity of adenosine deaminase and phosphodiesterase, enzymes causing accumulation of adenosine, cyclic adenosine monophosphate (AMP). **Therapeutic Effect:** Inhibits platelet aggregation; may cause coronary vasodilation.

PHARMACOKINETICS

Slowly, variably absorbed from the GI tract. Widely distributed. Protein binding: 91%–99%. Metabolized in liver. Primarily eliminated via biliary excretion. **Half-life:** 10–15 hrs.

USES

PO: Adjunct to warfarin (Coumadin) anticoagulant therapy in prevention of postop thromboembolic complications of cardiac valve replacement. **OFF-LABEL:** Stroke prevention (in combination with aspirin).

PRECAUTIONS

Contraindications: None known. **Cautions:** Hypotension, unstable angina, recent MI, hepatic impairment. Bronchospastic disease. Concomitant use of other antiplatelet medication or anticoagulation.

⧗ LIFESPAN CONSIDERATIONS

Pregnancy/Lactation: Distributed in breast milk. **Pregnancy Category B. Children:** Safety and efficacy not established. **Elderly:** No age-related precautions noted.

INTERACTIONS

DRUG: Anticoagulants, aspirin, heparin, salicylates, thrombolytics may increase risk of bleeding. **HERBAL:** Cat's claw, dong quai, evening primrose, garlic, ginseng may increase antiplatelet activity. **FOOD:** None known. **LAB VALUES:** May increase AST, ALT, bilirubin.

AVAILABILITY (Rx)

Tablets: 25 mg, 50 mg, 75 mg.

ADMINISTRATION/HANDLING

PO
• Best taken on empty stomach with full glass of water.

INDICATIONS/ROUTES/DOSAGE

Prevention of Thromboembolic Disorders
PO: ADULTS, ELDERLY: 75–100 mg 4 times a day in combination with other medica-

---

tions. **CHILDREN:** 3–6 mg/kg/day in 3 divided doses.

SIDE EFFECTS

Frequent (14%): Dizziness. **Occasional (6%–2%):** Abdominal distress, headache, rash. **Rare (less than 2%):** Diarrhea, vomiting, flushing, pruritus.

ADVERSE EFFECTS/ TOXIC REACTIONS

Overdose produces peripheral vasodilation, resulting in hypotension.

NURSING CONSIDERATIONS

BASELINE ASSESSMENT

Assess for presence of chest pain. Obtain baseline B/P, pulse. When used as antiplatelet, check hematologic status.

INTERVENTION/EVALUATION

Assist with ambulation if dizziness occurs. Assess B/P for hypotension. Monitor for change in heart rate. Assess skin for flushing, rash.

PATIENT/FAMILY TEACHING

• Avoid alcohol. • If nausea occurs, cola, unsalted crackers, dry toast may relieve effect. • Therapeutic response may not be achieved before 2–3 mos of continuous therapy. • Go from lying to standing slowly.

---

*DOBUTamine HIGH ALERT

doe-**bue**-ta-meen
(Dobutrex)
Do not confuse dobutamine with dopamine.

◆ CLASSIFICATION

PHARMACOTHERAPEUTIC: Sympathomimetic. **CLINICAL:** Cardiac stimulant.

ACTION

Direct-action inotropic agent acting primarily on beta$_1$-adrenergic receptors,

decreasing preload, afterload. **Therapeutic Effect:** Enhances myocardial contractility, stroke volume, cardiac output. Improves renal blood flow, urinary output.

PHARMACOKINETICS

Route	Onset	Peak	Duration
IV	1–2 min	10 min	Length of infusion

Metabolized in liver. Primarily excreted in urine. Not removed by hemodialysis. **Half-life:** 2 min.

USES

Short-term management of cardiac decompensation. **OFF-LABEL:** Positive inotropic agent in myocardial dysfunction or sepsis, stress echocardiography.

PRECAUTIONS

Contraindications: Idiopathic hypertrophic subaortic stenosis. **Cautions:** Atrial fibrillation, hypovolemia, post MI, concurrent use of MAOIs.

⧗ LIFESPAN CONSIDERATIONS

Pregnancy/Lactation: Unknown if drug crosses placenta or is distributed in breast milk. **Pregnancy Category B. Children/Elderly:** No age-related precautions noted.

INTERACTIONS

DRUG: Sympathomimetics may increase effects. **HERBAL:** None significant. **FOOD:** None known. **LAB VALUES:** May decrease serum potassium.

AVAILABILITY (Rx)

Infusion (Ready-to-Use): 1 mg/ml (250 ml), 2 mg/ml (250 ml), 4 mg/ml (250 ml). **Injection Solution:** 12.5-mg/ml vial.

ADMINISTRATION/HANDLING

◀ALERT▶ Correct hypovolemia with volume expanders before dobutamine infusion. Those with atrial fibrillation should be digitalized before infusion. Administer by IV infusion only.

IV

Reconstitution • Dilute vial in 0.9% NaCl or D$_5$W to maximum concentration of 5,000 mcg/ml (5 mg/ml).

Rate of Administration • Use infusion pump to control flow rate. • Titrate dosage to individual response. • Infiltration causes local inflammatory changes. • Extravasation may cause dermal necrosis.

Storage • Store at room temperature (freezing produces crystallization). • Pink discoloration of solution (due to oxidation) does not indicate loss of potency if used within recommended time period. • Further diluted solution for infusion is stable for 48 hrs at room temperature, 7 days if refrigerated.

IV INCOMPATIBILITIES

Acyclovir (Zovirax), alteplase (Activase), amphotericin B complex (Abelcet, AmBisome, Amphotec), bumetanide (Bumex), cefepime (Maxipime), foscarnet (Foscavir), furosemide (Lasix), heparin, piperacillin/tazobactam (Zosyn), sodium bicarbonate.

IV COMPATIBILITIES

Amiodarone (Cordarone), calcium chloride, calcium gluconate, diltiazem (Cardizem), dopamine (Intropin), enalapril (Vasotec), epinephrine, famotidine (Pepcid), hydromorphone (Dilaudid), insulin (regular), lidocaine, lorazepam (Ativan), magnesium sulfate, midazolam (Versed), milrinone (Primacor), morphine, nitroglycerin, nitroprusside (Nipride), norepinephrine (Levophed), potassium chloride, propofol (Diprivan).

INDICATIONS/ROUTES/DOSAGE

◄**ALERT**► Dosage determined by pt response to drug.

Management of Cardiac Decompensation
IV Infusion: ADULTS, ELDERLY, CHILDREN: 2.5–20 mcg/kg/min titrated to desired response. May be infused at a rate of up to 40 mcg/kg/min to increase cardiac output. **NEONATES:** 2–20 mcg/kg/min titrated to desired response.

SIDE EFFECTS

Frequent (greater than 5%): Increased heart rate, B/P. **Occasional (5%–3%):** Pain at injection site. **Rare (3%–1%):** Nausea, headache, anginal pain, shortness of breath, fever.

ADVERSE EFFECTS/TOXIC REACTIONS

Overdose may produce marked increase in heart rate (30 beats/min or higher), marked increase in B/P (50 mm Hg or higher), anginal pain, premature ventricular contractions (PVCs).

NURSING CONSIDERATIONS

BASELINE ASSESSMENT

Pt must be on continuous cardiac monitoring. Determine weight (for dosage calculation). Obtain initial B/P, heart rate, respirations. Correct hypovolemia before drug therapy.

INTERVENTION/EVALUATION

Continuously monitor for cardiac rate, arrhythmias. Maintain accurate I&O; measure urinary output frequently. Assess serum potassium, plasma dobutamine (therapeutic range: 40–190 ng/ml). Monitor B/P continuously (hypertension risk greater in pts with preexisting hypertension). Check cardiac output, pulmonary wedge pressure/central venous pressure (CVP) frequently. Immediately notify physician of decreased urinary output, cardiac arrhythmias, significant increase in B/P, heart rate, or less commonly, hypotension.

---

docetaxel

doe-se-**tax**-el
(Docefrez, <u>Taxotere</u>)

BLACK BOX ALERT Pts with hepatic impairment are at increased risk for grade 4 neutropenia, infections, severe thrombocytopenia, severe stomatitis, skin toxicity, death. Severe hypersensitivity reaction (rash, hy-

---

potension, bronchospasm, anaphylaxis) may occur. Fluid retention syndrome (pleural effusions, ascites, edema, dyspnea at rest) has been reported.

Do not confuse docetaxel with paclitaxel or Taxotere with Taxol.

◆ CLASSIFICATION

PHARMACOTHERAPEUTIC: Antimitotic agent, taxoid. **CLINICAL:** Antineoplastic (see p. 85C).

ACTION

Disrupts microtubular cell network, essential for cellular function. **Therapeutic Effect:** Inhibits cellular mitosis.

PHARMACOKINETICS

Widely distributed. Protein binding: 94%. Extensively metabolized in liver. Excreted in feces (75%), urine (6%). **Half-life:** 11.1 hrs.

USES

Treatment of locally advanced or metastatic breast carcinoma after failure of prior chemotherapy. Treatment of metastatic non–small-cell lung cancer. Treatment of metastatic prostate cancer, head and neck cancer (with prednisone). Treatment of advanced gastric adenocarcinoma. **OFF-LABEL:** Bladder, esophageal, ovarian, small-cell lung carcinoma, soft tissue carcinoma, cervical cancer, Ewing's sarcoma, osteosarcoma.

PRECAUTIONS

Contraindications: History of severe hypersensitivity to drugs formulated with polysorbate 80, neutrophil count less than 1,500 cells/mm³. **Cautions:** Hepatic impairment, myelosuppression, concomitant CYP3A4 inhibitors, fluid retention, pulmonary disease, HF, active infection.

⌛ LIFESPAN CONSIDERATIONS

Pregnancy/Lactation: May cause fetal harm. Unknown if distributed in breast milk. Breastfeeding not recommended. **Pregnancy Category D. Children:** Safety and efficacy not established in those younger than 16 yrs. **Elderly:** No age-related precautions noted.

INTERACTIONS

DRUG: CYP3A4 inhibitors (e.g., erythromycin, ketoconazole) may increase concentration/toxicity. **CYP3A4 inducers (e.g., rifampin)** may decrease concentration/effects. **Live virus vaccines** may potentiate replication, increase vaccine side effects, decrease pt's antibody response to vaccine. **HERBAL: Echinacea** may decrease concentration. **FOOD:** None known. **LAB VALUES:** May increase serum alkaline phosphatase, bilirubin, AST, ALT. Reduces neutrophil, platelet counts, Hgb, Hct.

AVAILABILITY (Rx)

Injection, Powder for Reconstitution: 20 mg, 80 mg. **Injection Solution:** 10 mg/ml, 20 mg/ml.

ADMINISTRATION/HANDLING

◀**ALERT**▶ Pt should be premedicated with oral corticosteroids (e.g., dexamethasone 16 mg/day for 5 days beginning day 1 before docetaxel therapy); reduces severity of fluid retention, hypersensitivity reaction.

 IV

Reconstitution (Solution) • Withdraw dose and add to 250–500 ml 0.9% NaCl or D₅W in glass or polyolefin container to provide a final concentration of 0.3–0.74 mg/ml. **(Powder)** Add 1 ml diluent provided to 20-mg vial to provide a concentration of 20 mg/0.8 ml (4 ml to 80-mg vial to provide a concentration of 24 mg/ml). Shake well. Further dilute in 250 ml NaCl or D₅W to a final concentration of 0.3–0.74 mg/ml. **Rate of Administration** • Administer as a 1-hr infusion. • Monitor closely for hypersensitivity reaction (flushing, localized skin reaction, bronchospasm [may occur within a few min after beginning infusion]).

Storage • Store vials between 36°F–77°F. • Protect from bright light. • If refrigerated, stand vial at room temperature for 5 min before administering (do not store in PVC bags). • Diluted solution should be used within 4 hrs.

🔲 IV INCOMPATIBILITIES

Amphotericin B (Fungizone), methylprednisolone (Solu-Medrol), nalbuphine (Nubain).

🔲 IV COMPATIBILITIES

Bumetanide (Bumex), calcium gluconate, dexamethasone (Decadron), diphenhydramine (Benadryl), dobutamine (Dobutrex), dopamine (Intropin), furosemide (Lasix), granisetron (Kytril), heparin, hydromorphone (Dilaudid), lorazepam (Ativan), magnesium sulfate, mannitol, morphine, ondansetron (Zofran), palonosetron (Aloxi), potassium chloride.

INDICATIONS/ROUTES/DOSAGE

◀ALERT▶ Not recommended with total bilirubin greater than upper limit of normal (ULN), or AST and/or ALT greater than 1.5 times ULN with alkaline phosphatase greater than 2.5 times ULN.

Breast Carcinoma
IV: **ADULTS:** 60–100 mg/m² given over 1 hr q3wks as a single agent. Operable, node positive: 75 mg/m² q3wks for 6 courses (in combination with doxorubicin and cyclophosphamide).

Non–Small-Cell Lung Carcinoma (NSCLC)
IV: **ADULTS:** 75 mg/m² q3wks (as monotherapy or in combination with cisplatin).

Prostate Cancer
IV: **ADULTS, ELDERLY:** 75 mg/m² q3wks with concurrent administration of prednisone.

Head/Neck Cancer
IV: **ADULTS, ELDERLY:** 75 mg/m² q3wks (in combination with cisplatin and fluorouracil) for 3–4 cycles, followed by radiation therapy.

Gastric Adenocarcinoma
IV: **ADULTS, ELDERLY:** 75 mg/m² q3wks (in combination with cisplatin and fluorouracil).

SIDE EFFECTS

Frequent: Alopecia (80%); asthenia (loss of strength, energy) (62%); hypersensitivity reaction (e.g., dermatitis) (59%), which decreases to 16% in those pretreated with oral corticosteroids; fluid retention (49%); stomatitis (43%); nausea, diarrhea (40%); fever (30%); nail changes (28%); vomiting (24%); myalgia (19%). **Occasional:** Hypotension, edema, anorexia, headache, weight gain, infection (urinary tract, injection site, indwelling catheter tip), dizziness. **Rare:** Dry skin, sensory disorders (vision, speech, taste), arthralgia, weight loss, conjunctivitis, hematuria, proteinuria.

ADVERSE EFFECTS/ TOXIC REACTIONS

In pts with normal hepatic function, neutropenia (neutrophil count less than 2,000 cells/mm³), leukopenia (WBC count less than 4,000 cells/mm³) occur in 96% of pts; anemia (hemoglobin level less than 11 g/dl) occurs in 90% of pts; thrombocytopenia (platelet count less than 100,000 cells/mm³) occurs in 8% of pts; infection occurs in 28% of pts. Neurosensory, neuromotor disturbances (distal paresthesia, weakness) occur in 54% and 13% of pts, respectively.

NURSING CONSIDERATIONS

BASELINE ASSESSMENT

Obtain baseline CBC, serum chemistries. Offer emotional support to pt, family. Antiemetics may be effective in preventing, treating nausea/vomiting. Pt should be pretreated with corticosteroids to reduce fluid retention, hypersensitivity reaction.

INTERVENTION/EVALUATION

Frequently monitor blood counts, particularly neutrophil count (less than 1,500 cells/mm^3 requires discontinuation of therapy). Monitor hepatic function tests, serum uric acid levels. Observe for cutaneous reactions (rash with eruptions, mainly on hands, feet). Assess for extravascular fluid accumulation: rales in lungs, dependent edema, dyspnea at rest, pronounced abdominal distention (due to ascites).

PATIENT/FAMILY TEACHING

• Hair loss is reversible, but new hair growth may have different color or texture. • New hair growth resumes 2–3 mos after last therapy dose. • Maintain strict oral hygiene. • Do not have immunizations without physician's approval (drug lowers resistance). • Avoid those who have recently taken any live virus vaccine. • Report persistent nausea, diarrhea, respiratory difficulty, chest pain, fever, chills, unusual bleeding, bruising.

---

docusate

dok-ue-sate
(Apo-Docusate ✤, Colace, Diocto, Docusoft-S, Novo-Docusate ✤, PMS-Docusate ✤, Regulex ✤, Selax ✤, Soflax ✤, Surfak)
Do not confuse Colace with Calan or Cozaar, or Surfak with Surbex.

FIXED COMBINATION(S)

Peri-Colace, Senokot-S: colace/senna (a laxative): 50 mg/8.6 mg.

◆CLASSIFICATION

PHARMACOTHERAPEUTIC: Bulk-producing laxative. **CLINICAL:** Stool softener (see p. 125C).

ACTION

Decreases surface film tension by mixing liquid with bowel contents. **Therapeutic Effect:** Increases infiltration of liquid to form softer stool.

PHARMACOKINETICS

Minimal absorption from GI tract. Acts in small and large intestines. Results usually occur 1–2 days after first dose but may take 3–5 days.

USES

Pts who need to avoid straining during defecation; constipation associated with hard, dry stools.

PRECAUTIONS

Contraindications: Acute abdominal pain, concomitant use of mineral oil, intestinal obstruction, nausea, vomiting. **Cautions:** Do not use for longer than 1 wk.

⌛ LIFESPAN CONSIDERATIONS

Pregnancy/Lactation: Unknown if drug is distributed in breast milk. **Pregnancy Category C. Children:** Not recommended in those younger than 6 yrs. **Elderly:** No age-related precautions noted.

INTERACTIONS

DRUG: None significant. **HERBAL:** None significant. **FOOD:** None known. **LAB VALUES:** None significant.

AVAILABILITY (OTC)

Capsules: 50 mg (Colace), 100 mg (Colace, Docusoft-S), 240 mg (Surfak). **Liquid (Colace, Diocto):** 50 mg/5 ml. **Syrup (Colace, Diocto):** 60 mg/15 ml.

ADMINISTRATION/HANDLING

• Drink 6–8 glasses of water a day (aids stool softening). • Give each dose with full glass of water, fruit juice. • Administer docusate liquid with milk, fruit juice, infant formula (masks bitter taste).

INDICATIONS/ROUTES/DOSAGE

Stool Softener
PO: ADULTS, ELDERLY, CHILDREN 12 YRS AND OLDER: 50–500 mg/day in 1–4 divided doses. **CHILDREN 6–11 YRS:** 40–150 mg/day in 1–4 divided doses. **CHILDREN 3–5 YRS:** 20–60 mg/day in 1–4 divided doses. **CHILDREN YOUNGER THAN 3 YRS:** 10–40 mg in 1–4 divided doses.

SIDE EFFECTS

Occasional: Mild GI cramping, throat irritation (with liquid preparation). **Rare:** Rash.

ADVERSE EFFECTS/ TOXIC REACTIONS

None known.

NURSING CONSIDERATIONS

INTERVENTION/EVALUATION

Encourage adequate fluid intake. Assess bowel sounds for peristalsis. Monitor daily pattern of bowel activity, stool consistency. Record time of evacuation.

PATIENT/FAMILY TEACHING

• Institute measures to promote defecation: increase fluid intake, exercise, high-fiber diet. • Do not use for longer than 1 wk.

dofetilide

doe-**fet**-i-lide
(Tikosyn)

BLACK BOX ALERT Pt must be placed in a setting with continuous EKG monitoring for minimum of 3 days and monitored by staff familiar with treatment of life-threatening arrhythmias.

◆ CLASSIFICATION

PHARMACOTHERAPEUTIC: Potassium channel blocker. **CLINICAL:** Antiarrhythmic: Class III (see p. 18C).

ACTION

Prolongs repolarization without affecting conduction velocity by blocking one or more time-dependent potassium currents. No effect on sodium channels, alpha-adrenergic, beta-adrenergic receptors. **Therapeutic Effect:** Terminates reentrant tachyarrhythmias, preventing reinduction.

PHARMACOKINETICS

Well absorbed following PO administration. 80% eliminated in urine as unchanged drug, 20% excreted as minimally active metabolites. Protein binding: 60%–70%. **Half-life:** 2–3 hrs.

USES

Maintenance of normal sinus rhythm (NSR) in pts with chronic atrial fibrillation/atrial flutter of longer than 1-wk duration who have been converted to NSR. Conversion of atrial fibrillation/flutter to NSR. **OFF-LABEL:** Treatment of atrial fibrillation in pts with hypertrophic cardiomyopathy.

PRECAUTIONS

Contraindications: Paroxysmal atrial fibrillation, congenital or acquired prolonged QT syndrome, severe renal impairment, concurrent use of drugs that may prolong QT interval, hypokalemia, hypomagnesemia, concurrent use with verapamil, itraconazole, ketoconazole, prochlorperazine, megestrol, cimetidine, hydrochlorothiazide, trimethoprim. Severe renal impairment. **Cautions:** Severe hepatic impairment, renal impairment, pts previously taking amiodarone.

⌛ LIFESPAN CONSIDERATIONS

Pregnancy/Lactation: Unknown if drug is distributed in breast milk. **Pregnancy Category C. Children:** No age-related precautions noted. **Elderly:** Age-related renal impairment may require dosage adjustment.

INTERACTIONS

DRUG: Cimetidine, verapamil, itracanazole, ketoconazole, trimethoprim, hydrochlorothiazide may increase concentration, toxicity. **HERBAL: St. John's wort** may decrease concentration. **Ephedra** may worsen arrhythmias. **FOOD:** None known. **LAB VALUES:** None significant.

AVAILABILITY (Rx)

Capsules: 125 mcg, 250 mcg, 500 mcg.

ADMINISTRATION/HANDLING

PO

• Give without regard to meals. • Do not open capsules.

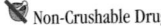

♣ Canadian trade name   🥄 Non-Crushable Drug   **HIGH ALERT** High Alert drug

INDICATIONS/ROUTES/DOSAGE

◄ALERT► EKG interval measurements, esp. QTc interval, must be determined prior to first dose.

Antiarrhythmias

PO: ADULTS, ELDERLY: Initially, 500 mcg twice daily. Modify dose in response to initial dose.

Dosage in Renal Impairment

Creatinine Clearance	Dosage
40–60 ml/min	250 mcg twice daily
20–39 ml/min	125 mcg twice daily

SIDE EFFECTS

Rare (less than 2%): Headache, chest pain, dizziness, dyspnea, nausea, insomnia, back/abdominal pain, diarrhea, rash.

ADVERSE EFFECTS/ TOXIC REACTIONS

Angioedema, bradycardia, cerebral ischemia, facial paralysis, serious arrhythmias (ventricular, various forms of block) have been noted.

NURSING CONSIDERATIONS

BASELINE ASSESSMENT

Prior to initiating treatment, QTc intervals must be determined. Do not use if heart rate less than 50 beats/min. Provide continuous EKG monitoring, calculation of creatinine clearance, equipment for resuscitation available for minimum of 3 days. Anticipate proarrhythmic events.

INTERVENTION/EVALUATION

Assess for conversion of cardiac dysrhythmias and absence of new arrhythmias. Constantly monitor EKG. Provide emotional support. Monitor renal function for electrolyte imbalance (prolonged or excessive diarrhea, sweating, vomiting, thirst).

PATIENT/FAMILY TEACHING

• Instruct pt on need for compliance and requirement for periodic monitoring of EKG and renal function.

dolasetron

doe-**las**-e-tron
(Anzemet)
Do not confuse Anzemet with Aldomet, Antivert, or Avandamet, or dolasetron with granisetron, ondansetron, or palonosetron.

◆CLASSIFICATION

PHARMACOTHERAPEUTIC: Selective 5-HT$_3$ receptor antagonist. **CLINICAL:** Antiemetic.

ACTION

Acts centrally in chemoreceptor trigger zone, peripherally at the vagal nerve terminals to antagonize 5-HT$_3$ receptors. **Therapeutic Effect:** Prevents nausea/vomiting.

PHARMACOKINETICS

Readily absorbed from GI tract after PO administration. Protein binding: 69%–77%. Metabolized in liver. Primarily excreted in urine. Unknown if removed by hemodialysis. **Half-life:** 5–10 hrs.

USES

PO: Prevention of nausea/vomiting associated with cancer chemotherapy, including high-dose cisplatin; prevention of postop nausea/vomiting. **Injection:** Treatment of postop nausea/vomiting. **OFF-LABEL:** Radiation therapy-induced nausea/vomiting.

PRECAUTIONS

Contraindications: Injection only: Prevention of chemotherapy-induced nausea and vomiting. **Cautions:** Pts who have or may have prolongation of cardiac conduction intervals, hypokalemia, hypomagnesemia, those taking diuretics with potential for inducing electrolyte disturbances, congenital prolonged QT interval syndrome, pts taking antiarrhythmics that may lead to QT prolongation, cumulative high-dose anthracycline therapy, allergy to other 5-HT₃ receptor antagonists.

⌛ LIFESPAN CONSIDERATIONS

Pregnancy/Lactation: Unknown if drug is distributed in breast milk. **Pregnancy Category B. Children:** Safety and efficacy not established in those younger than 2 yrs. **Elderly:** No age-related precautions noted.

INTERACTIONS

DRUG: Medications prolonging QT interval (e.g., clarithromycin, tricyclic antidepressants) may have additive effects. **HERBAL: St. John's wort** may decrease concentration. **FOOD:** None known. **LAB VALUES:** May transiently increase serum AST, ALT.

AVAILABILITY (Rx)

Injection, Solution: 20 mg/ml (0.625 ml, 5 ml, 25 ml).

🔖 Tablets: 50 mg, 100 mg.

ADMINISTRATION/HANDLING

 IV

Reconstitution • May dilute in 0.9% NaCl, D₅W, D₅W with 0.45% NaCl, D₅W with lactated Ringer's, lactated Ringer's, or 10% mannitol injection to 50 ml.
Rate of Administration • Can be given as IV push as rapidly as 100 mg/30 sec. • Intermittent IV infusion (piggyback) may be infused over 15 min.
Storage • Store vials at room temperature. • After dilution, solution is stable for 24 hrs at room temperature or 48 hrs if refrigerated.

PO

• May give with or without food. • Do not cut, break, open film-coated tablets.

Injection form may be mixed in juice for oral dosing. This dilution is stable for 2 hrs at room temperature.

🔲 IV COMPATIBILITIES

Azithromycin (Zithromax), dexmedetomidine (Precedex).

INDICATIONS/ROUTES/DOSAGE

Prevention of Chemotherapy-Induced Nausea/Vomiting
PO: ADULTS: 100 mg within 1 hr of chemotherapy. **CHILDREN 2–16 YRS:** 1.8 mg/kg within 1 hr of chemotherapy. **Maximum:** 100 mg.

Prevention of Postop Nausea/Vomiting
PO: ADULTS: 100 mg within 2 hrs of surgery. **CHILDREN 2–16 YRS:** 1.2 mg/kg within 2 hrs of surgery. **Maximum:** 100 mg.
IV: ADULTS: 12.5 mg 15 min before cessation of anesthesia or as soon as nausea occurs. **CHILDREN 2–16 YRS:** 0.35 mg/kg 15 min before cessation of anesthesia or as soon as nausea occurs. **Maximum:** 12.5 mg.

Treatment of Postop Nausea/Vomiting
IV: ADULTS, ELDERLY: 12.5 mg as soon as nausea or vomiting presents. **CHILDREN 2–16 YRS:** 0.35 mg/kg as soon as nausea or vomiting presents. **Maximum:** 12.5 mg.

SIDE EFFECTS

Frequent (10%–5%): Headache, diarrhea, fatigue. **Occasional (5%–1%):** Fever, dizziness, tachycardia, dyspepsia.

ADVERSE EFFECTS/ TOXIC REACTIONS

Overdose may produce a combination of CNS stimulant, depressant effects.

NURSING CONSIDERATIONS

BASELINE ASSESSMENT

Assess for dehydration if excessive vomiting occurs (poor skin turgor, dry mucous membranes, longitudinal furrows in tongue). Provide emotional support.

INTERVENTION/EVALUATION

Monitor electrolytes, EKG in high-risk pts. Observe for therapeutic relief from nausea/vomiting. Maintain quiet, supportive atmosphere.

dolutegravir

doe-loo-**teg**-ra-vir
(Tivicay)

◆**CLASSIFICATION**

PHARMACOTHERAPEUTIC: Integrase stand transfer inhibitor (INSTI). **CLINICAL:** Antiretroviral agent (see p. 121C).

ACTION

Inhibits HIV integrase by blocking strand transfer of retroviral DNA integration (essential for HIV replication cycle). **Therapeutic Effect:** Interferes with HIV replication, slowing progression of HIV infection.

PHARMACOKINETICS

Readily absorbed after PO administration. Peak plasma concentration: 2–3 hrs. Protein binding: 99%. Metabolized in liver. Excreted primarily unchanged in feces and as metabolite in urine. **Half-life:** 14 hrs.

USES

Treatment of HIV-1 infection in adults and children age 12 yrs and older and weighing at least 40 kg, in combination with at least two other antiretroviral agents.

PRECAUTIONS

Contraindications: Co-administration of dofetilide. **Cautions:** Diabetes mellitus, hepatic/renal impairment, history of hepatitis or tuberculosis, prior hypersensitivity reaction to INSTIs.

⧖ LIFESPAN CONSIDERATIONS

Pregnancy/Lactation: Breastfeeding not recommend due to risk of postnatal HIV transmission. Unknown if distributed in human breast milk. **Pregnancy Category B. Children:** Safety and efficacy not established in pts less than 12 yrs or weighing under 40 kg or who are INSTI-experienced with documented or clinically suspected resistance to other INSTIs. **Elderly:** May have increased risk of adverse effects or worsening hepatic, renal, cardiac function.

INTERACTIONS

DRUG: Medications containing aluminum, calcium, magnesium or iron; metabolic inducers (e.g., carbamazepine, phenytoin, phenobarbital, rifampin); nonnucleoside reverse transcriptase inhibitors (e.g., efavirenz, etravirine, nevirapine); protease inhibitors (e.g., fosamprenavir/ritonavir, tipranavir/ritonavir) may decrease concentration/effect. May increase concentration/effect of **metformin. HERBAL: St John's wort** may decrease effectiveness. **FOOD:** None known. **LAB VALUES:** May increase ALT, AST, serum bilirubin, cholesterol, creatinine, creatine kinase (CK), glucose, lipase, triglycerides. May decrease creatinine clearance, neutrophils.

AVAILABILITY (Rx)

Tablets: 50 mg.

ADMINISTRATION/HANDLING

PO

• Give without regard to meal. Administer at least 2 hrs before or at least 6 hrs after giving medications containing aluminum, calcium, iron, magnesium (supplements, antacids, laxatives).

INDICATIONS/ROUTES/DOSAGE

HIV Infection

PO: ADULTS/ELDERLY: Treatment naïve or treatment-experienced, INSTI naïve: 50 mg once daily. Increase to 50 mg twice daily if also receiving efavirenz, fosamprenavir/ritonavir, tipranavir/ritonavir, rifampin or INSTI-experienced with certain INSTI-associated resistance substitutions or clinically suspected INSTI resistance.

PO: CHILDREN: Treatment naïve: 50 mg once daily. Increase to 50 mg twice daily if also receiving **fosamprenavir/ritonavir, tipranavir/ritonavir, rifampin.**

SIDE EFFECTS

Rare (3%-1%): Insomnia, headache, nausea.

ADVERSE EFFECTS/ TOXIC REACTIONS

Hypersensitivity reaction including rash, fever, angioedema, difficulty breathing, skin blistering/peeling, arthralgia, lethargy reported. Pts co-infected with hepatitis B or C have increased risk for viral reactivation, worsening of hepatic function, and may experience hepatic decompensation and/or failure if therapy is discontinued. May cause redistribution/accumulation of body fat (lipodystrophy). May induce immune recovery syndrome (inflammatory response to dormant opportunistic infections such as *Mycobacterium avium,* cytomegalovirus, PCP, tuberculosis, or acceleration of autoimmune disorders such as Graves' disease, polymyositis, Guillain-Barré).

NURSING CONSIDERATIONS

BASELINE ASSESSMENT

Obtain CBC, CMP, CD4+ count, viral load, lipid panel, lipase. Screen all pts for hepatitis B or C co-infection. Receive full medication history including vitamins, minerals, herbal products. Question possibility of pregnancy.

INTERVENTION/EVALUATION

Monitor labs accordingly. Assess for hepatic impairment (bruising, hematuria, jaundice, right upper abdominal pain, nausea, vomiting, weight loss). Screen for immune recovery syndrome, hypersensitivity reaction.

PATIENT/FAMILY TEACHING

• Offer emotional support. • Blood levels will be monitored routinely. • Report any signs of abdominal pain, darkened urine, decreased urine output, yellowing of skin or eyes, clay-colored stools, weight loss. • Do not breastfeed. • Report any newly prescribed medications. • Dolutegravir does not cure HIV infection nor reduce risk of transmission. Practice safe sex with barrier methods or abstinence. • As immune system strengthens, it may respond to dormant infections hidden within the body. Report any new fever, chills, body aches, cough, night sweats, shortness of breath. • Antiretrovirals may cause excess body fat in upper back, neck, breast, trunk; and may cause decreased body fat in legs, arms, face. Drug resistance can form if therapy is interrupted for even a short time; do not run out of supply.

donepezil
TOP 200

doe-**nep**-e-zil
(Aricept, Aricept ODT)
Do not confuse Aricept with Aciphex, Ascriptin, or Azilect.

◆CLASSIFICATION

PHARMACOTHERAPEUTIC: Cholinesterase inhibitor. **CLINICAL:** Cholinergic.

ACTION

Inhibits enzyme acetylcholinesterase, increasing concentration of acetylcholine at cholinergic synapses, enhancing cholinergic function in CNS. **Therapeutic Effect:** Slows progression of Alzheimer's disease.

PHARMACOKINETICS

Well absorbed after PO administration. Protein binding: 96%. Extensively metabolized. Eliminated in urine, feces. **Half-life:** 70 hrs.

USES

Treatment of dementia of Alzheimer's disease. **OFF-LABEL:** Treatment of behavioral syndromes in dementia, dementia associated with Parkinson's disease, Lewy body dementia.

PRECAUTIONS

Contraindications: History of hypersensitivity to piperidine derivatives. **Cautions:** Asthma, COPD, bradycardia, bladder outflow obstruction, history of ulcer disease, those taking concurrent NSAIDs, supraventricular cardiac conduction disturbances (e.g., "sick sinus syndrome," Wolff-Parkinson-White syndrome), seizures.

⌛ LIFESPAN CONSIDERATIONS

Pregnancy/Lactation: Unknown if drug is distributed in breast milk. **Pregnancy Category C. Children:** Safety and efficacy not established. **Elderly:** No age-related precautions noted.

INTERACTIONS

DRUG: May decrease effect of **anticholinergic medications.** May increase synergistic effects of **cholinergic agonists, neuromuscular blockers, succinylcholine. Ketoconazole** may inhibit metabolism of donepezil. **CYP3A4 inducers (e.g., carbamazepine, rifampin)** may decrease concentration/effects. **HERBAL: St. John's wort** may decrease concentration. **Ginkgo** may increase adverse effects. **FOOD:** None known. **LAB VALUES:** None significant.

AVAILABILITY (Rx)

Tablets (Aricept): 5 mg, 10 mg, 23 mg. **Tablets (Orally Disintegrating [Aricept ODT]):** 5 mg, 10 mg.

ADMINISTRATION/HANDLING

PO
• May be given at bedtime without regard to meals. • Swallow whole; do not split or crush. • **ODT:** Allow to dissolve completely on tongue. • Follow dose with water.

INDICATIONS/ROUTES/DOSAGE

Alzheimer's Disease
PO: ADULTS, ELDERLY: Initially 5 mg/day at bedtime. May increase at 4- to 6-wk inter-

vals to 10 mg/day at bedtime. For moderate to severe Alzheimer's, a dose of 23 mg once daily can be administered once pt has been taking 10 mg once daily for at least 3 mos.

SIDE EFFECTS

Frequent (11%–8%): Nausea, diarrhea, headache, insomnia, nonspecific pain, dizziness. **Occasional (6%–3%):** Mild muscle cramps, fatigue, vomiting, anorexia, ecchymosis. **Rare (3%–2%):** Depression, abnormal dreams, weight loss, arthritis, drowsiness, syncope, frequent urination.

ADVERSE EFFECTS/ TOXIC REACTIONS

Overdose may result in cholinergic crisis (severe nausea, increased salivation, diaphoresis, bradycardia, hypotension, flushed skin, abdominal pain, respiratory depression, seizures, cardiorespiratory collapse). Increasing muscle weakness may occur, resulting in death if muscles of respiration become involved. **Antidote:** Atropine sulfate 1–2 mg IV with subsequent doses based on therapeutic response.

NURSING CONSIDERATIONS

BASELINE ASSESSMENT

Assess cognitive function (e.g., memory, attention, reasoning). Obtain baseline vital signs. Assess history for peptic ulcer, urinary obstruction, asthma, COPD, seizure disorder, cardiac conduction disturbances.

INTERVENTION/EVALUATION

Monitor behavior, mood/cognitive function, activities of daily living. Monitor for cholinergic reaction (GI discomfort/cramping, feeling of facial warmth, excessive salivation/diaphoresis), lacrimation, pallor, urinary urgency, dizziness. Monitor for nausea, diarrhea, headache, insomnia.

PATIENT/FAMILY TEACHING

• Report nausea, vomiting, diarrhea, diaphoresis, increased salivary secretions, severe abdominal pain, dizziness. • May take without regard to food (best taken at bedtime). • Not a cure for Alzheimer's disease but may slow progression of symptoms.

*DOPamine

dope-a-meen

BLACK BOX ALERT If extravasation occurs, infiltrate area with phentolamine (5–10 ml 0.9% NaCl) as soon as possible, no later than 12 hrs after extravasation.

Do not confuse dopamine with dobutamine or Dopram.

◆CLASSIFICATION

PHARMACOTHERAPEUTIC: Sympathomimetic (adrenergic agonist). **CLINICAL:** Cardiac stimulant, vasopressor.

ACTION

Stimulates adrenergic receptors. Effects are dose dependent. Lower dosage stimulates dopaminergic receptors, causing renal vasodilation. Higher doses stimulate both dopaminergic and beta$_1$-adrenergic receptors, causing cardiac stimulation and renal vasodilation. **Therapeutic Effect: Low dosage (1–3 mcg/kg/min):** Increases renal blood flow, urinary flow, sodium excretion. **Low to moderate dosage (4–10 mcg/kg/min):** Increases myocardial contractility, stroke volume, cardiac output. **High dosage (greater than 10 mcg/kg/min):** Increases peripheral resistance, vasoconstriction, B/P.

PHARMACOKINETICS

Route	Onset	Peak	Duration
IV	1–2 min	N/A	Less than 10 min

Widely distributed. Does not cross blood-brain barrier. Metabolized in liver, kidneys, plasma. Primarily excreted in urine. Not removed by hemodialysis. Half-life: 2 min.

USES

Adjunct in treatment of hypotension, shock (associated with MI, trauma, renal failure, cardiac decompensation, open heart surgery, persisting after adequate fluid volume replacement). **OFF-LABEL:** Symptomatic bradycardia or heart block unresponsive to atropine or cardiac pacing.

PRECAUTIONS

Contraindications: Pheochromocytoma, ventricular fibrillation. **Cautions:** Ischemic heart disease, occlusive vascular disease, hypovolemia, recent use of MAOIs (within 2–3 weeks), ventricular arrhythmias, post-MI pts.

⧗ LIFESPAN CONSIDERATIONS

Pregnancy/Lactation: Unknown if drug crosses placenta or is distributed in breast milk. **Pregnancy Category C. Children:** Recommended close hemodynamic monitoring (gangrene due to extravasation reported). **Elderly:** No age-related precautions noted.

INTERACTIONS

DRUG: May have increased effects with **vasopressors, vasoconstrictive agents. COMT inhibitors** may increase levels/effects. **HERBAL:** None significant. **FOOD:** None known. **LAB VALUES:** None significant.

AVAILABILITY (Rx)

Injection Solution: 40 mg/ml, 80 mg/ml, 160 mg/ml. **Injection (Premix with Dextrose):** 0.8 mg/ml (250 ml, 500 ml), 1.6 mg/ml (250 ml, 500 ml), 3.2 mg/ml (250 ml).

ADMINISTRATION/HANDLING

◄**ALERT**► Blood volume depletion must be corrected before administering dopamine (may be used concurrently with fluid replacement).

 IV

Reconstitution • Available prediluted in 250 or 500 ml D$_5$W or dilute in 250–500 ml 0.9% NaCl, D$_5$W, or lactated Ringer's to

 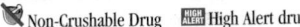

D

maximum concentration of 3,200 mcg/ml (3.2 mg/ml).

Rate of Administration • Administer into large vein (antecubital fossa, central line preferred) to prevent extravasation. • Use infusion pump to control flow rate. • Titrate drug to desired hemodynamic, renal response (optimum urinary flow determines dosage).

Storage • Do not use solutions darker than slightly yellow or discolored to yellow, brown, pink to purple (indicates decomposition of drug). • Stable for 24 hrs after dilution.

🔳 IV INCOMPATIBILITIES

Acyclovir (Zovirax), amphotericin B complex (Abelcet, AmBisome, Amphotec), cefepime (Maxipime), furosemide (Lasix), insulin, sodium bicarbonate.

🔳 IV COMPATIBILITIES

Amiodarone (Cordarone), calcium chloride, dexmedetomidine (Precedex), diltiazem (Cardizem), dobutamine (Dobutrex), enalapril (Vasotec), epinephrine, heparin, hydromorphone (Dilaudid), labetalol (Trandate), levofloxacin (Levaquin), lidocaine, lorazepam (Ativan), methylprednisolone (Solu-Medrol), midazolam (Versed), milrinone (Primacor), morphine, nicardipine (Cardene), nitroglycerin, norepinephrine (Levophed), piperacillin/tazobactam (Zosyn), potassium chloride, propofol (Diprivan).

INDICATIONS/ROUTES/DOSAGE

◄**ALERT►** Effects of dopamine are dose dependent. Titrate to desired response.

Acute Hypotension, Shock

IV Infusion: ADULTS, ELDERLY: Initially, 1–5 mcg/kg/min up to 20 mcg/kg/min. **Maximum:** 50 mcg/kg/min. Titrate to desired response. **CHILDREN:** Initially, 1–5 mcg/kg/min. Increase in 5–10 mcg/kg/min increments. Titrate to desired response. **Maximum:** 50 mcg/kg/min. **NEONATES:** 1–20 mcg/kg/min. Titrate to desired response.

SIDE EFFECTS

Frequent: Headache, arrhythmias, tachycardia, anginal pain, palpitations, vasoconstriction, hypotension, nausea, vomiting, dyspnea. **Occasional:** Piloerection (goose bumps), bradycardia, widening of QRS complex.

ADVERSE EFFECTS/ TOXIC REACTIONS

High doses may produce ventricular arrhythmias. Pts with occlusive vascular disease are at high risk for further compromise of circulation to extremities, which may result in gangrene. Tissue necrosis with sloughing may occur with extravasation of IV solution.

NURSING CONSIDERATIONS

BASELINE ASSESSMENT

Pt must be on continuous cardiac monitoring. Determine weight (for dosage calculation). Obtain initial B/P, heart rate, respirations. Assess potency of IV access.

INTERVENTION/EVALUATION

Continuously monitor for cardiac arrhythmias. Measure urinary output frequently. If extravasation occurs, immediately infiltrate affected tissue with 10–15 ml 0.9% NaCl solution containing 5–10 mg phentolamine mesylate. Monitor B/P, heart rate, respirations q15min during administration (more often if indicated). Assess cardiac output, pulmonary wedge pressure, or central venous pressure (CVP) frequently. Assess peripheral circulation (palpate pulses, note color/temperature of extremities). Immediately notify physician of decreased urinary output, cardiac arrhythmias, significant changes in B/P, heart rate, or failure to respond to increase or decrease in infusion rate, decreased peripheral circulation (cold, pale, mottled extremities). Taper dosage before discontinuing (abrupt cessation of therapy may result in marked hypotension). Be alert to excessive vasoconstriction (decreased urine output, increased heart rate, arrhythmias, disproportionate increase in diastolic B/P, decrease in pulse pressure); slow or temporarily stop infusion, notify physician.

doripenem

dor-i-**pen**-em
(Doribax)
Do not confuse Doribax with Zovirax, or doripenem with ertapenem, imipenem, or meropenem.

◆CLASSIFICATION

PHARMACOTHERAPEUTIC: Carbapenem. **CLINICAL:** Antibiotic.

ACTION

Inactivates penicillin-binding proteins, resulting in inhibition of cell wall synthesis. **Therapeutic Effect:** Produces bacterial cell death.

PHARMACOKINETICS

Penetrates into body fluids, tissues. Widely distributed. Protein binding: 8%. Primarily excreted in urine. Removed by dialysis. **Half-life:** 1 hr.

USES

Treatment of complicated intra-abdominal infections, complicated UTIs due to susceptible gram-positive, gram-negative (including *Pseudomonas aeruginosa*), and anaerobic bacteria. **OFF-LABEL:** Treatment of intravascular catheter-related bloodstream infection due to ESBL producing *Escherichia coli* and *Klebsiella* spp.

PRECAUTIONS

Contraindications: History of serious hypersensitivity to carbapenems (meropenem, imipenem-cilastin, ertapenem). Anaphylactic reactions to beta-lactam antibiotics. **Cautions:** Hypersensitivity to penicillins, cephalosporins.

LIFESPAN CONSIDERATIONS

Pregnancy/Lactation: Distributed in breast milk. **Pregnancy Category B. Children:** Safety and efficacy not established in those younger than 18 yrs. **Elderly:** Advanced renal insufficiency, end-stage renal insufficiency may require dosage adjustment.

INTERACTIONS

DRUG: Probenecid reduces renal excretion of doripenem. May decrease **valproic acid** concentrations (do not use concurrently). **HERBAL:** None significant. **FOOD:** None known. **LAB VALUES:** May increase serum alkaline phosphatase, AST, ALT. May decrease Hgb, Hct, platelet count, serum potassium.

AVAILABILITY (Rx)

Injection, Powder for Reconstitution: 250 mg, 500 mg.

ADMINISTRATION/HANDLING

IV

Reconstitution • Reconstitute 250-mg or 500-mg vial with 10 ml Sterile Water for Injection or 0.9% NaCl. • Shake well to dissolve. • Further dilute with 100 ml 0.9% NaCl or D₅W.
Rate of Administration • Give by intermittent IV infusion (piggyback). • Do not give IV push. • Infuse over 60 min.
Storage • Stable for 12 hrs at room temperature, 72 hrs if refrigerated when diluted in 0.9% NaCl; 4 hrs at room temperature, 24 hrs if refrigerated when diluted in D₅W.

IV INCOMPATIBILITIES

Diazepam (Valium), potassium phosphate, propofol (Diprivan).

IV COMPATIBILITIES

Amiodarone, bumetanide (Bumex), calcium gluconate, dexamethasone, diltiazem (Cardizem), diphenhydramine (Benadryl), furosemide (Lasix), heparin, hydrocortisone (Solu-Cortef), hydro-

 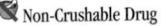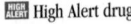

morphone (Dilaudid), insulin, labetalol (Trandate), lorazepam (Ativan), magnesium sulfate, methylprednisolone (Solu-Medrol), metoclopramide (Reglan), milrinone, morphine, ondansetron (Zofran), pantoprazole (Protonix), potassium chloride.

INDICATIONS/ROUTES/DOSAGE

Intra-Abdominal Infections
IV: **ADULTS, ELDERLY:** 500 mg q8h for 5–14 days.

Urinary Tract Infections
IV: **ADULTS, ELDERLY:** 500 mg q8h for 10–14 days.

Dosage in Renal Impairment

Creatinine Clearance	Dosage
30–50 ml/min	250 mg q8h
11–29 ml/min	250 mg q12h
Hemodialysis	250 mg q24h, if treating infection caused by *Pseudomonas aeruginosa:* 500 mg q12h on day 1, then 500 g q24h
Continuous renal replacement therapy	250 mg q12h

SIDE EFFECTS

Frequent (10%–6%): Diarrhea, nausea, headache. **Occasional (5%–2%):** Altered mental status, insomnia, rash, abdominal pain, constipation, vomiting, edema, fever. **Rare (less than 2%):** Dizziness, cough, oral candidiasis, anxiety, tachycardia, phlebitis at IV site.

ADVERSE EFFECTS/ TOXIC REACTIONS

Antibiotic-associated colitis, other super-infections (abdominal cramps, severe watery diarrhea, fever) may occur. Anaphylactic reactions in those receiving beta-lactams have occurred. Seizures may occur in those with CNS disorders (brain lesions, history of seizures) or with bacterial meningitis or severe impaired renal function.

NURSING CONSIDERATIONS

BASELINE ASSESSMENT

Question pt for history of allergies, particularly to beta-lactams, penicillins, cephalosporins. Inquire about history of seizures.

INTERVENTION/EVALUATION

Monitor for signs of hypersensitivity reaction during first dose. Monitor daily pattern of bowel activity, stool consistency. Monitor for nausea, vomiting. Evaluate hydration status. Evaluate for inflammation at IV injection site. Assess skin for rash. Check mental status; be alert to tremors, possible seizures. Assess sleep pattern for evidence of insomnia.

PATIENT/FAMILY TEACHING

• Report tremors, seizures, rash, diarrhea, or other new symptoms.

doxazosin

dox-a-**zoe**-sin
(Apo-Doxazosin ✲, Cardura, Cardura XL, Novo-Doxazosin ✲)
Do not confuse Cardura with Cardene, Cordarone, Coumadin, K-Dur, or Ridaura, or doxazosin with doxapram, doxepin, or doxorubicin.

◆CLASSIFICATION

PHARMACOTHERAPEUTIC: Alpha-adrenergic blocker. **CLINICAL:** Antihypertensive (see p. 61C).

ACTION

Selectively blocks alpha$_1$-adrenergic receptors, decreasing peripheral vascular resistance. **Therapeutic Effect:** Causes peripheral vasodilation, lowering B/P. Relaxes smooth muscle of bladder, prostate.

PHARMACOKINETICS

Route	Onset	Peak	Duration
PO (antihypertensive)	1–2 hrs	2–6 hrs	24 hrs

Well absorbed from GI tract. Protein binding: 98%–99%. Metabolized in liver. Primarily eliminated in feces. Not removed by hemodialysis. **Half-life:** 19–22 hrs.

USES

Cardura: Treatment of mild to moderate hypertension. Used alone or in combination with other antihypertensives. Treatment of benign prostatic hyperplasia. **Cardura XL:** Treatment of benign prostatic hyperplasia. **OFF-LABEL:** Pediatric hypertension.

PRECAUTIONS

Contraindications: Hypersensitivity to other quinazolines (prazosin, terazosin). **Cautions:** Constipation, ileus, GI obstruction, hepatic impairment.

⌛ LIFESPAN CONSIDERATIONS

Pregnancy/Lactation: Unknown if drug crosses placenta or is distributed in breast milk. **Pregnancy Category C. Children:** Safety and efficacy not established. **Elderly:** May be more sensitive to hypotensive effects.

INTERACTIONS

DRUG: NSAIDs may decrease effect. **Hypotension-producing medications** (e.g., **antihypertensives, diuretics**) may increase effect. **CYP3A4 inhibitors** (e.g., **atanazavir, ketoconazole**) may increase hypotensive effect. **HERBAL: Ephedra, ginseng, yohimbe** may worsen hypertension. **Garlic** may increase antihypertensive effect. Avoid **saw palmetto** (limited experience with this combination). **FOOD:** None known. **LAB VALUES:** None significant.

AVAILABILITY (Rx)

Tablets: 1 mg, 2 mg, 4 mg, 8 mg.
🦃 Tablets, Extended-Release: 4 mg, 8 mg.

ADMINISTRATION/HANDLING

PO
• Give without regard to food. • Do not crush, cut, divide extended-release tablet. • Immediate-release tablets given morning or evening; extended-release tablets given with morning meal.

INDICATIONS/ROUTES/DOSAGE

Hypertension
PO (Immediate-Release): ADULTS: Initially, 1 mg once a day. May increase upward over several weeks to a maximum of 16 mg/day. **ELDERLY:** Initially, 0.5 mg once a day. May increase upward over several weeks.

Benign Prostatic Hyperplasia
PO (Immediate-Release): ADULTS, ELDERLY: Initially, 1 mg/day. May increase q1–2wks. **Maximum:** 8 mg/day. **(Extended-Release):** Initially, 4 mg/day. May increase to 8 mg in 3–4 wks. Note: When switching to extended-release, omit evening dose prior to starting morning dose.

SIDE EFFECTS

Frequent (20%–10%): Dizziness, asthenia (loss of strength, energy), headache, edema. **Occasional (9%–3%):** Nausea, pharyngitis, rhinitis, pain in extremities, drowsiness. **Rare (2%–1%):** Palpitations, diarrhea, constipation, dyspnea, myalgia, altered vision, anxiety.

ADVERSE EFFECTS/ TOXIC REACTIONS

First-dose syncope (hypotension with sudden loss of consciousness) may occur 30–90 min following initial dose of 2 mg or greater, too-rapid increase in dosage, addition of another antihypertensive agent to therapy. First-dose syncope may be preceded by tachycardia (pulse rate 120–160 beats/min).

NURSING CONSIDERATIONS

BASELINE ASSESSMENT
Give first dose at bedtime. If initial dose is given during daytime, pt must remain

D

recumbent for 3–4 hrs. Assess B/P, pulse immediately before each dose, and q15–30min until B/P is stabilized (be alert to fluctuations).

INTERVENTION/EVALUATION

Monitor B/P, I/O. Monitor pulse diligently (first-dose syncope may be preceded by tachycardia). Assess for edema, headache. Assist with ambulation if dizziness, light-headedness occurs.

PATIENT/FAMILY TEACHING

• Full therapeutic effect may not occur for 3–4 wks. • May cause syncope (fainting); rise slowly from sitting/lying position. • Avoid tasks that require alertness, motor skills until response to drug is established.

---

doxepin

dox-eh-pin
(Apo-Doxepin ✦, Novo-Doxepin ✦, Prudoxin, Silenor, Sinequan ✦, Zonalon)

BLACK BOX ALERT Increased risk of suicidal ideation and behavior in children, adolescents, young adults 18–24 yrs with major depressive disorder, other psychiatric disorders.

Do not confuse doxepin with digoxin, doxapram, doxazosin, Doxidan, or doxycycline, or Sinequan with Seroquel, or Singulair.

◆CLASSIFICATION

PHARMACOTHERAPEUTIC: Tricyclic. **CLINICAL:** Antidepressant, antianxiety, antineuralgic, antiulcer, antipruritic.

ACTION

Increases synaptic concentrations of norepinephrine, serotonin. **Therapeutic Effect:** Produces antidepressant, anxiolytic effects.

PHARMACOKINETICS

PO: Rapidly absorbed from GI tract. Protein binding: 80%–85%. Metabolized in liver. Primarily excreted in urine. Not removed by hemodialysis. **Half-life:** 6–8 hrs. **Topical:** Absorbed through skin. Distributed to body tissues. Metabolized to active metabolite. Excreted in urine.

USES

Treatment of depression, often in conjunction with psychotherapy. **Silenor:** Treatment of insomnia in pts with difficulty staying asleep. **Topical:** Treatment of pruritus associated with atopic dermatitis. **OFF-LABEL:** Treatment of neurogenic pain, treatment of anxiety.

PRECAUTIONS

Contraindications: Narrow-angle glaucoma, hypersensitivity to other tricyclic antidepressants, urinary retention, use of MAOIs within 14 days. **Cautions:** Cardiac/hepatic/renal disease, pts at risk for suicidal ideation, respiratory compromise, sleep apnea, history of bowel obstruction, increased IOP, glaucoma, history of seizures, history of urinary retention/obstruction, hyperthyroidism, prostatic hypertrophy, hiatal hernia.

⌛ LIFESPAN CONSIDERATIONS

Pregnancy/Lactation: Crosses placenta. Distributed in breast milk. **Pregnancy Category C (B for topical form). Children:** Safety and efficacy not established in those younger than 12 yrs. **Elderly:** Increased risk of toxicity (lower dosages recommended).

INTERACTIONS

DRUG: Alcohol, other CNS depressants may increase CNS, respiratory depression, hypotensive effects. **Cimetidine** may increase concentration, risk of toxicity. **MAOIs** may increase risk of seizures, hyperpyrexia, hypertensive crisis (discontinue at least 2 wks prior to starting doxepin). **Phenothiazines** may increase anticholinergic, sedative effects.

HERBAL: Kava kava, SAMe, St. John's wort, valerian may increase sedation, risk of serotonin syndrome. **St. John's wort** may decrease concentration/effects. **FOOD:** None known. **LAB VALUES:** May alter serum glucose, EKG readings. **Therapeutic serum level:** 110–250 ng/ml; **toxic serum level:** greater than 300 ng/ml.

AVAILABILITY (Rx)

Capsules: 10 mg, 25 mg, 50 mg, 75 mg, 100 mg, 150 mg. **Cream (Prudoxin, Zonalon):** 5%. **Oral Concentrate:** 10 mg/ml. **Tablets (Silenor):** 3 mg, 6 mg.

ADMINISTRATION/HANDLING

PO
• Give with food, milk if GI distress occurs. • Dilute concentrate in 4-oz glass of water, milk, orange, tomato, prune, pineapple juice. Incompatible with carbonated drinks. • Give larger portion of daily dose at bedtime. • **Silenor:** Give within 30 min of bedtime but not within 3 hrs of a meal.

Topical
• Apply thin film of cream on affected areas of skin. • Do not use for more than 8 days. • Do not use occlusive dressing.

INDICATIONS/ROUTES/DOSAGE

Depression, Anxiety
PO: ADULTS: 25–150 mg/day at bedtime or in 2–3 divided doses. May increase gradually to 300 mg/day (single dose should not exceed 150 mg). **ELDERLY:** Initially, 10–25 mg at bedtime. May increase by 10–25 mg/day every 3–7 days. **Maximum:** 75 mg/day. **ADOLESCENTS:** Initially, 25–50 mg/day as a single dose or in divided doses. May increase to 100 mg/day. **CHILDREN 12 YRS AND YOUNGER:** 1–3 mg/kg/day.

Insomnia
PO: ADULTS: 3–6 mg. **ELDERLY:** 3 mg (give within 30 min of bedtime). May increase to 6 mg once daily.

Pruritus Associated with Atopic Dermatitis
Topical: ADULTS, ELDERLY: Apply thin film 4 times a day at 3- to 4-hr intervals. Not recommended for more than 8 days.

SIDE EFFECTS

Frequent: PO: Orthostatic hypotension, drowsiness, dry mouth, headache, increased appetite, weight gain, nausea, unusual fatigue, unpleasant taste. **Topical:** Edema, increased pruritus, eczema, burning, tingling, stinging at application site, altered taste, dizziness, drowsiness, dry skin, dry mouth, fatigue, headache, thirst. **Occasional: PO:** Blurred vision, confusion, constipation, hallucinations, difficult urination, eye pain, irregular heartbeat, fine muscle tremors, nervousness, impaired sexual function, diarrhea, diaphoresis, heartburn, insomnia. **Silenor:** Nausea, upper respiratory infection. **Topical:** Anxiety, skin irritation/cracking, nausea. **Rare: PO:** Allergic reaction, alopecia, tinnitus, breast enlargement. **Topical:** Fever, photosensitivity.

ADVERSE EFFECTS/ TOXIC REACTIONS

Abrupt or too-rapid withdrawal may result in headache, malaise, nausea, vomiting, vivid dreams. Overdose may produce confusion, severe drowsiness, agitation, tachycardia, arrhythmias, shortness of breath, vomiting.

NURSING CONSIDERATIONS

BASELINE ASSESSMENT
Assess B/P, pulse, EKG (those with history of cardiovascular disease). Perform CBC, serum electrolyte tests before long-term therapy. Assess pt's appearance, behavior, level of interest, mood, suicidal ideation, sleep pattern.

INTERVENTION/EVALUATION
Monitor B/P, pulse, weight. Perform CBC, serum electrolyte tests periodically to assess renal/hepatic function. Monitor mental status, suicidal ideation. Supervise sui-

cidal-risk pt closely during early therapy (as depression lessens, energy level improves, increasing suicide potential). Assess appearance, behavior, speech pattern, level of interest, mood. **Therapeutic serum level:** 110–250 ng/ml; **toxic serum level:** greater than 300 ng/ml.

PATIENT/FAMILY TEACHING

• Do not discontinue abruptly. • Change positions slowly to avoid dizziness. • Avoid tasks that require alertness, motor skills until response to drug is established. • Do not cover affected area with occlusive dressing after applying cream. • May cause dry mouth. • Avoid alcohol, limit caffeine. • May increase appetite. • Avoid exposure to sunlight/artificial light source. • Therapeutic effect may be noted within 2–5 days, maximum effect within 2–3 wks. • Report worsening depression, suicidal ideation, unusual changes in behavior (esp. at initiation of therapy or with changes in dosage).

---

*DOXOrubicin

dox-oh-**rue**-bi-sin
(Adriamycin, Caelyx 🍁, <u>Doxil</u>)

BLACK BOX ALERT May cause concurrent or cumulative myocardial toxicity. Acute allergic or anaphylaxis-like infusion reaction may be life-threatening. Severe myelosuppresion may occur. Must be administered by personnel trained in administration/handling of chemotherapeutic agents. Secondary acute myelogenous leukemia and myelodysplastic syndrome have been reported.

Do not confuse doxorubicin with dactinoycin, daunorubicin, doxazosin, epirubicin, idarubicin, or valrubicin, or Adriamycin with Aredia or idamycin.

◆CLASSIFICATION

PHARMACOTHERAPEUTIC: Anthracycline antibiotic. **CLINICAL:** Antineoplastic (see p. 85C).

ACTION

Inhibits DNA, DNA-dependent RNA synthesis by binding with DNA strands. Liposomal encapsulation increases uptake by tumors, prolongs drug action, may decrease toxicity. **Therapeutic Effect:** Prevents cell division.

PHARMACOKINETICS

Widely distributed. Protein binding: 74%–76%. Does not cross blood-brain barrier. Metabolized in liver. Primarily eliminated by biliary system. Not removed by hemodialysis. **Half-life:** 20–48 hrs.

USES

Adriamycin: Treatment of acute lymphocytic leukemia (ALL), acute myeloid leukemia (AML), Hodgkin's disease, malignant lymphoma, breast, gastric, small-cell lung, ovarian, epithelial, thyroid, bladder carcinomas, neuroblastoma, Wilms tumor, osteosarcoma, soft tissue sarcoma. **Doxil:** Treatment of AIDS-related Kaposi's sarcoma, metastatic ovarian cancer. Used with bortezomib to treat multiple myeloma in pts who have not previously received bortezomib and have received at least one previous treatment. **OFF-LABEL: Adriamycin:** Multiple myeloma, endometrial carcinoma, uterine sarcoma, head and neck cancer, liver, kidney cancer. **Doxil:** Metastatic breast cancer, Hodgkin's lymphoma, cutaneous T-cell lymphomas, advanced soft tissue sarcomas, recurrent or metastatic cervical cancer, advanced or metastatic uterine sarcoma.

PRECAUTIONS

Contraindications: Adriamycin: Severe hepatic impairment, recent MI, severe arrhythmias. Previous or concomitant treatment with high accumulative doses of doxorubicin, daunorubicin, idarubicin, or other anthracyclines or anthracenediones; baseline neutrophil count less than 1,500/mm³. **Doxil:** Breastfeeding (Canada). **Cautions:** Hepatic impairment. Cardiomyopathy; preexisting myelosuppression; severe HF.

⧗ LIFESPAN CONSIDERATIONS

Pregnancy/Lactation: If possible, avoid use during pregnancy, esp. first trimester. Breastfeeding not recommended. **Pregnancy Category D. Children/Elderly:** Cardiotoxicity may be more frequent in those younger than 2 yrs or older than 70 yrs.

INTERACTIONS

DRUG: Cyclosporine may increase risk of hematologic toxicity. **Bone marrow depressants** may increase myelosuppression. **Daunorubicin** may increase risk of cardiotoxicity. **Live virus vaccines** may potentiate virus replication, increase vaccine side effects, decrease pt's antibody response to vaccine. **HERBAL: St. John's wort** may decrease concentration. Avoid **black cohosh, dong quai** in estrogen-dependent tumors. **FOOD:** None known. **LAB VALUES:** May cause EKG changes, increase serum uric acid. May reduce neutrophil, RBC counts.

AVAILABILITY (Rx)

Injection, Powder for Reconstitution: 10 mg (Adriamycin), 50 mg (Adriamycin RDF). **Injection Solution (Adriamycin):** 2 mg/ml (5-ml, 10-ml, 25-ml, 100-ml vial). **Lipid Complex (Doxil):** 2 mg/ml (10 ml, 25 ml).

ADMINISTRATION/HANDLING

◀ALERT▶ Wear gloves. If powder or solution comes in contact with skin, wash thoroughly. Avoid small veins; swollen/edematous extremities; areas overlying joints, tendons. **Doxil:** Do not use with in-line filter or mix with any diluent except D₅W. May be carcinogenic, mutagenic, teratogenic. Handle with extreme care during preparation/administration.

 IV

Reconstitution • Reconstitute vials of powder with 0.9% NaCl to provide concentration of 2 mg/ml. • Shake vial; allow contents to dissolve. • Withdraw appropriate volume of air from vial during reconstitution (avoids excessive pressure buildup). • May be further diluted with 50–1,000 ml D₅W or 0.9% NaCl and given as continuous infusion. **Doxil:** Dilute each dose in 250 ml D₅W (doses greater than 90 mg in 500 ml D₅W).

Rate of Administration • For IV push, administer into tubing of freely running IV infusion of D₅W or 0.9% NaCl, preferably via butterfly needle over 3–5 min (avoids local erythematous streaking along vein and facial flushing). • Must test for flashback q30sec to be certain needle remains in vein during injection. IV piggyback over 15–60 min or continuous infusion. • Extravasation produces immediate pain, severe local tissue damage. Terminate administration immediately; withdraw as much medication as possible, obtain extravasation kit, follow protocol. **Doxil:** Give as infusion over 60 min. Do not use in-line filter.

Storage • **Adriamycin powder:** Store at room temperature. • Reconstituted vials stable for 7 days at room temperature, 15 days if refrigerated. Infusions stable for 48 hrs at room temperature. • Protect from prolonged exposure to sunlight; discard unused solution. • **Adriamycin solution:** Refrigerate vials. Solutions diluted in D₅W or 0.9% NaCl stable for 48 hrs at room temperature. • **Doxil:** Refrigerate unopened vials. After solution is diluted, use within 24 hrs.

⧈ IV INCOMPATIBILITIES

Doxorubicin: Allopurinol (Aloprim), amphotericin B complex (Abelcet, AmBisome, Amphotec), cefepime (Maxipime), furosemide (Lasix), ganciclovir (Cytovene), heparin, piperacillin/tazobactam (Zosyn), propofol (Diprivan). **Doxil:** Do not mix with any other medications.

⧈ IV COMPATIBILITIES

Dexamethasone (Decadron), diphenhydramine (Benadryl), granisetron (Kytril), hydromorphone (Dilaudid), lorazepam (Ativan), morphine, ondansetron (Zofran).

---

* "Tall Man" lettering   ♣ Canadian trade name   ⟍ Non-Crushable Drug   ▦ High Alert drug

D

INDICATIONS/ROUTES/DOSAGE

◄ALERT► Refer to individual protocols.

Usual Dosage

IV *(Adriamycin)*: **ADULTS:** 60–75 mg/m² as a single dose every 21 days, 20 mg/m² once weekly, or 20–30 mg/m²/day on 2–3 successive days q4wks. Because of risk of cardiotoxicity, do not exceed cumulative dose of 550 mg/m² (400–450 mg/m² for those previously treated with related compounds or irradiation of cardiac region). **CHILDREN:** 35–75 mg/m² as a single dose q3wks or 20–30 mg/m² weekly, or 60–90 mg/m² as continuous infusion over 96 hrs q3–4wks.

Kaposi's Sarcoma

IV *(Doxil)*: **ADULTS:** 20 mg/m² q3wks infused over 30 min.

Ovarian Cancer

IV *(Doxil)*: **ADULTS:** 50 mg/m² q4wks.

Multiple Myeloma

IV *(Doxil)*: **ADULTS:** 30 mg/m²/dose every 3 wks (with bortezomib).

Dosage in Hepatic Impairment
ADRIAMYCIN

Hepatic Function	Dosage
ALT/AST 2–3 times ULN	75% of normal dose
ALT/AST greater than 3 times ULN or bilirubin 1.2–3 mg/dl	50% of normal dose
Bilirubin 3.1–5 mg/dl	25% of normal dose
Bilirubin greater than 5 mg/dl	Not recommended

ULN = upper limit of normal.

DOXIL

Hepatic Function	Dosage
Bilirubin 1.2–3 mg/dl	50% of normal dose
Bilirubin greater than 3 mg/dl	25% of normal dose

SIDE EFFECTS

Frequent: Complete alopecia (scalp, axillary, pubic hair), nausea, vomiting, stomatitis, esophagitis (esp. if drug is given on several successive days), reddish urine. **Doxil:** Nausea. **Occasional:** Anorexia, diarrhea; hyperpigmentation of nailbeds, phalangeal, dermal creases. **Rare:** Fever, chills, conjunctivitis, lacrimation.

ADVERSE EFFECTS/ TOXIC REACTIONS

Myelosuppression manifested as hematologic toxicity (principally leukopenia and, to lesser extent, anemia, thrombocytopenia) generally occurs within 10–15 days, returns to normal levels by third wk. Cardiotoxicity (either acute, manifested as transient EKG abnormalities, or chronic, manifested as HF) may occur.

NURSING CONSIDERATIONS

BASELINE ASSESSMENT

Obtain WBC, platelet, erythrocyte counts before and at frequent intervals during therapy. Obtain EKG before therapy, hepatic function studies before each dose. Antiemetics may be effective in preventing, treating nausea.

INTERVENTION/EVALUATION

Monitor for stomatitis (burning or erythema of oral mucosa at inner margin of lips, difficulty swallowing). Observe IV injection site for infiltration, vein irritation. May lead to ulceration of mucous membranes within 2–3 days. Assess dermal creases, nailbeds for hyperpigmentation. Monitor hematologic status, renal/hepatic function studies, serum uric acid levels. Monitor daily pattern of bowel activity, stool consistency. Monitor for hematologic toxicity (fever, sore throat, signs of local infection, unusual bruising/bleeding from any site), symptoms of anemia (excessive fatigue, weakness).

PATIENT/FAMILY TEACHING

• Hair loss is reversible, but new hair growth may have different color, texture.

---

* "Tall Man" lettering   <u>underlined</u> – top prescribed drug

D

New hair growth resumes 2–3 mos after last therapy dose. • Maintain strict oral hygiene. • Do not have immunizations without physician's approval (drug lowers resistance). • Avoid contact with those who have recently received live virus vaccine. • Promptly report fever, sore throat, signs of local infection, unusual bruising/bleeding from any site. • Report persistent nausea/vomiting. • Avoid alcohol (may cause GI irritation, a common side effect with liposomal doxorubicin).

---

doxycycline `TOP 200`

dox-i-**sye**-kleen
(Adoxa, Apo-Doxy ✽, Doryx, Doxy-100, Doxycin ✽, Monodox, Novo-Doxylin ✽, Oracea, Oraxyl, Periostat, Vibramycin, Vibra-Tabs ✽).
Do not confuse doxycycline with dicyclomine or doxepin, Monodox with Maalox, Oracea with Orencia, Vibramycin with Vancomycin or Vibativ, or Vibra-Tabs with Vibativ.

◆CLASSIFICATION

PHARMACOTHERAPEUTIC: Tetracycline. **CLINICAL:** Antibiotic.

ACTION

Inhibits bacterial protein synthesis by binding to ribosomes. **Therapeutic Effect:** Bacteriostatic.

PHARMACOKINETICS

Rapidly absorbed after PO administration. Protein binding: 90%. Partially excreted in urine; partially eliminated in bile. **Half-life:** 15–24 hrs.

USES

Treatment of susceptible infections due to *H. ducreyi, Pasteurella pestis, P. tularensis, Bacteroides* spp., *V. cholerae, Brucella* spp., *Rickettsiae, Y. pestis, Fran-*cisella tularensis, M. pneumoniae including brucellosis, chlamydia, cholera, granuloma inguinale, lymphogranuloma venereum, malaria prophylaxis, nongonococcal urethritis, pelvic inflammatory disease (PID), plague, psittacosis, relapsing fever, rickettsia infections, primary and secondary syphilis, tularemia. Treatment of inflammatory lesions in adults with rosacea. **OFF-LABEL:** Sclerosing agent for pleural effusion; vancomycin-resistant enterococci (VRE); alternative for MRSA, treatment of refractory periodontis, juvenile periodontis.

PRECAUTIONS

Contraindications: Hypersensitivity to tetracyclines. **Cautions:** Renal impairment; history or predisposition to oral candidiasis. Avoid use during pregnancy, during tooth development in children.

⧗ LIFESPAN CONSIDERATIONS

Pregnancy/Lactation: Crosses placenta; distributed in breast milk. **Pregnancy Category D. Children:** May cause permanent discoloration of teeth, enamel hypoplasia. **Elderly:** No age-related precautions noted.

INTERACTIONS

DRUG: Antacids containing aluminum, calcium, magnesium; laxatives containing magnesium, oral iron preparations decrease absorption. **Barbiturates, carbamazepine, phenytoin** may decrease concentration. **Cholestyramine, colestipol** may decrease absorption. May decrease effects of **oral contraceptives. HERBAL: Dong quai, St. John's wort** may increase photosensitization. **St. John's wort** may decrease concentration/effects. **FOOD:** None known. **LAB VALUES:** May increase serum alkaline phosphatase, amylase, bilirubin, AST, ALT. May alter CBC.

AVAILABILITY (Rx)

Capsules: 20 mg (Oraxyl), 40 mg (Oracea), 50 mg (Monodox), 75 mg (Monodox), 100 mg (Doryx, Monodox, Vibramy-

---

✽ "Tall Man" lettering   ✽ Canadian trade name   🔔 Non-Crushable Drug   🔲 High Alert drug

cin). **Injection, Powder for Reconstitution (Doxy-100):** 100 mg. **Oral Suspension (Vibramycin):** 25 mg/5 ml. **Syrup (Vibramycin):** 50 mg/5 ml. **Tablets:** 20 mg (Periostat), 50 mg (Adoxa), 75 mg (Adoxa), 100 mg (Adoxa, Vibra-Tabs), 150 mg (Adoxa).

ADMINISTRATION/HANDLING

◀**ALERT**▶ Do not administer IM or subcutaneous. Space doses evenly around clock.

 IV

Reconstitution • Reconstitute each 100-mg vial with 10 ml Sterile Water for Injection for concentration of 10 mg/ml. • Further dilute each 100 mg with at least 100 ml D₅W, 0.9% NaCl, lactated Ringer's. **Rate of Administration** • Give by intermittent IV infusion (piggyback). • Infuse over 1–4 hrs.
Storage • After reconstitution, IV infusion (piggyback) is stable for 12 hrs at room temperature or 72 hrs if refrigerated. • Protect from direct sunlight. Discard if precipitate forms.

PO
• Store capsules, tablets at room temperature. • Oral suspension is stable for 2 wks at room temperature. • Give with full glass of fluid. • Instruct pt to sit up for 30 min after taking to reduce risk of esophageal irritation and ulceration. • Give without regard to food. Oracea should be given 1 hr before or 2 hrs after meals. • Avoid concurrent use of antacids, milk; separate by 2 hrs.

💠 IV INCOMPATIBILITIES

Allopurinol (Aloprim), heparin, piperacillin/tazobactam (Zosyn).

💠 IV COMPATIBILITIES

Acyclovir (Zovirax), amiodarone (Cordarone), dexmedetomidine (Precedex), diltiazem (Cardizem), granisetron (Kytril), hydromorphone (Dilaudid), magnesium sulfate, meperidine (Demerol), morphine, ondansetron (Zofran), propofol (Diprivan).

INDICATIONS/ROUTES/DOSAGE

Usual Dosage
IV/PO: ADULTS, ELDERLY, CHILDREN OLDER THAN 8 YRS; GREATER THAN 45 KG: 100–200 mg/day in 1–2 divided doses. **CHILDREN OLDER THAN 8 YRS 45 KG OR LESS:** 2–5 mg/kg/day (**maximum:** 200 mg/day) in 1–2 divided doses.

Rosacea
PO: ADULTS, ELDERLY: 40 mg (Oracea) once daily.

Periodontitis
PO: ADULTS: 20 mg twice a day.

SIDE EFFECTS

Frequent: Anorexia, nausea, vomiting, diarrhea, dysphagia, photosensitivity (may be severe). **Occasional:** Rash, urticaria.

ADVERSE EFFECTS/ TOXIC REACTIONS

Superinfection (esp. fungal), benign intracranial hypertension (headache, visual changes) may occur. Hepatotoxicity, fatty degeneration of liver, pancreatitis occur rarely.

NURSING CONSIDERATIONS

BASELINE ASSESSMENT
Question for history of allergies, esp. to tetracyclines, sulfites.

INTERVENTION/EVALUATION
Monitor daily pattern of bowel activity, stool consistency. Assess skin for rash. Monitor LOC due to potential for increased intracranial pressure (ICP). Be alert for superinfection: fever, vomiting, diarrhea, anal/genital pruritus, oral mucosal changes (ulceration, pain, erythema). Monitor CBC, renal/hepatic function tests.

PATIENT/FAMILY TEACHING
• Avoid unnecessary exposure to sunlight. • Do not take with antacids, iron products. • Complete full course of therapy. • After application of dental gel, avoid

brushing teeth, flossing the treated areas for 7 days. • Report severe diarrhea.

---

dronabinol

droe-**nab**-i-nol
(Marinol ✦)
Do not confuse dronabinol with droperidol.

◆ CLASSIFICATION

PHARMACOTHERAPEUTIC: Controlled substance **(Schedule III).**
CLINICAL: Antinausea, antiemetic, appetite stimulant.

ACTION

Inhibits vomiting control mechanisms in medulla oblongata. **Therapeutic Effect:** Inhibits nausea/vomiting, stimulates appetite.

PHARMACOKINETICS

Well absorbed after PO administration, only 10%–20% reaches systemic circulation. Protein binding: 97%. Undergoes first-pass metabolism. Highly lipid soluble. Primarily excreted in feces. **Half-life:** 25–36 hrs.

USES

Prevention, treatment of nausea/vomiting due to cancer chemotherapy; appetite stimulant in AIDS. **OFF-LABEL:** Cancer-related anorexia.

PRECAUTIONS

Contraindications: Hypersensitivity to sesame oil, tetrahydrocannabinol products, marijuana, history of schizophrenia. **Cautions:** History of psychiatric illness, history of substance abuse, mania, depression, seizure disorder, hepatic impairment, elderly.

⌛ LIFESPAN CONSIDERATIONS

Pregnancy/Lactation: Unknown if drug crosses placenta. Distributed in breast milk. **Pregnancy Category C. Children:** Not recommended. **Elderly:** Monitor carefully during therapy.

INTERACTIONS

DRUG: Alcohol, other CNS suppressants may increase CNS depression. **Sympathomimetics, tricyclic antidepressants** may increase risk of hypertension, tachycardia. **Anticholinergics** may increase drowsiness, tachycardia. **HERBAL: St. John's wort** may decrease concentration. **FOOD:** None known. **LAB VALUES:** None significant.

AVAILABILITY (Rx)

Capsules (Gelatin [Marinol]): 2.5 mg, 5 mg, 10 mg.

ADMINISTRATION/HANDLING

PO
• Store in cool environment. May refrigerate capsules. • May administer without regard to meals. Give before meals if used for appetite stimulant.

INDICATIONS/ROUTES/DOSAGE

Prevention of Chemotherapy-Induced Nausea and Vomiting
PO: ADULTS, CHILDREN: Initially, 5 mg/m^2 1–3 hrs before chemotherapy, then q2–4h after chemotherapy for total of 4–6 doses a day. May increase by 2.5 mg/m^2 up to 15 mg/m^2 per dose.

Appetite Stimulant
PO: ADULTS: Initially, 2.5 mg twice a day (before lunch and dinner). Range: 2.5–20 mg/day.

SIDE EFFECTS

Frequent (24%–3%): Euphoria, dizziness, paranoid reaction, drowsiness. **Occasional (less than 3%–1%):** Asthenia (loss of strength, energy), ataxia, confusion, abnormal thinking, depersonalization. **Rare (less than 1%):** Diarrhea, depression, nightmares, speech difficulties, headache, anxiety, tinnitus, flushed skin.

✦ Canadian trade name   🗱 Non-Crushable Drug   🔲 High Alert drug

ADVERSE EFFECTS/ TOXIC REACTIONS

Mild intoxication may produce increased sensory awareness (taste, smell, sound), altered time perception, reddened conjunctiva, dry mouth, tachycardia. Moderate intoxication may produce memory impairment, urinary retention. Severe intoxication may produce lethargy, decreased motor coordination, slurred speech, orthostatic hypotension.

NURSING CONSIDERATIONS

BASELINE ASSESSMENT

Assess dehydration status if excessive vomiting occurs (skin turgor, mucous membranes, urinary output).

INTERVENTION/EVALUATION

Supervise closely for serious mood, behavior responses, esp. in pts with history of psychiatric illness. Monitor B/P, heart rate.

PATIENT/FAMILY TEACHING

• Change positions slowly to avoid dizziness. • Relief from nausea/vomiting generally occurs within 15 min of drug administration. • Do not take any other medications, including OTC, without physician approval. • Avoid alcohol, barbiturates. • Avoid tasks that require alertness, motor skills until response to drug is established. • For appetite stimulation, take before lunch and dinner.

---

dronedarone

droe-**ne**-da-rone
(Multaq)

BLACK BOX ALERT Contraindicated in those with Class II–III congestive heart failure (HF) with recent decompensation requiring hospitalization or referral to specialized HF clinic or with Class IV HF (over 2-fold increased mortality risk).

Do not confuse dronedarone with amiodarone, dexamethasone, methyltrexone, milrinone, prednisone, or risperidone, or Multaq with Adalat, Atarax, Betaloc, Carac, or Titralac.

◆CLASSIFICATION

PHARMACOTHERAPEUTIC: Cardiac agent. **CLINICAL:** Antiarrhythmic (see p. 18C).

ACTION

Exact mechanism unknown. Has antiarrhythmic properties of all 4 Vaughan-Williams classes, but contribution of each of these to clinical effect unknown. **Therapeutic Effect:** Suppresses arrhythmias.

PHARMACOKINETICS

Derivative of amiodarone. Protein binding: 98%. Metabolized extensively in liver. Eliminated mainly in feces, with smaller amount excreted in urine. **Half-life:** 13–19 hrs.

USES

Outpatient management to reduce cardiovascular hospitalization in pts with persistent or paroxysmal atrial fibrillation, atrial flutter in those in sinus rhythm. **OFF-LABEL:** Treatment of atrial fibrillation in pts with hypertrophic cardiomyopathy.

PRECAUTIONS

Contraindications: Class II–III HF with recent decompensation requiring hospitalization or referral to specialized HF clinic, Class IV HF, sick sinus syndrome without pacemaker, bradycardia less than 50 beats/min, concurrent use of drugs that prolong QT interval (QTc interval equal to or greater than 500 ms or PR interval greater than 280 ms), pregnancy, breastfeeding, severe hepatic impairment. Concomitant use of strong CYP3A4 inhibitors (e.g., ketoconazole, cyclosporine, clarithromycin). **Cautions:** Mild to moderate hepatic impairment, hypomagnesemia, hypokalemia. May increase risk of serious cardiovascular events in pts with permanent atrial fibrillation. Renal impairment, women of childbearing potential.

⌛ LIFESPAN CONSIDERATIONS

Pregnancy/Lactation: May be distributed in breast milk. May cause fetal harm; teratogenic. **Pregnancy Category X. Children:** Safety and efficacy not established in those younger than 18 yrs. **Elderly:** No age-related precautions noted.

INTERACTIONS

DRUG: Drugs prolonging QT interval (e.g., **tricyclic antidepressants, macrolide antibiotics, class I and III antiarrhythmics**) are contraindicated. **Calcium channel blockers, beta blockers** that depress SA/AV node function may increase effects. May increase concentration, toxicity of **digoxin. Simvastatin** may increase risk of myopathy, rhabdomyolysis. **CYP3A4 inducers** (e.g., **rifampin**) may increase risk for torsades. **CYP3A4 inhibitors** (e.g., **ketoconazole**) may increase concentration. May increase concentration of **tacrolimus, sirolimus. HERBAL: St. John's wort** may decrease effect. **FOOD: Grapefruit products** may decrease effect. **LAB VALUES:** May increase serum alkaline phosphatase, AST, ALT, ANA titer. May cause changes in EKG, thyroid function tests. Expected to increase serum creatinine by about 0.1 mg/dl; elevation has rapid onset, reaches plateau after 7 days, and is reversible after discontinuation.

AVAILABILITY (Rx)

🔖 Tablets (Film-Coated): 400 mg.

ADMINISTRATION/HANDLING

PO
• Give with meals to reduce risk of GI distress. • Do not break, cut, crush, or divide film-coated tablets.

INDICATIONS/ROUTES/DOSAGE

◀ALERT▶ Should only be used in pts who can be converted to normal sinus rhythm.

Atrial Fibrillation/Atrial Flutter
PO: ADULTS, ELDERLY: 400 mg twice daily: 1 tablet with morning meal, 1 tablet with evening meal.

SIDE EFFECTS

Frequent (9%–5%): Diarrhea, asthenia (lack of strength, weakness), nausea, rash (including pruritus, dermatitis, eczema). **Occasional (4%–3%):** Abdominal pain, bradycardia. **Rare (2%–1%):** Vomiting, dyspepsia, photosensitivity reaction, dysgeusia (distortion or loss of taste).

ADVERSE EFFECTS/TOXIC REACTIONS

Overdose manifested as arrhythmias, B/P changes.

NURSING CONSIDERATIONS

BASELINE ASSESSMENT

Premenopausal women who have not undergone a hysterectomy or oophorectomy must use effective contraception (Pregnancy Category X). Obtain baseline pulmonary function tests, chest X-ray, AST, ALT, alkaline phosphatase, serum potassium, magnesium, creatinine. Potassium levels should be within normal range prior to administration and maintained in normal range during administration.

INTERVENTION/EVALUATION

If serum creatinine increases and plateaus, use increased value as pt's new baseline. Stop medication if QTc interval is equal to or greater than 500 ms. Assess pulse for strength/weakness, irregular rate, bradycardia. Monitor EKG for cardiac changes, particularly widening of QRS, prolongation of PR and QT intervals. Notify physician of any significant interval changes. Assess for diarrhea, nausea, rash, weakness.

PATIENT/FAMILY TEACHING

• Protect against photosensitivity reaction on skin exposed to sunlight. Wear protective clothing; avoid suntanning booths. • Report increased shortness of breath, cough, sudden weight gain, dependent edema. • Pt should monitor pulse before taking medication. • Compliance with therapy regimen is essential to control arrhythmias. • Use appropriate contraception to avoid pregnancy (Pregnancy Category X).

duloxetine

TOP 200

du-**lox**-e-teen
(Cymbalta)

BLACK BOX ALERT Increased risk of suicidal thinking and behavior in children, adolescents, young adults 18–24 yrs with major depressive disorder, other psychiatric disorders.

Do not confuse duloxetine with fluoxetine or paroxetine.

◆ CLASSIFICATION

PHARMACOTHERAPEUTIC: Serotonin norepinephrine reuptake inhibitor (SNRI). **CLINICAL:** Antidepressant (see p. 41C).

ACTION

Appears to inhibit serotonin and norepinephrine reuptake at CNS neuronal presynaptic membranes; is a less potent inhibitor of dopamine reuptake. **Therapeutic Effect:** Produces antidepressant effect.

PHARMACOKINETICS

Well absorbed from GI tract. Protein binding: greater than 90%. Metabolized in liver. Excreted in urine (70%), feces (20%). **Half-life:** 8–17 hrs.

USES

Treatment of major depression. Management of pain associated with diabetic neuropathy, fibromyalgia, or chronic musculoskeletal pain. Treatment of generalized anxiety disorder. **OFF-LABEL:** Treatment of stress incontinence, urinary incontinence.

PRECAUTIONS

Contraindications: Uncontrolled narrow-angle glaucoma, use within 14 days of MAOIs. Concomitant use with linezolid or IV methylene blue. **Cautions:** Renal impairment, history of alcoholism, chronic hepatic disease, history of seizures, history of mania, pts with suicidal ideation and behavior. Inhibitors of CYP1A2 or thioridazine, hypertension. Controlled narrow-angle glaucoma, pts with impaired GI motility. Concomitant use of NSAIDs (may increase risk of bleeding). Use of medications that lower seizure threshold.

⌧ LIFESPAN CONSIDERATIONS

Pregnancy/Lactation: May produce neonatal adverse reactions (constant crying, feeding difficulty, hyperreflexia, irritability). Unknown if distributed in breast milk. Breastfeeding not recommended. **Pregnancy Category C. Children:** Safety and efficacy not established. **Elderly:** Caution required when increasing dosage.

INTERACTIONS

DRUG: Alcohol increases risk of hepatic injury. **CYP1A2** and **CYP2D6 inhibitors (e.g., fluoxetine, fluvoxamine, paroxetine, quinidine, quinolone antimicrobials)** may increase plasma concentration. **MAOIs** may cause serotonin syndrome (autonomic hyperactivity, coma, diaphoresis, excitement, hyperthermia, rigidity). **Aspirin, NSAIDs** may increase risk of bleeding. May increase concentration, potential toxicity of **tricyclic antidepressants.** Serotonergic drugs **(e.g., triptans, lithium, tramadol)** may increase risk of serotonin syndrome. **HERBAL: Gotu kola, kava kava, St. John's wort, valerian** may increase CNS depression. **St. John's wort** may increase risk of serotonin syndrome. **FOOD:** None known. **LAB VALUES:** May increase serum bilirubin, AST, ALT, alkaline phosphatase.

AVAILABILITY (Rx)

Capsules (Delayed-Release, Enteric-Coated Pellets): 20 mg, 30 mg, 60 mg.

ADMINISTRATION/HANDLING

◀ALERT▶ Allow at least 14 days to elapse between use of MAOIs and duloxetine.

PO
• Give without regard to meals. Give with food, milk if GI distress occurs. • Do not crush, cut delayed-release capsules. • Contents of capsule may be sprinkled on applesauce or mixed in apple juice and swallowed (without chewing) immediately.

INDICATIONS/ROUTES/DOSAGE

Fibromyalgia
PO: ADULTS: Initially, 30 mg/day for 1 wk. Increase to 60 mg/day.

Major Depressive Disorder
PO: ADULTS: Initially, 40–60 mg/day in 1 or 2 divided doses. For doses greater than 60 mg/day, titrate in increments of 30 mg/day over 1 wk. **Maximum:** 120 mg/day. **ELDERLY:** Initially, 20 mg 1–2 times day. May increase to 40–60 mg/day as single or divided doses.

Diabetic Neuropathy Pain
PO: ADULTS, ELDERLY: 60 mg once a day. **Maximum:** 120 mg/day.

Generalized Anxiety Disorder
PO: ADULTS, ELDERLY: Initially, 30–60 mg once daily. May increase up to 120 mg/day in 30-mg increments weekly.

Chronic Musculoskeletal Pain
PO: ADULTS, ELDERLY: 30 mg once daily for 1 wk, then increase to 60 mg once daily.

Dosage in Renal Impairment
Not recommended with creatinine clearance less than 30 ml/min or ESRD.

SIDE EFFECTS

Frequent (20%–11%): Nausea, dry mouth, constipation, insomnia. **Occasional (9%–5%):** Dizziness, fatigue, diarrhea, drowsiness, anorexia, diaphoresis, vomiting. **Rare (4%–2%):** Blurred vision, erectile dysfunction, delayed or failed ejaculation, anorgasmia, anxiety, decreased libido, hot flashes.

ADVERSE EFFECTS/ TOXIC REACTIONS

May slightly increase heart rate. Colitis, dysphagia, gastritis, irritable bowel syndrome occur rarely.

NURSING CONSIDERATIONS

BASELINE ASSESSMENT
Assess appearance, behavior, speech pattern, level of interest, mood, sleep pattern, suicidal tendencies. Question pain level, intensity, location of pain.

INTERVENTION/EVALUATION
For those on long-term therapy, serum chemistry profile to assess hepatic/renal function should be performed periodically. Supervise suicidal-risk pt closely during early therapy (as depression lessens, energy level improves, increasing suicide potential). Monitor B/P, mental status, anxiety, social functioning, serum glucose levels.

PATIENT/FAMILY TEACHING
• Therapeutic effect may be noted within 1–4 wks. • Do not abruptly discontinue medication. • Avoid tasks that require alertness, motor skills until response to drug is established. • Inform physician of intention of pregnancy or if pregnancy occurs. • Inform physician of anxiety, agitation, panic attacks, worsening of depression occurs. • Avoid heavy alcohol intake (associated with severe hepatic injury).

---

dutasteride
TOP 200

du-**tas**-ter-ide
(Avodart)

FIXED-COMBINATION(S)
Jalyn: dutasteride/tamsulosin (alpha-adrenergic blocker): 0.5 mg/0.4 mg.

◆CLASSIFICATION

PHARMACOTHERAPEUTIC: Androgen hormone inhibitor. **CLINICAL:** Benign prostatic hyperplasia (BPH) agent.

ACTION

Inhibits 5-alpha reductase, an intracellular enzyme that converts testosterone into dihydrotestosterone (DHT) in the prostate gland, reducing serum DHT level. **Therapeutic Effect:** Reduces enlarged prostate gland.

PHARMACOKINETICS

Route	Onset	Peak	Duration
PO	24 hrs	N/A	3–8 wks

Moderately absorbed after PO administration. Widely distributed. Protein binding: 99%. Metabolized in liver. Primarily excreted in feces. **Half-life:** Up to 5 wks.

USES

Treatment of benign prostatic hyperplasia (BPH), alone or in combination with tamsulosin (Flomax). **OFF-LABEL:** Treatment of hair loss.

PRECAUTIONS

Contraindications: Females who are pregnant or of childbearing potential, pediatric pts. **Cautions:** Obstructive uropathy, physical handling of tablets by those who are or may be pregnant, **Pregnancy Category X.**

INTERACTIONS

DRUG: **CYP3A4 inhibitors (e.g., ritonavir)** may increase concentration. **HERBAL:** Avoid **saw palmetto** (limited experience with this combination). **St. John's wort** may decrease concentration. **FOOD:** None known. **LAB VALUES:** Decreases serum prostate-specific antigen (PSA) level.

AVAILABILITY (Rx)

🍶 Capsules: 0.5 mg.

ADMINISTRATION/HANDLING

PO
• Swallow whole. Do not break, chew, crush, or divide capsules. • Give without regard to meals.

INDICATIONS/ROUTES/DOSAGE

Benign Prostatic Hyperplasia (BPH)
PO: ADULTS, ELDERLY (MEN ONLY): 0.5 mg once a day (alone or in combination with tamsulosin).

SIDE EFFECTS

Occasional (5%–3%): Impotence, decreased libido. **Rare (less than 2%):** Ejaculation disorders, gynecomastia.

ADVERSE EFFECTS/ TOXIC REACTIONS

Toxicity manifested as rash, diarrhea, abdominal pain.

NURSING CONSIDERATIONS

BASELINE ASSESSMENT

Serum prostate-specific antigen (PSA) determination should be performed in pts with benign prostatic hyperplasia (BPH) before beginning therapy and periodically thereafter. Question possibility of sexual dysfunction.

INTERVENTION/EVALUATION

Diligently monitor I&O. Assess for signs/symptoms of BPH (hesitancy, reduced force of urinary stream, postvoid dribbling, sensation of incomplete bladder emptying).

PATIENT/FAMILY TEACHING

• Take whole; do not break, chew, crush, or divide capsules. • Discuss potential for impotence; volume of ejaculate may be decreased during treatment. • May not notice improved urinary flow for up to 6 mos after beginning treatment. • Women who are or may be pregnant should not handle capsules (risk of fetal anomaly to male fetus). • Do not donate blood for at least 6 mos after last dose.

ecallantide

e-**kal**-an-tide
(Kalbitor)

BLACK BOX ALERT Risk of anaphylactic reaction. Must be administered by health care personnel with
appropriate support to manage
anaphylaxis, hereditary angioedema and an understanding of the
similarity of symptoms.

◆ CLASSIFICATION

PHARMACOTHERAPEUTIC: Plasma
kallikrein inhibitor. **CLINICAL:** Proteolytic complex.

ACTION

Blocks inflammatory and coagulation
pathways; converts kininogen to bradykinin by inactivating enzymatic active components. **Therapeutic Effect:** Reduces
conversion of kininogen to bradykinin,
thereby treating symptoms of hereditary
angioedema.

PHARMACOKINETICS

Half-life: 1.5–2.5 hrs.

USES

Treatment of acute attacks of hereditary
angioedema in pts 16 yrs and older.

PRECAUTIONS

Contraindications: Known hypersensitivity to other proteolytic medications or
to ecallantide. **Cautions:** Hepatic/renal
disease.

☒ LIFESPAN CONSIDERATIONS

Pregnancy/Lactation: Unknown if distributed in breast milk. **Pregnancy Category C. Children:** Safety and efficacy not
established in those younger than 16 yrs.
Elderly: Age-related renal, hepatic, cardiac impairment may require dosage adjustment. Initiate treatment at low end of
dosage range.

INTERACTIONS

DRUG: None significant. **HERBAL:** None
significant. **FOOD:** None known. **LAB VAL-
UES:** May prolong aPTT.

AVAILABILITY (Rx)

Single-Use Vial: 10 mg/ml. Dose supplied as three single-use vials in one
carton.

ADMINISTRATION/HANDLING

Subcutaneous
Reconstitution • Withdraw 1 ml (10
mg) from each vial.
Rate of Administration • Administer
as 3 subcutaneous injections. • Injection
site for each injection may be in same or
different anatomic locations (abdomen,
thigh, upper arm). There is no need for
site rotation. Injection sites should be
located at least 2 inches away from anatomic site of attack.
Storage • Refrigerate unused vials.
• Liquid appears as clear, colorless. Discard if solution contains particulate or is
discolored. • Vials kept at room temperature must be used within 14 days or
returned to refrigeration.

INDICATIONS/ROUTES/DOSAGE

Hereditary Angioedema
**Subcutaneous: ADULTS, ELDERLY, ADO-
LESCENTS 16 YRS AND OLDER:** 30 mg (3
ml) administered as three injections of
10 mg (1 ml) each. If attack persists, an
additional 30-mg dose may be administered within 24 hrs.

SIDE EFFECTS

Occasional (8%–3%): Headache, nausea,
diarrhea, fever, injection site reactions,
nasopharyngitis.

ADVERSE EFFECTS/ TOXIC REACTIONS

Symptoms associated with anaphylactic
reactions may include chest discomfort,
flushing, pharyngeal edema, pruritus,
rhinorrhea, sneezing, urticaria, rash,

E

E

wheezing, hypotension. Reactions occur within first hr after dosing.

NURSING CONSIDERATIONS

BASELINE ASSESSMENT

Assess for history of immediate hypersensitivity reactions, including anaphylaxis.

INTERVENTION/EVALUATION

Observe pt following drug administration. Given the similarity between hypersensitivity reactions and acute hereditary angioedema symptoms, pt should be monitored closely in the event of a hypersensitivity reaction.

PATIENT/FAMILY TEACHING

• Immediately report signs, symptoms of allergic reactions. Pt should be advised that medication may cause anaphylaxis, other hypersensitivity reactions. • A second 30-mg subcutaneous dose administered within 24 hrs following initial dose may be given if symptoms persist or relapse occurs.

---

eculizumab

e-kue-**liz**-ue-mab
(Soliris)

BLACK BOX ALERT Increased risk for meningococcal infections (septicemia, meningitis) in those with paroxysmal nocturnal hemoglobinemia. Meningococcal vaccination to be given 2 wks before initiation of treatment. Access restricted through a REMS program.

Do not confuse eculizumab with efalizumab or palivizumab, or Soliris with Synagis.

◆ CLASSIFICATION

PHARMACOTHERAPEUTIC: Monoclonal antibody. **CLINICAL:** Hemostatic agent.

ACTION

Binds to complement protein C5, preventing terminal intravascular hemolysis. **Therapeutic Effect:** Prevents intravascular hemolysis in paroxysmal nocturnal hemoglobinuria.

PHARMACOKINETICS

Route	Onset	Peak	Duration
IV	Rapid	End of infusion	1–2 wks

Complete bioavailablity. Unknown metabolism. **Half-life:** 11.3 days.

USES

Reduces hemolysis in pts with paroxysmal nocturnal hemoglobinuria. Treatment of atypical hemolytic uremic syndrome to inhibit complement-mediated thrombotic microangiopathy.

PRECAUTIONS

Contraindications: Unresolved serious *Neisseria meningitides* infection, pts not currently vaccinated against *N. meningitides*. **Cautions:** Systemic infection.

⧗ LIFESPAN CONSIDERATIONS

Pregnancy/Lactation: Crosses placenta. Distributed in breast milk. **Pregnancy Category C. Children:** Safety and efficacy not established in those younger than 18 yrs. **Elderly:** No age-related precautions noted.

INTERACTIONS

DRUG: May increase levels/effect of **leflunomide, natalizumab. Trastuzumab** may increase concentration/effect. **HERBAL:** **Echinacea** may decrease effects. **FOOD:** None known. **LAB VALUES:** Reduces serum LDH levels.

AVAILABILITY (Rx)

Injection, Solution: 10 mg/ml (30-ml vial).

ADMINISTRATION/HANDLING

◄ALERT► Vaccination with a meningococcal vaccine must be given at least 2 wks prior to receiving first dose of eculizumab. Must be given by IV infusion; do not give by bolus or IV push.

IV

Reconstitution • Withdraw required amount of eculizumab from vial and dilute with equal volume of 0.9% NaCl, D₅W, or lactated Ringer's to provide final concentration of 5 mg/ml. • Final admixture is 120 ml for 600-mg dose or 180 ml for 900-mg dose. • Gently invert bag to ensure thorough mixing. • Prior to administration, allow admixture to adjust to room temperature.

Rate of Administration • Administer over 35 min. • Total infusion time should not exceed 2 hrs.

Storage • Refrigerate vials. • Discard solution that is discolored or contains particulate matter. • Solution is stable for 24 hrs at room temperature or if refrigerated.

INDICATIONS/ROUTES/DOSAGE

Paroxysmal Nocturnal Hemoglobinuria
IV Infusion: ADULTS, ELDERLY: 600 mg every 7 days for 4 doses, followed by 900 mg 7 days later, then 900 mg every 14 days thereafter.

Atypical Hemolytic Uremic Syndrome
IV Infusion: ADULTS, ELDERLY: 900 mg every 7 days for 4 doses, followed by 1,200 mg 7 days later, then 1,200 mg every 14 days thereafter. **CHILDREN (based on body weight):**

Body Weight	Induction	Maintenance
40 kg and over	900 mg weekly × 4 doses	1,200 mg wk 5, then 1,200 mg q2wks
30–39 kg	600 mg weekly × 2 doses	900 mg wk 3, then 900 mg q2wks
20–29 kg	600 mg weekly × 2 doses	600 mg wk 3, then 600 mg q2wks
10–19 kg	600 mg weekly × 1 dose	300 mg wk 2, then 300 mg q2wks
5–9 kg	300 mg weekly × 1 dose	300 mg wk 2, then 300 mg q3wks

SIDE EFFECTS

Frequent (44%–23%): Headache, pharyngitis. **Occasional (19%–12%):** Back pain, nausea, cough, fatigue. **Rare (7%):** Constipation, myalgia, sinusitis, herpes simplex infection, extremity pain, influenza-like symptoms.

ADVERSE EFFECTS/TOXIC REACTIONS

Eculizumab increases susceptibility to serious meningococcal infections (septicemia, meningitis), encapsulated bacteria. Pts who discontinue treatment may be at increased risk for serious hemolysis.

NURSING CONSIDERATIONS

BASELINE ASSESSMENT

Obtain baseline laboratory studies. Vaccinate pts with meningococcal vaccine at least 2 wks prior to receiving first dose of eculizumab.

INTERVENTION/EVALUATION

Observe for infusion site reaction. Monitor CBC, LDH, AST, urinalysis results. Monitor for early signs of meningococcal infection (moderate to severe headache with nausea or vomiting; moderate to severe headache and fever; moderate to severe headache with stiff neck or stiff back; fever 103°F or higher; fever with rash, confusion, severe myalgia with flu-like symptoms, photosensitivity).

PATIENT/FAMILY TEACHING

• Vaccination may not prevent meningococcal infection.

---

efavirenz

e-**fav**-ir-enz
(<u>Sustiva</u>)

FIXED COMBINATION(S)

Atripla: efavirenz/emtricitabine (an antiretroviral)/tenofovir (an antiretroviral): 600 mg/200 mg/300 mg.

E

◆CLASSIFICATION

PHARMACOTHERAPEUTIC: Nonnucleoside reverse transcriptase inhibitor. **CLINICAL:** Antiretroviral (see pp. 69C, 119C).

ACTION

Inhibits activity of HIV-1 reverse transcriptase. **Therapeutic Effect:** Interrupts HIV replication, slowing progression of HIV infection.

PHARMACOKINETICS

Rapidly absorbed after PO administration. Protein binding: 99%. Metabolized in liver. Eliminated in feces (16%–61%), urine (14%–34%). **Half-life:** 40–55 hrs.

USES

Treatment of HIV infection in combination with at least two other appropriate antiretroviral agents in adults and children 3 mos and older.

PRECAUTIONS

Contraindications: Concurrent use with bepridil, ergot derivatives, midazolam, St. John's wort, triazolam. **Cautions:** History of mental illness, seizures, suspected hepatitis B or C, substance abuse, hepatic impairment (class A).

⧖ LIFESPAN CONSIDERATIONS

Pregnancy/Lactation: Breastfeeding not recommended. **Pregnancy Category C. Children:** Safety and efficacy not established in those younger than 3 yrs; may have increased incidence of rash. **Elderly:** No age-related precautions noted.

INTERACTIONS

DRUG: Ergot derivatives, midazolam, triazolam may cause serious or life-threatening reactions (cardiac arrhythmias, prolonged sedation, respiratory depression). Decreases plasma concentrations of **amprenavir, atazanavir, boceprevir, telaprevir, indinavir, saquinavir.** Increases plasma concentrations of **ritonavir. CYP3A4 inducers** (e.g., **phenobarbital, rifabutin, rifampin**) decrease concentration/effect. May alter **warfarin** plasma concentration. **HERBAL: St. John's wort** may decrease concentration/effect. **FOOD: High-fat meals** may increase drug absorption. **LAB VALUES:** May produce false-positive urine test results for cannabinoid. May increase serum AST, ALT. May decrease neutrophils.

AVAILABILITY (Rx)

Capsules: 50 mg, 200 mg.

Tablets: 600 mg.

ADMINISTRATION/HANDLING

PO

• Give with water at bedtime (decreases CNS adverse effects). • Avoid high-fat meals (may increase absorption) • Capsules may be opened and added to small amount of food/liquid. Administer within 30 min. • Do not break, cut, crush, or divide tablets.

INDICATIONS/ROUTES/DOSAGE

HIV Infection (in Combination with Other Antiretrovirals)

PO: ADULTS, ELDERLY, CHILDREN WEIGHING 40 KG OR MORE: 600 mg once a day at bedtime. **CHILDREN WEIGHING 32.5 KG–LESS THAN 40 KG:** 400 mg once a day. **CHILDREN WEIGHING 25 KG–LESS THAN 32.5 KG:** 350 mg once a day. **CHILDREN WEIGHING 20 KG–LESS THAN 25 KG:** 300 mg once a day. **CHILDREN WEIGHING 15 KG–LESS THAN 20 KG:** 250 mg once a day. **CHILDREN WEIGHING 7.5 KG–LESS THAN 15 KG:** 200 mg once a day. **CHILDREN WEIGHING 5 KG–LESS THAN 7.5 KG:** 150 mg once a day. **CHILDREN WEIGHING 3.5 KG–LESS THAN 5 KG:** 100 mg once a day.

Dosage: Concurrent Rifampin

PO: ONLY IF PT WEIGHS 50 KG OR GREATER: 800 mg once daily.

Dosage: Concurrent Voriconazole

PO: Reduce efavirenz to 300 mg once daily; increase voriconazole to 400 mg q12h.

SIDE EFFECTS

Frequent (52%): Mild to severe: Dizziness, vivid dreams, insomnia, confusion, impaired concentration, amnesia, agitation, depersonalization, hallucinations, euphoria. **Occasional: Mild to moderate:** Maculopapular rash (27%); nausea, fatigue, headache, diarrhea, fever, cough (less than 26%).

ADVERSE EFFECTS/ TOXIC REACTIONS

Serious adverse psychiatric experiences (aggressive reactions, agitation, delusions, emotional lability, mania, neurosis, paranoia, psychosis, suicide) have been reported.

NURSING CONSIDERATIONS

BASELINE ASSESSMENT

Offer emotional support. Obtain baseline AST, ALT in pts with history of hepatitis B or C; serum cholesterol or triglycerides before initiating therapy and at intervals during therapy. Obtain history of all prescription and OTC medications (high level of drug interaction).

INTERVENTION/EVALUATION

Monitor for CNS, psychological symptoms: severe acute depression (including suicidal ideation or attempts), dizziness, impaired concentration, drowsiness, abnormal dreams, insomnia (begins during first or second day of therapy, generally resolves in 2–4 wks). Assess for evidence of rash (common side effect). Monitor hepatic enzyme studies for abnormalities. Assess for headache, nausea, diarrhea.

PATIENT/FAMILY TEACHING

• Avoid high-fat meals during therapy. • If rash appears, contact physician immediately. • CNS, psychological symptoms occur in more than half of pts (dizziness, impaired concentration, delusions, depression). • Take medication every day as prescribed. • Do not alter dose or discontinue medication without informing physician. • Do not break, chew, crush, or divide tablets. • Avoid tasks that require alertness, motor skills until response to drug is established. • Avoid alcohol. • Efavirenz is not a cure for HIV infection, nor does it reduce risk of transmission to others.

eletriptan

el-e-**trip**-tan
(Relpax)

◆ **CLASSIFICATION**

PHARMACOTHERAPEUTIC: Serotonin receptor agonist. **CLINICAL:** Antimigraine (see p. 64C).

ACTION

Binds selectively to vascular receptors, producing vasoconstrictive effect on cranial blood vessels. **Therapeutic Effect:** Relieves migraine headache.

PHARMACOKINETICS

Well absorbed after PO administration. Metabolized by liver. Eliminated in urine. **Half-life:** 4.4 hrs (increased in hepatic impairment, elderly [older than 65 yrs]).

USES

Treatment of acute migraine headache with or without aura.

PRECAUTIONS

Contraindications: Arrhythmias associated with conduction disorders, cerebrovascular syndrome including strokes and transient ischemic attacks (TIAs), coronary artery disease, hemiplegic or basilar migraine, ischemic heart disease, peripheral vascular disease including ischemic bowel disease, severe hepatic impairment, uncontrolled hypertension; use within 24 hrs of treatment with another 5-HT1 agonist, an ergotamine-

---

✤ Canadian trade name   🦋 Non-Crushable Drug   🄷🄸 High Alert drug

containing or ergot-type medication such as dihydroergotamine (DHE) or methysergide. **Cautions:** Mild to moderate renal/hepatic impairment, controlled hypertension, history of CVA.

⧗ LIFESPAN CONSIDERATIONS

Pregnancy/Lactation: May decrease possibility of ovulation. Distributed in breast milk. **Pregnancy Category C. Children:** Safety and efficacy not established in those younger than 18 yrs. **Elderly:** Increased risk of hypertension in those older than 65 yrs.

INTERACTIONS

DRUG: CYP3A4 inhibitors (e.g., clarithromycin, itraconazole, ketoconazole, nefazodone, nelfinavir, ritonavir) may decrease metabolism. Ergotamine-containing medications may produce vasospastic reaction. **HERBAL:** None significant. **FOOD:** None known. **LAB VALUES:** None known.

AVAILABILITY (Rx)

💊 **Tablets:** 20 mg, 40 mg.

ADMINISTRATION/HANDLING

PO
• Do not crush, break film-coated tablets.

INDICATIONS/ROUTES/DOSAGE

Acute Migraine Headache
PO: ADULTS, ELDERLY: 20–40 mg. If headache improves but then returns, dose may be repeated after 2 hrs. **Maximum:** 80 mg/day.

SIDE EFFECTS

Occasional (6%–5%): Dizziness, drowsiness, asthenia (loss of strength, energy), nausea. **Rare (3%–2%):** Paresthesia, headache, dry mouth, warm or hot sensation, dyspepsia, dysphagia.

ADVERSE EFFECTS/ TOXIC REACTIONS

Cardiac reactions (ischemia, coronary artery vasospasm, MI), noncardiac vasospasm-related reactions (hemorrhage, CVA) occur rarely, particularly in pts with hypertension, obesity, diabetes, strong family history of coronary artery disease; smokers; males older than 40 yrs; postmenopausal women.

NURSING CONSIDERATIONS

BASELINE ASSESSMENT

Question pt regarding onset, location, duration of migraine, possible precipitating symptoms. Obtain baseline B/P for evidence of uncontrolled hypertension (contraindication).

INTERVENTION/EVALUATION

Assess for relief of migraine headache, potential for photophobia, phonophobia (sound sensitivity), nausea, vomiting.

PATIENT/FAMILY TEACHING

• Take a single dose as soon as symptoms of an actual migraine attack appear. • Medication is intended to relieve migraine headaches, not to prevent or reduce number of attacks. • Avoid tasks that require alertness, motor skills until response to drug is established. • Immediately report palpitations, pain/tightness in chest/throat, sudden or severe abdominal pain, pain/weakness of extremities.

eltrombopag

el-**trom**-boe-pag
(Promacta, Revolade ✦)

BLACK BOX ALERT May cause hepatotoxicity. Measure ALT, AST, and bilirubin prior to initiation of eltrombopag, every 2 wks during dose adjustment phase, and monthly following establishment of a stable dose. If bilirubin is elevated, perform fractionation. Discontinue eltrombopag if ALT levels increase to 3 times or greater upper limit of normal and are progressive, persistent for 4 or more wks, accompanied by increased direct bilirubin, clinical symptoms of hepatic injury, or evidence of hepatic decompensation.

◆ CLASSIFICATION

PHARMACOTHERAPEUTIC: Thrombopoietin receptor agonist. **CLINICAL:** Prevents thrombocytopenia.

ACTION

Interacts with the human thrombopoietin receptor and initiates signaling cascades. **Therapeutic Effect:** Induces proliferation and differentiation of megakaryocytes from bone marrow progenitor cells.

PHARMACOKINETICS

Readily absorbed from gastrointestinal tract. Primarily distributed in blood cells. Protein binding: 99%. Extensively metabolized including oxidation, conjugation with glucuronic acid or cysteine. Excreted primarily in feces. **Half-life:** 26–35 hrs.

USES

Treatment of thrombocytopenia in pts with chronic immune (idiopathic) thrombocytopenic purpura (ITP) with insufficient response with corticosteroids, immunoglobulins, or splenectomy. Use only in pts who are at increased risk for bleeding; should not be used to normalize platelet counts. Treatment of thrombocytopenia in pts with chronic hepatitis C to allow the initiation and maintenance of interferon-based therapy.

PRECAUTIONS

Contraindications: None known. **Cautions:** Preexisting hepatic impairment, renal impairment (any degree), myelodysplastic syndrome (may increase risk for hematologic malignancies). Pts with known risk for thromboembolism, risk for cataracts.

⧖ LIFESPAN CONSIDERATIONS

Pregnancy/Lactation: Unknown if distributed in breast milk. **Pregnancy Cate-** gory C. **Children:** Safety and efficacy not established. **Elderly:** Use caution due to increased frequency of hepatic, renal, cardiac dysfunction.

INTERACTIONS

DRUG: May increase concentration/toxicity of **atorvastatin, fluvastatin, methotrexate, nateglinide, pravastatin, repaglinide, rifampin, rosuvastatin. Aluminum, antacids, calcium, iron, magnesium** may decrease concentration/effect. **HERBAL:** None significant. **FOOD: Dairy products** may decrease concentration/effect. **LAB VALUES:** May increase serum ALT, AST.

AVAILABILITY (Rx)

Tablets: 12.5 mg, 25 mg, 50 mg, 75 mg.

ADMINISTRATION/HANDLING

PO
• Give on an empty stomach, either 1 hr before or 2 hrs after eating food.
• Give at least 4 hrs before or 4 hrs after ingestion of antacids, food high in calcium or minerals, or calcium-fortified juices.

INDICATIONS/ROUTES/DOSAGE

ITP
PO: ADULTS, ELDERLY: Initially, 50 mg once daily (25 mg for pts of East Asian ancestry or moderate to severe hepatic insufficiency). After initiating eltrombopag, adjust dose (25 mg to 75 mg once daily) to achieve and maintain platelet count of 50,000 mm^3 or greater as necessary to reduce risk of bleeding. **Maximum:** 75 mg once daily.

Chronic Hepatitis C–associated Thrombocytopenia
PO: ADULTS, ELDERLY: 25 mg once daily. **Maximum:** 100 mg once daily.

SIDE EFFECTS

Frequent (6%–4%): Nausea, vomiting, menorrhagia. **Occasional (3%–2%):** Myalgia, paresthesia, dyspepsia, ecchymosis, cataract, conjunctival hemorrhage.

E

ADVERSE EFFECTS/ TOXIC REACTIONS

May cause hepatotoxicity. Increases risk of reticulin fiber deposits within bone marrow (may lead to bone marrow fibrosis). May produce hematologic malignancies. May cause excessive increase in platelets, leading to thrombotic complications.

NURSING CONSIDERATIONS

BASELINE ASSESSMENT

Assess CBC and peripheral blood smears; hepatic function tests (ALT, AST, bilirubin) prior to initiating therapy. Examine peripheral blood smear to establish extent of RBC and WBC abnormalities. Obtain baseline ocular examination.

INTERVENTION/EVALUATION

Monitor CBC, platelet counts, peripheral blood smears, hepatic function tests (ALT, AST, bilirubin) throughout and following discontinuation of eltrombopag. Monitor for signs of cataracts during therapy.

PATIENT/FAMILY TEACHING

• Lab values will be closely monitored throughout therapy and for at least 4 wks following discontinuation of therapy. • Report any yellowing of the skin or whites of eyes, unusual darkening of the urine, unusual tiredness, pain in right upper stomach area.

---

emtricitabine TOP 200

em-tri-**sye**-ta-bine
(Emtriva)

BLACK BOX ALERT Serious, sometimes fatal, hypersensitivity reaction, lactic acidosis, severe hepatomegaly with steatosis (fatty liver) have occurred. May exacerbate hepatitis B following completion of emtricitabine therapy.

FIXED-COMBINATION(S)

Atripla: emtricitabine/efavirenz (an antiretroviral)/tenofovir (an antiretroviral): 200 mg/600 mg/300 mg. **Complera:** emtricitabine/rilpivirine (an antiretroviral)/tenofovir (an antiretroviral): 200 mg/25 mg/300 mg. **Truvada:** emtricitabine/tenofovir (an antiretroviral): 200 mg/300 mg. **Stribild:** emtricitabine/elvitegravir (an integrase inhibitor)/cobicistat (a pharmacokinetic enhancer)/tenofovir (a nucleotide reverse transcriptase inhibitor): 200 mg/150 mg/150 mg/ 300 mg.

◆CLASSIFICATION

PHARMACOTHERAPEUTIC: Nucleoside reverse transcriptase inhibitor. **CLINICAL:** Antiretroviral agent (see p. 117C).

ACTION

Inhibits HIV-1 reverse transcriptase by incorporating itself into viral DNA, resulting in chain termination. **Therapeutic Effect:** Impairs HIV replication, slowing progression of HIV infection.

PHARMACOKINETICS

Rapidly, extensively absorbed from GI tract. Protein binding: less than 4%. Excreted primarily in urine. **Half-life:** 10 hrs.

USES

Used in combination with at least two other antiretroviral agents for treatment of HIV-1 infection.

PRECAUTIONS

Contraindications: None known. **Cautions:** Renal impairment, history of hepatitis, diabetes.

⌛ LIFESPAN CONSIDERATIONS

Pregnancy/Lactation: Breastfeeding not recommended. **Pregnancy Category B. Children:** Safety and efficacy not established. **Elderly:** Age-related renal impairment may require dosage adjustment.

INTERACTIONS

DRUG: None known. **HERBAL:** None significant. **FOOD:** None known. **LAB VALUES:** May increase serum amylase, lipase, ALT, AST, triglycerides. May alter serum glucose.

AVAILABILITY (Rx)

Capsules: 200 mg. **Oral Solution:** 10 mg/ml.

ADMINISTRATION/HANDLING

PO
• Give without regard to food.

INDICATIONS/ROUTES/DOSAGE

HIV
Capsules
PO: ADULTS, ELDERLY, CHILDREN 3 MOS–17 YRS, WEIGHING MORE THAN 33 KG: 200 mg once daily.
Oral Solution
PO: ADULTS, ELDERLY: 240 mg once daily. **CHILDREN 3 MOS–17 YRS WEIGHING MORE THAN 33 KG:** 6 mg/kg once daily. **Maximum:** 240 mg once daily. **CHILDREN 0–3 MOS:** 3 mg/kg/day.

Dosage in Renal Impairment

Creatinine Clearance	Capsule	Oral Solution
30–49 ml/min	200 mg q48h	120 mg q24h
15–29 ml/min	200 mg q72h	80 mg q24h
Less than 15 ml/min; hemodialysis pts	200 mg q96h	60 mg q24h (administer after dialysis)

Administer after dialysis on dialysis days.

SIDE EFFECTS

Frequent (23%–13%): Headache, rhinitis, rash, diarrhea, nausea. **Occasional (14%–4%):** Cough, vomiting, abdominal pain, insomnia, depression, paresthesia, dizziness, peripheral neuropathy, dyspepsia, myalgia. **Rare (3%–2%):** Arthralgia, abnormal dreams.

ADVERSE EFFECTS/TOXIC REACTIONS

Lactic acidosis, hepatomegaly with steatosis (excess fat in liver) occur rarely; may be severe.

NURSING CONSIDERATIONS

BASELINE ASSESSMENT
Obtain baseline laboratory tests, esp. serum hepatic function, triglycerides before beginning and at periodic intervals during therapy. Offer emotional support.

INTERVENTION/EVALUATION
Monitor daily pattern of bowel activity, stool consistency. Question for evidence of nausea, pruritus. Assess skin for rash, urticaria. Monitor serum chemistry tests, hepatic function tests for marked abnormalities, signs/symptoms of lactic acidosis.

PATIENT/FAMILY TEACHING
• May cause redistribution of body fat. • Continue therapy for full length of treatment. • Emtricitabine is not a cure for HIV infection, nor does it reduce risk of transmission to others. • Pts may continue to acquire illnesses associated with advanced HIV infection. • Avoid tasks that require alertness, motor skills until response to drug is established. • Report persistent severe abdominal pain, nausea, vomiting, numbness.

enalapril
TOP 200

en-al-a-pril
(Apo-Enalapril ✤, Epaned, Novo-Enalapril ✤, Vasotec)
BLACK BOX ALERT May cause fetal injury, mortality if used during second or third trimester of pregnancy. **Do not confuse enalapril with Anafranil, Elavil, Eldepryl, or ramipril.**

FIXED-COMBINATION(S)
Lexxel: enalapril/felodipine (calcium channel blocker): 5 mg/2.5

mg, 5 mg/5 mg. **Teczem:** enalapril/ diltiazem (calcium channel blocker): 5 mg/180 mg. **Vaseretic:** enalapril/ hydrochlorothiazide (diuretic): 5 mg/ 12.5 mg, 10 mg/25 mg.

◆CLASSIFICATION

PHARMACOTHERAPEUTIC: Angiotensin-converting enzyme (ACE) inhibitor. **CLINICAL:** Antihypertensive, vasodilator (see pp. 9C, 61C).

ACTION

Suppresses renin-angiotensin-aldosterone system (prevents conversion of angiotensin I to angiotensin II, a potent vasoconstrictor; may inhibit angiotensin II at local vascular, renal sites). Decreases plasma angiotensin II, increases plasma renin activity, decreases aldosterone secretion. **Therapeutic Effect:** In hypertension, reduces peripheral arterial resistance. In HF, increases cardiac output; decreases peripheral vascular resistance, B/P, pulmonary capillary wedge pressure, heart size.

PHARMACOKINETICS

Route	Onset	Peak	Duration
PO	1 hr	4–6 hrs	24 hrs
IV	15 min	1–4 hrs	6 hrs

Readily absorbed from GI tract. Protein binding: 50%–60%. Primarily excreted in urine. Removed by hemodialysis. **Half-life:** 11 hrs (increased in renal impairment).

USES

Treatment of hypertension alone or in combination with other antihypertensives. Adjunctive therapy for symptomatic HF. Treatment of asymptomatic left ventricular dysfunction. **(Epaned):** Treatment of hypertension in adults and children older than 1 mo. **OFF-LABEL:** Hypertension due to scleroderma renal crisis, hypertensive crisis, idiopathic edema, renal artery stenosis, diagnosis of aldosteronism, post MI for prevention of ventricular failure. Delay progression of nephropathy and reduce risks of cardiovascular events in hypertensive pts with type 1 or 2 diabetes.

PRECAUTIONS

Contraindications: History of angioedema from previous treatment with ACE inhibitors. Idiopathic/hereditary angioedema. Concomitant use of aliskiren in pts with diabetes. **Cautions:** Renal impairment, pts with sodium depletion or on diuretic therapy, hypovolemia, severe HF, left ventricular outflow tract obstruction, unstented unilateral or bilateral renal artery stenosis.

⌛ LIFESPAN CONSIDERATIONS

Pregnancy/Lactation: Crosses placenta. Distributed in breast milk. May cause fetal/neonatal mortality, morbidity. **Pregnancy Category D (C if used in first trimester). Children:** Safety and efficacy not established. **Elderly:** May be more susceptible to hypotensive effects.

INTERACTIONS

DRUG: Alcohol, antihypertensive agents, diuretics may increase effect. **NSAIDs** may decrease antihypertensive effect, increase risk of possible acute renal failure. **Potassium-sparing diuretics, potassium supplements** may cause hyperkalemia. May increase **lithium** concentration, toxicity. **HERBAL: Ephedra, ginseng, yohimbe** may worsen hypertension. **Garlic** may increase antihypertensive effect. **Licorice** may cause sodium/water retention, loss of potassium. **FOOD:** None known. **LAB VALUES:** May increase BUN, serum alkaline phosphatase, bilirubin, creatinine, potassium, AST, ALT. May decrease serum sodium. May cause positive ANA titer.

AVAILABILITY (Rx)

Injection Solution: 1.25 mg/ml. **Powder for Oral Solution (Epaned):** 1 mg/ml (after reconstitution). **Tablets:** 2.5 mg, 5 mg, 10 mg, 20 mg.

ADMINISTRATION/HANDLING

 IV

Reconstitution • May give undiluted or dilute with D₅W or 0.9% NaCl.
Rate of Administration • For IV push, give undiluted over 5 min. • For IV piggyback, infuse over 10–15 min.
Storage • Store parenteral form at room temperature. • Use only clear, colorless solution. • Diluted IV solution is stable for 24 hrs at room temperature.

PO

• Give without regard to food. • Tablets may be crushed.

Epaned

• Reconstitute with 150 ml Ora-Sweet SF (provided) to produce a 1 mg/ml concentration.

🔲 IV INCOMPATIBILITIES

Amphotericin B (Fungizone), amphotericin B complex (Abelcet, AmBisome, Amphotec), cefepime (Maxipime), phenytoin (Dilantin).

🔲 IV COMPATIBILITIES

Calcium gluconate, dexmedetomidine (Precedex), dobutamine (Dobutrex), dopamine (Intropin), fentanyl (Sublimaze), heparin, lidocaine, magnesium sulfate, morphine, nitroglycerin, potassium chloride, potassium phosphate, propofol (Diprivan).

INDICATIONS/ROUTES/DOSAGE

Hypertension
PO: ADULTS, ELDERLY: Initially, 2.5–5 mg/day. May increase at 1–2 wk intervals. Range: 2.5–40 mg/day in 1–2 divided doses. **CHILDREN 1 MO–16 YRS:** 0.08 mg/kg/day in 1–2 divided doses. **Maximum:** 5 mg/day. **NEONATES:** 0.04–0.1 mg/kg/day given q24h. **Epaned: ADULTS, ELDERLY:** Initially, 5 mg once daily. **CHILDREN:** Initially, 0.08 mg/kg once daily. **Maximum:** 5 mg. **IV: ADULTS, ELDERLY:** 0.625–1.25 mg q6h up to 5 mg q6h. **CHILDREN, NEONATES:** 5–10 mcg/kg/dose q8–24h.

Adjunctive Therapy for HF
PO: ADULTS, ELDERLY: Initially, 2.5–5 mg/day. Titrate slowly at 1–2 wk intervals. Range: 5–40 mg/day in 2 divided doses.

Asymptomatic Left Ventricular Dysfunction
PO: ADULTS, ELDERLY: 2.5 mg twice daily. Titrate up to 20 mg/day.

Dosage in Renal Impairment

Creatinine Clearance	PO	IV
30 ml/min or greater	5 mg/day; titrate to maximum 40 mg/day	1.25 mg q6h; titrate to desired response
Less than 30 ml/min	2.5 mg/day; titrate to control B/P	0.626 mg q6h; titrate to desired response

Hemodialysis: Initially, 2.5 mg on dialysis days, adjust dose on non-dialysis days depending on B/P.

SIDE EFFECTS

Frequent (7%–5%): Headache, dizziness. **Occasional (3%–2%):** Orthostatic hypotension, fatigue, diarrhea, cough, syncope. **Rare (less than 2%):** Angina, abdominal pain, vomiting, nausea, rash, asthenia (loss of strength, energy).

ADVERSE EFFECTS/ TOXIC REACTIONS

Excessive hypotension ("first-dose syncope") may occur in pts with HF, severe salt or volume depletion. Angioedema (facial, lip swelling), hyperkalemia occur rarely. Agranulocytosis, neutropenia may be noted in pts with renal impairment, collagen vascular diseases (scleroderma, systemic lupus erythematosus). Nephrotic syndrome may be noted in those with history of renal disease.

NURSING CONSIDERATIONS

BASELINE ASSESSMENT

Obtain B/P immediately before each dose (be alert to fluctuations). In pts with renal impairment, autoimmune disease, or taking drugs that affect leukocytes/immune response, CBC should be performed before beginning therapy, q2wks for 3 mos, then periodically thereafter.

INTERVENTION/EVALUATION

Assist with ambulation if dizziness occurs. Monitor CBC, BUN, serum potassium, creatinine, B/P. Monitor daily pattern of bowel activity, stool consistency.

PATIENT/FAMILY TEACHING

• To reduce hypotensive effect, go from lying to standing slowly. • Several wks may be needed for full therapeutic effect of B/P reduction. • Skipping doses or voluntarily discontinuing drug may produce severe, rebound hypertension. • Limit alcohol intake. • Report vomiting, diarrhea, diaphoresis, persistent cough, swelling of face, lips, tongue, difficulty in breathing.

enfuvirtide

en-**fue**-veer-tide
(Fuzeon)

◆CLASSIFICATION

PHARMACOTHERAPEUTIC: Fusion inhibitor. **CLINICAL:** Antiretroviral agent (see p. 120C).

ACTION

Interferes with entry of HIV-1 into CD4$^+$ cells by inhibiting fusion of viral, cellular membranes. **Therapeutic Effect:** Impairs HIV replication, slowing progression of HIV infection.

PHARMACOKINETICS

Comparable absorption when injected into subcutaneous tissue of abdomen, arm, thigh. Protein binding: 92%. Undergoes catabolism to amino acids. **Half-life:** 3.8 hrs.

USES

Used in combination with other antiretroviral agents for treatment of HIV-1 infection in treatment-experienced pts with evidence of HIV-1 replication.

PRECAUTIONS

Contraindications: None known. **Cautions:** Not recommended in antiretroviral-naïve pts, those with coagulation disorders (e.g., hemophilia) or on anticoagulants.

⌛ LIFESPAN CONSIDERATIONS

Pregnancy/Lactation: Breastfeeding not recommended. **Pregnancy Category B. Children:** Safety and effectiveness not established in those 6 yrs and younger. **Elderly:** No age-related precautions noted.

INTERACTIONS

DRUG: May increase levels of **protease inhibitors. Protease inhibitors** may increase concentration. **HERBAL:** None significant. **FOOD:** None known. **LAB VALUES:** May elevate serum glucose, amylase, creatine kinase (CK), lipase, triglycerides, AST, ALT. May decrease Hgb.

AVAILABILITY (Rx)

Injection, Powder for Reconstitution: 108-mg vials (approximately 90 mg/ml when reconstituted).

ADMINISTRATION/HANDLING

Subcutaneous

Reconstitution • Reconstitute with 1.1 ml Sterile Water for Injection. • Visually inspect vial for particulate matter. Solution should appear clear, colorless (may take up to 45 min to form clear, colorless solution). • Discard unused portion.

Rate of Administration • Administer into upper arm, anterior thigh, abdomen. Rotate injection sites.

Storage • Store at room temperature. • Refrigerate reconstituted solution; use within 24 hrs. • Bring reconstituted solution to room temperature before injection.

INDICATIONS/ROUTES/DOSAGE

HIV Infection

Subcutaneous: ADULTS, ELDERLY: 90 mg (1 ml) twice a day. **CHILDREN 6–16 YRS:** 2 mg/kg twice a day. **Maximum:** 90 mg twice a day.

Pediatric Dosing Guidelines

Weight: kg (lb)	Dose: mg (ml)
11–15.5 (24–34)	27 (0.3)
15.6–20 (35–44)	36 (0.4)
20.1–24.5 (45–54)	45 (0.5)
24.6–29 (55–64)	54 (0.6)
29.1–33.5 (65–74)	63 (0.7)
33.6–38 (75–84)	72 (0.8)
38.1–42.5 (85–94)	81 (0.9)
Greater than 42.5 (greater than 94)	90 (1)

SIDE EFFECTS

Expected (98%): Local injection site reactions (pain, discomfort, induration, erythema, nodules, cysts, pruritus, ecchymosis). **Frequent (26%–16%):** Diarrhea, nausea, fatigue. **Occasional (11%–4%):** Insomnia, peripheral neuropathy, depression, cough, decreased appetite or weight loss, sinusitis, anxiety, asthenia (loss of strength, energy), myalgia, cold sores. **Rare (3%–2%):** Constipation, influenza, upper abdominal pain, anorexia, conjunctivitis.

ADVERSE EFFECTS/ TOXIC REACTIONS

May potentiate bacterial pneumonia. Hypersensitivity (rash, fever, chills, rigors, hypotension), thrombocytopenia, neutropenia, renal insufficiency/failure occur rarely.

NURSING CONSIDERATIONS

BASELINE ASSESSMENT

Obtain baseline laboratory tests, esp. CBC, serum hepatic function, triglycerides before beginning enfuvirtide therapy and at periodic intervals during therapy. Offer emotional support.

INTERVENTION/EVALUATION

Assess skin for local injection site hypersensitivity reaction. Question for evidence of nausea, fatigue. Assess sleep pattern. Monitor for insomnia, signs/symptoms of depression, pneumonia. Monitor CBC, serum chemistry tests for marked abnormalities.

PATIENT/FAMILY TEACHING

• Increased rate of bacterial pneumonia has occurred with enfuvirtide therapy; seek medical attention if cough with fever, rapid breathing occurs. • Continue therapy for full length of treatment. • Enfuvirtide is not a cure for HIV infection, nor does it reduce risk of transmission to others. • Notify physician if injection site reaction is severe.

---

enoxaparin

en-**ox**-a-par-in
(Lovenox)

BLACK BOX ALERT Epidural or spinal anesthesia greatly increases potential for spinal or epidural hematoma, subsequent long-term or permanent paralysis.

Do not confuse Lovenox with Lasix, Levaquin, Lotronex, or Protonix.

◆CLASSIFICATION

PHARMACOTHERAPEUTIC: Low-molecular-weight heparin. **CLINICAL:** Anticoagulant (see p. 32C).

ACTION

Potentiates action of antithrombin III, inactivates coagulation factor Xa. **Therapeutic Effect:** Produces anticoagulation. Does not significantly influence PT, aPTT.

PHARMACOKINETICS

Route	Onset	Peak	Duration
Subcutaneous	N/A	3–5 hrs	12 hrs

Well absorbed after subcutaneous administration. Eliminated primarily in

E

urine. Not removed by hemodialysis. **Half-life:** 4.5 hrs.

USES

Prevention of postop deep vein thrombosis (DVT) following hip or knee replacement surgery, abdominal surgery. Longterm DVT prevention following hip replacement surgery, nonsurgical acute illness. Treatment of acute coronary syndrome (ACS): unstable angina, non–Q-wave MI, acute ST-segment elevation MI (STEMI). Acute DVT (with warfarin). **OFF-LABEL:** Prophylaxis/treatment of thromboembolism in children. DVT prophylaxis following moderate-risk general surgery, gynecologic surgery; management of venous thromboembolism (VTE) during pregnancy.

PRECAUTIONS

Contraindications: Active major bleeding, concurrent heparin therapy, hypersensitivity to heparin, pork products, thrombocytopenia associated with positive in vitro test for antiplatelet antibodies. Not for IM use. **Cautions:** Conditions with increased risk of hemorrhage, platelet defects, renal impairment (renal failure), elderly, uncontrolled arterial hypertension, history of recent GI ulceration or hemorrhage. When neuraxial anesthesia (epidural or spinal anesthesia) or spinal puncture is used, pts anticoagulated or scheduled to be anticoagulated with enoxaparin for prevention of thromboembolic complications are at risk for developing an epidural or spinal hematoma that can result in long-term or permanent paralysis.

⏳ LIFESPAN CONSIDERATIONS

Pregnancy/Lactation: Use with caution, particularly during third trimester, immediate postpartum period (increased risk of maternal hemorrhage). Unknown if distributed in breast milk. **Pregnancy Category B. Children:** Safety and efficacy not established. **Elderly:** May be more susceptible to bleeding.

INTERACTIONS

DRUG: Antiplatelet agents, aspirin, NSAIDs, thrombolytics may increase risk of bleeding. **HERBAL: Cat's claw, dong quai, evening primrose, feverfew, garlic, ginger, ginkgo, ginseng** may increase antiplatelet action. **FOOD:** None known. **LAB VALUES:** Increases serum alkaline phosphatase, AST, ALT. May decrease Hgb, Hct, RBCs.

AVAILABILITY (Rx)

Injection Solution: 30 mg/0.3 ml, 40 mg/0.4 ml, 60 mg/0.6 ml, 80 mg/0.8 ml, 100 mg/ml, 120 mg/0.8 ml, 150 mg/ml in prefilled syringes.

ADMINISTRATION/HANDLING

◀**ALERT**▶ Do not mix with other injections, infusions. Do not give IM.

Subcutaneous

• Parenteral form appears clear, colorless to pale yellow. • Store at room temperature. • Instruct pt to lie down before administering by deep subcutaneous injection. • Inject between left and right anterolateral and left and right posterolateral abdominal wall. • Introduce entire length of needle (½ inch) into skin fold held between thumb and forefinger, holding skin fold during injection.

INDICATIONS/ROUTES/DOSAGE

Prevention of Deep Vein Thrombosis (DVT) After Hip and Knee Surgery
Subcutaneous: ADULTS, ELDERLY: 30 mg twice a day, generally for 7–10 days, with initial dose given within 12–24 hrs following surgery. Once-daily dosing following hip surgery: 40 mg with initial dose within 9–15 hrs before surgery.

Prevention of DVT After Abdominal Surgery
Subcutaneous: ADULTS, ELDERLY: 40 mg a day for 7–10 days, with initial dose given 2 hrs prior to surgery.

Prevention of DVT After Bariatric Surgery
BMI 50 or less (kg/m^2): 40 mg q12h.
BMI greater than 50 kg/m^2: 60 mg q12h.

Prevention of Long-Term DVT in Nonsurgical Acute Illness
Subcutaneous: ADULTS, ELDERLY: 40 mg once a day; continue until risk of DVT has diminished (usually 6–11 days).

Prevention of Ischemic Complications of Unstable Angina, Non–Q-Wave MI (with Oral Aspirin Therapy)
Subcutaneous: ADULTS, ELDERLY: 1 mg/kg q12h (with oral aspirin).

STEMI
Subcutaneous: ADULTS LESS THAN 75 YRS OF AGE: 30 mg IV once plus 1 mg/kg q12h (**maximum:** 100 mg first 2 doses only). **ADULTS 75 YRS OR GREATER:** 0.75 mg/kg (**maximum:** 75 mg first 2 doses only) q12h.

Acute DVT
Subcutaneous: ADULTS, ELDERLY: 1 mg/kg q12h or 1.5 mg/kg once daily.

Usual Pediatric Dosage
Subcutaneous: CHILDREN 2 MOS AND OLDER: 0.5 mg/kg q12h (prophylaxis); 1 mg/kg q12h (treatment). **NEONATES, INFANTS LESS THAN 2 MOS:** 0.75/mg/kg/dose q12h (prophylaxis); 1.5 mg/kg/dose q12h (treatment).

Dosage in Renal Impairment
Clearance is decreased when creatinine clearance is less than 30 ml/min. Monitor and adjust dosage as necessary.

Use	Dosage
Abdominal surgery, pts with acute illness	30 mg once/day
Hip, knee surgery	30 mg once/day
DVT, angina, MI	1 mg/kg once/day
STEMI: (<75 yrs)	30 mg IV once plus 1 mg/kg q24h
STEMI (75 yrs or greater)	1 mg/kg q24h
NSTEMI	1 mg/kg q24h

SIDE EFFECTS

Occasional (4%–1%): Injection site hematoma, nausea, peripheral edema.

ADVERSE EFFECTS/ TOXIC REACTIONS

May lead to bleeding complications ranging from local ecchymoses to major hemorrhage. May cause heparin-induced thrombocytopenia (HIT). **Antidote:** IV injection of protamine sulfate (1% solution) equal to dose of enoxaparin injected. One mg protamine sulfate neutralizes 1 mg enoxaparin. One additional dose of 0.5 mg protamine sulfate per 1 mg enoxaparin may be given if aPTT tested 2–4 hrs after first injection remains prolonged.

NURSING CONSIDERATIONS

BASELINE ASSESSMENT
Obtain baseline CBC. Note platelet count.

INTERVENTION/EVALUATION
Periodically monitor CBC, platelet count, stool for occult blood (no need for daily monitoring in pts with normal presurgical coagulation parameters). Assess for any sign of bleeding (bleeding at surgical site, hematuria, blood in stool, bleeding from gums, petechiae, bruising, bleeding from injection sites).

PATIENT/FAMILY TEACHING
• Usual length of therapy is 7–10 days.
• Do not take any OTC medication (esp. aspirin) without consulting physician.
• Report unusual bleeding or bruising.

entacapone

en-**tak**-a-pone
(Comtan)

FIXED-COMBINATION(S)

Stalevo: entacapone/carbidopa/levodopa (an antiparkinson agent): 200 mg/12.5 mg/50 mg, 200 mg/25 mg/100 mg, 200 mg/37.5 mg/150 mg.

E

◆CLASSIFICATION

PHARMACOTHERAPEUTIC: Enzyme inhibitor. **CLINICAL:** Antiparkinson agent (see p. 145C).

ACTION

Inhibits the enzyme catechol-*O*-methyltransferase (COMT), potentiating dopamine activity, increasing duration of action of levodopa. **Therapeutic Effect:** Decreases signs, symptoms of Parkinson's disease by enhancing effectiveness of levodopa/carbidopa in the brain.

PHARMACOKINETICS

Rapidly absorbed after PO administration. Protein binding: 98%. Metabolized in liver. Primarily eliminated by biliary excretion. Not removed by hemodialysis. **Half-life:** 2.4 hrs.

USES

◀ALERT▶ Adjunct to carbidopa/levodopa therapy when pts experience end-of-dose diminishing effectiveness.

PRECAUTIONS

Contraindications: None known. **Cautions:** Pts at risk for hypotension, preexisting dyskinesias, use of MAOIs within 14 days, hepatic impairment, severe renal impairment, lower GI disease.

⧗ LIFESPAN CONSIDERATIONS

Pregnancy/Lactation: Unknown if distributed in breast milk. **Pregnancy Category C. Children:** Not used in this pt population. **Elderly:** No age-related precautions noted.

INTERACTIONS

DRUG: Nonselective MAOIs (including phenelzine) may inhibit catecholamine metabolism. **HERBAL:** None significant. **FOOD:** None known. **LAB VALUES:** Serum iron may decrease.

AVAILABILITY (Rx)

Tablets: 200 mg.

ADMINISTRATION/HANDLING

PO
• Give without regard to food.

INDICATIONS/ROUTES/DOSAGE

◀ALERT▶ Always administer with levodopa/carbidopa.

Adjunctive Treatment of Parkinson's Disease
PO: ADULTS, ELDERLY: 200 mg concomitantly with each dose of carbidopa and levodopa up to a maximum of 8 times a day (1,600 mg).

SIDE EFFECTS

Frequent (greater than 10%): Dyskinesia (uncontrolled body movements), nausea, dark yellow or orange urine and sweat, diarrhea. **Occasional (9%–3%):** Abdominal pain, vomiting, constipation, dry mouth, fatigue, back pain. **Rare (less than 2%):** Anxiety, drowsiness, agitation, dyspepsia, flatulence, diaphoresis, asthenia (loss of strength, energy), dyspnea.

ADVERSE EFFECTS/ TOXIC REACTIONS

Hallucinations may be noted.

NURSING CONSIDERATIONS

INTERVENTION/EVALUATION

Monitor for evidence of dyskinesia (difficulty with movement). Assess for clinical reversal of symptoms (improvement of tremor of head and hands at rest, mask-like facial expression, shuffling gait, muscular rigidity). Monitor B/P, hepatic function tests. Assess for orthostatic hypotension, diarrhea.

PATIENT/FAMILY TEACHING

• Avoid tasks that require alertness, motor skills until response to drug is established.
• May cause color change in urine or sweat (dark yellow, orange). • Report any uncontrolled movement of face, eyelids, mouth, tongue, arms, hands, legs.

---

entecavir

en-tek-a-veer
(Baraclude)

BLACK BOX ALERT Serious, sometimes fatal, hypersensitivity reaction, lactic acidosis, severe hepatomegaly with steatosis (fatty liver) have occurred. May cause HIV resistance in chronic hepatitis B pts. Severe acute exacerbations of hepatitis B may occur upon discontinuation of entecavir.

◆CLASSIFICATION

PHARMACOTHERAPEUTIC: Reverse transcriptase inhibitor. **CLINICAL:** Antiretroviral agent.

ACTION

Inhibits hepatitis B viral polymerase, an enzyme blocking reverse transcriptase activity. **Therapeutic Effect:** Interferes with viral DNA synthesis.

PHARMACOKINETICS

Poorly absorbed from GI tract. Protein binding: 13%. Extensively distributed into tissues. Partially metabolized in liver. Eliminated mainly in urine. **Half-life:** 5–6 days (increased in renal impairment).

USES

Treatment of chronic hepatitis B infection with evidence of active viral replication and evidence of either persistent transaminase elevations or histologically active disease or evidence of decompensated hepatic disease. **OFF-LABEL:** HBV reinfection prophylaxis, post–liver transplant; HIV/HBV coinfection.

PRECAUTIONS

Contraindications: None known. **Cautions:** Renal impairment, pts receiving concurrent therapy that may reduce renal function.

⌛ LIFESPAN CONSIDERATIONS

Pregnancy/Lactation: Unknown if drug crosses placenta or is distributed in breast milk. **Pregnancy Category C. Children:** Safety and efficacy not established in those younger than 16 yrs. **Elderly:** Age-related renal impairment may require dosage adjustment.

INTERACTIONS

DRUG: Ganciclovir, ribavirin, valganciclovir may increase concentration. **HERBAL:** None significant. **FOOD:** Food delays absorption, decreases concentration. **LAB VALUES:** May increase serum amylase, lipase, bilirubin, ALT, AST, creatinine, glucose. May decrease serum albumin, platelets.

AVAILABILITY (Rx)

Oral Solution: 0.05 mg/ml. **Tablets:** 0.5 mg, 1 mg.

ADMINISTRATION/HANDLING

PO
• Administer tablets on an empty stomach (at least 2 hrs after a meal and 2 hrs before the next meal). • Do not dilute, mix oral solution with water or any other liquid. • Each bottle of oral solution is accompanied by a dosing spoon. Before administering, hold spoon in vertical position, fill it gradually to mark corresponding to prescribed dose.
Storage • Store tablets, oral solution at room temperature.

INDICATIONS/ROUTES/DOSAGE

Chronic Hepatitis B (No Previous Nucleoside Treatment)
PO: ADULTS, ELDERLY, CHILDREN 16 YRS AND OLDER: 0.5 mg once daily.

Chronic Hepatitis B (Receiving Lamivudine, Known Lamivudine Resistance, Decompensated Liver Disease)
PO: ADULTS, ELDERLY, CHILDREN 16 YRS AND OLDER: 1 mg once daily.

E

Dosage in Renal Impairment

Creatinine Clearance	Dosage
50 ml/min and greater	0.5 mg once daily
30–49 ml/min	0.25 mg once daily
10–29 ml/min	0.15 mg once daily
9 ml/min and less	0.05 mg once daily

SIDE EFFECTS

Occasional (4%–3%): Headache, fatigue.
Rare (less than 1%): Diarrhea, dyspepsia, nausea, vomiting, dizziness, insomnia.

ADVERSE EFFECTS/ TOXIC REACTIONS

Lactic acidosis, severe hepatomegaly with steatosis have been reported. Severe, acute exacerbations of hepatitis B have been reported in pts who have discontinued therapy; reinitiation of antihepatitis B therapy may be required. Hematuria occurs occasionally. May cause development of HIV resistance if HIV untreated.

NURSING CONSIDERATIONS

BASELINE ASSESSMENT

Obtain baseline laboratory tests, esp. hepatic function, before beginning therapy and at periodic intervals during therapy. Offer emotional support. Obtain full medication history.

INTERVENTION/EVALUATION

Hepatic function should be monitored closely with both clinical and laboratory follow-up for at least several mos in pts who discontinue antihepatitis B therapy. For pts on therapy, closely monitor serum amylase, lipase, bilirubin, ALT, AST, creatinine, glucose, albumin, platelet count. Assess for evidence of GI discomfort.

PATIENT/FAMILY TEACHING

• Take medication at least 2 hrs after a meal and 2 hrs before the next meal. • Avoid transmission of hepatitis B infection to others through sexual contact, blood contamination. • Immediately report unusual muscle pain, abdominal pain with nausea/vomiting, cold feeling in extremities, dizziness (signs and symptoms signaling onset of lactic acidosis).

enzalutamide

en-za-**loo**-ta-mide
(XTANDI)
Do not confuse enzalutamide with bicalutamide, flutamide, or nilutamide.

◆CLASSIFICATION

PHARMACOTHERAPEUTIC: Antiandrogen renal inhibitor. **CLINICAL:** Antineoplastic.

ACTION

Inhibits androgen binding to androgen receptors in target tissue, and inhibits interaction with DNA. **Therapeutic Effect:** Decreases proliferation, induces cell death of prostate cancer cells.

PHARMACOKINETICS

Readily absorbed in GI tract. Maximum plasma concentration achieved in 0.5–3 hrs. Metabolized in liver. Protein binding: (97%–98%). Primarily excreted in urine. **Half-life:** 5.8 days (Range: 2.8–10.2 days).

USES

Treatment of metastatic castration-resistant prostate cancer in pts who have previously received docetaxel.

PRECAUTIONS

Contraindications: Women who are pregnant or may become pregnant (not indicated in female population). **Cautions:** History of seizure, underlying brain injury with loss of consciousness, transient ischemic attack within past 12 mos, CVA, brain metastases, brain arteriovenous abnormality, use of concurrent medications that may lower seizure threshold.

⌛ LIFESPAN CONSIDERATIONS

Pregnancy/Lactation: Not used in female population. **Pregnancy Category X.** **Children:** Safety and efficacy not established. **Elderly:** No age-related precautions noted.

INTERACTIONS

DRUG: Strong CYP2C8, CYP3A4 inhibitors (e.g., gemfibrozil, itraconazole) may increase enzalutamide concentration. **Moderate or strong CYP3A4 inducers** may decrease concentration. **HERBAL:** None significant. **FOOD:** None known. **LAB VALUES:** May increase serum AST, ALT, bilirubin. May decrease Hgb, Hct, platelets, WBC count.

AVAILABILITY (Rx)

🔖 **Capsules:** 40 mg.

ADMINISTRATION/HANDLING

PO • Must be given on empty stomach. • No food is to be consumed 2 hrs before or 1 hr after each dose (food may increase absorption up to 10× normal limit). • Do not break, crush, dissolve, or open capsules.

INDICATIONS/ROUTES/DOSAGE

Metastatic Castration-Resistant Prostate Cancer
PO: ADULTS, ELDERLY: 160 mg (40 mg capsules) given once daily.

Dose Modification
If a grade 3 or greater toxicity or an intolerable side effect occurs, withhold dosing for 1 week or until symptoms improve to grade 2 or less, then resume at same dose or a reduced dose (120 mg or 80 mg). Concurrent use of strong CYP2C8 inhibitors (e.g., gemfibrozil) should be avoided if possible. If concurrent use is necessary, reduce the enzalutamide dose to 80 mg once daily.

SIDE EFFECTS

Common (51%): Asthenia (loss of strength, energy). **Frequent (26%–15%):** Back pain, diarrhea, arthralgia, hot flashes, peripheral edema, musculoskeletal pain. **Occasional (12%–6%):** Headache, dizziness, insomnia, hematuria, paresthesia, anxiety, hypertension. **Rare (4%–2%):** Mental impairment disorders (includes amnesia, memory impairment, cognitive disorder, attention deficit), hematuria (includes pollakiuria, pruritus, dry skin).

ADVERSE EFFECTS/ TOXIC REACTIONS

Upper respiratory tract infection occurs in 11% of pts; lower respiratory tract and lung infection (includes pneumonia, bronchitis) occur in slightly less (9%). Spinal cord compression and cauda equina syndrome occurs in 7% of pts.

NURSING CONSIDERATIONS

BASELINE ASSESSMENT

Offer emotional support. Obtain baseline CBC, ALT/AST, bilirubin periodically throughout therapy. Assess bowel activity, stool consistency. Pregnancy Category X. If coadministered with warfarin (CYP2C9 substrate), perform additional INR monitoring.

INTERVENTION/EVALUATION

Assess for peripheral edema behind medial malleolus (sacral area in bedridden patients). Question level of fatigue, weakness. Question presence of back pain, arthralgia, or headache. Assess level of anxiety. Monitor B/P for hypertension. Assess for hematuria. Question pt regarding sleeping pattern.

PATIENT/FAMILY TEACHING

• Sexually active men must wear condom during treatment and for 1 wk after treatment due to potential risks to fetus. • Women who are pregnant or are planning pregnancy may not touch medication without gloves. • Dizziness, headache, muscle weakness, leg swelling/discomfort should be reported. • Immediately report fever or cough. • Routine blood draws will occur during treatment.

✦ Canadian trade name · 🔖 Non-Crushable Drug · 🔲 High Alert drug

◄**ALERT**► Must be given on empty stomach. No food is to be consumed 2 hrs before or 1 hr after each dose. Food may increase absorption up to 10× normal limit.

epinephrine

ep-i-**nef**-rin
(Adrenalin, EpiPen, EpiPen Jr., Twinject)
Do not confuse epinephrine with ephedrine.

FIXED-COMBINATION(S)

LidoSite: epinephrine/lidocaine (anesthetic): 0.1%/10%.

◆ CLASSIFICATION

PHARMACOTHERAPEUTIC: Sympathomimetic (adrenergic agonist). **CLINICAL:** Antiglaucoma, bronchodilator, cardiac stimulant, antiallergic, antihemorrhagic, priapism reversal agent.

ACTION

Stimulates alpha-adrenergic receptors (vasoconstriction, pressor effects), beta$_1$-adrenergic receptors (cardiac stimulation), beta$_2$-adrenergic receptors (bronchial dilation, vasodilation). **Therapeutic Effect:** Relaxes smooth muscle of bronchial tree, produces cardiac stimulation, dilates skeletal muscle vasculature.

PHARMACOKINETICS

Route	Onset	Peak	Duration
IM	5–10 min	20 min	1–4 hrs
Subcutaneous	5–10 min	20 min	1–4 hrs
Inhalation	3–5 min	20 min	1–3 hrs

Well absorbed after parenteral administration; minimally absorbed after inhalation. Metabolized in liver, other tissues, sympathetic nerve endings. Excreted in urine. Ophthalmic form may be systemically absorbed as a result of drainage into nasal pharyngeal passages. Mydriasis occurs within several min and persists several hrs; vasoconstriction occurs within 5 min and lasts less than 1 hr.

USES

Treatment of asthma (acute exacerbation, reversible bronchospasm), anaphylaxis, hypersensitivity reaction, cardiac arrest. Added to local anesthetics to decrease systemic absorption and increase duration of activity of local anesthetic. Decreases superficial hemorrhage. **OFF-LABEL:** Ventricular fibrillation or pulseless ventricular tachycardia unresponsive to initial defibrillatory shocks; pulseless electrical activity, asystole, hypotension unresponsive to volume resuscitation; bradycardia/hypotension unresponsive to atropine or pacing; inotropic support.

PRECAUTIONS

Contraindications: Note: There are no absolute contraindications with injectable epinephrine in a life-threatening situation. **IV:** Narrow-angle glaucoma, shock, organic brain damage; during labor, heart failure; coronary insufficiency. **Inhalation:** Concurrent use or within 2 wks of MAOIs. **Cautions:** Elderly, diabetes mellitus, hypertension, Parkinson's disease, thyroid disease, cerebrovascular disease, concurrent use of tricyclic antidepressants.

⌛ LIFESPAN CONSIDERATIONS

Pregnancy/Lactation: Crosses placenta. Distributed in breast milk. **Pregnancy Category C. Children/Elderly:** No age-related precautions noted.

INTERACTIONS

DRUG: May decrease effects of **beta-blockers. Digoxin, sympathomimetics** may increase risk of arrhythmias. **Ergonovine, methergine, oxytocin** may increase vasoconstriction. **MAOIs, tricyclic antidepressants** may increase cardiovascular effects. **HERBAL:** **Ephedra, yohimbe** may increase CNS stimulation. **FOOD:** None known. **LAB VALUES:** May decrease serum potassium.

AVAILABILITY (Rx)

Injection, Solution (Prefilled Syringes):
(EpiPen): 0.3 mg/0.3 ml, *(EpiPen Jr.):* 0.15 mg/0.3 ml, *(Twinject):* 0.15 mg/0.15 ml. **Injection, Solution:** 0.1 mg/ml (1:10,000), 1 mg/ml (1:1,000).

Solution for Oral Inhalation
(Adrenalin): 2.25% (0.5 ml).

ADMINISTRATION/HANDLING

 IV

Reconstitution • For injection, dilute each 1 mg of 1:1,000 solution with 10 ml 0.9% NaCl to provide 1:10,000 solution and inject each 1 mg or fraction thereof over 1 min or more (except in cardiac arrest). • For infusion, further dilute with 250–500 ml D₅W. Maximum concentration 64 mcg/ml.
Rate of Administration • For IV infusion, give at 1–10 mcg/min (titrate to desired response).
Storage • Store parenteral forms at room temperature. • Do not use if solution appears discolored or contains a precipitate.

Subcutaneous
• Shake ampule thoroughly. • Use tuberculin syringe for injection into lateral deltoid region. • Massage injection site (minimizes vasoconstriction effect). Use only 1:1,000 solution.

Nebulizer
• No more than 10 drops Adrenalin Chloride solution 1:100 should be placed in reservoir of nebulizer. • Place nozzle just inside pt's partially opened mouth. • As bulb is squeezed once or twice, instruct pt to inhale deeply, drawing vaporized solution into lungs. • Rinse mouth with water immediately after inhalation (prevents mouth/throat dryness).

• When nebulizer is not in use, replace stopper, keep in upright position.

IV INCOMPATIBILITIES

Ampicillin, pantoprazole (Protonix), sodium bicarbonate.

IV COMPATIBILITIES

Calcium chloride, calcium gluconate, dexmedetomidine (Precedex), diltiazem (Cardizem), dobutamine (Dobutrex), dopamine (Intropin), fentanyl (Sublimaze), heparin, hydromorphone (Dilaudid), lorazepam (Ativan), midazolam (Versed), milrinone (Primacor), morphine, nitroglycerin, norepinephrine (Levophed), potassium chloride, propofol (Diprivan).

INDICATIONS/ROUTES/DOSAGE

Anaphylaxis
IM: **ADULTS, ELDERLY:** 0.2–0.5 mg (0.2–0.5 ml of 1:1,000 solution). May repeat if anaphylaxis persists. **CHILDREN WEIGHING 30 KG OR MORE:** 0.3 mg; may repeat in 5–15 min. **WEIGHING LESS THAN 30 KG:** 0.15 mg; may repeat in 5–15 min.

Asthma Bronchodilation
Subcutaneous: **ADULTS, ELDERLY:** 0.3–0.5 mg (0.3–0.5 ml of 1:1,000 solution) q20min times 3 doses. **CHILDREN:** 0.01 ml/kg/dose (1:1,000 solution); q20min times 3 doses.
Nebulization: **ADULTS, ELDERLY, CHILDREN 4 YRS OR OLDER:** Add 0.5 ml to hand bulb nebulizer: 1–3 inhalations up to q3h if needed.

Cardiac Arrest
IV: **ADULTS, ELDERLY:** Initially, 1 mg. May repeat q3–5min as needed. **CHILDREN:** Initially, 0.01 mg/kg (0.1 ml/kg of a 1:10,000 solution). May repeat q3–5min as needed.
Endotracheal: **ADULTS, ELDERLY:** 2–2.5 mg q3–5 min as needed. **CHILDREN:** 0.1 mg/kg (0.1 ml/kg of a 1:1,000 solution). May repeat q3–5min as needed.

Hypersensitivity Reaction
IM, Subcutaneous: **ADULTS, ELDERLY:** 0.2–0.5 mg (1:1,000) q15–20min.

 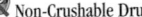

E

IV: 0.1 mg (1:10,000) over 5 min.
IM, Subcutaneous: CHILDREN: 0.01 mg/kg every 5–15 min. **Maximum single dose:** 0.3 mg.

SIDE EFFECTS

Frequent: Systemic: Tachycardia, palpitations, anxiety. **Ophthalmic:** Headache, eye irritation, watering of eyes. **Occasional: Systemic:** Dizziness, lightheadedness, facial flushing, headache, diaphoresis, increased B/P, nausea, trembling, insomnia, vomiting, fatigue. **Ophthalmic:** Blurred/decreased vision, eye pain. **Rare: Systemic:** Chest discomfort/pain, arrhythmias, bronchospasm, dry mouth/throat.

ADVERSE EFFECTS/ TOXIC REACTIONS

Excessive doses may cause acute hypertension, arrhythmias. Prolonged/excessive use may result in metabolic acidosis due to increased serum lactic acid. Metabolic acidosis may cause disorientation, fatigue, hyperventilation, headache, nausea, vomiting, diarrhea.

NURSING CONSIDERATIONS

INTERVENTION/EVALUATION

Monitor for vital sign changes. Assess lung sounds for rhonchi, wheezing, rales. Monitor ABGs. In cardiac arrest, adhere to ACLS protocols.

PATIENT/FAMILY TEACHING

• Avoid excessive use of caffeine. • Report any new symptoms (tachycardia, shortness of breath, dizziness) immediately: may be systemic effects.

---

epirubicin   `HIGH ALERT`

ep-i-**rue**-bi-sin
(Ellence, Pharmorubicin)
`BLACK BOX ALERT` Potential for cardiotoxicity, severe myelosuppre-

sion. May increase risk of secondary leukemias. With IV, severe local tissue damage, necrosis may occur. Must be administered by personnel trained in administration/handling of chemotherapeutic agents.

Do not confuse Ellence with Elase, or epirubicin with daunorubicin, doxorubicin, or idarubicin.

◆CLASSIFICATION

PHARMACOTHERAPEUTIC: Anthracycline antibiotic. **CLINICAL:** Antineoplastic (see p. 85C).

ACTION

May include formation of complex with DNA, subsequent inhibition of DNA, RNA, protein synthesis. Inhibits DNA helicase activity, preventing enzymatic separation of double-stranded DNA, interfering with replication, transcription. **Therapeutic Effect:** Produces antiproliferative, cytotoxic activity.

PHARMACOKINETICS

Widely distributed into tissues. Protein binding: 77%. Metabolized in liver and RBCs. Primarily eliminated through biliary excretion. Not removed by hemodialysis. **Half-life:** 33 hrs.

USES

Component of adjuvant therapy in pts with evidence of axillary node tumor involvement following resection of primary breast cancer. **OFF-LABEL:** Esophageal, gastric, soft tissue sarcoma; uterine sarcoma.

PRECAUTIONS

Contraindications: Hypersensitivity to epirubicin, previous treatment with anthracyclines up to maximum cumulative dose, recent MI, severe myocardial insufficiency, severe arrhythmias. **Cautions:** Renal/hepatic/cardiac impairment.

⌛ LIFESPAN CONSIDERATIONS

Pregnancy/Lactation: May cause fetal harm. Unknown if distributed in breast milk. **Pregnancy Category D. Children:**

Safety and efficacy not established. **Elderly:** No age-related precautions noted but monitor for toxicity.

INTERACTIONS

DRUG: Cytotoxic medications may increase risk of hematologic and GI effects. **Calcium channel blockers** may increase risk of developing heart failure. **Cimetidine** may increase serum concentration, toxicity. **Daunorubicin, doxorubicin, idarubicin, mitoxantrone** may increase risk of GI, hematologic, hepatic effects; cardiotoxicity. **Hepatotoxic medications** may increase risk of hepatotoxicity. **Live virus vaccines** may potentiate virus replication, increase vaccine side effects, decrease pt's antibody response to vaccine. **HERBAL: Echinacea** may decrease concentration. Avoid **black cohosh, dong quai** in estrogen-dependent tumors. **FOOD:** None known. **LAB VALUES:** May increase serum uric acid.

AVAILABILITY (Rx)

Injection Solution: 2-mg/ml single-use vials (25 ml, 100 ml). **Injection, Powder for Reconstitution:** 50 mg.

ADMINISTRATION/HANDLING

◀**ALERT**▶ Exclude pregnant staff from working with epirubicin; wear protective clothing. If accidental contact with skin or eyes occurs, flush area immediately with copious amounts of water.

 IV

Reconstitution • Ready-to-use vials require no reconstitution. **Powder:** Reconstitute with Sterile Water for Injection to final concentration of 2 mg/ml.
Rate of Administration • **IV Push:** Infuse medication into tubing of free-flowing IV of 0.9% NaCl or D₅W over 3–10 min. **IV Infusion:** Further dilute with 50–250 ml 0.9% NaCl or D₅W and infuse over 15–20 min.
Storage • Refrigerate vial of solution; store vials of powder at room temperature. • Protect from light. • Use within

24 hrs of first penetration of rubber stopper. • Discard unused portion.

🔅 IV INCOMPATIBILITIES

Fluorouracil (5-FU), heparin. Do not mix epirubicin in same syringe with other medications.

INDICATIONS/ROUTES/DOSAGE

◀**ALERT**▶ Avoid use of veins over joints or in extremities with compromised venous or lymphatic drainage.

Breast Cancer
IV: ADULTS: 60 mg/m² on days 1 and 8 q28days for 6 cycles or 100 mg/m² on day 1 q21days for 6 cycles in combination with 5-fluorouracil (5-FU) and Cytoxan. Dosage adjustment considered in pts with bone marrow depression or impaired renal function.

Dosage in Hepatic Impairment

Bilirubin 1.2–3 mg/dl or AST 2–4 times the upper limit of normal	50% of starting dose
Bilirubin >3 mg/dl or AST >4 times the upper limit of normal	25% of starting dose

SIDE EFFECTS

Frequent (83%–70%): Nausea, vomiting, alopecia, amenorrhea. **Occasional (9%–5%):** Stomatitis, diarrhea, hot flashes. **Rare (2%–1%):** Rash, pruritus, fever, lethargy, conjunctivitis.

ADVERSE EFFECTS/ TOXIC REACTIONS

Risk of cardiotoxicity (either acute, manifested as transient EKG abnormalities, or chronic, manifested as HF) increases when total cumulative dose exceeds 900 mg/m². Extravasation during administration may result in severe local tissue necrosis. Myelosuppression may produce hematologic toxicity, manifested principally as leukopenia and, to lesser extent, anemia, thrombocytopenia.

E

NURSING CONSIDERATIONS

BASELINE ASSESSMENT

Obtain CBC before and at frequent intervals during therapy. Obtain baseline serum chemistries before therapy. Obtain EKG before therapy, serum hepatic function studies before each dose. Antiemetics may be effective in preventing, treating nausea.

INTERVENTION/EVALUATION

Monitor for stomatitis (may lead to ulceration of mucous membranes within 2–3 days). Monitor blood counts for evidence of myelosuppression, renal/hepatic function studies. Assess cardiac function. Monitor daily pattern of bowel activity, stool consistency. Monitor for hematologic toxicity (fever, sore throat, signs of local infection, unusual bruising/bleeding from any site), symptoms of anemia (excessive fatigue, weakness). Monitor EKG changes. Assess injection site for extravasation, local skin reactions.

PATIENT/FAMILY TEACHING

• Hair loss is reversible, but new hair growth may have different color, texture. New hair growth resumes 2–3 mos after last therapy dose. • Maintain strict oral hygiene. • Do not have immunizations without physician's approval (drug lowers resistance). • Avoid contact with those who have recently received live virus vaccine. • Promptly report fever, sore throat, signs of local infection, unusual bruising/bleeding from any site.

eplerenone

ep-**ler**-e-none
(Inspra)
Do not confuse Inspra with Spiriva.

◆ CLASSIFICATION

PHARMACOTHERAPEUTIC: Aldosterone receptor antagonist. **CLINICAL:** Antihypertensive (see p. 105C).

ACTION

Binds to mineralocorticoid receptors in kidney, heart, blood vessels, brain, blocking binding of aldosterone. **Therapeutic Effect:** Reduces B/P.

PHARMACOKINETICS

Absorption unaffected by food. Protein binding: 50%. Metabolized in liver. Excreted in urine (67%), feces (32%). Not removed by hemodialysis. **Half-life:** 4–6 hrs.

USES

Treatment of hypertension alone or in combination with other antihypertensive agents. Treatment of HF following acute myocardial infarction (AMI).

PRECAUTIONS

Contraindications: Concurrent use with strong CYP3A4 inhibitors (e.g., ketoconazole, itraconazole), creatinine clearance less than 50 ml/min (30 ml/min or less in pts with hypertension), serum creatinine level greater than 2 mg/dl in males or 1.8 mg/dl in females, serum potassium level greater than 5.5 mEq/L, type 2 diabetes mellitus with microalbuminuria. Concomitant use with potassium supplements or potassium-sparing diuretics. **Cautions:** Hyperkalemia, HF, post MI, diabetes, mild renal impairment.

⧗ LIFESPAN CONSIDERATIONS

Pregnancy/Lactation: Unknown if drug crosses placenta or is distributed in breast milk. **Pregnancy Category B. Children:** Safety and efficacy not established. **Elderly:** No age-related precautions noted.

INTERACTIONS

DRUG: ACE inhibitors, angiotensin II antagonists potassium-sparing diuretics (e.g., **spironolactone**), **potassium supplements** increase risk of hyperkalemia. **CYP3A4 inhibitors** (e.g., **itraconazole, ketoconazole**) increase concentration five-fold (use is contraindicated). **NSAIDs** may decrease antihypertensive effect. **HERBAL:** **St. John's wort** decreases effectiveness. **FOOD:** **Grapefruit products** may increase potential for hyperkalemia, arrhythmias. **LAB VALUES:** May increase serum potassium, ALT, AST, cholesterol, triglycerides, serum creatinine, uric acid. May decrease serum sodium.

AVAILABILITY (Rx)

Tablets: 25 mg, 50 mg.

ADMINISTRATION/HANDLING

• Do not break, crush, cut film-coated tablets. • May give without regard to food.

INDICATIONS/ROUTES/DOSAGE

Hypertension
PO: ADULTS, ELDERLY: 50 mg once a day. If 50 mg once a day produces an inadequate B/P response, may increase dosage to 50 mg twice a day. If pt is concurrently receiving CYP3A4 inhibitors (e.g., erythromycin, saquinavir, verapamil, or fluconazole), reduce initial dose to 25 mg once a day.

HF Following MI
PO: ADULTS, ELDERLY: Initially, 25 mg once a day. If tolerated, titrate up to 50 mg once a day within 4 wks.

Dosage Adjustment for Serum Potassium Concentrations in HF
Less than 5 mEq/L: Increase dose from 25 mg daily to 50 mg daily or increase dose from 25 mg every other day to 25 mg daily.
5–5.4 mEq/L: No adjustment needed.
5.5–5.9 mEq/L: Decrease dose from 50 mg daily to 25 mg daily. Decrease dose from 25 mg daily to 25 mg every other day. Decrease dose from 25 mg every other day to withhold medication.
6 mEq/L or Greater: Withhold medication until potassium is less than 5.5 mEq/L, then restart at 25 mg every other day.

Dosage in Renal Impairment
Use is contraindicated in pts with hypertension with creatinine clearance less than 50 ml/min or serum creatinine greater than 2 mg/dl in males or greater than 1.8 mg/dl in females. All other indications, creatinine clearance less than 30 ml/min, use is contraindicated.

SIDE EFFECTS

Rare (3%–1%): Dizziness, diarrhea, cough, fatigue, flu-like symptoms, abdominal pain.

ADVERSE EFFECTS/ TOXIC REACTIONS

Hyperkalemia may occur, particularly in pts with type 2 diabetes mellitus and microalbuminuria.

NURSING CONSIDERATIONS

BASELINE ASSESSMENT

Obtain B/P, apical pulse immediately before each dose, in addition to regular monitoring (be alert to fluctuations). If excessive reduction in B/P occurs, place pt in supine position, feet slightly elevated.

INTERVENTION/EVALUATION

Assist with ambulation if dizziness occurs. Monitor serum potassium levels. Assess B/P for hypertension and hypotension. Monitor daily pattern of bowel activity, stool consistency. Assess for evidence of flu-like symptoms.

PATIENT/FAMILY TEACHING

• Avoid tasks that require alertness, motor skills until response to drug is established (possible dizziness effect). • Hypertension requires lifelong control. • Avoid exercising during hot weather (risk of dehydration, hypotension). • Do not use salt substitutes containing potassium.

epoetin alfa
TOP 200

e-**poe**-e-tin **al**-fa
(Epogen, Eprex ✤, Procrit)
BLACK BOX ALERT Increased risk of serious cardiovascular events,

---

thromboembolic events, mortality, time-to-tumor progression in pts with head and neck cancer, metastatic breast cancer, non–small-cell lung cancer when administered to a target hemoglobin of more than 11 g/dl. Increases rate of deep vein thrombosis in perioperative pts not receiving anticoagulant therapy. **Do not confuse epoetin with darbepoetin, or Epogen with Neupogen.**

♦**CLASSIFICATION**

PHARMACOTHERAPEUTIC: Glycoprotein. **CLINICAL:** Erythropoietin.

ACTION

Stimulates division, differentiation of erythroid progenitor cells in bone marrow. **Therapeutic Effect:** Induces erythropoiesis, releases reticulocytes from bone marrow.

PHARMACOKINETICS

Well absorbed after subcutaneous administration. Following administration, an increase in reticulocyte count occurs within 10 days, and increases in Hgb, Hct, and RBC count are seen within 2–6 wks. **Half-life:** 4–13 hrs.

USES

Treatment of anemia in pts receiving or who have received chemotherapy, pts with chronic renal failure to decrease need for RBC transfusion, HIV-infected pts on zidovudine (AZT) therapy when endogenous erythropoietin levels are 500 mUnits/ml or less, those scheduled for elective noncardiac, nonvascular surgery, reducing need for allogenic blood transfusions. **OFF-LABEL:** Anemia in myelodysplastic syndromes.

PRECAUTIONS

Contraindications: Pure red cell aplasia, uncontrolled hypertension. **Cautions:** History of seizures or hypertension. **Cancer pts:** Tumor growth, shortened survival may occur when Hgb levels of 11 g/dl or

greater are achieved with epoetin alfa. **Chronic kidney failure pts:** Increased risk for serious cardiovascular reactions (e.g., stroke, MI) when Hgb levels greater than 11 g/dl are achieved with epoetin alfa.

⚖ LIFESPAN CONSIDERATIONS

Pregnancy/Lactation: Unknown if drug crosses placenta or is distributed in breast milk. **Pregnancy Category C. Children:** Safety and efficacy not established in those 12 yrs and younger. **Elderly:** No age-related precautions noted.

INTERACTIONS

DRUG: None significant. **HERBAL:** None significant. **FOOD:** None known. **LAB VALUES:** May increase BUN, serum phosphorus, potassium, creatinine, uric acid, sodium. May decrease bleeding time, iron concentration, serum ferritin.

AVAILABILITY (Rx)

Injection Solution (Epogen, Procrit): 2,000 units/ml, 3,000 units/ml, 4,000 units/ml, 10,000 units/ml, 20,000 units/ml, 40,000 units/ml.

ADMINISTRATION/HANDLING

◀**ALERT**▶ Avoid excessive agitation of vial; do not shake (foaming).

 IV

Reconstitution • No reconstitution necessary.
Rate of Administration • May be given as an IV bolus.
Storage • Refrigerate. • Vigorous shaking may denature medication, rendering it inactive.

Subcutaneous
• Mix in syringe with bacteriostatic 0.9% NaCl with benzyl alcohol 0.9% (bacteriostatic saline) at a 1:1 ratio (benzyl alcohol acts as local anesthetic; may reduce injection site discomfort). • Use 1 dose per vial; do not reenter vial. Discard unused portion.

▨ IV INCOMPATIBILITIES

Do not mix injection form with other medications.

INDICATIONS/ROUTES/DOSAGE

Anemia Associated with Chemotherapy
◀ALERT▶ Begin therapy only if Hgb less than 10 g/dl and anticipated duration of myelosuppressive chemotherapy is greater than 2 months. Use minimum effective dose to maintain Hgb level that will avoid red blood cell transfusions. Discontinue upon completion of chemotherapy.
Subcutaneous: ADULTS, ELDERLY: Initially, 150 units/kg 3 times/wk (commonly used dose of 10,000 units 3 times/wk) or 40,000 units once weekly. **CHILDREN 5 YRS AND OLDER:** 600 units/kg once weekly. **Maximum:** 40,000 units.
Increase dose: (Adults, elderly): If Hgb does not increase by greater than 1 g/dl and remains below 10 g/dl after initial 4 wks may increase to 300 units/kg 3 times/wk or 60,000 units once weekly. *(Children):* If Hgb does not increase by greater than 1 g/dl and remains less than 10 g/dl after initial 4 wks of once-weekly dosing, may increase dose to 900 units/kg/wk. **Maximum:** 60,000 units once weekly.
Decrease dose: Decrease dose by 25% if Hgb increases greater than 1 g/dl in any 2-wk period or Hgb levels reaches level that will avoid red blood cell transfusions.

Reduction of Allogenic Blood Transfusions in Elective Surgery
Subcutaneous: ADULTS, ELDERLY: 300 units/kg/day for 10 days before and 4 days after surgery.

Anemia in Chronic Renal Failure
◀ALERT▶ Individualize dose, using lowest dose to reduce need for RBC transfusions. **ON DIALYSIS:** Initiate when Hgb less than 10 g/dl; reduce dose or discontinue if Hgb approaches or exceeds 11 g/dl. **NOT ON DIALYSIS:** Initiate when Hgb less than 10 g/dl; reduce dose or stop if Hgb exceeds 10 g/dl.
IV, Subcutaneous: ADULTS, ELDERLY: 50–100 units/kg 3 times/wk. **CHILDREN:** 50 units/kg 3 times/wk.
Maintenance:
Decrease dose by 25%: If Hgb increases greater than 1 g/dl in any 2-wk period.
Increase dose by 25%: If Hgb does not increase by greater than 1 g/dl after 4 wks of therapy. Do not increase dose more frequently than every 4 wks.
Note: If pt does not attain adequate response after appropriate dosing over 12 wks, do not continue to increase dose and use minimum effective dose to maintain Hgb level that will avoid red blood cell transfusions.

HIV Infection in Pts Treated with Zidovudine (AZT)
IV, Subcutaneous: ADULTS: Initially, 100 units/kg 3 times a wk for 8 wks; may increase by 50–100 units/kg 3 times a wk. Evaluate response q4–8wks thereafter. Adjust dosage by 50–100 units/kg 3 times a wk. If dosages larger than 300 units/kg 3 times a wk are not eliciting response, it is unlikely pt will respond. Maintenance: Titrate to maintain desired Hgb level. Hgb levels should not exceed 12 g/dl. If Hgb greater than 12 g/dl, resume treatment with 25% dose reduction when Hgb drops below 11 g/dl. Discontinue if Hgb increase not attained with 300 units/kg for 8 wks.

Anemia of Prematurity
Intravenous, Subcutaneous: 500–1,250 units/kg/wk divided in 2–5 doses for 10 doses.

SIDE EFFECTS

Pts Receiving Chemotherapy
Frequent (20%–17%): Fever, diarrhea, nausea, vomiting, edema. **Occasional (13%–11%):** Asthenia (loss of strength, energy), shortness of breath, paresthesia. **Rare (5%–3%):** Dizziness, trunk pain.

Pts with Chronic Renal Failure
Frequent (24%–11%): Hypertension, headache, nausea, arthralgia. **Occasional (9%–7%):** Fatigue, edema, diarrhea, vomiting, chest pain, skin reactions at administration site, asthenia (loss of strength, energy), dizziness.

Pts with HIV Infection Treated with AZT
Frequent (38%–15%): Fever, fatigue, headache, cough, diarrhea, rash, nausea. **Occasional (14%–9%):** Shortness of breath, asthenia (loss of strength, energy), skin reaction at injection site, dizziness.

ADVERSE EFFECTS/TOXIC REACTIONS

Hypertensive encephalopathy, thrombosis, cerebrovascular accident, MI, seizures occur rarely. Hyperkalemia occurs occasionally in pts with chronic renal failure, usually in those who do not comply with medication regimen, dietary guidelines, frequency of dialysis regimen.

NURSING CONSIDERATIONS

BASELINE ASSESSMENT

Assess B/P before drug initiation (80% of pts with chronic renal failure have history of hypertension). B/P often rises during early therapy in pts with history of hypertension. Consider that all pts eventually need supplemental iron therapy. Assess serum iron (should be greater than 20%), serum ferritin (should be greater than 100 ng/ml) before and during therapy. Establish baseline CBC (esp. note Hct).

INTERVENTION/EVALUATION

Assess CBC routinely. Monitor Hgb, Hct. Monitor aggressively for increased B/P (25% of pts on medication require antihypertensive therapy, dietary restrictions). Monitor temperature, esp. in cancer pts on chemotherapy and zidovudine-treated HIV pts. Monitor BUN, serum uric acid, creatinine, phosphorus, potassium, esp. in chronic renal failure pts.

PATIENT/FAMILY TEACHING

• Frequent laboratory assessments needed to determine correct dosage. • Immediately report any severe headache. • Avoid potentially hazardous activity during first 90 days of therapy (increased risk of seizures in pts with chronic renal failure during first 90 days). • Specific dietary regimen must be maintained.

eprosartan

ep-roe-**sar**-tan
(Teveten)

BLACK BOX ALERT May cause fetal injury, mortality if used during second or third trimester of pregnancy.

FIXED COMBINATION(S)

Teveten HCT: eprosartan/hydrochlorothiazide (a diuretic): 400 mg/12.5 mg.

◆CLASSIFICATION

PHARMACOTHERAPEUTIC: Angiotensin II receptor antagonist. **CLINICAL:** Antihypertensive (see p. 11C).

ACTION

Potent vasodilator. Blocks vasoconstrictor, aldosterone-secreting effects of angiotensin II, inhibiting binding of angiotensin II to AT_1 receptors. **Therapeutic Effect:** Causes vasodilation, decreases peripheral resistance, decreases B/P.

PHARMACOKINETICS

Rapidly absorbed after PO administration. Protein binding: 98%. Minimally metabolized in liver. Primarily excreted via urine, biliary system. Minimally removed by hemodialysis. **Half-life:** 5–9 hrs.

USES

Treatment of hypertension (alone or in combination with other medications).

PRECAUTIONS

Contraindications: Concomitant use with aliskiren in pts with diabetes. **Cautions:** Unstented renal artery stenosis, preexisting renal insufficiency, significant aortic/mitral stenosis, HF.

⌛ LIFESPAN CONSIDERATIONS

Pregnancy/Lactation: Has caused fetal and neonatal morbidity and mortality. Potential for adverse effects on breast-feeding infant. Breastfeeding not recommended. **Pregnancy Category C (D if used in second or third trimester).** **Children:** Safety and efficacy not established. **Elderly:** No age-related precautions noted.

INTERACTIONS

DRUG: Potassium-sparing diuretics, potassium supplements may increase risk of hyperkalemia. May produce additive effect with **antihypertensive agents. HERBAL: Ephedra, ginseng, yohimbe** may worsen hypertension. **Garlic** may increase antihypertensive effect. **FOOD:** None known. **LAB VALUES:** May increase BUN, serum alkaline phosphatase, bilirubin, creatinine, AST, ALT. May decrease Hgb, Hct.

AVAILABILITY (Rx)

🗡 **Tablets:** 400 mg, 600 mg.

ADMINISTRATION/HANDLING

PO
• Give without regard to food. • Do not break, cut, crush, or divide tablets.

INDICATIONS/ROUTES/DOSAGE

Hypertension
PO: ADULTS, ELDERLY: Initially, 600 mg/day. Range: 400–800 mg/day as single dose or 2 divided doses.

SIDE EFFECTS

Occasional (5%–2%): Headache, cough, dizziness. **Rare (less than 2%):** Muscle pain, fatigue, diarrhea, upper respiratory tract infection, dyspepsia.

ADVERSE EFFECTS/ TOXIC REACTIONS

Overdosage may manifest as hypotension, tachycardia. Bradycardia occurs less often.

NURSING CONSIDERATIONS

E

BASELINE ASSESSMENT

Obtain B/P, apical pulse immediately before each dose, in addition to regular monitoring (be alert to fluctuations). Question for possibility of pregnancy (see Pregnancy Category), history of hepatic/renal impairment, renal artery stenosis. Assess medication history (esp. diuretics).

INTERVENTION/EVALUATION

Monitor B/P, pulse, BUN, serum creatinine, electrolytes, urinalysis.

PATIENT/FAMILY TEACHING

• Inform female pt regarding consequences of second- and third-trimester exposure to medication. • Avoid tasks that require alertness, motor skills until response to drug is established. • Restrict sodium, alcohol intake. • Follow diet, control weight. • Do not stop taking medication; hypertension requires lifelong control. • Check B/P regularly. • Do not break, chew, crush, or divide tablets; take whole.

---

eptifibatide

ep-ti-**fye**-ba-tide
(<u>Integrilin</u>)

◆ CLASSIFICATION

PHARMACOTHERAPEUTIC: Glycoprotein IIb/IIIa inhibitor. **CLINICAL:** Antiplatelet, antithrombotic (see p. 34C).

ACTION

Produces rapid inhibition of platelet aggregation by preventing binding of fi-

---

brinogen to receptor sites on platelets. **Therapeutic Effect:** Prevents thrombus formation within coronary arteries. Prevents acute cardiac ischemic complications.

PHARMACOKINETICS

Protein binding: 25%. Excreted in urine. **Half-life:** 2.5 hrs.

USES

Treatment of pts with acute coronary syndrome (ACS), including those managed medically and those undergoing percutaneous coronary intervention (PCI). **OFF-LABEL:** Support PCI during ST-elevation myocardial infarction (STEMI).

PRECAUTIONS

Contraindications: Active abnormal bleeding within previous 30 days; history of bleeding diathesis; history of stroke within 30 days or history of hemorrhagic stroke; severe hypertension (SBP >200 mm Hg or DPB >110 mm Hg); major surgery within previous 6 wks, dependency on hemodialysis. **Cautions:** Impaired renal function, hemorrhagic retinopathy, platelet counts less than 100,000/mm³. **Pregnancy Category B.**

INTERACTIONS

DRUG: Anticoagulants, heparin, NSAIDs, antiplatelets, thrombolytic agents may increase risk of bleeding. **HERBAL: Cat's claw, dong quai, evening primrose, feverfew, garlic, ginger, ginkgo, ginseng** may increase antiplatelet effects. **FOOD:** None known. **LAB VALUES:** Increases PT, aPTT, clotting time. Decreases platelet count.

AVAILABILITY (Rx)

Injection Solution: 0.75 mg/ml, 2 mg/ml.

ADMINISTRATION/HANDLING

 IV

Reconstitution • Withdraw bolus dose from 10-ml vial (2 mg/ml); for IV infu-sion, withdraw from 100-ml vial (0.75 mg/ml). • IV push and infusion adminis-tration may be given undiluted.
Rate of Administration • Give bolus dose IV push over 1–2 min.
Storage • Store vials in refrigerator. • Solution appears clear, colorless. • Do not shake. • Discard any unused portion left in vial or if preparation contains *any* opaque particles.

▥ IV INCOMPATIBILITIES

Administer in separate line; do not add other medications to infusion solution.

▥ IV COMPATIBILITIES

Amiodarone (Cordarone), argatroban, bivalirudin, metoprolol (Lopressor).

INDICATIONS/ROUTES/DOSAGE

Adjunct to Percutaneous Coronary Intervention (PCI)
IV Bolus, IV Infusion: ADULTS, ELDERLY: 180 mcg/kg (**maximum: 22.6 mg**) be-fore PCI initiation; then continuous drip of 2 mcg/kg/min and a second 180 mcg/kg (**maximum: 22.6 mg**) bolus 10 min after the first. **Maximum:** 15 mg/hr. Continue until hospital discharge or for up to 18–24 hrs. Minimum 12 hrs is recommended. Concurrent aspirin and heparin therapy is recommended.

Acute Coronary Syndrome (ACS)
IV Bolus, IV Infusion: ADULTS, ELDERLY: 180 mcg/kg (**maximum: 22.6 mg**) bo-lus then 2 mcg/kg/min until discharge or coronary artery bypass graft, up to 72 hrs. **Maximum:** 15 mg/hr. Concurrent aspirin and heparin therapy is recom-mended.

Dosage in Renal Impairment
Creatinine Clearance Less than 50 ml/min: Use 180 mcg/kg bolus (**maxi-mum: 22.6 mg**) and 1 mcg/kg/min infu-sion (**maximum: 7.5 mg/hr**).

SIDE EFFECTS

Occasional (7%): Hypotension.

ADVERSE EFFECTS/ TOXIC REACTIONS

Minor to major bleeding complications may occur, most commonly at arterial access site for cardiac catheterization.

NURSING CONSIDERATIONS

BASELINE ASSESSMENT

Assess platelet count, Hgb, Hct before treatment and during therapy. If platelet count less than 90,000/mm^3, additional platelet counts should be obtained routinely to avoid thrombocytopenia.

INTERVENTION/EVALUATION

Diligently monitor for potential bleeding, particularly at other arterial, venous puncture sites. If possible, urinary catheters, nasogastric tubes should be avoided.

---

eribulin

er-i-bue-lin
(Halaven)
Do not confuse eribulin with epirubicin or erlotinib.

◆ CLASSIFICATION

PHARMACOTHERAPEUTIC: Microtubule inhibitor. **CLINICAL:** Antineoplastic.

ACTION

Binds directly on microtubules during active stage of G_2 and M phases of cell cycle, preventing formation of microtubules, an essential part of process of separation of chromosomes. **Therapeutic Effect:** Blocks cells in mitotic phase of cell division, leading to cell death.

PHARMACOKINETICS

Extensively metabolized in liver. Protein binding: 49%–65%. Excreted in feces (82%), urine (9%). **Half-life:** 40 hrs.

USES

Treatment of metastatic breast cancer in pts who previously received at least 2 chemotherapeutic regimens for treatment, including an anthracycline and a taxane agent.

PRECAUTIONS

Contraindications: None known. **Cautions:** Prolonged QTc (congenital, other medications that prolong QT interval), hepatic/ renal impairment, moderate to severe neuropathy, HF.

⧗ LIFESPAN CONSIDERATIONS

Pregnancy/Lactation: May cause embryo-fetal toxicity. Unknown if distributed in breast milk. **Pregnancy Category D. Children:** Safety and efficacy not established in those younger than 18 yrs. **Elderly:** No age-related precautions noted.

INTERACTIONS

DRUG: None significant. **FOOD:** None known. **HERBAL:** None significant. **LAB VALUES:** May decrease WBC, Hgb, Hct, platelet count, potassium. May increase ALT.

AVAILABILITY (Rx)

Injection, Solution: 1 mg/2 ml (0.5-mg/ ml).

ADMINISTRATION/HANDLING

 IV

Reconstitution • May administer undiluted or dilute in 100 ml 0.9% NaCl.
Rate of Administration • Administer over 2–5 min.
Storage • Store at room temperature. • Once diluted, syringe or diluted solution may be stored for up to 4 hrs at room temperature or up to 24 hrs if refrigerated.

▧ IV INCOMPATIBILITIES

Do not dilute with D$_5$W or administer through IV line containing solutions with dextrose or in same IV line with other medications.

INDICATIONS/ROUTES/DOSAGE

Metastatic Breast Cancer
IV: ADULTS, ELDERLY: 1.4 mg/m² over 2–5 min on days 1 and 8 of 21-day cycle.

Mild Hepatic/Renal Impairment
(Creatinine Clearance 30–50 ml/min)
IV: ADULTS, ELDERLY: 1.1 mg/m² over 2–5 min on days 1 and 8 of 21-day cycle.

Moderate Hepatic Impairment
IV: ADULTS, ELDERLY: 0.7 mg/m² over 2–5 min on days 1 and 8 of 21-day cycle.

Recommended Dose Delays
Do not administer day 1 or day 8 of treatment for any of the following: ANC less than 1,000/mm³, platelets less than 75,000/mm³, grade 3 or 4 nonhematologic toxicities. Day 8 dose may be delayed for maximum of 1 wk. If toxicities do not resolve or improve to grade 2 severity by day 15, omit dose. If toxicities resolve or improve to grade 2 severity by day 15, continue treatment at reduced dose and initiate next cycle no sooner than 2 wks later. Do not re-escalate dose after it has been reduced.

SIDE EFFECTS

Common (54%–35%): Fatigue, asthenia (loss of strength, energy), alopecia, peripheral sensory neuropathy, nausea. **Frequent (25%–18%):** Constipation, arthralgia/myalgia, decreased weight, anorexia, pyrexia, headache, diarrhea, vomiting. **Occasional (16%–9%):** Back pain, dyspnea, cough, bone pain, extremity pain, urinary tract infection, oral mucosal inflammation.

ADVERSE EFFECTS/ TOXIC REACTIONS

Neutropenia occurs in 82% of pts, with 57% developing grade 3 neutropenia. Severe neutropenia (ANC less than 500/mm³) lasting more than 1 wk occurred in 12%. Anemia occurs in 58% of pts. Peripheral neuropathy occurs in 8% of pts but is the most common adverse reaction requiring discontinuation of therapy. Prolonged QTc may be noted on day 8 of treatment.

NURSING CONSIDERATIONS

BASELINE ASSESSMENT
Question for possibility of pregnancy. Obtain baseline CBC, serum chemistries before treatment begins. Obtain CBC prior to each dose.

INTERVENTION/EVALUATION
Diligently monitor for neutropenia, peripheral neuropathy (most frequent cause of drug discontinuation). Monitor for symptoms of neuropathy (burning sensation, hyperesthesia, hypoesthesia, paresthesia, discomfort, neuropathic pain). Assess hands, feet for erythema. Monitor CBC for evidence of neutropenia, thrombocytopenia. Assess mouth for stomatitis (erythema, ulceration, mucosal burning).

PATIENT/FAMILY TEACHING
• Avoid crowds, those with known infection. • Avoid contact with anyone who recently received live virus vaccine. • Do not have immunizations without physician's approval (drug lowers body resistance). • Promptly report fever over 100.5°F, chills, cough, burning or pain urinating, numbness, tingling, burning sensation, erythema of hands/feet.

erlotinib

er-**loe**-tih-nib
(<u>Tarceva</u>)
Do not confuse erlotinib with dasatinib, eribulin, geftinib, imatinib, or lapatinib.

◆**CLASSIFICATION**

PHARMACOTHERAPEUTIC: Human epidermal growth factor. **CLINICAL:** Antineoplastic (see p. 85C).

ACTION

Inhibits tyrosine kinases (TK) associated with transmembrane cell surface receptors found on both normal and cancer cells. One such receptor is epidermal growth factor receptor (EGFR). **Therapeutic Effect:** TK activity appears to be vitally important to cell proliferation and survival.

PHARMACOKINETICS

About 60% is absorbed after PO administration; bioavailability is increased by food to almost 100%. Protein binding: 93%. Extensively metabolized in liver. Primarily eliminated in feces; minimal excretion in urine. **Half-life:** 24–36 hrs.

USES

Treatment of locally advanced or metastatic non–small-cell lung cancer (NSCLC) after failure of at least one prior chemotherapy regimen (as monotherapy). Treatment of locally advanced, unresectable, or metastatic pancreatic cancer (in combination with gemcitabine). Maintenance treatment of locally advanced or metastatic NSCLC that has not progressed after 4–6 cycles of first-line platinum-based chemotherapy. **OFF-LABEL:** Salvage therapy of advanced or metastatic breast, or head and neck tumors.

PRECAUTIONS

Contraindications: None known. **Cautions:** Severe hepatic/renal impairment, cardiovascular disease. Concurrent use of strong CYP3A4 inhibitors and inducers (see Appendix J).

⏳ LIFESPAN CONSIDERATIONS

Pregnancy/Lactation: Unknown if drug crosses placenta or is distributed in breast milk. **Pregnancy Category D. Children:** Safety and efficacy not established. **Elderly:** No age-related precautions noted.

INTERACTIONS

DRUG: CYP3A4 inhibitors (e.g., atanzavir, clarithromycin, indinavir, itraconazole, ketoconazole, nefazodone, nelfinavir, ritonavir, saquinavir) may increase concentration/effects. **CYP3A4**
inducers (e.g., carbamazepine, phenobarbital, phenytoin, rifampin)** may decrease concentration/effect. **Proton pump inhibitors (e.g., omeprazole), H_2 antagonists (e.g., ranitidine)** may decrease absorption/effect. **HERBAL: St. John's wort** may decrease concentration/effects. **FOOD: Grapefruit products** may increase potential for myelotoxicity. **LAB VALUES:** May increase serum bilirubin, ALT, AST.

AVAILABILITY (Rx)

Tablets: 25 mg, 100 mg, 150 mg.

ADMINISTRATION/HANDLING

PO
• Give at least 1 hr before or 2 hrs after ingestion of food. • Avoid grapefruit, grapefruit juice. • May dissolve in 3–4 oz water and give orally or via feeding tube.

INDICATIONS/ROUTES/DOSAGE

◀ALERT▶ Dosage adjustment for toxicity: Reduce dose in 50-mg increments.

Lung Cancer
PO: ADULTS, ELDERLY: 150 mg/day until disease progression or unacceptable toxicity occurs.

Pancreatic Cancer
PO: ADULTS, ELDERLY: 100 mg/day in combination with gemcitabine until disease progression or unacceptable toxicity occurs.

Dosage in Renal Impairment
Interrupt dosing for renal disease due to dehydration.

Dosage in Hepatic Impairment
Reduce starting dose to 75 mg and individualize dose escalation if tolerated.

SIDE EFFECTS

Frequent (greater than 10%): Fatigue, anxiety, headache, depression, insomnia, rash, pruritus, dry skin, erythema, diarrhea, anorexia, nausea, vomiting, mucositis, constipation, dyspepsia, weight loss, dysphagia, abdominal pain, arthralgia, dyspnea, cough. **Occasional (10%–1%):** Keratitis. **Rare (less than 1%):** Corneal ulceration.

ADVERSE EFFECTS/ TOXIC REACTIONS

UTI occurs occasionally. Pneumonitis, GI bleeding occur rarely.

NURSING CONSIDERATIONS

BASELINE ASSESSMENT

Obtain CBC, serum electrolytes, hepatic enzyme levels before beginning therapy.

INTERVENTION/EVALUATION

Assess hepatic enzyme levels, CBC, renal function, serum electrolytes, hydration status periodically.

PATIENT/FAMILY TEACHING

• Take drug on empty stomach. • Report rash, blood in stool, diarrhea, irritated eyes, fever. • Avoid grapefruit products.

ertapenem

er-ta-**pen**-em
(Invanz)
Do not confuse ertapenem with doripenem, imipenem, or meropenem, or Invanz with Avinza.

◆CLASSIFICATION

PHARMACOTHERAPEUTIC: Carbapenem. **CLINICAL:** Antibiotic.

ACTION

Penetrates bacterial cell wall of microorganisms, binds to penicillin-binding proteins, inhibiting cell wall synthesis. **Therapeutic Effect:** Produces bacterial cell death.

PHARMACOKINETICS

Almost completely absorbed after IM administration. Protein binding: 85%–95%. Widely distributed. Primarily excreted in urine (80%), feces (10%). Removed by hemodialysis. **Half-life:** 4 hrs.

USES

Treatment of susceptible infections due to *S. aureus* (methicillin-susceptible only), *S. agalactiae*, *S. pneumoniae* (penicillin-susceptible only), *S. pyogenes*, *E. coli*, *H. influenzae* (beta-lactamase negative strains only), *K. pneumoniae*, *M. catarrhalis*, *Bacteroides* spp., *C. clostridioforme*, *Peptostreptococcus* spp., including moderate to severe intra-abdominal, skin/skin structure infections; community-acquired pneumonia; complicated UTI; acute pelvic infection; adult diabetic foot infections without osteomyelitis. Prevention of surgical site infection.

PRECAUTIONS

Contraindications: History of anaphylactic hypersensitivity to beta-lactams (e.g., imipenem and cilastin, meropenem), hypersensitivity to amide-type local anesthetics (IM). **Cautions:** Hypersensitivity to penicillins, cephalosporins, renal impairment, CNS disorders, esp. brain lesions or history of seizures.

⌛ LIFESPAN CONSIDERATIONS

Pregnancy/Lactation: Distributed in breast milk. **Pregnancy Category B. Children:** Safety and efficacy not established in those younger than 18 yrs. **Elderly:** Advanced or end-stage renal insufficiency may require dosage adjustment.

INTERACTIONS

DRUG: Probenecid may increase concentration/effect. May decrease concentration/effect of **valproic acid. HERBAL:** None significant. **FOOD:** None known. **LAB VALUES:** May increase serum alkaline phosphatase, AST, ALT, bilirubin, BUN, creatinine, glucose, PT, aPTT, sodium. May decrease platelet count, Hgb, Hct, WBC.

AVAILABILITY (Rx)

Injection, Powder for Reconstitution: 1 g.

ADMINISTRATION/HANDLING

 IV

Reconstitution • Dilute 1-g vial with 10 ml 0.9% NaCl or Bacteriostatic Water for Injection. • Shake well to dissolve. • Further dilute with 50 ml 0.9% NaCl (**maximum concentration:** 20 mg/ml). **Rate of Administration** • Give by intermittent IV infusion (piggyback). Do not give IV push. • Infuse over 30 min. **Storage** • Solution appears colorless to yellow (variation in color does not affect potency). • Discard if solution contains precipitate. • Reconstituted solution is stable for 6 hrs at room temperature or 24 hrs if refrigerated.

IM

• Reconstitute with 3.2 ml 1% lidocaine HCl injection (without epinephrine). • Shake vial thoroughly. • Inject deep in large muscle mass (gluteal or lateral part of thigh). • Administer suspension within 1 hr after preparation.

🔳 IV INCOMPATIBILITIES

Do not mix or infuse with any other medications. Do not use diluents or IV solutions containing dextrose.

🔳 IV COMPATIBILITIES

Heparin, potassium chloride, tigecycline (Tygacil), Sterile Water for Injection, 0.9% NaCl.

INDICATIONS/ROUTES/DOSAGE

Usual Dosage Range
IM, IV: ADULTS, ELDERLY, CHILDREN 13 YRS AND OLDER: 1 g/day. **CHILDREN 3 MOS–12 YRS:** 15 mg/kg 2 times/day. **Maximum:** 1 g/day.

Intra-Abdominal Infection
IV, IM: ADULTS, ELDERLY, CHILDREN 13 YRS AND OLDER: 1 g/day for 5–14 days. **CHILDREN 3 MOS–12 YRS:** 15 mg/kg 2 times/day. **Maximum:** 1 g/day.

Skin/Skin Structure Infection
IV, IM: ADULTS, ELDERLY, CHILDREN 13 YRS AND OLDER: 1 g/day for 7–14 days. **CHILDREN 3 MOS–12 YRS:** 15 mg/kg 2 times/day. **Maximum:** 1 g/day.

Pneumonia, UTI
IV, IM: ADULTS, ELDERLY, CHILDREN 13 YRS AND OLDER: 1 g/day for 10–14 days. **CHILDREN 3 MOS–12 YRS:** 15 mg/kg 2 times/day. **Maximum:** 1 g/day.

Pelvic Infection
IV, IM: ADULTS, ELDERLY, CHILDREN 13 YRS AND OLDER: 1 g/day for 3–10 days. **CHILDREN 3 MOS–12 YRS:** 15 mg/kg 2 times/day. **Maximum:** 1 g/day.

Diabetic Foot Infection
IV, IM: ADULTS, ELDERLY: 1 g/day for 7–14 days.

Prevention of Surgical Site Infection
IV: ADULTS, ELDERLY: 1 g given 1 hr preoperatively.

Dosage in Renal Impairment

Creatinine clearance 30 ml/min or less	500 mg once daily
Hemodialysis	If daily dose given within 6h prior to HD, give 150 mg dose after HD.
Peritoneal dialysis	500 mg once daily

SIDE EFFECTS

Frequent (10%–6%): Diarrhea, nausea, headache. **Occasional (5%–2%):** Altered mental status, insomnia, rash, abdominal pain, constipation, chest pain, vomiting, edema, fever. **Rare (less than 2%):** Dizziness, cough, oral candidiasis, anxiety, tachycardia, phlebitis at IV site.

ADVERSE EFFECTS/ TOXIC REACTIONS

Antibiotic-associated colitis, other superinfections (abdominal cramps, severe watery diarrhea, fever) may result from altered bacterial balance. Anaphylactic reactions have been reported. Seizures may occur in those with CNS disorders (brain lesions, history of seizures), bacterial meningitis, severe renal impairment.

NURSING CONSIDERATIONS

BASELINE ASSESSMENT

Question for history of allergies, particularly to beta-lactams, penicillins, cephalosporins. Inquire about history of seizures. Monitor WBC count.

INTERVENTION/EVALUATION

Monitor renal/hepatic function. Monitor daily pattern of bowel activity, stool consistency. Monitor for nausea, vomiting. Evaluate hydration status. Evaluate for inflammation at IV injection site. Assess skin for rash. Observe mental status; be alert to tremors, possible seizures. Assess sleep pattern for evidence of insomnia.

PATIENT/FAMILY TEACHING

• Notify physician in event of tremors, seizures, rash, prolonged diarrhea, chest pain, other new symptoms.

erythromycin

er-**ith**-roe-**mye**-sin
(Akne-Mycin, Apo-Erythro Base ✦, EES, Erybid ✦, Eryc, EryDerm, EryPed, Ery-Tab, Erythrocin, PCE Dispertab)
Do not confuse Eryc with Emcyt, or erythromycin with azithromycin or clarithromycin.

FIXED-COMBINATION(S)

Eryzole, Pediazole: erythromycin/sulfisoxazole (sulfonamide): 200 mg/600 mg per 5 ml.

◆CLASSIFICATION

PHARMACOTHERAPEUTIC: Macrolide. **CLINICAL:** Antibiotic, antiacne (see p. 27C).

ACTION

Penetrates bacterial cell membranes, reversibly binds to bacterial ribosomes, inhibiting protein synthesis. **Therapeutic Effect:** Bacteriostatic.

PHARMACOKINETICS

Variably absorbed from GI tract (depending on dosage form used). Protein binding: 70%–90%. Widely distributed. Metabolized in liver. Primarily eliminated in feces by bile. Not removed by hemodialysis. **Half-life:** 1.4–2 hrs (increased in renal impairment).

USES

Treatment of susceptible infections due to *S. pyogenes, S. pneumoniae, S. aureus, M. pneumoniae, Legionella, Chlamydia, N. gonorrheae, E. histolytica,* including syphilis, nongonococcal urethritis, diphtheria, pertussis, chancroid, *Campylobacter* gastroenteritis. **Topical:** Treatment of acne vulgaris. **Ophthalmic:** Prevention of gonococcal ophthalmia neonatorum, superficial ocular infections. **OFF-LABEL: Systemic:** Treatment of acne vulgaris, chancroid, *Campylobacter* enteritis, gastroparesis, Lyme disease, preoperative gut sterilization. **Topical:** Treatment of minor bacterial skin infections. **Ophthalmic:** Treatment of blepharitis, conjunctivitis, keratitis, chlamydial trachoma.

PRECAUTIONS

Contraindications: Hepatic impairment. Concomitant administration with ergot derivatives, lovastatin, simvastatin. **Cautions:** Elderly, myasthenia gravis. CYP3A4 inhibitors.

⌛ LIFESPAN CONSIDERATIONS

Pregnancy/Lactation: Crosses placenta. Distributed in breast milk. Erythromycin estolate may increase hepatic enzymes in pregnant women. **Pregnancy Category B. Children/Elderly:** No age-related precautions noted. High dosage in those with decreased hepatic/renal function increases risk of hearing loss.

INTERACTIONS

DRUG: May increase concentration of **buspirone, cyclosporine, calcium channel blockers, statins.** May inhibit metabolism of **carbamazepine. Hepatotoxic medications** may increase risk of hepatotoxicity. May increase risk of **theophylline** toxicity. May increase effects of **warfarin. HERBAL: St. John's wort** may decrease concentration. **FOOD: Grapefruit** may increase potential for torsades. **LAB VALUES:** May increase serum alkaline phosphatase, bilirubin, AST, ALT.

AVAILABILITY (Rx)

Gel, Topical: 2%. **Ointment, Ophthalmic:** 0.5%. **Ointment, Topical (Akne-Mycin):** 2%. **Oral Suspension (EES, EryPed):** 100 mg/2.5 ml, 200 mg/5 ml, 400 mg/5ml. **Tablet as Base:** 250 mg, 333 mg, 500 mg. **Tablet as Ethylsuccinate (EES):** 400 mg. **Tablet as Stearate (Erythrocin):** 250 mg, 500 mg.

 Capsules, Delayed-Release (Eryc): 250 mg. **Tablets, Delayed-Release (Ery-Tab):** 250 mg, 333 mg, 500 mg.

ADMINISTRATION/HANDLING

 IV

Reconstitution • Reconstitute each 500 mg with 10 ml Sterile Water for Injection without preservative to provide a concentration of 50 mg/ml. • Further dilute with 100–250 ml D_5W or 0.9% NaCl to maximum concentration of 5 mg/ml.

Rate of Administration • For intermittent IV infusion (piggyback), infuse over 20–60 min.

Storage • Store parenteral form at room temperature. • Initial reconstituted solution in vial is stable for 2 wks refrigerated or 24 hrs at room temperature. • Diluted IV solution stable for 8 hrs at room temperature or 24 hrs if refrigerated. • Discard if precipitate forms.

PO

• Store capsules, tablets at room temperature. • Oral suspension is stable for 14 days at room temperature. • Adminis-

ter erythromycin base, stearate 1 hr before or 2 hrs following ingestion of food. Erythromycin estolate, ethylsuccinate may be given without regard to meals, but optimal absorption occurs when given on empty stomach. • Give with 8 oz water. • If swallowing difficulties occur, sprinkle capsule contents on teaspoon of applesauce, follow with water. • Do not crush delayed-release capsules, tablets.

Ophthalmic

• Place gloved finger on lower eyelid and pull out until a pocket is formed between eye and lower lid. • Place ¼–½ inch of ointment into pocket. • Instruct pt to close eye gently for 1–2 min (so medication will not be squeezed out of the sac) and to roll eyeball to increase contact area of drug to eye.

⊞ IV INCOMPATIBILITIES

Fluconazole (Diflucan), furosemide (Lasix), heparin, metoclopramide (Reglan).

⊞ IV COMPATIBILITIES

Amiodarone (Cordarone), diltiazem (Cardizem), hydromorphone (Dilaudid), lidocaine, lorazepam (Ativan), magnesium sulfate, midazolam (Versed), morphine, multivitamins, potassium chloride.

INDICATIONS/ROUTES/DOSAGE

Mild to Moderate Infections of Upper and Lower Respiratory Tract, Pharyngitis, Skin Infections

PO: ADULTS, ELDERLY: BASE: 250–500 mg q6–12h. **CHILDREN:** 30–50 mg/kg/day in 2–4 divided doses. **Maximum:** 2 g/day. **ETHYLSUCCINATE:** 400–800 mg q6–12h. **Maximum:** 4 g/day. **CHILDREN:** 30–50 mg/kg/day in divided doses. **Maximum:** 3.2 g/day. **NEONATES:** 10 mg/kg/dose q8–12h.

IV: ADULTS, ELDERLY: 15–20 mg/kg/day divided q6h. **Maximum:** 4 g/day. **CHILDREN, INFANTS:** 15–50 mg/kg/day divided q6h. **Maximum:** 4 g /day.

Preop Intestinal Antisepsis
PO: ADULTS, ELDERLY: 1 g at 1 PM, 2 PM, and 11 PM on day before surgery (with neomycin). **CHILDREN:** 20 mg/kg at 1 PM, 2 PM, and 11 PM on day before surgery (with neomycin).

Acne Vulgaris
Topical: ADULTS: Apply thin layer to affected area twice a day.

Gonococcal Ophthalmia Neonatorum
Ophthalmic: NEONATES: 0.5–2 cm no later than 1 hr after delivery.

SIDE EFFECTS

Frequent: IV: Abdominal cramping/discomfort, phlebitis/thrombophlebitis. **Topical:** Dry skin (50%). **Occasional:** Nausea, vomiting, diarrhea, rash, urticaria. **Rare: Ophthalmic:** Sensitivity reaction with increased irritation, burning, itching, inflammation. **Topical:** Urticaria.

ADVERSE EFFECTS/ TOXIC REACTIONS

Antibiotic-associated colitis, other super-infections (abdominal cramps, severe watery diarrhea, fever), reversible cholestatic hepatitis may occur. High dosage in pts with renal impairment may lead to reversible hearing loss. Anaphylaxis occurs rarely. Ventricular arrhythmias, prolonged QT interval occur rarely with IV form.

NURSING CONSIDERATIONS

BASELINE ASSESSMENT

Question for history of allergies (particularly erythromycins), hepatitis.

INTERVENTION/EVALUATION

Monitor daily pattern of bowel activity, stool consistency. Assess skin for rash. Assess for hepatotoxicity (malaise, fever, abdominal pain, GI disturbances). Be alert for superinfection: fever, vomiting, diarrhea, anal/genital pruritus, oral mucosal changes (ulceration, pain, erythema). Check for phlebitis (heat, pain, red streaking over vein). Monitor for high-dose hearing loss.

PATIENT/FAMILY TEACHING

• Continue therapy for full length of treatment. • Doses should be evenly spaced. • Take medication with 8 oz water 1 hr before or 2 hrs following food or beverage. • **Ophthalmic:** Report burning, itching, inflammation. • **Topical:** Report excessive skin dryness, itching, burning. • Improvement of acne may not occur for 1–2 mos; maximum benefit may take 3 mos; therapy may last mos or yrs. • Use caution if using other topical acne preparations containing peeling or abrasive agents, medicated or abrasive soaps, cosmetics containing alcohol (e.g., astringents, aftershave lotion).

escitalopram   TOP 200

es-sye-**tal**-o-pram
(Cipralex ✦, <u>Lexapro</u>)
BLACK BOX ALERT Increased risk of suicidal ideation and behavior in children, adolescents, young adults 18–24 yrs with major depressive disorder, other psychiatric disorders.

◆CLASSIFICATION

PHARMACOTHERAPEUTIC: Serotonin reuptake inhibitor. **CLINICAL:** Antidepressant (see p. 40C).

ACTION

Blocks uptake of neurotransmitter serotonin at neuronal presynaptic membranes, increasing its availability at postsynaptic receptor sites. **Therapeutic Effect:** Antidepressant effect.

PHARMACOKINETICS

Well absorbed after PO administration. Protein binding: 56%. Primarily metabolized in liver. Primarily excreted in feces, with a lesser amount eliminated in urine. **Half-life:** 35 hrs.

USES

Treatment of major depressive disorder. Treatment of generalized anxiety disorder (GAD). **OFF-LABEL:** Social anxiety disorders in children and adolescents, developmental disorders (including autism). Treatment of mild dementia-associated agitation in nonpsychotic pt.

PRECAUTIONS

Contraindications: Use within 14 days of MAOIs. **Cautions:** Hepatic/renal impairment, history of seizures, concurrent use of CNS depressants, pts at high risk of suicide, concomitant aspirin, NSAIDs, warfarin (may potentiate bleeding risk).

⌛ LIFESPAN CONSIDERATIONS

Pregnancy/Lactation: Distributed in breast milk. **Pregnancy Category C. Children:** May cause increased anticholinergic effects or hyperexcitability. **Elderly:** More sensitive to anticholinergic effects (e.g., dry mouth), more likely to experience dizziness, sedation, confusion, hypotension, hyperexcitability.

INTERACTIONS

DRUG: Alcohol, other CNS suppressants may increase CNS depression. **Linezolid, aspirin, NSAIDs, warfarin** may increase risk of bleeding. **MAOIs** may cause serotonin syndrome (autonomic hyperactivity, diaphoresis, excitement, hyperthermia, rigidity, neuroleptic malignant syndrome, coma). **Sumatriptan** may cause weakness, hyperreflexia, poor coordination. **HERBAL: Gotu kola, kava kava, SAMe, St. John's wort, valerian** may increase CNS depression. **Ginkgo biloba, St. John's wort** may increase risk of serotonin syndrome. **FOOD:** None known. **LAB VALUES:** May decrease serum sodium.

AVAILABILITY (Rx)

Oral Solution: 5 mg/5 ml.
🔖 **Tablets:** 5 mg, 10 mg, 20 mg.

ADMINISTRATION/HANDLING

PO
• Give without regard to food. • Do not crush, cut tablets.

INDICATIONS/ROUTES/DOSAGE

Depression
PO: ADULTS: Initially, 10 mg once a day in the morning or evening. May increase to 20 mg after a minimum of 1 wk. **ELDERLY:** 10 mg/day. **CHILDREN 12–17 YRS:** Initially, 10 mg once daily. May increase to 20 mg/day after at least 3 wks. **Maximum:** 20 mg once daily. Recommended: 10 mg once daily.

Generalized Anxiety Disorder
PO: ADULTS: Initially, 10 mg once a day in morning or evening. May increase to 20 mg after minimum of 1 wk. **ELDERLY:** 10 mg/day.

Dosage in Renal Impairment
Use caution in pts with creatinine clearance less than 20 ml/min.

Dosage in Hepatic Impairment
10 mg/day.

SIDE EFFECTS

Frequent (21%–11%): Nausea, dry mouth, drowsiness, insomnia, diaphoresis. **Occasional (8%–4%):** Tremor, diarrhea, abnormal ejaculation, dyspepsia, fatigue, anxiety, vomiting, anorexia. **Rare (3%–2%):** Sinusitis, sexual dysfunction, menstrual disorder, abdominal pain, agitation, decreased libido.

ADVERSE EFFECTS/ TOXIC REACTIONS

Overdose manifested as dizziness, drowsiness, tachycardia, confusion, seizures.

NURSING CONSIDERATIONS

BASELINE ASSESSMENT

For pts on long-term therapy, hepatic/renal function tests, blood counts should be performed periodically. Observe, record behavior. Assess psychological status, thought content, sleep pattern, appearance, interest in environment.

INTERVENTION/EVALUATION

Supervise suicidal-risk pt closely during early therapy (as depression lessens, energy level improves, suicide potential increases). Assess appearance, behavior, speech pattern, level of interest, mood. Monitor for suicidal ideation (esp. at beginning of therapy or when doses are increased or decreased), social interaction, mania, panic attacks.

PATIENT/FAMILY TEACHING

• Do not stop taking medication or increase dosage. • Avoid alcohol. • Avoid tasks that require alertness, motor skills until response to drug is established. • Report worsening depression, suicidal ideation, unusual changes in behavior.

---

esmolol

es-moe-lol
(Brevibloc)
Do not confuse Brevibloc with Bumex or Buprenex, or esmolol with Osmitrol.

◆CLASSIFICATION

PHARMACOTHERAPEUTIC: Beta₁-adrenergic blocker. **CLINICAL:** Antiarrhythmic (see p. 18C).

ACTION

Selectively blocks beta₁-adrenergic receptors. **Therapeutic Effect:** Slows sinus heart rate, decreases cardiac output, reducing B/P.

PHARMACOKINETICS

Rapidly metabolized primarily by esterase in cytosol of red blood cells. Protein binding: 55%. Less than 1%–2% excreted in urine. **Half-life:** 9 min.

USES

Rapid, short-term control of ventricular rate in supraventricular tachycardia (SVT), atrial fibrillation or flutter; treatment of tachycardia and/or hypertension (esp. in-

traop or postop). Treatment of noncompensatory sinus tachycardia. **OFF-LABEL:** Postoperative hypertension or SVT in children. Arrhythmia and/or rate control during ACS, intubation, thyroid storm, pheochromocytoma, electroconvulsive therapy.

PRECAUTIONS

Contraindications: Cardiogenic shock, uncompensated cardiac failure, second- or third-degree heart block (except in pts with pacemaker), sinus bradycardia. **Cautions:** Pts with sick sinus syndrome; compensated heart failure; concurrent use of digoxin, verapamil, diltiazem; diabetes; myasthenia gravis; renal impairment; history of anaphylaxis to allergens.

⌛ LIFESPAN CONSIDERATIONS

Pregnancy/Lactation: Crosses placenta; distributed in breast milk. **Pregnancy Category C. Children:** Safety and efficacy not established. **Elderly:** No age-related precautions noted.

INTERACTIONS

DRUG: Opioids, calcium channel blockers, MAOIs may increase level/effects. **HERBAL: Yohimbe** may decrease effects. **FOOD:** None known. **LAB VALUES:** None significant.

AVAILABILITY (Rx)

Injection Solution: 10 mg/ml (250 ml), 20 mg/ml (100 ml).

ADMINISTRATION/HANDLING

◀**ALERT**▶ Give by IV infusion. Avoid butterfly needles, very small veins (can cause thrombophlebitis).

 IV

Rate of Administration • Administer by controlled infusion device; titrate to tolerance and response. • Infuse IV loading dose over 1–2 min. • Hypotension (systolic B/P less than 90 mm Hg) is greatest during first 30 min of IV infusion.

Storage • Use only clear and colorless to light yellow solution. • Discard solution if discolored or precipitate forms.

IV INCOMPATIBILITIES

Amphotericin B complex (Abelcet, AmBisome, Amphotec), furosemide (Lasix).

IV COMPATIBILITIES

Amiodarone (Cordarone), dexmedetomidine (Precedex), diltiazem (Cardizem), dopamine (Intropin), heparin, magnesium, midazolam (Versed), potassium chloride, propofol (Diprivan).

INDICATIONS/ROUTES/DOSAGE

Rate Control in Supraventricular Arrhythmias
IV: ADULTS, ELDERLY: Initially, loading dose of 500 mcg/kg/min for 1 min, followed by 50 mcg/kg/min for 4 min. If optimum response is not attained in 5 min, give second loading dose of 500 mcg/kg/min for 1 min, followed by infusion of 100 mcg/kg/min for 4 min. A third (and final) loading dose can be given and infusion increased by 50 mcg/kg/min, up to 200 mcg/kg/min, for 4 min. Once desired response is attained, increase infusion by no more than 25 mcg/kg/min. Infusion usually administered over 24–48 hrs in most pts. Range: 50–200 mcg/kg/min (average dose 100 mcg/kg/min).

Intraop/Postop Tachycardia Hypertension (Immediate Control)
IV: ADULTS, ELDERLY: Initially, 80 mg over 30 sec, then 150 mcg/kg/min infusion up to 300 mcg/kg/min.

SIDE EFFECTS

Generally well tolerated, with transient, mild side effects. **Frequent:** Hypotension (systolic B/P less than 90 mm Hg) manifested as dizziness, nausea, diaphoresis, headache, cold extremities, fatigue. **Occasional:** Anxiety, drowsiness, flushed skin, vomiting, confusion, inflammation at injection site, fever.

ADVERSE EFFECTS/ TOXIC REACTIONS

Overdose may produce profound hypotension, bradycardia, dizziness, syncope, drowsiness, breathing difficulty, bluish fingernails or palms of hands, seizures. May potentiate insulin-induced hypoglycemia in diabetic pts.

NURSING CONSIDERATIONS

BASELINE ASSESSMENT

Assess B/P, apical pulse immediately before drug is administered (if pulse is 60 or less/min or systolic B/P is 90 mm Hg or less, withhold medication, contact physician).

INTERVENTION/EVALUATION

Monitor B/P for hypotension, EKG, heart rate, respiratory rate, development of diaphoresis, dizziness (usually first sign of impending hypotension). Assess pulse for quality, irregular rate, bradycardia, extremities for coldness. Assist with ambulation if dizziness occurs. Assess for nausea, diaphoresis, headache, fatigue.

---

esomeprazole `TOP 200`

es-o-**mep**-ra-zole
(Nexium)
Do not confuse esomeprazole with aripiprazole or omeprazole, or Nexium with Nexavar.

FIXED-COMBINATION(S)

Vimovo: esomeprazole/naproxen (NSAID): 20 mg/375 mg, 20 mg/500 mg.

◆CLASSIFICATION

PHARMACOTHERAPEUTIC: Proton pump inhibitor. **CLINICAL:** Gastric acid inhibitor (see p. 147C).

ACTION

Converted to active metabolites that irreversibly bind to, inhibit enzymes on surface of gastric parietal cells. Inhibits hydrogen ion transport into gastric lumen. **Therapeutic Effect:** Increases gastric pH; reduces gastric acid production.

PHARMACOKINETICS

Well absorbed after PO administration. Protein binding: 97%. Extensively metabolized in liver. Primarily excreted in urine. **Half-life:** 1–1.5 hrs.

USES

PO: Short-term treatment (4–8 wks) of erosive esophagitis (diagnosed by endoscopy); symptomatic gastroesophageal reflux disease (GERD). Treatment of Zollinger-Ellison syndrome. Used in triple therapy with amoxicillin and clarithromycin for treatment of *H. pylori* infection in pts with duodenal ulcer. Reduces risk of NSAID-induced gastric ulcer. **IV:** Treatment of GERD with erosive esophagitis. Short-term treatment of GERD when oral therapy is not appropriate. **OFF-LABEL:** Prevent recurrent peptic ulcer bleeding postendoscopy.

PRECAUTIONS

Contraindications: Hypersensitivity to benzimidazoles. **Cautions:** May increase risk of hip, wrist, spine fractures; hepatic impairment; elderly; Asian populations. Concurrent use of CYP3A4 inducers (e.g., rifampin).

⌛ LIFESPAN CONSIDERATIONS

Pregnancy/Lactation: Unknown if drug crosses placenta or is distributed in breast milk. **Pregnancy Category B. Children:** Safety and efficacy not established. **Elderly:** No age-related precautions noted.

INTERACTIONS

DRUG: May decrease concentration/effects of **atazanavir, digoxin, iron, ketoconazole.** May increase effect of **warfarin.** May decrease effect of **clopidogrel.** CYP3A4 inducers (e.g., rifampin) may decrease concentration/effect. **HERBAL:** St. John's wort may decrease concentration/effects. **FOOD:** None known. **LAB VALUES:** None significant.

AVAILABILITY (Rx)

Injection, Powder for Reconstitution: 20 mg, 40 mg. **Oral Suspension, Delayed-Release Packets:** 10 mg, 20 mg, 40 mg.

 Capsules (Delayed-Release [Nexium]): 20 mg, 40 mg.

ADMINISTRATION/HANDLING

🖢 IV

Reconstitution • For IV push, add 5 ml of 0.9% NaCl to esomeprazole vial.
Infusion • For IV infusion, dissolve content of one vial in 50 ml 0.9% NaCl, or D_5W.
Rate of Administration • For IV push, administer over not less than 3 min. For intermittent infusion (piggyback) infuse over 10–30 min. • Flush line with 0.9% NaCl, or D_5W, both before and after administration.
Storage • Use only clear and colorless to very slightly yellow solution. • Discard solution if particulate forms. • IV infusion stable for 12 hrs in 0.9% NaCl or lactated Ringer's; 6 hrs in D_5W.

PO (Capsules)

• Give 1 hr or more before eating (best before breakfast). • Do not crush, cut capsule; administer whole. • For those with difficulty swallowing capsules, open capsule and mix pellets with 1 tbsp applesauce. Swallow spoonful without chewing.

PO (Oral Suspension)

• Empty contents into 15 ml water and stir. • Let stand 2–3 min to thicken. • Stir and drink within 30 min.

🖳 IV INCOMPATIBILITIES

Do not mix esomeprazole with any other medications through the same IV line or tubing.

🖳 IV COMPATIBILITIES

Ceftaroline (Teflaro), doripenem (Doribax).

INDICATIONS/ROUTES/DOSAGE

Erosive Esophagitis
PO: ADULTS, ELDERLY, CHILDREN 12 YRS AND OLDER: 20–40 mg once daily for 4–8 wks. May continue for additional 4–8 wks. **CHILDREN 1–11 YRS, WEIGHING 20 KG OR MORE:** 10–20 mg/day for up to 8 wks. **WEIGHING LESS THAN 20 KG:** 10 mg/day for up to 8 wks.

Maintenance Therapy for Erosive Esophagitis
PO: ADULTS, ELDERLY: 20 mg/day.

Treatment of NSAID-Induced Gastric Ulcers
PO: ADULTS, ELDERLY: 20 mg/day for 4–8 wks.

Prevention of NSAID-Induced Gastric Ulcer
PO: ADULTS, ELDERLY: 20–40 mg once a day for up to 6 mos.

Gastroesophageal Reflux Disease (GERD)
IV: ADULTS, ELDERLY: 20 or 40 mg once daily for up to 10 days. **CHILDREN 1–17 YRS, WEIGHING 55 KG OR MORE:** 20 mg once daily; **1–17 YRS, WEIGHING LESS THAN 55 KG:** 10 mg once daily; **1 MO TO LESS THAN 1 YR:** 0.5 mg/kg once daily.
PO: ADULTS, ELDERLY, CHILDREN, 12–17 YRS: 20 mg once daily. **CHILDREN 1–11 YRS:** 10 mg/day for up to 8 wks.

Zollinger-Ellison Syndrome
PO: ADULTS, ELDERLY: 40 mg 2 times a day. Doses up to 240 mg/day have been used.

Duodenal Ulcer Caused by *Helicobacter Pylori*
PO: ADULTS, ELDERLY: 40 mg (esomeprazole) once a day, with amoxicillin 1,000 mg and clarithromycin 500 mg twice a day for 10 days.

Dosage Hepatic Impairment
SEVERE: Doses should not exceed 20 mg/day.

SIDE EFFECTS

Frequent (7%): Headache. **Occasional (3%–2%):** Diarrhea, abdominal pain, nausea. **Rare (less than 2%):** Dizziness, asthenia (loss of strength, energy), vomiting, constipation, rash, cough.

ADVERSE EFFECTS/ TOXIC REACTIONS

Pancreatitis, hepatotoxicity, interstitial nephritis occur rarely.

NURSING CONSIDERATIONS

BASELINE ASSESSMENT
Assess epigastric/abdominal pain.

INTERVENTION/EVALUATION
Evaluate for therapeutic response (relief of GI symptoms). Question if GI discomfort, nausea, diarrhea occur. Monitor for occult blood, observe for hemorrhage in pts with peptic ulcer.

PATIENT/FAMILY TEACHING
• Report headache. • Take at least 1 hr before eating. • If swallowing capsules is difficult, open capsule and mix pellets with 1 tbsp applesauce. Swallow spoonful without chewing.

estradiol

es-tra-**dye**-ole
(Alora, Climara, Delestrogen, Depo-Estradiol, Divigel, Elestrin, Estrace, Estraderm, Estrasorb, Estring, Estrogel, Evamist, Femring, Femtrace, Menostar, Vagifem, Vivelle Dot)

BLACK BOX ALERT Increased risk of dementia when given to women 65 yrs and older. Use of estrogen without progestin increases risk of endometrial cancer in postmenopausal women with intact uterus. Do not use to prevent cardiovascular disease or dementia.

Do not confuse Alora with Aldara, or Estraderm with Testoderm.

E

E

FIXED-COMBINATION(S)

Activella: estradiol/norethindrone (hormone): 1 mg/0.5 mg. **Climara PRO:** estradiol/levonorgestrel (progestin): 0.045 mg/24 hr, 0.015 mg/24 hr. **Combi-patch:** estradiol/norethindrone (hormone): 0.05 mg/0.14 mg, 0.05 mg/0.25 mg. **Femhrt:** estradiol/norethindrone (hormone): 5 mcg/1 mg. **Lunelle:** estradiol/medroxy-progesterone (progestin): 5 mg/25 mg per 0.5 ml.

◆CLASSIFICATION

PHARMACOTHERAPEUTIC: Estrogen. **CLINICAL:** Estrogen, antineoplastic.

ACTION

Increases synthesis of DNA, RNA, proteins in target tissues; reduces release of gonadotropin-releasing hormone from hypothalamus; reduces follicle-stimulating hormone (FSH), luteinizing hormone (LH) release from pituitary. **Therapeutic Effect:** Promotes normal growth/development of female sex organs, maintains GU function, vasomotor stability. Prevents accelerated bone loss by inhibiting bone resorption, restoring balance of bone resorption, formation. Inhibits LH, decreases serum testosterone concentration.

PHARMACOKINETICS

Well absorbed from GI tract. Widely distributed. Protein binding: 50%–80%. Metabolized in liver. Primarily excreted in urine. **Half-life:** Unknown.

USES

Treatment of moderate to severe vasomotor symptoms, vulvar and vaginal atrophy associated with menopause, hypoestrogenism (due to hypogonadism, primary ovarian failure), metastatic breast cancer (palliation) in men and post-menopausal women, advanced prostate cancer (palliation), prevention of osteoporosis in menopausal women.

PRECAUTIONS

Contraindications: Hepatic dysfunction or disease, undiagnosed abnormal vaginal bleeding, active or history of arterial thrombosis, estrogen-dependent cancer, known or suspected breast cancer (except for pts being treated for metastatic disease), pregnancy, thrombophlebitis or thromboembolic disorders (current or history of). **Cautions:** Renal insufficiency, diabetes mellitus, endometriosis, hypercalcemia, hyperlipidemias, asthma, epilepsy, migraines, SLE, hypertension, hypocalcemia, hypothyroidism, history of jaundice due to past estrogen use or pregnancy, cardiovascular disease, obesity, porphyria.

⧗ LIFESPAN CONSIDERATIONS

Pregnancy/Lactation: Distributed in breast milk. May be harmful to infant. Breastfeeding not recommended. **Pregnancy Category X. Children:** Caution in those for whom bone growth is not complete (may accelerate epiphyseal closure). **Elderly:** No age-related precautions noted.

INTERACTIONS

DRUG: CYP3A4 inducers (e.g., carbamazepine, rifampin) may decrease concentration/effect. **CYP3A4 inhibitors (e.g., ketoconazole, ritonavir)** may increase concentration/effect. **HERBAL:** Avoid **black cohosh, dong quai, saw palmetto;** may enhance toxic/adverse effects. **St. John's wort** may decrease concentration/effects of estrogens. **FOOD:** None known. **LAB VALUES:** May increase serum glucose, calcium, HDL, triglycerides. May decrease serum cholesterol, LDL. May affect metapyrone testing, thyroid function tests.

AVAILABILITY (Rx)

Emulsion, Topical (Estrasorb): 4.35 mg estradiol/1.74 g pouch (contents of 2 pouches deliver estradiol 0.05 mg/day). **Gel, Topical: (Divigel):** 0.1% (0.25-g packet delivers estradiol 0.25 mg, 0.5 g-packet delivers estradiol 0.5 mg, 1-g packet delivers 1 mg). (Elestrin): 0.06% delivers 0.52 mg estradiol/actuation. (Estrogel): 0.06% delivers 0.75 mg/actuation. Injection (Cypionate): Depo-Estradiol: 5 mg/ml. (Valerate): Delestrogen: 10 mg/ml, 20 mg/ml, 40 mg/ml. Tablets: (Estrace): 0.5 mg, 1 mg, 2 mg. (Femtrace): 0.9 mg. Topical Spray (Evamist): 1.53 mg/spray. Transdermal System (Alora): twice weekly: 0.025 mg/24 hrs, 0.05 mg/24 hrs, 0.075 mg/24 hrs, 0.1 mg/24 hrs. Transdermal System (Climara): once weekly: 0.025 mg/24 hrs, 0.0375 mg/24 hrs, 0.05 mg/24 hrs, 0.06 mg/24 hrs, 0.075 mg/24 hrs, 0.1 mg/24 hrs. Transdermal System (Menostar): once weekly: 0.014 mg/24 hrs. Transdermal System (Vivelle Dot): twice weekly: 0.025 mg/24 hrs, 0.0375 mg/24 hrs, 0.05 mg/24 hrs, 0.075 mg/24 hrs, 0.1 mg/24 hrs. Vaginal Cream (Estrace): 0.1 mg/g. Vaginal Ring (Estring): 2 mg (releases 7.5 mcg/day over 90 days). Vaginal Ring (Femring): 0.05 mg/day (total estradiol 12.4 mg-release 0.05 mg/day over 3 mos); 0.1 mg/day (total estradiol 24.8 mg-release 0.1 mg/day over 3 mos). Vaginal Tablet (Vagifem): 10 mcg.

ADMINISTRATION/HANDLING

IM
• Rotate vial to disperse drug in solution.
• Inject deep IM in large muscle mass.

PO
• Administer at same time each day.
• Administer with food.

Transdermal
• Remove old patch; select new site (buttocks are alternative application site). • Peel off protective strip to expose adhesive surface. • Apply to clean, dry, intact skin on trunk of body (area with as little hair as possible). • Press in place for at least 10 sec (do not apply to breasts or waistline).

Vaginal
• Apply at bedtime for best absorption.
• Insert end of filled applicator into vagina, directed slightly toward sacrum; push plunger down completely. • Avoid skin contact with cream (prevents skin absorption).

INDICATIONS/ROUTES/DOSAGE

Prostate Cancer
IM *(Delestrogen)*: **ADULTS, ELDERLY:** 30 mg or more q1–2wks.
PO: ADULTS, ELDERLY: 1–2 mg tid for at least 3 mos.

Breast Cancer
PO: ADULTS, ELDERLY: 10 mg 3 times a day for at least 3 mos.

Osteoporosis Prophylaxis in Postmenopausal Females
PO: ADULTS, ELDERLY: 0.45–0.5 mg/day cyclically (3 wks on, 1 wk off).
Transdermal *(Climara)*: **ADULTS, ELDERLY:** Initially, 0.025 mg/24 hrs weekly, adjust dose as needed.
Transdermal *(Alora, Vivelle Dot)*: **ADULTS, ELDERLY:** Initially, 0.025 mg/24 hrs patch twice weekly, adjust dose as needed.
Transdermal *(Menostar)*: **ADULTS, ELDERLY:** 0.014 mg/24 hrs patch weekly.

Female Hypoestrogenism
PO: ADULTS, ELDERLY: 0.9–2 mg/day, adjust dose as needed.
IM *(Depo-Estradiol)*: **ADULTS, ELDERLY:** 1.5–2 mg monthly.
IM *(Delestrogen)*: **ADULTS, ELDERLY:** 10–20 mg q4wks.

Vasomotor Symptoms Associated with Menopause
PO: ADULTS, ELDERLY: 0.9–2 mg/day cyclically (3 wks on, 1 wk off), adjust dose as needed.
IM *(Depo-Estradiol)*: **ADULTS, ELDERLY:** 1–5 mg q3–4wks.
IM *(Delestrogen)*: **ADULTS, ELDERLY:** 10–20 mg q4wks.
Topical Emulsion *(Estrasorb)*: **ADULTS, ELDERLY:** 3.48 g (contents of 2 pouches) once a day in the morning.

E

Topical Gel *(Estrogel)*: **ADULTS, ELDERLY:** 1.25 g/day.

Transdermal Spray *(Evamist)*: Initially, 1 spray daily. May increase to 2–3 sprays daily.

Transdermal *(Climara)*: **ADULTS, ELDERLY:** 0.025 mg/24 hrs weekly. Adjust dose as needed.

Transdermal *(Alora, Vivelle Dot)*: **ADULTS, ELDERLY:** 0.05 mg/24 hrs twice a wk.

Vaginal Ring *(Femring)*: **ADULTS, ELDERLY:** 0.05 mg. May increase to 0.1 mg if needed.

Vaginal Atrophy

Vaginal Ring *(Estring)*: **ADULTS, ELDERLY:** 2 mg.

Vaginal Cream *(Estrace)*: Insert 2–4 g/day intravaginally for 2 wks, then reduce dose by ½ initial dose for 2 wks, then maintenance dose of 1 g 1–3 times a wk.

Atrophic Vaginitis

Vaginal Tablet *(Vagifem)*: **ADULTS, ELDERLY:** Initially, 1 tablet/day for 2 wks. Maintenance: 1 tablet twice a wk.

SIDE EFFECTS

Frequent: Anorexia, nausea, swelling of breasts, peripheral edema marked by swollen ankles and feet. **Transdermal:** Skin irritation, redness. **Occasional:** Vomiting (esp. with high doses), headache (may be severe), intolerance to contact lenses, hypertension, glucose intolerance, brown spots on exposed skin. **Vaginal:** Local irritation, vaginal discharge, changes in vaginal bleeding (spotting, breakthrough, prolonged bleeding). **Rare:** Chorea (involuntary movements), hirsutism (abnormal hairiness), loss of scalp hair, depression.

ADVERSE EFFECTS/ TOXIC REACTIONS

Prolonged administration increases risk of gallbladder disease, thromboembolic disease, breast/cervical/vaginal/endometrial/hepatic carcinoma. Cholestatic jaundice occurs rarely.

NURSING CONSIDERATIONS

BASELINE ASSESSMENT

Assess frequency/severity of vasomotor symptoms. Question for hypersensitivity to estrogen, previous jaundice, thromboembolic disorders associated with pregnancy, estrogen therapy. Question for possibility of pregnancy (Pregnancy Category X).

INTERVENTION/EVALUATION

Monitor B/P, weight, serum calcium, glucose, hepatic enzymes. Monitor for loss of vision, sudden onset of proptosis, diplopia, migraine, thromboembolic disorders.

PATIENT/FAMILY TEACHING

• Limit alcohol, caffeine. • Avoid grapefruit products. • Immediately report sudden headache, vomiting, disturbance of vision/speech, numbness/weakness of extremities, chest pain, calf pain, shortness of breath, severe abdominal pain, mental depression, unusual bleeding. • Avoid smoking. • Report abnormal vaginal bleeding. • Never place patch on breast or waistline.

---

estramustine

es-tra-**mus**-teen
(Emcyt)
Do not confuse Emcyt with Eryc, or estramustine with exemestane.

◆CLASSIFICATION

PHARMACOTHERAPEUTIC: Alkylating agent, estrogen/nitrogen mustard. **CLINICAL:** Antineoplastic (see p. 85C).

ACTION

Binds to microtubule-associated proteins, causing their disassembly. **Therapeutic Effect:** Reduces serum testosterone concentration.

PHARMACOKINETICS

Well absorbed from GI tract. Highly localized in prostatic tissue. Metabolized in liver. Primarily eliminated in feces by biliary system. **Half-life:** 20 hrs.

USES

Treatment of metastatic or progressive carcinoma of prostate gland.

PRECAUTIONS

Contraindications: Active thrombophlebitis or thromboembolic disorders (unless tumor is cause of thromboembolic disorder and benefits outweigh risk), hypersensitivity to estradiol, nitrogen mustard. **Cautions:** History of thrombophlebitis, thrombosis, thromboembolic disorders; cerebrovascular, coronary artery disease; hepatic impairment; renal insufficiency; migraine, seizure disorder; hypertension.

⌛ LIFESPAN CONSIDERATIONS

Pregnancy/Lactation: Not indicated for use in women. **Children:** Not used in this pt population. **Elderly:** Age-related renal impairment and/or peripheral vascular disease may require dosage adjustment.

INTERACTIONS

DRUG: Hepatotoxic medications may increase risk of hepatotoxicity. **HERBAL: Echinacea** may decrease concentration/effects. **FOOD: Milk, dairy products, other calcium-rich foods** may impair absorption. **LAB VALUES:** May increase serum glucose, bilirubin, cortisol, LDH, phospholipid, prolactin, AST, sodium, triglyceride. May decrease serum phosphate. May alter thyroid function test results.

AVAILABILITY (Rx)

Capsules: 140 mg.

ADMINISTRATION/HANDLING

PO
• Refrigerate capsules (may remain at room temperature for 24–48 hrs without loss of potency). • Give with water 1 hr before or 2 hrs after meals.

INDICATIONS/ROUTES/DOSAGE

Prostatic Carcinoma
PO: ADULTS, ELDERLY: 10–16 mg/kg/day (most common: 14 mg/kg/day) in 3–4 divided doses.

SIDE EFFECTS

Frequent: Peripheral edema (esp. lower extremities), breast tenderness/enlargement, diarrhea, flatulence, nausea. **Occasional:** Increase in B/P, thirst, dry skin, ecchymosis, flushing, alopecia, night sweats. **Rare:** Headache, rash, fatigue, insomnia, vomiting.

ADVERSE EFFECTS/TOXIC REACTIONS

May exacerbate HF; increased risk of pulmonary emboli, thrombophlebitis, CVA.

NURSING CONSIDERATIONS

INTERVENTION/EVALUATION

Monitor serum calcium, hepatic function tests, B/P periodically.

PATIENT/FAMILY TEACHING

• Do not take with milk, milk products, calcium-rich food, calcium-containing antacids. • Use contraceptive measures during therapy. • If headache (migraine or severe), vomiting, disturbed speech/vision, dizziness, numbness, shortness of breath, calf pain, chest pain/pressure, unexplained cough occurs, contact physician.

eszopiclone TOP 200

e-**zop**-i-klone
(Lunesta)
Do not confuse Lunesta with Neulasta.

◆ CLASSIFICATION

PHARMACOTHERAPEUTIC: Nonbenzodiazepine **(Schedule IV). CLINICAL:** Hypnotic (see p. 149C).

E

ACTION

May interact with GABA-receptor complexes at binding domains located close to or allosterically coupled to benzodiazepine receptors. **Therapeutic Effect:** Prevents insomnia, difficulty maintaining normal sleep.

PHARMACOKINETICS

Rapidly absorbed following PO administration. Protein binding: 52%–59%. Metabolized in liver. Excreted in urine. **Half-life:** 5–6 hrs.

USES

Treatment of insomnia in pts who experience difficulty falling asleep or are unable to sleep through the night (sleep maintenance difficulty).

PRECAUTIONS

Contraindications: None known. **Cautions:** Hepatic impairment, compromised respiratory function, clinical depression; concomitant CNS depressants, strong CYP3A4 inhibitors (e.g., ketoconazole); elderly.

⧗ LIFESPAN CONSIDERATIONS

Pregnancy/Lactation: Unknown if drug crosses placenta or is distributed in breast milk. **Pregnancy Category C. Children:** Safety and efficacy not established. **Elderly:** Those with impaired motor or cognitive performance may require dosage adjustment.

INTERACTIONS

DRUG: Alcohol, anticonvulsants, antihistamines, other CNS depressants may increase CNS depression. **CYP3A4 inhibitors (e.g., clarithromycin, itraconazole, ketoconazole, nelfinavir, ritonavir)** may increase concentration/toxicity. **HERBAL: Gotu kola, kava kava, St. John's wort, valerian** may increase CNS depression. **FOOD:** Onset of action may be reduced if taken with or immediately after a **high-fat meal. LAB VALUES:** None known.

AVAILABILITY (Rx)

◈ **Tablets, Film-Coated:** 1 mg, 2 mg, 3 mg.

ADMINISTRATION/HANDLING

PO
• Should be administered immediately before bedtime. • Do not give with or immediately following a high-fat or heavy meal. • Do not break, cut, crush, or divide tablet.

INDICATIONS/ROUTES/DOSAGE

Insomnia
PO: ADULTS: 2 mg before bedtime. **Maximum:** 3 mg. **Concurrent use with CYP3A4 inhibitors** (e.g., clarithromycin, erythromycin, azole antifungals): 1 mg before bedtime; if needed, dose may be increased to 2 mg. **ELDERLY:** Initially, 1 mg before bedtime. **Maximum:** 2 mg.

Sleep Maintenance Difficulty
PO: ADULTS: 2 mg before bedtime.

Dosage in Hepatic Impairment
SEVERE: 1 mg; **maximum:** 2 mg.

SIDE EFFECTS

Frequent (34%–21%): Unpleasant taste, headache. **Occasional (10%–4%):** Drowsiness, dry mouth, dyspepsia, dizziness, nervousness, nausea, rash, pruritus, depression, diarrhea. **Rare (3%–2%):** Hallucinations, anxiety, confusion, abnormal dreams, decreased libido, neuralgia.

ADVERSE EFFECTS/ TOXIC REACTIONS

Chest pain, peripheral edema occur occasionally.

NURSING CONSIDERATIONS

BASELINE ASSESSMENT

Assess B/P, pulse, respirations. Raise bed rails, provide call light. Provide environment conducive to sleep (quiet environment, low or no lighting, TV off).

INTERVENTION/EVALUATION

Assess sleep pattern of pt. Evaluate for therapeutic response (decrease in number of nocturnal awakenings, increase in length of sleep).

PATIENT/FAMILY TEACHING

• Take only when experiencing insomnia. Do not take when insomnia is not present. • Do not break, chew, crush, or divide tablet. Take whole. • Avoid alcohol. • At least 8 hrs must be devoted for sleep time before daily activity begins. • Take immediately before bedtime. • Report insomnia that worsens or persists longer than 7–10 days; abnormal thoughts or behavior, memory loss, anxiety.

etanercept
TOP 200

e-tan-er-sept
(Enbrel)
BLACK BOX ALERT Serious, potentially fatal, infections, including bacterial sepsis, tuberculosis, have occurred. Lymphomas, other malignancies may occur (reported in children/adolescents).
Do not confuse Enbrel with Levbid.

◆ CLASSIFICATION

PHARMACOTHERAPEUTIC: Protein.
CLINICAL: Antiarthritic.

ACTION

Binds to tumor necrosis factor (TNF), blocking its interaction with cell surface receptors. Elevated levels of TNF, involved in inflammatory and immune responses, are found in synovial fluid of rheumatoid arthritis pts. **Therapeutic Effect:** Relieves symptoms of rheumatoid arthritis.

PHARMACOKINETICS

Well absorbed after subcutaneous administration. **Half-life:** 72–132 hrs.

USES

Treatment of moderate to severely active rheumatoid arthritis (RA). Treatment of moderately to severely active polyarticular juvenile idiopathic arthritis (JIA), ankylosing spondylitis, psoriatic arthritis. Treatment of chronic, moderate to severe plaque psoriasis.

PRECAUTIONS

Contraindications: Serious active infection or sepsis. **Cautions:** History of recurrent infections, illnesses that predispose to infection (e.g., diabetes). Pts with HF, decreased left ventricular function, history of significant hematologic abnormalities; moderate to severe alcoholic hepatitis, elderly, preexisting or recent-onset CNS demyelinating disorder.

⌛ LIFESPAN CONSIDERATIONS

Pregnancy/Lactation: Unknown if distributed in breast milk. **Pregnancy Category B. Children:** No age-related precautions noted in those 4 yrs and older. **Elderly:** No age-related precautions noted.

INTERACTIONS

DRUG: Anakinra may increase risk of infection. Use of **live virus vaccines** may potentiate virus replication, increase vaccine side effect, decrease pt's antibody response to vaccine. **HERBAL: Echinacea** may decrease effects. **FOOD:** None known. **LAB VALUES:** May increase serum alkaline phosphatase, AST, ALT, bilirubin.

AVAILABILITY (Rx)

Injection, Powder for Reconstitution: 25 mg. **Injection, Solution (Prefilled Syringe):** 50 mg/ml. **Injection, Solution (Autoinjector):** 50 mg/ml.

ADMINISTRATION/HANDLING

◄ALERT► Do not add other medications to solution. Do not use filter during reconstitution or administration.

♣ Canadian trade name   🐄 Non-Crushable Drug   🄷 High Alert drug

Subcutaneous

• Refrigerate prefilled syringes, powder for reconstitution. • Reconstitute with 1 ml Bacteriostatic Water for Injection (0.9% benzyl alcohol). Do not reconstitute with other diluents. • Slowly inject diluent into vial. Some foaming will occur. To avoid excessive foaming, slowly swirl contents until powder is dissolved (less than 5 min). • Visually inspect solution for particles, discoloration. Reconstituted solution should appear clear, colorless. If discolored, cloudy, or particles remain, discard solution; do not use. • Withdraw all of the solution into syringe. Final volume should be approximately 1 ml. • Inject into thigh, abdomen, upper arm. Rotate injection sites. • Give new injection at least 1 inch from an old site and never into area where skin is tender, bruised, red, hard. • Once reconstituted, may be stored in vial for up to 14 days refrigerated.

INDICATIONS/ROUTES/DOSAGE

Rheumatoid Arthritis (RA), Psoriatic Arthritis, Ankylosing Spondylitis
Subcutaneous: ADULTS, ELDERLY: 25 mg twice weekly given 72–96 hrs apart or 50 mg once weekly. **Maximum:** 50 mg/wk.

Juvenile Rheumatoid Arthritis (JIA)
Subcutaneous: CHILDREN 2–17 YRS: Twice weekly: 0.4 mg/kg 2 times/wk given 72–96 hrs apart. **Maximum dose:** 25 mg. Once weekly: 0.8 mg/kg/dose. **Maximum dose:** 50 mg.

Plaque Psoriasis
Subcutaneous: ADULTS, ELDERLY: 50 mg twice a wk (give 3–4 days apart) for 3 mos. Maintenance: 50 mg once a wk.

SIDE EFFECTS

Frequent (37%): Injection site erythema, pruritus, pain, swelling; abdominal pain, vomiting (more common in children than adults). **Occasional (16%–4%):**

Headache, rhinitis, dizziness, pharyngitis, cough, asthenia (loss of strength, energy), abdominal pain, dyspepsia. **Rare (less than 3%):** Sinusitis, allergic reaction.

ADVERSE EFFECTS/ TOXIC REACTIONS

Infection (pyelonephritis, cellulitis, osteomyelitis, wound infection, leg ulcer, septic arthritis, diarrhea, bronchitis, pneumonia) occurs in 29%–38% of pts. Rare adverse effects include heart failure, hypertension, hypotension, pancreatitis, GI hemorrhage.

NURSING CONSIDERATIONS

BASELINE ASSESSMENT

Assess onset, type, location, duration of pain, inflammation. If significant exposure to varicella virus has occurred during treatment, therapy should be temporarily discontinued and treatment with varicella-zoster immune globulin should be considered.

INTERVENTION/EVALUATION

Assess for improvement of joint swelling, pain, tenderness. Monitor erythrocyte sedimentation rate (ESR), C-reactive protein level, CBC with differential, platelet count. Observe for signs of infection.

PATIENT/FAMILY TEACHING

• Instruct pt in subcutaneous injection technique, including areas of body acceptable as injection sites. • Injection site reaction generally occurs in first mo of treatment and decreases in frequency during continued therapy. • Do not receive live vaccines during treatment. • Report persistent fever, bruising, bleeding, pallor.

ethambutol

eth-**am**-bue-tol
(Etibi ✤, Myambutol)

◆CLASSIFICATION

PHARMACOTHERAPEUTIC: Isonicotinic acid derivative. **CLINICAL:** Antitubercular.

ACTION

Interferes with RNA synthesis. **Therapeutic Effect:** Suppresses multiplication of mycobacteria.

PHARMACOKINETICS

Rapidly, well absorbed from GI tract. Protein binding: 20%–30%. Widely distributed. Metabolized in liver. Primarily excreted in urine. Removed by hemodialysis. **Half-life:** 3–4 hrs (increased in renal impairment).

USES

In conjunction with other antitubercular agents for treatment of pulmonary tuberculosis. **OFF-LABEL:** Treatment of atypical mycobacterial infections (e.g., *Mycobacterium avium* complex [MAC]).

PRECAUTIONS

Contraindications: Optic neuritis. Use in young children, unconscious pts, or anyone unable to report visual changes. **Cautions:** Renal dysfunction, ocular defects (diabetic retinopathy, cataracts), recurrent ocular inflammatory conditions. Not recommended for children 13 yrs and younger (unless benefit outweighs risk).

⧗ LIFESPAN CONSIDERATIONS

Pregnancy/Lactation: Crosses placenta. Distributed in breast milk. **Pregnancy Category B. Children:** Safety and efficacy not established in those younger than 13 yrs. **Elderly:** Age-related renal impairment may require dosage adjustment.

INTERACTIONS

DRUG: Aluminum hydroxide may decrease concentration/effect. **HERBAL:** None significant. **FOOD:** None known.

LAB VALUES: May increase serum uric acid.

AVAILABILITY (Rx)

Tablets: 100 mg, 400 mg.

ADMINISTRATION/HANDLING

PO
• May be crushed and mixed with apple juice or applesauce. • Administer at least 4 hrs before giving aluminum hydroxide. • Give with food (decreases GI upset).

INDICATIONS/ROUTES/DOSAGE

Tuberculosis
PO: ADULTS, ELDERLY: Initially, 15 mg/kg once daily (**maximum:** 1.5 g/day). **RETREATMENT:** 25 mg/kg once daily (**maximum:** 2.5 g/day) for 60 days or until cultures become negative, then 15 mg/kg daily. **CHILDREN:** 15–20 mg/kg/day (**maximum:** 1 g/day) or 50 mg/kg twice weekly (**maximum:** 2.5 g/dose).

Dosage in Renal Impairment
Dosage interval is modified based on creatinine clearance.

Creatinine Clearance	Dosage
10–50 ml/min	q24–36h
Less than 10 ml/min	q48h
Hemodialysis	Administer post HD
Peritoneal dialysis	Administer q48h
Continuous renal replacement therapy	Administer q24–36h

SIDE EFFECTS

Occasional: Acute gouty arthritis (chills, pain, swelling of joints with hot skin), confusion, abdominal pain, nausea, vomiting, anorexia, headache. **Rare:** Rash, fever, blurred vision, red-green color blindness.

ADVERSE EFFECTS/ TOXIC REACTIONS

Optic neuritis (more common with high-dosage, long-term therapy), peripheral neuritis, thrombocytopenia, anaphylactoid reaction occur rarely.

NURSING CONSIDERATIONS

BASELINE ASSESSMENT

Evaluate baseline CBC, renal/hepatic function test results, and monitor periodically.

INTERVENTION/EVALUATION

Assess for vision changes (altered color perception, decreased visual acuity may be first signs). Give with food if GI distress occurs. Monitor serum uric acid. Assess for hot, painful, swollen joints, esp. great toe, ankle, knee (gout). Report numbness, tingling, burning of extremities (peripheral neuritis).

PATIENT/FAMILY TEACHING

• Do not skip doses; take for full length of therapy (may take mos or yrs). • Immediately report any visual problem (visual effects generally reversible with discontinuation of ethambutol but in rare cases may take up to 1 yr to disappear or may be permanent). • Promptly report swelling or pain of joints, numbness or tingling/burning of extremities, fever, chills.

---

etodolac

e-**toe**-doe-lak
(Apo-Etodolac ✢, Ultradol ✢)

BLACK BOX ALERT Increased risk of serious cardiovascular thrombotic events, including myocardial infarction, CVA. Increased risk of severe GI reactions, including ulceration, bleeding, perforation of stomach, intestines.

◆CLASSIFICATION

PHARMACOTHERAPEUTIC: NSAID. **CLINICAL:** NSAID, analgesic (see p. 129C).

ACTION

Produces analgesic, anti-inflammatory effects by inhibiting prostaglandin synthesis. **Therapeutic Effect:** Reduces inflammatory response, intensity of pain.

PHARMACOKINETICS

Route	Onset	Peak	Duration
PO (analgesic)	2–4 hrs	N/A	4–12 hrs

Completely absorbed from GI tract. Protein binding: greater than 99%. Widely distributed. Metabolized in liver. Primarily excreted in urine. Not removed by hemodialysis. **Half-life:** 6–7 hrs. **Extended-release:** 12 hrs.

USES

Acute and long-term treatment of osteoarthritis, management of pain, treatment of rheumatoid arthritis (RA), juvenile idiopathic arthritis (JIA).

PRECAUTIONS

Contraindications: Perioperative pain in setting of CABG surgery, history of hypersensitivity to aspirin, NSAIDs. **Cautions:** Renal/hepatic impairment, history of GI tract disease, predisposition to fluid retention, HF. Active peptic ulcer disease, chronic inflammation of GI tract, GI bleeding/ulceration. Cardiovascular disease; concurrent use of aspirin, anticoagulants; smoking; elderly; use of alcohol; debilitated pts; asthma.

⏳ LIFESPAN CONSIDERATIONS

Pregnancy/Lactation: Unknown if drug crosses placenta or is distributed in breast milk. Avoid use during third trimester (may adversely affect fetal cardiovascular system: premature closure of ductus arteriosus). **Pregnancy Category C (D if used in third trimester or near delivery). Children:** Safety and efficacy not established. **Elderly:** GI bleeding, ulceration more likely to cause serious adverse effects. Age-related renal impairment may increase risk of hepatic/renal toxicity; decreased dosage recommended.

INTERACTIONS

DRUG: May decrease antihypertensive effect of **ACE inhibitors. Aspirin, other salicylates** may increase risk of GI side effects, bleeding. May increase concentration/toxicity of **cyclosporine, digoxin, methotrexate, lithium. HERBAL: Cat's claw, dong quai, evening primrose, feverfew, garlic, ginger, ginkgo, ginseng** may increase antiplatelet action, risk of bleeding. **FOOD:** None known. **LAB VALUES:** May increase bleeding time, serum creatinine, alkaline phosphatase, AST, ALT, bilirubin. May decrease serum uric acid.

AVAILABILITY (Rx)

Tablets: 400 mg, 500 mg.
Capsules: 200 mg, 300 mg. Tablets (Extended-Release): 400 mg, 500 mg, 600 mg.

ADMINISTRATION/HANDLING

PO
• Do not break, crush, dissolve, or divide capsules, extended-release tablets.
• May give with food, milk, antacids if GI distress occurs.

INDICATIONS/ROUTES/DOSAGE

Osteoarthritis, Rheumatoid Arthritis (RA)
PO (Immediate-Release): ADULTS, ELDERLY: Initially, 300 mg 2–3 times a day or 400 mg twice a day.
PO (Extended-Release): ADULTS, ELDERLY: 400–1,000 mg once daily.

Juvenile Idiopathic Arthritis (JIA)
PO (Extended-Release): CHILDREN 6–16 YRS: 1,000 mg in children weighing more than 60 kg, 800 mg once daily in children weighing 46–60 kg, 600 mg once daily in children weighing 31–45 kg, 400 mg once daily in children weighing 20–30 kg.

Analgesia
PO (Immediate-Release): ADULTS, ELDERLY: 200–400 mg q6–8h as needed. **Maximum:** 1,000 mg/day.

SIDE EFFECTS

Occasional (9%–4%): Dizziness, headache, abdominal pain/cramping, bloated feeling, diarrhea, nausea, indigestion. **Rare (3%–1%):** Constipation, rash, pruritus, visual disturbances, tinnitus.

ADVERSE EFFECTS/TOXIC REACTIONS

Overdose may result in acute renal failure. Increased risk of cardiovascular events (MI, CVA) and serious, potentially life-threatening GI bleeding. Rare reactions with long-term use include peptic ulcer, gastritis, jaundice, nephrotoxicity (hematuria, dysuria, proteinuria), severe hypersensitivity reaction (bronchospasm, angioedema).

NURSING CONSIDERATIONS

BASELINE ASSESSMENT

Assess onset, type, location, duration of pain/inflammation. Inspect appearance of affected joints for immobility, deformities, skin condition.

INTERVENTION/EVALUATION

Monitor CBC, hepatic/renal function tests. Observe for bleeding/ecchymosis. Evaluate for therapeutic response: relief of pain, stiffness, swelling; increased joint mobility; reduced joint tenderness; improved grip strength.

PATIENT/FAMILY TEACHING

• Swallow capsule whole; do not break, crush, dissolve, or divide. • Avoid aspirin, alcohol (increases risk of GI bleeding). • Report GI distress, visual disturbances, rash, edema, headache. • Report any signs of bleeding. • Take with food, milk, antacid if GI distress occurs. • Avoid tasks that require alertness, motor skills until response to drug is established.

E

etoposide, VP-16

e-**toe**-poe-side
(Etopophos, Toposar, VePesid ❧)

BLACK BOX ALERT Severe myelosuppression with resulting infection, bleeding may occur. Must be administered by personnel trained in administration/handling of chemotherapeutic agents.

Do not confuse etoposide with etidronate, or VePesid with Pepcid or Versed.

◆ CLASSIFICATION

PHARMACOTHERAPEUTIC: Epipodophyllotoxin. **CLINICAL:** Antineoplastic (see p. 85C).

ACTION

Induces single- and double-stranded breaks in DNA. Cell cycle-dependent and phase-specific; most effective in S and G_2 phases of cell division. **Therapeutic Effect:** Inhibits, alters DNA synthesis.

PHARMACOKINETICS

Variably absorbed from GI tract. Rapidly distributed, low concentrations in CSF. Protein binding: 97%. Metabolized in liver. Primarily excreted in urine. Not removed by hemodialysis. **Half-life:** 3–12 hrs.

USES

Treatment of refractory testicular tumors, small-cell lung carcinoma. **OFF-LABEL:** Acute lymphocytic, acute nonlymphocytic leukemias; Ewing's and Kaposi's sarcoma; Hodgkin's and non-Hodgkin's lymphomas; endometrial, gastric, non–small-cell lung carcinomas; multiple myeloma; myelodysplastic syndromes; neuroblastoma; osteosarcoma; ovarian germ cell tumors; primary brain, gestational trophoblastic tumors; soft tissue sarcomas; Wilms tumor.

PRECAUTIONS

Contraindications: None known. **Cautions:** Hepatic/renal impairment, myelosuppression, elderly, pts with low serum albumin.

🕰 LIFESPAN CONSIDERATIONS

Pregnancy/Lactation: If possible, avoid use during pregnancy, esp. first trimester. May cause fetal harm. Breastfeeding not recommended. **Pregnancy Category D. Children:** Safety and efficacy not established. **Elderly:** Age-related renal impairment may require dosage adjustment.

INTERACTIONS

DRUG: Bone marrow depressants may increase myelosuppression. **Live-virus vaccines** may potentiate virus replication, increase vaccine side effects, decrease pt's antibody response to vaccine. **HERBAL: Echinacea, St. John's wort** may decrease concentration. **FOOD:** None known. **LAB VALUES:** Expected decrease of leukocytes, platelets, RBC, Hgb, Hct.

AVAILABILITY (Rx)

Capsules: 50 mg. **Injection, Powder for Reconstitution (Water-Soluble [Etopophos]):** 100 mg. **Injection Solution (Toposar):** 20 mg/ml (5 ml, 25 ml, 50 ml).

ADMINISTRATION/HANDLING

◀ **ALERT** ▶ Administer by slow IV infusion. Wear gloves when preparing solution. If powder or solution comes in contact with skin, wash immediately and thoroughly with soap, water. May be carcinogenic, mutagenic, teratogenic. Handle with extreme care during preparation, administration.

 IV

Reconstitution
Vepesid • Dilute each 100 mg (5 ml) with at least 250 ml D_5W or 0.9% NaCl to provide concentration of 0.4 mg/ml (500 ml for concentration of 0.2 mg/ml).
Etopophos • Reconstitute each 100 mg with 5–10 ml Sterile Water for Injection, D_5W, or 0.9% NaCl to provide concentration of 20 mg/ml or 10 mg/ml, respectively. • May give without

further dilution or further dilute to concentration as low as 0.1 mg/ml with 0.9% NaCl or D₅W.

Rate of administration

Vepesid • Infuse slowly, at least 30–60 min (rapid IV may produce marked hypotension) at a rate not to exceed 100 mg/m²/hr. • Monitor for anaphylactic reaction during infusion (chills, fever, dyspnea, diaphoresis, lacrimation, sneezing, throat, back, chest pain).

Etopophos • May give over as little as 5 min up to 210 min.

Storage

Vepesid • Store injection at room temperature before dilution. • Concentrate for injection is clear, yellow. • Diluted solution is stable at room temperature for 96 hrs at 0.2 mg/ml, 24 hrs at 0.4 mg/ml. • Discard if crystallization occurs.

Etopophos • Refrigerate vials. • Stable at room temperature for 24 hrs or for 7 days if refrigerated after reconstitution.

PO

Storage • Refrigerate gelatin capsules.

🔲 IV INCOMPATIBILITIES

VePesid: Cefepime (Maxipime), filgrastim (Neupogen). **Etopophos:** Amphotericin B (Fungizone), cefepime (Maxipime), chlorpromazine (Thorazine), methylprednisolone (Solu-Medrol), prochlorperazine (Compazine).

🔲 IV COMPATIBILITIES

VePesid: Carboplatin (Paraplatin), cisplatin (Platinol), cytarabine (Cytosar), daunorubicin (Cerubidine), doxorubicin (Adriamycin), granisetron (Kytril), mitoxantrone (Novantrone), ondansetron (Zofran). **Etopophos:** Carboplatin (Paraplatin), cisplatin (Platinol), cytarabine (Cytosar), dacarbazine (DTIC-Dome), daunorubicin (Cerubidine), dexamethasone (Decadron), diphenhydramine (Benadryl), doxorubicin (Adriamycin), granisetron (Kytril), magnesium sulfate, mannitol, mitoxantrone (Novantrone), ondansetron (Zofran), potassium chloride.

INDICATIONS/ROUTES/DOSAGE

◄ **ALERT** ► Dosage individualized based on clinical response, tolerance to adverse effects. Treatment repeated at 3- to 4-wk intervals. Refer to individual protocols.

Refractory Testicular Tumors

IV: ADULTS: 50–100 mg/m²/day on days 1–5, or 100 mg/m²/day on days 1, 3, 5 (as combination therapy). Give q3–4wks for 3–4 courses.

Small-Cell Lung Carcinoma

PO: ADULTS: Twice the IV dose rounded to nearest 50 mg. Give once a day for doses 400 mg or less, in divided doses for dosages greater than 400 mg.

IV: ADULTS: 35 mg/m²/day for 4 consecutive days up to 50 mg/m²/day for 5 consecutive days q3–4wks (as combination therapy).

Dosage in Renal Impairment

Creatinine Clearance	Dosage
15–50 ml/min	75% of normal dose
Less than 15 ml/min	Consider further dose reduction.

SIDE EFFECTS

Frequent (66%–43%): Mild to moderate nausea/vomiting, alopecia. **Occasional (13%–6%):** Diarrhea, anorexia, stomatitis. **Rare (2% or less):** Hypotension, peripheral neuropathy.

ADVERSE EFFECTS/ TOXIC REACTIONS

Myelosuppression manifested as hematologic toxicity, principally anemia, leukopenia (occurring 7–14 days after drug administration), thrombocytopenia (occurring 9–16 days after administration), and, to lesser extent, pancytopenia. Bone marrow recovery occurs by day 20. Hepatotoxicity occurs occasionally.

NURSING CONSIDERATIONS

BASELINE ASSESSMENT
Obtain hematologic tests before and at frequent intervals during therapy. Antiemetics readily control nausea, vomiting.

INTERVENTION/EVALUATION
Monitor Hgb, Hct, WBC, platelet count, B/P, hepatic/renal function tests. Monitor daily pattern of bowel activity, stool consistency. Monitor for hematologic toxicity (fever, sore throat, signs of local infection, unusual bruising/bleeding from any site), symptoms of anemia (excessive fatigue, weakness). Assess for paresthesia (peripheral neuropathy). Monitor for stomatitis.

PATIENT/FAMILY TEACHING
• Hair loss is reversible, but new hair growth may have different color, texture. • Do not have immunizations without physician's approval (drug lowers resistance). • Avoid contact with those who have recently received live virus vaccine. • Promptly report fever, sore throat, signs of local infection, unusual bruising or bleeding from any site, burning or pain with urination, numbness in extremities, yellowing of skin, whites of eyes.

---

etravirine

e-tra-**veer**-een
(Intelence)

◆CLASSIFICATION
PHARMACOTHERAPEUTIC: Nonnucleoside reverse transcriptase inhibitor. **CLINICAL:** Antiretroviral agent (see pp. 70C, 119C).

ACTION
Binds directly to human immunodeficiency virus type 1 (HIV-1) reverse transcriptase, changing shape of enzyme, blocking RNA-, DNA-dependent DNA polymerase activity. **Therapeutic Effect:** Interferes with HIV replication, slowing progression of HIV infection.

PHARMACOKINETICS
Well absorbed following PO administration if given following a meal. Protein binding: 99.6%. Metabolized in liver. Eliminated in feces and urine. **Half-life:** 41 hrs.

USES
Used in combination with at least two other antiretroviral agents for treatment of HIV-1 infection in antiretroviral treatment-experienced adults and children aged 6 yrs of age and older weighing at least 16 kg.

PRECAUTIONS
Contraindications: None known. **Cautions:** Severe hepatic impairment, renal impairment, elderly.

⌛ LIFESPAN CONSIDERATIONS
Pregnancy/Lactation: Unknown if distributed in breast milk. **Pregnancy Category B. Children:** Safety and efficacy not established. **Elderly:** Age-related hepatic, renal, cardiac impairment may require dosage adjustment.

INTERACTIONS
DRUG: CYP3A4 inducers (e.g., rifampin, carbamazepine, phenytoin) may decrease concentration. **CYP3A4 inhibitors (e.g., clarithromycin, ketoconazole)** may increase concentration. May decrease effects of **cyclosporine, sirolimus, tacrolimus.** May alter **warfarin** plasma concentrations. **HERBAL: Gotu kola, kava kava, St. John's wort, valerian** may increase CNS depressant effects. **St. John's wort** may decrease concentration/effects. **FOOD:** None known. **LAB VALUES:** May increase serum amylase, cholesterol, lipase, creatinine, triglycerides, glucose, ALT, AST. May decrease Hgb, neutrophil, platelet count.

AVAILABILITY (Rx)

Tablets: 25 mg, 100 mg, 200 mg.

ADMINISTRATION/HANDLING

PO

• Give following a meal. • Tablets may be dissolved in water. • Stir dispersion well and instruct pt to swallow immediately after dispersion. • Glass should be rinsed several times with water and each rinse swallowed to ensure entire dose is consumed.

INDICATIONS/ROUTES/DOSAGE

HIV-1 Infection

PO: ADULTS: 200 mg (one 200-mg or two 100-mg tablets) twice daily following a meal. **CHILDREN 6–18 YRS, WEIGHING 30 KG OR GREATER:** 200 mg twice daily. **WEIGHING 25–29 KG:** 150 mg twice daily. **WEIGHING 20–24 KG:** 125 mg twice daily. **WEIGHING 16–19 KG:** 100 mg twice daily.

SIDE EFFECTS

Occasional (17%–16%): Rash (mild to moderate, occurring primarily during wk 2 of therapy and infrequently after wk 4), nausea. **Rare (6%–3%):** Diarrhea, fatigue, abdominal pain, hypertension, peripheral neuropathy, headache.

ADVERSE EFFECTS/ TOXIC REACTIONS

Severe/life-threatening rash presenting as Stevens-Johnson syndrome, hypersensitivity reaction, erythema multiforme occurs rarely.

NURSING CONSIDERATIONS

BASELINE ASSESSMENT

Obtain baseline lab tests before beginning therapy and at periodic intervals thereafter. Offer emotional support.

INTERVENTION/EVALUATION

Closely monitor for evidence of rash (usually appears on trunk, face, extremities during second wk of drug initiation). Rash generally resolves within 1–2 wks on continued therapy.

PATIENT/FAMILY TEACHING

• Do not take any medications, including OTC drugs, without consulting physician. • Small, frequent meals may offset anorexia, nausea. • Etravirine is not a cure for HIV infection, nor does it reduce risk of transmission to others. • If rash appears, contact physician before continuing therapy.

E

everolimus

e-**veer**-oh-li-mus
(Afinitor, Afinitor Disperz, Zortress)
Do not confuse Afinitor with Lipitor, or everolimus with sirolimus, tacrolimus, or temsirolimus.

BLACK BOX ALERT Immunosuppressant (may result in infection, malignancy including lymphoma or skin cancer); increased risk of nephrotoxicity in renal transplants (avoid standard doses of cyclosporine); increased risk of renal thrombosis in renal transplants.

◆CLASSIFICATION

PHARMACOTHERAPEUTIC: Enzyme inhibitor. **CLINICAL:** Antineoplastic, immunosuppressant (see p. 85C).

ACTION

Prevents activation of rapamycin (MTOR) kinase activity. **Therapeutic Effect:** Reduces cell proliferation, produces cell death.

PHARMACOKINETICS

Peak concentration occurs in 1–2 hrs following administration, with steady-state levels achieved in 2 wks. Undergoes extensive hepatic metabolism. Protein binding: 74%. Eliminated in feces (80%), urine (5%). **Half-life:** 30 hrs.

E

USES

Afinitor: Treatment of advanced renal cell carcinoma after failure of treatment with sunitinib or sorafenib. Treatment of subependymal giant cell astrocytoma (SEGA) associated with tuberous sclerosis. Advanced pancreatic neuroendocrine tumors (PNET). Treatment of breast cancer in postmenopausal women. Treatment of tuberous sclerosis complex (TSC) not requiring immediate surgery. **Afinitor Disperz:** Treatment of SEGA associated with TSC requiring intervention but that cannot be curatively resected. **Zortress:** Prophylaxis of organ rejection after kidney transplant at low to moderate immunologic risk. **OFF-LABEL:** Relapsed or refractory Waldenström's macroglobulinemia.

PRECAUTIONS

Contraindications: Hypersensitivity to everolimus, sirolimus, other rapamycin derivatives. **Cautions:** Noninfectious pneumonitis; viral, fungal, or bacterial infection; oral ulceration; mucositis; current immunosuppression; hereditary galactose intolerance; hepatic impairment; hyperlipidemia; concurrent use of CYP3A4 inducers and inhibitors (see Interactions).

⌛ LIFESPAN CONSIDERATIONS

Pregnancy/Lactation: May cause fetal harm. Unknown if distributed in breast milk. **Pregnancy Category D. Children:** Safety and efficacy not established. **Elderly:** No age-related precautions noted.

INTERACTIONS

DRUG: **CYP3A4 inhibitors** (e.g., **atazanavir, clarithromycin, indinavir, itraconazole, ketoconazole, nefazodone, nelfinavir, ritonavir, saquinavir, voriconazole**) may increase concentration. **CYP3A4 inducers** (e.g., **carbamazepine, dexamethasone, phenobarbital, phenytoin, rifabutin, rifampin, rifapentine**) may decrease concentration. **P-gp inhibitors** (e.g., **cyclosporine**) may increase everolimus concentrations,

toxicity. **Statins** may increase risk of rhabdomyolysis. **FOOD:** **High-fat meals** may reduce plasma concentration. **Grapefruit products** may increase concentration (potential for meylotoxicity, nephrotoxicity). **HERBAL:** **St. John's wort** may decrease plasma concentration. **LAB VALUES:** May increase BUN, serum creatinine, glucose, triglycerides, lipids. May decrease WBCs, neutrophils, Hgb, platelets.

AVAILABILITY (Rx)

▨ Tablets (Zortress): 0.25 mg, 0.5 mg, 0.75 mg. ▨ Tablets (Afinitor): 2.5 mg, 5 mg, 10 mg. **Tablets for Oral Suspension (Afinitor Disperz):** 2 mg, 3 mg, 5 mg.

ADMINISTRATION/HANDLING

• Give without regard to food. • Do not crush/cut Afinitor or Zortress. • Avoid direct contact of crushed tablets with skin or mucous membranes. If unable to swallow, disperse in 30 ml water with gentle stirring, give immediately.

INDICATIONS/ROUTES/DOSAGE

◀ALERT▶ If pt requires coadministration of a strong CYP3A4 inducer (carbamazepine, dexamethasone, phenobarbital, phenytoin, rifabutin, rifampin), consider doubling the dose. If strong inducer is discontinued, reduce everolimus to dose used prior to initiation. If moderate CYP3A4 inhibitors are required, reduce dose by 50%.

Renal Carcinoma, Pancreatic Neuroendocrine Tumors, Breast Cancer, TSC

PO: ADULTS, ELDERLY: (Afinitor): 10 mg once daily at same time every day. Coadministration with CYP3A4 inhibitors or P-gp inhibitors: 2.5 mg once daily. May increase to 5 mg/day. Coadministration with CYP3A4 inducers: Increase by 5-mg increments up to 20 mg/day.

SEGA with TSC

PO: ADULTS, CHILDREN: 4.5 mg/m^2 once daily.

Transplant Prophylaxis

PO: ADULTS, ELDERLY: (Zortress): Initially, 0.75 mg 2 times/day. Give in combination with basiliximab and concurrent with reduced doses of cyclosporine and corticosteroids.

Astrocytoma

PO: ADULTS, ELDERLY: Initial dose based on body surface area (BSA), titrated to attain trough concentration of 5–15 ng/ml.

BSA	Dose
2.2 m² or greater	7.5 mg/day
1.3–2.1 m²	5 mg/day
0.5–1.2 m²	2.5 mg/day

SIDE EFFECTS

Common (44%–26%): Stomatitis, asthenia (loss of strength, energy), diarrhea, cough, rash, nausea. **Frequent (25%–20%):** Peripheral edema, anorexia, dyspnea, vomiting, pyrexia. **Occasional (19%–10%):** Mucosal inflammation, headache, epistaxis, pruritus, dry skin, epigastric distress, extremity pain. **Rare (less than 10%):** Abdominal pain, insomnia, dry mouth, dizziness, paresthesia, eyelid edema, hypertension, nail disorder, chills.

ADVERSE EFFECTS/ TOXIC REACTIONS

Noninfectious pneumonitis characterized as hypoxia, pleural effusion, cough, or dyspnea was reported in 14% of pts; grade 3 noninfectious pneumonitis reported in 4%. Localized and systemic infections, including pneumonia, other bacterial infections, and invasive fungal infections, have occurred due to everolimus immunosuppressive properties. Renal failure occurs in 3% of pts.

NURSING CONSIDERATIONS

BASELINE ASSESSMENT

Assess medical history, esp. renal function, use of other immunosuppressants. Obtain baseline CBC, serum chemistries including hepatic function tests, BUN,

creatinine before treatment begins and routinely thereafter.

INTERVENTION/EVALUATION

Offer antiemetics to control nausea, vomiting. Monitor daily pattern of bowel activity, stool consistency. Assess skin for evidence of rash, edema. Monitor CBC, particularly Hgb, platelet, neutrophil count, BUN, creatinine, hepatic function tests (AST, ALT, total bilirubin). Monitor for shortness of breath, fatigue, hypertension. Assess mouth for stomatitis, mucositis.

PATIENT/FAMILY TEACHING

• Take dose at same time each day. • Avoid crowds, those with known infection. • Avoid contact with anyone who recently received live virus vaccine. • Do not have immunizations without physician's approval (drug lowers body resistance). • Promptly report fever, unusual bruising/bleeding from any site. • Swallow tablet whole. Do not crush, avoid direct contact of crushed tablets with skin or mucous membrane (wash thoroughly if contact occurs). • Do not drink grapefruit juice or eat grapefruit.

exemestane

ex-e-**mes**-tane
(Aromasin)
Do not confuse Aromasin with Arimidex, or exemestane with estramustine.

◆ CLASSIFICATION

PHARMACOTHERAPEUTIC: Hormone. **CLINICAL:** Antineoplastic (see p. 85C).

ACTION

Inactivates aromatase, the principal enzyme that converts androgens to estrogens in both premenopausal and postmenopausal women, lowering circulating estrogen level. **Therapeutic Effect:** Inhibits growth of breast cancers stimulated by estrogens.

PHARMACOKINETICS

Rapidly absorbed after PO administration. Protein binding: 90%. Distributed extensively into tissues. Metabolized in liver; eliminated in urine and feces. **Half-life:** 24 hrs.

USES

Treatment of advanced breast cancer in postmenopausal women whose disease has progressed following tamoxifen therapy. Adjuvant treatment of postmenopausal women with estrogen-receptor positive early breast cancer after 2–3 yrs of tamoxifen therapy for completion of 5 consecutive yrs of adjuvant hormonal therapy. **OFF-LABEL:** Reduces risk of invasive breast cancer in postmenopausal women; treatment of endometrial cancer, uterine sarcoma.

PRECAUTIONS

Contraindications: Women who are pregnant or may become pregnant; use in premenopausal women. **Cautions:** Concomitant use of estrogen-containing agents, CYP3A4 inducers (e.g., phenobarbital, rifampin).

⌛ LIFESPAN CONSIDERATIONS

Pregnancy/Lactation: Indicated for postmenopausal women. **Pregnancy Category D. Children:** Not indicated for use in this pt population. **Elderly:** No age-related precautions noted.

INTERACTIONS

DRUG: **CYP3A4 inducers (e.g., phenobarbital, rifampin)** may decrease concentration/effect. **HERBAL: St. John's wort** may decrease concentration. Avoid **black cohosh, dong quai** in estrogen-dependent tumors. **FOOD:** None known. **LAB VALUES:** May increase serum alkaline phosphatase, AST, ALT.

AVAILABILITY (Rx)

Tablets: 25 mg.

ADMINISTRATION/HANDLING

PO
• Give after meals.

INDICATIONS/ROUTES/DOSAGE

Breast Cancer
PO: ADULTS, ELDERLY: 25 mg once a day after a meal. 50 mg/day when used concurrently with potent CYP3A4 inducers (e.g., rifampin, phenytoin).

SIDE EFFECTS

Frequent (22%–10%): Fatigue, nausea, depression, hot flashes, pain, insomnia, anxiety, dyspnea. **Occasional (8%–5%):** Headache, dizziness, vomiting, peripheral edema, abdominal pain, anorexia, flu-like symptoms, diaphoresis, constipation, hypertension. **Rare (4%):** Diarrhea.

ADVERSE EFFECTS/ TOXIC REACTIONS

MI has been noted.

NURSING CONSIDERATIONS

INTERVENTION/EVALUATION

Monitor for onset of depression. Assess sleep pattern. Monitor for and assist with ambulation if dizziness occurs. Assess for headache. Offer antiemetic for nausea/vomiting.

PATIENT/FAMILY TEACHING

• Notify physician if nausea, hot flashes become unmanageable. • Avoid tasks that require alertness, motor skills until response to drug is established. • Best taken after meals and at same time each day.

---

exenatide   TOP 200   HIGH ALERT

ex-**en**-a-tide
(Bydureon, <u>Byetta</u>)
BLACK BOX ALERT (Bydureon): Risk of thyroid C-cell tumors.

◆CLASSIFICATION

PHARMACOTHERAPEUTIC: Incretin mimetic. **CLINICAL:** Antidiabetic (see p. 45C).

ACTION

Stimulates release of insulin from beta cells of pancreas, mimics enhancement of glucose-dependent insulin secretion, suppresses elevated glucagon secretion, slows gastric emptying (central action increases satiety). **Therapeutic Effect:** Improves glycemic control by increasing postmeal insulin secretion, decreasing postmeal glucagon levels, delaying gastric emptying, and increasing satiety.

PHARMACOKINETICS

Minimal systemic metabolism. Eliminated by glomerular filtration with subsequent proteolytic degradation. **Half-life:** 2.4 hrs.

USES

Adjunct to diet, exercise to improve glycemic control in pts with type 2 diabetes mellitus.

PRECAUTIONS

Contraindications: Bydureon: History of medullary thyroid carcinoma. Pts with multiple endocrine neoplasia syndrome type 2 (MEN2). **Cautions:** Diabetic ketoacidosis, type 1 diabetes mellitus. Not recommended in severe renal impairment, severe GI disease, pancreatitis, gastroparesis.

⌛ LIFESPAN CONSIDERATIONS

Pregnancy/Lactation: Unknown if distributed in breast milk. **Pregnancy Category C. Children:** Safety and efficacy not established. **Elderly:** No age-related precautions noted.

INTERACTIONS

DRUG: May decrease effects of **digoxin, lovastatin.** May increase bleeding time, risk of bleeding when used with **warfa-**rin. **HERBAL:** None significant. **FOOD:** None known. **LAB VALUES:** None known.

AVAILABILITY (Rx)

Injection, Solution (Prefilled Pen): (Byetta) 250 mcg/ml (1.2 ml provides 5 mcg/dose; 2.4 ml provides 10 mcg/dose). **Injection, Suspension** (Bydureon): 2 mg.

ADMINISTRATION/HANDLING

Subcutaneous
• May be given in thigh, abdomen, upper arm. • Rotation of injection sites is essential; maintain careful injection site record. • Give within 60 min before morning and evening meals. Give suspension immediately after powder is suspended.
Storage • Refrigerate prefilled pens. • Discard if freezing occurs. • May be stored at room temperature after first use. • Discard pen 30 days after initial use.

INDICATIONS/ROUTE/DOSAGE

Diabetes Mellitus
Subcutaneous: ADULTS, ELDERLY: (Byetta) 5 mcg per dose given twice a day at any time within the 60-min period before the morning and evening meals. Dose may be increased to 10 mcg twice a day after 1 mo of therapy. (Bydureon): 2 mg once q7days.
◀ALERT▶ Not recommended in pts with creatinine clearance less than 30 ml/min.

SIDE EFFECTS

(Byetta) **Frequent (44%):** Nausea. **Occasional (13%–6%):** Diarrhea, vomiting, dizziness, anxiety, dyspepsia. **Rare (less than 6%):** Weakness. (Bydureon) **5% or greater:** Nausea, diarrhea, headache, constipation, vomiting, dyspepsia, injection site pruritus or nodule.

ADVERSE EFFECTS/ TOXIC REACTIONS

With concurrent sulfonylurea, hypoglycemia occurs in 36% when given a 10-mcg dose of exenatide, 16% when given a 5-mcg dose. May cause acute pancreatitis.

NURSING CONSIDERATIONS

BASELINE ASSESSMENT

Check serum glucose before administration. Discuss lifestyle to determine extent of learning, emotional needs. Ensure follow-up instruction if pt or family does not thoroughly understand diabetes management, glucose-testing technique. At least 1 mo should elapse to assess response to drug before new dose adjustment is made.

INTERVENTION/EVALUATION

Monitor serum glucose, food intake, renal function. Assess for hypoglycemia (cool wet skin, tremors, dizziness, anxiety, headache, tachycardia, numbness in mouth, hunger, diplopia), hyperglycemia (polyuria, polyphagia, polydipsia, nausea, vomiting, dim vision, fatigue, deep rapid breathing). Be alert to conditions that alter glucose requirements (fever, increased activity or stress, surgical procedure).

PATIENT/FAMILY TEACHING

• Diabetes mellitus requires lifelong control. • Prescribed diet and exercise are principal parts of treatment. Do not skip, delay meals. • Continue to adhere to dietary instructions, regular exercise program, regular testing of serum glucose. • When taking combination therapy with a sulfonylurea, have source of glucose available to treat symptoms of hypoglycemia. • Report any unexplained severe abdominal pain with or without nausea and vomiting.

---

ezetimibe

e-**zet**-i-mib
(Ezetrol ✤, Zetia)
Do not confuse Zetia with Zebeta or Zestril.

FIXED-COMBINATION(S)

Vytorin: ezetimibe/simvastatin (hydroxymethyglutaryl-CoA [HMG-CoA] reductase inhibitor): 10 mg/10 mg, 10 mg/20 mg, 10 mg/40 mg, 10 mg/80 mg.

◆CLASSIFICATION

PHARMACOTHERAPEUTIC: Antihyperlipidemic. **CLINICAL:** Anticholesterol agent (see p. 57C).

ACTION

Inhibits cholesterol absorption in small intestine, leading to decrease in delivery of intestinal cholesterol to liver. **Therapeutic Effect:** Reduces total serum cholesterol, LDL, triglyceride; increases HDL.

PHARMACOKINETICS

Well absorbed following PO administration. Protein binding: greater than 90%. Metabolized in small intestine and liver. Excreted by kidneys and bile. **Half-life:** 22 hrs.

USES

Adjunct to diet for treatment of primary hypercholesterolemia (monotherapy or in combination with HMG-CoA reductase inhibitors [statins]), homozygous sitosterolemia, homozygous familial hypercholesterolemia (combined with atrovastatin or simvastatin). Mixed hyperlipidemia (in combination with fenofibrate).

PRECAUTIONS

Contraindications: Concurrent use of an HMG-CoA reductase inhibitor (atorvastatin, fluvastatin, lovastatin, pravastatin, simvastatin) in pts with active hepatic disease or unexplained persistent elevations in serum transaminase; pregnancy; breast-feeding. **Cautions:** Severe renal or mild hepatic impairment. Not recommended in those with moderate or severe hepatic impairment.

⧗ LIFESPAN CONSIDERATIONS

Pregnancy/Lactation: Unknown if drug crosses placenta or is distributed in breast milk. **Pregnancy Category C. Children:** Safety and efficacy not established in those 10 yrs or younger. **Elderly:** Age-related mild hepatic impairment may require dosage adjustment.

INTERACTIONS

DRUG: Antacids containing aluminum or magnesium, cyclosporine, fenofibrate, gemfibrozil increase concentration. **Cholestyramine resin** decreases effectiveness. **HERBAL:** None significant. **FOOD:** None known. **LAB VALUES:** May increase serum alkaline phosphatase, bilirubin, AST, ALT.

AVAILABILITY (Rx)

Tablets: 10 mg.

ADMINISTRATION/HANDLING

• Give without regard to food. • May give at same time as statins. Give at least 2 hrs before or 4 hrs after cholestyramine, colestipol, colesevelam.

INDICATIONS/ROUTES/DOSAGE

Hypercholesterolemia
PO: ADULTS, ELDERLY, CHILDREN, 10 YRS AND OLDER: Initially, 10 mg once a day, given with or without food. If pt is also receiving a bile acid sequestrant, give ezetimibe at least 2 hrs before or at least 4 hrs after bile acid sequestrant.

Sitosterolemia
PO: ADULTS, ELDERLY: 10 mg/day.

SIDE EFFECTS

Occasional (4%–3%): Back pain, diarrhea, arthralgia, sinusitis, abdominal pain. **Rare (2%):** Cough, pharyngitis, fatigue, depression.

ADVERSE EFFECTS/ TOXIC REACTIONS

Hepatitis, hypersensitivity reaction, myopathy, rhabdomyolysis occur rarely.

NURSING CONSIDERATIONS

BASELINE ASSESSMENT
Obtain diet history, esp. fat consumption. Obtain serum cholesterol, triglycerides, hepatic function tests, blood counts during initial therapy and periodically during treatment. Treatment should be discontinued if hepatic enzyme levels persist more than 3 times normal limit.

INTERVENTION/EVALUATION
Monitor daily pattern of bowel activity, stool consistency. Question pt for signs/ symptoms of back pain, abdominal disturbances. Monitor serum cholesterol, triglycerides for therapeutic response.

PATIENT/FAMILY TEACHING
• Periodic laboratory tests are essential part of therapy. • Do not stop medication without consulting physician. • Report muscular or bone pain. • May give at same time as statins. Give at least 2 hrs before or 4 hrs after cholestyramine, colestipol, colesevelam.

ezogabine

e-**zog**-a-bine
(Potiga)

◆ CLASSIFICATION

PHARMACOTHERAPEUTIC: Potassium channel opener **(Schedule V).** **CLINICAL:** Anticonvulsant (see p. 35C).

ACTION

Reduces brain excitability and stabilizes resting membrane potentials by augmenting GABA-mediated currents, the major inhibitory neurotransmitter in CNS. **Therapeutic Effect:** Enhances transmembrane currents of potassium ion channels.

PHARMACOKINETICS

Rapidly absorbed after PO administration. Peak concentration: 0.5–2 hrs. Protein binding: 80%. Metabolized by glucuronidation and acetylation. Primarily excreted in urine (85%), feces (14%). **Half-life:** 7–11 hrs.

USES

Adjunctive therapy for treatment of partial-onset seizures in pts 18 yrs of age and older.

PRECAUTIONS

Contraindications: None known. **Cautions:** Hepatic/renal impairment, BPH, chronic cognitive impairment, psychiatric history, prolonged QT interval, those at risk for suicide.

⌛ LIFESPAN CONSIDERATIONS

Pregnancy/Lactation: Unknown if drug crosses placenta or is distributed in breast milk. Must either discontinue breastfeeding or discontinue drug regimen. **Pregnancy Category C. Children:** Safety and efficacy not established in pts under 18 yrs of age. **Elderly:** Dosage adjustment recommended for pts older than 65 yrs.

INTERACTIONS

DRUG: Phenytoin, carbamazepine may decrease plasma concentration/effect. **Alcohol** may increase concentration/adverse effects. May inhibit clearance of **digoxin. HERBAL:** None known. **FOOD:** None significant. **LAB VALUES:** May create falsely elevated urine bilirubin level.

AVAILABILITY (Rx)

Tablets: 50 mg, 200 mg, 300 mg, 400 mg.

ADMINISTRATION/HANDLING

• May give without regard to food.

INDICATIONS/ROUTES/DOSAGE

Partial Seizures
◄**ALERT**► Increase at weekly intervals by no more than 50 mg 3 times daily (150 mg per day).
PO: ADULTS: Initially, 100 mg 3 times daily for 7 days. Increase to maintenance dose of 200–400 mg 3 times daily (600–1,200 mg daily). **Maximum:** 1,200 mg per day. **ELDERLY:** Initially, 50 mg 3 times a day for 7 days. Then increase weekly to therapeutic level. **Maximum:** 250 mg 3 times a day (750 mg per day).

Dosage Modification
Renal Impairment (CrCl less than 50 ml/min or ESRD): 50 mg 3 times a day for 7 days. Then increase to therapeutic level. **Maximum:** 200 mg 3 times a day (600 mg per day). **Hepatic Impairment (Child-Pugh score less than 9):** Initially, 50 mg 3 times a day for 7 days. Then increase to therapeutic level. **Maximum:** 250 mg 3 times a day (750 mg per day). **Hepatic Impairment (Child-Pugh score greater than 9):** Initially, 50 mg 3 times a day for 7 days. Then increase to therapeutic level. **Maximum:** 200 mg 3 times a day (600 mg per day). **Discontinuation:** Reduce gradually over period of at least 3 wks.

SIDE EFFECTS

Frequent (23%–15%): Dizziness, somnolence, fatigue. **Occasional (8%–4%):** Tremor, vertigo, abnormal coordination, nausea, diplopia, attention disturbance, memory impairment, asthenia (loss of strength, energy), blurred vision, gait disturbance, aphasia, dysarthria, balance disorder. **Rare (3%–1%):** Constipation, anxiety, weight gain, dyspepsia, amnesia, dysphasia, disorientation, dysuria, urinary hesitation, hematuria, urine discoloration, psychotic behavior.

ADVERSE EFFECTS/ TOXIC REACTIONS

Urinary retention requiring catheterization, prolonged QT interval, myoclonus, peripheral edema, hypokinesia, dysphasia, hyperhydrosis, malaise reported in less than 2% of pts. Hydronephrosis associated with baseline renal impairment, increased risk of psychosis, hallucinations, suicidal ideation, depression, aggression, mania noted.

NURSING CONSIDERATIONS

BASELINE ASSESSMENT

Review history of seizure disorder (intensity, frequency, duration, LOC). Question history of BPH, urinary retention, cognitive impairment, psychiatric disorder, hepatic/renal impairment, alcoholism, prolonged QT syndrome. Obtain full medication history including digoxin, antiarrhythmics, adjunct anticonvulsant therapy. Obtain baseline EKG, digoxin level if applicable. Question possibility of pregnancy or current breast-feeding.

INTERVENTION/EVALUATION

Initiate seizure precautions and observe for seizure activity. Assist with ambulation if dizziness occurs. Monitor for depression, suicidal ideation, unusual behavior, mania, anxiety. Routinely monitor digoxin levels. Monitor QT interval for pts with HF, ventricular hypertrophy, hypokalemia, hypomagnesemia.

PATIENT/FAMILY TEACHING

• Monitor closely for seizure activity. • Immediately report any new medications, trouble urinating, palpitations, pregnancy, or plans to breast-feed. • Do not drink alcohol. • Report any thoughts of suicide, aggressive behavior, depression, anxiety, trouble sleeping, impulsiveness, unusual behavior. • Noncompliance may lead to increased risk of seizures.

E

famciclovir

fam-**sye**-klo-veer
(Apo-Famciclovir ✤, <u>Famvir</u>)
Do not confuse Famvir with Femara.

◆**CLASSIFICATION**

PHARMACOTHERAPEUTIC: Synthetic nucleoside. **CLINICAL:** Antiviral (see p. 70C).

ACTION

Inhibits viral DNA synthesis. **Therapeutic Effect:** Suppresses replication of herpes simplex virus, varicella-zoster virus.

PHARMACOKINETICS

Rapidly, extensively absorbed after PO administration. Protein binding: 20%–25%. Rapidly metabolized to penciclovir by enzymes in GI tract, liver, plasma. Eliminated unchanged in urine. Removed by hemodialysis. **Half-life:** 2–3 hrs (increased in severe renal failure).

USES

Treatment of acute herpes zoster (shingles), treatment and suppression of recurrent genital herpes in immunocompetent pts, treatment of recurrent mucocutaneous herpes simplex in HIV-infected pts. Treatment of recurrent herpes labialis (cold sores) in immunocompetent pts.

PRECAUTIONS

Contraindications: Hypersensitivity to penciclovir cream. **Cautions:** Renal impairment. Avoid use in galactose intolerance, severe lactose deficiency, or glucose-galactose malabsorption syndromes.

⌛ LIFESPAN CONSIDERATIONS

Pregnancy/Lactation: Unknown if excreted in breast milk. **Pregnancy Cate-** gory B. **Children:** Safety and efficacy not established. **Elderly:** Age-related renal impairment may require dosage adjustment.

INTERACTIONS

DRUG: None significant. **HERBAL:** None significant. **FOOD:** None known. **LAB VALUES:** May increase ALT, AST, amylase, bilirubin, lipase.

AVAILABILITY (Rx)

Tablets: 125 mg, 250 mg, 500 mg.

ADMINISTRATION/HANDLING

PO
• Give without regard to meals. • Give with food to decrease GI distress.

INDICATIONS/ROUTES/DOSAGE

Acute Herpes Zoster (Shingles)
PO: ADULTS: 500 mg q8h for 7 days. Begin within 72 hrs of rash onset.

Initial Genital Herpes
PO: ADULTS: 250 mg 3 times/day for 7–10 days.

Recurrent Genital Herpes
PO: ADULTS: 1,000 mg twice a day for 1 day.

Suppression of Recurrent Genital Herpes
PO: ADULTS: 250 mg twice a day for up to 1 yr.

Recurrent Mucotaneous/Genital Herpes Simplex in HIV Pts
PO: ADULTS: 500 mg twice a day for 7 days or 5–10 days.

Herpes Labialis (Cold Sores)
PO: ADULTS, ELDERLY: 1,500 mg as a single dose. Initiate at first sign or symptom.

Dosage in Renal Impairment
Dosage and frequency are modified based on creatinine clearance and disease process.

F

Creatinine Clearance	Herpes Zoster	Recurrent Genital Herpes (single-day regimen)	Recurrent Genital Herpes (suppression)	Recurrent Herpes Labialis Treatment (single-day regimen)	Recurrent Orolabial or Genital Herpes in HIV Pts
40–59 ml/min	500 mg q12h	500 mg q12h	—	750 mg	—
20–39 ml/min	500 mg q24h	500 mg	125 mg q12h	500 mg	500 mg q24h
Less than 20 ml/min	250 mg q24h	250 mg	125 mg q24h	250 mg	250 mg q24h
Hemodialysis	250 mg after each hemodialysis session	250 mg after each hemodialysis session	125 mg after each hemodialysis session	250 mg after each hemodialysis session	250 mg after each hemodialysis session

Dosage in Hemodialysis Pts

For adults with herpes zoster, give 250 mg after each dialysis treatment; for adults with genital herpes, give 125 mg after each dialysis treatment.

SIDE EFFECTS

Frequent: Headache (23%), nausea (12%). **Occasional (10%–2%):** Dizziness, drowsiness, paresthesia (esp. feet), diarrhea, vomiting, constipation, decreased appetite, fatigue, fever, pharyngitis, sinusitis, pruritus. **Rare (less than 2%):** Insomnia, abdominal pain, dyspepsia, flatulence, back pain, arthralgia.

ADVERSE EFFECTS/ TOXIC REACTIONS

Urticaria, hallucinations, confusion (delirium, disorientation occur predominantly in elderly) has been reported.

NURSING CONSIDERATIONS

BASELINE ASSESSMENT

Obtain baseline chemistry tests, esp. renal function.

INTERVENTION/EVALUATION

Evaluate cutaneous lesions. Be alert to neurologic effects: headache, dizziness. Provide analgesics, comfort measures; esp. exhausting in elderly. Monitor renal function, hepatic enzymes, CBC.

PATIENT/FAMILY TEACHING

• Drink adequate fluids. • Fingernails should be kept short, hands clean. • Do not touch lesions with fingers to avoid spreading infection to new site. • **Genital herpes:** Continue therapy for full length of treatment. • Avoid contact with lesions during duration of outbreak to prevent cross-contamination. • Notify physician if lesions recur or do not improve. • Change position slowly from sitting/lying to standing to avoid dizziness. • Avoid tasks that require alertness, motor skills until response to drug is established.

famotidine

 TOP 200

fa-**moe**-ta-deen
(Apo-Famotidine ✤, Novo-Famotidine ✤, Pepcid, Pepcid AC, Pepcid AC Maximum Strength, Ulcidine ✤)

Do not confuse famotidine with fluoxetine or furosemide.

FIXED-COMBINATION(S)

Duexis: famotidine/ibuprofen (an NSAID): 26.6 mg/800 mg. **Pepcid Complete:** famotidine/calcium chloride/magnesium hydroxide (antacids): 10 mg/800 mg/165 mg.

◆CLASSIFICATION

PHARMACOTHERAPEUTIC: H_2 receptor antagonist. **CLINICAL:** Antiulcer, gastric acid secretion inhibitor (see p. 111C).

ACTION

Inhibits histamine action of H_2 receptors of parietal cells. **Therapeutic Effect:** Inhibits gastric acid secretion (fasting, nocturnal, or stimulated by food, caffeine, insulin).

PHARMACOKINETICS

Route	Onset	Peak	Duration
PO	1 hr	1–4 hrs	10–12 hrs
IV	0.5 hr	0.5–3 hrs	10–12 hrs

Rapidly, incompletely absorbed from GI tract. Protein binding: 15%–20%. Partially metabolized in liver. Primarily excreted in urine. Not removed by hemodialysis. **Half-life:** 2.5–3.5 hrs (increased in renal impairment).

USES

Short-term treatment of active duodenal ulcer. Prevention, maintenance of duodenal ulcer recurrence. Treatment of active benign gastric ulcer, pathologic GI hypersecretory conditions. Short-term treatment of gastroesophageal reflux disease (GERD), including erosive esophagitis. OTC formulation for relief of heartburn, acid indigestion, sour stomach. **OFF-LABEL:** *H. pylori* eradication, risk reduction of duodenal ulcer recurrence (part of multidrug regimen), stress ulcer prophylaxis in critically ill pts, relief of gastritis.

PRECAUTIONS

Contraindications: Hypersensitivity to other H_2 antagonists. **Cautions:** Renal/hepatic impairment, elderly, thrombocytopenia.

⌛ LIFESPAN CONSIDERATIONS

Pregnancy/Lactation: Unknown if drug crosses placenta or is distributed in breast milk. **Pregnancy Category B. Children:** No age-related precautions noted. **Elderly:** Confusion more likely to occur, esp. in those with renal/hepatic impairment.

INTERACTIONS

DRUG: May decrease absorption of **atazanavir, itraconazole, ketoconazole.** **HERBAL:** None significant. **FOOD:** None known. **LAB VALUES:** Interferes with skin tests using allergen extracts. May increase serum alkaline phosphatase, AST, ALT. May decrease platelet count.

AVAILABILITY (Rx)

Infusion, Premix: 20 mg in 50 ml 0.9% NaCl. **Injection, Solution (Pepcid):** 10 mg/ml. **Powder for Oral Suspension (Pepcid):** 40 mg/5 ml. **Tablets: (Pepcid AC):** 10 mg. (Pepcid): 20 mg, 40 mg. **Tablets, Chewable (Pepcid AC Maximum Strength):** 20 mg.

ADMINISTRATION/HANDLING

 IV

Reconstitution • For IV push, dilute 20 mg with 5–10 ml 0.9% NaCl. • For intermittent IV infusion (piggyback), dilute with 50–100 ml D_5W, or 0.9% NaCl.
Rate of Administration • Give IV push over at least 2 min. • Infuse piggyback over 15–30 min.
Storage • Refrigerate unreconstituted vials. • IV solution appears clear, colorless. • After dilution, IV solution is stable for 48 hrs if refrigerated.

PO

• Store tablets, suspension at room temperature. • Following reconstitution, oral suspension is stable for 30 days at room temperature. • Give without regard to meals. • Shake suspension well before use.

▦ IV INCOMPATIBILITIES

Amphotericin B complex (Abelcet, AmBisome, Amphotec), piperacillin/tazobactam (Zosyn).

▦ IV COMPATIBILITIES

Calcium gluconate, dexamethasone (Decadron), dexmedetomidine (Precedex), dobutamine (Dobutrex), dopamine (Intropin), doxorubicin (Adriamycin), furosemide (Lasix), heparin, hydromorphone (Dilaudid), insulin (regular), lidocaine, lorazepam (Ativan), magnesium sulfate, midazolam (Versed), morphine, nitroglycerin, norepinephrine (Levophed), ondansetron (Zofran), potassium chloride, potassium phosphate, propofol (Diprivan).

INDICATIONS/ROUTES/DOSAGE

Duodenal Ulcer
PO: ADULTS, ELDERLY: Acute therapy: 40 mg/day at bedtime or 20 mg twice daily for 4–8 wks. **Maintenance:** 20 mg/day at bedtime.

Peptic Ulcer
PO: CHILDREN 1–16 YRS: 0.5 mg/kg/day at bedtime or 2 divided doses. **Maximum:** 40 mg/day.

Gastric Ulcer
PO: ADULTS, ELDERLY: 40 mg/day at bedtime.

Gastroesophageal Reflux Disease (GERD)
PO: ADULTS, ELDERLY: 20 mg twice a day for 6 wks. **CHILDREN 1–16 YRS:** 1 mg/kg/day in 2 divided doses. **Maximum:** 40 mg 2 times/day. **CHILDREN 3 MOS–11 MOS:** 0.5 mg/kg/dose twice a day. **CHILDREN YOUNGER THAN 3 MOS, NEONATES:** 0.5 mg/kg/dose once a day.

Esophagitis
PO: ADULTS, ELDERLY, CHILDREN 12 YRS AND OLDER: 20–40 mg twice a day for up to 12 wks.

Hypersecretory Conditions
PO: ADULTS, ELDERLY, CHILDREN 12 YRS AND OLDER: Initially, 20 mg q6h. May increase up to 160 mg q6h.

Acid Indigestion, Heartburn (OTC Use)
PO: ADULTS, ELDERLY, CHILDREN 12 YRS AND OLDER: 10–20 mg q12h. May take 15–60 min before eating. **Maximum:** 2 doses per day.

Usual Parenteral Dosage
IV: ADULTS, ELDERLY, CHILDREN OLDER THAN 12 YRS: 20 mg q12h. **CHILDREN 1–12 YRS:** 0.25–0.5 mg/kg q12h. **Maximum:** 40 mg/day.

Dosage in Renal Impairment

Creatinine Clearance	Dosage
Less than 50 ml/min	50% normal dose or increase dosing interval to 36–48 hrs

SIDE EFFECTS

Occasional (5%): Headache. **Rare (2% or less):** Confusion, constipation, diarrhea, dizziness.

ADVERSE EFFECTS/ TOXIC REACTIONS

Agranulocytosis, pancytopenia, thrombocytopenia occur rarely.

NURSING CONSIDERATIONS

BASELINE ASSESSMENT
Assess epigastric/abdominal pain.

INTERVENTION/EVALUATION
Monitor daily pattern of bowel activity, stool consistency. Monitor for diarrhea, constipation, headache. Assess for confusion in elderly.

PATIENT/FAMILY TEACHING
• May take without regard to meals, antacids. • Report headache. • Avoid excessive amounts of coffee, aspirin. • If symptoms of heartburn, acid indigestion, sour stomach persist with medication, consult physician.

febuxostat

fe-**bux**-oh-stat
(Uloric)
Do not confuse febuxostat with Femstat.

 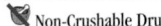

F

◆CLASSIFICATION

PHARMACOTHERAPEUTIC: Xanthine oxidase inhibitor. **CLINICAL:** Antigout agent.

ACTION

Decreases uric acid production by inhibiting the enzyme xanthine oxidase. **Therapeutic Effect:** Reduces uric acid concentrations in serum and urine.

PHARMACOKINETICS

Well absorbed from GI tract. Widely distributed. Protein binding: 99%. Metabolized in liver. Eliminated in urine (49%), feces (45%). Removed by hemodialysis. **Half-life:** 5–8 hrs.

USES

Management of hyperuricemia in pts with gout. Not recommended for treatment of asymptomatic hyperuricemia.

PRECAUTIONS

Contraindications: Concurrent use with azathioprine, mercaptopurine. **Canada:** Concomitant use with theophylline. **Cautions:** Severe renal/hepatic impairment, history of heart disease or stroke.

⌛ LIFESPAN CONSIDERATIONS

Pregnancy/Lactation: Unknown if drug crosses placenta or is distributed in breast milk. **Pregnancy Category C. Children:** Safety and efficacy not established. **Elderly:** No age-related precautions noted.

INTERACTIONS

DRUG: May increase concentration, toxicity of **azathioprine, mercaptopurine, theophylline. HERBAL:** None significant. **FOOD:** None known. **LAB VALUES:** May increase serum alkaline phosphatase, AST, ALT, LDH, amylase, sodium, potassium, cholesterol, triglycerides, BUN, creatinine. May decrease platelet count, Hgb, Hct, neutrophil count. May prolong prothrombin time.

AVAILABILITY (Rx)

Tablets: 40 mg, 80 mg.

ADMINISTRATION/HANDLING

PO

• May give without regard to meals or antacids.

INDICATIONS/ROUTES/DOSAGE

◀**ALERT**▶ Recommended to take an NSAID or colchicine with initiation of therapy and continue for up to 6 mos to prevent exacerbations of gout.

Hyperuricemia

PO: ADULTS, ELDERLY: 40 mg once daily. If pt does not achieve serum uric acid level less than 6 mg/dl after 2 wks with 40 mg, may give 80 mg once daily.

SIDE EFFECTS

Rare (1%): Nausea, arthralgia, rash, dizziness.

ADVERSE EFFECTS/ TOXIC REACTIONS

Hepatic function abnormalities occur in 6% of pts.

NURSING CONSIDERATIONS

BASELINE ASSESSMENT

Assess baseline renal/hepatic function; concomitant medication (azathioprine, mercaptopurine, theophylline) contraindicated.

INTERVENTION/EVALUATION

Discontinue medication immediately if rash appears. Encourage high fluid intake (3,000 ml/day). Monitor I&O (output should be at least 2,000 ml/day). Monitor CBC, serum uric acid, renal/hepatic function levels. Assess urine for cloudiness, unusual color, odor. Assess for therapeutic response (reduced joint tenderness, swelling, redness, limitation of motion).

PATIENT/FAMILY TEACHING

• Encourage drinking 8–10 glasses (8 oz) of fluid daily while taking medication. • Report rash, chest pain, shortness of breath, symptoms suggestive of stroke. • Gout attacks may occur for several months after starting treatment (medication is not a pain reliever). • Continue taking even if gout attack occurs.

felodipine

fe-**loe**-di-peen
(Plendil ✦, Renedil ✦)
Do not confuse Plendil with Isordil, Pletal, Prilosec, or Prinivil, or Renedil with Prinivil.

FIXED-COMBINATION(S)

Lexxel: felodipine/enalapril (ACE inhibitor): 2.5 mg/5 mg, 5 mg/5 mg.

◆CLASSIFICATION

PHARMACOTHERAPEUTIC: Calcium channel blocker. **CLINICAL:** Antihypertensive, antianginal (see pp. 62C, 79C).

ACTION

Inhibits calcium movement across cardiac, vascular smooth muscle cell membranes (does not depress SA, AV nodes). Potent peripheral vasodilator. **Therapeutic Effect:** Increases myocardial contractility, heart rate, cardiac output; decreases peripheral vascular resistance, B/P.

PHARMACOKINETICS

Route	Onset	Peak	Duration
PO	2–5 hrs	N/A	24 hrs

Rapidly, completely absorbed from GI tract. Protein binding: greater than 99%. Metabolized in liver. Primarily excreted in urine. Not removed by hemodialysis. **Half-life:** 11–16 hrs.

USES

Management of hypertension. May be used alone or with other antihyperten-

sives. **OFF-LABEL:** Management of pediatric hypertension.

PRECAUTIONS

Contraindications: Hypersensitivity to felodipine or other calcium channel blocker. **Cautions:** Severe left ventricular dysfunction, HF, hepatic impairment, hypertrophic cardiomyopathy with outflow tract obstruction, edema, severe aortic stenosis. Concomitant CYP3A4 inhibitors (see Appendix J).

⌛ LIFESPAN CONSIDERATIONS

Pregnancy/Lactation: Unknown if drug crosses placenta or is distributed in breast milk. **Pregnancy Category C. Children:** Safety and efficacy not established. **Elderly:** May experience greater hypotensive response. Constipation may be more problematic.

INTERACTIONS

DRUG: CYP3A4 inhibitors (e.g., ketoconazole, erythromycin, cimetidine) may increase concentration. **HERBAL: St. John's wort** may decrease concentration. **Ephedra, ginseng, yohimbe** may worsen hypertension. **Garlic** may increase antihypertensive effect. **FOOD: Grapefruit products** may increase absorption, concentration. **LAB VALUES:** None significant.

AVAILABILITY (Rx)

🌱 Tablets (Extended-Release): 2.5 mg, 5 mg, 10 mg.

ADMINISTRATION/HANDLING

PO
• Give without food. • Do not cut, crush, break extended-release tablets. Swallow whole.

INDICATIONS/ROUTES/DOSAGE

Hypertension
PO: ADULTS: Initially, 5 mg/day as single dose. Increase by 5 mg at 2-wk intervals. **Maximum:** 20 mg/day. **ELDERLY, PTS WITH HEPATIC IMPAIRMENT:** Initially, 2.5

mg/day. Adjust dosage at no less than 2-wk intervals. Range: 2.5–20 mg/day. **CHILDREN:** Initially, 2.5 mg once daily. **Maximum:** 10 mg/day.

SIDE EFFECTS

Frequent (22%–18%): Headache, peripheral edema. **Occasional (6%–4%):** Flushing, respiratory infection, dizziness, lightheadedness, asthenia (loss of strength, energy). **Rare (less than 3%):** Angina, gingival hyperplasia, paresthesia, abdominal discomfort, anxiety, muscle cramping, cough, diarrhea, constipation.

ADVERSE EFFECTS/ TOXIC REACTIONS

Overdose produces nausea, drowsiness, confusion, slurred speech, hypotension, bradycardia.

NURSING CONSIDERATIONS

BASELINE ASSESSMENT

Assess B/P, apical pulse immediately before drug administration (if pulse is 60 or less/min or systolic B/P is less than 90 mm Hg, withhold medication, contact physician).

INTERVENTION/EVALUATION

Assist with ambulation if dizziness occurs. Assess for peripheral edema behind media malleolus (sacral area in bedridden pts). Monitor pulse rate for bradycardia. Assess skin for flushing. Monitor hepatic function. Question for headache, asthenia (loss of strength, energy).

PATIENT/FAMILY TEACHING

• Do not abruptly discontinue medication. • Compliance with therapy regimen is essential to control hypertension. • To avoid hypotensive effect, go from lying to standing slowly. • Avoid tasks that require alertness, motor skills until response to drug is established. • Contact physician if palpitations, shortness of breath, pronounced dizziness, nausea occur. • Swallow tablet whole; do not crush, chew. • Avoid grapefruit products, alcohol. • Report exacerbation of angina.

---

fenofibrate   TOP 200

fen-oh-**fye**-brate
(Antara, Apo-Fenofibrate ✦, Fenoglide, Lipofen, Lofibra, Novo-Fenofibrate ✦, Tricor, Triglide)
Do not confuse Tricor with Fibricor or Tracleer.

◆CLASSIFICATION

PHARMACOTHERAPEUTIC: Fibric acid derivative. **CLINICAL:** Antihyperlipidemic (see p. 57C).

ACTION

Enhances synthesis of lipoprotein lipase (VLDL). **Therapeutic Effect:** Increases VLDL catabolism, reduces total plasma cholesterol, LDL, VLDL, triglycerides.

PHARMACOKINETICS

Well absorbed from GI tract. Absorption increased when given with food. Protein binding: 99%. Metabolized in liver. Excreted in urine (60%), feces (25%). Not removed by hemodialysis. **Half-life:** 10–35 hrs.

USES

Adjunct to diet for reduction of low-density lipoprotein cholesterol (LDL-C), total cholesterol, triglycerides (types IV and V hyperlipidemia), apo-lipoprotein B, and to increase high-density lipoprotein cholesterol (HDL-C) in pts with primary hypercholesterolemia, mixed dyslipidemia.

PRECAUTIONS

Contraindications: Gallbladder disease, severe renal/hepatic dysfunction (including primary biliary cirrhosis, unexplained persistent hepatic function abnormality), breast-feeding (Fenoglide,

Lipofen, Tricor, Triglide). **Cautions:** Anticoagulant therapy (e.g., warfarin), history of hepatic disease, renal impairment, substantial alcohol consumption, statin or colchicine therapy (increased risk of myopathy, rhabdomyolysis).

⧗ LIFESPAN CONSIDERATIONS

Pregnancy/Lactation: Safety in pregnancy not established. Breastfeeding not recommended. **Pregnancy Category C. Children:** Safety and efficacy not established. **Elderly:** No age-related precautions noted.

INTERACTIONS

DRUG: Potentiates effects of **anticoagulants (e.g., warfarin). Bile acid sequestrants** may impede absorption. **Cyclosporine** may increase concentration/risk of nephrotoxicity. **Colchicine, HMG-CoA reductase inhibitors (statins)** may increase risk of severe myopathy, rhabdomyolysis, acute renal failure. **HERBAL:** None significant. **FOOD: All foods** increase absorption. **LAB VALUES:** May increase serum creatine kinase (CK), AST, ALT. May decrease Hgb, Hct, serum uric acid, WBC count.

AVAILABILITY (Rx)

Capsules: *(Antara):* 43 mg, 130 mg. *(Lipofen):* 50 mg, 150 mg. *(Lofibra):* 67 mg, 134 mg, 200 mg. **Tablets:** *(Fenoglide):* 40 mg, 120 mg. *(Lofibra):* 54 mg, 160 mg. *(Tricor):* 48 mg, 145 mg. *(Triglide):* 50 mg, 160 mg.

ADMINISTRATION/HANDLING

PO
• Give Fenoglide, Lipofen, Lofibra with meals. • Antara, Tricor, and Triglide may be given without regard to food.

INDICATIONS/ROUTES/DOSAGE

Hypertriglyceridemia
PO *(Antara):* **ADULTS, ELDERLY:** 43–130 mg/day.
PO *(Fenoglide):* **ADULTS, ELDERLY:** 40–120 mg/day with meals.

PO *(Lipofen):* **ADULTS, ELDERLY:** 50–150 mg/day with meals.
PO *(Lofibra):* **ADULTS, ELDERLY:** 67–200 mg/day with meals.
PO *(Tricor):* **ADULTS, ELDERLY:** 48–145 mg/day.
PO *(Triglide):* **ADULTS, ELDERLY:** 50–160 mg/day.

Hypercholesterolemia, Mixed Hyperlipidemia
PO *(Antara):* **ADULTS, ELDERLY:** 130 mg/day.
PO *(Fenoglide):* **ADULTS, ELDERLY:** 120 mg/day with meals.
PO *(Lipofen):* **ADULTS, ELDERLY:** 150 mg/day with meals.
PO *(Lofibra):* **ADULTS, ELDERLY:** 200 mg/day with meals.
PO *(Tricor):* **ADULTS, ELDERLY:** 145 mg/day.
PO *(Triglide):* **ADULTS, ELDERLY:** 160 mg/day.

Dosage in Renal Impairment
Monitor renal function/lipid profile before adjusting dose. Decrease dose or increase dosing interval for pts with renal failure.

Initial doses:	Antara: 43 mg/day	Lofibra: 67 mg/day
	Fenoglide: 40 mg/day	Tricor: 48 mg/day
	Lipofen: 50 mg/day	Triglide: 50 mg/day

SIDE EFFECTS

Frequent (8%–4%): Pain, rash, headache, asthenia (loss of strength, energy), fatigue, flu-like symptoms, dyspepsia, nausea/vomiting, rhinitis. **Occasional (3%–2%):** Diarrhea, abdominal pain, constipation, flatulence, arthralgia, decreased libido, dizziness, pruritus. **Rare (less than 2%):** Increased appetite, insomnia, polyuria, cough, blurred vision, eye floaters, earache.

ADVERSE EFFECTS/ TOXIC REACTIONS

May increase cholesterol excretion into bile, leading to cholelithiasis. Pancreatitis, hepatitis, thrombocytopenia, agranulocytosis occur rarely.

NURSING CONSIDERATIONS

BASELINE ASSESSMENT

Obtain diet history, esp. fat consumption. Obtain serum cholesterol, triglycerides, hepatic function tests, blood counts during initial therapy and periodically during treatment. Treatment should be discontinued if hepatic enzyme levels persist greater than 3 times normal limit.

INTERVENTION/EVALUATION

For pts on concurrent therapy with HMG-CoA reductase inhibitors, monitor for complaints of myopathy (muscle pain, weakness). Monitor serum creatine kinase (CK). Monitor serum cholesterol, triglyceride for therapeutic response.

PATIENT/FAMILY TEACHING

• Report severe diarrhea, constipation, nausea. • Report skin rash/irritation, insomnia, muscle pain, tremors, dizziness.

---

fenofibric acid `TOP 200`

fen-oh-**fye**-brick as-id
(Fibricor, Trilipix)
Do not confuse Fibricor with Tricor or Trilipix with Trileptal.

◆ CLASSIFICATION

PHARMACOTHERAPEUTIC: Fibric acid derivative. **CLINICAL:** Antihyperlipidemic (see p. 57C).

ACTION

Increases lipolysis and elimination of triglyceride-rich particles from plasma by activating lipoprotein lipase, reducing lipase activity. **Therapeutic Effect:** Produces alteration in size, composition of LDL allowing for greater affinity for catabolism, decreasing plasma triglycerides, cholesterol.

PHARMACOKINETICS

Well absorbed from GI tract. Protein binding: 99%. Does not undergo oxidative metabolism. Excreted primarily in urine. **Half-life:** 20 hrs.

USES

Fibricor, Trilipix: Adjunct to diet for treatment of severely elevated serum triglycerides; adjunct for reduction of LDL-C, total cholesterol, triglycerides, apoprotein B, and increased HDL-C in primary hypercholesterolemia or mixed hyperlipidemia. **Trilipix:** With statin to reduce triglycerides, elevate HDL-C in pts with mixed lipidemia and/or at risk for coronary heart disease.

PRECAUTIONS

Contraindications: Severe renal impairment, primary biliary cirrhosis, active hepatic disease, gallbladder disease, nursing mothers. **Cautions:** Anticoagulant therapy, history of hepatic disease, substantial alcohol consumption.

⏳ LIFESPAN CONSIDERATIONS

Pregnancy/Lactation: Safety in pregnancy not established. Avoid use in nursing mothers. **Pregnancy Category C. Children:** Safety and efficacy not established. **Elderly:** Age-related renal impairment may require monitoring.

INTERACTIONS

DRUG: Potentiates effects of **anticoagulants (e.g., warfarin)**. Bile acid sequestrants (cholestyramine, colestipol) may impede absorption; give Trilipix 1 hr before or 4–6 hrs after dosing. Cyclosporine may increase risk of nephrotoxicity. **HMG-CoA reductase inhibitors (statins)** may increase risk of severe myopathy, rhabdomyolysis, acute renal failure. **HERBAL:** None significant. **FOOD: All foods** increase absorption. **LAB VALUES:** May increase serum creatine kinase (CK), AST, ALT. May decrease Hgb, Hct, serum uric acid, WBC count.

AVAILABILITY (Rx)

Delayed-Release Capsules (Trilipix): 45 mg, 135 mg. Tablets (Fibricor): 35 mg, 105 mg.

ADMINISTRATION/HANDLING

PO

• Give without regard to meals. • Do not break, crush, or cut capsule. • May be given at the same time as a statin.

INDICATIONS/ROUTE/DOSAGE

Mixed Dyslipidemia, Primary Hypercholesterolemia
PO: ADULTS, ELDERLY: (Trilipix): 135 mg once daily. **(Fibricor):** 105 mg once daily.

Hypertriglyceridemia
PO: ADULTS, ELDERLY: (Trilipix): 45–135 mg once daily. **(Fibricor):** 35–105 mg once daily.

Mixed Lipidemia (with Statin)
PO: ADULTS, ELDERLY: (Trilipix): 135 mg once daily.

Renal Impairment (Creatinine Clearance: 30–80 ml/min)
PO: ADULTS, ELDERLY: (Trilipix): 45 mg once daily. **(Fibricor):** 35 mg once daily. (Contraindicated with creatinine clearance less than 30 ml/min.)

SIDE EFFECTS

Frequent (13%): Headache. **Occasional (6%–4%):** Back pain, upper respiratory tract infection, extremity pain, nausea, dizziness, diarrhea, arthralgia, dyspepsia, nasopharyngitis. **Rare (3%–2%):** Constipation, sinusitis, myalgia, fatigue, muscle spasm.

ADVERSE EFFECTS/TOXIC REACTIONS

Increased risk for myopathy, rhabdomyolysis, particularly in elderly, those with diabetes, renal failure, hypothyroidism. May increase cholesterol excretion into the bile, leading to cholelithiasis. Pancreatitis, hepatitis, thrombocytopenia, agranulocytosis occur rarely.

NURSING CONSIDERATIONS

BASELINE ASSESSMENT

Assess baseline cholesterol, triglycerides, hepatic function tests, blood counts during initial therapy and periodically during treatment.

INTERVENTION/EVALUATION

For those on concurrent therapy with HMG-CoA reductase inhibitors, monitor for complaints of myopathy (muscle pain, weakness), including serum creatine kinase levels. Monitor cholesterol, triglyceride concentrations for therapeutic response.

PATIENT/FAMILY TEACHING

• Periodic lab tests are essential part of therapy. • Follow special diet (important part of treatment). • Report severe diarrhea, constipation, nausea. • Report muscle pain, back/extremity pain, dizziness.

---

fentanyl   TOP 200   HIGH ALERT

fen-ta-nil
(Abstral, <u>Actiq</u>, <u>Duragesic</u>, Fentora, Lazanda, Novo-Fentanyl ✦, Onsolis, Subsys)

BLACK BOX ALERT Physical and psychological dependence may occur with prolonged use. Must be alert to abuse, misuse, or diversion. May cause life-threatening hypoventilation, respiratory depression, or death. Use with strong or moderate CYP3A4 inhibitors may result in potentially fatal respiratory depression. **Buccal:** Tablet and lozenge contain enough medication that may be fatal to children. **Transdermal patch:** Serious or life-threatening hypoventilation has occurred. Limit use to children 2 yrs of age and older. Exposure to direct heat source increases drug release, resulting in overdose/death.
Do not confuse fentanyl with alfentanil or sufentanil.

F

◆CLASSIFICATION

PHARMACOTHERAPEUTIC: Opioid, narcotic agonist **(Schedule II)**. **CLINICAL:** Analgesic.

ACTION

Binds to opioid receptors in CNS, reducing stimuli from sensory nerve endings, inhibits ascending pain pathways. **Therapeutic Effect:** Alters pain reception, increases pain threshold.

PHARMACOKINETICS

Route	Onset	Peak	Duration
IV	1–2 min	3–5 min	0.5–1 hr
IM	7–15 min	20–30 min	1–2 hrs
Trans-dermal	6–8 hrs	24 hrs	72 hrs
Trans-mucosal	5–15 min	20–30 min	1–2 hrs

Well absorbed after IM or topical administration. Transmucosal form absorbed through buccal mucosa and GI tract. Protein binding: 80%–85%. Metabolized in liver. Primarily eliminated by biliary system. **Half-life:** 2–4 hrs IV; 17 hrs transdermal; 6.6 hrs transmucosal.

USES

Injection: pain relief, preop medication; adjunct to general or regional anesthesia. **Abstral:** Treatment of breakthrough pain in cancer pts 18 yrs of age and older. **Duragesic:** Management of chronic pain *(transdermal)*. **Actiq:** Treatment of breakthrough pain in chronic cancer or AIDS-related pain. **Fentora:** Breakthrough pain in pts on chronic opioids. **Onsolis:** Breakthrough pain in pts with cancer currently receiving opioids and tolerant to opioid therapy. **Lazanda:** Management of breakthrough pain in cancer. **Subsys:** Treatment of breakthrough cancer pain.

PRECAUTIONS

Contraindications: Transdermal: Severe respiratory disease/depression, paralytic ileus; short term therapy; intermittent pain. **Transdermal, transmucosal,** **lozenges, buccal films:** Management of acute or postoperative pain, pts not opioid tolerant. **Cautions:** Bradycardia; renal, hepatic, respiratory disease; head injuries; altered LOC; biliary tract disease; acute pancreatitis; cor pulmonale; significant COPD; increased ICP; use of MAOIs within 14 days; elderly; morbid obesity.

⧗ LIFESPAN CONSIDERATIONS

Pregnancy/Lactation: Readily crosses placenta. Unknown if distributed in breast milk. May prolong labor if administered in latent phase of first stage of labor or before cervical dilation of 4–5 cm has occurred. Respiratory depression may occur in neonate if mother received opiates during labor. **Pregnancy Category C (D if used for prolonged periods or at high dosages at term). Children:** Patch: Safety and efficacy not established in those younger than 12 yrs. Neonates more susceptible to respiratory depressant effects. **Elderly:** May be more susceptible to respiratory depressant effects. Age-related renal impairment may require dosage adjustment.

INTERACTIONS

DRUG: CYP3A4 inducers (e.g., rifampin, modafanil) may decrease concentration/effect. **Alcohol, CNS depressant medications** may increase CNS depression. **CYP3A4 inhibitors (e.g., erythromycin, itraconazole, ketoconazole, protease inhibitors [e.g., ritonavir])** may increase effect and potential of respiratory depression. **HERBAL: Gotu kola, kava kava, St. John's wort, valerian** may increase CNS depression. **St. John's wort** may decrease concentration/effects. **FOOD: Grapefruit products** may increase potential for respiratory depression with oral, transmucosal forms. **LAB VALUES:** May increase serum amylase, lipase.

AVAILABILITY (Rx)

Buccal Tablet (Fentora): 100 mcg, 200 mcg, 400 mcg, 600 mcg, 800 mcg. **Buccal Soluble Film (Onsolis):** 200 mcg, 400 mcg, 600 mcg, 800 mcg, 1,200 mcg. **Injection Solution:** 50 mcg/ml. **Nasal Spray (Lazanda):** 100 mcg/spray, 400 mcg/spray. **Sublingual Tablets (Abstral):** 100 mcg, 200 mcg, 300 mcg, 400 mcg, 600 mcg, 800 mcg. **Sublingual Spray (Subsys):** 100 mcg, 200 mcg, 400 mcg, 600 mcg, 800 mcg. **Transdermal Patch (Duragesic):** 12 mcg/hr, 25 mcg/hr, 50 mcg/hr, 75 mcg/hr, 100 mcg/hr. **Transmucosal Lozenges (Actiq):** 200 mcg, 400 mcg, 600 mcg, 800 mcg, 1,200 mcg, 1,600 mcg.

ADMINISTRATION/HANDLING

 IV

Rate of Administration • Give by slow IV injection (over 1–2 min). • Too-rapid IV increases risk of severe adverse reactions (skeletal/thoracic muscle rigidity resulting in apnea, laryngospasm, bronchospasm, peripheral circulatory collapse, anaphylactoid effects, cardiac arrest).
Storage • Store parenteral form at room temperature. • Opiate antagonist (naloxone) should be readily available.

Transdermal
• Apply to hairless area of intact skin of upper torso. • Use flat, nonirritated site. • Firmly press evenly and hold for 30 sec, ensuring adhesion is in full contact with skin and edges are completely sealed. • Use only water to cleanse site before application (soaps, oils may irritate skin). • Rotate sites of application. • Carefully fold used patches so that system adheres to itself; discard in toilet.

Buccal Film
• Wet inside of cheek. • Place film inside mouth with pink side of unit against cheek. • Press film against cheek and hold for 5 sec. • Leave in place until dissolved (15–30 min). • Do not chew, swallow, cut film. • Liquids may be given after 5 min of application; food after film dissolves.

Buccal Tablets
• Place tablet above a rear molar between upper cheek and gum. • Dissolve over 30 min. • Swallow remaining pieces with water. • Do not split tablet.

Sublingual Spray
• Open blister pack with scissors immediately prior to use. • Spray contents underneath tongue.

Sublingual Tablets
• Place under tongue. • Dissolves rapidly. • Do not suck, chew, or swallow tablet.

Nasal
• Prime device before use by spraying into pouch. • Insert nozzle about ½ inch into nose, pointing toward bridge of nose, tilting bottle slightly. • Press down firmly until hearing a "click" and number on counting window advances by one.

Transmucosal
• Suck lozenge vigorously. • Allow to dissolve over 15 min. • Do not chew.

IV INCOMPATIBILITIES

Azithromycin (Zithromax), pantoprazole (Protonix), phenytoin (Dilantin).

IV COMPATIBILITIES

Atropine, bupivacaine (Marcaine, Sensorcaine), clonidine (Duraclon), dexmedetomidine (Precedex), diltiazem (Cardizem), diphenhydramine (Benadryl), dobutamine (Dobutrex), dopamine (Intropin), droperidol (Inapsine), heparin, hydromorphone (Dilaudid), ketorolac (Toradol), lorazepam (Ativan), metoclopramide (Reglan), midazolam (Versed), milrinone (Primacor), morphine, nitroglycerin, norepinephrine (Levophed), ondansetron (Zofran), potassium chloride, propofol (Diprivan).

INDICATIONS/ROUTES/DOSAGE

Note: Doses titrated to desired effect dependent upon degree of analgesia, pt status.
Acute Pain Management
IM/IV: ADULTS, ELDERLY: 25–100 mcg/dose q1–2h as needed. **CHILDREN:** 0.5–2 mcg/kg/dose q1–2h as needed.

F

Continuous IV Infusion
ADULTS, ELDERLY: 1–2 mcg/kg/hr. **CHILDREN:** 0.5–2 mcg/kg/hr.

Premedication
IV, IM: ADULTS, ELDERLY, CHILDREN 12 YRS AND OLDER: 50–100 mcg/dose 30–60 min prior to surgery.

Adjunct to Regional Anesthesia
IV: ADULTS, ELDERLY, CHILDREN 12 YRS AND OLDER: 25–100 mcg/dose over 1–2 min.

Adjunct to General Anesthesia
IV: ADULTS, ELDERLY, CHILDREN 12 YRS AND OLDER: 2–50 mcg/kg.

Usual Buccal Dose
ADULTS, ELDERLY: Initially, 100 mcg. Titrate dose, providing adequate analgesia with tolerable side effects.

Usual Buccal Soluble Film Dose
Note: All pts must initiate with 200 mcg.
ADULTS, ELDERLY: Initially, 200 mcg up to 1,200 mcg. **Maximum:** No more than 4 doses per day, separate by at least 2 hrs.

Usual Nasal Dose
Nasal: ADULTS, ELDERLY: Initially, 100 mcg. Titrate from 100 mcg to 200 mcg to 400 mcg to 800 mcg **(maximum)**. Wait at least 2 hrs between doses; no more than 4 doses in 24 hrs.

Usual Sublingual Tablet Dose
ADULTS, ELDERLY: Initially, 100 mcg, then titrate to desired dose/effect. Wait at least 2 hrs between doses; no more than 4 doses in 24 hrs.

Usual Sublingual Spray Dose
ADULTS, ELDERLY: Initially, 100 mcg. May repeat in 30 min if pain not relieved. Must wait at least 4 hours before treating another episode of pain.

Usual Transdermal Dose
ADULTS, ELDERLY, CHILDREN 12 YRS AND OLDER: Initially, 12–25 mcg/hr. May increase after 3 days.

Usual Transmucosal Dose
ADULTS, CHILDREN: 200–400 mcg for breakthrough pain. Limit to 4 units/day.

Dosage in Renal Impairment
Dosage is modified based on creatinine clearance.

Creatinine Clearance	Dosage
10–50 ml/min	75% of usual dose
Less than 10 ml/min	50% of usual dose

SIDE EFFECTS

Frequent: IV: Postop drowsiness, nausea, vomiting. **Transdermal (10%–3%):** Headache, pruritus, nausea, vomiting, diaphoresis, dyspnea, confusion, dizziness, drowsiness, diarrhea, constipation, decreased appetite. **Occasional: IV:** Postop confusion, blurred vision, chills, orthostatic hypotension, constipation, difficulty urinating. **Transdermal (3%–1%):** Chest pain, arrhythmias, erythema, pruritus, syncope, agitation, skin irritations.

ADVERSE EFFECTS/ TOXIC REACTIONS

Overdose or too-rapid IV administration may produce severe respiratory depression, skeletal/thoracic muscle rigidity (may lead to apnea, laryngospasm, bronchospasm, cold/clammy skin, cyanosis, coma). Tolerance to analgesic effect may occur with repeated use. **Antidote:** Naloxone (see Appendix K for dosage).

NURSING CONSIDERATIONS

BASELINE ASSESSMENT

Resuscitative equipment, opiate antagonist (naloxone 0.5 mcg/kg) must be available for initial input use. Establish baseline B/P, respirations. Assess type, location, intensity, duration of pain.

INTERVENTION/EVALUATION

Assist with ambulation. Encourage post-op pt to turn, cough, deep breathe q2h.

Monitor respiratory rate, B/P, heart rate, oxygen saturation. Assess for relief of pain.

PATIENT/FAMILY TEACHING

• Avoid alcohol; do not take other medications without consulting physician. • Avoid tasks that require alertness, motor skills until response to drug is established. • Teach pt proper transdermal, buccal, lozenge administration. **Transdermal:** Avoid saunas (increases drug release time). • Use as directed to avoid overdosage; potential for physical dependence with prolonged use. • Report absence of pain relief, constipation. • After long-term use, must be discontinued slowly.

---

ferric carboxymaltose

fer-ik car-**box**-ee-**mal**-tose
(Injectafer)

◆CLASSIFICATION

PHARMACOTHERAPEUTIC: Iron preparation. **CLINICAL:** Iron replacement.

ACTION

Essential component in formation of Hgb, myoglobin, essential enzymes. Necessary for effective erythropoiesis, transport, utilization of oxygen. **Therapeutic Effect:** Replenishes iron stores.

PHARMACOKINETICS

Iron is protein-bound to form hemosiderin, ferritin, or transferrin. No physiologic system of elimination. Small amounts are lost in daily shedding of skin, hair, nails, with trace elimination in feces, urine. **Half-life:** 7–12 hrs.

USES

Treatment of iron deficiency anemia in adults who are intolerant to oral iron or have had an unsatisfactory response to oral iron, or who have non–dialysis-dependent chronic kidney disease.

PRECAUTIONS

Contraindications: Hypersensitivity to ferric carboxymaltose, oral iron supplements, history of hemochromatosis, non–iron deficiency anemia. **Cautions:** Pts with history of significant allergies, asthma, severe hepatic impairment, hypertension.

⧗ LIFESPAN CONSIDERATIONS

Pregnancy/Lactation: Distributed in breast milk. **Pregnancy Category C. Children:** Safety and efficacy not established. **Elderly:** No age-related precautions noted.

INTERACTIONS

DRUG: Oral iron supplements may increase risk of hemosiderosis (iron overload). **HERBAL:** None significant. **FOOD:** None known. **LAB VALUES:** May decrease serum phosphate. May increase serum ALT.

AVAILABILITY (Rx)

Injection Solution: 750 mg/15 ml.

ADMINISTRATION/HANDLING

🝪 IV

Reconstitution • May give either as undiluted slow IV push or IV infusion. • When administering as IV infusion, dilute 750 mg dose in maximum of 250 ml 0.9% NaCl for concentration no less than 2 mg/ml. • Inspect for particulate matter. Solution will appear dark to light brown. **Rate of Administration** • For IV push, administer at maximum rate of 100 mg/min. For IV infusion, administer over at least 15 min. Monitor for extravasation. **Storage** • Following dilution, stable at room temperature for up to 72 hrs.

INDICATIONS/ROUTES/DOSAGE

Iron Deficiency Anemia
Dosage expressed in mg of elemental iron (50 mg iron per ml).

IV: **ADULTS/ELDERLY:** **(WEIGHING 50 KG OR MORE):** 750 mg times 2 doses, separated by at least 7 days. **Maximum dose:** 1500 mg/treatment course. **(WEIGHING LESS THAN 50 KG):** 15 mg/kg times 2 doses, separated by at least 7 days. **Maximum dose:** 1500 mg/treatment course.

SIDE EFFECTS

Occasional (7%–2%): Nausea, hypertension, flushing, dizziness. **Rare (less than 2%):** Vomiting, headache, dysgeusia, hypotension, constipation.

ADVERSE EFFECTS/ TOXIC REACTIONS

Hypersensitivity reaction including angioedema, chills, erythema, hypotension, pruritus, syncope, urticaria, wheezing reported in 1.5% of pts. Anaphylaxis was noted in less than 1% of pts. Transient hypertension reported in 4% of pts. Hemosiderosis (iron overload) may present with joint disorder, gait disturbance, asthenia. Extravasation may cause injection site discoloration.

NURSING CONSIDERATIONS

BASELINE ASSESSMENT

Obtain baseline Hgb, serum ferritin, phosphate, hepatic function test. Obtain baseline B/P. Assess patency of IV site; do not administer if infiltration is suspected. Question history of hepatic impairment. Question use of oral iron medication.

INTERVENTION/EVALUATION

Monitor Hgb, serum ferritin, phosphate. Monitor for hypersensitivity reaction, hypertension for at least 30 min after administration. Assess IV site for extravasation.

PATIENT/FAMILY TEACHING

• Pain and brown staining may occur at IV site. • Do not take oral iron while receiving intravenous iron (may increase risk of iron overload). • Stools frequently becomes black with iron therapy; this is harmless unless accompanied by red streaking, sticky consistency of stool, abdominal pain, or cramping. • Oral hygiene, hard candy, gum may reduce unpleasant taste caused by therapy. • Report signs of allergic reaction.

ferrous fumarate

fer-us **fue**-ma-rate
(Femiron, Ferro-Sequels, Palafer ✦)

ferrous gluconate

fer-us **gloo**-koe-nate
(Apo-Ferrous Gluconate ✦, Fergon)

ferrous sulfate

fer-us **sul**-fate
(Apo-Ferrous Sulfate ✦, Fer-In-Sol, Fer-Iron, Slow-Fe)

FIXED-COMBINATION(S)

Ferro-Sequels: ferrous fumarate/docusate (stool softener): 150 mg/100 mg.

◆CLASSIFICATION

PHARMACOTHERAPEUTIC: Enzymatic mineral. **CLINICAL:** Iron preparation (see p. 112C).

ACTION

Essential component in formation of Hgb, myoglobin, enzymes. Promotes effective erythropoiesis and transport, utilization of oxygen. **Therapeutic Effect:** Prevents iron deficiency.

PHARMACOKINETICS

Absorbed in duodenum and upper jejunum. Ten percent absorbed in pts with normal iron stores; increased to 20%–30% in those with inadequate iron stores. Primarily bound to serum transferrin. Excreted in urine, sweat, sloughing of intestinal mucosa, by menses. Half-life: 6 hrs.

USES

Prevention, treatment of iron deficiency anemia due to inadequate diet, malabsorption, pregnancy, blood loss.

PRECAUTIONS

Contraindications: Hemochromatosis, hemolytic anemias. **Cautions:** Peptic ulcer, regional enteritis, ulcerative colitis.

⧖ LIFESPAN CONSIDERATIONS

Pregnancy/Lactation: Crosses placenta; distributed in breast milk. **Pregnancy Category A. Children/Elderly:** No age-related precautions noted.

INTERACTIONS

DRUG: Antacids, calcium supplements, pancreatin, pancrelipase may decrease absorption of ferrous compounds. May decrease absorption of **etidronate, quinolones, tetracyclines.** **HERBAL:** None significant. **FOOD: Cereal, coffee, dietary fiber, eggs, milk, tea** decrease absorption. **LAB VALUES:** May increase serum bilirubin, iron. May decrease serum calcium.

AVAILABILITY (OTC)

Ferrous Fumarate
Tablets (Femiron): 63 mg (20 mg elemental iron), 324 mg (106 mg elemental iron).

🏷 Tablets (Timed-Release [Ferro-Sequels]): 150 mg (50 mg elemental iron).

Ferrous Gluconate
Tablets: 240 mg (27 mg elemental iron) (Fergon), 325 mg (36 mg elemental iron).

Ferrous Sulfate
Oral Drops (Fer-In-Sol, Fer-Iron): 75 mg/0.6 ml (15 mg/0.6 ml elemental iron). Tablets: 325 mg (65 mg elemental iron). Elixir: 220 mg/5 ml (44 mg elemental iron per 5 ml).

🏷 Tablets (Timed-Release [Slow-Fe]): 160 mg (50 mg elemental iron).

ADMINISTRATION/HANDLING

PO
• Store all forms (tablets, capsules, suspension, drops) at room temperature.
• Ideally, give between meals with water or juice but may give with meals if GI discomfort occurs. • Transient staining of mucous membranes, teeth occurs with liquid iron preparation. To avoid staining, place liquid on back of tongue with dropper or straw.
• Do not give with milk or milk products.
• Do not crush timed-release preparations.

INDICATIONS/ROUTES/DOSAGE

Iron Deficiency Anemia
Dosage is expressed in terms of milligrams of elemental iron, degree of anemia, pt weight, presence of any bleeding. Expect to use periodic hematologic determinations as guide to therapy.
PO (Ferrous Fumarate): ADULTS, ELDERLY: 60–100 mg twice a day. **CHILDREN:** 3–6 mg/kg/day in 2–3 divided doses.
PO (Ferrous Gluconate): ADULTS, ELDERLY: 60 mg 2–4 times a day. **CHILDREN:** 3–6 mg/kg/day in 2–3 divided doses.
PO (Ferrous Sulfate): ADULTS, ELDERLY: 65 mg 2–4 times a day. **CHILDREN:** 3–6 mg/kg/day in 2–3 divided doses.

Prevention of Iron Deficiency
PO (Ferrous Fumarate): ADULTS, ELDERLY: 60–100 mg/day. **CHILDREN:** 1–2 mg/kg/day.
PO (Ferrous Gluconate): ADULTS, ELDERLY: 60 mg/day. **CHILDREN:** 1–2 mg/kg/day.
PO (Ferrous Sulfate): ADULTS, ELDERLY: 65 mg/day. **CHILDREN:** 1–2 mg/kg/day.

SIDE EFFECTS

Occasional: Mild, transient nausea. **Rare:** Heartburn, anorexia, constipation, diarrhea.

ADVERSE EFFECTS/ TOXIC REACTIONS

Large doses may aggravate existing GI tract disease (peptic ulcer, regional enteritis, ulcerative colitis). Severe iron poisoning occurs most often in children,

---

✤ Canadian trade name   🏷 Non-Crushable Drug   🔺 High Alert drug

manifested as vomiting, severe abdominal pain, diarrhea, dehydration, followed by hyperventilation, pallor, cyanosis, cardiovascular collapse.

NURSING CONSIDERATIONS

BASELINE ASSESSMENT

Assess nutritional status, dietary history. To prevent mucous membrane and teeth staining with liquid preparation, use dropper or straw and allow solution to drop on back of tongue.

INTERVENTION/EVALUATION

Monitor serum iron, total iron-binding capacity, reticulocyte count, Hgb, ferritin. Monitor daily pattern of bowel activity, stool consistency. Assess for clinical improvement, record relief of iron deficiency symptoms (fatigue, irritability, pallor, paresthesia of extremities, headache).

PATIENT/FAMILY TEACHING

• Expect stool color to darken. • Oral liquid may stain teeth. • If GI discomfort occurs, take after meals or with food. • Do not take within 2 hrs of other medication or eggs, milk, tea, coffee, cereal.

fesoterodine

fes-oh-**ter**-oh-deen
(Toviaz)
Do not confuse fesoterodine with fexofenadine or tolteradine.

◆CLASSIFICATION

PHARMACOTHERAPEUTIC: Muscarinic receptor antagonist. **CLINICAL:** Antispasmodic.

ACTION

Exhibits antimuscarinic activity by interceding via cholinergic muscarinic receptors, thereby inhibiting urinary bladder contraction. **Therapeutic Effect:** Decreases urinary frequency, urgency.

PHARMACOKINETICS

Well absorbed following PO administration. Protein binding: 50%. Rapidly and extensively hydrolyzed to its active metabolite. Primarily excreted in urine. **Half-life:** 7 hours.

USES

Treatment of overactive bladder with symptoms including urinary incontinence, urgency, frequency.

PRECAUTIONS

Contraindications: Gastric retention, uncontrolled narrow-angle glaucoma, urinary retention. **Cautions:** Severe renal impairment, severe hepatic impairment, clinically significant bladder outflow obstruction (risk of urinary retention), GI obstructive disorders (e.g., pyloric stenosis [risk of gastric retention], treated narrow-angle glaucoma, myasthenia gravis, concurrent therapy with strong CYP3A4 inhibitors.

⧗ LIFESPAN CONSIDERATIONS

Pregnancy/Lactation: Unknown if distributed in breast milk. **Pregnancy Category C. Children:** Safety and efficacy not established. **Elderly:** Increased incidence of antimuscarinic adverse events including dry mouth, constipation, dyspepsia, increase in residual urine, dizziness, urinary tract infections higher in pts 75 yrs of age and older.

INTERACTIONS

DRUG: CYP3A4 inhibitors (e.g., clarithromycin, erythromycin, itraconazole, ketoconazole, miconazole) may increase concentration. **HERBAL:** None significant. **FOOD: Grapefruit products** may increase potential for urinary retention, constipation. **LAB VALUES:** May increase serum ALT, GGT.

AVAILABILITY (Rx)

▓ **Tablets, Extended-Release:** 4 mg, 8 mg.

ADMINISTRATION/HANDLING

PO
• Take with liquid and swallow whole.
• May be administered with or without food. • Do not break, crush, dissolve, or divide tablet.

INDICATIONS/ROUTES/DOSAGE

Overactive Bladder
PO: ADULTS, ELDERLY: Initially, 4 mg once daily. May increase to 8 mg once daily. Maximum dose for pts with creatinine clearance less than 30 ml/min or concurrent use of strong CYP3A4 inhibitors (e.g., erythromycin, ketoconazole) is 4 mg once daily. Not recommended for use in severe hepatic impairment.

Dosage in Renal Impairment
PO: ADULTS, ELDERLY: Maximum dose: 4 mg with creatinine clearance less than 30 ml/min.

SIDE EFFECTS

Frequent: Dry mouth (34%–18%), constipation (6%–4%), urinary tract infection (4.2%–3.2%), dry eyes (3.7%–1.4%). **Occasional (2% or less):** Nausea, dysuria, back pain, rash, insomnia, peripheral edema.

ADVERSE EFFECTS/ TOXIC REACTIONS

Severe anticholinergic effects including abdominal cramps, facial warmth, excessive salivation/lacrimation, diaphoresis, pallor, urinary urgency, blurred vision.

NURSING CONSIDERATIONS

BASELINE ASSESSMENT
Assess urinary pattern (e.g., urinary frequency, urgency). Obtain baseline chemistries.

INTERVENTION/EVALUATION
Assist with ambulation if dizziness occurs. Question for visual changes. Monitor incontinence, postvoid residuals.

PATIENT/FAMILY TEACHING
• May produce constipation and urinary retention. • Blurred vision may occur, use caution until drug effects have been determined. • Heat prostration (due to decreased sweating) can occur if used in a hot environment.

F

---

fexofenadine TOP 200

fex-**oh**-fen-a-deen
(Allegra, Allegra Children's Allergy ODT)
Do not confuse Allegra with Viagra, or fexofenadine with fesoterodine.

FIXED-COMBINATION(S)

Allegra-D 12 Hour: fexofenadine/ pseudoephedrine (sympathomimetic): 60 mg/120 mg. **Allegra-D 24 Hour:** fexofenadine/pseudoephedrine (sympathomimetic): 180 mg/240 mg.

◆CLASSIFICATION

PHARMACOTHERAPEUTIC: Piperidine. **CLINICAL:** Antihistamine (see p. 55C).

ACTION

Prevents, antagonizes most histamine effects (urticaria, pruritus). **Therapeutic Effect:** Relieves allergic rhinitis symptoms.

PHARMACOKINETICS

	Onset	Peak	Duration
PO	60 min	—	12 hrs or greater

Rapidly absorbed after PO administration. Protein binding: 60%–70%. Does not cross blood-brain barrier. Minimally metabolized. Eliminated in feces (80%), urine (11%). Not removed by hemodialysis. **Half-life:** 14.4 hrs (increased in renal impairment).

USES

Relief of seasonal allergic rhinitis, chronic idiopathic urticaria.

PRECAUTIONS

Contraindications: None known. **Cautions:** Severe renal impairment.

⧗ LIFESPAN CONSIDERATIONS

Pregnancy/Lactation: Unknown if drug crosses placenta or is distributed in breast milk. **Pregnancy Category C. Children:** Safety and efficacy not established in those younger than 12 yrs. **Elderly:** No age-related precautions noted.

INTERACTIONS

DRUG: Aluminum- and **magnesium-containing antacids** may decrease absorption if given within 15 min of fexofenadine. May increase concentrations of **erythromycin, ketoconazole. HERBAL: St. John's wort** may decrease concentration. **FOOD: Fruit juices** may decrease bioavailability. **LAB VALUES:** May suppress wheal, flare reactions to antigen skin testing unless drug is discontinued at least 4 days before testing.

AVAILABILITY (Rx)

Oral Suspension: 6 mg/ml. **Tablets:** 30 mg, 60 mg, 180 mg. **Tablets (Orally Disintegrating):** 30 mg.

ADMINISTRATION/HANDLING

PO
• Give without regard to food. • Avoid giving with fruit juices (apple, grapefruit, orange).

PO (Orally Disintegrating Tablet)
• Take on empty stomach. • Remove from blister pack; immediately place on tongue. • May take with or without liquid. • Do not split or cut.

INDICATIONS/ROUTES/DOSAGE

Allergic Rhinitis
PO: ADULTS, ELDERLY, CHILDREN 12 YRS AND OLDER: 60 mg twice a day or 180 mg once a day. **CHILDREN 2–11 YRS:** 30 mg twice a day.

Urticaria
PO: ADULTS, ELDERLY, CHILDREN 12 YRS AND OLDER: 60 mg twice a day or 180 mg once a day. **CHILDREN 2–11 YRS:** 30 mg twice a day. **CHILDREN 6 MOS–LESS THAN 2 YRS:** 15 mg twice a day.

Dosage in Renal Impairment (Creatinine Clearance Less Than 80 ml/min)
PO: ADULTS, ELDERLY, CHILDREN 12 YRS AND OLDER: 60 mg once daily. **CHILDREN 2–11 YRS:** 30 mg once daily. **CHILDREN 6 MOS–LESS THAN 2 YRS:** 15 mg once daily.

SIDE EFFECTS

Rare (less than 2%): Drowsiness, headache, fatigue, nausea, vomiting, abdominal distress, dysmenorrhea.

ADVERSE EFFECTS/ TOXIC REACTIONS

Hypersensitivity reaction occurs rarely.

NURSING CONSIDERATIONS

BASELINE ASSESSMENT

If pt is having an allergic reaction, obtain history of recently ingested foods, drugs, environmental exposure, emotional stress. Monitor rate, depth, rhythm, type of respiration; quality, rate of pulse. Assess lung sounds for rhonchi, wheezing, rales.

INTERVENTION/EVALUATION

Assess for therapeutic response; relief from allergy: itching, red, watery eyes, rhinorrhea, sneezing.

PATIENT/FAMILY TEACHING

• Avoid tasks that require alertness, motor skills until response to drug is established. • Avoid alcohol during antihistamine therapy. • Coffee, tea may help reduce drowsiness. • Do not take with any fruit juices.

fidaxomicin

fye-**dax**-oh-**mye**-sin
(Dificid)

◆CLASSIFICATION

PHARMACOTHERAPEUTIC: Macrolide. **CLINICAL:** Antibiotic.

ACTION

Binds to ribosomal sites of susceptible organisms, inhibiting RNA-dependent protein synthesis by RNA polymerase. **Therapeutic Effect:** Bactericidal against *Clostridium difficile*.

PHARMACOKINETICS

Minimal systemic absorption following PO administration. Mainly confined to GI tract. Excreted primarily in feces (92%). **Half-life:** 9 hrs.

USES

Treatment of *C. difficile*–associated diarrhea.

PRECAUTIONS

Contraindications: None known. **Cautions:** History of anemia, neutropenia.

⌛ LIFESPAN CONSIDERATIONS

Pregnancy/Lactation: Unknown if distributed in breast milk. **Pregnancy Category B. Children:** Safety and efficacy not established. **Elderly:** No age-related precautions noted.

INTERACTIONS

DRUG: Cyclosporine may increase serum concentration/effect. **HERBAL:** None known. **FOOD:** None significant. **LAB VALUES:** May increase serum AST, ALT, bilirubin, alkaline phosphatase.

AVAILABILITY (Rx)

Tablets: 200 mg.

ADMINISTRATION/HANDLING

• Give without regard to food.

INDICATIONS/ROUTES/DOSAGE

Clostridium Difficile–Associated Diarrhea
PO: ADULTS: 200 mg twice daily for 10 days.

SIDE EFFECTS

Frequent (62%–33%): Nausea, vomiting, abdominal pain. **Rare (less than 2%):** Pruritus, rash.

ADVERSE EFFECTS/ TOXIC REACTIONS

Less than 2% reported events most likely related to diarrhea-associated illness including volume loss, dehydration, GI bleeding, bloating, megacolon, abdominal distention/tenderness, flatulence, dyspepsia, dysphasia, intestinal obstruction, bicarbonate loss, hyperglycemia, metabolic acidosis, and increased hepatic function tests. GI tract infection may cause bleeding, decreased platelets, decreased RBC count.

NURSING CONSIDERATIONS

BASELINE ASSESSMENT

Verify positive C-Diff toxin test before initiating treatment. Implement infection control measures. Baseline CBC, electrolytes, renal function, fecal occult blood test. Assess abdominal pain, bowel sounds, and stool characteristics (color, frequency, consistency). Assess hydration status.

INTERVENTION/EVALUATION

Monitor for volume loss, dehydration, hypotension. Encourage nutrition/fluid intake. Routinely assess bowel sounds. Screen for intestinal obstruction (increased nausea, abdominal pain, hyperactive bowel sounds) and consider abdominal X-ray if suspected.

PATIENT/FAMILY TEACHING

• Complete drug therapy, despite symptom improvement. Early discontinuation may result in antibacterial resistance and increased risk of recurrent infection.
• Notify physician of weakness, fatigue, pale skin, dizziness, or red/dark, tarry stools relating to GI bleeding.

F

filgrastim

`TOP 200`

fil-**gras**-tim
(Neupogen)
Do not confuse Neupogen with Epogen, Neulasta, Neumega, or Nutramigen.

◆CLASSIFICATION

PHARMACOTHERAPEUTIC: Biologic modifier. **CLINICAL:** Granulocyte colony-stimulating factor (G-CSF).

ACTION

Stimulates production, maturation, activation of neutrophils. **Therapeutic Effect:** Increases migration, activation of neutrophils.

PHARMACOKINETICS

Readily absorbed after subcutaneous administration. Onset of action: 24 hrs (plateaus in 3–5 days). White counts return to normal in 4–7 days. Not removed by hemodialysis. **Half-life:** 3.5 hrs.

USES

Decreases infection incidence in pts with malignancies receiving chemotherapy associated with severe neutropenia, fever. Reduces neutropenia duration, sequelae in pts with nonmyeloid malignancies having myeloablative therapy followed by bone marrow transplant (BMT). Mobilization of hematopoietic progenitor cells into peripheral blood for collection by leukapheresis. Treatment of chronic, severe neutropenia. **OFF-LABEL:** Treatment of AIDS-related neutropenia in pts receiving zidovudine, drug-induced neutropenia, treatment of anemia in myelodysplastic syndrome. Treatment of hepatitis C treatment-associated neutropenia.

PRECAUTIONS

Contraindications: Hypersensitivity to *Escherichia coli*–derived proteins. **Cautions:** Malignancy with myeloid characteristics (due to G-CSF's potential to act as growth factor), gout, psoriasis, 24 hrs before or after cytotoxic chemotherapy, concurrent use of other drugs that may result in lowered platelet count. Neutrophil count greater than 50,000/mm³, pts with sickle cell disease.

⧖ LIFESPAN CONSIDERATIONS

Pregnancy/Lactation: Unknown if drug crosses placenta or is distributed in breast milk. **Pregnancy Category C. Children/Elderly:** No age-related precautions noted.

INTERACTIONS

DRUG: None significant. **HERBAL:** None significant. **FOOD:** None known. **LAB VALUES:** May increase LDH, leukocyte alkaline phosphatase (LAP) scores, serum alkaline phosphatase, uric acid.

AVAILABILITY (Rx)

Injection Solution: 300 mcg/ml (1 ml, 1.6 ml) vial, 600 mcg/ml (0.5 ml, 0.8 ml) prefilled syringe.

ADMINISTRATION/HANDLING

◀ALERT▶ May be given by subcutaneous injection, short IV infusion (15–30 min), or continuous IV infusion.

 IV

Reconstitution • Use single-dose vial; do not reenter vial. • Do not shake. • Dilute with 10–50 ml D₅W to concentration of 15 mcg/ml or greater. For concentration from 5–14 mcg/ml, add 2 ml of 5% albumin to each 50 ml D₅W to provide a final concentration of 2 mg/ml. Do not dilute to final concentration less than 5 mcg/ml.

Rate of Administration • For intermittent infusion (piggyback), infuse over 15–30 min. • For continuous infusion, give single dose over 4–24 hrs. • In all situations, flush IV line with D₅W before and after administration.

Storage • Refrigerate vials. • Stable for up to 24 hrs at room temperature (provided vial contents are clear and contain no particulate matter). Remains stable if accidentally exposed to freezing temperature.

Subcutaneous
• Aspirate syringe before injection (avoid intra-arterial administration).

Storage • Store in refrigerator, but remove before use and allow to warm to room temperature.

🌐 IV INCOMPATIBILITIES

Amphotericin (Fungizone), cefepime (Maxipime), cefotaxime (Claforan), cefoxitin (Mefoxin), ceftizoxime (Cefizox), ceftriaxone (Rocephin), clindamycin (Cleocin), dactinomycin (Cosmegen), etoposide (VePesid), fluorouracil, furosemide (Lasix), heparin, mannitol, methylprednisolone (Solu-Medrol), mitomycin (Mutamycin), prochlorperazine (Compazine).

🌐 IV COMPATIBILITIES

Bumetanide (Bumex), calcium gluconate, hydromorphone (Dilaudid), lorazepam (Ativan), morphine, potassium chloride.

INDICATIONS/ROUTES/DOSAGE

◄ALERT► Begin therapy at least 24 hrs after last dose of chemotherapy and at least 24 hrs after bone marrow infusion. Dosing based on actual body weight.

Chemotherapy-Induced Neutropenia
IV or Subcutaneous Infusion, Subcutaneous Injection: ADULTS, ELDERLY, CHILDREN: Initially, 5 mcg/kg/day. May increase by 5 mcg/kg for each chemotherapy cycle based on duration/severity of neutropenia; continue for up to 14 days or until absolute neutrophil count (ANC) reaches 10,000/mm³.

Bone Marrow Transplant
IV or Subcutaneous Infusion: ADULTS, ELDERLY, CHILDREN: 5–10 mcg/kg/day. Adjust dosage daily during period of neutrophil recovery based on neutrophil response.

Mobilization of Progenitor Cells
IV or Subcutaneous Infusion: ADULTS: 10 mcg/kg/day in donors beginning at least 4 days before first leukapheresis and continuing until last leukapheresis (usually for 6–7 days).

Chronic Neutropenia,
Congenital Neutropenia
Subcutaneous: ADULTS, CHILDREN: 6 mcg/kg/dose twice a day.

Idiopathic or Cyclic Neutropenia
Subcutaneous: ADULTS, CHILDREN: 5 mcg/kg/dose once a day.

SIDE EFFECTS

Frequent: Nausea/vomiting (57%), mild to severe bone pain (22%) (more frequent with high-dose IV form, less frequent with low-dose subcutaneous form), alopecia (18%), diarrhea (14%), fever (12%), fatigue (11%). **Occasional (9%–5%):** Anorexia, dyspnea, headache, cough, rash. **Rare (less than 5%):** Psoriasis, hematuria, proteinuria, osteoporosis.

ADVERSE EFFECTS/ TOXIC REACTIONS

Long-term administration occasionally produces chronic neutropenia, splenomegaly. Thrombocytopenia, MI, arrhythmias occur rarely. Adult respiratory distress syndrome may occur in septic pts.

NURSING CONSIDERATIONS

BASELINE ASSESSMENT
CBC, platelet count should be obtained before therapy initiation and twice weekly thereafter.

INTERVENTION/EVALUATION
In septic pts, be alert for adult respiratory distress syndrome. Closely monitor those with preexisting cardiac conditions. Monitor B/P (transient decrease in B/P may occur), temperature, CBC with differential, platelet count, Hct, serum uric acid, hepatic function tests.

PATIENT/FAMILY TEACHING
• Report fever, chills, severe bone pain, chest pain, palpitations.

---

finasteride

fin-**as**-ter-ide
(Apo-Finasteride ✥, Propecia,
<u>Proscar</u>)
**Do not confuse finasteride with
furosemide, or Proscar with
ProSom, Provera, or Prozac.**

◆CLASSIFICATION

PHARMACOTHERAPEUTIC: Androgen
hormone inhibitor. **CLINICAL:** Benign
prostatic hyperplasia agent.

ACTION

Inhibits 5-alpha reductase, an intracellular enzyme that converts testosterone into dihydrotestosterone (DHT) in prostate gland, resulting in decreased serum DHT. **Therapeutic Effect:** Reduces size of prostate gland.

PHARMACOKINETICS

Route	Onset	Peak	Duration
PO (reduction of DHT)	8 hrs	—	24 hrs

Rapidly absorbed from GI tract. Protein binding: 90%. Widely distributed. Metabolized in liver. **Half-life:** 6–8 hrs. Onset of clinical effect: 3–6 mos of continued therapy.

USES

Proscar: Reduces risk of acute urinary retention, need for surgery in symptomatic benign prostatic hyperplasia (BPH) alone or in combination with doxazosin (Carura). Most improvement noted in urinary hesitancy, feeling of incomplete bladder emptying, interruption of urinary stream, difficulty initiating flow, dysuria, impaired volume, force of urinary stream. **Propecia:** Treatment of hair loss. **OFF-LABEL:** Treatment of female hirsutism.

PRECAUTIONS

Contraindications: Pregnancy, use in children. **Cautions:** Hepatic function abnormalities. Pregnant women, those attempting to conceive should not handle; pts with large residual urine volume, severe diminished urine flow.

⌛ LIFESPAN CONSIDERATIONS

Pregnancy/Lactation: Physical handling of tablet by those who are or may become pregnant may produce abnormalities of external genitalia of male fetus. **Pregnancy Category X. Children:** Not indicated for use in children. **Elderly:** No age-related precautions noted.

INTERACTIONS

DRUG: None known. **HERBAL: St. John's wort** may decrease concentration. Avoid concurrent use with **saw palmetto** (not adequately studied). **FOOD:** None known. **LAB VALUES:** Decreases serum prostate-specific antigen (PSA) level, even in presence of prostate cancer. Decreases dihydrotestosterone (DHT). Increases follicle-stimulating hormone (FSH), luteinizing hormone (LH), testosterone.

AVAILABILITY (Rx)

Tablets: 1 mg (Propecia), 5 mg (Proscar).

ADMINISTRATION/HANDLING

PO
• Do not break, crush film-coated tablets. • Give without regard to meals.

INDICATIONS/ROUTES/DOSAGE

Benign Prostatic Hyperplasia (BPH)
PO: ADULTS, ELDERLY: (Proscar): 5 mg once a day (for minimum of 6 mos).

Hair Loss
PO: ADULTS: (Propecia): 1 mg/day.

SIDE EFFECTS

Rare (4%–2%): Gynecomastia, sexual dysfunction (impotence, decreased libido, decreased volume of ejaculate).

ADVERSE EFFECTS/
TOXIC REACTIONS

Hypersensitivity reaction, circumoral swelling, testicular pain occur rarely.

NURSING CONSIDERATIONS

BASELINE ASSESSMENT

Digital rectal exam, serum prostate-specific antigen (PSA) determination should be performed in pts with benign prostatic hyperplasia (BPH) before initiating therapy and periodically thereafter.

INTERVENTION/EVALUATION

Diligent monitoring of I&O, esp. in pts with large residual urinary volume, severely diminished urinary flow, or obstructive uropathy.

PATIENT/FAMILY TEACHING

• Pt should be aware of potential for impotence. • May not notice improved urinary flow even if prostate gland shrinks. • Must take medication longer than 6 mos, and it is unknown if medication decreases need for surgery. • Because of potential risk to male fetus, women who are or may become pregnant should not handle tablets or be exposed to pt's semen. • Volume of ejaculate may be decreased during treatment.

---

fingolimod   `TOP 200`

fin-**goe**-li-mod
(Gilenya)

◆ CLASSIFICATION

PHARMACOTHERAPEUTIC: Immunomodulator. **CLINICAL:** Multiple sclerosis agent.

ACTION

Blocks capacity of lymphocytes to move out from lymph nodes, reducing number of lymphocytes in peripheral blood. **Therapeutic Effect:** May involve reduction of lymphocyte migration into central nervous system.

PHARMACOKINETICS

Metabolized by the enzyme sphingosine kinase to active metabolite. Highly distributed in red blood cells (85%). Minimally metabolized in liver. Protein binding: 99.7%. Primarily excreted in urine. **Half-life:** 6–9 days.

USES

Treatment of pts with relapsing forms of multiple sclerosis (MS) to reduce frequency of clinical exacerbations, delay accumulation of physical disability.

PRECAUTIONS

Contraindications: Sick sinus syndrome, second-degree or higher conduction block. Baseline QT interval 500 msec or greater. Concurrent use of class 1a or 111 antiarrhythmic. Recent (within 6 mos) MI, unstable angina, stroke, TIA, decompensated heart failure requiring hospitalization. **Cautions:** Antiarrhythmic drugs, beta-blockers, calcium channel blockers, those with low heart rate, history of syncope, ischemic heart disease, congestive heart failure, pts at increased risk for developing bradycardia or heart blocks. Severe hepatic impairment. Concomitant administration of immunosuppressants, immune modulating or antineoplastic medications. History of diabetes or uveitis. Prolonged QT interval at baseline.

⧗ LIFESPAN CONSIDERATIONS

Pregnancy/Lactation: May cause fetal harm. Unknown if distributed in breast milk. **Pregnancy Category C. Children:** Safety and efficacy not established in those younger than 18 yrs. **Elderly:** Age-related severe hepatic impairment may increase risk of adverse reactions.

INTERACTIONS

DRUG: Antineoplastics, immunosuppressives, immunomodulators in-

---

crease risk of immunosuppression. **Ketoconazole** increases concentration/adverse effects. May decrease effect of **vaccines.** May increase effects of **QT-prolonging medications.** HERBAL: **Echinacea** may decrease concentration. FOOD: None known. LAB VALUES: Expect decrease in neutrophil count. May increase serum alkaline phosphatase, AST, ALT, bilirubin, triglycerides.

AVAILABILITY (Rx)

Capsules: 0.5 mg.

ADMINISTRATION/HANDLING

PO
• May give without regard to food.

INDICATIONS/ROUTES/DOSAGE

Multiple Sclerosis
PO: ADULTS 18 YRS AND OLDER, ELDERLY: 0.5 mg once daily.

SIDE EFFECTS

Frequent (25%–10%): Headache, diarrhea, back pain, cough. Occasional (8%–5%): Dyspnea, clinical depression, dizziness, hypertension, migraine, paresthesia, decreased weight. Rare (4%–2%): Blurred vision, alopecia, eye pain, asthenia (loss of strength, energy), eczema, pruritus.

ADVERSE EFFECTS/ TOXIC REACTIONS

May increase risk of infections (influenza, herpes viral infection, bronchitis, sinusitis, gastroenteritis, ear infection) in 13%–4% of pts. Pts with diabetes or history of uveitis are at increased risk for developing macular edema.

NURSING CONSIDERATIONS

BASELINE ASSESSMENT

Obtain baseline CBC, serum chemistries prior to initial treatment. At initial treatment (within first 4–6 hrs after dose), medication reduces heart rate, AV conduction, followed by progressive increase after first day of treatment. Obtain baseline vitals, with particular attention to pulse rate. Perform ophthalmologic evaluation prior to treatment and 3–4 mos after initiation of treatment.

INTERVENTION/EVALUATION

Monitor for bradycardia for 6 hrs after first dose, followed by progressive improvement in heart rate after first day of treatment. Periodically monitor CBC, serum chemistries, particularly lymphocyte count (expected to decrease approximately 80% from baseline with continued treatment). Monitor for signs of systemic or local infection.

PATIENT/FAMILY TEACHING

• Obtain regular eye examinations during and for 2 mos following treatment. • Use effective methods of contraception during and for 3 mos following treatment. • Report fever, chills, aches, weakness, cough, nausea, symptoms of infection, visual changes, yellowing of skin, eyes, dark urine.

---

fluconazole   TOP 200

flu-**con**-a-zole
(Apo-Fluconazole ✦, Diflucan, Novo-Fluconazole ✦)
Do not confuse Diflucan with diclofenac, Diprivan, or disulfiram, or fluconazole with fluoxetine, furosemide, or itraconazole.

◆CLASSIFICATION

PHARMACOTHERAPEUTIC: Synthetic azole. CLINICAL: Systemic antifungal (see p. 48C).

ACTION

Interferes with cytochrome P-450, an enzyme necessary for ergosterol formation. **Therapeutic Effect:** Directly damages fungal membrane, altering its function. Fungistatic.

PHARMACOKINETICS

Well absorbed from GI tract. Widely distributed, including to CSF. Protein binding: 11%. Partially metabolized in liver. Excreted unchanged primarily in urine. Partially removed by hemodialysis. **Half-life:** 20–30 hrs (increased in renal impairment).

USES

Candidiasis prophylaxis in pts undergoing bone marrow transplant, receiving chemotherapy and/or radiation therapy; treatment of esophageal, oropharyngeal, disseminated, vulvovaginal, urinary tract, systemic, peritonitis, pneumonia, candidiasis; treatment and suppression of cryptococcal meningitis. **OFF-LABEL:** Cryptococcal pneumonia, candidal intertrigo.

PRECAUTIONS

Contraindications: Concomitant administration of QT-prolonging medications. **Cautions:** Hepatic/renal impairment, hypersensitivity to other triazoles (e.g., itraconazole, terconazole), imidazoles (e.g., butoconazole, ketoconazole).

⧖ LIFESPAN CONSIDERATIONS

Pregnancy/Lactation: Unknown if distributed in breast milk. **Pregnancy Category C. Children:** No age-related precautions noted. **Elderly:** Age-related renal impairment may require dosage adjustment.

INTERACTIONS

DRUG: High fluconazole dosages increase **cyclosporine, sirolimus, tacrolimus** concentrations. **Isoniazid, rifampin** may increase drug metabolism. May increase concentration/effects of **oral antidiabetic medication.** May decrease metabolism of **phenytoin, warfarin.** **HERBAL:** None significant. **FOOD:** None known. **LAB VALUES:** May increase serum alkaline phosphatase, bilirubin, AST, ALT.

AVAILABILITY (Rx)

Injection, Solution, Pre-Mix: 200 mg (100 ml); 400 mg (200 ml). **Powder for Oral** **Suspension:** 10 mg/ml, 40 mg/ml. **Tablets:** 50 mg, 100 mg, 150 mg, 200 mg.

ADMINISTRATION/HANDLING

 IV

Rate of Administration • Do not exceed maximum flow rate of 200 mg/hr. **Storage** • Store at room temperature. • Do not remove from outer wrap until ready to use. • Squeeze inner bag to check for leaks. • Do not use parenteral form if solution is cloudy, precipitate forms, seal is not intact, or it is discolored. • Do not add supplementary medication.

PO

• Give without regard to meals. • PO and IV therapy equally effective; IV therapy for pt intolerant of drug or unable to take orally. Oral suspension stable for 14 days at room temperature or refrigerated.

▦ IV INCOMPATIBILITIES

Amphotericin B (Fungizone), amphotericin B complex (Abelcet, AmBisome, Amphotec), ampicillin (Polycillin), calcium gluconate, cefotaxime (Claforan), ceftriaxone (Rocephin), cefuroxime (Zinacef), chloramphenicol (Chloromycetin), clindamycin (Cleocin), co-trimoxazole (Bactrim), diazepam (Valium), digoxin (Lanoxin), erythromycin (Erythrocin), furosemide (Lasix), haloperidol (Haldol), hydroxyzine (Vistaril), imipenem and cilastatin (Primaxin).

▦ IV COMPATIBILITIES

Dexmedetomidine (Precedex), diltiazem (Cardizem), dobutamine (Dobutrex), dopamine (Intropin), heparin, lipids, lorazepam (Ativan), midazolam (Versed), propofol (Diprivan).

INDICATIONS/ROUTES/DOSAGE

Usual Dosage
PO/IV: ADULTS, ELDERLY: 150 mg once or **loading dose:** 200–800 mg. **Maintenance dose:** 200–800 mg once daily. **CHILDREN AND NEONATES: Loading dose:** 6–12 mg/kg. **Maintenance dose:**

3–12 mg/kg once daily. **Maximum:** 600 mg/day.

Oropharyngeal Candidiasis

PO, IV: ADULTS, ELDERLY: 200 mg once, then 100 mg/day for at least 14 days. **CHILDREN:** 6 mg/kg/day once, then 3 mg/kg/day for at least 14 days.

Esophageal Candidiasis

PO, IV: ADULTS, ELDERLY: 200 mg once, then 100 mg/day (up to 400 mg/day) for 21 days and at least 14 days following resolution of symptoms. **CHILDREN:** 6 mg/kg/day once, then 3 mg/kg/day (up to 12 mg/kg/day) for 21 days and at least 14 days following resolution of symptoms. **Maximum:** 600 mg/day.

Urinary Candidiasis

PO, IV: ADULTS, ELDERLY: 200–400 mg/day for 1–2 wks.

Vaginal Candidiasis

PO: ADULTS: (Uncomplicated): 150 mg once. (Complicated): 150 mg q72h for 3 doses.

Candidiasis Prophylaxis

PO: ADULTS: 400 mg/day. Begin 3 days before onset of neutropenia and continue for 7 days after neutrophils greater than 10,000 cells/mm^3.

Systemic Candidiasis

PO, IV: ADULTS, ELDERLY: 400–800 mg/day for at least 28 days and at least 14 days following resolution of symptoms. **CHILDREN:** 12 mg/kg/dose once daily for 21 days. **Maximum:** 600 mg/day.

Cryptococcal Meningitis

PO, IV: ADULTS, ELDERLY: 400 mg once, then 200 mg/day (up to 800 mg/day) for 10–12 wks after CSF becomes negative (200 mg/day for suppression of relapse in pts with AIDS). **CHILDREN:** 12 mg/kg/day once, then 6–12 mg/kg/day for 10–12 wks. **Maximum:** 800 mg/day. (6 mg/kg/day for suppression of relapse). **Maximum:** 200 mg/day.

Dosage in Renal Impairment

After a loading dose of 400 mg, daily dosage is based on creatinine clearance.

Creatinine Clearance	Dosage
Greater than 50 ml/min	100%
50 ml/min or less	50%
Dialysis	50%
CCRT	400–800 mg as loading dose
CVVH	then 200–800 mg/day
CVVHDF	400–800 mg as loading dose, then 400–800 mg/day

SIDE EFFECTS

Occasional (4%–1%): Hypersensitivity reaction (chills, fever, pruritus, rash), dizziness, drowsiness, headache, constipation, diarrhea, nausea, vomiting, abdominal pain.

ADVERSE EFFECTS/ TOXIC REACTIONS

Exfoliative skin disorders, serious hepatic effects, blood dyscrasias (eosinophilia, thrombocytopenia, anemia, leukopenia) have been reported rarely.

NURSING CONSIDERATIONS

BASELINE ASSESSMENT

Assess infected area. Establish baselines for CBC, serum potassium, hepatic function.

INTERVENTION/EVALUATION

Assess for hypersensitivity reaction (chills, fever). Monitor serum hepatic/renal function tests, potassium, CBC, platelet count. Report rash, itching promptly. Monitor temperature at least daily. Monitor daily pattern of bowel activity, stool consistency. Assess for dizziness; provide assistance as needed.

PATIENT/FAMILY TEACHING

• Avoid tasks that require alertness, motor skills until response to drug is established. • Report dark urine, pale stool, jaundiced skin or sclera of eyes, rash, pruritus. • Pts with oropharyngeal infections should maintain fastidious oral hygiene. • Consult physician before taking any other medication.

fludarabine

HIGH ALERT

floo-**dar**-a-been
(Fludara)

BLACK BOX ALERT Must be administered by certified chemotherapy personnel. Severe neurologic toxicity reported. Life-threatening hemolytic anemia, autoimmune thrombocytopenic purpura, hemophilia have occurred. Risk of severe myelosuppression (anemia, thrombocytopenia, neutropenia). Concurrent use with pentostatin may produce severe/fatal pulmonary toxicity.

Do not confuse Fludara with FUDR, or fludarabine with cladribine or Flumadine.

◆CLASSIFICATION

PHARMACOTHERAPEUTIC: Antimetabolite. **CLINICAL:** Antineoplastic (see p. 86C).

ACTION

Inhibits DNA synthesis by interfering with DNA polymerase alpha, ribonucleotide reductase, DNA primase. **Therapeutic Effect:** Induces cell death.

PHARMACOKINETICS

Rapidly dephosphorylated in serum, then phosphorylated intracellularly to active triphosphate. Primarily excreted in urine. **Half-life:** 7–20 hrs.

USES

Treatment of chronic lymphocytic leukemia (CLL) in pts who have not responded to or have not progressed with another standard alkylating agent. **Tablets:** Treatment of CLL. **OFF-LABEL:** Treatment of non-Hodgkin's lymphoma, acute leukemias in children, Waldenström's macroglobulinemia, reduced-intensity conditioning regimens prior to allogeneic hematopoietic stem-cell transplantation.

PRECAUTIONS

Contraindications: None known. (Canada): Severe renal impairment. Concurrent use with pentostatin. **Cautions:** Renal insufficiency, preexisting hematological disorders (e.g., granulocytopenia), seizure disorder, spasticity, peripheral neuropathy, infection, fever, immunodeficiency.

⧗ LIFESPAN CONSIDERATIONS

Pregnancy/Lactation: If possible, avoid use during pregnancy, esp. first trimester. May cause fetal harm. Not known whether distributed in breast milk. Breastfeeding not recommended. **Pregnancy Category D. Children:** Safety and efficacy not established. **Elderly:** Age-related renal impairment may require dosage adjustment.

INTERACTIONS

DRUG: Pentostatin may increase risk of pulmonary toxicity. **Bone marrow depressants** may increase risk of myelosuppression. **Live virus vaccines** may potentiate virus replication, increase vaccine side effects, decrease pt's antibody response to vaccine. **HERBAL:** None significant. **FOOD:** None known. **LAB VALUES:** May increase serum alkaline phosphatase, uric acid, AST.

AVAILABILITY (Rx)

Injection, Powder for Reconstitution (Fludara): 50 mg. Injection, Solution: 25 mg/ml.

Tablets: 10 mg.

ADMINISTRATION/HANDLING

◀**ALERT**▶ Give by IV infusion. Do not add to other IV infusions. Avoid small veins; swollen, edematous extremities; areas overlying joints, tendons.

IV

Reconstitution • Reconstitute 50-mg vial with 2 ml Sterile Water for Injection to provide concentration of 25 mg/ml. • Further dilute with 100–125 ml 0.9% NaCl or D$_5$W.

Rate of Administration • Infuse over 30 min.

Storage • Store in refrigerator. • Handle with extreme care during preparation/administration. If contact with skin or mucous membranes occurs, wash thoroughly with soap and water; rinse eyes profusely with plain water. • Reconstituted vials stable for 16 days at room temperature or refrigerated. • Diluted solutions stable for 48 hrs at room temperature or refrigerated.

PO

• May give with or without food. • Swallow whole; do not cut, break, or crush tablets.

⬛ IV INCOMPATIBILITIES

Acyclovir (Zovirax), amphotericin B (Fungizone), daunorubicin, hydroxyzine (Vistaril), prochlorperazine (Compazine).

⬛ IV COMPATIBILITIES

Heparin, hydromorphone (Dilaudid), lorazepam (Ativan), magnesium sulfate, morphine, multivitamins, potassium chloride.

INDICATIONS/ROUTES/DOSAGE

Chronic Lymphocytic Leukemia (CLL), Non-Hodgkin's Lymphoma

IV: ADULTS: 25 mg/m^2 daily for 5 consecutive days. Continue for up to 3 additional cycles. Begin each course of treatment every 28 days.

CLL

PO: ADULTS, ELDERLY: 40 mg/m^2 once daily for 5 days every 28 days.

Dosage in Renal Impairment

Creatinine Clearance	Dosage
PO	
30–70 ml/min	Decrease dose by 50%
Less than 30 ml/min	Not recommended

Creatinine Clearance	Dosage
IV	
50–79 ml/min	20 mg/m^2
30–49 ml/min	15 mg/m^2
Less than 30 ml/min	Not recommended

SIDE EFFECTS

Frequent: Fever (60%), nausea/vomiting (36%), chills (11%). **Occasional (20%–10%):** Fatigue, generalized pain, rash, diarrhea, cough, asthenia (loss of strength, energy), stomatitis, dyspnea, peripheral edema. **Rare (7%–3%):** Anorexia, sinusitis, dysuria, myalgia, paresthesia, headache, visual disturbances.

ADVERSE EFFECTS/ TOXIC REACTIONS

Pneumonia occurs frequently. Severe hematologic toxicity (anemia, thrombocytopenia, neutropenia), GI bleeding may occur. Tumor lysis syndrome may begin with flank pain, hematuria; may also include hypercalcemia, hyperphosphatemia, hyperuricemia, resulting in renal failure. High-dosage therapy may produce acute leukemia, blindness, coma. Neurotoxicity (progressive demyelinating encephalopathy, mental status deterioration) occurs rarely.

NURSING CONSIDERATIONS

BASELINE ASSESSMENT

Assess baseline CBC, serum creatinine, Hgb, AST, ALT, electrolytes, uric acid and monitor during treatment. Drug should be discontinued if intractable vomiting, diarrhea, stomatitis, GI bleeding occurs.

INTERVENTION/EVALUATION

Assess for fatigue, visual disturbances, peripheral edema. Assess for onset of pneumonia. Monitor for dyspnea, cough, rapid decrease in WBC count, intractable vomiting, diarrhea, GI bleeding (bright red or tarry stool). Assess oral mucosa for erythema, ulceration at inner margin of lips, sore throat, difficulty swallowing (stomatitis). Assess skin for rash. Be alert to possible tumor lysis syndrome (onset of flank pain, hematuria), signs of neurotoxicity.

PATIENT/FAMILY TEACHING
• Avoid crowds, exposure to infection. • Maintain strict oral hygiene. • Promptly report fever, sore throat, signs of local infection, unusual bruising/bleeding from any site. • Report persistent nausea/vomiting.

flunisolide

floo-**niss**-oh-lyde
(Apo-Flunisolide ✦, Nasalide ✦, Rhinalar ✦)
Do not confuse flunisolide with fluocinonide.

◆ CLASSIFICATION

PHARMACOTHERAPEUTIC: Adrenocorticosteroid. **CLINICAL:** Antiasthmatic, anti-inflammatory (see pp. 2C, 100C).

ACTION

Controls rate of protein synthesis, depresses migration of polymorphonuclear leukocytes, reverses capillary permeability, stabilizes lysosomal membranes. **Therapeutic Effect:** Prevents, controls inflammation.

PHARMACOKINETICS

Rapidly absorbed from lungs and GI tract following inhalation. About 50% of dose is absorbed from nasal mucosa following intranasal administration. Metabolized in liver. Partially excreted in urine and feces. **Half-life:** 1–2 hrs.

USES

Relieves symptoms of seasonal, perennial rhinitis.

PRECAUTIONS

Contraindications: Hypersensitivity to any corticosteroid, untreated nasal mucosal infection. **Cautions:** Respiratory tuberculosis, untreated systemic infections, ocular herpes simplex.

⌛ LIFESPAN CONSIDERATIONS

Pregnancy/Lactation: Unknown if distributed in breast milk. **Pregnancy Category C. Children:** Safety and efficacy not established. **Elderly:** No age-related precautions noted.

INTERACTIONS

DRUG: None significant. **HERBAL:** None significant. **FOOD:** None known. **LAB VALUES:** None significant.

AVAILABILITY (Rx)

Nasal Spray: 25 mcg/activation.

ADMINISTRATION/HANDLING

Intranasal
• Instruct pt to clear nasal passages as much as possible before use (topical nasal decongestants may be needed 5–15 min before use). • Tilt head slightly forward. • Insert spray tip into nostril, pointing toward inflamed nasal turbinates, away from nasal septum. • Pump medication into one nostril while pt holds other nostril closed, concurrently inspires through nose. • Discard opened nasal solution after 3 mos.

INDICATIONS/ROUTES/DOSAGE

Usual Intranasal Dosage
◀ **ALERT** ▶ Improvement usually seen within a few days; may take up to 3 wks. Discontinue use after 3 wks if no significant improvement occurs.
Intranasal: ADULTS, ELDERLY, CHILDREN 15 YRS AND OLDER: Initially, 2 sprays each nostril twice a day, may increase at 4- to 7-day intervals to 2 sprays 3 times a day. **Maximum:** 8 sprays in each nostril daily. **CHILDREN 6–14 YRS:** Initially, 1 spray 3 times a day or 2 sprays twice a day. **Maximum:** 4 sprays in each nostril daily. Maintenance: 1 spray into each nostril daily.

SIDE EFFECTS

Frequent: Inhalation (25%–10%): Unpleasant taste, nausea, vomiting, sore throat, diarrhea, cold symptoms, nasal congestion. **Occasional: Inhalation (9%–3%):** Dizziness, irritability, anxiety, tremors, abdominal pain, heartburn, oropharyngeal candidiasis, edema. **Nasal:** Mild nasopharyngeal irritation/dryness, rebound congestion, bronchial asthma, rhinorrhea, altered taste.

ADVERSE EFFECTS/ TOXIC REACTIONS

Acute hypersensitivity reaction (urticaria, angioedema, severe bronchospasm) occurs rarely. Transfer from systemic to local steroid therapy may unmask previously suppressed bronchial asthma condition.

NURSING CONSIDERATIONS

BASELINE ASSESSMENT

Establish baseline assessment of asthma, rhinitis.

INTERVENTION/EVALUATION

Advise pts receiving bronchodilators by inhalation concomitantly with steroid inhalation therapy to use bronchodilator several min before corticosteroid aerosol (enhances penetration of steroid into bronchial tree). Monitor rate, depth, rhythm, type of respiration; quality/rate of pulse. Assess lung sounds for rhonchi, wheezing, rales. Monitor ABGs.

PATIENT/FAMILY TEACHING

• Notify physician if exposed to measles, chickenpox. • Do not change dose/schedule or stop taking drug; must taper off gradually under medical supervision. • Maintain strict oral hygiene. • Rinse mouth with water immediately after inhalation (prevents mouth/throat dryness, oral fungal infection). • Increase fluid intake (decreases lung secretion viscosity). • **Intranasal:** Clear nasal passages before use. • Contact physician if no improvement in symptoms, sneezing or nasal irritation occurs. • Improvement usually noted in several days.

fluorouracil, 5-FU [HIGH ALERT]

flore-oh-**yer**-a-sil
(Adrucil, Carac, Efudex, Fluoroplex)

BLACK BOX ALERT Must be administered by personnel trained in administration/handling of chemotherapeutic agents.
Do not confuse Efudex with Efidac.

◆CLASSIFICATION

PHARMACOTHERAPEUTIC: Antimetabolite. **CLINICAL:** Antineoplastic (see p. 86C).

ACTION

Blocks formation of thymidylic acid. Cell cycle–specific for S phase of cell division. **Therapeutic Effect:** Inhibits DNA, RNA synthesis. **Topical:** Destroys rapidly proliferating cells.

PHARMACOKINETICS

Widely distributed. Crosses blood-brain barrier. Metabolized in liver. Primarily excreted by lungs as carbon dioxide. Removed by hemodialysis. **Half-life:** 16 min.

USES

Parenteral: Treatment of carcinoma of: colon, rectum, breast, stomach, pancreas. **Topical:** Treatment of multiple actinic or solar keratoses, superficial basal cell carcinomas. **OFF-LABEL: Parenteral:** Treatment of carcinoma of: bladder, cervical, endometrial, head/neck, anal, esophageal, renal cell, unknown primary cancer.

PRECAUTIONS

Contraindications: Myelosuppression, poor nutritional status, potentially serious infections. **Cautions:** History of high-dose pelvic irradiation, hepatic/renal impairment, palmar-plantar erythrodysesthia syndrome (hand and foot syndrome), previous use of alkylating agents.

⌛ LIFESPAN CONSIDERATIONS

Pregnancy/Lactation: If possible, avoid use during pregnancy, esp. first trimester. May cause fetal harm. Unknown if distributed in breast milk. Breastfeeding not recommended. **Pregnancy Category D. Topical: Pregnancy Category X. Children:** No age-related precautions noted. **Elderly:** Age-related renal impairment may require dosage adjustment.

INTERACTIONS

DRUG: Bone marrow depressants may increase risk of myelosuppression. **Live virus vaccines** may potentiate virus replication, increase vaccine side effects, decrease pt's antibody response to vaccine. **HERBAL: Echinacea** may decrease effect. Avoid use of **black cohosh, dong quai** in pts with estrogen-dependent tumors. **FOOD:** None known. **LAB VALUES:** May decrease serum albumin. **Topical:** May cause eosinophilia, leukocytosis, thrombocytopenia, toxic granulation.

AVAILABILITY (Rx)

Cream, Topical (Carac): 0.5%: **(Efudex):** 5%: **(Fluoroplex):** 1%. **Injection Solution (Adrucil):** 50 mg/ml. **Solution, Topical (Efudex):** 2%, 5%.

ADMINISTRATION/HANDLING

◀**ALERT**▶ Give by IV injection or IV infusion. Do not add to other IV infusions. Avoid small veins, swollen/edematous extremities, areas overlying joints, tendons. May be carcinogenic, mutagenic, teratogenic. Handle with extreme care during preparation/administration.

💉 IV

Reconstitution • IV push does not need to be diluted or reconstituted. • Inject through Y-tube or 3-way stopcock of free-flowing solution. • For IV infusion, further dilute with 50–1,000 ml D_5W or 0.9% NaCl.
Rate of Administration • Give IV push slowly over 1–2 min. • IV infusion is administered over 30 min–24 hrs. • Extravasation produces immediate pain,

severe local tissue damage. • Follow protocol.
Storage • Solution appears colorless to faint yellow. Slight discoloration does not adversely affect potency or safety. • If precipitate forms, redissolve by heating, shaking vigorously; allow to cool to body temperature. • Diluted solutions stable for 72 hrs at room temperature.

🔲 IV INCOMPATIBILITIES

Amphotericin B complex (Abelcet, AmBisome, Amphotec), filgrastim (Neupogen), ondansetron (Zofran), vinorelbine (Navelbine).

🔲 IV COMPATIBILITIES

Granisetron (Kytril), heparin, hydromorphone (Dilaudid), leucovorin, morphine, potassium chloride, propofol (Diprivan).

INDICATIONS/ROUTES/DOSAGE

Refer to individual protocols.

Usual Therapy
IV Bolus: ADULTS, ELDERLY: 500 mg/m² once weekly.
IV Infusion: ADULTS, ELDERLY: 1,000 mg/m²/day for 4–5 days every 3–4 wks, or 2,600 mg/m² every wk or 1,600 mg/m²/day for 2 days q2wks, or 400 mg/m² bolus, then 1,200 mg/m² for 2 days q2wks.

Multiple Actinic or Solar Keratoses
Topical (Carac): ADULTS, ELDERLY: Apply once a day for up to 4 wks.
Topical (Efudex): ADULTS, ELDERLY: Apply twice a day for 2–4 wks.
Topical (Fluoroplex): Apply twice daily for 2–6 wks.

Basal Cell Carcinoma
Topical (Efudex 5%): ADULTS, ELDERLY: Apply twice a day for 3–6 wks up to 10–12 wks.

SIDE EFFECTS

Parenteral: Frequent (greater than 10%): Alopecia, dermatitis, anorexia, diarrhea, esophagitis, dyspepsia, stomatitis. Occasional (10%–1%): Cardiotoxicity (angina,

EKG changes), skin dryness, epithelial fissuring, nausea, vomiting, excessive lacrimation, blurred vision. **Rare (less than 1%):** Headache, photosensitivity, somnolence, allergic reaction, dyspnea, hypotension, MI, pulmonary edema. **Topical: Occasional:** Erythema, skin ulceration, pruritus, hyperpigmentation, dermatitis, insomnia, stomatitis, irritability, photosensitivity, excessive lacrimation, blurred vision.

ADVERSE EFFECTS/ TOXIC REACTIONS

Earliest sign of toxicity (4–8 days after beginning therapy) is stomatitis (dry mouth, burning sensation, mucosal erythema, ulceration at inner margin of lips). Most common dermatologic toxicity is pruritic rash (generally on extremities, less frequently on trunk). Leukopenia generally occurs within 9–14 days after drug administration but may occur as late as 25th day. Thrombocytopenia occasionally occurs within 7–17 days after administration. Pancytopenia, agranulocytosis occur rarely.

NURSING CONSIDERATIONS

BASELINE ASSESSMENT

Obtain baseline CBC with differential, serum renal/hepatic function tests and monitor during therapy.

INTERVENTION/EVALUATION

Monitor for rapidly falling WBC, platelet count, intractable diarrhea, GI bleeding (bright red or tarry stool). Assess oral mucosa for stomatitis. Drug should be discontinued if intractable diarrhea, stomatitis, GI bleeding occurs. Assess skin for rash.

PATIENT/FAMILY TEACHING

• Maintain strict oral hygiene. • Inform physician of signs/symptoms of infection, unusual bruising/bleeding, visual changes, nausea, vomiting, diarrhea, chest pain, palpitations. • Avoid sunlight, artificial light sources; wear protective clothing, sunglasses, sunscreen. • **Topical:** Apply only to affected area. • Do not

use occlusive coverings. • Be careful near eyes, nose, mouth. • Wash hands thoroughly after application. • Treated areas may be unsightly for several weeks after therapy.

fluoxetine TOP 200

floo-**ox**-e-teen
(Apo-Fluoxetine ♦, Novo-Fluoxetine ♦, Prozac, Prozac Weekly, Sarafem)

BLACK BOX ALERT Increased risk of suicidal thinking and behavior in children, adolescents, young adults 18–24 yrs of age with major depressive disorder, other psychiatric disorders.

Do not confuse fluoxetine with duloxetine, famotidine, fluconazole, fluvastatin, fluvoxamine, fosinopril, furosemide, or paroxetine, or Prozac with Paxil, Prilosec, Prograf, Proscar, or ProSom, or Sarafem with Serophene.

FIXED-COMBINATION(S)

Symbyax: fluoxetine/olanzapine (an antipsychotic): 25 mg/6 mg, 25 mg/12 mg, 50 mg/6 mg, 50 mg/12 mg.

◆CLASSIFICATION

PHARMACOTHERAPEUTIC: Selective serotonin reuptake inhibitor (SSRI). **CLINICAL:** Antidepressant, antiobsessional agent, antibulimic (see p. 40C).

ACTION

Selectively inhibits serotonin uptake in CNS, enhancing serotonergic function. **Therapeutic Effect:** Relieves depression; reduces obsessive-compulsive, bulimic behavior.

PHARMACOKINETICS

Well absorbed from GI tract. Crosses blood-brain barrier. Protein binding: 94%. Metabolized in liver. Primarily excreted in urine. Not removed by hemodialysis. **Half-life:** 2–3 days; metabolite, 7–9 days.

USES

Treatment of major depressive disorder (MDD), obsessive-compulsive disorder (OCD), bulimia nervosa, premenstrual dysphoric disorder (PMDD), panic disorder. Treatment of resistant or bipolar 1 depression (with olanzapine). **OFF-LABEL:** Treatment of fibromyalgia, post-traumatic stress disorder (PTSD), Raynaud's phenomena, social anxiety disorder, selective mutism.

PRECAUTIONS

Contraindications: Use within 14 days of MAOIs or thioridazine. **Cautions:** Seizure disorder, cardiac dysfunction (e.g., history of MI), diabetes, third-trimester pregnancy, impaired platelet aggregation, use of aspirin or NSAIDs, renal/hepatic impairment, pts at high risk for suicide, in pts where weight-loss is undesirable, elderly. Pts at risk of acute narrow-angle glaucoma or with increased intraocular pressure.

⌛ LIFESPAN CONSIDERATIONS

Pregnancy/Lactation: Unknown whether drug crosses placenta or is distributed in breast milk. **Pregnancy Category C. Children:** May be more sensitive to behavioral side effects (e.g., insomnia, restlessness). **Elderly:** No age-related precautions noted.

INTERACTIONS

DRUG: NSAIDS, antiplatelets, anticoagulants may increase risk of bleeding. **Alcohol, other CNS depressants** may increase CNS depression. **MAOIs** may produce serotonin syndrome and neuroleptic malignant syndrome. May increase concentration/toxicity of **phenytoin, tricyclic antidepressants. HERBAL: Gotu kola, kava kava, St. John's wort, valerian** may increase CNS depression. **St. John's wort** may increase effect, risk of serotonin syndrome. **FOOD:** None known. **LAB VALUES:** May decrease serum sodium. May increase AST, ACT.

AVAILABILITY (Rx)

Capsules: 10 mg (Prozac, Sarafem), 20 mg (Prozac, Sarafem), 40 mg (Prozac), 60 mg. **Oral Solution (Prozac):** 20 mg/5 ml. **Tablets (Sarafem):** 10 mg, 15 mg, 20 mg.

🍃**Capsules (Delayed-Release [Prozac Weekly]):** 90 mg.

ADMINISTRATION/HANDLING

PO
• Give without regard to food, but give with food, milk if GI distress occurs.
• **Bipolar disorder:** Give once daily in evening. • **Depression OCD:** Give once daily in morning or twice daily (morning and noon). • **Bulimia:** Give once daily in morning.

INDICATIONS/ROUTES/DOSAGE

◀**ALERT**▶ Use lower or less frequent doses in pts with renal/hepatic impairment, those with concurrent disease or multiple medications, the elderly.

Depression
PO: ADULTS: Initially, 20 mg each morning. If therapeutic improvement does not occur after 2 wks, gradually increase to maximum of 80 mg/day in 2 equally divided doses in morning and at noon. **ELDERLY:** Initially, 10 mg/day. May increase by 10–20 mg q2wks. **Prozac Weekly:** 90 mg/wk, begin 7 days after last dose of 20 mg. **CHILDREN 8–18 YRS:** Initially, 5–10 mg/day. Titrate upward as needed. Usual dosage: 20 mg/day.

Panic Disorder
PO: ADULTS, ELDERLY: Initially, 10 mg/day. May increase to 20 mg/day after 1 wk. **Maximum:** 60 mg/day.

Bulimia Nervosa
PO: ADULTS: 60 mg each morning.

Obsessive-Compulsive Disorder (OCD)
PO: ADULTS, ELDERLY: 20–60 mg/day. **CHILDREN 7–18 YRS:** Initially, 10 mg/day. May increase to 20 mg/day after 2 wks. Range: 10–60 mg/day.

Depression Associated with Bipolar Disorder
PO: **ADULTS, ELDERLY** *(with olanzapine)*: Initially, 20 mg/day. May increase after several wks. Range: 20–50 mg/day.

Premenstrual Dysphoric Disorder (PMDD) (Sarafem)
PO: **ADULTS**: 20 mg/day **or** 20 mg/day beginning 14 days prior to menstruation and continuing through first full day of menses (repeated with each cycle).

SIDE EFFECTS

Frequent (greater than 10%): Headache, asthenia (loss of strength, energy), insomnia, anxiety, drowsiness, nausea, diarrhea, decreased appetite. **Occasional (9%–2%):** Dizziness, tremor, fatigue, vomiting, constipation, dry mouth, abdominal pain, nasal congestion, diaphoresis, rash. **Rare (less than 2%):** Flushed skin, light-headedness, impaired concentration.

ADVERSE EFFECTS/ TOXIC REACTIONS

Overdose may produce seizures, nausea, vomiting, excessive agitation, restlessness.

NURSING CONSIDERATIONS

BASELINE ASSESSMENT
Assess appearance, behavior, mood, suicidal tendencies. For pts on long-term therapy, baseline hepatic/renal function tests, blood counts should be performed at baseline and periodically thereafter.

INTERVENTION/EVALUATION
Supervise suicidal-risk pt closely during early therapy (as depression lessens, energy level improves, increasing suicide potential). Monitor mental status, anxiety, social functioning, appetite, nutritional intake. Monitor daily pattern of bowel activity, stool consistency. Assess skin for rash. Monitor serum hepatic function tests, glucose, sodium, weight.

PATIENT/FAMILY TEACHING
• Maximum therapeutic response may require 4 or more wks of therapy. • Do not abruptly discontinue medication. • Avoid tasks that require alertness, motor skills until response to drug is established. • Avoid alcohol. • To avoid insomnia, take last dose of drug before 4 PM.

fluphenazine

floo-**fen**-a-zeen
(Apo-Fluphenazine ✤, Modecate ✤)
BLACK BOX ALERT Increased mortality in elderly with dementia-related psychosis.
Do not confuse fluphenazine with fluvoxamine.

◆CLASSIFICATION

PHARMACOTHERAPEUTIC: Phenothiazine. **CLINICAL:** Antipsychotic (see p. 66C).

ACTION

Antagonizes dopamine neurotransmission at synapses by blocking postsynaptic dopaminergic receptors in brain. **Therapeutic Effect:** Decreases psychotic behavior. Produces weak anticholinergic, sedative, antiemetic effects; strong extrapyramidal effects.

PHARMACOKINETICS

Erratic absorption. Protein binding: greater than 90%. Metabolized in liver. Excreted in urine. **Half-life:** 33 hrs (Decanoate: 163–232 hrs).

USES

Management of psychotic disturbances (schizophrenia, delusions, hallucinations). **OFF-LABEL:** Psychosis/agitation related to Alzheimer's dementia.

PRECAUTIONS

Contraindications: Myelosuppression, coma, severe CNS depression, receiving large doses of hypnotics, hepatic disease, subcortical brain damage. **Cautions:** Elderly, seizures, Parkinson's disease, severe cardiac disease, renal impairment, pts at risk for pneumonia, pts at risk for hypotension, decreased GI motility, urinary retention, BPH, narrow-angle glaucoma, myasthenia gravis, visual problems.

⌛ LIFESPAN CONSIDERATIONS

Pregnancy/Lactation: Crosses placenta; distributed in breast milk. **Pregnancy Category C. Children:** Pts with acute illnesses (e.g., chickenpox, measles, gastroenteritis, CNS infection) are at risk for developing neuromuscular, extrapyramidal symptoms (EPS), particularly dystonias. **Elderly:** Susceptible to anticholinergic effects.

INTERACTIONS

DRUG: Alcohol, other CNS depressants may increase hypotensive, CNS, respiratory depressant effects. EPS may increase with **medications producing EPS. Antihypertensive medications, hypotensive agents** may worsen hypotension. **Lithium** may decrease absorption, produce adverse neurologic effects. **MAOIs, tricyclic antidepressants** may increase anticholinergic, sedative effects. **Medications prolonging QT interval (e.g., erythromycin)** may have additive effect. **HERBAL: Dong quai, St. John's wort** may increase photosensitization. **Gotu kola, kava kava, St. John's wort, valerian** may increase CNS depression. **FOOD:** None known. **LAB VALUES:** May produce false-positive pregnancy, phenylketonuria test results. May cause EKG changes, including Q- and T-wave disturbances.

AVAILABILITY (Rx)

Elixir: 2.5 mg/5 ml. **Injection (Decanoate):** 25 mg/ml. **Injection Solution: Hydrochloride** 2.5 mg/ml. **Oral Concentrate:** 5 mg/ml. **Tablets:** 1 mg, 2.5 mg, 5 mg, 10 mg.

ADMINISTRATION/HANDLING

• Avoid skin contact with fluphenazine solution (may cause contact dermatitis).

• Dilute oral liquid only with water, milk, juice. Do not dilute with caffeine-containing beverages.

INDICATIONS/ROUTES/DOSAGE

Psychosis
PO: ADULTS: 2.5–10 mg/day in divided doses q6–8h. Maintenance: 1–5 mg/day. **Maximum:** 40 mg/day. **ELDERLY:** Initially, 1–2.5 mg/day. Titrate gradually.
IM (Hydrochloride): ADULTS, ELDERLY: 1.25 mg as single dose. May need 2.5–10 mg/day in divided doses q6–8h. **(Decanoate):** Initially, 12.5–25 mg q2–4wks. May increase in 12.5-mg increments. **Maximum dose:** 100 mg.

SIDE EFFECTS

Frequent: Hypotension, dizziness, syncope (occur frequently after first injection, occasionally after subsequent injections, rarely with oral doses). **Occasional:** Drowsiness (during early therapy), dry mouth, blurred vision, lethargy, constipation or diarrhea, nasal congestion, peripheral edema, urinary retention. **Rare:** Ocular changes, altered skin pigmentation (with prolonged use of high doses).

ADVERSE EFFECTS/ TOXIC REACTIONS

EPS appears dose–related (particularly high dosage), divided into 3 categories: akathisia (inability to sit still, tapping of feet, urge to move around), parkinsonian symptoms (hypersalivation, mask-like facial expression, shuffling gait, tremors), acute dystonias (torticollis [neck muscle spasm], opisthotonos [rigidity of back muscles], oculogyric crisis [rolling back of eyes]). Dystonic reaction may produce diaphoresis, pallor. Tardive dyskinesia (tongue protrusion, puffing of cheeks, chewing/puckering of the mouth) occurs rarely but may be irreversible. Abrupt withdrawal after long-term therapy may precipitate dizziness, gastritis, nausea, vomiting, tremors. Blood dyscrasias, particularly agranulocytosis, mild leukopenia, may occur. May lower seizure threshold.

NURSING CONSIDERATIONS

BASELINE ASSESSMENT

Obtain baseline CBC. Assess behavior, appearance, emotional status, response to environment, speech pattern, thought content.

INTERVENTION/EVALUATION

Monitor B/P for hypotension. Monitor CBC for blood dyscrasias. Monitor for fine tongue movement (may be early sign of tardive dyskinesia). Supervise suicidal-risk pt closely during early therapy (as depression lessens, energy level improves, increasing suicide potential). Assess for therapeutic response (interest in surroundings, improvement in self-care, increased ability to concentrate, relaxed facial expression).

PATIENT/FAMILY TEACHING

• Full therapeutic effect may take up to 6 wks. • Avoid skin contact with solution (may cause contact dermatitis). • Urine may darken. • Do not abruptly withdraw from long-term drug therapy. • Avoid tasks that require alertness, motor skills until response to drug is established. • Drowsiness generally subsides during continued therapy.

flurazepam

flure-**az**-e-pam
(Apo-Flurazepam ✦, Dalmane)
Do not confuse Dalmane with Dialume, or flurazepam with temazepam.

◆CLASSIFICATION

PHARMACOTHERAPEUTIC: Benzodiazepine (**Schedule IV**). **CLINICAL:** Sedative-hypnotic (see p. 148C).

ACTION

Enhances action of inhibitory neurotransmitter gamma-aminobutyric acid (GABA). **Therapeutic Effect:** Produces hypnotic effect due to CNS depression.

PHARMACOKINETICS

Route	Onset	Peak	Duration
PO	15–20 min	3–6 hrs	7–8 hrs

Well absorbed from GI tract. Protein binding: 97%. Crosses blood-brain barrier. Widely distributed. Metabolized in liver. Primarily excreted in urine. Not removed by hemodialysis. **Half-life:** 2.3 hrs; metabolite, 40–114 hrs.

USES

Short-term treatment of insomnia (4 wks or less). Reduces sleep-induction time, number of nocturnal awakenings; increases length of sleep.

PRECAUTIONS

Contraindications: Respiratory depression, preexisting CNS depression, hypersensitivity to other benzodiazepines, pregnancy, breastfeeding, narrow-angle glaucoma. **Cautions:** Renal/hepatic impairment, depression, chronic pulmonary insufficiency, low albumin, history of drug dependence.

⧗ LIFESPAN CONSIDERATIONS

Pregnancy/Lactation: Crosses placenta; may be distributed in breast milk. Chronic ingestion during pregnancy may produce withdrawal symptoms, CNS depression in neonates. **Pregnancy Category X. Children:** Safety and efficacy not established in those younger than 15 yrs. **Elderly:** Use small initial doses with gradual dose increases to avoid ataxia, excessive sedation.

INTERACTIONS

DRUG: Alcohol, CNS depressants may increase CNS depression. **CYP3A4 inhibitors (e.g., azole antifungals)** may increase concentration, risk of toxicity. **HERBAL: Gotu kola, kava kava, St. John's wort, valerian** may increase CNS depression. **FOOD:** None known. **LAB VALUES:** None significant.

AVAILABILITY (Rx)

Capsules: 15 mg, 30 mg.

ADMINISTRATION/HANDLING

PO

• Give without regard to meals. • Capsules may be emptied and mixed with food.

INDICATIONS/ROUTES/DOSAGE

Insomnia

PO: ELDERLY, DEBILITATED, HEPATIC DISEASE, LOW SERUM ALBUMIN: 15 mg at bedtime. **ADULTS:** 15–30 mg at bedtime. **CHILDREN OLDER THAN 15 YRS:** 15 mg at bedtime.

SIDE EFFECTS

Frequent: Drowsiness, dizziness, ataxia, sedation. Morning drowsiness occurs initially. **Occasional:** GI disturbances, anxiety, blurred vision, dry mouth, headache, confusion, skin rash, irritability, slurred speech. **Rare:** Paradoxical CNS excitement, restlessness (esp. in elderly, debilitated).

ADVERSE EFFECTS/ TOXIC REACTIONS

Abrupt or too-rapid withdrawal after long-term use may result in pronounced restlessness/irritability, insomnia, hand tremors, abdominal/muscle cramps, vomiting, diaphoresis, seizures. Overdose results in drowsiness, confusion, diminished reflexes, coma. **Antidote:** Flumazenil (see Appendix K for dosage).

NURSING CONSIDERATIONS

BASELINE ASSESSMENT

Assess B/P, pulse, respirations immediately before administration. Provide safe environment conducive to sleep (back rub, quiet environment, low lighting, raise bed rails).

INTERVENTION/EVALUATION

Assess for paradoxical reaction, particularly during early therapy. Evaluate for therapeutic response (decrease in number of nocturnal awakenings, increase in sleep duration).

PATIENT/FAMILY TEACHING

• Smoking reduces drug effectiveness. • Do not abruptly withdraw medication after long-term use. • May have disturbed sleep pattern 1–2 nights after discontinuing. • Notify physician if pregnant or planning to become pregnant (Pregnancy Category X). • Avoid alcohol, other CNS depressants. • May be habit forming.

F

---

flutamide
HIGH ALERT

flew-ta-mide
(Apo-Flutamide ✿, Euflex ✿, Eulexin ✿, Novo-Flutamide ✿)

BLACK BOX ALERT Hospitalization and, rarely, death due to flutamide-associated hepatic failure have been reported.

Do not confuse Eulexin with Edecrin, or flutamide with Flumadine.

◆ **CLASSIFICATION**

PHARMACOTHERAPEUTIC: Antiandrogen, hormone. **CLINICAL:** Antineoplastic (see p. 86C).

ACTION

Inhibits androgen uptake and/or binding of androgen in target tissue. Used in conjunction with leuprolide to inhibit stimulant effects of flutamide on serum testosterone. **Therapeutic Effect:** Suppresses testicular androgen production, decreases growth of prostate carcinoma.

PHARMACOKINETICS

Completely absorbed from GI tract. Protein binding: 94%–96%. Metabolized in liver. Primarily excreted in urine. Not removed by hemodialysis. **Half-life:** 6 hrs (increased in elderly).

✿ Canadian trade name   🜊 Non-Crushable Drug   **HIGH ALERT** High Alert drug

USES

Treatment of metastatic carcinoma of prostate (in combination with luteinizing hormone-releasing hormone [LHRH] analogues, e.g., leuprolide). **OFF-LABEL:** Female hirsutism.

PRECAUTIONS

Contraindications: Severe hepatic impairment, pregnancy. **Cautions:** Diabetes mellitus.

⏳ LIFESPAN CONSIDERATIONS

Pregnancy/Lactation: Not used in this pt population. **Pregnancy Category D. Children:** Not used in children. **Elderly:** No age-related precautions noted.

INTERACTIONS

DRUG: May increase effects of **warfarin. HERBAL: St. John's wort** may decrease concentration. **FOOD:** None known. **LAB VALUES:** May increase serum glucose, estradiol, testosterone, bilirubin, creatinine, alkaline phosphatase, BUN, AST, ALT. May decrease Hgb, WBC.

AVAILABILITY (Rx)

Capsules: 125 mg.

ADMINISTRATION/HANDLING

PO
• Give without regard to food. • May open and mix with soft food (e.g., applesauce, pudding).

INDICATIONS/ROUTES/DOSAGE

Prostatic Carcinoma
PO: ADULTS, ELDERLY: 250 mg q8h.

SIDE EFFECTS

Frequent (50%–11%): Hot flashes, decreased libido, diarrhea, generalized pain, asthenia (loss of strength, energy), constipation, nausea, nocturia. **Occasional (8%–6%):** Dizziness, paresthesia, insomnia, impotence, peripheral edema, gynecomastia. **Rare (5%–4%):** Rash, diaphoresis, hypertension, hematuria, vomiting, urinary incontinence, headache, flu-like syndrome, photosensitivity.

ADVERSE EFFECTS/ TOXIC REACTIONS

Hepatotoxicity (including hepatic encephalopathy), hemolytic anemia may occur.

NURSING CONSIDERATIONS

INTERVENTION/EVALUATION

Obtain baseline hepatic function tests and periodically during long-term therapy.

PATIENT/FAMILY TEACHING

• Do not stop taking medication (both drugs must be continued). • Urine color may change to amber or yellow-green. • Avoid prolonged exposure to sun, tanning beds. Wear clothing to protect from ultraviolet exposure until tolerance is determined.

---

fluticasone

floo-**tik**-a-sone
(Apo-Fluticasone 🍁, Cutivate, <u>Flonase</u>, Flovent Diskus, Flovent HFA, Veramyst)
Do not confuse Cutivate with Ultravate, or Flonase with Flovent.

FIXED-COMBINATION(S)

Advair, Advair Diskus, Advair HFA: fluticasone/salmeterol (bronchodilator): 100 mcg/50 mcg, 250 mcg/50 mcg, 500 mcg/50 mcg. **Dymista:** Fluticasone/azelastine (an antihistamine): 50 mcg/137 mcg per spray.

◆CLASSIFICATION

PHARMACOTHERAPEUTIC: Corticosteroid. **CLINICAL:** Anti-inflammatory, antipruritic (see pp. 3C, 77C, 100C, 102C).

ACTION

Controls rate of protein synthesis, depresses migration of polymorphonuclear leukocytes, reverses capillary permeabil-

---

ity, stabilizes lysosomal membranes. **Therapeutic Effect:** Prevents, controls inflammation.

PHARMACOKINETICS

Inhalation/intranasal: Protein binding: 91%. Metabolized in liver. Excreted in urine. Half-life: 3–7.8 hrs. **Topical:** Amount absorbed depends on affected area and skin condition (absorption increased with fever, hydration, inflamed or denuded skin).

USES

Nasal: Relief of seasonal/perennial allergic rhinitis. **Topical:** Relief of inflammation/pruritus associated with steroid-responsive disorders (e.g., contact dermatitis, eczema), atopic dermatitis. **Inhalation:** Maintenance treatment of bronchial asthma. Assists in reducing, discontinuing oral corticosteroid therapy.

PRECAUTIONS

Contraindications: Inhalation: Primary treatment of status asthmaticus, acute excacerbation of asthma, other acute asthmatic conditions. **Cautions:** Untreated systemic ocular herpes simplex; untreated fungal, bacterial infection; active or quiescent tuberculosis. Thyroid disease, cardiovascular disease, diabetes, glaucoma, hepatic/renal impairment, cataracts, myasthenia gravis, seizures, GI disease, risk for osteoporosis, untreated localized infection of nasal mucosa.

⌛ LIFESPAN CONSIDERATIONS

Pregnancy/Lactation: Unknown if drug crosses placenta or is distributed in breast milk. **Pregnancy Category C. Children:** Safety and efficacy not established in those younger than 4 yrs. Children 4 yrs and older may experience growth suppression with prolonged or high doses. **Elderly:** No age-related precautions noted.

INTERACTIONS

DRUG: CYP3A4 inhibitors (ritonavir, nelfinavir, clarithromycin, itraconazole, ketoconazole) may increase concentration. **Ritonavir** may reduce serum cortisol concentration. **HERBAL: Echinacea, St. John's wort** may decrease concentration/effect. **FOOD:** None known. **LAB VALUES:** None known.

AVAILABILITY (Rx)

Aerosol for Oral Inhalation (Flovent HFA): 44 mcg/inhalation, 110 mcg/inhalation, 220 mcg/inhalation. **Cream (Cutivate):** 0.05%. **Ointment (Cutivate):** 0.005%. **Powder for Oral Inhalation (Flovent Diskus):** 50 mcg, 100 mcg, 250 mcg. **Suspension Intranasal Spray: (Flonase):** 50 mcg/inhalation. **(Veramyst):** 27.5 mcg/spray.

ADMINISTRATION/HANDLING

Inhalation

• Shake container well. Instruct pt to exhale completely. Place mouthpiece fully into mouth, inhale, hold breath as long as possible before exhaling. • Allow at least 1 min between inhalations. • Rinsing mouth after each use decreases dry mouth, hoarseness.

Intranasal

• Instruct pt to clear nasal passages as much as possible before use (topical nasal decongestants may be needed 5–15 min before use). • Tilt head slightly forward. • Insert spray tip into 1 nostril, pointing toward inflamed nasal turbinates, away from nasal septum. • Pump medication into 1 nostril while pt holds other nostril closed, concurrently inspires through nose.

INDICATIONS/ROUTES/DOSAGE

Allergic Rhinitis

Intranasal: *(Flonase)*: **ADULTS, ELDERLY:** Initially, 200 mcg (2 sprays in each nostril once daily or 1 spray in each nostril q12h). Maintenance: 1 spray in each nostril once daily. May increase to 100 mcg (2 sprays) in each nostril. **Maximum:** 200 mcg/day. **CHILDREN 4 YRS AND**

OLDER: Initially, 100 mcg (1 spray in each nostril once daily). **Maximum:** 200 mcg/day (2 sprays each nostril).
(Veramyst): **ADULTS, ELDERLY, CHILDREN 12 YRS AND OLDER:** 110 mcg (2 sprays in each nostril) once daily. Maintenance: 55 mcg (1 spray in each nostril) once daily. **CHILDREN 2–11 YRS:** 55 mcg (1 spray in each nostril) once daily. May increase to 110 mcg (2 sprays each nostril) once daily.

Usual Topical Dosage
Topical: **ADULTS, ELDERLY, CHILDREN 3 MOS AND OLDER:** Apply sparingly to affected area once or twice a day.

Maintenance Treatment for Asthma (Previously Treated with Bronchodilators)
Inhalation Powder *(Flovent Diskus):* **ADULTS, ELDERLY, CHILDREN 12 YRS AND OLDER:** Initially, 100 mcg q12h. **Maximum:** 500 mcg/twice a day.
Inhalation *(Oral):* **ADULTS, ELDERLY, CHILDREN 12 YRS AND OLDER:** 88 mcg twice a day. **Maximum:** 440 mcg twice a day.

Maintenance Treatment for Asthma (Previously Treated with Inhaled Steroids)
Inhalation Powder *(Flovent Diskus):* **ADULTS, ELDERLY, CHILDREN 12 YRS AND OLDER:** Initially, 100–250 mcg q12h. **Maximum:** 500 mcg q12h.
Inhalation *(Oral):* **ADULTS, ELDERLY, CHILDREN 12 YRS AND OLDER:** 88–220 mcg twice a day. **Maximum:** 440 mcg twice a day.

Maintenance Treatment for Asthma (Previously Treated with Oral Steroids)
Inhalation Powder *(Flovent Diskus):* **ADULTS, ELDERLY, CHILDREN 12 YRS AND OLDER:** 500–1,000 mcg twice a day.
Inhalation *(Oral):* **ADULTS, ELDERLY, CHILDREN 12 YRS AND OLDER:** 440–880 mcg twice a day.

Usual Pediatric Dose (4–11 Yrs)
Flovent Diskus: Initially, 50 mcg twice a day. May increase to 100 mcg twice a day. **Flovent HFA:** Initially, 88 mcg twice daily.

SIDE EFFECTS

Frequent: Inhalation: Throat irritation, hoarseness, dry mouth, cough, temporary wheezing, oropharyngeal candidiasis (particularly if mouth is not rinsed with water after each administration). **Intranasal:** Mild nasopharyngeal irritation, nasal burning, stinging, dryness, rebound congestion, rhinorrhea, altered sense of taste. **Occasional: Inhalation:** Oral candidiasis. **Intranasal:** Nasal/pharyngeal candidiasis, headache. **Topical:** Stinging, burning of skin.

ADVERSE EFFECTS/ TOXIC REACTIONS

None known.

NURSING CONSIDERATIONS

BASELINE ASSESSMENT
Establish baseline history of skin disorder, asthma, rhinitis.

INTERVENTION/EVALUATION
Monitor rate, depth, rhythm, type of respiration; quality/rate of pulse. Assess lung sounds for rhonchi, wheezing, rales. Monitor ABGs. Assess oral mucous membranes for evidence of candidiasis. Monitor growth in pediatric pts. **Topical:** Assess involved area for therapeutic response to irritation.

PATIENT/FAMILY TEACHING
• Pts receiving bronchodilators by inhalation concomitantly with steroid inhalation therapy should use bronchodilator several min before corticosteroid aerosol (enhances penetration of steroid into bronchial tree). • Do not change dose/schedule or stop taking drug; must taper off gradually under medical supervision. • Maintain strict oral hygiene. • Rinse mouth with water immediately after inhalation (prevents mouth/throat dryness, oral fungal infection). • Increase fluid intake (decreases lung secretion viscosity).

underlined – top prescribed drug

• **Intranasal:** • Clear nasal passages before use. • Contact physician if no improvement in symptoms or sneezing/nasal irritation occurs. • Improvement noted in several days. • **Topical:** Rub thin film gently into affected area. • Use only for prescribed area and no longer than ordered. • Avoid contact with eyes.

fluvastatin

floo-va-**sta**-tin
(Lescol, <u>Lescol XL</u>)
**Do not confuse fluvastatin
with fluoxetine, nystatin,
or pitavastatin.**

◆ CLASSIFICATION

PHARMACOTHERAPEUTIC: Hydroxymethylglutaryl-CoA (HMG-CoA) reductase inhibitor. **CLINICAL:** Antihyperlipidemic (see p. 58C).

ACTION

Inhibits hydroxymethylglutaryl-CoA (HMG-CoA) reductase, the enzyme that catalyzes cholesterol synthesis. **Therapeutic Effect:** Decreases LDL cholesterol, VLDL, plasma triglyceride. Slightly increases HDL.

PHARMACOKINETICS

Well absorbed from GI tract. Unaffected by food. Does not cross blood-brain barrier. Protein binding: greater than 98%. Primarily eliminated in feces. **Half-life:** 3 hrs; extended-release, 9 hrs.

USES

Adjunct to diet therapy to reduce elevated total cholesterol (TC), low-density lipoprotein (LDL), apo-protein B, and triglycerides (TG) and increase high-density lipoprotein (HDL) in primary hypercholesterolemia and mixed dyslipidemia; reduce elevated TC, LDL, ApoB in children 10–16 yrs of age with heterozygous familial hypercholesterolemia

(HFH); reduce need for revascularization procedures in pts with coronary artery disease (CAD); slow progression of atherosclerosis in pts with CAD.

PRECAUTIONS

Contraindications: Active hepatic disease, breastfeeding, pregnancy, unexplained increased serum transaminase. **Cautions:** Hepatic impairment; concurrent use with colchicine, gemfibrozil, fibric acid derivatives, or niacin; those at risk for rhabdomyolysis; heavy alcohol consumption; elderly.

⏳ LIFESPAN CONSIDERATIONS

Pregnancy/Lactation: Contraindicated in pregnancy (suppression of cholesterol biosynthesis may cause fetal toxicity), lactation. Unknown if drug is distributed in breast milk. **Pregnancy Category X. Children:** Safety and efficacy not established. **Elderly:** No age-related precautions noted.

INTERACTIONS

DRUG: Increased risk of acute renal failure, rhabdomyolysis with **cyclosporine, colchicine, gemfibrozil, niacin.** May increase concentration/toxicity of **digoxin. HERBAL:** None significant. **FOOD:** None known. **LAB VALUES:** May increase serum creatine kinase (CK), ALT, AST.

AVAILABILITY (Rx)

Capsules (Lescol): 20 mg, 40 mg.

⚕ **Tablets (Extended-Release [Lescol XL]):** 80 mg.

ADMINISTRATION/HANDLING

PO
• Give without regard to food. • Do not break, crush, dissolve, or divide extended-release tablets. • Do not open capsules.

INDICATIONS/ROUTES/DOSAGE

Hyperlipoproteinemia
PO: ADULTS, ELDERLY, PATIENTS REQUIRING 25% OR LESS DECREASE IN LDL: Initially, 20

mg/day (capsule) in the evening. May increase up to 80 mg/day given as 40 mg 2 times/day (immediate-release) or 80 mg once daily (extended-release). **PATIENTS REQUIRING MORE THAN 25% DECREASE IN LDL:** 40 mg 1–2 times a day or 80-mg extended-release tablet once a day.

Heterozygous Familial Hypercholesterolemia
PO: CHILDREN 10–16 YRS: Initially, 20 mg/day. May increase q6wks to maximum dose of 80 mg/day, given in 2 divided doses or a single daily dose (extended-release).

SIDE EFFECTS

Frequent (8%–5%): Headache, dyspepsia, back pain, myalgia, arthralgia, diarrhea, abdominal cramping, rhinitis. **Occasional (4%–2%):** Nausea, vomiting, insomnia, constipation, flatulence, rash, pruritus, fatigue, cough, dizziness.

ADVERSE EFFECTS/ TOXIC REACTIONS

Myositis (inflammation of voluntary muscle) with or without increased creatine kinase (CK), muscle weakness occur rarely. May progress to frank rhabdomyolysis, renal impairment, renal failure.

NURSING CONSIDERATIONS

BASELINE ASSESSMENT

Question for possibility of pregnancy before initiating therapy (Pregnancy Category X). Assess baseline lab results (serum cholesterol, triglycerides, hepatic function test, CPK).

INTERVENTION/EVALUATION

Monitor daily pattern of bowel activity, stool consistency. Assess for headache, dizziness. Assess for rash, pruritus. Monitor serum cholesterol, triglyceride lab results for therapeutic response. Be alert for malaise, muscle cramping, weakness.

PATIENT/FAMILY TEACHING

• Follow special diet (important part of treatment). • Periodic lab tests are es-

sential part of therapy. • Do not open capsules; do not break, crush, or dissolve tablets. • Report promptly vision changes, unusual bruising, yellowing of skin or eyes, any muscle pain/weakness, esp. if accompanied by fever, malaise.

fluvoxamine

floo-**vox**-a-meen
(Apo-Fluvoxumine ✲, Luvox CR, Novo-Fluvoxamine ✲)

BLACK BOX ALERT Increased risk of suicidal ideation and behavior in children, adolescents, young adults 18–24 yrs with major depressive disorder, other psychiatric disorders.

Do not confuse fluvoxamine with flavoxate or fluoxetine, or Luvox with Lasix, Levoxyl, or Lovenox.

◆CLASSIFICATION

PHARMACOTHERAPEUTIC: Serotonin reuptake inhibitor. **CLINICAL:** Antidepressant, antiobsessive (see p. 40C).

ACTION

Selectively inhibits neuronal reuptake of serotonin. **Therapeutic Effect:** Relieves depression, symptoms of obsessive-compulsive disorder (OCD).

PHARMACOKINETICS

Well absorbed following PO administration. Protein binding: 77%. Metabolized in liver. Excreted in urine. **Half-life:** 15–20 hrs.

USES

Immediate-Release: Treatment of obsessive-compulsive disorder (OCD) in adults and children 8 yrs and older. **Luvox CR:** Treatment of OCD in adults. **OFF-LABEL:** Treatment of anxiety disorders in children, depression, panic disorder, social anxiety disorder (SAD), mild dementia-associated agitation in nonpsychotic pts, post-traumatic stress disorder (PTSD).

PRECAUTIONS

Contraindications: Use within 14 days of MAOIs. Concomitant use with alosetron, pimozide, ramelteon, thioridazine, or tizanidine. **Cautions:** Renal/hepatic impairment; elderly; impaired platelet aggregation; concurrent use of NSAIDs, aspirin; seizure disorder; pts that are volume depleted; third trimester of pregnancy; pts with high suicide risk.

⧖ LIFESPAN CONSIDERATIONS

Pregnancy/Lactation: Unknown if drug crosses the placenta; distributed in breast milk. **Children:** Safety and efficacy not established in those younger than 8 yrs. **Elderly:** Potential for reduced serum clearance; maintain caution.

INTERACTIONS

DRUG: May increase concentration, risk of toxicity of **benzodiazepines, carbamazepine, clozapine, theophylline. Lithium, tryptophan** may enhance fluvoxamine's serotonergic effects. **MAOIs** may produce serious reactions (hyperthermia, rigidity, myoclonus). **Tricyclic antidepressants** may increase concentration. May increase effects of **warfarin. HERBAL:** Valerian, St. John's wort, SAMe, kava kava may increase risk of serotonin syndrome or CNS depression. Avoid **herbs with antiplatelet activity (e.g., cat's claw, feverfew, ginger). FOOD:** None known. **LAB VALUES:** May decrease serum sodium.

AVAILABILITY (Rx)

Tablets: 25 mg, 50 mg, 100 mg.

🗲 **Capsules (Extended-Release [Luvox CR]):** 100 mg, 150 mg.

ADMINISTRATION/HANDLING

• Do not break, crush, dissolve, or divide extended-release capsules. • May give with or without food.

INDICATIONS/ROUTES/DOSAGE

Obsessive-Compulsive Disorder (OCD)
PO *(Immediate-Release):* **ADULTS:** 50 mg at bedtime; may increase by 50 mg every 4–7 days. Dosages greater than 100 mg/day should be given in 2 divided doses. **Maximum:** 300 mg/day. *(Extended-Release)* Initially, 100 mg once daily at bedtime. May increase by 50 mg at no less than 1-wk intervals. **Maximum:** 300 mg/day. **CHILDREN 8–17 YRS (IMMEDIATE-RELEASE):** 25 mg at bedtime; may increase by 25 mg every 4–7 days. Dosages greater than 50 mg/day should be given in 2 divided doses. **Maximum: (CHILDREN 8–11 YRS):** 200 mg/day. **(CHILDREN 12–17 YRS):** 300 mg/day.

OCD, Social Anxiety Disorder
PO *(Extended-Release): (Luvox CR):* **ADULTS, ELDERLY:** Initially, 100 mg once daily. May increase by 50 mg at weekly intervals. Range: 100–300 mg/day.

SIDE EFFECTS

Frequent (40%–21%): Nausea, headache, drowsiness, insomnia. **Occasional (14%–8%):** Dizziness, diarrhea, dry mouth, asthenia (loss of strength, energy), dyspepsia, constipation, abnormal ejaculation. **Rare (6%–3%):** Anorexia, anxiety, tremor, vomiting, flatulence, urinary frequency, sexual dysfunction, altered taste.

ADVERSE EFFECTS/ TOXIC REACTIONS

Overdose may produce seizures, nausea, vomiting, excessive agitation, extreme restlessness.

NURSING CONSIDERATIONS

BASELINE ASSESSMENT

Obtain baseline chemistries, esp. renal/hepatic function tests.

INTERVENTION/EVALUATION

Supervise suicidal-risk pt closely during early therapy (as depression lessens, energy level improves, increasing suicide potential). Assess appearance, behavior, speech pattern, level of interest, mood. Assist with ambulation if dizziness, drowsiness occurs. Monitor daily pattern of bowel activity, stool consistency.

PATIENT/FAMILY TEACHING

• Maximum therapeutic response may require 4 wks or more of therapy. • Dry mouth may be relieved by sugarless gum, sips of water. • Do not abruptly discontinue medication. • Avoid tasks that require alertness, motor skills until response to drug is established.

folic acid

foe-lik as-id
(Apo-Folic ✦, Folacin-800)
Do not confuse folic acid with folinic acid.

◆CLASSIFICATION

PHARMACOTHERAPEUTIC: Coenzyme. **CLINICAL:** Nutritional supplement.

ACTION

Stimulates production of platelets, RBCs, WBCs. **Therapeutic Effect:** Essential for nucleoprotein synthesis, maintenance of normal erythropoiesis.

PHARMACOKINETICS

PO form almost completely absorbed from GI tract (upper duodenum). Protein binding: High. Metabolized in liver. Excreted in urine. Removed by hemodialysis.

USES

Treatment of megaloblastic and macrocytic anemias due to folate deficiency (e.g., pregnancy, inadequate dietary intake). Supplement to prevent fetal neural tube defects. **OFF-LABEL:** Adjunct cofactor therapy in methanol toxicity.

PRECAUTIONS

Contraindications: None known. **Cautions:** Anemias (aplastic, normocytic, pernicious, refractory).

⌛ LIFESPAN CONSIDERATIONS

Pregnancy/Lactation: Distributed in breast milk. **Pregnancy Category A (C if more than recommended daily allowance). Children/Elderly:** No age-related precautions noted.

INTERACTIONS

DRUG: May decrease effects of **phenobarbital, phenytoin, primidone, raltitrexed. HERBAL: Green tea** may increase concentration. **FOOD:** None known. **LAB VALUES:** May decrease vitamin B_{12} concentration.

AVAILABILITY (Rx)

Injection Solution: 5 mg/ml. **Tablets:** 0.4 mg (OTC), 0.8 mg (OTC), 1 mg.

ADMINISTRATION/HANDLING

PO
• May give without regard to food.
◀ALERT▶ Parenteral form used in acutely ill, parenteral/enteral alimentation, those unresponsive to oral route in GI malabsorption syndrome. Dosage greater than 0.1 mg/day may conceal pernicious anemia.

INDICATIONS/ROUTES/DOSAGE

Anemia
IM/IV/Subcutaneous/PO: ADULTS, ELDERLY, CHILDREN 4 YRS AND OLDER: 0.4 mg/day. **CHILDREN YOUNGER THAN 4 YRS:** Up to 0.3 mg/day. **INFANTS:** 0.1 mg/day. **PREGNANT/LACTATING WOMEN:** 0.8 mg/day.

Prevention of Neural Tube Defects
PO: WOMEN OF CHILDBEARING AGE: 400–800 mcg/day. **WOMEN AT HIGH RISK OR FAMILY HISTORY OF NEURAL TUBE DEFECTS:** 4 mg/day.

SIDE EFFECTS

None known.

ADVERSE EFFECTS/ TOXIC REACTIONS

Allergic hypersensitivity occurs rarely with parenteral form. Oral folic acid is nontoxic.

NURSING CONSIDERATIONS

BASELINE ASSESSMENT

Pernicious anemia should be ruled out with Schilling test and vitamin B_{12} blood level before initiating therapy (may produce irreversible neurologic damage). Resistance to treatment may occur if decreased hematopoiesis, alcoholism, antimetabolic drugs, deficiency of vitamin B_6, B_{12}, C, E is evident.

INTERVENTION/EVALUATION

Assess for therapeutic improvement: improved sense of well-being, relief from iron deficiency symptoms (fatigue, shortness of breath, sore tongue, headache, pallor).

PATIENT/FAMILY TEACHING

• Eat foods rich in folic acid, including fruits, vegetables, organ meats.

---

fondaparinux   **HIGH ALERT**

fon-**dap**-a-rin-ux
(Arixtra)

BLACK BOX ALERT Epidural or spinal anesthesia greatly increases potential for spinal or epidural hematoma, subsequent long-term or permanent paralysis.

◆ CLASSIFICATION

PHARMACOTHERAPEUTIC: Factor Xa inhibitor. **CLINICAL:** Antithrombotic (see p. 33C).

ACTION

Factor Xa inhibitor and pentasaccharide that selectively binds to antithrombin and increases its affinity for factor Xa, inhibiting factor Xa, stopping blood coagulation cascade. **Therapeutic Effect:** Indirectly prevents formation of thrombin and subsequently fibrin clot.

PHARMACOKINETICS

Well absorbed after subcutaneous administration. Undergoes minimal, if any, metabolism. Highly bound to antithrombin III. Distributed mainly in blood and to a minor extent in extravascular fluid. Excreted unchanged in urine. Removed by hemodialysis. **Half-life:** 17–21 hrs (increased in renal impairment).

USES

Prevention of venous thromboembolism in pts undergoing total hip replacement, hip fracture surgery, knee replacement surgery, abdominal surgery. Treatment of acute deep vein thrombosis (DVT), acute pulmonary embolism. **OFF-LABEL:** Prophylaxis of DVT in pts with history of heparin-induced thrombocytopenia, acute symptomatic superficial vein thrombosis of the legs.

PRECAUTIONS

Contraindications: Active major bleeding, bacterial endocarditis, prophylaxis treatment in pts with body weight less than 50 kg, severe renal impairment (creatinine clearance less than 30 ml/min), thrombocytopenia associated with antiplatelet antibody formation in presence of fondaparinux. **Cautions:** Conditions with increased risk of hemorrhage (GI ulceration, hemophilia, concurrent use of antiplatelet agents, severe uncontrolled hypertension, history of CVA), history of heparin-induced thrombocytopenia, renal/hepatic impairment, elderly, indwelling epidural catheter use.

⧗ LIFESPAN CONSIDERATIONS

Pregnancy/Lactation: Use with caution, particularly during third trimester, immediate postpartum period (increased risk of maternal hemorrhage). Unknown if excreted in breast milk. **Pregnancy Category B. Children:** Safety and efficacy

---

not established. **Elderly:** Age-related renal impairment may increase risk of bleeding.

INTERACTIONS

DRUG: **Anticoagulants, antiplatelet medications, aspirin, drotrecogin alfa, NSAIDs, thrombolytics** may increase risk of bleeding. **HERBAL: Cat's claw, dong quai, evening primrose, feverfew, garlic, ginger, ginkgo, ginseng, horse chestnut, red clover, Omega-3** may increase antiplatelet activity. **FOOD:** None known. **LAB VALUES:** May cause reversible increases in serum creatinine, AST, ALT. May decrease Hgb, Hct, platelet count.

AVAILABILITY (Rx)

Injection, Solution: 2.5 mg/0.5 ml, 5 mg/0.4 ml, 7.5 mg/0.6 ml, 10 mg/0.8 ml.

ADMINISTRATION/HANDLING

Subcutaneous
• Parenteral form appears clear, colorless. Discard if discoloration or particulate matter is noted. • Store at room temperature. • Do not expel air bubble from prefilled syringe before injection. • Pinch fold of skin at injection site between thumb and forefinger. Introduce entire length of subcutaneous needle into skin fold during injection. Inject into fatty tissue between left and right anterolateral or left and right posterolateral abdominal wall. • Rotate injection sites.

INDICATIONS/ROUTES/DOSAGE

◄**ALERT**► For subcutaneous administration only.

Prevention of Venous Thromboembolism
Subcutaneous: ADULTS: 2.5 mg once a day for 5–9 days after surgery (up to 10 days following abdominal surgery; 11 days following hip or knee replacement). Initial dose should be given 6–8 hrs after surgery. Dosage should be adjusted in elderly and those with renal impairment.

Treatment of Venous Thromboembolism, Pulmonary Embolism
Note: Start warfarin on first treatment day and continue fondaparinux until INR reaches 2 to 3 for at least 24 hr.
Subcutaneous: ADULTS, ELDERLY WEIGHING GREATER THAN 100 KG: 10 mg once daily. **ADULTS, ELDERLY WEIGHING 50–100 KG:** 7.5 mg once daily. **ADULTS, ELDERLY WEIGHING LESS THAN 50 KG:** 5 mg once daily.

Dosage in Renal Impairment
Creatinine clearance 30–50 ml/min: Use caution (50% dose reduction or use of low-dose heparin). **Creatinine clearance less than 30 ml/min:** Contraindicated.

SIDE EFFECTS

Frequent (19%–11%): Anemia, fever, nausea. **Occasional (10%–4%):** Edema, constipation, rash, vomiting, insomnia, increased wound drainage, hypokalemia. **Rare (less than 4%):** Dizziness, hypotension, confusion, urinary retention, injection site hematoma, diarrhea, dyspepsia, headache.

ADVERSE EFFECTS/ TOXIC REACTIONS

Accidental overdose may lead to bleeding complications ranging from local ecchymoses to major hemorrhage. Thrombocytopenia occurs rarely.

NURSING CONSIDERATIONS

BASELINE ASSESSMENT
Assess CBC, including renal function.

INTERVENTION/EVALUATION
Periodically monitor CBC, esp. platelet count, stool for occult blood (no need for daily monitoring in pts with normal presurgical coagulation parameters). Assess for any signs of bleeding: bleeding at surgical site, hematuria, blood in stool, bleeding from gums, petechiae, ecchymosis, bleeding from injection sites. Monitor B/P, pulse; hypotension,

tachycardia may indicate bleeding, hypovolemia.

PATIENT/FAMILY TEACHING

• Usual length of therapy is 5–9 days.
• Do not take any OTC medication (esp. aspirin, NSAIDs). • Consult physician if swelling of hands/feet, unusual back pain, unusual bleeding/bruising, weakness, sudden or severe headache occurs.

---

formoterol

TOP 200

for-**moe**-ter-all
(Foradil Aerolizer, Oxeze ✤, Perforomist)

BLACK BOX ALERT Long-acting beta-agonists (salmeterol, formoterol) increase risk of asthma-related deaths. May increase asthma-related hospitalizations in children.

Do not confuse formoterol or Foradil with toradol.

FIXED COMBINATION(S)

Dulera: formoterol/mometasone (a corticosteroid): 5 mcg/100 mcg, 5 mcg/200 mcg. **Symbicort:** formoterol/budesonide (a glucocorticoid): 4.5 mcg/80 mcg, 4.5 mcg/160 mcg.

◆CLASSIFICATION

PHARMACOTHERAPEUTIC: Sympathomimetic (beta$_2$-adrenergic agonist). **CLINICAL:** Bronchodilator (see pp. 76C, 77C).

ACTION

Stimulates beta$_2$-adrenergic receptors in lungs, resulting in relaxation of bronchial smooth muscle. Inhibits release of mediators from various cells in lungs, including mast cells, with little effect on heart rate. **Therapeutic Effect:** Relieves bronchospasm, reduces airway resistance. Improves bronchodilation, nighttime asthma control, peak flow rates.

PHARMACOKINETICS

Route	Onset	Peak	Duration
Inhalation	1–3 min	15 min	12 hrs

Absorbed from bronchi after inhalation. Protein binding: 61%–64%. Metabolized in liver. Primarily excreted in urine. Unknown if removed by hemodialysis. **Half-life:** 10–14 hrs.

USES

Foradil: For long-term maintenance treatment of asthma (only as concomitant therapy with inhaled corticosteroid), prevention of exercise-induced bronchospasm, treatment of bronchoconstriction in pts with COPD. Can be used concomitantly with short-acting beta-agonists, inhaled or systemic corticosteroids, theophylline therapy. **Perforomist:** Maintenance treatment of bronchoconstriction in pts with COPD.

PRECAUTIONS

Contraindications: Monotherapy for asthma, acute episodes of asthma or COPD. **Cautions:** Hypertension, cardiovascular disease, seizure disorder, hyperthyroidism, glaucoma, diabetes, hepatic impairment, hypokalemia. May increase risk of severe exacerbation of asthma.

⊠ LIFESPAN CONSIDERATIONS

Pregnancy/Lactation: Unknown if drug crosses placenta or is distributed in breast milk. **Pregnancy Category C. Children:** Safety and efficacy not established in those younger than 5 yrs. **Elderly:** May be more sensitive to tremor, tachycardia due to age-related increased sympathetic sensitivity.

INTERACTIONS

DRUG: Beta-blockers may decrease bronchodilating effects. **Diuretics, steroids, xanthine derivatives** may increase risk of hypokalemia. **Drugs that can prolong QT interval (e.g., erythromycin, quinidine, thioridazine),**

F

MAOIs, tricyclic antidepressants may potentiate cardiovascular effects. **HERBAL:** None significant. **FOOD:** None known. **LAB VALUES:** May decrease serum potassium. May increase serum glucose.

AVAILABILITY (Rx)

Inhalation Powder (Foradil): 12 mcg. Inhalation Solution for Nebulization (Performist): 20 mcg/2 ml.

ADMINISTRATION/HANDLING

Inhalation
• Pull off Aerolizer Inhaler cover, twisting mouthpiece in direction of arrow to open. • Place capsule in chamber. Capsule is pierced by pressing and releasing buttons on side of Aerolizer, once only. • Instruct pt to exhale completely; place mouthpiece into mouth, close lips and inhale quickly, deeply through mouth (this causes capsule to spin, dispensing the drug). Pt should hold breath as long as possible before exhaling slowly. • Check capsule to ensure all the powder is gone. If not, pt should inhale again to receive rest of the dose. Rinse mouth with water immediately after inhalation (prevents mouth/throat dryness).
Storage • Maintain capsules in individual blister pack until immediately before use. • Do not swallow capsules. • Do not use with a spacer.

Nebulization
• No diluent necessary. • Protect from heat. • Remove from foil pouch immediately before use. • Do not mix with other medications.

INDICATIONS/ROUTES/DOSAGE

Asthma (not Monotherapy)
Inhalation Powder: ADULTS, ELDERLY, CHILDREN 5 YRS AND OLDER: 12 mcg capsule inhaled q12h.

COPD (Maintenance)
Inhalation Powder: ADULTS, ELDERLY, CHILDREN 5 YRS AND OLDER: 12 mcg capsule q12h.

Inhalation Solution for Nebulization: ADULTS, ELDERLY: 20 mcg q12h. **Maximum dose:** 40 mcg.

Exercise-Induced Bronchospasm
Inhalation Powder: ADULTS, ELDERLY, CHILDREN 5 YRS AND OLDER: 12 mcg capsule inhaled at least 15 min before exercise. Do not repeat for another 12 hrs.

SIDE EFFECTS

Occasional (less than 5%): Tremor, muscle cramps, tachycardia, insomnia, headache, irritability, mouth/throat irritation, diarrhea, nausea, vomiting, dizziness, nasopharyngitis.

ADVERSE EFFECTS/ TOXIC REACTIONS

Excessive sympathomimetic stimulation may produce palpitations, extrasystoles, chest pain.

NURSING CONSIDERATIONS

INTERVENTION/EVALUATION

Assess rate, depth, rhythm, type of respiration; quality/rate of pulse. Monitor EKG, serum potassium, ABG determinations. Assess lung sounds for wheezing (bronchoconstriction), rales, pulmonary function tests.

PATIENT/FAMILY TEACHING

• Follow manufacturer guidelines for proper use of inhaler. • Increase fluid intake (decreases lung secretion viscosity). • Rinsing mouth with water immediately after inhalation may prevent mouth/throat irritation. • Avoid excessive use of caffeine derivatives (chocolate, coffee, tea, cola).

fosamprenavir

foss-am-**pren**-a-veer
(Lexiva, Telzir ✦)
Do not confuse Lexiva with Levitra.

CLASSIFICATION

PHARMACOTHERAPEUTIC: Protease inhibitor. **CLINICAL:** Antiviral (see p. 120C).

ACTION

Rapidly converted to amprenavir, inhibiting HIV-1 protease by binding to enzyme's active site, preventing processing of viral precursors, forming immature, noninfectious viral particles. **Therapeutic Effect:** Impairs HIV replication, proliferation.

PHARMACOKINETICS

Rapidly absorbed after PO administration. Protein binding: 90%. Metabolized in liver. Primarily excreted in feces. **Half-life:** 7.7 hrs.

USES

Treatment of HIV infection in combination with at least 2 other antiretroviral agents.

PRECAUTIONS

Contraindications: Concurrent use of alfuzosin, delavirdine, dihydroergotamine, ergonovine, ergotamine, lovastatin, methylergonovine, midazolam, pimozide, rifampin, sildenafil (when used for pulmonary arterial hypertension), simvastatin, St. John's wort, triazolam, concurrent therapy with CYP3A4 substrates with a narrow therapeutic window. If fosamprenavir is given concurrently with ritonavir, then flecainide and propafenone are also contraindicated. **Caution:** Hepatic impairment. Diabetes mellitus, elderly, known sulfonamide allergy, hemophilia, hepatitis B or C.

⌛ LIFESPAN CONSIDERATIONS

Pregnancy/Lactation: Unknown if drug crosses placenta or is distributed in breast milk. **Pregnancy Category C. Children:** Safety and efficacy not established in those younger than 4 yrs. **Elderly:** Age-related hepatic impairment may require decreased dosage.

INTERACTIONS

DRUG: May interfere with metabolism of **amiodarone, bepridil, ergotamine, lidocaine, midazolam, oral contraceptives, quinidine, triazolam, tricyclic antidepressants. Carbamazepine, phenobarbital, phenytoin, rifampin** may decrease concentration. May increase concentrations of **colchicine, calcium channel blockers, bosentan, cyclosporine, tacrolimus, sirolimus, HMG-CoA reductase inhibitors (statins), warfarin. HERBAL:** St. John's wort may decrease concentration. **FOOD:** None known. **LAB VALUES:** May increase serum lipase, triglycerides, AST, ALT. May decrease neutrophil count.

AVAILABILITY (Rx)

Oral Suspension: 50 mg/ml.

Tablets: 700 mg (equivalent to 600 mg amprenavir).

ADMINISTRATION/HANDLING

PO
- Give tablets without regard to meals.
- Do not crush, break, dissolve, or divide film-coated tablets. • Adults should take oral suspension without food. Children should take oral suspension with food.
- Shake suspension vigorously prior to use.

INDICATIONS/ROUTES/DOSAGE

HIV Infection without Previous Protease Inhibitor Therapy

PO: ADULTS, ELDERLY: (Unboosted regimen) 1,400 mg twice daily without ritonavir; or (Ritonavir boosted regimen) 1,400 mg once daily plus ritonavir 100 mg or 200 mg once daily; or 700 mg twice daily plus ritonavir 100 mg twice daily. **CHILDREN (Unboosted): 2 YRS OR OLDER AND 47 KG OR GREATER:** Use adult regimen. **2 YRS OR OLDER AND LESS THAN 47 KG:** 30 mg/kg/dose. **Maximum:** 1,400 mg. **(Boosted): 4 WKS OR OLDER AND 20 KG OR GREATER:** 18 mg/kg/dose twice daily plus ritonavir 3 mg/kg/dose. **15–19 KG:** 23 mg/kg/dose twice daily plus ritonavir 3 mg/kg/dose. **11–14 KG:** 30 mg/kg/dose twice daily plus ritonavir 3 mg/kg/dose. **LESS THAN 11**

KG: 45 mg/kg/dose twice daily plus ritonavir 7 mg/kg/dose.

HIV Infection with Previous Protease Inhibitor Therapy

PO: ADULTS, ELDERLY: 700 mg twice daily plus ritonavir 100 mg twice daily. **CHILDREN 6 MOS OR OLDER AND 20 KG OR GREATER:** 18 mg/kg/dose twice daily plus ritonavir 3 mg/kg/dose. **15–19 KG:** 23 mg/kg/dose twice daily plus ritonavir 3 mg/kg/dose. **11–14 KG:** 30 mg/kg/dose twice daily plus ritonavir 3 mg/kg/dose. **LESS THAN 11 KG:** 45 mg/kg/dose twice daily plus ritonavir 7 mg/kg/dose.

Concurrent Therapy with Efavirenz (600 mg)

PO: ADULTS, ELDERLY: Once-daily regimen: 1,400 mg plus 300 mg ritonavir. Twice-daily regimen: 700 mg twice daily plus ritonavir 100 mg twice daily.

Dosage in Hepatic Impairment

Mild to moderate impairment: Reduce fosamprenavir to 700 mg twice daily (without concurrent ritonavir). **Severe impairment:** Reduce fosamprenavir to 350 mg twice daily (without ritonavir).

SIDE EFFECTS

Frequent (39%–35%): Nausea, rash, diarrhea. **Occasional (19%–8%):** Headache, vomiting, fatigue, depression. **Rare (7%–2%):** Pruritus, abdominal pain, perioral paresthesia.

ADVERSE EFFECTS/ TOXIC REACTIONS

Severe or life-threatening dermatologic reactions, including Stevens-Johnson syndrome, occur rarely.

NURSING CONSIDERATIONS

BASELINE ASSESSMENT

Obtain baseline lab testing, esp. hepatic function tests, before beginning therapy and at periodic intervals during therapy. Offer emotional support. Obtain full medication history.

INTERVENTION/EVALUATION

Closely monitor for evidence of GI discomfort. Monitor daily pattern of bowel activity, stool consistency. Assess skin for rash. Monitor serum chemistry tests for marked abnormalities, particularly hepatic function, glucose, triglycerides, cholesterol. Assess for opportunistic infections (onset of fever, oral mucosa changes, cough, other respiratory symptoms).

PATIENT/FAMILY TEACHING

• Eat small, frequent meals to offset nausea, vomiting. • Continue therapy for full length of treatment. • Doses should be evenly spaced. • Fosamprenavir is not a cure for HIV infection, nor does it reduce risk of transmission to others. • Pt may continue to experience illnesses, including opportunistic infections. • Diarrhea can be controlled with OTC medication. • Report new-onset rash development.

foscarnet

foss-**kar**-net
(Foscavir)

BLACK BOX ALERT Renal toxicity occurs to some degree in majority of pts. For use only in immunocompromised pts with CMV retinitis and mucocutaneous acyclovir-resistant HSV infection. Seizures due to electrolyte/mineral imbalance may occur.

◆ CLASSIFICATION

PHARMACOTHERAPEUTIC: Phosphonic acid derivative. **CLINICAL:** Antiviral (see p. 70C).

ACTION

Selectively inhibits binding sites on virus-specific DNA polymerase, reverse transcriptase. **Therapeutic Effect:** Inhibits replication of herpes virus.

PHARMACOKINETICS

Sequestered into bone, cartilage. Protein binding: 14%–17%. Primarily excreted unchanged in urine. Removed by hemodialysis. **Half-life:** 3.3–6.8 hrs (increased in renal impairment).

USES

Treatment of herpes virus infections suspected to be caused by acyclovir-resistant or ganciclovir-resistant strains. Treatment of cytomegalovirus (CMV) retinitis. Treatment of HIV/AIDS-related CMV infections and herpes. **OFF-LABEL:** Other CMV infections (e.g., colitis, esophagitis); CMV prophylaxis for cancer pts receiving alemtuzumab or allogenic stem cell transplant.

PRECAUTIONS

Contraindications: None known. **Cautions:** Neurologic/cardiac abnormalities, history of hepatic/renal impairment, altered calcium, other electrolyte imbalances.

⏳ LIFESPAN CONSIDERATIONS

Pregnancy/Lactation: Unknown if distributed in breast milk. **Pregnancy Category C. Children:** Safety and efficacy not established. **Elderly:** Age-related renal impairment may require dosage adjustment.

INTERACTIONS

DRUG: Nephrotoxic medications may increase risk of renal toxicity. **Pentamidine (IV)** may cause reversible hypocalcemia, hypomagnesemia, nephrotoxicity. **HERBAL:** None significant. **FOOD:** None known. **LAB VALUES:** May increase serum alkaline phosphatase, bilirubin, creatinine, AST, ALT. May decrease serum magnesium, potassium. May alter serum calcium, phosphate concentrations.

AVAILABILITY (Rx)

Injection Solution: 24 mg/ml.

ADMINISTRATION/HANDLING

💧 IV

Reconstitution • Standard 24 mg/ml solution may be used without dilution when central venous catheter is used for infusion; 24 mg/ml solution *must* be diluted to maximum concentration of 12 mg/ml when peripheral vein catheter is being used. • Dilute only with D₅W or 0.9% NaCl solution.

Rate of Administration • Because dosage is calculated on body weight, unneeded quantity may be removed before start of infusion to avoid overdosage. Aseptic technique must be used and solution administered within 24 hrs of first entry into sealed bottle. • Do not give by IV injection or rapid infusion (increases toxicity). • Administer at rate not faster than 1 hr for doses up to 60 mg/kg and 2 hrs for doses greater than 60 mg/kg. • To minimize toxicity and phlebitis, use central venous lines or veins with adequate blood flow to permit rapid dilution, dissemination. • Use IV infusion pump to prevent accidental overdose.

Storage • Store parenteral vials at room temperature. • After dilution, stable for 24 hrs at room temperature. • Do not use if solution is discolored or particulate forms.

💉 IV INCOMPATIBILITIES

Acyclovir (Zovirax), amphotericin B (Fungizone), calcium, co-trimoxazole (Bactrim), diazepam (Valium), digoxin (Lanoxin), diphenhydramine (Benadryl), dobutamine (Dobutrex), ganciclovir (Cytovene), haloperidol (Haldol), leucovorin, magnesium, midazolam (Versed), pentamidine (Pentam IV), prochlorperazine (Compazine), vancomycin (Vancocin).

💉 IV COMPATIBILITIES

Dopamine (Intropin), heparin, hydromorphone (Dilaudid), lorazepam (Ativan), morphine, potassium chloride.

INDICATIONS/ROUTES/DOSAGE

Cytomegalovirus (CMV) Retinitis
IV: ADULTS, ELDERLY: Initially, 60 mg/kg q8h or 90 mg/kg q12h for 2–3 wks. Maintenance: 90–120 mg/kg/day as a single IV infusion.

Herpes Simplex Infection
IV: ADULTS: 40 mg/kg q8–12h for 2–3 wks or until healed.

Dosage in Renal Impairment
Dosages are individualized based on creatinine clearance. Refer to dosing guide provided by manufacturer.

SIDE EFFECTS

Frequent (65%–30%): Fever, nausea, vomiting, diarrhea. **Occasional (29%–5%):** Anorexia, pain/inflammation at injection site, rigors, malaise, altered B/P, headache, paresthesia, dizziness, rash, diaphoresis, abdominal pain. **Rare (4%–1%):** Back/chest pain, edema, flushing, pruritus, constipation, dry mouth.

ADVERSE EFFECTS/ TOXIC REACTIONS

Nephrotoxicity occurs to some extent in most pts. Seizures, serum mineral/electrolyte imbalances may be life-threatening.

NURSING CONSIDERATIONS

BASELINE ASSESSMENT

Obtain baseline CBC, serum electrolyte levels, renal function tests, vital signs. Risk of renal impairment can be reduced by sufficient fluid intake to ensure diuresis prior to and during therapy.

INTERVENTION/EVALUATION

Monitor serum chemistries, renal function tests. Assess for signs of hypocalcemia (perioral paresthesia, paresthesia of extremities), hypokalemia (weakness, muscle cramps, paresthesia of extremities, irritability). Assess for tremors; provide safety measures for potential seizures. Assess for bleeding, anemia, developing superinfections. Obtain periodic ophthalmologic exams.

PATIENT/FAMILY TEACHING

• Report perioral tingling, numbness in extremities, paresthesia during or following infusion (may indicate electrolyte abnormalities). • Tremors should be reported promptly due to potential for seizures.

fosinopril

foe-**sin**-oh-pril
(Apo-Fosinopril ✦, Monopril ✦, Novo-Fosinopril ✦)

BLACK BOX ALERT May cause fetal injury, mortality if used during second or third trimester of pregnancy. **Do not confuse fosinopril with Fosamax, or lisinopril, or Monopril with Accupril, minoxidil, moexipril, or ramipril.**

◆CLASSIFICATION

PHARMACOTHERAPEUTIC: ACE inhibitor. **CLINICAL:** Antihypertensive (see p. 9C).

ACTION

Suppresses renin-angiotensin-aldosterone system (prevents conversion of angiotensin I to angiotensin II, a potent vasoconstrictor; may inhibit angiotensin II at local vascular, renal sites). Decreases plasma angiotensin II, increases plasma renin activity, decreases aldosterone secretion. **Therapeutic Effect:** Reduces peripheral arterial resistance, pulmonary capillary wedge pressure; improves cardiac output, exercise tolerance.

PHARMACOKINETICS

Route	Onset	Peak	Duration
PO	1 hr	2–6 hrs	24 hrs

Slowly absorbed from GI tract. Protein binding: 97%–98%. Metabolized in liver and GI mucosa. Primarily excreted in urine. Minimal removal by hemodialysis. **Half-life:** 11.5 hrs.

USES

Treatment of hypertension, used alone or in combination with other antihypertensives. Treatment of heart failure.

PRECAUTIONS

Contraindications: Idiopathic or hereditary angioedema, history of angioedema from previous treatment with ACE inhibitors. Concomitant use with aliskiren in pts with diabetes. **Cautions:** Renal impairment, pts with sodium depletion or on diuretic therapy, dialysis, hypovolemia, hypertrophic cardiomyopathy, hyperkalemia, unstented unilateral/bilateral renal stenosis.

⧗ LIFESPAN CONSIDERATIONS

Pregnancy/Lactation: Crosses placenta. Distributed in breast milk. May cause fetal or neonatal mortality or morbidity. **Pregnancy Category C (D if used in second or third trimester). Children:** Safety and efficacy not established. Neonates, infants may be at increased risk for oliguria, neurologic abnormalities. **Elderly:** May be more sensitive to hypotensive effects.

INTERACTIONS

DRUG: Alcohol, antihypertensive agents, diuretics, NSAIDs may increase effect. **Potassium-sparing diuretics, potassium supplements** may cause hyperkalemia. May increase **lithium** concentration/toxicity. **Antacids** may decrease absorption. **HERBAL: Ephedra, ginseng, yohimbe** may worsen hypertension. **Garlic** may increase antihypertensive effect. **Licorice** may cause sodium/water retention, loss of potassium. **FOOD:** None known. **LAB VALUES:** May increase BUN, serum alkaline phosphatase, bilirubin, creatinine, potassium, AST, ALT. May decrease serum sodium. May cause positive antinuclear antibody titer (ANA).

AVAILABILITY (Rx)

Tablets: 10 mg, 20 mg, 40 mg.

ADMINISTRATION/HANDLING

PO
• Give without regard to food. • Tablets may be crushed.

INDICATIONS/ROUTES/DOSAGE

Hypertension
PO: ADULTS, ELDERLY: Initially, 10 mg/day. Maintenance: 20–40 mg/day as a single dose or 2 divided doses. **Maximum:** 80 mg/day. **CHILDREN 6–16 YRS WEIGHING MORE THAN 50 KG:** Initially, 5–10 mg/day. **Maximum:** 40 mg/day.

Heart Failure
PO: ADULTS, ELDERLY: Initially, 5–10 mg/day. Maintenance: 20–40 mg/day. **Maximum:** 40 mg/day.

SIDE EFFECTS

Frequent (12%–9%): Dizziness, cough. **Occasional (4%–2%):** Hypotension, nausea, vomiting, upper respiratory tract infection.

ADVERSE EFFECTS/TOXIC REACTIONS

Excessive hypotension ("first-dose syncope") may occur in pts with HF, severely salt/volume depleted. Angioedema (swelling of face/lips), hyperkalemia occur rarely. Agranulocytosis, neutropenia may be noted in those with renal impairment, collagen vascular disease (scleroderma, systemic lupus erythematosus). Nephrotic syndrome may be noted in those with history of renal disease.

NURSING CONSIDERATIONS

BASELINE ASSESSMENT
Obtain B/P immediately before each dose, in addition to regular monitoring (be alert to fluctuations). Renal function tests should be performed before beginning therapy. In pts with renal impairment, autoimmune disease, or taking drugs that affect leukocytes or immune response, CBC, differential count should be performed before therapy begins and q2wks for 3 mos, then periodically thereafter.

INTERVENTION/EVALUATION
If excessive reduction in B/P occurs, place pt in supine position with legs ele-

 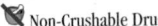

vated. Assist with ambulation if dizziness occurs. Assess for urinary frequency. Auscultate lung sounds for rales, wheezing in those with HF. Monitor renal function tests, CBC, urinalysis for proteinuria. Observe for angioedema (circumoral swelling, edema around eyes). Monitor serum potassium in those on concurrent diuretic therapy.

PATIENT/FAMILY TEACHING

• Report any sign of infection (sore throat, fever). • Several wks may be needed for full therapeutic effect of B/P reduction. • Skipping doses or voluntarily discontinuing drug may produce severe, rebound hypertension. • To reduce hypotensive effect, go from lying to standing slowly. • Immediately report swelling of face, lips, tongue, difficulty breathing, vomiting, excessive perspiration, persistent cough. • Avoid potassium salt substitutes.

fosphenytoin

fos-**fen**-i-toyn
(<u>Cerebyx</u>)
Do not confuse Cerebyx with Celebrex or Celexa, or fosphenytoin with fospropofol.

◆CLASSIFICATION

PHARMACOTHERAPEUTIC: Hydantoin. **CLINICAL:** Anticonvulsant (see p. 36C).

ACTION

Stabilizes neuronal membranes, limits spread of seizure activity. Decreases sodium, calcium ion influx into neurons. Decreases post-tetanic potentiation, repetitive discharge. **Therapeutic Effect:** Decreases seizure activity.

PHARMACOKINETICS

Completely absorbed after IM administration. Protein binding: 95%–99%. Rapidly and completely hydrolyzed to phenytoin after IM or IV administration. Time of complete conversion to phenytoin: 4 hrs after IM injection; 2 hrs after IV infusion. **Half-life:** 8–15 min (for conversion to phenytoin).

USES

Acute treatment, control of generalized convulsive status epilepticus; prevention, treatment of seizures occurring during neurosurgery; short-term substitution for oral phenytoin.

PRECAUTIONS

Contraindications: Adams-Stokes syndrome; hypersensitivity to phenytoin, other hydantoins; second- or third-degree AV block; sinus bradycardia; SA block; occurrence of rash during treatment; treatment of absence seizures; concurrent use of delavirdine. **Cautions:** Porphyria, diabetes, hypothyroidism, hypotension, severe myocardial insufficiency, renal/hepatic disease, hypoalbuminemia.

⌛ LIFESPAN CONSIDERATIONS

Pregnancy/Lactation: May increase frequency of seizures during pregnancy. Increased risk of congenital malformations. Unknown if excreted in breast milk. **Pregnancy Category D. Children:** Safety not established. **Elderly:** Lower dosage recommended.

INTERACTIONS

DRUG: Alcohol, other CNS depressants may increase CNS depression. **Amiodarone, anticoagulants, cimetidine, disulfiram, fluoxetine, isoniazid, sulfonamides** may increase concentration/effects, risk of toxicity. **CYP3A4 inhibitors** (e.g., **fluconazole, ketoconazole, miconazole**) may increase concentration. **HERBAL:** None significant. **FOOD:** None known. **LAB VALUES:** May increase serum glucose, GGT, alkaline phosphatase.

AVAILABILITY (Rx)

Injection Solution: 75 mg/ml (equivalent to 50 mg PE/ml phenytoin).

ADMINISTRATION/HANDLING

🖫 IV

Reconstitution • Dilute in D₅W or 0.9% NaCl to a concentration ranging from 1.5–25 mg phenytoin equivalents (PE)/ml.
Rate of Administration • Administer at rate less than 150 mg PE/min (decreases risk of hypotension, arrhythmias). Children: 1–3 mg PE/kg/min.
Storage • Refrigerate. • Do not store at room temperature for longer than 48 hrs. • After dilution, solution is stable for 8 hrs at room temperature or 24 hrs if refrigerated.

🖫 IV INCOMPATIBILITY

Midazolam (Versed).

🖫 IV COMPATIBILITIES

Lorazepam (Ativan), phenobarbital, potassium chloride.

INDICATIONS/ROUTES/DOSAGE

◀**ALERT**▶ 150 mg fosphenytoin yields 100 mg phenytoin. Dosage, concentration solution, infusion rate of fosphenytoin are expressed in terms of phenytoin equivalents (PE).

Status Epilepticus
IV: ADULTS: Loading dose: 15–20 mg PE/kg infused at rate of 100–150 mg PE/min.

Nonemergent Seizures
IV, IM: ADULTS: Loading dose: 10–20 mg PE/kg. Maintenance: 4–6 mg PE/kg/day.

Short-Term Substitution for Oral Phenytoin
IV, IM: ADULTS: May substitute for oral phenytoin at same total daily dose.

SIDE EFFECTS

Frequent: Dizziness, paresthesia, tinnitus, pruritus, headache, drowsiness. **Occasional:** Morbilliform rash.

ADVERSE EFFECTS/TOXIC REACTIONS

Toxic fosphenytoin blood concentration may produce ataxia (muscular incoordination), nystagmus (rhythmic oscillation of eyes), diplopia, lethargy, slurred speech, nausea, vomiting, hypotension. As drug level increases, extreme lethargy may progress to coma.

NURSING CONSIDERATIONS

BASELINE ASSESSMENT
Review history of seizure disorder (intensity, frequency, duration, LOC). Initiate seizure precautions. Obtain vital signs, medication history (esp. use of phenytoin, other anticonvulsants). Observe clinically.

INTERVENTION/EVALUATION
Monitor EKG, measure cardiac function, respiratory function, B/P during and immediately following infusion (10–20 min). Discontinue if skin rash appears. Interrupt or decrease rate if hypotension, arrhythmias are detected. Assess pt postinfusion (may feel dizzy, ataxic, drowsy). Monitor free and total dilatin levels (2 hrs post IV infusion or 4 hrs post IM injection).

PATIENT/FAMILY TEACHING
• If noncompliance is cause of acute seizures, discuss and address reasons for noncompliance. • Avoid tasks that require alertness, motor skills until response to drug is established.

frovatriptan

froe-va-**trip**-tan
(Frova)

◆CLASSIFICATION

PHARMACOTHERAPEUTIC: Serotonin receptor agonist. **CLINICAL:** Antimigraine (see p. 64C).

ACTION

Binds selectively to vascular receptors, producing vasoconstrictive effect on cranial blood vessels. **Therapeutic Effect:** Relieves migraine headache.

PHARMACOKINETICS

Well absorbed after PO administration. Protein binding: 15%. Metabolized in liver. Primarily eliminated in feces (62%), urine (32%). **Half-life:** 26 hrs (increased in hepatic impairment).

USES

Treatment of acute migraine headache with or without aura in adults. **OFF-LABEL:** Short-term prevention of menstruation-associated migraines.

PRECAUTIONS

Contraindications: Management of basilar or hemiplegic migraine, cerebrovascular or peripheral vascular disease, coronary artery disease, ischemic heart disease (angina pectoris, history of MI, silent ischemia, Prinzmetal's angina), severe hepatic impairment (Child-Pugh grade C), uncontrolled hypertension, use within 24 hrs of ergotamine-containing preparations or another serotonin receptor agonist. **Cautions:** Mild to moderate hepatic impairment, pt profile suggesting cardiovascular risks. History of seizures or structural brain lesions.

⚖ LIFESPAN CONSIDERATIONS

Pregnancy/Lactation: Unknown if drug is excreted in breast milk. **Pregnancy Category C. Children:** Safety and efficacy not established. **Elderly:** Not recommended for use in this pt population.

INTERACTIONS

DRUG: Ergotamine-containing medications may produce vasospastic reaction. **SSRI, SNRI (e.g., duloxetine, fluoxetine, fluvoxamine, paroxetine, sertraline, venlafaxine)** may produce weakness, hyperreflexia, uncoordination. **HERBAL:** None significant. **FOOD:** None known. **LAB VALUES:** None significant.

AVAILABILITY (Rx)

▣ **Tablets:** 2.5 mg.

ADMINISTRATION/HANDLING

PO
• Give with fluids. • Do not crush, chew film-coated tablets.

INDICATIONS/ROUTES/DOSAGE

Acute Migraine Headache
PO: ADULTS, ELDERLY: Initially, 2.5 mg. If headache improves but then returns, dose may be repeated after at least 2 hrs. **Maximum:** 7.5 mg/day.

SIDE EFFECTS

Occasional (8%–4%): Dizziness, paresthesia, fatigue, flushing. **Rare (3%–2%):** Hot/cold sensation, dry mouth, dyspepsia (heartburn, epigastric distress).

ADVERSE EFFECTS/ TOXIC REACTIONS

Cardiac reactions (ischemia, coronary artery vasospasm, MI), noncardiac vasospasm-related reactions (cerebral hemorrhage, CVA) occur rarely, particularly in pts with hypertension, obesity, smokers, diabetes, strong family history of coronary artery disease; males older than 40 yrs; postmenopausal women.

NURSING CONSIDERATIONS

BASELINE ASSESSMENT

Question for history of peripheral vascular disease, renal/hepatic impairment, possibility of pregnancy. Question regarding onset, location, duration of migraine, possible precipitating factors.

INTERVENTION/EVALUATION

Assess for relief of migraine headache, potential for photophobia, phonophobia (sound sensitivity), nausea, vomiting.

PATIENT/FAMILY TEACHING

• Take a single dose as soon as symptoms of an actual migraine attack appear. • Medication is intended to relieve migraine headaches, not to prevent or reduce number of attacks. • Avoid tasks that require alertness, motor skills until response to drug is established. • Immediately report palpitations, pain, tightness in chest or throat, sudden or severe abdominal pain, pain or weakness of extremities.

fulvestrant HIGH ALERT

ful-**vest**-rant
(Faslodex)
Do not confuse Faslodex with Fosamax.

◆ CLASSIFICATION

PHARMACOTHERAPEUTIC: Estrogen antagonist. **CLINICAL:** Antineoplastic (see p. 86C).

ACTION

Competes with endogenous estrogen at estrogen receptor binding sites. **Therapeutic Effect:** Inhibits tumor growth.

PHARMACOKINETICS

Extensively, rapidly distributed after IM administration. Protein binding: 99%. Metabolized in liver. Eliminated by hepatobiliary route; excreted in feces. **Half-life:** 40 days in postmenopausal women. Peak serum levels occur in 7–9 days.

USES

Treatment of hormone receptor–positive metastatic breast cancer in postmenopausal women with disease progression following antiestrogen therapy.

PRECAUTIONS

Contraindications: None known. **Cautions:** Thrombocytopenia, bleeding diathesis, anticoagulant therapy, hepatic disease, reduced hepatic blood flow, pregnancy.

 LIFESPAN CONSIDERATIONS

Pregnancy/Lactation: Do not administer to pregnant women. Unknown if excreted in breast milk. May cause fetal harm. **Pregnancy Category D. Children:** Not used in this pt population. **Elderly:** No age-related precautions noted.

INTERACTIONS

DRUG: None significant. **HERBAL:** None significant. **FOOD:** None known. **LAB VALUES:** May increase ALT, AST.

AVAILABILITY (Rx)

Injection, Solution: 50 mg/ml.

ADMINISTRATION/HANDLING

IM
• Administer slowly into upper, outer quadrant or ventrogluteal area of buttock as two injections, one in each buttock over 1–2 min.

INDICATIONS/ROUTES/DOSAGE

Breast Cancer
IM: ADULTS, ELDERLY: 500 mg (two 250-mg injections) on days 1, 15, and 29, and 500 mg once monthly thereafter.

SIDE EFFECTS

Frequent (26%–13%): Nausea, hot flashes, pharyngitis, asthenia (loss of strength, energy), vomiting, vasodilation, headache. **Occasional (12%–5%):** Injection site pain, constipation, diarrhea, abdominal pain, anorexia, dizziness, insomnia, paresthesia, bone/back pain, depression, anxiety, peripheral edema, rash, diaphoresis, fever. **Rare (2%–1%):** Vertigo, weight gain.

ADVERSE EFFECTS/ TOXIC REACTIONS

UTI occurs occasionally. Vaginitis, anemia, thromboembolic phenomena, leukopenia occur rarely.

F

NURSING CONSIDERATIONS

BASELINE ASSESSMENT
Estrogen receptor assay should be done before beginning therapy. Baseline CT should be performed initially and periodically thereafter for evidence of tumor regression.

INTERVENTION/EVALUATION
Monitor blood chemistry, plasma lipids. Be alert to increased bone pain, ensure adequate pain relief. Check for edema, esp. of dependent areas. Monitor for and assist with ambulation if asthenia (loss of strength, energy) or dizziness occurs. Assess for headache. Offer antiemetic for nausea/vomiting.

PATIENT/FAMILY TEACHING
• Notify physician if nausea/vomiting, asthenia (loss of strength, energy), hot flashes become unmanageable.

---

furosemide

TOP 200

fur-**oh**-se-myde
(Apo-Furosemide ♦, Lasix, Novo-Semide ♦)

BLACK BOX ALERT Large amounts can lead to profound diuresis with water and electrolyte depletion.
Do not confuse furosemide with famotidine, finasteride, fluconazole, fluoxetine, loperamide, or torsemide, or Lasix with Lidex, Lovenox, Luvox, or Luxiq.

◆CLASSIFICATION
PHARMACOTHERAPEUTIC: Loop diuretic. **CLINICAL:** Diuretic (see p. 104C).

ACTION
Enhances excretion of sodium, chloride, potassium by direct action at ascending limb of loop of Henle. **Therapeutic Effect:** Produces diuresis, lowers B/P.

PHARMACOKINETICS

Route	Onset	Peak	Duration
PO	30–60 min	1–2 hrs	6–8 hrs
IV	5 min	20–60 min	2 hrs
IM	30 min	N/A	N/A

Well absorbed from GI tract. Protein binding: greater than 98%. Partially metabolized in liver. Primarily excreted in urine (nonrenal clearance increases in severe renal impairment). Not removed by hemodialysis. **Half-life:** 30–90 min (increased in renal/hepatic impairment, neonates).

USES
Treatment of edema associated with HF, chronic renal failure (including nephrotic syndrome), hepatic cirrhosis, acute pulmonary edema. Treatment of hypertension, either alone or in combination with other antihypertensives.

PRECAUTIONS
Contraindications: Anuria. **Cautions:** Hepatic cirrhosis, hepatic coma, severe electrolyte depletion, prediabetes, diabetes, systemic lupus erythematosus.

⏳ LIFESPAN CONSIDERATIONS
Pregnancy/Lactation: Crosses placenta. Distributed in breast milk. **Pregnancy Category C. Children:** Half-life increased in neonates; may require increased dosage interval. **Elderly:** May be more sensitive to hypotensive, electrolyte effects, developing circulatory collapse, thromboembolic effect. Age-related renal impairment may require dosage adjustment.

INTERACTIONS
DRUG: Amphotericin B, nephrotoxic, ototoxic medications may increase risk of nephrotoxicity, ototoxicity. May increase risk of **lithium** toxicity. **Other medications causing hypokalemia** may increase risk of hypokalemia. **HERBAL: Ephedra, ginseng, yohimbe** may worsen hypertension. **Garlic** may increase antihypertensive effect. **FOOD:** None

known. **LAB VALUES:** May increase serum glucose, BUN, uric acid. May decrease serum calcium, chloride, magnesium, potassium, sodium.

AVAILABILITY (Rx)

Injection Solution: 10 mg/ml. **Oral Solution:** 10 mg/ml, 40 mg/5 ml. **Tablets:** 20 mg, 40 mg, 80 mg.

ADMINISTRATION/HANDLING

 IV

Rate of Administration • May give undiluted but is compatible with D₅W or 0.9% NaCl. • Mlay be diluted for infusion to 1–2 mg/ml (**maximum:** 10 mg/ml). • Administer each 40 mg or fraction by IV push over 1–2 min. Do not exceed administration rate of 4 mg/min for short-term intermittent infusion.

Storage • Solution appears clear, colorless. • Discard yellow solutions. • Stable for 24 hrs at room temperature when mixed with 0.9% NaCl or D₅W.

IM

• Temporary pain at injection site may be noted.

PO

• Administer on empty stomach. • Give with food to avoid GI upset, preferably with breakfast (may prevent nocturia). • Food may decrease diuretic effect.

IV INCOMPATIBILITIES

Ciprofloxacin (Cipro), diltiazem (Cardizem), dobutamine (Dobutrex), dopamine (Intropin), doxorubicin (Adriamycin), droperidol (Inapsine), esmolol (Brevibloc), famotidine (Pepcid), filgrastim (Neupogen), fluconazole (Diflucan), gemcitabine (Gemzar), gentamicin (Garamycin), idarubicin (Idamycin), labetalol (Trandate), metoclopramide (Reglan), midazolam (Versed), milrinone (Primacor), nicardipine (Cardene), ondansetron (Zofran), quinidine, thiopental (Pentothal), vinblastine (Velban), vincristine (Oncovin), vinorelbine (Navelbine).

IV COMPATIBILITIES

Amiodarone (Cordarone), bumetanide (Bumex), calcium gluconate, cimetidine (Tagamet), dexmedetomidine (Precedex), heparin, hydromorphone (Dilaudid), lidocaine, lipids, morphine, nitroglycerin, norepinephrine (Levophed), potassium chloride, propofol (Diprivan).

INDICATIONS/ROUTES/DOSAGE

Edema, Heart Failure, Hypertension
PO: ADULTS, ELDERLY: Initially, 20–80 mg/dose; may increase by 20–40 mg/dose q6–8h. May titrate up to 600 mg/day in severe edematous states. **CHILDREN:** Initially, 2 mg/kg/dose. May increase by 1–2 mg/kg/dose at 6–8 hr intervals. **Maximum:** 6 mg/kg/dose. **NEONATES:** 1 mg/kg/dose 1–2 times a day.
IV, IM: ADULTS, ELDERLY: 20–40 mg/dose; may increase by 20 mg/dose q1–2h. **Maximum single dose:** 160–200 mg. **CHILDREN:** Initially, 1 mg/kg/dose. May increase by 1 mg/kg/dose no sooner than 2 hrs after previous dose. **Maximum:** 6 mg/kg/dose. **NEONATES:** 1–2 mg/kg/dose q12–24h.
IV Infusion: ADULTS, ELDERLY: Bolus of 20–40 mg, followed by infusion of 10–40 mg/hr; may double q2h. **Maximum:** 80–160 mg/hr. **CHILDREN:** 0.05 mg/kg/hr; titrate to desired effect. **NEONATES:** Initially, 0.2 mg/kg/hr. May increase by 0.1 mg/kg/hr q12–24h. **Maximum:** 0.4 mg/kg/hr.

SIDE EFFECTS

Expected: Increased urinary frequency/volume. **Frequent:** Nausea, dyspepsia, abdominal cramps, diarrhea or constipation, electrolyte disturbances. **Occasional:** Dizziness, light-headedness, headache, blurred vision, paresthesia, photosensitivity, rash, fatigue, bladder spasm, restlessness, diaphoresis. **Rare:** Flank pain.

ADVERSE EFFECTS/ TOXIC REACTIONS

Vigorous diuresis may lead to profound water loss/electrolyte depletion, resulting in hypokalemia, hyponatremia, dehydration. Sudden volume depletion may result in increased risk of thrombosis, circulatory collapse, sudden death. Acute hypotensive episodes may occur, sometimes several days after beginning therapy. Ototoxicity (deafness, vertigo, tinnitus) may occur, esp. in pts with severe renal impairment. Can exacerbate diabetes mellitus, systemic lupus erythematosus, gout, pancreatitis. Blood dyscrasias have been reported.

NURSING CONSIDERATIONS

BASELINE ASSESSMENT

Check vital signs, esp. B/P, pulse, for hypotension before administration. Assess baseline serum electrolytes, esp. for hypokalemia. Assess skin turgor, mucous membranes for hydration status; observe for edema. Assess muscle strength, mental status. Note skin temperature, moisture. Obtain baseline weight. Initiate I&O monitoring.

INTERVENTION/EVALUATION

Monitor B/P, vital signs, serum electrolytes, I&O, weight. Note extent of diuresis. Watch for changes from initial assessment (hypokalemia may result in changes in muscle strength, tremor, muscle cramps, altered mental status, cardiac arrhythmias). Hyponatremia may result in confusion, thirst, cold/clammy skin.

PATIENT/FAMILY TEACHING

• Expect increased frequency, volume of urination. • Report palpitations, signs of electrolyte imbalances (noted previously), hearing abnormalities (sense of fullness in ears, tinnitus). • Eat foods high in potassium such as whole grains (cereals), legumes, meat, bananas, apricots, orange juice, potatoes (white, sweet), raisins. • Avoid sunlight, sunlamps.

gabapentin

ga-ba-**pen**-tin
(Apo-Gabapentin ♣, Gralise,
Horizant, <u>Neurontin</u>)
**Do not confuse Neurontin with
Motrin, Neoral, nitrofurantoin,
Noroxin, or Zarontin.**

◆CLASSIFICATION

PHARMACOTHERAPEUTIC: Gamma-aminobutyric acid analogue. **CLINICAL:** Anticonvulsant, antineuralgic (see p. 36C).

ACTION

May increase synthesis or accumulation of gamma-aminobutyric acid (GABA) by binding to as-yet-undefined receptor sites in brain tissue. **Therapeutic Effect:** Reduces seizure activity, neuropathic pain.

PHARMACOKINETICS

Well absorbed from GI tract (not affected by food). Protein binding: less than 5%. Widely distributed. Crosses blood-brain barrier. Primarily excreted unchanged in urine. Removed by hemodialysis. **Half-life:** 5–7 hrs (increased in renal impairment, elderly).

USES

Neurontin: Adjunct in treatment of partial seizures (with or without secondary generalized seizures) in children 13 yrs and older and adults. Adjunct to treatment of partial seizures in children 3–12 yrs; management of postherpetic neuralgia. **Horizant:** Treatment of moderate to severe primary restless legs syndrome (RLS). **Gralise:** Management of postherpetic neuralgia. **OFF-LABEL:** Treatment of neuropathic pain, diabetic peripheral neuropathy, vasomotor symptoms, fibromyalgia, postoperative pain.

PRECAUTIONS

Contraindications: None known. **Cautions:** Severe renal impairment.

⧖ LIFESPAN CONSIDERATIONS

Pregnancy/Lactation: Unknown if distributed in breast milk. **Pregnancy Category C. Children:** Safety and efficacy not established in those 3 yrs and younger. **Elderly:** Age-related renal impairment may require dosage adjustment.

INTERACTIONS

DRUG: Antacids decrease absorption. **Morphine** may increase CNS depression. **HERBAL: Evening primrose** may decrease seizure threshold. **Gotu kola, kava kava, St. John's wort, valerian** may increase CNS depression. **FOOD:** None known. **LAB VALUES:** May alter serum glucose, WBC count. May increase serum alkaline phosphatase, ALT, AST, bilirubin.

AVAILABILITY (Rx)

Capsules (Neurontin): 100 mg, 300 mg, 400 mg. **Oral Solution (Neurontin):** 250 mg/5 ml. **Tablets (Neurontin):** 600 mg, 800 mg. **Tablets (Gralise):** 300 mg, 600 mg.

🐾**Tablets, Extended-Release:** (Horizant) 600 mg.

ADMINISTRATION/HANDLING

PO
• Give without regard to meals; may give with food to avoid, reduce GI upset. • If treatment is discontinued or anticonvulsant therapy is added, do so gradually over at least 1 wk (reduces risk of loss of seizure control). Swallow extended-release tablets whole; do not break, crush, dissolve, or divide.

INDICATIONS/ROUTES/DOSAGE

Note: When given 3 times/day, maximum time between doses should not exceed 12 hrs.

Adjunctive Therapy for Seizure Control
PO: ADULTS, ELDERLY, CHILDREN 13 YEARS AND OLDER: Initially, 300 mg 3 times a day. May titrate dosage. Range: 900–1,800 mg/day in 3 divided doses. **Maximum:** 3,600 mg/day. **CHILDREN 3–12 YRS:** Initially, 10–15 mg/kg/day in 3 divided doses. May titrate up to 25–35 mg/kg/day (for children 5–12 yrs) and 40 mg/kg/day (for children 3–4 yrs). **Maximum:** 50 mg/kg/day.

Adjunctive Therapy for Neuropathic Pain
PO: ADULTS, ELDERLY: Initially, 100 mg 3 times a day; may increase by 300 mg/day at weekly intervals. **Maximum:** 3,600 mg/day in 3 divided doses. **CHILDREN:** Initially, 5 mg/kg/dose at bedtime, followed by 5 mg/kg/dose for 2 doses on day 2, then 5 mg/kg/dose for 3 doses on day 3. **Maximum:** 300 mg. Range: 8–35 mg/kg/day in 3 divided doses.

Postherpetic Neuralgia
PO: ADULTS, ELDERLY: *(Neurontin):* 300 mg once on day 1, 300 mg twice a day on day 2, and 300 mg 3 times a day on day 3 as needed. Range: 1,800–3,600 mg/day. *(Gralise):* 300 mg once on day 1; 600 mg once on day 2; 900 mg once daily on days 3–6; 1,200 mg once daily on days 7–10; 1,500 mg once daily on days 11–14; then 1,800 mg once daily.

RLS
PO: ADULTS, ELDERLY (HORIZANT): 600 mg once daily at 5 PM.

Dosage in Renal Impairment
Dosage and frequency are modified based on creatinine clearance:

Horizant not recommended in pts with creatinine clearance less than 30 ml/min or pts on hemodialysis.

SIDE EFFECTS

Frequent (19%–10%): Fatigue, drowsiness, dizziness, ataxia. **Occasional (8%–3%):** Nystagmus (rapid eye movements), tremor, diplopia (double vision), rhinitis, weight gain. **Rare (less than 2%):** Anxiety, dysarthria (speech difficulty), memory loss, dyspepsia, pharyngitis, myalgia.

ADVERSE EFFECTS/ TOXIC REACTIONS

Abrupt withdrawal may increase seizure frequency, increased risk of suicidal behavior/thoughts. Overdosage may result in slurred speech, drowsiness, lethargy, diarrhea.

NURSING CONSIDERATIONS

BASELINE ASSESSMENT
Review history of seizure disorder (type, onset, intensity, frequency, duration, LOC). Assess location, intensity of neuralgia/neuropathic pain.

INTERVENTION/EVALUATION
Provide safety measures as needed. Monitor seizure frequency/duration, renal function, weight, behavior in children. Monitor signs/symptoms of depression, suicidal tendencies, other unusual behavior.

PATIENT/FAMILY TEACHING
• Use only as prescribed; do not abruptly stop taking drug (may increase seizure frequency). • Avoid tasks that require

Creatinine Clearance	Dosage (Immediate-release)	(Extended-release)
60 ml/min or higher	300–1,200 mg tid	1,800 mg once/day
30–59 ml/min	200–700 mg q12h	600–1,800 mg once/day
16–29 ml/min	200–700 mg once daily	Not recommended
Less than 16 ml/min	100–300 mg once daily	Not recommended
Hemodialysis	125–350 mg after each 4-hr hemodialysis session	

alertness, motor skills until response to drug is established. • Avoid alcohol. • Carry identification card/bracelet to note seizure disorder/anticonvulsant therapy. • Report suicidal ideation, depression, unusual behavioral changes (esp. with changes in dosage), worsening of seizure activity or loss of seizure control.

galantamine

gal-**an**-ta-meen
(Razadyne, Razadyne ER, Reminyl ✦, Reminyl ER ✦)
Do not confuse Razadyne with Rozerem, or Reminyl with Amaryl.

◆CLASSIFICATION

PHARMACOTHERAPEUTIC: Cholinesterase inhibitor. **CLINICAL:** Antidementia.

ACTION

Elevates acetylcholine concentrations by slowing degeneration of acetylcholine released by still intact cholinergic neurons (Alzheimer's disease involves degeneration of cholinergic neuronal pathways). **Therapeutic Effect:** Slows progression of Alzheimer's disease.

PHARMACOKINETICS

Rapidly, completely absorbed from GI tract. Protein binding: 18%. Distributed to blood cells; binds to plasma proteins, mainly albumin. Metabolized in liver. Excreted in urine. **Half-life:** 7 hrs.

USES

Treatment of mild to moderate dementia of Alzheimer's type. **OFF-LABEL:** Severe dementia associated with Alzheimer's disease, mild to moderate dementia associated with Parkinson's disease, Lewy body dementia.

PRECAUTIONS

Contraindications: None known. **Cautions:** Moderate renal/hepatic impairment (not recommended in severe impairment), history of ulcer disease, asthma, COPD, bladder outflow obstruction, supraventricular cardiac conduction conditions (except with pacemaker), seizure disorder, concurrent medications that slow cardiac conduction through SA or AV node.

⏳ LIFESPAN CONSIDERATIONS

Pregnancy/Lactation: Unknown if drug crosses placenta or is distributed in breast milk. **Pregnancy Category B. Children:** Not prescribed for this pt population. **Elderly:** No age-related precautions noted, but use is not recommended in those with severe hepatic/renal impairment (creatinine clearance less than 9 ml/min).

INTERACTIONS

DRUG: May interfere with the effects of **bethanechol, succinylcholine. Cimetidine, ketoconazole, paroxetine** may increase concentration/effect. **HERBAL: St. John's wort** may decrease concentration. **FOOD:** None known. **LAB VALUES:** None significant.

AVAILABILITY (Rx)

Oral Solution (Razadyne): 4 mg/ml. **Tablets (Razadyne):** 4 mg, 8 mg, 12 mg.

🥄 **Capsules (Extended-Release [Razadyne ER]):** 8 mg, 16 mg, 24 mg.

ADMINISTRATION/HANDLING

PO
• Give tablet or solution with morning and evening meals. • Mix oral solution with nonalcoholic beverage, take immediately. • Capsule should be given at breakfast.

INDICATIONS/ROUTES/DOSAGE

Alzheimer's Disease
PO *(Immediate-Release Tablets, Oral Solution)*: **ADULTS, ELDERLY:** Initially, 4 mg twice a day (8 mg/day). After

a minimum of 4 wks (if well tolerated), may increase to 8 mg twice a day (16 mg/day). After another 4 wks, may increase to 12 mg twice daily (24 mg/day). Range: 16–24 mg/day in 2 divided doses.

PO *(Extended-Release):* **ADULTS, ELDERLY:** Initially, 8 mg once daily for 4 wks; then increase to 16 mg once daily for 4 wks or longer. If tolerated, may increase to 24 mg once daily. Range: 16–24 mg once daily.

Dosage in Renal/Hepatic Impairment
For moderate impairment, maximum dosage is 16 mg/day. Drug is not recommended for pts with severe impairment.

SIDE EFFECTS

Frequent (17%–7%): Nausea, vomiting, diarrhea, anorexia, weight loss. **Occasional (5%–4%):** Abdominal pain, insomnia, depression, headache, dizziness, fatigue, rhinitis. **Rare (less than 3%):** Tremors, constipation, confusion, cough, anxiety, urinary incontinence.

ADVERSE EFFECTS/ TOXIC REACTIONS

Overdose may cause cholinergic crisis (increased salivation, lacrimation, urination, defecation, bradycardia, hypotension, muscle weakness). Treatment aimed at generally supportive measures, use of anticholinergics (e.g., atropine).

NURSING CONSIDERATIONS

BASELINE ASSESSMENT
Assess cognitive, behavioral, functional deficits of pt. Obtain baseline serum hepatic/renal function tests.

INTERVENTION/EVALUATION
Monitor cognitive, behavioral, functional status of pt. Evaluate EKG, periodic rhythm strips in pts with underlying arrhythmias. Assess for evidence of GI disturbances (nausea, vomiting, diarrhea, anorexia, weight loss).

PATIENT/FAMILY TEACHING
• Take with meals (reduces risk of nausea). • Avoid tasks that require alertness, motor skills until response to drug is established. • Report persistent GI disturbances, excessive salivation, diaphoresis, excessive tearing, excessive fatigue, insomnia, depression, dizziness, increased muscle weakness.

ganciclovir

gan-**sye**-kloe-veer
(Cytovene, Zirgan)

BLACK BOX ALERT Toxicity presents as neutropenia, thrombocytopenia, anemia. Studies suggest carcinogenic and teratogenic effects, inhibition of spermatogenesis.
Do not confuse Cytovene with Cytosar, or ganciclovir with acyclovir.

◆CLASSIFICATION

PHARMACOTHERAPEUTIC: Synthetic nucleoside. **CLINICAL:** Antiviral (see p. 70C).

ACTION

Competes with viral DNA polymerase and incorporation into growing viral DNA chains. **Therapeutic Effect:** Interferes with DNA synthesis, viral replication.

PHARMACOKINETICS

Widely distributed (including CSF and ocular tissue). Protein binding: 1%–2%. Excreted primarily in urine. Removed by hemodialysis. **Half-life:** 1.7–5.8 hrs (increased in renal impairment).

USES

Parenteral: Treatment of cytomegalovirus (CMV) retinitis in immunocompromised pts (e.g., HIV), prophylaxis of CMV infection in transplant pts. **Ophthalmic:** Treatment of acute herpetic keratitis. **OFF-LABEL:** CMV retinitis.

PRECAUTIONS

Contraindications: Absolute neutrophil count less than 500/mm³, platelet count less than 25,000/mm³, hypersensitivity to acyclovir, ganciclovir. **Cautions:** Neutropenia, thrombocytopenia, renal impairment; children (long-term safety not determined due to potential for long-term carcinogenic, adverse reproductive effects).

⚕ LIFESPAN CONSIDERATIONS

Pregnancy/Lactation: Effective contraception should be used during therapy; ganciclovir should not be used during pregnancy. Breastfeeding should be discontinued; may be resumed no sooner than 72 hrs after the last dose. **Pregnancy Category C. Children:** Safety and efficacy not established in those younger than 12 yrs. **Elderly:** Age-related renal impairment may require dosage adjustment.

INTERACTIONS

DRUG: Bone marrow depressants may increase myelosuppression. **Imipenem** may increase risk for generalized seizures. **HERBAL:** None significant. **FOOD:** None known. **LAB VALUES:** May increase BUN, serum creatinine, alkaline phosphatase, bilirubin, AST, ALT.

AVAILABILITY (Rx)

Injection, Powder for Reconstitution (Cytovene): 500 mg. **Ophthalmic Gel (Zirgan):** 0.15%.

ADMINISTRATION/HANDLING

 IV

Reconstitution • Reconstitute 500-mg vial with 10 ml Sterile Water for Injection to provide concentration of 50 mg/ml; do **not** use Bacteriostatic Water (contains parabens, which is incompatible with ganciclovir). • Further dilute with 250–1,000 ml D₅W, 0.9% NaCl to provide a concentration of 10 mg/ml or less for infusion.

Rate of Administration • Administer only by IV infusion over at least 1 hr. • Do not give by IV push or rapid IV infusion (increases risk of toxicity); protect from infiltration (high pH causes severe tissue irritation). • Use large veins to permit rapid dilution, dissemination of ganciclovir (minimizes phlebitis); central venous ports may reduce catheter-associated infection.

Storage • Store vials at room temperature. Do not refrigerate. • Reconstituted solution in vial is stable for 12 hrs at room temperature. • After dilution, stable for 5 days at room temperature or if refrigerated. • Discard if precipitate forms, discoloration occurs. • Avoid exposure to skin, eyes, mucous membranes. • Use latex gloves, safety glasses during preparation/handling of solution. • Avoid inhalation. • If solution contacts skin or mucous membranes, wash thoroughly with soap and water; rinse eyes thoroughly with plain water.

⚕ IV INCOMPATIBILITIES

Aldesleukin (Proleukin), amifostine (Ethyol), aztreonam (Azactam), cefepime (Maxipime), cytarabine (ARA-C), doxorubicin (Adriamycin), fludarabine (Fludara), foscarnet (Foscavir), gemcitabine (Gemzar), ondansetron (Zofran), piperacillin and tazobactam (Zosyn), sargramostim (Leukine), vinorelbine (Navelbine).

⚕ IV COMPATIBILITIES

Amphotericin B, enalapril (Vasotec), filgrastim (Neupogen), fluconazole (Diflucan), granisetron (Kytril), propofol (Diprivan).

INDICATIONS/ROUTES/DOSAGE

Cytomegalovirus (CMV) Retinitis
IV: ADULTS, CHILDREN 3 MOS AND OLDER: 5 mg/kg/dose q12h for 14–21 days, then 5 mg/kg/day as a single daily dose or 6 mg/kg 5 days a wk.

Prevention of CMV in Transplant Pts
IV: **ADULTS, CHILDREN:** 5 mg/kg/dose q12h for 7–14 days, then 5 mg/kg/day as a single daily dose dependent on clinical condition and degree of immunosuppression.

Congenital CMV
IV: **NEONATES:** 6 mg/kg/dose q12h for 6 wks (if HIV positive, longer duration considered).

Acute Herpetic Keratitis
Ophthalmic: **ADULTS, ELDERLY:** 1 drop 5 times/day until ulcer heals, then 1 drop 3 times/day for 7 days.

Dosage in Renal Impairment
Dosage and frequency are modified based on creatinine clearance (see table).

SIDE EFFECTS

Frequent (41%–13%): Diarrhea, fever, nausea, abdominal pain, vomiting. **Occasional (11%–6%):** Diaphoresis, infection, paresthesia, flatulence, pruritus. **Rare (4%–2%):** Headache, stomatitis, dyspepsia, phlebitis.

ADVERSE EFFECTS/ TOXIC REACTIONS

Hematologic toxicity occurs commonly: leukopenia (41%–29%), anemia (25%–19%). Intraocular implant occasionally results in visual acuity loss, vitreous hemorrhage, retinal detachment. GI hemorrhage occurs rarely.

NURSING CONSIDERATIONS

BASELINE ASSESSMENT
Evaluate hematologic baseline. Perform baseline ophthalmic exam. Obtain specimens for support of differential diagnosis (urine, feces, blood, throat) since retinal infection is usually due to hematogenous dissemination.

INTERVENTION/EVALUATION
Monitor I&O, ensure adequate hydration (minimum 1,500 ml/24 hrs). Diligently evaluate hematology reports for neutropenia, thrombocytopenia, leukopenia. Obtain periodic ophthalmic examinations. Question pt regarding visual acuity, therapeutic improvement, complications. Assess for rash, pruritus.

PATIENT/FAMILY TEACHING
• Ganciclovir provides suppression, not cure, of cytomegalovirus (CMV) retinitis. • Frequent blood tests, eye exams are necessary during therapy due to toxic nature of drug. • Report any new symptom promptly. • May temporarily or permanently inhibit sperm production in men, suppress fertility in women. • Barrier contraception should be used during and for 90 days after therapy due to mutagenic potential.

| | Dosage | |
Creatinine Clearance	IV Induction	IV Maintenance
50–69 ml/min	2.5 mg/kg q12h	2.5 mg/kg q24h
25–49 ml/min	2.5 mg/kg q24h	1.25 mg/kg q24h
10–24 ml/min	1.25 mg/kg q24h	0.625 mg/kg q24h
Less than 10 ml/min	1.25 mg/kg 3 times/wk	0.625 mg/kg 3 times/wk
Hemodialysis (give after HD on HD days)	1.25 mg/kg q48–72h	0.625 mg/kg q48–72h
Peritoneal dialysis	1.25 mg/kg 3 times/wk	0.625 mg/kg 3 times/wk
Continuous renal replacement therapy		
Continuous venovenous hemofiltration	2.5 mg/kg q24h	1.25 mg/kg q24h
Continuous venovenous hemodialysis/ continuous venovenous hemodiafiltration	2.5 mg/kg q12h	2.5 mg/kg q24h

gefitinib

ge-fi-ti-nib
(Iressa)
Do not confuse gefitinib with erlotinib, dasatinib, imatinib, or lapatinib.

◆CLASSIFICATION

PHARMACOTHERAPEUTIC: Tyrosine kinase inhibitor. **CLINICAL:** Antineoplastic (see p. 86C).

ACTION

Inhibits epidermal growth factor receptor–tyrosine kinase (EGFR-TK), a key driver in tumor cell growth. Interrupts angiogenesis and metastasis. **Therapeutic Effect:** Inhibits tumor cell proliferation and survival.

PHARMACOKINETICS

Slowly absorbed after PO administration. Peak plasma levels in 3–7 hrs. Protein binding: 90%. Metabolized in liver. Excreted primarily in feces (86%). **Half-life:** 48 hrs.

USES

Treatment of locally advanced or metastatic non–small-cell lung cancer (NSCLC) after failure with platinum-based or docetaxel therapies. **OFF-LABEL:** First-line treatment of NSCLC with known EGFR mutation.

PRECAUTIONS

◄ALERT► Product contains lactose. Not recommended for pts who are lactose intolerant.
Contraindications: None known. **Cautions:** Hepatic impairment, lung disease, ocular disease, concurrent administration of CYP3A4 inducers and inhibitors.

⌛ LIFESPAN CONSIDERATIONS

Pregnancy/Lactation: Avoid pregnancy. Unknown if crosses placenta or is distributed in breast milk. Nursing mothers must either discontinue breast-feeding or discontinue therapy. **Pregnancy Category D. Children:** Safety and efficacy not established in those younger than 18 yrs. **Elderly:** No age-related precautions noted.

INTERACTIONS

DRUG: CYP3A4 inhibitors (e.g., **clarithromycin, ketoconazole**) may increase concentration. **CYP3A4 inducers** (e.g., **phenytoin, rifampin**) may decrease concentration. **H₂ antagonists** (e.g., **ranitidine**) may decrease concentration. May increase bleeding risk with **warfarin. HERBAL: St. John's wort** may decrease effectiveness. **FOOD:** Avoid **grapefruit products. LAB VALUES:** May increase serum AST, ALT, bilirubin, urine protein.

AVAILABILITY (Rx)

Tablets: 250 mg.

ADMINISTRATION/HANDLING

• May give without regard to meals.
• Avoid grapefruit products. • Do not crush or cut. Swallow whole or administer as dispersion in water. Gently swirl glass for up to 20 min and immediately ingest once dispersed.

INDICATIONS/ROUTES/DOSAGE

Non–Small-Cell Lung Cancer
PO: ADULTS: 250 mg daily. (Concomitant CYP3A4 inducers: consider increasing dose to 500 mg daily.)

SIDE EFFECTS

Frequent: Diarrhea, anorexia, hematuria, epistaxis, vomiting, nausea, stomatitis, rash, pruritus, asthenia (loss of strength, energy). **Occasional:** Conjunctivitis, blepharitis, dry eye, dehydration, dry mouth, alopecia, pyrexia. **Rare:** Aberrant eyelash growth, urticaria.

ADVERSE EFFECTS/ TOXIC REACTIONS

Hepatotoxicity, pancreatitis, Stevens-Johnson syndrome (toxic epidermal necrolysis), cutaneous vasculitis, cystitis, corneal ulcer/erosion, ocular bleeding, hypothyroidism was reported. Interstitial lung disease (ILD) reported in 1.3% of pts; must consider interrupting treatment and promptly investigate. Allergic reactions including angioedema, urticaria reported in 1.5%.

NURSING CONSIDERATIONS

BASELINE ASSESSMENT

Obtain baseline CBC with differential, serum chemistries, hepatic function test, thyroid function test, PT/INR (if taking warfarin), EGRF mutation serostatus. Question possibility of pregnancy or plans of breastfeeding. Receive full medication history including vitamins, minerals, herbal products. Assess visual acuity.

INTERVENTION/EVALUATION

Assess vital signs, O_2 saturation routinely. Routinely monitor CBC with differential, hepatic function tests. Worsening cough, fever, or shortness of breath may indicate interstitial lung disease. Consider ophthalmologic evaluation for vision changes. Monitor for bruising, hematuria, jaundice, right upper abdominal pain, weight loss, or acute infection (fever, diaphoresis, lethargy, productive cough). Monitor for skin lesions.

PATIENT/FAMILY TEACHING

• Blood levels will be drawn routinely. • Report urine changes, bloody or clay-colored stools, upper abdominal pain, nausea, vomiting, bruising, fever, cough, difficulty breathing. • Immediately report any newly prescribed medications, suspected pregnancy, vision changes (eye pain, bleeding, sensitivity to light), or persistent diarrhea, dehydration. • Avoid alcohol. • Avoid grapefruit products.

---

gemcitabine

jem-**sye**-ta-been
(Gemzar)

Do not confuse gemcitabine with gemtuzumab, Gemzar with Zinecard.

◆CLASSIFICATION

PHARMACOTHERAPEUTIC: Antimetabolite. **CLINICAL:** Antineoplastic (see p. 86C).

ACTION

Inhibits ribonucleotide reductase, the enzyme necessary for catalyzing DNA synthesis. **Therapeutic Effect:** Produces death of cells undergoing DNA synthesis.

PHARMACOKINETICS

Not extensively distributed after IV infusion (increased with length of infusion). Protein binding: less than 10%. Metabolized intracellularly by nucleoside kinases. Excreted primarily in urine. **Half-life:** Influenced by duration of infusion. Infusion 1 hr or less: 42–94 min; infusion 3–4 hrs: 4–10.5 hrs.

USES

Metastatic breast cancer in combination with paclitaxel. Treatment of locally advanced (stage II, III) or metastatic (stage IV) adenocarcinoma of pancreas. Indicated for pts previously treated with 5-fluorouracil. Monotherapy or in combination with cisplatin for treatment of locally advanced or metastatic non–small-cell lung cancer (NSCLC), ovarian cancer. **OFF-LABEL:** Treatment of biliary tract carcinoma, bladder carcinoma, germ cell tumors (e.g., testicular), Hodgkin's lymphoma, non-Hodgkin's lymphoma, acute leukemia; cervical, head, and neck cancer.

PRECAUTIONS

Contraindications: None known. **Cautions:** Renal/hepatic impairment, pregnancy, elderly, concurrent radiation therapy.

⚖ LIFESPAN CONSIDERATIONS

Pregnancy/Lactation: If possible, avoid use during pregnancy, esp. first trimester. May cause fetal harm. Unknown if distributed in breast milk. Breastfeeding not recommended. **Pregnancy Category D. Children:** Safety and efficacy not established. **Elderly:** Increased risk of hematologic toxicity.

INTERACTIONS

DRUG: Bone marrow depressants may increase risk of myelosuppression. **Live virus vaccines** may potentiate virus replication, increase vaccine side effects, decrease pt's antibody response to vaccine. **HERBAL: Echinacea** may decrease effects. **FOOD:** None known. **LAB VALUES:** May increase BUN, serum alkaline phosphatase, bilirubin, creatinine, AST, ALT. May decrease Hgb, Hct, leukocyte count, platelet count.

AVAILABILITY (Rx)

Injection, Powder for Reconstitution: 200-mg, 1-g, 2-g vials. **Injection, Solution:** 38 mg/ml.

ADMINISTRATION/HANDLING

 IV

Reconstitution • Use gloves when handling/preparing gemcitabine. • Reconstitute 200-mg or 1-g vial with 0.9% NaCl injection without preservative (5 ml or 25 ml, respectively) to provide concentration of 38 mg/ml. • Shake to dissolve. **Rate of Administration** • May give without further dilution. • May be further diluted with 50–500 ml 0.9% NaCl to a concentration as low as 0.1 mg/ml. • Infuse over 30 min. • Infusion time greater than 60 min increases toxicity. **Storage** • Store at room temperature (refrigeration may cause crystallization). • Reconstituted solution is stable for 24 hrs at room temperature. Do not refrigerate.

▓ IV INCOMPATIBILITIES

Acyclovir (Zovirax), amphotericin B (Fungizone), cefotaxime (Claforan), furosemide (Lasix), ganciclovir (Cytovene), imipenem and cilastatin (Primaxin), irinotecan (Camptosar), methotrexate, methylprednisolone (Solu-Medrol), mitomycin (Mutamycin), piperacillin/tazobactam (Zosyn), prochlorperazine (Compazine).

▓ IV COMPATIBILITIES

Bumetanide (Bumex), calcium gluconate, dexamethasone (Decadron), diphenhydramine (Benadryl), dobutamine (Dobutrex), dopamine (Intropin), granisetron (Kytril), heparin, hydrocortisone (Solu-Cortef), lorazepam (Ativan), ondansetron (Zofran), potassium chloride.

INDICATIONS/ROUTES/DOSAGE

◀ALERT▶ Dosage is individualized based on clinical response, tolerance to adverse effects. When used in combination therapy, consult specific protocols for optimum dosage, sequence of drug administration.

Breast Cancer
IV: ADULTS, ELDERLY: (in combination with paclitaxel): 1,250 mg/m² over 30 min on days 1 and 8 of each 21-day cycle.

Non–Small-Cell Lung Cancer (NSCLC)
IV: ADULTS, ELDERLY, CHILDREN: (in combination with cisplatin): 1,000 mg/m² on days 1, 8, and 15, repeated every 28 days; or 1,250 mg/m² on days 1 and 8. Repeat every 21 days.

Ovarian Cancer
IV: ADULTS, ELDERLY: (in combination with carboplatin): 1,000 mg/m² on days 1 and 8 of each 21-day cycle.

Pancreatic Cancer
IV: ADULTS: 1,000 mg/m² once weekly for up to 7 wks or until toxicity necessitates decreasing dosage or withholding the dose, followed by 1 wk of rest. Subsequent cycles should consist of once-weekly dose for 3 consecutive wks out of every 4 wks. For pts completing cycles at 1,000 mg/m², increase dose to 1,250 mg/m² as tolerated. Dose for next cycle may be increased to 1,500 mg/m².

G

Dosage Reduction Guidelines
Pancreatic Cancer, Non–Small-Cell Lung Cancer (NSCLC)
Dosage adjustments should be based on granulocyte count and platelet count, as follows:

Absolute Granulocyte Counts (cells/mm³)	Platelet Count (cells/mm³)	% of Full Dose
1,000 and	100,000	100
500–999 or	50,000–99,000	75
Less than 500 or	Less than 50,000	Hold

Breast Cancer

Absolute Granulocyte Counts (cells/mm³)	Platelet Count (cells/mm³)	% of Full Dose
Equal to or greater than 1,200 and	Greater than 75,000	100
1,000–1,199 or	50,000–75,000	75
700–999 and	Equal to or greater than 50,000	50
Less than 700 or	Less than 50,000	Hold

Ovarian Cancer

Absolute Granulocyte Counts (cells/mm³)	Platelet Count (cells/mm³)	% of Full Dose
1,500 or greater and	100,000 or greater	100
1,000–1,499 and/or	75,000–99,999	50
Less than 1,000 and/or	Less than 75,000	Hold

SIDE EFFECTS

Frequent (69%–20%): Nausea, vomiting, generalized pain, fever, mild to moderate pruritic rash, mild to moderate dyspnea, constipation, peripheral edema. **Occasional (19%–10%):** Diarrhea, petechiae, alopecia, stomatitis, infection, drowsi-ness, paresthesia. **Rare:** Diaphoresis, rhinitis, insomnia, malaise.

ADVERSE EFFECTS/ TOXIC REACTIONS

Severe myelosuppression (anemia, thrombocytopenia, leukopenia) occurs commonly.

NURSING CONSIDERATIONS

BASELINE ASSESSMENT

Obtain baseline CBC, renal/hepatic function tests and periodically thereafter (CBC, platelets before each dose). Drug should be suspended or dosage modified if myelosuppression is detected.

INTERVENTION/EVALUATION

Assess all lab results prior to each dose. Monitor for dyspnea, fever, pruritic rash, dehydration. Assess oral mucosa for erythema, ulceration at inner margin of lips, sore throat, difficulty swallowing (stomatitis). Assess skin for rash. Monitor for, report diarrhea. Provide antiemetics as needed.

PATIENT/FAMILY TEACHING

• Avoid crowds, exposure to infection. • Maintain strict oral hygiene. • Promptly report fever, sore throat, signs of local infection, easy bruising, rash, yellowing of skin or eyes. • Report nausea or vomiting that continues at home.

gemfibrozil

jem-**fye**-broe-zil
(Apo-Gemfibrozil ✤, Lopid, Novo-Gemfibrozil ✤)
Do not confuse Lopid with Levbid, Lipitor, Lodine, or Slo-Bid.

◆CLASSIFICATION

PHARMACOTHERAPEUTIC: Fibric acid derivative. **CLINICAL:** Antihyperlipidemic (see p. 57C).

ACTION

Inhibits lipolysis of fat in adipose tissue; decreases hepatic uptake of free fatty acids (reduces hepatic triglyceride production). Inhibits synthesis of VLDL carrier apolipoprotein B. **Therapeutic Effect:** Lowers serum cholesterol, triglycerides (decreases VLDL, LDL; increases HDL).

PHARMACOKINETICS

Well absorbed from GI tract. Protein binding: 99%. Metabolized in liver. Primarily excreted in urine. Not removed by hemodialysis. **Half-life:** 1.5 hrs.

USES

Treatment of hypertriglyceridemia in types IV and V hyperlipidemia in pts who are at greater risk for pancreatitis and those who have not responded to dietary intervention. Reduce risk of coronary heart disease (CHD) development in pts without symptoms who have decreased HDL, increased LDL, increased triglycerides.

PRECAUTIONS

Contraindications: Hepatic dysfunction (including primary biliary cirrhosis), preexisting gallbladder disease, severe renal dysfunction, concurrent use with repaglinide. **Cautions:** Concurrent use with statins, mild to moderate renal impairment. anticoagulant therapy (e.g., warfarin).

⧖ LIFESPAN CONSIDERATIONS

Pregnancy/Lactation: Unknown if drug crosses placenta or is distributed in breast milk. Decision to discontinue nursing or drug should be based on potential for serious adverse effects. **Pregnancy Category C. Children:** Not recommended in pts younger than 2 yrs (cholesterol necessary for normal development). **Elderly:** Age-related renal impairment may require dosage adjustment.

INTERACTIONS

DRUG: Statins may increase risk for myopathy/rhabdomyolysis. May increase effect of **repaglinide, warfarin. Bile acid–binding resins (e.g., colestipol)** may decrease concentration. **HERBAL:** None significant. **FOOD:** None known. **LAB VALUES:** May increase serum alkaline phosphatase, bilirubin, creatine kinase, LDH, AST, ALT. May decrease Hgb, Hct, leukocyte counts, serum potassium.

AVAILABILITY (Rx)

Tablets: 600 mg.

ADMINISTRATION/HANDLING

PO
• Give 30 min before morning and evening meals.

INDICATIONS/ROUTES/DOSAGE

Hyperlipidemia
PO: ADULTS, ELDERLY: 600 mg twice daily 30 min before breakfast and dinner.

SIDE EFFECTS

Frequent (20%): Dyspepsia. **Occasional (10%–2%):** Abdominal pain, diarrhea, nausea, vomiting, fatigue. **Rare (less than 2%):** Constipation, acute appendicitis, vertigo, headache, rash, pruritus, altered taste.

ADVERSE EFFECTS/ TOXIC REACTIONS

Cholelithiasis, cholecystitis, acute appendicitis, pancreatitis, malignancy occur rarely.

NURSING CONSIDERATIONS

BASELINE ASSESSMENT

Obtain diet history, esp. fat/alcohol consumption. Obtain baseline lab results: serum glucose, triglyceride, cholesterol, hepatic function tests, CBC.

INTERVENTION/EVALUATION

Monitor daily pattern of bowel activity, stool consistency. Monitor LDL, VLDL, serum triglycerides, cholesterol lab results for therapeutic response. Assess for rash, pruritus. Question for headache, dizziness. Monitor hepatic function, hematology tests. Assess for abdominal pain, esp. right upper quadrant or epigastric pain suggestive of adverse gallbladder effects. Monitor serum glucose in those receiving insulin, oral antihyperglycemics.

PATIENT/FAMILY TEACHING

• Follow special diet (important part of treatment). • Take before meals. • Periodic lab tests are essential part of therapy. • Report pronounced dizziness, blurred vision, abdominal pain, diarrhea, nausea, vomiting.

gemifloxacin

jem-i-**flox**-a-sin
(Factive)

BLACK BOX ALERT Increased risk of tendonitis, tendon rupture (with corticosteroids, organ transplant recipients, pts greater than 60 yrs of age).

◆CLASSIFICATION

PHARMACOTHERAPEUTIC: Fluoroquinolone. **CLINICAL:** Antibiotic (see p. 26C).

ACTION

Inhibits the enzyme DNA gyrase in susceptible microorganisms, interfering with bacterial cell replication, repair. **Therapeutic Effect:** Bactericidal.

PHARMACOKINETICS

Rapidly, well absorbed from GI tract. Protein binding: 70%. Widely distributed. Penetrates well into lung tissue and fluid. Metabolized in liver. Excreted in feces (61%), urine (36%). Partially removed by hemodialysis. **Half-life:** 4–12 hrs.

USES

Treatment of susceptible infections due to *S. pneumoniae, H. influenzae, H. parainfluenzae, M. catarrhalis, M. pneumoniae, C. pneumoniae, K. pneumoniae* including acute bacterial exacerbation of chronic bronchitis, community-acquired pneumonia of mild to moderate severity. **OFF-LABEL:** Acute sinusitis.

PRECAUTIONS

Contraindications: Hypersensitivity to other fluroquinolones. **Cautions:** Renal impairment, rheumatoid arthritis, history of QT prolongation, hypokalemia, hypomagnesemia, concurrent medications that prolong QT interval, seizure disorder, significant bradycardia, acute myocardial ischemia.

⧗ LIFESPAN CONSIDERATIONS

Pregnancy/Lactation: Has potential for teratogenic effects. Substitute formula feedings for breastfeeding. **Pregnancy Category C. Children:** Safety and efficacy not established in those 18 yrs and younger. **Elderly:** Age-related renal impairment may require dosage adjustment.

INTERACTIONS

DRUG: Aluminum-, magnesium-containing antacids, didanosine, iron preparations, sucralfate may decrease absorption. **Antipsychotics, class IA and class III antiarrhythmics, erythromycin, tricyclic antidepressants** may increase risk of prolonged QT interval, life-threatening arrhythmias. **HERBAL: Dong quai, St. John's wort** may increase risk of photosensitization. **FOOD:** None known. **LAB VALUES:** May increase BUN, serum alkaline phosphatase, bilirubin, LDH, creatinine, AST, ALT. May alter platelets, neutrophils, Hgb, Hct, RBCs.

AVAILABILITY (Rx)

▽ **Tablets:** 320 mg.

ADMINISTRATION/HANDLING

PO

• Give without regard to meals, milk, or calcium supplements. • Do not crush, break tablets. • Take 3 hrs before or 2 hrs after supplements containing iron, zinc, or magnesium.

INDICATIONS/ROUTES/DOSAGE

Acute Bacterial Exacerbation of Chronic Bronchitis
PO: ADULTS, ELDERLY: 320 mg once a day for 5 days.

Community-Acquired Pneumonia
PO: ADULTS, ELDERLY: 320 mg once a day for 5–7 days.

Dosage in Renal Impairment
Dosage and frequency are modified based on creatinine clearance.

Creatinine Clearance	Dosage
Greater than 40 ml/min	320 mg once a day
40 ml/min or less	160 mg once a day

SIDE EFFECTS

Occasional (4%–2%): Diarrhea, rash, nausea. **Rare (1% or less):** Headache, abdominal pain, dizziness.

ADVERSE EFFECTS/ TOXIC REACTIONS

Antibiotic-associated colitis, other superinfections (abdominal cramps, severe watery diarrhea, fever) may result from altered bacterial balance. Hypersensitivity reaction, including photosensitivity (rash, pruritus, blisters, edema, burning skin) may occur.

NURSING CONSIDERATIONS

BASELINE ASSESSMENT
Question for history of hypersensitivity to fluoroquinolone antibiotics.

INTERVENTION/EVALUATION
Monitor for signs/symptoms of infection. Assess WBC count, renal/hepatic function tests. Encourage adequate fluid intake. Monitor daily pattern of bowel activity, stool consistency. Assess skin for rash. Be alert for superinfection: fever, vomiting, diarrhea, anal/genital pruritus, oral mucosal changes (ulceration, pain, erythema).

PATIENT/FAMILY TEACHING

• Take with 8 oz of water, without regard to food. • Drink several glasses of water between meals. • Complete full course of therapy. • Take 3 hrs before or 2 hrs after supplements containing iron, zinc, magnesium, or antacids.

gentamicin

G

jen-ta-**mye**-sin
(Gentak)
BLACK BOX ALERT Aminoglycoside antibiotics may cause neurotoxicity, nephrotoxicity. Risk of ototoxicity directly proportional to dosage, duration of treatment; ototoxicity usually is irreversible, precipitated by tinnitus, vertigo.
Do not confuse gentamicin with vancomycin.

◆CLASSIFICATION

PHARMACOTHERAPEUTIC: Aminoglycoside. **CLINICAL:** Antibiotic (see p. 22C).

ACTION

Irreversibly binds to protein of bacterial ribosomes. **Therapeutic Effect:** Interferes with protein synthesis of susceptible microorganisms. Bactericidal.

PHARMACOKINETICS

Rapid, complete absorption after IM administration. Protein binding: less than 30%. Widely distributed (does not cross blood-brain barrier, low concentrations in CSF). Excreted unchanged in urine. Removed by hemodialysis. **Half-life:** 2–4 hrs (increased in renal impairment, neonates; decreased in cystic fibrosis, burn, or febrile pts).

USES

Parenteral: Treatment of infections susceptible to *Pseudomonas, Proteus, Serratia,* and other gram-negative organisms and gram-positive *Staphylococcus* includ-

G

ing skin/skin structure, bone, joint, respiratory tract, intra-abdominal, complicated urinary tract, acute pelvic infections; burns; septicemia; meningitis. **Ophthalmic:** Ophthalmic infections caused by susceptible bacteria.

PRECAUTIONS

Contraindications: Hypersensitivity to other aminoglycosides (cross-sensitivity) or their components. **Cautions:** Elderly, neonates due to renal insufficiency or immaturity; neuromuscular disorders (potential for respiratory depression), prior hearing loss, vertigo, renal impairment, hypocalcemia, myasthenia gravis. Pediatric pts on extracorporeal membrane oxygenation.

⏳ LIFESPAN CONSIDERATIONS

Pregnancy/Lactation: Readily crosses placenta; unknown if distributed in breast milk. **Pregnancy Category C. Children:** Caution in neonates: Immature renal function increases half-life and toxicity. **Elderly:** Age-related renal impairment may require dosage adjustment.

INTERACTIONS

DRUG: Nephrotoxic, ototoxic medications may increase risk of nephrotoxicity, ototoxicity. May increase neuromuscular blockade with concurrent use of **neuromuscular blockers. HERBAL:** None significant. **FOOD:** None known. **LAB VALUES:** May increase BUN, serum creatinine, bilirubin, LDH, AST, ALT. May decrease serum calcium, magnesium, potassium, sodium. **Therapeutic serum level:** peak: 4–10 mcg/ml; trough: 0.5–2 mcg/ml. **Toxic serum level:** peak: greater than 10 mcg/ml; trough: greater than 2 mcg/ml.

AVAILABILITY (Rx)

Injection, Infusion: 60 mg/50 ml, 80 mg/50 ml, 80 mg/100 ml, 100 mg/50 ml, 100 mg/100 ml, 120 mg/100 ml. **Injection, Solution:** 10 mg/ml, 40 mg/ml. **Ointment, Ophthalmic:** 0.3%. **Solution, Ophthalmic (Gentak):** 0.3%.

ADMINISTRATION/HANDLING

 IV

Reconstitution • Dilute with 50–100 ml D₅W or 0.9% NaCl. Amount of diluent for infants, children depends on individual needs.
Rate of Administration • Infuse over 30–60 min for adults, older children; over 60–120 min for infants, young children.
Storage • Store vials at room temperature. • Solution appears clear or slightly yellow. • Intermittent IV infusion (piggyback) is stable for 24 hrs at room temperature. • Discard if precipitate forms.

IM
• To minimize discomfort, give deep IM slowly. • Less painful if injected into gluteus maximus than lateral aspect of thigh.

Ophthalmic
• Place gloved finger on lower eyelid and pull out until a pocket is formed between eye and lower lid. • Place prescribed number of drops or ¼–½ inch ointment into pocket. Instruct pt to close eye gently for 1–2 min (so medication will not be squeezed out of the sac). • **Solution:** Instruct pt to apply digital pressure to lacrimal sac at inner canthus for 1 min to minimize systemic absorption. • **Ointment:** Instruct pt to roll eyeball to increase contact area of drug to eye. • Remove excess solution or ointment around eye with tissue.

🔲 IV INCOMPATIBILITIES

Allopurinol (Aloprim), amphotericin B complex (Abelcet, AmBisome, Amphotec), furosemide (Lasix), heparin, hetastarch (Hespan), idarubicin (Idamycin), indomethacin (Indocin), propofol (Diprivan).

🔲 IV COMPATIBILITIES

Amiodarone (Cordarone), dexmedetomidine (Precedex), diltiazem (Cardizem), enalapril (Vasotec), filgrastim

(Neupogen), hydromorphone (Dilaudid), insulin, lorazepam (Ativan), magnesium sulfate, midazolam (Versed), morphine, multivitamins.

INDICATIONS/ROUTES/DOSAGE

◄**ALERT**► Space parenteral doses evenly around the clock. Dosage based on ideal body weight. Peak, trough levels are determined periodically to maintain desired serum concentrations and minimize risk of toxicity.

Usual Parenteral Dosage

IM, IV: ADULTS, ELDERLY: (Conventional): 1–2.5 mg/kg/dose q8–12h. (Once Daily): 4–7 mg/kg/dose q24h. **CHILDREN 5 YRS AND OLDER:** 2–2.5 mg/kg/dose q8h. **INFANTS, CHILDREN YOUNGER THAN 5 YRS:** 2.5 mg/kg/dose q8h. **NEONATES (GREATER THAN 2 KG) PNA 8–28 days:** 4 mg/kg/dose q12–24h; **PNA 7 days or less:** 4 mg/kg/dose q24h. **(1–2 KG) PNA 8–28 days:** 4–5 mg/kg/dose q24–48h; **PNA 7 days or less:** 5 mg/kg/dose q48h. **(LESS THAN 1 KG) PNA 15–28 days:** 4–5 mg/kg/dose q24–48h; **PNA 14 days or less:** 5 mg/kg/dose q48h.

Hemodialysis (HD)

Note: Administer after HD on dialysis days.

Loading dose: 2–3 mg/kg, then 1 mg/kg q48–72h for mild UTI or synergy (consider redose for pre- or post-HD concentrations less than 1 mg/L); 1–1.5 mg/kg q48–72h for moderate to severe UTI (consider redose for pre-HD concentration less than 1.5–2 mg/L or post-HD concentrations less than 1 mg/L); 1.5–2 mg/kg q48–72h for systemic gram-negative rod infection (consider redose for pre-HD concentration less than 3–5 mg/L or post-HD concentrations less than 2 mg/L).

Continuous Renal Replacement Therapy (CRRT)

Loading dose of 2–3 mg/kg, then 1 mg/kg q24–36h for mild UTI or synergy (redose when concentration less than 1

mg/L); 1–1.5 mg/kg q24–36h for moderate to severe UTI (redose when concentration less than 1.5–2 mg/L; 1.5–2 mg/kg q24–48h for systemic gram-negative infection (redose when concentration less than 3–5 mg/L).

Usual Ophthalmic Dosage

Ophthalmic Ointment: ADULTS, ELDERLY: Apply ½-inch strip to conjunctival sac 2–4 times/day.

Ophthalmic Solution: ADULTS, ELDERLY, CHILDREN: 1–2 drops q2–4h up to 2 drops/hr.

Dosage in Renal Impairment
Conventional Dosing:

Creatinine Clearance	Dosage
Greater than 60 ml/mil	q8h
41–60 ml/min	q12h
20–40 ml/min	q24h
Less than 20 ml/min	Loading dose, then monitor levels to determine dosage interval

SIDE EFFECTS

Occasional: IM: Pain, induration at injection site. **IV:** Phlebitis, thrombophlebitis, hypersensitivity reactions (fever, pruritus, rash, urticaria). **Ophthalmic:** Burning, tearing, itching, blurred vision. **Rare:** Alopecia, hypertension, fatigue.

ADVERSE EFFECTS/ TOXIC REACTIONS

Nephrotoxicity (increased BUN, serum creatinine; decreased creatinine clearance) may be reversible if drug is stopped at first sign of symptoms. Irreversible ototoxicity (tinnitus, dizziness, diminished hearing), neurotoxicity (headache, dizziness, lethargy, tremor, visual disturbances) occur occasionally. Risk increases with higher dosages, prolonged therapy, or if solution is applied directly to mucosa. Superinfections, particularly with fungi, may result from bacterial imbalance via any route of administration. Ophthalmic application may cause paresthesia of conjunctiva, mydriasis.

NURSING CONSIDERATIONS

BASELINE ASSESSMENT

Dehydration must be treated before beginning parenteral therapy. Establish baseline hearing acuity. Question for history of allergies, esp. aminoglycosides, sulfites (parabens for topical/ophthalmic routes).

INTERVENTION/EVALUATION

Monitor I&O (maintain hydration), urinalysis (casts, RBCs, WBCs, decrease in specific gravity). Be alert to ototoxic, neurotoxic symptoms (see Adverse Effects/Toxic Reactions). Check IM injection site for induration. Evaluate IV site for phlebitis (heat, pain, red streaking over vein). Assess for rash (**Ophthalmic:** redness, burning, itching, tearing). Be alert for superinfection (genital/anal pruritus, changes in oral mucosa, diarrhea). When treating pts with neuromuscular disorders, assess respiratory response carefully. **Therapeutic serum level:** peak: 4–10 mcg/ml; peak levels are 2–3 times greater with once-daily dosing trough: 0.5–2 mcg/ml. **Toxic serum level:** peak: greater than 10 mcg/ml; trough: greater than 2 mcg/ml.

PATIENT/FAMILY TEACHING

• Discomfort may occur with IM injection. • Blurred vision, tearing may occur briefly after each ophthalmic dose. • Report any hearing, visual, balance, urinary problems, even after therapy is completed. • **Ophthalmic:** Report if tearing, redness, irritation continues.

---

glatiramer

```
TOP
200
```

gla-**tir**-a-mer
(Copaxone)
Do not confuse Copaxone with Compazine.

◆CLASSIFICATION

PHARMACOTHERAPEUTIC: Immunosuppressive. **CLINICAL:** Neurologic agent for multiple sclerosis.

ACTION

May act by modifying immune processes thought to be responsible for pathogenesis of multiple sclerosis. **Therapeutic Effect:** Slows progression of multiple sclerosis.

PHARMACOKINETICS

Substantial fraction of glatiramer is hydrolyzed locally. Some fraction of injected material enters lymphatic circulation, reaching regional lymph nodes; some may enter systemic circulation intact.

USES

Treatment of relapsing, remitting multiple sclerosis.

PRECAUTIONS

Contraindications: Hypersensitivity to glatiramer, mannitol. **Cautions:** Pts exhibiting immediate postinjection reaction (flushing, chest pain, palpitations, anxiety, dyspnea, urticaria).

⚖ LIFESPAN CONSIDERATIONS

Pregnancy/Lactation: Unknown if distributed in breast milk. **Pregnancy Category B. Children:** Safety and efficacy not established. **Elderly:** Information not available.

INTERACTIONS

DRUG: None significant. **HERBAL: Echinacea** may decrease effects. **FOOD:** None known. **LAB VALUES:** None significant.

AVAILABILITY (Rx)

Injection Solution: 20 mg/ml in prefilled syringes.

ADMINISTRATION/HANDLING

Subcutaneous
• Refrigerate syringes (bring to room temperature before use). • May be

stored at room temperature for up to 1 mo. • Avoid heat, intense light. • Inject into deltoid region, abdomen, gluteus maximus, or lateral aspect of thigh. • Prefilled syringe suitable for single use only; discard unused portions.

INDICATIONS/ROUTES/DOSAGE

Multiple Sclerosis
Subcutaneous: ADULTS, ELDERLY: 20 mg once a day.

SIDE EFFECTS

Expected (73%–40%): Pain, erythema, inflammation, pruritus at injection site, asthenia (loss of strength, energy). **Frequent (27%–18%):** Arthralgia, vasodilation, anxiety, hypertonia, nausea, transient chest pain, dyspnea, flu-like symptoms, rash, pruritus. **Occasional (17%–10%):** Palpitations, back pain, diaphoresis, rhinitis, diarrhea, urinary urgency. **Rare (less than 9%):** Anorexia, fever, neck pain, peripheral edema, ear pain, facial edema, vertigo, vomiting.

ADVERSE EFFECTS/ TOXIC REACTIONS

Infection occurs commonly. Lymphadenopathy occurs occasionally.

NURSING CONSIDERATIONS

BASELINE ASSESSMENT

Establish baseline neurologic function.

INTERVENTION/EVALUATION

Observe injection site for reaction. Monitor for fever, chills (evidence of infection). Observe for improvement in neurologic function.

PATIENT/FAMILY TEACHING

• Report difficulty in breathing/swallowing, rash, itching, swelling of lower extremities, fatigue. • Avoid pregnancy.

glimepiride

glye-**mep**-ir-ide
(Amaryl, Apo-Glimepiride ✤,
Novo-Glimepiride ✤)
Do not confuse Amaryl with Altace, Amerge, or Reminyl, Avandaryl with Benadryl, or glimepiride with glipizide or glyburide.

FIXED-COMBINATION(S)

Avandaryl: glimepiride/rosiglitazone (an antidiabetic): 1 mg/4 mg, 2 mg/4 mg, 4 mg/4 mg.
Duetact: glimepiride/pioglitazone (an antidiabetic): 2 mg/30 mg, 4 mg/30 mg.

◆CLASSIFICATION

PHARMACOTHERAPEUTIC: Third-generation sulfonylurea. **CLINICAL:** Antidiabetic agent (see p. 44C).

ACTION

Promotes release of insulin from beta cells of pancreas, increases insulin sensitivity at peripheral sites. **Therapeutic Effect:** Lowers serum glucose.

PHARMACOKINETICS

Route	Onset	Peak	Duration
PO	N/A	2–3 hrs	24 hrs

Completely absorbed from GI tract. Protein binding: greater than 99%. Metabolized in liver. Excreted in urine, eliminated in feces. **Half-life:** 5–9.2 hrs.

USES

Adjunct to diet, exercise in management of non–insulin-dependent diabetes mellitus (type 2, NIDDM). Use in combination with insulin or metformin in pts whose diabetes is not controlled by diet, exercise in conjunction with a single oral hypoglycemic agent.

G

PRECAUTIONS

Contraindications: Diabetic complications (diabetic ketoacidosis). **Cautions:** Renal impairment, stress (fever, trauma, infection), G6PD deficiency.

⌛ LIFESPAN CONSIDERATIONS

Pregnancy/Lactation: Avoid pregnancy. Unknown if distributed in breast milk. **Pregnancy Category C. Children:** Safety and efficacy not established. **Elderly:** Hypoglycemia may be difficult to recognize. Age-related renal impairment may increase sensitivity to glucose-lowering effect.

INTERACTIONS

DRUG: Beta-blockers may increase hypoglycemic effect, mask signs of hypoglycemia. **Cimetidine, ciprofloxacin, fluconazole, ranitidine, large doses of salicylates** may increase effect. **Corticosteroids, thiazide diuretics** may decrease effect. **HERBAL: Garlic** may worsen hypoglycemia. **FOOD:** None known. **LAB VALUES:** May increase LDH concentrations, serum alkaline phosphatase, AST, ALT, bilirubin, C-peptide.

AVAILABILITY (Rx)

Tablets: 1 mg, 2 mg, 4 mg.

ADMINISTRATION/HANDLING

PO
• Give with breakfast or first main meal.

INDICATIONS/ROUTES/DOSAGE

Diabetes Mellitus
PO: ADULTS: Initially, 1–2 mg once a day with breakfast or first main meal. May increase by 1–2 mg q1–2wks, based on serum glucose response. **Maximum:** 8 mg/day. **ELDERLY:** Initially, 1 mg/day. Titrate dose to avoid hypoglycemia.

Dosage in Renal Impairment
Creatinine clearance less than 22 ml/min: Initially, 1 mg/day, then titrate dose based on fasting serum glucose levels.

SIDE EFFECTS

Rare (less than 3%): Altered taste, dizziness, drowsiness, weight gain, constipation, diarrhea, heartburn, nausea, vomiting, stomach fullness, headache, photosensitivity, peeling of skin, pruritus, rash.

ADVERSE EFFECTS/TOXIC REACTIONS

Overdose or insufficient food intake may produce hypoglycemia (esp. with increased glucose demands). GI hemorrhage, cholestatic hepatic jaundice, leukopenia, thrombocytopenia, pancytopenia, agranulocytosis, aplastic or hemolytic anemia occur rarely.

NURSING CONSIDERATIONS

BASELINE ASSESSMENT

Check serum glucose level. Discuss lifestyle to determine extent of learning, emotional needs. Ensure follow-up instruction if pt or family does not thoroughly understand diabetes management or serum glucose testing technique.

INTERVENTION/EVALUATION

Monitor serum glucose level, food intake. Assess for hypoglycemia (cool/wet skin, tremors, dizziness, anxiety, headache, tachycardia, perioral numbness, hunger, diplopia), hyperglycemia (polyuria, polyphagia, polydipsia, nausea, vomiting, dim vision, fatigue, deep or rapid breathing). Be alert to conditions that alter glucose requirements (fever, increased activity or stress, trauma, surgical procedure).

PATIENT/ FAMILY TEACHING

• Prescribed diet is principal part of treatment; do not skip or delay meals. • Avoid alcohol. • Carry candy, sugar packets, other quick-acting sugar supplements for immediate response to hypoglycemia. • Wear medical alert identification. • Check with physician when glucose demands are altered (fever, infection, trauma, stress, heavy physical activity). • Avoid direct exposure to sunlight.

*glipiZIDE   [TOP 200] [HIGH ALERT]

glip-i-zide
(Glucotrol, Glucotrol XL)
**Do not confuse glipizide with
glimepiride or glyburide, or
Glucotrol with Glucophage or
Glucotrol XL.**

FIXED-COMBINATION(S)

Metaglip: glipizide/metformin (an
antidiabetic): 2.5 mg/250 mg, 2.5
mg/500 mg, 5 mg/500 mg.

◆CLASSIFICATION

PHARMACOTHERAPEUTIC: Second-
generation sulfonylurea. **CLINICAL:**
Antidiabetic agent (see p. 44C).

ACTION

Promotes release of insulin from beta
cells of pancreas, increases insulin sensitivity at peripheral sites. **Therapeutic
Effect:** Lowers serum glucose.

PHARMACOKINETICS

Route	Onset	Peak	Duration
PO	15–30 min	2–3 hrs	12–24 hrs
Extended-release	2–3 hrs	6–12 hrs	24 hrs

Well absorbed from GI tract. Protein
binding: 92%–99%. Metabolized in liver.
Excreted in urine. **Half-life:** 2–4 hrs.

USES

Adjunct to diet, exercise in management
of stable, mild to moderately severe non–
insulin-dependent diabetes mellitus (type
2, NIDDM). May be used concomitantly
with insulin or metformin to improve
glycemic control.

PRECAUTIONS

Contraindications: Diabetic ketoacidosis
with or without coma, type 1 diabetes mellitus. **Cautions:** Adrenal/pituitary insufficiency, hypoglycemic reactions, hepatic/
renal impairment.

⏳ LIFESPAN CONSIDERATIONS

Pregnancy/Lactation: Insulin is drug of
choice during pregnancy; glipizide given
within 1 mo of delivery may produce
neonatal hypoglycemia. Drug crosses placenta. Distributed in breast milk. **Pregnancy Category C. Children:** Safety and
efficacy not established. **Elderly:** Hypoglycemia may be difficult to recognize. Age-
related renal impairment may increase
sensitivity to glucose-lowering effect.

INTERACTIONS

DRUG: Beta-blockers may increase hypoglycemic effect, mask signs of hypoglycemia. **Corticosteroids, thiazide diuretics** may decrease the effect. **HERBAL:
Garlic** may worsen hypoglycemia. **FOOD:**
None known. **LAB VALUES:** May increase
serum alkaline phosphatase, LDH, AST,
ALT, bilirubin, C-peptide.

AVAILABILITY (Rx)

Tablets (Glucotrol): 5 mg, 10 mg.

Tablets (Extended-Release [Glucotrol
XL]): 2.5 mg, 5 mg, 10 mg.

ADMINISTRATION/HANDLING

PO
• Give immediate-release tablets 30 min
before meals. Give extended-release tablets with breakfast. • Do not crush extended-release tablets.

INDICATIONS/ROUTES/DOSAGE

Diabetes Mellitus
PO: ADULTS: (Immediate-Release): Initially, 5 mg/day. Adjust dosage in 2.5- to
5-mg increments at intervals of several
days. Immediate-release tablet: **Maximum single dose: 15 mg. Maximum
dose/day: 40 mg. (Extended-Release):**
Initially, 5 mg/day. May increase dose no
more frequently than q7days. **Maximum
dose: 20 mg/day. ELDERLY: (Immediate-
Release):** Initially, 2.5–5 mg/day. May
increase by 2.5–5 mg/day q1–2wks. **(Extended-Release):** Dosing should be on
lower end of adult dosing.

---

* "Tall Man" lettering   ◆ Canadian trade name   Non-Crushable Drug   [HIGH ALERT] High Alert drug

Dosage in Renal Impairment
For creatinine clearance of 50 or less, reduce dose by 50%.

Dosage in Hepatic Impairment
(**Immediate-Release**): Initial dose: 2.5 mg/day.

SIDE EFFECTS

Rare (less than 3%): Altered taste, dizziness, drowsiness, weight gain, constipation, diarrhea, heartburn, nausea, vomiting, headache, photosensitivity, peeling of skin, pruritus, rash.

ADVERSE EFFECTS/ TOXIC REACTIONS

Overdose or insufficient food intake may produce hypoglycemia (esp. with increased glucose demands). GI hemorrhage, cholestatic hepatic jaundice, leukopenia, thrombocytopenia, pancytopenia, agranulocytosis, aplastic or hemolytic anemia occur rarely.

NURSING CONSIDERATIONS

BASELINE ASSESSMENT

Check serum glucose level. Discuss lifestyle to determine extent of learning, emotional needs. Ensure follow-up instruction if pt or family does not thoroughly understand diabetes management or serum glucose testing technique.

INTERVENTION/EVALUATION

Monitor serum glucose level, food intake. Assess for hypoglycemia (cool/wet skin, tremors, dizziness, anxiety, headache, tachycardia, perioral numbness, hunger, diplopia), hyperglycemia (polyuria, polyphagia, polydipsia, nausea, vomiting, dim vision, fatigue, deep or rapid breathing). Be alert to conditions that alter glucose requirements (fever, increased activity or stress, trauma, surgical procedure).

PATIENT/ FAMILY TEACHING

• Prescribed diet is principal part of treatment; do not skip or delay meals. • Avoid alcohol. • Carry candy, sugar packets, other quick-acting sugar supplements for immediate response to hypoglycemia. • Wear medical alert identification. • Check with physician when glucose demands are altered (fever, infection, trauma, stress, heavy physical activity). • Avoid direct exposure to sunlight.

glucagon

gloo-ka-gon
(GlucaGen, GlucaGen Diagnostic Kit, Glucagon Emergency Kit)

◆CLASSIFICATION

PHARMACOTHERAPEUTIC: Glucose elevating agent. **CLINICAL:** Antihypoglycemic, antispasmodic, antidote.

ACTION

Promotes hepatic glycogenolysis, gluconeogenesis. Stimulates cAMP, an enzyme, resulting in increased serum glucose concentration, smooth muscle relaxation, and exerts inotropic myocardial effect. **Therapeutic Effect:** Increases serum glucose level.

PHARMACOKINETICS

Route	Onset	Peak	Duration
IV	5–20 min	—	60–90 min
IM	30 min	—	60–90 min
Subcutaneous	30–45 min	—	60–90 min

Metabolized in liver. **Half-life:** 3–10 min.

USES

Treatment of severe hypoglycemia in diabetic pts. Diagnostic aid in radiographic examination to temporarily inhibit GI tract movement. **OFF-LABEL:** Treatment of esophageal obstruction due to foreign bodies; toxicity associated with beta-blockers, calcium channel blockers.

---

glucagon **553**

PRECAUTIONS

Contraindications: Hypersensitivity to glucagon, insulinoma, known pheochromocytoma. **Cautions:** History of insulinoma, pheochromocytoma, prolonged fasting, starvation, adrenal insufficiency, chronic hypoglycemia.

🔳 LIFESPAN CONSIDERATIONS

Pregnancy/Lactation: Unknown if drug crosses placenta or is distributed in breast milk. **Pregnancy Category B. Children/Elderly:** No age-related precautions noted.

INTERACTIONS

DRUG: May increase effects of **anticoagulants. HERBAL:** None significant. **FOOD:** None known. **LAB VALUES:** May decrease serum potassium.

AVAILABILITY (Rx)

Injection Powder (GlucaGen, GlucaGen Diagnostic Kit, Glucagon Emergency Kit): 1 mg.

ADMINISTRATION/HANDLING

◄**ALERT**► Place pt in side-lying position to prevent aspiration (glucagon, hypoglycemia may produce nausea/vomiting).

IV, IM, Subcutaneous
Reconstitution • Reconstitute with 1 ml sterile diluent to provide concentration of 1 mg/ml.
Rate of Administration • Pt usually awakens in 5–20 min. Although 1–2 additional doses may be administered, concern for effects of continuing cerebral hypoglycemia requires consideration of parenteral glucose. • When pt awakens, give supplemental carbohydrate to restore hepatic glycogen and prevent secondary hypoglycemia. If pt fails to respond to glucagon, IV dextrose is necessary.
Storage • Store vial at room temperature. • After reconstitution, is stable for 48 hrs if refrigerated. If reconstituted with Sterile Water for Injection, use immediately. Do not use glucagon solution unless clear.

🔳 IV INCOMPATIBILITIES

Do not mix glucagon with any other medications.

INDICATIONS/ROUTES/DOSAGE

Hypoglycemia
◄**ALERT**► Administer IV dextrose if pt fails to respond to glucagon.
IV, IM, Subcutaneous: ADULTS, ELDERLY, CHILDREN WEIGHING MORE THAN 20 KG: 1 mg. May repeat in 20 min. **CHILDREN WEIGHING 20 KG OR LESS:** 0.5 mg. May repeat in 20 min.

Diagnostic Aid
IV: ADULTS, ELDERLY: 0.25–2 mg 10 min prior to procedure. **IM:** 1–2 mg 10 minutes prior to procedure.

SIDE EFFECTS

Occasional: Nausea, vomiting. **Rare:** Allergic reaction (urticaria, respiratory distress, hypotension).

ADVERSE EFFECTS/ TOXIC REACTIONS

Overdose may produce persistent nausea/vomiting, hypokalemia (severe fatigue, decreased appetite, palpitations, muscle cramps).

NURSING CONSIDERATIONS

BASELINE ASSESSMENT

Obtain immediate assessment, including history, clinical signs/symptoms. If presence of hypoglycemic coma is established, give glucagon promptly.

INTERVENTION/EVALUATION

Monitor serum glucose, B/P, pulse, mental status. Monitor response time carefully. Have IV dextrose readily available in event pt does not respond. Assess for possible allergic reaction (urticaria, respiratory difficulty, hypotension). When pt is conscious, give oral carbohydrate.

G

✦ Canadian trade name   🌿 Non-Crushable Drug   🔲 High Alert drug

PATIENT/FAMILY TEACHING

• Recognize significance of identifying symptoms of hypoglycemia: pale, cool skin; anxiety; difficulty concentrating; headache; hunger; nausea; shakiness; diaphoresis; unusual fatigue; unusual weakness; unconsciousness. • If symptoms of hypoglycemia develop, give sugar form first (orange juice, honey, hard candy, sugar cubes, table sugar dissolved in water or juice) followed by cheese and crackers, half a sandwich, glass of milk.

---

glyBURIDE   `TOP 200` `HIGH ALERT`

glye-bue-ride
(Apo-Glyburide ✤, DiaBeta, Euglucon ✤, Glynase Pres-Tab, Novo-Glyburide ✤)

Do not confuse DiaBeta with Zebeta, glyburide with glimepiride, glipizide, or Glucotrol.

FIXED-COMBINATION(S)

Glucovance: glyburide/metformin (an antidiabetic): 1.25 mg/250 mg, 2.5 mg/500 mg, 5 mg/500 mg.

◆CLASSIFICATION

PHARMACOTHERAPEUTIC: Second-generation sulfonylurea. **CLINICAL:** Antidiabetic agent (see p. 44C).

ACTION

Promotes release of insulin from beta cells of pancreas, increases insulin sensitivity at peripheral sites. **Therapeutic Effect:** Lowers serum glucose level.

PHARMACOKINETICS

Route	Onset	Peak	Duration
PO	0.25–1 hr	1–2 hrs	12–24 hrs

Well absorbed from GI tract. Protein binding: 99%. Metabolized in liver. Primarily excreted in urine. Not removed by hemodialysis. **Half-life:** 5–16 hrs.

USES

Adjunct to diet, exercise in management of stable, mild to moderately severe non–insulin-dependent diabetes mellitus (type 2, NIDDM). May be used concomitantly with insulin or metformin to improve glycemic control. **OFF-LABEL:** Alternative to insulin in women for treatment of gestational diabetes mellitus.

PRECAUTIONS

Contraindications: Diabetic ketoacidosis with or without coma, type 1 diabetes mellitus, concurrent use with bosentan. **Cautions:** Adrenal or pituitary insufficiency, hypoglycemic reactions (more likely in elderly, debilitated, malnourished), hepatic/renal impairment, G6PD deficiency.

⌛ LIFESPAN CONSIDERATIONS

Pregnancy/Lactation: Crosses placenta. Distributed in breast milk. May produce neonatal hypoglycemia if given within 2 wks of delivery. **Pregnancy Category C. Children:** Safety and efficacy not established. **Elderly:** Hypoglycemia may be difficult to recognize. Age-related renal impairment may increase sensitivity to glucose-lowering effect.

INTERACTIONS

DRUG: Beta-blockers may increase hypoglycemic effect, mask signs of hypoglycemia. **Corticosteroids, thiazide diuretics** may decrease effect. **HERBAL: Garlic,** other herbs with hypoglycemic properties may enhance effect. **FOOD:** None known. **LAB VALUES:** May increase serum alkaline phosphatase, LDH, AST, ALT, bilirubin, C-peptide.

AVAILABILITY (Rx)

Tablets (DiaBeta): 1.25 mg, 2.5 mg, 5 mg. **Tablets, Micronized (Glynase Pres-Tab):** 1.5 mg, 3 mg, 6 mg.

ADMINISTRATION/HANDLING

PO
• May give with food (response better if taken 15–30 min before meals).

INDICATIONS/ROUTES/DOSAGE

Diabetes Mellitus

PO *(Diabeta)*: **ADULTS:** Initially, 1.25–5 mg. May increase by 2.5 mg/day at weekly intervals. Maintenance: 1.25–20 mg/day. **Maximum:** 20 mg/day. **ELDERLY:** Initially, 1.25–2.5 mg/day. May increase by 1.25–2.5 mg/day at 1- to 3-wk intervals.

PO *(Glynase)*: **ADULTS, ELDERLY:** Initially 0.75–3 mg/day. May increase by 1.5 mg/day at weekly intervals. Maintenance: 0.75–12 mg/day as a single dose or in divided doses.

Dosage in Renal Impairment

Not recommended for pts with creatinine clearance less than 50 ml/min.

SIDE EFFECTS

Rare (less than 3%): Altered taste, dizziness, drowsiness, weight gain, constipation, diarrhea, heartburn, nausea, vomiting, headache, photosensitivity, peeling of skin, pruritis, rash.

ADVERSE EFFECTS/ TOXIC REACTIONS

Overdose or insufficient food intake may produce hypoglycemia (esp. in pts with increased glucose demands). Cholestatic jaundice, leukopenia, thrombocytopenia, pancytopenia, agranulocytosis, aplastic or hemolytic anemia occur rarely.

NURSING CONSIDERATIONS

BASELINE ASSESSMENT

Check serum glucose level. Discuss lifestyle to determine extent of learning, emotional needs. Ensure follow-up instruction if pt or family does not thoroughly understand diabetes management or glucose testing technique.

INTERVENTION/EVALUATION

Monitor serum glucose level, food intake. Assess for hypoglycemia (cool/wet skin, tremors, dizziness, anxiety, headache, tachycardia, perioral numbness, hunger, diplopia), hyperglycemia (polyuria, polyphagia, polydipsia, nausea, vomiting, dim vision, fatigue, deep or rapid breathing). Be alert to conditions that alter glucose requirements (fever, increased activity or stress, trauma, surgical procedure).

PATIENT/ FAMILY TEACHING

• Prescribed diet is principal part of treatment; do not skip or delay meals. • Avoid alcohol. • Carry candy, sugar packets, other quick-acting sugar supplements for immediate response to hypoglycemia. • Wear medical alert identification. • Check with physician when glucose demands are altered (fever, infection, trauma, stress, heavy physical activity). • Avoid direct exposure to sunlight.

golimumab

goe-li-**mue**-mab
(Simponi, Simponi Aria)
Do not confuse Simponi (subcutaneous) with Simponi Aria (intravenous).

BLACK BOX ALERT Tuberculosis (TB), invasive fungal infections, other opportunistic infections reported. Discontinue treatment if active infection or sepsis occurs. Test for TB prior to and during treatment, regardless of initial result; if positive, start treatment for TB prior to initiating therapy. Lymphoma, other malignancies reported in pts treated with tumor necrosis factor blockers.

◆CLASSIFICATION

PHARMACOTHERAPEUTIC: Monoclonal antibody. **CLINICAL:** Immune modulator, antirheumatic, tumor necrosis factor (TNF) blocking agent.

ACTION

Binds specifically to tumor necrosis factor (TNF) alpha, blocking its interaction with cell surface TNF receptors. **Thera-**

---

* "Tall Man" lettering   ✦ Canadian trade name   🚫 Non-Crushable Drug   🔺 High Alert drug

peutic Effect: Alters biologic activity of TNF alpha, reduces inflammation, may alter pathophysiology of rheumatoid arthritis.

PHARMACOKINETICS

Serum concentration reaches steady state by wk 12. Elimination pathway not specified. **Half-life:** 12–14 days.

USES

Simponi: Used alone or in combination with methotrexate for the treatment of adult pts with active psoriatic arthritis. Used in combination with methotrexate for the treatment of adult pts with moderately to severely active rheumatoid arthritis. Used alone for the treatment of adult pts with active ankylosing spondylitis. Treatment of moderate to severe ulcerative colitis.
Simponi Aria: Used in combination with methotrexate for treatment of adult pts with moderately to severely active rheumatoid arthritis.

PRECAUTIONS

Contraindications: None known. **Cautions:** Elderly, concomitant immunosuppressants, comorbid conditions predisposing to infections (e.g., diabetes). Residence or travel from areas of endemic mycosis, tuberculosis, underlying hematologic disorders, preexisting or recent-onset demyelinating disorders (e.g., multiple sclerosis, polyneuropathy), pts with HF or decreased left ventricular function. Avoid concomitant use with live vaccines, abatacept, or anakinra (increased incidence of serious infections). Concomitant use of live vaccines.

⌛ LIFESPAN CONSIDERATIONS

Pregnancy/Lactation: Unknown if distributed in breast milk. Must either discontinue drug or discontinue breastfeeding. **Pregnancy Category B. Children:** Safety and efficacy not established in those younger than 18 yrs. **Elderly:** May have increased risk of serious infections, malignancy.

INTERACTIONS

DRUG: Anakinra, abatacept, rituximab, natalizumab, immunosuppressive therapy may increase risk of infections. May decrease efficacy of immune response with **live vaccines.** **HERBAL: Echinacea** may decrease effects. **FOOD:** None known. **LAB VALUES:** May increase ALT, AST. May decrease Hgb, leukocytes, neutrophils, platelets.

AVAILABILITY (Rx)

Injection Solution (Simponi): 50 mg/0.5 ml, 100 mg/ml in single-dose prefilled autoinjector or prefilled syringe. **Injection Solution (Simponi Aria):** 50 mg/4 ml per single-use vial (12.5 mg/ml).

ADMINISTRATION/HANDLING

Simponi
SUBCUTANEOUS
• Remove prefilled syringe or autoinjector from refrigerator. Allow to sit at room temperature for 30 min; do not warm in any other way. • Avoid areas where skin is scarred, tender, bruised, red, scaly, hard. Recommended injection site is front of middle thighs, although lower abdomen 2 in below naval or outer, upper arms are acceptable. • Inject within 5 min after cap has been removed.
Autoinjector: • Push open end of autoinjector firmly against skin at 90-degree angle. • Do not pull autoinjector away from skin until a first "click" sound is heard and then a second "click" sound (injection is finished and needle is pulled back). This usually takes 3 to 6 sec but may take up to 15 sec for the second "click" to be heard. If autoinjector is pulled away from skin before injection is completed, full dose may not be administered.
Prefilled Syringe: • Gently pinch skin and hold firmly. Use a quick, dart-like motion to insert needle into pinched skin at a 45-degree angle.
Storage: • Refrigerate; do not freeze. Do not shake. • Solution appears slightly opalescent, colorless to light yellow. Discard if cloudy or contains particulate.

Simponi Aria

◄ **ALERT** ► Use in-line 0.22 micron filter.

 IV

Reconstitution • Calculate dosage and number of vials needed based on pt weight. • Visually inspect for particulate matter. • Dilute in 100 ml 0.9% NaCl. • Prior to mixing, withdraw and discard volume of NaCl equal to the volume of patient-dosed solution. • Slowly inject solution into bag and gently mix. • Do not shake.

Rate of Administration • Infuse over 30 min.

Storage • Vial solution should be colorless to light yellow and opalescent. • It is normal for solution to develop fine translucent particles since drug is a protein. • Do not use if opaque particles, discoloration, or other foreign particles present. • May store diluted solution at room temperature up to 4 hrs.

🕮 IV INCOMPATIBILITIES

Do not infuse concomitantly with other drugs.

INDICATIONS/ROUTES/DOSAGE

Active Psoriatic Arthritis
Subcutaneous: ADULTS, ELDERLY: 50 mg once monthly. Use alone or in combination with methotrexate.

Moderate to Severe Active Rheumatoid Arthritis
Subcutaneous: ADULTS, ELDERLY: (Simponi): 50 mg once monthly. Use in combination with methotrexate.
IV Infusion: ADULTS, ELDERLY: (Simponi Aria): 2 mg/kg at wk 0 and wk 4. Then decrease frequency to every 8 wks. (Use in combination with methotrexate.)

Active Ankylosing Spondylitis
Subcutaneous: ADULTS, ELDERLY: 50 mg once monthly.

Ulcerative Colitis
Subcutaneous: ADULTS, ELDERLY: Initially, 200 mg; then 100 mg 2 wks later, and then 100 mg q4wks thereafter.

SIDE EFFECTS

Frequent (13%): Laryngitis, nasopharyngitis, pharyngitis, rhinitis, upper respiratory tract infection. **Occasional (3%–2%):** Bronchitis, hypertension, rash, pyrexia. **Rare (less than 1%):** Dizziness, paresthesia, constipation.

ADVERSE EFFECTS/ TOXIC REACTIONS

Neutropenia, lymphopenia may increase risk of infection. New-onset psoriasis, exacerbation of preexisting psoriasis have been reported. Serious infections including sepsis, pneumonia, cellulitis, TB, invasive fungal infections reported. May increase risk of lymphoma, melanoma, new malignancies. New onset or exacerbation of CNS demyelinating disorders, including multiple sclerosis, or worsening of HF have occurred. Viral reactivation of herpes zoster, HIV, hepatitis B may occur. Pts who receive TNF blockers have risk of autoantibody formation (immunogenicity). Hypersensitivity reactions including anaphylaxis reported. May induce lupus-like symptoms (butterfly rash, new joint pain, peripheral edema, UV sensitivity).

NURSING CONSIDERATIONS

BASELINE ASSESSMENT

Obtain baseline hepatic function test, CBC, vital signs, urine pregnancy. Obtain B-type natriuretic peptide (BNP) level and review echocardiogram for pts with history of HF. Do not initiate therapy if active infection suspected. Evaluate for active TB and test for latent infection prior to and during treatment. Induration of 5 mm or greater with tuberculin skin test should be considered a positive result when assessing for latent TB. Antifungal therapy should be considered for those who reside or travel to regions where mycoses are endemic. Question history of anemia, HF, CNS disorders, hepatic impairment, HIV, malignancies. Assess skin for moles, lesions. Receive full medication history including vitamins, herbal products.

INTERVENTION/EVALUATION

Monitor CBC, hepatic function test every 4–8 wks, then periodically. Screen pts for TB (night sweats, hemoptysis, weight loss, fever) regardless of baseline tuberculin skin test result. Monitor hepatitis B carriers during treatment and several mos after treatment. If any viral reactivation occurs, interrupt treatment and consider antiviral therapy. Discontinue treatment if acute infection, opportunistic infection, sepsis occur and initiate appropriate antimicrobial therapy. Routinely assess skin for new lesions. Peripheral edema, difficulty breathing, course crackles on lung auscultation, elevated BNP may indicate worsening HF. Monitor for hypersensitivity reactions.

PATIENT/FAMILY TEACHING

• Therapy may lower immune system response. Do not receive live vaccines.
• Report history of HIV, fungal infections, HF, hepatitis B, multiple sclerosis, TB, or close relatives who have active TB. Report travel plans to possible endemic areas. Blood levels, TB screening will be routinely monitored. • Hives, swelling of face, difficulty breathing may indicate allergic reaction. • Do not breastfeed.
• Abdominal pain, yellowing of skin or eyes, dark-amber urine, clay-colored stools, fatigue, loss of appetite may indicate liver problems. • Decreased platelet count may increase risk of bleeding.
• Swelling of hands or feet, difficulty breathing may indicate HF.

---

goserelin   HIGH ALERT

goe-se-**rel**-in
(Zoladex, Zoladex LA ✦)

◆CLASSIFICATION

PHARMACOTHERAPEUTIC: Gonadotropin-releasing hormone analogue.
CLINICAL: Antineoplastic (see pp. 86C, 108C).

ACTION

Stimulates release of luteinizing hormone (LH) and follicle-stimulating hormone (FSH) from anterior pituitary. **Therapeutic Effect:** In females, reduces ovarian, uterine, mammary gland size, regresses hormone-responsive tumors. In males, decreases testosterone level, reduces growth of abnormal prostate tissue.

PHARMACOKINETICS

Protein binding: 27%. Metabolized in liver. Excreted in urine. **Half-life:** 4.2 hrs (male); 2.3 hrs (female).

USES

Treatment of locally confined prostate cancer. Palliative treatment of advanced carcinoma of prostate as alternative when orchiectomy, estrogen therapy is either not indicated or unacceptable. In combination with flutamide before and during radiation therapy for early stages of prostate cancer. Management of endometriosis. Treatment of advanced breast cancer in premenopausal and perimenopausal women. Endometrial thinning before ablation for dysfunctional uterine bleeding.

PRECAUTIONS

Contraindications: Pregnancy (except when used for palliative treatment of advanced breast cancer). **Cautions:** Women of childbearing potential until pregnancy has been excluded.

LIFESPAN CONSIDERATIONS

Pregnancy/Lactation: Crosses placenta; unknown if distributed in breast milk. **Pregnancy Category D (advanced breast cancer), X (endometriosis, endometrial thinning). Children:** Safety and efficacy not established. **Elderly:** No age-related precautions noted.

INTERACTIONS

DRUG: None significant. **HERBAL:** None significant. **FOOD:** None known. **LAB VALUES:** May increase serum prostatic acid phosphatase, testosterone, calcium.

AVAILABILITY (Rx)

Injection, Solution (Zoladex): 3.6 mg, 10.8 mg.

ADMINISTRATION/HANDLING

Subcutaneous

• Clean area of skin on upper abdominal wall with alcohol swab. • Stretch or pinch skin with one hand, and insert needle into subcutaneous tissue. • Direct needle so that it parallels the abdominal wall. Push needle in until barrel hub touches pt's skin. Withdraw needle 1 cm to create a space to discharge goserelin. Fully depress plunger. • Withdraw needle, bandage site.

INDICATIONS/ROUTES/DOSAGE

Prostatic Carcinoma, Advanced

Subcutaneous: ADULTS OLDER THAN 18 YRS, ELDERLY: 3.6 mg every 28 days or 10.8 mg q12wks subcutaneously into upper abdominal wall.

Prostate Carcinoma, Locally Confined

Subcutaneous: ADULTS, ELDERLY: (in combination with an antiestrogen and radiotherapy, begin 8 wks prior to radiotherapy): 3.6 mg once. Report in 28 days with 10.8 mg or 3.6 mg q28days for 4 doses.

Breast Carcinoma, Endometriosis

Subcutaneous: ADULTS: 3.6 mg every 28 days subcutaneously into upper abdominal wall.

Endometrial Thinning

Subcutaneous: ADULTS: 3.6 mg subcutaneously into upper abdominal wall as a single dose or in 2 doses 4 wks apart.

Endometriosis

Subcutaneous: ADULTS: 3.6 mg every 28 days for 6 mos.

SIDE EFFECTS

Frequent (60%–13%): Headache, hot flashes, depression, diaphoresis, sexual dysfunction, impotence, lower urinary tract symptoms. **Occasional (10%–5%):** Pain, lethargy, dizziness, insomnia, anorexia, nausea, rash, upper respiratory tract infection, hirsutism, abdominal pain. **Rare:** Pruritus.

ADVERSE EFFECTS/ TOXIC REACTIONS

Arrhythmias, HF, hypertension occur rarely. Ureteral obstruction, spinal cord compression observed (immediate orchiectomy may be necessary).

NURSING CONSIDERATIONS

INTERVENTION/EVALUATION

Monitor pt closely for worsening signs/ symptoms of prostatic cancer, esp. during first mo of therapy.

PATIENT/FAMILY TEACHING

• Use nonhormonal methods of contraception during therapy. • Report suspected pregnancy or regular menstruation persists. • Breakthrough menstrual bleeding may occur if dose is missed.

G

granisetron

gra-**nis**-e-tron
(Granisol, Kytril ♣, Sancuso)
Do not confuse granisetron with dolasetron, ondansetron, or palonosetron.

◆CLASSIFICATION

PHARMACOTHERAPEUTIC: Serotonin receptor antagonist (5-HT$_3$). **CLINICAL:** Antiemetic.

ACTION

Selectively blocks serotonin stimulation at receptor sites at chemoreceptor trigger zone, vagal nerve terminals. **Therapeutic Effect:** Prevents nausea/ vomiting.

♣ Canadian trade name   🗌 Non-Crushable Drug   🗌 High Alert drug

PHARMACOKINETICS

Route	Onset	Peak	Duration
IV	1–3 min	N/A	24 hrs

Rapidly, widely distributed to tissues. Protein binding: 65%. Metabolized in liver. Eliminated in urine (48%), feces (38%). **Half-life:** 10–12 hrs (increased in elderly).

USES

Prevention of nausea/vomiting associated with emetogenic cancer therapy and cancer radiation therapy. Prevention, treatment of postop nausea, vomiting. **OFF-LABEL: PO:** Breakthrough treatment of chemotherapy-associated nausea/vomiting.

PRECAUTIONS

Contraindications: None known. **Cautions:** Hypersensitivity to other 5-HT$_3$ receptor antagonists, congenital QT prolongation, concomitant administration of medications that prolong QT interval, following abdominal surgery or in chemotherapy-induced nausea, vomiting (may mask progressive ileus or gastric distention), hepatic disease.

⧗ LIFESPAN CONSIDERATIONS

Pregnancy/Lactation: Unknown if distributed in breast milk. **Pregnancy Category B. Children:** Safety and efficacy not established in those younger than 2 yrs. **Elderly:** No age-related precautions noted.

INTERACTIONS

DRUG: None significant. **HERBAL:** None significant. **FOOD:** None known. **LAB VALUES:** May increase serum AST, ALT.

AVAILABILITY (Rx)

Injection Solution: 0.1 mg/ml, 1 mg/ml. **Oral Solution (Granisol):** 2 mg/10 ml. **Tablets:** 1 mg. **Transdermal Patch (Sancuso):** 52-cm^2 patch containing 34.3 mg granisetron delivering 3.1 mg/24 hrs.

ADMINISTRATION/HANDLING

 IV

Reconstitution • May be given undiluted or dilute with 20–50 ml 0.9% NaCl or D$_5$W. Do not mix with other medications.

Rate of Administration • May give undiluted as IV push over 30 sec. • For IV piggyback, infuse over 5–20 min depending on volume of diluent used.

Storage • Appears as a clear, colorless solution. • Store at room temperature. • After dilution, stable for 3 days at room temperature or 7 days if refrigerated. • Inspect for particulates, discoloration.

PO

• Give 30 min to 1 hr prior to initiating chemotherapy.

Transdermal

• Apply to clean, dry, intact skin on upper outer arm. • Remove immediately from pouch before application. • Do not cut patch.

▦ IV INCOMPATIBILITY

Amphotericin B (Fungizone).

▦ IV COMPATIBILITIES

Allopurinol (Aloprim), bumetanide (Bumex), calcium gluconate, carboplatin (Paraplatin), cisplatin (Platinol), cyclophosphamide (Cytoxan), cytarabine (Ara-C), dacarbazine (DTIC-Dome), dexamethasone (Decadron), dexmedetomidine (Precedex), diphenhydramine (Benadryl), docetaxel (Taxotere), doxorubicin (Adriamycin), etoposide (VePesid), gemcitabine (Gemzar), magnesium, mitoxantrone (Novantrone), paclitaxel (Taxol), potassium.

INDICATIONS/ROUTES/DOSAGE

Prevention of Chemotherapy-Induced Nausea/Vomiting
PO: ADULTS, ELDERLY: 2 mg 1 hr before chemotherapy or 1 mg 1 hr before and 12 hrs after chemotherapy.

IV: **ADULTS, ELDERLY, CHILDREN 2 YRS AND OLDER:** 10 mcg/kg/dose (**maximum:** 1 mg/dose) within 30 min of chemotherapy. **Maximum:** 1 mg.

Transdermal: ADULTS, ELDERLY: Apply 24–48 hrs prior to chemotherapy. Remove minimum 24 hrs after completion of chemotherapy. May be worn up to 7 days, depending on chemotherapy duration.

Prevention of Radiation-Induced Nausea/ Vomiting
PO: **ADULTS, ELDERLY:** 2 mg once a day, given 1 hr before radiation therapy.

Postop Nausea/Vomiting
IV: **ADULTS, ELDERLY:** 1 mg as a single postop dose. **CHILDREN OLDER THAN 4 YRS:** 20–40 mcg/kg. **Maximum:** 1 mg.

SIDE EFFECTS

Frequent (21%–14%): Headache, constipation, asthenia (loss of strength, energy). **Occasional (8%–6%):** Diarrhea, abdominal pain. **Rare (less than 2%):** Altered taste, fever.

ADVERSE EFFECTS/ TOXIC REACTIONS

Hypersensitivity reaction, hypertension, hypotension, arrhythmias (sinus bradycardia, atrial fibrillation, AV block, ventricular ectopy), EKG abnormalities occur rarely.

NURSING CONSIDERATIONS

BASELINE ASSESSMENT

Assess hydration status. Ensure that granisetron is given within 30 min of starting chemotherapy.

INTERVENTION/EVALUATION

Monitor for therapeutic effect. Assess for headache. Monitor for dehydration due to recurrent vomiting. Monitor daily pattern of bowel activity, stool consistency.

PATIENT/FAMILY TEACHING

• Granisetron is effective shortly following administration; prevents nausea/vomiting.
• Transitory taste disorder may occur.

griseofulvin

gris-ee-oh-**ful**-vin
(Grifulvin V, Gris-PEG)

◆CLASSIFICATION

PHARMACOTHERAPEUTIC: Antifungal antibiotic. **CLINICAL:** Antifungal.

ACTION

Inhibits fungal cell mitosis by disrupting mitotic spindle structure. **Therapeutic Effect:** Fungistatic.

PHARMACOKINETICS

Ultramicrosize is almost completely absorbed. Absorption is significantly enhanced after a fatty meal. Metabolized in liver. Minimal excretion in urine. **Half-life:** 9–22 hrs.

USES

Treatment of susceptible tinea (ringworm) infections of the skin, hair caused by susceptible species of *Microsporum, Epidermophyton,* or *Trichophyton.*

PRECAUTIONS

Contraindications: Hepatocellular failure, porphyria, pregnancy. **Cautions:** Exposure to sun/ultraviolet light (photosensitivity), hypersensitivity to penicillins.

⌛ LIFESPAN CONSIDERATIONS

Pregnancy/Lactation: Crosses placenta; unknown if distributed in breast milk. **Pregnancy Category C. Children:** Safety and efficacy not established in those younger than 2 yrs. **Elderly:** No age-related precautions noted.

INTERACTIONS

DRUG: May decrease effects of **oral contraceptives, warfarin. HERBAL:** None significant. **FOOD:** High-fat foods enhance absorption. **LAB VALUES:** May increase AST, ALT, bilirubin.

G

AVAILABILITY (Rx)

Oral Suspension (Grifulvin V): 125 mg/5 ml.
Tablets (Microsize Grifulvin V): 500 mg.
Tablets (Ultramicrosize, Gris-PEG): 125 mg, 250 mg.

ADMINISTRATION/HANDLING

• Administer with fatty meal to increase absorption. • Take with food or milk to reduce GI irritation. • Ultramicrosize tablets may be crushed and sprinkled on applesauce. • Shake suspension well before use.

INDICATIONS/ROUTES/DOSAGE

Usual Dosage
◄**ALERT**► Duration of therapy depends on site of infection.
PO *(Microsize Tablets, Oral Suspension)*: **ADULTS:** 500–1,000 mg as a single dose or in divided doses. **CHILDREN 2 YRS AND OLDER:** 10–20 mg/kg/day in single or divided doses.
PO *(Ultramicrosize Tablets)*: **ADULTS:** 375–750 mg/day as a single dose or in divided doses. **CHILDREN 2 YRS AND OLDER:** 5–15 mg/kg/day in single or divided doses. **Maximum:** 750 mg/day in 2 divided doses.

SIDE EFFECTS

Occasional: Hypersensitivity reaction (pruritus, rash, urticaria), headache, nausea, diarrhea, excessive thirst, flatulence, oral thrush, dizziness, insomnia. **Rare:** Paresthesia of hands/feet, proteinuria, photosensitivity reaction.

ADVERSE EFFECTS/ TOXIC REACTIONS

Granulocytopenia occurs rarely and should necessitate discontinuation of drug.

NURSING CONSIDERATIONS

BASELINE ASSESSMENT

Question for history of allergies, esp. to griseofulvin, penicillins, or hepatic impairment.

INTERVENTION/EVALUATION

Assess skin for rash, response to therapy. Monitor daily pattern of bowel activity, stool consistency. Question presence of headache: onset, location, type of discomfort. Assess for dizziness.

PATIENT/FAMILY TEACHING

• Prolonged therapy (wks or mos) is usually necessary. • Do not miss a dose; continue therapy as long as ordered. • Avoid alcohol (may produce tachycardia, flushing). • May cause photosensitivity reaction; avoid exposure to sunlight. • Maintain good hygiene (prevents superinfection). • Separate personal items in direct contact with affected areas. • Keep affected areas dry; wear light clothing for ventilation. • Take with foods high in fat such as milk, ice cream (reduces GI upset, assists absorption).

guaifenesin

gwye-**fen**-e-sin
(Mucinex, Organidin, Robitussin ✦)
Do not confuse guaifenesin with guanfacine, or Mucinex with Mucomyst.

FIXED-COMBINATION(S)

Mucinex D: guaifenesin/pseudoephedrine (a sympathomimetic): 600 mg/60 mg, 1,200 mg/120 mg. **Mucinex DM:** guaifenesin/dextromethorphan (a cough suppressant): 600 mg/30 mg, 1,200 mg/60 mg. **Robitussin AC:** guaifenesin/codeine (a narcotic analgesic): 100 mg/10 mg, 75 mg/2.5 mg per 5 ml. **Robitussin DM:** guaifenesin/dextromethorphan (a cough suppressant): 100 mg/10 mg per 5 ml.

◆CLASSIFICATION

PHARMACOTHERAPEUTIC: Respiratory expectorant. **CLINICAL:** Expectorant.

ACTION

Stimulates respiratory tract secretions by decreasing adhesiveness, viscosity of mucus. **Therapeutic Effect:** Promotes removal of viscous mucus.

PHARMACOKINETICS

Well absorbed from GI tract. Metabolized in liver. Excreted in urine. **Half-life:** 1 hr.

USES

Expectorant for symptomatic treatment of productive coughs.

PRECAUTIONS

Contraindications: None known. **Cautions:** None known.

⧖ LIFESPAN CONSIDERATIONS

Pregnancy/Lactation: Unknown if drug crosses placenta or is distributed in breast milk. **Pregnancy Category C. Children:** Caution advised in those younger than 2 yrs with persistent cough. **Elderly:** No age-related precautions noted.

INTERACTIONS

DRUG: None significant. **HERBAL:** None significant. **FOOD:** None known. **LAB VALUES:** None significant.

AVAILABILITY (OTC)

Liquid: 100 mg/5 ml. **Syrup:** 100 mg/5 ml. **Tablets:** 200 mg, 400 mg.

Tablets, Extended-Release: (Mucinex): 600 mg, 1,200 mg.

ADMINISTRATION/HANDLING

PO

• Store syrup, liquid, tablets at room temperature. • Give without regard to meals. • Do not crush, break extended-release tablet.

INDICATIONS/ROUTES/DOSAGE

Expectorant
PO: ADULTS, ELDERLY, CHILDREN OLDER THAN 12 YRS: 200–400 mg q4h. **Extended-Release:** 600–1,200 mg q12h.

Maximum: 2.4 g/day. **CHILDREN 6–12 YRS:** 100–200 mg q4h. **Maximum:** 1.2 g/day. **CHILDREN 2–5 YRS:** 50–100 mg q4h. **Maximum:** 600 mg/day. **CHILDREN 6 MOS–2 YRS:** 25–50 mg q4h. **Maximum:** 300 mg/day.
PO *(Extended-Release)*: **ADULTS, ELDERLY, CHILDREN OLDER THAN 12 YRS:** 600–1,200 mg q12h. **Maximum:** 2.4 g/day. **CHILDREN 6–12 YRS:** 600 mg q12h. **Maximum:** 1.2 g/day.

SIDE EFFECTS

Rare: Dizziness, headache, rash, diarrhea, nausea, vomiting, abdominal pain.

ADVERSE EFFECTS/TOXIC REACTIONS

Overdose may produce nausea, vomiting.

NURSING CONSIDERATIONS

BASELINE ASSESSMENT

Assess type, severity, frequency of cough. Increase fluid intake, environmental humidity to lower viscosity of lung secretions.

INTERVENTION/EVALUATION

Initiate deep breathing, coughing exercises, particularly in pts with pulmonary impairment. Assess for clinical improvement; record onset of relief of cough.

PATIENT/FAMILY TEACHING

• Avoid tasks that require alertness, motor skills until response to drug is established. • Do not take for chronic cough. • Report persistent cough if fever, rash, headache, sore throat is present with cough. • Maintain adequate hydration.

guanfacine

gwan-fah-seen
(Intuniv)
Do not confuse guanfacine with guaifenesin or guanidine.

G

◆CLASSIFICATION

PHARMACOTHERAPEUTIC: Alpha$_{2A}$-adrenergic agonist. **CLINICAL:** Psychotherapeutic agent.

ACTION

Not a CNS stimulant. Interacts with alpha$_{2A}$-adrenergic receptors in prefrontal cortex of brain. Behaviors (inattention, hyperactivity, impulsiveness) related to attention-deficit hyperactivity disorder (ADHD) may be controlled in this part of the brain. **Therapeutic Effect:** Improves symptoms of ADHD.

PHARMACOKINETICS

Readily absorbed from GI tract. Protein binding: 70%. Metabolized in liver. Excreted in urine. **Half-life:** 14–22 hrs.

USES

Treatment of ADHD. **OFF-LABEL:** Tic disorder, aggression, Tourette's syndrome.

PRECAUTIONS

Contraindications: None known. **Cautions:** Renal/hepatic impairment.

⧗ LIFESPAN CONSIDERATIONS

Pregnancy/Lactation: Unknown if distributed in breast milk. **Pregnancy Category B. Children:** Safety and efficacy not established in pts younger than 6 yrs. Efficacy beyond 9 wks and safety beyond 2 yrs of treatment not established for children and adolescents older than 6 yrs. **Elderly:** Safety and efficacy not established. Not used in this pt population.

INTERACTIONS

DRUG: CYP3A4 inhibitors (e.g., **atazanavir, clarithromycin, indinavir, itraconazole, ketoconazole, nefazodone, nelfinavir, ritonavir, saquinavir**) may increase risk of hypotension, bradycardia, sedation. **Rifampin** decreases guanfacine concentration. May increase **valproic acid** concentration. Increased risk of cardiovascular effects with **antihypertensives.** Alcohol, **antipsychotics, barbiturates, benzodiazepines, sedative/hypnotics** may produce additive sedative effects. **HERBAL:** None significant. **FOOD:** High-fat meals may increase concentration. **LAB VALUES:** None known.

AVAILABILITY (Rx)

⬛ **Tablets:** 1 mg, 2 mg. **Tablets, Extended-Release:** 1 mg, 2 mg, 3 mg, 4 mg.

ADMINISTRATION/HANDLING

PO
• Do not give with high-fat meal. • Do not break, crush, dissolve or divide extended-release tablets.

INDICATIONS/ROUTES/DOSAGE

◀**ALERT**▶ Dosing should be considered on a mg/kg basis.

ADHD
PO: CHILDREN 6 YRS AND OLDER, (IMMEDIATE-RELEASE) GREATER THAN 45 KG: Initially, 1 mg once daily at bedtime. May increase by 1 mg/day q3–4 days. **Maximum:** 4 mg/day. **45 KG OR LESS:** Initially, 0.5 mg once daily at bedtime. May increase by 0.5 mg/day q3–4 days. **Maximum:** 27–40.5 kg: 2 mg/day; 40.6–45 kg: 3 mg/day. **(EXTENDED-RELEASE):** Begin at dose of 1 mg/day and adjust in increments of no more than 1 mg/wk until clinical response and tolerability are observed. Maintain dose within range of 1–4 mg once daily. If switching from immediate-release guanfacine, discontinue that treatment and titrate with extended-release guanfacine. When discontinuing, taper dose in decrements of no more than 1 mg every 3–7 days.

SIDE EFFECTS

Frequent (38%–10%): Lethargy, headache, fatigue, upper abdominal pain. **Occasional (6%–3%):** Nausea, lethargy, dizziness, irritability, hypotension or decreased B/P, decreased appetite, dry mouth, constipation. **Rare (2%–1%):** Dyspepsia, asthenia (loss of strength, energy), increased B/P, increased weight, orthostatic hypotension, increased urinary frequency.

ADVERSE EFFECTS/ TOXIC REACTIONS

Abrupt discontinuation may produce infrequent, transient elevations in B/P above original baseline (taper dose in decrements of no more than 1 mg every 3–7 days). Abrupt withdrawal following prolonged administration of high dosage may produce extreme fatigue (may last for wks). Prolonged administration to children may produce suppression of weight and/or height patterns. AV block, bradycardia, arrhythmias occur rarely.

NURSING CONSIDERATIONS

BASELINE ASSESSMENT

Obtain baseline vital signs, serum chemistries. Measure pulse, B/P prior to initiation of therapy, following dose increases, and periodically during therapy.

INTERVENTION/EVALUATION

Assist with ambulation if sedation, dizziness, fatigue, lethargy occur. Be alert to mood changes. Assess for nausea, headache. Monitor B/P, blood serum chemistries, particularly renal/hepatic function studies for change from baseline. Monitor daily pattern of bowel activity, stool consistency.

PATIENT/FAMILY TEACHING

• Avoid tasks that require alertness, motor skills until response to drug is established.
• Avoid alcohol. • Dry mouth may be relieved with sugarless gum, sips of water.
• Advise pts to avoid becoming dehydrated, overheated. • Do not substitute for immediate-release guanfacine tablets.
• Swallow whole; do not chew, crush, dissolve, or divide. • Do not take with high-fat meal.

G

haloperidol

hal-o-**per**-i-dol
(Apo-Haloperidol ✹, Haldol, Haldol Decanoate, Novo-Peridol ✹)

BLACK BOX ALERT Increased risk of mortality in elderly pts with dementia-related psychosis with use of injections.
Do not confuse Haldol with Halcion or Stadol.

◆CLASSIFICATION

PHARMACOTHERAPEUTIC: Butyrophenone antpsychotic. **CLINICAL:** Antipsychotic, antiemetic, antidyskinetic (see p. 66C).

ACTION

Competitively blocks postsynaptic dopamine receptors, interrupts nerve impulse movement, increases turnover of dopamine in brain. **Therapeutic Effect:** Produces tranquilizing effect. Strong extrapyramidal, antiemetic effects; weak anticholinergic, sedative effects.

PHARMACOKINETICS

Readily absorbed from GI tract. Protein binding: 92%. Metabolized in liver. Excreted in urine. Not removed by hemodialysis. **Half-life:** 20 hrs.

USES

Treatment of schizophrenia, Tourette's disorder (controls tics and vocal utterances), severe behavioral problems in children. **OFF-LABEL:** Treatment of nonschizophrenic psychosis, alcohol dependence, psychosis/agitation related to Alzheimer's dementia, emergency sedation of severely agitated/psychotic pts.

PRECAUTIONS

Contraindications: Narrow-angle glaucoma, CNS depression, coma, myelosuppression, Parkinson's disease, severe cardiac/hepatic disease. **Cautions:** Renal/hepatic impairment, cardiovascular disease, history of seizures, prolonged QT syndrome, medications that prolong QT interval, hypothyroidism, thyrotoxicosis, electrolyte imbalance (e.g., hypokalemia, hypomagnesemia), EEG abnormalities, elderly, pts at risk for pneumonia, decreased GI motility, urinary retention, BPH, visual disturbances, myasthenia gravis.

⧗ LIFESPAN CONSIDERATIONS

Pregnancy/Lactation: Crosses placenta. Distributed in breast milk. **Pregnancy Category C. Children:** More susceptible to dystonias; not recommended in those younger than 3 yrs. **Elderly:** More susceptible to orthostatic hypotension, anticholinergic effects, sedation; increased risk for extrapyramidal effects. Decreased dosage recommended.

INTERACTIONS

DRUG: Alcohol, other CNS depressants may increase CNS depression. **CYP3A4 inducers (e.g., carbamazepine)** may decrease concentration. **Medications prolonging QT interval** may increase risk of QT prolongation. **Medications producing extrapyramidal symptoms (EPS)** may increase EPS. **HERBAL: Gotu kola, kava kava, St. John's wort, valerian** may increase CNS depression. **FOOD:** None known. **LAB VALUES:** None significant. **Therapeutic serum level:** 0.2–1 mcg/ml; **toxic serum level:** greater than 1 mcg/ml.

AVAILABILITY (Rx)

Injection, Oil (Decanoate [Haldol Decanoate]): 50 mg/ml, 100 mg/ml. **Injection, Solution (Lactate [Haldol]):** 5 mg/ml. **Oral Concentrate:** 2 mg/ml. **Tablets (Haldol):** 0.5 mg, 1 mg, 2 mg, 5 mg, 10 mg, 20 mg.

ADMINISTRATION/HANDLING

 IV

◄ALERT► Only haloperidol lactate is given IV.
Reconstitution • May give undiluted.
• May add to 50–100 ml of D₅W.

Rate of Administration • Give IV push at rate of 5 mg/min. • Infuse IV piggyback over 30 min. • For IV infusion, up to 25 mg/hr has been used (titrated to pt response).

Storage • Discard if precipitate forms, discoloration occurs. • Store at room temperature; do not freeze. • Protect from light.

IM

Parenteral Administration • Pt should remain recumbent for 30–60 min to minimize hypotensive effect. • Prepare Decanoate IM injection using 21-gauge needle. • Do not exceed maximum volume of 3 ml per IM injection site. • Inject slow, deep IM into upper outer quadrant of gluteus maximus.

PO

• Give without regard to meals. • Scored tablets may be crushed. • Dilute oral concentrate with water or juice. • Avoid skin contact with oral concentrate; may cause contact dermatitis.

🔲 IV INCOMPATIBILITIES

Allopurinol (Aloprim), amphotericin B complex (Abelcet, AmBisome, Amphotec), cefepime (Maxipime), fluconazole (Diflucan), foscarnet (Foscavir), heparin, nitroprusside (Nipride), piperacillin/tazobactam (Zosyn).

🔲 IV COMPATIBILITIES

Dobutamine (Dobutrex), dopamine (Intropin), fentanyl (Sublimaze), hydromorphone (Dilaudid), lidocaine, lorazepam (Ativan), midazolam (Versed), morphine, nitroglycerin, norepinephrine (Levophed), propofol (Diprivan).

INDICATIONS/ROUTES/DOSAGE

Usual Dosage

IM *(Lactate)*: **ADULTS, ELDERLY:** 2–5 mg q4–8h as needed. **CHILDREN 6–12 YRS:** 1–3 mg/dose q4–8h as needed. **Maximum:** 0.15 mg/kg/day. *(Decanoate)*: **ADULTS, ELDERLY:** 10–20 times stabilized oral dose, given at 4-wk intervals.

PO: **ADULTS, ELDERLY:** 0.5–5 mg 2–3 times/day. **Maximum:** 30 mg/day. **CHILDREN 3–12 YRS (15–40 KG):** 0.25–0.5 mg/day. May increase by 0.25–0.5 mg q5–7days. **Maximum:** 0.15 mg/kg/day.

SIDE EFFECTS

Frequent: Blurred vision, constipation, orthostatic hypotension, dry mouth, swelling or soreness of female breasts, peripheral edema. **Occasional:** Allergic reaction, difficulty urinating, decreased thirst, dizziness, diminished sexual function, drowsiness, nausea, vomiting, photosensitivity, lethargy.

ADVERSE EFFECTS/ TOXIC REACTIONS

Extrapyramidal symptoms (EPS) appear to be dose related and typically occur in first few days of therapy. Marked drowsiness/lethargy, excessive salivation, fixed stare may be mild to severe in intensity. Less frequently noted are severe akathisia (motor restlessness), acute dystonias: torticollis (neck muscle spasm), opisthotonos (rigidity of back muscles), oculogyric crisis (rolling back of eyes). Tardive dyskinesia (tongue protrusion, puffing of cheeks, chewing/puckering of the mouth) may occur during long-term therapy or after drug discontinuance and may be irreversible. Elderly female pts have greater risk of developing this reaction.

NURSING CONSIDERATIONS

BASELINE ASSESSMENT

Assess behavior, appearance, emotional status, response to environment, speech pattern, thought content.

INTERVENTION/EVALUATION

Monitor B/P, heart rate. Supervise suicidal-risk pt closely during early therapy (as depression lessens, energy level improves, increasing suicide potential). Monitor for rigidity, tremor, mask-like facial expression, fine tongue movement. Assess for therapeutic response (interest

H

in surroundings, improvement in self-care, increased ability to concentrate, relaxed facial expression). Monitor EKG and QT interval. **Therapeutic serum level:** 0.2–1 mcg/ml; **toxic serum level:** greater than 1 mcg/ml.

PATIENT/FAMILY TEACHING

• Full therapeutic effect may take up to 6 wks. • Do not abruptly withdraw from long-term drug therapy. • Sugarless gum, sips of water may relieve dry mouth. • Drowsiness generally subsides during continued therapy. • Avoid tasks that require alertness, motor skills until response to drug is established. • Avoid alcohol. • Report muscle stiffness. • Avoid exposure to sunlight, overheating, dehydration (increased risk of heatstroke).

---

heparin

hep-a-rin
(Hepalean ✤, Hepalean Leo ✤, Hep-Lock)
Do not confuse heparin with Hespan.

◆CLASSIFICATION

PHARMACOTHERAPEUTIC: Sulfated polysaccharide; blood modifier. **CLINICAL:** Anticoagulant (see p. 32C).

ACTION

Interferes with blood coagulation by blocking conversion of prothrombin to thrombin and fibrinogen to fibrin. **Therapeutic Effect:** Prevents further extension of existing thrombi or new clot formation. No effect on existing clots.

PHARMACOKINETICS

Well absorbed following subcutaneous administration. Protein binding: Very high. Metabolized in liver. Removed from circulation via uptake by reticuloendothelial system. Primarily excreted in urine. Not removed by hemodialysis. **Half-life:** 1–6 hrs.

USES

Prophylaxis and treatment of thromboembolic disorders; anticoagulant for extracorporeal and dialysis procedures; maintain patency of IV devices. **OFF-LABEL:** STEMI, non-STEMI, unstable angina, anticoagulant used during percutaneous coronary intervention.

PRECAUTIONS

Contraindications: Severe thrombocytopenia, uncontrolled active bleeding (unless secondary to DIC). **Cautions:** IM injections, peptic ulcer disease, menstruation, recent surgery or invasive procedures, severe hepatic/renal/biliary disease, indwelling catheters. Pts at risk for bleeding (e.g., bacterial endocarditis, uncontrolled hypertension, platelet defects).

⌛ LIFESPAN CONSIDERATIONS

Pregnancy/Lactation: Use with caution, particularly during last trimester, immediate postpartum period (increased risk of maternal hemorrhage). Does not cross placenta. Not distributed in breast milk. **Pregnancy Category C. Children:** No age-related precautions noted. Benzyl alcohol preservative may cause gasping syndrome in infants. **Elderly:** More susceptible to hemorrhage. Age-related renal impairment may increase risk of bleeding.

INTERACTIONS

DRUG: Other anticoagulants, platelet aggregation inhibitors, thrombolytics may increase risk of bleeding. **HERBAL: Cat's claw, dong quai, evening primrose, feverfew, garlic, ginkgo, ginseng, horse chestnut, red clover** have additional antiplatelet activity. **FOOD:** None known. **LAB VALUES:** May increase free fatty acids, serum AST, ALT, aPPT. May decrease serum cholesterol.

AVAILABILITY (Rx)

Injection Solution: 10 units/ml (Hep-Lock), 100 units/ml, 1,000 units/ml,

5,000 units/ml, 10,000 units/ml, 20,000 units/ml. **Premix Solution for Infusion:** 25,000 units/250 ml infusion, 25,000 units/500 ml infusion.

ADMINISTRATION/HANDLING

◄**ALERT**► Do **not** give by IM injection (pain, hematoma, ulceration, erythema).

 IV

◄**ALERT**► Used in full-dose therapy. Intermittent IV dosage produces higher incidence of bleeding abnormalities. Continuous IV route preferred.
Reconstitution • Premix solution requires no reconstitution.
Rate of Administration • Use constant-rate IV infusion pump.
Storage • Store at room temperature.

Subcutaneous
◄**ALERT**► Used in low-dose therapy. • After withdrawal of heparin from vial, change needle before injection (prevents leakage along needle track). • Inject above iliac crest or in abdominal fat layer. Do not inject within 2 inches of umbilicus or any scar tissue. • Withdraw needle rapidly, apply prolonged pressure at injection site. Do not massage. • Rotate injection sites.

⊞ IV INCOMPATIBILITIES

Amiodarone (Cordarone), amphotericin B complex (Abelcet, AmBisome, Amphotec), ciprofloxacin (Cipro), dacarbazine (DTIC), diazepam (Valium), dobutamine (Dobutrex), doxorubicin (Adriamycin), filgrastim (Neupogen), gentamicin (Garamycin), haloperidol (Haldol), idarubicin (Idamycin), labetalol (Trandate), nicardipine (Cardene), phenytoin (Dilantin), quinidine, tobramycin (Nebcin), vancomycin (Vancocin).

⊞ IV COMPATIBILITIES

Ampicillin/sulbactam (Unasyn), aztreonam (Azactam), calcium gluconate, cefazolin (Ancef), ceftazidime (Fortaz), ceftriaxone (Rocephin), dexmedetomidine (Precedex), digoxin (Lanoxin), diltiazem (Cardizem), dopamine (Intropin), enalapril (Vasotec), famotidine (Pepcid), fentanyl (Sublimaze), furosemide (Lasix), hydromorphone (Dilaudid), insulin, lidocaine, lorazepam (Ativan), magnesium sulfate, methylprednisolone (Solu-Medrol), midazolam (Versed), milrinone (Primacor), morphine, nitroglycerin, norepinephrine (Levophed), oxytocin (Pitocin), piperacillin/tazobactam (Zosyn), procainamide (Pronestyl), propofol (Diprivan).

INDICATIONS/ROUTES/DOSAGE

Line Flushing
IV: ADULTS, ELDERLY, CHILDREN: 100 units q6–8h. **INFANTS WEIGHING LESS THAN 10 KG:** 10 units q6–8h.

Unstable Angina, NSTEMI, Acute Coronary Syndrome
IV Infusion: ADULTS, ELDERLY: 60 units/kg bolus (**maximum:** 4,000 units), then 12 units/kg/hr (**maximum:** 1,000 units/hr).

Treatment of DVT/PE
IV Infusion: ADULTS, ELDERLY: 80 units/kg bolus (**maximum:** 5,000 units), then 18 units/kg/hr adjusted according to aPTT.

Usual Pediatric/Neonatal Dose
IV Infusion: 75 units/kg bolus over 10 min, then initial maintenance dose of 28 units/kg/hr. Adjust to maintain aPTT of 60–85 sec.

Prevention of Thromboembolic Disorders
Subcutaneous: ADULTS, ELDERLY: 5,000 units q8–12h.

SIDE EFFECTS

Occasional: Pruritus, burning (particularly on soles of feet) caused by vasospastic reaction. **Rare:** Pain, cyanosis of extremity 6–10 days after initial therapy lasting 4–6 hrs, hypersensitivity reaction (chills, fever, pruritus, urticaria, asthma, rhinitis, lacrimation, headache).

ADVERSE EFFECTS/ TOXIC REACTIONS

Bleeding complications ranging from local ecchymoses to major hemorrhage occur more frequently in high-dose therapy, intermittent IV infusion, women 60 yrs and older. **Antidote:** Protamine sulfate 1–1.5 mg IV for every 100 units heparin subcutaneous within 30 min of overdose, 0.5–0.75 mg for every 100 units heparin subcutaneous if within 30–60 min of overdose, 0.25–0.375 mg for every 100 units heparin subcutaneous if 2 hrs have elapsed since overdose, 25–50 mg if heparin was given by IV infusion.

NURSING CONSIDERATIONS

BASELINE ASSESSMENT

Cross-check dose with co-worker. Determine aPTT before administration and 24 hrs following initiation of therapy, then q24–48hrs for first wk of therapy or until maintenance dose is established. Follow with aPTT determinations 1–2 times weekly for 3–4 wks. In long-term therapy, monitor 1–2 times a mo.

INTERVENTION/EVALUATION

Monitor aPTT (therapeutic range at 1.5–2.5 times normal) diligently. Assess Hct, platelet count, AST, ALT. Monitor urine and stool for occult blood. Assess for decrease in B/P, increase in pulse rate, complaint of abdominal/back pain, severe headache (may be evidence of hemorrhage). Question for increase in amount of discharge during menses. Assess peripheral pulses; skin for ecchymosis, petechiae. Check for excessive bleeding from minor cuts, scratches. Assess gums for erythema, gingival bleeding. Assess urine output for hematuria. Avoid IM injections due to potential for hematomas. When converting to warfarin (Coumadin) therapy, monitor PT results (will be 10%–20% higher while heparin is given concurrently).

PATIENT/FAMILY TEACHING

• Use electric razor, soft toothbrush to prevent bleeding. • Report any sign of red or dark urine, black or red stool, coffee-ground vomitus, blood-tinged mucus from cough. • Do not use any OTC medication without physician approval (may interfere with platelet aggregation). • Wear or carry identification that notes anticoagulant therapy. • Inform dentist, other physicians of heparin therapy. • Limit alcohol.

*hydrALAZINE

hye-**dral**-a-zeen
(Apo-Hydralazine ✤, Apresoline ✤, Novo-Hylazin ✤)
Do not confuse hydralazine with hydroxyzine.

FIXED-COMBINATION(S)

Apresazide: hydralazine/hydrochlorothiazide (a diuretic): 25 mg/25 mg, 50 mg/50 mg, 100 mg/50 mg. **BiDil:** hydralazine/isosorbide (a nitrate): 37.5 mg/20 mg.

◆CLASSIFICATION

PHARMACOTHERAPEUTIC: Vasodilator. **CLINICAL:** Antihypertensive (see p. 63C).

ACTION

Direct vasodilating effects on arterioles. **Therapeutic Effect:** Decreases B/P, systemic vascular resistance.

PHARMACOKINETICS

Route	Onset	Peak	Duration
PO	20–30 min	N/A	Up to 8 hrs
IV	5–20 min	N/A	1–4 hrs

Well absorbed from GI tract. Widely distributed. Protein binding: 85%–90%. Metabolized in liver. Primarily excreted in urine. Not removed by hemodialysis. **Half-life:** 3–7 hrs (increased in renal impairment).

H

USES

Management of moderate to severe hypertension. **OFF-LABEL:** Hypertension secondary to eclampsia, preeclampsia. Treatment of HF.

PRECAUTIONS

Contraindications: Coronary artery disease, mitral valvular rheumatic heart disease, dissecting aortic aneurysm. **Cautions:** Renal impairment, cerebrovascular disease, positive ANA titer.

⏳ LIFESPAN CONSIDERATIONS

Pregnancy/Lactation: Drug crosses placenta. Unknown if distributed in breast milk. Thrombocytopenia, leukopenia, petechial bleeding, hematomas have occurred in newborns (resolved within 1–3 wks). **Pregnancy Category C. Children:** No age-related precautions noted. **Elderly:** More sensitive to hypotensive effects. Age-related renal impairment may require dosage adjustment.

INTERACTIONS

DRUG: Diuretics, other antihypertensives may increase hypotensive effect. **HERBAL: Ephedra, ginseng, yohimbe** may worsen hypertension. **Garlic** may increase antihypertensive effect. **FOOD:** Any **foods** may increase absorption. **LAB VALUES:** May produce positive direct Coombs' test.

AVAILABILITY (Rx)

Injection Solution: 20 mg/ml. **Tablets:** 10 mg, 25 mg, 50 mg, 100 mg.

ADMINISTRATION/HANDLING

 IV

Rate of Administration • May give undiluted. • Administer slowly: maximum rate 5 mg/min (0.2 mg/kg/min for children).
Storage • Store at room temperature.

PO
• Best given with food at regularly spaced meals. • Tablets may be crushed.

🔲 IV INCOMPATIBILITIES

Ampicillin (Polycillin), furosemide (Lasix).

🔲 IV COMPATIBILITIES

Dobutamine (Dobutrex), heparin, hydrocortisone (Solu-Cortef), nitroglycerin, potassium chloride.

INDICATIONS/ROUTES/DOSAGE

Hypertension
PO: ADULTS: Initially, 10 mg 4 times a day for first 2–4 days. May increase to 25 mg 4 times/day balance of first wk. May increase by 10–25 mg/dose gradually to 50 mg 4 times/day. Usual range: 25–100 mg in 2–3 divided doses. **Maximum:** 300 mg/day. **ELDERLY:** Initially, 10 mg 2–3 times a day. May increase by 10–25 mg q2–5 days. **CHILDREN:** Initially, 0.75–1 mg/kg/day in 2–4 divided doses, not to exceed 25 mg/dose. May increase over 3–4 wks. **Maximum:** 7.5 mg/kg/day (5 mg/kg/day in infants). **Maximum daily dose:** 200 mg.
IV, IM: ADULTS, ELDERLY: Initially, 10–20 mg/dose q4–6h. May increase to 40 mg/dose. **CHILDREN:** Initially, 0.1–0.2 mg/kg/dose (**maximum:** 20 mg) q4–6h, as needed, up to 1.7–3.5 mg/kg/day in 4–6 divided doses.

HF
PO: ADULTS, ELDERLY: Initially, 10–25 mg 3–4 times/day up to 225–300 mg/day in combination with isosorbide dinitrate.

Dosage in Renal Impairment
Dosage interval is based on creatinine clearance.

Creatinine Clearance	Dosage
10–50 ml/min	q8h
Less than 10 ml/min	q8–24h

SIDE EFFECTS

Occasional: Headache, anorexia, nausea, vomiting, diarrhea, palpitations, tachycardia, angina pectoris. **Rare:** Constipation, ileus, edema, peripheral neuritis (paresthesia), dizziness, muscle cramps,

H

 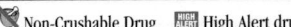

anxiety, hypersensitivity reactions (rash, urticaria, pruritus, fever, chills, arthralgia), nasal congestion, flushing, conjunctivitis.

ADVERSE EFFECTS/ TOXIC REACTIONS

High dosage may produce lupus erythematosus–like reaction (fever, facial rash, muscle/joint aches, glomerulonephritis, splenomegaly). Severe orthostatic hypotension, skin flushing, severe headache, myocardial ischemia, cardiac arrhythmias may develop. Profound shock may occur with severe overdosage.

NURSING CONSIDERATIONS

BASELINE ASSESSMENT

Obtain B/P, pulse immediately before each dose, in addition to regular monitoring (be alert to fluctuations).

INTERVENTION/EVALUATION

Monitor B/P, pulse, ANA titer. Monitor for headache, palpitations, tachycardia. Assess for peripheral edema of hands, feet. Monitor daily pattern of bowel activity, stool consistency.

PATIENT/FAMILY TEACHING

• To reduce hypotensive effect, go from lying to standing slowly. • Report muscle/joint aches, fever (lupus-like reaction), flu-like symptoms. • Limit alcohol use.

TOP 200

hydrochlorothiazide

hye-dro-**klor**-oh-**thy**-ah-zide
(Apo-Hydro ✦, Microzide, Novo-Hydrazide ✦)
Do not confuse Microzide with Maxzide.

FIXED-COMBINATION(S)

Accuretic: hydrochlorothiazide/quinapril (an angiotensin-converting enzyme [ACE] inhibitor): 12.5 mg/10 mg, 12.5 mg/20 mg, 25 mg/20 mg. **Aldactazide:** hydrochlorothiazide/spironolactone (a potassium-sparing diuretic): 25 mg/25 mg, 50 mg/50 mg. **Aldoril:** hydrochlorothiazide/methyldopa (an antihypertensive): 15 mg/250 mg, 25 mg/250 mg, 30 mg/500 mg, 50 mg/500 mg. **Amturnide:** hydrochlorothiazide/aliskiren (renin inhibitor)/amlodipine (calcium channel blocker): 12.5 mg/150 mg/5 mg, 12.5 mg/300 mg/5 mg, 25 mg/300 mg/5 mg, 12.5 mg/300 mg/10 mg, 25 mg/300 mg/10 mg. **Apresazide:** hydrochlorothiazide/hydralazine (a vasodilator): 25 mg/25 mg, 50 mg/50 mg, 50 mg/100 mg. **Atacand HCT:** hydrochlorothiazide/candesartan (an angiotensin II receptor antagonist): 12.5 mg/16 mg, 12.5 mg/32 mg. **Avalide:** hydrochlorothiazide/irbesartan (an angiotensin II receptor antagonist): 12.5 mg/150 mg, 12.5 mg/300 mg, 25 mg/300 mg. **Benicar HCT:** hydrochlorothiazide/olmesartan (an angiotensin II receptor antagonist): 12.5 mg/20 mg, 12.5 mg/40 mg, 25 mg/40 mg. **Capozide:** hydrochlorothiazide/captopril (an ACE inhibitor): 15 mg/25 mg, 15 mg/50 mg, 25 mg/25 mg, 25 mg/50 mg. **Diovan HCT:** hydrochlorothiazide/valsartan (an angiotensin II receptor antagonist): 12.5 mg/80 mg, 12.5 mg/160 mg. **Dutoprol:** hydrochlorothiazide/metoprolol (a beta blocker): 12.5 mg/25 mg, 12.5 mg/50 mg, 12.5 mg/100 mg. **Dyazide/Maxide:** hydrochlorothiazide/triamterene (a potassium-sparing diuretic): 25 mg/37.5 mg, 25 mg/50 mg, 50 mg/75 mg. **Exforge HCT:** hydrochlorothiazide/amlodipine (a calcium channel blocker)/valsartan (an angiotensin II receptor blocker): 12.5 mg/5 mg/160 mg, 25 mg/5 mg/160 mg, 12.5 mg/10 mg/160 mg, 25 mg/10 mg/160 mg, 25 mg/10 mg/320 mg. **Hyzaar:** hydrochlorothiazide/losartan (an angiotensin II receptor

H

antagonist): 12.5 mg/50 mg, 12.5 mg/100 mg, 25 mg/100 mg. **Inderide:** hydrochlorothiazide/propranolol (a beta-blocker): 25 mg/40 mg, 25 mg/80 mg, 50 mg/80 mg, 50 mg/120 mg, 50 mg/160 mg. **Lopressor HCT:** hydrochlorothiazide/metoprolol (a beta-blocker): 25 mg/50 mg, 25 mg/100 mg, 50 mg/100 mg. **Lotensin HCT:** hydrochlorothiazide/bepridil (a calcium channel blocker): 6.25 mg/5 mg, 12.5 mg/10 mg, 12.5 mg/20 mg, 25 mg/20 mg. **Micardis HCT:** hydrochlorothiazide/telmisartan (an angiotensin II receptor antagonist): 12.5 mg/40 mg, 12.5 mg/80 mg. **Moduretic:** hydrochlorothiazide/amiloride (a potassium-sparing diuretic): 50 mg/5 mg. **Normozide:** hydrochlorothiazide/labetalol (a beta-blocker): 25 mg/100 mg, 25 mg/300 mg. **Prinzide/Zestoretic:** hydrochlorothiazide/lisinopril (an ACE inhibitor): 12.5 mg/10 mg, 12.5 mg/20 mg, 25 mg/20 mg. **Tekturna HCT:** hydrochlorothiazide/aliskiren (a renin inhibitor): 12.5 mg/150 mg, 25 mg/300 mg. **Teveten HCT:** hydrochlorothiazide/eprosartan (an angiotensin II receptor antagonist): 12.5 mg/600 mg, 25 mg/600 mg. **Timolide:** hydrochlorothiazide/timolol (a beta-blocker): 25 mg/10 mg. **Tribenzor:** hydrochlorothiazide/olmesartan/amlodipine: 12.5 mg/20 mg/5 mg, 12.5 mg/40 mg/5 mg, 25 mg/40 mg/5 mg, 12.5 mg/40 mg/10 mg, 25 mg/40 mg/10 mg. **Uniretic:** hydrochlorothiazide/moexipril (an ACE inhibitor): 12.5 mg/7.5 mg, 25 mg/15 mg. **Vaseretic:** hydrochlorothiazide/enalapril (an ACE inhibitor): 12.5 mg/5 mg, 25 mg/10 mg. **Ziac:** hydrochlorothiazide/bisoprolol (a beta-blocker): 6.25 mg/5 mg, 6.25 mg/10 mg.

◆CLASSIFICATION

PHARMACOTHERAPEUTIC: Sulfonamide derivative. **CLINICAL:** Thiazide diuretic, antihypertensive (see pp. 63C, 104C).

ACTION

Diuretic: Blocks reabsorption of water, sodium, potassium at cortical diluting segment of distal tubule. **Antihypertensive:** Reduces plasma, extracellular fluid volume, peripheral vascular resistance by direct effect on blood vessels. **Therapeutic Effect:** Promotes diuresis; reduces B/P.

PHARMACOKINETICS

Route	Onset	Peak	Duration
PO (diuretic)	2 hrs	4–6 hrs	6–12 hrs

Variably absorbed from GI tract. Primarily excreted unchanged in urine. Not removed by hemodialysis. **Half-life:** 5.6–14.8 hrs.

USES

Treatment of mild to moderate hypertension, edema in HF, nephrotic syndrome. **OFF-LABEL:** Treatment of lithium-induced diabetes insipidus.

PRECAUTIONS

Contraindications: Anuria, history of hypersensitivity to sulfonamides or thiazide diuretics. **Cautions:** Severe renal/hepatic impairment, diabetes mellitus, elderly or debilitated, history of gout, moderate to high cholesterol, hypercalcemia.

⏳ LIFESPAN CONSIDERATIONS

Pregnancy/Lactation: Crosses placenta. Small amount distributed in breast milk. Breastfeeding not recommended. **Pregnancy Category B (D if used in pregnancy-induced hypertension). Children:** No age-related precautions noted, except jaundiced infants may be at risk for hyperbilirubinemia. **Elderly:** May be more sensitive to hypotensive, electrolyte effects. Age-related renal impairment may require dosage adjustment.

INTERACTIONS

DRUG: Cholestyramine, colestipol may decrease absorption, effects. May increase risk of **digoxin** toxicity associated with hydrochlorothiazide-induced hypokalemia. May increase risk of **lithium** toxicity. **HERBAL: Ephedra, ginseng, yohimbe** may diminish effect. **Black cohosh, periwinkle** may increase antihypertensive effect. **FOOD:** None known. **LAB VALUES:** May increase serum glucose, cholesterol, LDL, bilirubin, calcium, creatinine, uric acid, triglycerides. May decrease urinary calcium, serum magnesium, potassium, sodium.

AVAILABILITY (Rx)

Capsules (Microzide): 12.5 mg. Tablets: 12.5 mg, 25 mg, 50 mg.

ADMINISTRATION/HANDLING

PO
• If GI upset occurs, give with food or milk, preferably with breakfast (may prevent nocturia). • Give last dose no later than 6 PM unless instructed otherwise.

INDICATIONS/ROUTES/DOSAGE

Edema
PO: **ADULTS:** 25–100 mg/day in 1–2 divided doses. **Maximum:** 200 mg/day.

Hypertension
PO: **ADULTS:** 12.5–50 mg/day.

Usual Elderly Dosage
PO: 12.5–25 mg once daily.

Usual Pediatric Dosage
PO: **CHILDREN 2–17 YRS:** Initially, 1 mg/kg/day. **Maximum:** 3 mg/kg/day (50 mg). **CHILDREN 6 MOS TO 2 YRS:** 1–3 mg/kg/day in 1–2 divided doses. **Maximum:** 37.5 mg/day. **CHILDREN YOUNGER THAN 6 MOS:** 1–3 mg/kg/day in 2 divided doses.

Dosage in Renal Impairment
Creatinine clearance less than 30 ml/min—generally not effective. Avoid use with creatinine clearance less than 10 ml/min.

SIDE EFFECTS

Expected: Increased urinary frequency, urine volume. **Frequent:** Potassium depletion. **Occasional:** Orthostatic hypotension, headache, GI disturbances, photosensitivity.

ADVERSE EFFECTS/TOXIC REACTIONS

Vigorous diuresis may lead to profound water loss/electrolyte depletion, resulting in hypokalemia, hyponatremia, dehydration. Acute hypotensive episodes may occur. Hyperglycemia may occur during prolonged therapy. Pancreatitis, blood dyscrasias, pulmonary edema, allergic pneumonitis, dermatologic reactions occur rarely. Overdose can lead to lethargy, coma without changes in electrolytes or hydration.

NURSING CONSIDERATIONS

BASELINE ASSESSMENT
Check vital signs, esp. B/P for hypotension before administration. Assess baseline electrolytes, esp. for hypokalemia. Evaluate skin turgor, mucous membranes for hydration status. Evaluate for peripheral edema. Assess muscle strength, mental status. Note skin temperature, moisture. Obtain baseline weight. Monitor I&O.

INTERVENTION/EVALUATION
Continue to monitor B/P, vital signs, electrolytes, I&O, daily weight. Note extent of diuresis. Watch for changes from initial assessment (hypokalemia may result in weakness, tremor, muscle cramps, nausea, vomiting, altered mental status, tachycardia; hyponatremia may result in confusion, thirst, cold/clammy skin). Be esp. alert for potassium depletion in pts taking digoxin (cardiac arrhythmias). Potassium supplements are frequently ordered. Check for constipation (may occur with exercise diuresis).

PATIENT/FAMILY TEACHING
• Expect increased frequency, volume of urination. • To reduce hypotensive effect, go from lying to standing slowly. • Eat foods high in potassium, such as whole grains (cereals), legumes, meat, bananas, apricots, orange juice, potatoes (white, sweet), raisins. • Protect skin from sun, ultraviolet light (photosensitivity may occur).

hydrocodone

hye-droe-**koe**-done
(Hycodan ✤, Robidone ✤,
Zohydro ER)
**Do not confuse Hycodan with
Vicodin.**

FIXED-COMBINATION(S)

Anexsia: hydrocodone/acetamin-
ophen (a non-narcotic analgesic): 5
mg/500 mg, 7.5 mg/650 mg, 10
mg/650 mg. **Duocet:** hydrocodone/
acetaminophen: 5 mg/500 mg. **Hycet:**
hydrocodone/acetaminophen: 7.5 mg/
325 mg per 15 ml. **Hycodan:** hydro-
codone/homatropine (an anticholinergic): 5 mg/1.5 mg. **Hycotuss, Vitus-
sin:** hydrocodone/guaifenesin (an
expectorant): 5 mg/100 mg. **Lorcet:**
hydrocodone/acetaminophen: 7.5 mg/
650 mg, 10 mg/650 mg. **Lortab:** hy-
drocodone/acetaminophen: 2.5 mg/
500 mg, 5 mg/500 mg, 7.5 mg/500 mg,
10 mg/500 mg. **Lortab Elixir:** hydro-
codone/acetaminophen: 2.5 mg/167
mg per 5 ml. **Lortab with ASA:** hydro-
codone/aspirin: 5 mg/500 mg. **Norco:**
hydrocodone/acetaminophen: 10 mg/
325 mg. **Reprexain CIII:** hydroco-
done/ibuprofen (an NSAID): 5 mg/200
mg. **Rezira:** hydrocodone/pseudo-
ephedrine (a nasal decongestant): 5
mg/60 mg per 5 ml. **Tussend:** hydro-
codone/pseudoephedrine (a sympathomimetic)/guaifenesin (an expectorant): 2.5 mg/30 mg/100 mg per 5 ml.
Vicodin: hydrocodone/acetaminophen:
5 mg/500 mg. **Vicodin ES:** hydro-
codone/acetaminophen: 7.5 mg/750 mg.
Vicodin HP: hydrocodone/acetamino-
phen: 10 mg/650 mg. **Vicoprofen:** hy-
drocodone/ibuprofen (an NSAID): 7.5
mg/200 mg. **Xodol:** hydrocodone/acet-
aminophen: 5 mg/300 mg. **Zutripto:**
hydrocodone/chlorpheniramine (an
antihistamine)/pseudoephedrine (a nasal decongestant): 5 mg/4 mg/60 mg.
Zydone: hydrocodone/acetaminophen:
5 mg/400 mg, 7.5 mg/400 mg, 10
mg/400 mg.

◆CLASSIFICATION

PHARMACOTHERAPEUTIC: Opioid
agonist **(Schedule III). CLINICAL:**
Narcotic analgesic, antitussive.

ACTION

Binds with opioid receptors in CNS. **Therapeutic Effect:** Reduces intensity of incoming pain stimuli from sensory nerve
endings, altering pain perception, emotional response to pain; suppresses cough
reflex.

PHARMACOKINETICS

Route	Onset	Peak	Duration
PO (analgesic)	10–20 min	30–60 min	4–6 hrs
PO (antitussive)	N/A	N/A	4–6 hrs

Well absorbed from GI tract. Metabolized
in liver. Primarily excreted in urine.
Half-life: 3.8 hrs (increased in elderly).

USES

Relief of moderate to moderately severe
pain, nonproductive cough. **Zohydro
ER:** Around-the-clock management of
moderate to severe chronic pain.

PRECAUTIONS

Contraindications: Significant respiratory
depression, acute or severe bronchial
asthma or hypercarbia, paralytic ileus.
Cautions: Concomitant use of CYP3A4 inhibitors, CNS depressants, elderly, ca-
chectic, debilitated, chronic pulmonary
disease, head injury or increased intracranial pressure, GI obstruction, impaired mental/physical abilities.

⧗ LIFESPAN CONSIDERATIONS

Pregnancy/Lactation: Readily crosses
placenta. Distributed in breast milk. May
prolong labor if administered in latent
phase of first stage of labor or before

H

cervical dilation of 4–5 cm has occurred. Respiratory depression may occur in neonate if mother received opiates during labor. Regular use of opiates during pregnancy may produce withdrawal symptoms (irritability, excessive crying, tremors, hyperactive reflexes, fever, vomiting, diarrhea, yawning, sneezing, seizures) in the neonate. **Pregnancy Category C (D if used for prolonged periods or at high dosages at term). Children:** Those younger than 2 yrs may be more susceptible to respiratory depression. **Elderly:** May be more susceptible to respiratory depression, may cause paradoxical excitement. Age-related renal impairment, prostatic hypertrophy or obstruction may increase risk of urinary retention; dosage adjustment recommended.

INTERACTIONS

DRUG: Alcohol, other CNS depressants may increase CNS or respiratory depression, hypotension. **MAOIs, tricyclic antidepressants** may alter effect of hydrocodone. **CYP3A4 inhibitors** may increase or prolong opioid effects. **HERBAL: Gotu kola, kava kava, St. John's wort, valerian** may increase CNS depression. **FOOD:** None known. **LAB VALUES:** May increase serum amylase, lipase.

AVAILABILITY (Rx)

Capsules, Extended-Release (Zohydro ER): 10 mg, 15 mg, 20 mg, 30 mg, 40 mg, 50 mg.

ADMINISTRATION/HANDLING

PO
• Give without regard to meals. • Capsules must be swallowed whole. Do not cut, crush, or dissolve.

INDICATIONS/ROUTES/DOSAGE

Analgesia
PO: ADULTS, CHILDREN WEIGHING 50 KG OR MORE: Initially, 5–10 mg q3–4h as needed. **ADULTS, CHILDREN WEIGHING LESS THAN 50 KG:** Initially, 0.1–0.2 mg/kg

q3–4h as needed. **ELDERLY:** 2.5–5 mg q4–6h.

Analgesia (Zohydro ER)
PO: ADULTS, ELDERLY: Initially, 10 mg q12h. May increase by 10 mg q12h q3–7 days to achieve adequate analgesia.

Cough
PO: ADULTS, ELDERLY: 5–10 mg q4–6h as needed. **Maximum:** 15 mg/dose. **CHILDREN:** 0.6 mg/kg/day in 3–4 divided doses at intervals of at least 4 hrs. **Maximum single dose:** 10 mg (children older than 12 yrs), 5 mg (children 2–12 yrs), 1.25 mg (children younger than 2 yrs).

SIDE EFFECTS

Frequent: Lethargy, hypotension, diaphoresis, facial flushing, dizziness, drowsiness. **Occasional:** Urine retention, blurred vision, constipation, dry mouth, headache, nausea, vomiting, difficult/painful urination, euphoria, dysphoria.

ADVERSE EFFECTS/ TOXIC REACTIONS

Overdose results in respiratory depression, skeletal muscle flaccidity, cold/clammy skin, cyanosis, extreme drowsiness progressing to seizures, stupor, coma. Tolerance to analgesic effect, physical dependence may occur with repeated use. Prolonged duration of action, cumulative effect may occur in those with hepatic/renal impairment. **Antidote:** Naloxone (see Appendix K).

NURSING CONSIDERATIONS

BASELINE ASSESSMENT

Obtain vital signs. If respirations are 12/min or less (20/min or less in children), withhold medication, contact physician. **Analgesic:** Assess onset, type, location, duration of pain. Effect of medication is reduced if full pain recurs before next dose. **Antitussive:** Assess type, severity, frequency of cough.

INTERVENTION/EVALUATION

Palpate bladder for urinary retention. Monitor daily pattern of bowel activity, stool consistency. Initiate deep breathing and coughing exercises, particularly in pts with pulmonary impairment. Assess for clinical improvement; record onset of relief of pain, cough.

PATIENT/FAMILY TEACHING

• Change positions slowly to avoid orthostatic hypotension. • Avoid tasks that require alertness, motor skills until response to drug is established. • Avoid alcohol. • Tolerance or dependence may occur with prolonged use at high dosages. • Report nausea, vomiting, constipation, shortness of breath, difficulty breathing. • May take with food.

hydrocortisone

hye-droe-**kor**-ti-sone
(Anusol HC, Caldecort, Colocort, Cortaid, Cortef, Cortenema, Cortizone-10, Preparation H Hydrocortisone, Proctocort, Solu-Cortef, Westcort).
Do not confuse hydrocortisone with hydrochlorothiazide, hydrocodone, or hydroxychloroquine, Cortef with Coreg, or Solu-Cortef with Solu-Medrol.

FIXED-COMBINATION(S)

Cortisporin: hydrocortisone/neomycin/polymyxin (an anti-infective): 5 mg/10,000 units/5 mg, 10 mg/10,000 units/5 mg. **Liposivir:** hydrocortisone/acyclovir (an antiviral): 1%/5%.

◆CLASSIFICATION

PHARMACOTHERAPEUTIC: Adrenal corticosteroid. **CLINICAL:** Glucocorticoid (see pp. 100C, 102C).

ACTION

Inhibits accumulation of inflammatory cells at inflammation sites, phagocytosis, lysosomal enzyme release, synthesis and/or release of mediators of inflammation. **Therapeutic Effect:** Prevents/suppresses cell-mediated immune reactions. Decreases/prevents tissue response to inflammatory process.

PHARMACOKINETICS

Route	Onset	Peak	Duration
IV	N/A	4–6 hrs	8–12 hrs

Well absorbed after IM administration. Widely distributed. Metabolized in liver. **Half-life:** Plasma, 1.5–2 hrs; biologic, 8–12 hrs.

USES

Systemic: Management of adrenocortical insufficiency, antiinflammatory, immunosuppressive. **Topical:** Inflammatory dermatoses, adjunctive treatment of ulcerative colitis, atopic dermatitis, inflamed hemorrhoids. **OFF-LABEL:** Management of septic shock. Treatment of thyroid storm.

PRECAUTIONS

Contraindications: Fungal, tuberculosis, viral skin lesions; serious infections, IM administration in idiopathic thrombocytopenia purpura. **Cautions:** Thyroid dysfunction, cirrhosis, hypertension, osteoporosis, thromboembolic tendencies or thrombophlebitis, HF, seizure disorders, diabetes, respiratory tuberculosis, untreated systemic infections, renal/hepatic impairment, acute MI, myasthenia gravis, glaucoma, cataracts, increased intraocular pressure.

⧗ LIFESPAN CONSIDERATIONS

Pregnancy/Lactation: Crosses placenta; distributed in breast milk. May produce cleft palate if used chronically during first trimester. Breastfeeding not recommended. **Pregnancy Category C (D if used in first trimester). Children:** Prolonged treatment or high dosages may decrease short-term growth rate, cortisol secretion. **Elderly:** May be more susceptible to developing hypertension or osteoporosis.

H

INTERACTIONS

DRUG: May decrease effects of **diuretics, insulin, oral hypoglycemics, potassium supplements. Hepatic enzyme inducers** may decrease effects. **Live virus vaccines** may decrease pt's antibody response to vaccine, increase vaccine side effects, potentiate virus replication. **HERBAL: St. John's wort** may decrease concentration. **Cat's claw, echinacea** may increase immunostimulant properties. **FOOD:** None known. **LAB VALUES:** May increase serum glucose, lipids, sodium. May decrease serum calcium, potassium, thyroxine, WBC count.

AVAILABILITY (Rx)

Cream, Rectal (Cortizone-10, Preparation H Hydrocortisone): 1%, 2.5%. **Cream, Topical:** 0.5%, 1%, 2.5%. **Injection, Powder for Reconstitution (Solu-Cortef):** 100 mg, 250 mg, 500 mg, 1 g. **Ointment, Topical:** 0.5%, 1%, 2.5%. **Suppository (Anusol HC):** 25 mg. **Suspension, Rectal (Colocort, Cortenema):** 100 mg/60 ml. **Tablets (Cortef):** 5 mg, 10 mg, 20 mg.

ADMINISTRATION/HANDLING

 IV

Hydrocortisone Sodium Succinate
Reconstitution • Initially, reconstitute vial per manufacturer's instructions. • May further dilute with D_5W or 0.9% NaCl. For IV push, dilute to 50 mg/ml; for intermittent infusion, dilute to 1 mg/ml. Note: 100–3,000 mg may be added to 50 ml D_5W or 0.9% NaCl.
Rate of Administration • Administer IV push over 3–5 min (over 10 min for doses 500 mg or greater). Give intermittent infusion over 20–30 min.
Storage • Store at room temperature. • Once reconstituted, stable for 3 days at room temperature. Once further diluted with 0.9% NaCl or D_5W stability concentration dependent: 1 mg/ml (24 hrs) 2 mg/ml to 60 mg/ml (4 hrs).

PO
• Give with food or milk if GI distress occurs.

Rectal
• Shake homogeneous suspension well. • Instruct pt to lie on left side with left leg extended, right leg flexed. • Gently insert applicator tip into rectum, pointed slightly toward navel (umbilicus). Slowly instill medication.

Topical
• Gently cleanse area before application. • Use occlusive dressings only as ordered. • Apply sparingly; rub into area thoroughly.

IV INCOMPATIBILITIES

Ciprofloxacin (Cipro), diazepam (Valium), midazolam (Versed), phenytoin (Dilantin).

IV COMPATIBILITIES

Amphotericin, calcium gluconate, cefepime (Maxipime), digoxin (Lanoxin), diltiazem (Cardizem), diphenhydramine (Benadryl), dopamine (Intropin), insulin, lidocaine, lorazepam (Ativan), magnesium sulfate, morphine, norepinephrine (Levophed), procainamide (Pronestyl), potassium chloride, propofol (Diprivan).

INDICATIONS/ROUTES/DOSAGE

Acute Adrenal Insufficiency
IV: ADULTS, ELDERLY: 100 mg IV bolus, then 300 mg/day in divided doses q8h. **CHILDREN:** 1–2 mg/kg IV bolus, then 150–250 mg/day in divided doses q6–8h. **INFANTS:** 1–2 mg/kg/dose IV bolus, then 25–150 mg/day in divided doses q6–8h.

Anti-Inflammation, Immunosuppression
IV, IM: ADULTS, ELDERLY: 15–240 mg q12h. **CHILDREN:** 1–5 mg/kg/day in divided doses q12h.
PO: ADULTS, ELDERLY: 15–240 mg q12h. **CHILDREN:** 2.5–10 mg/kg/day in divided doses q6–8h.

Physiologic Replacement
PO: CHILDREN: 8–10 mg/m²/day in 3 divided doses.

Status Asthmaticus
IV: ADULTS, ELDERLY, CHILDREN: 1–2 mg/kg/dose q6h for 24 hrs. Maintenance: 0.5–1 mg/kg q6h.

Anaphylactic Shock
IV: ADULTS, ELDERLY, CHILDREN 12 YRS AND OLDER: 500 mg–2 g q2–6h. **CHILDREN YOUNGER THAN 12 YRS:** 50 mg/kg. May repeat in 4 hrs, then q24h as needed.

Adjunctive Treatment of Ulcerative Colitis
Rectal (Enema): ADULTS, ELDERLY: 100 mg at bedtime for 21 nights or until clinical and proctologic remission occurs (may require 2–3 mos of therapy).
Rectal: ADULTS, ELDERLY: 1 applicator 1–2 times a day for 2–3 wks, then every second day until therapy ends.
Usual Topical Dosage: ADULTS, ELDERLY: Apply sparingly 2–4 times a day.

SIDE EFFECTS

Frequent: Insomnia, heartburn, anxiety, abdominal distention, diaphoresis, acne, mood swings, increased appetite, facial flushing, delayed wound healing, increased susceptibility to infection, diarrhea or constipation. **Occasional:** Headache, edema, change in skin color, frequent urination. **Topical:** Pruritus, redness, irritation. **Rare:** Tachycardia, allergic reaction (rash, hives), psychological changes, hallucinations, depression. **Topical:** Allergic contact dermatitis, purpura. **Systemic:** Absorption more likely with use of occlusive dressings or extensive application in young children.

ADVERSE EFFECTS/ TOXIC REACTIONS

Long-term therapy: Hypocalcemia, hypokalemia, muscle wasting (esp. arms, legs), osteoporosis, spontaneous fractures, amenorrhea, cataracts, glaucoma, peptic ulcer, HF. **Abrupt withdrawal after long-term therapy:** Nausea, fever, headache, sudden severe joint pain, rebound inflammation, fatigue, weakness, lethargy, dizziness, orthostatic hypotension.

NURSING CONSIDERATIONS

BASELINE ASSESSMENT

Obtain baseline values for weight, B/P, serum glucose, cholesterol, electrolytes. Check results of initial tests (tuberculosis [TB] skin test, X-rays, EKG).

INTERVENTION/EVALUATION

Assess for edema. Be alert to infection (reduced immune response): sore throat, fever, vague symptoms. Monitor daily pattern of bowel activity, stool consistency. Monitor electrolytes, B/P, weight, serum glucose. Watch for hypocalcemia (muscle twitching, cramps), hypokalemia (weakness, paresthesia [esp. lower extremities], nausea/vomiting, irritability, EKG changes). Assess emotional status, ability to sleep.

PATIENT/FAMILY TEACHING

• Report fever, sore throat, muscle aches, sudden weight gain, swelling, visual disturbances, behavioral changes. • Do not take aspirin or any other medication without consulting physician. • Limit caffeine, avoid alcohol. • Inform dentist, other physicians of cortisone therapy now or within past 12 mos. • Caution against overusing joints injected for symptomatic relief. • **Topical:** Apply after shower or bath for best absorption. • Do not cover or use occlusive dressings unless ordered by physician; do not use tight diapers, plastic pants, coverings. • Avoid contact with eyes.

---

hydromorphone

hye-droe-**mor**-fone
(Dilaudid, Dilaudid HP, Exalgo, Hydromorph Contin ❋)

BLACK BOX ALERT High abuse potential, respiratory depression risk. Other opioids, alcohol, CNS depressants increase risk of potentially fatal respiratory depression. Highly

---

concentrated (Dilaudid HP, 10 mg/ml) form not to be interchanged with less concentrated (Dilaudid) form; overdose, death may result. **Do not confuse Dilaudid with demerol or Dilantin, or hydromorphone with hydrocodone or morphine.**

♦ **CLASSIFICATION**

PHARMACOTHERAPEUTIC: Opioid agonist **(Schedule II). CLINICAL:** Narcotic analgesic, antitussive.

ACTION

Binds to opioid receptors in CNS, reducing intensity of pain stimuli from sensory nerve endings. **Therapeutic Effect:** Alters perception, emotional response to pain; suppresses cough reflex.

PHARMACOKINETICS

Route	Onset	Peak	Duration
PO	30 min	90–120 min	4 hrs
IV	10–15 min	15–30 min	2–3 hrs
IM	15 min	30–60 min	4–5 hrs
Subcutaneous	15 min	30–90 min	4 hrs
Rectal	15–30 min	N/A	N/A

Well absorbed from GI tract after IM administration. Widely distributed. Metabolized in liver. Excreted in urine. **Half-life:** 2.6–4 hrs.

USES

Relief of moderate to severe pain. Extended-release tablet (Exalgo): Around the clock, continuous analgesia for extended period.

PRECAUTIONS

Contraindications: Acute or severe asthma, severe respiratory depression. **Dilaudid liquids and tablets:** Obstetric analgesia. **Dilaudid injection:** Opioid-intolerant pts, pts at risk of developing GI obstruction. **Exalgos:** Opioid-intolerant pts, preexisting GI surgery/diseases causing GI narrowing, GI obstruction. **Cautions:** Severe hepatic, renal, respiratory disease; hypothyroidism, myxedema, respiratory depression, adrenal cortical insufficiency, seizures, acute abdominal conditions, acute alcoholism, head injury, intracranial lesions, prostatic hypertrophy, Addison's disease, urethral stricture, pancreatitis, biliary tract disease.

⧖ LIFESPAN CONSIDERATIONS

Pregnancy/Lactation: Readily crosses placenta. Unknown if distributed in breast milk. May prolong labor if administered in latent phase of first stage of labor or before cervical dilation of 4–5 cm has occurred. Respiratory depression may occur in neonate if mother receives opiates during labor. Regular use of opiates during pregnancy may produce withdrawal symptoms in the neonate (irritability, excessive crying, tremors, hyperactive reflexes, fever, vomiting, diarrhea, yawning, sneezing, seizures). **Pregnancy Category C (D if used for prolonged periods or at high dosages at term). Children:** Those younger than 2 yrs may be more susceptible to respiratory depression. **Elderly:** May be more susceptible to respiratory depression, may cause paradoxical excitement. Age-related renal impairment, prostatic hypertrophy or obstruction may increase risk of urinary retention; dosage adjustment recommended.

INTERACTIONS

DRUG: Alcohol, other CNS depressants may increase CNS, respiratory depression, hypotension. **HERBAL: Gotu kola, kava kava, St. John's wort, valerian** may increase CNS depression. **FOOD:** None known. **LAB VALUES:** May increase serum amylase, lipase.

AVAILABILITY (Rx)

Injection, Powder for Reconstitution (Dilaudid HP): 250 mg. **Injection, Solution (Dilaudid):** 1 mg/ml, 2 mg/ml, 4 mg/ml, 10 mg/ml. **Liquid, Oral:** 1 mg/ml. **Suppository (Dilaudid):** 3 mg. **Tablets (Dilaudid):** 2 mg, 4 mg, 8 mg.

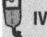 Tablets, Extended-Release (Exalgo): 8 mg, 12 mg, 16 mg, 32 mg.

ADMINISTRATION/HANDLING
IV

◀ALERT▶ High concentration injection (10 mg/ml) should be used only in those tolerant to opiate agonists, currently receiving high doses of another opiate agonist for severe, chronic pain due to cancer.

Reconstitution • May give undiluted. • May further dilute with 5 ml Sterile Water for Injection or 0.9% NaCl.

Rate of Administration • Administer IV push very slowly (over 2–3 min). • Rapid IV increases risk of severe adverse reactions (chest wall rigidity, apnea, peripheral circulatory collapse, anaphylactoid effects, cardiac arrest).

Storage • Store at room temperature; protect from light. • Slight yellow discoloration of parenteral form does not indicate loss of potency.

IM, Subcutaneous

• Use short 25- to 30-gauge needle for subcutaneous injection. • Administer slowly; rotate injection sites. • Pts with circulatory impairment experience higher risk of overdosage due to delayed absorption of repeated administration.

PO

• Give without regard to meals. • Tablets may be crushed. • Extended-release tablets must be swallowed whole; do not break, crush, dissolve, or inject.

Rectal

• Refrigerate suppositories. • Moisten suppository with cold water before inserting well up into rectum.

▦ IV INCOMPATIBILITIES

Amphotericin B complex (Abelcet, AmBisome, Amphotec), cefazolin (Ancef, Kefzol), diazepam (Valium), phenobarbital, phenytoin (Dilantin).

▦ IV COMPATIBILITIES

Dexmedetomidine (Precedex), diltiazem (Cardizem), diphenhydramine (Benadryl), dobutamine (Dobutrex), dopamine (Intropin), fentanyl (Sublimaze), furosemide (Lasix), heparin, lorazepam (Ativan), magnesium sulfate, metoclopramide (Reglan), midazolam (Versed), milrinone (Primacor), morphine, propofol (Diprivan).

INDICATIONS/ROUTES/DOSAGE

Analgesia
PO: ADULTS, ELDERLY: 2–4 mg q3–4h. Range: 2–8 mg/dose. **CHILDREN, ADOLESCENTS WEIGHING MORE THAN 50 KG:** 1–2 mg q3–4h. **CHILDREN OLDER THAN 6 MOS AND WEIGHING LESS THAN 50 KG:** 0.03–0.08 mg/kg/dose q3–4h.

Extended-Release: ADULTS, ELDERLY: Range: 8–64 mg once daily.

IV: ADULTS, ELDERLY, CHILDREN WEIGHING MORE THAN 50 KG (FOR OPIATE-NAIVE PT): 0.2–0.6 mg q2–3h. **USUAL DOSAGE:** 1–2 mg q3–4h. **CHILDREN WEIGHING 50 KG OR LESS:** 0.015 mg/kg/dose q3–6h as needed.

Rectal: ADULTS, ELDERLY: 3 mg q6–8h.

Patient-Controlled Analgesia (PCA)
IV: ADULTS, ELDERLY: (Usual concentration: 0.2 mg/ml). Initially, 0.1–0.2 mg. Range: 0.05–0.4 mg. Lockout interval: 6 min. Range: 5–10 min.

Epidural: ADULTS, ELDERLY: Bolus dose of 0.4–1 mg; infusion rate: 0.03–0.3 mg/hr; demand dose: 0.02–0.05 mg. Lockout interval: 10–15 min.

SIDE EFFECTS

Frequent: Drowsiness, dizziness, hypotension (including orthostatic hypotension), decreased appetite. **Occasional:** Confusion, diaphoresis, facial flushing, urinary retention, constipation, dry mouth, nausea, vomiting, headache, pain at injection site. **Rare:** Allergic reaction, depression.

ADVERSE EFFECTS/ TOXIC REACTIONS

Overdose results in respiratory depression, skeletal muscle flaccidity, cold/

H

clammy skin, cyanosis, extreme drowsiness progressing to seizures, stupor, coma. Tolerance to analgesic effect, physical dependence may occur with repeated use. Prolonged duration of action, cumulative effect may occur in those with hepatic/renal impairment. **Antidote:** Naloxone (see Appendix K).

NURSING CONSIDERATIONS

BASELINE ASSESSMENT

Obtain vital signs. If respirations are 12/min or less (20/min or less in children), withhold medication, contact physician. **Analgesic:** Assess onset, type, location, duration of pain. Effect of medication is reduced if full pain recurs before next dose. **Antitussive:** Assess type, severity, frequency of cough.

INTERVENTION/EVALUATION

Monitor vital signs; assess for pain relief, cough. To prevent pain cycles, instruct pt to request pain medication as soon as discomfort begins. Monitor daily pattern of bowel activity, stool consistency (esp. in long-term use). Initiate deep breathing and coughing exercises, particularly in pts with pulmonary impairment. Assess for clinical improvement; record onset of relief of pain, cough.

PATIENT/FAMILY TEACHING

• Avoid alcohol. • Avoid tasks that require alertness/motor skills until response to drug is established. • Tolerance or dependence may occur with prolonged use at high dosages. • Change positions slowly to avoid orthostatic hypotension. • Do not break, crush, chew, dissolve extended-release tablets.

hydroxychloroquine

hye-drox-ee-**klor**-oh-kwin
(Apo-Hydroxyquine ✦, Plaquenil)

BLACK BOX ALERT Should be given by physicians familiar with prescribing information before use. **Do not confuse hydroxychloroquine with hydrocortisone or hydroxyzine, or Plaquenil with Platinol.**

◆CLASSIFICATION

PHARMACOTHERAPEUTIC: Aminoquinoline antimalarial. **CLINICAL:** Antimalarial, antirheumatic.

ACTION

Concentrates in parasite acid vesicles, interfering with parasite protein (DNA/RNA) synthesis. Antirheumatic action may involve suppressing formation of antigens responsible for hypersensitivity reactions. **Therapeutic Effect:** Inhibits parasite growth.

PHARMACOKINETICS

Variable rate of absorption. Widely distributed in body tissues (eyes, kidneys, liver, lungs). Protein binding: 45%. Partially metabolized in liver. Partially excreted in urine. **Half-life:** 32 days (in plasma), 50 days (in blood).

USES

Suppression and treatment of acute attacks of malaria. Treatment of systematic lupus erythematosus, rheumatoid arthritis (RA). **OFF-LABEL:** Porphyria.

PRECAUTIONS

Contraindications: Long-term therapy for children, psoriasis, retinal or visual field changes, porphyria. **Cautions:** Alcoholism, hepatic disease, G6PD deficiency. Concurrent medications that are hepatotoxic. Children are esp. susceptible to hydroxychloroquine fatalities.

⌛ LIFESPAN CONSIDERATIONS

Pregnancy/Lactation: Crosses placenta; distributed in breast milk. **Pregnancy Category C. Children:** Long-term therapy not recommended. **Elderly:** No age-related precautions noted.

INTERACTIONS

DRUG: May increase concentration of **dapsone. HERBAL: Echinacea** may decrease concentration. **FOOD:** None known. **LAB VALUES:** None significant.

AVAILABILITY (Rx)

Tablets: 200 mg (155 mg base).

ADMINISTRATION/HANDLING

PO
• Give with food or milk.

INDICATIONS/ROUTES/DOSAGE

Treatment of Acute Malaria
PO:

Dose	Times	Adults	Children
Initial	Day 1	800 mg	13 mg/kg
Second	6 hrs later	400 mg	6.5 mg/kg
Third	Day 2	400 mg	6.5 mg/kg
Fourth	Day 3	400 mg	6.5 mg/kg

Suppression of Malaria
PO: ADULTS: 400 mg base weekly on same day each wk, beginning 2 wks before entering an endemic area and continuing for 4–6 wks after leaving the area. **CHILDREN:** 6.5 mg/kg/wk, beginning 2 wks before entering an endemic area and continuing for 4–6 wks after leaving the area. If therapy is not begun before exposure, administer a loading dose of 13 mg/kg in 2 equally divided doses 6 hrs apart, followed by the usual dosage regimen.

Rheumatoid Arthritis (RA)
PO: ADULTS: Initially, 400–600 mg (310–465 mg base) daily for 5–10 days, gradually increased to optimum response level. Maintenance (usually within 4–12 wks): Dosage decreased by 50% and then continued at maintenance dose of 200–400 mg (155–310 mg base) daily. Maximum effect may not be seen for several mos.

Lupus Erythematosus
PO: ADULTS: Initially, 400 mg (310 mg base) once or twice a day for several wks or mos. Maintenance: 200–400 mg/day (155–310 mg base).

SIDE EFFECTS

Frequent: Transient headache, anorexia, nausea, vomiting. **Occasional:** Visual disturbances, anxiety, fatigue, pruritus (esp. palms, soles, scalp), irritability, personality changes, diarrhea, photosensitivity. **Rare:** Stomatitis, dermatitis, impaired hearing.

ADVERSE EFFECTS/ TOXIC REACTIONS

Ocular toxicity (esp. retinopathy) may progress even after drug is discontinued. **Prolonged therapy:** Peripheral neuritis, neuromyopathy, hypotension, EKG changes, agranulocytosis, aplastic anemia, thrombocytopenia, seizures, psychosis. **Overdosage:** Headache, vomiting, visual disturbances, drowsiness, seizures, hypokalemia followed by cardiovascular collapse, death.

NURSING CONSIDERATIONS

BASELINE ASSESSMENT
Evaluate CBC, hepatic function tests, vision.

INTERVENTION/EVALUATION
Monitor CBC. Observe for muscular weakness. Evaluate for GI distress. Monitor hepatic function tests. Assess skin/buccal mucosa; inquire about pruritus. Report impaired vision/hearing immediately.

PATIENT/FAMILY TEACHING
• Avoid exposure to direct sunlight. • Avoid alcohol. • Explain need for eye exams q3mos with prolonged therapy. • Immediately report **any** new visual difficulties, muscular weakness, impaired hearing, tinnitus, numbness, tremors, rash, persistent diarrhea, emotional changes.

hydroxyurea · HIGH ALERT

hye-**drox**-ee-yoo-**ree**-a
(Apo-Hydroxyurea ✤, Droxia, Hydrea)

✤ Canadian trade name   Non-Crushable Drug   HIGH ALERT High Alert drug

BLACK BOX ALERT Must be administered by personnel trained in administration/handling of chemotherapeutic agents or in treatment of sickle cell anemia. Carcinogenic risk; secondary leukemias reported with long-term treatment.

Do not confuse hydroxyurea with hydroxyzine.

◆CLASSIFICATION

PHARMACOTHERAPEUTIC: Synthetic urea analogue. **CLINICAL:** Antineoplastic (see p. 86C).

ACTION

Inhibits DNA synthesis without interfering with RNA synthesis or protein. **Therapeutic Effect:** Interferes with normal repair process of cancer cells damaged by irradiation.

PHARMACOKINETICS

Well absorbed from GI tract. Protein binding: 75%–80%. Metabolized in liver. Excreted in urine as urea and unchanged drug. **Half-life:** 3–4 hrs.

USES

Treatment of melanoma, resistant chronic myelocytic leukemia, recurrent, metastatic, inoperable ovarian carcinoma. Used in combination with radiation therapy for local control of primary squamous cell carcinoma of head/neck, excluding lip. Treatment of sickle cell anemia with at least 3 painful crises in previous 12 mos. **OFF-LABEL:** Treatment of hematologic conditions (e.g., polycythemia vera), cervical cancer, essential thrombocythemia, hyperleukocytosis due to AML, treatment of meningiomas.

PRECAUTIONS

Contraindications: WBC count less than 2,500/mm³ or platelet count less than 100,000/mm³, severe anemia in sickle cell anemia. **Cautions:** Previous irradiation therapy, concurrent use with other cytoxic drugs, renal/hepatic impairment.

⌛ LIFESPAN CONSIDERATIONS

Pregnancy/Lactation: Crosses placenta; distributed in breast milk. May cause fetal harm. **Pregnancy Category D. Children:** Safety and efficacy not established. **Elderly:** More sensitive to hydroxyurea effects; may require lower dosage.

INTERACTIONS

DRUG: Bone marrow depressants may increase myelosuppression. **Live virus vaccines** may potentiate virus replication, increase vaccine side effects, decrease the pt's antibody response to vaccine. **HERBAL: Echinacea** may decrease effect. **FOOD:** None known. **LAB VALUES:** May increase BUN, serum creatinine, uric acid.

AVAILABILITY (Rx)

Capsules: 200 mg (Droxia), 300 mg (Droxia), 400 mg (Droxia), 500 mg (Hydrea).

ADMINISTRATION/HANDLING

Capsules may be opened and emptied into water (will not dissolve completely).

INDICATIONS/ROUTES/DOSAGE

◀**ALERT**▶ Therapy interrupted when platelet count falls below 100,000/mm³ or WBC count falls below 2,500/mm³. Resume when counts return to normal.

Melanoma; Recurrent, Metastatic, Inoperable Ovarian Carcinoma
PO: ADULTS, ELDERLY: 80 mg/kg every 3 days or 20–30 mg/kg/day as a single dose.

Control of Primary Squamous Cell Carcinoma of Head/Neck, Excluding Lips (in Combination with Radiation Therapy)
PO (Intermittent Therapy): ADULTS, ELDERLY: 80 mg/kg every 3 days, beginning at least 7 days before starting radiation therapy. **(Continuous Therapy):** 20–30 mg/kg once daily.

Resistant Chronic Myelocytic Leukemia
PO: ADULTS, ELDERLY: 20–30 mg/kg once a day.

Sickle Cell Anemia
PO: ADULTS, ELDERLY: Initially, 15 mg/kg once a day. May increase by 5 mg/kg/day every 12 wks. **Maximum:** 35 mg/kg/day. **CHILDREN:** 20 mg/kg/dose once daily; increase by 5 mg/kg/dose q2–6mos. **Maximum:** 35 mg/kg/day (2,000 mg).

SIDE EFFECTS

Frequent: Nausea, vomiting, anorexia, constipation or diarrhea. Occasional: Mild, reversible rash; facial flushing; pruritus; fever; chills; malaise. Rare: Alopecia, headache, drowsiness, dizziness, disorientation.

ADVERSE EFFECTS/ TOXIC REACTIONS

Myelosuppression manifested as hematologic toxicity (leukopenia and, to a lesser extent, thrombocytopenia, anemia).

NURSING CONSIDERATIONS

BASELINE ASSESSMENT

Obtain bone marrow studies, hepatic/renal function tests before therapy begins, periodically thereafter. Obtain Hgb, WBC, platelet count, serum uric acid at baseline and weekly during therapy. Pts with marked renal impairment may develop visual or auditory hallucinations, marked hematologic toxicity.

INTERVENTION/EVALUATION

Monitor daily pattern of bowel activity, stool consistency. Monitor for hematologic toxicity (fever, sore throat, signs of local infection, unusual bleeding/bruising at any site), symptoms of anemia (excessive fatigue, weakness). Assess skin for rash, erythema. Monitor CBC with differential, renal/hepatic function, uric acid.

PATIENT/FAMILY TEACHING

• Promptly report fever, sore throat, signs of local infection, unusual bleeding/bruising at any site.

*hydrOXYzine

hye-**drox**-ee-zeen
(Apo-Hydroxyzine ✤, Atarax ✤, Novo-Hydroxyzin ✤, Vistaril)
Do not confuse hydroxyzine with hydralazine or hydroxyurea, or Vistaril with Restoril, Versed, or Zestril.

◆CLASSIFICATION

PHARMACOTHERAPEUTIC: Piperazine derivative. **CLINICAL:** Antihistamine, antianxiety, antispasmodic, antiemetic, antipruritic (see pp. 15C, 55C).

ACTION

Competes with histamine for receptor sites in GI tract, blood vessels, respiratory tract. Diminishes vestibular stimulation, depresses labyrinthine function. **Therapeutic Effect:** Produces anxiolytic, anticholinergic, antihistaminic, analgesic effects; relaxes skeletal muscle; controls nausea, vomiting.

PHARMACOKINETICS

Route	Onset	Peak	Duration
PO	15–30 min	N/A	4–6 hrs

Well absorbed from GI tract and after parenteral administration. Metabolized in liver. Primarily excreted in urine. Not removed by hemodialysis. **Half-life:** 3–7 hrs (increased in elderly).

USES

Antiemetic, treatment of anxiety, preop sedation, antipruritic.

PRECAUTIONS

Contraindications: Early pregnancy; subcutaneous, intravenous administration.

H

---

* "Tall Man" lettering   ✤ Canadian trade name   🏴 Non-Crushable Drug   🔲 High Alert drug

Cautions: Narrow-angle glaucoma, prostatic hypertrophy, bladder neck obstruction, asthma, COPD.

⌛ LIFESPAN CONSIDERATIONS

Pregnancy/Lactation: Unknown if drug crosses placenta or is distributed in breast milk. **Pregnancy Category C. Children:** Not recommended in newborns or premature infants (increased risk of anticholinergic effects). Paradoxical excitement may occur. **Elderly:** Increased risk of dizziness, sedation, confusion. Hypotension, hyperexcitability may occur.

INTERACTIONS

DRUG: Alcohol, other CNS depressants may increase CNS depressant effects. **HERBAL: Gotu kola, kava kava, St. John's wort, valerian** may increase CNS depression. **FOOD:** None known. **LAB VALUES:** May cause false-positive urine 17-hydroxycorticosteroid determinations.

AVAILABILITY (Rx)

Injection Solution (Vistaril): 25 mg/ml, 50 mg/ml. **Oral Solution (Vistaril):** 10 mg/5 ml. **Syrup:** 10 mg/5 ml. **Tablets:** 10 mg, 25 mg, 50 mg.

Capsules (Vistaril): 25 mg, 50 mg, 100 mg.

ADMINISTRATION/HANDLING

IM

◀ALERT▶ Significant tissue damage, thrombosis, gangrene may occur if injection is given subcutaneous, intra-arterial, or by IV.
• IM may be given undiluted. • Use Z-track technique of injection to prevent subcutaneous infiltration. • Inject deep IM into gluteus maximus or midlateral thigh in adults, midlateral thigh in children.

PO

• May give without regard to food. • Shake oral suspension well. • Scored tablets may be crushed; do not crush/break capsule.

INDICATIONS/ROUTES/DOSAGE

Anxiety

PO: ADULTS, ELDERLY: 50–100 mg 4 times a day. **Maximum:** 600 mg/day. **CHILDREN 6 YRS AND OLDER:** 50–100 mg/day in divided doses. **CHILDREN YOUNGER THAN 6 YRS:** 50 mg/day in divided doses.

Nausea/Vomiting

IM: ADULTS, ELDERLY: 25–100 mg/dose q4–6h.

Pruritus

PO: ADULTS, ELDERLY: 25 mg 3–4 times a day. **CHILDREN 6 YRS AND OLDER:** 50–100 mg/day in divided doses. **CHILDREN YOUNGER THAN 6 YRS:** 50 mg/day in divided doses.

Preop Sedation

PO: ADULTS, ELDERLY: 50–100 mg. **CHILDREN:** 0.6 mg/kg/dose.
IM: ADULTS, ELDERLY: 25–100 mg. **CHILDREN:** 1.1 mg/kg/dose.

SIDE EFFECTS

Side effects are generally mild, transient. **Frequent:** Drowsiness, dry mouth, marked discomfort with IM injection. **Occasional:** Dizziness, ataxia, asthenia (loss of strength, energy), slurred speech, headache, agitation, increased anxiety. **Rare:** Paradoxical reactions (hyperactivity, anxiety in children; excitement, restlessness in elderly or debilitated pts) generally noted during first 2 wks of therapy, particularly in presence of uncontrolled pain.

ADVERSE EFFECTS/ TOXIC REACTIONS

Hypersensitivity reaction (wheezing, dyspnea, chest tightness) may occur.

NURSING CONSIDERATIONS

BASELINE ASSESSMENT

Anxiety: Offer emotional support. Assess motor responses (agitation, trembling, tension), autonomic responses (cold/clammy hands, diaphoresis). **Antiemetic:**

Assess for dehydration (poor skin turgor, dry mucous membranes, longitudinal furrows in tongue).

INTERVENTION/EVALUATION

For pts on long-term therapy, hepatic/renal function tests, blood counts should be performed periodically. Monitor lung sounds for signs of hypersensitivity reaction. Monitor serum electrolytes in pts with severe vomiting. Assess for paradoxical reaction, particularly during early therapy. Assist with ambulation if drowsiness, light-headedness occur.

PATIENT/FAMILY TEACHING

• Marked discomfort may occur with IM injection. • Sugarless gum, sips of water may relieve dry mouth. • Drowsiness usually diminishes with continued therapy. • Avoid tasks that require alertness, motor skills until response to drug is established.

hyoscyamine

hye-oh-sye-a-meen
(Anaspaz, Hyosyne, Levbid, Levsin, Levsin S/L, Nu-Lev, Symax SL, Symax SR)
Do not confuse Anaspaz with Anaprox, or Levbid with Lithobid or Lopid.

FIXED COMBINATIONS

Donnatal: hyoscyamine/atropine (anticholinergic)/phenobarbital (sedative)/scopolamine (anticholinergic): 0.1037 mg/0.0194 mg/16.2 mg/0.0065 mg.

◆CLASSIFICATION

PHARMACOTHERAPEUTIC: Anticholinergic. **CLINICAL:** Antimuscarinic, antispasmodic.

ACTION

Inhibits action of acetylcholine at postganglionic (muscarinic) receptor sites. **Therapeutic Effect:** Decreases secretions (bronchial, salivary, sweat gland, gastric juices). Reduces motility of GI, urinary tracts.

PHARMACOKINETICS

Route	Onset	Peak	Duration
PO	15–30 min	—	4–6 hrs

Well absorbed following PO administration. Protein binding: 50%. Metabolized in liver. Excreted in urine. Removed by hemodialysis. **Half-life:** 3.5 hrs (immediate-release); 7 hrs (sustained-release).

USES

PO: Adjunctive therapy for peptic ulcer disease, irritable bowel syndrome, neurogenic bladder or bowel; treatment of infantile colic, GI tract disorders caused by spasm, hypermotility of lower urinary tract; reduce abdominal rigidity; reduce tremors associated with Parkinson's disease; drying agent in acute rhinitis. **Parenteral:** Preoperatively to reduce secretions, block cardiac vagal inhibitory reflexes; relief of biliary, renal colic; reduce GI motility to facilitate diagnostic procedures; reduce pain, hypersecretion in pancreatitis; reversal of neuromuscular blockade.

PRECAUTIONS

Contraindications: GI/GU obstruction, myasthenia gravis, narrow-angle glaucoma, paralytic ileus, severe ulcerative colitis. **Cautions:** Hyperthyroidism, HF, cardiac arrhythmias, prostatic hypertrophy, neuropathy, chronic lung disease, biliary tract disease.

⌛ LIFESPAN CONSIDERATIONS

Pregnancy/Lactation: Crosses placenta; distributed in breast milk. **Pregnancy Category C. Children:** Safety and efficacy not established. **Elderly:** No age-related precautions noted.

INTERACTIONS

DRUG: Antacids may decrease absorption. **Other anticholinergics** may increase effects. **HERBAL:** None significant.

FOOD: None known. **LAB VALUES:** None significant.

AVAILABILITY (Rx)

Capsules, Timed-Release: 0.375 mg.
Elixir (Hyosyne, Levsin): 0.125 mg/5 ml.
Injection, Solution (Levsin): 0.5 mg/ml.
Solution, Oral Drops (Hyosyne, Levsin): 0.125 mg/ml. **Tablets (Anaspaz, Levsin):** 0.125 mg. **Tablets, Orally Disintegrating (Anaspaz):** 0.125 mg. **Tablets, Sublingual (Levsin S/L, Symax SL):** 0.125 mg.

Tablets, Extended-Release (Levbid, Symax SR): 0.375 mg.

ADMINISTRATION/HANDLING

PO
• Give before meals. • Immediate-release tablets may be crushed, chewed. • Extended-release tablet should be administered whole. • Allow orally disintegrating tablet placed on tongue to dissolve before swallowing; may give with or without water.
• Sublingual: Place under tongue.

Parenteral
• May give undiluted.

INDICATIONS/ROUTES/DOSAGE

GI Tract Disorders
PO *(Sublingual):* **ADULTS, ELDERLY, CHILDREN 12 YRS AND OLDER:** 0.125–0.25 mg q4h as needed. **CHILDREN 2–11 YRS:** 0.0625–0.125 mg q4h as needed. **Maximum:** 0.75 mg/day. **ADULTS, ELDERLY:** *(Extended-Release):* 0.375–0.75 mg q12h. **Maximum:** 1.5 mg/day.
IV, IM: ADULTS, ELDERLY, CHILDREN 12 YRS AND OLDER: 0.25–0.5 mg. May repeat as needed up to 4 times/day at 4-hr intervals.

Hypermotility of Lower Urinary Tract
PO *(Sublingual):* **ADULTS, ELDERLY:** 0.15–0.3 mg 4 times a day. **(EXTENDED-RELEASE):** 0.375 mg q12h.

Infant Colic
PO: INFANTS: Drops dosed q4h as needed (based on weight): 2.3 kg: 3 drops; 3.4 kg: 4 drops; 5 kg: 5 drops; 7 kg: 6 drops; 10 kg: 8 drops; 15 kg: 11 drops.

SIDE EFFECTS

Frequent: Dry mouth, decreased diaphoresis, constipation. **Occasional:** Blurred vision, bloated feeling, urinary hesitancy, drowsiness (with high dosage), headache, intolerance to light, loss of taste, anxiety, flushing, insomnia, impotence, mental confusion or excitement (particularly in elderly, children), temporary light-headedness (with parenteral form), local irritation (with parenteral form). **Rare:** Dizziness, faintness.

ADVERSE EFFECTS/ TOXIC REACTIONS

Overdose may produce temporary paralysis of ciliary muscle, pupillary dilation, tachycardia, palpitations, hot/dry/flushed skin, absence of bowel sounds, hyperthermia, increased respiratory rate, EKG abnormalities, nausea, vomiting; rash over face/upper trunk, CNS stimulation, psychosis (agitation, restlessness, rambling speech, visual hallucinations, paranoid behavior, delusions) followed by depression.

NURSING CONSIDERATIONS

BASELINE ASSESSMENT
Before giving medication, instruct pt to void (reduces risk of urinary retention).

INTERVENTION/EVALUATION
Monitor daily pattern of bowel activity, stool consistency. Palpate bladder for urinary retention. Monitor changes in B/P, temperature. Assess skin turgor, mucous membranes to evaluate hydration status (encourage adequate fluid intake), bowel sounds for peristalsis. Be alert for fever (increased risk of hyperthermia).

PATIENT/FAMILY TEACHING
• May cause dry mouth; maintain proper oral hygiene habits (lack of saliva may increase risk of cavities). • Report rash, eye pain, difficulty in urinating, constipation. • Avoid tasks that require alertness, motor skills until response to drug is established. • Avoid hot baths, saunas.

ibandronate

eye-**ban**-droe-nate
(Boniva)

◆CLASSIFICATION

PHARMACOTHERAPEUTIC: Bisphosphonate. **CLINICAL:** Calcium regulator (see p. 142C).

ACTION

Binds to bone hydroxyapatite (part of mineral matrix of bone), inhibits osteoclast activity. **Therapeutic Effect:** Reduces rate of bone turnover, bone resorption, resulting in net gain in bone mass.

PHARMACOKINETICS

Absorbed in upper GI tract. Extent of absorption impaired by food, beverages (other than plain water). Protein binding: 85%–99%. Rapidly binds to bone. Unabsorbed portion eliminated in urine. **Half-life: PO:** 37–157 hrs; **IV:** 5–25 hrs.

USES

Treatment/prevention of osteoporosis in postmenopausal women. **OFF-LABEL:** Hypercalcemia of malignancy; reduces bone pain from metastatic bone disease.

PRECAUTIONS

Contraindications: Hypersensitivity to other bisphosphonates (e.g., alendronate, etidronate, pamidronate, risedronate, tiludronate); inability to stand or sit upright for at least 60 min; abnormalities of the esophagus that would delay emptying, hypocalcemia. **Cautions:** GI diseases (duodenitis, dysphagia, esophagitis, gastritis, ulcers [drug may exacerbate these conditions]); renal impairment with creatinine clearance less than 30 ml/min.

⏳ LIFESPAN CONSIDERATIONS

Pregnancy/Lactation: Potential for teratogenic effects. Unknown if distributed in breast milk. Breastfeeding not recommended. **Pregnancy Category C. Children:** Safety and efficacy not established. **Elderly:** No age-related precautions noted.

INTERACTIONS

DRUG: Antacids containing aluminum, calcium, magnesium; vitamin D decrease absorption. **Aspirin, NSAIDs** may increase GI irritation. **HERBAL:** None significant. **FOOD: Beverages (other than plain water), dietary supplements, food** interfere with absorption. **LAB VALUES:** May decrease serum alkaline phosphatase. May increase serum cholesterol.

AVAILABILITY (Rx)

Injection Solution: 3 mg/3 ml syringe.
Tablets: 150 mg.

ADMINISTRATION/HANDLING

PO
• Give 60 min before first food, beverage of the day, on an empty stomach with 6–8 oz plain water (not mineral water) while pt is standing or sitting in upright position. • Pt cannot lie down for 60 min following drug administration. • Instruct pt to swallow whole; do not chew, suck tablet (potential for oropharyngeal ulceration).

 IV

• Give over 15–30 sec.

INDICATIONS/ROUTES/DOSAGE

Osteoporosis
PO *(Prevention/Treatment)*: **ADULTS, ELDERLY:** 150 mg once monthly.
IV *(Treatment)*: **ADULTS, ELDERLY:** 3 mg q3mos.

Dosage in Renal Impairment
Not recommended for pts with creatinine clearance less than 30 ml/min.

SIDE EFFECTS

Frequent (13%–6%): Back pain, dyspepsia (epigastric distress, heartburn), peripheral discomfort, diarrhea, headache, myalgia. **IV:** Abdominal pain, dyspepsia, constipation, nausea, diarrhea. **Occasional**

(4%–3%): Dizziness, arthralgia, asthenia (loss of strength, energy). **Rare (2% or less):** Vomiting, hypersensitivity reaction.

ADVERSE EFFECTS/ TOXIC REACTIONS

Upper respiratory infection occurs occasionally. Overdose results in hypocalcemia, hypophosphatemia, significant GI disturbances.

NURSING CONSIDERATIONS

BASELINE ASSESSMENT

Hypocalcemia, vitamin D deficiency must be corrected before beginning therapy. Obtain laboratory baselines, esp. serum chemistries, renal function. Obtain results of bone density study.

INTERVENTION/EVALUATION

Monitor electrolytes, esp. serum calcium, alkaline phosphatase. Monitor renal function tests.

PATIENT/FAMILY TEACHING

• Expected benefits occur only when medication is taken with full glass (6–8 oz) of plain water, first thing in the morning and at least 60 min before first food, beverage, medication of the day. Any other beverage (mineral water, orange juice, coffee) significantly reduces absorption of medication. • Do not lie down for at least 60 min after taking medication (potentiates delivery to stomach, reduces risk of esophageal irritation). • Report swallowing difficulties, pain when swallowing, chest pain, new/worsening heartburn. • Consider weight-bearing exercises; modify behavioral factors (e.g., cigarette smoking, alcohol consumption). • Calcium and vitamin D supplements should be taken if dietary intake inadequate.

ibritumomab

ib-rye-**tyoo**-mo-mab
(Zevalin)

BLACK BOX ALERT Severe, potentially fatal infusion reactions (angioedema, hypoxia, marked hypotension, myocardial infarction) reported, usually within 30–130 min of rituximab infusion (cotherapy). Prolonged, severe cytopenia occurs in most pts. Severe cutaneous, mucocutaneous reactions (including fatalities) have been reported. Must be administered by personnel trained in administration/handling of radioisotopes.

◆CLASSIFICATION

PHARMACOTHERAPEUTIC: Monoclonal antibody. **CLINICAL:** Antineoplastic (see p. 86C).

ACTION

Combines targeting power of monoclonal antibodies (MAbs) with cancer-killing ability of radiation. **Therapeutic Effect:** Targets CD antigen (present in greater than 90% of pts with B-cell non-Hodgkin's lymphoma), inducing cellular damage.

PHARMACOKINETICS

Tumor uptake is greater than normal tissue in non-Hodgkin's lymphoma. Most of dose cleared by binding to tumor. Minimally excreted in urine. **Half-life:** 27–30 hrs.

USES

Treatment of non-Hodgkin's lymphoma (NHL) in combination with rituximab in pts with relapsed or refractory low-grade, follicular, or CD20-positive transformed B-cell non-Hodgkin's lymphoma. Pts with previously untreated follicular NHL who achieve a partial or complete response to first-line chemotherapy.

PRECAUTIONS

Contraindications: None known. **Cautions:** Platelet count less than 100,000 cells/mm³, neutrophil count less than 1,500 cells/mm³, history of failed stem cell collection.

⌛ LIFESPAN CONSIDERATIONS

Pregnancy/Lactation: May cause fetal harm. Pts with childbearing potential should use contraceptive methods during and up to 12 mos after therapy. **Pregnancy Category D. Children:** Safety and efficacy not established. **Elderly:** No age-related precautions noted.

INTERACTIONS

DRUG: Antiplatelets, anticoagulants increase potential for prolonged/severe thrombocytopenia. **HERBAL: Cat's claw, dong quai, evening primrose, fever-few, garlic, ginkgo, ginseng, horse chestnut, red clover** may increase antiplatelet activity. **Echinacea** may decrease effect. **FOOD:** None known. **LAB VALUES:** May decrease platelet count, neutrophil count, Hgb, Hct.

AVAILABILITY (Rx)

Injection Solution: 3.2-mg vial (1.6 mg/ml).

ADMINISTRATION/HANDLING

Rate of Administration • Give IV push over 10 min through a 0.22-micron, low protein-binding in-line filter. After injection, flush line with 10 ml 0.9% NaCl.

▧ IV INCOMPATIBILITIES

Do not mix with any medications.

INDICATIONS/ROUTES/DOSAGE

Non-Hodgkin's Lymphoma
IV: ADULTS, ELDERLY: Regimen consists of two steps: Step 1: Single infusion of 250 mg/m^2 rituximab at initial rate of 50 mg/hr. Increase infusion by 50 mg/hr q30min up to a maximum of 400 mg/hr. Step 2: Follows step 1 by 7–9 days and consists of a second infusion of 250 mg/m^2 rituximab preceding (4 hrs or less) a fixed dose of 0.4 mCi/kg of Y-90 ibritumomab administered IV push over 10 min. ◀ALERT▶ Reduce dosage to 0.3 mCi/kg if platelet count is 100,000–149,000 cells/mm^3. Do not administer if platelet count is less than 100,000 cells/mm^3.

SIDE EFFECTS

Frequent (43%–24%): Asthenia (loss of strength, energy), nausea, chills. **Occa-**sional (17%–10%): Fever, abdominal pain, dyspnea, headache, vomiting, dizziness, cough, oral candidiasis. **Rare (9%–5%):** Pruritus, diarrhea, back pain, peripheral edema, anorexia, rash, flushing, arthralgia, myalgia, ecchymosis, rhinitis, constipation, insomnia.

ADVERSE EFFECTS/ TOXIC REACTIONS

Thrombocytopenia (95%), neutropenia (77%), anemia (61%) may be severe and prolonged; may be followed by infection (29%). Hypersensitivity reaction produces hypotension, bronchospasm, angioedema. Severe cutaneous or mucocutaneous reactions (erythema multiforme, Stevens-Johnson syndrome, toxic epidermal necrolysis) have been noted.

NURSING CONSIDERATIONS

BASELINE ASSESSMENT

Pretreatment with acetaminophen and diphenhydramine before each infusion may prevent infusion-related effects. Offer emotional support. Use strict asepsis. Obtain baseline CBC, serum chemistries. Absolute neutrophil count (ANC) nadir is 62 days before recovery begins.

INTERVENTION/EVALUATION

Diligently monitor lab values for possibly severe/prolonged thrombocytopenia, neutropenia, anemia. Monitor for hematologic toxicity (fever, sore throat, signs of local infections, unusual bruising/bleeding), symptoms of anemia (excessive fatigue, weakness), infusion-related allergic reaction. Assess for GI symptoms (nausea, vomiting, abdominal pain, diarrhea).

PATIENT/FAMILY TEACHING

• Do not have immunizations without physician's approval (drug lowers resistance). • Avoid crowds, persons with known infections. • Report signs of infection at once (fever, flu-like symptoms). • Report if nausea/vomiting continues at home. • Avoid pregnancy during therapy.

ibrutinib

eye-**broo**-ti-nib
(Imbruvica)
**Do not confuse ibrutinib with
axitinib, dasatinib, erlotinib,
gefitinib, imatinib, nilotinib,
ponatinib, sorafenib, sunitinib,
or vandetanib.**

◆CLASSIFICATION

PHARMACOTHERAPEUTIC: Kinase inhibitor. **CLINICAL:** Antineoplastic.

ACTION

Inhibits enzymatic activity of Bruton's tyrosine kinase (BTK), a signaling molecule that promotes malignant B-cell proliferation and survival. **Therapeutic Effect:** Inhibits tumor cell growth and metastasis.

PHARMACOKINETICS

Readily absorbed following PO. Metabolized in liver. Peak plasma concentration: 1–2 hrs. Protein binding: 97%. Excreted in feces (80%), urine (10%). **Half-life:** 4–6 hrs.

USES

Treatment of pts with mantle cell lymphoma (MCL) who have received at least one prior therapy.

PRECAUTIONS

Contraindications: None known. **Cautions:** Baseline anemia, neutropenia, thrombocytopenia, hepatic/renal impairment, HF, hypertension, hypovolemia, open wounds, pregnancy, recent surgery or dental procedure, concurrent antiplatelet or anticoagulant therapy.

⌛ LIFESPAN CONSIDERATIONS

Pregnancy/Lactation: May cause fetal harm. Avoid pregnancy. Unknown if distributed in breast milk. Must either discontinue drug or discontinue breast-feeding. **Pregnancy Category D. Children:** Safety and efficacy not established. **Elderly:** Increased risk of cardiac events (atrial fibrillation, hypertension), infections (pneumonia, cellulitis), GI events (diarrhea, dehydration, bleeding).

INTERACTIONS

DRUG: Strong CYP3A4 inhibitors (e.g., ketoconazole, clarithromycin) may increase plasma concentration/effect; avoid use. **Strong CYP3A4 inducers (e.g., rifampin, phenytoin)** may decrease plasma concentration/effect; avoid use. **Anticoagulants, antiplatelets, NSAIDS** may increase risk of bleeding. **HERBAL: St John's wort** may decrease concentration/effect. **FOOD: Grapefruit products, Seville oranges** may increase concentration/effect. **All foods** may increase absorption/concentration. **LAB VALUES:** May decrease Hgb, Hct, neutrophils, platelets.

AVAILABILITY (Rx)

💊 **Capsules:** 140 mg.

ADMINISTRATION/HANDLING

PO
• Give with water. • Do not break, crush, dissolve, or open capsule.

INDICATIONS/ROUTES/DOSAGE

Mantle Cell Lymphoma
PO: ADULTS/ELDERLY: 560 mg (4 × 140-mg capsules) once daily.

Dose Modification
Based on Common Terminology Criteria for Adverse Events (CTCAE).

Any Grade 3 or Greater Nonhematologic Event, Grade 3 or Greater Neutropenia with Infection or Fever, or Any Grade 4 Hematologic Toxicities
Interrupt treatment until resolution to grade 1 or baseline, then restart at initial dose. If toxicity reoccurs, interrupt treatment until resolution to grade 1 or baseline, then reduce dose to 420 mg daily (one capsule less). If toxicity reoccurs, interrupt treatment until resolution to

grade 1 or baseline, then reduce dose to 280 mg once daily (one capsule less). If toxicity still occurs at 280 mg dose, discontinue treatment.

Concomitant Use of Moderate CYP3A4 Inhibitors (e.g., Fluconazole, Diltiazem, Verapamil)

Start at reduced dose of 140 mg daily. If toxicity occurs, either discontinue treatment or find alternate agent with less CYP3A inhibition.

Concomitant Short-Term Use of Strong CYP3A4 Inhibitors (≤7 days) (e.g., Antifungals, Antibiotics)

Interrupt treatment until strong CYP3A medications no longer needed.

Concomitant Chronic Use of Strong CYP3A4 Inhibitors or Inducers

Treatment not recommended.

SIDE EFFECTS

Frequent (51%–23%): Diarrhea, fatigue, musculoskeletal pain, peripheral edema, nausea, bruising, dyspnea, constipation, rash, abdominal pain, vomiting. **Occasional (21%–11%):** Decreased appetite, cough, pyrexia, stomatitis, asthenia, dizziness, muscle spasms, dehydration, headache, dyspepsia, petechiae, arthralgia.

ADVERSE EFFECTS/ TOXIC REACTIONS

Anemia, lymphopenia, neutropenia, thrombocytopenia is expected response to therapy. Treatment-emergent myelosuppression (grade 3–4 CTCAE) reported in 41% of pts: neutropenia (29%), thrombocytopenia (17%), anemia (9%). Infections including upper respiratory tract infection, UTI, pneumonia, skin infection, sinusitis were reported. Hemorrhagic events including epistaxis, GI bleeding, hematuria, intracranial hemorrhage, subdural hematoma reported in 5% of pts. Serious and fatal cases of renal toxicity reported: increased serum creatinine 1.5 times upper limit of normal (ULN) (67% of pts), increased serum creatinine 1.53

times UNL (9% of pts). Second primary malignancies including skin cancer (4%), other carcinomas (1%) occurred.

NURSING CONSIDERATIONS

BASELINE ASSESSMENT

Obtain baseline vital signs, CBC, serum chemistries, liver function test, PT/INR if on anticoagulants. Question history of arrhythmias, HF, GI bleed, hepatic/renal impairment, peripheral edema, pulmonary disease. Obtain negative urine pregnancy before initiating treatment. Assess hydration status. Receive full medication history including vitamins, herbal products. Assess skin for open/unhealed wounds, lesions, moles. Conduct baseline neurologic exam.

INTERVENTION/EVALUATION

Monitor CBC monthly; liver function tests, serum chemistries, renal panel routinely. Monitor stool frequency, consistency, characteristics. Immediately report hemorrhagic events: epistaxis, hematuria, hemoptysis, melena. Encourage PO intake. Obtain EKG for arrhythmias, dyspnea, palpitations. Screen for possible intracranial hemorrhage: altered mental status, aphasia, hemiparesis, unequal pupils, homonymous hemianopsia (blindness of one half of vision on same side of both eyes). Monitor for renal toxicity (anuria, hypertension, generalized edema, flank pain). Assess skin for new lesions.

PATIENT/FAMILY TEACHING

• Blood levels will be monitored routinely. • Difficulty breathing, fever, cough, burning with urination, body aches, chills may indicate an acute infection. • Avoid pregnancy. • Report any black/tarry stools, bruising, nausea, RUQ abdominal pain, yellowing of skin or eyes, palpitations, nose bleeds, blood in urine or stool, decreased urine output. • Avoid alcohol. • Do not take herbal products. • Do not ingest grapefruit products. • Severe diarrhea may lead to dehydration. • Contact doctor before any planned surgical/dental procedures. • Immediately report neurological changes: confusion, one-sided paralysis, difficulty speaking, partial blindness. • Do not receive live vaccines. • Do not break, crush, dissolve, or open capsule.

ibuprofen

eye-bue-**pro**-fen
(Advil, Advil Children's, Advil Infants', Advil Junior, Advil Migraine, Apo-Ibuprofen ✦, Caldolor, Ibu-200, Motrin, Motrin Children's, Motrin IB, Motrin Infants', Motrin Junior Strength, NeoProfen, Novoprofen ✦)

BLACK BOX ALERT Increased risk of serious cardiovascular thrombotic events, including myocardial infarction, CVA. Increased risk of severe GI reactions, including ulceration, bleeding, perforation.
Do not confuse Motrin with Neurontin.

FIXED-COMBINATION(S)

Children's Advil Cold: ibuprofen/pseudoephedrine (a nasal decongestant): 100 mg/15 mg per 5 ml. **Combunox:** ibuprofen/oxycodone (a narcotic analgesic): 400 mg/5 mg. **Duexis:** ibuprofen/famotidine (an H₂ antagonist): 800 mg/26.6 mg. **Reprexain CIII:** ibuprofen/hydrocodone (a narcotic analgesic): 200 mg/5 mg. **Vicoprofen:** ibuprofen/hydrocodone (a narcotic analgesic): 200 mg/7.5 mg.

◆CLASSIFICATION

PHARMACOTHERAPEUTIC: NSAID. **CLINICAL:** Antirheumatic, analgesic, antipyretic, antidysmenorrheal, vascular headache suppressant (see p. 129C).

ACTION

Inhibits prostaglandin synthesis. Produces vasodilation acting on heat-regulating center of hypothalamus. **Therapeutic Effect:** Produces analgesic, anti-inflammatory effects; decreases fever.

PHARMACOKINETICS

Route	Onset	Peak	Duration
PO (analgesic)	0.5 hr	N/A	4–6 hrs
PO (anti-rheumatic)	2 days	1–2 wks	N/A

Rapidly absorbed from GI tract. Protein binding: 90%–99%. Metabolized in liver. Primarily excreted in urine. Not removed by hemodialysis. **Half-life:** 2–4 hrs.

USES

Treatment of fever, juvenile rheumatoid arthritis (JRA), osteoarthritis, minor to moderate pain, primary dysmenorrhea. **Caldolor:** Mild to moderate pain; severe pain in combination with an opioid analgesic; fever. **NeoProfen:** Closes clinically significant patent ductus arteriosus (PDA) in premature infants weighing between 500 and 1,500 g who are no more than 32 wks gestational age when usual medical management is ineffective. **OFF-LABEL:** Treatment of gout, migraine headaches, migraine prophylaxis, cystic fibrosis, ankylosing spondylitis.

PRECAUTIONS

Contraindications: History of hypersensitivity to aspirin, NSAIDs (asthma, urticaria, allergic-type reaction). Treatment of perioperative pain in coronary artery bypass graft (CABG) surgery. **NeoProfen:** Infants with proven or suspected untreated infection, elevated total bilirubin, congenital heart disease in whom patency of the patent ductus arteriosus is necessary for satisfactory pulmonary or systemic blood flow (e.g., pulmonary atresia), bleeding, thrombocytopenia, coagulation defects, suspected necrotizing enterocolitis, significant renal impairment. **Cautions:** Active peptic ulcer, chronic inflammation of GI tract, GI bleeding disorders, smoking, alcohol use, HF, hypertension, renal/hepatic impairment, dehydration, asthma, concurrent aspirin, anticoagulant use, elderly, debilitated.

⏳ LIFESPAN CONSIDERATIONS

Pregnancy/Lactation: Unknown if drug crosses placenta or is distributed in breast milk. Avoid use during third trimester (may adversely affect fetal cardiovascular system: premature closure of ductus arteriosus). **Pregnancy Category B (D if used in third trimester or near delivery). Children:** Safety and efficacy not established in those younger than 6 mos. **Elderly:** GI bleeding, ulceration more likely to cause serious adverse effects. Age-related renal impairment may increase risk of hepatic/renal toxicity; reduced dosage recommended.

INTERACTIONS

DRUG: May decrease effects of **antihypertensives, diuretics. Aspirin, other salicylates** may increase risk of GI side effects, bleeding. May increase effects of **oral anticoagulants.** May increase concentration, risk of toxicity of **lithium, methotrexate. HERBAL: Cat's claw, dong quai, evening primrose, feverfew, garlic, ginkgo, ginseng, horse chestnut, red clover** may increase antiplatelet activity. **FOOD:** None known. **LAB VALUES:** May prolong bleeding time. May alter serum glucose level. May increase BUN, serum creatinine, potassium, AST, ALT. May decrease serum calcium, glucose, Hgb, Hct, platelets.

AVAILABILITY (Rx)

Caplets (Advil, Ibu-200, Motrin IB): 200 mg. **Capsules (Advil, Advil Migraine):** 200 mg. **Gelcaps (Advil):** 200 mg. **Injection, Solution (NeoProfen):** 10 mg/ml. **(Caldolor):** 100 mg/ml. **Suspension, Oral (Advil Children's, Motrin Children's):** 100 mg/5 ml. **Suspension, Oral Drops (Advil Infants', Motrin Infants'):** 40 mg/ml. **Tablets:** 200 mg, 400 mg, 600 mg, 800 mg. **Tablets, Chewable (Motrin Junior Strength):** 100 mg.

ADMINISTRATION/HANDLING

 IV (Caldolor)

Reconstitution • Dilute with D₅W or 0.9% NaCl to final concentration of 4 mg/ml or less.
Rate of Administration • Infuse over at least 30 min.
Storage • Store at room temperature. • Stable for 24 hrs after dilution.

 IV (NeoProfen)

Reconstitution • Dilute to appropriate volume with D₅W or 0.9% NaCl. • Discard any remaining medication after first withdrawal from vial.
Rate of Administration • Administer via IV port nearest the insertion site. • Infuse continuously over 15 min.
Storage • Store at room temperature. • Stable for 30 min after dilution.

PO
• Give with food, milk, antacids if GI distress occurs.

INDICATIONS/ROUTES/DOSAGE

Fever
PO: ADULTS, ELDERLY, CHILDREN 12 YRS AND OLDER: 200–400 mg q4–6h prn. **Maximum:** 1,200 mg/day. **CHILDREN 6 MOS–11 YRS:** 5–10 mg/kg/dose q6–8h prn. **Maximum:** 40 mg/kg/day.
IV: ADULTS, ELDERLY: 400 mg q4–6h or 100–200 mg q4h prn. **Maximum:** 3.2 g/day.

Osteoarthritis, Rheumatoid Arthritis (RA)
PO: ADULTS, ELDERLY: 400–800 mg/dose 3–4 times/day. **Maximum:** 3.2 g/day.

Pain
PO: ADULTS, ELDERLY, CHILDREN 12 YRS AND OLDER: 200–400 mg q4–6h prn. **Maximum:** 1,200 mg/day. **CHILDREN 6 MOS–11 YRS:** 4–10 mg/kg q6–8h prn. **Maximum:** 40 mg/kg/day.

I

Primary Dysmenorrhea
PO: ADULTS: 200–400 mg q4–6h prn. **Maximum:** 1,200 mg/day.

Juvenile Rheumatoid Arthritis (JRA)
PO: CHILDREN: 30–50 mg/kg/day in 3–4 divided doses. **Maximum:** 2.4 g/day.

Patent Ductus Arteriosus (PDA)
IV: INFANTS: Initially, 10 mg/kg then 2 doses of 5 mg/kg, after 24 hrs and 48 hrs. All doses based on birth weight.

SIDE EFFECTS

Occasional (9%–3%): Nausea, vomiting, dyspepsia, dizziness, rash. **Rare (less than 3%):** Diarrhea or constipation, flatulence, abdominal cramps or pain, pruritus, increased B/P.

ADVERSE EFFECTS/ TOXIC REACTIONS

Overdose may result in metabolic acidosis. Rare reactions with long-term use include peptic ulcer, GI bleeding, gastritis, severe hepatic reaction (cholestasis, jaundice), nephrotoxicity (dysuria, hematuria, proteinuria, nephrotic syndrome), severe hypersensitivity reaction (particularly in pts with systemic lupus erythematosus or other collagen diseases). **NeoProfen:** Hypoglycemia, hypocalcemia, respiratory failure, UTI, edema, atelectasis may occur. **Caldolor:** Abdominal pain, anemia, cough, dizziness, dyspnea, edema, hypertension, nausea, vomiting.

NURSING CONSIDERATIONS

BASELINE ASSESSMENT

Assess onset, type, location, duration of pain, inflammation. Inspect appearance of affected joints for immobility, deformities, skin condition. Assess temperature.

INTERVENTION/EVALUATION

Monitor for evidence of nausea, dyspepsia. Monitor CBC, hepatic/renal function tests. Assess skin for rash. Observe for bleeding, bruising, occult blood loss.

Evaluate for therapeutic response: relief of pain, stiffness, swelling; increased joint mobility; reduced joint tenderness; improved grip strength. Monitor for fever.

PATIENT/FAMILY TEACHING

• Avoid aspirin, alcohol during therapy (increases risk of GI bleeding). • If GI upset occurs, take with food, milk, antacids. • May cause dizziness. • Report ringing in ears, persistent stomach pain, respiratory difficulty, unusual bruising/bleeding, swelling of extremities, chest pain/palpitations.

icatibant

eye-**kat**-i-bant
(Firazyr)

◆CLASSIFICATION

PHARMACOTHERAPEUTIC: Bradykinin B_2 receptor antagonist. **CLINICAL:** Angioedema agent.

ACTION

Inhibits bradykinin from binding to B_2 receptor. Inhibits effects of hereditary angioedema (HAE), an autosomal dominant disorder that causes rapid inflammation of skin and mucosal membranes. **Therapeutic Effect:** Reduces rapid swelling of submucosal tissues during episodic attack of HAE.

PHARMACOKINETICS

Metabolized by proteolytic enzymes into inactive enzymes. Primarily excreted in urine. **Peak plasma:** 45 min. **Half-life:** 1.4 hrs.

USES

Treatment of acute attacks related to hereditary angioedema.

PRECAUTIONS

Contraindications: None known. **Cautions:** Airway obstruction during acute laryngeal HAE attack may occur.

⧗ LIFESPAN CONSIDERATIONS

Pregnancy/Lactation: Unknown if drug crosses placenta or is distributed in breast milk. Use caution when administering to nursing mothers. **Pregnancy Category C. Children:** Safety and efficacy not established in those younger than 18 yrs. **Elderly:** Increased risk of higher systemic exposure due to lower medication clearance.

INTERACTIONS

DRUG: May decrease effectiveness of **ACE inhibitors. HERBAL:** None significant. **FOOD:** None known. **LAB VALUES:** May increase serum AST, ALT.

AVAILABILITY (Rx)

Injection Solution: 30 mg/3 ml in pre-filled syringes.

ADMINISTRATION/HANDLING

Subcutaneous
• Inject into left or right anterolateral abdominal wall. • Introduce entire length of needle (1/2 inch) into skin fold between thumb and forefinger, holding skin fold during injection. • Rotate injection sites if applicable. • Inject over 30 sec.
Storage • Refrigerate until time of use. • Visually inspect syringe for particulate matter. • Solution should appear clear, colorless. • Do not freeze.

INDICATIONS/ROUTES/DOSAGE

Acute Hereditary Angioedema
Subcutaneous: ADULTS, ELDERLY: Initially, 30 mg once. May repeat 30 mg dose at intervals of at least 6 hrs. **Maximum:** 90 mg/24 hrs.

SIDE EFFECTS

Frequent (97%): Injection site reactions: bruising, hematoma, burning, erythema, hypoesthesia, irritation, numbness, edema, pain, pressure sensation, pruritus, urticaria. **Rare (3%):** Dizziness, allergic reaction, nausea, vomiting, rash, headache, pyrexia.

ADVERSE EFFECTS/ TOXIC REACTIONS

Positive anti-icatibant antibodies reported in 4% of pts.

NURSING CONSIDERATIONS

BASELINE ASSESSMENT

Assess characteristics of inflammatory attacks (location, severity, history of drooling, difficulty breathing/swallowing). Question history of laryngeal-associated angioedema. Question possibility of pregnancy or plans of breastfeeding. Assess full medication history, esp. ACE inhibitors.

INTERVENTION/EVALUATION

Assess O_2 saturation, airway patency for mouth, tongue, throat inflammation. If applicable, monitor ACE inhibitor effectiveness, B/P. Frequently monitor for symptom improvement after injection. Notify physician if inflammation remains after 3 doses.

PATIENT/FAMILY TEACHING

• Avoid tasks that require alertness, motor skills until response to drug is established. • Instruct proper self-administration techniques. • If applicable, inform pt of decreased ACE inhibitor effectiveness. • Report suspected pregnancy. • Seek medical attention immediately if throat swelling, drooling, difficulty breathing occurs during acute attacks. • Symptoms that do not improve or recur will require additional interval doses. • Do not use more than 3 doses in 24 hrs. • Educate pt about common injection site reactions. Seek medical attention in health care facility if laryngeal symptoms occur after administration of icatibant.

---

icosapent

eye-**koe**-sa-pent
(Vascepa)
Do not confuse icosapent with icatibant or Vascepa with Vaseretic.

◆ CLASSIFICATION

PHARMACOTHERAPEUTIC: Omega-3 fatty acid. **CLINICAL:** Antihypertriglyceride agent (see p. 59C).

ACTION

Potential mechanisms of action include increased B-oxidation, decreased lipogenesis in liver, increased plasma lipoprotein lipase activity. **Therapeutic Effect:** Reduces hepatic very-low density lipoprotein triglyceride (VLOL-TG) synthesis.

PHARMACOKINETICS

Absorbed in small intestine; enters systemic circulation via thoracic duct lymphatic system. Protein binding: 99%. Metabolized in liver. **Half-life:** 89 hrs.

USES

Adjunct to diet to reduce serum triglyceride levels in adult pts with serum hypertriglyceridemia (500 mg/dl or greater).

PRECAUTIONS

Contraindications: None known. **Cautions:** Known sensitivity or allergy to fish, shellfish; hepatic impairment, coagulopathy, pts receiving therapeutic anticoagulation.

⏳ LIFESPAN CONSIDERATIONS

Pregnancy/Lactation: Distributed in breast milk. **Pregnancy Category C. Children:** Safety and efficacy in children younger than 18 yrs not established. **Elderly:** No age-related precautions noted.

INTERACTIONS

DRUG: None significant. **HERBAL:** None significant. **FOOD:** None known. **LAB VALUES:** May increase serum ALT, AST, low-density lipoprotein (LDL) cholesterol. May alter bleeding time.

AVAILABILITY (Rx)

🔖 **Capsules, Soft Gelatin:** 1 g.

ADMINISTRATION/HANDLING

PO
• Give with food. • Capsule(s) should be swallowed whole. • Instruct pt not to chew capsule. • Do not break open, crush, or dissolve medication.

INDICATIONS/ROUTES/DOSAGE

◄**ALERT**► Before initiating therapy, pt should be on appropriate cholesterol-lowering diet and regimen of physical activity. Continue diet and activity program throughout therapy.

Usual Dosage
PO: ADULTS, ELDERLY: 4 g per day, given as 2 capsules twice daily with food.

SIDE EFFECTS

Rare (2%): Arthralgia. **(Less Than 1%):** Oropharyngeal pain.

ADVERSE EFFECTS/ TOXIC REACTIONS

Increased bleeding time has been noted.

NURSING CONSIDERATION

BASELINE ASSESSMENT

Obtain diet history. Obtain baseline chemistries, hepatic function tests, fasting lipid profile. In patients with hepatic impairment, ALT, AST, serum triglyceride, and lipid levels should be monitored periodically.

INTERVENTION/EVALUATION

Monitor serum triglyceride level for therapeutic response. Monitor LDL cholesterol periodically. For those taking antiplatelets, monitor bleeding time. Discontinue therapy if no response after 3 mos of treatment.

PATIENT/FAMILY TEACHING

• Continue to adhere to lipid-lowering diet (important part of treatment). • Periodic lab tests are essential part of therapy to determine drug effectiveness.

idarubicin
HIGH ALERT

eye-da-**roo**-bi-sin
(Idamycin PFS)

BLACK BOX ALERT Cardiotoxicity may occur (HF, arrhythmias, cardiomyopathy). Severe myelosuppressant. Must be administered by personnel trained in administration/handling of chemotherapeutic agents. Severe local tissue damage, necrosis if extravasation occurs.
Do not confuse Idamycin with Adriamycin, or idarubicin with daunorubicin, doxorubicin, or epirubicin.

◆CLASSIFICATION

PHARMACOTHERAPEUTIC: Anthracycline antibiotic. **CLINICAL:** Antineoplastic (see p. 87C).

ACTION

Inhibits nucleic acid synthesis by interacting with enzyme topoisomerase II, promoting DNA strand supercoiling. **Therapeutic Effect:** Produces death of rapidly dividing cells.

PHARMACOKINETICS

Widely distributed. Protein binding: 97%. Rapidly metabolized in liver. Primarily eliminated by biliary excretion. Not removed by hemodialysis. **Half-life:** 12–27 hrs.

USES

Treatment of acute myeloid leukemia (AML). **OFF-LABEL:** Acute lymphocytic leukemia (ALL).

PRECAUTIONS

Contraindications: Arrhythmias, cardiomyopathy, preexisting myelosuppression, pregnancy, severe HF, bilirubin greater than 5 mg/dL. **Cautions:** Renal/hepatic impairment, concurrent radiation therapy.

⧗ LIFESPAN CONSIDERATIONS

Pregnancy/Lactation: If possible, avoid use during pregnancy (may be embryotoxic). Unknown if drug is distributed in breast milk (advise to discontinue breastfeeding before drug initiation). **Pregnancy Category D. Children:** Safety and efficacy not established. **Elderly:** Cardiotoxicity may be more prevalent. Caution in pts with inadequate bone marrow reserves. Age-related renal impairment may require dosage adjustment.

INTERACTIONS

DRUG: May decrease effects of **antigout medications. Bone marrow depressants** may increase myelosuppression. **Live virus vaccines** may potentiate virus replication, increase vaccine side effects, decrease pt's antibody response to vaccine. **HERBAL:** None significant. **FOOD:** None known. **LAB VALUES:** May increase serum alkaline phosphatase, bilirubin, uric acid, AST, ALT. May cause EKG changes.

AVAILABILITY (Rx)

Injection Solution: 1 mg/ml in 5-ml, 10-ml, 20-ml vials.

ADMINISTRATION/HANDLING

◀**ALERT**▶ Give by free-flowing IV infusion (**never** subcutaneous or IM). Gloves, gowns, eye goggles recommended during preparation/administration of medication. If powder/solution comes in contact with skin, wash thoroughly. Avoid small veins, swollen/edematous extremities, areas overlying joints/tendons.

 IV

Reconstitution • May give undiluted or dilute with 0.9% NaCl or D₅W.
Rate of Administration • Administer IV push into tubing of freely running IV infusion of D₅W or 0.9% NaCl, preferably via butterfly needle, **slowly** over 3–5

min. • May give intermittent infusion over 10–15 min. • Extravasation produces immediate pain, severe local tissue damage. Terminate infusion immediately. Apply cold compresses for 30 min immediately, then q30min 4 times a day for 3 days. Keep extremity elevated.

Storage • Refrigerate vials. • Diluted solutions in 0.9% NaCl or D_5W are stable for 72 hrs at room temperature or 7 days if refrigerated.

⚙ IV INCOMPATIBILITIES

Acyclovir (Zovirax), allopurinol (Aloprim), ampicillin and sulbactam (Unasyn), cefazolin (Ancef, Kefzol), cefepime (Maxipime), ceftazidime (Fortaz), clindamycin (Cleocin), dexamethasone (Decadron), furosemide (Lasix), hydrocortisone (Solu-Cortef), lorazepam (Ativan), methotrexate, piperacillin and tazobactam (Zosyn), sodium bicarbonate, teniposide (Vumon), vancomycin (Vancocin), vincristine (Oncovin).

⚙ IV COMPATIBILITIES

Diphenhydramine (Benadryl), granisetron (Kytril), magnesium, potassium.

INDICATIONS/ROUTES/DOSAGE

◄**ALERT**► Refer to individual protocols.

AML
IV: ADULTS, ELDERLY: (Induction): 12 mg/m²/day for 3 days. **(Consolidation):** 10–12 mg/m²/day for 2 days.

Dosage in Renal Impairment
ADULTS: Creatinine clearance 10–50 ml/min: Give 75% of dose. Creatinine clearance less than 10 ml/min: Give 50% of dose. **CHILDREN:** Creatinine clearance less than 50 ml/min: Give 75% of dose.
Hemodialysis, Peritoneal Dialysis, Continuous Renal Replacement Therapy: Administer 75% of dose.

Dosage in Hepatic Impairment
Bilirubin 2.6–5 mg/dl: Give 50% of dose. **Bilirubin greater than 5 mg/dl:** Avoid use.

SIDE EFFECTS

Frequent (82%–50%): Nausea, vomiting, complete alopecia (scalp, axillary, pubic hair), abdominal cramping, diarrhea, mucositis. **Occasional (46%–20%):** Hyperpigmentation of nailbeds, phalangeal, dermal creases, fever, headache. **Rare:** Conjunctivitis, neuropathy.

ADVERSE EFFECTS/ TOXIC REACTIONS

Myelosuppression (principally leukopenia and, to lesser extent, anemia, thrombocytopenia) generally occurs within 10–15 days after starting therapy, returns to normal levels by third wk. Cardiotoxicity (either acute, manifested as transient EKG abnormalities, or chronic, manifested as HF) may occur.

NURSING CONSIDERATIONS

BASELINE ASSESSMENT
Determine baseline renal/hepatic function, CBC results. Obtain EKG before therapy. Antiemetic medication before and during therapy may prevent or relieve nausea, vomiting. Inform pt of high potential for alopecia.

INTERVENTION/EVALUATION
Monitor CBC, serum electrolytes, EKG, renal/hepatic function tests. Monitor for hematologic toxicity (fever, sore throat, signs of local infection, unusual bruising/bleeding from any site), symptoms of anemia (excessive fatigue, weakness). Avoid IM injections, rectal temperatures, other trauma that may precipitate bleeding. Check infusion site frequently for extravasation (causes severe local necrosis). Assess for potentially fatal HF (dyspnea, rales, pulmonary edema), life-threatening arrhythmias.

PATIENT/FAMILY TEACHING
• Total body hair loss is frequent but reversible. • New hair growth resumes 2–3 mos after last therapy dose and may have different color, texture. • Maintain strict oral hygiene. • Avoid crowds, those with

infections. • Inform physician of fever, sore throat, bruising/bleeding. • Urine may turn pink or red. • Frequent lab testing (CBC, hepatic/renal function) is a normal part of therapy. • Use contraceptive measures.

ifosfamide

HIGH ALERT

eye-**fos**-fa-mide
(Ifex)

BLACK BOX ALERT Hemorrhagic cystitis may occur. Severe myelosuppressant. May cause CNS toxicity, including confusion, coma. Must be administered by personnel trained in administration/handling of chemotherapeutic agents.
Do not confuse ifosfamide with cyclophosphamide.

◆CLASSIFICATION

PHARMACOTHERAPEUTIC: Alkylating agent. **CLINICAL:** Antineoplastic (see p. 87C).

ACTION

Inhibits DNA, RNA protein synthesis by cross-linking with DNA, RNA strands, preventing cell growth. Cell cycle–phase nonspecific. **Therapeutic Effect:** Interferes with DNA, RNA function.

PHARMACOKINETICS

Metabolized in liver. Protein binding: Negligible. Crosses blood-brain barrier (to a limited extent). Primarily excreted in urine. Removed by hemodialysis. **Half-life:** 11–15 hrs (high dose); 4–7 hrs (low dose).

USES

Treatment of germ cell testicular carcinoma (used in combination with agents that protect against hemorrhagic cystitis). **OFF-LABEL:** Small cell lung, non–small-cell lung, ovarian, cervical, bladder, soft tissue sarcomas, Hodgkin's, non-Hodgkin's lymphomas, osteosarcoma, head and neck, Ewing's sarcoma.

PRECAUTIONS

Contraindications: Urinary outflow obstruction. **Cautions:** Renal/hepatic impairment, compromised bone marrow function, active urinary tract infection, preexisting cardiac disease, prior radiation therapy.

⧗ LIFESPAN CONSIDERATIONS

Pregnancy/Lactation: If possible, avoid use during pregnancy, esp. first trimester. May cause fetal harm. Distributed in breast milk. Breastfeeding not recommended. **Pregnancy Category D. Children:** Not intended for this pt population. **Elderly:** Age-related renal impairment may require dosage adjustment.

INTERACTIONS

DRUG: Bone marrow depressants may increase myelosuppression. **Live virus vaccines** may potentiate virus replication, increase vaccine side effects, decrease pt's antibody response to vaccine. **HERBAL: St. John's wort** may decrease concentration. **FOOD:** None known. **LAB VALUES:** May increase BUN, serum bilirubin, creatinine, uric acid, AST, ALT.

AVAILABILITY (Rx)

Injection, Powder for Reconstitution (Ifex): 1 g, 3 g. **Injection, Solution:** 50 mg/ml.

ADMINISTRATION/HANDLING

◀**ALERT**▶ Hemorrhagic cystitis occurs if mesna is not given concurrently. Mesna should always be given with ifosfamide.

 IV

Reconstitution • Reconstitute vial with Sterile Water for Injection or Bacteriostatic Water for Injection to provide concentration of 50 mg/ml. Shake to dissolve. • Further dilute with 50–1,000 ml D5W or 0.9% NaCl to provide concentration of 0.6–20 mg/ml.

Rate of Administration • Infuse over minimum of 30 min. • Give with at least 2,000 ml PO or IV fluid (prevents bladder toxicity). • Give with protectant against hemorrhagic cystitis (i.e., mesna).

Storage • Store vials of powder at room temperature. • Refrigerate vials of solution. • After reconstitution with Bacteriostatic Water for Injection, solution is stable for 3 wks if refrigerated (further diluted solution is stable for 7 days at room temperature or 6 wks if refrigerated).

🔷 IV INCOMPATIBILITIES

Cefepime (Maxipime), methotrexate.

🔷 IV COMPATIBILITIES

Granisetron (Kytril), ondansetron (Zofran).

INDICATIONS/ROUTES/DOSAGE

◀ALERT▶ Dosage individualized based on clinical response, tolerance to adverse effects. When used in combination therapy, consult specific protocols for optimum dosage, sequence of drug administration.

Germ Cell Testicular Carcinoma
IV: ADULTS: 1,200 mg/m²/day for 5 consecutive days. Repeat q3–4wks or after recovery from hematologic toxicity. Administer with mesna.

SIDE EFFECTS

Frequent (83%–58%): Alopecia, nausea, vomiting. **Occasional (15%–5%):** Confusion, drowsiness, hallucinations, infection. **Rare (less than 5%):** Dizziness, seizures, disorientation, fever, malaise, stomatitis (mucosal irritation, glossitis, gingivitis).

ADVERSE EFFECTS/ TOXIC REACTIONS

Hemorrhagic cystitis with hematuria, dysuria occurs frequently if protective agent (mesna) is not used. Myelosuppression (leukopenia, thrombocytopenia) occurs frequently. Pulmonary toxicity, hepatotox- icity, nephrotoxicity, cardiotoxicity, CNS toxicity (confusion, hallucinations, drowsiness, coma) may require discontinuation of therapy.

NURSING CONSIDERATIONS

BASELINE ASSESSMENT

Obtain urinalysis before each dose. If hematuria occurs (greater than 10 RBCs per field), therapy should be withheld until resolution occurs. Obtain WBC, platelet count, Hgb before each dose.

INTERVENTION/EVALUATION

Monitor hematologic studies, urinalysis, renal/hepatic function tests. Assess for fever, sore throat, signs of local infection, unusual bruising/bleeding from any site, symptoms of anemia (excessive fatigue, weakness).

PATIENT/FAMILY TEACHING

• Alopecia is reversible, but new hair growth may have a different color or texture. • Maintain copious daily fluid intake (protects against cystitis). • Do not have immunizations without physician's approval (drug lowers resistance). • Avoid contact with those who have recently received live virus vaccine. • Avoid crowds, those with infections. • Report unusual bleeding/bruising, fever, chills, sore throat, joint pain, sores in mouth or on lips, yellowing skin or eyes.

iloperidone

eye-loe-**per**-i-doan
(Fanapt)
BLACK BOX ALERT Elderly pts with dementia-related psychosis are at increased risk for mortality due to cerebrovascular events.
Do not confuse iloperidone with amiodarone or dronedarone.

◆ CLASSIFICATION

PHARMACOTHERAPEUTIC: Piperidi-nyl-benzisoxazole derivative. **CLINICAL:** Antipsychotic (see p. 66C).

ACTION

Exact mechanism unknown; may be mediated through combination of dopamine type 2 (D_2) and serotonin type 2 (5-HT_2) antagonisms. **Therapeutic Effect:** Diminishes symptoms of schizophrenia.

PHARMACOKINETICS

Steady-state concentration occurs in 3–4 days. Well absorbed from GI tract (unaffected by food). Protein binding: 95%. Metabolized in liver. Primarily excreted in urine, with a lesser amount eliminated in feces. **Half-life:** 18–33 hrs.

USES

Acute treatment of schizophrenia in adults.

PRECAUTIONS

Contraindications: None known. **Cautions:** Cardiovascular disease (heart failure, history of MI, ischemia, cardiac conduction abnormalities), cerebrovascular disease (increases risk of CVA in pts with dementia, seizure disorders). Pts with bradycardia, hypokalemia, hypomagnesemia may be at greater risk for torsade de pointes. History of seizures, conditions lowering seizure threshold, high risk of suicide, risk of aspiration pneumonia, congenital QT syndrome, concurrent use of medications that prolong QT interval, decreased GI motility, urinary retention, BPH, xerostomia, visual problems, hepatic impairment, narrow-angle glaucoma, diabetes.

⌛ LIFESPAN CONSIDERATIONS

Pregnancy/Lactation: Unknown if drug crosses placenta or is excreted in breast milk. Breastfeeding not recommended. **Pregnancy Category C. Children:** Safety and efficacy not established. **Elderly:** More susceptible to postural hypotension. Increased risk of cerebrovascular events, mortality, including stroke in elderly pts with psychosis.

INTERACTIONS

DRUG: Alcohol, CNS depressants may increase CNS depression. Strong **CYP3A4 inhibitors (e.g., clarithromycin, ketoconazole)** or strong **CYP2D6 inhibitors (e.g., fluoxetine, paroxetine)** may increase concentration. **Medications causing prolongation of QT interval (amiodarone, dofetilide, sotalol)** may increase effects on cardiac conduction, leading to malignant arrhythmias (torsade de pointes). **HERBAL: Gotu kola, kava kava, St. John's wort, valerian** may increase CNS depression. **St. John's wort** may decrease concentration. **FOOD:** None known. **LAB VALUES:** May increase serum prolactin levels.

AVAILABILITY (Rx)

Tablets: 1 mg, 2 mg, 4 mg, 6 mg, 8 mg, 10 mg, 12 mg.

ADMINISTRATION/HANDLING

PO

• Give without regard to food. • Tablets may be crushed.

INDICATIONS/ROUTES/DOSAGE

Schizophrenia

PO: ADULTS: To avoid orthostatic hypotension, begin with 1 mg twice daily, then adjust dosage to 2 mg twice daily, 4 mg twice daily, 6 mg twice daily, 8 mg twice daily, 10 mg twice daily, and 12 mg twice daily on days 2, 3, 4, 5, 6, and 7, respectively, to reach target daily dose of 12–24 mg, given twice daily. Note: Reduce dose by 50% when receiving strong CYP2D6 or CYP3A4 inhibitors or poor metabolizers of CYP2D6 (see Interactions).

SIDE EFFECTS

Frequent (20%–12%): Dizziness, drowsiness, tachycardia. **Occasional (10%–4%):** Nausea, dry mouth, nasal congestion, weight increase, diarrhea, fatigue, orthostatic hypotension. **Rare (3%–1%):** Arthralgia, musculoskeletal stiffness, abdominal discomfort, nasopharyngitis, tremor, hypotension, rash, ejaculatory failure, dyspnea, blurred vision, lethargy.

ADVERSE EFFECTS/ TOXIC REACTIONS

Extrapyramidal disorders, including tardive dyskinesia (protrusion of tongue, puffing of cheeks, chewing/puckering of the mouth), occur in 4% of pts. Upper respiratory infection occurs in 3% of pts. QT interval prolongation may produce torsade de pointes, a form of ventricular tachycardia. Neuroleptic malignant syndrome (e.g., hyperpyrexia, muscle rigidity, altered mental status, irregular pulse or B/P) has been noted.

NURSING CONSIDERATIONS

BASELINE ASSESSMENT

Assess pt's behavior, appearance, emotional status, response to environment, speech pattern, thought content. EKG should be obtained to assess for QT prolongation before instituting medication.

INTERVENTION/EVALUATION

Monitor for orthostatic hypotension; assist with ambulation. Monitor for fine tongue movement (may be first sign of tardive dyskinesia, possibly irreversible). Monitor serum potassium, magnesium in pts at risk for electrolyte disturbances. Assess for therapeutic response (greater interest in surroundings, improved self-care, increased ability to concentrate, relaxed facial expression).

PATIENT/FAMILY TEACHING

• Avoid tasks that require alertness, motor skills until response to drug is established. • Be alert to symptoms of orthostatic hypotension; rise slowly from sitting or lying position. • Report if feeling faint, experience heart palpitations or if fever or muscle rigidity occurs. • Report extrapyramidal symptoms (e.g., involuntary muscle movements, tics) immediately.

iloprost

eye-loe-prost
(Ventavis)

◆CLASSIFICATION

PHARMACOTHERAPEUTIC: Prostaglandin. **CLINICAL:** Vasodilator.

ACTION

Dilates systemic, pulmonary arterial vascular beds, alters pulmonary vascular resistance, suppresses vascular smooth muscle proliferation. **Therapeutic Effect:** Improves symptoms, exercise tolerance in pts with pulmonary hypertension; delays deterioration of condition.

PHARMACOKINETICS

Protein binding: 60%. Metabolized in liver. Excreted in urine (68%), feces (12%). **Half-life:** 20–30 min.

USES

Treatment of pulmonary arterial hypertension (WHO group I) in pts with NYHA class III, IV symptoms. May be used in combination with bosentan for treatment of pulmonary arterial hypertension. **OFF-LABEL:** WHO group III and IV pulmonary arterial hypertension.

PRECAUTIONS

Contraindications: None known. **Cautions:** Hepatic impairment, concurrent conditions or medications that may increase risk of syncope.

⌛ LIFESPAN CONSIDERATIONS

Pregnancy/Lactation: Unknown if drug crosses placenta or is distributed in breast milk. **Pregnancy Category C. Children:** Safety and efficacy not established. **Elderly:** No age-related precautions noted.

INTERACTIONS

DRUG: Anticoagulants, antiplatelet agents may increase risk of bleeding. **Antihypertensives, other vasodilators** may increase hypotensive effects.

HERBAL: None significant. **FOOD:** None known. **LAB VALUES:** May increase serum alkaline phosphatase, GGT.

AVAILABILITY (Rx)

Solution for Oral Inhalation: 10 mcg/ml, 20 mcg/ml.

ADMINISTRATION/HANDLING

Oral Inhalation
• For inhalation only, using Prodose ADD system. • Transfer entire contents of ampule into the medication chamber. • After use, discard remainder of medicine.

INDICATIONS/ROUTES/DOSAGE

◀**ALERT**▶ The 20 mcg/ml concentration is used for pts experiencing extended treatment times.

Pulmonary Hypertension
Oral Inhalation: ADULTS: Initially, 2.5 mcg/dose; if tolerated, increase to 5 mcg/dose. Administer 6–9 times a day at intervals of 2 hrs or longer while pt is awake. Maintenance: 2.5–5 mcg/dose. **Maximum daily dose:** 45 mcg.

SIDE EFFECTS

Frequent (39%–27%): Increased cough, headache, flushing. **Occasional (13%–11%):** Flu-like symptoms, nausea, lockjaw, jaw pain, hypotension. **Rare (8%–2%):** Insomnia, syncope, palpitations, vomiting, back pain, muscle cramps.

ADVERSE EFFECTS/ TOXIC REACTIONS

Hemoptysis, pneumonia occur occasionally. HF, renal failure, dyspnea, chest pain occur rarely.

NURSING CONSIDERATIONS

BASELINE ASSESSMENT
Assess B/P, pulse.

INTERVENTION/EVALUATION
Monitor pulse, B/P during therapy. Assess for signs of pulmonary venous hypertension.

PATIENT/FAMILY TEACHING
• Follow manufacturer guidelines for proper administration of medication using supplied inhalation system. • Discard any remaining solution in the medication chamber after each inhalation session.

imatinib

im-**at**-in-ib
(Gleevec)
Do not confuse imatinib with dasatinib, erlotinib, lapatinib, nilotinib, sorafenib, or sunitinib.

◆CLASSIFICATION

PHARMACOTHERAPEUTIC: Protein tyrosine kinase inhibitor. **CLINICAL:** Antineoplastic (see p. 87C).

ACTION

Inhibits Bcr-Abl tyrosine kinase, an enzyme created by Philadelphia chromosome abnormality found in pts with chronic myeloid leukemia (CML). **Therapeutic Effect:** Suppresses tumor growth during the three stages of CML: blast crisis, accelerated phase, chronic phase.

PHARMACOKINETICS

Well absorbed after PO administration. Protein binding: 95%. Metabolized in liver. Eliminated in feces (68%), urine (13%). **Half-life:** 18 hrs; metabolite, 40 hrs.

USES

Newly diagnosed chronic-phase Philadelphia chromosome positive chronic myeloid leukemia (Ph+ CML) in children and adults. Pts in blast crisis, accelerated phase, or chronic phase Ph+ CML who have already failed interferon therapy. Adults with relapsed or refractory Ph+ acute lymphoblastic leukemia (ALL). Adults with myelodysplastic/myeloproliferative disease (MDS/MPD) associated with platelet-derived growth factor receptor (PDGFR) gene rearrangements. Adults with aggressive systemic mastocytosis (ASM) without mutation of the D816V c-Kit or unknown mutation status of the c-Kit. Adults with hypereosinophilic syndrome (HES) and/or chronic eosinophilic leukemia (CEL) with positive, negative, or unknown FIP1L1-PDGFR fusion kinase. Adults with dermatofibrosarcoma protuberans (DFSP) that is unresectable, recurrent, and/or metastatic. Pts with malignant gastrointestinal stromal tumors (GIST) that are unresectable and/or metastatic. Prevention of cancer recurrence in pts following surgical removal of GIST. Treatment in children with Ph+ acute lymphoblastic leukemia (ALL) (Ph+ALL). **OFF-LABEL:** Treatment of desmoid tumors (soft tissue sarcoma). Post stem cell transplant (allogenic), follow-up treatment in recurrent CML. Treatment of Ph+ acute lymphoblastic lymphoma.

PRECAUTIONS

Contraindications: None known. **Cautions:** Hepatic/renal impairment, thyroidectomy pts, hypothyroidism, gastric surgery pts.

⌛ LIFESPAN CONSIDERATIONS

Pregnancy/Lactation: May cause fetal harm. Breastfeeding not recommended. **Pregnancy Category D. Children:** Safety and efficacy not established. **Elderly:** Increased frequency of fluid retention.

INTERACTIONS

DRUG: **CYP3A4 inducers** (e.g., **carbamazepine, phenobarbital, phenytoin, rifampin**) may decrease concentration. **CYP3A4 inhibitors** (e.g., **clarithromycin, erythromycin, ketoconazole**) may increase concentration. **Bone marrow depressants** may increase myelosuppression. **Live virus vaccines** may potentiate virus replication, increase vaccine side effects, decrease pt's antibody response to vaccine. May reduce effect of **warfarin**. **HERBAL: St. John's wort** decreases concentration. **FOOD: Grapefruit products** may increase concentration. **LAB VALUES:** May increase serum bilirubin, AST, ALT, creatinine. May decrease platelet count, WBC count, serum potassium, albumin, calcium, RBC.

AVAILABILITY (Rx)

Tablets: 100 mg, 400 mg.

ADMINISTRATION/HANDLING

PO
• Give with a meal and large glass of water.
• Tablets may be dispersed in water or apple juice.

INDICATIONS/ROUTES/DOSAGE

Ph+ Chronic Myeloid Leukemia (CML) (Chronic Phase)
PO: ADULTS, ELDERLY: 400 mg once daily; may increase to 600 mg/day.

Ph+ CML (Accelerated Phase)
PO: ADULTS, ELDERLY: 600 mg once daily. May increase to 800 mg/day in 2 divided doses (400 mg twice daily).

Ph+ Acute Lymphoblastic Leukemia (ALL)
PO: ADULTS, ELDERLY: 600 mg once daily.

Gastrointestinal Stromal Tumors (GIST) (Following Complete Resection)
PO: ADULTS, ELDERLY: 400–600 mg/day.

GIST (Unresectable)
PO: ADULTS, ELDERLY: 400–800 mg/day.

Aggressive Systemic Mastocytosis (ASM) with Eosinophilia
PO: ADULTS, ELDERLY: Initially, 100 mg/day. May increase up to 400 mg/day.

ASM without Mutation of the D816V C-Kit or Unknown Mutation Status of C-Kit
PO: ADULTS, ELDERLY: 400 mg once daily.

Dermatofibrosarcoma Protuberans (DFSP)
PO: ADULTS, ELDERLY: 400 mg twice a day.

**Hypereosinophilic Syndrome (HES)/
Chronic Eosinophilic Leukemia (CEL)**
PO: ADULTS, ELDERLY: 400 mg once daily.

**HES/CEL with Positive or Unknown
FIP1L1-PDGFR Fusion Kinase**
PO: ADULTS, ELDERLY: Initially, 100 mg/day. May increase up to 400 mg/day.

**Myelodysplastic/Myeloproliferative
Disease (MDS/MPD)**
PO: ADULTS, ELDERLY: 400 mg once daily.

Usual Dosage for Children (2 Yrs and Older)
Ph+ CML (Chronic Phase, Recurrent or Resistant): 340 mg/m^2/day. **Maximum:** 600 mg/day.
Ph+ CML (Chronic Phase, Newly Diagnosed, Ph+ ALL): 340 mg/m^2/day. **Maximum:** 600 mg/day.

Dosage in Hepatic Impairment (Severe)
Reduce dosage by 25%.

Dosage with Strong CYP3A4 Inducers
Increase dose by 50% with careful monitoring.

SIDE EFFECTS

Frequent (68%–24%): Nausea, diarrhea, vomiting, headache, fluid retention, rash, musculoskeletal pain, muscle cramps, arthralgia. **Occasional (23%–10%):** Abdominal pain, cough, myalgia, fatigue, fever, anorexia, dyspepsia, constipation, night sweats, pruritus, dizziness, blurred vision, somnolence. **Rare (less than 10%):** Nasopharyngitis, petechiae, asthenia (loss of strength, energy), epistaxis.

ADVERSE EFFECTS/ TOXIC REACTIONS

Severe fluid retention (pleural effusion, pericardial effusion, pulmonary edema, ascites), hepatotoxicity occur rarely. Neu-tropenia, thrombocytopenia are expected responses to the therapy. Respiratory toxicity is manifested as dyspnea, pneumonia. Heart damage (left ventricular dysfunction, HF) may occur.

NURSING CONSIDERATIONS

BASELINE ASSESSMENT
Obtain baseline CBC, serum chemistries, renal function. Monitor hepatic function tests before beginning treatment, monthly thereafter.

INTERVENTION/EVALUATION
Assess periorbital area, lower extremities for early evidence of fluid retention. Monitor for unexpected, rapid weight gain. Offer antiemetics to control nausea, vomiting. Monitor daily pattern of bowel activity, stool consistency. Monitor CBC weekly for first mo, biweekly for second mo, periodically thereafter for evidence of neutropenia, thrombocytopenia; assess hepatic function tests for hepatotoxicity. Monitor renal function, serum electrolytes. Duration of neutropenia or thrombocytopenia ranges from 2–4 wks.

PATIENT/FAMILY TEACHING
• Avoid crowds, those with known infection. • Avoid contact with anyone who recently received live virus vaccine; do not receive vaccinations. • Take with food and a full glass of water. • Avoid grapefruit products. • Notify physician if chest pain, swelling of extremities, weight gain greater than 5 lb, easy bruising/bleeding occur. • Avoid tasks requiring alertness, motor skills, including driving or operating machinery, until response to drug is established.

imipenem/cilastatin

im-i-**pen**-em/sye-la-**stat**-in
(Primaxin)

Do not confuse imipenem with doripenem, ertapenem, or meropenem, or Primaxin with Premarin or Primacor.

◆CLASSIFICATION

PHARMACOTHERAPEUTIC: Fixed-combination carbapenem. **CLINICAL:** Antibiotic.

ACTION

Imipenem: Penetrates bacterial cell membrane, inhibiting cell wall synthesis. **Cilastatin:** Competitively inhibits the enzyme dehydropeptidase, preventing renal metabolism of imipenem. **Therapeutic Effect:** Produces bacterial cell death.

PHARMACOKINETICS

Readily absorbed after IM administration. Protein binding: **Imipenem:** 20%; **Cilastatin:** 40%. Widely distributed. Metabolized in kidneys. Primarily excreted in urine. Removed by hemodialysis. **Half-life:** 1 hr (increased in renal impairment).

USES

Treatment of susceptible infections due to gram-negative (ESBL *Escherichia coli* and *Klebsiella, Enterobacter* spp. PsAs), gram-positive (MSSA, *Streptococcus* spp.), anaerobic organisms including respiratory tract, skin/skin structure, gynecologic, bone, joint, intra-abdominal, complicated or uncomplicated UTIs; endocarditis (caused by *S. aureus*); polymicrobic infections; septicemia; serious nosocomial infections. **OFF-LABEL:** Hepatic abscess, neutropenic fever, melioidosis.

PRECAUTIONS

Contraindications: None known. **Cautions:** History of seizures, sensitivity to penicillins, renal impairment.

⚖ LIFESPAN CONSIDERATIONS

Pregnancy/Lactation: Crosses placenta. Distributed in cord blood, amniotic fluid, breast milk. **Pregnancy Cate-**gory C. **Children:** No precautions noted. **Elderly:** Age-related renal impairment may require dosage adjustment.

INTERACTIONS

DRUG: May decrease concentration of **valproic acid. HERBAL:** None significant. **FOOD:** None known. **LAB VALUES:** May increase BUN, serum alkaline phosphatase, bilirubin, creatinine, LDH, AST, ALT. May decrease Hgb, Hct.

AVAILABILITY (Rx)

Injection, Powder for Reconstitution (Primaxin): 250 mg, 500 mg.

ADMINISTRATION/HANDLING

 IV

Reconstitution • Dilute each 250- or 500-mg vial with 100–250 ml D₅W or 0.9% NaCl. Final concentration not to exceed 5 mg/ml.

Rate of Administration • Give by intermittent IV infusion (piggyback). • Do not give IV push. • Infuse over 15–30 min (doses greater than 500 mg over 40–60 min). • Observe pt during initial 30 min of first-time infusion for possible hypersensitivity reaction.

Storage • Solution appears colorless to yellow; discard if solution turns brown. • IV infusion (piggyback) is stable for 4 hrs at room temperature, 24 hrs if refrigerated. • Discard if precipitate forms.

IM

• Prepare 500-mg vial with 2 ml 1% lidocaine without epinephrine • Administer suspension within 1 hr of preparation. • Do not mix with any other medications. • Inject deep in large muscle mass.

▓ IV INCOMPATIBILITIES

Allopurinol (Aloprim), amphotericin B complex (Abelcet, AmBisome, Amphotec), fluconazole (Diflucan).

▓ IV COMPATIBILITIES

Diltiazem (Cardizem), insulin, propofol (Diprivan).

Creatinine Clearance (ml/min)	70 kg or greater	60–69 kg	50–59 kg	40–49 kg	30–39 kg
41–70	250 mg q8h–750 mg q8h	125 mg q6h–750 mg q8h	125 mg q6h–500 mg q6h	125 mg q6h–500 mg q8h	125 mg q8h–250 mg q6h
21–40	250 mg q12h–500 mg q6h	250 mg q12h–500 mg q8h	125 mg q8h–500 mg q8h	125 mg q12h–250 mg q6h	125 mg q12h–250 mg q8h
6–20	250 mg q12h–500 mg q12h	125 mg q12h–500 mg q12h	125 mg q12h–500 mg q12h	125 mg q12h–250 mg q12h	125 mg q12h–250 mg q12h

INDICATIONS/ROUTES/DOSAGE

◄ALERT► Only IM formulation can be used for IM administration. Limit IM use to mild-moderate infection. Dosage based on imipenem content.

Usual Dosage Ranges
IV/IM: ADULTS, ELDERLY, WEIGHING 70 KG OR MORE: 250 mg q6h up to 1,000 mg q6h. **60–69 KG:** 250 mg q8h up to 1 g q8h. **50–59 KG:** 125 mg q6h up to 750 mg q8h. **40–49 KG:** 125 mg q6h up to 500 mg q6h. **30–39 KG:** 125 mg q8h up to 500 mg q8h. **CHILDREN OLDER THAN 3 MOS–12 YRS:** 60–100 mg/kg/day in 4 divided doses q6h. **Maximum:** 4 g/day. **CHILDREN 1–3 MOS:** 100 mg/kg/day in 4 divided doses q6h. **CHILDREN 1–4 WKS:** 20–25 mg/kg q8h. **CHILDREN YOUNGER THAN 1 WK:** 20–25 mg/kg q12h.

Dosage in Renal Impairment
Dosage and frequency are modified based on creatinine clearance and severity of infection.

SIDE EFFECTS

Occasional (3%): Diarrhea, nausea, vomiting. **Rare (1%):** Rash.

ADVERSE EFFECTS/ TOXIC REACTIONS

Antibiotic-associated colitis, other superinfections (abdominal cramps, severe watery diarrhea, fever) may result from altered bacterial balance in GI tract. Anaphylactic reactions have been reported.

NURSING CONSIDERATIONS

BASELINE ASSESSMENT
Question for history of allergies, particularly to beta-lactams, penicillins, cephalosporins. Inquire about history of seizures.

INTERVENTION/EVALUATION
Monitor renal, hepatic, hematologic function tests. Evaluate for phlebitis (heat, pain, red streaking over vein), pain at IV injection site. Assess for GI discomfort, nausea, vomiting. Monitor daily pattern of bowel activity, stool consistency. Assess skin for rash. Be alert to tremors, possible seizures.

imipramine

i-**mip**-ra-meen
(Apo-Imipramine ❖, Novo-Pramine ❖, Tofranil, Tofranil-PM)
BLACK BOX ALERT Increased risk of suicidal ideation and behavior in children, adolescents, young adults 18–24 yrs with major depressive disorder, other psychiatric disorders.
Do not confuse imipramine with amitriptyline, desipramine, or Norpramin.

◆CLASSIFICATION

PHARMACOTHERAPEUTIC: Tricyclic antidepressant. **CLINICAL:** Antidepressant, antineuritic, antipanic, antineuralgic, antinarcoleptic adjunct, anticataplectic, antibulimic (see p. 39C).

ACTION

Blocks reuptake of neurotransmitters (norepinephrine, serotonin) at presynaptic membranes, increasing concentration at postsynaptic receptor sites. **Therapeutic Effect:** Relieves depression, controls nocturnal enuresis.

USES

Treatment of depression, often in conjunction with psychotherapy. Treatment of nocturnal enuresis in children older than 6 yrs. **OFF-LABEL:** Treatment of ADHD, post-traumatic stress disorder (PTSD), neurogenic pain, panic disorder.

PRECAUTIONS

Contraindications: Acute recovery period after MI, use within 14 days of MAOIs, pregnancy, concurrent use with linezolid or methylene blue. **Cautions:** Prostatic hypertrophy, history of urinary retention, obstruction, glaucoma, diabetes mellitus, history of seizures, hyperthyroidism; cardiac, hepatic, renal disease; increased intraocular pressure, hiatal hernia, pts with high risk for suicide. Decreased GI motility, paralytic ileus, visual problems, respiratory disease, sleep apnea. **Pregnancy Category D.**

INTERACTIONS

DRUG: Alcohol, other CNS depressants may increase hypotensive effects, CNS, respiratory depression. **Cimetidine, fluoxetine** may increase concentration, risk of toxicity. **Phenytoin, barbiturates** may decrease concentration. **HERBAL: Kava kava, SAMe, St. John's wort, valerian** may increase risk of serotonin syndrome, CNS depression. **St. John's wort** may decrease concentration. **FOOD: Grapefruit products** may increase concentration/toxicity. **LAB VALUES:** May alter serum glucose, EKG readings. **Therapeutic serum level:** 225–300 ng/ml; **toxic serum level:** greater than 500 ng/ml.

AVAILABILITY (Rx)

Capsules (Tofranil-PM): 75 mg, 100 mg, 125 mg, 150 mg. **Tablets (Tofranil):** 10 mg, 25 mg, 50 mg.

ADMINISTRATION/HANDLING

PO

• Give with food, milk if GI distress occurs.

INDICATIONS/ROUTES/DOSAGE

Depression

PO: ADULTS: Initially, 75–100 mg/day in 3–4 divided doses. May gradually increase to maximum of 200 mg/day (outpatient) or 300 mg/day (inpatient). **ELDERLY, ADOLESCENTS:** Initially, 25–50 mg/day at bedtime. May increase by 10–25 mg every 3–7 days. **Maximum:** 100 mg/day. **CHILDREN:** 1.5 mg/kg/day. May increase by 1 mg/kg every 3–4 days. **Maximum:** 5 mg/kg/day in 1–4 divided doses.

Enuresis

PO: CHILDREN, 6 YRS AND OLDER: Initially, 10–25 mg 1 hr before bedtime. May increase by 25 mg if inadequate response seen after 1 wk. **Maximum:** 2.5 mg/kg/day or 50 mg at bedtime for ages 6–12 yrs; 75 mg at bedtime for ages over 12 yrs.

SIDE EFFECTS

Frequent: Drowsiness, fatigue, dry mouth, blurred vision, constipation, delayed micturition, orthostatic hypotension, diaphoresis, impaired concentration, increased appetite, urinary retention, photosensitivity. **Occasional:** GI disturbances (nausea, metallic taste). **Rare:** Paradoxical reactions (agitation, restlessness, nightmares, insomnia), extrapyramidal symptoms (EPS) (particularly fine hand tremor).

ADVERSE EFFECTS/ TOXIC REACTIONS

Overdose may produce seizures; cardiovascular effects (severe orthostatic hypotension, dizziness, tachycardia, palpitations, arrhythmias). May result in altered temperature regulation (hyperpyrexia, hypothermia). Abrupt withdrawal from prolonged therapy may produce headache, malaise, nausea, vomiting, vivid dreams.

NURSING CONSIDERATIONS

BASELINE ASSESSMENT

Assess appearance, behavior, speech pattern, level of interest, mood. Obtain baseline CBC, hepatic/renal function tests.

INTERVENTION/EVALUATION

Supervise suicidal-risk pt closely during early therapy (as depression lessens, energy level improves, increasing suicide potential). Monitor appearance, behavior, speech pattern, level of interest, mood. For pts on long-term therapy, hepatic/renal function tests, blood counts should be performed periodically. Monitor daily pattern of bowel activity, stool consistency. Monitor B/P, pulse for hypotension, arrhythmias. Assess for urinary retention by bladder palpation. **Therapeutic serum level:** 225–300 ng/ml; **toxic serum level:** greater than 500 ng/ml.

PATIENT/FAMILY TEACHING

• Notify physician if depression worsens, thoughts of suicide, agitation, irritability occur. • Change positions slowly to avoid hypotensive effect. • Tolerance to postural hypotension, sedative, anticholinergic effects usually develops during early therapy. • Avoid tasks that require alertness, motor skills until response to drug is established. • Therapeutic effect may be noted within 2–5 days, maximum effect within 2–3 wks. • Sugarless gum, sips of water may relieve dry mouth. • Do not abruptly discontinue medication. • Limit caffeine; avoid alcohol.

---

immune globulin IV (IGIV)

im-**mune glob**-u-lin
(Carimune NF, Flebogamma DIF, Gammagard Liquid, Gammagard S/D, Gammaplex, Gamunex-C, Hizentra, Octagam 5%, Privigen)

BLACK BOX ALERT Acute renal impairment characterized by increased serum creatinine, oliguria, acute renal failure, osmotic nephrosis, particularly pts with any degree of renal insufficiency, diabetes mellitus, volume depletion, sepsis, and those older than age 65 yrs.

◆CLASSIFICATION

PHARMACOTHERAPEUTIC: Immune globulins, blood product. **CLINICAL:** Immunizing agent.

ACTION

Blocks Fc receptor on macrophages in pts with idiopathic thrombocytopenia purpura (ITP). Immunomodulatory effects on T cells and macrophages, esp. cytokine synthesis, B-cell immune function. Provides antibodies that neutralize bacteria, viral toxins. **Therapeutic Effect:** Provides passive immunity against infection; induces rapid increase in platelet count; produces anti-inflammatory effect.

PHARMACOKINETICS

Evenly distributed between intravascular and extravascular space. **Half-life:** 21–23 days.

USES

Treatment of pts with primary humoral immunodeficiency syndromes, acute/chronic immune idiopathic thrombocytopenic purpura (ITP), prevention of coronary artery aneurysms associated with Kawasaki disease, prevention of recurrent bacterial infections in pts with hypogammaglobulinemia associated with B-cell chronic lymphocytic leukemia (CLL). Treatment of chronic inflammatory demyelinating polyneuropathies. Provide passive immunity in pts with hepatitis A, measles, rubella, varicella. **OFF-LABEL:** Guillain-Barré syndrome; myasthenia gravis; prevention of acute infections in immunosuppressed pts; prevention, treatment of infection in high-risk, preterm, low birth-weight neonates; treatment of multiple sclerosis; HIV-associated thrombocytopenia.

PRECAUTIONS

Contraindications: Selective IgA deficiency, hyperprolinemia (Hizentra, Privigen), severe thrombocytopenia, coagulation disorders where IM injections contraindicated. **Cautions:** Cardiovascular disease, history of thrombosis.

⌛ LIFESPAN CONSIDERATIONS

Pregnancy/Lactation: Unknown if drug crosses placenta or is distributed in breast milk. **Pregnancy Category C. Children/Elderly:** No age-related precautions noted.

INTERACTIONS

DRUG: Live virus vaccines may increase vaccine side effects, potentiate virus replication, decrease pt's antibody response to vaccine. **HERBAL:** None significant. **FOOD:** None known. **LAB VALUES:** None significant.

AVAILABILITY (Rx)

Injection, Powder for Reconstitution (Carimune NF): 3 g, 6 g, 12 g. **(Gammagard S/D):** 2.5 g, 5 g, 10 g. **Injection, Solution (Flebogamma DIF 5%, 10%, Gammagard Liquid 10%, Gammaplex 5%, Gamunex-C 10%, Octagam 5%, Privigen):** 10%.

ADMINISTRATION/HANDLING

 IV

◀**ALERT**▶ Monitor vital signs, B/P diligently during and immediately after IV administration (precipitous fall in B/P may indicate anaphylactic reaction). Stop infusion immediately. Epinephrine should be readily available.

Reconstitution • Reconstitute only with diluent provided by manufacturer. • Discard partially used or turbid preparations. **Rate of Administration** • Give by infusion only. • After reconstitution, administer via separate tubing. • Avoid mixing with

other medication or IV infusion fluids. • Rate of infusion varies with product used. **Storage** • Refer to individual IV preparations for storage requirements, stability after reconstitution.

▦ IV INCOMPATIBILITIES

Do not mix with any other medications.

INDICATIONS/ROUTES/DOSAGE

Primary Immunodeficiency Syndrome
IV: ADULTS, ELDERLY, CHILDREN: *(Privigen):* 200–800 mg/kg q3–4wks. *(Carimune NF):* 400–800 mg/kg q3–4 wks. *(Flebogamma DIF, Gammagard, Gamunex-C, Octagam):* 300–600 mg/kg/ q3–4wks. *(Gammaplex):* 300–800 mg/kg q3–4wks.

Idiopathic Thrombocytopenic Purpura (ITP)
IV: ADULTS, ELDERLY, CHILDREN: *(Carimune NF):* 400 mg/kg/day for 2–5 days. Maintenance: 400–1,000 mg/kg/dose to maintain platelet count or control bleeding. *(Gammagard):* **1,000 MG/KG:** up to 3 additional doses may be given. *(Privigen):* 1,000 mg/kg/day for 2 consecutive days.

Kawasaki Disease
IV: ADULTS, ELDERLY, CHILDREN: *(Gammagard):* 2,000 mg/kg as a single dose given over 10–12 hrs within 10 days of disease onset. Must be used in combination with aspirin.

Chronic Leukocytic Leukemia (CLL)
IV: ADULTS, ELDERLY, CHILDREN: *(Gammagard):* 400 mg/kg/dose q3–4wks.

Chronic Inflammatory Demyelinating Polyneuropathy
IV: ADULTS, ELDERLY, CHILDREN: *(Gamunex-C):* 2,000 mg/kg divided over 2–4 days (consecutive). Maintenance: 1,000 mg/kg/day q3wks or 500 mg/kg for 2 consecutive days q3wks.

Passive Immunity (Measles)
Subcutaneous Infusion: ADULTS, ELDERLY, CHILDREN: Pre-exposure: 200

mg/kg/dose (or greater) once weekly for 2 doses for pts at risk for measles. **Post-exposure:** 200 mg/kg/dose as soon as possible following exposure.

SIDE EFFECTS

Frequent: Tachycardia, backache, headache, arthralgia, myalgia. **Occasional:** Fatigue, wheezing, injection site rash/pain, leg cramps, urticaria, bluish color of lips/nailbeds, light-headedness.

ADVERSE EFFECTS/ TOXIC REACTIONS

Anaphylactic reactions occur rarely but incidence increases with repeated injections. Epinephrine should be readily available. Overdose may produce chest tightness, chills, diaphoresis, dizziness, facial flushing, nausea, vomiting, fever, hypotension. Hypersensitivity reaction (anxiety, arthralgia, dizziness, flushing, myalgia, palpitations, pruritus) occurs rarely.

NURSING CONSIDERATIONS

BASELINE ASSESSMENT

Inquire about exposure history to disease for pt/family as appropriate. Have epinephrine readily available. Pt should be well hydrated prior to administration.

INTERVENTION/EVALUATION

Control rate of IV infusion carefully; too-rapid infusion increases risk of precipitous fall in B/P, signs of anaphylaxis (facial flushing, chest tightness, chills, fever, nausea, vomiting, diaphoresis). Assess pt closely during infusion, esp. first hr; monitor vital signs continuously. Stop infusion if aforementioned signs noted. For treatment of idiopathic thrombocytopenic purpura (ITP), monitor platelet count.

PATIENT/FAMILY TEACHING

• Explain rationale for therapy. • Inform physician if sudden weight gain, fluid retention, edema, decreased urine output, shortness of breath occur.

indacaterol

in-da-**ka**-ter-ol
(Arcapta Neohaler, Onbrez Breezhaler ✦)

BLACK BOX ALERT Long-acting beta$_2$-adrenergic agonists (LABAs) have an increased risk of asthma-related deaths. Not indicated for treatment of asthma or acute deterioration of COPD.

◆CLASSIFICATION

PHARMACOTHERAPEUTIC: Long-acting beta$_2$-adrenergic agonist. **CLINICAL:** Bronchodilator (see p. 76C).

ACTION

Stimulates beta$_2$-adrenergic receptors in lungs, resulting in relaxation of bronchial smooth muscle. **Therapeutic Effect:** Relieves bronchospasm, reduces airway resistance, improves bronchodilation.

PHARMACOKINETICS

Extensive activation of systemic beta-adrenergic receptors; acts primarily in lungs. Protein binding: 94%–95%. Metabolized in liver by hydroxylation. Steady-state level: 12–15 days. Primarily excreted in feces. **Half-life:** 45–126 hrs.

USES

Long-term maintenance treatment of airflow obstruction in pts with chronic obstructive pulmonary disease (COPD), including chronic bronchitis and emphysema.

PRECAUTIONS

◀**ALERT**▶ Not indicated for the treatment of asthma.
Contraindications: Asthma without use of long-term asthma control medication, acutely deteriorating COPD. **Cautions:** Pts with cardiovascular disease (coronary insufficiency, arrhythmias, hypertension, history of hypersensitivity to sympathomimetics), seizure disorders, hyperthyroidism, hypokalemia, diabetes mellitus. May

cause paradoxical bronchospasm, severe asthma.

⏳ LIFESPAN CONSIDERATIONS

Pregnancy/Lactation: Unknown if drug crosses placenta or is distributed in breast milk. **Pregnancy Category C. Children:** Safety and efficacy not established. **Elderly:** May be more sensitive to tremor, tachycardia due to age-related increased sympathetic sensitivity.

INTERACTIONS

DRUG: May decrease effectiveness of **beta-adrenergic blocking agents (beta-blockers). Diuretics, steroids, xanthine derivatives** may increase risk of hypokalemia. **Drugs that can prolong QT interval (e.g., erythromycin, quinidine, thioridazine), antiarrhythmics, MAOIs, tricyclic antidepressants** may potentiate cardiovascular effects (increased risk of ventricular arrhythmias). **Erythromycin, ketoconazole, ritonavir, verapamil** may increase serum concentration. **HERBAL:** None known. **FOOD:** None significant. **LAB VALUES:** May decrease serum potassium. May increase serum glucose.

AVAILABILITY (Rx)

Powder for Inhalation: 75 mcg (in blister packs).

ADMINISTRATION/HANDLING

Inhalation
• Open cap of Neohaler by pulling upward, then open mouthpiece. • Remove capsule from blister package and place in center of chamber. Firmly close until click is heard. • Hold inhaler upright and pierce capsule by pressing side buttons once only. • Instruct pt to exhale completely. Place mouthpiece into mouth, close lips, and inhale quickly and deeply through mouth (this causes capsule to spin, dispensing the drug). A slight whirring noise should occur. If not, this may indicate capsule is stuck. Gently tap inhaler to loosen and re-attempt. • Pt should hold breath as long as possible before exhaling. • Check capsule to ensure all the powder is gone. Instruct pt to reinhale if powder remains.
Storage • Store at room temperature. • Maintain capsules within individual blister pack until time of use. • Do not store capsules in Neohaler device.

INDICATIONS/ROUTES/DOSAGE

Maintenance Therapy and Prevention of COPD
Inhalation: ADULTS, ELDERLY: 75 mcg (1 capsule) once daily via Neohaler inhalation device.

SIDE EFFECTS

Occasional (7%–5%): Cough, nasopharyngitis, headache. **Rare (2%):** Oropharyngeal pain, nausea.

ADVERSE EFFECTS/ TOXIC REACTIONS

Peripheral edema, diabetes mellitus, hyperglycemia, sinusitis, URI reported in greater than 2% of pts. Excessive sympathomimetic stimulation, hypokalemia may produce palpitations, arrhythmias, angina pectoris, tachycardia, muscle cramps, weakness. Hyperglycemia symptoms present with increased thirst, polyuria, dry mouth, drowsiness/confusion, blurred vision. Severe shortness of breath may indicate paradoxical bronchospasm, deteriorating COPD. Serious asthma-related events including death reported.

NURSING CONSIDERATIONS

BASELINE ASSESSMENT

Assess rate, depth, rhythm, type of respirations. Monitor EKG, serum potassium, ABG determinations, O_2 saturation, pulmonary function test. Assess lung sounds for wheezing (bronchoconstriction), rales. Obtain baseline electrolytes, capillary blood glucose. Receive full medication history and screen for possible drug interactions. Question for history of asthma, angina pectoris, diabetes mellitus, peripheral edema.

INTERVENTION/EVALUATION

Routinely monitor serum electrolytes, blood glucose, O_2 saturation. Recommend discontinuation of short-acting beta$_2$-agonists (use only for symptomatic relief of acute respiratory symptoms). Monitor for palpitations, tachycardia, serum hypokalemia. Inspect oropharyngeal cavity for irritation.

PATIENT/FAMILY TEACHING

• Follow manufacturer guidelines for proper use of inhaler. • Increase fluid intake (decreases lung secretion viscosity). • Rinse mouth with water after inhalation to decrease mouth/throat irritation. • Avoid excessive use of caffeine derivatives (chocolate, coffee, tea, cola). • An immediate cough lasting 15 sec may occur after inhaler use. • Report any fever, productive cough, body aches, difficulty breathing.

indapamide

in-**dap**-a-mide
(Apo-Indapamide ✦, Lozide ✦,
Novo-Indapamide ✦)
**Do not confuse indapamide
with Iopidine.**

◆CLASSIFICATION

PHARMACOTHERAPEUTIC: Thiazide.
CLINICAL: Diuretic, antihypertensive
(see p. 104C).

ACTION

Diuretic: Blocks reabsorption of water, sodium, potassium at cortical diluting segment of distal tubule. **Antihypertensive:** Reduces plasma, extracellular fluid volume, and peripheral vascular resistance by direct effect on blood vessels. **Therapeutic Effect:** Promotes diuresis, reduces B/P.

PHARMACOKINETICS

Almost completely absorbed following PO administration. Protein binding: 71%–

79%. Metabolized in liver. Excreted in urine. **Half-life:** 14–18 hrs.

USES

Management of hypertension. Treatment of edema associated with HF. **OFF-LABEL:** Nephrotic syndrome.

PRECAUTIONS

Contraindications: Anuria. **Canada:** Renal decompensation, hepatic impairment, breastfeeding. **Cautions:** History of hypersensitivity to sulfonamides or thiazide diuretics. Severe renal disease, hepatic impairment, prediabetes, diabetes mellitus, elderly, debilitated pts, thyroid disorders, severe hyponatremia, high cholesterol.

⧖ LIFESPAN CONSIDERATIONS

Pregnancy/Lactation: Unknown if drug crosses placenta or is distributed in breast milk. **Pregnancy Category B (D if used in pregnancy-induced hypertension). Children:** Safety and efficacy not established. **Elderly:** May be more sensitive to hypotensive, electrolyte effects.

INTERACTIONS

DRUG: May increase risk of **lithium** toxicity. **HERBAL: Ephedra, ginseng, licorice, yohimbe** may worsen hypertension. **Black cohosh** may increase antihypertensive effect. **FOOD:** None known. **LAB VALUES:** May increase plasma renin activity. May decrease protein-bound iodine, serum calcium, potassium, sodium.

AVAILABILITY (Rx)

Tablets: 1.25 mg, 2.5 mg.

ADMINISTRATION/HANDLING

PO
• Give with food, milk if GI upset occurs, preferably with breakfast (may prevent nocturia).

INDICATIONS/ROUTES/DOSAGE

Edema
PO: ADULTS: Initially, 2.5 mg/day, may increase to 5 mg/day after 1 wk.

Hypertension

PO: ADULTS, ELDERLY: Initially, 1.25 mg. May increase to 2.5 mg/day after 4 wks or 5 mg/day after additional 4 wks.

SIDE EFFECTS

Frequent (5% and greater): Fatigue, paresthesia of extremities, tension, irritability, agitation, headache, dizziness, lightheadedness, insomnia, muscle cramps. **Occasional (less than 5%):** Urinary frequency, urticaria, rhinorrhea, flushing, weight loss, orthostatic hypotension, depression, blurred vision, nausea, vomiting, diarrhea, constipation, dry mouth, impotence, rash, pruritus.

ADVERSE EFFECTS/ TOXIC REACTIONS

Vigorous diuresis may lead to profound water and electrolyte depletion, resulting in hypokalemia, hyponatremia, dehydration. Acute hypotensive episodes may occur. Hyperglycemia may be noted during prolonged therapy. Pancreatitis, blood dyscrasias, pulmonary edema, allergic pneumonitis, dermatologic reactions occur rarely. Overdose can lead to lethargy, coma without changes in electrolytes or hydration.

NURSING CONSIDERATIONS

BASELINE ASSESSMENT

Check vital signs, esp. B/P for hypotension, before administration. Assess baseline electrolytes, particularly check for hypokalemia. Observe for edema; assess skin turgor, mucous membranes for hydration status. Assess muscle strength, mental status. Note skin temperature, moisture. Obtain baseline weight. Initiate I&O.

INTERVENTION/EVALUATION

Continue to monitor B/P, vital signs, electrolytes, I&O, weight. Note extent of diuresis. Watch for electrolyte disturbances (hypokalemia may result in weakness, tremor, muscle cramps, nausea, vomiting, altered mental status, tachycardia; hyponatremia may result in confusion, thirst, cold/clammy skin).

PATIENT/FAMILY TEACHING

• Expect increased frequency, volume of urination. • To reduce hypotensive effect, go from lying to standing slowly. • Eat foods high in potassium such as whole grains (cereals), legumes, meat, bananas, apricots, orange juice, potatoes (white, sweet), raisins. • Take early in the day to avoid nocturia.

---

indinavir

in-**din**-ah-veer
(Crixivan)
Do not confuse indinavir with Denavir.

◆ CLASSIFICATION

PHARMACOTHERAPEUTIC: Protease inhibitor. **CLINICAL:** Antiviral (see pp. 70C, 120C).

ACTION

Suppresses HIV protease, an enzyme necessary for splitting viral polyprotein precursors into mature infectious viral particles. **Therapeutic Effect:** Interrupts HIV replication, slowing progression of HIV infection.

PHARMACOKINETICS

Rapidly absorbed after PO administration. Protein binding: 60%. Metabolized in liver. Primarily eliminated in feces. Unknown if removed by hemodialysis. **Half-life:** 1.4–2.2 hrs (increased in hepatic impairment).

USES

Treatment of HIV infection as part of a multidrug regimen (at least 3 antiretroviral agents). **OFF-LABEL:** Prophylaxis following occupational exposure to HIV.

PRECAUTIONS

Contraindications: Concurrent use with alfuzosin, alprazolam, amiodarone, ergot derivatives, midazolam, pimozide, silde-nafil (when used for pulmonary arterial hypertension), simvastatin, St. John's wort, triazolam. **Cautions:** Hepatic impairment, hemophilia.

⧗ LIFESPAN CONSIDERATIONS

Pregnancy/Lactation: Unknown if excreted in breast milk. Breastfeeding not recommended in HIV-infected women. **Pregnancy Category C. Children:** Safety and efficacy not established. **Elderly:** Information not available.

INTERACTIONS

DRUG: Note: See Contraindications. May increase concentration/toxicity of **mid-azolam, sildenafil, triazolam. Ri-fabutin, rifampin** may decrease concentration/effects. **HMG-CoA inhibitors (e.g., lovastatin, simvastatin)** may increase risk of myopathy. **Itracon-azole, ketoconazole** may increase concentration. **HERBAL: St. John's wort, garlic** may decrease concentration/effects. **FOOD: Grapefruit products** may decrease concentration/effects. **High-fat, high-calorie, high-protein meals** may decrease concentration. **LAB VAL-UES:** May increase serum bilirubin, amylase, glucose, AST, ALT. May alter serum triglycerides, cholesterol.

AVAILABILITY (Rx)

Capsules: 200 mg, 400 mg.

ADMINISTRATION/HANDLING

PO

• Store at room temperature. • Protect from moisture (capsules sensitive to moisture; keep in original bottle). • Best given without food 1 hr before or 2 hrs following a meal but may give with water, skim milk, juice, coffee, tea, light meal (e.g., dry toast with jelly). • Do not give with meal high in fat, calories, protein. • If indinavir and didanosine are given concurrently, give at least 1 hr apart on an empty stomach. • May be taken with food when administered with ritonavir.

INDICATIONS/ROUTES/DOSAGE

HIV Infection (in Combination with Other Antiretrovirals)
PO: ADULTS (UNBOOSTED WITH RITONAVIR): 800 mg (two 400-mg capsules) q8h. **(BOOSTED WITH RITONAVIR):** 100–200 mg twice a day and indinavir 800 mg twice a day.
Dosage Adjustments When Given Concomitantly: DELAVIRDINE, ITRACON-AZOLE, KETOCONAZOLE: Reduce dose to 600 mg q8h. **EFAVIRENZ:** Increase dose to 1,000 mg q8h. **LOPINAVIR/RITONAVIR:** Reduce dose to 600 mg twice a day. **NEVI-RAPINE:** Increase dose to 1,000 mg q8h. **RIFABUTIN:** Reduce rifabutin by ½ and increase indinavir to 1,000 mg q8h.

HIV Infection in Pts with Hepatic Insufficiency
PO: ADULTS: 600 mg q8h.

SIDE EFFECTS

Frequent (12%–5%): Nausea, abdominal pain, headache, diarrhea. **Occasional (4%):** Vomiting, asthenia (loss of strength, energy), fatigue, insomnia, accumulation of fat in waist, abdomen, back of neck. **Rare:** Altered taste, heartburn, symptomatic urinary tract disease, transient renal dysfunction.

ADVERSE EFFECTS/ TOXIC REACTIONS

Nephrolithiasis (flank pain with or without hematuria) occurs in 4% of pts.

NURSING CONSIDERATIONS

BASELINE ASSESSMENT

Offer emotional support. Obtain baseline lab values. Emphasize need for close monitoring of renal function (urinalysis, serum creatinine) during therapy.

INTERVENTION/EVALUATION

Encourage adequate hydration. Pt should drink 48 oz (1.5 L) of liquid for each 24 hrs during therapy. Monitor for evidence of nephrolithiasis (flank pain, hematuria); contact physician if symptoms occur (therapy should be interrupted for 1–3 days). Monitor daily pattern of bowel activity, stool consistency. Assess for abdominal discomfort, headache. Monitor serum bilirubin, glucose, cholesterol, triglycerides, amylase, lipase, hepatic function tests, CD4 cell count, CBC.

PATIENT/FAMILY TEACHING

• Indinavir is not a cure for HIV infection, nor does it reduce risk of transmission to others. Condition may progress despite treatment. • If dose is missed, take next dose at regularly scheduled time (do **not** double the dose). • Best taken without food but water only (optimal absorption) 1 hr before or 2 hrs following a meal; may take with water, skim milk, juice, coffee, tea, light carbohydrate meal. • Avoid St. John's wort, grapefruit products.

---

indomethacin

in-doe-**meth**-a-sin
(Apo-Indomethacin ✽, Indocid ✽, Indocin, Indocin IV, Novo-Methacin ✽)

BLACK BOX ALERT Increased risk of serious cardiovascular thrombotic events, including myocardial infarction, CVA. Increased risk of severe GI reactions, including ulceration, bleeding, perforation.

Do not confuse Indocin with Imodium, Minocin, or Vicodin.

◆CLASSIFICATION

PHARMACOTHERAPEUTIC: NSAID. **CLINICAL:** Anti-inflammatory, analgesic (see p. 130C).

ACTION

Produces analgesic, anti-inflammatory effects by inhibiting prostaglandin synthesis. Increases sensitivity of premature ductus to dilating effects of prostaglandins. **Therapeutic Effect:** Reduces inflammatory response, intensity of pain. Closure of patent ductus arteriosus.

PHARMACOKINETICS

Route	Onset	Peak	Duration
PO	30 min	—	4–6 hrs

Well absorbed from GI tract. Protein binding: 99%. Metabolized in liver. Excreted in urine. **Half-life:** 4.5 hrs.

USES

Treatment of active stages of rheumatoid arthritis, osteoarthritis, ankylosing spondylitis, acute gouty arthritis. Relieves acute bursitis, tendonitis. **(IV Form):** For closure of hemodynamically significant patent ductus arteriosus of premature infants. **OFF-LABEL:** Management of preterm labor.

PRECAUTIONS

Contraindications: Hypersensitivity to aspirin, indomethacin, other NSAIDs. Perioperative pain in setting of CABG surgery. History of proctitis or recent rectal bleeding. **Injection:** In preterm infants with untreated/systemic infection or congenital heart disease where patency of PDA necessary for pulmonary or systemic blood flow; bleeding; thrombocytopenia; coagulation defects; necrotizing enterocolitis; significant renal dysfunction. **Cautions:** Cardiac dysfunction, hypertension, renal/hepatic impairment, epilepsy, concurrent anticoagulant therapy. Treatment of juvenile rheumatoid arthritis in children.

⌛ LIFESPAN CONSIDERATIONS

Pregnancy/Lactation: Crosses placenta; distributed in breast milk. **Pregnancy Category C (D if used after 34 wks' gestation, close to delivery, or for longer than 48 hrs). Children:** Safety and efficacy not established in those younger than 14 yrs. **Elderly:** GI bleeding, ulceration increase risk of serious adverse effects.

INTERACTIONS

DRUG: May decrease effects of **antihypertensives, diuretics. Aspirin, other salicylates** may increase risk of GI side effects, bleeding. **Bone marrow depres-**

sants may increase risk of hematologic reactions. May increase risk of bleeding with **heparin, anticoagulants, thrombolytics.** May increase concentration, risk of toxicity of **lithium.** May increase risk of **cyclosporine, methotrexate** toxicity. **HERBAL: Cat's claw, dong quai, evening primrose, feverfew, garlic, ginkgo, ginseng, horse chestnut, red clover** may increase antiplatelet activity. **FOOD:** None known. **LAB VALUES:** May prolong bleeding time. May alter serum glucose. May increase BUN, serum creatinine, potassium, AST, ALT. May decrease serum sodium, platelet count, leukocytes.

AVAILABILITY (Rx)

Capsules (Indocin): 25 mg, 50 mg. Injection, Powder for Reconstitution (Indocin IV): 1 mg. Oral Suspension (Indocin): 25 mg/5 ml. Suppository: 50 mg.

 Capsules, Extended-Release: 75 mg.

ADMINISTRATION/HANDLING
IV

Reconstitution • To 1-mg vial, add 1–2 ml preservative-free Sterile Water for Injection or 0.9% NaCl to provide concentration of 1 mg/ml or 0.5 mg/ml, respectively. • Do not further dilute.
Rate of Administration • Administer over 20–30 min.
Storage • IV solutions made without preservatives should be used immediately. • Use IV solution immediately following reconstitution. • IV solution appears clear; discard if cloudy or precipitate forms. • Discard unused portion.

PO

• Give after meals or with food, antacids.
• Do not crush, break extended-release capsule. Swallow whole.
◀**ALERT**▶ IV injection preferred for patent ductus arteriosus in neonate (but may give dose PO via NG tube or rectally).

IV INCOMPATIBILITIES

Amino acid injection, calcium gluconate, dobutamine (Dobutrex), dopamine (Intropin), gentamicin (Garamycin), tobramycin (Nebcin).

IV COMPATIBILITIES

Insulin, potassium.

INDICATIONS/ROUTES/DOSAGE

Moderate to Severe Rheumatoid Arthritis (RA), Osteoarthritis, Ankylosing Spondylitis
PO: ADULTS, ELDERLY (IMMEDIATE-RELEASE): Initially, 25–50 mg 2–3 times a day; increased by 25–50 mg/wk up to 200 mg/day.
Extended-Release: 75–150 mg/day in 1–2 doses/day. **Maximum:** 150 mg/day.
CHILDREN 2 YRS AND OLDER (IMMEDIATE-RELEASE): 1–2 mg/kg/day in 2–4 divided doses. **Maximum:** 4 mg/kg/day not to exceed 150–200 mg/day.

Acute Gouty Arthritis
PO: ADULTS, ELDERLY (IMMEDIATE-RELEASE): 50 mg 3 times a day for 3–5 days.

Acute Bursitis, Tendonitis
PO: ADULTS, ELDERLY (IMMEDIATE-RELEASE): 75–150 mg/day in 3–4 divided doses for 7–14 days. **Extended-Release:** 75–150 mg/day in 1–2 doses/day.

Patent Ductus Arteriosus
IV: NEONATES: Initially, 0.2 mg/kg. Subsequent doses are based on age, as follows: **NEONATES OLDER THAN 7 DAYS:** 0.25 mg/kg for 2nd and 3rd doses. **NEONATES 2–7 DAYS:** 0.2 mg/kg for 2nd and 3rd doses. **NEONATES LESS THAN 48 HRS:** 0.1 mg/kg for 2nd and 3rd doses. In general, dosing interval is 12 hrs if urine output is greater than 1 ml/kg/hr after prior dose, 24 hrs if urine output is less than 1 ml/kg/hr but greater than 0.6 ml/kg/hr. Dose is held if urine output is less than 0.6. ml/kg/hr or if neonate is anuric.

SIDE EFFECTS

Frequent (11%–3%): Headache, nausea, vomiting, dyspepsia (heartburn, indigestion, epigastric pain), dizziness. **Occasional (less than 3%):** Depression, tinnitus, diaphoresis, drowsiness, constipation, diarrhea. **Patent ductus arteriosus:** Bleeding abnormalities. **Rare:** Hypertension, confusion, urticaria, pruritus, rash, blurred vision.

ADVERSE EFFECTS/ TOXIC REACTIONS

Paralytic ileus, ulceration of esophagus, stomach, duodenum, small intestine may occur. Pts with renal impairment may develop hyperkalemia with worsening of renal impairment. May aggravate depression or other psychiatric disturbances, epilepsy, parkinsonism. Nephrotoxicity (dysuria, hematuria, proteinuria, nephrotic syndrome) occurs rarely. Metabolic acidosis/alkalosis, bradycardia occur rarely in pts with patent ductus arteriosus.

NURSING CONSIDERATIONS

BASELINE ASSESSMENT

Assess onset, type, location, duration of pain, fever, inflammation. Inspect appearance of affected joints for immobility, deformities, skin condition.

INTERVENTION/EVALUATION

Monitor for evidence of nausea, dyspepsia. Assist with ambulation if dizziness occurs. Evaluate for therapeutic response: relief of pain, stiffness, swelling; increased joint mobility; reduced joint tenderness; improved grip strength. Monitor BUN, serum creatinine, potassium, hepatic function tests. Observe for weight gain, edema, bleeding, bruising. In neonates, also monitor heart rate, heart sounds for murmur, B/P, urine output, EKG, serum sodium, glucose, platelets.

PATIENT/FAMILY TEACHING

• Avoid aspirin, alcohol during therapy (increases risk of GI bleeding). • If GI upset occurs, take with food, milk. • Avoid tasks that require alertness, motor skills until response to drug is established. • Report ringing in ears, persistent stomach pain, unusual bruising/bleeding.

infliximab

in-**flix**-i-mab
(<u>Remicade</u>)

BLACK BOX ALERT Risk of severe/ fatal opportunistic infections (tuberculosis, sepsis, fungal), reactivation of latent infections. Rare cases of very aggressive, usually fatal hepatosplenic T-cell lymphoma reported in adolescents, young adults with Crohn's disease. **Do not confuse infliximab with rituximab, or Remicade with Reminyl.**

◆CLASSIFICATION

PHARMACOTHERAPEUTIC: Monoclonal antibody. **CLINICAL:** GI antiinflammatory.

ACTION

Binds to tumor necrosis factor (TNF), inhibiting functional activity of TNF. Reduces infiltration of inflammatory cells. **Therapeutic Effect:** Decreases inflamed areas of intestine.

PHARMACOKINETICS

Absorbed into GI tissue; primarily distributed in vascular compartment. **Half-life:** 8–9.5 days.

USES

In combination with methotrexate, reduces signs/symptoms, inhibits progression of structural damage, improves physical function in moderate to severe active rheumatoid arthritis (RA), psoriatic arthritis. Reduces signs/symptoms, induces and maintains remission in moderate to severe active Crohn's disease. Reduces number of draining enterocutaneous/rectovaginal fistulas, maintains fistula closure in fistulizing Crohn's disease. Reduces sign/ symptoms of active ankylosing spondylitis. Treatment of chronic severe plaque psoriasis in pts who are candidates for systemic therapy. Reduces sign/symptoms, induces and maintains clinical remission and mucosal healing, eliminates corticosteroid use in moderate to severe active ulcerative colitis.

PRECAUTIONS

Contraindications: Moderate to severe HF (doses greater than 5 mg/kg should be avoided). Sensitivity to murine proteins, sepsis, serious active infection. **Cautions:** Hematological abnormalities, history of COPD, preexisting or recent onset CNS demyelinating disorders, seizures, mild HF, history of recurrent infections, conditions predisposing pt to infections (e.g., diabetes).

⌛ LIFESPAN CONSIDERATIONS

Pregnancy/Lactation: Unknown if distributed in breast milk. **Pregnancy Category B. Children:** Safety and efficacy not established. **Elderly:** Use cautiously due to higher rate of infection.

INTERACTIONS

DRUG: Anakinra, abatacept may increase risk of infection. **Immunosuppressants** may reduce frequency of infusion reactions, antibodies to infliximab. **Live virus vaccines** may decrease immune response (do not give concurrently). **HERBAL: Echinacea** may decrease effect. **FOOD:** None known. **LAB VALUES:** May increase serum alkaline phosphatase, AST, ALT, bilirubin.

AVAILABILITY (Rx)

Injection, Powder for Reconstitution: 100 mg.

ADMINISTRATION/HANDLING
💉 IV

Reconstitution • Reconstitute each vial with 10 ml Sterile Water for Injection, using 21-gauge or smaller needle. Direct stream of Sterile Water for Injection to glass wall of vial. • Swirl vial gently to dissolve contents (do not shake). • Allow solution to stand for 5 min and inject into 250-ml bag 0.9% NaCl; gently mix. Concentration should range between 0.4 and 4 mg/ml. • Begin infusion within 3 hrs after reconstitution.

Rate of Administration • Administer IV infusion over at least 2 hrs using a low protein-binding filter.

Storage • Refrigerate vials. • Solution should appear colorless to light yellow and opalescent; do not use if discolored or particulate forms.

🚫 IV INCOMPATIBILITIES

Do not infuse in same IV line with other agents.

INDICATIONS/ROUTES/DOSAGE

◄ALERT► Premedicate with antihistamines, acetaminophen, steroids to prevent/manage infusion reactions.

Rheumatoid Arthritis (RA)
IV Infusion: ADULTS, ELDERLY: (in combination with methotrexate): 3 mg/kg followed by additional doses at 2 and 6 wks after first infusion, then q8wks thereafter. Range: 3–10 mg/kg at 4- to 8-wk intervals.

Crohn's Disease
IV Infusion: ADULTS, ELDERLY, CHILDREN 6 YRS AND OLDER: 5 mg/kg followed by additional doses at 2 and 6 wks after first infusion, then q8wks thereafter. For adults who respond then lose response, consideration may be given to treatment with 10 mg/kg.

Fistulizing Crohn's Disease
IV Infusion: ADULTS, ELDERLY: 5 mg/kg followed by additional doses at 2 and 6 wks after first infusion, then q8wks thereafter. For pts who respond then lose response, consideration may be given to treatment with 10 mg/kg.

Ankylosing Spondylitis
IV Infusion: ADULTS, ELDERLY: 5 mg/kg followed by additional doses at 2 and 6 wks after first infusion, then q6wks thereafter.

Psoriatic Arthritis
IV Infusion: ADULTS, ELDERLY: 5 mg/kg followed by additional doses at 2 and 6

wks after first infusion, then q8wks thereafter. May be used with or without methotrexate.

Plaque Psoriasis
IV Infusion: ADULTS, ELDERLY: 5 mg/kg followed by additional doses at 2 and 6 wks after first infusion, then q8wks thereafter.

Ulcerative Colitis
IV Infusion: ADULTS, ELDERLY, CHILDREN 6 YRS AND OLDER: 5 mg/kg followed by additional doses at 2 and 6 wks after first infusion, then q8wks thereafter.

SIDE EFFECTS

Frequent (22%–10%): Headache, nausea, fatigue, fever. **Occasional (9%–5%):** Fever/chills during infusion, pharyngitis, vomiting, pain, dizziness, bronchitis, rash, rhinitis, cough, pruritus, sinusitis, myalgia, back pain. **Rare (4%–1%):** Hypotension or hypertension, paresthesia, anxiety, depression, insomnia, diarrhea, UTI.

ADVERSE EFFECTS/ TOXIC REACTIONS

Serious infections, including sepsis, occur rarely. Potential for hypersensitivity reaction, lupus-like syndrome, severe hepatic reaction, HF.

NURSING CONSIDERATIONS

BASELINE ASSESSMENT

Check baseline hydration status (skin turgor for tenting mucous membranes, urinary status).

INTERVENTION/EVALUATION

Monitor urinalysis, erythrocyte sedimentation rate (ESR), B/P. Monitor for signs of infection. Monitor daily pattern of bowel activity, stool consistency. **Crohn's disease:** Monitor C-reactive protein, frequency of stools. Assess for abdominal pain. **Rheumatoid arthritis (RA):** Monitor C-reactive protein. Assess for decreased pain, swollen joints, stiffness.

PATIENT/FAMILY TEACHING

• Report persistent fever, cough, abdominal pain, swelling of ankles/feet.

---

insulin

in-su-lin
Rapid-acting: INSULIN ASPART: (Novolog), **INSULIN GLULISINE:** (Apidra), **INSULIN LISPRO:** (Humalog)
Short-acting: REGULAR INSULIN: (Humulin R, Novolin R)
Intermediate-acting: NPH: (Humulin N, Novolin N)
Long-acting: INSULIN DETEMIR: (Levemir), **INSULIN GLARGINE:** (Lantus)
Do not confuse Novolog with Humalog or Novolin.

FIXED-COMBINATION(S)

Humalog Mix 75/25: lispro suspension 75% and lispro solution 25%. **Humulin Mix 50/50:** NPH 50% and regular 50%. **Humulin 70/30, Novolin 70/30:** NPH 70% and rapid-acting regular 30%. **Novolog Mix 70/30:** aspart suspension 70% and aspart solution 30%.

◆CLASSIFICATION

PHARMACOTHERAPEUTIC: Exogenous insulin. **CLINICAL:** Antidiabetic (see p. 43C).

ACTION

Facilitates passage of glucose, potassium, magnesium across cellular membranes of skeletal/cardiac muscle, adipose tissue. Controls storage, metabolism of carbohydrates, protein, fats. Promotes conversion of glucose to glycogen in liver. **Therapeutic Effect:** Controls glucose levels in diabetic pts.

PHARMACOKINETICS

Rapid-Acting

	Onset (min)	Peak (hrs)	Duration (hrs)
Aspart (Novolog)	10–20	1–3	3–5
Glulisine (Apidra)	5–15	0.75–1.25	2–4
Lispro (Humalog)	15–30	0.5–2.5	3–6.5

Short-Acting

	Onset (min)	Peak (hrs)	Duration (hrs)
Regular (Humulin R)	30–60	1–5	6–10
Regular (Novolin R)	30–60	1–5	6–10

Intermediate-Acting

	Onset (hrs)	Peak (hrs)	Duration (hrs)
NPH (Humulin N)	1–2	6–14	16–24+
NPH (Novolin N)	1–2	6–14	16–24+

Long-Acting

	Onset (hrs)	Peak (hrs)	Duration (hrs)
Detemir (Levemir)	3–4 hrs	3–9 hrs	6–23 hrs
Glargine (Lantus)	3–4 hrs	No peak	24

USES

Treatment of insulin-dependent type 1 diabetes mellitus; non–insulin-dependent type 2 diabetes mellitus (NIDDM) when diet and weight control therapy have failed to maintain satisfactory serum glucose levels or in event of pregnancy, surgery, trauma, infection, fever, severe renal, hepatic, endocrine dysfunction. Regular insulin used for emergency treatment of ketoacidosis, to promote passage of glucose across cell membrane in hyperalimentation, to facilitate intracellular shift of potassium in hyperkalemia. **OFF-LABEL:** Insulin aspart, insulin lispro,

insulin regular: Gestational diabetes, mild to moderate diabetic ketoacidosis, mild to moderate hyperosmolar hyperglycemic state. **Insulin NPH:** Gestational diabetes.

PRECAUTIONS

Contraindications: Hypersensitivity, hypoglycemia.

⧖ LIFESPAN CONSIDERATIONS

Pregnancy/Lactation: Insulin is drug of choice for diabetes in pregnancy; close medical supervision is needed. Following delivery, insulin needs may drop for 24–72 hrs, then rise to pre-pregnancy levels. Not distributed in breast milk; lactation may decrease insulin requirements. **Pregnancy Category B:** Aspart, Lispro, Regular, NPH; **Pregnancy Category C:** Detemir, Glargine, Glulisine. **Children:** No age-related precautions noted. **Elderly:** Decreased vision, fine motor tremors may lead to inaccurate self-dosing.

INTERACTIONS

DRUG: Alcohol may increase risk of hypoglycemia. **Beta-adrenergic blockers** may alter effects; may mask signs, prolong periods of hypoglycemia. **Glucocorticoids, thiazide diuretics** may increase serum glucose. **HERBAL: Garlic, ginger, ginseng** may increase risk of hypoglycemia. **FOOD:** None known. **LAB VALUES:** May decrease serum magnesium, phosphate, potassium.

AVAILABILITY

Rapid-Acting
Aspart (Novolog): 100 units/ml vial, 3 ml cartridge, 3 ml Flex-Pen. **Glulisine (Apidra):** 100 units/ml vial, 3 ml cartridge. **Lispro (Humalog):** 100 units/ml vial, 3 ml cartridge, 3 ml pen.

Short-Acting
Regular (Humulin R): 100 units/ml vial. **Regular (Novolin R):** 100 units/ml vial, 3 ml cartridge, 3 ml Innolet prefilled syringe.

Intermediate-Acting
NPH (Humulin N): 100 units/ml vial, 3 ml pen. **NPH (Novolin N):** 100 units/ml vial, 3 ml cartridge, 3 ml Innolet prefilled syringe.

Long-Acting
Detemir (Levemir): 100 units/ml vial, 3 ml Flex-Pen. **Glargine (Lantus):** 100 units/ml vial, 3 ml cartridge.

Intermediate- and Short-Acting Mixtures
Humulin 50/50, Humulin 70/30, Humalog Mix 75/25, Humalog Mix 50/50, Novolin 70/30, Novolog Mix 70/30.

ADMINISTRATION/HANDLING

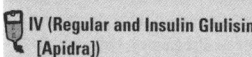 **IV (Regular and Insulin Glulisine [Apidra])**

• Use only if solution is clear. • May give undiluted.

Rapid-Acting
Aspart (Novolog) • May give subcutaneous, IV infusion. • Can mix with NPH (draw aspart into syringe first; inject immediately after mixing). • After first use, stable at room temperature for 28 days. • Administer 5–10 min before meals.
Glulisine (Apidra) • May mix with NPH (draw glulisine into syringe first; inject immediately after mixing). • After first use, stable at room temperature for 28 days. • Administer 15 min before or within 20 min after starting a meal.
Lispro (Humalog) • For subcutaneous use only. • May mix with NPH. Stable for 28 days at room temperature; syringe is stable for 14 days if refrigerated. • After first use, stable at room temperature for 28 days. • Administer 15 min before or immediately after meals.

Short-Acting
Regular (Humulin R, Novolin R) • May give subcutaneous, IM, IV. • May mix with NPH for immediate use or for storage for future use. Stable for 1 mo at room temperature, 3 mos if refrigerated.

• Can mix with Sterile Water for Injection or 0.9% NaCl. • After first use, stable at room temperature for 28 days. • Administer 30 min before meals.

Intermediate-Acting
NPH (Humulin N, Novolin N) • For subcutaneous use only. • May mix with aspart (Novolog) or lispro (Humalog). Draw aspart or lispro first and use immediately. • May mix with regular (Humulin R, Novolin R) insulin. Draw regular insulin first, use immediately or may store for future use (up to 28 days). • After first use, stable at room temperature for 28 days. • Administer 15 min before meals when mixed with aspart or lispro; 30 min before meals when mixed with regular.

Long-Acting
Detemir (Levemir) • For subcutaneous use only. • Do not mix with other insulins. • After first use, stable at room temperature for 42 days. • Evening dose given at dinner or at bedtime. Twice-daily regimens can be given 12 hrs after morning dose.
Glargine (Lantus) • For subcutaneous use only. • Do not mix with other insulins. • After first use, stable at room temperature for 28 days. • Administer once daily at same time. Meal timing is not applicable.

Subcutaneous
• Check serum glucose concentration before administration; dosage highly individualized. • Subcutaneous injections may be given in thigh, abdomen, upper arm, buttocks, upper back if there is adequate adipose tissue. • Rotation of injection sites is essential; maintain careful record. • Prefilled syringes should be stored in vertical or oblique position to avoid plugging; plunger should be pulled back slightly and syringe rocked to remix solution before injection.

IV INCOMPATIBILITIES
Diltiazem (Cardizem), dopamine (Intropin), nafcillin (Nafcil).

✦ IV COMPATIBILITIES

Amiodarone (Cordarone), ampicillin/sulbactam (Unasyn), cefazolin (Ancef), digoxin (Lanoxin), dobutamine (Dobutrex), famotidine (Pepcid), gentamicin, heparin, magnesium sulfate, metoclopramide (Reglan), midazolam (Versed), milrinone (Primacor), morphine, nitroglycerin, potassium chloride, propofol (Diprivan), vancomycin (Vancocin).

INDICATIONS/ROUTES/DOSAGE

Usual Dosage

◀ALERT▶ Adjust dosage to achieve premeal and bedtime serum glucose of 80–140 mg/dl (children younger than 5 yrs: 100–200 mg/dl).

**Total Units/kg/Day of All Insulin
Formulations Combined**
Type 1 Diabetes
Subcutaneous: ADULTS, ADOLESCENTS, CHILDREN: Initially, 0.2–0.6 units/kg/day in divided doses. **Maintenance:** 0.5–1 unit/kg/day in divided doses. **Note:** Needs may be based on wgt and/or activity. **ADOLESCENTS:** 1.2 unit/kg/day. **NON-OBESE:** 0.4–0.6 units/kg/day. **OBESE:** 0.8–1.2 units/kg/day.

Type 2 Diabetes
Subcutaneous: ADULTS: 0.2 units/kg/day or 10 units/day of an intermediate- or long-acting insulin at bedtime.

Diabetic Ketoacidosis
IV Infusion: ADULTS, ELDERLY: 0.1 unit/kg/hr. Titration based on serum glucose level. **CHILDREN:** 0.05–0.1 units/kg/hr.

SIDE EFFECTS

Occasional: Localized redness, swelling, itching (due to improper insulin injection technique), allergy to insulin cleansing solution. **Infrequent:** Somogyi effect (rebound hyperglycemia) with chronically excessive insulin dosages. Systemic allergic reaction (rash, angioedema, anaphylaxis), lipodystrophy (depression at injection site due to breakdown of adipose tissue), lipohypertrophy (accumulation of subcutaneous tissue at injection site due to inadequate site rotation). **Rare:** Insulin resistance.

ADVERSE EFFECTS/TOXIC REACTIONS

Severe hypoglycemia (due to hyperinsulinism) may occur with insulin overdose, decrease/delay of food intake, excessive exercise, pts with brittle diabetes. Diabetic ketoacidosis may result from stress, illness, omission of insulin dose, long-term poor insulin control.

NURSING CONSIDERATIONS

BASELINE ASSESSMENT

Check serum glucose level. Discuss lifestyle to determine extent of learning, emotional needs. If given IV, obtain serum chemistries (esp. serum potassium).

INTERVENTION/EVALUATION

Assess for hypoglycemia (refer to pharmacokinetics table for peak times and duration): cool, wet skin, tremors, dizziness, headache, anxiety, tachycardia, numbness in mouth, hunger, diplopia. Assess sleeping pt for restlessness, diaphoresis. Check for hyperglycemia: polyuria (excessive urine output), polyphagia (excessive food intake), polydipsia (excessive thirst), nausea/vomiting, dim vision, fatigue, deep and rapid breathing (Kussmaul respirations). Be alert to conditions altering glucose requirements: fever, trauma, increased activity/stress, surgical procedure.

PATIENT/FAMILY TEACHING

• Instruct on proper technique for drug administration, testing of glucose, signs/symptoms of hypoglycemia and hyperglycemia. • Prescribed diet is an essential part of treatment; do not skip/delay meals. • Carry candy, sugar packets, other sugar supplements for immediate response to hypoglycemia. • Wear or carry medical alert identification. • Check with physician when insulin demands are altered (e.g., fever, infection, trauma, stress, heavy physical activity). • Do not take other medication without consulting physician. • Weight control, exercise, hygiene (including foot care), not smoking are integral parts of therapy. • Protect skin, limit sun exposure. • Inform dentist, physician, surgeon of medication before any treatment is given.

interferon alfa-2b HIGH ALERT

in-ter-**feer**-on
(Intron-A)

BLACK BOX ALERT May cause or aggravate fatal or life-threatening autoimmune disorders, ischemia, neuropsychiatric symptoms (profound depression, suicidal thoughts/behaviors), infectious disorders.

Do not confuse interferon alfa-2b with interferon alfa-2a, interferon alfa-n3, or peginterferon alfa-2b, or Intron with Peg-Intron.

FIXED-COMBINATION(S)

Rebetron: interferon alfa-2b/ribavirin (an antiviral): 3 million units/200 mg.

◆CLASSIFICATION

PHARMACOTHERAPEUTIC: Biologic response modifier. **CLINICAL:** Antineoplastic (see p. 87C).

ACTION

Inhibits viral replication in virus-infected cells, suppresses cell proliferation, augments specific cytotoxicity of lymphocytes. **Therapeutic Effect:** Prevents rapid growth of malignant cells; inhibits hepatitis virus.

PHARMACOKINETICS

Well absorbed after IM, subcutaneous administration. Undergoes proteolytic degradation during reabsorption in kidneys. **Half-life:** 2–3 hrs.

USES

Treatment of hairy cell leukemia, condylomata acuminata (genital, venereal warts), malignant melanoma, AIDS-related Kaposi's sarcoma, chronic hepatitis C (including children 3 yrs of age and older), chronic hepatitis B (including children 1 yr and older), follicular non-Hodgkin's lymphoma. **OFF-LABEL:** Treatment of bladder, cervical, renal carcinoma; chronic myelocytic leukemia; laryngeal papillomatosis; multiple myeloma; cutaneous T-cell lymphoma; mycosis fungoides; West Nile virus.

PRECAUTIONS

Contraindications: Decompensated hepatic disease, autoimmune hepatitis. **Cautions:** Renal/hepatic impairment, seizure disorder, compromised CNS function, cardiac diseases, history of cardiac abnormalities, myelosuppression, pulmonary impairment, multiple sclerosis, diabetes, thyroid disease, coagulopathy, hypertension, preexisting eye disorders.

⧗ LIFESPAN CONSIDERATIONS

Pregnancy/Lactation: If possible, avoid use during pregnancy. Breastfeeding not recommended. **Pregnancy Category C (X in combination with ribavirin). Children:** Safety and efficacy not established. **Elderly:** Neurotoxicity, cardiotoxicity may occur more frequently. Age-related renal impairment may require dosage adjustment.

INTERACTIONS

DRUG: Bone marrow depressants may increase myelosuppression. **HERBAL:** None significant. **FOOD:** None known. **LAB VALUES:** May increase PT, aPTT, LDH, alkaline phosphatase, AST, ALT. May decrease Hgb, Hct, leukocyte, platelet counts.

AVAILABILITY (Rx)

Injection, Powder for Reconstitution: 10 million units, 18 million units, 50 million units. **Injection, Solution (Multidose Prefilled Pen):** 3 million units/0.2 ml (6 doses-18 million units), 5 million units/0.2 ml (6 doses-30 million units), 10 million units/0.2 mg (6 doses-60 million units). **Injection, Solution (Multidose Vial):** 6 million units/ml, 10 million units/ml.

ADMINISTRATION/HANDLING

 IV

Reconstitution • Prepare immediately before use. • Reconstitute with diluent provided by manufacturer. • Withdraw desired dose and further dilute with 100 ml 0.9% NaCl to provide final concentration of at least 10 million international units/100 ml.
Rate of Administration • Administer over 20 min.
Storage • Refrigerate unopened vials. • Following reconstitution, stable for 24 hrs if refrigerated.

IM, Subcutaneous
• **IM:** Administer in evening (if possible). • **Subcutaneous:** Reconstitute with recommended amount of Sterile Water for Injection. Agitate gently; do not shake.

IV INCOMPATIBILITIES

D₅W. Do not mix with other medications via Y-site administration.

IV COMPATIBILITIES

0.9% NaCl, lactated Ringer's.

INDICATIONS/ROUTES/DOSAGE

Hairy Cell Leukemia
IM, Subcutaneous: ADULTS: 2 million units/m² 3 times a wk for 2–6 mos. If severe adverse reactions occur, modify dose or temporarily discontinue drug.

Condylomata Acuminata
Intralesional: ADULTS: 1 million units/lesion 3 times a wk for 3 wks. May administer a 2nd course at 12–16 wks. Use only 10-million-unit vial, and reconstitute with no more than 1 ml diluent. **Maximum:** 5 lesions per treatment.

AIDS-Related Kaposi's Sarcoma
IM, Subcutaneous: ADULTS: 30 million units/m² 3 times a wk. Use only 50-million-unit vials. If severe adverse reactions occur, modify dose or temporarily discontinue drug.

Chronic Hepatitis C
IM, Subcutaneous: ADULTS: 3 million units 3 times a wk for up to 6 mos. For pts who tolerate therapy and whose ALT level normalizes within 16 wks, therapy may be extended for up to 18–24 mos. May be used in combination with ribavirin. **CHILDREN, 3–17 YRS (WITH HIV CO-INFECTION):** 3–5 million units/m² 3 times/wk with ribavirin for 48 wks.

Chronic Hepatitis B
IM, Subcutaneous: ADULTS: 30–35 million units weekly, either as 5 million units/day or 10 million units 3 times a wk for 16 wks.
Subcutaneous: CHILDREN 1–17 YRS: 3 million units/m² 3 times/wk for 1 wk, then 6 million units/m² 3 times/wk for 16–24 wks. **Maximum:** 10 million units 3 times/wk.

Malignant Melanoma
IV: ADULTS: Initially, 20 million units/m² 5 times a wk for 4 wks. Maintenance: 10 million units subcutaneously 3 times a wk for 48 wks.

Follicular Non-Hodgkin's Lymphoma
Subcutaneous: ADULTS: 5 million units 3 times a wk for up to 18 mos.

SIDE EFFECTS

Frequent: Flu-like symptoms (fever, fatigue, headache, myalgia, anorexia, chills), rash (hairy cell leukemia, Kaposi's sarcoma only). **Pts with Kaposi's sarcoma:** All previously mentioned side effects plus depression, dyspepsia, dry mouth or thirst, alopecia, rigors. **Occasional:** Dizziness, pruritus, dry skin, dermatitis, altered taste. **Rare:** Confusion, leg cramps, back pain, gingivitis, flushing, tremor, anxiety, eye pain.

ADVERSE EFFECTS/ TOXIC REACTIONS

Hypersensitivity reactions occur rarely. Severe flu-like symptoms appear dose-related.

NURSING CONSIDERATIONS

BASELINE ASSESSMENT

CBC, blood chemistries, urinalysis, renal/hepatic function tests, should be performed before initial therapy and routinely thereafter.

INTERVENTION/EVALUATION

Offer emotional support. Monitor all levels of clinical function (numerous side effects). Encourage PO intake, particularly during early therapy. Monitor for worsening depression, suicidal ideation, associated behaviors.

PATIENT/FAMILY TEACHING

• Clinical response occurs in 1–3 mos. • Flu-like symptoms tend to diminish with continued therapy. • Some symptoms may be alleviated or minimized by bedtime doses. • Do not have immunizations without physician's approval (drug lowers resistance). • Avoid contact with those who have recently received live virus vaccine. • Avoid tasks that require alertness, motor skills until response to drug is established. • Sips of tepid water may relieve dry mouth. • Report depression, thoughts of suicide, unusual behavior.

TOP 200

interferon beta-1a

in-ter-**feer**-on
(Avonex), Rebif)
Do not confuse Avonex with Avelox, or interferon beta-1a with interferon beta-1b.

◆CLASSIFICATION

PHARMACOTHERAPEUTIC: Biologic response modifier. **CLINICAL:** Multiple sclerosis agent.

ACTION

Interacts with specific cell receptors found on surface of cells. **Therapeutic Effect:** Produces antiviral, immunoregulatory effects.

PHARMACOKINETICS

Peak serum levels attained 3–15 hrs after IM administration. Biologic markers increase within 12 hrs and remain elevated for 4 days. **Half-life:** 10 hrs (Avonex); 69 hrs (Rebif).

USES

Treatment of relapsing multiple sclerosis to slow progression of physical disability, decrease frequency of clinical exacerbations.

PRECAUTIONS

Contraindications: Hypersensitivity to natural or recombinant interferon, human albumin. **Cautions:** Chronic progressive multiple sclerosis, children younger than 18 yrs, depression, severe psychiatric disorders, hepatic impairment, alcohol abuse, cardiovascular disease, seizure disorders, myelosuppression.

⧗ LIFESPAN CONSIDERATIONS

Pregnancy/Lactation: Has abortifacient potential. Unknown if distributed in breast milk. **Pregnancy Category C. Children:** Safety and efficacy not established. **Elderly:** No information available.

INTERACTIONS

DRUG: Alcohol, hepatotoxic drugs may increase risk of hepatic injury. **HERBAL:** None significant. **FOOD:** None known. **LAB VALUES:** May increase serum glucose, BUN, alkaline phosphatase, bilirubin, calcium, AST, ALT. May decrease Hgb, neutrophil, platelet, WBC counts.

AVAILABILITY (Rx)

Injection, Powder for Reconstitution (Avonex): 30 mcg. Injection Solution (Prefilled Syringe): 22 mcg/0.5 ml (Rebif), 30 mcg/0.5 ml (Avonex Prefilled Syringe), 44 mcg/0.5 ml (Rebif). Titration Pack (Prefilled Syringe [Rebif]): 8.8 mcg/0.2 ml, 22 mcg/0.5 ml.

ADMINISTRATION/HANDLING

IM (Avonex) Syringe

• Refrigerate syringe. • Allow to warm to room temperature before use. • May store up to 7 days at room temperature.

IM (Avonex) Vial

• Refrigerate vials (may store at room temperature up to 30 days). • Following reconstitution, may refrigerate again but use within 6 hrs if refrigerated. • Reconstitute 30-mcg *MicroPin* (6.6 million international units) vial with 1.1 ml diluent (supplied by manufacturer). • Gently swirl to dissolve medication; do not shake. • Discard if discolored or particulate forms. • Discard unused portion (contains no preservative).

Subcutaneous (Rebif)

• Refrigerate. May store at room temperature up to 30 days. Avoid heat, light. • Administer at same time of day 3 days each wk. Separate doses by at least 48 hrs.

INDICATIONS/ROUTES/DOSAGE

Relapsing Multiple Sclerosis

IM *(Avonex)*: ADULTS: 30 mcg once weekly.
Subcutaneous *(Rebif)*: ADULTS: **(Target dose 44 mcg 3 times a wk):** Initially, 8.8 mcg 3 times a wk for 2 wks, then 22 mcg 3 times a wk for 2 wks, then 44 mcg 3 times a wk thereafter. **(Target dose 22 mcg 3 times a wk):** Initially, 4.4 mcg 3 times a wk for 2 wks, then 11 mcg 3 times a wk for 2 wks, then 22 mcg 3 times a wk thereafter.

Dosage in Hepatic Impairment (Rebif)

Increased hepatic function test results, leukopenia: Decrease dose 20%–50% until toxicity resolves.

SIDE EFFECTS

Frequent (67%–11%): Headache, flu-like symptoms, myalgia, upper respiratory tract infection, depression with suicidal ideation, generalized pain, asthenia (loss of strength, energy), chills, sinusitis, infection. Occasional (9%–4%): Abdominal pain, arthralgia, chest pain, dyspnea, malaise, syncope. Rare (3%): Injection site reaction, hypersensitivity reaction.

ADVERSE EFFECTS/ TOXIC REACTIONS

Anemia occurs in 8% of pts. Hepatic failure has been reported.

NURSING CONSIDERATIONS

BASELINE ASSESSMENT

Obtain CBC, blood chemistries including hepatic function tests. Assess home situation for support of therapy.

INTERVENTION/EVALUATION

Assess for headache, flu-like symptoms, myalgia. Periodically monitor lab results, re-evaluate injection technique. Assess for depression, suicidal ideation.

PATIENT/FAMILY TEACHING

• Do not change schedule, dosage without consulting physician. • Follow guidelines for reconstitution of product and administration, including aseptic technique. • Use puncture-resistant container for used needles, syringes; dispose of used needles, syringes properly. • Injection site reactions may occur. These do not require discontinuation of therapy, but type and extent should be carefully noted.

TOP
200

interferon beta-1b

in-ter-**feer**-on
(Betaseron, Extavia)
Do not confuse interferon beta-1b with interferon beta-1a.

◆CLASSIFICATION

PHARMACOTHERAPEUTIC: Biologic response modifier. **CLINICAL:** Multiple sclerosis agent.

ACTION

Interacts with specific cell receptors found on surface of cells. **Therapeutic Effect:** Produces antiviral, immunoregulatory effects.

PHARMACOKINETICS

Slowly absorbed following subcutaneous administration. **Half-life:** 8 min–4.3 hrs.

USES

Reduces frequency of clinical exacerbations in pts with relapsing-remitting multiple sclerosis (recurrent attacks of neurologic dysfunction). Treatment of early stages of multiple sclerosis.

PRECAUTIONS

Contraindications: Hypersensitivity to albumin, *Escherichia coli*–derived products, interferon. **Cautions:** Chronic progressive multiple sclerosis, children younger than 18 yrs, severe psychiatric disorders, hepatic/renal impairment, alcohol abuse, cardiovascular disease, seizure disorders, myelosuppression, pulmonary disease.

⧗ LIFESPAN CONSIDERATIONS

Pregnancy/Lactation: Unknown if distributed in breast milk. **Pregnancy Category C. Children:** Safety and efficacy not established. **Elderly:** No information available.

INTERACTIONS

DRUG: None significant. **HERBAL:** None significant. **FOOD:** None known. **LAB VALUES:** May increase bilirubin, AST, ALT. May decrease neutrophil, lymphocyte, WBC counts.

AVAILABILITY (Rx)

Injection, Powder for Reconstitution: 0.3 mg (9.6 million units).

ADMINISTRATION/HANDLING

Subcutaneous
• Store vials at room temperature. • After reconstitution, stable for 3 hrs if refrigerated. • Use within 3 hrs of reconstitution. • Discard if discolored or precipitate forms. • Reconstitute 0.3-mg (9.6 million international units) vial with 1.2 ml diluent (supplied by manufacturer) to provide concentration of 0.25 mg/ml (8 million units/ml). • Gently swirl to dissolve medication; do not shake. • Withdraw 1 ml solution and inject subcutaneous into arms, abdomen, hips, thighs using 27-gauge needle. • Discard unused portion (contains no preservative).

INDICATIONS/ROUTES/DOSAGE

Relapsing-Remitting Multiple Sclerosis
Subcutaneous: **ADULTS:** Initially, 0.0625 mg (2 million units) every other day; gradually increase by 0.0625 mg every 2 wks. Target dose: 0.25 mg (8 million units) every other day.

SIDE EFFECTS

Frequent (85%–21%): Injection site reaction, headache, flu-like symptoms, fever, asthenia (loss of strength, energy), myalgia, sinusitis, diarrhea, dizziness, altered mental status, constipation, diaphoresis, vomiting. **Occasional (15%–4%):** Malaise, drowsiness, alopecia.

ADVERSE EFFECTS/ TOXIC REACTIONS

Seizures occur rarely.

NURSING CONSIDERATIONS

BASELINE ASSESSMENT

Obtain CBC, blood chemistries (including hepatic function tests). Assess home situation for support of therapy.

INTERVENTION/EVALUATION

Periodically monitor lab results, re-evaluate injection technique. Assess for nausea (high incidence). Monitor sleep pattern. Monitor daily pattern of bowel activity, stool consistency. Assist with ambulation if dizziness occurs. Monitor food intake.

PATIENT/FAMILY TEACHING

• Report flu-like symptoms (occur commonly but decrease over time). • Wear sunscreen, protective clothing if exposed to sunlight, ultraviolet light until tolerance known.

interferon gamma-1b

in-ter-**feer**-on
(Actimmune)

◆CLASSIFICATION

PHARMACOTHERAPEUTIC: Biologic response modifier. **CLINICAL:** Immunologic agent.

ACTION

Induces activation of macrophages in blood monocytes to phagocytes (necessary in cellular immune response to intracellular, extracellular pathogens). Enhances phagocytic function, antimicrobial activity of monocytes. **Therapeutic Effect:** Decreases signs/symptoms of serious infections in chronic granulomatous disease.

PHARMACOKINETICS

Slowly absorbed after subcutaneous administration. **Half-life:** 3–6 hrs.

USES

Reduces frequency, severity of serious infections due to chronic granulomatous disease. Delays time to disease progression in pts with severe, malignant osteopetrosis.

PRECAUTIONS

Contraindications: Hypersensitivity to *Escherichia coli*–derived products. **Cautions:** Seizure disorders, compromised CNS function, preexisting cardiac disease (e.g., ischemia, HF, arrhythmias), hepatic disease, myelosuppression.

⧗ LIFESPAN CONSIDERATIONS

Pregnancy/Lactation: Unknown if drug crosses placenta or is distributed in breast milk. **Pregnancy Category C. Children:** Safety and efficacy not established in those younger than 1 yr. Flu-like symptoms may occur more frequently. **Elderly:** No information available.

INTERACTIONS

DRUG: Bone marrow depressants may increase myelosuppression. **HERBAL:** None significant. **FOOD:** None known. **LAB VALUES:** May increase serum ALT, AST, alkaline phosphatase, LDH, triglycerides, cortisol concentrations. May decrease leukocytes, neutrophils, platelets.

AVAILABILITY (Rx)

Injection Solution: 100 mcg/0.5 ml (2 million units).

ADMINISTRATION/HANDLING

◀ALERT▶ Avoid excessive agitation of vial; do not shake.

Subcutaneous

• Refrigerate vials. Do not freeze. • Do not keep at room temperature for more than 12 hrs; discard after 12 hrs. • Vials are single dose; discard unused portion. • Solution is clear, colorless. Do not use if discolored or precipitate forms. • When given 3 times a wk, rotate injection sites.

INDICATIONS/ROUTES/DOSAGE

Chronic Granulomatous Disease; Severe, Malignant Osteopetrosis
Subcutaneous: ADULTS, ELDERLY, CHILDREN OLDER THAN 1 YR: 50 mcg/m^2 (1 million units/m^2) 3 times/wk in pts with body surface area (BSA) greater than 0.5 m^2; 1.5 mcg/kg/dose 3 times/wk in pts with BSA 0.5 m^2 or less.

SIDE EFFECTS

Frequent: Fever (52%), headache (33%), rash (17%), chills, fatigue, diarrhea (14%). **Occasional (13%–10%):** Vomiting, nausea. **Rare (6%–3%):** Weight loss, myalgia, anorexia.

ADVERSE EFFECTS/ TOXIC REACTIONS

May exacerbate preexisting CNS dysfunction (manifested as decreased mental status, gait disturbance, dizziness), cardiac abnormalities.

NURSING CONSIDERATIONS

BASELINE ASSESSMENT

CBC, blood chemistries, urinalysis, renal/hepatic function tests should be performed before initial therapy and at 3-mo intervals during course of treatment.

INTERVENTION/EVALUATION

Monitor for flu-like symptoms (fever, chills, fatigue, myalgia). Assess skin for evidence of rash.

PATIENT/FAMILY TEACHING

• Flu-like symptoms (fever, chills, fatigue, muscle aches) are generally mild and tend to disappear as treatment continues. Symptoms may be minimized with bedtime administration. • Avoid tasks that require alertness, motor skills until response to drug is established. • If home use prescribed, follow guidelines for proper technique of administration; care in proper disposal of needles, syringes. • Vials should remain refrigerated.

interleukin-2 (aldesleukin)   HIGH ALERT

in-ter-**loo**-kin
(Proleukin)

BLACK BOX ALERT High-dose therapy is associated with capillary leak syndrome resulting in significant hypotension and reduced organ perfusion. Use restricted to pts with normal cardiac/pulmonary function. Increased risk of disseminated infection (sepsis, bacterial endocarditis). Withhold treatment for pts developing moderate-to-severe lethargy or drowsiness (continued treatment may result in coma). Must be administered by personnel trained in administration/handling of chemotherapeutic agents.
Do not confuse aldesleukin with oprelvekin.

◆CLASSIFICATION

PHARMACOTHERAPEUTIC: Biologic response modifier. **CLINICAL:** Antineoplastic.

ACTION

Promotes proliferation, differentiation, recruitment of T and B cells, lymphokine-activated and natural killer cells, thymocytes. **Therapeutic Effect:** Enhances cytolytic activity in lymphocytes.

PHARMACOKINETICS

Primarily distributed into plasma, lymphocytes, lungs, liver, kidney, spleen. Metabolized to amino acids in cells lining the kidneys. **Half-life:** 80–120 min.

USES

Treatment of metastatic renal cell carcinoma, metastatic melanoma. **OFF-LABEL:** Treatment of AML.

PRECAUTIONS

Contraindications: Abnormal pulmonary function or thallium stress test results, bowel ischemia or perforation, coma or toxic psychosis lasting longer than 48 hrs, GI bleeding requiring surgery, intubation lasting more than 72 hrs, organ allografts, pericardial tamponade, renal dysfunction requiring dialysis for longer than 72 hrs, repetitive or difficult-to-control seizures; retreatment in those who experience any of the following toxicities: angina, MI, recurrent chest pain with EKG changes, sustained ventricular tachycardia, uncontrolled or unresponsive cardiac rhythm disturbances. **Extreme Caution:** Pts with normal thallium stress tests and pulmonary function tests who have history of cardiac or pulmonary disease. **Cautions:** Pts with fixed requirements for large volumes of fluid (e.g., those with hypercalcemia), history of seizures, renal/hepatic impairment, autoimmune disease, inflammatory disorders.

⌛ LIFESPAN CONSIDERATIONS

Pregnancy/Lactation: Avoid use in those of either sex not practicing effective contraception. **Pregnancy Category C. Children:** Safety and efficacy not established. **Elderly:** Age-related renal impairment may require dosage adjustment; will not tolerate toxicity.

INTERACTIONS

DRUG: Antihypertensives may increase hypotensive effect. **Cardiotoxic, hepatotoxic, myelotoxic, nephrotoxic medications** may increase risk of toxicity. **Glucocorticoids** may decrease effects. **HERBAL:** None significant. **FOOD:** None known. **LAB VALUES:** May increase BUN, serum alkaline phosphatase, bilirubin, creatinine, AST, ALT. May decrease serum calcium, magnesium, phosphorus, potassium, sodium.

AVAILABILITY (Rx)

Injection, Powder for Reconstitution (Proleukin): 22 million units (1.3 mg) (18 million units/ml = 1.1 mg/ml when reconstituted).

ADMINISTRATION/HANDLING

◀ALERT▶ Hold administration in pts who develop moderate to severe lethargy or drowsiness (continued administration may result in coma).

 IV

Reconstitution • Reconstitute 22 million units vial with 1.2 ml Sterile Water for Injection to provide concentration of 18 million units/ml (1.1 mg/ml). • Bacteriostatic Water for Injection or NaCl should not be used to reconstitute because of increased aggregation. • During reconstitution, direct Sterile Water for Injection at the side of vial. Swirl contents gently to avoid foaming. Do not shake.

Rate of Administration • Further dilute dose in 50 ml D₅W to a final concentration between 0.49 and 1.1 million international units/ml (30–70 mcg/ml) and infuse over 15 min. Do not use an in-line filter. • Solution should be warmed to room temperature before infusion. • Monitor diligently for drop in mean arterial B/P (sign of capillary leak syndrome [CLS]). Continued treatment may result in significant hypotension (less than 90 mm Hg or a 20 mm Hg drop from baseline systolic pressure), edema, pleural effusion, altered mental status.

Storage • Refrigerate vials; do not freeze. • Reconstituted solution is stable for 48 hrs refrigerated or at room temperature (refrigeration preferred).

🚫 IV INCOMPATIBILITIES

Ganciclovir (Cytovene), pentamidine (Pentam), prochlorperazine (Compazine), promethazine (Phenergan).

🔀 IV COMPATIBILITIES

Calcium gluconate, dopamine (Intropin), heparin, lorazepam (Ativan), magnesium, potassium.

INDICATIONS/ROUTES/DOSAGE

Metastatic Melanoma, Metastatic Renal Cell Carcinoma

IV: ADULTS 18 YRS AND OLDER: 600,000 units/kg q8h for 14 doses; followed by 9 days of rest, then another 14 doses for a total of 28 doses per course. Course may be repeated after rest period of at least 7 wks from date of hospital discharge.

SIDE EFFECTS

Side effects are generally self-limited and resolve within 2–3 days after discontinuing therapy. **Frequent (89%–48%):** Fever, chills, nausea, vomiting, hypotension, diarrhea, oliguria/anuria, altered mental status, irritability, confusion, depression, sinus tachycardia, pain (abdominal, chest, back), fatigue, dyspnea, pruritus. **Occasional (47%–17%):** Edema, erythema, rash, stomatitis, anorexia, weight gain, infection (UTI, injection site, catheter tip), dizziness. **Rare (15%–4%):** Dry skin, sensory disorders (vision, speech, taste), dermatitis, headache, arthralgia, myalgia, weight loss, hematuria, conjunctivitis, proteinuria.

ADVERSE EFFECTS/ TOXIC REACTIONS

Anemia, thrombocytopenia, leukopenia occur commonly. GI bleeding, pulmonary edema occur occasionally. Capillary leak syndrome (CLS) results in hypotension (systolic pressure less than 90 mm Hg or a 20 mm Hg drop from baseline systolic pressure), extravasation of plasma proteins and fluid into extravascular space, loss of vascular tone. May result in cardiac arrhythmias, angina, MI, respiratory insufficiency. Fatal malignant hyperthermia, cardiac arrest, CVA, pulmonary emboli, bowel perforation/gangrene, severe depression leading to suicide occur in less than 1% of pts.

NURSING CONSIDERATIONS

BASELINE ASSESSMENT

Pts with bacterial infection and with indwelling central lines should be treated with antibiotic therapy before treatment begins. All pts should be neurologically stable with a negative CT scan before treatment begins. CBC, blood chemistries, renal/hepatic function tests, chest X-ray should be performed before therapy begins and daily thereafter.

INTERVENTION/EVALUATION

Monitor CBC with differential, amylase, electrolytes, renal/hepatic function tests, weight, pulse oximetry. Discontinue medication at first sign of hypotension and hold for moderate to severe lethargy (physician must decide whether therapy should continue). Assess for altered mental status (irritability, confusion, depression), weight gain/loss. Maintain strict I&O. Assess for extravascular fluid accumulation (rales in lungs, edema in dependent areas).

PATIENT/FAMILY TEACHING

• Nausea may decrease during therapy. • At home, increase fluid intake (protects against renal impairment). • Do not have immunizations without physician's approval (drug lowers resistance). • Avoid exposure to persons with infection. • Report fever, chills, lower back pain, difficulty with urination, unusual bleeding/bruising, black tarry stools, blood in urine, petechial rash (pinpoint red spots on skin). • Report symptoms of depression or suicidal ideation immediately.

ipilimumab

ip-i-**lim**-ue-mab
(Yervoy)

BLACK BOX ALERT Severe and fatal immune-mediated adverse reactions due to T-cell activation and proliferation are capable of involving any organ system. Specific reactions include enterocolitis, hepatitis, dermatitis, neuropathy, endocrinopathy. Majority of immune-mediated reactions may initially manifest during treatment or weeks to months after treatment. Permanently discontinue treatment and initiate high-dose corticosteroid therapy for severe immune-mediated adverse reactions. Assess all pts for signs/symptoms of enterocolitis, hepatitis, dermatitis (including toxic epidermal necrolysis), neuropathy, endocrinopathy and evaluate clinical chemistries including hepatic function tests and thyroid tests at baseline and before each treatment.

◆CLASSIFICATION

PHARMACOTHERAPEUTIC: Human cytotoxic T-lymphocyte antigen 4 (CTLA-4)-blocking antibody. **CLINICAL:** Antineoplastic (see p. 87C).

ACTION

Augments T-cell activation and proliferation. Binds to cytotoxic T-lymphoctye-associated antigen 4 (CTLA-4) and blocks interaction of CTLA-4 with its ligands. **Therapeutic Effect:** Inhibits tumor cell growth.

PHARMACOKINETICS

Metabolized in liver. Steady state reached by third dose. **Half-life:** 14.7 days.

USES

Treatment of unresectable or metastatic melanoma.

PRECAUTIONS

Contraindications: None known. **Cautions:** Hepatic impairment, chronic peripheral neuropathy, thyroid/adrenal/pituitary dysfunction, autoimmune disorders (ulcerative colitis, Crohn's disease, lupus, sarcoidosis).

⧗ LIFESPAN CONSIDERATIONS

Pregnancy/Lactation: May cause fetal harm. Unknown if distributed in breast milk. Must decide to discontinue either breastfeeding or drug regimen due to potential fetal harm. **Pregnancy Category C. Children:** Safety and efficacy not established. **Elderly:** No age-related precautions noted.

INTERACTIONS

DRUG: None significant. **HERBAL:** None significant. **FOOD:** None known. **LAB VALUES:** May increase serum AST, ALT, bilirubin, eosinophils.

AVAILABILITY (Rx)

Injection, Solution: 5 mg/ml (10 ml, 40 ml vials).

ADMINISTRATION/HANDLING
💧 IV

◀**ALERT**▶ Use sterile, nonpyrogenic, low protein-binding in-line filter. Use dedicated line only.

Reconstitution • Calculate number of vials needed for injection. • Inspect for particulate matter or discoloration. • Allow vials to stand at room temperature for approximately 5 min. • Withdraw proper volume and transfer to infusion bag. Dilute in NaCl or D₅W with final concentration ranging from 1–2 mg/ml. • Mix diluted solution by gentle inversion. Do not shake or agitate.

Rate of Administration • Infuse over 90 min.

Storage • Solution should be translucent to white or pale yellow with amorphous particles. • Discard vial if cloudy or discolored. • Refrigerate vials until time of use. • May store diluted solution either under refrigeration or at room temperature for no more than 24 hrs.

INDICATIONS/ROUTES/DOSAGE

Metastatic Melanoma

IV: ADULTS: 3 mg/kg q3wks for 4 doses. ◀**ALERT**▶ Pts who are presenting with severe immune-mediated adverse reactions must immediately discontinue drug therapy and start prednisone 1 mg/kg/day.

Dosage Modification: Hold scheduled dose for moderate immune-mediated adverse reactions. Pts with complete or partial resolution of adverse reactions and who are receiving less than 7.5 mg/day of prednisone may resume scheduled doses. Permanently discontinue for persistent moderate adverse reactions or inability to reduce corticosteroid dose to 7.5 mg/day, failure to complete full treatment course in 16 wks, any severe or life-threatening adverse reactions.

SIDE EFFECTS

Frequent (42%): Fatigue. **Occasional (32%–29%):** Diarrhea, pruritus, rash, colitis.

ADVERSE EFFECTS/TOXIC REACTIONS

Severe and fatal immune-mediated adverse reactions have occurred. Enterocolitis (7% of pts) may present with fever, ileus, abdominal pain, GI bleeding, intestinal perforation, severe dehydrating diarrhea. Endocrinopathies (4% of pts), including hypopituitarism, adrenal insufficiency, hypogonadism, hypothyroidism may present with fatigue, headache, mental status change, unusual bowel habits, hypotension and may require emergent hormone replacement therapy. Dermatitis including toxic epidermal necrolysis (2% of pts) may present with full-thickness ulceration or necrotic, bullous, hemorrhagic manifestations. Hepatotoxicity (1% of pts), defined as hepatic function tests greater than 2.5–5 times upper normal limit, may present with right upper abdominal pain, jaundice, black/tarry stools, bruising, dark-colored urine, nausea, vomiting. Neuropathy (1% of pts), including Guillain-Barré syndrome or myasthenia gravis, may present with weakness, sensory alterations, paresthesia, paralysis. Other serious adverse reactions such as pneumonitis, meningitis, nephritis, eosinophilia, pericarditis, myocarditis, angiopathy, temporal arteritis, vasculitis, polymyalgia rheumatica, conjunctivitis, blepharitis, episcleritis, scleritis, leukocytoclastic vasculitis, erythema multiforme, psoriasis, pancreatitis, arthritis, autoimmune thyroiditis reported. Anti-ipilimumab antibodies reported in 1.1% of pts. All severe immune-mediated adverse reactions require immediate high-dose corticoid steroid therapy.

NURSING CONSIDERATIONS

BASELINE ASSESSMENT

Obtain baseline CBC, complete metabolic profile, hepatic panel, TSH, free T4, urine pregnancy. Screen for history of hepatic impairment, chronic neuropathy, thyroid/adrenal/pituitary dysfunction, autoimmune disorders. Focused assessment relating to possible adverse reactions includes abdominal area (inspection, auscultation, percussion, palpation, bowel pattern, symmetry), skin (color, lesions, mucosal inspection, edema), neurologic (mental status, gait, numbness, tingling, pain, strength, visual acuity), hormonal glands (lymph node inspection/palpation, pyrexia, goiter, palpitations). Question possibility of pregnancy or plans of breastfeeding. Receive full medication history including vitamins, minerals, herbal products.

INTERVENTION/EVALUATION

Monitor vital signs, hepatic function, thyroid panel before each dose. Continue focused assessment and screen for life-threatening immune-mediated adverse reactions. If adverse reactions occur, immediately notify physician and initiate proper treatment. Report suspected pregnancy. Obtain CBC, blood cultures for fever, suspected infection. EKG for palpitations, chest pain, difficulty breathing, dizziness. If prednisone therapy initiated, monitor capillary blood glucose and screen for side effects.

PATIENT/FAMILY TEACHING

• Inform pt that serious and fatal adverse reactions indicate inflammation to certain systems: intestines (diarrhea, dark/tarry stools, abdominal pain), liver (yellowing of the skin, dark-colored urine, right upper quadrant pain, bruising), skin (rash, mouth sores, blisters, ulcers), nerves (weakness, numbness, tingling, difficulty breathing, paralysis), hormonal glands (headaches, weight gain, palpitations, changes in mood or behavior, dizziness), eyes (blurry vision, double vision, eye pain/redness). • Prednisone therapy may be started if adverse reactions occur. • May cause fatal harm, stillbirth, premature delivery. • Blood levels will be drawn before each dose.

• Report any chest pain, palpitations, fever, swollen glands, stomach pain, vomiting, or any sign of adverse reactions.

ipratropium

ip-ra-**troe**-pee-um
(Atrovent, Atrovent HFA, Novo-Ipramide ✦, Nu-Ipratropium ✦, PMS-Ipratropium ✦)
Do not confuse Atrovent with Alupent or Serevent, or ipratropium with tiotropium.

FIXED-COMBINATION(S)

Combivent, DuoNeb: ipratropium/albuterol (a bronchodilator): *Aerosol:* 18 mcg/90 mcg per actuation. *Solution:* 0.5 mg/2.5 mg per 3 ml.

◆CLASSIFICATION

PHARMACOTHERAPEUTIC: Anticholinergic. **CLINICAL:** Bronchodilator (see pp. 4C, 75C).

ACTION

Blocks action of acetylcholine at parasympathetic sites in bronchial smooth muscle. **Therapeutic Effect:** Causes bronchodilation, inhibits nasal secretions.

PHARMACOKINETICS

Route	Onset	Peak	Duration
Inhalation	1–3 min	1.5–2 hrs	Up to 4 hrs
Nasal	5 min	1–4 hrs	4–8 hrs

Minimal systemic absorption after inhalation. Metabolized in liver (systemic absorption). Primarily eliminated in feces. **Half-life:** 1.5–4 hrs (nasal).

USES

Inhalation, Nebulization: Maintenance treatment of bronchospasm due to COPD, bronchitis, emphysema, asthma. Not indicated for immediate broncho-spasm relief. **Nasal Spray:** Symptomatic relief of rhinorrhea associated with the common cold and allergic/nonallergic rhinitis.

PRECAUTIONS

Contraindications: History of hypersensitivity to atropine. **Cautions:** Narrow-angle glaucoma, prostatic hypertrophy, bladder neck obstruction, myasthenia gravis.

⌛ LIFESPAN CONSIDERATIONS

Pregnancy/Lactation: Unknown if distributed in breast milk. **Pregnancy Category B. Children/Elderly:** No age-related precautions noted.

INTERACTIONS

DRUG: Anticholinergics, medications with anticholinergic properties may increase toxicity. **HERBAL:** None significant. **FOOD:** None known. **LAB VALUES:** None known.

AVAILABILITY (Rx)

Aerosol for Oral Inhalation (Atrovent HFA): 17 mcg/actuation. **Solution, Intranasal Spray:** 0.03%; 0.06%. **Solution for Nebulization:** 0.02% (500 mcg).

ADMINISTRATION/HANDLING

Inhalation
• Shake container well. • Instruct pt to exhale completely, place mouthpiece between lips, inhale deeply through mouth while fully depressing top of canister. Hold breath as long as possible before exhaling slowly. • Allow at least 1 minute between inhalations. • Rinse mouth with water immediately after inhalation (prevents mouth/throat dryness).

Nebulization
• May be administered with or without dilution in 0.9% NaCl. • Stable for 1 hr when mixed with albuterol. • Give over 5–15 min.

Nasal
• Store at room temperature. • Initial pump priming requires 7 actuations of

pump. • If used regularly as recommended, no further priming is required. If not used for more than 4 hrs, pump will require 2 actuations, or if not used for more than 7 days, the pump will require 7 actuations to reprime.

INDICATIONS/ROUTES/DOSAGE

Bronchodilator for COPD
Inhalation: ADULTS, ELDERLY, CHILDREN OLDER THAN 12 YRS: 2 inhalations 4 times a day. **Maximum:** 12 inhalations/day.
Nebulization: ADULTS, ELDERLY, CHILDREN OLDER THAN 12 YRS: 500 mcg (one unit dose vial) 3–4 times a day (doses 6–8 hrs apart).

Asthma Exacerbation
Note: Should be given in combination with a short-acting beta-adrenergic agonist.
Inhalation: ADULTS, ELDERLY, CHILDREN OLDER THAN 12 YRS: 8 inhalations q20min as needed for up to 3 hrs. **CHILDREN 12 YRS OR LESS:** 4–8 inhalations q20min as needed for up to 3 hrs.
Nebulization: ADULTS, ELDERLY, CHILDREN OLDER THAN 12 YRS: 500 mcg q20min for 3 doses, then as needed. **CHILDREN 12 YRS OR LESS:** 250–500 mcg q20min for 3 doses, then as needed.

Rhinorrhea (Perennial Allergic/ Nonallergic Rhinitis)
Intranasal *(0.03%)*: **ADULTS, ELDERLY, CHILDREN 6 YRS AND OLDER:** 2 sprays per nostril 2–3 times a day.

Rhinorrhea (Common Cold)
Intranasal *(0.06%)*: **ADULTS, ELDERLY, CHILDREN 12 YRS AND OLDER:** 2 sprays per nostril 3–4 times a day for up to 4 days. **CHILDREN 5–11 YRS:** 2 sprays per nostril 3 times a day for up to 4 days.

Rhinorrhea (Seasonal Allergy)
Intranasal *(0.06%)*: **ADULTS, ELDERLY, CHILDREN 5 YRS AND OLDER:** 2 sprays per nostril 4 times a day for up to 3 wks.

SIDE EFFECTS

Frequent: Inhalation (6%–3%): Cough, dry mouth, headache, nausea. **Nasal:** Dry nose/mouth, headache, nasal irritation. **Occasional: Inhalation (2%):** Dizziness, transient increased bronchospasm. **Rare (less than 1%): Inhalation:** Hypotension, insomnia, metallic/unpleasant taste, palpitations, urinary retention. **Nasal:** Diarrhea, constipation, dry throat, abdominal pain, nasal congestion.

ADVERSE EFFECTS/ TOXIC REACTIONS

Worsening of angle-closure glaucoma, acute eye pain, hypotension occur rarely.

NURSING CONSIDERATIONS

BASELINE ASSESSMENT
Offer emotional support (high incidence of anxiety due to difficulty in breathing, sympathomimetic response to drug).

INTERVENTION/EVALUATION
Monitor rate, depth, rhythm, type of respiration; quality, rate of pulse. Assess lung sounds for rhonchi, wheezing, rales. Monitor ABGs. Observe lips, fingernails for cyanosis (blue or dusky color in light-skinned pts; gray in dark-skinned pts). Observe for retractions (clavicular, sternal, intercostal), hand tremor. Evaluate for clinical improvement (quieter, slower respirations, relaxed facial expression, cessation of retractions). Monitor for improvement of rhinorrhea.

PATIENT/ FAMILY TEACHING
• Increase fluid intake (decreases lung secretion viscosity). • Do not take more than 2 inhalations at any one time (excessive use may produce paradoxical bronchoconstriction, decreased bronchodilating effect). • Rinsing mouth with water immediately after inhalation may prevent mouth and throat dryness. • Avoid excessive use of caffeine derivatives (chocolate, coffee, tea, cola, cocoa).

irbesartan

ir-be-**sar**-tan
(Avapro)

BLACK BOX ALERT May cause fetal injury, mortality if used during second or third trimester of pregnancy. **Do not confuse Avapro with Anaprox.**

FIXED-COMBINATION(S)

Avalide: irbesartan/hydrochlorothiazide (a diuretic): 150 mg/12.5 mg, 300 mg/12.5 mg, 300 mg/25 mg.

◆CLASSIFICATION

PHARMACOTHERAPEUTIC: Angiotensin II receptor antagonist. **CLINICAL:** Antihypertensive (see p. 11C).

ACTION

Blocks vasoconstriction, aldosterone-secreting effects of angiotensin II, inhibiting binding of angiotensin II to AT_1 receptors. **Therapeutic Effect:** Produces vasodilation, decreases peripheral resistance, decreases B/P.

PHARMACOKINETICS

Route	Onset	Peak	Duration
PO	—	1–2 hrs	Greater than 24 hrs

Rapidly, completely absorbed after PO administration. Protein binding: 90%. Metabolized in liver. Recovered primarily in feces and, to a lesser extent, in urine. Not removed by hemodialysis. **Half-life:** 11–15 hrs.

USES

Treatment of hypertension alone or in combination with other antihypertensives. Treatment of diabetic nephropathy in pts with type 2 diabetes. **OFF-LABEL:** Slow rate of progression of aortic root dilation in children with Marfan's syndrome.

PRECAUTIONS

Contraindications: Concomitant use with aliskiren in pts with diabetes. **Cautions:** Impaired renal function, unstented unilateral or bilateral renal artery stenosis, sodium/water depletion.

⧖ LIFESPAN CONSIDERATIONS

Pregnancy/Lactation: Unknown if distributed in breast milk. May cause fetal or neonatal morbidity or mortality. **Pregnancy Category C (D if used in second or third trimester). Children:** Safety and efficacy not established. **Elderly:** No age-related precautions noted.

INTERACTIONS

DRUG: Diuretics produce additive hypotensive effects. Potassium-sparing **diuretics, potassium supplements** may increase risk of hyperkalemia. **NSAIDs** may decrease antihypertensive effect. **HERBAL: Ephedra, ginseng, yohimbe** may worsen hypertension. **Garlic** may increase antihypertensive effect. **FOOD:** None known. **LAB VALUES:** May slightly increase BUN, serum creatinine. May decrease Hgb.

AVAILABILITY (Rx)

Tablets: 75 mg, 150 mg, 300 mg.

ADMINISTRATION/HANDLING

PO

• Give without regard to meals.

INDICATIONS/ROUTES/DOSAGE

Hypertension
PO: ADULTS, ELDERLY, CHILDREN 13 YRS AND OLDER: Initially, 75–150 mg/day. May increase to 300 mg/day. **CHILDREN 6–12 YRS:** Initially, 75 mg/day. May increase to 150 mg/day.

Nephropathy
PO: ADULTS, ELDERLY: Target dose of 300 mg once daily.

SIDE EFFECTS

Occasional (9%–3%): Upper respiratory tract infection, fatigue, diarrhea, cough.

Rare (2%–1%): Heartburn, dizziness, headache, nausea, rash.

ADVERSE EFFECTS/ TOXIC REACTIONS

Overdose may manifest as hypotension, syncope, tachycardia. Bradycardia occurs less often.

NURSING CONSIDERATIONS

BASELINE ASSESSMENT

Obtain B/P, apical pulse immediately before each dose, in addition to regular monitoring (be alert to fluctuations). If excessive reduction in B/P occurs, place pt in supine position, feet slightly elevated. Question possibility of pregnancy (see Pregnancy Category). Assess medication history (esp. diuretic therapy).

INTERVENTION/EVALUATION

Maintain hydration (offer fluids frequently). Assess for evidence of upper respiratory infection. Assist with ambulation if dizziness occurs. Monitor electrolytes, renal/hepatic function tests, urinalysis, B/P, pulse. Assess for hypotension.

PATIENT/ FAMILY TEACHING

• May cause fetal or neonatal morbidity or mortality. • Avoid tasks that require alertness, motor skills until response to drug is established (possible dizziness effect); ensure appropriate birth control measures are in place. • Report any sign of infection (sore throat, fever). • Avoid exercising during hot weather (risk of dehydration, hypotension).

---

irinotecan

eye-rin-**oh**-tee-kan
(Camptosar)

BLACK BOX ALERT Can induce both early and late forms of severe diarrhea. Early diarrhea (during or shortly after administration) accompanied by salivation, rhinitis, lacri-mation, diaphoresis, flushing. Late diarrhea (occurring more than 24 hrs after administration) can be prolonged and life-threatening. May produce severe, profound myelosuppression. Administer under supervision of experienced cancer chemotherapy physician.

◆CLASSIFICATION

PHARMACOTHERAPEUTIC: DNA to-poisomerase inhibitor. **CLINICAL:** Antineoplastic (see p. 87C).

ACTION

Interacts with topoisomerase I, an enzyme that relieves torsional strain in DNA by inducing reversible single-strand breaks. Prevents religation of these single-stranded breaks resulting in damage to double-strand DNA, cell death. **Therapeutic Effect:** Produces cytotoxic effect on cancer cells.

PHARMACOKINETICS

Metabolized in liver. Protein binding: 95% (metabolite). Excreted in urine and eliminated by biliary route. **Half-life:** 6–12 hrs; metabolite, 10–20 hrs.

USES

Treatment of metastatic carcinoma of colon, rectum in pts whose disease has recurred or progressed after 5-fluoro-uracil-based therapy. **OFF-LABEL:** Non–small-cell lung cancer; small-cell lung cancer; refractory solid tumor configuration; untreated rhabdomyosarcoma; cervical, gastric, pancreatic, ovarian, esophageal cancer; Ewing's sarcoma; brain tumor.

PRECAUTIONS

Contraindications: None known. **Cautions:** Pt previously receiving pelvic, abdominal irradiation (increased risk of myelosuppression), pts older than 65 yrs, hepatic dysfunction, hyperbilirubine-mia, renal impairment.

⧖ LIFESPAN CONSIDERATIONS

Pregnancy/Lactation: May cause fetal harm. Unknown if distributed in breast milk. Breastfeeding not recommended. **Pregnancy Category D. Children:** Safety and efficacy not established. **Elderly:** Risk of diarrhea significantly increased.

INTERACTIONS

DRUG: CYP3A4 inducers (e.g., phenytoin, phenobarbital, carbamazepine) decrease concentration/effects. **CYP3A4 inhibitors (e.g., ketoconazole)** increase concentration. Avoid **live vaccines** during treatment. **HERBAL: St. John's wort** may decrease irinotecan effectiveness. **FOOD:** None known. **LAB VALUES:** May increase serum alkaline phosphatase, AST. May decrease Hgb, leukocytes, platelets.

AVAILABILITY (Rx)

Injection Solution: 20 mg/ml (2 ml, 5 ml, 25 ml).

ADMINISTRATION/HANDLING

 IV

Reconstitution • Dilute in D₅W (preferred) or 0.9% NaCl to concentration of 0.12–2.8 mg/ml.
Rate of Administration • Administer all doses as IV infusion over 30–90 min. • Assess for extravasation (flush site with Sterile Water for Injection, apply ice if extravasation occurs).
Storage • Store vials at room temperature, protect from light. • Solution diluted with D₅W is stable for 24 hrs at room temperature or 48 hrs if refrigerated. • Solution diluted with 0.9% NaCl is stable for 24 hrs at room temperature. • Do not refrigerate solution if diluted with 0.9% NaCl.

▦ IV INCOMPATIBILITY

Gemcitabine (Gemzar).

INDICATIONS/ROUTES/DOSAGE

Note: Genotyping of UGTIAI available. Pts who are homozygous for the UGTIAI*28 allele are at increased risk for neutropenia. Decreased dose is recommended.

Carcinoma of the Colon, Rectum
IV *(Single-Agent Therapy)***: ADULTS, ELDERLY: (WEEKLY REGIMEN):** Initially, 125 mg/m² once weekly for 4 wks, followed by a rest period of 2 wks. Additional courses may be repeated q6wks. Dosage may be adjusted in 25–50 mg/m² increments to as high as 150 mg/m² or as low as 50 mg/m². **(THREE-WEEK REGIMEN):** 350 mg/m² q3wks. Dosage may be adjusted to as low as 200 mg/m².
*(In Combination with Leucovorin and 5-Fluorouracil)***: REGIMEN ONE:** 125 mg/m² on days 1, 8, 15, 22. **REGIMEN TWO:** 180 mg/m² on days 1, 15, 29.

SIDE EFFECTS

Expected (64%–32%): Nausea, alopecia, vomiting, diarrhea. **Frequent (29%–22%):** Constipation, fatigue, fever, asthenia (loss of strength, energy), skeletal pain, abdominal pain, dyspnea. **Occasional (19%–16%):** Anorexia, headache, stomatitis, rash.

ADVERSE EFFECTS/ TOXIC REACTIONS

Myelosuppression characterized as neutropenia occurs in 97% of pts; neutrophil count less than 50/mm³ occurs in 78% of pts. Thrombocytopenia, anemia, sepsis occur frequently.

NURSING CONSIDERATIONS

BASELINE ASSESSMENT

Offer emotional support. Assess hydration status, electrolytes, CBC before each dose. Premedicate with antiemetics on day of treatment, starting at least 30 min before administration. Inform pt of possibility of alopecia.

INTERVENTION/EVALUATION

Assess for early signs of diarrhea. Monitor hydration status, I&O, electrolytes, CBC, renal/hepatic function tests. Monitor infusion site for signs of inflammation. Assess skin for rash.

PATIENT/ FAMILY TEACHING

• Report diarrhea, vomiting, fever, lightheadedness, dizziness. • Do not have immunizations without physician's approval (drug lowers resistance). • Avoid contact with those who have recently received live virus vaccine. • Avoid crowds, those with infections.

---

iron dextran

iron **dex**-tran
(DexFerrum, Dexiron ✦, Infed, Infufer ✦)

BLACK BOX ALERT Potentially fatal anaphylactic-type reaction has been associated with parenteral administration.
Do not confuse DexFerrum with Desferal, or iron dextran with iron sucrose.

◆ CLASSIFICATION

PHARMACOTHERAPEUTIC: Trace element. **CLINICAL:** Hematinic iron preparation.

ACTION

Essential component in formation of Hgb. Necessary for effective erythropoiesis, transport and utilization of oxygen. Serves as cofactor of several essential enzymes. **Therapeutic Effect:** Replenishes Hgb, depleted iron stores.

PHARMACOKINETICS

Readily absorbed after IM administration. Most absorption occurs within 72 hrs; remainder within 3–4 wks. Bound to protein to form hemosiderin, ferritin, or transferrin. No physiologic system of elimination. Small amounts lost daily in shedding of skin, hair, nails and in feces, urine, perspiration. **Half-life:** 5–20 hrs.

USES

Treatment of anemia, iron deficiency. Use only when PO administration is not feasible or when rapid replenishment of iron is warranted. **OFF-LABEL:** Cancer chemotherapy-associated anemia.

PRECAUTIONS

Contraindications: All anemias not associated with iron deficiency anemia (pernicious, aplastic, normocytic, refractory). **Caution:** Serious hepatic impairment. History of allergies, bronchial asthma, rheumatoid arthritis, preexisting cardiac disease. Avoid use during acute kidney infection.

⌛ LIFESPAN CONSIDERATIONS

Pregnancy/Lactation: May cross placenta in some form (unknown). Trace distributed in breast milk. **Pregnancy Category C. Children/Elderly:** No age-related precautions noted.

INTERACTIONS

DRUG: None significant. **HERBAL:** None significant. **FOOD:** None known. **LAB VALUES:** None significant.

AVAILABILITY (Rx)

Injection Solution (DexFerrum, Infed): 50 mg/ml.

ADMINISTRATION/HANDLING

◄ALERT► Test dose is generally given before full dosage; monitor pt for several min after injection due to potential for anaphylactic reaction.

 IV

Reconstitution • May give undiluted or dilute in 250–1,000 ml 0.9% NaCl for infusion. • Avoid dilution in dextrose (increased pain/phlebitis).
Rate of Administration • Do not exceed IV administration rate of 50 mg/min (1 ml/min). Too-rapid IV rate may produce flushing, chest pain, hypotension, tachycardia, shock. • Infuse diluted solution over 1–6 hrs. • Pt must remain recumbent 30–45 min after IV

administration (minimizes postural hypotension).

Storage • Store at room temperature.

IM
• Draw up medication with one needle; use new needle for injection (minimizes skin staining). • Administer deep IM in upper outer quadrant of buttock only. • Use Z-tract technique (displacement of subcutaneous tissue lateral to injection site before inserting needle) to minimize skin staining.

⊞ IV INCOMPATIBILITIES

Do not mix with other medications.

INDICATIONS/ROUTES/DOSAGE

0.5-ml test dose (0.25 ml in infants). Give prior to initiating iron dextran therapy.
◄ALERT► Discontinue oral iron preparations before administering iron dextran. Dosage expressed in terms of milligrams of elemental iron. Dosage individualized based on degree of anemia, pt weight, presence of any bleeding. Use periodic hematologic determinations as guide to therapy.
◄ALERT► Not normally given in first 4 mos of life.

Iron Deficiency Anemia
IV, IM: ADULTS, ELDERLY, CHILDREN WEIGHING MORE THAN 15 KG: Dose in ml (50 mg elemental iron/ml) = 0.0442 (desired Hgb less observed Hgb) × lean body weight (in kg) + (0.26 × lean body weight). Give 2 ml or less once daily until total dose reached. **CHILDREN WEIGHING 5–15 KG:** Dose in ml (50 mg elemental iron/ml) = 0.0442 (desired Hgb less observed Hgb) × body weight (in kg) + (0.26 × body weight). Give 2 ml or less once daily until total dose reached.

Maximum Daily Dosages
ADULTS WEIGHING MORE THAN 50 KG: 100 mg. **CHILDREN WEIGHING MORE THAN 15 KG:** 100 mg. **CHILDREN WEIGHING 5–15 KG:** 50 mg. **CHILDREN WEIGHING LESS THAN 5 KG:** 25 mg.

SIDE EFFECTS
Frequent: Allergic reaction (rash, pruritus), backache, myalgia, chills, dizziness, headache, fever, nausea, vomiting, flushed skin, pain/redness at injection site, brown discoloration of skin, metallic taste.

ADVERSE EFFECTS/ TOXIC REACTIONS
Anaphylaxis occurs rarely in first few min following injection. Leukocytosis, lymphadenopathy occur rarely.

NURSING CONSIDERATIONS

BASELINE ASSESSMENT
Do not give concurrently with oral iron form (excessive iron may produce excessive iron storage [hemosiderosis]). Be alert to pts with rheumatoid arthritis (RA), iron deficiency anemia (acute exacerbation of joint pain, swelling may occur). Inguinal lymphadenopathy may occur with IM injection. Assess for adequate muscle mass before injecting medication.

INTERVENTION/EVALUATION
Monitor IM site for abscess formation, necrosis, atrophy, swelling, brownish color of skin. Question pt regarding soreness, pain, inflammation at/near IM injection site. Check IV site for phlebitis. Monitor serum ferritin. Monitor daily pattern of bowel activity, stool consistency.

PATIENT/FAMILY TEACHING
• Pain, brown staining may occur at injection site. • Oral iron should not be taken when receiving iron injections. • Stools often become black with iron therapy but is harmless unless accompanied by red streaking, sticky consistency of stool, abdominal pain/cramping, which should be reported to physician. • Oral hygiene, hard candy, gum may reduce metallic taste. • Immediately report fever, back pain, headache.

iron sucrose

iron **soo**-krose
(Venofer)
Do not confuse iron sucrose with iron dextran.

♦CLASSIFICATION

PHARMACOTHERAPEUTIC: Trace element. **CLINICAL:** Hematinic iron preparation.

ACTION

Essential component in formation of Hgb. Necessary for effective erythropoiesis, transport and utilization of oxygen. Serves as cofactor of several essential enzymes. **Therapeutic Effect:** Replenishes body iron stores in pts on chronic hemodialysis who have iron deficiency anemia and are receiving erythropoietin.

PHARMACOKINETICS

Distributed mainly in blood and to some extent in extravascular fluid. Iron sucrose is dissociated into iron and sucrose by reticuloendothelial system. Sucrose component is eliminated mainly by urinary excretion. **Half-life:** 6 hrs.

USES

Treatment of iron deficiency anemia in pts undergoing chronic hemodialysis or peritoneal dialysis who are receiving supplemental erythropoietin therapy. Treatment of iron deficiency anemia in pts with chronic kidney disease who are not undergoing dialysis (with or without erythropoietin therapy). **OFF-LABEL:** Chemotherapy-associated anemia.

PRECAUTIONS

Contraindications: All anemias except iron deficiency anemia (pernicious, aplastic, normocytic, refractory anemia), evidence of iron overload. **Cautions:** History of allergies, bronchial asthma; hepatic dysfunction, rheumatoid arthritis, preexisting cardiac disease.

⧗ LIFESPAN CONSIDERATIONS

Pregnancy/Lactation: Unknown if drug crosses placenta or is distributed in breast milk. **Pregnancy Category B. Children:** Safety and efficacy not established. **Elderly:** Age-related renal impairment may require dosage adjustment.

INTERACTIONS

DRUG: None significant. **HERBAL:** None significant. **FOOD:** None known. **LAB VALUES:** Increases Hgb, Hct, serum ferritin, transferrin.

AVAILABILITY (Rx)

Injection Solution: 20 mg of elemental iron/ml in 2.5-ml, 5-ml, 10-ml vials.

ADMINISTRATION/HANDLING

◄**ALERT**► Administer directly into dialysis line during hemodialysis.

 IV

Reconstitution • May give undiluted as slow IV injection or IV infusion. For IV infusion, dilute 100-mg (5-ml) vial in maximum of 100 ml 0.9% NaCl immediately before infusion. • Dilute large doses in maximum of 250 ml 0.9% NaCl. **Rate of Administration** • For IV injection, administer 100–200 mg (5–10 ml) over 2–5 min. • For IV infusion, administer 100 mg over at least 15 min; 300 mg over 1.5 hrs; 400 mg over 2.5 hrs; 500 mg over 3.5 hrs. **Storage** • Store at room temperature. • Following dilution, stable for 48 hrs at room temperature or if refrigerated.

▦ IV INCOMPATIBILITIES

Do not mix with other medications or add to parenteral nutrition solution for IV infusion.

INDICATIONS/ROUTES/DOSAGE

Iron Deficiency Anemia
Dosage is expressed in terms of milligrams of elemental iron.
IV: ADULTS, ELDERLY (HEMODIALYSIS-DEPENDENT PTS): 5 ml iron sucrose (100 mg elemental iron) delivered during di-

alysis; administer 1–3 times a wk to total dose of 1,000 mg in 10 doses. Give no more than 3 times a wk. **(PERITONEAL DIALYSIS-DEPENDENT PTS):** Two infusions of 300 mg over 90 min 14 days apart followed by a single 400-mg dose over 2½ hrs 14 days later. **(NON-DIALYSIS-DEPENDENT PTS):** 200 mg over 2–5 min on 5 different occasions within 14 days.

SIDE EFFECTS

Frequent (36%–23%): Hypotension, leg cramps, diarrhea.

ADVERSE EFFECTS/ TOXIC REACTIONS

Too-rapid IV administration may produce severe hypotension, headache, vomiting, nausea, dizziness, paresthesia, abdominal/muscle pain, edema, cardiovascular collapse. Hypersensitivity reaction occurs rarely.

NURSING CONSIDERATIONS

INTERVENTION/EVALUATION

Initially, monitor Hgb, Hct, serum ferritin, transferrin monthly, then q2–3mos thereafter. Reliable serum iron values can be obtained 48 hrs following administration.

---

isoniazid

eye-**soe**-nye-a-zid
(Isotamine ♣, PMS Isoniazid ♣)
BLACK BOX ALERT Severe, potentially fatal hepatitis may occur.

FIXED-COMBINATION(S)

Rifamate: isoniazid/rifampin (antitubercular): 150 mg/300 mg.
Rifater: isoniazid/pyrazinamide/rifampin (antitubercular): 50 mg/300 mg/120 mg.

◆ CLASSIFICATION

PHARMACOTHERAPEUTIC: Isonicotinic acid derivative. **CLINICAL:** Antitubercular.

ACTION

Inhibits mycolic acid synthesis. Causes disruption of bacterial cell wall, loss of acid-fast properties in susceptible mycobacteria. Active only during bacterial cell division. **Therapeutic Effect:** Bactericidal against actively growing intracellular, extracellular susceptible mycobacteria.

PHARMACOKINETICS

Readily absorbed from GI tract. Protein binding: 10%–15%. Widely distributed (including to CSF). Metabolized in liver. Primarily excreted in urine. Removed by hemodialysis. **Half-life:** 0.5–5 hrs.

USES

Treatment of susceptible mycobacterial infection due to *Mycobacterium tuberculosis*. Drug of choice in tuberculosis prophylaxis. Used in combination with one or more other antitubercular agents for treatment of active tuberculosis.

PRECAUTIONS

Contraindications: Acute hepatic disease, hepatic injury or severe adverse reactions with previous isoniazid therapy. **Cautions:** Chronic hepatic disease, alcoholism, severe renal impairment. Pregnancy, pts at risk for peripheral neuropathy, history of hypersensitivity reactions to latent TB infection medications.

⧗ LIFESPAN CONSIDERATIONS

Pregnancy/Lactation: Prophylaxis usually postponed until after delivery. Crosses placenta. Distributed in breast milk. **Pregnancy Category C. Children:** No age-related precautions noted. **Elderly:** More susceptible to developing hepatitis.

INTERACTIONS

DRUG: Alcohol may increase isoniazid metabolism, risk of hepatotoxicity. May increase toxicity of **carbamazepine, phenytoin. Hepatotoxic medications** may increase risk of hepatotoxicity. May decrease **ketoconazole** concentration. **HERBAL:** None significant. **FOOD: Foods containing tyramine** may cause hypertensive crisis. **LAB VALUES:** May increase serum bilirubin, AST, ALT.

AVAILABILITY (Rx)

Oral Solution: 50 mg/5 ml. **Solution, Injection:** 100 mg/ml. **Tablets:** 100 mg, 300 mg.

ADMINISTRATION/HANDLING

PO

• Give 1 hr before or 2 hrs following meals (may give with food to decrease GI upset, but will delay absorption). • Administer at least 1 hr before antacids, esp. those containing aluminum.

INDICATIONS/ROUTES/DOSAGE

Active Tuberculosis (in Combination with One or More Antituberculars)
IM/PO: ADULTS, ELDERLY: 5 mg/kg/day as a single daily dose. Usual dose: 300 mg/day or 15 mg/kg 2–3 times/wk. **Maximum:** 900 mg/dose. **CHILDREN:** 10–15 mg/kg/day as a single daily dose. **Maximum:** 300 mg/day or 20–40 mg/kg 2–3 times/wk. **Maximum:** 900 mg/dose.

Tuberculosis Prophylaxis
IM/PO: ADULTS, ELDERLY: 5 mg/kg/day (**maximum:** 300 mg) or 15 mg/kg twice weekly (**maximum:** 900 mg). **CHILDREN:** 10–20 mg/kg/day as a single daily dose. **Maximum:** 300 mg/day or 20–40 mg/kg 2 times/wk. **Maximum:** 900 mg/dose.

SIDE EFFECTS

Frequent: Nausea, vomiting, diarrhea, abdominal pain. **Rare:** Pain at injection site, hypersensitivity reaction.

ADVERSE EFFECTS/ TOXIC REACTIONS

Neurotoxicity (ataxia, paresthesia), optic neuritis, hepatotoxicity occur rarely.

NURSING CONSIDERATIONS

BASELINE ASSESSMENT

Question for history of hypersensitivity reactions, hepatic injury or disease, sensitivity to nicotinic acid or chemically related medications. Ensure collection of specimens for culture, sensitivity. Evaluate initial hepatic function results.

INTERVENTION/EVALUATION

Monitor hepatic function test results, assess for hepatitis: anorexia, nausea, vomiting, weakness, fatigue, dark urine, jaundice (hold concurrent INH therapy and inform physician promptly). Assess for paresthesia of extremities (those esp. at risk for neuropathy may be given pyridoxine prophylactically: malnourished, elderly, diabetics, pts with chronic hepatic disease [including alcoholics]). Be alert for fever, skin eruptions (hypersensitivity reaction).

PATIENT/FAMILY TEACHING

• Do not skip doses; continue taking isoniazid for full length of therapy (6–24 mos). • Take preferably 1 hr before or 2 hrs following meals (with food if GI upset). • Avoid alcohol during treatment. • Do not take any other medications, including antacids, without consulting physician. • Must take isoniazid at least 1 hr before antacid. • Avoid tuna, sauerkraut, aged cheeses, smoked fish (consult list of tyramine-containing foods) that may cause hypertensive reaction (red/itching skin, palpitations, light-headedness, hot or clammy feeling, headache). • Report any new symptom, immediately for vision difficulties, nausea/vomiting, dark urine, yellowing of skin/eyes (jaundice), fatigue, paresthesia of extremities.

isosorbide dinitrate

TOP 200

eye-soe-**sor**-bide
(ISDN ✦, Dilatrate-SR, Isordil, Novo-Sorbide ✦)

isosorbide mononitrate

(Apo-ISMO ✦, Imdur)

Do not confuse Imdur with Imuran, Inderal, or K-Dur, Isordil with Inderal, Isuprel, or Plendil.

FIXED-COMBINATION(S)

BiDil: isosorbide dinitrate/hydralazine (a vasodilator): 20 mg/37.5 mg.

◆CLASSIFICATION

PHARMACOTHERAPEUTIC: Nitrate.
CLINICAL: Antianginal (see p. 127C).

ACTION

Stimulates intracellular cyclic guanosine monophosphate. **Therapeutic Effect:** Relaxes vascular smooth muscle of arterial, venous vasculature. Decreases preload, afterload.

PHARMACOKINETICS

Route	Onset	Peak	Duration
Dinitrate			
Sublingual	3 min	N/A	1–2 hrs
PO	45–60 min	N/A	up to 8 hrs
Mononitrate			
PO (extended-release)	30–60 min	N/A	12–24 hrs

Dinitrate poorly absorbed and metabolized in liver to its active metabolite isosorbide mononitrate. Mononitrate well absorbed after PO administration. Excreted in urine and feces. **Half-life:** Dinitrate, 1–4 hrs; mononitrate, 4 hrs.

USES

Dinitrate: Prevention and treatment of angina. **Mononitrate:** Prevention of angina pectoris. **OFF-LABEL:** Esophageal spastic disorders, HF.

PRECAUTIONS

Contraindications: Hypersensitivity to nitrates, concurrent use of sildenafil, tadalafil, vardenafil. **Cautions:** Inferior wall MI, head trauma, increased intracranial pressure (ICP), orthostatic hypotension, blood volume depletion from diuretic therapy, systolic B/P less than 90 mm Hg, hypertrophic cardiomyopathy.

⧗ LIFESPAN CONSIDERATIONS

Pregnancy/Lactation: Unknown if drug crosses placenta or is distributed in breast milk. **Pregnancy Category C. Children:** Safety and efficacy not established. **Elderly:** May be more sensitive to hypotensive effects. Age-related renal impairment may require dosage adjustment.

INTERACTIONS

DRUG: Alcohol, antihypertensives, vasodilators may increase risk of orthostatic hypotension. **Sildenafil, tadalafil, vardenafil** may potentiate hypotensive effects (concurrent use of these agents is contraindicated). **HERBAL:** None significant. **FOOD:** None known. **LAB VALUES:** May increase urine catecholamine, urine vanillylmandelic acid levels.

AVAILABILITY (Rx)

Dinitrate
Tablets (Isordil): 5 mg, 10 mg, 20 mg, 30 mg, 40 mg.

🗹Capsules, Sustained-Release (Dilatrate-SR): 40 mg. 🗹Tablets, Extended-Release: 40 mg. 🗹Tablets, Sublingual (Isordil): 2.5 mg, 5 mg.

Mononitrate
Tablets: 10 mg, 20 mg.

🗹Tablets, Extended-Release (Imdur): 30 mg, 60 mg, 120 mg.

ADMINISTRATION/HANDLING

PO
• Best if taken on an empty stomach. • Do not administer around the clock. • Oral tablets may be crushed. • Do not crush/break sustained-, extended-release form. • Do not crush chewable form before administering.

Sublingual
• Do not crush/chew sublingual tablets. • Dissolve tablets under tongue; do not swallow.

◆ Canadian trade name   🗹 Non-Crushable Drug   **HIGH ALERT** High Alert drug

INDICATIONS/ROUTES/DOSAGE

Angina

PO *(Isosorbide Dinitrate) (Immediate-Release)*: **ADULTS, ELDERLY:** 5–40 mg 2–3 times a day.
Sublingual: ADULTS, ELDERLY: 2.5–5 mg, q5–10 min. **Maximum:** 3 doses in 15–30 min.
Sustained-Release: ADULTS, ELDERLY: 40 mg 1–2 times/day.
PO *(Isosorbide Mononitrate) (Immediate-Release)*: **ADULTS, ELDERLY:** 5–20 mg twice a day given 7 hrs apart.
Sustained-Release: Initially, 30–60 mg/day in morning as a single dose. May increase dose at 3-day intervals. **Maximum daily single dose:** 240 mg.

SIDE EFFECTS

Frequent: Headache (may be severe) occurs mostly in early therapy, diminishes rapidly in intensity, usually disappears during continued treatment. **Occasional:** Transient flushing of face/neck, dizziness, weakness, orthostatic hypotension, nausea, vomiting, restlessness. GI upset, blurred vision, dry mouth. **Sublingual: Frequent:** Burning, tingling at oral point of dissolution.

ADVERSE EFFECTS/ TOXIC REACTIONS

Discontinue if blurred vision occurs. Severe orthostatic hypotension manifested by syncope, pulselessness, cold/clammy skin, diaphoresis has been reported. Tolerance may occur with repeated, prolonged therapy, but may not occur with extended-release form. Minor tolerance with intermittent use of sublingual tablets. High dosage tends to produce severe headache.

NURSING CONSIDERATIONS

BASELINE ASSESSMENT

Record onset, type (sharp, dull, squeezing), radiation, location, intensity, duration of anginal pain; precipitating factors (exertion, emotional stress). If headache occurs during management therapy, administer medication with meals.

INTERVENTION/EVALUATION

Assist with ambulation if light-headedness, dizziness occurs. Assess for facial/neck flushing. Monitor number of anginal episodes, orthostatic B/P.

PATIENT/FAMILY TEACHING

• Do not chew/crush sublingual, extended-release, sustained-release forms. • Take sublingual tablets while sitting down. • Go from lying to standing slowly (prevents dizziness effect). • Take oral form on empty stomach (however, if headache occurs during management therapy, take medication with meals). • Dissolve sublingual tablet under tongue; do not swallow. • Avoid alcohol (intensifies hypotensive effect). • If alcohol is ingested soon after taking nitrates, possible acute hypotensive episode (marked drop in B/P, vertigo, pallor) may occur. • Report signs/symptoms of hypotension, angina.

isotretinoin

eye-so-**tret**-i-noyn
(Absorica, Myorisan, Accutane ✤, Amnesteem, Claravis, Sotret)
BLACK BOX ALERT High risk of teratogenic effects; Pregnancy Category X. Obtain two negative pregnancy tests prior to treatment. All pts (male and female) must register and be active in the IPLEDGE™ risk management program.
Do not confuse Accutane with Accolate or Accupril, Claravis with Cleviprex, or isotretinoin with tretinoin.

◆CLASSIFICATION

PHARMACOTHERAPEUTIC: Keratinization stabilizer. **CLINICAL:** Antiacne, antirosacea agent.

ACTION

Reduces sebaceous gland size, inhibiting gland activity. **Therapeutic Effect:** Produces antikeratinizing, anti-inflammatory effects.

USES

Treatment of severe, recalcitrant cystic acne unresponsive to conventional acne therapies. **OFF-LABEL:** Treatment of children with metastatic neuroblastoma or leukemia not responding to conventional therapy.

PRECAUTIONS

Contraindications: Hypersensitivity to isotretinoin, parabens (component of capsules), vitamin A supplements, pregnancy, breast-feeding. **Cautions:** Hepatic dysfunction. Diabetes; hypertriglyceridemia; history of childhood osteoporosis; osteomalacia, other disorders of bone metabolism; psychiatric disorders.

⧗ LIFESPAN CONSIDERATIONS

Pregnancy/Lactation: Contraindicated in females who are or may become pregnant (very high risk of fetal harm, major fetal birth defects/deformities). Unknown if distributed in breast milk. Breastfeeding contraindicated. **Pregnancy Category X. Children:** Safety and efficacy not established in those younger than 12 yrs. Careful consideration must be given to those 12–17 yrs, esp. children with known metabolic disease, structural bone disease. **Elderly:** No age-related precautions noted.

INTERACTIONS

DRUG: Vitamin A may increase toxic effects. **Tetracycline** may increase potential for pseudotumor cerebri. **HERBAL: Dong quai, St. John's wort** may cause photosensitization. **FOOD:** None known. **LAB VALUES:** May increase serum triglycerides, cholesterol, AST, ALT, alkaline phosphatase, LDH, fasting serum glucose, uric acid, sedimentation rate. May decrease HDL.

AVAILABILITY (Rx)

Capsules: (Amnesteem, Myorisan): 10 mg, 20 mg, 40 mg. **(Absorica, Claravis, Sotret):** 10 mg, 20 mg, 30 mg, 40 mg.

ADMINISTRATION/HANDLING

PO
• Give with food. Give whole with full glass of water. • May chew or open capsule with large needle, place on applesauce, cottage cheese, pudding, oatmeal, or ice cream.

INDICATIONS/ROUTES/DOSAGE

Recalcitrant Cystic Acne
PO: ADULTS, CHILDREN 12–17 YRS: Initially, 0.5–1 mg/kg/day divided in 2 doses for 15–20 wks or until total cyst count decreases by 70%, whichever is sooner. Adults may require doses up to 2 mg/kg/day. May repeat after at least 2 mos off therapy.

Dosage in Hepatic Disease
Dose reductions recommended.

SIDE EFFECTS

Frequent (90%–20%): Cheilitis (inflammation of lips), skin/mucous membrane dryness, skin fragility, pruritus, epistaxis, dry nose/mouth, conjunctivitis, hypertriglyceridemia, nausea, vomiting, abdominal pain. **Occasional (16%–5%):** Musculoskeletal symptoms including bone/joint pain, arthralgia, generalized muscle aches; photosensitivity . **Rare:** Diminished night vision, depression.

ADVERSE EFFECTS/ TOXIC REACTIONS

Inflammatory bowel disease, pseudotumor cerebri (benign intracranial hypertension) have been associated with isotretinoin therapy.

NURSING CONSIDERATIONS

BASELINE ASSESSMENT
Assess baseline serum glucose, lipids, triglycerides. Obtain two negative preg-

nancy tests prior to treatment (Pregnancy Category X).

INTERVENTION/EVALUATION

Assess acne for decreased cysts. Evaluate skin/mucous membranes for excessive dryness. Monitor serum glucose, lipids, triglycerides.

PATIENT/FAMILY TEACHING

• Transient exacerbation of acne may occur during initial period. • May have decreased tolerance to contact lenses during and following therapy. • Do not take vitamin supplements with vitamin A due to additive effects. • Immediately report onset of abdominal pain, severe diarrhea, rectal bleeding (possible inflammatory bowel disease), headache, nausea/vomiting, visual disturbances (possible pseudotumor cerebri). • Diminished night vision may occur suddenly; take caution with night driving. • Avoid prolonged exposure to sunlight; use sunscreens, protective clothing. • Do not donate blood during or for 1 mo following treatment. • **Women:** Explain serious risk to fetus if pregnancy occurs (give both oral and written warnings, with pt acknowledging in writing that she understands the warnings and consents to treatment). • Must have negative serum pregnancy test within 2 wks before starting therapy; therapy will begin on the second or third day of next normal menstrual period. • Two reliable forms of contraception must be used for at least 1 mo before, during, and for at least 1 mo after therapy.

---

isradipine

is-**ra**-di-peen
(DynaCirc ✶)
Do not confuse DynaCirc with Dynabac or Dynacin.

◆**CLASSIFICATION**

PHARMACOTHERAPEUTIC: Calcium channel blocker. **CLINICAL:** Antihypertensive (see p. 79C).

ACTION

Inhibits calcium movement across cardiac, vascular smooth-muscle cell membranes. Potent peripheral vasodilator (does not depress SA, AV nodes). **Therapeutic Effect:** Produces relaxation of coronary vascular smooth muscle; produces coronary vasodilation. Increases myocardial oxygen delivery in pts with vasospastic angina.

PHARMACOKINETICS

Route	Onset	Peak	Duration
PO (immediate-release hypertension)	1 hr	2–3 hrs	Greater than 12 hrs

Well absorbed from GI tract. Protein binding: 95%. Metabolized in liver. Primarily excreted in urine. Not removed by hemodialysis. **Half-life:** 8 hrs.

USES

Management of hypertension. May be used alone or with other antihypertensives. **OFF-LABEL:** Treatment of pediatric hypertension.

PRECAUTIONS

Contraindications: None known. **Cautions:** HF, hepatic dysfunction, severe GI narrowing (for controlled-release tablets).

⧗ LIFESPAN CONSIDERATIONS

Pregnancy/Lactation: Unknown if drug crosses placenta or is distributed in breast milk. **Pregnancy Category C. Children:** Safety and efficacy not established. **Elderly:** Age-related renal impairment may require dosage adjustment.

INTERACTIONS

DRUG: Cimetidine may increase concentration. **Rifampin** may decrease concentration. **HERBAL: Ephedra, ginseng, yohimbe** may worsen hypertension. **Garlic** may increase antihypertensive effect. **FOOD: Grapefruit products** may increase absorption. **LAB VALUES:** None significant.

AVAILABILITY (Rx)

Capsules, Immediate-Release: 2.5 mg, 5 mg.

ADMINISTRATION/HANDLING

PO
* May give without regard to food.
* Swallow controlled-release tablet whole; do not crush, break, cut, divide.

INDICATIONS/ROUTES/DOSAGE

Hypertension
PO: ADULTS, ELDERLY (IMMEDIATE-RELEASE): Initially 2.5 mg twice a day. May increase by 5 mg/day at 2- to 4-wk intervals. Range: 2.5–10 mg in 2 divided doses.

SIDE EFFECTS

Frequent (7%–4%): Peripheral edema, palpitations (higher frequency in females). **Occasional (3%):** Facial flushing, cough. **Rare (2%–1%):** Angina, tachycardia, rash, pruritus.

ADVERSE EFFECTS/ TOXIC REACTIONS

Overdose produces nausea, drowsiness, confusion, slurred speech. HF occurs rarely.

NURSING CONSIDERATIONS

BASELINE ASSESSMENT

Obtain baseline renal/hepatic function tests. Assess B/P, apical pulse immediately before drug is administered (if pulse is 60 beats/min or less or systolic B/P is less than 90 mm Hg, withhold medication, contact physician).

INTERVENTION/EVALUATION

Assess for peripheral edema behind medial malleolus (sacral area in bedridden pts). Monitor pulse rate for bradycardia. Monitor B/P; observe for signs, symptoms of HF. Assess skin for flushing.

PATIENT/FAMILY TEACHING

* Do not abruptly discontinue medication. Compliance with therapy regimen is essential to control hypertension. * To avoid hypotensive effect, go from lying to standing slowly. * Report palpitations, shortness of breath, pronounced dizziness, nausea, chest pain, swelling in extremities. * Avoid grapefruit products.

itraconazole

eye-tra-**con**-ah-zoll
(Onmel, Sporanox)

BLACK BOX ALERT Serious cardiovascular events, including HF, ventricular tachycardia, torsade de pointes, death, have occurred due to concurrent use with pimozide, quinidine, dofetilide, ergot alkaloids, felodipine, lovastatin, methadone, midazolam (oral), simvastatin, triazolam, or levomethadyl.
Do not confuse itraconazole with fluconazole, or Sporanox with Suprax or Topamax.

◆CLASSIFICATION

PHARMACOTHERAPEUTIC: Imidazole/triazole type antifungal. **CLINICAL:** Antifungal (see p. 48C).

ACTION

Inhibits synthesis of ergosterol (vital component of fungal cell formation). **Therapeutic Effect:** Damages fungal cell membrane, altering its function. Fungistatic.

PHARMACOKINETICS

Moderately absorbed from GI tract. Absorption is increased when taken with food. Protein binding: 99%. Widely distributed, primarily in fatty tissue, liver, kidneys. Metabolized in liver. Primarily excreted in urine. Not removed by hemodialysis. **Half-life:** 16–26 hrs.

USES

Oral capsules: Treatment of aspergillosis, blastomycosis, esophageal and oropharyngeal candidiasis, empiric treatment in febrile neutropenia, histoplasmosis, onychomycosis. **Oral solution:** Treatment of oral and esophageal candidiasis.

PRECAUTIONS

Contraindications: Hypersensitivity to fluconazole, ketoconazole, miconazole. Left ventricular dysfunction; history of HF; concurrent use of dofetilide, ergot derivatives, lovastatin, methadone, felodipine, midazolam (oral), quinidine, simvastatin, triazolam; pregnancy or intending to become pregnant. **Cautions:** Hepatic impairment, renal impairment, pts with risk factors for HF (e.g., COPD, myocardial ischemia).

⌛ LIFESPAN CONSIDERATIONS

Pregnancy/Lactation: Distributed in breast milk. **Pregnancy Category C. Children:** Safety and efficacy not established. **Elderly:** Age-related renal impairment may require dosage adjustment.

INTERACTIONS

DRUG: May increase concentration/toxicity of **calcium channel-blocking agents (e.g., felodipine, nifedipine), carbamazepine, cyclosporine, digoxin, ergot alkaloids, HMG-CoA reductase inhibitors (e.g., lovastatin, simvastatin), midazolam, oral antidiabetic agents (e.g., glyburide, glipizide), protease inhibitors (e.g., indinavir, ritonavir, saquinavir), sirolimus, tacrolimus, triazolam, warfarin.** CYP3A4 inducers (e.g., **carbamazepine, isoniazid, phenobarbital, phenytoin, rifampin**) may decrease concentration/effects. May inhibit metabolism of **busulfan, docetaxel, vinca alkaloids.** **Erythromycin** may increase risk of cardiac toxicity. **Antacids, H₂ antagonists,**

proton pump inhibitors may decrease absorption. **HERBAL: St. John's wort** may decrease concentration. **FOOD: Grapefruit products** may alter absorption. **LAB VALUES:** May increase serum alkaline phosphatase, bilirubin, AST, ALT, LDH. May decrease serum potassium.

AVAILABILITY (Rx)

Capsules: 100 mg. **Oral Solution:** 10 mg/ml.

ADMINISTRATION/HANDLING

PO

• Give capsules with food (increases absorption). • Give solution on empty stomach.

INDICATIONS/ROUTES/DOSAGE

Usual Dosage Range
PO: ADULTS, ELDERLY: 100–800 mg/day. Doses greater than 200 mg given in 2 divided doses. Length of therapy ranges from 1 day to more than 6 mos.

Blastomycosis, Histoplasmosis
PO: ADULTS, ELDERLY: Initially, 200 mg 3 times/day for 3 days, then 400 mg/day in 2 divided doses for 6–12 mos (6–12 wks for histoplasmosis).

Aspergillosis (Invasive)
PO: ADULTS, ELDERLY: 600 mg/day in 3 divided doses for 3–4 days, then 200–400 mg/day in 2 divided doses.

Esophageal Candidiasis
PO: ADULTS, ELDERLY: Swish 100–200 mg (10–20 ml) in mouth for several seconds, then swallow once daily for a minimum of 3 wks. Continue for 2 wks after resolution of symptoms. **Maximum:** 200 mg/day.

Oropharyngeal Candidiasis
PO: ADULTS, ELDERLY: 200 mg (10 ml) oral solution, swish and swallow once a day for 7–14 days.

Onychomycosis (Fingernail)
PO: ADULTS, ELDERLY: 200 mg twice a day for 7 days, off for 21 days, repeat 200 mg twice a day for 7 days.

Onychomycosis (Toenail)
PO: ADULTS, ELDERLY: 200 mg once daily for 12 wks.

SIDE EFFECTS

Frequent (11%–9%): Nausea, rash. **Occasional (5%–3%):** Vomiting, headache, diarrhea, hypertension, peripheral edema, fatigue, fever. **Rare (2% or less):** Abdominal pain, dizziness, anorexia, pruritus.

ADVERSE EFFECTS/ TOXIC REACTIONS

Hepatitis (anorexia, abdominal pain, unusual fatigue/weakness, jaundiced skin/ sclera, dark urine) occurs rarely.

NURSING CONSIDERATIONS

BASELINE ASSESSMENT

Determine baseline temperature, hepatic function tests. Assess allergies. Receive full medication history (numerous contraindications/cautions).

INTERVENTION/EVALUATION

Assess for signs, symptoms of hepatic dysfunction. Monitor hepatic function results in pts with preexisting hepatic impairment.

PATIENT/ FAMILY TEACHING

• Take capsules with food, liquids if GI distress occurs. • Therapy will continue for at least 3 mos, until lab tests, clinical presentation indicate infection is controlled. • Immediately report unusual fatigue, yellow skin, dark urine, pale stool, anorexia, nausea, vomiting. • Avoid grapefruit products.

ivacaftor

eye-va-**kaf**-tor
(Kalydeco)

◆CLASSIFICATION

PHARMACOTHERAPEUTIC: Cystic fibrosis transmembrane conductance regulator potentiator. **CLINICAL:** Cystic fibrosis agent.

ACTION

Potentiates a specific protein to facilitate, regulate chloride ions, water transport. In cystic fibrosis pts with a specific gene mutation (G551D), a defect in chloride and water transport results in formation of thick mucus in lungs. **Therapeutic Effect:** Improves lung function, noted fewer respiratory exacerbations.

PHARMACOKINETICS

Readily absorbed. Peak concentration occurs in 4 hrs. Metabolized in liver. Protein binding: 99%. Primarily excreted in feces. **Half-life:** 12 hrs.

USES

Treatment of cystic fibrosis in pts age 6 yrs and older who have a G551D mutation in the cystic fibrosis transmembrane conductance regulator *(CFTR)* gene.

PRECAUTIONS

Contraindications: None known. **Cautions:** Severe hepatic/renal impairment.

⌛ LIFESPAN CONSIDERATIONS

Pregnancy/Lactation: Distributed in breast milk. **Pregnancy Category B. Children:** Safety and efficacy in children younger than 6 yrs not established. **Elderly:** No age-related precautions noted.

INTERACTIONS

DRUG: Strong CYP3A4 inducers (e.g., **carbamazepine, rifampin**) substantially decreases concentration/effects. Concurrent use not recommended. **Strong CYP3A4 inhibitors (e.g., clarithromycin, ketoconazole)** significantly increases concentration. **Moderate CYP3A4 inhibitors (e.g., erythromycin, fluconazole)** may increase concentration and should not be given concurrently. **HERBAL: St. John's wort** decreases concentration/ effect. **FOOD: Grapefruit products, Seville oranges** should be avoided (increases concentration). **LAB VALUES:** May increase serum ALT, AST.

AVAILABILITY (Rx)

Tablets, Film-Coated: 150 mg.

ADMINISTRATION/HANDLING

PO
• Give with a fat-containing meal (e.g., eggs, butter, peanut butter, cheese pizza).

INDICATIONS/ROUTES/DOSAGE

Cystic Fibrosis
PO: ADULTS, CHILDREN 6 YRS AND OLDER: One 150-mg tablet every 12 hrs with fat-containing food. **Total daily dose:** 300 mg.

Moderate Hepatic Impairment, Concurrent Use with Moderate CYP3A4 Inhibitors (e.g., fluconazole)
PO: ADULTS, CHILDREN 6 YRS AND OLDER: 150 mg once daily.

Severe Hepatic Impairment
PO: ADULTS, CHILDREN 6 YRS AND OLDER: 150 mg once daily or less frequently.

Concurrent Use with Strong CYP3A4 Inhibitors (e.g., ketoconazole)
PO: ADULTS, CHILDREN 6 YRS AND OLDER: 150 mg twice weekly.

SIDE EFFECTS

Frequent (24%–10%): Headache, nasal congestion, abdominal discomfort, diarrhea, nausea, rash. **Occasional (6%–5%):** Rhinitis, dizziness, arthralgia, bacteria in sputum. **Rare (4% and Less):** Myalgia, wheezing, acne.

ADVERSE EFFECTS/TOXIC REACTIONS

Upper respiratory infections occurs in 22% of pts, nasopharyngitis in 15%. Increase in ALT, AST occurs in 6% of pts.

NURSING CONSIDERATIONS

BASELINE ASSESSMENT
If the pt's genotype is unknown, an FDA-cleared CF mutation test should be used to detect presence of the G551D mutation. Assess hepatic function prior to and periodically during therapy.

INTERVENTION/EVALUATION
Patients who develop increased ALT, AST levels should be closely monitored until the abnormalities resolve. Dosing should be interrupted if transaminases (ALT or AST) are greater than 5 times upper limit normal. Transaminases should be obtained every 3 mos during the first year of treatment, and annually thereafter.

PATIENT/FAMILY TEACHING
• Always take medication with fatty food. • Avoid grapefruit products and Seville oranges. • Adhere to routine laboratory testing as a part of treatment regimen. • Report headache, diarrhea, rash, signs and symptoms of respiratory infection.

ixabepilone

ix-ab-**ep**-i-lone
(Ixempra)
BLACK BOX ALERT Combination therapy with capecitabine is contraindicated in pts with AST or ALT greater than 2.5 times upper limit of normal (ULN) or bilirubin greater than 1 times ULN. Increased risk of toxicity, neutropenia-related mortality.

◆CLASSIFICATION

PHARMACOTHERAPEUTIC: Epothilone microtubule inhibitor, antimitotic agent. **CLINICAL:** Antineoplastic (see p. 87C).

ACTION

Binds directly on microtubules during active stage of G2 and M phases of cell cycle, preventing formation of microtubules, an essential part of the process of separation of chromosomes. **Therapeutic Effect:** Blocks cells in mitotic phase of cell division, leading to cell death.

PHARMACOKINETICS

Metabolized in liver. Protein binding: 77%. Excreted in feces (65%), urine (21%). **Half-life:** 52 hrs.

USES

Combination therapy with capecitabine for treatment of metastatic or locally advanced breast cancer in pts after failure of anthracycline, taxane therapy. As monotherapy, treatment of metastatic or locally advanced breast cancer in pts after failure of anthracycline, taxane, and capecitabine therapy. **OFF-LABEL:** Treatment of endometrial cancer.

PRECAUTIONS

Contraindications: Severe hypersensitivity reaction to Cremophor, baseline neutrophil count less than 1,500/mm³, platelet count less than 100,000 cells/mm³. **Combination Capecitabine Therapy:** AST or ALT greater than 2.5 times normal range, bilirubin greater than 1 times normal range. **Cautions:** Diabetes mellitus, existing moderate to severe neuropathy, history of cardiovascular disease. **Monotherapy:** AST or ALT greater than 5 times normal range, bilirubin greater than 3 times normal range.

⌛ LIFESPAN CONSIDERATIONS

Pregnancy/Lactation: May cause fetal harm. Unknown if distributed in breast milk. **Pregnancy Category D. Children:** Safety and efficacy not established. **Elderly:** Higher incidence of severe adverse reactions in those older than 65 yrs.

INTERACTIONS

DRUG: CYP3A4 inhibitors (e.g., atazanavir, clarithromycin, indinavir, itraconazole, ketoconazole, nefazodone, ritonavir, voriconazole) may increase concentration. **CYP3A4 inducers (e.g., carbamazepine, dexamethasone, phenobarbital, phenytoin, rifabutin, rifampin, rifapentin)** may decrease concentration. **HERBAL: St. John's wort** may decrease plasma concentration. **FOOD: Grapefruit, grapefruit juice** may increase plasma concentration. **LAB VALUES:** May increase serum ALT, AST, bilirubin. May decrease WBCs, Hgb, platelets.

AVAILABILITY (Rx)

Injection, Solution: Kit: 15 mg kit supplied with diluent for Ixempra, 8 ml; 45 mg supplied with diluent for Ixempra, 23.5 ml.

ADMINISTRATION/HANDLING

 IV

Reconstitution • Withdraw diluent and slowly inject into vial. • Gently swirl and invert until powder is completely dissolved. • Further dilute with 250 ml lactated Ringer's. • Solution may be stored in vial for a maximum of 1 hr at room temperature. • Final concentration for infusion must be between 0.2 mg/ml and 0.6 mg/ml. • Mix infusion bag by manual rotation.

Rate of Administration • Administer through an in-line filter of 0.2 to 1.2 microns. • Infuse over 3 hrs. Administration must be completed within 6 hrs of reconstitution.

Storage • Refrigerate kit. • Prior to reconstitution, kit should be removed from refrigerator and allowed to stand at room temperature for approximately 30 min. • When vials are initially removed from refrigerator, a white precipitate may be observed in the diluent vial. • This precipitate will dissolve to form a clear solution once diluent warms to room temperature. • Once diluted with lactated Ringer's, solution is stable at room temperature and room light for a maximum of 6 hrs.

INDICATIONS/ROUTES/DOSAGE

◄ALERT► An H₁ antagonist (diphenhydramine 50 mg PO or equivalent) and an H₂ antagonist (ranitidine 150–300 mg PO or equivalent) must be given prior to beginning treatment with ixabepilone. Those who experienced a previous hypersensitivity reaction to ixabepilone require pretreatment with corticosteroids (e.g., dexamethasone 20 mg IV, 30 min before infusion or PO, 1 hr before infusion) in addition to pretreatment with H_1 and H_2 antagonists.

Breast Cancer

IV: ADULTS, ELDERLY: 40 mg/m^2 infused over 3 hrs, every 3 wks. **Maximum:** 88 mg.

Monotherapy Dosage Adjustments for Hepatic Impairment

Mild Hepatic Impairment (AST and ALT Less Than 2.5 Times Upper Limit of Normal (ULN) and Bilirubin Less Than 1 Time ULN)

IV: ADULTS, ELDERLY: 40 mg/m^2 infused over 3 hrs, every 3 wks.

Mild Hepatic Impairment (AST and ALT Greater Than 2.5 Times ULN and Less Than 10 Times ULN and Bilirubin Greater Than 1 Time ULN and Less Than 1.5 Times ULN)

IV: ADULTS, ELDERLY: 32 mg/m^2 infused over 3 hrs, every 3 wks.

Moderate Hepatic Impairment (AST and ALT Less Than 10 Times ULN and Bilirubin Greater Than 1.5 Times ULN and Less Than 3 Times ULN)

IV Infusion: ADULTS, ELDERLY: 20–30 mg/m^2 infused over 3 hrs, every 3 wks.

Dose Modification

Dosage adjustment based on grade of neuropathy, hematologic conditions.

SIDE EFFECTS

Common (62%): Peripheral sensory neuropathy. **Frequent (56%–46%):** Fatigue, asthenia (loss of strength, energy), myalgia, arthralgia, alopecia, nausea. **Occasional (29%–11%):** Vomiting, stomatitis, mucositis, diarrhea, musculoskeletal pain, anorexia, constipation, abdominal pain, headache. **Rare (9%–5%):** Skin rash, nail disorder, edema, hand-foot syndrome (blistering/rash/peeling of skin on palms of hands, soles of feet), pyrexia, dizziness, pruritus, gastroesophageal reflux disease (GERD), hot flashes, taste disorder, insomnia.

ADVERSE EFFECTS/TOXIC REACTIONS

Neuropathy occurs early during treatment; 75% of new onset or worsening neuropathy occurred during first 3 cycles. Diabetics may be at increased risk for severe neuropathy manifested as grade 4 neutropenia. Neutropenia, leukopenia occurs commonly; anemia, thrombocytopenia occur rarely.

NURSING CONSIDERATIONS

BASELINE ASSESSMENT

Question possibility of pregnancy. Obtain baseline CBC, serum chemistries, hepatic function tests before treatment begins as baseline and monitor for hepatotoxicity, peripheral neuropathy (most frequent cause of drug discontinuation).

INTERVENTION/EVALUATION

Monitor for symptoms of neuropathy (burning sensation, hyperesthesia, hypoesthesia, paresthesia, discomfort, neuropathic pain). Assess hands and feet for erythema. Monitor CBC for evidence of neutropenia, thrombocytopenia; hepatic function tests for hepatotoxicity. Assess mouth for stomatitis, mucositis.

PATIENT/FAMILY TEACHING

• Avoid crowds, those with known infection. • Avoid contact with those who have recently received live virus vaccine. • Do not have immunizations without physician's approval (drug lowers resistance). • Promptly report fever over 100.5°F, chills, numbness, tingling, burning sensation, erythema of hands/feet.

ketoconazole

kee-toe-kon-a-zol
(Apo-Ketoconazole ✤, Extina,
Nizoral, Nizoral AD,
Novo-Ketoconazole ✤, Xolegel)

BLACK BOX ALERT Potentially fatal
hepatotoxicity has occurred. Concurrent cisapride, terfenadine, astemizole contraindicated; serious
cardiovascular events (QT prolongation, torsade de pointes, ventricular tachycardia, ventricular fibrillation, fatalities) have occurred.
**Do not confuse Nizoral with
Nasarel, Neoral, or Nitrol.**

◆CLASSIFICATION

PHARMACOTHERAPEUTIC: Imidazole
derivative. **CLINICAL:** Antifungal (see
pp. 48C, 49C).

ACTION

Inhibits synthesis of ergosterol, a vital
component of fungal cell formation.
Therapeutic Effect: Damages fungal
cell membrane, altering its function. Fungistatic.

PHARMACOKINETICS

Well absorbed from GI tract following PO
administration. Protein binding: 93%–
96%. Metabolized in liver. Primarily excreted in bile with minimal elimination in
urine. Negligible systemic absorption following topical administration. Ketoconazole
is not detected in plasma after shampooing, topical administration. **Half-life:**
8 hrs.

USES

PO: Treatment of susceptible fungal infections including histoplasmosis, blastomycosis, candidiasis, chronic mucocutaneous candidiasis, coccidioidomycosis,
paracoccidioidomycosis, chromomycosis, oral thrush, candiduria. **Shampoo:**
Treatment of dandruff. Treatment of tinea
versicolor. **Topical:** Treatment of tineas,
pityriasis versicolor, cutaneous candidiasis, seborrhea dermatitis, dandruff. **Xolegel:** Treatment of seborrheic dermatitis. **OFF-LABEL: Systemic:** Treatment of
prostate cancer.

PRECAUTIONS

Contraindications: Concurrent use with
ergot derivatives, triazolam, CNS fungal
infections. **Cautions:** Hepatic impairment.

⧗ LIFESPAN CONSIDERATIONS

Pregnancy/Lactation: Oral form distributed in breast milk. Unknown if topical form crosses placenta or is distributed in breast milk. **Pregnancy Category
C. Children: Cream, shampoo:** Safety
and efficacy not established. **Oral form:**
Safety and efficacy not established in
those younger than 2 yrs. **Elderly:** No
age-related precautions noted.

INTERACTIONS

DRUG: May increase concentration/toxicity
of **cyclosporine, digoxin, ergot alkaloids, midazolam, protease inhibitors (e.g., indinavir, ritonavir, saquinavir), sirolimus, tacrolimus,
triazolam, warfarin.** Isoniazid, rifampin may decrease concentration/
effects. **Antacids, H₂ antagonists, proton pump inhibitors (e.g., omeprazole)** may decrease absorption. **HERBAL:
St. John's wort** may decrease concentration. **FOOD:** None known. **LAB VALUES:**
May increase serum alkaline phosphatase,
bilirubin, AST, ALT. May decrease serum
corticosteroid, testosterone.

AVAILABILITY (Rx)

Foam (Extina): 2%. **Gel (Xolegel):** 2%.
Shampoo (Nizoral AD [OTC]): 1%. **Tablets
(Nizoral):** 200 mg.

ADMINISTRATION/HANDLING

PO
• Give with food to minimize GI irritation. • Tablets may be crushed. • Ketoconazole requires acidity; give antacids,
anticholinergics, H₂ blockers **at least**
2 hrs following dosing.

✤ Canadian trade name   🖤 Non-Crushable Drug   **HIGH ALERT** High Alert drug

K

Shampoo

• Apply to wet hair, massage for 1 min, rinse thoroughly, reapply for 3 min, rinse.

Topical

• Apply, rub gently into affected/surrounding area.

INDICATIONS/ROUTES/DOSAGE

Usual Dosage

PO: ADULTS, ELDERLY: 200–400 mg/day. **Maximum:** 800 mg/day in 2 divided doses. **CHILDREN 2 YRS AND OLDER:** 3.3–6.6 mg/kg/day.

Topical: ADULTS, ELDERLY: Apply to affected area 1–2 times a day for 2–4 wks.

Shampoo: ADULTS, ELDERLY: Use twice weekly for 4 wks, allowing at least 3 days between shampooing. Use intermittently to maintain control.

SIDE EFFECTS

Occasional (10%–3%): Nausea, vomiting. **Rare (less than 2%):** Abdominal pain, diarrhea, headache, dizziness, photophobia. **Topical:** Burning, irritation, pruritus.

ADVERSE EFFECTS/ TOXIC REACTIONS

Hematologic toxicity (thrombocytopenia, hemolytic anemia, leukopenia) occurs occasionally. Hepatotoxicity may occur within first wk to several mos after starting therapy. Anaphylaxis occurs rarely.

NURSING CONSIDERATIONS

BASELINE ASSESSMENT

Confirm culture or histologic test for accurate diagnosis; therapy may begin before results known. Receive full medication history and screen for contraindications.

INTERVENTION/EVALUATION

Monitor hepatic function tests; be alert for hepatotoxicity: dark urine, pale stools, jaundice, fatigue, anorexia, nausea, or vomiting (unrelieved by giving medication with food). Monitor CBC for hematologic toxicity. Monitor daily pattern of bowel activity, stool consistency. Assess for dizziness, provide assistance as needed. Evaluate skin for rash, urticaria, pruritus. **Topical:** Check for localized burning, pruritus, irritation.

PATIENT/FAMILY TEACHING

• Prolonged therapy (wks or mos) is usually necessary. • Avoid alcohol. • May cause dizziness; avoid tasks that require alertness, motor skills until response to drug is established. • Take antacids, antiulcer medications at least 2 hrs after ketoconazole. • Report dark urine, pale stool, yellow skin or eyes, vomiting, increased irritation in topical use, onset of other new symptoms. • **Topical:** Rub well into affected areas. • Avoid contact with eyes. • Keep skin clean, dry; wear light clothing for ventilation. • Separate personal items in direct contact with affected area. • **Shampoo:** Initially, use 2 times a wk for 4 wks with at least 3 days between shampooing; frequency then determined by response to medication.

ketoprofen

kee-toe-**proe**-fen
(Apo-Keto ✦)

BLACK BOX ALERT Increased risk of serious cardiovascular thrombotic events, including myocardial infarction, CVA. Increased risk of severe GI reactions, including ulceration, bleeding, perforation.

◆CLASSIFICATION

PHARMACOTHERAPEUTIC: NSAID. **CLINICAL:** Antirheumatic, analgesic, antidysmenorrheal, vascular headache suppressant (see p. 130C).

ACTION

Produces analgesic, anti-inflammatory effects by inhibiting prostaglandin synthesis. **Therapeutic Effect:** Reduces inflammatory response, intensity of pain.

PHARMACOKINETICS

Immediate-release capsules are rapidly absorbed following PO administration; extended-release capsules are well absorbed. Protein binding: 99%. Metabolized in liver. Excreted in urine; less than 10% excreted as unchanged (unconjugated) drug. **Half-life:** 2–4 hrs; extended-release: 3–7.5 hrs.

USES

Symptomatic treatment of acute and chronic rheumatoid arthritis (RA), osteoarthritis. Relief of mild to moderate pain, primary dysmenorrhea.

PRECAUTIONS

Contraindications: Perioperative pain in setting of CABG surgery, history of hypersensitivity to aspirin, NSAIDs. **Cautions:** Renal/hepatic impairment, history of GI tract disease (bleeding or ulcers), predisposition to fluid retention, asthma.

⧖ LIFESPAN CONSIDERATIONS

Pregnancy/Lactation: Crosses placenta; unknown if distributed in breast milk. Avoid during late pregnancy (ductus arteriosus). **Pregnancy Category C. (D if used in third trimester or near delivery). Children:** Safety and efficacy not established. **Elderly:** Age-related renal impairment may require dosage adjustment.

INTERACTIONS

DRUG: May decrease effects of **antihypertensives, diuretics. Aspirin, other salicylates** may increase risk of GI side effects, bleeding. May increase risk of bleeding with **heparin, oral anticoagulants, thrombolytics.** May increase concentration, risk of toxicity of **lithium, methotrexate. Probenecid** may increase concentration. **HERBAL: Cat's claw, dong quai, evening primrose, feverfew, garlic, ginkgo, ginseng, horse chestnut, red clover** may in-

crease antiplatelet activity, risk of bleeding. **FOOD:** None known. **LAB VALUES:** May prolong bleeding time. May increase serum alkaline phosphatase, AST, ALT, bilirubin. May decrease Hgb, Hct, serum sodium.

AVAILABILITY (OTC)

Capsules: 50 mg, 75 mg.

⧖ **Capsules, Extended-Release:** 200 mg.

ADMINISTRATION/HANDLING

PO
• May give with food, milk, full glass of water (minimizes potential GI distress).
• Do not break, cut extended-release capsules.

INDICATIONS/ROUTES/DOSAGE

Acute or Chronic Rheumatoid Arthritis and Osteoarthritis
PO: ADULTS: Initially, 75 mg 3 times a day or 50 mg 4 times a day. **ELDERLY:** Initially, 25–50 mg 3–4 times a day. Maintenance: 150–300 mg/day in 3–4 divided doses.
PO *(Extended-Release)*: **ADULTS, ELDERLY:** 200 mg once a day.

Mild to Moderate Pain, Dysmenorrhea
PO: ADULTS, ELDERLY: 25–50 mg q6–8h. **Maximum:** 300 mg/day.

Dosage in Renal Impairment
Mild: 150 mg/day maximum. **Severe** *(creatinine clearance less than 25 ml/min)*: 100 mg/day maximum.

SIDE EFFECTS

Frequent (11%): Dyspepsia (heartburn, indigestion, epigastric pain). **Occasional (more than 3%):** Nausea, diarrhea/constipation, flatulence, abdominal cramps, headache. **Rare (less than 2%):** Anorexia, vomiting, visual disturbances, fluid retention.

ADVERSE EFFECTS/ TOXIC REACTIONS

Peptic ulcer, GI bleeding, gastritis, severe hepatic reaction (cholestasis, jaundice) oc-

K

cur rarely. Nephrotoxicity (dysuria, hematuria, proteinuria, nephrotic syndrome), severe hypersensitivity reaction (bronchospasm, angioedema) occur rarely.

NURSING CONSIDERATIONS

BASELINE ASSESSMENT

Assess onset, type, location, duration of pain/inflammation. Inspect appearance of affected joints for immobility, deformities, skin condition.

INTERVENTION/EVALUATION

Monitor for evidence of nausea, dyspepsia. Monitor for therapeutic response: relief of pain, improved range of motion, grip strength, mobility. Monitor renal/hepatic function tests, occult blood loss, mental status.

PATIENT/FAMILY TEACHING

• Avoid aspirin, alcohol (increases risk of GI bleeding). • If GI upset occurs, take with food, milk. • Swallow capsule whole; do not crush/chew.

---

ketorolac

kee-toe-role-ak
(Acular, Acular LS, Acuvail, Apo-Ketorolac ✱, Novo-Ketorolac ✱, Sprix, <u>Toradol</u> ✱)

BLACK BOX ALERT Increased risk of serious cardiovascular thrombotic events, including myocardial infarction, CVA. Increased risk of severe GI reactions, including ulceration, bleeding, perforation.
Do not confuse Acular with Acthar or Ocular, ketorolac with Ketalar, or Toradol with Foradil, Inderal, Tegretol, or tramadol.

◆CLASSIFICATION

PHARMACOTHERAPEUTIC: NSAID.
CLINICAL: Analgesic, intraocular anti-inflammatory (see p. 130C).

ACTION

Inhibits prostaglandin synthesis, reduces prostaglandin levels in aqueous humor. **Therapeutic Effect:** Reduces intensity of pain stimulus, reduces intraocular inflammation.

PHARMACOKINETICS

Readily absorbed from GI tract after IM administration. Protein binding: 99%. Metabolized in liver. Primarily excreted in urine. Not removed by hemodialysis. **Half-life:** 2–8 hrs (increased in renal impairment, in elderly).

USES

PO, injection, nasal: Short-term (5 days or less) relief of mild to moderate pain. **Ophthalmic:** Relief of ocular itching due to seasonal allergic conjunctivitis. Treatment postop for inflammation following cataract extraction, pain following incisional refractive surgery. **OFF-LABEL:** Prevention, treatment of ocular inflammation (ophthalmic form).

PRECAUTIONS

Contraindications: Intracranial bleeding, hemorrhagic diathesis, high risk of bleeding, concomitant use of probenecid or pentoxifylline, labor and delivery, breastfeeding, advanced renal impairment, active peptic ulcer disease, chronic inflammation of GI tract, GI bleeding/ulceration, history of hypersensitivity to aspirin, NSAIDs. Perioperative pain in setting of CABG surgery. **Cautions:** Hepatic impairment, history of GI tract disease, asthma, coagulation disorders, receiving anticoagulants.

⏳ LIFESPAN CONSIDERATIONS

Pregnancy/Lactation: Unknown if distributed in breast milk. Avoid use during third trimester (may adversely affect fetal cardiovascular system: premature closure of ductus arteriosus). **Pregnancy Category C (D if used in third trimester).** **Children:** Safety and efficacy not established, but doses of 0.5 mg/kg have been used. **Elderly:** GI bleeding, ulceration more likely to cause serious adverse effects. Age-related renal impairment may increase risk of hepatic/renal toxicity; decreased dosage recommended.

INTERACTIONS

DRUG: May decrease effects of **antihypertensives, diuretics. Aspirin, NSAIDs, other salicylates** may increase risk of GI side effects, bleeding. May increase risk of bleeding with **heparin, oral anticoagulants, thrombolytics.** May increase concentration, risk of toxicity of **lithium.** May increase risk of **methotrexate** toxicity. **Probenecid** may increase concentration. **HERBAL: Cat's claw, dong quai, evening primrose, feverfew, garlic, ginkgo, ginseng, horse chestnut, red clover** may decrease antiplatelet activity, risk of bleeding. **FOOD:** None known. **LAB VALUES:** May prolong bleeding time. May increase hepatic function test results, BUN, potassium, creatinine.

AVAILABILITY (Rx)

Injection Solution (Toradol): 15 mg/ml, 30 mg/ml. **Nasal Spray (Sprix):** 1.7-g bottle provides 8 sprays (15.75 mg/spray). **Ophthalmic Solution:** 0.4% (Acular LS), 0.45% (Acuvail), 0.5% (Acular). **Tablets (Toradol):** 10 mg.

ADMINISTRATION/HANDLING

 IV

• Give undiluted as IV push. • Give over at least 15 sec.

IM
• Give deep IM slowly into large muscle mass.

PO
• Give with food, milk, antacids if GI distress occurs.

Ophthalmic
• Place gloved finger on lower eyelid and pull out until pocket is formed between eye and lower lid. Place prescribed number of drops into pocket. • Instruct pt to close eye gently for 1–2 min (so medication will not be squeezed out of the sac) and to apply digital pressure to lacrimal sac at inner canthus for 1 min to minimize system absorption.

🔲 IV INCOMPATIBILITY

Promethazine (Phenergan).

🔲 IV COMPATIBILITIES

Fentanyl (Sublimaze), hydromorphone (Dilaudid), morphine, nalbuphine (Nubain).

INDICATIONS/ROUTES/DOSAGE

Short-Term Relief of Mild to Moderate Pain (Multiple Doses)
PO: ADULTS, ELDERLY: Initially, 20 mg (10 mg for elderly), then 10 mg q4–6h. **Maximum:** 40 mg/24 hrs.
IV, IM: ADULTS YOUNGER THAN 65 YRS: 30 mg q6h. **Maximum:** 120 mg/24 hrs. **ADULTS 65 YRS AND OLDER, THOSE WITH RENAL IMPAIRMENT, THOSE WEIGHING LESS THAN 50 KG:** 15 mg q6h. **Maximum:** 60 mg/24 hrs.
Nasal Spray: ADULTS, ELDERLY YOUNGER THAN 65 YRS: 31.5 mg (1 spray each nostril) q6–8h. **Maximum daily dose:** 126 mg. **ADULTS 65 YRS AND OLDER, PTS WEIGHING LESS THAN 50 KG:** 15.75 (1 spray in one nostril) mg q6–8h. **Maximum daily dose:** 63 mg.

Short-Term Relief of Mild to Moderate Pain (Single Dose)
IV: ADULTS YOUNGER THAN 65 YRS, CHILDREN 17 YRS AND OLDER WEIGHING MORE THAN 50 KG: 30 mg. **ADULTS 65 YRS AND OLDER, WITH RENAL IMPAIRMENT, WEIGHING LESS THAN 50 KG:** 15 mg. **CHILDREN 2–16 YRS:** 0.5 mg/kg. **Maximum:** 15 mg.
IM: ADULTS YOUNGER THAN 65 YRS, CHILDREN 17 YRS AND OLDER, WEIGHING MORE THAN 50 KG: 60 mg. **ADULTS 65 YRS AND OLDER, WITH RENAL IMPAIRMENT, WEIGHING LESS THAN 50 KG:** 30 mg. **CHILDREN 2–16 YRS:** 1 mg/kg. **Maximum:** 30 mg.

K

Allergic Conjunctivitis
Ophthalmic: ADULTS, ELDERLY, CHILDREN 3 YRS AND OLDER: 1 drop 4 times a day.

Cataract Extraction
Ophthalmic: ADULTS, ELDERLY: 1 drop 4 times a day. Begin 24 hrs after surgery and continue for 2 wks.

Refractive Surgery
Ophthalmic: ADULTS, ELDERLY: 1 drop 4 times a day for 3 days.

SIDE EFFECTS

Frequent (17%–12%): Headache, nausea, abdominal cramps/pain, dyspepsia (heartburn, indigestion, epigastric pain). **Occasional (9%–3%):** Diarrhea. **Nasal:** Nasal discomfort, rhinalgia, increased lacrimation, throat irritation, rhinitis. **Ophthalmic:** Transient stinging, burning. **Rare (3%–1%):** Constipation, vomiting, flatulence, stomatitis. **Ophthalmic:** Ocular irritation, allergic reactions (manifested by pruritus, stinging), superficial ocular infection, keratitis.

ADVERSE EFFECTS/ TOXIC REACTIONS

Peptic ulcer, GI bleeding, gastritis, severe hepatic reaction (cholestasis, jaundice) occur rarely. Nephrotoxicity (glomerular nephritis, interstitial nephritis, nephrotic syndrome) may occur in pts with preexisting renal impairment. Acute hypersensitivity reaction (fever, chills, joint pain) occurs rarely.

NURSING CONSIDERATIONS

BASELINE ASSESSMENT

Assess onset, type, location, duration of pain. Obtain baseline renal/hepatic function tests.

INTERVENTION/EVALUATION

Monitor renal/hepatic function tests, urinary output. Monitor daily pattern of bowel activity, stool consistency. Observe for occult blood loss. Assess for therapeutic response: relief of pain, stiffness, swelling; increased joint mobility; reduced joint tenderness; improved grip strength. Monitor for bleeding (may also occur with ophthalmic route due to systemic absorption).

PATIENT/ FAMILY TEACHING

• Avoid aspirin, alcohol. • Report abdominal pain, bloody stools, or vomiting blood. • If GI upset occurs, take with food, milk. • **Ophthalmic:** Transient stinging, burning may occur upon instillation. • Do not administer while wearing soft contact lenses.

labetalol

la-**bay**-ta-lol
(Apo-Labetalol ♣, Normodyne ♣, Trandate)
Do not confuse labetalol with betaxolol, metoprolol or propranolol, or Trandate with tramadol or Trental.

FIXED-COMBINATION(S)

Normozide: labetalol/hydrochlorothiazide (a diuretic): 100 mg/25 mg, 200 mg/25 mg, 300 mg/25 mg.

◆CLASSIFICATION

PHARMACOTHERAPEUTIC: Alpha-, beta-adrenergic blocker. **CLINICAL:** Antihypertensive (see p. 73C).

ACTION

Blocks alpha$_1$-, beta$_1$-, beta$_2$- (large doses) adrenergic receptor sites. Large doses increase airway resistance. **Therapeutic Effect:** Slows sinus heart rate; decreases peripheral vascular resistance, cardiac output, B/P.

PHARMACOKINETICS

Route	Onset	Peak	Duration
PO	0.5–2 hrs	2–4 hrs	8–12 hrs
IV	2–5 min	5–15 min	2–4 hrs

Completely absorbed from GI tract. Protein binding: 50%. Metabolized in liver. Primarily excreted in urine. Not removed by hemodialysis. **Half-life:** 2.5–8 hrs.

USES

Management of mild to severe hypertension. May be used alone or in combination with other antihypertensives. **OFF-LABEL:** Management of preeclampsia, severe hypertension in pregnancy, hypertension during acute ischemic stroke, pediatric hypertension.

PRECAUTIONS

Contraindications: Bronchial asthma, cardiogenic shock, uncompensated HF, second- or third-degree heart block (except in pts with functioning pacemaker), severe bradycardia, conditions associated with severe, prolonged hypotension. **Cautions:** Compensated HF, severe anaphylaxis to allergens, myasthenia gravis, psychiatric disease, hepatic impairment, pheochromocytoma, diabetes mellitus; concurrent use with digoxin, verapamil, or diltiazem; arterial obstruction.

⧗ LIFESPAN CONSIDERATIONS

Pregnancy/Lactation: Drug crosses placenta. Small amount distributed in breast milk. **Pregnancy Category C (D if used in second or third trimester).** **Children:** Safety and efficacy not established. **Elderly:** Age-related peripheral vascular disease may increase susceptibility to decreased peripheral circulation.

INTERACTIONS

DRUG: May decrease effects of **beta$_2$ agonists, theophylline. Beta blockers, digoxin** may increase risk of bradycardia. **HERBAL: Ephedra, ginseng, yohimbe** may worsen hypertension. **Garlic** may increase antihypertensive effect. **Licorice** may cause water retention, increased serum sodium, decreased serum potassium. **FOOD:** None known. **LAB VALUES:** May increase serum antinuclear antibody titer (ANA), BUN, LDH, alkaline phosphatase, bilirubin, creatinine, potassium, triglycerides, lipoprotein, uric acid, AST, ALT.

AVAILABILITY (Rx)

Injection Solution (Trandate): 5 mg/ml. **Tablets (Trandate):** 100 mg, 200 mg, 300 mg.

ADMINISTRATION/HANDLING

 IV

◀ALERT▶ Pt must be in supine position for IV administration and for 3 hrs after initially receiving medication (substantial drop in B/P upon standing should be expected).
Reconstitution • For IV infusion, dilute in D$_5$W to provide concentration of 1–2 mg/ml.

♣ Canadian trade name　　🗣 Non-Crushable Drug　　**HIGH ALERT** High Alert drug

L

Rate of Administration • For IV push, give over 2–3 min at 10-min intervals. • Do not administer faster than 2 mg/min. • For IV infusion, administer at rate of 2 mg/min initially. Rate is adjusted according to B/P. • Monitor B/P immediately before and q5–10min during IV administration (maximum effect occurs within 5 min).

Storage • Store at room temperature. • After dilution, IV solution is stable for 24 hrs. • Solution appears clear, colorless to light yellow. • Discard if discolored or precipitate forms.

PO
• Give without regard to food. • Tablets may be crushed.

▦ IV INCOMPATIBILITIES

Amphotericin B complex (Abelcet, AmBisome, Amphotec), ceftaroline (Teflaro), ceftriaxone (Rocephin), furosemide (Lasix), heparin, nafcillin (Nafcil).

▦ IV COMPATIBILITIES

Amiodarone (Cordarone), calcium gluconate, dexmedetomidine (Precedex), diltiazem (Cardizem), dobutamine (Dobutrex), dopamine (Intropin), enalapril (Vasotec), fentanyl (Sublimaze), hydromorphone (Dilaudid), lidocaine, lorazepam (Ativan), magnesium sulfate, midazolam (Versed), milrinone (Primacor), morphine, nitroglycerin, norepinephrine (Levophed), potassium chloride, potassium phosphate, propofol (Diprivan).

INDICATIONS/ROUTES/DOSAGE

Hypertension
PO: ADULTS: Initially, 100 mg twice a day. Adjust in increments of 100 mg twice a day q2–3days. **Maintenance:** 100–400 mg twice a day. **Maximum:** 2.4 g/day. **ELDERLY:** Initially, 100 mg 1–2 times a day. May increase as needed. **Maintenance:** 100–200 mg twice daily. **CHILDREN:** 1–3 mg/kg/day in 2 divided doses. **Maximum:** 10–12 mg/kg/day up to 1,200 mg/day.

Severe Hypertension, Hypertensive Crisis
IV: ADULTS: Initially, 20 mg. Additional doses of 40–80 mg may be given at 10-min intervals, up to total dose of 300 mg. **IV Infusion: ADULTS:** Initially, 2 mg/min up to total dose of 300 mg. **CHILDREN:** 0.4–1 mg/kg/hr. **Maximum:** 3 mg/kg/hr.

SIDE EFFECTS

Frequent (20%–11%): Drowsiness, dizziness, excessive fatigue. **Occasional (10% or less):** Dyspnea, peripheral edema, depression, anxiety, constipation, diarrhea, nasal congestion, weakness, diminished sexual function, transient scalp tingling, insomnia, nausea, vomiting, abdominal discomfort. **Rare:** Altered taste, dry eyes, increased urination, paresthesia.

ADVERSE EFFECTS/ TOXIC REACTIONS

May precipitate, aggravate HF due to decreased myocardial stimulation. Abrupt withdrawal may precipitate myocardial ischemia, producing chest pain, diaphoresis, palpitations, headache, tremor. May mask signs, symptoms of acute hypoglycemia (tachycardia, B/P changes) in diabetic pts.

NURSING CONSIDERATIONS

BASELINE ASSESSMENT

Assess baseline renal/hepatic function tests. Assess B/P, apical pulse immediately before drug administration (if pulse is 60/min or less or systolic B/P is lower than 90 mm Hg, withhold medication, contact physician).

INTERVENTION/EVALUATION

Monitor B/P for hypotension. Assess pulse for quality, irregular rate, bradycardia. Monitor EKG for cardiac arrhythmias. Monitor daily pattern of bowel activity, stool consistency. Assist with ambulation if dizziness occurs. Assess for evidence of HF: dyspnea (particularly on exertion or lying down), night cough, peripheral edema, distended neck veins. Monitor I&O (increase in weight, decrease in urine output may indicate HF).

PATIENT/FAMILY TEACHING

• Do not discontinue drug except upon advice of physician (abrupt discontinuation may precipitate heart failure). • Rise slowly from sitting position. • Compliance with therapy regimen is essential to control hypertension, arrhythmias. • Avoid tasks that require alertness, motor skills until response to drug is established. • Report shortness of breath, excessive fatigue, weight gain, prolonged dizziness, headache. • Do not use nasal decongestants, OTC cold preparations (stimulants) without physician approval. • Limit alcohol.

lacosamide

la-**koe**-sa-myde
(Vimpat)
Do not confuse lacosamide with zonisamide.

◆ CLASSIFICATION

PHARMACOTHERAPEUTIC: Succinimide **(Schedule V). CLINICAL:** Anticonvulsant (see p. 36C).

ACTION

Selectively enhances slow inactivation of sodium channels, stabilizing hyperexcitable neuronal membranes and inhibits neuronal firing. **Therapeutic Effect:** Produces anticonvulsant effect.

PHARMACOKINETICS

Completely absorbed following PO administration. Protein binding: 15%. Peak plasma concentration: 1–4 hrs after oral dosing and is reached at the end of IV infusion. Primarily excreted in urine. Steady-state levels achieved in 3 days. Removed by hemodialysis. **Half-life:** 13 hrs.

USES

Tablets used as adjunctive therapy for treatment of partial-onset seizures in pts 17 yrs and older with epilepsy. Injection form indicated as adjunctive therapy for treatment of partial-onset seizures in pts 17 years and older with epilepsy when oral administration is temporarily not feasible.

PRECAUTIONS

Contraindications: None known. **Cautions:** Renal/hepatic impairment, cardiac conduction problems (e.g., marked first-degree AV block, second-degree or higher AV block, sick sinus syndrome without pacemaker), myocardial ischemia, HF, high risk of suicide.

⧗ LIFESPAN CONSIDERATIONS

Pregnancy/Lactation: Unknown if distributed in breast milk. **Pregnancy Category C. Children:** Safety and efficacy not established in pts younger than 17 yrs. **Elderly:** No age-related precautions noted.

INTERACTIONS

DRUG: None significant. **HERBAL:** None significant. **FOOD:** None known. **LAB VALUES:** May increase serum ALT, proteinuria.

AVAILABILITY (Rx)

Injection Solution: 10 mg/ml (20 ml).
Oral Solution: 10 mg/ml.
▧ **Tablets:** 50 mg, 100 mg, 150 mg, 200 mg.

ADMINISTRATION/HANDLING

PO

• Give without regard to meals. • Do not crush or break film-coated tablets. • Oral solution should be administered with a calibrated measuring device. • Discard any unused portion after 7 wks.

IV

• Appears as a clear, colorless solution. • Discard unused portion or if precipitate or discoloration is present. • If mixing with diluent, may be stored for 24 hrs at room temperature. Infuse over 30–60 min.

▥ IV COMPATIBILITIES

0.9% NaCl, D₅W, lactated Ringer's.

INDICATIONS/ROUTES/DOSAGE

Note: IV dose is same as oral dose.

Partial-Onset Seizures
PO: ADULTS, CHILDREN 17 YRS AND OLDER:
Initially, 50 mg twice daily (100 mg/day).
May increase by 100 mg/day at weekly
intervals, given as 2 daily divided doses
up to maintenance dose of 200–400 mg/
day, based on pt response, tolerability.
IV: ADULTS, CHILDREN 17 YRS AND OLDER:
May be given undiluted or mixed in compatible diluent and given as 30- to 60-
min infusion.

Switch from IV to PO
When switching from IV to PO form, use
same equivalent daily dosage and frequency as IV administration.

Switch from PO to IV
When switching from PO to IV form, initial total daily IV dosage should be equivalent to total daily dosage and frequency
of PO form and should be infused IV over
30–60 min.

**Severe Renal Impairment (Creatinine
Clearance 30 ml/min or Less, Pts With
End-Stage Renal Disease)**
**PO/IV: ADULTS, ELDERLY, CHILDREN 17 YRS
AND OLDER: Maximum:** 300 mg/day.
Hemodialysis: Supplement dose of up
to 50% may be given after 4-hr HD treatment.

Mild to Moderate Hepatic Impairment
**PO/IV: ADULTS, ELDERLY, CHILDREN 17 YRS
AND OLDER: Maximum:** 300 mg/day.

SIDE EFFECTS

Frequent (31%–13%): Dizziness, headache.
Occasional (11%–5%): Nausea, double vision, vomiting, fatigue, blurred vision,
ataxia (difficulty with balance, coordination, slurred speech), tremor, nystagmus
(involuntary horizontal movement of eyeball). **Rare (4%–2%):** Vertigo, diarrhea, gait

disturbances, memory impairment, depression, pruritus, injection site discomfort.

ADVERSE EFFECTS/
TOXIC REACTIONS

Increased risk of suicidal ideation, behavior. Dose-dependent prolongations in
PR interval noted. Leukopenia, anemia,
thrombocytopenia occur rarely.

NURSING CONSIDERATIONS

BASELINE ASSESSMENT
Review history of seizure disorder (intensity, frequency, duration, level of consciousness). Initiate seizure precautions.
Hepatic/renal function tests, CBC should
be performed before therapy begins and
periodically during therapy.

INTERVENTION/EVALUATION
Observe for recurrence of seizure activity. Assess for clinical improvement (decrease in intensity/frequency of seizures). Assist with ambulation if dizziness
occurs. Assess for suicidal ideation, depression, behavioral changes. Drug
should be withdrawn gradually (over a
minimum of 1 wk) to minimize potential
for increased seizure frequency.

PATIENT/FAMILY TEACHING
• Strict maintenance of drug therapy is
essential for seizure control. • Avoid
tasks that require alertness, motor skills
until response to drug is established.
• Avoid alcohol. • Report depression,
suicidal ideation, unusual behavioral
changes.

lactulose

lak-too-lohs
(Acilac ✦, Apo-Lactulose ✦,
Constulose, Enulose, Generlac,
Kristalose, Laxilose ✦)
**Do not confuse lactulose with
lactose.**

◆ **CLASSIFICATION**

PHARMACOTHERAPEUTIC: Lactose derivative. **CLINICAL:** Hyperosmotic laxative, ammonia detoxicant (see p. 126C).

ACTION

Prevents reabsorption of ammonia, producing osmotic effect. **Therapeutic Effect:** Promotes increased peristalsis, bowel evacuation; decreases serum ammonia concentration.

PHARMACOKINETICS

Poorly absorbed from GI tract. Extensively metabolized in colon. Primarily excreted in feces.

USES

Prevention, treatment of portal-systemic encephalopathy (including hepatic precoma, coma); treatment of chronic constipation.

PRECAUTIONS

Contraindications: Pts requiring a low-galactose diet. **Cautions:** Diabetes mellitus, hepatic impairment, dehydration.

⌛ LIFESPAN CONSIDERATIONS

Pregnancy/Lactation: Unknown if drug crosses placenta or is distributed in breast milk. **Pregnancy Category B. Children:** Avoid use in those younger than 6 yrs (usually unable to describe symptoms). **Elderly:** No age-related precautions noted.

INTERACTIONS

DRUG: None significant. **HERBAL:** None significant. **FOOD:** None known. **LAB VALUES:** May decrease serum potassium (GI loss).

AVAILABILITY (Rx)

Packets (Kristalose): 10 g, 20 g. **Solution, Oral (Constulose, Enulose, Generlac):** 10 g/15 ml.

ADMINISTRATION/HANDLING

PO

• Store solution at room temperature.
• Solution appears pale yellow to yellow, viscous liquid. Cloudiness, darkened solution does not indicate potency loss.
• Drink water, juice, milk with each dose (aids stool softening, increases palatability). • Mix packets with 4 oz water.

Rectal

• Lubricate anus with petroleum jelly before enema insertion. • Insert carefully (prevents damage to rectal wall) with nozzle toward navel. • Squeeze container until entire dose expelled. • Instruct pt to retain 30–60 min in divided doses. **Maximum:** 60 ml/day (40 g/day).

INDICATIONS/ROUTES/DOSAGE

Constipation

PO: ADULTS, ELDERLY: 15–30 ml (10–20 g)/day, up to 60 ml (40 g)/day. **CHILDREN:** 1–3 ml/kg/day (0.7–2 g/kg/day).

Prevention of Portal-Systemic Encephalopathy

ADULTS, ELDERLY: 30–45 ml 3–4 times/day. **CHILDREN:** 40–90 ml/day in divided doses 3–4 times a day. **INFANTS:** 2.5–10 ml/day in 3–4 divided doses. Adjust dose q1–2 days to produce 2–3 soft stools/day.

Treatment of Portal-Systemic Encephalopathy

PO: ADULTS, ELDERLY: Initially, 30–45 ml (20–30 g) every hr to induce rapid laxation. Then, 30–45 ml 3–4 times a day. Adjust dose q1–2days to produce 2–3 soft stools a day.

Rectal Administration (as Retention Enema)

200 g (300 ml) diluted with 700 ml water or NaCl via rectal balloon catheter. Retain 30–60 min q4–6h. (Transition to oral prior to stopping rectal administration.)

SIDE EFFECTS

Occasional: Abdominal cramping, flatulence, increased thirst, abdominal discomfort. **Rare:** Nausea, vomiting.

L

ADVERSE EFFECTS/ TOXIC REACTIONS

Severe diarrhea indicates overdose. Long-term use may result in laxative dependence, chronic constipation, loss of normal bowel function.

NURSING CONSIDERATIONS

INTERVENTION/EVALUATION

Encourage adequate fluid intake. Assess bowel sounds for peristalsis. Monitor daily pattern of bowel activity, stool consistency; record time of evacuation. Assess for abdominal disturbances. Monitor serum electrolytes in pts with prolonged, frequent, excessive use of medication.

PATIENT/FAMILY TEACHING

• Evacuation occurs in 24–48 hrs of initial dose. • Institute measures to promote defecation: increase fluid intake, exercise, high-fiber diet.

lamivudine

la-**miv**-yoo-deen
(Epivir, Epivir-HBV, Heptovir ✦)

BLACK BOX ALERT Serious, sometimes fatal lactic acidosis, severe hepatomegaly with steatosis (fatty liver) have occurred. Pts must be monitored for chronic hepatitis B for several months following therapy.
Do not confuse Epivir with Combivir, or lamivudine with lamotrigine.

FIXED-COMBINATION(S)

Combivir: lamivudine/zidovudine (an antiviral): 150 mg/300 mg. **Epzicom:** lamivudine/abacavir (an antiviral): 300 mg/600 mg. **Trizivir:** lamivudine/zidovudine/abacavir (an antiviral): 150 mg/300 mg/300 mg.

◆ CLASSIFICATION

PHARMACOTHERAPEUTIC: Nucleoside reverse transcriptase inhibitor. **CLINICAL:** Antiviral (see pp. 70C, 118C).

ACTION

Inhibits HIV reverse transcriptase by viral DNA chain termination. Inhibits RNA-, DNA-dependent DNA polymerase, an enzyme necessary for HIV replication. **Therapeutic Effect:** Slows HIV replication, reduces progression of HIV infection.

PHARMACOKINETICS

Rapidly, completely absorbed from GI tract. Protein binding: less than 36%. Widely distributed (crosses blood-brain barrier). Primarily excreted unchanged in urine. Not removed by hemodialysis or peritoneal dialysis. **Half-life: Children:** 2 hrs. **Adults:** 5–7 hrs.

USES

Epivir: Treatment of HIV infection in combination with at least two other antiretroviral agents. **Epivir-HBV:** Treatment of chronic hepatitis B associated with evidence of hepatitis B viral replication and active liver inflammation. **OFF-LABEL:** Prophylaxis in health care workers at risk of acquiring HIV after occupational exposure to virus. Use as part of multidrug regimen.

PRECAUTIONS

Contraindications: None known. **Cautions:** Use in children with history of pancreatitis or risk factors for developing pancreatitis. Use in combination with interferon alfa with or without ribavirin in HIV/HBV coinfected pts, renal/hepatic impairment.

⌛ LIFESPAN CONSIDERATIONS

Pregnancy/Lactation: Drug crosses placenta. Unknown if distributed in breast milk. Breastfeeding not recommended (possibility of HIV transmission). **Pregnancy Category C. Children:** Safety and efficacy not established in those younger than 3 mos. **Elderly:** Age-related renal impairment may require dosage adjustment.

INTERACTIONS

DRUG: Zalcitabine may inhibit absorption of both drugs; avoid concurrent administration. **HERBAL:** None significant.

FOOD: None known. **LAB VALUES:** May increase Hgb, neutrophil count, serum amylase, AST, ALT, bilirubin.

AVAILABILITY (Rx)

Oral Solution: 5 mg/ml (Epivir-HBV), 10 mg/ml (Epivir). **Tablets:** 100 mg (Epivir-HBV), 150 mg (Epivir), 300 mg (Epivir).

ADMINISTRATION/HANDLING

PO

• Give without regard to meals.

INDICATIONS/ROUTES/DOSAGE

HIV Infection
PO: ADULTS WEIGHING 50 KG OR MORE: 150 mg twice a day or 300 mg once a day. **ADULTS WEIGHING LESS THAN 50 KG:** 4 mg/kg twice a day (up to 150 mg/dose). **CHILDREN 4 MOS–16 YRS:** 4 mg/kg twice a day (up to 150 mg/dose). **INFANTS 1–3 MOS:** 4 mg/kg twice/day. **NEONATES YOUNGER THAN 30 DAYS:** 2 mg/kg twice/day.

Chronic Hepatitis B
PO: ADULTS: 100 mg/day. **CHILDREN 2–17 YRS:** 3 mg/kg/day. **Maximum:** 100 mg/day.

Dosage in Renal Impairment
Dosage and frequency are modified based on creatinine clearance.

Creatinine Clearance	Dosage HIV	Dosage Hepatitis B
30–49 ml/min	150 mg once a day	100 mg first dose, then 50 mg once a day
15–29 ml/min	150 mg first dose, then 100 mg once a day	100 mg first dose, then 25 mg once a day
5–14 ml/min	150 mg first dose, then 50 mg once a day	35 mg first dose, then 15 mg once a day
Less than 5 ml/min	50 mg first dose, then 25 mg once a day	35 mg first dose, then 10 mg once a day

Hemodialysis: Dosing post-HD recommended.

SIDE EFFECTS

Frequent (35%–10%): Headache, nausea, malaise, fatigue, nasal disturbances, diarrhea, cough, musculoskeletal pain, neuropathy, insomnia, anorexia, dizziness, fever, chills. **Occasional (9%–5%):** Depression, myalgia, abdominal cramps, dyspepsia, arthralgia.

ADVERSE EFFECTS/ TOXIC REACTIONS

Pancreatitis occurs in 13% of pediatric pts. Anemia, neutropenia, thrombocytopenia occur rarely. Lactic acidosis, severe hepatomegaly with steatosis have been reported.

NURSING CONSIDERATIONS

BASELINE ASSESSMENT

Establish baseline lab values, esp. renal function. Screen HIV pt for hepatitis B infection before initiating therapy.

INTERVENTION/EVALUATION

Monitor BUN, serum creatinine, amylase, lipase, ALT, AST, bilirubin. Assess for headache, nausea, cough. Monitor daily pattern of bowel activity, stool consistency. Modify diet or administer laxative as needed. Assess for dizziness, sleep pattern. If pancreatitis in children occurs, movement aggravates abdominal pain; sitting up, flexing at the waist relieves the pain.

PATIENT/FAMILY TEACHING

• Continue therapy for full length of treatment. • Doses should be evenly spaced. • Lamivudine is not a cure for HIV infection, nor does it reduce risk of transmission to others. • Avoid tasks requiring alertness, motor skills until response to drug is established. • Avoid alcohol. • Closely monitor for symptoms of pancreatitis (severe, steady abdominal pain often radiating to the back, clammy skin, hypotension; nausea/vomiting may accompany abdominal pain).

lamotrigine

la-**moe**-tri-jeen
(Apo-Lamotrigine ✚, Lamictal, Lamictal ODT, Lamictal XR, Novo-Lamotrigine ✚)

BLACK BOX ALERT Severe, potentially life-threatening skin rashes have been reported, including Stevens-Johnson syndrome. Risk increased with coadministration with valproic acid and rapid-dose titration.

Do not confuse Lamictal with Lamisil or Lomotil, or lamotrigine with labetalol or lamivudine.

◆CLASSIFICATION

PHARMACOTHERAPEUTIC: Phenyltriazine. **CLINICAL:** Anticonvulsant (see p. 36C).

ACTION

May block voltage-sensitive sodium channels, stabilizing neuronal membranes, regulating presynaptic transmitter release of excitatory amino acids. **Therapeutic Effect:** Produces anticonvulsant activity. Delays time to occurrence of acute mood episodes (mania, depression, hypomania).

USES

Adjunctive therapy in adults and children with generalized tonic-clonic seizures and partial seizures, treatment of adults and children with generalized seizures of Lennox-Gastaut syndrome. Conversion to monotherapy in adults treated with another enzyme-inducing antiepileptic drug (EIAED) (e.g., valproic acid, carbamazepine, phenytoin, phenobarbital, primidone). Long-term maintenance treatment of bipolar disorder. Treatment of pts 2 yrs and older with primary generalized tonic-clonic seizures. **Extended-release:** Adjunctive therapy for primary generalized tonic-clonic and partial onset seizures in pts 13 yrs and older. Conversion to monotherapy in pt 13 yrs and older with partial seizures receiving treatment with a single antiepileptic drug (AED).

PRECAUTIONS

Contraindications: None known. **Cautions:** Renal, hepatic, cardiac impairment, pts at high risk of suicide, pts taking estrogen-containing oral contraceptives.

⧗ LIFESPAN CONSIDERATIONS

Pregnancy/Lactation: Distributed in breast milk. Breastfeeding not recommended. Increased fetal risk of oral cleft formation has been noted with use during pregnancy. **Pregnancy Category C.** **Children:** Safety and efficacy in those 18 yrs and younger with bipolar disorder, younger than 13 yrs with epilepsy not established. **Elderly:** Age-related renal impairment may require dosage adjustment.

INTERACTIONS

DRUG: Carbamazepine, phenobarbital, primidone, phenytoin, rifampin may decrease concentration. **Valproic acid** may increase concentration/effects. **Oral contraceptives** may decrease concentration. **HERBAL: Evening primrose** may decrease seizure threshold. **FOOD:** None known. **LAB VALUES:** None significant.

AVAILABILITY (Rx)

Tablets: 25 mg, 100 mg, 150 mg, 200 mg.
Tablets (Chewable): 2 mg, 5 mg, 25 mg.
Tablets (Orally Disintegrating): 25 mg, 50 mg, 100 mg, 200 mg.
 Tablets (Extended-Release): 25 mg, 50 mg, 100 mg, 200 mg, 250 mg, 300 mg.

ADMINISTRATION/HANDLING
PO

• Give without regard to food. • Chewable tablets may be dispensed in water or diluted fruit juice, or swallowed whole.

• Extended-release tablets must be swallowed whole; do not break, cut, crush, or divide. • Place orally disintegrating tablet on tongue, allow to dissolve. Pt must not break, cut, or chew. Can be swallowed without regard to food or water.

INDICATIONS/ROUTES/DOSAGE

Lennox-Gastaut, Primary Generalized Tonic-Clonic Seizures, Partial Seizures
PO: ADULTS, ELDERLY, CHILDREN OLDER THAN 12 YRS: Initially, 25 mg/day for 2 wks, then increase to 50 mg/day for 2 wks. After 4 wks, may increase by 50 mg/day at 1- to 2-wk intervals. **Maintenance:** 225–375 mg/day in 2 divided doses. **CHILDREN 2–12 YRS:** Initially, 0.3 mg/kg/day in 1–2 divided doses for 2 wks, then increase to 0.6 mg/kg/day in 1–2 divided doses for 2 wks. After 4 wks, may increase by 0.6 mg/kg/day at 1- to 2-wk intervals. **Maintenance:** 4.5–7.5 mg/kg/day in 2 divided doses. **Maximum:** 300 mg/day in 2 divided doses.

Adjusted Dosage with Antiepileptic Drugs Containing Valproic Acid
PO: ADULTS, ELDERLY, CHILDREN OLDER THAN 12 YRS: Initially, 25 mg every other day for 2 wks, then increase to 25 mg/day for 2 wks. After 4 wks, may increase by 25–50 mg/day at 1- to 2-wk intervals. **Maintenance:** 100–400 mg/day in 2 divided doses (100–200 mg/day when taking lamotrigine with valproic acid alone). **CHILDREN 2–12 YRS:** Initially, 0.15 mg/kg/day in 1–2 divided doses for 2 wks, then increase to 0.3 mg/kg/day in 1–2 divided doses for 2 wks. After 4 wks, may increase by 0.3 mg/kg/day at 1- to 2-wk intervals. **Maintenance:** 1–5 mg/kg/day in 2 divided doses. **Maximum:** 200 mg/day in 2 divided doses.

Adjusted Dosage with EIAED without Valproic Acid
PO: ADULTS, ELDERLY, CHILDREN OLDER THAN 12 YRS: Initially, 50 mg/day for 2 wks, then increase to 100 mg/day in 2 divided doses for 2 wks. After 4 wks, may increase by 100 mg/day at 1- to 2-wk intervals. **Maintenance:** 300–500 mg/day in 2 divided doses. **CHILDREN 2–12 YRS:** Initially, 0.6 mg/kg/day in 1–2 divided doses for 2 wks, then increase to 1.2 mg/kg/day in 1–2 divided doses for 2 wks. After 4 wks, may increase by 1.2 mg/kg/day at 1- to 2-wk intervals. **Maintenance:** 5–15 mg/kg/day in 2 divided doses. **Maximum:** 400 mg/day in 2 divided doses.

Usual Maintenance Range for Extended-Release Tablets
PT TAKING VALPROIC ACID: 200–250 mg once daily. **PT TAKING EIAED WITHOUT VALPROIC ADIC:** 400–600 mg once daily. **PT NOT TAKING EIAED:** 300–400 mg once daily.

Conversion to Monotherapy for Pts Receiving EIAEDs
PO: ADULTS, ELDERLY, CHILDREN 16 YRS AND OLDER: 500 mg/day in 2 divided doses. Titrate to desired dose while maintaining EIAED at fixed level, then withdraw EIAED by 20% each wk over a 4-wk period.

Conversion to Monotherapy for Pts Receiving Valproic Acid
PO: ADULTS, ELDERLY, CHILDREN 16 YRS AND OLDER: Titrate lamotrigine to 200 mg/day, maintaining valproic acid dose. Maintain lamotrigine dose and decrease valproic acid to 500 mg/day, no greater than 500 mg/day/wk, then maintain 500 mg/day for 1 wk. Increase lamotrigine to 300 mg/day and decrease valproic acid to 250 mg/day. Maintain for 1 wk, then discontinue valproic acid and increase lamotrigine by 100 mg/day each wk until maintenance dose of 500 mg/day reached.

Bipolar Disorder
PO: ADULTS, ELDERLY: Initially, 25 mg/day for 2 wks, then 50 mg/day for 2 wks, then 100 mg/day for 1 wk, then 200 mg/day beginning with wk 6.

Bipolar Disorder in Pts Receiving EIAEDs
PO: ADULTS, ELDERLY: 50 mg/day for 2 wks, then 100 mg/day for 2 wks, then

L

200 mg/day for 1 wk, then 300 mg/day for 1 wk, then up to usual maintenance dose 400 mg/day in divided doses.

Bipolar Disorder in Pts Receiving Valproic Acid
PO: ADULTS, ELDERLY: 25 mg/day every other day for 2 wks, then 25 mg/day for 2 wks, then 50 mg/day for 1 wk, then 100 mg/day. Usual maintenance dose with valproic acid: 100 mg/day.

Usual Dosage for Lamictal XR
Adjunct Therapy: Range: 200–600 mg/day.
Conversion to Monotherapy: Range: 250–500 mg/day.

Discontinuation Therapy
◀ALERT▶ A dosage reduction of approximately 50% per wk over at least 2 wks is recommended.

Dosage in Renal Impairment
◀ALERT▶ Decreased dosage may be effective in pts with significant renal impairment.

Dosage in Hepatic Impairment
Moderate to severe without ascites: Reduce dose by 25%. **Severe with ascites:** Reduce dose by 50%.

SIDE EFFECTS

Frequent (38%–14%): Dizziness, headache, diplopia (double vision), ataxia, nausea, blurred vision, drowsiness, rhinitis. **Occasional (10%–5%):** Rash, pharyngitis, vomiting, cough, flu-like symptoms, diarrhea, dysmenorrhea, fever, insomnia, dyspepsia. **Rare:** Constipation, tremor, anxiety, pruritus, vaginitis, hypersensitivity reaction.

ADVERSE EFFECTS/ TOXIC REACTIONS

Abrupt withdrawal may increase seizure frequency. Serious rashes, including Stevens-Johnson syndrome, have been reported.

NURSING CONSIDERATIONS

BASELINE ASSESSMENT
Review history of seizure disorder (type, onset, intensity, frequency, duration, LOC), medication history (esp. other anticonvulsants), other medical conditions (e.g., renal impairment). Provide safety precautions; quiet, dark environment. Assess baseline mood, behavior.

INTERVENTION/EVALUATION
Report occurrence of rash (drug discontinuation may be necessary). Assist with ambulation if dizziness, ataxia occurs. Assess for clinical improvement (decreased intensity/frequency of seizures). Assess for visual abnormalities, headache. Monitor for suicidal ideation, depression, behavioral changes.

PATIENT/ FAMILY TEACHING
• Take medication only as prescribed; do not abruptly discontinue medication after long-term therapy. • Avoid alcohol. • Avoid tasks that require alertness, motor skills until response to drug is established. • Carry identification card/bracelet to note anticonvulsant therapy. • Strict maintenance of drug therapy is essential for seizure control. • Report any rash, fever, swelling of glands, worsening depression, suicidal ideation, unusual changes in behavior, worsening of seizure control. • May cause photosensitivity reaction; avoid exposure to sunlight, artificial light.

lansoprazole   TOP 200

lan-**soe**-pra-zol
(Apo-Lansoprazole ✤, First Lansoprazole, <u>Prevacid</u>, Prevacid Solu-Tab, Prevacid 24HR)
Do not confuse lansoprazole with aripiprazole or dexlansoprazole, or Prevacid with Pravachol, Prilosec, or Prinivil.

FIXED-COMBINATION(S)

Prevacid NapraPac: lansoprazole/naproxen (an NSAID): 15 mg/375 mg, 15 mg/500 mg. **Prevpac:** Combination card containing amoxicillin 500 mg (4 capsules), lansoprazole 30 mg (2 capsules), clarithromycin 500 mg (2 tablets).

◆CLASSIFICATION

CLINICAL: Proton pump inhibitor (see p. 147C).

ACTION

Selectively inhibits gastric parietal cell membrane enzyme system (hydrogen-potassium adenosine triphosphatase, proton pump). **Therapeutic Effect:** Suppresses gastric acid secretion.

PHARMACOKINETICS

Rapid, complete absorption (food may decrease absorption) once drug has left stomach. Protein binding: 97%. Distributed primarily to gastric parietal cells. Metabolized in liver. Eliminated in bile and urine. Not removed by hemodialysis. **Half-life:** 1.5 hrs (increased in hepatic impairment, elderly).

USES

Short-term treatment (4 wks and less) of healing, symptomatic relief of active duodenal ulcer; short-term treatment (8 wks and less) for healing, symptomatic relief of erosive esophagitis. Long-term treatment of pathologic hypersecretory conditions, including Zollinger-Ellison syndrome. Short-term treatment (8 wks and less) of active benign gastric ulcer, *H. pylori*–associated duodenal ulcer (part of multidrug regimen), maintenance treatment for healed duodenal ulcer. Treatment of gastroesophageal reflux disease (GERD), NSAID-associated gastric ulcer. **OTC:** Relief of frequent heartburn (2 or more days/wk). **IV:** Short-term treatment of erosive esophagitis.

PRECAUTIONS

Contraindications: None known. **Cautions:** Hepatic impairment. May increase risk of hip, wrist, spine fractures; GI infections.

⌛ LIFESPAN CONSIDERATIONS

Pregnancy/Lactation: Unknown if distributed in breast milk. **Pregnancy Category B. Children:** Safety and efficacy not established. **Elderly:** No age-related precautions noted but doses greater than 30 mg not recommended.

INTERACTIONS

DRUG: May decrease concentration of **atazanavir.** May interfere with absorption of **ampicillin, digoxin, iron salts, ketoconazole. Sucralfate** may delay absorption. May increase effect of **warfarin.** May decrease effect of **clopidogrel. HERBAL: St. John's wort** may decrease concentration/effects. **FOOD: Food** may decrease absorption. **LAB VALUES:** May increase LDH, serum alkaline phosphatase, bilirubin, cholesterol, creatinine, AST, ALT, triglycerides, uric acid, Hgb, Hct. May produce abnormal albumin/globulin ratio, electrolyte balance, platelet, RBC, WBC count.

AVAILABILITY (Rx)

Tablets, Orally Disintegrating (Prevacid Solu-Tab): 15 mg, 30 mg. **Powder for Oral Suspension (First Lansoprazole):** 3 mg/ml.

🐍 **Capsules (Delayed-Release): (Prevacid):** 15 mg, 30 mg. **(Prevacid 24HR):** 15 mg.

ADMINISTRATION/HANDLING

PO
• Give while fasting or before meals (food diminishes absorption). • Do not cut/crush delayed-release capsules. • If pt has difficulty swallowing capsules, open capsules, sprinkle granules on 1 tbsp of applesauce, give immediately.

PO (Solu-Tab)
• Place tablet on tongue; allow to dissolve, then swallow. • May give via oral syringe

L

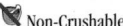

or nasogastric tube. • May dissolve in 4 ml (15 mg) or 10 ml (30 mg) water.

INDICATIONS/ROUTES/DOSAGE

Duodenal Ulcer
PO: ADULTS, ELDERLY: 15 mg/day, before morning meal for up to 4 wks. Maintenance: 15 mg/day.

Erosive Esophagitis
PO: ADULTS, ELDERLY: 30 mg/day, before morning meal for up to 8 wks. If healing does not occur within 8 wks (in 5%–10% of cases), may give for additional 8 wks. Maintenance: 15 mg/day. **CHILDREN 1–11 YRS, WEIGHING GREATER THAN 30 KG:** 30 mg/day; **WEIGHING 30 KG OR LESS:** 15 mg/day.

Gastric Ulcer
PO: ADULTS: 30 mg/day for up to 8 wks.

NSAID Gastric Ulcer
PO: ADULTS, ELDERLY: (Healing): 30 mg/day for up to 8 wks. (Prevention): 15 mg/day for up to 12 wks.

Gastroesophageal Reflux Disease (GERD)
PO: ADULTS: 15 mg/day for up to 8 wks. **CHILDREN 12–17 YRS:** 30 mg/day up to 8 wks. **CHILDREN 1–11 YRS, WEIGHING GREATER THAN 30 KG:** 30 mg/day; **WEIGHING 30 KG OR LESS:** 15 mg/day.

H. Pylori Infection
PO: ADULTS, ELDERLY: (triple drug therapy including amoxicillin, clarithromycin) 30 mg q12h for 10–14 days.

Pathologic Hypersecretory Conditions (Including Zollinger-Ellison Syndrome)
PO: ADULTS, ELDERLY: 60 mg/day. Individualize dosage according to pt needs and for as long as clinically indicated. Administer up to 120 mg/day in divided doses.

Heartburn (OTC)
PO: ADULTS, ELDERLY: 15 mg once daily for 14 days. May repeat q4mos.

SIDE EFFECTS

Occasional (3%–2%): Diarrhea, abdominal pain, rash, pruritus, altered appetite. **Rare (1%):** Nausea, headache.

ADVERSE EFFECTS/ TOXIC REACTIONS

Bilirubinemia, eosinophilia, hyperlipemia occur rarely.

NURSING CONSIDERATIONS

BASELINE ASSESSMENT
Obtain baseline lab values. Assess for epigastric/abdominal pain, evidence of GI bleeding, ecchymosis.

INTERVENTION/EVALUATION
Monitor CBC, hepatic/renal function tests. Assess for therapeutic response (relief of GI symptoms). Question if diarrhea, abdominal pain, nausea occurs.

PATIENT/ FAMILY TEACHING
• Do not chew, crush delayed-release capsules. • For pts who have difficulty swallowing capsules, open capsules, sprinkle granules on 1 tbsp of applesauce, swallow immediately.

lanthanum

lan-tha-num
(Fosrenol)
Do not confuse lanthanum with lithium.

◆CLASSIFICATION

PHARMACOTHERAPEUTIC: Detoxifying agent. **CLINICAL:** Phosphate regulator.

ACTION

Dissociates in acidic environment of upper GI tract to lanthanum ions that bind to dietary phosphate released from food during digestion, forming highly insoluble lanthanum phosphate complexes. **Therapeutic Effect:** Reduces phosphate absorption.

PHARMACOKINETICS

Very low absorption following PO administration. Protein binding: greater than 99%. Not metabolized. Phosphate complexes are eliminated in urine. **Half-life:** 53 hrs (in plasma); 2–3.6 yrs (from bone).

USES

Hyperphosphatemia. Reduces serum phosphate levels in pts with end-stage renal disease. Renal failure (GFR less than 15 ml/min).

PRECAUTIONS

Contraindications: None known. **Cautions:** Acute peptic ulcer disease, ulcerative colitis, Crohn's disease, bowel obstruction.

⊠ LIFESPAN CONSIDERATIONS

Pregnancy/Lactation: Unknown if drug crosses placenta or is distributed in breast milk. Breastfeeding not recommended. **Pregnancy Category C. Children:** Safety and efficacy not established; not recommended for children. **Elderly:** No age-related precautions noted.

INTERACTIONS

DRUG: May decrease concentrations of **captopril, simvastatin, antacids, levothyroxine, oral quinolones;** separate antacid administration by 2 hrs. Administer oral quinolones 1 hr before or 4 hrs after lanthanum. **HERBAL:** None significant. **FOOD:** None known. **LAB VALUES:** None known.

AVAILABILITY (Rx)

Tablets, Chewable: 500 mg, 750 mg, 1 g.

ADMINISTRATION/HANDLING

PO
• Tablets should be chewed thoroughly before swallowing. • Give during or immediately after meals.

INDICATIONS/ROUTES/DOSAGE

Phosphate Control/Hyperphosphatemia
PO: ADULTS, ELDERLY: 750 mg–1,500 mg in divided doses, taken with or immediately after a meal. Dose can be titrated at 2- to 3-wk intervals in 750-mg increments, based on serum phosphate levels. Usual dosage range: 1,500–3,000 mg/day.

SIDE EFFECTS

Frequent (11%–5%): Nausea, vomiting, dialysis graft occlusion, abdominal pain. Nausea, vomiting decrease over time.

ADVERSE EFFECTS/ TOXIC REACTIONS

None known.

NURSING CONSIDERATIONS

BASELINE ASSESSMENT
Obtain baseline serum phosphate level.

INTERVENTION/EVALUATION
Monitor serum phosphate (target concentration is less than 6 mg/dl).

PATIENT/FAMILY TEACHING
• Take with or immediately after a meal.
• Do not take lanthanum within 2 hrs of antacids. • Nausea, vomiting usually diminish over time.

---

lapatinib

la-**pa**-tin-ib
(Tykerb)

BLACK BOX ALERT Hepatotoxicity, possibly severe, has occurred.
Do not confuse lapatinib with dasatinib, erlotinib, or imatinib.

◆ CLASSIFICATION

PHARMACOTHERAPEUTIC: Tyrosine kinase inhibitor. **CLINICAL:** Antineoplastic (see p. 87C).

ACTION

Inhibitory action against kinases targeting intracellular components of epidermal growth factor receptor ErbB1 and a second receptor, human epidermal receptor (HER2 [ErbB2]). **Therapeutic**

✦ Canadian trade name   🦅 Non-Crushable Drug   🔲 High Alert drug

Effect: Inhibits ErbB-driven tumor cell growth, produces tumor regression, inhibits metastasis.

PHARMACOKINETICS

Route	Onset	Peak	Duration
PO	30 min	4 hrs	—

Steady-state level occurs within 6–7 days. Incomplete and variable oral absorption. Undergoes extensive metabolism. Protein binding: 99%. Minimally excreted in feces and plasma. **Half-life:** 24 hrs.

USES

Combination treatment with capecitabine for advanced or metastatic breast cancer in pts who have received prior therapy including an anthracycline, a taxane, and trastuzumab. Combination treatment with letrozole for treatment of postmenopausal women with hormone receptor-positive metastatic breast cancer for whom hormonal therapy is indicated. **OFF-LABEL:** Treatment (in combination with trastuzumab) of HER2-overexpressing metastatic breast cancer that progressed on prior trastuzumab-containing therapy.

PRECAUTIONS

Contraindications: None known. **Cautions:** Left ventricular function abnormalities, prolonged QT interval or medications known to prolong QT interval, hepatic impairment. Avoid concurrent use with strong CYP3A4 inhibitors or inducers.

⌛ LIFESPAN CONSIDERATIONS

Pregnancy/Lactation: May cause fetal harm. Unknown if distributed in breast milk. **Pregnancy Category D. Children:** Safety and efficacy not established. **Elderly:** No age-related precautions noted.

INTERACTIONS

DRUG: May increase **digoxin** levels. **CYP3A4 inhibitors (e.g., clarithromycin, indinavir, itraconazole, ketoconazole, nefazodone, ritonavir, saquinavir)** may increase plasma concentration. **CYP3A4 inducers (e.g.,** **carbamazepine, dexamethasone, phenobarbital, phenytoin, rifampin)** may decrease plasma concentration. **HERBAL:** St. John's **wort** decreases plasma concentration. **FOOD:** **Grapefruit products** may increase plasma concentration (potential for torsades, myelotoxicity). **LAB VALUES:** May increase serum ALT, AST, bilirubin. May decrease neutrophils, Hgb, platelets.

AVAILABILITY (Rx)

▼ **Tablets:** 250 mg.

ADMINISTRATION/HANDLING

PO
• Do not break, chew, crush, or divide film-coated tablets. • Give at least 1 hr before or 1 hr after food.

INDICATIONS/ROUTES/DOSAGE

Breast Cancer
PO: ADULTS, ELDERLY: (With capecitabine): 1,250 mg (5 tablets) once daily. **(With letrozole):** 1,500 mg once daily continuously with letrozole.

Dose Modification
PO: ADULTS, ELDERLY: (Cardiac toxicity): Discontinue with decreased left ventricular ejection fraction grade 2 or higher, or in pts with an ejection fraction that drops to lower limit of normal. May be started at a reduced dose (1,000 mg/day) at a minimum of 2 wks when ejection fraction returns to normal and pt is asymptomatic. **(Pulmonary toxicity):** Discontinue with symptoms indicative of interstitial lung disease or pneumonitis grade 3 or higher. **(Severe hepatic impairment): (with capecitabine):** 750 mg/day. **(With letrozole):** 1,000 mg/day. **(CYP3A4 inhibitors/inducers):** Concomitant CYP3A4 inhibitors may require dose reduction of lapatinib; CYP3A4 inducers may require dose increase of lapatinib.

SIDE EFFECTS

Common (65%–44%): Diarrhea, hand-foot syndrome (blistering/rash/peeling of skin on palms of hands, soles of feet), nausea. **Frequent (28%–26%):** Rash, vomiting. **Occasional (15%–10%):** Mucosal inflammation, stomatitis, extremity pain, back pain, dry skin, insomnia.

ADVERSE EFFECTS/ TOXIC REACTIONS

Decreases in left ventricular ejection grade 3 or higher have been observed; 20% decrease relative to baseline is considered toxic.

NURSING CONSIDERATIONS

BASELINE ASSESSMENT

Question for possibility of pregnancy. Obtain baseline CBC, serum chemistries before treatment begins and monthly thereafter.

INTERVENTION/EVALUATION

Offer antiemetics to control nausea, vomiting. Monitor daily pattern of bowel activity, stool consistency. Monitor CBC (particularly Hgb, platelets, neutrophil count), hepatic function tests. Assess hands and feet for erythema/blistering/ peeling. Monitor for shortness of breath, palpitations, fatigue (decreased cardiac ejection fraction).

PATIENT/FAMILY TEACHING

• Avoid crowds, those with known infection. • Avoid contact with those who recently received live virus vaccine. • Do not have immunizations without physician's approval (drug lowers resistance). • Promptly report fever, unusual bruising/bleeding from any site. • Assure use of appropriate birth control measures in women.

leflunomide

lee-**floo**-noe-mide
(Apo-Leflunomide ✤, Arava, Novo-Leflunomide ✤)
BLACK BOX ALERT Do not use during pregnancy (Pregnancy Category X). Women of childbearing potential must be counseled regarding fetal risk, use of reliable contraceptives confirmed, possibility of pregnancy excluded. Severe hepatic injury may occur.

◆CLASSIFICATION

PHARMACOTHERAPEUTIC: Immunomodulatory agent. **CLINICAL:** Antiinflammatory.

ACTION

Inhibits dihydroorotate dehydrogenase, the enzyme involved in autoimmune process that leads to rheumatoid arthritis (RA). **Therapeutic Effect:** Reduces signs/symptoms of RA, retards structural damage.

PHARMACOKINETICS

Well absorbed after PO administration. Protein binding: greater than 99%. Metabolized in GI wall, liver. Excreted through renal, biliary systems. Not removed by hemodialysis. **Half-life:** 16 days.

USES

Treatment of active rheumatoid arthritis (RA). Improve physical function in pts with rheumatoid arthritis. **OFF-LABEL:** Treatment of cytomegalovirus (CMV) disease. Prevention of acute/chronic rejection in recipients of solid organ transplants.

PRECAUTIONS

Contraindications: Pregnancy or plans for pregnancy. **Cautions:** Hepatic/renal impairment, positive hepatitis B or C serology, those with immunodeficiency or bone marrow dysplasias, breast-feeding mothers, history of new/recurrent infections, significant hematologic abnormalities, diabetes.

⌛ LIFESPAN CONSIDERATIONS

Pregnancy/Lactation: Can cause fetal harm. Unknown if distributed in breast milk. Breastfeeding not recommended. **Pregnancy Category X. Children:** Safety and efficacy not established in those younger than 18 yrs. **Elderly:** No age-related precautions noted.

INTERACTIONS

DRUG: Rifampin may increase concentration/effects. **Hepatotoxic medications** may increase risk of side effects, hepatotoxicity. Use of **live virus vaccine** not recommended. **HERBAL: Echinacea** may decrease effect. **FOOD:** None known. **LAB VALUES:** May increase serum AST, ALT, alkaline phosphatase, bilirubin.

AVAILABILITY (Rx)

Tablets: 10 mg, 20 mg.

ADMINISTRATION/HANDLING

PO

• Give without regard to food.

INDICATIONS/ROUTES/DOSAGE

Rheumatoid Arthritis (RA)
PO: ADULTS, ELDERLY: Initially, 100 mg/day for 3 days, then 10–20 mg/day. (Loading dose may be omitted in pts at increased risk of hepatitis or toxicity.)

Dosage Adjustment in Hepatic Toxicity
ALT 2–3 Times Upper Limit of Normal (ULN): Not recommended. **Persistent ALT Level Greater Than 3 Times ULN:** Discontinue and initiate cholestyramine (8 g 3 times/day for 1–3 days) or activated charcoal (50 g q6h for 24 hrs) to accelerate elimination.

SIDE EFFECTS

Frequent (20%–10%): Diarrhea, respiratory tract infection, alopecia, rash, nausea.

ADVERSE EFFECTS/TOXIC REACTIONS

May cause immunosuppression. Transient thrombocytopenia, leukopenia, hepatotoxicity occur rarely.

NURSING CONSIDERATIONS

BASELINE ASSESSMENT
Question for possibility of pregnancy (Pregnancy Category X). Obtain baseline CBC, hepatic function tests. Assess limitations in activities of daily living due to rheumatoid arthritis (RA).

INTERVENTION/EVALUATION
Monitor tolerance to medication. Assess symptomatic relief of RA (relief of pain; improved range of motion, grip strength, mobility). Monitor hepatic function tests.

PATIENT/FAMILY TEACHING
• May take without regard to food.
• Improvement may take longer than 8 wks. • Avoid pregnancy (Pregnancy Category X).

lenalidomide

len-a-**lid**-o-mide
(Revlimid)

BLACK BOX ALERT Pregnancy Category X. Analogue to thalidomide. High potential for significant birth defects. Hematologic toxicity (thrombocytopenia, neutropenia) occurs in 80% of pts. Greatly increases risk for DVT, pulmonary embolism in multiple myeloma pts. **Do not confuse lenalidomide with thalidomide.**

◆CLASSIFICATION

PHARMACOTHERAPEUTIC: Isoxazole immunomodulator. **CLINICAL:** Immunosuppressive agent.

ACTION

Inhibits secretion of pro-inflammatory cytokines, increases secretion of anti-inflammatory cytokines. **Therapeutic Effect:** Prevents growth of B-cell lymphoma cell line, myeloblastic cell line.

PHARMACOKINETICS

Well absorbed following PO administration. Protein binding: 30%. Eliminated in urine. **Half-life:** 3 hrs (increased in renal impairment).

USES

Treatment of low- to intermediate-risk myelodysplastic syndrome (MDS) in pts with deletion 5q cytogenetic abnormality with

---

underlined – top prescribed drug

transfusion-dependent anemia. Treatment of multiple myeloma (in combination with dexamethasone). Treatment of relapsed or refractory mantle cell lymphoma. **OFF-LABEL:** Systemic amyloidosis, lower-risk myelodysplastic syndrome, non-Hodgkin's lymphoma, maintenance treatment for multiple myeloma (following autologous stem cell transplant).

PRECAUTIONS

Contraindications: Pregnancy (**Pregnancy Category X**), women capable of becoming pregnant. **Cautions:** Renal impairment.

⌛ LIFESPAN CONSIDERATIONS

Pregnancy/Lactation: Contraindicated in women who are or may become pregnant, who are not using two reliable forms of contraception, or who are not abstinent. Can cause severe birth defects, fetal death. Unknown if distributed in breast milk; breastfeeding not recommended. **Pregnancy Category X. Children:** Safety and efficacy not established in those younger than 18 yrs. **Elderly:** Age-related renal impairment may require caution in dosage selection. Risk of toxic reactions greater in those with renal insufficiency.

INTERACTIONS

DRUG: Erythropoietin, dexamethasone, oral contraceptives may increase risk of deep vein thrombosis, pulmonary embolism. May increase concentration of digoxin. **HERBAL:** Avoid **echinacea** (has immunostimulant properties). **FOOD:** None known. **LAB VALUES:** May decrease WBC count, Hgb, Hct platelets, troponin I, serum creatinine, sodium, T_3, T_4. May decrease serum bilirubin, glucose, potassium, magnesium.

AVAILABILITY (Rx)

💊 **Capsules:** 2.5 mg, 5 mg, 10 mg, 15 mg, 25 mg.

ADMINISTRATION/HANDLING

• Store at room temperature. • Do not break, chew, crush, or divide capsules. • Swallow whole with water.

INDICATIONS/ROUTES/DOSAGE

Myelodysplastic Syndrome
PO: ADULTS, ELDERLY: 10 mg once daily.

Dosage Adjustments for Myelodysplastic Syndrome
Platelets:
Thrombocytopenia within 4 wks with 10 mg/day
Baseline platelets 100,000/mm³ or greater: Platelets less than 50,000/mm³, hold treatment. Resume at 5 mg/day when platelets return to 50,000/mm³ or greater.
Baseline platelets less than 100,000/mm³: Platelets fall to 50% of baseline, hold treatment. Resume at 5 mg/day if baseline is 60,000/mm³ or greater and platelets return to 50,000/mm³ or greater. Resume at 5 mg/day if baseline is less than 60,000/mm³ and platelets return to 30,000/mm³ or greater.
Thrombocytopenia after 4 wks with 10 mg/day: Platelets less than 30,000/mm³ OR less than 50,000/mm³ with platelet transfusion, hold treatment. Resume at 5 mg/day when platelets return to 30,000/mm³ or greater.
Thrombocytopenia developing with 5 mg/day: Platelets less than 30,000/mm³ OR less than 50,000/mm³ with platelet transfusion, hold treatment. Resume at 5 mg every other day when platelets return to 30,000/mm³ or greater.

Neutrophils:
Neutropenia within 4 wks with 10 mg/day
Baseline absolute neutrophil count (ANC) 1,000/mcl or greater: ANC less than 750/mm³, hold treatment. Resume at 5 mg/day when ANC 1,000/mm³ or greater. **Baseline ANC less than 1,000/mm³:** ANC less than 500/mm³, hold treatment. Resume at 5 mg/day when ANC 500/mm³ or greater.
Neutropenia after 4 wks with 10 mg/day: ANC less than 500/mm³ for 7 days or longer or associated with fever, hold treatment. Resume at 5 mg/day when ANC 500/mm³ or greater.

L

Neutropenia developing with 5 mg/day: ANC less than 500/mm^3 for 7 days or longer or associated with fever, hold treatment. Resume at 5 mg every other day when ANC 500/mm^3 or greater.

Mantle Cell Lymphoma

PO: ADULTS, ELDERLY: 25 mg once daily on days 1–21 of repeated 28-day cycle.

Multiple Myeloma

PO: ADULTS, ELDERLY: 25 mg/day on days 1–21 of repeated 28-day cycle. (Dexamethasone 40 mg/day on days 1–4, 9–12, 17–20 of each 28-day cycle for first 4 cycles, then 40 mg/day on days 1–4 every 28 days.)

Dosage Adjustments for Multiple Myeloma
Platelets:

Thrombocytopenia: Platelets fall to less than 30,000/mm^3, hold treatment, monitor CBC. Resume at 15 mg/day when platelets 30,000/mm^3 or greater. For each subsequent fall to less than 30,000/mm^3, hold treatment and resume at 5 mg/day less than previous dose when platelets return to 30,000/mm^3 or greater. Do not dose to less than 5 mg/day.

Neutrophils:

Neutropenia: Neutrophils fall to less than 1,000/mm^3, hold treatment, add G-CSF, follow CBC weekly. Resume at 25 mg/day when neutrophils return to 1,000/mm^3 and neutropenia is the only toxicity. Resume at 15 mg/day if other toxicity is present. For each subsequent fall to less than 1,000/mm^3, hold treatment and resume at 5 mg/day less than previous dose when neutrophils return to 1,000/mm^3 or greater. Do not dose to less than 5 mg/day.

Dosage in Renal Impairment

SIDE EFFECTS

Frequent (49%–31%): Diarrhea, pruritus, rash, fatigue. **Occasional (24%–12%):** Constipation, nausea, arthralgia, fever, back pain, peripheral edema, cough, dizziness, headache, muscle cramps, epistaxis, asthenia (loss of strength, energy), dry skin, abdominal pain. **Rare (10%–5%):** Extremity pain, vomiting, generalized edema, anorexia, insomnia, night sweats, myalgia, dry mouth, ecchymosis, rigors, depression, dysgeusia, palpitations.

ADVERSE EFFECTS/TOXIC REACTIONS

Significant increased risk of deep vein thrombosis (DVT), pulmonary embolism. Thrombocytopenia occurs in 62% of pts, neutropenia in 59% of pts, and anemia in 12% of pts. Upper respiratory infection (nasopharyngitis, pneumonia, sinusitis, bronchitis, rhinitis), UTI occur occasionally. Cellulitis, peripheral neuropathy, hypertension, hypothyroidism occur in approximately 6% of pts.

NURSING CONSIDERATIONS

BASELINE ASSESSMENT

Obtain baseline CBC. Due to high potential for human birth defects/fetal death, female pts must avoid pregnancy 4 wks before therapy, during therapy, during dose interruptions, and 4 wks following therapy. Two reliable forms of contraception must be used even if pt has history of infertility unless it is due to hysterectomy or menopause that has occurred for at least 24 consecutive mos. Confirm two negative pregnancy tests before therapy initiation.

	Creatinine Clearance 30–59 ml/min	Creatinine Clearance Less Than 30 ml/min (Nondialysis Dependent)	Creatinine Clearance Less Than 30 ml/min (Dialysis Dependent)
Myelodysplastic syndrome	5 mg once daily	2.5 mg once daily	2.5 mg once daily (give after dialysis)
Multiple myeloma	10 mg once daily	15 mg q48h	5 mg once daily (give after dialysis)

underlined – top prescribed drug

INTERVENTION/EVALUATION

Perform pregnancy tests on women of childbearing potential: weekly during the first 4 wks, then at 4-wk intervals in pts with regular menstrual cycles or q2wks in pts with irregular menstrual cycles. Monitor for hematologic toxicity; obtain CBC weekly during first 8 wks of therapy and at least monthly thereafter. Observe for signs, symptoms of thromboembolism (shortness of breath, chest pain, extremity pain, swelling, stroke-like symptoms).

PATIENT/FAMILY TEACHING

• Two reliable forms of birth control must be used before, during, and after therapy for female pts. • A pregnancy test must be performed within 10–14 days and 24 hrs before therapy begins. • Males must always use a latex condom during any sexual contact with females of childbearing potential even if they have undergone a successful vasectomy.

---

letrozole

let-roe-zole
(Femara)
Do not confuse Femara with Famvir, Femhrt, or Provera, or letrozole with anastrozole.

◆CLASSIFICATION

PHARMACOTHERAPEUTIC: Aromatase inhibitor, hormone. **CLINICAL:** Antineoplastic (see p. 87C).

ACTION

Decreases circulating estrogen by inhibiting aromatase, an enzyme that catalyzes the final step in estrogen production. **Therapeutic Effect:** Inhibits growth of breast cancers stimulated by estrogens.

PHARMACOKINETICS

Rapidly, completely absorbed. Metabolized in liver. Primarily eliminated by kid-

neys. Unknown if removed by hemodialysis. **Half-life:** Approximately 2 days.

USES

First-line treatment of locally advanced or metastatic breast cancer. Treatment of advanced breast cancer in postmenopausal women with disease progression following antiestrogen therapy. Postsurgical treatment for postmenopausal women with hormone sensitive early breast cancer. Extended treatment of early breast cancer after 5 yrs of tamoxifen. **OFF-LABEL:** Treatment of ovarian, endometrial cancer.

PRECAUTIONS

Contraindications: Use in women who are or may become pregnant. **Cautions:** Hepatic impairment.

⚖ LIFESPAN CONSIDERATIONS

Pregnancy/Lactation: Unknown if distributed in breast milk. May cause fetal harm. **Pregnancy Category X. Children:** Safety and efficacy not established. **Elderly:** No age-related precautions noted.

INTERACTIONS

DRUG: Tamoxifen may reduce concentration. **HERBAL:** None significant. **FOOD:** None known. **LAB VALUES:** May increase serum calcium, cholesterol, GGT, AST, ALT, bilirubin.

AVAILABILITY (Rx)

Tablets: 2.5 mg.

ADMINISTRATION/HANDLING

PO
• Give without regard to food.

INDICATIONS/ROUTES/DOSAGE

Breast Cancer
PO: ADULTS, ELDERLY: 2.5 mg/day. Continue until tumor progression is evident.

Dosage in Severe Hepatic Impairment
PO: ADULTS, ELDERLY: 2.5 mg every other day.

 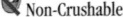

SIDE EFFECTS

Frequent (21%–9%): Musculoskeletal pain (back, arm, leg), nausea, headache. **Occasional (8%–5%):** Constipation, arthralgia, fatigue, vomiting, hot flashes, diarrhea, abdominal pain, cough, rash, anorexia, hypertension, peripheral edema. **Rare (4%–1%):** Asthenia (loss of strength, energy), drowsiness, dyspepsia (heartburn, indigestion, epigastric pain), weight gain, pruritus.

ADVERSE EFFECTS/ TOXIC REACTIONS

Pleural effusion, pulmonary embolism, bone fracture, thromboembolic disorder, MI occur rarely.

NURSING CONSIDERATIONS

BASELINE ASSESSMENT

Obtain baseline CBC, chemistries, hepatic/renal function tests. Obtain pregnancy test prior to beginning therapy.

INTERVENTION/EVALUATION

Monitor for, assist with ambulation if asthenia (loss of strength, energy), dizziness occurs. Assess for headache. Offer antiemetic for nausea, vomiting. Monitor CBC, thyroid function, electrolytes, hepatic/renal function tests. Monitor for evidence of musculoskeletal pain; offer analgesics for pain relief.

PATIENT/FAMILY TEACHING

• Report if nausea, asthenia (loss of strength, energy), hot flashes become unmanageable. • Discuss importance of negative pregnancy test prior to beginning therapy and nonhormonal methods of birth control. • Explain possible risk to fetus if pt is or becomes pregnant before or during therapy.

leucovorin calcium (folinic acid, citrovorum factor)

loo-**koe**-vor-in

Do not confuse folinic acid with folic acid, or leucovorin with Leukeran.

◆CLASSIFICATION

PHARMACOTHERAPEUTIC: Folic acid antagonist. **CLINICAL:** Antidote.

ACTION

Competes with methotrexate for same transport processes into cells (limits methotrexate action on normal cells). **Therapeutic Effect:** Reverses toxic effects of folic acid antagonists. Reverses folic acid deficiency.

PHARMACOKINETICS

Readily absorbed from GI tract. Widely distributed. Metabolized in liver, intestinal mucosa. Primarily excreted in urine. **Half-life:** 15 min; metabolite, 30–35 min.

USES

Antidote for folic acid antagonists (methotrexate, trimethoprim, pyrimethamine). Treatment of megaloblastic anemias when folate deficient (e.g., infancy, celiac disease, pregnancy, when oral therapy not possible). Treatment of colon cancer (with fluorouracil). Rescue therapy after high-dose methotrexate for osteosarcoma. **OFF-LABEL:** Adjunctive cofactor therapy in methanol toxicity. Prevents pyrimethamine hematologic toxicity in HIV-positive pts.

PRECAUTIONS

Contraindications: Pernicious anemia, other megaloblastic anemias secondary to vitamin B_{12} deficiency. **Cautions:** None known.

⌛ LIFESPAN CONSIDERATIONS

Pregnancy/Lactation: Unknown if drug crosses placenta or is distributed in breast milk. **Pregnancy Category C. Children:** May increase risk of seizures by counteracting anticonvulsant effects of barbiturate, hydantoins. **Elderly:** Age-related renal impairment may require dosage adjustment when used for rescue from effects of high-dose methotrexate therapy.

INTERACTIONS

DRUG: May decrease effects of **anticonvulsants (e.g., phenytoin).** May increase **5-fluorouracil** toxicity/effect when taken in combination. **HERBAL:** None significant. **FOOD:** None known. **LAB VALUES:** May decrease platelets, WBCs (when used in combination with 5-fluorouracil).

AVAILABILITY (Rx)

Injection, Powder for Reconstitution: 50 mg, 100 mg, 200 mg, 350 mg, 500 mg. **Injection, Solution:** 10 mg/ml. **Tablets:** 5 mg, 10 mg, 15 mg, 25 mg.

ADMINISTRATION/HANDLING

 IV

◀ALERT▶ Strict adherence to timing of 5-fluorouracil following leucovorin therapy must be maintained.

Reconstitution • Reconstitute each 50-mg vial with 5 ml Sterile Water for Injection or Bacteriostatic Water for Injection containing benzyl alcohol to provide concentration of 10 mg/ml. • Due to benzyl alcohol in 1-mg ampule and in Bacteriostatic Water for Injection, reconstitute doses greater than 10 mg/m² with Sterile Water for Injection. • Further dilute with 100–1,000 ml D₅W or 0.9% NaCl.

Rate of Administration • Do not exceed 160 mg/min if given by IV infusion (due to calcium content).

Storage • Store powdered vials for parenteral use at room temperature. • Refrigerate solution for injection vials. • Injection appears as clear, yellowish solution. • Use immediately if reconstituted with Sterile Water for Injection; stable for 7 days if reconstituted with Bacteriostatic Water for Injection.

PO
• Scored tablets may be crushed.

▦ IV INCOMPATIBILITIES

Amphotericin B complex (Abelcet, AmBisome, Amphotec), droperidol (Inapsine), foscarnet (Foscavir).

▦ IV COMPATIBILITIES

Cisplatin (Platinol AQ), cyclophosphamide (Cytoxan), doxorubicin (Adriamycin), etoposide (VePesid), filgrastim (Neupogen), 5-fluorouracil, gemcitabine (Gemzar), granisetron (Kytril), heparin, methotrexate, metoclopramide (Reglan), mitomycin (Mutamycin), piperacillin and tazobactam (Zosyn), vinblastine (Velban), vincristine (Oncovin).

INDICATIONS/ROUTES/DOSAGE

Conventional Rescue Dosage in High-Dose Methotrexate Therapy

PO, IV, IM: ADULTS, ELDERLY, CHILDREN: 15 mg (approximately 10 mg/m²) IM or IV one time, then PO q6h until serum methotrexate level is less than 0.05 micromole/L. If 24-hr serum creatinine level increases by 50% or greater over baseline or methotrexate level exceeds 5 micromole/L, increase to 150 mg q3h until methotrexate level is less than 1 micromole/L, then 15 mg q3h until methotrexate level is less than 0.05 micromole/L.

Folic Acid Antagonist Overdose

PO: ADULTS, ELDERLY, CHILDREN: 5–15 mg/day.

Megaloblastic Anemia Secondary to Folate Deficiency

IM: ADULTS, ELDERLY, CHILDREN: 1 mg or less per day.

Colon Cancer

◀ALERT▶ For rescue therapy in cancer chemotherapy, refer to specific protocols used for optimal dosage and sequence of leucovorin administration.

L

IV: ADULTS, ELDERLY: 200 mg/m² followed by 370 mg/m² fluorouracil daily for 5 days. Repeat course at 4-wk intervals for 2 courses, then 4- to 5-wk intervals or 20 mg/m² followed by 425 mg/m² fluorouracil daily for 5 days. Repeat course at 4-wk intervals for 2 courses, then 4- to 5-wk intervals.

SIDE EFFECTS

Frequent: When combined with chemotherapeutic agents: diarrhea, stomatitis, nausea, vomiting, lethargy, malaise, fatigue, alopecia, anorexia. **Occasional:** Urticaria, dermatitis.

ADVERSE EFFECTS/ TOXIC REACTIONS

Excessive dosage may negate chemotherapeutic effects of folic acid antagonists. Anaphylaxis occurs rarely. Diarrhea may cause rapid clinical deterioration.

NURSING CONSIDERATIONS

BASELINE ASSESSMENT

Give as soon as possible, preferably within 1 hr, for treatment of accidental overdosage of folic acid antagonists. Obtain baseline CBC, liver function test, renal function.

INTERVENTION/EVALUATION

Monitor for vomiting (may need to change from oral to parenteral therapy). Observe elderly, debilitated closely due to risk for severe toxicities. Assess CBC with differential (also electrolytes, hepatic function tests if used in combination with chemotherapeutic agents).

PATIENT/FAMILY TEACHING

• Explain purpose of medication in treatment of cancer. • Report allergic reaction, vomiting.

---

leuprolide   **HIGH ALERT**

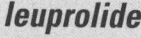

loo-proe-lide

(Eligard, Lupron , <u>Lupron Depot</u>, Lupron Depot-Ped)

◆CLASSIFICATION

PHARMACOTHERAPEUTIC: Gonadotropin-releasing hormone (GnRH) analogue. **CLINICAL:** Antineoplastic (see pp. 87C, 109C).

ACTION

Stimulates release of luteinizing hormone (LH), follicle-stimulating hormone (FSH) from anterior pituitary gland, stimulating production of estrogen, testosterone. **Therapeutic Effect:** Produces pharmacologic castration, decreases growth of abnormal prostate tissue in males; causes endometrial tissue to become inactive, atrophic in females; decreases rate of pubertal development in children with central precocious puberty.

PHARMACOKINETICS

Rapidly, well absorbed after subcutaneous administration. Absorbed slowly after IM administration. Protein binding: 43%–49%. **Half-life:** 3–4 hrs.

USES

Palliative treatment of advanced prostate carcinoma. Management of endometriosis. Treatment of anemia caused by uterine leiomyomata (fibroids). Treatment of central precocious puberty. **OFF-LABEL:** Treatment of breast cancer, infertility.

PRECAUTIONS

Contraindications: Pregnancy, breastfeeding, undiagnosed vaginal bleeding. Eligard 7.5 mg is contraindicated in women, children; pts with hypersensitivity to GnRH, GnRH agonist analogues, or any of its components. 22.5 mg, 30 mg, 45 mg Lupron Depot contraindicated in women. **Cautions:** History of psychiatric illness.

☒ LIFESPAN CONSIDERATIONS

Pregnancy/Lactation: Depot: Contraindicated in pregnancy. May cause spontaneous abortion. **Pregnancy Category X.**

<u>underlined</u> – top prescribed drug

Children: Long-term safety not established. **Elderly:** No age-related precautions noted.

INTERACTIONS

DRUG: None significant. **HERBAL:** None significant. **FOOD:** None known. **LAB VALUES:** May increase serum prostatic acid phosphatase (PAP). Initially increases, then decreases, serum testosterone. May increase serum ALT, AST, alkaline phosphatase, glucose, LDH, LDL, cholesterol, triglycerides. May decrease platelets, WBC.

AVAILABILITY (Rx)

Injection Depot Formulation: Eligard: 7.5 mg, 22.5 mg, 30 mg, 45 mg. **Lupron Depot-Ped:** 7.5 mg, 11.25 mg (3-month), 11.25 (monthly), 15 mg, 30 mg. **Lupron Depot:** 3.75 mg, 7.5 mg, 11.25 mg, 22.5 mg, 30 mg, 45 mg. **Injection Solution (Lupron):** 5 mg/ml.

ADMINISTRATION/HANDLING

◄**ALERT**► May be carcinogenic, mutagenic, teratogenic. Handle with extreme care during preparation/administration.

IM
Lupron Depot • Store at room temperature. • Protect from light, heat. • Do not freeze vials. • Reconstitute only with diluent provided. Follow manufacturer's instructions for mixing.
• Do not use needles less than 22 gauge; use syringes provided by the manufacturer (0.5-ml low-dose insulin syringes may be used as an alternative). • Administer immediately.
Eligard • Refrigerate. • Allow to warm to room temperature before reconstitution. • Follow manufacturer's instructions for mixing. • Following reconstitution, administer within 30 min.

Subcutaneous
Lupron • Refrigerate vials. • Injection appears clear, colorless. • Discard if discolored or precipitate forms. • Administer into deltoid muscle, anterior thigh, abdomen.

INDICATIONS/ROUTES/DOSAGE

Advanced Prostatic Carcinoma
IM *(Lupron Depot)*: **ADULTS, ELDERLY:** 7.5 mg every mo, 22.5 mg q3mos, 30 mg q4mos, or 45 mg q6mos.
Subcutaneous *(Eligard)*: **ADULTS, ELDERLY:** 7.5 mg every mo, 22.5 mg q3mos, 30 mg q4mos, or 45 mg q6mos.
Subcutaneous *(Lupron)*: **ADULTS, ELDERLY:** 1 mg/day.

Endometriosis
IM *(Lupron Depot)*: **ADULTS, ELDERLY:** 3.75 mg/mo for up to 6 mos or 11.25 mg q3mos for up to 2 doses.

Uterine Leiomyomata
IM *(with Iron [Lupron Depot])*: **ADULTS, ELDERLY:** 3.75 mg/mo for up to 3 mos or 11.25 mg as a single injection.

Precocious Puberty
IM *(Lupron Depot-Ped)*: **CHILDREN GREATER THAN 37.5 KG:** 15 mg q month. **GREATER THAN 25 KG TO 37.5 KG:** 11.25 mg q month. **25 KG OR LESS:** 7.5 mg q month. Titrate dose upward by 3.75 mg/mo if down regulation not achieved. **LUPRON DEPOT-PED (3 MOS):** 11.25 mg or 30 mg q12wks. **Subcutaneous** *(Lupron)*: **CHILDREN:** Initially, 50 mcg/kg/day. Titrate upward by 10 mcg/kg/day if down regulation is not achieved.

SIDE EFFECTS

Frequent: Hot flashes (ranging from mild flushing to diaphoresis), migraines, hyperhidrosis. **Females:** Amenorrhea, spotting. **Occasional:** Arrhythmias, palpitations, blurred vision, dizziness, edema, headache, burning, pruritus, swelling at injection site, nausea, insomnia, weight gain. **Females:** Deepening voice, hirsutism, decreased libido, increased breast tenderness, vaginitis, altered mood. **Males:** Constipation, decreased testicle size, gynecomastia, impotence, decreased appetite, angina. **Rare: Males:** Thrombophlebitis.

L

ADVERSE EFFECTS/ TOXIC REACTIONS

Occasionally, signs/symptoms of prostatic carcinoma worsen 1–2 wks after initial dosing (subsides during continued therapy). Increased bone pain and, less frequently, dysuria, hematuria, weakness, paresthesia of lower extremities may be noted. MI, pulmonary embolism occur rarely.

NURSING CONSIDERATIONS

BASELINE ASSESSMENT

Question for possibility of pregnancy before initiating therapy (Pregnancy Category X). Obtain serum testosterone, prostatic acid phosphates (PAP) periodically during therapy. Serum testosterone, PAP should increase during first wk of therapy. Serum testosterone then should decrease to baseline level or less within 2 wks, PAP within 4 wks.

INTERVENTION/EVALUATION

Monitor for arrhythmias, palpitations. Assess for peripheral edema. Assess sleep pattern. Monitor for visual difficulties. Assist with ambulation if dizziness occurs. Offer antiemetics if nausea occurs.

PATIENT/ FAMILY TEACHING

• Hot flashes tend to decrease during continued therapy. • Temporary exacerbation of signs/symptoms of disease may occur during first few wks of therapy. • Use contraceptive measures. • Inform physician immediately if regular menstruation persists, pregnancy occurs. • Avoid tasks that require alertness, motor skills until response to drug is established (potential for dizziness).

levalbuterol

```
TOP
200
```

lee-val-**bue**-ter-all
(<u>Xopenex</u>, Xopenex HFA)
Do not confuse Xopenex with Xanax.

◆CLASSIFICATION

PHARMACOTHERAPEUTIC: Sympathomimetic. **CLINICAL:** Bronchodilator (see p. 76C).

ACTION

Stimulates beta$_2$-adrenergic receptors in lungs, resulting in relaxation of bronchial smooth muscle. **Therapeutic Effect:** Relieves bronchospasm, reduces airway resistance.

PHARMACOKINETICS

Route	Onset	Peak	Duration
Inhalation	5–10 min	1.5 hrs	5–6 hrs
Nebulization	10–17 min	1.5 hrs	5–8 hrs

Half-life: 3.3–4 hrs.

USES

Treatment, prevention of bronchospasm due to reversible obstructive airway disease (e.g., asthma, bronchitis, emphysema).

PRECAUTIONS

Contraindications: History of hypersensitivity to albuterol or levalbuterol. **Cautions:** Cardiovascular disorders (cardiac arrhythmias), seizures, hypertension, hyperthyroidism, diabetes mellitus, hypokalemia.

⌛ LIFESPAN CONSIDERATIONS

Pregnancy/Lactation: Crosses placenta. Unknown if distributed in breast milk. **Pregnancy Category C. Children:** Safety and efficacy not established in those younger than 12 yrs. **Elderly:** Lower initial dosages recommended.

INTERACTIONS

DRUG: Beta-adrenergic blocking agents (beta-blockers) antagonize effects; may produce severe bronchospasm. May decrease **digoxin** concentration. **MAOIs, tricyclic antidepressants** may potentiate cardiovascular effects. **Diuretics** may increase hypokalemia. **HERBAL:** None significant. **FOOD:** None known. **LAB VALUES:** May decrease serum potassium.

AVAILABILITY (Rx)

Inhalation Aerosol: 45 mcg/activation. **Solution for Nebulization:** 0.31 in 3-ml vials, 0.63 mg in 3-ml vials, 1.25 mg in 3-ml vials, 1.25 mg in 0.5-ml vials.

ADMINISTRATION/HANDLING

Nebulization
• No diluent necessary. • Protect from light, excessive heat. Store at room temperature. • Once foil is opened, use within 2 wks. • Use within 1 wk and protect from light after removal from pouch.• Discard if solution is not colorless. • Do not mix with other medications. • Concentrated solution (1.25 mg in 0.5 ml) should be diluted with 2.5 ml 0.9% NaCl prior to use. • Give over 5–15 min.

Inhalation
• Shake well before inhalation. • Following first inhalation, wait 2 min before inhaling second dose (allows for deeper bronchial penetration). • Rinsing mouth with water immediately after inhalation prevents mouth/throat dryness.

INDICATIONS/ROUTES/DOSAGE

Treatment/Prevention of Bronchospasm
Nebulization: ADULTS, ELDERLY, CHILDREN 12 YRS AND OLDER: Initially, 0.63 mg 3 times a day 6–8 hrs apart. May increase to 1.25 mg 3 times a day with dose monitoring. **CHILDREN 5–11 YRS:** Initially, 0.31 mg 3 times a day. **Maximum:** 0.63 mg 3 times a day. **CHILDREN 4 YRS OR YOUNGER:** 0.31– 1.25 mg q4–6h as needed.
Inhalation: ADULTS, ELDERLY, CHILDREN 4 YRS AND OLDER: 1–2 inhalations q4–6h.

Acute Asthma Exacerbation
Nebulization: ADULTS, ELDERLY: 1.25– 2.5 mg q20min for 3 doses, then 1.25–5 mg q1–4h as needed. **CHILDREN:** 0.075 mg/kg (minimum dose: 1.25 mg) q20min for 3 doses, then 0.075–0.15 mg/kg q1–4h as needed.

Inhalation: ADULTS, ELDERLY: 4–8 puffs q20min for up to 4 hrs, then q1–4h. **CHILDREN:** 4–8 puffs q20min for 3 doses, then q1–4h.

SIDE EFFECTS

Occasional (11%–4%): Nervousness, tremor, rhinitis, flu-like illness. **Rare (less than 3%):** Tachycardia, dizziness, anxiety, viral infection, dyspepsia, dry mouth, headache, chest pain.

ADVERSE EFFECTS/ TOXIC REACTIONS

Excessive sympathomimetic stimulation may produce palpitations, premature heart contraction, tachycardia, chest pain, slight increase in B/P followed by substantial decrease, chills, diaphoresis, blanching of skin. Too-frequent or excessive use may decrease bronchodilating effectiveness, lead to severe, paradoxical broncho-constriction.

NURSING CONSIDERATIONS

BASELINE ASSESSMENT
Offer emotional support (high incidence of anxiety due to difficulty in breathing, sympathomimetic response to drug). Assess lung sounds, pulse, B/P. Note color, amount of sputum.

INTERVENTION/EVALUATION
Monitor rate, depth, rhythm, type of respiration; quality/rate of pulse, EKG, serum potassium, ABG determinations. Assess lung sounds for wheezing (bronchoconstriction), rales. Observe for paradoxical bronchospasm.

PATIENT/ FAMILY TEACHING
• Increase fluid intake (decreases lung secretion viscosity). • Rinsing mouth with water immediately after inhalation may prevent mouth/throat dryness. • Avoid excessive use of caffeine derivatives (chocolate, coffee, tea, cola, cocoa). • Report if palpitations, tachycardia, chest pain, tremors, dizziness, headache occurs or shortness of breath is not relieved.

levetiracetam

lee-ve-tye-**ra**-see-tam
(Apo-Levetiracetam ✦, <u>Keppra</u>,
Keppra XR)
**Do not confuse Keppra with
Kaletra, Keflex, or Keppra XR,
or levetiracetam with levo-
floxacin.**

◆CLASSIFICATION

PHARMACOTHERAPEUTIC: Pyrro-
lidine derivative. **CLINICAL:** Anticonvulsant (see p. 36C).

ACTION

Inhibits burst firing without affecting normal neuronal excitability. **Therapeutic
Effect:** Prevents seizure activity.

PHARMACOKINETICS

Rapidly, completely absorbed following
PO administration. Protein binding: less
than 10%. Metabolized primarily by
enzymatic hydrolysis. Primarily excreted
in urine as unchanged drug. **Half-life:**
6–8 hrs.

USES

PO: Adjunctive treatment of partial-onset seizures in pts 1 mo and older with
epilepsy. Adjunctive treatment of myoclonic seizures in adults and children
12 yrs of age and older. Adjunctive treatment of primary generalized tonic-
clonic seizures in pts 6 yrs and older
with idiopathic generalized seizures.
Keppra XR: Adjunctive treatment of
partial-onset seizures in pts 16 yrs of
age and older. **Injection:** Treatment of
partial-onset seizures in adults. **OFF-LA-
BEL:** Bipolar disorder.

PRECAUTIONS

Contraindications: None known. **Cautions:** Renal impairment. Pts with depression at high risk for suicide.

⏳ LIFESPAN CONSIDERATIONS

Pregnancy/Lactation: Distributed in
breast milk. Breastfeeding not recommended. **Pregnancy Category C. Children:** Safety and efficacy not established
in children 4 yrs or younger. **Elderly:**
Age-related renal impairment may require dosage adjustment.

INTERACTIONS

DRUG: None significant. **HERBAL:** None
significant. **FOOD:** None known. **LAB VAL-
UES:** May decrease Hgb, Hct, RBC, WBC
counts.

AVAILABILITY (Rx)

Injection, Solution: 100 mg/ml. **Oral Solution:** 100 mg/ml. **Tablets:** 250 mg, 500
mg, 750 mg, 1,000 mg.

 Tablets, Extended-Release: 500 mg,
750 mg.

ADMINISTRATION/HANDLING
💧 IV

Rate of Infusion • Infuse over 15 min.
Reconstitution • Dilute with 100 ml
0.9% NaCl or D₅W.
Storage • Store at room temperature.
• Stable for 24 hrs following dilution.

🔲 IV INCOMPATIBILITY

Data not available.

🔲 IV COMPATIBILITIES

Diazepam (Valium), lorazepam (Ativan),
valproate (Depacon).

PO
• Give without regard to food. • Use oral
solution for pts weighing 20 kg or less.
• Use tablets or oral solution for pts
weighing more than 20 kg. • Oral solution should be administered with a calibrated measuring device. • Swallow extended-release and immediate-release
tablets whole; do not cut, break, or
crush.

INDICATIONS/ROUTES/DOSAGE

Partial-Onset Seizures

IV/PO: ADULTS, ELDERLY, CHILDREN 17 YRS AND OLDER: Initially, 500 mg q12h. May increase by 1,000 mg/day q2wks. **Maximum:** 3,000 mg/day. **Keppra XR:** 1,000 mg once daily. May increase in increments of 1,000 mg every 2 wks. **Maximum:** 3,000 mg daily.

PO: CHILDREN 4–16 YRS: 20 mg/kg/day in 2 divided doses. May increase q2wks by 10 mg/kg/dose. **Maximum:** 60 mg/kg/day in 2 divided doses. **CHILDREN 6 MOS TO YOUNGER THAN 4 YRS:** 20 mg/kg/day in 2 divided doses. May increase q2wks by 10 mg/kg/dose. **Maximum:** 50 mg/kg/day in 2 divided doses. **CHILDREN 1 MO TO YOUNGER THAN 6 MOS (ORAL SOLUTION):** 14 mg/kg/day in 2 divided doses. May increase q2wks by 7 mg/kg/dose. **Maximum:** 42 mg/kg/day in 2 divided doses.

Myoclonic Seizures

PO: ADULTS, ELDERLY, CHILDREN 12 YRS AND OLDER: Initially, 500 mg q12h. May increase by 1,000 mg/day q2wks. **Maximum:** 3,000 mg/day.

Tonic-Clonic Seizures

PO: ADULTS, ELDERLY, CHILDREN 16 YRS AND OLDER: Initially, 500 mg twice a day. May increase by 1,000 mg/day q2wks until dose of 3,000 mg/day attained. **CHILDREN 6–15 YRS:** Initially, 10 mg/kg twice a day. May increase by 20 mg/kg/day q2wks until dose of 60 mg/kg/day attained.

Dosage in Renal Impairment

Dosage is modified based on creatinine clearance.

Creatinine Clearance	Dosage (Immediate-Release, IV)	Dosage (Extended-Release)
Greater than 80 ml/min	500–1,500 mg q12h	1,000–3,000 mg q24h
50–80 ml/min	500–1,000 mg q12h	1,000–2,000 mg q24h
30–49 ml/min	250–750 mg q12h	500–1,500 mg q24h
Less than 30 ml/min	250–500 mg q12h	500–1,000 mg q24h
End-stage renal disease using dialysis	500–1,000 mg q24h, after dialysis, a 250- to 500-mg supplemental dose is recommended	NA
CRRT	250–750 mg q12h	

SIDE EFFECTS

Frequent (15%–10%): Drowsiness, asthenia (loss of strength, energy), headache, infection. **Occasional (9%–3%):** Dizziness, pharyngitis, pain, depression, anxiety, vertigo, rhinitis, anorexia. **Rare (less than 3%):** Amnesia, emotional lability, cough, sinusitis, anorexia, diplopia.

ADVERSE EFFECTS/TOXIC REACTIONS

Acute psychosis, seizures have been reported. Sudden discontinuance increases risk of seizure activity. Serious dermatological reactions, including Steven-Johnson syndrome and toxic epidermal necrolysis have been reported.

NURSING CONSIDERATIONS

BASELINE ASSESSMENT

Review history of seizure disorder (intensity, frequency, duration, LOC). Initiate seizure precautions. Assess for hypersensitivity to levetiracetam, renal function tests.

INTERVENTION/EVALUATION

Observe for recurrence of seizure activity. Assess for clinical improvement (decrease in intensity/frequency of seizures). Monitor renal function tests. Observe for suicidal ideation, depression, behavioral changes. Assist with ambulation if dizziness occurs.

L

PATIENT/ FAMILY TEACHING
• Drowsiness usually diminishes with continued therapy. • Avoid tasks that require alertness, motor skills until response to drug is established. • Avoid alcohol. • Do not abruptly discontinue medication (may precipitate seizures). • Strict maintenance of drug therapy is essential for seizure control. • Report mood swings, hostile behavior, suicidal ideation, unusual changes in behavior.

levocetirizine

lee-voe-se-**tir**-i-zeen
(Xyzal)
Do not confuse levocetirizine with cetirizine.

◆CLASSIFICATION
PHARMACOTHERAPEUTIC: Second-generation piperazine. **CLINICAL:** Antihistamine (see p. 55C).

ACTION
Competes with histamine for H_1-receptor sites on effector cells in GI tract, blood vessels, respiratory tract. **Therapeutic Effect:** Relieves allergic response (sneezing, rhinorrhea, postnasal discharge, nasal pruritus, ocular pruritus, tearing), allergic rhinitis (hay fever), mediated by histamine (urticaria, pruritus).

PHARMACOKINETICS
Rapidly, almost completely absorbed from GI tract. Protein binding: 92%. Excreted primarily unchanged in urine. **Half-life:** 8 hrs (increased in renal impairment).

USES
Relief of symptoms of allergic rhinitis (seasonal, perennial) and uncomplicated skin manifestations of chronic idiopathic urticaria.

PRECAUTIONS
Contraindications: Hypersensitivity to hydroxyzine, end-stage renal disease, children 6–11 yrs with renal impairment, pts undergoing dialysis. **Cautions:** Mild to moderate renal impairment.

⌛ LIFESPAN CONSIDERATIONS
Pregnancy/Lactation: Distributed in breast milk. **Pregnancy Category B. Children:** Less likely to cause anticholinergic effects (e.g., dry mouth, urinary retention). Safety and efficacy not established in pts younger than 6 yrs. **Elderly:** More sensitive to anticholinergic effects (e.g., dry mouth, urinary retention). Age-related renal impairment may require dosage adjustment.

INTERACTIONS
DRUG: Ritonavir may increase concentration/effect. **HERBAL:** None significant. **FOOD:** None known. **LAB VALUES:** May suppress wheal and flare reactions to antigen skin testing, unless antihistamines are discontinued 4 days before testing.

AVAILABILITY (Rx)
Oral Solution: 0.5 mg/ml. **Tablets:** 5 mg.

ADMINISTRATION/HANDLING
PO
• Give without regard to food. Tablets may be crushed.

INDICATIONS/ROUTES/DOSAGE
Allergic Rhinitis, Chronic Urticaria
PO: ADULTS, ELDERLY, CHILDREN 12 YRS AND OLDER: 5 mg once daily in the evening. **CHILDREN 6–11 YRS:** 2.5 mg once daily in the evening. **CHILDREN 6 MOS– 5 YRS:** 1.25 mg once daily in the evening.

Dosage in Renal Impairment
◀**ALERT**▶ **CHILDREN 6 MOS TO 5 YRS:** Avoid use.
Mild renal function impairment (creatinine clearance 50–80 ml/min): 2.5 mg once daily. **Moderate renal function impairment (creatinine clearance 30–49 ml/min):** 2.5 mg every other day. **Severe renal function impairment (creatinine clearance 10–29 ml/min):** 2.5 mg twice weekly (once every 3–4 days).

SIDE EFFECTS

Adults: Occasional (6%–4%): Drowsiness, nasopharyngitis, fatigue. **Rare (2%–1%):** Dry mouth, pharyngitis. **Children 6–12 yrs: Rare (4%–2%):** Fever, cough, fatigue, epistaxis.

ADVERSE EFFECTS/ TOXIC REACTIONS

None significant.

NURSING CONSIDERATIONS

BASELINE ASSESSMENT

Assess severity of rhinitis, urticaria, other symptoms. Obtain baseline renal function tests.

INTERVENTION/EVALUATION

For upper respiratory allergies, increase fluids to maintain thin secretions and offset thirst. Monitor symptoms for therapeutic response.

PATIENT/FAMILY TEACHING

• Avoid tasks that require alertness, motor skills until response to drug is established. • Avoid alcohol.

---

levofloxacin

lee-voe-**flox**-a-sin
(Apo-Levofloxacin ✤, Iquix,
Levaquin, Novo-Levofloxacin ✤,
Quixin)

BLACK BOX ALERT May increase risk of tendonitis, tendon rupture. (Risk increased with concurrent corticosteroids, organ transplant, pts older than 60 yrs.) May exacerbate myasthenia gravis.

Do not confuse Levaquin with Levoxyl, Levsin/SL, or Lovenox, or levofloxacin with levetiracetam or levothyroxine.

◆CLASSIFICATION

PHARMACOTHERAPEUTIC: Fluoroquinolone. **CLINICAL:** Antibiotic (see p. 26C).

ACTION

Inhibits DNA enzyme gyrase in susceptible microorganisms, interfering with bacterial cell replication, repair. **Therapeutic Effect:** Bactericidal.

PHARMACOKINETICS

Well absorbed after PO, IV administration. Protein binding: 50%. Widely distributed. Eliminated unchanged in urine. Partially removed by hemodialysis. **Half-life:** 6–8 hrs.

USES

Treatment of susceptible infections due to *S. pneumoniae, S. aureus, E. faecalis, H. influenzae, M. catarrhalis, Serratia marcescens, K. pneumoniae, E. coli, P. mirabilis, P. aeruginosa, C. pneumoniae, Legionella pneumophila, Mycoplasma pneumoniae,* including acute bacterial exacerbation of chronic bronchitis, acute bacterial sinusitis, community-acquired pneumonia, nosocomial pneumonia, complicated and uncomplicated UTI, acute pyelonephritis, complicated and uncomplicated mild to moderate skin/skin structure infections, prostatitis. Inhalation anthrax (post-exposure); plague. **Ophthalmic:** Treatment of superficial infections to conjunctiva (0.5%), cornea (1.5%). **OFF-LABEL:** Urethritis, traveler's diarrhea, diverticulitis, enterocolitis, Legionnaire's disease, peritonitis.

PRECAUTIONS

Contraindications: Hypersensitivity to other fluoroquinolones. **Cautions:** Known or suspected CNS disorders, seizure disorder, renal impairment, bradycardia, cardiomyopathy, hypokalemia, hypomagnesemia, myasthenia gravis, severe cerebral arteriosclerosis, prolonged QT interval, medications that potentiate QT interval prolongation, diabetes.

⧗ LIFESPAN CONSIDERATIONS

Pregnancy/Lactation: Distributed in breast milk. Avoid use in pregnancy. **Pregnancy Category C. Children:** Safety and efficacy not established in those

L

✤ Canadian trade name   ⬛ Non-Crushable Drug   ⬛ High Alert drug

younger than 18 yrs. **Elderly:** Age-related renal impairment may require dosage adjustment.

INTERACTIONS

DRUG: Antacids, iron preparations, sucralfate, zinc decrease absorption. **NSAIDs** may increase risk of CNS stimulation, seizures. **Medications that prolong QT interval** may increase risk of arrhythmias. May increase effect of **warfarin. HERBAL:** None significant. **FOOD:** None known. **LAB VALUES:** May alter serum glucose.

AVAILABILITY (Rx)

Infusion Premix: 250 mg/50 ml, 500 mg/100 ml, 750 mg/150 ml. **Injection, Solution:** 25 mg/ml. **Ophthalmic Solution: (Iquix):** 1.5%. **(Quixin):** 0.5%. **Oral Solution:** 25 mg/ml. **Tablets:** 250 mg, 500 mg, 750 mg.

ADMINISTRATION/HANDLING

💧 IV

Reconstitution • For infusion using single-dose vial, withdraw desired amount (10 ml for 250 mg, 20 ml for 500 mg). Dilute each 10 ml (250 mg) with minimum 40 ml 0.9% NaCl, D₅W, providing a concentration of 5 mg/ml.
Rate of Administration • Administer no less than 60 min for 250 mg or 500 mg; 90 min for 750 mg.
Storage • Available in single-dose 20-ml (500-mg) vials and premixed with D₅W, ready to infuse. • Diluted vials stable for 72 hrs at room temperature, 14 days if refrigerated.

PO

• Do not administer antacids (aluminum, magnesium), sucralfate, iron or multivitamin preparations with zinc within 2 hrs of administration (significantly reduces absorption). • Give tablets without regard to food. • Give oral solution 1 hr before or 2 hrs after meals.

Ophthalmic

• Place a gloved finger on lower eyelid and pull out until a pocket is formed between eye and lower lid. • Place prescribed number of drops into pocket. • Instruct pt to close eye gently (so medication will not be squeezed out of the sac) and to apply digital pressure to lacrimal sac for 1–2 min to minimize systemic absorption.

🔲 IV INCOMPATIBILITIES

Furosemide (Lasix), heparin, insulin, nitroglycerin, propofol (Diprivan).

🔲 IV COMPATIBILITIES

Dexmedetomidine (Precedex), dobutamine (Dobutrex), dopamine (Intropin), fentanyl (Sublimaze), lidocaine, lorazepam (Ativan), magnesium, morphine.

INDICATIONS/ROUTES/DOSAGE

Usual Dosage Range
IV/PO: ADULTS, ELDERLY: 250–500 mg q24h; 750 mg q24h for severe or complicated infections.

Bronchitis
PO, IV: ADULTS, ELDERLY: 500 mg q24h for 7 days.

Community-Acquired Pneumonia
PO: ADULTS, ELDERLY: 750 mg/day for 5 days or 500 mg q24h for 7–14 days.

Pneumonia, Nosocomial
PO, IV: ADULTS, ELDERLY: 750 mg q24h for 7–14 days.

Skin/Skin Structure Infections
PO, IV: ADULTS, ELDERLY: (Uncomplicated) 500 mg q24h for 7–10 days. (Complicated) 750 mg q24h for 7–14 days.

Prostatitis
IV, PO: ADULTS, ELDERLY: 500 mg q24h for 28 days.

Uncomplicated UTI
IV, PO: ADULTS, ELDERLY: 250 mg q24h for 3 days.

Complicated UTI, Acute Pyelonephritis
PO, IV: ADULTS, ELDERLY: 250 mg q24h for 10 days or 750 mg q24h for 5 days.

Bacterial Conjunctivitis
Ophthalmic: ADULTS, ELDERLY, CHILDREN 1 YR AND OLDER (QUIXIN) (0.5%): 1–2 drops q2h for 2 days (up to 8 times a day), then 1–2 drops q4h for 5 days.

Corneal Ulcer
Ophthalmic: ADULTS, ELDERLY, CHILDREN OLDER THAN 5 YRS (IQUIX) (1.5%): Days 1–3: Instill 1–2 drops q30min to 2 hrs while awake and 4–6 hrs after retiring. **Days 4 through completion:** 1–2 drops q1–4h while awake.

Dosage in Renal Impairment
Normal renal function dosage of 500 mg/day:

Creatinine Clearance	Dosage
50–80 ml/min	No change
20–49 ml/min	500 mg initially, then 250 mg q24h
10–19 ml/min	500 mg initially, then 250 mg q48h

For pts undergoing dialysis, 500 mg initially, then 250 mg q48h.

Normal renal function dosage of 250 mg/day:

Creatinine Clearance	Dosage
20–49 ml/min	No change
10–19 ml/min	250 mg initially, then 250 mg q48h

Normal renal function dosage of 750 mg/day:

Creatinine Clearance	Dosage
50–80 ml/min	No change
20–49 ml/min	Initially, 750 mg, then 750 mg q48h
10–19 ml/min	Initially, 750 mg, then 500 mg q48h

Creatinine Clearance	Dosage
Dialysis	500 mg q48h (administer after dialysis on dialysis days)
Continuous Renal Replacement Therapy	
CVVH	500–750 mg once, then 250 mg q24h
CVVHD	500–750 mg once, then 250–500 mg q24h
CVVHDT	500–750 mg once, then 250–750 mg q24h

SIDE EFFECTS

Occasional (3%–1%): Diarrhea, nausea, abdominal pain, dizziness, drowsiness, headache. **Ophthalmic:** Local burning/discomfort, margin crusting, crystals/scales, foreign body sensation, ocular itching, altered taste. **Rare (less than 1%):** Flatulence; pain, inflammation, swelling in calves, hands, shoulder; chest pain; difficulty breathing; palpitations; edema; tendon pain. **Ophthalmic:** Corneal staining, keratitis, allergic reaction, eyelid swelling, tearing, reduced visual acuity.

ADVERSE EFFECTS/ TOXIC REACTIONS

Antibiotic-associated colitis, other superinfections (abdominal cramps, severe watery diarrhea, fever) may occur. Superinfection (genital/anal pruritus, ulceration/changes in oral mucosa, moderate to severe diarrhea) may occur from altered bacterial balance in GI tract. Hypersensitivity reactions, including photosensitivity (rash, pruritus, blisters, edema, sensation of burning skin) have occurred in pts receiving fluoroquinolones.

NURSING CONSIDERATIONS

BASELINE ASSESSMENT
Question for hypersensitivity to levofloxacin, other fluoroquinolones.

INTERVENTION/EVALUATION

Monitor serum glucose, renal/hepatic function tests. Monitor daily pattern of bowel activity, stool consistency. Report hypersensitivity reaction: skin rash, urticaria, pruritus, photosensitivity promptly. Be alert for superinfection: fever, vomiting, diarrhea, anal/genital pruritus, oral mucosal changes (ulceration, pain, erythema). Provide symptomatic relief for nausea. Evaluate food tolerance, altered taste.

PATIENT/ FAMILY TEACHING

• Drink 6–8 glasses of fluid a day (prevents formation of urine crystals). • Avoid tasks that require alertness, motor skills until response to drug is established (may cause dizziness, drowsiness). • Notify physician if tendon pain/swelling, palpitations, chest pain, difficulty breathing, persistent diarrhea occurs. • Avoid exposure to direct sunlight. • Report use of warfarin.

levomilnacipran

lee-voe-mil-**na**-si-pran
(Fetzima)
Do not confuse milnacipran with levomilnacipran.

BLACK BOX ALERT Increased risk of suicidal ideation and behavior in children, adolescents, and young adults 18–24 yrs with major depressive disorder, other psychiatric disorders. Not approved for pediatric use.

◆CLASSIFICATION

PHARMACOTHERAPEUTIC: Serotonin, norepinephrine reuptake inhibitor. **CLINICAL:** Antidepressant.

ACTION

Blocks reuptake of the neurotransmitter serotonin and norepinephrine at CNS neuronal presynaptic membranes, increasing availability at postsynaptic receptor sites. **Therapeutic Effect:** Relieves depression.

PHARMACOKINETICS

Readily absorbed following oral administration. Widely distributed. Metabolized in liver. Protein binding: 22%. Peak plasma concentration: 6–8 hrs. Primarily excreted in urine (58%). **Half-life:** 12 hrs.

USES

Treatment of major depressive disorder (MDD).
◄ALERT► Not indicated for management of fibromyalgia.

PRECAUTIONS

Contraindications: Hypersensitivity reactions to levomilnacipran or milnacipran, concomitant use or within 14 days of MAOIs, uncontrolled narrow-angle glaucoma. **Cautions:** Renal impairment, pts with increase risk of suicide, hypertension, tachycardia, history of seizures, alcohol abuse, dysuria (e.g., prostatic hypertrophy, prostatitis), controlled narrow-angle glaucoma.

⧗ LIFESPAN CONSIDERATIONS

Pregnancy/Lactation: Increased risk of fetal complications, including respiratory support if drug is given during third trimester of pregnancy. Unknown if distributed in breast milk. **Pregnancy Category C. Children:** Safety and efficacy not established in pts younger than 17 yrs. **Elderly:** No age-related precautions noted.

INTERACTIONS

DRUG: **Buspirone, fentanyl, linezolid, lithium, MAOIs, methylene blue, tramadol** may induce serotonin syndrome. **NSAIDs, anticoagulants, antiplatelets** may increase risk of bleeding. **Strong CYP3A4 inhibitors (e.g., ketoconazole, ritonavir)** may increase concentration/effects. **HERBAL:** St John's wort may increase risk of serotonin syndrome. **FOOD:** None known. **LAB VALUES:** May decrease serum sodium. May increase serum cholesterol.

AVAILABILITY (Rx)

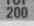 **Capsules (Extended-Release):** 20 mg, 40 mg, 80 mg, 120 mg.

ADMINISTRATION/HANDLING

PO

• Give without regard to meals. • Administer whole; do not crush, cut, or open capsule.

INDICATIONS/ROUTES/DOSAGE

Major Depressive Disorder

PO: ADULTS/ELDERLY: Initially, 20 mg once daily for 2 days, then increase to 40 mg once daily. Based on tolerability, may increase dose at 40-mg increments at intervals of 2 or more days. **Maximum dose:** 120 mg once daily. **Moderate Renal Impairment: Maximum dose:** 80 mg once daily. **Severe Renal Impairment: Maximum dose:** 40 mg once daily.

SIDE EFFECTS

Frequent (17%–9%): Nausea, constipation, hyperhidrosis. **Occasional (6%–3%):** Tachycardia, erectile dysfunction, vomiting, palpitations, ejaculation disorder, testicular pain, urinary hesitation, hypertension, flushing, anorexia, postural hypotension. **Rare (less than 2%):** Rash, dry eye, blurry vision, abdominal pain, migraine, urticaria.

ADVERSE EFFECTS/ TOXIC REACTIONS

May increase suicidal ideation in adolescents and young adults. Serotonin syndrome may include mental status changes (agitation, hallucinations, delirium), autonomic instability (tachycardia, labile blood pressure, dizziness, hyperthermia), neuromuscular symptoms (tremor, myoclonus, hyperreflexia, incoordination). May increase risk of bleeding (e.g., ecchymosis, hematoma, epistaxis, petechiae, GI bleeding). May worsen conditions of narrow-angle glaucoma. Abrupt discontinuation may induce withdrawal symptoms (dysphoria, irritability, agitation, dizziness, paresthesia, anxiety, confusion, headache, lethargy, emotional lability, tinnitus, seizures). Urinary hesitation or retention reported in 5% of pts. Activation of mania/hypomania reported in fewer than 1% of pts. Hyponatremia (including cases of serum sodium <110 mmol/L) may result in syncope, seizures, respiratory arrest, coma.

NURSING CONSIDERATIONS

BASELINE ASSESSMENT

Baseline vital signs, BMP. Receive full medication history including herbal products (esp. MAOIs). Screen for history of bipolar disorder, suicide ideation, seizures, alcohol dependency, narrow-angle glaucoma, urinary retention or benign prostatic hypertrophy. Baseline visual acuity.

INTERVENTION/EVALUATION

Monitor adolescents and young adults for suicidal ideation or behavior (esp. during initial mos of treatment or any dosage change). Monitor vital signs, serum sodium routinely. Obtain bladder scan for pts with urinary retention. Monitor for symptoms of serotonin syndrome.

PATIENT/FAMILY TEACHING

• Do not crush or chew capsule. • Avoid tasks that require alertness, motor skills until response to drug is established. • Do not abruptly discontinue medication. • Altered mood, agitation, insomnia, sweating, palpitations may indicate an overproduction of serotonin. • Report any changes in urinary frequency. • Report any newly prescribed medications. • Males may experience erectile dysfunction.

levothyroxine ⬛TOP 200

lee-voe-thy-**rox**-een
(Eltroxin ❋, Levothroid, Levoxyl, Synthroid, Tirosent, Unithroid)

BLACK BOX ALERT Ineffective, potentially toxic for weight reduction. High doses increase risk of serious, life-threatening toxic effects, especially when used with some anorectic drugs.

Do not confuse levothyroxine with levofloxacin or liothyronine, Levoxyl with Lanoxin or Luvox, or Synthroid with Symmetrel.

FIXED-COMBINATION(S)

With liothyronine, T₃ **(Thyrolar).**

◆CLASSIFICATION

PHARMACOTHERAPEUTIC: Synthetic isomer of thyroxine. **CLINICAL:** Thyroid hormone (T₄).

ACTION

Involved in normal metabolism, growth, development, esp. of CNS in infants. Possesses catabolic, anabolic effects. **Therapeutic Effect:** Increases basal metabolic rate, enhances gluconeogenesis, stimulates protein synthesis.

PHARMACOKINETICS

Variable, incomplete absorption from GI tract. Protein binding: greater than 99%. Widely distributed. Deiodinated in peripheral tissues, minimal metabolism in liver. Eliminated by biliary excretion. **Half-life:** 6–7 days.

USES

PO: Treatment of hypothyroidism, pituitary thyroid-stimulating hormone (TSH) suppression. **IV:** Myxedema coma.

PRECAUTIONS

Contraindications: Acute MI, thyrotoxicosis of any etiology, uncorrected adrenal insufficiency. **Capsule:** Inability to swallow capsules. **Cautions:** Elderly, angina pectoris, hypertension, other cardiovascular disease, adrenal insufficiency, myxedema, diabetes mellitus and insipidus, swallowing disorders.

⧖ LIFESPAN CONSIDERATIONS

Pregnancy/Lactation: Does not cross placenta. Minimal distribution in breast milk. **Pregnancy Category A. Children:** No age-related precautions noted. Caution in neonates in interpreting thyroid function tests. **Elderly:** May be more sensitive to thyroid effects; individualized dosage recommended.

INTERACTIONS

DRUG: Cholestyramine, colestipol, aluminum- and magnesium-containing antacids may decrease absorption. **Estrogens** may cause decrease in serum-free thyroxine. May enhance effect of **oral anticoagulants (e.g, warfarin). Sympathomimetics** may increase risk of coronary insufficiency, effects of levothyroxine. May decrease effect of **insulin, oral hypoglycemic agents. HERBAL:** None significant. **FOOD:** None known. **LAB VALUES:** None known.

AVAILABILITY (Rx)

Capsules (Tirosint): 13 mcg, 25 mcg, 50 mcg, 75 mcg, 88 mcg, 100 mcg, 112 mcg, 125 mcg, 137 mcg, 150 mcg. **Injection, Powder for Reconstitution (Synthroid):** 100 mcg, 500 mcg. **Tablets (Levothroid, Levoxyl, Synthroid, Unithroid):** 25 mcg, 50 mcg, 75 mcg, 88 mcg, 100 mcg, 112 mcg, 125 mcg, 137 mcg, 150 mcg, 175 mcg, 200 mcg, 300 mcg.

ADMINISTRATION/HANDLING

◀**ALERT**▶ Do not interchange brands (problems with bioequivalence between manufacturers).

 IV

Reconstitution • Reconstitute 200-mcg or 500-mcg vial with 5 ml 0.9% NaCl to provide concentration of 40 or 100 mcg/ml, respectively; shake until clear.
Rate of Administration • Use immediately; discard unused portions. • Give each 100 mcg or less over 1 min.
Storage • Store vials at room temperature.

PO

• Administer in the morning on an empty stomach, 30 min before food. • Administer before breakfast to prevent insomnia. • Tablets may be crushed. • Take 4 hrs apart from antacids, iron, calcium supplements.

⊞ IV INCOMPATIBILITIES

Do not use or mix with other IV solutions.

INDICATIONS/ROUTES/DOSAGE

Note: IV dose is 50% of oral dose.

Hypothyroidism

PO: ADULTS, GROWTH AND PUBERTY COMPLETE: 1.7 mcg/kg/day as single daily dose. Usual maintenance: 100–125 mcg/day. **ELDERLY (OLDER THAN 50 YRS):** Initially, 12.5–50 mcg/day. Adjust dose by 12.5–25 mcg/day at 4–8 wk intervals. **CHILDREN OLDER THAN 12 YRS, GROWTH AND PUBERTY INCOMPLETE:** 2–3 mcg/kg/day. **CHILDREN 6–12 YRS:** 4–5 mcg/kg/day. **CHILDREN 1–5 YRS:** 5–6 mcg/kg/day. **CHILDREN 6–12 MOS:** 6–8 mcg/kg/day. **CHILDREN 3–5 MOS:** 8–10 mcg/kg/day. **CHILDREN YOUNGER THAN 3 MOS:** 10–15 mcg/kg/day.

Myxedema Coma

IV: ADULTS, ELDERLY: Initially, 200–500 mcg, then 100–300 mcg next day if necessary.

Pituitary Thyroid-Stimulating Hormone (TSH) Suppression

PO: ADULTS, ELDERLY: Doses greater than 2 mcg/kg/day usually required to suppress TSH below 0.1 milliunits/L.

SIDE EFFECTS

Occasional: Reversible hair loss at start of therapy in children. **Rare:** Dry skin, GI intolerance, rash, urticaria, pseudotumor cerebri, severe headache in children.

ADVERSE EFFECTS/ TOXIC REACTIONS

Excessive dosage produces signs/symptoms of hyperthyroidism (weight loss, palpitations, increased appetite, tremors, anxiety, tachycardia, hypertension, headache, insomnia, menstrual irregularities). Cardiac arrhythmias occur rarely.

NURSING CONSIDERATIONS

BASELINE ASSESSMENT

Obtain baseline TSH, T_3, T_4, weight, vital signs. Signs/symptoms of diabetes mellitus, diabetes insipidus, adrenal insufficiency, hypopituitarism may become intensified. Treat with adrenocortical steroids before thyroid therapy in coexisting hypothyroidism and hypoadrenalism.

INTERVENTION/EVALUATION

Monitor pulse for rate, rhythm (report pulse greater than 100 or marked increase). Observe for tremors, anxiety. Assess appetite, sleep pattern. **Children: (Undertreatment):** May decrease intellectual development, linear growth. **(Overtreatment):** Adversely affects brain maturation, accelerates bone age. Monitor thyroid function test.

PATIENT/ FAMILY TEACHING

• Do not discontinue drug therapy; replacement for hypothyroidism is lifelong. • Follow-up office visits, thyroid function tests are essential. • Take medication at the same time each day, preferably in the morning. • Monitor pulse for rate, rhythm; report irregular rhythm or pulse rate over 100 beats/min. • Notify physician promptly of chest pain, weight loss, anxiety, tremors, insomnia. • Children may have reversible hair loss, increased aggressiveness during first few mos of therapy. • Full therapeutic effect may take 1–3 wks.

---

lidocaine

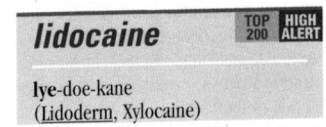

lye-doe-kane
(Lidoderm, Xylocaine)

FIXED-COMBINATION(S)

EMLA: lidocaine/prilocaine (an anesthetic): 2.5%/2.5%. **Lidosite:** lidocaine/epinephrine (a sympathomimetic): 10%/0.1%. **Lidocaine with epinephrine** (a sympathomimetic): 2%/1:50,000, 1%/1:100,000, 1%/1:200,000, 0.5%/1:200,000. **Synera:** lidocaine/tetracaine (an anesthetic): 70 mg/70 mg.

◆CLASSIFICATION

PHARMACOTHERAPEUTIC: Amide anesthetic. **CLINICAL:** Antiarrhythmic, anesthetic (see pp. 7C, 8C, 17C).

ACTION

Anesthetic: Inhibits conduction of nerve impulses. **Therapeutic Effect:** Causes temporary loss of feeling/sensation. **Antiarrhythmic:** Decreases depolarization, automaticity, excitability of ventricle during diastole by direct action. **Therapeutic Effect:** Inhibits ventricular arrhythmias.

PHARMACOKINETICS

Route	Onset	Peak	Duration
IV	30–90 sec	N/A	10–20 min
Local anesthetic	2.5 min	N/A	30–60 min

Completely absorbed after IM administration. Protein binding: 60%–80%. Widely distributed. Metabolized in liver. Primarily excreted in urine. Minimally removed by hemodialysis. **Half-life:** 1–2 hrs.

USES

Antiarrhythmic: Rapid control of acute ventricular arrhythmias following MI, cardiac catheterization, cardiac surgery, digitalis-induced ventricular arrhythmias. **Local Anesthetic:** Infiltration/nerve block for dental/surgical procedures, childbirth. **Topical Anesthetic:** Local skin disorders (minor burns, insect bites, prickly heat, skin manifestations of chickenpox, abrasions). Mucous membranes (local anesthesia of oral, nasal, laryngeal mucous membranes; local anesthesia of respiratory, urinary tracts; relief of discomfort of pruritus ani, hemorrhoids, pruritus vulvae). **Dermal patch:** Relief of chronic pain in post-herpetic neuralgia, allodynia (painful hypersensitivity). **OFF-LABEL:** IV infusion for chronic pain syndrome.

PRECAUTIONS

Contraindications: Adams-Stokes syndrome, hypersensitivity to amide-type local anesthetics, supraventricular arrhythmias, Wolff-Parkinson-White syndrome. Severe degree of SA, AV, or intraventricular heart block (except in pts with functioning pacemaker). **Cautions:** Hepatic disease, marked hypoxia, severe respiratory depression, hypovolemia, incomplete heart block, bradycardia, atrial fibrillation, heart failure.

⊠ LIFESPAN CONSIDERATIONS

Pregnancy/Lactation: Crosses placenta. Distributed in breast milk. **Pregnancy Category B. Children:** No age-related precautions noted. **Elderly:** More sensitive to adverse effects. Dose, rate of infusion should be reduced. Age-related renal impairment may require dosage adjustment.

INTERACTIONS

DRUG: Class 1 antiarrhythmics may increase cardiac effects. **HERBAL: St. John's wort** may decrease concentration. **FOOD:** None known. **LAB VALUES:** IM lidocaine may increase creatine kinase (CK) level (used to diagnose acute MI). **Therapeutic serum level:** 1.5 to 6 mcg/ml; **toxic serum level:** greater than 6 mcg/ml.

AVAILABILITY (Rx)

Cream, Topical: 4%. **Infusion Premix:** 0.4% (4 mg/ml in 250 ml, 500 ml); 0.8% (8 mg/ml in 250 ml, 500 ml). **Injection, Solution:** 0.5% (5 mg/ml), 1% (10 mg/ml), 2% (20 mg/ml). **Jelly, Topical:** 2%. **Solution, Topical:** 4%. **Solution, Viscous:** 2%. **Transdermal, Topical (Lidoderm):** 5%.

ADMINISTRATION/HANDLING

◀**ALERT**▶ Resuscitative equipment, drugs (including O_2) must always be

L

readily available when administering lidocaine by any route.

IV

◀ **ALERT** ▶ Use only lidocaine without preservative, clearly marked **for IV use.**
Reconstitution • For IV infusion, prepare solution by adding 2 g to 250–500 ml D_5W or 0.9% NaCl to provide concentration of 8 mg/ml or 4 mg/ml, respectively. • Commercially available preparations of 0.4% and 0.8% may be used for IV infusion. **Maximum concentration:** 4 g/ 250 ml (16 mg/ml).
Rate of Administration • For IV push, use 1% (10 mg/ml) or 2% (20 mg/ml). • Administer IV push at rate of 25–50 mg/min. • Administer for IV infusion at rate of 1–4 mg/min (1–4 ml); use volume control IV set.
Storage • Store premix solutions at room temperature.

IM

• Use 10% (100 mg/ml); clearly identify lidocaine that is **for IM use.** • Give in deltoid muscle (serum level is significantly higher than if injection is given in gluteus muscle or lateral thigh).

Topical

• Not for ophthalmic use. • For skin disorders, apply directly to affected area or put on gauze or bandage, which is then applied to the skin. • For mucous membrane use, apply to desired area per manufacturer's insert. • Administer lowest dosage possible that still provides anesthesia.

Dermal Patch

Patch may be cut to appropriate size.

IV INCOMPATIBILITIES

Amphotericin B complex (Abelcet, AmBisome, Amphotec).

IV COMPATIBILITIES

Amiodarone (Cordarone), calcium gluconate, dexmedetomidine (Precedex), digoxin (Lanoxin), diltiazem (Cardizem),

dobutamine (Dobutrex), dopamine (Intropin), enalapril (Vasotec), furosemide (Lasix), heparin, insulin, nitroglycerin, potassium chloride.

INDICATIONS/ROUTES/DOSAGE

Ventricular Arrhythmias

IM: ADULTS, ELDERLY: 300 mg (or 4.3 mg/ kg). May repeat in 60–90 min.
IV: ADULTS, ELDERLY: Initially, 1–1.5 mg/ kg. Refractory ventricular tachycardia, fibrillation: Repeat dose at 0.5–0.75 mg/kg q10–15min after initial dose for a maximum of 3 doses. Total dose not to exceed 3 mg/kg. Follow with continuous infusion (1–4 mg/min) after return of perfusion. Reappearance of arrhythmia during infusion: 0.5 mg/kg, reassess infusion. **CHILDREN, INFANTS:** Initially, 1 mg/kg (**maximum:** 100 mg). May repeat second dose of 0.5–1 mg/kg if start of infusion longer than 15 min. Maintenance: 20–50 mcg/ kg/min as IV infusion.

Local Anesthesia

Infiltration, Nerve Block: ADULTS: Local anesthetic dosage varies with procedure, degree of anesthesia, vascularity, duration. **Maximum dose:** 4.5 mg/kg. Do not repeat within 2 hrs.

Topical Local Anesthesia

Topical: ADULTS, ELDERLY: Apply to affected areas as needed.

Treatment of Post-Herpetic Neuralgia

◀ **ALERT** ▶ Transdermal patch may contain conducting metal (e.g., aluminum). Remove patch prior to MRI.
Topical *(Dermal Patch):* **ADULTS, ELDERLY:** Apply to intact skin over most painful area (up to 3 applications once for up to 12 hrs in a 24-hr period).

SIDE EFFECTS

CNS effects generally dose-related and of short duration. **Occasional: IM:** Pain at injection site. **Topical:** Burning, stinging, tenderness at application site. **Rare:** Generally associated with high dose: Drowsiness; dizziness; disorientation; light-headedness;

tremors; apprehension; euphoria; sensation of heat, cold, numbness; blurred or double vision; tinnitus (ringing in ears); nausea.

ADVERSE EFFECTS/ TOXIC REACTIONS

Serious adverse reactions to lidocaine are uncommon, but high dosage by any route may produce cardiovascular depression, bradycardia, hypotension, arrhythmias, heart block, cardiovascular collapse, cardiac arrest. Potential for malignant hyperthermia, CNS toxicity may occur, esp. with regional anesthesia use, progressing rapidly from mild side effects to tremors, drowsiness, seizures, vomiting, respiratory depression. Methemoglobinemia (evidenced by cyanosis) has occurred following topical application of lidocaine for teething discomfort and laryngeal anesthetic spray.

NURSING CONSIDERATIONS

BASELINE ASSESSMENT

Question for hypersensitivity to lidocaine, amide anesthetics. Obtain baseline B/P, pulse, respiratory rate, EKG, serum electrolytes.

INTERVENTION/EVALUATION

Monitor EKG, vital signs closely during and following drug administration for cardiac performance. If EKG shows arrhythmias, prolongation of PR interval or QRS complex, inform physician immediately. Assess pulse for rhythm, rate, quality. Assess B/P for evidence of hypotension. Monitor for therapeutic serum level (1.5–6 mcg/ml). For lidocaine given by all routes, monitor vital signs, LOC. Drowsiness should be considered a warning sign of high serum levels of lidocaine. **Therapeutic serum level:** 1.5–6 mcg/ml; **toxic serum level:** greater than 6 mcg/ml.

PATIENT/ FAMILY TEACHING

• **Local anesthesia:** Due to loss of feeling/sensation, protective measures may be needed until anesthetic wears off (no ambulation, including special positions for some regional anesthesia). • **Oral mucous membrane anesthesia:** Do not eat, drink, chew gum for 1 hr after application (swallowing reflex may be impaired, increasing risk of aspiration; numbness of tongue, buccal mucosa may lead to bite trauma). • **IV infusions:** Report dizziness, numbness, double vision, nausea, pain/burning, respiratory difficulty. • **Topical:** Report irritation, pain, numbness, swelling, blurred vision, tinnitus, respiratory difficulty.

linaclotide

lin-a-**kloe**-tide
(Linzess)

BLACK BOX ALERT Contraindicated in pediatric pts 6 yrs of age and younger. Avoid use in pediatric patients 7 yrs through 17 yrs old.

◆CLASSIFICATION

PHARMACOTHERAPEUTIC: Guanylate cyclase-C (cGMP) agonist. **CLINICAL:** Anti-constipation agent.

ACTION

Binds on the luminal surface of GI epithelium. Increase cGMP which stimulates chloride and bicarbonate into intestinal lumen. **Therapeutic Effect:** Increase intestinal fluid, accelerates transit.

PHARMACOKINETICS

Metabolized within GI tract. Minimal distribution beyond GI tissue. Minimal systemic absorption. **Half-life:** N/A.

USES

Treatment of irritable bowel syndrome with constipation, chronic idiopathic constipation.

PRECAUTIONS

Contraindications: Pediatric patients 6 yrs and younger, known or suspected mechanical GI obstruction. **Cautions:** Diarrhea.

⧗ LIFESPAN CONSIDERATIONS

Pregnancy/Lactation: Unknown if distributed in breast milk. **Pregnancy Category C. Children:** Avoid use in pediatric pts 7 yrs through 17 yrs. Contraindicated in pediatric pts 6 yrs of age and younger. **Elderly:** No age-related precautions noted.

INTERACTIONS

DRUG: None significant. **HERBAL:** None significant. **FOOD:** None known. **LAB VALUES:** None significant.

AVAILABILITY (Rx)

💊 **Capsules:** 145 mcg, 290 mcg.

ADMINISTRATION/HANDLING

PO
• Do not break, crush, dissolve, or divide capsule.

INDICATIONS/ROUTES/DOSAGE

Irritable Bowel Syndrome With Constipation
PO: ADULTS 18 YRS AND OLDER, ELDERLY: 290 mcg once daily. • Give on empty stomach at least 30 min prior to first meal of day.

Chronic Idiopathic Constipation
PO: ADULTS 18 YRS AND OLDER, ELDERLY: 145 mcg once daily.

SIDE EFFECTS

Frequent (16%): Diarrhea (may begin within first 2 wks of initiation of treatment). **Occasional (7%–2%):** Abdominal pain, flatulence, headache, abdominal distention. **Rare (1% and Less):** Gastroesophageal reflux, vomiting.

ADVERSE EFFECTS/TOXIC REACTIONS

Severe diarrhea was reported in 2% of pts. Viral gastroenteritis was noted in 3% of pts. Fecal incontinence, dehydration

was reported in 1%. Dose reduced or suspended secondary to diarrhea, other GI adverse reaction.

NURSING CONSIDERATIONS

BASELINE ASSESSMENT
Encourage adequate fluid intake. Assess bowel sounds for peristalsis. Monitor daily bowel activity, stool consistency (watery, loose, soft, semisolid, solid) and record time of evacuation. Assess for abdominal disturbances. Monitor serum electrolytes in pts with prolonged, frequent, or excessive use of medication.

INTERVENTION/EVALUATION
For pts with irritable bowel syndrome, assess for improvement in symptoms (relief from bloating, cramping, urgency, abdominal discomfort).

PATIENT/FAMILY TEACHING
• Institute measures to promote defecation: increase fluid intake, exercise, high-fiber diet. • Report new/worsening episodes of abdominal pain, severe diarrhea. • Do not break, crush, dissolve, or divide capsule. Take whole.

L

linagliptin

lin-a-**glip**-tin
(Tradjenta)
Do not confuse linagliptin with saxagliptin or sitagliptin.

FIXED-COMBINATION(S)

Jentadueto: linagliptin/metformin (an antidiabetic): 2.5 mg/500 mg; 2.5 mg/850 mg; 2.5 mg/1,000 mg.

◆CLASSIFICATION

PHARMACOTHERAPEUTIC: Dipeptidyl peptidase-4 (DDP-4) inhibitor (gliptan). **CLINICAL:** Antidiabetic agent (see p. 44C).

ACTION

Slows inactivation of incretin hormones by inhibiting DDP-4 enzyme. **Therapeutic Effect:** Incretin hormones increase insulin synthesis/release from pancreas and decrease glucagon secretion. Lowers serum glucose levels.

PHARMACOKINETICS

Rapidly absorbed following PO administration. Peak plasma concentration: 1.5 hrs. Extensive tissue distribution. Protein binding: 70%–99%. Minimal metabolism (90% excreted as unchanged metabolite). Excreted primarily in enterohepatic system (80%), urine (5%). **Half-life:** 12 hrs.

USES

Adjunctive treatment to diet and exercise to improve glycemic controls in pts with type 2 diabetes mellitus alone or in combination with insulin.

PRECAUTIONS

Contraindications: History of hypersensitive reactions to DD4 inhibitors. **Cautions:** Concurrent use of other hypoglycemics. Not recommended for use in Type 1 diabetes, diabetic ketoacidosis.

⌛ LIFESPAN CONSIDERATIONS

Pregnancy/Lactation: Unknown if distributed in breast milk. **Pregnancy Category B. Children:** Safety and efficacy not established. **Elderly:** No age-related precautions noted.

INTERACTIONS

DRUG: CYP3A4 inducers (e.g., rifampin) may decrease concentration. **Insulin, metformin, saxagliptin, sitagliptin, sulfonylureas** may increase risk of hypoglycemia. **HERBAL: Ginseng, ginger, other herbs with hypoglycemic activity** may increase risk of hypoglycemia. **FOOD:** None known. **LAB VALUES:** Decreases serum glucose. May increase serum uric acid.

AVAILABILITY (Rx)

Tablets: 5 mg.

ADMINISTRATION/HANDLING

PO
• May give without regard to food.

INDICATIONS/ROUTES/DOSAGE

Type 2 Diabetes Mellitus
PO: ADULTS, ELDERLY: 5 mg once daily.

SIDE EFFECTS

Occasional (5%): Nasopharyngitis. **Rare (less than 2%):** Cough, headache.

ADVERSE EFFECTS/ TOXIC REACTIONS

Hypoglycemia reported in 7% of pts. Concomitant use of hypoglycemic medication may increase hypoglycemic risk. Pancreatitis, hypersensitivity reactions (angioedema, rash, urticaria, pruritus, bronchospasm) occur rarely.

NURSING CONSIDERATIONS

BASELINE ASSESSMENT

Check blood glucose, hemoglobin A_{1c} level. Assess pt's understanding of diabetes management, routine glucose monitoring. Receive full medication history including vitamins, minerals, herbal products.

INTERVENTION/EVALUATION

Monitor blood glucose, hemoglobin A_{1c} level. Assess for hypoglycemia (diaphoresis, tremors, dizziness, anxiety, headache, tachycardia, perioral numbness, hunger, diplopia, difficulty concentrating), hyperglycemia (polyuria, polyphagia, polydipsia, nausea, vomiting, fatigue, Kussmaul breathing). Screen for glucose-altering conditions: fever, increased activity or stress, surgical procedures. Dietary consult for nutritional education.

PATIENT/FAMILY TEACHING

• Diabetes mellitus requires lifelong control. • Diet and exercise is principal part of treatment; do not skip or delay meals. • Test blood glucose regularly. • When taking combination drug therapy or when glucose demands are altered (fever, infection, trauma, stress, heavy physical activity), have hypoglycemic treatment available (glucagon, oral dextrose). • Monitor daily calorie intake.

linezolid

lin-**ez**-oh-lid
(<u>Zyvox</u>, Zyvoxam ✤)
Do not confuse Zyvox with Zosyn or Zovirax.

◆CLASSIFICATION

PHARMACOTHERAPEUTIC: Oxazolidinone. **CLINICAL:** Antibiotic.

ACTION

Binds to bacterial ribosomal RNA sites preventing formation of a complex essential for bacterial translation. **Therapeutic Effect:** Bacteriostatic against enterococci, staphylococci; bactericidal against streptococci.

PHARMACOKINETICS

Rapidly, extensively absorbed after PO administration. Protein binding: 31%. Metabolized in liver by oxidation. Excreted in urine. **Half-life:** 4–5.4 hrs.

USES

Treatment of susceptible infections due to aerobic and facultative, gram-positive microorganisms, including *E. faecium* (vancomycin-resistant strains only), *S. aureus* (including methicillin-resistant strains), *S. agalactiae*, *S. pneumoniae* (including multidrug-resistant strains), *S. pyogenes*. Treatment of pneumonia (community-acquired and hospital acquired), skin, soft tissue infections (including diabetic foot infections), bacteremia caused by susceptible vancomycin-resistant organisms.

PRECAUTIONS

Contraindications: Concurrent use or within 2 wks of MAOIs; uncontrolled hypertension, pheochromocytoma, thyrotoxicosis, concurrent sympathomimetic, vasopressive, or dopaminergic agents (unless closely monitored); carcinoid syndrome, concurrent use with SSRIs, tricyclic antidepressants, 5-HT agonists, or buspirone. **Cautions:** Severe renal/hepatic impairment, untreated hyperthyroidism. History of seizures, preexisting myelosuppression, other medications that may cause bone marrow depression.

⧗ LIFESPAN CONSIDERATIONS

Pregnancy/Lactation: Unknown if distributed in breast milk. **Pregnancy Category C. Children:** Safety and efficacy not established. **Elderly:** No age-related precautions noted.

INTERACTIONS

DRUG: CYP3A4 inducers (e.g., carbamazepine, phenytoin) may decrease concentration/effects. **Adrenergic medications (sympathomimetics)** may increase effect. **SSRIs** may increase risk of serotonin syndrome. **HERBAL:** Supplements containing **caffeine, tyrosine,** or **tryptophan** may precipitate hypertensive crisis. **FOOD:** Excessive amounts of **tyramine-containing foods, beverages** may cause significant hypertension. **LAB VALUES:** May decrease Hgb, neutrophils, platelets, WBC. May increase serum ALT, AST, alkaline phosphatase, amylase, bilirubin, BUN, creatinine, LDH, lipase.

AVAILABILITY (Rx)

Injection Premix: 2 mg/ml in 100-ml, 300-ml bags. **Powder for Oral Suspension:** 100 mg/5 ml. **Tablets:** 600 mg.

ADMINISTRATION/HANDLING
🖲 IV

Rate of Administration • Infuse over 30–120 min. • Should be administered without further dilution.
Storage • Store at room temperature. • Protect from light. • Yellow color does not affect potency.

PO

• Give without regard to meals. • Use suspension within 21 days after reconstitution. Gently invert 3–5 times before administration. • Do not shake.

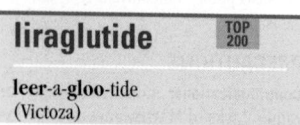 IV INCOMPATIBILITIES

Amphotericin B complex (Abelcet, AmBisome, Amphotec), co-trimoxazole (Bactrim), diazepam (Valium), erythromycin (Erythrocin), pentamidine (Pentam IV), phenytoin (Dilantin).

IV COMPATIBILITIES

Calcium gluconate, dexmedetomidine (Precedex), heparin, magnesium, potassium chloride.

INDICATIONS/ROUTES/DOSAGE

Vancomycin-Resistant Infections (VRI)
PO, IV: ADULTS, ELDERLY, CHILDREN OLDER THAN 11 YRS: 600 mg q12h for 14–28 days. **CHILDREN 11 YRS AND YOUNGER:** 10 mg/kg q8–12h for 14–28 days.

Nosocomial Pneumonia, Community-Acquired Pneumonia, Complicated Skin/Skin Structure Infections
PO, IV: ADULTS, ELDERLY, CHILDREN OLDER THAN 11 YRS: 600 mg q12h for 10–14 days. **CHILDREN 11 YRS AND YOUNGER:** 10 mg/kg q8h for 10–14 days.

Uncomplicated Skin/Skin Structure Infections
PO: ADULTS, ELDERLY: 400 mg q12h for 10–14 days. **CHILDREN OLDER THAN 11 YRS:** 600 mg q12h for 10–14 days. **CHILDREN 5–11 YRS:** 10 mg/kg/dose q12h for 10–14 days. **CHILDREN YOUNGER THAN 5 YRS:** 10 mg/kg q8h for 10–14 days.

MRSA
PO, IV: ADULTS, ELDERLY: 600 mg q12h.

Usual Neonate Dosage
PO, IV: NEONATES: 10 mg/kg/dose q8–12h.

SIDE EFFECTS

Occasional (9%–2%): Diarrhea, nausea, vomiting, insomnia, constipation, rash, dizziness, fever, headache. **Rare (less than 2%):** Altered taste, vaginal candidiasis, fungal infection, tongue discoloration.

ADVERSE EFFECTS/ TOXIC REACTIONS

Thrombocytopenia, myelosuppression occur rarely. Antibiotic-associated colitis, other superinfections (abdominal cramps, severe watery diarrhea, fever) may result from altered bacterial balance in GI tract.

NURSING CONSIDERATIONS

BASELINE ASSESSMENT

Obtain appropriate culture specimens for sensitivity testing prior to therapy. Obtain baseline CBC, chemistries.

INTERVENTION/EVALUATION

Monitor daily pattern of bowel activity, stool consistency. Mild GI effects may be tolerable, but increasing severity may indicate onset of antibiotic-associated colitis. Be alert for superinfection: fever, vomiting, diarrhea, anal/genital pruritus, oral mucosal changes (ulceration, pain, erythema). Monitor CBC, platelets, Hgb, chemistries.

PATIENT/ FAMILY TEACHING

• Continue therapy for full length of treatment. • Doses should be evenly spaced. • May cause GI upset (may take with food, milk). • Excessive amounts of tyramine-containing foods (red wine, aged cheese) may cause severe reaction (severe headache, neck stiffness, diaphoresis, palpitations). • Avoid alcohol. • Report persistent diarrhea, nausea, vomiting.

liraglutide

leer-a-**gloo**-tide
(Victoza)

BLACK BOX ALERT Causes dose-dependent and treatment duration–dependent thyroid C-cell tumors, including medullary thyroid cancer.

◆CLASSIFICATION

PHARMACOTHERAPEUTIC: Antihyperglycemic (glucagon-like peptide-1 [GLP-1] receptor agonist. **CLINICAL:** Antidiabetic agent (see p. 45C).

ACTION

Stimulates release of insulin from pancreatic beta cells, mimics enhancement of glucose-dependent insulin secretion, suppresses elevated glucagon secretion, slows gastric emptying. **Therapeutic Effect:** Improves glycemic control by increasing postmeal insulin secretion, emptying, increasing satiety.

PHARMACOKINETICS

Maximum concentration achieved in 8–12 hrs. Protein binding: 98%. Metabolized to large proteins without a specific organ as major route of elimination. **Half-life:** 13 hrs.

USES

Adjunct to diet and exercise to improve glycemic control in adult pts with type 2 diabetes mellitus.

PRECAUTIONS

Contraindications: Personal or family history of medullary thyroid carcinoma, pts with multiple endocrine neoplasia syndrome type 2. **Cautions:** History of pancreatitis, cholelithiasis, alcohol abuse, renal/hepatic impairment. History of angioedema to other GLP-1 receptor agonists. Do not use in type 1 diabetes or diabetic ketoacidosis.

☒ LIFESPAN CONSIDERATIONS

Pregnancy/Lactation: Unknown if distributed in breast milk. **Pregnancy Category C. Children:** Safety and efficacy not established. **Elderly:** No age-related precautions noted.

INTERACTIONS

DRUG: Liraglutide has potential to alter absorption of concurrently administered **oral medications. HERBAL:** None significant. **FOOD:** None known. **LAB VALUES:** Decreases glucose serum levels (when used in combination with insulin secretagogues [e.g., sulfonylureas]).

AVAILABILITY (Rx)

Subcutaneous, Solution (Prefilled Pen): 6 mg/ml.

ADMINISTRATION/HANDLING

Subcutaneous
• May be given in thigh, abdomen, upper arm. • Rotation of injection sites is essential; maintain careful records. • Give at any time without regard to meals.
Storage • Refrigerate prefilled pens. • Discard if freezing occurs. • Discard pen 30 days after initial use.

INDICATIONS/ROUTES/DOSAGE

Diabetes Mellitus
Subcutaneous: ADULTS, ELDERLY: Initial dose: 0.6 mg subcutaneously once per day for at least 1 wk. This dose is intended to reduce GI symptoms during initial titration; it is not effective for glycemic control. After 1 wk, increase dose to 1.2 mg. If 1.2-mg dose does not result in acceptable glycemic control, dose can be increased to 1.8 mg.

SIDE EFFECTS

Frequent (greater than 13%): Headache, nausea, diarrhea, liraglutide antibody resistance. **Occasional (13%–6%):** Diarrhea, vomiting, dizziness, jitteriness, dyspepsia. **Rare (less than 6%):** Weakness, decreased appetite.

ADVERSE EFFECTS/ TOXIC REACTIONS

Serious hypoglycemia may occur when used concurrently with insulin analogue (e.g., sulfonylurea); consider lowering dose.

L

NURSING CONSIDERATIONS

BASELINE ASSESSMENT

Check blood glucose concentration before administration. Discuss pt's lifestyle to determine extent of learning, emotional needs. Ensure follow-up instruction if pt/family does not thoroughly understand diabetes management or glucose testing technique. Dose is gradually increased to improve GI tolerance.

INTERVENTION/EVALUATION

Monitor blood glucose level, food intake. Assess for hypoglycemia (cool wet skin, tremors, dizziness, anxiety, headache, tachycardia, numbness in mouth, hunger, diplopia) or hyperglycemia (polyuria, polyphagia, polydipsia, nausea, vomiting, dim vision, fatigue, deep rapid breathing). Be alert to conditions that alter glucose requirements (fever, increased activity/stress, surgical procedures). Consider lowering dose of insulin analogue to reduce risk of hypoglycemia.

PATIENT/FAMILY TEACHING

• Diabetes mellitus requires lifelong control. • Prescribed diet, exercise are principal parts of treatment; do not skip/delay meals. • Continue following dietary instructions, regular exercise program, regular testing of blood glucose level. • Serious hypoglycemia may occur when used concurrently with insulin analogue (e.g., sulfonylurea). • Have source of glucose available to treat symptoms of low blood sugar.

TOP 200

lisdexamfetamine

lis-dex-am-**fet**-a-meen
(Vyvanse)

BLACK BOX ALERT Associated with serious cardiovascular events in pts with preexisting structural cardiac abnormalities or other serious heart problems. Potential for drug dependency exists.

Do not confuse lisdexamfetamine with dextroamphetamine, or Vyvanse with Glucovance, Vivactil, or Vytorin.

◆ CLASSIFICATION

PHARMACOTHERAPEUTIC: Amphetamine **(Schedule II). CLINICAL:** CNS stimulant.

ACTION

Enhances action of dopamine, norepinephrine by blocking reuptake from synapses, increasing levels in extraneuronal space. **Therapeutic Effect:** Improves attention span in ADHD.

PHARMACOKINETICS

Rapidly absorbed. Converted to dextroamphetamine. Excreted in urine. **Half-life:** Less than 1 hr.

USES

Treatment of ADHD.

PRECAUTIONS

Contraindications: Concurrent use or within 2 wks of use of MAOI. **Cautions:** Hyperthyroidism, glaucoma, agitated states, cardiovascular conditions (hypertension, recent MI, ventricular arrhythmias), elderly, psychiatric/seizures.

⏳ LIFESPAN CONSIDERATIONS

Pregnancy/Lactation: Has potential for fetal harm. Unknown if distributed in breast milk. **Pregnancy Category C. Children:** Safety and efficacy not established in those younger than 6 yrs. **Elderly:** No age-related precautions noted.

INTERACTIONS

DRUG: MAOIs may prolong/intensify effects. May decrease sedative effect of **antihistamines.** May decrease hypotensive effects of **antihypertensives.** Effects may be decreased by **chlorpromazine, haloperidol, lithium, urinary**

acidifying agents (**ammonium chloride, sodium acid phosphate**). May increase absorption of **phenobarbital, phenytoin.** Tricyclic antidepressants may increase cardiovascular effects. **HERBAL:** None significant. **FOOD:** None known. **LAB VALUES:** May increase plasma corticosteroid.

AVAILABILITY (Rx)

Capsules: 20 mg, 30 mg, 40 mg, 50 mg, 60 mg, 70 mg.

ADMINISTRATION/HANDLING

PO

• May be given in the morning without regard to food. • Administer capsule whole; pt must not chew. • Capsules may be opened and dissolved in water and taken immediately.

INDICATIONS/ROUTES/DOSAGE

ADHD

PO: ADULTS, CHILDREN 6 YRS AND OLDER: Initially, 30 mg once daily in the morning. May increase dosage in increments of 10 or 20 mg/day at weekly intervals. **Maximum:** 70 mg/day.

SIDE EFFECTS

Frequent (39%): Decreased appetite. **Occasional (19%–9%):** Insomnia, upper abdominal pain, headache, irritability, vomiting, weight decrease. **Rare (6%–2%):** Nausea, dry mouth, dizziness, rash, affect change, fatigue, tic.

ADVERSE EFFECTS/ TOXIC REACTIONS

Abrupt withdrawal following prolonged administration of high dosage may produce extreme fatigue (may last for wks). Prolonged administration to children with ADHD may produce a suppression of weight and/or height patterns. May produce cardiac irregularities, psychotic syndrome.

NURSING CONSIDERATIONS

BASELINE ASSESSMENT

Assess attention span, impulse control, interaction with others.

INTERVENTION/EVALUATION

Monitor for CNS stimulation, increase in B/P, weight loss, pulse, sleep pattern, appetite. Observe for signs of hostility, aggression, depression.

PATIENT/FAMILY TEACHING

• Take early in day. • May mask extreme fatigue. • Report pronounced dizziness, decreased appetite, dry mouth, weight loss, new or worsened psychiatric problems, palpitations, dyspnea.

---

lisinopril `TOP 200`

lye-**sin**-o-pril
(Apo-Lisinopril ✷, Prinivil, <u>Zestril</u>)

BLACK BOX ALERT May cause fetal injury, mortality if used during second or third trimester of pregnancy. **Do not confuse lisinopril with fosinopril, or Prinivil with Plendil, Pravachol, Prevacid, Prilosec, Proventil, or Restoril, or Zestril with Desyrel, Restoril, Vistaril, Zetia, or Zostrix. Do not confuse lisinopril's combination form Zestoretic with Prilosec.**

FIXED-COMBINATION(S)

Prinzide/Zestoretic: lisinopril/hydrochlorothiazide (a diuretic): 10 mg/12.5 mg, 20 mg/12.5 mg, 20 mg/25 mg.

✦CLASSIFICATION

PHARMACOTHERAPEUTIC: ACE inhibitor. **CLINICAL:** Antihypertensive (see p. 9C, 61C).

ACTION

Suppresses renin-angiotensin-aldosterone system (prevents conversion of angiotensin

---

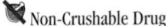 ✷ Canadian trade name   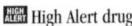 Non-Crushable Drug   **HIGH ALERT** High Alert drug

I to angiotensin II, a potent vasoconstrictor; may inhibit angiotensin II at local vascular, renal sites). Decreases plasma angiotensin II, increases plasma renin activity, decreases aldosterone secretion. **Therapeutic Effect:** Reduces peripheral arterial resistance, B/P (afterload), pulmonary capillary wedge pressure (preload), pulmonary vascular resistance. In those with heart failure, decreases heart size, increases cardiac output, exercise tolerance time.

PHARMACOKINETICS

Route	Onset	Peak	Duration
PO	1 hr	6 hrs	24 hrs

Incompletely absorbed from GI tract. Protein binding: 25%. Primarily excreted unchanged in urine. Removed by hemodialysis. **Half-life:** 12 hrs (increased in renal impairment).

USES

Treatment of hypertension. Used alone or in combination with other antihypertensives. Adjunctive therapy in management of heart failure. Treatment of acute MI within 24 hrs in hemodynamically stable pts to improve survival. Treatment of left ventricular dysfunction following MI.

PRECAUTIONS

Contraindications: History of angioedema from treatment with ACE inhibitors, idiopathic or hereditary angioedema. Concomitant use with aliskiren in pts with diabetes. **Cautions:** Renal impairment, unstented unilateral/bilateral renal artery stenosis, volume depletion, ischemic heart disease, cerebrovascular disease, severe aortic stenosis, hypertrophic cardiomyopathy.

⌛ LIFESPAN CONSIDERATIONS

Pregnancy/Lactation: Crosses placenta. Unknown if distributed in breast milk. **Pregnancy Category C (D if used in second or third trimester). Children:** Safety and efficacy not established. **Elderly:** May be more sensitive to hypotensive effects.

INTERACTIONS

DRUG: Diuretics may increase effects. May increase concentration, risk of toxicity of **lithium. NSAIDs** may decrease effects. **Potassium-sparing diuretics, potassium supplements** may cause hyperkalemia. May increase hypoglycemic effect of **oral hypoglycemic agents. HERBAL: Ephedra, ginseng, licorice, yohimbe** may worsen hypertension. **Black cohosh, periwinkle** may increase antihypertensive effect. **FOOD:** None known. **LAB VALUES:** May increase BUN, serum alkaline phosphatase, bilirubin, creatinine, potassium, AST, ALT. May decrease serum sodium. May cause positive ANA titer.

AVAILABILITY (Rx)

Tablets (Prinivil, Zestril): 2.5 mg, 5 mg, 10 mg, 20 mg, 30 mg, 40 mg.

ADMINISTRATION/HANDLING

PO
• Give without regard to food. • Tablets may be crushed.

INDICATIONS/ROUTES/DOSAGE

Hypertension (Used Alone)
PO: ADULTS: Initially, 10 mg/day. May increase by 5–10 mg/day at 1- to 2-wk intervals. Range: 10–40 mg/day. **ELDERLY:** Initially, 2.5–5 mg/day. May increase by 2.5–5 mg/day at 1- to 2-wk intervals. **Maximum:** 40 mg/day. **CHILDREN 6 YRS OR OLDER:** Initially, 0.07 mg/kg once daily (up to 5 mg). Titrate at 1- to 2-wk intervals. **Maximum:** 40 mg/day.

Hypertension (in Combination with Other Antihypertensives)
◀**ALERT▶** If possible, discontinue diuretics 48–72 hrs prior to initiating lisinopril therapy.
PO: ADULTS: Initially, 2.5–5 mg/day titrated to pt's needs. Range: 10–40 mg/day.

Adjunctive Therapy for Management of Heart Failure
PO: ADULTS, ELDERLY: Initially, 2.5–5 mg/day. May increase by no more than 10

mg/day at intervals of at least 2 wks. Maintenance: 5–40 mg/day.

Improve Survival in Pts after MI

PO: ADULTS, ELDERLY: Initially, 5 mg, then 5 mg after 24 hrs, 10 mg after 48 hrs, then 10 mg/day for 6 wks. For pts with low systolic B/P, give 2.5 mg/day for 5 days, then 2.5–5 mg/day. Pt should continue with thrombolytics, aspirin, beta-blockers.

Dosage in Renal Impairment

Titrate to pt's needs after giving the following initial dose:

Hypertension

Creatinine Clearance	Dosage
10–30 ml/min	5 mg
Dialysis	2.5 mg

HF

Creatinine clearance less than 30 ml/min or serum creatinine greater than 3 mg/dl: Initial dose: 2.5 mg.

SIDE EFFECTS

Frequent (12%–5%): Headache, dizziness, postural hypotension. **Occasional (4%–2%):** Chest discomfort, fatigue, rash, abdominal pain, nausea, diarrhea, upper respiratory infection. **Rare (1% or less):** Palpitations, tachycardia, peripheral edema, insomnia, paresthesia, confusion, constipation, dry mouth, muscle cramps.

ADVERSE EFFECTS/ TOXIC REACTIONS

Excessive hypotension ("first-dose syncope") may occur in pts with HF, severe salt/volume depletion. Angioedema (swelling of face and lips) occur rarely. Agranulocytosis, neutropenia may be noted in pts with collagen vascular disease (scleroderma, systemic lupus erythematosus). Nephrotic syndrome may be noted in pts with history of renal disease.

NURSING CONSIDERATIONS

BASELINE ASSESSMENT

Obtain B/P, apical pulse immediately before each dose, in addition to regular monitoring (be alert to fluctuations). In pts with renal impairment, autoimmune disease, taking drugs that affect leukocytes or immune response, CBC and differential count should be performed before beginning therapy and q2wks for 3 mos, then periodically thereafter.

INTERVENTION/EVALUATION

Assess for edema. Auscultate lungs for rales. Monitor I&O; weigh daily. Monitor daily pattern of bowel activity, stool consistency. Assist with ambulation if dizziness occurs. Monitor B/P, renal function tests, WBC, serum potassium. If excessive reduction in B/P occurs, place pt in supine position, feet slightly elevated.

PATIENT/ FAMILY TEACHING

• To reduce hypotensive effect, go from lying to standing slowly. • Limit alcohol intake. • Report vomiting, diarrhea, diaphoresis, swelling of face/lips/tongue, difficulty in breathing, persistent cough. • Limit salt intake.

L

lithium

lith-ee-um
(Apo-Lithium ✦, Duralith ✦, Lithobid)

BLACK BOX ALERT Lithium toxicity is closely related to serum lithium levels and can occur at therapeutic doses. Routine determination of serum lithium levels is essential during therapy.

Do not confuse Lithobid with Levbid or Lithostat.

◆ CLASSIFICATION

PHARMACOTHERAPEUTIC: Psychotherapeutic. **CLINICAL:** Antimanic, antidepressant, vascular headache prophylactic.

ACTION

Affects storage, release, reuptake of neurotransmitters. Antimanic effect may result from increased norepinephrine reuptake, serotonin receptor sensitivity. **Therapeutic Effect:** Produces antimanic, antidepressant effects.

PHARMACOKINETICS

Rapidly, completely absorbed from GI tract. Protein binding: None. Primarily excreted unchanged in urine. Removed by hemodialysis. **Half-life:** 18–24 hrs (increased in elderly).

USES

Prophylaxis, treatment of acute mania, manic phase of bipolar disorder (manic depressive illness). **OFF-LABEL:** Aggression, post-traumatic stress disorder, conduct disorder in children. Augmenting agent for depression.

PRECAUTIONS

Contraindications: Debilitated pts, severe cardiovascular disease, severe dehydration, severe renal disease, severe sodium depletion or dehydration, pregnancy. **Cautions:** Mild to moderate cardiovascular disease, thyroid disease, elderly, mild to moderate renal impairment, medications altering sodium excretion, pts at risk for suicide.

⧗ LIFESPAN CONSIDERATIONS

Pregnancy/Lactation: Freely crosses placenta. Distributed in breast milk. **Pregnancy Category D. Children:** May increase bone formation or density (alter parathyroid hormone concentrations). **Elderly:** More susceptible to develop lithium-induced goiter or clinical hypothyroidism, CNS toxicity. Increased thirst, urination noted more frequently; lower dosage recommended.

INTERACTIONS

DRUG: Diuretics, NSAIDs, metronidazole, ACE inhibitors, angiotensin II antagonists, SSRIs, calcium channel blockers may increase lithium concentration, risk of toxicity. **HERBAL:** None significant. **FOOD:** None known. **LAB VALUES:** May increase serum glucose, immunoreactive parathyroid hormone, calcium. **Therapeutic serum level:** 0.6–1.2 mEq/L; **toxic serum level:** greater than 1.5 mEq/L.

AVAILABILITY (Rx)

Capsules: 150 mg, 300 mg, 600 mg. **Oral Solution:** 300 mg/5 ml. **Tablets:** 300 mg, 600 mg.

Tablets (Extended-Release): 300 mg, 450 mg.

ADMINISTRATION/HANDLING

PO
• Administer with meals, milk to decrease GI upset. • Do not crush, cut, break extended-release tablets.

INDICATIONS/ROUTES/DOSAGE

◀**ALERT**▶ During acute phase, a therapeutic serum lithium concentration of 0.6–1.2 mEq/L is required. For long-term control, desired level is 0.8–1 mEq/L. Monitor serum drug concentration, clinical response to determine proper dosage.

Usual Dosage
PO: ADULTS: 300 mg 3–4 times a day or 450–900 mg extended-release form twice a day. **Maximum:** 2.4 g/day. **ELDERLY:** 900–1,200 mg/day. Maintenance: 300 mg twice a day. May increase by 300 mg/day q1wk. **CHILDREN 12 YRS AND OLDER:** 600–1,800 mg/day in 3–4 divided doses (2 doses/day for extended-release). **CHILDREN 6–11 YRS:** 15–60 mg/kg/day in 3–4 divided doses not to exceed usual adult dose.

Dosage in Renal Impairment

Creatinine Clearance	Dosage
10–50 ml/min	50%–75% normal dose
Less than 10 ml/min	25%–50% normal dose

SIDE EFFECTS

◄ALERT► Side effects are dose related and seldom occur at lithium serum levels less than 1.5 mEq/L. **Occasional:** Fine hand tremor, polydipsia, polyuria, mild nausea. **Rare:** Weight gain, bradycardia, tachycardia, acne, rash, muscle twitching, peripheral cyanosis, pseudotumor cerebri (eye pain, headache, tinnitus, vision disturbances).

ADVERSE EFFECTS/ TOXIC REACTIONS

Lithium serum concentration of 1.5–2.0 mEq/L may produce vomiting, diarrhea, drowsiness, confusion, incoordination, coarse hand tremor, muscle twitching, T-wave depression on EKG. Lithium serum concentration of 2.0–2.5 mEq/L may result in ataxia, giddiness, tinnitus, blurred vision, clonic movements, severe hypotension. Acute toxicity may be characterized by seizures, oliguria, circulatory failure, coma, death.

NURSING CONSIDERATIONS

BASELINE ASSESSMENT

Assess mental status (e.g., mood, behavior). Serum lithium levels should be tested q3–4days during initial phase of therapy, q1–2mos thereafter, and weekly if there is no improvement of disorder or adverse effects occur.

INTERVENTION/EVALUATION

Clinical assessment of therapeutic effect, tolerance to drug effect is necessary for correct dosing-level management. Assess behavior, appearance, emotional status, response to environment, speech pattern, thought content. Monitor serum lithium concentrations, CBC with differential, urinalysis, creatinine clearance. Monitor renal, hepatic, thyroid, cardiovascular function; serum electrolytes. Assess for increased urinary output, persistent thirst. Report polyuria, prolonged vomiting, diarrhea, fever to physician (may need to temporarily reduce or discontinue dosage). Monitor for signs of lithium toxicity. Assess for therapeutic response (interest in surroundings, improvement in self-care, increased ability to concentrate, relaxed facial expression). Monitor lithium levels q3–4days at initiation of therapy (then q1–2mos). Obtain lithium levels 8–12 hrs postdose. **Therapeutic serum level:** 0.6–1.2 mEq/L; **toxic serum level:** greater than 1.5 mEq/L.

PATIENT/ FAMILY TEACHING

• Limit alcohol, caffeine intake. • Avoid tasks requiring coordination until CNS effects of drug are known. • May cause dry mouth. • Maintain steady salt, fluid intake (avoid dehydration). • Inform physician if vomiting, diarrhea, muscle weakness, tremors, drowsiness, ataxia occur. • Serum level monitoring is necessary to determine proper dose.

lomitapide

lom-i-**ta**-pide
(Juxtapid)
Do not confuse lomitapide with loperamide.

BLACK BOX ALERT May cause hepatotoxicity. May cause hepatic steatosis (increase in hepatic fat) regardless of ALT, AST elevation; may be risk factor for progressive hepatic disease, including steatohepatitis and cirrhosis. Treatment only available through restricted program under the Risk Evaluation and Mitigation Strategy (REMS) named JUXTAPID REMS PROGRAM.

◆CLASSIFICATION

PHARMACOTHERAPEUTIC: Microsomal triglyceride transfer protein inhibitor. **CLINICAL:** Antihyperlipidemic.

ACTION

Inhibits microsomal triglyceride transfer protein in lumen of endoplasmic reticulum. Prevents assembly of apo-B-containing lipoproteins in enterocytes, hepatocytes; inhibits synthesis of chylomicrons, very low-density lipoprotein (VLDL). **Therapeutic Effect:** Decreases plasma low-density lipoprotein cholesterol (LDL-C).

PHARMACOKINETICS

Well absorbed in GI tract. Metabolized in liver. Protein binding: 99%. Peak plasma concentration: 6 hrs. Primarily excreted in feces. **Half-life:** 40 hrs.

USES

Treatment of homozygous familial hypercholesterolemia (HoFH) in combination with low-fat diet and other lipid-lowering therapies, including LDL-cholesterol apheresis, to reduce LDL, total cholesterol, apoprotein B, non–HDL-C.

PRECAUTIONS

Contraindications: Pregnancy (Pregnancy Category X), breastfeeding, moderate to severe hepatic impairment, concomitant use of strong CYP3A4 inhibitors (e.g., ketoconazole, protease inhibitors). **Cautions:** End-stage renal disease, mild hepatic impairment, alcohol consumption, avoid use in pts with history of glucose-galactose malabsorption, concurrent use of warfarin, other agents having hepatotoxic potential (e.g., acetaminophen). Concomitant use of weak CYP3A4 inhibitors, anticoagulants.

⧖ LIFESPAN CONSIDERATIONS

Pregnancy/Lactation: Contraindicated in pregnancy. May cause fetal harm. Must use effective contraception in addition to barrier methods. Unknown if distributed in breast milk. Must either discontinue breastfeeding or discontinue therapy. **Pregnancy Category X. Children:** Safety and efficacy not established. **Elderly:** Increased risk for side effects, adverse reactions.

INTERACTIONS

DRUG: Acetaminophen, amiodarone, isotretinoin, methotrexate, tamoxifen, tetracycline may increase risk for hepatotoxicity. **Strong CYP3A4 inhibitors (e.g., ketoconazole, protease inhibitors)** contraindicated due to increased risk for myopathy, rhabdomyolysis. Moderate **CYP3A4 inhibitors (e.g., atorvastatin, oral contraceptives)** may increase concentration. May increase concentration of **warfarin.** May increase effects of **P-glycoprotein substrates (e.g., digoxin, sitagliptin). HERBAL:** None known. **FOOD: Grapefruit products** may increase absorption, toxicity. **LAB VALUES:** May increase serum alkaline phosphatase, bilirubin, ALT, AST.

AVAILABILITY (Rx)

Capsules: 5 mg, 10 mg, 20 mg.

ADMINISTRATION/HANDLING

PO

• Give with water only. • Administer without food (at least 2 hrs after evening meal). • Administer whole; do not break, crush, dissolve, or divide capsules.

INDICATIONS/ROUTES/DOSAGE

◀ALERT▶ To reduce risk for fat-soluble nutrient deficiency, recommend supplemental coadministration: vitamin E 400 international units PO daily, linoleic acid 200 mg PO daily, alpha-linolenic acid (ALA) 210 mg PO daily, eicosapentaenoic acid (EPA) 110 mg PO daily, docosahexaenoic acid (DHA) 80 mg PO daily. Because of risk for myopathy, concurrent use of simvastatin should not exceed 20–40 mg/day.

Homozygous Familial Hypercholesterolemia

PO: ADULTS, ELDERLY: Initially, 5 mg once daily for minimum of 2 wks. Gradually increase dose at 4-wk (minimum) intervals to 10 mg once daily, then 20 mg once daily, then 40 mg once daily, then 60 mg once daily based on tolerability. **Maximum:** 60 mg/day.

Dose Modification

Elevated Hepatic Enzymes

If ALT, AST is between 3–5 times upper limit normal (ULN), reduce dose until ALT, AST less than 3 times ULN. If ALT, AST is greater than 5 times ULN, withhold dose until less than 3 times ULN, then restart at reduced dose. If hepatotoxicity occurs or bilirubin level rises greater than 2 times ULN, discontinue treatment.

End-Stage Renal Disease Receiving Dialysis, Mild Hepatic Impairment

Do not exceed 40 mg/day.

Concurrent Use of Weak CYP3A4 Inhibitors

Do not exceed 30 mg/day.

Concurrent Use of Oral Contraception

Do not exceed 30 mg/day.

SIDE EFFECTS

Frequent (79%–65%): Diarrhea, nausea. **Occasional (38%–10%):** Dyspepsia, vomiting, abdominal pain, weight loss, abdominal distention, constipation, flatulence, fatigue, back pain, gastric reflux, headache, dizziness.

ADVERSE EFFECTS/ TOXIC REACTIONS

Progressive hepatic disease including steatohepatitis, cirrhosis has been reported in 6% of pts due to increased hepatic fat. May reduce absorption of fat-soluble nutrients; recommend daily supplemental replacement. Increased risk for myopathy including rhabdomyolysis (muscle pain/tenderness, weakness, dark or decreased urine output, elevated serum creatinine, CPK) when used with other antihyperlipidemics. May increase risk for supratherapeutic INR

with warfarin. Infections including influenza, nasopharyngitis, gastroenteritis reported in 5% of pts. Palpitations, angina pectoris report in 3% of pts. Increased risk for dehydration/malabsorption with galactose intolerance hereditary disorder, pancreatic disease, diarrhea.

NURSING CONSIDERATIONS

BASELINE ASSESSMENT

Obtain detailed dietary history, esp. fat consumption. Confirm negative pregnancy test before initiating treatment (Pregnancy Category X). Obtain baseline laboratory studies: ALT, AST, alkaline phosphatase, bilirubin, serum cholesterol, triglycerides, PT/INR (if pt is on warfarin). Confirm positive history of HoFH. Receive full medication history including vitamins, minerals, herbal products. Screen for history of galactose intolerance, renal/hepatic impairment, angina.

INTERVENTION/EVALUATION

Maintain hydration; offer fluids frequently. Monitor INR routinely (with anticoagulants). Monitor alkaline phosphatase, ALT, AST, bilirubin with any dosage change, then every month for first year when maintenance goal reached, then every 3 mos. Obtain EKG for palpitations, shortness of breath, dizziness. Monitor for bruising, hematuria, jaundice, right upper abdominal pain, fever, lethargy, melena.

PATIENT/FAMILY TEACHING

• Avoid pregnancy. • Use appropriate contraception measures, including barrier precautions (Pregnancy Category X). • If pregnancy occurs, inform physician immediately. • Diarrhea may decrease effectiveness of oral contraception. • Do not breast-feed. • Maintain low-fat diet. • Report yellowing of skin, bruising, black/tarry stool, right upper quadrant pain, fever, lethargy, chest pain, palpitations. • Avoid alcohol. • Do not ingest grapefruit products. • Do not chew, crush, dissolve, or divide capsule. • Report any newly prescribed medications.

✚ Canadian trade name   🅝 Non-Crushable Drug   🅷🅐 High Alert drug

lomustine

loe-mus-teen
(CeeNU)

BLACK BOX ALERT Must be administered by certified chemotherapy personnel. Severe myelosuppressant (notably thrombocytopenia, leukopenia). May lead to bleeding, overwhelming infection.

Do not confuse lomustine with bendamustine or carmustine.

◆CLASSIFICATION

PHARMACOTHERAPEUTIC: Alkylating agent (nitrosourea). **CLINICAL:** Antineoplastic (see p. 88C).

ACTION

Inhibits DNA, RNA protein synthesis by cross-linking with DNA and RNA strands, preventing cell division. Cell cycle–phase nonspecific. **Therapeutic Effect:** Interferes with DNA, RNA function.

PHARMACOKINETICS

Rapidly, completely absorbed following PO administration. Highly lipid soluble. Metabolized in liver. Excreted in urine. **Half-life:** 16–72 hrs.

USES

Treatment of primary/metastatic brain tumors (after surgery and/or radiation therapy), disseminated Hodgkin's lymphoma (as part of combination chemotherapy). **OFF-LABEL:** Treatment of gastric cancer, metastatic melanoma.

PRECAUTIONS

Contraindications: None known. **Cautions:** Depressed platelet, leukocyte, erythrocyte counts; renal/hepatic impairment.

⧗ LIFESPAN CONSIDERATIONS

Pregnancy/Lactation: May be harmful to fetus. Distributed in breast milk. Breastfeeding not recommended. **Pregnancy Category D. Children:** Safety and efficacy not established. **Elderly:** Age-related renal impairment may require dosage adjustment.

INTERACTIONS

DRUG: Bone marrow depressants may increase myelosuppression. **Live virus vaccines** may potentiate virus replication, increase vaccine side effects, decrease pt's antibody response to vaccine. **HERBAL:** None significant. **FOOD:** None known. **LAB VALUES:** May increase serum hepatic function test results.

AVAILABILITY (Rx)

Capsules: 10 mg, 40 mg, 100 mg.

ADMINISTRATION/HANDLING

PO
• Give with fluids on an empty stomach (decreases nausea, vomiting). • Do not break capsules. • No food or drink for 2 hrs after administration.

INDICATIONS/ROUTES/DOSAGE

◄ALERT► Dosage is individualized based on clinical response and tolerance of adverse effects. When used in combination therapy, consult specific protocols for optimum dosage, sequence of drug administration. Should only be given q6wks.

Usual Dosage

PO: ADULTS, ELDERLY: 100–130 mg/m^2 as single dose. Repeat dose at intervals of at least 6 wks but not until circulating blood elements have returned to acceptable levels. Adjust dose based on hematologic response to previous dose. **CHILDREN:** 75–130 mg/m^2 as a single dose every 6 wks.

Dosage in Renal Impairment

Creatinine Clearance	Dosage
10–50 ml/min	75% of normal dose
Less than 10 ml/min	25%–50% of normal dose

SIDE EFFECTS

Frequent: Nausea, vomiting (occurs 45 min–6 hrs after dose, lasts 12–24 hrs);

anorexia (often follows for 2–3 days). **Occasional:** Neurotoxicity (confusion, slurred speech), stomatitis, darkening of skin, diarrhea, rash, pruritus, alopecia.

ADVERSE EFFECTS/ TOXIC REACTIONS

Myelosuppression may result in hematologic toxicity (principally leukopenia, mild anemia, thrombocytopenia). Leukopenia occurs about 6 wks after a dose, thrombocytopenia about 4 wks after a dose; both persist for 1–2 wks. Refractory anemia, thrombocytopenia occur commonly if lomustine therapy continues for more than 1 yr. Hepatotoxicity occurs infrequently. Large cumulative doses of lomustine may result in renal damage.

NURSING CONSIDERATIONS

BASELINE ASSESSMENT

Recommend weekly CBC with differential, experts recommend first CBC with differential obtained 2–3 wks following initial therapy, subsequent CBC with differential, indicated by prior toxicity. Obtain baseline serum chemistries. Antiemetics can reduce duration, frequency of nausea, vomiting.

INTERVENTION/EVALUATION

Monitor CBC with differential, hepatic, renal, pulmonary function tests. Observe for stomatitis. Monitor for hematologic toxicity (fever, sore throat, signs of local infection, unusual bruising/bleeding from any site), symptoms of anemia (excessive fatigue, weakness).

PATIENT/FAMILY TEACHING

• Nausea, vomiting generally resolves in less than 1 day. • Fasting before therapy can reduce frequency/duration of GI effects. • Maintain strict oral hygiene. • Do not have immunizations without physician's approval (drug lowers resistance). • Avoid crowds, those with known illness. • Promptly report fever, sore throat, signs of local infection, unusual

bruising/bleeding from any site, swelling of legs or feet, jaundice (yellowing of eyes, skin).

loperamide

loe-**per**-a-mide
(Apo-Loperamide ✤, Diamode, Diarr-Eze ✤, Imodium, Imodium A-D, Loperacap ✤, Novo-Loperamide ✤)
Do not confuse Imodium with Indocin, or loperamide with furosemide.

FIXED-COMBINATION(S)

Imodium Advanced: loperamide/simethicone (an antiflatulant): 2 mg/125 mg.

◆CLASSIFICATION

PHARMACOTHERAPEUTIC: Antidiarrheal agent. **CLINICAL:** Antidiarrheal (see p. 46C).

ACTION

Directly affects intestinal wall muscles. **Therapeutic Effect:** Slows intestinal motility, prolongs transit time of intestinal contents by reducing fecal volume, diminishing loss of fluid, electrolytes, increasing viscosity, bulk of stool.

PHARMACOKINETICS

Poorly absorbed from GI tract. Protein binding: 97%. Metabolized in liver. Eliminated in feces; excreted in urine. Not removed by hemodialysis. **Half-life:** 7–14 hrs.

USES

Controls, provides symptomatic relief of acute nonspecific diarrhea, chronic diarrhea associated with inflammatory bowel disease, traveler's diarrhea. **OFF-LABEL:** Chemotherapy-induced diarrhea, chronic diarrhea caused by bowel resection.

L

PRECAUTIONS

Contraindications: Abdominal pain in presence of diarrhea, children younger than 2 yrs of age, bloody diarrhea. **Cautions:** Hepatic impairment.

⧗ LIFESPAN CONSIDERATIONS

Pregnancy/Lactation: Unknown if drug crosses placenta or is distributed in breast milk. **Pregnancy Category C. Children:** Not recommended for those younger than 6 yrs (infants younger than 3 mos more susceptible to CNS effects). **Elderly:** May mask dehydration, electrolyte depletion.

INTERACTIONS

DRUG: Ritonavir may increase levels/side effects. May decrease concentration of **saquinavir. HERBAL:** None significant. **FOOD:** None known. **LAB VALUES:** None significant.

AVAILABILITY (Rx)

Caplets: 2 mg. **Capsules:** 2 mg. **Liquid:** 1 mg/5 ml, 1 mg/7.5 ml. **Solution, Oral:** 1 mg/5 ml. **Tablet, Chewable:** 2 mg.

ADMINISTRATION/HANDLING

Liquid

• When administering to children, use accompanying plastic dropper to measure the liquid.

INDICATIONS/ROUTES/DOSAGE

Acute Diarrhea

PO *(Capsules)*: **ADULTS, ELDERLY:** Initially, 4 mg, then 2 mg after each unformed stool. **Maximum:** 16 mg/day. **CHILDREN 9–12 YRS, WEIGHING MORE THAN 30 KG:** Initially, 2 mg 3 times a day for 24 hrs. **CHILDREN 6–8 YRS, WEIGHING 20–30 KG:** Initially, 2 mg twice a day for 24 hrs. **CHILDREN 2–5 YRS, WEIGHING 13–20 KG:** Initially, 1 mg 3 times a day for 24 hrs. Maintenance: 1 mg/10 kg only after loose stool but not exceeding initial dose.

Chronic Diarrhea

PO: ADULTS, ELDERLY: Initially, 4 mg, then 2 mg after each unformed stool until diarrhea is controlled. Average maintenance dose: 4–8 mg/day. **Maximum:** 16 mg/day. **CHILDREN:** 0.08–0.24 mg/kg/day in 2–3 divided doses. **Maximum:** 2 mg/dose.

Traveler's Diarrhea

PO: ADULTS, ELDERLY: Initially, 4 mg, then 2 mg after each loose bowel movement (LBM). **Maximum:** 8 mg/day for 2 days. **CHILDREN 9–11 YRS:** Initially, 2 mg, then 1 mg after each LBM. **Maximum:** 6 mg/day for 2 days. **CHILDREN 6–8 YRS:** Initially, 2 mg, then 1 mg after each LBM. **Maximum:** 4 mg/day for 2 days.

SIDE EFFECTS

Rare: Dry mouth, drowsiness, abdominal discomfort, allergic reaction (rash, pruritus).

ADVERSE EFFECTS/ TOXIC REACTIONS

Toxicity results in constipation, GI irritation (nausea, vomiting), CNS depression. Activated charcoal is used to treat loperamide toxicity.

NURSING CONSIDERATIONS

BASELINE ASSESSMENT

Do not administer in presence of bloody diarrhea, temperature greater than 101°F.

INTERVENTION/EVALUATION

Encourage adequate fluid intake. Assess bowel sounds for peristalsis. Monitor daily pattern of bowel activity, stool consistency. Withhold drug, notify physician promptly in event of abdominal pain, distention, fever.

PATIENT/FAMILY TEACHING

• Do not exceed prescribed dose. • May cause dry mouth. • Avoid alcohol. • Avoid tasks that require alertness, motor skills until response to drug is established. • Notify physician if diarrhea does not stop within 3 days; abdominal distention, pain occurs; fever develops.

lopinavir/ritonavir

loe-**pin**-ah-veer/rye-**toe**-na-veer
(<u>Kaletra</u>)
**Do not confuse Kaletra with
Keppra.**

◆CLASSIFICATION

PHARMACOTHERAPEUTIC: Protease
inhibitor combination. **CLINICAL:** Antiretroviral (see pp. 70C, 120C).

ACTION

Lopinavir inhibits activity of protease,
an enzyme, late in HIV replication process; ritonavir increases plasma levels
of lopinavir. **Therapeutic Effect:** Formation of immature, noninfectious viral
particles.

PHARMACOKINETICS

Readily absorbed after PO administration
(absorption increased when taken with
food). Protein binding: 98%–99%. Metabolized in liver. Eliminated primarily in
feces. Not removed by hemodialysis.
Half-life: 5–6 hrs.

USES

In combination with other antiretroviral
agents for treatment of HIV infection.

PRECAUTIONS

Contraindications: Concomitant use of alfuzosin, ergot derivatives (causes vasospasm, peripheral ischemia of extremities), lovastatin, midazolam (oral),
pimozide, rifampin, sildenafil (for treatment of pulmonary arterial hypertension),
simvastatin, St. John's wort, triazolam (increased sedation, respiratory depression);
hypersensitivity to lopinavir, ritonavir. **Cautions:** Hepatic impairment, hepatitis B or
C, cardiac disease with underlying conduction abnormalities or structural heart
defects, ischemic heart disease, cardiomy-
opathies, congenital long QT syndrome or
medications that prolong QT interval, hypokalemia, history of pancreatitis.

⌛ LIFESPAN CONSIDERATIONS

Pregnancy/Lactation: Unknown if distributed in breast milk. Breastfeeding by
HIV-infected mothers not recommended.
Pregnancy Category C. Children: Safety
and efficacy not established in those
younger than 6 mos. **Elderly:** Age-related renal/hepatic/cardiac impairment
requires caution.

INTERACTIONS

DRUG: May increase concentration/toxic-
ity of **amiodarone, atorvastatin, bepridil, clarithromycin, cyclosporine,
felodipine, fluticasone, ketoconazole, lidocaine, lovastatin, midazolam, nelfinavir, nicardipine,
nifedipine, sildenafil, simvastatin,
tacrolimus, trazodone, triazolam,
warfarin.** May decrease concentration/
effects of **oral contraceptives. CYP3A4
inducers (e.g., carbamazepine, phenytoin, rifampin)** may decrease con-
centration/effects. May cause disulfiram-
like reaction with **metronidazole.**
HERBAL: St. John's wort may decrease
concentration/effects. **FOOD:** None
known. **LAB VALUES:** May increase serum glucose, GGT, amylase, bilirubin,
total cholesterol, triglycerides, uric acid,
AST, ALT. May decrease platelets, serum
sodium.

AVAILABILITY (Rx)

Oral Solution: 80 mg/ml lopinavir/20 mg/
ml ritonavir.

Tablets: 100 mg lopinavir/25 mg
ritonavir, 200 mg lopinavir/50 mg ritonavir.

ADMINISTRATION/HANDLING

PO

• Give tablets whole; do not break, cut,
crush, or divide. • Does not require refrigeration. • Give tablets without regard
to food. • Solution should be given with
food. • Administer solution using calibrated oral syringe.

L

INDICATIONS/ROUTES/DOSAGE

HIV Infection

Doses based on lopinavir component.
PO: ADULTS: 800 mg once daily or 400 mg twice daily. **CHILDREN 6 MOS–18 YRS, WEIGHING GREATER THAN 40 KG:** 400 mg twice daily. **WEIGHING 15–40 KG:** 10 mg/kg twice a day. **WEIGHING LESS THAN 15 KG:** 12 mg/kg twice daily. **CHILDREN 14 DAYS–6 MOS:** 16 mg/kg twice daily.

Dosage Adjustment for Combination Therapy

Efavirenz, Fosamprenavir, Nelfinavir, Nevirapine: ADULTS, CHILDREN 6 MOS–18 YRS, WEIGHING GREATER THAN 45 KG: 500 mg (533-mg solution) twice daily. **WEIGHING 15–45 KG:** 11 mg/kg twice daily. **WEIGHING LESS THAN 15 KG:** 13 mg/kg twice daily. **Maraviroc, Saquinavir: ADULTS:** 400 mg twice daily.

SIDE EFFECTS

Frequent (14%): Mild to moderate diarrhea. **Occasional (6%–2%):** Nausea, asthenia (loss of strength, energy), abdominal pain, headache, vomiting. **Rare (less than 2%):** Insomnia, rash.

ADVERSE EFFECTS/ TOXIC REACTIONS

Anemia, leukopenia, lymphadenopathy, deep vein thrombosis (DVT), Cushing's syndrome, pancreatitis, hemorrhagic colitis occur rarely.

NURSING CONSIDERATIONS

BASELINE ASSESSMENT

Obtain baseline CBC, renal/hepatic function tests, viral load, CD4 count, cell count. Obtain baseline weight.

INTERVENTION/EVALUATION

Monitor daily pattern of bowel activity, stool consistency. Assess for opportunistic infections: onset of fever, oral mucosa changes, cough, other respiratory symptoms. Check weight at least 2 times a wk. Assess for nausea, vomiting. Observe for signs/symptoms of pancreatitis (nausea, vomiting, abdominal pain). Monitor electrolytes, serum glucose, cholesterol, hepatic function, CBC with differential, CD4 cell count, viral load.

PATIENT/ FAMILY TEACHING

• Explain correct administration of medication. • Eat small, frequent meals to offset nausea, vomiting. • Lopinavir/ritonavir is not a cure for HIV infection, nor does it reduce risk of transmission to others. • Pt must continue practices to prevent HIV transmission. • Illnesses, including opportunistic infections, may still occur.

loratadine

lor-**at**-ah-deen
(Alavert, Apo-Loratadine ✦, Claritin, Loradamed)
Do not confuse Claritin with clarithromycin.

FIXED-COMBINATION(S)

Alavert Allergy and Sinus, Claritin-D: loratadine/pseudoephedrine (a sympathomimetic): 5 mg/120 mg, 10 mg/240 mg.

◆CLASSIFICATION

PHARMACOTHERAPEUTIC: H_1 antagonist. **CLINICAL:** Antihistamine (see p. 55C).

ACTION

Competes with histamine for H_1 receptor sites on effector cells. **Therapeutic Effect:** Prevents allergic responses mediated by histamine (e.g., rhinitis, urticaria, pruritus).

PHARMACOKINETICS

Route	Onset	Peak	Duration
PO	1–3 hrs	8–12 hrs	Longer than 24 hrs

Rapidly, almost completely absorbed from GI tract. Protein binding: 97%; metabolite, 73%–77%. Distributed mainly to liver, lungs, GI tract, bile. Metabolized in liver. Eliminated in urine and feces. Not removed by hemodialysis. **Half-life:** 8.4 hrs; metabolite, 28 hrs (increased in elderly, hepatic impairment).

USES

Relief of nasal, non-nasal symptoms of seasonal allergic rhinitis (hay fever). Treatment of idiopathic chronic urticaria (hives).

PRECAUTIONS

Contraindications: None known. **Cautions:** Renal/hepatic impairment, breast-feeding women.

⌛ LIFESPAN CONSIDERATIONS

Pregnancy/Lactation: Distributed in breast milk. **Pregnancy Category B. Children:** Safety and efficacy not established in those younger than 2 yrs. **Elderly:** More sensitive to anticholinergic effects (e.g., dry mouth, nose, throat).

INTERACTIONS

DRUG: Clarithromycin, erythromycin, fluconazole, ketoconazole may increase concentration. **HERBAL: St. John's wort** may decrease concentration/effects. **FOOD: All foods** delay absorption. **LAB VALUES:** May suppress wheal, flare reactions to antigen skin testing unless drug is discontinued 4 days before testing.

AVAILABILITY (Rx)

Solution, Oral: 5 mg/5 ml. **Syrup:** 5 mg/5 ml. **Tablets (Alavert, Claritin, Loradamed):** 10 mg. **Tablets, Chewable (Claritin):** 5 mg. **Tablets (Orally Disintegrating [Alavert]):** 10 mg.

ADMINISTRATION/HANDLING

PO
• Preferably give on empty stomach (food delays absorption).

Orally Disintegrating Tablets
• Place under tongue. • Disintegration occurs within seconds, after which tablet contents may be swallowed with or without water.

INDICATIONS/ROUTES/DOSAGE

Allergic Rhinitis, Urticaria
PO: ADULTS, ELDERLY, CHILDREN 6 YRS AND OLDER: 10 mg once a day. **CHILDREN 2–5 YRS:** 5 mg once a day.

Dosage in Renal (Creatinine Clearance Less Than 30 ml/min)/Hepatic Impairment
PO: ADULTS, ELDERLY, CHILDREN 6 YRS AND OLDER: 10 mg every other day. **CHILDREN 2–5 YRS:** 5 mg every other day.

SIDE EFFECTS

Frequent (12%–8%): Headache, fatigue, drowsiness. **Occasional (3%):** Dry mouth, nose, throat. **Rare:** Photosensitivity.

ADVERSE EFFECTS/ TOXIC REACTIONS

None significant.

NURSING CONSIDERATIONS

BASELINE ASSESSMENT

Assess lung sounds for wheezing, skin for urticaria, other allergy symptoms.

INTERVENTION/EVALUATION

For upper respiratory allergies, increase fluids to decrease viscosity of secretions, offset thirst, replenish loss of fluids from increased diaphoresis. Monitor symptoms for therapeutic response.

PATIENT/FAMILY TEACHING

• Drink plenty of water (may cause dry mouth). • Avoid alcohol. • Avoid tasks that require alertness, motor skills until response to drug is established (may cause drowsiness). • May cause photosensitivity reactions (avoid direct exposure to sunlight).

L

lorazepam

TOP
200

lor-a-ze-pam
(Apo-Lorazepam ✦, Ativan, Lorazepam Intensol, Novo-Lorazem ✦)
Do not confuse Ativan with Ambien or Atarax, or lorazepam with alprazolam, diazepam, Lovaza, temazepam, or Zolpidem.

◆ CLASSIFICATION

PHARMACOTHERAPEUTIC: Benzodiazepine (**Schedule IV**). **CLINICAL:** Antianxiety, sedative-hypnotic, antiemetic, skeletal muscle relaxant, amnesiac, anticonvulsant, antitremor (see p. 15C).

ACTION

Enhances action of inhibitory neurotransmitter gamma-aminobutyric acid (GABA) in CNS, affecting memory, motor, sensory, cognitive function. **Therapeutic Effect:** Produces anxiolytic, anticonvulsant, sedative, muscle relaxant, antiemetic effects.

PHARMACOKINETICS

Route	Onset	Peak	Duration
PO	30–60 min	N/A	6–8 hrs
IV	5–20 min	N/A	6–8 hrs
IM	20–30 min	N/A	6–8 hrs

Well absorbed after PO, IM administration. Protein binding: 85%. Widely distributed. Metabolized in liver. Primarily excreted in urine. Not removed by hemodialysis. **Half-life:** 10–20 hrs.

USES

PO: Management of anxiety disorders, short-term relief of symptoms of anxiety, anxiety associated with depressive symptoms. Insomnia due to anxiety or transient stress; adjunct to antiemetics. **IV:** Status epilepticus, preanesthesia for amnesia, sedation. **OFF-LABEL:** Treatment of alcohol withdrawal, psychogenic catatonia, partial complex seizures, agitation (IV administration only), antiemetic for chemotherapy; rapid tranquilization of agitated pt.

PRECAUTIONS

Contraindications: Acute narrow-angle glaucoma, IV administration in pts with sleep apnea, severe respiratory depression (except during mechanical ventilation). **Cautions:** Neonates, renal/hepatic impairment, compromised pulmonary function, concomitant CNS depressant use. Depression, history of drug dependence, alcohol abuse, or significant personality disorder.

⧗ LIFESPAN CONSIDERATIONS

Pregnancy/Lactation: May cross placenta. May be distributed in breast milk. May increase risk of fetal abnormalities if administered during first trimester of pregnancy. Chronic ingestion during pregnancy may produce fetal toxicity, withdrawal symptoms, CNS depression in neonates. **Pregnancy Category D. Children:** Safety and efficacy not established in those younger than 12 yrs. **Elderly:** Use small initial doses with gradual increases to avoid ataxia, excessive sedation, or paradoxical CNS restlessness, excitement.

INTERACTIONS

DRUG: Valproic acid may increase concentration/effects. **Alcohol, other CNS depressants** may increase CNS depression. **HERBAL: Gotu kola, kava kava, St. John's wort, valerian** may increase CNS depression. **FOOD:** None known. **LAB VALUES:** None known. **Therapeutic serum level:** 50–240 ng/ml; **toxic serum level:** unknown.

AVAILABILITY (Rx)

Injection Solution: 2 mg/ml, 4 mg/ml. **Oral Solution (Lorazepam Intensol):** 2 mg/ml. **Tablets:** 0.5 mg, 1 mg, 2 mg.

ADMINISTRATION/HANDLING

 IV

Reconstitution • Dilute with equal volume of Sterile Water for Injection, D$_5$W, or 0.9% NaCl.

Rate of Administration • Give by IV push into tubing of free-flowing IV infusion (0.9% NaCl, D₅W) at a rate not to exceed 2 mg/min.
Storage • Refrigerate parenteral form. • Do not use if discolored or precipitate forms. • Avoid freezing.

IM
• Give deep IM into large muscle mass.

PO
• Give with food. • Tablets may be crushed. • Dilute oral solution in water, juice, soda, or semisolid food.

🔲 IV INCOMPATIBILITIES

Aztreonam (Azactam), ondansetron (Zofran).

🔲 IV COMPATIBILITIES

Bumetanide (Bumex), cefepime (Maxipime), dexmedetomidine (Precedex), diltiazem (Cardizem), dobutamine (Dobutrex), dopamine (Intropin), heparin, labetalol (Normodyne, Trandate), milrinone (Primacor), norepinephrine (Levophed), piperacillin and tazobactam (Zosyn), potassium, propofol (Diprivan).

INDICATIONS/ROUTES/DOSAGE

Anxiety
PO: ADULTS: 1–10 mg/day in 2–3 divided doses. Average: 2–6 mg/day. **ELDERLY:** Initially, 0.5–1 mg/day. May increase gradually. Range: 0.5–4 mg.
IV: ADULTS, ELDERLY: 0.02–0.06 mg/kg q2–6h.
IV Infusion: ADULTS, ELDERLY: 0.01–0.1 mg/kg/h.
PO, IV: CHILDREN: 0.05 mg/kg/dose q4–8h. Range: 0.02–0.1 mg/kg. **Maximum:** 2 mg/dose.

Insomnia Due to Anxiety
PO: ADULTS: 2–4 mg at bedtime. **ELDERLY:** 0.5–1 mg at bedtime.

Antiemetic
IV: ADULTS, ELDERLY: 0.5–2 mg q4–6h as needed. **CHILDREN 2–15 YRS:** 0.05 mg/kg (up to 2 mg) prior to chemotherapy.
PO: ADULTS, ELDERLY: 0.5–2 mg q4–6h as needed.

Status Epilepticus
IV: ADULTS, ELDERLY: 4 mg over 2–5 min. May repeat in 10–15 min. **Usual maximum:** 8 mg in 12-hr period. **CHILDREN:** 0.05–0.1 mg/kg over 2–5 min. **Maximum:** 4 mg. May repeat in 10–15 min. **NEONATES:** 0.05 mg/kg over 2–5 min. May repeat in 10–15 min.

SIDE EFFECTS

Frequent (16%–7%): Drowsiness, dizziness. **Rare (less than 4%):** Weakness, ataxia, headache, hypotension, nausea, vomiting, confusion, injection site reaction.

ADVERSE EFFECTS/ TOXIC REACTIONS

Abrupt or too-rapid withdrawal may result in pronounced restlessness, irritability, insomnia, hand tremor, abdominal cramping, muscle cramps, diaphoresis, vomiting, seizures. Overdose results in drowsiness, confusion, diminished reflexes, coma. **Antidote:** Flumazenil (see Appendix K for dosage).

NURSING CONSIDERATIONS

BASELINE ASSESSMENT

Offer emotional support to anxious pt. Pt must remain recumbent following parenteral administration to reduce hypotensive effect. Assess motor responses (agitation, trembling, tension), autonomic responses (cold or clammy hands, diaphoresis).

INTERVENTION/EVALUATION

Monitor B/P, respiratory rate, heart rate. For those on long-term therapy, hepatic/renal function tests, CBC should be performed periodically. Assess for paradoxical reaction, particularly during early therapy. Evaluate for therapeutic response: calm facial expression, decreased restlessness, insomnia. **Therapeutic serum level:** 50–240 ng/ml; **toxic serum level:** N/A.

PATIENT/ FAMILY TEACHING

• Drowsiness usually subsides during continued therapy. • Avoid tasks that require alertness, motor skills until response to drug is established. • Smoking reduces drug effectiveness. • Do not abruptly discontinue medication after long-term therapy. • Do not use alcohol, CNS depressants. • Contraception recommended for long-term therapy. • Notify physician at once if pregnancy is suspected.

lorcaserin

lor-ca-ser-in
(Belviq)

◆CLASSIFICATION

PHARMACOTHERAPEUTIC: Serotonin receptor agonist. **CLINICAL:** Weight loss agent (see p. 138C).

ACTION

Activates $5HT_{2C}$ receptors on anorexigenic neurons located in the hypothalamus. **Therapeutic Effect:** Decreases food consumption, promotes satiety.

PHARMACOKINETICS

Rapidly absorbed from GI tract. Peak plasma concentration: 1.5–2h. Distributed in cerebrospinal fluid and CNS. Protein binding: 70%. Metabolized in liver. Primarily excreted in urine with minimal amount eliminated in feces.

USES

Adjunct to reduced-calorie diet and increased physical activity for chronic weight management in adults with an initial body mass index (BMI) of 30 kg/m^2 or greater (obese), or 27 kg/m^2 or greater (overweight) with at least one weight-re-

lated comorbid condition (e.g., hypertension, dyslipidemia, type 2 diabetes).

PRECAUTIONS

Contraindications: Pregnancy (Pregnancy Category X). **Cautions:** Use in those with severe renal impairment, end-stage renal disease is not recommended. Concurrent use with medications that affect serotonergic neurotransmitter system (particularly during initiation of therapy and dose increases). Moderate renal impairment, severe hepatic impairment, HF, pts predisposed to priapism (e.g., leukemia). Pts at high risk for suicidal thoughts, behavior. Bradycardia, heart block, diabetes.

⌛ LIFESPAN CONSIDERATIONS

Pregnancy/Lactation: May cause fetal harm. Unknown if distributed in breast milk. **Pregnancy Category X. Children:** Not for use in this age group. **Elderly:** Age-related renal impairment may require dose adjustment.

INTERACTIONS

DRUG: May increase concentration/effects of **CYP3D6 substrates** (e.g., **amitriptyline, metoprolol, venlafaxine**). **Triptans, monoamine oxidase inhibitors (MAOIs, including linezolid), selective serotonin reuptake inhibitors (SSRIs), selective serotonin-norepinephrine reuptake inhibitors, dextromethorphan, tricyclic antidepressants, bupropion, lithium, tramadol, tryptophan** may increase risk for serotonergic syndrome. **HERBAL: St. John's wort** increases potential for serotonin syndrome. **FOOD:** None known. **ALTERED LAB VALUES:** May lower Hgb, neutrophil count. May increase serum prolactin.

AVAILABILITY (Rx)

▼ **Tablets, Film-Coated:** 10 mg.

ADMINISTRATION/HANDLING

• Do not break, crush, dissolve, or divide film-coated tablet. May give without regard to food.

INDICATIONS/ROUTES/DOSAGE

Weight Management
PO: ADULTS, ELDERLY: 10 mg twice daily. Do not exceed 10 mg twice daily. Belviq should be discontinued if 5% weight loss is not achieved by week 12 of therapy.

SIDE EFFECTS

Note: Side effects tend to be mild and transient in nature, gradually diminishing during treatment. **Frequent (16%–5%):** Headache, dizziness, fatigue, diarrhea, nausea, dry mouth, constipation. **Type 2 Diabetic Pts (29%–7%):** Hypoglycemia, headache, back pain, nasopharyngitis, nausea, cough, fatigue, dizziness. **Occasional (6%–2%):** Cough, oropharyngeal pain, sinus congestion, musculoskeletal pain, rash. **Rare (4%–2%): Type 2 Diabetic Pts:** Muscle spasm, peripheral edema, anxiety, insomnia, seasonal allergy, gastroenteritis, toothache, decreased appetite, depression.

ADVERSE EFFECTS/ TOXIC REACTIONS

Potential for Serotonin Syndrome Serotonin syndrome symptoms including mental status changes (e.g., agitation, hallucinations, coma), autonomic instability (e.g., tachycardia, labile B/P, hyperthermia), neuromuscular changes (e.g., hyperreflexia, incoordination), and/or GI symptoms (e.g., nausea, vomiting, diarrhea) have been observed. Serotonin syndrome, in its most severe form, can resemble neuroleptic malignant syndrome, which includes hyperthermia, muscle rigidity, autonomic instability with possible rapid fluctuation of vital signs, and mental status changes. Urinary tract infection occurs in 9% of type 2 diabetic pts.

NURSING CONSIDERATIONS

BASELINE ASSESSMENT

Ensure negative pregnancy test prior to initiating treatment. Obtain baseline chemistries, particularly renal/hepatic function tests. Obtain weight, BMI.

INTERVENTION/EVALUATION

In trials, most patients lost at least 5% of their body weight over a year, and a further one third lost at least 10%. Most pts who develop signs or symptoms of valvular cardiac disease, including dyspnea, dependent edema, HF, or a new cardiac murmur while on medication; pts should be consistently monitored; discontinuation of treatment may be necessary.

PATIENT/FAMILY TEACHING

• Discontinue therapy if 5% weight loss has not been achieved by 12 wks of treatment. • High-fiber, low-fat diet decreases fat evacuation. • Avoid tasks that require alertness, motor skills until response to drug is established. • Swallow whole. Do not break, chew, crush, or divide tablets.

---

losartan

`TOP 200`

loe-**sar**-tan
(Apo-Losartan ♣, <u>Cozaar</u>)

BLACK BOX ALERT May cause fetal injury, mortality if used during second or third trimester of pregnancy. **Do not confuse Cozaar with Colace, Coreg, Hyzaar, or Zocor, or losartan with locaserin, valsartan.**

FIXED-COMBINATION(S)

Hyzaar: losartan/hydrochlorothiazide (a diuretic): 50 mg/12.5 mg, 100 mg/12.5 mg, 100 mg/25 mg.

◆CLASSIFICATION

PHARMACOTHERAPEUTIC: Angiotensin II receptor antagonist. **CLINICAL:** Antihypertensive (see p. 11C, 62C).

ACTION

Potent vasodilator. Blocks vasoconstrictor, aldosterone-secreting effects of angiotensin II, inhibiting binding of angiotensin II to AT_1 receptors. **Therapeutic Effect:** Causes vasodilation, decreases peripheral resistance, decreases B/P.

PHARMACOKINETICS

Route	Onset	Peak	Duration
PO	N/A	6 hrs	24 hrs

Well absorbed after PO administration. Protein binding: 98%. Metabolized in liver. Excreted in urine and via the biliary system. Not removed by hemodialysis. **Half-life:** 2 hrs; metabolite, 6–9 hrs.

USES

Treatment of hypertension. Used alone or in combination with other antihypertensives. Treatment of diabetic nephropathy (in pts with type 2 diabetes and hypertension), prevention of stroke in pts with hypertension and left ventricular hypertrophy. **OFF-LABEL:** Slow rate of progression of aortic root dilation in children with Marfan's syndrome.

PRECAUTIONS

Contraindications: Concomitant use of aliskiren in pts with diabetes. **Cautions:** Renal/hepatic impairment, unstented renal arterial stenosis, significant aortic/mitral stenosis.

⌛ LIFESPAN CONSIDERATIONS

Pregnancy/Lactation: Has caused fetal/neonatal morbidity, mortality. Potential for adverse effects on breast-fed infant. Breastfeeding not recommended. **Pregnancy Category C (D if used in second or third trimester). Children:** Safety and efficacy not established. **Elderly:** No age-related precautions noted.

INTERACTIONS

DRUG: NSAIDs may decrease effect. **Potassium-sparing diuretics, potassium supplements** may increase serum potassium. **Diuretics, other antihypertensive medications** may produce additive hypotension. **HERBAL: Ephedra, ginseng, licorice, yohimbe** may worsen hypertension. **Black cohosh, periwinkle** may increase antihypertensive effect. **Garlic, ginger, ginseng** may increase hypoglycemic effect. **FOOD:** None known. **LAB VALUES:** May increase serum bilirubin, AST, ALT, Hgb, Hct. May decrease serum glucose.

AVAILABILITY (Rx)

Tablets: 25 mg, 50 mg, 100 mg.

ADMINISTRATION/HANDLING

PO
• May give without regard to food.

INDICATIONS/ROUTES/DOSAGE

Hypertension
PO: ADULTS, ELDERLY: Initially, 50 mg once a day. **Maximum:** May be given once or twice a day, with total daily doses ranging from 25–100 mg. **CHILDREN 6–16 YRS:** 0.7 mg/kg once daily. **Maximum:** 50 mg/day.

Nephropathy
PO: ADULTS, ELDERLY: Initially, 50 mg/day. May increase to 100 mg/day based on B/P response.

Stroke Prevention
PO: ADULTS, ELDERLY: 50 mg/day. **Maximum:** 100 mg/day.

Hepatic Impairment
PO: ADULTS, ELDERLY: Initially, 25 mg/day. May increase up to 100 mg/day.

Renal Impairment
Not recommended if glomerular filtration rate (GFR) less than 30 ml/min.

SIDE EFFECTS

Frequent (8%): Upper respiratory tract infection. **Occasional (4%–2%):** Dizziness, diarrhea, cough. **Rare (1% or less):** Insomnia, dyspepsia, heartburn, back/leg pain, muscle cramps, myalgia, nasal congestion, sinusitis, depression.

ADVERSE EFFECTS/ TOXIC REACTIONS

Overdosage may manifest as hypotension and tachycardia. Bradycardia occurs less often. Institute supportive measures.

NURSING CONSIDERATIONS

BASELINE ASSESSMENT

Obtain B/P, apical pulse immediately before each dose, in addition to regular monitoring (be alert to fluctuations). Question for possibility of pregnancy (see Pregnancy/Lactation). Assess medication history (esp. diuretic).

INTERVENTION/EVALUATION

Maintain hydration (offer fluids frequently). Assess for evidence of upper respiratory infection, cough. Monitor B/P, pulse. If excessive reduction in B/P occurs, place pt in supine position, feet slightly elevated. Assist with ambulation if dizziness occurs. Monitor daily pattern of bowel activity, stool consistency.

PATIENT/FAMILY TEACHING

• Pts should take measures to avoid pregnancy. • Report pregnancy to physician as soon as possible. • Avoid tasks that require alertness, motor skills until response to drug is established (possible dizziness effect). • Report any sign of infection (sore throat, fever), chest pain. • Do not take OTC cold preparations, nasal decongestants. • Do not stop taking medication. • Limit salt intake.

---

lovastatin

loe-va-stat-in
(Altoprev, Apo-Lovastatin ✤, Mevacor, Novo-Lovastatin ✤)
Do not confuse lovastatin with atorvastatin, Leustatin, Lotensin, nystatin, pitavastatin, or pravastatin, or Mevacor with Benicar or Lipitor.

FIXED-COMBINATION(S)

Advicor: lovastatin/niacin: 20 mg/500 mg, 20 mg/750 mg, 20 mg/1,000 mg.

◆CLASSIFICATION

PHARMACOTHERAPEUTIC: HMG-CoA reductase inhibitor. **CLINICAL:** Antihyperlipidemic (see p. 58C).

ACTION

Inhibits HMG-CoA reductase, the enzyme that catalyzes the early step in cholesterol synthesis. **Therapeutic Effect:** Decreases LDL, VLDL, triglycerides; increases HDL.

PHARMACOKINETICS

Route	Onset	Peak	Duration
PO (LDL, cholesterol reduction)	3 days	N/A	N/A

Incompletely absorbed from GI tract (increased on empty stomach). Protein binding: 95%. Hydrolyzed in liver. Primarily eliminated in feces. Not removed by hemodialysis. **Half-life:** 1.1–1.7 hrs.

USES

Decreases elevated serum total and LDL cholesterol in primary hypercholesterolemia; primary prevention of coronary artery disease. Slows progression of coronary atherosclerosis in pts with coronary heart disease. Adjunct to diet in adolescent pts (10–17 yrs) with heterozygous familial hypercholesterolemia.

PRECAUTIONS

Contraindications: Active hepatic disease, pregnancy, unexplained elevated hepatic function tests. Pregnancy, breastfeeding. Concomitant use of strong CYP3A4 inhibitors. **Cautions:** History of heavy/chronic alcohol use, renal impairment, previous history of hepatic disease; concomitant use of amiodarone, cyclosporine, fibrates, gemfibrozil, niacin, verapamil.

⌛ LIFESPAN CONSIDERATIONS

Pregnancy/Lactation: Contraindicated in pregnancy (suppression of cholesterol biosynthesis may cause fetal toxicity) and

---

lactation. Unknown if drug is distributed in breast milk. **Pregnancy Category X. Children:** Safety and efficacy not established. **Elderly:** No age-related precautions noted.

INTERACTIONS

DRUG: CYP3A4 inhibitors (e.g., keto-conazole, clarithromycin) may increase concentration, risk of myopathy, rhabdomyolysis. **Cyclosporine, fibrates, gemfibrozil, niacin, amiodarone, verapamil** may increase risk of rhabdomyolysis, acute renal failure. **HERBAL: St. John's wort** may decrease concentration/effects. **FOOD:** Large amounts of **grapefruit juice** may increase risk of side effects (e.g., myalgia, weakness). **Red yeast rice** may increase concentration (2.4 mg lovastatin/600 mg rice). **LAB VALUES:** May increase serum creatine kinase (CK), transaminase.

AVAILABILITY (Rx)

Tablets (Mevacor): 10 mg, 20 mg, 40 mg.
Tablets (Extended-Release [Altoprev]): 20 mg, 40 mg, 60 mg.

ADMINISTRATION/HANDLING

PO
• Immediate-release tablet given with meals; extended-release at bedtime.
• Avoid intake of large quantities of grapefruit juice (greater than 1 quart).
• Do not crush extended-release tablets.

INDICATIONS/ROUTES/DOSAGE

Atherosclerosis, Coronary Artery Disease
PO *(Immediate-Release):* **ADULTS, EL-DERLY:** Initially, 20 mg/day. **Maintenance:** 10–80 mg once daily or in 2 divided doses. **Maximum:** 80 mg/day.

Hypercholesterolemia
PO *(Immediate-Release):* **ADULTS, EL-DERLY:** Initially, 20 mg/day. **Maintenance:** 10–80 mg once daily or in 2 divided doses. **Maximum:** 80 mg/day.
PO *(Extended-Release):* **ADULTS, EL-DERLY:** Initially, 20–60 mg once daily at

bedtime. **Maximum:** 60 mg once daily at bedtime.

Heterozygous Familial Hypercholesterolemia
PO *(Immediate-Release):* **CHILDREN 10–17 YRS:** Initially, 10–20 mg/day. Range: 10–40 mg daily.

Dosage with Concurrent Medication
Cyclosporine: Initially, 10 mg/day. **Maximum:** 20 mg/day. **Fibrates, niacin** (1 gram or more): **Maximum:** 20 mg/day. **Amiodarone, verapamil: Maximum:** 40 mg/day (immediate-release); 20 mg/day (extended-release).

SIDE EFFECTS

Generally well tolerated. Side effects usually mild and transient. **Frequent (9%–5%):** Headache, flatulence, diarrhea, abdominal pain, abdominal cramping, rash, pruritus. **Occasional (4%–3%):** Nausea, vomiting, constipation, dyspepsia. **Rare (2%–1%):** Dizziness, heartburn, myalgia, blurred vision, eye irritation.

ADVERSE EFFECTS/TOXIC REACTIONS

Potential for cataract development. Occasionally produces myopathy manifested as muscle pain, tenderness, weakness with elevated creatine kinase (CK). Severe myopathy may lead to rhabdomyolysis.

NURSING CONSIDERATIONS

BASELINE ASSESSMENT
Obtain dietary history. Question for possibility of pregnancy before initiating therapy (Pregnancy Category X). Assess baseline lab results: serum cholesterol, triglycerides, hepatic function tests.

INTERVENTION/EVALUATION
Monitor daily pattern of bowel activity, stool consistency. Monitor for headache, dizziness, blurred vision. Assess for rash, pruritus. Monitor serum cholesterol, triglycerides for therapeutic response. Be

alert for malaise, muscle cramping/weakness. Monitor hepatic function tests.

PATIENT/FAMILY TEACHING
• Follow special diet (important part of treatment). • Periodic lab tests are essential part of therapy. • Maintain appropriate birth control measures (Pregnancy Category X). • Avoid grapefruit juice, alcohol. • Inform physician of severe gastric upset, vision changes, myalgia, weakness, changes in color of urine/stool, yellowing of eyes/skin, unusual bruising.

---

lubiprostone

loo-bi-**pros**-tone
(Amitiza)

◆CLASSIFICATION
PHARMACOTHERAPEUTIC: Chloride channel activator. **CLINICAL:** Constipation agent.

ACTION
Secretes fluid into abdominal lumen through activation of chloride channels in apical membranes of GI epithelium. **Therapeutic Effect:** Increases intestinal motility, thereby increasing passage of stool, alleviating symptoms associated with chronic idiopathic constipation.

PHARMACOKINETICS
Rapidly, extensively metabolized within stomach and jejunum. Minimal distribution beyond GI tissue. Protein binding: 94%. Excreted in urine (60%), feces (30%). **Half-life:** 0.9–1.4 hrs.

USES
Treatment of chronic idiopathic constipation in adults. Treatment of opioid-induced constipation. Treatment of irritable bowel syndrome (IBS) with constipation in women 18 yrs and older.

PRECAUTIONS
Contraindications: History of mechanical GI obstruction. **Cautions:** Severe diarrhea.

⧗ LIFESPAN CONSIDERATIONS
May have potential for teratogenic effects. **Pregnancy/Lactation:** Unknown if distributed in breast milk. **Pregnancy Category C. Children:** Safety and efficacy not established. **Elderly:** No age-related precautions noted.

INTERACTIONS
DRUG: None significant. **HERBAL:** None significant. **FOOD:** None known. **LAB VALUES:** None significant.

AVAILABILITY (Rx)
Capsules: 8 mcg, 24 mcg.

ADMINISTRATION/HANDLING
PO
• Give with food and water.

INDICATIONS/ROUTES/DOSAGE
Chronic Idiopathic Constipation, Opioid-Induced Constipation
PO: ADULTS, ELDERLY: 24 mcg twice daily with food.

IBS
PO: ADULTS, ELDERLY (FEMALES): 8 mcg twice daily with food.

SIDE EFFECTS
Frequent (31%): Nausea. **Occasional (13%–4%):** Headache, diarrhea, abdominal distention, abdominal pain, flatulence, vomiting, peripheral edema, dizziness. **Rare (3%–2%):** Dyspepsia (heartburn, indigestion, epigastric distress), loose stools, fatigue, dry mouth, arthralgia, back pain, cough.

ADVERSE EFFECTS/ TOXIC REACTIONS
UTI, upper respiratory tract infection occurs in 4% of pts.

NURSING CONSIDERATIONS

BASELINE ASSESSMENT

Confirm negative pregnancy test prior to beginning therapy and comply with effective contraceptive measures during therapy. Assess for diarrhea (avoid use in these pts).

INTERVENTION/EVALUATION

Assess for improvement in symptoms (relief from bloating, cramping, urgency, abdominal discomfort). Monitor daily pattern of bowel activity, stool consistency.

PATIENT/FAMILY TEACHING

• Inform physician of new/worsening episodes of abdominal pain, severe diarrhea.
• Avoid tasks that require alertness, motor skills until response to drug is established.

---

lucinactant

loo-sin-**ak**-tant
(Surfaxin)
Do not confuse Surfaxin with Surfak.

◆CLASSIFICATION

PHARMACOTHERAPEUTIC: Synthetic peptide-containing surfactant. **CLINICAL:** Pulmonary surfactant.

ACTION

Lowers surface tension at air-liquid interface of alveoli during respiration. Stabilizes alveoli versus collapse trans-pulmonary pressure. **Therapeutic Effect:** Improves lung compliance, gas exchange.

PHARMACOKINETICS

Absorbed directly at terminal bronchiole and alveolar surface. No distribution, metabolism, elimination noted. **Half-life:** N/A.

USES

Prevention of respiratory distress syndrome (RDS) in high-risk premature infants.

PRECAUTIONS

Contraindications: None known. **Cautions:** Infants at high-risk for rapid deoxygenation, difficult intubation.

⌛ LIFESPAN CONSIDERATIONS

Used only in infants. No age-related precautions noted.

INTERACTIONS

DRUG: None known. **HERBAL:** None significant. **FOOD:** None known. **LAB VALUES:** None significant.

AVAILABILITY (Rx)

Intratracheal Suspension: 8.5 ml/vial.

ADMINISTRATION/HANDLING

Drug Preparation
• Warm glass vial for 15 min on block heater set at 44°C. • Once warmed, vigorously shake suspension until fluidity achieved. • Record warming date/time on specified carton space. • Visually inspect before use. • Suspension should appear opaque to off-white once warmed. • Slowly draw into syringe using 16- to 18-gauge needle.

Patient Preparation
• Assess satisfactory placement, position, patency of endotracheal (ET) tube. • May suction ET tube prior to administration. • Allow oxygenation to stabilize before proceeding.
Rate of Administration • Raise head of bed to 30 degrees and place infant in right lateral decubitus position. • Attach syringe to 5-French instillation catheter. • Thread catheter into endotracheal access device and advance to position slightly past the distal end of ET tube. • Instill one fourth of suspension as bolus. • Repeat procedure in left lateral decubitus position, then repeat in right lateral decubitus position, then repeat in left lateral decubitus position for total of 4 separate instillations. • If appropriate, do not suction ET tube for 1 hr after administration.
Storage • Refrigerate unused vials. • Protect from light. • Do not freeze.

• May store warmed suspension at room temperature for 2 hrs only. • Do not refrigerate warmed suspension. • Discard if not used within 2 hrs.

INDICATIONS/ROUTES/DOSAGE

Respiratory Distress Syndrome
Endotracheal: INFANTS: 5.8 ml/kg, up to 4 doses within first 48 hrs of life. Do not administer more frequently than every 6 hrs.

ADVERSE EFFECTS/ TOXIC REACTIONS

Adverse reactions are mainly attributed to administration, including bradycardia, oxygen desaturation, cyanosis, apnea, airway/ET tube obstruction, reflux into ET tube. Suctioning and/or reintubation may be necessary if airway obstruction occurs.

NURSING CONSIDERATIONS

BASELINE ASSESSMENT

Must be administered by or under the close supervision of clinicians experienced in ventilator management, intubation, resuscitation, general care of premature infants.

INTERVENTION/EVALUATION

Frequently assess vital signs, airway patency, lung sounds, oxygen saturation, end-tidal CO_2. Modify ventilator settings if adverse reaction, sustained oxygen desaturation occurs. Maintain positive end-expiratory pressure of 4–5 cm H_2O during administration.

PATIENT/FAMILY TEACHING

• Offer emotional support to parents.
• Explain role of surfactant in infants.

lurasidone

loo-**ras**-i-done
(Latuda)
BLACK BOX ALERT Elderly pts with dementia-related psychosis are at increased risk for mortality due to cardiovascular events, infectious diseases.

◆CLASSIFICATION

PHARMACOTHERAPEUTIC: Dopamine, serotonin receptor antagonist. **CLINICAL:** Antipsychotic.

ACTION

Antagonizes central dopamine type 2 and serotonin type 2 receptors. **Therapeutic Effect:** Diminishes symptoms of schizophrenia.

PHARMACOKINETICS

Absorbed in 1–3 hrs. Steady-state concentration occurs in 7 days. Well absorbed from GI tract (unaffected by food). Protein binding: 99%. Metabolized in liver. Primarily excreted in urine, with lesser amount eliminated in feces. **Half-life:** 28–36 hrs.

USES

Treatment of schizophrenia. Depression associated with bipolar-1 disorder.

PRECAUTIONS

Contraindications: Strong CYP3A4 inhibitors (e.g., ketoconazole) and inducers (e.g., rifampin). **Cautions:** Cardiovascular disease (HF, history of MI, ischemia, conduction abnormalities), cerebrovascular disease (history of CVA in pts with dementia, seizure disorders). Pts with an established diagnosis of diabetes mellitus. Parkinson's disease, renal/hepatic impairment, pts at risk for aspiration pneumonia, those at risk for suicide.

⧖ LIFESPAN CONSIDERATIONS

Pregnancy/Lactation: Unknown if distributed in breast milk. Breastfeeding not recommended. **Pregnancy Category B. Children:** Safety and efficacy not established. **Elderly:** More susceptible to postural hypotension. Increased risk of cerebrovascular events, mortality, including stroke, in elderly pts with psychosis.

INTERACTIONS

DRUG: Alcohol, CNS depressants may increase CNS depression. **Rifampin** decreases concentration/effects. **Diltiazem, ketoconazole, ritonavir** may increase concentration/effects. **HERBAL: Gotu kola, kava kava, St. John's wort, valerian** may increase CNS depression. **FOOD: Grapefruit, grapefruit juice** may increase risk of torsades, orthostatic hypotension. **LAB VALUES:** May increase prolactin levels.

AVAILABILITY (Rx)

Tablets: 20 mg, 40 mg, 80 mg, 120 mg.

ADMINISTRATION/HANDLING

PO
• Give with food. • Tablets may be crushed.

INDICATIONS/ROUTES/DOSAGE

Schizophrenia
PO: ADULTS, ELDERLY: 40 mg once daily with food. **Maximum:** 160 mg once daily with food. In those with moderate to severe hepatic/renal impairment, do not exceed 40 mg daily.

Concomitant CYP3A4 Inhibitors/Inducers
PO: ADULTS, ELDERLY: Initially, 20 mg/day. **Maximum:** 80 mg/day.

Renal Impairment (Less Than 50 ml/min)
PO: ADULTS, ELDERLY: Initially, 20 mg/day. **Maximum:** 80 mg/day.

Hepatic Impairment
PO: ADULTS, ELDERLY: (Moderate): Initially, 20 mg/day. **Maximum:** 80 mg/day. **(Severe):** Initially, 20 mg/day. **Maximum:** 40 mg/day.

Depressive Episode Associated with Bipolar Disorder
PO: ADULTS, ELDERLY: Initially, 20 mg once daily. **Maximum:** 120 mg/day.

SIDE EFFECTS

Frequent (15%–7%): Drowsiness, sedation, insomnia (paradoxical reaction). **Occasional (6%–3%):** Nausea, vomiting, dyspepsia (heartburn, GI upset), fatigue, back pain, akathisia, dizziness, agitation, anxiety. **Rare (2%–1%):** Restlessness, salivary hypersecretion, tongue spasm, torticollis, trismus.

ADVERSE EFFECTS/TOXIC REACTIONS

Extrapyramidal disorder (including cogwheel rigidity, drooling, bradykinesia, tardive dyskinesia, tremors) occurs in 5% of pts. Neuroleptic malignant syndrome (fever, muscle rigidity, irregular B/P or pulse, altered mental status) occurs rarely.

NURSING CONSIDERATIONS

BASELINE ASSESSMENT

Assess behavior, appearance, emotional status, response to environment, speech pattern, thought content. Renal/hepatic function tests should be obtained before therapy as dose adjustment is required when initiating therapy.

INTERVENTION/EVALUATION

Supervise suicidal risk pt closely during early therapy (as depression lessens, energy level improves, increasing suicide potential). Monitor for potential neuroleptic malignant syndrome (fever, muscle rigidity, irregular B/P or pulse, altered mental status, visual changes, dyspnea). Assess for therapeutic response (greater interest in surroundings, improved self-care, increased ability to concentrate, relaxed facial expression).

PATIENT/FAMILY TEACHING

• Avoid tasks that may require alertness, motor skills until response to drug is established (may cause drowsiness, dizziness). • Avoid alcohol. • Inform physician of trembling in fingers, altered gait, unusual muscle/skeletal movements, palpitations, severe dizziness, fainting, visual changes, rash, difficulty breathing. • Report suicidal ideation, unusual changes in behavior.

lymphocyte immune globulin N

lim-foe-site ih-**myoon glah**-bue-lin **N**
(Atgam)

BLACK BOX ALERT Use only by physicians experienced in immunosuppressive therapy for treatment of renal transplant or aplastic anemia pts.
Do not confuse Atgam with Ativan.

◆CLASSIFICATION

PHARMACOTHERAPEUTIC: Biologic response modifier. **CLINICAL:** Immunosuppressant.

ACTION

Acts as lymphocyte selective immunosuppressant, reducing number/altering function of T lymphocytes, which are responsible for cell-mediated and humoral immunity. Stimulates release of hematopoietic growth factors. **Therapeutic Effect:** Prevents allograft rejection; treats aplastic anemia.

PHARMACOKINETICS

Unknown absorption, metabolism, elimination. **Half-life:** Approximately 5–7 days.

USES

Prevention/treatment of renal allograft rejection. Treatment of moderate to severe aplastic anemia in pts not candidates for bone marrow transplant. **OFF-LABEL:** Prevention/treatment of other solid organ allograft rejection, prevent graft-vs-host disease following stem cell transplantation, myelodysplastic syndrome.

PRECAUTIONS

Contraindications: Systemic hypersensitivity reaction to previous injection of lymphocyte immune globulin N. **Cautions:** Concurrent immunosuppressive therapy.

⏳ LIFESPAN CONSIDERATIONS

Pregnancy/Lactation: Unknown if drug crosses placenta or is distributed in breast milk. **Pregnancy Category C. Children:** Safety and efficacy not established. **Elderly:** No age-related precautions noted.

INTERACTIONS

DRUG: Reduction of **corticosteroids, other immunosuppressants** may unmask reactions to lymphocyte immune globulin. **HERBAL:** **Echinacea** may decrase levels/effects. **FOOD:** None known. **LAB VALUES:** May alter BUN, serum creatinine.

AVAILABILITY

Injection Solution: 50 mg/ml.

ADMINISTRATION/HANDLING

 IV

Reconstitution • Total daily dose must be further diluted with 0.9% NaCl (do not use D₅W). • Gently rotate diluted solution. Do not shake. • Final concentration must not exceed 4 mg/ml.
Rate of Administration • Use 0.2- to 1-micron filter. • Give total daily dose over minimum of 4 hrs.
Storage • Keep refrigerated before and after dilution. • Discard diluted solution after 24 hrs.

🚫 IV INCOMPATIBILITIES

No information is available for Y-site administration.

INDICATIONS/ROUTES/DOSAGE

◀ **ALERT** ▶ Skin test recommended prior to initial dose. Use 0.1 ml of fresh 1:1,000 dilution. Observe q15–20min for 1 hr.

Prevention of Renal Allograft Rejection
IV: ADULTS, ELDERLY, CHILDREN: 15 mg/kg/day for 14 days, then every other day for 14 days. First dose within 24 hrs before or after transplantation.

Treatment of Renal Allograft Rejection
IV: **ADULTS, ELDERLY, CHILDREN**: 10–15 mg/kg/day for 14 days, then every other day for 14 more days. **Maximum**: 21 doses in 28 days.

Aplastic Anemia
IV: **ADULTS, ELDERLY, CHILDREN**: 10–20 mg/kg once a day for 8–14 days, then every other day. **Maximum**: 21 doses.

SIDE EFFECTS

Frequent (51%–13%): Fever, thrombocytopenia, rash, chills, leukopenia, systemic infection. **Occasional (10%–5%)**: Serum sickness-like reaction, dyspnea, apnea, arthralgia, chest pain, back pain, flank pain, nausea, vomiting, diarrhea, phlebitis.

ADVERSE EFFECTS/ TOXIC REACTIONS

Thrombocytopenia may occur but is generally transient. Severe hypersensitivity reaction, including anaphylaxis, occurs rarely.

NURSING CONSIDERATIONS

BASELINE ASSESSMENT
Use of high-flow vein (CVL, PICC, Groshong catheter) may prevent chemical phlebitis that may occur if peripheral vein is used.

INTERVENTION/EVALUATION
Monitor frequently for chills, fever, erythema, pruritus. Obtain order for prophylactic antihistamines or corticosteroids.

L

macitentan

ma-si-**ten**-tan
(Opsumit)

BLACK BOX ALERT Do not administer during pregnancy. May cause fetal harm. Exclude pregnancy before, during, and at least 1 mo after treatment. Treatment of female pts only available through restricted program called OPSUMIT Risk Evaluation and Mitigation Strategy (REMS).

◆CLASSIFICATION

PHARMACOTHERAPEUTIC: Endothelial receptor antagonist. **CLINICAL:** Pulmonary vasodilator.

ACTION

Prevents binding of endothelin (ET-1) and its receptors. Decreases occurrence of vasoconstriction, fibrosis, hypertrophy, and inflammation in pulmonary smooth muscle cells. **Therapeutic Effect:** Improves exercise ability, slows clinical worsening of pulmonary arterial hypertension (PAH).

PHARMACOKINETICS

Metabolized in liver. Protein binding: 99%. Peak plasma concentration: 8 hrs. Excreted in urine (50%), feces (24%). **Half-life:** 16 hrs.

USES

Treatment of pulmonary arterial hypertension (PAH, World Health Organization Group I) to delay disease progression.

PRECAUTIONS

Contraindications: Pregnancy (Category X). **Cautions:** Hepatic impairment, anemia, pulmonary edema, HF, pulmonary edema with pulmonary veno-occlusive disease.

⧗ LIFESPAN CONSIDERATIONS

Pregnancy/Lactation: May cause fetal harm. Recommend either intrauterine device (IUD) or oral contraceptive, plus barrier methods. Unknown if distributed in breast milk. Must either discontinue drug or discontinue breastfeeding. **Males:** May induce atrophy of seminiferous tubules of the testes, reduced sperm count, male infertility. **Pregnancy Category X. Children:** Safety and efficacy not established. **Elderly:** No age-related precautions noted.

INTERACTIONS

DRUG: Strong **CYP3A4 inducers (e.g., rifampin)** may decrease concentration/effect. Strong **CYP3A4 inhibitors (e.g., ketoconazole, ritonavir)** may increase concentration/effect. **HERBAL:** None significant. **FOOD:** None known. **LAB VALUES:** May increase serum AST, ALT, bilirubin. May decrease Hgb, Hct.

AVAILABILITY (Rx)

🗋 **Tablets:** 10 mg.

ADMINISTRATION/HANDLING

PO
• Give without regard to meals. • Swallow whole; do not split, crush, or break.

INDICATIONS/ROUTES/DOSAGE

Pulmonary Arterial Hypertension
PO: ADULTS/ELDERLY: 10 mg once daily.

SIDE EFFECTS

Frequent (20%): Nasopharyngitis, pharyngitis. **Occasional (14%–6%):** Headache, anemia, bronchitis, urinary tract infection.

ADVERSE EFFECTS/ TOXIC REACTIONS

Hepatotoxicity, hepatic failure reported in 3% of pts. Decreased Hgb level below 10 g/dL occurred in 9% of pts. May decrease sperm count in males. May increase risk of influenza infection.

NURSING CONSIDERATIONS

BASELINE ASSESSMENT

Obtain baseline CBC, hepatic function test. Confirm negative pregnancy status before

M

initiating treatment. Receive full medication history.

INTERVENTION/EVALUATION

Monitor hepatic/renal function test, Hgb, Hct, renal panel routinely. Monitor pregnancy status every mo during treatment and for 1 mo after discontinuation. Notify physician to obtain CXR if difficulty in breathing occurs and screen for veno-occlusive disease or pulmonary embolism. Monitor for jaundice, right upper abdominal pain, amber-colored urine, bruising.

PATIENT/FAMILY TEACHING

• May cause fetal harm. Immediately report suspected pregnancy. • Do not breastfeed. • Do not have unprotected sexual intercourse if taking only oral hormonal birth control. Consult with gynecologist for appropriate birth control methods. • Report any yellowing of skin or eyes, abdominal pain, bruising, black/tarry stools, dark urine, decreased urine output. • Swallow tablets whole; do not crush or chew.

magnesium   `HIGH ALERT`

mag-**nee**-zee-um

magnesium chloride

(Mag-Delay, Slow-Mag)

magnesium citrate

(Citroma, Citro-Mag ✤)

magnesium hydroxide

(Phillips Milk of Magnesia)

magnesium oxide

(Mag-Ox 400, Uro-Mag)

magnesium protein complex

(Mg-PLUS)

magnesium sulfate

(Epsom salt, magnesium sulfate injection)

Do not confuse magnesium sulfate with morphine sulfate.

FIXED-COMBINATION(S)

With aluminum, an antacid (**Aludrox, Delcid, Gaviscon, Maalox**); with aluminum and simethicone, an antiflatulent (**Di-Gel, Gelusil, Maalox Plus, Mylanta**); with aluminum and calcium, an antacid (**Camalox**); with mineral oil, a lubricant laxative (**Haley's MO**); with magnesium oxide and aluminum oxide, an antacid (**Riopan**).

◆CLASSIFICATION

CLINICAL: Antacid, anticonvulsant, electrolyte, laxative (see pp. 13C, 125C).

ACTION

Antacid: Acts in stomach to neutralize gastric acid. **Therapeutic Effect:** Increases pH. **Laxative:** Osmotic effect primarily in small intestine, draws water into intestinal lumen. **Therapeutic Effect:** Promotes peristalsis, bowel evacuation. **Systemic (dietary supplement replacement):** Found primarily in intracellular fluids. **Therapeutic Effect:** Essential for enzyme activity, nerve conduction, muscle contraction. Maintains and restores magnesium levels. **Anticonvulsant:** Blocks neuromuscular transmission, amount of acetylcholine released at motor end plate. **Therapeutic Effect:** Produces seizure control.

PHARMACOKINETICS

Antacid, laxative: Minimal absorption through intestine. Absorbed dose primarily excreted in urine. **Systemic:** Widely distributed. Primarily excreted in urine.

USES

Magnesium chloride: Dietary supplement. **Magnesium citrate:** Evacuation of bowel before surgical, diagnostic procedures. **Magnesium hydroxide:** Short-term treatment of constipation, symptoms of hyperacidity. **Magnesium oxide:** Magnesium replacement. **Magnesium sulfate:** Treatment/prevention of hypomagnesemia; prevention and treatment of seizures in eclampsia; treatment of seizures associated with acute nephritis; torsade de pointes (atypical ventricular tachycardia); treatment of arrhythmias due to hypomagnesemia (ventricular tachycardia/ventricular fibrillation). **OFF-LABEL: Magnesium sulfate:** Premature labor, acute asthma, MI, tocolysis.

PRECAUTIONS

Contraindications: Antacid: Appendicitis, symptoms of appendicitis, ileostomy, intestinal obstruction, severe renal impairment. **Laxative:** Appendicitis, HF, colostomy, hypersensitivity, ileostomy, intestinal obstruction, undiagnosed rectal bleeding. **Systemic:** Heart block, myocardial damage, renal failure. **Cautions:** Safety in children younger than 6 yrs not known. **Antacids:** Undiagnosed GI/rectal bleeding, ulcerative colitis, colostomy, diverticulitis, chronic diarrhea. **Laxative:** Diabetes mellitus, pts on low-salt diet (some products contain sugar, sodium). **Systemic:** Severe renal impairment.

⚗ LIFESPAN CONSIDERATIONS

Pregnancy/Lactation: Antacid: Unknown if distributed in breast milk. **Parenteral:** Readily crosses placenta. Distributed in breast milk for 24 hrs after magnesium therapy is discontinued. Continuous IV infusion increases risk of magnesium toxicity in neonate. IV administration should not be used 2 hrs preceding delivery. **Pregnancy Category B. Children:** No age-related precautions noted. **Elderly:** Increased risk of developing magnesium deficiency (e.g., poor diet, decreased absorption, medications).

INTERACTIONS

DRUG: May decrease absorption of **quinolones, tetracycline, bisphospho-**

nates. May increase effects of **antihypertensives. HERBAL:** None significant. **FOOD:** None known. **LAB VALUES: Antacid:** May increase gastrin production, pH. **Laxative:** May decrease serum potassium. **Systemic:** None significant.

AVAILABILITY

MAGNESIUM CHLORIDE
Tablets (Mag Delay, Slow-Mag): 64 mg.
MAGNESIUM CITRATE
Oral Solution (Citroma): 290 mg/5 ml.
MAGNESIUM HYDROXIDE
Oral Liquid (Phillips Milk of Magnesia): 400 mg/5 ml, 800 mg/5 ml.
Tablets (Chewable [Phillips Milk of Magnesia]): 311 mg.
MAGNESIUM OXIDE
Capsules (Uro-Mag): 140 mg. **Tablets (Mag-Ox 400):** 400 mg.
MAGNESIUM SULFATE
Infusion Solution: 10 mg/ml, 20 mg/ml, 40 mg/ml, 80 mg/ml. **Injection Solution:** 125 mg/ml, 500 mg/ml.

ADMINISTRATION/HANDLING

 IV

Reconstitution • Must dilute to maximum concentration of 20%.
Rate of Administration • For IV infusion, maximum rate of infusion is 2 g/hr.
Storage • Store at room temperature.

IM
• For adults, elderly, use 250 mg/ml (25%) or 500 mg/ml (50%) magnesium sulfate concentration. • For infants, children, do not exceed 200 mg/ml (20%).

PO (Antacid)
• Shake suspension well before use.
• Chewable tablets should be chewed thoroughly before swallowing, followed by full glass of water.

PO (Laxative)
• Drink full glass of liquid (8 oz) with each dose (prevents dehydration). • Flavor may be improved by following with fruit juice, citrus carbonated beverage.

• Refrigerate citrate of magnesia (retains potency, palatability).

🔷 IV INCOMPATIBILITIES

Amphotericin B complex (Abelcet, AmBisome, Amphotec), cefepime (Maxipime), lansoprazole (Prevacid), pantoprazole (Protonix).

🔷 IV COMPATIBILITIES

Amikacin (Amikin), cefazolin (Ancef), ciprofloxacin (Cipro), dexmedetomidine (Precedex), dobutamine (Dobutrex), enalapril (Vasotec), gentamicin, heparin, hydromorphone (Dilaudid), insulin, linezolid (Zyvox), metoclopramide (Reglan), milrinone (Primacor), morphine, piperacillin/tazobactam (Zosyn), potassium chloride, propofol (Diprivan), tobramycin (Nebcin), vancomycin (Vancocin).

INDICATIONS/ROUTES/DOSAGE

Hypomagnesemia
Magnesium sulfate

Mild Deficiency
IM: ADULTS, ELDERLY: 1 g q6h for 4 doses.

Severe Deficiency
IM: ADULTS, ELDERLY: Up to 250 mg/kg over 4 hrs.
IV: ADULTS, ELDERLY: 1–2 g/hr for 3–6 hrs, then 0.5–1 g/hr as needed to correct deficiency. **CHILDREN:** 25–50 mg/kg/dose q4–6h for 3–4 doses.

Symptomatic Deficiency
IV: ADULTS, ELDERLY: 1–2 g over 5–60 min.

Usual Dose for Children
IM/IV: 25–50 mg/kg/dose q4–6h for 3–4 doses. **Maximum single dose:** 2 g.

Usual Dose for Neonates
IM/IV: 25–50 mg/kg/dose q8–12h for 2–3 doses.

Eclampsia
IV: ADULTS: 4–5 g infusion, then 1–2 g/hr continuous infusion. **Maximum:** 40 g/24 hrs.

Hypertension, Seizures
IV, IM *(Magnesium Sulfate)*: **ADULTS, ELDERLY:** 1 g q6h for 4 doses as needed. **CHILDREN:** 20–100 mg/kg/dose q4–6h as needed.

Arrhythmias, Torsade de Pointes
IV *(Magnesium Sulfate)*: **ADULTS, ELDERLY:** Initially, 1–2 g over 15 min. **CHILDREN:** 25–50 mg/kg/dose.

Bronchodilation
IV *(Magnesium Sulfate)*: **ADULTS, ELDERLY:** 2 g as a single dose. **CHILDREN:** 25–75 mg/kg/dose as a single dose.

Constipation
PO *(Magnesium Hydroxide)*: **ADULTS, ELDERLY, CHILDREN 12 YRS AND OLDER:** 6–8 tablets or 30–60 ml/day (400 mg/5 ml). **CHILDREN 6–11 YRS:** 3–4 tablets or 15–30 ml/day (400 mg/5 ml). **CHILDREN 2–5 YRS:** 1–2 tablets or 5–15 ml/day (400 mg/5 ml).

Hyperacidity
PO *(Magnesium Hydroxide)*: **ADULTS, ELDERLY, CHILDREN 12 YRS AND OLDER:** 2–4 tablets or 5–15 ml as needed up to 4 times a day.

Magnesium Deficiency
PO *(Magnesium Oxide)*: **ADULTS, ELDERLY:** 1–2 tablets 2–3 times a day.

Dietary Supplement
PO *(Magnesium Chloride)*: **ADULTS, ELDERLY:** 2 tablets daily.

Cathartic
PO *(Magnesium Citrate)*: **ADULTS, ELDERLY, CHILDREN 12 YRS AND OLDER:** 120–300 ml. **CHILDREN 6–11 YRS:** 100–150 ml. **CHILDREN YOUNGER THAN 6 YRS:** 0.5 ml/kg up to maximum of 200 ml.

SIDE EFFECTS

Frequent: **Antacid:** Chalky taste, diarrhea, laxative effect. Occasional: **Antacid:** Nausea, vomiting, stomach cramps. **Antacid, laxative:** Prolonged use or large doses in renal impairment may cause hypermagnesemia (dizziness, palpitations, altered mental status, fatigue, weakness). **Laxative:** Cramping, diarrhea, increased thirst, flatulence. **Systemic (dietary supplement, electrolyte replacement):** Reduced respiratory rate, decreased reflexes, flushing, hypotension, decreased heart rate.

ADVERSE EFFECTS/ TOXIC REACTIONS

Magnesium as antacid, laxative has no known adverse reactions. Systemic use may produce prolonged PR interval, widening of QRS interval. Magnesium toxicity may cause loss of deep tendon reflexes, heart block, respiratory paralysis, cardiac arrest. **Antidote:** 10–20 ml 10% calcium gluconate (5–10 mEq of calcium).

NURSING CONSIDERATIONS

BASELINE ASSESSMENT

Assess sensitivity to magnesium. **Antacid:** Assess GI pain (duration, location, quality, time of occurrence, relief with food, causative/exacerbative factors). **Laxative:** Assess for weight loss, nausea, vomiting, history of recent abdominal surgery. **Systemic:** Assess renal function, serum magnesium.

INTERVENTION/EVALUATION

Antacid: Assess for relief of gastric distress. Monitor renal function (esp. if dosing is long term or frequent). **Laxative:** Monitor daily pattern of bowel activity, stool consistency. Maintain adequate fluid intake. **Systemic:** Monitor renal function, magnesium levels, EKG for cardiac function. Test patellar reflexes (knee jerk reflexes) before giving repeat parenteral doses (used as indication of CNS depression; suppressed reflexes may be sign of impending respiratory arrest). Patellar reflex must be present, respiratory rate should be 16/min or over before each parenteral dose. Initiate seizure precautions.

PATIENT/FAMILY TEACHING

• **Antacid:** Take at least 2 hrs apart from other medication. • Do not take longer than 2 wks unless directed by physician. • For peptic ulcer, take 1 and 3 hrs after meals and at bedtime for 4–6 wks. • Chew tablets thoroughly, followed by 8 oz of water; shake suspensions well. • Repeat dosing or large doses may have laxative effect. • **Laxative:** Drink full glass (8 oz) liquid to aid stool softening. • Use only for short term. Do not use if abdominal pain, nausea, vomiting is present. • **Systemic:** Inform physician of any signs of hypermagnesemia (dizziness, palpitations, altered mental status, fatigue, weakness).

mannitol

man-it-ol
(Aridol, Osmitrol)
Do not confuse Osmitrol with esmolol.
BLACK BOX ALERT May result in severe bronchospasm. Not recommended in pts with asthma.

◆CLASSIFICATION

PHARMACOTHERAPEUTIC: Polyol (sugar alcohol). **CLINICAL:** Osmotic diuretic, antiglaucoma, antihemolytic.

ACTION

Elevates osmotic pressure of glomerular filtrate, inhibiting tubular reabsorption of water and electrolytes, resulting in increased flow of water into interstitial fluid/plasma. **Therapeutic Effect:** Produces diuresis; reduces intraocular pressure (IOP), intracranial pressure (ICP), cerebral edema.

PHARMACOKINETICS

Route	Onset	Peak	Duration
IV (diuresis)	1–3 hrs	N/A	—
IV (reduced ICP)	15–30 min	N/A	1.5–6 hrs

M

Remains in extracellular fluid. Primarily excreted unchanged in urine. Removed by hemodialysis. **Half-life:** 4.7 hrs.

USES

Prevention, treatment of oliguric phase of acute renal failure (before evidence of permanent renal failure). Reduces increased ICP due to cerebral edema, IOP due to acute glaucoma. Promotes urinary excretion of toxic substances. **OFF-LABEL:** Improve renal transplant function.

PRECAUTIONS

Contraindications: Dehydration, intracranial bleeding, severe pulmonary edema, congestion, severe renal disease (anuria), progressive HF. **Cautions:** Concurrent nephrotoxic agents, conditions increasing sensitivity to bronchoconstriction.

⏳ LIFESPAN CONSIDERATIONS

Pregnancy/Lactation: Unknown if drug crosses placenta or is distributed in breast milk. **Pregnancy Category C. Children:** Safety and efficacy not established in those younger than 12 yrs. **Elderly:** Age-related renal impairment may require dosage adjustment.

INTERACTIONS

DRUG: None significant. **HERBAL:** Yohimbe may decrease effects. **FOOD:** None known. **LAB VALUES:** May decrease serum phosphate, potassium, sodium.

AVAILABILITY (Rx)

Injection Solution (Osmitrol): 20%, 25%.

ADMINISTRATION/HANDLING

◀**ALERT**▶ Assess IV site for patency before each dose. Pain, thrombosis noted with extravasation. In-line filter (less than 5 microns) used for concentrations over 20%.

 IV

Rate of Administration • Administer test dose for pts with oliguria. • Give IV

push over 3–5 min; over 20–30 min for cerebral edema, elevated ICP. Maximum concentration: 25%. • Do not add KCl or NaCl to mannitol 20% or greater. Do not add to whole blood for transfusion. **Storage** • Store at room temperature. • If crystals are noted in solution, warm bottle in hot water, shake vigorously at intervals. Cool to body temperature before administration. Do not use if crystals remain after warming procedure.

🖥 IV INCOMPATIBILITIES

Cefepime (Maxipime), filgrastim (Neupogen), imipenem-cilastatin (Primaxin).

🖥 IV COMPATIBILITIES

Cisplatin (Platinol), furosemide (Lasix), linezolid (Zyvox), ondansetron (Zofran), propofol (Diprivan).

INDICATIONS/ROUTES/DOSAGE

Usual Dosage
Elevated Intracranial Pressure
IV: ADULTS, ELDERLY: 0.25–1 g/kg/dose. May repeat q6–8h as needed. **CHILDREN:** 0.25–1 g/kg/dose; repeat to maintain serum osmolality <300–320 mOsm/kg.

SIDE EFFECTS

Frequent: Dry mouth, thirst. **Occasional:** Blurred vision, increased urinary frequency/volume, headache, arm pain, backache, nausea, vomiting, urticaria, dizziness, hypotension, hypertension, tachycardia, fever, angina-like chest pain.

ADVERSE EFFECTS/ TOXIC REACTIONS

Fluid, electrolyte imbalance may occur due to rapid administration of large doses or inadequate urine output resulting in overexpansion of extracellular fluid. Circulatory overload may produce pulmonary edema, HF. Excessive diuresis may produce hypokalemia, hyponatremia. Fluid loss in excess of electrolyte excretion may produce hypernatremia, hyperkalemia.

NURSING CONSIDERATIONS

BASELINE ASSESSMENT

Obtain baseline B/P, pulse. Assess skin turgor, mucous membranes, mental status, muscle strength. Obtain baseline weight, chemistry studies. Assess I&O.

INTERVENTION/EVALUATION

Monitor urinary output to ascertain therapeutic response. Monitor serum electrolytes, serum osmolarity, ICP, renal/hepatic function tests. Assess vital signs, skin turgor, mucous membranes. Weigh daily. Signs of hyponatremia include confusion, drowsiness, thirst, dry mouth, cold/clammy skin. Signs of hypokalemia include changes in muscle strength, tremors, muscle cramps, altered mental status, cardiac arrhythmias. Signs of hyperkalemia include colic, diarrhea, muscle twitching followed by weakness, paralysis, arrhythmias.

PATIENT/FAMILY TEACHING

• Expect increased urinary frequency/volume. • May cause dry mouth.

---

maraviroc

ma-**ra**-veer-ock
(Celsentri ✦, Selzentry)

BLACK BOX ALERT Possible drug-induced hepatotoxicity with allergic-type features reported.

◆ CLASSIFICATION

PHARMACOTHERAPEUTIC: Chemokine receptor 5 (CCR5) co-receptor antagonist. **CLINICAL:** Antiretroviral (see pp. 70C, 121C).

ACTION

Binds to human chemokine receptor (CCR5), present on CD-4 and T-cell membranes, preventing interaction of HIV-1 and CCR5, necessary for HIV-1 to enter cells. **Therapeutic Effect:** Decreased invasion of HIV-1 virus into cells.

PHARMACOKINETICS

Variably absorbed following PO administration. Protein binding: 76%. Metabolized in liver. Eliminated in feces (76%), urine (20%). **Half-life:** 14–18 hrs.

USES

Treatment of HIV infection in pts infected only with detectable chemokine receptor 5 (CCR5)-tropic HIV-1, with evidence of viral replication; HIV-1 strains resistant to multiple antiretroviral agents. Used in combination with at least two other antiretroviral agents.

PRECAUTIONS

Contraindications: Severe renal impairment or ESRD (CrCl less than 30 ml/min) who are taking potent CYP3A4 inhibitors or inducers. **Cautions:** Mild to moderate hepatic/renal impairment, history of orthostatic hypotension, hepatitis B or C, concurrent medication known to lower B/P, pts at increased risk for cardiovascular events.

⌛ LIFESPAN CONSIDERATIONS

Pregnancy/Lactation: Unknown if drug crosses placenta or is distributed in breast milk. Breastfeeding not recommended. **Pregnancy Category B. Children:** Safety and efficacy not established in those younger than 16 yrs. **Elderly:** Age-related hepatic/renal impairment requires close monitoring.

INTERACTIONS

DRUG: CYP3A4 inhibitors (e.g., **atazanavir, atazanavir/ritonavir, ketoconazole, lopinavir, ritonavir, saquinavir/ritonavir**) may increase concentration. **CYP3A4 inducers (e.g., efavirenz, rifampin)** may decrease concentration. **HERBAL: St. John's wort** may lead to loss of virologic response, potential resistance to maraviroc. **FOOD: Grapefruit products** may increase orthostatic hypotension. **LAB VALUES:** May increase serum AST, ALT, bilirubin, amylase, lipase. May decrease lymphocytes/neutrophil count.

M

AVAILABILITY (Rx)

Tablets: 150 mg, 300 mg.

ADMINISTRATION/HANDLING

PO

• Give without regard to food. • Do not break, crush, dissolve, or divide film-coated tablets.

INDICATIONS/ROUTES/DOSAGE

HIV Infection

PO: ADULTS, ELDERLY, CHILDREN OVER 16 YRS WITH CONCURRENT ANTIRETROVIRAL AGENTS: 300 mg twice a day. **With CYP3A4 inhibitors: (e.g., clarithromycin, delavirdine, itraconazole, ketoconazole):** 150 mg twice a day. **With CYP3A4 inducers: (e.g., carbamazepine, efavirenz, phenobarbital, phenytoin, rifampin):** 600 mg twice a day.

Dosage in Renal Impairment

Creatinine clearance 30 ml/min or greater	
CYP3A4 inhibitors	150 mg twice daily
CYP3A4 inducers	600 mg twice daily
Creatinine clearance less than 30 ml/min: 150 mg twice daily	
CYP3A4 inhibitors	Not recommended
Postural hypotension	150 mg twice daily

SIDE EFFECTS

Common (20%): Upper respiratory tract infection. **Frequent (13%–7%):** Cough, fever, rash, musculoskeletal pain, abdominal pain, dizziness, appetite change, herpes simplex infection, sleep disturbances. **Occasional (6%–4%):** Sinusitis, joint pain, bronchitis, constipation, bladder infection, paresthesia, sensory abnormalities. **Rare (3% or less):** Sleep disturbances, pruritus, peripheral neuropathy, dermatitis, dyspepsia.

ADVERSE EFFECTS/ TOXIC REACTIONS

Cardiovascular events (MI, ischemia, unstable angina, coronary artery occlusion/ disease), CVA, hepatic failure/cirrhosis, neoplasms were reported.

NURSING CONSIDERATIONS

BASELINE ASSESSMENT

Obtain baseline laboratory testing, esp. hepatic function tests, before beginning therapy and at periodic intervals during therapy. Offer emotional support. Obtain medication history.

INTERVENTION/EVALUATION

Closely monitor for evidence of GI discomfort. Monitor daily pattern of bowel activity, stool consistency. Assess skin for evidence of rash. Monitor serum chemistry tests for marked laboratory abnormalities, particularly hepatic profile. Assess for opportunistic infections: onset of fever, cough, or other respiratory symptoms.

PATIENT/FAMILY TEACHING

• Report fever, abdominal pain, jaundice, dark urine. • Avoid tasks that require alertness, motor skills until response to drug is established. • Maraviroc is not a cure for HIV infection, nor does it reduce risk of transmission to others. • May continue to experience illnesses, including opportunistic infections.

meclizine

mek-li-zeen
(Antivert, Bonine, Dramamine Less Drowsy Formula)
Do not confuse Antivert with Alavert or Axert.

◆ CLASSIFICATION

PHARMACOTHERAPEUTIC: Anticholinergic. **CLINICAL:** Antiemetic, antivertigo.

ACTION

Reduces labyrinthine excitability, diminishes vestibular stimulation of labyrinth, affecting chemoreceptor trigger zone. **Therapeutic Effect:** Reduces nausea, vomiting, vertigo.

PHARMACOKINETICS

Route	Onset	Peak	Duration
PO	30–60 min	N/A	8–24 hrs

Well absorbed from GI tract. Widely distributed. Metabolized in liver. Primarily excreted in urine. **Half-life:** 6 hrs.

USES

Prevention/treatment of nausea, vomiting, vertigo due to motion sickness. Treatment of vertigo associated with diseases affecting vestibular system.

PRECAUTIONS

Contraindications: None known. **Cautions:** Narrow-angle glaucoma, obstructive diseases of GI/GU tract, asthma, prostatic hyperplasia, CNS disorders where CNS depression is present.

⧗ LIFESPAN CONSIDERATIONS

Pregnancy/Lactation: Unknown if drug crosses placenta or is distributed in breast milk (may produce irritability in nursing infants). **Pregnancy Category B. Children/Elderly:** May be more sensitive to anticholinergic effects (e.g., dry mouth).

INTERACTIONS

DRUG: Alcohol, CNS depressants may increase CNS depressant effect. **HERBAL:** None significant. **FOOD:** None known. **LAB VALUES:** May produce false-negative results in antigen skin testing unless meclizine is discontinued 4 days before testing.

AVAILABILITY (Rx)

Tablets (Antivert): 12.5 mg, 25 mg, 50 mg. **(Dramamine Less Drowsy Formula):** 25 mg. **Tablets (Chewable):** 25 mg.

ADMINISTRATION/HANDLING

PO

• Give without regard to meals. • Scored tablets may be crushed.

INDICATIONS/ROUTES/DOSAGE

Motion Sickness
PO: ADULTS, ELDERLY, CHILDREN 12 YRS AND OLDER: 25–50 mg 1 hr before travel. May repeat q12–24h.

Vertigo
PO: ADULTS, ELDERLY, CHILDREN 12 YRS AND OLDER: 25–100 mg/day in divided doses, as needed.

SIDE EFFECTS

Frequent: Drowsiness. **Occasional:** Blurred vision, dry mouth, nose, throat.

ADVERSE EFFECTS/ TOXIC REACTIONS

Hypersensitivity reaction (eczema, pruritus, rash, cardiac disturbances, photosensitivity) may occur. Overdose may vary from CNS depression (sedation, apnea, cardiovascular collapse, death) to severe paradoxical reaction (hallucinations, tremor, seizures). Children may experience paradoxical reaction (restlessness, insomnia, euphoria, anxiety, tremors). Overdose in children may result in hallucinations, seizures, death.

NURSING CONSIDERATIONS

BASELINE ASSESSMENT

Assess degree of nausea/vomiting, degree of vertigo.

INTERVENTION/EVALUATION

Monitor B/P, esp. in elderly (increased risk of hypotension). Monitor children closely for paradoxical reaction. Monitor serum electrolytes in pts with severe vomiting. Assess skin turgor, mucous membranes to evaluate hydration status.

PATIENT/FAMILY TEACHING

• Tolerance to sedative effect may occur. • Avoid tasks that require alertness, motor skills until response to drug is established. • Dry mouth, drowsiness, dizziness may be an expected response to drug. • Avoid alcohol. • Sugarless gum, sips of water may relieve dry mouth.

M

• Coffee, tea may help reduce drowsiness.

*medroxy-PROGESTERone

me-**drox**-e-proe-**jes**-te-rone
(Apo-Medroxy ♣, Depo-Provera, Depo-Provera Contraceptive, Depo-SubQ Provera 104, Novo-Medrone ♣, Provera)

BLACK BOX ALERT Prolonged use (over 2 yrs) of contraceptive injection form may result in loss of bone mineral density. May increase risk of dementia in postmenopausal women. Increased risk of invasive breast cancer in postmenopausal women in combination with conjugated estrogens.

Do not confuse medroxyprogesterone with hydroxyprogesterone, methylprednisolone, or methyltestosterone, or Provera with Covera, Femara, Parlodel, or Premarin.

◆CLASSIFICATION

PHARMACOTHERAPEUTIC: Hormone.
CLINICAL: Progestin, antineoplastic.

ACTION

Transforms endometrium from proliferative to secretory (in estrogen-primed endometrium). Inhibits secretion of pituitary gonadotropins. **Therapeutic Effect:** Prevents follicular maturation, ovulation. Stimulates growth of mammary alveolar tissue; relaxes uterine smooth muscle. Corrects hormonal imbalance.

PHARMACOKINETICS

Well absorbed after PO administration. Slowly absorbed after IM administration. Protein binding: 90%. Metabolized in liver. Primarily excreted in urine. **Half-life: PO:** 12–17 hrs. **IM:** 40–50 days.

USES

PO: Reduction of endometrial hyperplasia in nonhysterectomized postmenopausal women (concurrently given with estrogen to women with intact uterus), treatment of secondary amenorrhea, abnormal uterine bleeding due to hormonal imbalance. **IM:** Adjunctive therapy, palliative treatment of inoperable, recurrent, metastatic endometrial carcinoma; prevention of pregnancy; endometriosis-associated pain. **OFF-LABEL:** Treatment of endometrial, stromal carcinoma.

PRECAUTIONS

Contraindications: Carcinoma of breast, estrogen-dependent neoplasm, history of or active thrombotic disorders (cerebral apoplexy, thrombophlebitis, thromboembolic disorders), known or suspected pregnancy, missed abortion, severe hepatic dysfunction, undiagnosed abnormal vaginal bleeding, cerebrolvascular disease, use as pregnancy test. **Cautions:** Those with conditions aggravated by fluid retention (asthma, seizures, migraine, cardiac/renal dysfunction), diabetes, history of mental depression, preexisting hypertriglyceremia.

⧖ LIFESPAN CONSIDERATIONS

Pregnancy/Lactation: Avoid use during pregnancy, esp. first 4 mos (congenital heart, limb reduction defects may occur). Distributed in breast milk. **Pregnancy Category X. Children:** Safety and efficacy not established. **Elderly:** No age-related precautions noted.

INTERACTIONS

DRUG: CYP3A inducers (e.g., **carbamazepine, phenytoin, rifampin**) may decrease effect. **HERBAL: St. John's wort** may decrease effect of progestin contraceptive. **FOOD:** None known. **LAB VALUES:** May alter serum thyroid, hepatic function tests, PT, metapyrone test, HDL, total cholesterol, triglycerides. May increase LDL.

M

AVAILABILITY (Rx)

Injection Suspension: 104 mg/0.65 ml prefilled syringe (Depo-SubQ Provera 104), 150 mg/ml (Depo-Provera Contraceptive), 400 mg/ml (Depo-Provera). **Tablets (Provera):** 2.5 mg, 5 mg, 10 mg.

ADMINISTRATION/HANDLING

IM
• Shake vial immediately before administering (ensures complete suspension).
• Administer deep IM into gluteal or deltoid muscle.

SUBCUTANEOUS
• Shake vigorously prior to administration. • Inject in upper thigh or abdomen (avoid bony areas and umbilicus). • Give over 5–7 sec; do not rub injection area.

PO
• Give with food.

INDICATIONS/ROUTES/DOSAGE

Endometrial Hyperplasia
PO: ADULTS: 2.5–10 mg/day for 12–14 consecutive days each month starting on day 1 or 16 of cycle.

Secondary Amenorrhea
PO: ADULTS: 5–10 mg/day for 5–10 days, beginning at any time during menstrual cycle.

Abnormal Uterine Bleeding
PO: ADULTS: 5–10 mg/day for 5–10 days, beginning on calculated day 16 or day 21 of menstrual cycle.

Endometrial Carcinoma
IM: ADULTS, ELDERLY: Initially, 400–1,000 mg; repeat at 1-wk intervals. If improvement occurs and disease is stabilized, begin maintenance with as little as 400 mg/mo.

Pregnancy Prevention
IM (Depo-Provera Contraceptive): ADULTS: 150 mg q3mos.
Subcutaneous (Depo-Subq Provera 104): ADULTS: 104 mg q3mos (q12–14wks).

Endometriosis-Associated Pain
Subcutaneous (Depo-Subq Provera 104): ADULTS: 104 mg q3mos (q12–14 wks) for up to 2 yrs.

SIDE EFFECTS

Frequent: Transient menstrual abnormalities (spotting, change in menstrual flow/cervical secretions, amenorrhea) at initiation of therapy. **Occasional:** Edema, weight change, breast tenderness, anxiety, insomnia, fatigue, dizziness. **Rare:** Alopecia, depression, dermatologic changes, headache, fever, nausea.

ADVERSE EFFECTS/ TOXIC REACTIONS

Thrombophlebitis, pulmonary/cerebral embolism, retinal thrombosis occur rarely.

NURSING CONSIDERATIONS

BASELINE ASSESSMENT
Obtain usual menstrual history. Question for hypersensitivity to progestins, possibility of pregnancy before initiating therapy (Pregnancy Category X). Obtain baseline weight, serum glucose, B/P.

INTERVENTION/EVALUATION
Check weight daily; report weekly gain of 5 lb or more. Assess B/P periodically. Assess skin for rash, urticaria. Report development of chest pain, sudden shortness of breath, sudden decrease in vision, migraine headache, pain (esp. with swelling, warmth, redness) in calves, numbness of arm/leg (thrombotic disorders) immediately.

PATIENT/FAMILY TEACHING
• Inform physician of sudden loss of vision, severe headache, chest pain, coughing up of blood (hemoptysis), numbness in arm/leg, severe pain/swelling in calf, unusual heavy vaginal bleeding, severe abdominal pain/tenderness.
• Depo-Provera Contraceptive injection should be used as long-term birth control method (e.g., longer than 2 yrs) only

---

* "Tall Man" lettering ✦ Canadian trade name   Non-Crushable Drug **HIGH ALERT** High Alert drug

if other birth control methods are inadequate.

megestrol

meh-**jes**-trol
(Apo-Megestrol ✦, Megace, Megace ES, Megace OS ✦)
Do not confuse megestrol with mesalamine.

◆ CLASSIFICATION

PHARMACOTHERAPEUTIC: Synthetic hormone. **CLINICAL:** Antineoplastic (see p. 88C).

ACTION

Suppresses release of luteinizing hormone (LH) from anterior pituitary gland by inhibiting pituitary function. **Therapeutic Effect:** Reduces tumor size. Increases appetite.

PHARMACOKINETICS

Well absorbed from GI tract. Metabolized in liver. Excreted in urine. **Half-life:** 13–105 hrs (mean 34 hrs).

USES

Palliative management of recurrent, inoperable, metastatic endometrial or breast carcinoma; treatment of anorexia, cachexia, unexplained significant weight loss in pts with AIDS.

PRECAUTIONS

Contraindications: Suspension: Known or suspected pregnancy, concomitant use with doffilide. **Cautions:** History of thrombophlebitis, diabetes.

⧖ LIFESPAN CONSIDERATIONS

Pregnancy/Lactation: If possible, avoid use during pregnancy, esp. first 4 mos. Breastfeeding not recommended. **Pregnancy Category D (tablets), X (suspension). Children:** Safety and efficacy not established. **Elderly:** No age-related precautions noted.

INTERACTIONS

DRUG: None significant. **HERBAL:** Avoid **black cohosh, dong quai** in estrogen-dependent tumors. Avoid **herbs with progestogenic properties (e.g., chasteberry);** may increase adverse effects. **FOOD:** None known. **LAB VALUES:** May alter serum thyroid, hepatic function tests, PT, HDL, total cholesterol, triglycerides. May increase LDL.

AVAILABILITY (Rx)

Oral Suspension: 40 mg/ml (Megace), 125 mg/ml (Megace ES). **Tablets** (Megace): 20 mg, 40 mg.

ADMINISTRATION/HANDLING

PO
• Store tablets, oral suspension at room temperature. • Shake suspension well before use. • Oral suspension compatible with water, orange juice, apple juice. • Administer without regard to food.

INDICATIONS/ROUTES/DOSAGE

Palliative Treatment of Advanced Breast Cancer
PO: ADULTS, ELDERLY: 160 mg/day in 4 equally divided doses.

Palliative Treatment of Advanced Endometrial Carcinoma
PO: ADULTS, ELDERLY: 40–320 mg/day in divided doses. **Maximum:** 800 mg/day in divided doses.

Anorexia, Cachexia, Weight Loss
PO *(Megace)*: ADULTS, ELDERLY: 800 mg (20 ml)/day.
PO *(Megace ES)*: ADULTS, ELDERLY: 625 mg/day.

SIDE EFFECTS

Frequent: Weight gain secondary to increased appetite. **Occasional:** Nausea, breakthrough menstrual bleeding, backache, headache, breast tenderness, carpal tunnel syndrome. **Rare:** Feeling of coldness.

M

ADVERSE EFFECTS/ TOXIC REACTIONS

Thrombophlebitis, pulmonary embolism occur rarely.

NURSING CONSIDERATIONS

BASELINE ASSESSMENT

Question for possibility of pregnancy (Pregnancy Category D [tablets]; X [suspension]). Provide support to pt, family, recognizing this drug is palliative, not curative.

INTERVENTION/EVALUATION

Monitor for tumor response. Monitor pt weight, caloric intake (appetite stimulant).

PATIENT/FAMILY TEACHING

• Contraception is imperative. • Report lower leg (calf) pain, difficulty breathing, vaginal bleeding. • May cause headache, nausea, vomiting, breast tenderness, backache.

---

meloxicam

mel-**ox**-i-kam
(Apo-Meloxicam ✤, Mobic, Novo-Meloxicam ✤)

BLACK BOX ALERT Increased risk of serious cardiovascular thrombotic events, including myocardial infarction, CVA. Increased risk of severe GI reactions, including ulceration, bleeding, GI perforation.

◆CLASSIFICATION

PHARMACOTHERAPEUTIC: NSAID. **CLINICAL:** Anti-inflammatory, analgesic (see p. 130C).

ACTION

Produces analgesic, anti-inflammatory effects by inhibiting prostaglandin synthesis. **Therapeutic Effect:** Reduces inflammatory response, intensity of pain.

PHARMACOKINETICS

Route	Onset	Peak	Duration
PO (analgesic)	30 min	4–5 hrs	N/A

Well absorbed after PO administration. Protein binding: 99%. Metabolized in liver. Eliminated in urine, feces. Not removed by hemodialysis. **Half-life:** 15–20 hrs.

USES

Relief of signs/symptoms of osteoarthritis, rheumatoid arthritis (RA). Treatment of juvenile rheumatoid arthritis (JRA).

PRECAUTIONS

Contraindications: History of asthma, urticaria with NSAIDs, perioperative pain in setting of CABG surgery. **Cautions:** Renal/hepatic impairment, asthma, coagulation disorders, hypertension, history of GI disease. Concurrent use of anticoagulants.

⧗ LIFESPAN CONSIDERATIONS

Pregnancy/Lactation: Distributed in breast milk. **Pregnancy Category C (D if used in third trimester or near delivery). Children:** Safety and efficacy not established. **Elderly:** Age-related renal impairment may require dosage adjustment. More susceptible to GI toxicity; lower dosage recommended.

INTERACTIONS

DRUG: May decrease antihypertensive effects of **ACE inhibitors.** May increase risk of nephrotoxicity with **cyclosporine. Aspirin** may increase risk of epigastric distress (heartburn, indigestion). **Warfarin, aspirin** may increase risk of bleeding. May increase concentration, risk of toxicity of **lithium. HERBAL: Cat's claw, dong quai, evening primrose, feverfew, garlic, ginger, ginkgo, green tea, red clover, SAMe** may increase antiplatelet activity, risk of bleeding. **FOOD:** None known. **LAB VALUES:** May increase serum creatinine, AST, ALT.

AVAILABILITY (Rx)

Oral Suspension: 7.5 mg/5 ml. **Tablets:** 7.5 mg, 15 mg.

✤ Canadian trade name   Non-Crushable Drug   **HIGH ALERT** High Alert drug

M

ADMINISTRATION/HANDLING

PO
• Give with food or milk to minimize GI irritation. Shake oral suspension gently before administering.

INDICATIONS/ROUTES/DOSAGE

Osteoarthritis, Rheumatoid Arthritis (RA)
PO: ADULTS, ELDERLY: Initially, 7.5 mg/day. **Maximum:** 15 mg/day (7.5 mg for pts on dialysis).

Juvenile Rheumatoid Arthritis (JRA)
PO: CHILDREN, 2 YRS AND OLDER: 0.125 mg/kg once daily. **Maximum:** 7.5 mg.

SIDE EFFECTS

Frequent (9%–7%): Dyspepsia, headache, diarrhea, nausea. **Occasional (4%–3%):** Dizziness, insomnia, rash, pruritus, flatulence, constipation, vomiting. **Rare (less than 2%):** Drowsiness, urticaria, photosensitivity, tinnitus.

ADVERSE EFFECTS/ TOXIC REACTIONS

In pts treated chronically, peptic ulcer, GI bleeding, gastritis, severe hepatic reaction (jaundice), nephrotoxicity (hematuria, dysuria, proteinuria), severe hypersensitivity reaction (bronchospasm, angioedema) occur rarely.

NURSING CONSIDERATIONS

BASELINE ASSESSMENT
Assess onset, type, location, duration of pain/inflammation. Inspect appearance of affected joints for immobility, deformities, skin condition.

INTERVENTION/EVALUATION
Monitor CBC, hepatic/renal function tests. Assess skin for petechiae. Assess for therapeutic response: relief of pain, stiffness, swelling; increased joint mobility; reduced joint tenderness; improved grip strength.

PATIENT/FAMILY TEACHING
• Take with food, milk to reduce GI upset. • Report tinnitus, persistent abdominal pain/cramping, severe nausea, vomiting, difficulty breathing, unusual bruising or bleeding, rash, peripheral edema, chest pain, palpitations.

---

melphalan

mel-fa-lan
(Alkeran)

BLACK BOX ALERT Myelosuppression is common. Potentially mutagenic, leukemogenic. Hypersensitivity noted with IV administration. Must be administered by certified chemotherapy personnel.
Do not confuse Alkeran with Leukeran or Myleran, or melphalan with Mephyton or Myleran.

◆CLASSIFICATION

PHARMACOTHERAPEUTIC: Alkylating agent. **CLINICAL:** Antineoplastic (see p. 88C).

ACTION

Inhibits protein synthesis primarily by cross-linking strands of DNA, RNA. Cell cycle–phase nonspecific. **Therapeutic Effect:** Disrupts nucleic acid function, producing cell death.

PHARMACOKINETICS

Oral administration is highly variable. Incomplete intestinal absorption, variable first-pass metabolism, rapid hydrolysis may result. Protein binding: 60%–90%. Extensively metabolized in blood. Eliminated from plasma primarily by chemical hydrolysis. Partially excreted in feces; minimal elimination in urine. **Half-life: PO:** 1–1.25 hrs. **IV:** 1.5 hrs.

USES

Treatment of nonresectable epithelial ovarian carcinoma, multiple myeloma. **OFF-LABEL:** Hodgkin's lymphoma, malignant melanoma, neuroblastoma, induction regimen for bone marrow and stem cell transplantation.

PRECAUTIONS

Contraindications: Resistance to prior melphalan therapy. **Cautions:** Bone marrow suppression, renal impairment, pregnancy, prior chemotherapy or irradiation.

⧗ LIFESPAN CONSIDERATIONS

Pregnancy/Lactation: May cause fetal harm. Unknown if distributed in breast milk. **Pregnancy Category D. Children:** Safety and efficacy not established. **Elderly:** Age-related renal impairment may require dosage adjustment.

INTERACTIONS

DRUG: Bone marrow depressants may increase myelosuppression. **Live virus vaccines** may potentiate virus replication, increase vaccine side effects, decrease pt's antibody response to vaccine. **HERBAL: Echinacea** may decrease effects. **FOOD:** None known. **LAB VALUES:** May increase serum uric acid.

AVAILABILITY (Rx)

Injection, Powder for Reconstitution: 50 mg. **Tablets (Alkeran):** 2 mg.

ADMINISTRATION/HANDLING
💊 IV

Reconstitution • Reconstitute 50-mg vial with diluent supplied by manufacturer to yield 5 mg/ml solution. • Further dilute with 0.9% NaCl to final concentration not exceeding 0.45 mg/ml.
Rate of Administration • Infuse over 15–30 min at rate not to exceed 10 mg/min (total infusion should be administered within 1 hr).
Storage • Store at room temperature; protect from light. • Once reconstituted, complete administration within 60 min.

PO
• Store tablets in refrigerator; protect from light. • Give on empty stomach (1 hr before or 2 hrs after meals).

▨ IV INCOMPATIBILITIES

Amphotericin B complex (Abelcet, AmBisome, Amphotec).

▨ IV COMPATIBILITIES

Acyclovir, dexamethasone (Decadron), famotidine (Pepcid), furosemide (Lasix), lorazepam (Ativan), morphine.

INDICATIONS/ROUTES/DOSAGE
Ovarian Carcinoma
PO: ADULTS, ELDERLY: 0.2 mg/kg/day for 5 successive days. Repeat at 4- to 5-wk intervals.

Multiple Myeloma
PO: ADULTS: Initially, 6 mg once a day for 2–3 wks, followed by up to 4 wks rest, then maintenance dose of 2 mg daily; or 0.15 mg/kg/day for 7 days with 2–6 wks rest, then maintenance dose of 0.05 mg/kg/day; or 0.25 mg/kg/day for 4 days, repeat at 4- to 6-wk intervals.
IV: ADULTS: 16 mg/m²/dose every 2 wks for 4 doses, then repeat monthly after hematologic recovery.

Dosage in Renal Impairment
IV: BUN LEVEL GREATER THAN 30 MG/DL: Decrease melphalan dosage by 50%.

SIDE EFFECTS
Frequent: Nausea, vomiting (may be severe with large dose). **Occasional:** Diarrhea, stomatitis, rash, pruritus, alopecia.

ADVERSE EFFECTS/ TOXIC REACTIONS

Myelosuppression manifested as hematologic toxicity (principally leukopenia, thrombocytopenia, and, to lesser extent, anemia, pancytopenia, agranulocytosis). Leukopenia may occur as early as 5 days after drug initiation. WBC, platelet counts return to normal during 5th wk after therapy, but leukopenia, thrombocytopenia may last more than 6 wks after discontinuing drug. Hyperuricemia noted by hematuria, crystalluria, flank pain.

M

NURSING CONSIDERATIONS

BASELINE ASSESSMENT

Obtain baseline CBC, then weekly thereafter. Dosage may be decreased or discontinued if WBC falls below 3,000/mm³ or platelet count falls below 100,000/mm³. Antiemetics may be effective in preventing/treating nausea, vomiting.

INTERVENTION/EVALUATION

Monitor CBC with diffferential, serum electrolytes, Hgb. Monitor for stomatitis. Monitor for hematologic toxicity (fever, sore throat, signs of local infection, unusual bruising/bleeding from any site), symptoms of anemia (excessive fatigue, weakness), signs of hyperuricemia (hematuria, flank pain). Avoid IM injections, rectal temperatures, other traumas that may induce bleeding.

PATIENT/FAMILY TEACHING

• Increase fluid intake (may protect against hyperuricemia). • Maintain strict oral hygiene. • Hair loss is reversible, but new hair growth may have different color, texture. • Avoid crowds, those with infections. • Report fever, shortness of breath, cough, sore throat, bleeding, bruising occurs.

---

memantine

TOP 200

meh-**man**-teen
(Apo-Memantine , Ebixa , Namenda, Namenda XR)

◆ CLASSIFICATION

PHARMACOTHERAPEUTIC: Neurotransmitter inhibitor. **CLINICAL:** Anti-Alzheimer's agent.

ACTION

Decreases effects of glutamate, the principal excitatory neurotransmitter in the brain. Persistent CNS excitation by glutamate is thought to cause symptoms of Alzheimer's disease. **Therapeutic Effect:** May inhibit clinical deterioration in moderate to severe Alzheimer's disease.

PHARMACOKINETICS

Rapidly, completely absorbed after PO administration. Protein binding: 45%. Undergoes little metabolism; most of dose is excreted unchanged in urine. **Half-life:** 60–80 hrs.

USES

Treatment of moderate to severe dementia of Alzheimer's type. **OFF-LABEL:** Treatment of mild to moderate vascular dementia.

PRECAUTIONS

Contraindications: None known. **Cautions:** Moderate to severe renal impairment, severe hepatic impairment, cardiovascular disease, seizure disorder, GU conditions that raise urine pH level.

⏳ LIFESPAN CONSIDERATIONS

Pregnancy/Lactation: Unknown if drug crosses placenta or is distributed in breast milk. **Pregnancy Category B. Children:** Not prescribed for this pt population. **Elderly:** No age-related precautions noted, but use is not recommended in those with severe renal impairment (creatinine clearance less than 9 ml/min).

INTERACTIONS

DRUG: Urine alkalinizers (e.g., carbonic anhydrase inhibitors, sodium bicarbonate) may decrease renal elimination. **HERBAL:** None significant. **FOOD:** None known. **LAB VALUES:** None known.

AVAILABILITY (Rx)

Oral Solution: 2 mg/ml. **Tablets:** 5 mg, 10 mg.

Capsules (Extended-Release [Namenda XR]): 7 mg, 14 mg, 21 mg, 28 mg.

ADMINISTRATION/HANDLING

PO

• Give without regard to food. • Administer oral solution using syringe provided. Do not dilute or mix with other fluids. • Give extended-release capsules whole. Do not crush. May open capsule and sprinkle on applesauce.

INDICATIONS/ROUTES/DOSAGE

Alzheimer's Disease

PO: ADULTS, ELDERLY (Immediate-Release): Initially, 5 mg once a day. May increase dosage at intervals of at least 1 wk in 5-mg increments to 10 mg/day (5 mg twice a day), then 15 mg/day (5 mg and 10 mg as separate doses), and finally 20 mg/day (10 mg twice a day). Target dose: 20 mg/day. **(Extended-Release):** Initially, 7 mg once daily. May increase at intervals of at least 7 days in increments of 7 mg. **Maximum:** 28 mg once daily. Switching from immediate-release to extended-release: Begin the day following last dose of immediate release.

10 mg twice a day: 28 mg once daily.

5 mg twice a day: 14 mg once daily.

Dosage in Renal Impairment

Creatinine Clearance	Dosage Immediate-Release	Extended-Release
30 ml/min or greater	No adjustments	No adjustments
5–29 ml/min	5 mg twice daily	14 mg once daily

SIDE EFFECTS

Occasional (7%–4%): Dizziness, headache, confusion, constipation, hypertension, cough. **Rare (3%–2%):** Back pain, nausea, fatigue, anxiety, peripheral edema, arthralgia, insomnia.

ADVERSE EFFECTS/ TOXIC REACTIONS

None known.

NURSING CONSIDERATIONS

BASELINE ASSESSMENT

Assess cognitive, behavioral, functional deficits of pt. Assess renal function.

INTERVENTION/EVALUATION

Monitor cognitive, behavioral, functional status of pt. Monitor urine pH (alterations of urine pH toward the alkaline condition may lead to accumulation of the drug with possible increase in side effects). Monitor BUN, creatinine clearance lab values.

PATIENT/FAMILY TEACHING

• Do not reduce or stop medication; do not increase dosage without physician direction. • Ensure adequate fluid intake. • If therapy is interrupted for several days, restart at lowest dose, titrate to current dose at minimum of 1-wk intervals. • Local chapter of Alzheimer's Disease Association can provide a guide to services.

M

meperidine

me-**per**-i-deen
(Demerol)
Do not confuse Demerol with Demulen, Desyrel, Dilaudid, or Pamelor, or meperidine with meprobamate.

◆CLASSIFICATION

PHARMACOTHERAPEUTIC: Narcotic agonist **(Schedule II). CLINICAL:** Opiate analgesic.

ACTION

Binds to opioid receptors within CNS. **Therapeutic Effect:** Alters pain perception, emotional response to pain.

♣ Canadian trade name   🔪 Non-Crushable Drug   🔲 High Alert drug

PHARMACOKINETICS

Route	Onset	Peak	Duration
PO	15 min	120 min	2–4 hrs
IV	Less than 5 min	5–7 min	2–3 hrs
IM	10–15 min	30–50 min	2–4 hrs
Subcutaneous	10–15 min	60 min	2–4 hrs

Variably absorbed from GI tract; absorption erratic and highly variable after IM administration. Protein binding: 15%–30%. Widely distributed. Metabolized in liver. Primarily excreted in urine. Not removed by hemodialysis. **Half-life:** 2.4–4 hrs; metabolite, 15–30 hrs (increased in hepatic impairment/disease).

USES

◄**ALERT**► Not considered an opioid of choice for treatment of pain. Relief of moderate to severe pain. **OFF-LABEL:** Reduces postop shivering. Reduces rigors from amphotericin.

PRECAUTIONS

Contraindications: Use of MAOIs within 14 days, severe respiratory insufficiency. **Cautions:** Renal/hepatic impairment, elderly, debilitated, supraventricular tachycardia, cor pulmonale, history of seizures, acute abdominal conditions, increased intracranial pressure (ICP), respiratory abnormalities, sickle cell anemia, Addison's disease, hypothyroidism, prostatic hypertrophy, urethral stricture, pheochromocytoma.

⧖ LIFESPAN CONSIDERATIONS

Pregnancy/Lactation: Crosses placenta. Distributed in breast milk. Respiratory depression may occur in neonate if mother received opiates during labor. Regular use of opiates during pregnancy may produce withdrawal symptoms in neonate (irritability, excessive crying, tremors, hyperactive reflexes, fever, vomiting, diarrhea, yawning, sneezing, seizures). **Pregnancy Category B (D if used for prolonged periods or at high dosages at term). Children:** Paradoxical excitement may occur. Those younger than 2 yrs more susceptible to respiratory depressant effects. **Elderly:** More susceptible to respiratory depressant effects. Age-related renal impairment may increase risk of urinary retention.

INTERACTIONS

DRUG: Alcohol, other CNS depressants may increase CNS, respiratory depression, hypotension. **MAOIs** may produce severe, sometimes fatal reaction; meperidine use is contraindicated. **HERBAL: Gotu kola, kava kava, St. John's wort, valerian** may increase CNS depression, sedation. **FOOD:** None known. **LAB VALUES:** May increase serum amylase, lipase. **Therapeutic serum level:** 100–550 ng/ml; **toxic serum level:** greater than 1,000 ng/ml.

AVAILABILITY (Rx)

Injection, Solution: 25 mg/ml, 50 mg/ml, 75 mg/ml, 100 mg/ml. **Injection, Solution (Patient-Controlled Analgesia [PCA]):** 10 mg/ml. **Solution, Oral (Demerol):** 50 mg/5 ml. **Tablets (Demerol):** 50 mg, 100 mg.

ADMINISTRATION/HANDLING

 IV

Reconstitution • May give undiluted or dilute in D_5W, dextrose-saline combination (2.5%, 5%, 10% dextrose in water—0.45%, 0.9% NaCl), Ringer's, lactated Ringer's, molar sodium lactate diluent for IV injection or infusion.
Rate of Administration • IV dosage must always be administered very slowly, over 2–3 min. • Rapid IV increases risk of severe adverse reactions (chest wall rigidity, apnea, peripheral circulatory collapse, anaphylactoid effects, cardiac arrest).
Storage • Store at room temperature.

IM, Subcutaneous
◄**ALERT**► IM preferred over subcutaneous route (subcutaneous produces pain, local irritation, induration). • Ad-

minister slowly. • Pts with circulatory impairment at higher risk for overdosage due to delayed absorption of repeated administration.

PO

• Give without regard to meals. • Dilute syrup in glass of water (prevents anesthetic effect on mucous membranes).

IV INCOMPATIBILITIES

Amphotericin B complex (Abelcet, AmBisome, Amphotec), cefepime (Maxipime), furosemide (Lasix), heparin, phenytoin (Dilantin), sodium bicarbonate.

IV COMPATIBILITIES

Atropine, bumetanide (Bumex), diltiazem (Cardizem), diphenhydramine (Benadryl), dobutamine (Dobutrex), dopamine (Intropin), glycopyrrolate (Robinul), hydroxyzine (Vistaril), insulin, lidocaine, magnesium, midazolam (Versed), oxytocin (Pitocin), potassium, total parenteral nutrition (TPN).

INDICATIONS/ROUTES/DOSAGE

Analgesia

◄**ALERT**► Avoid use in elderly.

PO, IM, Subcutaneous: ADULTS: 50–150 mg/dose q3–4h as needed. **CHILDREN**: 1.1–1.8 mg/kg/dose q3–4h as needed. **Maximum dose:** 50–150 mg.

Dosage in Renal Impairment

Avoid use in renal impairment.

SIDE EFFECTS

Frequent: Sedation, hypotension (including orthostatic hypotension), diaphoresis, facial flushing, dizziness, nausea, vomiting, constipation. **Occasional:** Confusion, arrhythmias, tremors, urinary retention, abdominal pain, dry mouth, headache, irritation at injection site, euphoria, dysphoria. **Rare:** Allergic reaction (rash, pruritus), insomnia.

ADVERSE EFFECTS/ TOXIC REACTIONS

Overdose results in respiratory depression, skeletal muscle flaccidity, cold/clammy skin, cyanosis, extreme drowsiness progressing to seizures, stupor, coma. **Antidote:** 0.4 mg naloxone (Narcan). Tolerance to analgesic effect, physical dependence may occur with repeated use.

NURSING CONSIDERATIONS

BASELINE ASSESSMENT

Pt should be in recumbent position before drug is administered by parenteral route. Assess onset, type, location, duration of pain. Obtain vital signs before giving medication. If respirations are 12/min or less (20/min or less in children), withhold medication, contact physician. Effect of medication is reduced if full pain recurs before next dose.

INTERVENTION/EVALUATION

Monitor vital signs 15–30 min after subcutaneous/IM dose, 5–10 min after IV dose (monitor for hypotension, change in rate/quality of pulse). Monitor pain level, sedation response. Monitor daily pattern of bowel activity, stool consistency; avoid constipation. Check for adequate voiding. Initiate deep breathing, coughing exercises, particularly in pts with pulmonary impairment. **Therapeutic serum level:** 100–550 ng/ml; **toxic serum level:** greater than 1,000 ng/ml.

PATIENT/FAMILY TEACHING

• Medication should be taken before pain fully returns, within ordered intervals. • Discomfort may occur with injection. • Change positions slowly to avoid orthostatic hypotension. • Increase fluids, bulk to prevent constipation. • Tolerance, dependence may occur with prolonged use of high doses. • Avoid alcohol, other CNS depressants. • Avoid tasks requiring mental alertness, motor skills until response to drug is established.

M

meropenem

mer-oh-**pen**-em
(Merrem IV)
**Do not confuse meropenem
with doripenem, ertapenem, or
imipenem.**

◆CLASSIFICATION

PHARMACOTHERAPEUTIC: Carbapenem. **CLINICAL:** Antibiotic.

ACTION

Binds to penicillin-binding proteins. Inhibits bacterial cell wall synthesis. **Therapeutic Effect:** Bactericidal.

PHARMACOKINETICS

After IV administration, widely distributed into tissues and body fluids, including CSF. Protein binding: 2%. Primarily excreted unchanged in urine. Removed by hemodialysis. **Half-life:** 1 hr.

USES

Treatment of multidrug-resistant infections; meningitis in children 3 mos and older; intra-abdominal infections; complicated skin/skin structure infections caused by susceptible *S. aureus, S. pyogenes, S. agalactiae, S. pneumoniae, H. influenzae, N. meningitidis, M. catarrhalis, E. coli, Klebsiella, Enterobacter, Serratia, P. aeruginosa, B. fragilis.* **OFF-LABEL:** Febrile neutropenia, liver abscess, otitis externa.

PRECAUTIONS

Contraindications: Anaphylactic reaction to other beta-lactams. **Cautions:** Renal impairment, CNS disorders, particularly with history of seizures, concurrent use with valproic acid.

⧗ LIFESPAN CONSIDERATIONS

Pregnancy/Lactation: Unknown if distributed in breast milk. **Pregnancy Category B. Children:** Safety and efficacy not

established in those younger than 3 mos. **Elderly:** Age-related renal impairment may require dosage adjustment.

INTERACTIONS

DRUG: None significant. **HERBAL:** None significant. **FOOD:** None known. **LAB VALUES:** May increase BUN, serum alkaline phosphatase, LDH, AST, ALT, bilirubin. May decrease Hgb, Hct, WBC.

AVAILABILITY (Rx)

Injection, Powder for Reconstitution: 500 mg, 1 g.

ADMINISTRATION/HANDLING
 IV

Reconstitution • Reconstitute each 500 mg with 10 ml Sterile Water for Injection, 0.9% NaCl, or D₅W to provide concentration of 50 mg/ml. • Shake to dissolve until clear. • May further dilute with 0.9% NaCl or D₅W to a concentration of 1–20 mg/ml.
Rate of Administration • May give by IV push or IV intermittent infusion (piggyback). • If administering as IV intermittent infusion (piggyback), give over 15–30 min (at a concentration of 1–20 mg/ml); if administered by IV push, give over 3–5 min (at a concentration not greater than 50 mg/ml).
Storage • Store vials at room temperature. • After reconstitution of vials with 0.9% NaCl, stable for 2 hrs at room temperature or 18 hrs if refrigerated (with D₅W, stable for 1 hr at room temperature, 8 hrs if refrigerated). IV infusion with 0.9% NaCl stable for 4 hrs at room temperature or 24 hrs if refrigerated (with D₅W, 1 hr at room temperature or 4 hrs if refrigerated).

⊞ IV INCOMPATIBILITIES

Acyclovir (Zovirax), amphotericin B (Fungizone), diazepam (Valium), doxycycline (Vibramycin), metronidazole (Flagyl), ondansetron (Zofran).

▓ IV COMPATIBILITIES

Dexamethasone (Decadron), dobutamine (Dobutrex), dopamine (Intropin), furosemide (Lasix), heparin, magnesium, morphine.

INDICATIONS/ROUTES/DOSAGE

Usual Dosage
IV: ADULTS, ELDERLY: 1.5–6 g/day in divided doses q8h. **CHILDREN 3 MOS AND OLDER:** 30–120 mg/kg/day in divided doses q8h. **Maximum:** 6 g/day. **NEONATES:** 20 mg/kg/dose q8–12h.

Meningitis
IV: ADULTS, ELDERLY, CHILDREN WEIGHING 50 KG OR MORE: 2 g q8h. **CHILDREN 3 MOS AND OLDER WEIGHING LESS THAN 50 KG:** 40 mg/kg q8h. **Maximum:** 2 g/dose.

Dosage in Renal Impairment
Dosage and frequency are modified based on creatinine clearance.

Creatinine Clearance	Dosage	Interval
26–49 ml/min	Normal dose (1,000 mg)	q12h
10–25 ml/min	50% of normal dose	q12h
Less than 10 ml/min	50% of normal dose	q24h
Hemodialysis:	500 mg	q24h
Peritoneal dialysis:	Recommended dose (based on indication)	q24h

Continuous renal replacement therapy

Continuous venovenous hemofiltration	1 gram then 500 mg 1 gram	q8h OR q12h
Continuous venovenous hemodialysis/ continuous venovenous hemodiafiltration	1 gram then 500 mg 1 gram	q6–8h OR q8–12h

SIDE EFFECTS

Frequent (5%–3%): Diarrhea, nausea, vomiting, headache, inflammation at injection site. **Occasional (2%):** Oral candidiasis, rash, pruritus. **Rare (less than 2%):** Constipation, glossitis.

ADVERSE EFFECTS/ TOXIC REACTIONS

Antibiotic-associated colitis, other superinfections (abdominal cramps, severe watery diarrhea, fever) may result from altered bacterial balance in GI tract. Anaphylactic reactions have been reported. Seizures may occur in those with CNS disorders (e.g., brain lesions, history of seizures), bacterial meningitis, renal impairment.

NURSING CONSIDERATIONS

BASELINE ASSESSMENT
Question history of hypersensitivity, allergic reaction to penicillins, cephalosporins. Inquire about history of seizures.

INTERVENTION/EVALUATION
Monitor daily pattern of bowel activity, stool consistency. Monitor for nausea, vomiting. Evaluate for inflammation at IV injection site. Assess skin for rash. Evaluate hydration status. Monitor I&O, renal/hepatic function tests. Check mental status; be alert to tremors, possible seizures. Assess temperature, B/P twice a day, more often if necessary. Monitor serum electrolytes, esp. potassium.

PATIENT/FAMILY TEACHING
• Report persistent diarrhea, abdominal cramps, fever.

mesalamine (5-aminosalicylic acid, 5-ASA)

me-**sal**-a-meen
(Apriso, Asacol, Asacol HD, Canasa, Delzicol, Lialda, Mesasal ♣, Pentasa, Rowasa, Salofalk ♣, sfRowasa)

TOP 200

M

Do not confuse Asacol with Os-Cal, Lialda with Aldara, or mesalamine with megestrol, memantine, or methenamine.

◆CLASSIFICATION

PHARMACOTHERAPEUTIC: Salicylic acid derivative. **CLINICAL:** Anti-inflammatory agent.

ACTION

Locally inhibits arachidonic acid metabolite production (increased in chronic inflammatory bowel disease). **Therapeutic Effect:** Blocks prostaglandin production, diminishes inflammation in colon.

PHARMACOKINETICS

Poorly absorbed from colon. Moderately absorbed from GI tract. Metabolized in liver. Unabsorbed portion eliminated in feces; absorbed portion excreted in urine. Unknown if removed by hemodialysis. **Half-life:** 0.5–1.5 hrs; metabolite, 5–10 hrs.

USES

PO: Treatment, maintenance of remission of mild to moderate active ulcerative colitis. **Rectal:** Treatment of active mild to moderate distal ulcerative colitis, proctosigmoiditis or proctitis.

PRECAUTIONS

Contraindications: None known. **Cautions:** Sulfasalazine, salicylate sensitivity, active peptic ulcer, pyloric stenosis, pericarditis, myocarditis, renal/hepatic impairment.

⌛ LIFESPAN CONSIDERATIONS

Pregnancy/Lactation: Unknown if drug crosses placenta or is distributed in breast milk. **Pregnancy Category B. Children:** Safety and efficacy not established. **Elderly:** Age-related renal impairment may require dosage adjustment.

INTERACTIONS

DRUG: None known. **HERBAL:** None significant. **FOOD:** None known. **LAB VAL-** UES: May increase serum alkaline phosphatase, AST, ALT, bilirubin.

AVAILABILITY (Rx)

Rectal Suspension (Rowasa, sfRowasa): 4 g/60 ml. **Suppositories (Canasa):** 1 g. 🦃 **Capsules (Controlled-Release [Pentasa]):** 250 mg, 500 mg. **Capsules (Delayed-Release [Delzicol]):** 400 mg. 🦃 **Capsules (Extended-Release [Apriso]):** 375 mg. 🦃 **Tablets (Delayed-Release [Asacol]):** 400 mg. **(Asacol HD):** 800 mg. **(Lialda):** 1.2 g.

ADMINISTRATION/HANDLING

◄**ALERT►** Store rectal suspension, suppository, oral forms at room temperature.

PO

• Have pt swallow whole; do not break outer coating of tablet. • Give without regard to food. **Apriso:** Do not administer with antacids. **Lialda:** Administer once daily with meal.

Rectal

• Shake bottle well. • Instruct pt to lie on left side with lower leg extended, upper leg flexed forward. • Knee-chest position may also be used. • Insert applicator tip into rectum, pointing toward umbilicus. • Squeeze bottle steadily until contents are emptied. • Store suppositories at room temperature. Do not refrigerate.

INDICATIONS/ROUTES/DOSAGE

Treatment of Ulcerative Colitis
PO *(Capsule [Pentasa]):* **ADULTS, ELDERLY:** 1 g 4 times a day. **CHILDREN:** 30–60 mg/kg/day divided q6–12h.
PO *(Capsule [Delzicol]):* **ADULTS, ELDERLY:** 800 mg 3 times daily.
PO *(Tablet [Asacol]):* **ADULTS, ELDERLY:** 800 mg 3 times a day. **CHILDREN:** 30–60 mg/kg/day divided q8–12h.
PO *(Tablet [Lialda]):* **ADULTS, ELDERLY:** 2.4–4.8 g once daily.

Maintenance of Remission in Ulcerative Colitis

PO *(Capsule [Pentasa])*: **ADULTS, ELDERLY**: 1 g 4 times a day.

PO *(Capsule [Delzicol])*: **ADULTS, ELDERLY**: 1.6 g/day in divided doses.

PO *(Capsule, Extended-Release [Apriso])*: **ADULTS, ELDERLY**: 1,500 mg once daily in the morning.

PO *(Tablet [Asacol])*: **ADULTS, ELDERLY**: 1.6 g/day in divided doses.

PO *(Tablet [Lialda])*: **ADULTS, ELDERLY**: 2.4 g once daily with food.

Distal Ulcerative Colitis, Proctosigmoiditis, Proctitis

Rectal *(Retention Enema)*: **ADULTS, ELDERLY**: 60 ml (4 g) at bedtime; retained overnight for approximately 8 hrs for 3–6 wks.

Rectal *(1 G Suppository)*: **ADULTS, ELDERLY**: Once daily at bedtime. Continue therapy for 3–6 wks.

◀**ALERT**▶ Suppository should be retained for 1–3 hrs for maximum benefit.

SIDE EFFECTS

Mesalamine is generally well tolerated, with only mild, transient effects. **Frequent (greater than 6%): PO:** Abdominal cramps/pain, diarrhea, dizziness, headache, nausea, vomiting, rhinitis, unusual fatigue. **Rectal:** Abdominal/stomach cramps, flatulence, headache, nausea. **Occasional (6%–2%): PO:** Hair loss, decreased appetite, back/joint pain, flatulence, acne. **Rectal:** Alopecia. **Rare (less than 2%): Rectal:** Anal irritation.

ADVERSE EFFECTS/ TOXIC REACTIONS

Sulfite sensitivity may occur in susceptible pts, manifested as cramping, headache, diarrhea, fever, rash, urticaria, pruritus, wheezing. Discontinue drug immediately. Hepatitis, pancreatitis, pericarditis occur rarely with oral forms.

NURSING CONSIDERATIONS

BASELINE ASSESSMENT

Obtain baseline chemistries, esp. BUN, creatinine, hepatic function tests. Assess for abdominal pain, discomfort.

INTERVENTION/EVALUATION

Encourage adequate fluid intake. Assess bowel sounds for peristalsis. Monitor daily pattern of bowel activity, stool consistency; record time of evacuation. Assess for abdominal disturbances. Assess skin for rash, urticaria. Discontinue medication if rash, fever, cramping, diarrhea occurs.

PATIENT/FAMILY TEACHING

• Report rash, fever, abdominal pain, significant diarrhea to physician. • Avoid tasks that require alertness, motor skills until response to drug is established. • May discolor urine yellow-brown. • Suppositories stain fabrics.

M

mesna

mess-na
(Mesnex, Uromitexan ✺)

◆CLASSIFICATION

PHARMACOTHERAPEUTIC: Cytoprotective agent. **CLINICAL:** Antineoplastic adjunct, antidote.

ACTION

Binds with, detoxifies urotoxic metabolites of ifosfamide/cyclophosphamide. **Therapeutic Effect:** Inhibits ifosfamide/cyclophosphamide-induced hemorrhagic cystitis.

PHARMACOKINETICS

Rapidly metabolized after IV administration to mesna disulfide, which is reduced to mesna in kidneys. Protein binding: 69%–75%. Excreted in urine. **Half-life:** 24 min; metabolite: 72 min.

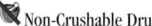 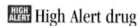

USES

Detoxifying agent used as protectant against hemorrhagic cystitis induced by ifosfamide. **OFF-LABEL:** Reduce incidence of cyclophosphamide-induced hemorrhagic cystitis with high-dose cyclophosphamide.

PRECAUTIONS

Contraindications: None known. **Cautions:** None known.

⧗ LIFESPAN CONSIDERATIONS

Pregnancy/Lactation: Unknown if drug crosses placenta or is distributed in breast milk. **Pregnancy Category B. Children:** Safety and efficacy not established. **Elderly:** Information not available.

INTERACTIONS

DRUG: None significant. **HERBAL:** None significant. **FOOD:** None known. **LAB VALUES:** May produce false-positive test result for urinary ketones.

AVAILABILITY (Rx)

Injection Solution: 100 mg/ml. **Tablets:** 400 mg.

ADMINISTRATION/HANDLING

 IV

Reconstitution • May dilute with D₅W or 0.9% NaCl to concentration of 1–20 mg/ml. • May add to solutions containing ifosfamide or cyclophosphamide.
Rate of Administration • Administer by IV infusion over 15–30 min or by continuous infusion.
Storage • Store parenteral form at room temperature. • After dilution, in 0.9% NaCl or D₅W, stable for 48 hrs at room temperature (solutions of mesna and cyclophosphamide in D₅W stable for 48 hrs if refrigerated or 6 hrs at room temperature). Discard unused medication.

PO
• Administer orally in either tablet formulation or parenteral solution. • Dilute mesna solution before PO administration to decrease sulfur odor. Can be diluted (1:1 to 1:10) in carbonated cola drinks, fruit juices, milk.

▦ IV INCOMPATIBILITIES

Amphotericin B complex (Abelcet, AmBisome, Amphotec), cisplatin (Platinol).

▦ IV COMPATIBILITIES

Allopurinol (Aloprim), docetaxel (Taxotere), doxorubicin (Adriamycin), etoposide (VePesid), gemcitabine (Gemzar), granisetron (Kytril), methotrexate, ondansetron (Zofran), paclitaxel (Taxol), vinorelbine (Navelbine).

INDICATIONS/ROUTES/DOSAGE

Prevention of Hemorrhagic Cystitis in Pts Receiving Ifosfamide
IV: ADULTS, ELDERLY: 20% of ifosfamide dose at time of ifosfamide administration and 4 and 8 hrs after each dose of ifosfamide. Total dose: 60% of ifosfamide dosage. Range: 60%–160% of the daily ifosfamide dose.
IV/PO: 100% of ifosfamide dose, given as 20% at start time followed by 40% given orally 2 and 6 hrs after start of ifosfamide.

SIDE EFFECTS

Frequent (greater than 17%): Altered taste, soft stools. **Large doses:** Diarrhea, myalgia, headache, fatigue, nausea, hypotension, allergic reaction.

ADVERSE EFFECTS/ TOXIC REACTIONS

Hematuria occurs rarely.

NURSING CONSIDERATIONS

BASELINE ASSESSMENT
◀**ALERT**▶ Each dose must be administered with ifosfamide therapy.

INTERVENTION/EVALUATION
Assess morning urine specimen for hematuria. If such occurs, dosage reduction or discontinuation may be necessary. Monitor daily pattern of bowel activity, stool consistency; record time of evacuation. Monitor B/P for hypotension.

PATIENT/FAMILY TEACHING

• Report headache, myalgia, nausea.

---

metaxalone

me-**tax**-a-lone
(Skelaxin)
**Do not confuse metaxalone with
mesalamine or metolazone, or
Skelaxin with Robaxin.**

◆CLASSIFICATION

PHARMACOTHERAPEUTIC: Autonomic agent. **CLINICAL:** Skeletal muscle relaxant (see p. 151C).

ACTION

Skeletal muscle relaxant action may be related to its CNS depressant effects. Does not directly relax skeletal muscle, motor end plate, or nerve fiber. **Therapeutic Effect:** Relieves musculoskeletal pain.

PHARMACOKINETICS

Rapidly absorbed from GI tract. Extensively distributed in tissues. Metabolized in liver. Excreted in urine. **Half-life:** 9 hrs.

USES

Adjunct to rest and physical therapy to decrease musculoskeletal pain, muscle spasm associated with strains, sprains, other muscle injuries.

PRECAUTIONS

Contraindications: Severe renal/hepatic impairment, drug-induced anemia, hemolytic anemia. **Cautions:** Mild to moderate hepatic/renal impairment, elderly, debilitated pts.

⧖ LIFESPAN CONSIDERATIONS

Pregnancy/Lactation: Unknown if distributed in breast milk. **Pregnancy Category B. Children:** Safety and efficacy not established in those 12 yrs and younger. **Elderly:** May be more susceptible to CNS effects.

INTERACTIONS

DRUG: CNS depressants, including **alcohol, benzodiazepines, opioids, tricyclic antidepressants** may increase sedative effects. **HERBAL: St. John's wort, kava kava, gotu kola, valerian** may increase CNS depression. **FOOD: High-fat meal** may increase concentration. **LAB VALUES:** May decrease WBC, RBC, platelet count.

AVAILABILITY (Rx)

Tablets: 800 mg.

ADMINISTRATION/HANDLING

• Give without regard to food. • May break, crush, dissolve, or divide tablets.

INDICATIONS/ROUTES/DOSAGE

PO: ADULTS, ELDERLY, CHILDREN 12 YRS AND OLDER: 800 mg 3–4 times daily.

SIDE EFFECTS

Occasional: Dizziness, drowsiness, headache, irritability, nausea, nervousness, dyspepsia (indigestion, heartburn, epigastric distress), vomiting.

ADVERSE EFFECTS/ TOXIC REACTIONS

Severe allergic reaction (rash, pruritus, urticaria, circumoral swelling). Overdosage produces progressive sedation, hypnosis, respiratory failure, but emetic action begins 15–30 min after increasingly higher doses are taken. Leukopenia, hemolytic anemia, hepatobiliary abnormalities occur rarely.

NURSING CONSIDERATIONS

BASELINE ASSESSMENT

Record onset, type, location, duration of musculoskeletal pain, inflammation. Inspect appearance of affected joints for immobility, stiffness, swelling.

INTERVENTION/EVALUATION

Assist with ambulation at all times. Evaluate for therapeutic response: relief of pain, stiffness, swelling; improved mobil-

M

ity; reduced joint tenderness; improved grip strength.

PATIENT/FAMILY TEACHING

• Avoid tasks that require alertness, motor skills until response to drug is established. • Avoid alcohol. • Medication intended for short-term use (3 wks). • If no improvement noted, contact physician.

---

metformin

met-**for**-min
(Apo-Metformin ❖, Fortamet, <u>Glucophage</u>, <u>Glucophage XR</u>, Glumetza, Glycon ❖, Novo-Metformin ❖, Riomet)

BLACK BOX ALERT Lactic acidosis occurs very rarely, but mortality rate is 50%. Risk increases with degree of renal impairment, pt's age, those with diabetes, unstable or acute HF.

Do not confuse Glucophage with Glucotrol, or metformin with metronidazole.

FIXED-COMBINATION(S)

Actoplus Met: metformin/pioglitazone (an antidiabetic): 500 mg/15 mg, 850 mg/15 mg. **Avandamet:** metformin/rosiglitazone (an antidiabetic): 500 mg/1 mg, 500 mg/2 mg, 500 mg/4 mg, 1,000 mg/2 mg, 1,000 mg/4 mg. **Glucovance:** metformin/glyburide (an antidiabetic): 250 mg/1.25 mg, 500 mg/2.5 mg, 500 mg/5 mg. **Janumet, Janumet XR:** metformin/sitagliptin (an antidiabetic): 500 mg/50 mg, 1,000 mg/50 mg. **Jentadueto:** metformin/linagliptin (an antidiabetic): 500 mg/2.5 mg; 1,000 mg/2.5 mg. **Kazano:** metformin/alogliptin (an antidiabetic): 500 mg/12.5 mg; 1,000 mg/12.5 mg. **Kombiglyze XR:** metformin/saxagliptin (an antidiabetic): 500 mg/5 mg, 1,000 mg/5 mg, 1,000 mg/2.5 mg. **Metaglip:** metformin/glipizide (an antidiabetic): 250 mg/2.5 mg, 500 mg/2.5 mg, 500 mg/5 mg.

PrandiMet: metformin/repaglinide (an antidiabetic): 500 mg/1 mg, 500 mg/2 mg.

◆CLASSIFICATION

PHARMACOTHERAPEUTIC: Antihyperglycemic. **CLINICAL:** Antidiabetic agent (see p. 44C).

ACTION

Decreases hepatic production of glucose. Decreases absorption of glucose, improves insulin sensitivity. **Therapeutic Effect:** Improves glycemic control, stabilizes/decreases body weight, improves lipid profile.

PHARMACOKINETICS

Slowly, incompletely absorbed after PO administration. Food delays, decreases extent of absorption. Protein binding: Negligible. Primarily distributed to intestinal mucosa, salivary glands. Primarily excreted unchanged in urine. Removed by hemodialysis. **Half-life:** 9–17 hrs.

USES

Management of type 2 diabetes mellitus as monotherapy or concomitantly with oral sulfonylurea or insulin. **OFF-LABEL:** Polycystic ovarian syndrome, gestational diabetes mellitus. Prevention of type 2 diabetes.

PRECAUTIONS

◀ALERT▶ Lactic acidosis is a rare but potentially severe consequence of metformin therapy. Withhold in pts with conditions that may predispose to lactic acidosis (e.g., hypoxemia, dehydration, hypoperfusion, sepsis).

Contraindications: Renal disease/dysfunction; abnormal creatinine clearance from any cause including MI, acute HF, septicemia, or shock; acute or chronic metabolic acidosis. **Cautions:** HF, impaired hepatic function, excessive acute/chronic alcohol intake.

⌛ LIFESPAN CONSIDERATIONS

Pregnancy/Lactation: Insulin is drug of choice during pregnancy. Distributed in breast milk in animals. **Pregnancy Category B. Children:** Safety and efficacy not established. **Elderly:** Age-related renal impairment or peripheral vascular disease may require dosage adjustment or discontinuation.

INTERACTIONS

DRUG: Furosemide may increase concentration. **Cationic medications (e.g., digoxin, morphine, quinine, ranitidine, vancomycin)** may increase concentration/effects. **Contrast agents** may increase risk of metformin-induced lactic acidosis, acute renal failure (discontinue metformin 24–48 hrs prior to and up to 72 hrs after contrast exposure). **HERBAL: Garlic** may cause hypoglycemia. **FOOD:** None known. **LAB VALUES:** May alter cholesterol, LDL, triglycerides, HDL.

AVAILABILITY (Rx)

Oral Solution (Riomet): 100 mg/ml. **Tablets (Glucophage):** 500 mg, 850 mg, 1,000 mg.

Tablets (Extended-Release): 500 mg (Fortamet, Glucophage XR, Glumetza), 750 mg (Glucophage XR), 1,000 mg (Fortamet, Glumetza).

ADMINISTRATION/HANDLING

PO
• Give extended-release tablets whole. Do not break, crush, dissolve, or divide extended-release tablets. • Give with meals (to decrease GI upset). Give Fortamet with glass of water.

INDICATIONS/ROUTES/DOSAGE

◀ALERT▶ Allow 1–2 wks between dose titrations.
Diabetes Mellitus
PO *(Immediate-Release Tablets, Solution):* **ADULTS, ELDERLY:** Initially, 500 mg twice a day or 850 mg once daily. **Maintenance:** 1,000–2,550 mg/day in 2–3 divided doses. **Maximum:** 2,550 mg/day. **CHILDREN 10–16 YRS:** Initially, 500 mg twice a day. **Maintenance:** Titrate in 500-mg increments weekly. **Maximum:** 2,000 mg/day.

PO *(Extended-Release Tablets [Glucophage XR]):* **ADULTS, ELDERLY:** Initially, 500 mg once daily. May increase by 500 mg at 1-wk intervals. **Maintenance:** 1,000–2,000 mg daily. **Maximum:** 2,000 mg/day.
PO *(Extended-Release Tablets [Glumetza]):* **ADULTS, ELDERLY:** Initially, 1,000 mg once daily. May increase by 500 mg at 1-wk intervals. **Maximum:** 2,000 mg/day.
[Fortamet]: Initially, 500–1,000 mg once daily. May increase by 500 mg at 1-wk intervals. **Maximum:** 2,500 mg/day.

Dosage in Renal Impairment
Contraindicated in pts with serum creatinine greater than 1.5 mg/dl (males) or greater than 1.4 mg/dl (females). Clinically not recommended in pts with creatinine clearance less than 60–70 ml/min.

SIDE EFFECTS

Occasional (greater than 3%): GI disturbances (diarrhea, nausea, vomiting, abdominal bloating, flatulence, anorexia) that are transient and resolve spontaneously during therapy. **Rare (3%–1%):** Unpleasant/metallic taste that resolves spontaneously during therapy.

ADVERSE EFFECTS/ TOXIC REACTIONS

Lactic acidosis occurs rarely (0.03 cases/1,000 pts) but is a serious and often fatal (50%) complication. Lactic acidosis is characterized by increase in blood lactate levels (greater than 5 mmol/L), decrease in blood pH, electrolyte disturbances. Symptoms include unexplained hyperventilation, myalgia, malaise, drowsiness. May advance to cardiovascular collapse (shock), acute HF, acute MI, prerenal azotemia.

NURSING CONSIDERATIONS

BASELINE ASSESSMENT
Assess baseline glucose, Hgb A1c, CBC, renal function tests.

INTERVENTION/EVALUATION
Monitor fasting serum glucose, Hgb A1c, renal function, CBC. Monitor folic acid,

M

renal function tests for evidence of early lactic acidosis. If pt is on concurrent oral sulfonylureas, assess for hypoglycemia (cool/wet skin, tremors, dizziness, anxiety, headache, tachycardia, numbness in mouth, hunger, diplopia). Be alert to conditions that alter glucose requirements: fever, increased activity, stress, surgical procedure.

PATIENT/FAMILY TEACHING

• Discontinue metformin, report immediately if evidence of lactic acidosis appears (unexplained hyperventilation, muscle aches, extreme fatigue, unusual drowsiness). • Prescribed diet is principal part of treatment; do not skip, delay meals. • Diabetes mellitus requires lifelong control. • Avoid alcohol. • Report persistent headache, nausea, vomiting, diarrhea or if skin rash, unusual bruising/bleeding, change in color of urine or stool occurs.

methadone

meth-a-done
(Dolophine, Metadol ❖, Methadone Disket, Methadone Intensol, Methadose)
BLACK BOX ALERT Potential to prolong QT interval. May cause respiratory depression.
Do not confuse methadone with Mephyton, Metadate CD, Metadate ER, methylphenidate, or morphine.

◆CLASSIFICATION

PHARMACOTHERAPEUTIC: Narcotic agonist **(Schedule II). CLINICAL:** Opioid analgesic.

ACTION

Binds with opioid receptors within CNS. **Therapeutic Effect:** Alters processes affecting analgesia, emotional response to pain; reduces withdrawal symptoms from other opioid drugs.

PHARMACOKINETICS

Route	Onset	Peak	Duration
PO	0.5–1 hr	1.5–2 hrs	6–8 hrs
IM	10–20 min	1–2 hrs	4–5 hrs
IV	N/A	15–30 min	3–4 hrs

Well absorbed after IM injection. Protein binding: 85%–90%. Metabolized in liver. Primarily excreted in urine. Not removed by hemodialysis. **Half-life:** 7–59 hrs.

USES

Relief of severe pain, detoxification, temporary maintenance treatment of narcotic abstinence syndrome.

PRECAUTIONS

Contraindications: Severe respiratory depression; acute or severe asthma, hypercarbia, paralytic ileus, concurrent use of selegiline. **Caution:** Renal/hepatic impairment, elderly/debilitated, risk for QT prolongation, medications that prolong QT interval, conduction abnormalities, severe volume depletion, cardiovascular disease, depression, suicidal tendencies, history of drug abuse, respiratory disease, biliary tract dysfunction, acute pancreatitis, hypothyroidism, Addison's disease, head injury, increased intracranial pressure.

⌛ LIFESPAN CONSIDERATIONS

Pregnancy/Lactation: Crosses placenta. Distributed in breast milk. Respiratory depression may occur in neonate if mother received opiates during labor. Regular use of opiates during pregnancy may produce withdrawal symptoms in neonate (irritability, excessive crying, tremors, hyperactive reflexes, fever, vomiting, diarrhea, yawning, sneezing, seizures). **Pregnancy Category B (D if used for prolonged periods or at high dosages at term). Children:** Paradoxical excitement may occur. Pts younger than 2 yrs more susceptible to respiratory depressant effects. **Elderly:** More susceptible to respiratory depressant effects. Age-related renal impairment may increase risk of urinary retention.

INTERACTIONS

DRUG: Alcohol, other CNS depressants may increase CNS effects, respiratory depression, hypotension. **CYP3A4 inducers (e.g., carbamazepine, phenobarbital)** may decrease concentration/effects. **CYP3A4 inhibitors (e.g., rifampin, clarithromycin)** may increase methadone levels. **Amiodarone, erythromycin** may prolong QT interval. **MAOIs** may produce severe, sometimes fatal reaction (reduce dose to ¼ of usual methadone dose). **HERBAL: Gotu kola, kava kava, St. John's wort, valerian** may increase CNS depression. **St. John's wort** may decrease concentration/effects. **FOOD: Grapefruit products** may alter concentration/effects. **LAB VALUES:** May increase serum amylase, lipase.

AVAILABILITY (Rx)

Injection Solution (Dolophine): 10 mg/ml. **Oral Concentrate (Methadone Intensol, Methadose):** 10 mg/ml. **Oral Solution:** 5 mg/5 ml, 10 mg/5 ml. **Tablets (Dispersible [Methadose, Methadone Disket]):** 40 mg. **Tablets (Dolophine):** 5 mg, 10 mg.

ADMINISTRATION/HANDLING

IM, Subcutaneous
◄**ALERT**► IM preferred over subcutaneous route (subcutaneous produces pain, local irritation, induration). • Do not use if solution appears cloudy or contains a precipitate. • Administer slowly. • Those with circulatory impairment experience higher risk of overdosage due to delayed absorption of repeated administration.

PO
• Give without regard to meals. • Oral dose for detoxification and maintenance may be given in fruit juice or water. • Dispersible tablet should not be chewed or swallowed; add to liquid, allow to dissolve before swallowing.

INDICATIONS/ROUTES/DOSAGE

Analgesia
PO: ADULTS, ELDERLY: Initially, 2.5–10 mg q4–12h. **CHILDREN:** 0.1–0.2 mg/kg/dose q4–8h for 2–3 doses then q6–12h as needed. **Maximum dose:** 10 mg.
IV, IM, Subcutaneous: ADULTS, ELDERLY: Initially, 2.5 mg q8–12h, then titrate slowly to desired effect. **CHILDREN:** 0.1 mg/kg q4–8h for 2–3 doses, then q4–12h. **Maximum:** 10 mg/dose.

Renal/Hepatic Impairment
Creatinine clearance less than 10 ml/min: 50–75% normal dose. Avoid in severe hepatic disease.

Detoxification
PO: ADULTS, ELDERLY: Initially, dose should not exceed 30 mg. An additional 5–10 mg may be provided if withdrawal symptoms have not been suppressed or if symptoms reappear after 2–4 hrs. Total daily dose not to exceed 40 mg. Maintenance range: 80–120 mg/day with titration occurring cautiously. Withdrawal should be less than 10% of the maintenance dose every 10–14 days. **Short-term:** Initially, titrate to 40 mg/day in 2 divided doses. Continue 40-mg dose for 2–3 days. Decrease dose every day or every other day.

SIDE EFFECTS

Frequent: Sedation, decreased B/P (orthostatic hypotension), diaphoresis, facial flushing, constipation, dizziness, nausea, vomiting. **Occasional:** Confusion, urinary retention, palpitations, abdominal cramps, visual changes, dry mouth, headache, decreased appetite, anxiety, insomnia. **Rare:** Allergic reaction (rash, pruritus).

ADVERSE EFFECTS/ TOXIC REACTIONS

Overdose results in respiratory depression, skeletal muscle flaccidity, cold/clammy skin, cyanosis, extreme drowsiness progressing to seizures, stupor, coma. Early sign of toxicity presents as increased sedation after being on a stable dose. Cardiac toxicity manifested as QT prolongation, torsade de pointes. Tolerance to analgesic effect, physical dependence may

M

occur with repeated use. **Antidote:** Naloxone (see Appendix K for dosage).

NURSING CONSIDERATIONS

BASELINE ASSESSMENT

Assess type, location, intensity of pain. **Detoxification:** Assess pt for opioid withdrawal. Pt should be in recumbent position before drug administration by parenteral route. Obtain vital signs before giving medication. If respirations are 12/min or less (20/min or less in children), withhold medication, contact physician.

INTERVENTION/EVALUATION

Monitor vital signs 15–30 min after subcutaneous/IM dose, 5–10 min following IV dose. Oral medication is 50% as potent as parenteral. Assess for adequate voiding. Assess for clinical improvement, record onset of relief of pain. Provide support to pt in detoxification program; monitor for withdrawal symptoms.

PATIENT/FAMILY TEACHING

• Methadone may produce drug dependence, has potential for being abused. • Avoid alcohol. • Do not stop taking abruptly after prolonged use. • May cause dry mouth, drowsiness. • Avoid tasks that require alertness, motor skills until response to drug is established. • Report severe drowsiness, respiratory depression.

methocarbamol

meth-oh-**kar**-ba-mal
(Robaxin)
Do not confuse Robaxin with Skelaxin.

◆CLASSIFICATION

PHARMACOTHERAPEUTIC: Autonomic agent, carbamate derivative of guaifenesin. **CLINICAL:** Skeletal muscle relaxant (see p. 152C).

ACTION

Skeletal muscle relaxant action may be related to its CNS depressant effects. Does not directly relax skeletal muscle, motor end plate, or nerve fiber. **Therapeutic Effect:** Relieves musculoskeletal pain.

PHARMACOKINETICS

Extensively distributed in tissues. Protein binding: 46%–50%. Converts to metabolites. Metabolized by dealkylation, hydroxylation; excreted in urine. **Half-life:** 1–2 hrs.

USES

Adjunct to rest and physical therapy for relief of discomfort associated with acute, painful musculoskeletal conditions (e.g., tetanus).

PRECAUTIONS

Contraindications: Renal impairment (injectable formulation). **Cautions:** Myasthenia gravis pts receiving pyridostigmine, hepatic impairment, seizure disorders (injectable formulation).

⏳ LIFESPAN CONSIDERATIONS

Pregnancy/Lactation: Unknown if distributed in breast milk. **Pregnancy Category C. Children:** Safety and efficacy not established in those 16 yrs and younger. **Elderly:** May be more susceptible to CNS effects.

INTERACTIONS

DRUG: CNS depressants, including **alcohol, benzodiazepines, opioids, tricyclic antidepressants,** may increase sedative effects. May inhibit effect of **pyridostigmine. HERBAL: St. John's wort, valerian, kava kava, gotu kola** may increase CNS depression. **FOOD: High-fat meal** may increase concentration. **LAB VALUES:** May decrease WBC counts.

AVAILABILITY (Rx)

Injection, Solution: <u>100 mg/ml.</u>

🦷 **Tablets, Film-Coated:** 500 mg, 750 mg.

ADMINISTRATION/HANDLING

IM/IV

(IM) • Maximum of 5 ml can be given into each gluteal region.

(IV) • May give undiluted at maximum rate of 3 ml/min. • May dilute with D₅W or 0.9% NaCl to concentration of 4 mg/ml. • Administer in recumbent position and remain in position for 10–15 min after IV administration.

PO

• Give without regard to food. • May crush or break tablets and mix with food or liquid if needed.

INDICATIONS/ROUTES/DOSAGE

Muscle Spasm
PO: ADULTS, ELDERLY, CHILDREN 16 YRS AND OLDER: 1.5 g 4 times/day for 2–3 days, then 4–4.5 g/day in 3–6 divided doses.

Usual Parenteral Dose
IM/IV: ADULTS, ELDERLY: 1 g q8h for up to 3 days.

Tetanus
◀ALERT▶ Do not use for longer than 72 hrs.
IV: ADULTS, ELDERLY: Initially, 1–2 g by direct IV injection, then 1–2 g by IV infusion q6h until oral therapy possible. **CHILDREN:** 15 mg/kg/dose. May repeat q6h if needed. **Maximum:** 1.8 g/m²/day.

SIDE EFFECTS

Occasional: Dizziness, drowsiness, confusion, double vision, insomnia, headache, irritability, nausea, nervousness, dyspepsia (including nausea, vomiting), vomiting, metallic taste.

ADVERSE EFFECTS/ TOXIC REACTIONS

Anaphylactic reaction (rash, pruritus, urticaria, angioneurotic edema, fever, bradycardia, hypotension, syncope) has occurred. Leukopenia, cholestatic jaundice, seizure occur rarely.

NURSING CONSIDERATIONS

BASELINE ASSESSMENT

Record onset, type, location, duration of musculoskeletal pain, inflammation. Inspect appearance of affected joints for immobility, stiffness, swelling.

INTERVENTION/EVALUATION

Assist with ambulation at all times. Evaluate for therapeutic response: relief of pain, stiffness, swelling; improved mobility; reduced joint tenderness; improved grip strength.

PATIENT/FAMILY TEACHING

• Avoid tasks that require alertness, motor skills until response to drug is established. • Avoid alcohol. • May color urine brown, black, or green. • Medication intended for short-term use (3 wks). • If no improvement noted, contact physician. • Report severe sedation.

M

methotrexate

meth-oh-**trex**-ate
(Apo-Methotrexate ✤, Rheumatrex, Trexall)
BLACK BOX ALERT Pregnancy Category X. May cause fetal abnormalities, death. May produce potentially fatal chronic hepatotoxicity, dermatologic reactions, acute renal failure, pneumonitis, myelosuppression, malignant lymphoma, aplastic anemia, GI toxicity.
Do not confuse methotrexate with metolazone, methylprednisolone, or mitoxantrone. MTX is an error-prone abbreviation; do not use as an abbreviation.

◆CLASSIFICATION

PHARMACOTHERAPEUTIC: Antimetabolite. **CLINICAL:** Antineoplastic, antiarthritic, antipsoriatic (see p. 88C).

✤ Canadian trade name   ⬛ Non-Crushable Drug   ⬛ High Alert drug

M

ACTION

Competes with enzymes necessary to reduce folic acid to tetrahydrofolic acid, a component essential to DNA, RNA, protein synthesis. **Therapeutic Effect:** Inhibits DNA, RNA, protein synthesis.

PHARMACOKINETICS

Variably absorbed from GI tract. Completely absorbed after IM administration. Protein binding: 50%–60%. Widely distributed. Metabolized in liver. Primarily excreted in urine. Removed by hemodialysis but not by peritoneal dialysis. Half-life: 3–10 hrs (large doses, 8–15 hrs).

USES

Oncology-related: Treatment of breast, head/neck, non–small-cell lung, small cell lung carcinomas; trophoblastic tumors, acute lymphocytic, meningeal leukemias; non-Hodgkin's lymphomas (lymphosarcoma, Burkitt's lymphoma), carcinoma of gastrointestinal tract, mycosis fungoides, osteosarcoma. **Non-Oncology uses:** Psoriasis, rheumatoid arthritis (including juvenile rheumatoid arthritis). **OFF-LABEL:** Treatment of acute myelocytic leukemia; bladder, carcinoma, ectopic pregnancy, management of abortion, systemic lupus erythematosus, treatment of and maintenance of remission in Crohn's disease.

PRECAUTIONS

Contraindications: Breastfeeding. **For pts with psoriasis or rheumatoid arthritis:** Pregnancy, hepatic disease, alcoholism, immunodeficiency syndrome, preexisting blood dyscrasias. **Cautions:** Peptic ulcer, ulcerative colitis, preexisting myelosuppression, history of chronic hepatic disease.

⧗ LIFESPAN CONSIDERATIONS

Pregnancy/Lactation: Avoid pregnancy during methotrexate therapy and minimum 3 mos after therapy in males or at least one ovulatory cycle after therapy in females. May cause fetal death, congenital anomalies. Distributed in breast milk. Breastfeeding not recommended. **Pregnancy Category D (X for patients with psoriasis or rheumatoid arthritis). Children/Elderly:** Renal/hepatic impairment may require dosage adjustment.

INTERACTIONS

DRUG: Alcohol, hepatotoxic medications may increase risk of hepatotoxicity. **Bone marrow depressants** may increase myelosuppression. **Live virus vaccines** may potentiate virus replication, increase vaccine side effects, decrease pt's antibody response to vaccine. **NSAIDs** may increase risk of toxicity. **Probenecid, salicylates** may increase concentration, risk of toxicity. **HERBAL: Cat's claw, echinacea** possess immunostimulant properties. **FOOD:** None known. **LAB VALUES:** May increase serum uric acid, AST.

AVAILABILITY (Rx)

Injection, Powder for Reconstitution: 1 g. **Injection Solution:** 25 mg/ml. **Tablets:** 2.5 mg (Rheumatrex), 5 mg (Trexall), 7.5 mg (Trexall), 10 mg (Trexall), 15 mg (Trexall).

ADMINISTRATION/HANDLING

◄**ALERT**► May be carcinogenic, mutagenic, teratogenic. Handle with extreme care during preparation/administration. Wear gloves when preparing solution. If powder or solution comes in contact with skin, wash immediately, thoroughly with soap, water. May give IM, IV, intra-arterially, intrathecally.

 IV

Reconstitution • Reconstitute powder with D₅W or 0.9% NaCl to provide concentration of 50 mg/ml. • For intrathecal use, dilute with preservative-free 0.9% NaCl to provide a concentration not greater than 2–4 mg/ml.
Rate of Administration • Give IV push at rate of 10 mg/min. • Give IV infusion at rate of 4–20 mg/hr.
Storage • Store vials at room temperature. Diluted solutions stable for 24 hrs at room temperature.

IV INCOMPATIBILITIES

Droperidol (Inapsine), gemcitabine (Gemzar), idarubicin (Idamycin), midazolam (Versed), nalbuphine (Nubain).

IV COMPATIBILITIES

Cisplatin (Platinol AQ), cyclophosphamide (Cytoxan), daunorubicin (DaunoXome), doxorubicin (Adriamycin), etoposide (VePesid), 5-fluorouracil, granisetron (Kytril), leucovorin, mitomycin (Mutamycin), ondansetron (Zofran), paclitaxel (Taxol), vinblastine (Velban), vincristine (Oncovin), vinorelbine (Navelbine).

INDICATIONS/ROUTES/DOSAGE

◄ALERT► Refer to individual specific protocols for optimum dosage, sequence of administration.

Antineoplastic Dosage Range
IV: ADULTS, ELDERLY: 30–40 mg/m^2/wk up to 100–12,000 mg/m^2 with leucovorin rescue.

Trophoblastic Neoplasms
PO, IM: ADULTS, ELDERLY: 15–30 mg/day for 5 days; repeat in 7 days for 3–5 courses.
IV: 11 mg/m^2 on days 1–5, repeat every 3 wks.

Head/Neck Cancer
PO, IV, IM: ADULTS, ELDERLY: 25–50 mg/m^2 once weekly.

Breast Cancer
IV: ADULTS, ELDERLY: 30–60 mg/m^2 days 1 and 8 q3–4wks.

Bladder Cancer (Off-Label)
IV: ADULTS, ELDERLY: 30 mg/m^2 days 1 and 8 q3wks.

Mycosis Fungoides
IM, PO: ADULTS, ELDERLY: 5–50 mg once weekly or 15–37.5 mg twice a wk.

Rheumatoid Arthritis (RA)
PO: ADULTS: 7.5 mg once weekly or 2.5 mg q12h for 3 doses once weekly. **EL-**
DERLY: Initially, 5–7.5 mg/wk. **Maximum:** 20 mg/wk.

Juvenile Rheumatoid Arthritis (JRA)
PO, IM, Subcutaneous: CHILDREN: Initially, 10 mg/m^2 once weekly, then 5–15 mg/m^2/wk as a single dose or in 3 divided doses given q12h.

Psoriasis
PO: ADULTS, ELDERLY: 10–25 mg once weekly or 2.5–5 mg q12h for 3 doses once weekly.
IM/Subcutaneous: ADULTS, ELDERLY: 10–25 mg once weekly.

Dosage in Renal Impairment

Creatinine Clearance	Reduce Dose to
61–80 ml/min	75% of normal
51–60 ml/min	70% of normal
10–50 ml/min	30–50% of normal
Less than 10 ml/min	Avoid use

SIDE EFFECTS

Frequent (10%–3%): Nausea, vomiting, stomatitis, burning/erythema at psoriatic site (in pts with psoriasis). **Occasional (3%–1%):** Diarrhea, rash, dermatitis, pruritus, alopecia, dizziness, anorexia, malaise, headache, drowsiness, blurred vision.

ADVERSE EFFECTS/ TOXIC REACTIONS

High potential for various, severe toxicities. GI toxicity may produce gingivitis, glossitis, pharyngitis, stomatitis, enteritis, hematemesis. Hepatotoxicity more likely to occur with frequent small doses than with large intermittent doses. Pulmonary toxicity characterized by interstitial pneumonitis. Hematologic toxicity, resulting from marked myelosuppression, may manifest as leukopenia, thrombocytopenia, anemia, hemorrhage. Dermatologic toxicity may produce rash, pruritus, urticaria, pigmentation, photosensitivity, petechiae, ecchymosis, pustules. Severe nephrotoxicity produces azotemia, hematuria, renal failure.

M

NURSING CONSIDERATIONS

BASELINE ASSESSMENT

Rheumatoid arthritis: Assess pain, range of motion. **Psoriasis:** Assess skin lesions. Question for possibility of pregnancy (Pregnancy Category X) in pts with psoriasis, rheumatoid arthritis (RA). Obtain all functional tests before therapy, repeat throughout therapy. Antiemetics may prevent nausea, vomiting.

INTERVENTION/EVALUATION

Monitor hepatic/renal function tests, CBC, urinalysis, chest X-rays, serum uric acid. Monitor for hematologic toxicity (fever, sore throat, signs of local infection, unusual bruising/bleeding from any site), symptoms of anemia (excessive fatigue, weakness). Assess skin for evidence of dermatologic toxicity. Keep pt well hydrated, urine alkaline. Avoid rectal temperatures, traumas that induce bleeding. Apply 5 full min of pressure to IV sites.

PATIENT/FAMILY TEACHING

• Maintain strict oral hygiene. • Do not have immunizations without physician's approval (drug lowers resistance). • Avoid crowds, those with infection. • Avoid alcohol, aspirin. • Avoid sunlamp, sunlight exposure. • Use contraceptive measures during therapy and for 3 mos (males) or 1 ovulatory cycle (females) after therapy. • Promptly report fever, sore throat, signs of local infection, unusual bruising/bleeding from any site, diarrhea. • Hair loss is reversible, but new hair growth may have different color, texture. • Report persistent nausea/vomiting.

methylergonovine

meth-il-er-**goe**-noe-veen
(Methergine ✦)

◆ CLASSIFICATION

PHARMACOTHERAPEUTIC: Ergot alkaloid. **CLINICAL:** Oxytoxic agent, uterine stimulant.

ACTION

Stimulates alpha-adrenergic, serotonin receptors, producing arterial vasoconstriction. Causes vasospasm of coronary arteries. Directly stimulates uterine muscle. **Therapeutic Effect:** Increases strength, frequency of uterine contractions, decreases uterine bleeding.

PHARMACOKINETICS

Route	Onset	Peak	Duration
PO	5–10 min	N/A	3 hrs
IV	Immediate	N/A	45 min
IM	2–5 min	N/A	3 hrs

Rapidly absorbed from GI tract after IM administration. Distributed rapidly to plasma, extracellular fluid, tissues. Metabolized in liver. Primarily excreted in urine. **Half-life:** 0.5–2 hrs.

USES

Management of uterine atony, hemorrhage and subinvolution of uterus following delivery of placenta. Control uterine hemorrhage following delivery of anterior shoulder in second stage of labor.

PRECAUTIONS

Contraindications: Hypertension, pregnancy, toxemia. **Cautions:** Renal/hepatic impairment, cardiovascular disease, concurrent use with CYP3A4 inhibitors (e.g., protease inhibitors), occlusive peripheral vascular disease, sepsis, second stage of labor.

⧖ LIFESPAN CONSIDERATIONS

Pregnancy/Lactation: Contraindicated during pregnancy. Small amounts distributed in breast milk. **Pregnancy Category C. Children/Elderly:** No information available.

INTERACTIONS

DRUG: Vasoconstrictors, vasopressors may increase effects. **HERBAL:** None significant. **FOOD:** None known. **LAB VALUES:** May decrease serum prolactin.

AVAILABILITY (Rx)

Injection Solution: 0.2 mg/ml. **Tablets:** 0.2 mg.

ADMINISTRATION/HANDLING

Reconstitution • Dilute with 0.9% NaCl to volume of 5 ml.
Rate of Administration • Give over at least 1 min, carefully monitoring B/P.
Storage • Refrigerate ampules. • Initial dose may be given parenterally, followed by oral regimen. • IV use in life-threatening emergencies only.

🔲 IV INCOMPATIBILITIES

None known.

🔲 IV COMPATIBILITIES

Heparin, potassium.

INDICATIONS/ROUTES/DOSAGE

Prevention/Treatment of Postpartum, Postabortion Hemorrhage
PO: ADULTS: 0.2 mg 3–4 times a day. Continue for up to 7 days.
IV, IM: ADULTS: Initially, 0.2 mg after delivery of anterior shoulder, after delivery of placenta, or during puerperium. May repeat q2–4h as needed.

SIDE EFFECTS

Frequent: Nausea, uterine cramping, vomiting. **Occasional:** Abdominal pain, diarrhea, dizziness, diaphoresis, tinnitus, bradycardia, chest pain. **Rare:** Allergic reaction (rash, pruritus), dyspnea; severe or sudden hypertension.

ADVERSE EFFECTS/ TOXIC REACTIONS

Severe hypertensive episodes may result in CVA, serious arrhythmias, seizures. Hypertensive effects are more frequent with pt susceptibility, rapid IV administration, concurrent use of regional anesthesia, vasoconstrictors. Peripheral ischemia may lead to gangrene.

NURSING CONSIDERATIONS

BASELINE ASSESSMENT

Determine baseline serum calcium level, B/P, pulse. Assess for any evidence of bleeding before administration.

INTERVENTION/EVALUATION

Monitor uterine tone, bleeding, B/P, pulse q15min until stable (about 1–2 hrs). Assess extremities for color, warmth, movement, pain. Report chest pain promptly. Provide support with ambulation if dizziness occurs.

PATIENT/FAMILY TEACHING

• Avoid smoking: causes increased vasoconstriction. • Report increased cramping, bleeding, foul-smelling lochia. • Report pale, cold hands/feet (possibility of diminished circulation).

M

methylnaltrexone

meth-il-nal-**trex**-own
(Relistor)
Do not confuse methylnaltrexone with naltrexone.

◆CLASSIFICATION

PHARMACOTHERAPEUTIC: Opioid receptor antagonist. **CLINICAL:** Constipation agent.

ACTION

Blocks binding of opioids to peripheral opioid receptors within GI tract. **Therapeutic Effect:** Decreases constipating effect of opioids without reducing analgesic effect.

PHARMACOKINETICS

Absorbed rapidly. Undergoes moderate tissue distribution. Protein binding: 11%–15%. Excreted primarily in urine, with lesser amount eliminated in feces. **Half-life:** 8 hrs.

USES

Treatment of opioid-induced constipation in pts with advanced illness who are receiving palliative care when response to laxative therapy is insufficient.

PRECAUTIONS

Contraindications: Known or suspected mechanical GI obstruction. **Cautions:** Severe renal impairment, history of GI tract lesions.

⧖ LIFESPAN CONSIDERATIONS

Pregnancy/Lactation: Unknown if distributed in breast milk. **Pregnancy Category B. Children:** Safety and efficacy not established. **Elderly:** No age-related precautions noted.

INTERACTIONS

DRUG: None significant. **HERBAL:** None significant. **FOOD:** None known. **LAB VALUES:** None significant.

AVAILABILITY (Rx)

Injection, Solution: 8 mg/0.4 ml, 12 mg/0.6 ml.

ADMINISTRATION/HANDLING

Subcutaneous
• Inject into upper arm, abdomen, or thigh. Do not inject in tender, bruised, red, or hard areas. **Storage** • Solution appears as clear and colorless to pale yellow. • If particulate matter is noted, discard. • Once solution is drawn into syringe, may be stored at room temperature. • Administer within 24 hrs.

INDICATIONS/ROUTES/DOSAGE

◀**ALERT**▶ Usual schedule is once every other day, as needed, but no more frequently than once every 24 hrs.

Constipation
Subcutaneous: ADULTS, ELDERLY WEIGHING 38 KG TO LESS THAN 62 KG: 8 mg. **ADULTS, ELDERLY WEIGHING 62–114 KG:** 12

mg. **ADULTS, ELDERLY WHOSE WEIGHT FALLS OUTSIDE THESE RANGES:** Dose at 0.15 mg/kg (round dose up to nearest 0.1 ml of volume).

Severe Renal Impairment (Creatinine Clearance Less Than 30 ml/min)
Subcutaneous: ADULTS, ELDERLY: Administer 50% of recommended dose.

SIDE EFFECTS

Frequent (29%–12%): Abdominal pain, flatulence, nausea. **Occasional (7%–5%):** Diarrhea, dizziness.

ADVERSE EFFECTS/TOXIC REACTIONS

None known.

NURSING CONSIDERATIONS

BASELINE ASSESSMENT

30% of pts report defecation within 30 min after drug administration.

INTERVENTION/EVALUATION

Encourage fluid intake. Assess bowel sounds for peristalsis. Monitor daily pattern of bowel activity, stool consistency. If opioid medication is stopped, drug should be discontinued. Assess for abdominal disturbances.

PATIENT/FAMILY TEACHING

• Laxative effect usually occurs within 30 min but may take up to 24 hrs after medication administration. • Common side effects include transient abdominal pain, nausea, vomiting. • Contact physician if any of these symptoms persist or worsen, or if severe or persistent diarrhea occurs.

TOP 200

methylphenidate

meth-il-**fen**-i-date
(Apo-Methylphenidate ✦, <u>Concerta</u>, Daytrana, Metadate CD, Metadate ER, Methylin, Methylin ER, PMS-

Methylphenidate ✣, Quillivant XR, Ritalin, Ritalin LA, Ritalin SR)

BLACK BOX ALERT Chronic abuse can lead to marked tolerance, psychological dependence. Abrupt withdrawal from prolonged use may lead to severe depression, psychosis.

Do not confuse Metadate ER with Metadate CD, Methylphenidate with methadone, or Ritalin with Rifadin.

◆ CLASSIFICATION

PHARMACOTHERAPEUTIC: CNS stimulant **(Schedule II). CLINICAL:** CNS stimulant.

ACTION

Blocks reuptake of norepinephrine, dopamine into presynaptic neurons. **Therapeutic Effect:** Decreases motor restlessness, fatigue. Increases motor activity, attention span, mental alertness. Produces mild euphoria.

PHARMACOKINETICS

Onset	Peak	Duration
Immediate-release	2 hrs	3–6 hrs
Sustained-release	4–7 hrs	8 hrs
Extended-release	N/A	12 hrs
Transdermal	2 hrs	N/A

Slowly, incompletely absorbed from GI tract. Protein binding: 15%. Metabolized in liver. Eliminated in urine, in feces by biliary system. Unknown if removed by hemodialysis. **Half-life:** 2–4 hrs.

USES

Treatment of attention-deficit hyperactivity disorder (ADHD). Management of narcolepsy. **OFF-LABEL:** Secondary mental depression (especially elderly, medically ill).

PRECAUTIONS

Contraindications: Use of MAOIs within 14 days, marked anxiety, tension, agitation, motor tics, family history or diagnosis of Tourette's syndrome, glaucoma. **Meta-**date **(additional):** Severe hypertension, heart failure, arrhythmia, hyperthyroidism, recent MI or angina. **Cautions:** Hypertension, seizures, acute stress reaction, emotional instability, history of drug dependence, HF, recent MI, hyperthyroidism, known structural cardiac abnormality, bipolar disorder.

⌛ LIFESPAN CONSIDERATIONS

Pregnancy/Lactation: Unknown if drug crosses placenta or is distributed in breast milk. **Pregnancy Category C. Children:** May be more susceptible to developing anorexia, insomnia, stomach pain, decreased weight. Chronic use may inhibit growth. **Elderly:** No age-related precautions noted.

INTERACTIONS

DRUG: MAOIs may increase effects. **Other CNS stimulants** may have additive effect. May inhibit metabolism of **warfarin, anticonvulsants, antidepressants. HERBAL: Ephedra** may cause hypertension, arrhythmias. **Yohimbe** may increase CNS stimulation. **FOOD:** None known. **LAB VALUES:** None known.

AVAILABILITY (Rx)

Oral Solution (Methylin): 5 mg/5 ml, 10 mg/5 ml, 10 mg/1 ml. **Tablets (Chewable [Methylin]):** 2.5 mg, 5 mg, 10 mg. **Tablets (Methylin, Ritalin):** 5 mg, 10 mg, 20 mg. **Topical Patch (Daytrana):** 10 mg/9 hrs, 15 mg/9 hrs, 20 mg/9 hrs, 30 mg/9 hrs. **Powder for Suspension, Extended-Release (Quillivant XR):** 25 mg/5 ml.

🍇 **Capsules (Extended-Release [Metadate CD]):** 10 mg, 20 mg, 30 mg, 40 mg, 50 mg, 60 mg. 🍇 **Capsules (Extended-Release [Ritalin LA]):** 10 mg, 20 mg, 30 mg, 40 mg. 🍇 **Tablets (Extended-Release [Concerta]):** 18 mg, 27 mg, 36 mg, 54 mg, 72 mg. 🍇 **Tablets (Extended-Release [Metadate ER, Methylin ER]):** 10 mg, 20 mg. 🍇 **Tablets (Sustained-Release [Ritalin SR]):** 20 mg.

ADMINISTRATION/HANDLING

◄ **ALERT** ► Sustained-release, extended-release tablets may be given in place of

M

regular tablets, once daily dose is titrated using regular tablets, and titrated dosage corresponds to sustained-release or extended-release tablet strength.

PO

• Do not give in afternoon or evening (may cause insomnia). • Do not crush, break extended-release capsules, extended- or sustained-release tablets. • Immediate-release tablets may be crushed. • Give dose 30–45 min before meals.

• **Concerta:** Administer once daily in morning. May take without regard to food but must be taken with water, milk, or juice.

• **Methylin Chewable:** Give with at least 8 oz of water or other fluid.

• **Metadate CD, Ritalin LA:** • May be opened, sprinkled on applesauce. • Instruct pt to swallow applesauce without chewing. Do not crush or chew capsule contents.

Patch

• To be worn daily for 9 hrs. • Replace daily in morning. • Apply to dry, clean area of hip. • Avoid applying to waistline (clothing may cause patch to rub off). • Alternate application site daily. • Press firmly in place for 30 sec to ensure patch is in good contact with skin. • Do not cut patch.

INDICATIONS/ROUTES/DOSAGE

ADHD

PO: ADULTS: 5 mg twice daily, before breakfast and lunch. May increase by 5–10 mg/day at weekly intervals. **Maximum:** 60 mg/day in 2–3 divided doses. **CHILDREN 6 YRS AND OLDER:** Initially, 0.3 mg/kg/dose or 2.5–5 mg before breakfast and lunch. May increase by 0.1 mg/kg/dose or by 5–10 mg/day at weekly intervals. **Usual dose:** 0.5–1 mg/kg/day. **Maximum:** 2 mg/kg/day or 60 mg/day if 50 kg or less; 100 mg if greater than 50 kg.

PO (Concerta): CHILDREN 6 YRS AND OLDER, ADULTS UP TO 65 YRS OF AGE: Initially, 18 mg once a day; may increase by 18 mg/day at weekly intervals. **Maximum:** 72 mg/day.

PO (Metadate CD): CHILDREN 6 YRS AND OLDER: Initially, 20 mg/day. May increase by 10–20 mg/day at weekly intervals. **Maximum:** 60 mg/day.

PO (Quillivant XR): CHILDREN 6 YRS AND OLDER: Initially, 20 mg once daily in the morning. May increase in increments of 10–20 mg per day at weekly increments. **Maximum:** 60 mg/day.

PO (Ritalin LA): CHILDREN 6 YRS AND OLDER: Initially, 20 mg/day. May increase by 10 mg/day at weekly intervals. **Maximum:** 60 mg/day.

PO (Metadate ER, Methylin ER, Ritalin SR): CHILDREN 6 YRS AND OLDER: May replace regular tablets after daily dose is titrated and 8-hr dosage corresponds to sustained-release or extended-release tablet strength. **Maximum:** 60 mg/day.

PATCH (Daytrana): CHILDREN 6–12 YRS, ADOLESCENTS: Initially, 10 mg daily (applied and worn for 9 hrs). Dosage is titrated to desired effect. May increase dose no more frequently than every wk.

Narcolepsy

PO: ADULTS, ELDERLY: Initially, 5 mg twice daily, before breakfast and lunch. May increase by 5–10 mg/day at weekly intervals. **Maximum:** 60 mg/day in 2–3 divided doses.

SIDE EFFECTS

Frequent: Anxiety, insomnia, anorexia. **Occasional:** Dizziness, drowsiness, headache, nausea, abdominal pain, fever, rash, arthralgia, vomiting. **Rare:** Blurred vision, Tourette's syndrome (uncontrolled vocal outbursts, repetitive body movements, tics), palpitations.

ADVERSE EFFECTS/ TOXIC REACTIONS

Prolonged administration to children with ADHD may delay normal weight gain pattern. Overdose may produce tachycardia, palpitations, arrhythmias, chest pain, psychotic episode, seizures, coma. Hypersensitivity reactions, blood dyscrasias occur rarely.

NURSING CONSIDERATIONS

BASELINE ASSESSMENT

ADHD: Assess attention span, impulsivity, interaction with others, distractibility. **Narcolepsy:** Observe/assess frequency of episodes.

INTERVENTION/EVALUATION

Monitor B/P, pulse, changes in ADHD symptoms. CBC with differential should be performed routinely during therapy. If paradoxical return of attention-deficit occurs, dosage should be reduced or discontinued. Monitor growth.

PATIENT/FAMILY TEACHING

• Avoid tasks that require alertness, motor skills until response to drug is established. • Sugarless gum, sips of water may relieve dry mouth. • Report any increase in seizures. • Take daily dose early in morning to avoid insomnia. • Report anxiety, palpitations, fever, vomiting, skin rash. • Report new or worsened symptoms (e.g., behavior, hostility, concentration ability). • Avoid caffeine. • Do not stop taking abruptly after prolonged use.

---

*methylPREDNISolone

(Medrol)

*methylPREDNISolone acetate

(DepoMedrol)

*methylPREDNISolone sodium succinate

(Solu-Medrol)
meth-il-pred-**niss**-oh-lone
Do not confuse DepoMedrol with Solu-Medrol, Medrol with Mebaral, or methylpredniso-

lone with medroxyprogesterone or prednisolone.

◆ CLASSIFICATION

PHARMACOTHERAPEUTIC: Adrenal corticosteroid. **CLINICAL:** Anti-inflammatory (see p. 100C).

ACTION

Suppresses migration of polymorphonuclear leukocytes, reverses increased capillary permeability. **Therapeutic Effect:** Decreases inflammation.

PHARMACOKINETICS

Route	Onset	Peak	Duration
PO	Rapid	1–2 hrs	30–36 hrs
IM	Rapid	4–8 days	1–4 wks
IV	Rapid	N/A	N/A

Well absorbed from GI tract after IM administration. Widely distributed. Metabolized in liver. Excreted in urine. Removed by hemodialysis. **Half-life:** 3.5 hrs.

USES

Endocrine disorders: Substitution therapy for deficiency states (acute or chronic adrenal insufficiency, congenital adrenal hyperplasia, adrenal insufficiency secondary to pituitary insufficiency). **Nonendocrine disorders:** Arthritis, rheumatic carditis, allergic reaction; collagen, intestinal tract, hepatic, ocular, renal, skin diseases; bronchial asthma, cerebral edema, malignancies, spinal cord injury.

PRECAUTIONS

Contraindications: Administration of live virus vaccines, systemic fungal infection. **IM (additional):** Idiopathic thrombocytopenia purpura. **Cautions:** Respiratory tuberculosis, untreated systemic infections, hypertension, HF, diabetes, GI disease (e.g., peptic ulcer), myasthenia gravis, renal/hepatic impairment, seizures, cataracts, glaucoma, following acute MI, thyroid disorder, thromboembolic tendencies, diabetes.

M

⏳ LIFESPAN CONSIDERATIONS

Pregnancy/Lactation: Crosses placenta. Distributed in breast milk. May cause cleft palate (chronic use in first trimester). Breastfeeding not recommended. **Pregnancy Category C. Children:** Prolonged treatment or high dosages may decrease short-term growth rate, cortisol secretion. **Elderly:** No age-related precautions noted.

INTERACTIONS

DRUG: May alter effects of **warfarin. Hepatic enzyme inducers (e.g., phenytoin, rifampin)** may decrease effects. **Live virus vaccines** may decrease pt's antibody response to vaccine, increase vaccine side effects, potentiate virus replication. **HERBAL: Cat's claw, echinacea** possess immunostimulant properties. **St. John's wort** may decrease concentration. **FOOD:** None known. **LAB VALUES:** May increase serum glucose, cholesterol, lipids, amylase, sodium. May decrease serum calcium, potassium, thyroxine, hypothalmic-pituitary-adrenal (HPA) axis.

AVAILABILITY (Rx)

Injection, Powder for Reconstitution (Solu-Medrol): 40 mg, 125 mg, 500 mg, 1 g. **Injection Suspension:** 40 mg/ml, 80 mg/ml. **Tablets (Medrol):** 2 mg, 4 mg, 8 mg, 16 mg, 32 mg. **(Medrol Dosepak):** 4 mg (21 tablets).

ADMINISTRATION/HANDLING

◄**ALERT**► Do **not** give methylprednisolone acetate IV.

 IV

Reconstitution • For infusion, add to D₅W, 0.9% NaCl.
Rate of Administration • Give IV push over 3–15 min. • Give IV piggyback. Dose of 250 mg over 15–30 min; dose of 500–999 mg over at least 30 min; dose of 1g or greater over 1 hr.
Storage • Store vials at room temperature.

IM
• Methylprednisolone acetate should not be further diluted. • Methylprednisolone sodium succinate should be reconstituted with Bacteriostatic Water for Injection. • Give deep IM in gluteus maximus (avoid injection into deltoid muscle).

PO
• Give with food, milk.

🚫 IV INCOMPATIBILITIES

Ciprofloxacin (Cipro), diltiazem (Cardizem), potassium chloride, propofol (Diprivan).

🟦 IV COMPATIBILITIES

Dexmedetomidine (Precedex), dopamine (Intropin), heparin, midazolam (Versed), theophylline.

INDICATIONS/ROUTES/DOSAGE

Anti-Inflammatory, Immunosuppressive
IV: ADULTS, ELDERLY: 10–40 mg. May repeat q4–6h as needed. **CHILDREN:** 0.5–1.7 mg/kg/day or 5–25 mg/m²/day in 2–4 divided doses.
PO: ADULTS, ELDERLY: 2–60 mg/day in 1–4 divided doses. **CHILDREN:** 0.5–1.7 mg/kg/day or 5–25 mg/m²/day in 2–4 divided doses.
IM *(Methylprednisolone Acetate)*:
ADULTS, ELDERLY: 10–80 mg q1–2wks.
Intra-Articular, Intralesional: ADULTS, ELDERLY: 20–60 mg q1–5wks.

Status Asthmaticus
IV: ADULTS, ELDERLY, CHILDREN: Initially, 2 mg/kg/dose, then 0.5–1 mg/kg/dose q6h.

Spinal Cord Injury
IV Bolus: ADULTS, ELDERLY, CHILDREN: 30 mg/kg over 15 min, followed by 5.4 mg/kg/hr over 23 hrs, to be given within 45 min of bolus dose.

SIDE EFFECTS

Frequent: Insomnia, heartburn, anxiety, abdominal distention, diaphoresis, acne, mood swings, increased appetite, facial flushing, GI distress, delayed wound healing, increased susceptibility to infection, diarrhea, constipation. **Occasional:** Headache, edema, tachycardia, change in skin color, frequent urination, depression. **Rare:** Psychosis, increased blood coagulability, hallucinations.

ADVERSE EFFECTS/ TOXIC REACTIONS

Long-term therapy: Hypocalcemia, hypokalemia, muscle wasting (esp. in arms, legs), osteoporosis, spontaneous fractures, amenorrhea, cataracts, glaucoma, peptic ulcer, HF. **Abrupt withdrawal after long-term therapy:** Anorexia, nausea, fever, headache, severe arthralgia, rebound inflammation, fatigue, weakness, lethargy, dizziness, orthostatic hypotension.

NURSING CONSIDERATIONS

BASELINE ASSESSMENT

Question for hypersensitivity to any of the corticosteroids, components. Obtain baselines for height, weight, B/P, serum glucose, electrolytes. Check results of initial tests (tuberculosis [TB] skin test, X-rays, EKG).

INTERVENTION/EVALUATION

Monitor I&O, daily weight; assess for edema. Monitor daily pattern of bowel activity, stool consistency. Check vital signs at least twice a day. Be alert for infection (sore throat, fever, vague symptoms). Monitor serum electrolytes, including B/P, glucose. Monitor for hypocalcemia (muscle twitching, cramps, positive Trousseau's or Chvostek's signs), hypokalemia (weakness, muscle cramps, numbness, tingling [esp. lower extremities], nausea/vomiting, irritability, EKG changes). Assess emotional status, ability to sleep. Check lab results for blood coagulability, clinical evidence of thromboembolism.

PATIENT/FAMILY TEACHING

• Take oral dose with food, milk. • Do not change dose/schedule or stop taking drug; must taper off gradually under medical supervision. • Notify physician of fever, sore throat, muscle aches, sudden weight gain or loss, edema, loss of appetite, fatigue. • Maintain strict personal hygiene, avoid exposure to disease, trauma. • Severe stress (serious infection, surgery, trauma) may require increased dosage. • Follow-up visits, lab tests are necessary. • Children must be assessed for growth retardation. • Inform dentist, other physicians of methylprednisolone therapy now or within past 12 mos.

metoclopramide

met-oh-**kloe**-pra-myde
(Apo-Metoclop ✦, Metozolv ODT, Reglan)

BLACK BOX ALERT Prolonged use may cause tardive dyskinesia.
Do not confuse metoclopramide with metolazone or metoprolol, or Reglan with Renagel.

◆CLASSIFICATION

PHARMACOTHERAPEUTIC: Dopamine receptor antagonist. **CLINICAL:** GI emptying adjunct, peristaltic stimulant, antiemetic.

ACTION

Stimulates motility of upper GI tract. Decreases reflux into esophagus. Raises threshold activity in chemoreceptor trigger zone. **Therapeutic Effect:** Accelerates intestinal transit, gastric emptying. Relieves nausea, vomiting.

PHARMACOKINETICS

Route	Onset	Peak	Duration
PO	30–60 min	N/A	1–2 hrs
IV	1–3 min	N/A	1–2 hrs
IM	10–15 min	N/A	1–2 hrs

Well absorbed from GI tract. Metabolized in liver. Protein binding: 30%. Primarily excreted in urine. Not removed by hemodialysis. **Half-life:** 4–6 hrs.

* "Tall Man" lettering ✦ Canadian trade name Non-Crushable Drug High Alert drug

USES

Facilitates placement of enteral feeding tubes; stimulates gastric emptying, intestinal transit in conjunction with radiography; symptomatic treatment of gastroparesis, gastroesophageal reflux disease (GERD); prevents or treats chemotherapy-induced nausea, vomiting; prevents or treats postop nausea, vomiting. **Orally disintegrating tablets:** Treatment of gastroparesis, GERD.

PRECAUTIONS

Contraindications: Concurrent use of medications likely to produce extrapyramidal reactions, GI hemorrhage, GI obstruction/ perforation, history of seizure disorder, pheochromocytoma. **Cautions:** Renal impairment, HF, cirrhosis, hypertension, depression, Parkinson's disease.

⌛ LIFESPAN CONSIDERATIONS

Pregnancy/Lactation: Crosses placenta. Distributed in breast milk. **Pregnancy Category B. Children:** More susceptible to having dystonic reactions. **Elderly:** More likely to have parkinsonian dyskinesias after long-term therapy.

INTERACTIONS

DRUG: Alcohol, other CNS depressants may increase CNS depressant effect. **Anticholinergics, opioid analgesics** may decrease effects on GI motility. **HERBAL:** None significant. **FOOD:** None known. **LAB VALUES:** May increase serum aldosterone, prolactin.

AVAILABILITY (Rx)

Injection Solution: 5 mg/ml. **Syrup:** 5 mg/ 5 ml. **Tablets:** 5 mg, 10 mg.

Tablets, Orally Disintegrating: 5 mg, 10 mg.

ADMINISTRATION/HANDLING

 IV

Reconstitution • Dilute doses greater than 10 mg in 50 ml D$_5$W or 0.9% NaCl.

Rate of Administration • Infuse over 15–30 min. • May give undiluted slow IV push at rate of 10 mg over 1–2 min. • Too-rapid IV injection may produce intense feeling of anxiety, restlessness, followed by drowsiness.

Storage • Store vials at room temperature. • After dilution, IV infusion (piggyback) is stable for 24 hrs.

PO

• Give 30 min before meals and at bedtime. • Tablets may be crushed. • Do not cut, divide, break orally disintegrating tablets. Place on tongue, swallow with saliva.

🔲 IV INCOMPATIBILITIES

Allopurinol (Aloprim), cefepime (Maxipime), furosemide (Lasix), propofol (Diprivan).

🔲 IV COMPATIBILITIES

Dexamethasone, dexmedetomidine (Precedex), diltiazem (Cardizem), diphenhydramine (Benadryl), fentanyl (Sublimaze), heparin, hydromorphone (Dilaudid), morphine, potassium chloride.

INDICATIONS/ROUTES/DOSAGE

Prevention of Chemotherapy-Induced Nausea/Vomiting
IV: ADULTS, ELDERLY, CHILDREN: 1–2 mg/ kg 30 min before chemotherapy; repeat q2h for 2 doses, then q3h as needed for total of 5 doses/day.

Postop Nausea/Vomiting
IV: ADULTS, ELDERLY: 10–20 mg near end of surgery.

Gastroparesis
PO, IV: ADULTS: 10 mg 30 min before meals and at bedtime for 2–8 wks.
PO: ELDERLY: Initially, 5 mg 30 min before meals and at bedtime. May increase to 10 mg.
IV: ELDERLY: 5 mg over 1–2 min. May increase to 10 mg.

M

Symptomatic Gastroesophageal Reflux Disease (GERD)

PO: ADULTS: 10–15 mg up to 4 times a day, or single doses up to 20 mg as needed. **ELDERLY:** Initially, 5 mg 4 times a day. May increase to 10 mg. **CHILDREN:** 0.1–0.2 mg/kg/dose 4 times/day.

Facilitate Small Bowel Intubation (Single Dose)

IV: ADULTS, ELDERLY: 10 mg as a single dose. **CHILDREN 6–14 YRS:** 2.5–5 mg as a single dose. **CHILDREN YOUNGER THAN 6 YRS:** 0.1 mg/kg as a single dose.

Dosage in Renal Impairment

Dosage is modified based on creatinine clearance.

Creatinine Clearance	Dosage
Less than 40 ml/min	50% of normal dose

SIDE EFFECTS

◀ALERT▶ Doses of 2 mg/kg or greater, or increased length of therapy, may result in a greater incidence of side effects. **Frequent (10%):** Drowsiness, restlessness, fatigue, lethargy. **Occasional (3%):** Dizziness, anxiety, headache, insomnia, breast tenderness, altered menstruation, constipation, rash, dry mouth, galactorrhea, gynecomastia. **Rare (less than 3%):** Hypotension, hypertension, tachycardia.

ADVERSE EFFECTS/ TOXIC REACTIONS

Extrapyramidal reactions occur most frequently in children, young adults (18–30 yrs) receiving large doses (2 mg/kg) during chemotherapy and usually are limited to akathisia (involuntary limb movement, facial grimacing, motor restlessness). Neuroleptic malignant syndrome (diaphoresis, fever, unstable B/P, muscular rigidity).

NURSING CONSIDERATIONS

BASELINE ASSESSMENT

Antiemetic: Assess for dehydration (poor skin turgor, dry mucous membranes, longitudinal furrows in tongue). Assess for nausea, vomiting, abdominal distention, bowel sounds.

INTERVENTION/EVALUATION

Monitor for anxiety, restlessness, extrapyramidal symptoms (EPS) during IV administration. Monitor daily pattern of bowel activity, stool consistency. Assess skin for rash. Evaluate for therapeutic response from gastroparesis (nausea, vomiting, bloating). Monitor renal function, B/P, heart rate.

PATIENT/FAMILY TEACHING

• Avoid tasks that require alertness, motor skills until response to drug is established. • Report involuntary eye, facial, limb movement (extrapyramidal reaction). • Avoid alcohol.

M

metolazone

meh-**toe**-la-zone
(Zaroxolyn)
Do not confuse metolazone with metaxolone, methotrexate, metoclopramide, or metoprolol, or Zaroxolyn with Zarontin.

◆CLASSIFICATION

PHARMACOTHERAPEUTIC: Thiazide diuretic. **CLINICAL:** Diuretic, antihypertensive (see p. 104C).

ACTION

Diuretic: Blocks reabsorption of sodium, potassium, chloride at distal convoluted tubule, promoting delivery of sodium to potassium side, increasing sodium-potassium (Na-K) exchange. **Therapeutic Effect:** Produces renal excretion. **Antihypertensive:** Reduces plasma and extracellular fluid volume, peripheral vascular resistance. **Therapeutic Effect:** Reduces B/P.

PHARMACOKINETICS

Route	Onset	Peak	Duration
PO (diuretic)	1 hr	—	24 hrs

✢ Canadian trade name   🦺 Non-Crushable Drug   📛 High Alert drug

Incompletely absorbed from GI tract. Protein binding: 95%. Primarily excreted unchanged in urine. Not removed by hemodialysis. **Half-life:** 20 hrs.

USES

Treatment of mild to moderate essential hypertension, edema due to HF, nephrotic syndrome or impaired renal function.

PRECAUTIONS

Contraindications: Anuria, hepatic coma/precoma, history of hypersensitivity to sulfonamides, thiazide diuretics. **Cautions:** Severe renal disease, severe hepatic impairment, gout, lupus erythematosus, prediabetes or diabetes, elevated serum cholesterol, triglycerides.

⌛ LIFESPAN CONSIDERATIONS

Pregnancy/Lactation: Crosses placenta. Small amount distributed in breast milk. Breastfeeding not recommended. **Pregnancy Category B (D if used in pregnancy-induced hypertension). Children:** No age-related precautions noted. **Elderly:** May be more sensitive to hypotensive or electrolyte effects. Age-related renal impairment may require dosage adjustment.

INTERACTIONS

DRUG: May increase risk of **digoxin** toxicity associated with metolazone-induced hypokalemia. May increase risk of **lithium** toxicity. **HERBAL: Ephedra, ginseng, licorice** may decrease effect. **Black cohosh, periwinkle** may enhance effect. **FOOD:** None known. **LAB VALUES:** May increase serum glucose, cholesterol, LDL, bilirubin, calcium, creatinine, uric acid, triglycerides. May decrease urinary calcium, serum magnesium, potassium, sodium.

AVAILABILITY (Rx)

Tablets: 2.5 mg, 5 mg, 10 mg.

ADMINISTRATION/HANDLING

PO
• May give with food, milk if GI upset occurs, preferably with breakfast (may prevent nocturia).

INDICATIONS/ROUTES/DOSAGE

Edema
PO: ADULTS: 2.5–10 mg/day. May increase to 20 mg/day in edema associated with renal disease or heart failure.

Hypertension
PO: ADULTS: 2.5–5 mg/day.

Usual Elderly Dosage
PO: Initially, 2.5 mg/day or every other day.

Usual Pediatric Dosage
PO: 0.2–0.4 mg/kg/day in 1–2 divided doses.

SIDE EFFECTS

Expected: Increased urinary frequency/volume. **Frequent (10%–9%):** Dizziness, lightheadedness, headache. **Occasional (6%–4%):** Muscle cramps/spasm, drowsiness, fatigue, lethargy. **Rare (less than 2%):** Asthenia (loss of strength, energy), palpitations, depression, nausea, vomiting, abdominal bloating, constipation, diarrhea, urticaria.

ADVERSE EFFECTS/TOXIC REACTIONS

Vigorous diuresis may lead to profound water loss and electrolyte depletion, resulting in hypokalemia, hyponatremia, dehydration. Acute hypotensive episodes may occur. Hyperglycemia may occur during prolonged therapy. Pancreatitis, paresthesia, blood dyscrasias, pulmonary edema, allergic pneumonitis, dermatologic reactions occur rarely. Overdose can lead to lethargy, coma without changes in electrolytes, hydration.

NURSING CONSIDERATIONS

BASELINE ASSESSMENT

Check vital signs, esp. B/P for hypotension, before administration. Assess baseline serum electrolytes, particularly check for hypokalemia. Assess skin turgor, mucous membranes for hydration status. Assess for peripheral edema. Assess muscle strength, mental status. Note skin temperature, moisture. Obtain baseline weight. Monitor I&O.

INTERVENTION/EVALUATION

Continue to monitor B/P, vital signs, serum electrolytes, I&O, weight. Note extent of diuresis. Monitor for electrolyte disturbances (hypokalemia may result in weakness, tremors, muscle cramps, nausea, vomiting, altered mental status, tachycardia; hyponatremia may result in confusion, thirst, cold/clammy skin).

PATIENT/FAMILY TEACHING

• Expect increased urinary frequency/volume. • Rise slowly from lying to sitting position, permit legs to dangle momentarily before standing to reduce hypotensive effect. • Avoid tasks requiring motor skills, mental alertness until response to drug is established. • Eat foods high in potassium, such as whole grains (cereals), legumes, meat, bananas, apricots, orange juice, potatoes (white, sweet), raisins.

---

metoprolol

me-**toe**-pro-lol
(Apo-Metoprolol ❧, Betaloc ❧, Lopressor, Nu-Metop ❧, Toprol XL)

BLACK BOX ALERT Abrupt withdrawal can produce acute tachycardia, hypertension, ischemia. Drug should be gradually tapered over 1–2 wks.

Do not confuse metoprolol with atenolol, labetolol, nadolol, or stanozolol, or Toprol XL with Tegretol, Tegretol XR, or Topamax.

FIXED-COMBINATION(S)

Dutoprol: metoprolol/hydrochlorothiazide (a diuretic): 25 mg/12.5 mg, 50 mg/12.5 mg, 100 mg/12.5 mg. **Lopressor HCT:** metoprolol/hydrochlorothiazide (a diuretic): 50 mg/25 mg, 100 mg/25 mg, 100 mg/50 mg.

◆CLASSIFICATION

PHARMACOTHERAPEUTIC: Beta₁-adrenergic blocker. **CLINICAL:** Antianginal, antihypertensive, MI adjunct (see p. 62C, 73C).

ACTION

Selectively blocks beta₁-adrenergic receptors; high dosages may block beta₂-adrenergic receptors. Decreases oxygen requirements. Large doses increase airway resistance. **Therapeutic Effect:** Slows heart rate, decreases cardiac output, reduces B/P. Decreases myocardial ischemia severity.

PHARMACOKINETICS

Route	Onset	Peak	Duration
PO	10–15 min	1–2 hrs	N/A
PO (extended-release)	N/A	6–12 hrs	N/A
IV	Immediate	20 min	N/A

Well absorbed from GI tract. Protein binding: 12%. Widely distributed. Metabolized in liver. Primarily excreted in urine. Removed by hemodialysis. **Half-life:** 3–7 hrs.

USES

Lopressor: Treatment of hemodynamically stable acute myocardial infarction (AMI), angina pectoris, hypertension. **Toprol XL:** Treatment of angina pectoris, to reduce mortality or hospitalization in pts with HF, already receiving ACE inhibitors, diuretics, and/or digoxin, hypertension. **OFF-LABEL:** Treatment of ventricular arrhythmias, migraine prophylaxis, essential tremor, aggressive behavior, prevent reinfarction post MI, prevent/treat atrial fibrillation/atrial flutter, hypertrophic cardiomyopathy, thyrotoxicosis.

PRECAUTIONS

Contraindications: **MI:** Cardiogenic shock, MI with heart rate less than 45 beats/min or systolic B/P less than 100

M

---

mm Hg, overt HF, second- or third-degree heart block, sinus bradycardia. **HTN/Angina:** Sinus bradycardia, second- or third-degree heart block, overt HF, sick sinus syndrome (except with pacemaker), severe peripheral arterial disease, pheochromocytoma. **Extended-Release:** Severe bradycardia, second- or third-degree heart block, cardiogenic shock, decompensated HF, sick sinus syndrome (except with functioning pacemaker). **Cautions:** Bronchospastic disease, renal impairment, peripheral vascular disease, hyperthyroidism, diabetes mellitus, myasthenia gravis, psychiatric disease. **Extended-Release:** Compensated heart failure.

⧖ LIFESPAN CONSIDERATIONS

Pregnancy/Lactation: Crosses placenta; distributed in breast milk. Avoid use during first trimester. May produce bradycardia, apnea, hypoglycemia, hypothermia during delivery, low birth-weight infants. **Pregnancy Category C (D if used in second or third trimester). Children:** Safety and efficacy not established. **Elderly:** Age-related peripheral vascular disease may increase susceptibility to decreased peripheral circulation.

INTERACTIONS

DRUG: **Diuretics, other antihypertensives** may increase hypotensive effect. May mask symptoms of hypoglycemia, prolong hypoglycemic effect of **insulin, oral hypoglycemics. NSAIDs** may decrease antihypertensive effect. **Sympathomimetics, xanthines** may mutually inhibit effects. Potent **CYP2D6 inhibitors (e.g., fluoxetine, cimetidine)** may increase concentration. **Digoxin, verapamil, diltiazem** may increase risk of bradycardia/heart block. **HERBAL:** **Ephedra, ginseng, yohimbe** may worsen hypertension. **Garlic** may increase antihypertensive effect. **FOOD:** None known. **LAB VALUES:** May increase serum antinuclear antibody titer (ANA), BUN, serum lipoprotein, LDH, alkaline phosphatase, bilirubin, creatinine, potassium, uric acid, AST, ALT, triglycerides.

AVAILABILITY (Rx)

Injection Solution (Lopressor): 1 mg/ml. **Tablets (Lopressor):** 25 mg, 50 mg, 100 mg.

 Tablets (Extended-Release [Toprol XL]): 25 mg, 50 mg, 100 mg, 200 mg.

ADMINISTRATION/HANDLING

IV

Rate of Administration • May give undiluted. • Administer IV injection over 1 min. • May give by IV piggyback (in 50 ml D₅W or 0.9% NaCl) over 30–60 min. • Monitor EKG, B/P during administration.
Storage • Store at room temperature.

PO

• Tablets may be crushed; do not crush/break extended-release tablets. • Extended-release tablets may be divided in half. • Give at same time each day. • May be given with or immediately after meals (enhances absorption).

▦ IV INCOMPATIBILITY

Amphotericin B complex (Abelcet, AmBisome, Amphotec), lidocaine, nitroglycerin.

▦ IV COMPATIBILITIES

Amiodarone, diltiazem, furosemide, heparin, morphine.

INDICATIONS/ROUTES/DOSAGE

Hypertension
PO: ADULTS: Initially, 50 mg twice daily. Increase at weekly (or longer) intervals. **Maintenance:** 100–450 mg/day. **ELDERLY:** Initially, 25 mg/day. Range: 25–300 mg/day. **CHILDREN:** Initially, 1–2 mg/kg/day in 2 divided doses. **Maximum:** 6 mg/kg/day in 2 divided doses.
PO *(Extended-Release)***: ADULTS:** 25–100 mg/day as single dose. May increase at least at weekly intervals until optimum

B/P attained. **Maximum:** 400 mg/day. **ELDERLY:** Initially, 25–50 mg/day as a single dose. May increase at 1- to 2-wk intervals. **CHILDREN:** Initially, 1 mg/kg once daily. **Maximum:** 50 mg. May increase to 2 mg/kg/day. **Maximum:** 200 mg/day.

Angina Pectoris

PO: ADULTS: Initially, 50 mg twice daily. Increase at weekly (or longer) intervals. **Usual range:** 50–200 mg twice daily. **Maximum:** 400 mg/day.

PO *(Extended-Release)*: **ADULTS:** Initially, 100 mg/day as single dose. May increase at least at weekly intervals until optimum clinical response achieved. **Maximum:** 400 mg/day.

HF

PO *(Extended-Release)*: **ADULTS:** Initially, 25 mg/day. May double dose q2wks. **Maximum:** 200 mg/day.

Early Treatment of MI

IV: ADULTS: 5 mg q2min for 3 doses, followed by 50 mg orally q6h for 48 hrs. Begin oral dose 15 min after last IV dose. In pts who do not tolerate full IV dose, give 25–50 mg orally q6h, 15 min after last IV dose, then 100 mg twice a day for at least 3 mos.

SIDE EFFECTS

Metoprolol is generally well tolerated, with transient and mild side effects. **Frequent:** Diminished sexual function, drowsiness, insomnia, unusual fatigue/weakness. **Occasional:** Anxiety, diarrhea, constipation, nausea, vomiting, nasal congestion, abdominal discomfort, dizziness, difficulty breathing, cold hands/feet. **Rare:** Altered taste, dry eyes, nightmares, paresthesia, allergic reaction (rash, pruritus).

ADVERSE EFFECTS/ TOXIC REACTIONS

Overdose may produce profound bradycardia, hypotension, bronchospasm. Abrupt withdrawal may result in dia-phoresis, palpitations, headache, tremulousness, exacerbation of angina, MI, ventricular arrhythmias. May precipitate HF, MI in pts with heart disease; thyroid storm in those with thyrotoxicosis; peripheral ischemia in those with existing peripheral vascular disease. Hypoglycemia may occur in pts with previously controlled diabetes mellitus (may mask signs of hypoglycemia). **Antidote:** Glucagon (see Appendix K for dosage).

NURSING CONSIDERATIONS

BASELINE ASSESSMENT

Assess baseline renal/hepatic function tests. Assess B/P, apical pulse immediately before drug administration (if pulse is 60/min or less or systolic B/P is less than 90 mm Hg, withhold medication, contact physician). **Antianginal:** Record onset, type (sharp, dull, squeezing), radiation, location, intensity, duration of anginal pain, precipitating factors (exertion, emotional stress).

INTERVENTION/EVALUATION

Measure B/P near end of dosing interval (determines whether B/P is controlled throughout day). Monitor B/P for hypotension, respiration for shortness of breath. Assess pulse for quality, rate, rhythm. Assess for evidence of HF: dyspnea (esp. on exertion, lying down), night cough, peripheral edema, distended neck veins. Monitor I&O (increased weight, decreased urinary output may indicate HF). Therapeutic response to hypertension noted in 1–2 wks.

PATIENT/FAMILY TEACHING

• Do not abruptly discontinue medication. • Compliance with therapy regimen is essential to control hypertension, arrhythmias. • If dose is missed, take next scheduled dose (do not double dose). • Go from lying to standing slowly. • Report excessive fatigue, dizziness. • Avoid tasks that require alertness, motor skills

M

until response to drug is established. • Do not use nasal decongestants, OTC cold preparations (stimulants) without physician approval. • Monitor B/P, pulse before taking medication. • Restrict salt, alcohol intake.

metronidazole `TOP 200`

me-troe-**nye**-da-zole
(Apo-Metronidazole ✦, Flagyl, Flagyl ER, <u>Flagyl 375</u>, MetroCream, MetroGel, MetroGel-Vaginal, NidaGel ✦, Noritate, Vandazole)
Do not confuse metronidazole with meropenum, metformin, methotrexate, or miconazole.

FIXED-COMBINATION(S)

Helidac: metronidazole/bismuth/tetracycline (an anti-infective): 250 mg/262 mg/500 mg. **Pylera:** metronidazole/bismuth/tetracycline (an anti-infective): 125 mg/140 mg/125 mg.

◆CLASSIFICATION

PHARMACOTHERAPEUTIC: Nitroimidazole derivative. **CLINICAL:** Antibacterial, antiprotozoal.

ACTION

Disrupts DNA, inhibiting nucleic acid synthesis. **Therapeutic Effect:** Produces bactericidal, antiprotozoal, amebicidal, trichomonacidal effects. Produces anti-inflammatory, immunosuppressive effects when applied topically.

PHARMACOKINETICS

Well absorbed from GI tract; minimally absorbed after topical application. Protein binding: less than 20%. Widely distributed; crosses blood-brain barrier. Metabolized in liver. Primarily excreted in urine; partially eliminated in feces. Removed by hemodialysis. **Half-life:** 8 hrs (increased in alcoholic hepatic disease, neonates).

USES

Treatment of anaerobic infections (skin/skin structure, CNS, lower respiratory tract, bone/joints, intra-abdominal, gynecologic, endocarditis, septicemia). Treatment of *H. pylori* (part of multidrug regimen); surgical prophylaxis (colorectal), trichomoniasis, amebiasis, antibiotic-associated pseudomembranous colitis (AAPC). Topical treatment of acne rosacea. **Vaginal gel:** Treatment of bacterial vaginosis. **OFF-LABEL:** Crohn's disease.

PRECAUTIONS

Contraindications: Pregnancy (first trimester). **Cautions:** Blood dyscrasias, severe hepatic dysfunction, CNS disease, predisposition to edema, concurrent corticosteroid therapy.

⧗ LIFESPAN CONSIDERATIONS

Pregnancy/Lactation: Readily crosses placenta. Distributed in breast milk. Contraindicated during first trimester in those with trichomoniasis. Topical use during pregnancy, lactation discouraged. **Pregnancy Category B. Children:** Safety and efficacy of topical administration not established in those younger than 21 yrs. **Elderly:** Age-related hepatic impairment may require dosage adjustment.

INTERACTIONS

DRUG: Alcohol may cause disulfiram-type reaction (e.g., abdominal cramps, nausea, vomiting, headache, psychotic reactions). **Disulfiram** may increase risk of toxicity. May increase effects of **oral anticoagulants. HERBAL:** None significant. **FOOD:** None known. **LAB VALUES:** May increase serum LDH, AST, ALT.

AVAILABILITY (Rx)

Capsules (Flagyl 375): 375 mg. **Injection (Infusion):** 500 mg/100 ml. **Tablets (Flagyl):** 250 mg, 500 mg. **Topical Cream:** 0.75% (MetroCream), 1% (Noritate). **Topical Gel (MetroGel):** 0.75%, 1%. **Vaginal Gel (MetroGel-Vaginal, Vandazole):** 0.75%.

Tablets (Extended-Release [Flagyl ER]): 750 mg.

ADMINISTRATION/HANDLING

IV

Rate of Administration • Infuse IV over 30–60 min. Do not give by IV bolus.
Storage • Store at room temperature (ready-to-use infusion bags).

PO

• Give without regard to meals. Give with food to decrease GI irritation. • Extended-release tablet should be given on an empty stomach (1 hr before or 2 hrs after meals). • Do not crush extended-release tablets.

IV INCOMPATIBILITIES

Amphotericin B complex (Abelcet, AmBisome, Amphotec).

IV COMPATIBILITIES

Dexmedetomidine (Precedex), diltiazem (Cardizem), dopamine (Intropin), heparin, hydromorphone (Dilaudid), lorazepam (Ativan), magnesium sulfate, midazolam (Versed), morphine.

INDICATIONS/ROUTES/DOSAGE

Anaerobic Infections
PO, IV: ADULTS, ELDERLY: 500 mg q6–8h. **Maximum:** 4 g/day.
PO: CHILDREN, INFANTS: 30–50 mg/kg/day in divided doses q8h. **Maximum:** 2,250 mg/day.
IV: CHILDREN, INFANTS: 22.5–40 mg/kg/day in 3 divided doses. **Maximum:** 1,500 mg/day.

Amebiasis
PO: ADULTS, ELDERLY: 500–750 mg 3 times a day for 5–10 days. **CHILDREN:** 35–50 mg/kg/day in 3 divided doses for 10 days. **Maximum:** 750 mg/dose.

Giardiasis
PO: ADULTS, ELDERLY: 500 mg 2 times per day for 5–7 days.

Pseudomembranous Colitis
PO: ADULTS, ELDERLY: 250–500 mg 3–4 times a day. **CHILDREN:** 30 mg/kg/day in divided doses q6h for 7–10 days. **Maximum:** 2 g/day.

Trichomoniasis
PO: ADULTS, ELDERLY: 250 mg 3 times a day or 375 mg twice a day or 500 mg twice a day or 2 g as a single dose. **CHILDREN:** 15–30 mg/kg/day in 3 divided doses for 7 days.

Bacterial Vaginosis
PO: ADULTS (NONPREGNANT): 500 mg twice a day for 7 days or 750 mg (extended-release) once daily for 7 days.
Intravaginal: ADULTS: 0.75% apply twice a day for 5 days.
◄**ALERT**► Centers for Disease Control and Prevention (CDC) does not recommend the use of topical agents during pregnancy.

Rosacea
Topical: ADULTS, ELDERLY: (1%): Apply to affected area once daily. **(0.75%):** Apply to affected area twice a day.

Dosage in Renal Impairment
Creatinine clearance less than 10 ml/min: Administer 50% of dose or q12h.

SIDE EFFECTS

Frequent: Systemic: Anorexia, nausea, dry mouth, metallic taste. **Vaginal:** Symptomatic cervicitis/vaginitis, abdominal cramps, uterine pain. **Occasional: Systemic:** Diarrhea, constipation, vomiting, dizziness, erythematous rash, urticaria, reddish-brown urine. **Topical:** Transient erythema, mild dryness, burning, irritation, stinging, tearing when applied too close to eyes. **Vaginal:** Vaginal, perineal, vulvar itching; vulvar swelling. **Rare:** Mild, transient leukopenia; thrombophlebitis with IV therapy.

ADVERSE EFFECTS/TOXIC REACTIONS

Oral therapy may result in furry tongue, glossitis, cystitis, dysuria, pancreatitis.

M

Peripheral neuropathy (manifested as numbness, tingling of hands/feet) usually is reversible if treatment is stopped immediately upon appearance of neurologic symptoms. Seizures occur occasionally.

NURSING CONSIDERATIONS

BASELINE ASSESSMENT
Question for history of hypersensitivity to metronidazole, other nitroimidazole derivatives (and parabens with topical). Obtain specimens for diagnostic tests, cultures before giving first dose (therapy may begin before results are known).

INTERVENTION/EVALUATION
Monitor daily pattern of bowel activity, stool consistency. Monitor I&O, assess for urinary problems. Be alert to neurologic symptoms (dizziness, paresthesia of extremities). Assess for rash, urticaria. Watch for onset of superinfection (ulceration/change of oral mucosa, furry tongue, vaginal discharge, genital/anal pruritus).

PATIENT/FAMILY TEACHING
• Urine may be red-brown or dark. • Avoid alcohol, alcohol-containing preparations (cough syrups, elixirs) for at least 48 hrs after last dose. • Avoid tasks that require alertness, motor skills until response to drug is established. • If taking metronidazole for trichomoniasis, refrain from sexual intercourse until full treatment is completed. • For amebiasis, frequent stool specimen checks will be necessary. • **Topical:** Avoid contact with eyes. • May apply cosmetics after application. • Metronidazole acts on erythema, papules, pustules but has no effect on rhinophyma (hypertrophy of nose), telangiectasia, ocular problems (conjunctivitis, keratitis, blepharitis). • Other recommendations for rosacea include avoidance of hot/spicy foods, alcohol, extremes of hot/cold temperatures, excessive sunlight.

micafungin
mye-ka-**fun**-jin
(Mycamine)

◆CLASSIFICATION
PHARMACOTHERAPEUTIC: Echinocandin antifungal. **CLINICAL:** Antifungal (see p. 48C).

ACTION
Inhibits synthesis of glucan (vital component of fungal cell formation), damaging fungal cell membrane. **Therapeutic Effect:** Decreased glucan content leads to cellular lysis.

PHARMACOKINETICS
Slowly metabolized in liver. Protein binding: greater than 99%. Primarily excreted in feces and, to a lesser extent, in urine. Not removed by hemodialysis. **Half-life:** 11–21 hrs.

USES
Treatment of esophageal candidiasis, candidemia, candida peritonitis, abscesses, acute disseminated candidiasis, prophylaxis of *Candida* infection in pts undergoing hematopoietic stem cell transplant. **OFF-LABEL:** Prophylaxis of HIV-related esophageal candidiasis. Treatment of infections due to *Aspergillus* spp.

PRECAUTIONS
Contraindications: None known. **Cautions:** Hepatic/renal impairment, concomitant hepatotoxic medications.

⌛ LIFESPAN CONSIDERATIONS
Pregnancy/Lactation: May reduce sperm count. May be embryotoxic. Unknown if distributed in breast milk. **Pregnancy Category C. Children:** Safety and efficacy not established. **Elderly:** No age-related precautions noted.

INTERACTIONS

DRUG: May increase concentration of **nifedipine, sirolimus, itraconazole.** **HERBAL:** None significant. **FOOD:** None known. **LAB VALUES:** May increase serum creatinine, alkaline phosphatase, LDH, AST, ALT.

AVAILABILITY (Rx)

Injection, Powder for Reconstitution: 50 mg, 100 mg.

ADMINISTRATION/HANDLING

 IV

Reconstitution • Add 5 ml 0.9% NaCl (without bacteriostatic agent) to each 50-mg vial (10 ml to 100-mg vial) to yield micafungin 10 mg/ml. • Gently swirl to dissolve; do not shake. • Further dilute in 0.9% NaCl or D₅W to final concentration of 0.5–1.5 mg/ml. • Alternatively, D₅W may be used for reconstitution and dilution. • Flush existing IV line with 0.9% NaCl or D₅W before infusion.
Rate of Administration • Infuse over 60 min.
Storage • Reconstituted solution is stable for 24 hrs at room temperature. • Discard if precipitate is present.

🔅 IV INCOMPATIBILITIES

Amiodarone, nicardipine.

🔅 IV COMPATIBILITIES

Bumetanide (Bumex), calcium gluconate, heparin.

INDICATIONS/ROUTES/DOSAGE

Esophageal Candidiasis
IV: ADULTS, ELDERLY: 150 mg/day for 10–30 days. **CHILDREN (GREATER THAN 30 KG):** 2.5 mg/kg/day. (**Maximum:** 150 mg daily.) **(30 KG OR LESS):** 3 mg/kg/day.

Candida Prophylaxis in Stem Cell Pts
IV: ADULTS, ELDERLY: 50 mg/day. **CHILDREN:** 1 mg/kg/day. **Maximum:** 50 mg/day.

Candidemia, Disseminated Candidiasis, Peritonitis, Abscesses
IV: ADULTS, ELDERLY: 100 mg/day for 15 days. **CHILDREN:** 2 mg/kg/day. **Maximum:** 100 mg daily.

SIDE EFFECTS

Occasional (3%–2%): Nausea, headache, diarrhea, vomiting, fever. **Rare (1%):** Dizziness, drowsiness, pruritus, abdominal pain, dyspepsia (heartburn, indigestion, epigastric pain).

ADVERSE EFFECTS/ TOXIC REACTIONS

Hypersensitivity reaction characterized by rash, pruritus, facial edema occurs rarely. Anaphylaxis, hemoglobinuria, hemolytic anemia have been reported.

NURSING CONSIDERATIONS

BASELINE ASSESSMENT

Determine baseline hepatic/renal function tests and periodically thereafter.

INTERVENTION/EVALUATION

Monitor serum chemistry results for evidence of hepatic/renal impairment.

M

miconazole

mye-**kon**-a-zoll
(Baza Antifungal, Lotrimin, Micaderm, Micatin, Micozole ✤, Mitrazol, Monistat, Monistat 3, Monistat 7)
Do not confuse Lotrimin with Lotrisone, Micatin with Miacalcin, or miconazole with metronidazole or Micronase.

◆CLASSIFICATION

PHARMACOTHERAPEUTIC: Imidazole derivative. **CLINICAL:** Antifungal (see p. 49C).

ACTION

Inhibits synthesis of ergosterol (vital component of fungal cell formation), damaging fungal cell membrane. **Therapeutic Effect:** Fungistatic; may be fungicidal, depending on concentration.

PHARMACOKINETICS

Small amounts absorbed systemically after vaginal administration. Widely distributed. Protein binding: 91%–93%. Metabolized in liver. Primarily excreted in feces. **Half-life:** 24 hrs.

USES

Vaginal: Vulvovaginal candidiasis. **Topical:** Cutaneous candidiasis, tinea cruris, t. corporis, t. pedis, t. versicolor.

PRECAUTIONS

Contraindications: Avoid vaginal preparations during first trimester of pregnancy (unless essential to pt's welfare). **Cautions:** Sensitivity to other antifungals (clotrimazole, ketoconazole).

⧗ LIFESPAN CONSIDERATIONS

Pregnancy/Lactation: Unknown if drug crosses placenta or is distributed in breast milk. **Pregnancy Category C. Children:** Safety not established in those younger than 1 yr. **Elderly:** No age-related precautions noted.

INTERACTIONS

DRUG: None significant. **HERBAL:** None significant. **FOOD:** None known. **LAB VALUES:** None significant.

AVAILABILITY (Rx)

Cream (Topical): Baza, Micaderm, Micatin: 2%. **Cream (Vaginal):** Monistat 7: 2%; Monistat 3: 2%, 4%. **Topical Powder:** Mitrazol: 2%. **Vaginal Suppository:** 100 mg, 200 mg.

INDICATIONS/ROUTES/DOSAGE

Vulvovaginal Candidiasis
Intravaginal Suppository: ADULTS, ELDERLY: 100-mg suppository at bedtime for 7 days, 200-mg suppository at bedtime for 3 days.
Intravaginal Cream: ADULTS, ELDERLY: 2% cream: 1 applicatorful at bedtime for

7 days. 4% cream: 1 applicatorful at bedtime for 3 days.

Topical Fungal Infections, Cutaneous Candidiasis
Topical: ADULTS, ELDERLY, CHILDREN: Apply liberally twice per day, morning and evening.

SIDE EFFECTS

Topical: Pruritus, burning, stinging, erythema, urticaria. **Vaginal (2%):** Vulvovaginal burning, pruritus, irritation; headache; skin rash.

ADVERSE EFFECTS/ TOXIC REACTIONS

None known.

NURSING CONSIDERATIONS

BASELINE ASSESSMENT

Topical: Avoid occlusive dressings. Apply only small amount to cover area completely.

INTERVENTION/EVALUATION

Topical/vaginal: Assess for burning, pruritus, irritation.

PATIENT/FAMILY TEACHING

• **Vaginal preparation:** Base interacts with certain latex products (e.g., condoms, contraceptive diaphragm). • Ask physician about douching, sexual intercourse. • **Topical:** Rub well into affected areas. • Avoid getting in eyes. • Keep areas clean, dry; wear light clothing for ventilation. • Separate personal items in contact with affected areas.

---

midazolam HIGH ALERT

mye-**da**-zoe-lam
(Apo-Midazolam , <u>Versed</u>)
BLACK BOX ALERT May cause severe respiratory depression, respiratory arrest, apnea. Avoid rapid injection, prolonged infusion (increases risk).

Do not confuse Versed with VePesid or Vistaril.

◆CLASSIFICATION

PHARMACOTHERAPEUTIC: Benzodiazepine **(Schedule IV)**. **CLINICAL:** Sedative, anxiolytic.

ACTION

Enhances action of gamma-aminobutyric acid (GABA), one of the major inhibitory neurotransmitters in the brain. **Therapeutic Effect:** Produces anxiolytic, hypnotic, anticonvulsant, muscle relaxant, amnestic effects.

PHARMACOKINETICS

Route	Onset	Peak	Duration
PO	10–20 min	N/A	N/A
IV	1–5 min	5–7 min	20–30 min
IM	5–15 min	30–60 min	2–6 hrs

Well absorbed after IM administration. Protein binding: 97%. Metabolized in liver. Primarily excreted in urine. Not removed by hemodialysis. **Half-life:** 1–5 hrs.

USES

Sedation, anxiolytic, amnesia before procedure or induction of anesthesia, conscious sedation before diagnostic/radiographic procedure, continuous IV sedation of intubated or mechanically ventilated pts. **OFF-LABEL:** Anxiety, status epilepticus, conscious sedation (intranasal route).

PRECAUTIONS

Contraindications: Acute narrow-angle glaucoma, concurrent use of potent CYP3A4 inhibitors (e.g., atazanavir). **Cautions:** Renal/hepatic/pulmonary impairment, impaired gag reflex, HF, treated open-angle glaucoma, obese pts, concurrent CNS depressants, alcohol dependency.

⌛ LIFESPAN CONSIDERATIONS

Pregnancy/Lactation: Crosses placenta. Unknown if drug is distributed in breast milk. **Pregnancy Category D. Children:** Neonates more likely to have respiratory depression. **Elderly:** Age-related renal impairment may require dosage adjustment.

INTERACTIONS

DRUG: Alcohol, other CNS depressants may increase CNS effects, respiratory depression, hypotensive effects. **CYP3A4 inhibitors (e.g., erythromycin)** may increase concentration/sedative effects. **HERBAL: Gotu kola, kava kava, St. John's wort, valerian** may increase CNS depression. **St. John's wort** may decrease concentration. **FOOD: Grapefruit products** increase oral absorption, systemic availability. **LAB VALUES:** None significant.

AVAILABILITY (Rx)

Injection Solution: 1 mg/ml, 5 mg/ml. **Syrup:** 2 mg/ml.

ADMINISTRATION/HANDLING

IV

Rate of Administration • May give undiluted or as infusion. • Resuscitative equipment, O₂ must be readily available before IV administration. • Administer by slow IV injection over at least 2–5 min at concentration of 1–5 mg/ml. • Reduce IV rate in those older than 60 yrs, debilitated pts with chronic disease states, pulmonary impairment. • Too-rapid IV rate, excessive doses, or single large dose increases risk of respiratory depression/arrest.
Storage • Store vials at room temperature.

IM
• Give deep IM into large muscle mass. **Maximum concentration:** 1 mg/ml.

PO
• Do not mix with grapefruit juice.

🔳 IV INCOMPATIBILITIES

Albumin, amphotericin B complex (Abelcet, AmBisome, Amphotec), ampicillin (Polycillin), ampicillin and sulbactam (Unasyn), bumetanide (Bumex), co-trimoxazole (Bactrim), dexamethasone

M

(Decadron), fosphenytoin (Cerebyx), furosemide (Lasix), hydrocortisone (Solu-Cortef), methotrexate, nafcillin (Nafcil), sodium bicarbonate.

▦ IV COMPATIBILITIES

Amiodarone (Cordarone), atropine, calcium gluconate, dexmedetomidine (Precedex), diltiazem (Cardizem), diphenhydramine (Benadryl), dobutamine (Dobutrex), dopamine (Intropin), etomidate (Amidate), fentanyl (Sublimaze), glycopyrrolate (Robinul), heparin, hydromorphone (Dilaudid), hydroxyzine (Vistaril), insulin, lorazepam (Ativan), milrinone (Primacor), morphine, nitroglycerin, norepinephrine (Levophed), potassium chloride, propofol (Diprivan).

INDICATIONS/ROUTES/DOSAGE

Preop Sedation
PO: CHILDREN: 0.25–0.5 mg/kg. **Maximum:** 20 mg.
IV: ADULTS, ELDERLY: 0.02–0.05 mg/kg. **CHILDREN 6–12 YRS:** 0.025–0.05 mg/kg. **CHILDREN 6 MOS–5 YRS:** 0.05–0.1 mg/kg.
IM: ADULTS, ELDERLY: 0.07–0.08 mg/kg 30–60 min before surgery. Usual dose: 5 mg. **CHILDREN:** 0.1–0.15 mg/kg 30–60 min before surgery. **Maximum:** 10 mg.

Continuous Sedation During Mechanical Ventilation
IV: ADULTS, ELDERLY: Initially, 0.02–0.08 mg/kg (1–5 mg in 70-kg adult). May repeat at 5- to 15-min intervals until adequate sedation achieved or continuous infusion rate of 0.04–0.2 mg/kg/hr and titrated to desired effect. **CHILDREN:** Initially, 0.05–0.2 mg/kg followed by continuous infusion of 0.06–0.12 mg/kg/hr (1–2 mcg/kg/min) titrated to desired effect. Usual range: 0.4–6 mcg/kg/min.

SIDE EFFECTS

Frequent (10%–4%): Decreased respiratory rate, tenderness at IM or IV injection site, pain during injection, oxygen desaturation, hiccups. **Occasional (3%–2%):** Hypotension, paradoxical CNS reaction. **Rare (less than 2%):** Nausea, vomiting, headache, coughing.

ADVERSE EFFECTS/ TOXIC REACTIONS

Inadequate or excessive dosage, improper administration may result in cerebral hypoxia, agitation, involuntary movements, hyperactivity, combativeness. Too-rapid IV rate, excessive doses, or single large dose increases risk of respiratory depression/arrest. Respiratory depression/apnea may produce hypoxia, cardiac arrest.

NURSING CONSIDERATIONS

BASELINE ASSESSMENT
Resuscitative equipment, oxygen must be available. Obtain vital signs before administration.

INTERVENTION/EVALUATION
Monitor respiratory rate, oxygen saturation continuously during parenteral administration for underventilation, apnea. Monitor vital signs, level of sedation q3–5min during recovery period.

midodrine

mye-doe-dreen
(Amatine ✤, Apo-Midodrine ✤)
BLACK BOX ALERT Can cause marked rise in supine blood pressure; use in pts for whom orthostatic hypotension significantly impairs daily life.
Do not confuse Amatine with amantadine or protamine, or midodrine with Midrin.

◆ CLASSIFICATION

PHARMACOTHERAPEUTIC: Vasopressor. **CLINICAL:** Orthostatic hypotension adjunct.

ACTION

Forms active metabolite desglymidodrine, an alpha$_1$ agonist, activating alpha receptors of arteriolar, venous vasculature. **Therapeutic Effect:** Increases vascular tone, B/P.

PHARMACOKINETICS

Route	Onset	Peak	Duration
PO	1 hr	—	2–3 hrs

Rapid absorption from GI tract following PO administration. Protein binding: Low. Undergoes enzymatic hydrolysis (deglycination) in systemic circulation. Excreted in urine. **Half-life:** 0.5 hr.

USES

Treatment of symptomatic orthostatic hypotension. **OFF-LABEL:** Vasovagal syncope, prevention of dialysis-induced hypotension, urinary incontinence.

PRECAUTIONS

Contraindications: Acute renal impairment, persistent supine hypertension, pheochromocytoma, severe cardiac disease, thyrotoxicosis, urinary retention. **Cautions:** Renal/hepatic impairment, history of visual problems, diabetes; concurrent administration with digoxin, beta blockers.

⧗ LIFESPAN CONSIDERATIONS

Pregnancy/Lactation: Unknown if drug crosses placenta or is distributed in breast milk. **Pregnancy Category C. Children:** Safety and efficacy not established. **Elderly:** Age-related renal impairment may require dosage adjustment.

INTERACTIONS

DRUG: Digoxin may have additive bradycardic effects. **Sodium-retaining steroids (e.g., fludrocortisone)** may increase sodium retention. **Vasoconstrictors** may have additive effects. **HERBAL:** None significant. **FOOD:** None known. **LAB VALUES:** None significant.

AVAILABILITY (Rx)

Tablets: 2.5 mg, 5 mg, 10 mg.

ADMINISTRATION/HANDLING

• Give without regard to food. • Last dose of day should be given 3–4 hrs before bedtime.

INDICATIONS/ROUTES/DOSAGE

Orthostatic Hypotension
PO: ADULTS, ELDERLY: 10 mg 3 times a day. Give during the day when pt is upright, such as upon arising, midday, and late afternoon. Do not give later than 6 PM. **Maximum:** 40 mg/day.

Dosage in Renal Impairment
For adults and elderly pts, give 2.5 mg 3 times a day; increase gradually, as tolerated. **Hemodialysis:** Dose after HD unless used to prevent HD-induced hypotension.

SIDE EFFECTS

Frequent (20%–7%): Paresthesia, piloerection, pruritus, dysuria, supine hypertension. **Occasional (Less Than 7%–1%):** Pain, rash, chills, headache, facial flushing, confusion, dry mouth, anxiety.

ADVERSE EFFECTS/ TOXIC REACTIONS

Increased systolic arterial pressure has been noted.

NURSING CONSIDERATIONS

BASELINE ASSESSMENT

Assess sensitivity to midodrine, other medications (esp. digoxin, sodium-retaining vasoconstrictors). Assess medical history, esp. for renal impairment, severe hypertension, cardiac disease.

INTERVENTION/EVALUATION

Monitor B/P, renal, hepatic, cardiac function.

PATIENT/FAMILY TEACHING

• Do not take last dose of the day after evening meal or less than 4 hrs before bedtime. • Do not give if pt will be supine. • Use caution with OTC medications that may affect B/P (e.g., cough and cold, diet medications).

M

mifepristone

mif-**ep**-ris-tone
(Korlym, Mifeprex)

BLACK BOX ALERT Discuss medication guide, pt agreement, and expected effects before prescribing. Serious, sometimes fatal, infections, excessive bleeding have occurred following surgical and medical abortions, including following use of mifepristone.

Do not confuse Mifeprex with Mirapex, or mifepristone with misoprostol.

◆ CLASSIFICATION

PHARMACOTHERAPEUTIC: Antiprogestin. **CLINICAL:** Abortifacient.

ACTION

Has antiprogestational activity resulting from competitive interaction with progesterone. Inhibits activity of endogenous, exogenous progesterone. Has antiglucocorticoid, weak antiandrogenic activity. **Therapeutic Effect:** Terminates pregnancy.

PHARMACOKINETICS

Rapidly absorbed from GI tract. Protein binding: 98%. Metabolized in liver. Primarily eliminated in feces; minimal excretion in urine. **Half-life:** 18 hrs.

USES

Korlym: Control hyperglycemia secondary to hypercortisolism in adults with endogenous Cushing's syndrome. **Mifeprex:** Termination of intrauterine pregnancy through day 49 of pregnancy. **OFF-LABEL:** Breast/ovarian cancer, unresectable meningioma.

PRECAUTIONS

Contraindications: Mifeprex: Chronic adrenal failure, concurrent long-term steroid or anticoagulant therapy, confirmed or suspected ectopic pregnancy, intrauterine device (IUD) in place, hemorrhagic disorders, inherited porphyria, hypersensitivity to misoprostol or other prostaglandins, lack of access to emergency medical service, inability to understand or comply with treatment. **Korlym:** Concomitant use with lovastatin, simvastatin, or CYP3A substrates, corticosteroids for serious medical conditions, history of unexplained vaginal bleeding, pregnancy, endometrial hyperplasia, or carcinoma. **Cautions:** Treatment of women older than 35 yrs, smoking more than 10 cigarettes/day, cardiovascular disease, hypertension, use of medications that prolong QT interval. **Pregnancy Category X.**

INTERACTIONS

DRUG: CYP3A4 inducers (e.g., carbamazepine, phenobarbital, phenytoin, rifampin) may increase metabolism. **CYP3A4 inhibitors (e.g., erythromycin, itraconazole, ketoconazole)** may inhibit metabolism. **HERBAL: St. John's wort** may increase metabolism. **FOOD: Grapefruit products** may inhibit metabolism. **LAB VALUES:** May alter serum ALT, AST, alkaline phosphatase.

AVAILABILITY (Rx)

Tablets (Mifeprex): 200 mg. **Korlym:** 300 mg.

ADMINISTRATION/HANDLING

Korlym
• Take with a meal.

INDICATIONS/ROUTES/DOSAGE

◀ALERT▶ May be used in combination with misoprostol for termination of pregnancy.

Termination of Pregnancy (Mifeprex)
PO: ADULTS: Day 1: 600 mg as single dose. **Day 3:** 400 mcg misoprostol (unless termination of pregnancy has occurred). **Day 14:** Post-treatment examination.

Cushing Syndrome (Korlym)
PO: ADULTS, ELDERLY: Initially, 300 mg once daily. May increase in 300 mg increments to maximum of 1,200 mg/day or 20 mg/kg/day.

SIDE EFFECTS

Frequent (greater than 10%): Headache, dizziness, abdominal pain, nausea, vomiting, diarrhea, fatigue. **Occasional (10%–3%):** Uterine hemorrhage, insomnia, vaginitis, dyspepsia (heartburn, indigestion, epigastric pain), back pain, fever, viral infections, rigors. **Rare (2%–1%):** Anxiety, syncope, anemia, asthenia (loss of strength, energy), leg pain, sinusitis, leukorrhea.

ADVERSE EFFECTS/ TOXIC REACTIONS

None known.

NURSING CONSIDERATIONS

BASELINE ASSESSMENT

Assess for use of ketoconazole, itraconazole, erythromycin, rifampin, anticonvulsants (affects metabolism).

INTERVENTION/EVALUATION

◄**ALERT**► If mifepristone results in an incomplete abortion, surgical intervention may be necessary.
Monitor Hgb/Hct. Confirm pregnancy is completely terminated at approximately 14 days after drug administration. Assess degree of vaginal bleeding.

PATIENT/FAMILY TEACHING

• Advise pts of treatment procedure and effects, need for follow-up visit. • Vaginal bleeding, uterine cramping may occur.

milnacipran

mil-na-**sip**-ran
(Savella)
BLACK BOX ALERT Increased risk of suicidal ideation and behavior in children, adolescents, and young adults 18–24 yrs with major depressive disorder, other psychiatric disorders.

Do not confuse Savella with cevimeline or sevelamer.

◆**CLASSIFICATION**

PHARMACOTHERAPEUTIC: Serotonin, norepinephrine reuptake inhibitor. **CLINICAL:** Fibromyalgia agent.

ACTION

Appears to inhibit serotonin and norepinephrine reuptake at CNS neuronal presynaptic membranes. **Therapeutic Effect:** Reduces chronic pain, fatigue, depression, sleep disorders associated with fibromyalgia syndrome; improves physical function.

PHARMACOKINETICS

Well absorbed following PO administration. Protein binding: 13%. Eliminated unchanged in urine. Steady-state levels reached in 36–48 hrs. **Half-life:** 6–8 hrs.

USES

Management of fibromyalgia.

PRECAUTIONS

Contraindications: Concomitant use or within 14 days of MAOIs, uncontrolled narrow-angle glaucoma. **Cautions:** Pts with depression, pts at increased risk of suicide, other psychiatric disorders; elevated blood pressure or heart rate, history of seizures, pts with substantial alcohol use or chronic liver disease, pts with history of dysuria (e.g., prostatic hypertrophy, prostatitis, controlled narrow-angle glaucoma). Renal impairment, cardiovascular disease.

⌛ LIFESPAN CONSIDERATIONS

Pregnancy/Lactation: Increased risk of fetal complications, including need for respiratory support, if given during third trimester. Unknown if distributed in breast milk. **Pregnancy Category C. Children:** Safety and efficacy not established in pts younger than 18 yrs. **Elderly:** Severe renal impairment requires dosage adjustment.

INTERACTIONS

DRUG: Lithium, MAOIs may increase risk of serotonin syndrome. **Epinephrine, norepinephrine** may produce paroxys-

M

mal hypertension, arrhythmias. **Intravenous digoxin** may produce tachycardia, hypotension. May inhibit antihypertensive effect of **clonidine. HERBAL: Gotu kola, kava kava, St. John's wort, valerian** may increase CNS depression, increase risk of serotonin syndrome. **FOOD:** None known. **LAB VALUES:** May decrease serum sodium.

AVAILABILITY (Rx)

Tablets, Film-Coated: 12.5 mg, 25 mg, 50 mg, 100 mg.

ADMINISTRATION/HANDLING

• Give without regard to food. • Do not crush, break film-coated tablets.

INDICATIONS/ROUTES/DOSAGE

Fibromyalgia
PO: ADULTS, ELDERLY: Day 1: 12.5 mg once. **Days 2–3:** 25 mg/day (12.5 mg twice daily). **Days 4–7:** 50 mg/day (25 mg twice daily). **After Day 7:** 100 mg/day (50 mg twice daily). Dose may be increased to 200 mg/day (100 mg twice daily).

Severe Renal Impairment (Creatine Clearance 5–29 ml/min)
Reduce maintenance dose by 50% to 50 mg/day (25 mg twice daily). Based on pt response, dose may be increased to 100 mg/day (50 mg twice daily). Not recommended in end-stage renal disease.

SIDE EFFECTS

Frequent (37%–18%): Nausea, headache. **Occasional (16%–5%):** Constipation, insomnia, hot flashes, dizziness, hyperhidrosis, palpitations, vomiting, URI. **Rare (Less Than 5%):** Dry mouth, increased B/P, anxiety, skin flushing, rash, blurred vision, abdominal pain, chest pain, chills, pruritus, paresthesia, tachycardia.

ADVERSE EFFECTS/ TOXIC REACTIONS

Abrupt discontinuation may present withdrawal symptoms (dysphoria, irritability, agitation, dizziness, paresthesia, anxiety, confusion, headache, lethargy, emotional lability, tinnitus, seizures). Serotonin syndrome symptoms may include mental status changes (agitation, hallucinations), hyperreflexia, incoordination. May increase risk of bleeding events (e.g., ecchymoses, hematomas, epistaxis).

NURSING CONSIDERATIONS

BASELINE ASSESSMENT

Obtain baseline pain intensity scale, location(s) of pain, tenderness. Obtain baseline B/P, heart rate. Question for history of changes in day-to-day pain intensity.

INTERVENTION/EVALUATION

Control nausea with antiemetics. Treat complaint of headache, migraine with appropriate analgesics. Monitor for increase in B/P, pulse. Question for changes in visual acuity. Assess for clinical improvement and record onset of pain control, decreased fatigue, lessening of depressive symptoms, improvement in sleep pattern. Monitor for suicidal ideation.

PATIENT/FAMILY TEACHING

• Avoid tasks that require alertness, motor skills until response to drug is established. • Do not abruptly discontinue medication. • Increase fluids, bulk to prevent constipation. • Report if mental status changes occur (including thoughts of suicide, unusual behavior) or sweating, hot flushing become intolerable. • Caution about risk of bleeding associated with concomitant use of NSAIDs, aspirin.

milrinone
HIGH ALERT

mil-ri-none
(Primacor)
Do not confuse Primacor with Primaxin.

◆ CLASSIFICATION

PHARMACOTHERAPEUTIC: Cardiac inotropic agent. **CLINICAL:** Vasodilator.

ACTION

Inhibits phosphodiesterase, which increases cyclic adenosine monophosphate (cAMP), potentiating delivery of calcium to myocardial contractile systems. **Therapeutic Effect:** Relaxes vascular muscle, causing vasodilation. Increases cardiac output, decreases pulmonary capillary wedge pressure, vascular resistance.

PHARMACOKINETICS

Route	Onset	Peak	Duration
IV	5–15 min	N/A	N/A

Protein binding: 70%. Metabolized in liver. Primarily excreted in urine. **Half-life:** 1.7–2.7 hrs.

USES

Short-term management of HF. **OFF-LABEL:** Inotropic therapy for pts unresponsive to other therapy, heart transplant candidates, palliation of symptoms in end-stage HF.

PRECAUTIONS

Contraindications: None known. **Cautions:** Severe obstructive aortic or pulmonic valvular disease, history of ventricular arrhythmias, atrial fibrillation/flutter, renal impairment.

LIFESPAN CONSIDERATIONS

Pregnancy/Lactation: Unknown if drug crosses placenta or is distributed in breast milk. **Pregnancy Category C. Children:** Safety and efficacy not established. **Elderly:** Age-related renal impairment may require dosage adjustment.

INTERACTIONS

DRUG: None significant. **HERBAL:** None significant. **FOOD:** None known. **LAB VALUES:** None significant.

AVAILABILITY (Rx)

Injection Solution (Primacor): 1 mg/ml, 10-ml single-dose vial, 20-ml single-dose vial, 50-ml single-dose vial. **Injection So-**lution (Premix [Primacor]): 200 mcg/ml (100 ml, 200 ml).

ADMINISTRATION/HANDLING

IV

Reconstitution • For IV infusion, dilute 20-mg (20-ml) vial with 80 ml 0.9% NaCl or D₅W to provide concentration of 0.2 mg/ml (200 mcg/ml).

Rate of Administration • For IV injection (loading dose), administer undiluted slowly over 10 min. • Monitor for arrhythmias, hypotension during IV therapy; reduce or temporarily discontinue infusion until condition stabilizes.

Storage • Diluted solutions stable for 72 hrs at room temperature.

IV INCOMPATIBILITIES

Furosemide (Lasix), imipenem-cilastatin (Primaxin), procainamide (Pronestyl).

IV COMPATIBILITIES

Calcium gluconate, dexamethasone (Decadron), dexmedetomidine (Precedex), digoxin (Lanoxin), diltiazem (Cardizem), dobutamine (Dobutrex), dopamine (Intropin), heparin, hydromorphone (Dilaudid), lidocaine, magnesium, midazolam (Versed), morphine, nitroglycerin, potassium, propofol (Diprivan).

INDICATIONS/ROUTES/DOSAGE

Management of HF

IV: ADULTS: Initially, 50 mcg/kg over 10 min. Continue with maintenance infusion rate of 0.375–0.75 mcg/kg/min based on hemodynamic and clinical response.

Dosage in Renal Impairment

Creatinine Clearance	Dosage
50 ml/min	0.43 mcg/kg/min
40 ml/min	0.38 mcg/kg/min
30 ml/min	0.33 mcg/kg/min
20 ml/min	0.28 mcg/kg/min
10 ml/min	0.23 mcg/kg/min
5 ml/min	0.2 mcg/kg/min

M

SIDE EFFECTS

Occasional (3%–1%): Headache, hypotension. **Rare (less than 1%):** Angina, chest pain.

ADVERSE EFFECTS/ TOXIC REACTIONS

Supraventricular/ventricular arrhythmias (12%), nonsustained ventricular tachycardia (2%), sustained ventricular tachycardia (1%) may occur. Ventricular fibrillation (0.2%) has been documented.

NURSING CONSIDERATIONS

BASELINE ASSESSMENT

Obtain baseline lab studies, esp. BN peptide. Offer emotional support (difficulty breathing may produce anxiety). Assess B/P, apical pulse rate before treatment begins and during IV therapy. Assess lung sounds; observe for edema.

INTERVENTION/EVALUATION

Monitor B/P, heart rate, cardiac output, EKG, serum potassium, renal function, signs/symptoms of HF.

minocycline   TOP 200

mye-noe-**sye**-kleen
(Apo-Minocycline ✦, Dynacin, Minocin, Novo-Minocycline ✦, Solodyn)
Do not confuse Dynacin with Dyazide, DynaCirc, or Dynapen, or Minocin with Indocin, Mithracin, or niacin.

◆ CLASSIFICATION

PHARMACOTHERAPEUTIC: Tetracycline. **CLINICAL:** Antibiotic.

ACTION

Inhibits bacterial protein synthesis by binding to ribosomes. **Therapeutic Effect:** Bacteriostatic.

PHARMACOKINETICS

Well absorbed from GI tract. Protein binding: 70%–75%. Partial elimination in feces; minimal excretion in urine. Not removed by hemodialysis. **Half-life:** 11–23 hrs.

USES

Treatment of susceptible infections due to *Rickettsiae, M. pneumoniae, C. trachomatis, C. psittaci, H. ducreyi, Yersinia pestis, Francisella tularensis, Vibrio cholerae, Brucella* spp., gram-negative organisms, including prostate, urinary tract, CNS infections (not meningitis), uncomplicated gonorrhea, inflammatory acne, brucellosis, skin granulomas, cholera, trachoma, nocardiasis, yaws, syphilis (when penicillins are contraindicated). **Solodyn:** Treatment of inflammatory lesions of moderate to severe non-nodular acne. **OFF-LABEL:** Treatment of nocardiosis, community-acquired MRSA infection, rheumatoid arthritis (RA).

PRECAUTIONS

Contraindications: Hypersensitivity to tetracyclines. **Cautions:** Children younger than 8 yrs, last half of pregnancy, renal impairment, hepatic impairment, sun/ultraviolet exposure (severe photosensitivity reaction).

⌛ LIFESPAN CONSIDERATIONS

Pregnancy/Lactation: Readily crosses placenta; distributed in breast milk. May inhibit fetal skeletal growth. **Pregnancy Category D. Children:** May cause permanent discoloration of teeth, enamel hypoplasia. Not recommended in those younger than 8 yrs. **Elderly:** No age-related precautions noted.

INTERACTIONS

DRUG: Aluminum-, calcium-, magnesium-containing antacids may decrease absorption, effect. **Ergot** may increase risk of ergotism. May decrease the effects of **estrogen-containing oral contraceptives. HERBAL: Dong quai, St. John's wort** may increase risk of photosensitivity. **FOOD:** None known. **LAB VALUES:** May increase serum alkaline phosphatase, amylase, bilirubin, AST, ALT, BUN.

AVAILABILITY (Rx)

Capsules: 50 mg, 75 mg, 100 mg. **Tablets (Dynacin):** 50 mg, 75 mg, 100 mg.

Capsules (Pellet-Filled [Minocin]): 50 mg, 100 mg. **Tablets (Extended-Release [Solodyn]):** 45 mg, 55 mg, 65 mg, 80 mg, 90 mg, 105 mg, 115 mg, 135 mg.

ADMINISTRATION/HANDLING

PO
• Take without regard to food. • Give with adequate fluid (reduces risk of esophageal irritation and ulceration). • Give pellet-filled capsules, extended-release tablets whole; do not cut, crush, or split.

INDICATIONS/ROUTES/DOSAGE

Usual Dosage
PO: ADULTS, ELDERLY: Initially, 100–200 mg, then 100 mg q12h or 50 mg 4 times/day. **CHILDREN OLDER THAN 8 YRS:** Initially, 4 mg/kg, then 2 mg/kg q12h. **Maximum:** 400 mg/day.

Acne
PO (Solodyn): CHILDREN 12 YRS AND OLDER, WEIGHING 126–136 KG: 135 mg once daily; **WEIGHING 111–125 KG:** 115 mg once daily; **WEIGHING 97–110 KG:** 105 mg once daily; **WEIGHING 85–96 KG:** 90 mg once daily; **WEIGHING 72–84 KG:** 80 mg once daily; **WEIGHING 60–71 KG:** 65 mg once daily; **WEIGHING 50–59 KG:** 55 mg once daily; **WEIGHING 45–49 KG:** 45 mg once daily. **(Capsule or Immediate-Release Tablet): ADULTS, ELDERLY:** 50–100 mg/day.

SIDE EFFECTS

Frequent: Dizziness, light-headedness, diarrhea, nausea, vomiting, abdominal cramps, possibly severe photosensitivity, drowsiness, vertigo. **Occasional:** Altered pigmentation of skin, mucous membranes, rectal/genital pruritus, stomatitis.

ADVERSE EFFECTS/ TOXIC REACTIONS

Superinfection (esp. fungal), anaphylaxis, increased ICP may occur. Bulging fontanelles occur rarely in infants.

NURSING CONSIDERATIONS

BASELINE ASSESSMENT
Question for history of allergies, esp. tetracyclines, sulfite.

INTERVENTION/EVALUATION
Assess ability to ambulate (may cause vertigo, dizziness). Monitor daily pattern of bowel activity, stool consistency. Monitor hepatic/renal function tests with long-term therapy. Assess skin for rash. Observe for signs of increased intracranial pressure (altered LOC, widened pulse pressure). Be alert for superinfection: fever, vomiting, diarrhea, anal/genital pruritus, oral mucosal changes (ulceration, pain, erythema).

PATIENT/FAMILY TEACHING
• Continue antibiotic for full length of treatment. • Space doses evenly. • Drink full glass of water with capsules or tablets. • Avoid tasks that require alertness, motor skills until response to drug is established. • Report diarrhea, rash, other new symptoms. • Protect skin from sun exposure. • Advise female pts to use additional form of birth control (may decrease effectiveness of oral contraceptives).

minoxidil

min-**ox**-i-dill
(Apo-Gain ✦, Loniten ✦, Minox ✦, Rogaine, Rogaine Extra Strength)

BLACK BOX ALERT Can cause pericarditis and pericardial effusion, occasionally progressing to tamponade; can exacerbate angina pectoris.

Do not confuse Loniten with Lotensin, or minoxidil with metolazone, midodrine,

M

Minipress, Minocin, Monopril, or Noxafil.

◆ CLASSIFICATION

PHARMACOTHERAPEUTIC: Peripheral vasodilator. **CLINICAL:** Antihypertensive, hair growth stimulant (see p. 63C).

ACTION

Acts directly on vascular smooth muscle, producing vasodilation of arterioles. **Therapeutic Effect:** Decreases peripheral vascular resistance, B/P; increases cutaneous blood flow; stimulates hair follicle epithelium, hair follicle growth.

PHARMACOKINETICS

Route	Onset	Peak	Duration
PO	0.5 hr	2–8 hrs	2–5 days

Well absorbed from GI tract; minimal absorption after topical application. Protein binding: None. Widely distributed. Metabolized in liver. Primarily excreted in urine. Removed by hemodialysis. **Half-life:** 3.5 hrs.

USES

PO: Management of severe hypertension. **Topical:** Treatment of alopecia androgenetica (**males:** baldness of vertex of scalp; **females:** diffuse hair loss or thinning of frontoparietal areas).

PRECAUTIONS

Contraindications: Pheochromocytoma. **Cautions:** Severe renal impairment, chronic HF, coronary artery disease, recent MI, pulmonary hypertension.

⌛ LIFESPAN CONSIDERATIONS

Pregnancy/Lactation: Crosses placenta; distributed in breast milk. **Pregnancy Category C. Children:** No age-related precautions noted. **Elderly:** More sensitive to hypotensive effects. Age-related renal impairment may require dosage adjustment.

INTERACTIONS

DRUG: NSAIDs may decrease hypotensive effects. **HERBAL: Licorice** may cause increased serum sodium, water retention. **FOOD:** None known. **LAB VALUES:** May increase plasma renin activity, BUN, serum alkaline phosphatase, creatinine, sodium. May decrease Hgb, Hct, erythrocyte count.

AVAILABILITY

Tablets: 2.5 mg, 10 mg. **Topical Solution (OTC):** 2% (20 mg/ml) (Rogaine), 5% (50 mg/ml) (Rogaine Extra Strength). **Aerosol:** 5%.

ADMINISTRATION/HANDLING

PO
• Give without regard to food. Give with food if GI upset occurs. • Tablets may be crushed.

Topical
• Shampoo, dry hair before applying medication. • Wash hands immediately after application. • Do not use hair dryer after application (reduces effectiveness).

INDICATIONS/ROUTES/DOSAGE

Hypertension
PO: ADULTS, CHILDREN 12 YRS AND OLDER: Initially, 5 mg/day. Increase gradually in at least 3-day intervals. **Range:** 2.5–80 mg/day in 1–2 divided doses. **ELDERLY:** Initially, 2.5 mg/day. May increase gradually. **CHILDREN YOUNGER THAN 12 YRS:** Initially, 0.1–0.2 mg/kg (5 mg maximum) daily. Gradually increase at a minimum of 3-day intervals. Maintenance: 0.25–1 mg/kg/day in 1–2 doses. **Maximum:** 50 mg/day.

Hair Regrowth
Topical: ADULTS: Apply to affected areas of scalp 2 times per day. Four months of therapy may be needed for hair growth.

SIDE EFFECTS

Frequent: PO: Edema with concurrent weight gain, hypertrichosis (elongation, thickening, increased pigmentation of fine body hair; develops in 80% of pts within

3–6 wks after beginning therapy). **Occasional: PO:** EKG T-wave changes (usually revert to pretreatment state with continued therapy or drug withdrawal). **Topical:** Pruritus, rash, dry/flaking skin, erythema. **Rare: PO:** Breast tenderness, headache, photosensitivity reaction. **Topical:** Allergic reaction, alopecia, burning sensation at scalp, soreness at hair root, headache, visual disturbances.

ADVERSE EFFECTS/ TOXIC REACTIONS

Tachycardia, angina pectoris may occur due to increased oxygen demands associated with increased heart rate, cardiac output. Fluid/electrolyte imbalance, HF may occur, esp. if a diuretic is not given concurrently. Too-rapid reduction in B/P may result in syncope, CVA, MI, ocular/vestibular ischemia. Pericardial effusion, tamponade may be seen in pts with renal impairment not on dialysis.

NURSING CONSIDERATIONS

BASELINE ASSESSMENT

Assess B/P in both arms and take pulse for 1 full min immediately before giving medication. If pulse increases 20 beats/min or more over baseline or systolic or diastolic B/P decreases more than 20 mm Hg, withhold drug, contact physician.

INTERVENTION/EVALUATION

Monitor fluids/electrolytes, body weight, B/P. Assess for peripheral edema. Assess for signs of HF (cough, rales at base of lungs, cool extremities, dyspnea on exertion). Monitor fluid, serum electrolytes. Assess for distant or muffled heart sounds by auscultation (pericardial effusion, tamponade).

PATIENT/FAMILY TEACHING

• Maximum B/P response occurs in 3–7 days. • Rise slowly from sitting/lying position. • Reversible growth of fine body hair may begin 3–6 wks following initiation of treatment. • When used topically for stimulation of hair growth, treatment must continue on a permanent basis—cessation of treatment will begin reversal of new hair growth. • Avoid exposure to sunlight, artificial light sources.

mipomersen

mi-poe-**mer**-sen
(Kynamro)

BLACK BOX ALERT May cause hepatotoxicity. May cause hepatic steatosis (increase in hepatic fat) regardless of ALT, AST elevation; may be risk factor for progressive hepatic disease including steatohepatitis and cirrhosis. Monitor hepatic enzymes regularly. Treatment only available through restricted program under the Risk Evaluation and Mitigation Strategy (REMS) named KYNAMRO REMS PROGRAM.

◆CLASSIFICATION

PHARMACOTHERAPEUTIC: Oligonucleotide inhibitor. **CLINICAL:** Antihyperlipidemic.

ACTION

Prevents assembly of apo-B–containing lipoproteins by inhibiting translation of apo-B 100 human messenger ribonucleic acid (mRNA); the principle precursor of LDL. **Therapeutic Effect:** Decreases plasma low-density lipoprotein cholesterol (LDL-C) and total cholesterol.

PHARMACOKINETICS

Readily absorbed following SQ administration. Metabolized in tissues by endonucleases. Protein binding: greater than 90%. Peak plasma concentration: 3–4 hrs. Steady state reached within 6 mos. Excreted primarily in urine. **Half-life:** 1–2 mos.

USES

Adjunct to lipid-lowering medications and diet to reduce low-density lipopro-

---

tein cholesterol (LDL-C), apolipoprotein B (apo-B), total cholesterol (TC), and non–high-density lipoprotein cholesterol (non-HDL-C) in pts with homozygous familial hypercholesterolemia (HoFH).

PRECAUTIONS

Contraindications: Moderate to severe hepatic impairment, active hepatic disease, hepatitis, unexplained persistent elevations of serum transaminases. **Cautions:** Alcohol dependency.

⧗ LIFESPAN CONSIDERATIONS

Pregnancy/Lactation: Unknown if distributed in breast milk. Must either discontinue drug or discontinue breastfeeding. **Pregnancy Category B. Children:** Safety and efficacy not established. **Elderly:** May have increased risk of adverse reactions including hypertension, peripheral edema.

INTERACTIONS

DRUG: Avoid medications that may increase risk of hepatotoxicity. **HERBAL: Black cohosh, kava kava** may increase risk of hepatotoxicity. **FOOD:** None known. **LAB VALUES:** May increase serum alkaline phosphatase, ALT, AST, bilirubin, urine protein.

AVAILABILITY (Rx)

Single Use Vial: 200 mg/ml (1 ml). **Single Use Prefilled Syringe:** 200 mg/ml (1 ml).

ADMINISTRATION/HANDLING

SQ
• Allow syringe/vial to reach room temperature before administration. • Inspect for particulate matter. • Pinch approx. 1 inch of SQ tissue on abdomen, thigh, or upper arm between thumb and first finger. • Do not inject areas with sunburn, tattoos, psoriasis, or active inflammation. • Insert needle at proper angle and steadily inject. • Alternate injection sites.
Storage • Refrigerate until time of use.
• Solution stored at room temperature

expires after 14 days. • Solution should appear clear and colorless. • Protect from light.

INDICATIONS/ROUTES/DOSAGE

Homozygous Familial Hypercholesterolemia
SQ: ADULTS/ELDERLY: 200 mg once weekly. (If dose is missed, the dose should be given at least 3 days from the next weekly dose.)

Dose Modification
If ALT, AST greater than 3 times upper limit normal (ULN), withhold dose until resolution to below 3 times ULN and investigate for other causes. If treatment resumed, monitor hepatic function test every 1–2 wks. Discontinue if symptomatic hepatotoxicity occurs or elevated ALT, AST does not resolve.

SIDE EFFECTS

Frequent (84%): Injection site reactions (pain, swelling, erythema, pruritus, rash, induration, urticaria). **Occasional (14%–4%):** Fatigue, nausea, body aches, chills, headache, pyrexia, extremity pain, hypertension, chills, peripheral edema, vomiting, musculoskeletal pain. **Rare (3%):** Palpitations, abdominal pain, insomnia.

ADVERSE EFFECTS/ TOXIC REACTIONS

Increased risk of progressive hepatic disease including steatohepatitis, cirrhosis due to increased hepatic fat. Elevated transaminases reported in 12% of pts. Alcohol may exacerbate hepatotoxicity. Increased risk of myopathy including rhabdomyolysis (muscle pain/tenderness, weakness, dark or decreased urine output, elevated serum creatinine or CPK level) when used with other antihyperlipidemics (statins). Angina pectoris reported in 4% of pts. Immunogenicity (autoantibodies) reported in 38% of pts. Neoplasms (benign and malignant) reported in 4% of pts.

NURSING CONSIDERATIONS

BASELINE ASSESSMENT

Obtain baseline lipid panel, hepatic function test. Confirm positive history of HoFH. Receive full medication history including vitamins, minerals, herbal products. Screen for history of hepatic impairment, cardiovascular disease, alcohol dependency. Assess skin for appropriate injection sites.

INTERVENTION/EVALUATION

Monitor lipid panel every 3 mos; hepatic function every mo for 12 mos, then every 3 mos. If AST, ALT elevations occur, obtain PT/INR and monitor for bruising, hematuria, jaundice, right upper abdominal pain, fever, lethargy, melena. Offer antiemetics for nausea/vomiting. Obtain EKG for chest pain, palpitations. Assess extremities for edema.

PATIENT/FAMILY TEACHING

• Diet and exercise are essential to treatment. • Blood levels will be routinely monitored. • Report signs of liver problems (yellowing of skin, bruising, black/tarry stool, right upper quadrant pain, fever, lethargy), chest pain, palpitations. • Avoid alcohol. • Most pts experience injection site reactions. • Flu-like symptoms (chills, fatigue, nausea, muscle pain) most likely occur within 2 days. • Inject medication into fatty tissue of upper arm, abdomen, thigh; do not inject into muscle.

mirabegron

mir-a-**beg**-ron
(Myrbetriq)

◆CLASSIFICATION

PHARMACOTHERAPEUTIC: Beta$_3$-adrenergic agonist. **CLINICAL:** Smooth muscle relaxant.

ACTION

Relaxes detrusor smooth muscle of bladder through beta$_3$ stimulation during storage phase of urinary bladder fill–void cycle. **Therapeutic Effect:** Increases bladder capacity, reduces symptoms of urinary urgency, increased voiding frequency, urge incontinence, nocturia.

PHARMACOKINETICS

Readily absorbed following PO administration; widely distributed. Protein binding: 71%. Renal elimination primarily through active tubular secretion along with glomerular filtration. Eliminated in urine (55%), feces (35%). **Half-life:** 50 hrs.

USES

Treatment of overactive bladder with symptoms of urinary incontinence, urgency, frequency.

PRECAUTIONS

Contraindications: None known. **Cautions:** Bladder outlet obstruction, pts taking antimuscarinic medications (increases urinary retention), mild to moderate hepatic/renal impairment. Not recommended for use in pts with severe uncontrolled hypertension (SBP equal to or greater than 180 mm Hg and/or DBP equal to or greater than 110 mm Hg).

⧖ LIFESPAN CONSIDERATIONS

Pregnancy/Lactation: Unknown if distributed in breast milk. **Pregnancy Category C. Children:** Safety and efficacy not established. **Elderly:** No age-related precautions noted.

INTERACTIONS

DRUG: May increase concentration of **desipramine, digoxin, metoprolol, thioridazine, flecainide, propafenone. HERBAL:** None significant. **FOOD:** None known. **LAB VALUES:** May increase GGT, LDH; temporarily increase ALT, AST.

AVAILABILITY (RX)

🗟Tablets, Extended Release: 25 mg, 50 mg.

M

ADMINISTRATION/HANDLING

PO
• Give without regard to meals. • Administer with water; instruct pt to swallow whole. • Do not break, crush, dissolve or divide film-coated tablets.

INDICATIONS/ROUTES/DOSAGE

Overactive Bladder
PO: ADULTS, ELDERLY: Initially, 25 mg once daily. May increase to 50 mg once daily.

Dosage in Renal/Hepatic Impairment
PO: ADULTS, ELDERLY: 25 mg once daily.

SIDE EFFECTS

Occasional (9%–4%): Hypertension, headache, nasopharyngitis. **Rare (2%–1%):** Constipation, arthralgia, diarrhea, tachycardia, fatigue.

ADVERSE EFFECTS/ TOXIC REACTIONS

Worsening of preexisting hypertension reported infrequently. Urinary tract infection occurs in 6% of patients; influenza in 3%, and upper respiratory infection in 1.5%.

NURSING CONSIDERATIONS

BASELINE ASSESSMENT
Check B/P; assess for hypertension. Monitor EKG. Receive full medication history and screen for possible drug interactions. Monitor I&O (particularly in pts with history of urinary retention).

INTERVENTION/EVALUATION
Monitor ALT, AST, LDH, GGT periodically. Palpate bladder for urinary retention. Measure B/P near end of dosing interval (determines whether B/P is controlled throughout day). Periodic B/P determinations are recommended, especially in hypertensive pts. Titrate digoxin serum level for therapeutic effect (very narrow line between therapeutic and toxic level). Assess pulse for quality, irregular rate, bradycardia. Question for evidence of headache.

PATIENT/FAMILY TEACHING
• Report urinary retention to doctor/nurse. • Do not use nasal decongestants, over-the-counter cold preparations without doctor approval. Restrict salt, alcohol intake. • Take mirabegron with water; swallow tablet whole; do not chew, crush, dissolve, or divide tablet. • May take with or without food.

---

mirtazapine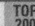

mir-**taz**-a-peen
(Apo-Mirtazapine ❖, Novo-Mirtazapine ❖, Remeron, Remeron Soltab)

BLACK BOX ALERT Increased risk of suicidal thinking and behavior in children, adolescents, young adults 18–24 yrs with major depressive disorder, other psychiatric disorders.
Do not confuse Remeron with Premarin, Rozerem, or Zemuron.

◆CLASSIFICATION

PHARMACOTHERAPEUTIC: Tetracyclic compound. **CLINICAL:** Antidepressant (see p. 41C).

ACTION

Acts as antagonist at presynaptic alpha$_2$-adrenergic receptors, increasing norepinephrine, serotonin neurotransmission. Has low anticholinergic activity. **Therapeutic Effect:** Relieves depression, produces sedative effects.

PHARMACOKINETICS

Rapidly, completely absorbed after PO administration; absorption not affected by food. Protein binding: 85%. Metabolized in liver. Primarily excreted in urine. Unknown if removed by hemodialysis. **Half-life:** 20–40 hrs (longer in males [37 hrs] than females [26 hrs]).

underlined – top prescribed drug

USES

Treatment of depression. **OFF-LABEL:** Post-traumatic stress disorder (PTSD), Alzheimer's dementia–related depression.

PRECAUTIONS

Contraindications: Use of MAOIs within 14 days. **Cautions:** Renal/hepatic impairment, elderly, high-risk pts for seizures, suicidal ideation or behavior.

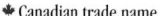 LIFESPAN CONSIDERATIONS

Pregnancy/Lactation: Unknown if distributed in breast milk. **Pregnancy Category C. Children:** Safety and efficacy not established. **Elderly:** Age-related renal impairment may require dosage adjustment.

INTERACTIONS

DRUG: Alcohol, CNS depressant medications may increase impairment of cognition, motor skills. **Serotonergic drugs (e.g., venlafaxine)** may increase risk of serotonin syndrome. **CYP3A4 inducers (e.g., phenytoin)** may decrease concentration/effects. **CYP3A4 inhibitors (e.g., ketoconazole)** may increase concentration/effects. **MAOIs** may increase risk of neuroleptic malignant syndrome, hypertensive crisis, severe seizures. **HERBAL: Gotu kola, kava kava, St. John's wort, valerian** may increase CNS depression. **St. John's wort** may decrease concentration/effects, may increase risk of serotonin syndrome. **FOOD:** None known. **LAB VALUES:** May increase serum cholesterol, triglycerides, ALT.

AVAILABILITY (Rx)

Tablets (Remeron): 7.5 mg, 15 mg, 30 mg, 45 mg. **Tablets (Orally Disintegrating [Remeron Soltab]):** 15 mg, 30 mg, 45 mg.

ADMINISTRATION/HANDLING

PO

• Give without regard to food. • May crush/break scored tablets.

Orally Disintegrating Tablets
• Do not split tablet. • Place on tongue; dissolves without water.

INDICATIONS/ROUTES/DOSAGE

Depression
PO: ADULTS: Initially, 15 mg at bedtime. May increase by 15 mg/day q1–2wks. **Maximum:** 45 mg/day. **ELDERLY:** Initially, 7.5 mg at bedtime. May increase by 7.5–15 mg/day q1–2wks. **Maximum:** 45 mg/day.

SIDE EFFECTS

Frequent (54%–12%): Drowsiness, dry mouth, increased appetite, constipation, weight gain. **Occasional (89%–4%):** Asthenia (loss of strength, energy), dizziness, flu-like symptoms, abnormal dreams. **Rare:** Abdominal discomfort, vasodilation, paresthesia, acne, dry skin, thirst, arthralgia.

ADVERSE EFFECTS/ TOXIC REACTIONS

Higher incidence of seizures than with tricyclic antidepressants (esp. in those with no history of seizures). Overdose may produce cardiovascular effects (severe orthostatic hypotension, dizziness, tachycardia, palpitations, arrhythmias). Abrupt discontinuation from prolonged therapy may produce headache, malaise, nausea, vomiting, vivid dreams. Agranulocytosis occurs rarely.

NURSING CONSIDERATIONS

BASELINE ASSESSMENT

Assess mental status, appearance, behavior, speech pattern, level of interest, mood. Obtain baseline weight. For pts on long-term therapy, hepatic/renal function tests, blood counts should be performed periodically.

INTERVENTION/EVALUATION

Supervise suicidal-risk pt closely during early therapy (as depression lessens, energy level improves, increasing suicide potential). Children, adolescents are at

M

 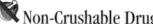

increased risk for suicidal thoughts/behavior and worsening of depression, esp. during first few mos of therapy. Assess appearance, behavior, speech pattern, level of interest, mood. Monitor for hypotension, arrhythmias.

PATIENT/FAMILY TEACHING

• Take as single bedtime dose. • Avoid alcohol, depressant/sedating medications. • Avoid tasks requiring alertness, motor skills until response to drug established. • Report worsening depression, suicidal ideation, unusual changes in behavior.

---

misoprostol

mis-oh-**pros**-tol
(Apo-Misoprostol ✤, Cytotec, Novo-Misoprostol ✤)

BLACK BOX ALERT Pregnancy Category X. Use during pregnancy can cause abortion, premature birth, birth defects. Not recommended in women of childbearing potential unless pt is capable of complying with effective contraception.
Do not confuse Cytotec with Cytoxan, or misoprostol with metoprolol or mifepristone.

FIXED-COMBINATION(S)

Arthrotec: misoprostol/diclofenac (an NSAID): 200 mcg/50 mg, 200 mcg/75 mg.

◆CLASSIFICATION

PHARMACOTHERAPEUTIC: Prostaglandin. **CLINICAL:** Antisecretory, gastric protectant.

ACTION

Replaces protective prostaglandins consumed with prostaglandin-inhibiting therapies (e.g., NSAIDs). **Therapeutic Effect:** Reduces acid secretion from gastric parietal cells, stimulates bicarbonate production from gastric/duodenal mucosa.

PHARMACOKINETICS

Route	Onset	Peak	Duration
PO	30 min	1–1.5 hrs	3–6 hrs

Rapidly absorbed from GI tract. Protein binding: 80%–90%. Rapidly converted to active metabolite. Primarily excreted in urine. Unknown if removed by hemodialysis. **Half-life:** 20–40 min.

USES

Prevention of NSAID-induced gastric ulcers and in pts at high risk for developing gastric ulcer/gastric ulcer complications. Medical termination of pregnancy (in conjunction with mifepristone). **OFF-LABEL:** Cervical ripening, labor induction, treatment/prevention of postpartum hemorrhage, treatment of incomplete or missed abortion.

PRECAUTIONS

Contraindications: Allergy to prostaglandins, pregnancy when used to reduce NSAID-induced ulcers (produces uterine contractions). **Cautions:** Renal impairment, cardiovascular disease, elderly.

⧗ LIFESPAN CONSIDERATIONS

Pregnancy/Lactation: Unknown if distributed in breast milk. Produces uterine contractions, uterine bleeding, expulsion of products of conception (abortifacient property). **Pregnancy Category X. Children:** Safety and efficacy not established. **Elderly:** No age-related precautions noted.

INTERACTIONS

DRUG: Antacids may increase levels. **HERBAL:** None significant. **FOOD:** None known. **LAB VALUES:** None significant.

AVAILABILITY (Rx)

Tablets: 100 mcg, 200 mcg.

ADMINISTRATION/HANDLING

PO

• Give with or after meals (minimizes diarrhea).

INDICATIONS/ROUTES/DOSAGE

Prevention of NSAID-Induced Gastric Ulcer

PO: ADULTS: 200 mcg 4 times a day with food (last dose at bedtime). Continue for duration of NSAID therapy. May reduce dosage to 100 mcg 4 times a day or 200 mcg 2 times a day with food. **ELDERLY:** 100–200 mcg 4 times a day with food.

Chemical Termination of Pregnancy
Refer to mifepristone monograph.

SIDE EFFECTS

Frequent (40%–20%): Abdominal pain, diarrhea. **Occasional (3%–2%):** Nausea, flatulence, dyspepsia, headache. **Rare (1%):** Vomiting, constipation.

ADVERSE EFFECTS/ TOXIC REACTIONS

Overdosage may produce sedation, tremor, seizures, dyspnea, palpitations, hypotension, bradycardia.

NURSING CONSIDERATIONS

BASELINE ASSESSMENT

Question for possibility of pregnancy before initiating therapy (Pregnancy Category X).

PATIENT/FAMILY TEACHING

• Avoid magnesium-containing antacids (minimizes potential for diarrhea).
• Women of childbearing potential must not be pregnant before or during medication therapy (may result in hospitalization, surgery, infertility, fetal death).
• Incidence of diarrhea may be lessened by taking immediately following meals.

mitomycin

mye-toe-**mye**-sin
(Mutamycin ✦)

BLACK BOX ALERT Potent vesicant. Marked myelosuppression. Infiltration produces ulceration, necrosis, cellulitis, tissue sloughing. Hemolytic-uremic syndrome reported. Must be administered by certified chemotherapy personnel.
Do not confuse mitomycin with mithramycin or mitoxantrone.

◆CLASSIFICATION

PHARMACOTHERAPEUTIC: Antibiotic. **CLINICAL:** Antineoplastic (see p. 88C).

ACTION

Alkylating agent, cross-linking with strands of DNA. **Therapeutic Effect:** Inhibits DNA, RNA synthesis.

PHARMACOKINETICS

Widely distributed. Does not cross blood-brain barrier. Primarily metabolized in liver. Excreted in urine. **Half-life:** 50 min.

USES

Treatment of disseminated adenocarcinoma of stomach, pancreas. **OFF-LABEL:** Treatment of bladder cancer, anal carcinoma, cervical, esophageal, gastric, non–small-cell lung cancer.

PRECAUTIONS

Contraindications: Coagulation disorders, bleeding tendencies, platelet count less than 75,000/mm^3. **Cautions:** Myelosuppression, renal (serum creatinine greater than 1.7 mg/dl)/hepatic impairment, pregnancy, prior radiation treatment.

⚕ LIFESPAN CONSIDERATIONS

Pregnancy/Lactation: If possible, avoid use during pregnancy, esp. first trimester. Breastfeeding not recommended. Safety in pregnancy not established. **Pregnancy Cat-**

M

 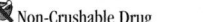

egory D. **Children:** No age-related precautions noted. **Elderly:** Age-related renal impairment may require dosage adjustment.

INTERACTIONS

DRUG: Bone marrow depressants may increase myelosuppression. **Live virus vaccines** may potentiate virus replication, increase vaccine side effects, decrease pt's antibody response to vaccine. **HERBAL:** Avoid **black cohosh, dong quai** in estrogen-dependent tumors. **FOOD:** None known. **LAB VALUES:** May increase BUN, serum creatinine.

AVAILABILITY (Rx)

Injection, Powder for Reconstitution: 5 mg, 20 mg, 40 mg.

ADMINISTRATION/HANDLING

◀**ALERT**▶ May be carcinogenic, mutagenic, teratogenic. Handle with extreme care during preparation/administration. Give via IV push, IV infusion. Extremely irritating to vein. Injection may produce pain with induration, thrombophlebitis, paresthesia.

 IV

Reconstitution • Reconstitute with Sterile Water for Injection to provide solution containing 0.5–1 mg/ml. • Do not shake vial to dissolve. • Allow vial to stand at room temperature until complete dissolution occurs. • For IV infusion, further dilute with 50–100 ml D₅W or 0.9% NaCl (concentration 20–40 mcg/ml).
Rate of Administration • Give slow IV push or by IV infusion over 15–30 min. • Extravasation may produce cellulitis, ulceration, tissue sloughing. Terminate administration immediately, inject ordered antidote. Apply ice intermittently for up to 72 hrs; keep area elevated.
Storage • Use only clear, blue-gray solutions. • Concentration of 0.5 mg/ml (reconstituted vial or syringe) is stable for 7 days at room temperature or 2 wks if refrigerated. Further diluted solution with D₅W is stable for 3 hrs, 12 hrs if di-

luted with 0.9% NaCl at room temperature.

🔳 IV INCOMPATIBILITIES

Aztreonam (Azactam), bleomycin (Blenoxane), cefepime (Maxipime), filgrastim (Neupogen), heparin, piperacillin/tazobactam (Zosyn), sargramostin (Leukine), vinorelbine (Navelbine).

🔳 IV COMPATIBILITIES

Cisplatin (Platinol AQ), cyclophosphamide (Cytoxan), doxorubicin (Adriamycin), 5-fluorouracil, granisetron (Kytril), leucovorin, methotrexate, ondansetron (Zofran), vinblastine (Velban), vincristine (Oncovin).

INDICATIONS/ROUTES/DOSAGE

Refer to individual protocols.

Usual Dosage
IV: ADULTS, ELDERLY, CHILDREN: Initially, 10–20 mg/m² as single dose. Repeat q6–8wks.

Dosage in Renal Impairment
Creatinine clearance less than 10 ml/min: Give 75% of normal dose.

SIDE EFFECTS

Frequent (Greater Than 10%): Fever, anorexia, nausea, vomiting. **Occasional (10%–2%):** Stomatitis, paresthesia, purple colored bands on nails; rash, alopecia, unusual fatigue. **Rare (Less Than 1%):** Thrombophlebitis, cellulitis with extravasation.

ADVERSE EFFECTS/ TOXIC REACTIONS

Marked myelosuppression results in hematologic toxicity manifested as leukopenia, thrombocytopenia, and, to a lesser extent, anemia (generally occurs within 2–4 wks after initial therapy). Renal toxicity may be evidenced by increased BUN, serum creatinine levels. Pulmonary toxicity manifested as dyspnea, cough, hemoptysis, pneumonia. Long-term therapy may produce hemolytic uremic syndrome, charac-

M

terized by hemolytic anemia, thrombocytopenia, renal failure, hypertension.

NURSING CONSIDERATIONS

BASELINE ASSESSMENT
Obtain CBC with differential, PT, bleeding time, before and periodically during therapy. Antiemetics before and during therapy may alleviate nausea/vomiting.

INTERVENTION/EVALUATION
Monitor hematologic status, renal function studies. Assess IV site for phlebitis, extravasation. Monitor for hematologic toxicity (fever, sore throat, signs of local infection, unusual bruising/bleeding from any site), symptoms of anemia (excessive fatigue, weakness). Assess for renal toxicity (foul odor from urine, elevated BUN, serum creatinine).

PATIENT/FAMILY TEACHING
• Maintain strict oral hygiene. • Immediately report stinging, burning, pain at injection site. • Do not have immunizations without physician's approval (drug lowers resistance to infection). • Avoid contact with those who have recently received live virus vaccine. • Hair loss is reversible, but new hair growth may have different color, texture. • Report nausea/vomiting, fever, sore throat, bruising, bleeding, shortness of breath, painful urination.

---

mitoxantrone

my-toe-**zan**-trone
(Novantrone)

BLACK BOX ALERT May cause cardiotoxicity, potentially fatal HF. Infiltration produces ulceration, necrosis, cellulitis, tissue sloughing. Secondary AML, myelodysplasia have occurred. Must be administered by certified chemotherapy personnel.

Do not confuse mitoxantrone with methotrexate, mitomycin, or Mutamycin.

◆CLASSIFICATION
PHARMACOTHERAPEUTIC: Anthracenedione. **CLINICAL:** Nonvesicant, antineoplastic (see p. 88C).

ACTION
Inhibits B-cell, T-cell, macrophage proliferation, DNA, RNA synthesis. Active throughout entire cell cycle. **Therapeutic Effect:** Causes cell death.

PHARMACOKINETICS
Protein binding: greater than 95%. Widely distributed. Metabolized in liver. Primarily eliminated in feces by biliary system. Not removed by hemodialysis. **Half-life:** 2.3–13 days.

USES
Treatment of acute, nonlymphocytic leukemia (monocytic, myelogenous, promyelocytic), late-stage hormone-resistant prostate cancer, secondary progressive or relapsing-remitting multiple sclerosis. **OFF-LABEL:** Treatment of acute lymphocytic leukemia, breast cancer, non-Hodgkin's lymphoma, pediatric acute leukemias, pediatric sarcoma, Hodgkin's lymphoma, myelodysplastic lymphoma.

PRECAUTIONS
Contraindications: None known. **Cautions:** Preexisting bone marrow suppression, previous treatment with cardiotoxic medications, hepatobiliary impairment. Baseline left ventricular ejection fraction less than 50%, cumulative lifetime mitoxantrone dose of 140 mg/m^2 or more, multiple sclerosis with hepatic impairment.

⧗ LIFESPAN CONSIDERATIONS
Pregnancy/Lactation: If possible, avoid use during pregnancy, esp. first trimester. May cause fetal harm. Breastfeeding not

M

recommended. **Pregnancy Category D.**
Children: Safety and efficacy not established. **Elderly:** No age-related precautions noted.

INTERACTIONS

DRUG: May decrease effect of **antigout**
medications. Bone marrow depressants may increase myelosuppression.
Live virus vaccines may potentiate virus replication, increase vaccine side effects, decrease pt's antibody response to
vaccine. **HERBAL:** Echinacea may decrease levels/effects. **FOOD:** None known.
LAB VALUES: May increase serum bilirubin, uric acid, AST, ALT.

AVAILABILITY (Rx)

Injection Solution: 2 mg/ml.

ADMINISTRATION/HANDLING

◀ALERT▶ May be carcinogenic, mutagenic, teratogenic. Handle with extreme
care during preparation/administration.
Give by IV injection, IV infusion. Must
dilute before administration.

 IV

Reconstitution • Dilute with at least 50
ml D_5W or 0.9% NaCl.
Rate of Administration • Do not administer by subcutaneous, IM, intrathecal, or intra-arterial injection. • Do not
give IV push over less than 3 min. • Give
IV bolus over at least 3 min, IV intermittent infusion over 15–60 min, or IV
continuous infusion (0.02–0.5 mg/ml)
in D_5W or 0.9% NaCl.
Storage • Store vials at room temperature. • Opened vials, diluted solutions stable for 7 days at room temperature or refrigerated.

▨ IV INCOMPATIBILITIES

Aztreonam (Azactam), cefepime (Maxipime), heparin, paclitaxel (Taxol), piperacillin/tazobactam (Zosyn).

▨ IV COMPATIBILITIES

Allopurinol (Aloprim), etoposide (VePesid), gemcitabine (Gemzar), granisetron

(Kytril), ondansetron (Zofran), potassium chloride.

INDICATIONS/ROUTES/DOSAGE

Refer to individual protocols.

Leukemias (In Combination With
Cytarabine)
IV: ADULTS, ELDERLY: 12 mg/m² once a
day for 2–3 days. **CHILDREN:** 10 mg/m²
once daily for 5 days.

Prostate Cancer
IV: ADULTS, ELDERLY: 12–14 mg/m² every
21 days.

Multiple Sclerosis
IV: ADULTS, ELDERLY: 12 mg/m²/dose
q3mos. **Maximum lifetime cumulative dose:** 140 mg/m².

SIDE EFFECTS

Frequent (Greater Than 10%): Nausea,
vomiting, diarrhea, cough, headache,
stomatitis, abdominal discomfort, fever,
alopecia. **Occasional (9%–4%):** Ecchymosis, fungal infection, conjunctivitis, UTI.
Rare (3%): Arrhythmias.

ADVERSE EFFECTS/
TOXIC REACTIONS

Myelosuppression may be severe, resulting in GI bleeding, sepsis, pneumonia.
Renal failure, seizures, jaundice, HF may
occur. Cardiotoxicity has been reported.

NURSING CONSIDERATIONS

BASELINE ASSESSMENT

Evaluate left ventricular ejection fraction
before initiating therapy and before administering each dose. Offer emotional
support. Establish baseline for CBC with
differential, temperature, pulse rate/
quality, respiratory status. Obtain pregnancy test prior to each dose for females
of childbearing age.

INTERVENTION/EVALUATION

Monitor hematologic status, pulmonary
function studies, hepatic/renal function

tests. Monitor for stomatitis, fever, signs of local infection, unusual bruising/bleeding from any site. Extravasation produces swelling, pain, burning, blue discoloration of skin.

PATIENT/FAMILY TEACHING

• Urine will appear blue-green for 24 hrs after administration. Blue tint to sclera may appear. • Maintain adequate daily fluid intake (may protect against renal impairment). • Do not have immunizations without physician's approval (drug lowers resistance to infection). • Avoid crowds, those with infection. • Contraceptive measures recommended during therapy. • Report chills, fever, sore throat, difficulty breathing, unusual bruising/bleeding.

---

modafinil

moe-**daf**-i-nil
(Alertec ♣, Apo-Modafinil ♣, Provigil)

◆CLASSIFICATION

PHARMACOTHERAPEUTIC: Alpha₁-agonist, CNS stimulant **(Schedule IV).** **CLINICAL:** Wakefulness-promoting agent, antinarcoleptic.

ACTION

Binds to dopamine reuptake carrier sites, increasing alpha activity, decreasing delta, theta, beta brain wave activity. **Therapeutic Effect:** Reduces number of sleep episodes, total daytime sleep.

PHARMACOKINETICS

Well absorbed from GI tract. Protein binding: 60%. Widely distributed. Metabolized in liver. Excreted by kidneys. Unknown if removed by hemodialysis. **Half-life:** 15 hrs.

USES

Treatment of excessive daytime sleepiness associated with narcolepsy, shift work sleep disorder, adjunct therapy for obstructive sleep apnea/hypopnea syndrome. **OFF-LABEL:** Treatment of ADHD, multiple sclerosis–related fatigue.

PRECAUTIONS

Contraindications: None known. **Cautions:** History of clinically significant mitral valve prolapse, left ventricular hypertrophy, renal/hepatic impairment, angina, cardiac disease, ischemia, recent MI, preexisting psychosis or bipolar disorder, Tourette's syndrome.

⌛ LIFESPAN CONSIDERATIONS

Pregnancy/Lactation: Unknown if drug is excreted in breast milk. Use caution if given to pregnant women. **Pregnancy Category C. Children:** Safety and efficacy not established in pts younger than 16 yrs. **Elderly:** Age-related renal/hepatic impairment may require decreased dosage.

INTERACTIONS

DRUG: May decrease concentrations of **cyclosporine, oral contraceptives.** May increase concentrations of **tricyclic antidepressants, warfarin. Other CNS stimulants** may increase CNS stimulation. **HERBAL:** None significant. **FOOD:** None known. **LAB VALUES:** None known.

AVAILABILITY (Rx)

Tablets (Provigil): 100 mg, 200 mg.

ADMINISTRATION/HANDLING

PO
• Give without regard to meals.

INDICATIONS/ROUTES/DOSAGE

Narcolepsy, Obstructive Sleep Apnea/Hypopnea Syndrome
PO: ADULTS: 200 mg/day in the morning. **ELDERLY:** Initially, 100 mg/day in the morning.

Shift Work Sleep Disorder
PO: ADULTS: 200 mg about 1 hr prior to start of work shift.

M

SIDE EFFECTS

Generally well tolerated. **Occasional (5%):** Headache, nausea, dizziness, insomnia, palpitations, diarrhea.

ADVERSE EFFECTS/ TOXIC REACTIONS

Agitation, excitation, increased B/P, insomnia may occur. Psychiatric disturbances (anxiety, hallucinations, suicidal ideation), serious allergic reactions (angioedema, Stevens-Johnson syndrome) may occur.

NURSING CONSIDERATIONS

BASELINE ASSESSMENT

Obtain baseline evidence of narcolepsy or other sleep disorders, including pattern, environmental situations, length of sleep episodes. Question for sudden loss of muscle tone (cataplexy) precipitated by strong emotional responses before sleep episode. Assess frequency/severity of sleep episodes before drug therapy.

INTERVENTION/EVALUATION

Monitor sleep pattern, evidence of restlessness during sleep, length of insomnia episodes at night. Assess for dizziness, anxiety; initiate fall precautions.

PATIENT/FAMILY TEACHING

• Avoid alcohol. • Sugarless gum, sips of water may relieve dry mouth. • Do not increase dose without physician approval. • Use alternative contraceptives during therapy and 1 mo after discontinuing modafinil (reduces effectiveness of oral contraceptives).

---

mometasone   `TOP 200`

moe-**met**-a-sone
(Elocon)

mometasone furoate

(Asmanex Twisthaler, <u>Nasonex</u>)

FIXED-COMBINATION(S)

Dulera: mometasone/formoterol (beta-adrenergic agonist): 100 mcg/ 5 mcg, 200 mcg/5 mcg.

◆CLASSIFICATION

PHARMACOTHERAPEUTIC: Adrenocorticosteroid. **CLINICAL:** Anti-inflammatory (see p. 3C, 78C, 102C).

ACTION

Inhibits release of inflammatory cells into nasal tissue, preventing early activation of allergic reaction. **Therapeutic Effect:** Decreases response to seasonal/perennial rhinitis.

PHARMACOKINETICS

Undetectable in plasma. Protein binding: 98%–99%. Swallowed portion undergoes extensive metabolism. Excreted primarily through bile and, to a lesser extent, urine. **Half-life:** 5 hrs.

USES

Nasal: Treatment of nasal symptoms of seasonal/perennial allergic rhinitis in adults, children over 2 yrs. Prophylaxis of nasal symptoms of seasonal allergic rhinitis in adults, adolescents over 12 yrs. Treatment of nasal polyps. **Inhalation:** Maintenance treatment of asthma as prophylactic therapy or supplement in pts requiring oral steroids for purpose of decreasing oral steroid requirement. **Topical:** Relief of inflammatory, pruritic manifestations of steroid-responsive dermatoses.

PRECAUTIONS

Contraindications: Hypersensitivity to milk proteins. Status asthmaticus or acute bronchospasm (inhalation). **Cautions:** Adrenal insufficiency, glaucoma, untreated infection, tuberculosis, ocular herpes simplex, *Candida albicans* infection of mouth/pharynx.

LIFESPAN CONSIDERATIONS

Pregnancy/Lactation: Unknown if drug crosses placenta or is distributed in breast milk. **Pregnancy Category C. Children:** Prolonged treatment/high doses may decrease short-term growth rate, cortisol secretion. **Elderly:** No age-related precautions noted.

INTERACTIONS

DRUG: Ketoconazole may increase concentration (inhalation). **HERBAL:** None significant. **FOOD:** None known. **LAB VALUES:** None known.

AVAILABILITY (Rx)

Cream (Elocon): 0.1%. **Lotion (Elocon):** 0.1%. **Nasal Spray (Nasonex):** 50 mcg/spray. **Ointment (Elocon):** 0.1%. **Powder for Oral Inhaler (Asmanex Twisthaler):** 110 mcg (delivers 100 mcg/actuation), 220 mcg (delivers 200 mcg/actuation).

ADMINISTRATION/HANDLING

Inhalation

• Hold twisthaler straight up with pink portion (base) on bottom, remove cap. • Exhale fully. • Firmly close lips around mouthpiece and inhale a fast, deep breath. • Hold breath for 10 sec.

Intranasal

• Instruct pt to clear nasal passages as much as possible before use. • Tilt head slightly forward. • Insert spray tip into nostril, pointing toward nasal passages, away from nasal septum. • Spray into one nostril while pt holds other nostril closed, concurrently inspires through nose to permit medication as high into nasal passages as possible.

Topical

• Apply thin layer of cream, lotion, ointment to cover affected area. Rub in gently. • Do not cover area with occlusive dressing.

INDICATIONS/ROUTES/DOSAGE

Allergic Rhinitis

Nasal Spray: ADULTS, ELDERLY, CHILDREN 12 YRS AND OLDER: 2 sprays in each nostril once a day. When used to prevent nasal rhinitis, begin 2–4 wks prior to start of pollen season. **CHILDREN 2–11 YRS:** 1 spray in each nostril once a day.

Asthma

Inhalation: ADULTS, ELDERLY, CHILDREN 12 YRS AND OLDER (Previous therapy with bronchodilators or inhaled corticosteroids): Initially, inhale 220 mcg (1 puff) once a day. **Maximum:** 440 mcg/day as single or 2 divided doses. **(Previous therapy with oral corticosteroids):** Initially, inhale 440 mcg (2 puffs) twice a day. Reduce prednisone no faster than 2.5 mg/day beginning after at least 1 wk of mometasone. **CHILDREN 4–11 YRS:** 110 mcg once daily in evening.

Skin Disease

Topical: ADULTS, ELDERLY, CHILDREN 12 YRS AND OLDER: Apply cream, lotion, or ointment to affected area once a day.

Nasal Polyp

Nasal Spray: ADULTS, ELDERLY: 2 sprays (100 mcg) in each nostril twice a day.

SIDE EFFECTS

Occasional: Inhalation: Headache, allergic rhinitis, upper respiratory infection, muscle pain, fatigue. **Nasal:** Nasal irritation, stinging. **Topical:** Burning. **Rare: Inhalation:** Abdominal pain, dyspepsia, nausea. **Nasal:** Nasal/pharyngeal candidiasis. **Topical:** Pruritus.

ADVERSE EFFECTS/TOXIC REACTIONS

Acute hypersensitivity reaction (urticaria, angioedema, severe bronchospasm) occurs rarely. Transfer from systemic to local steroid therapy may unmask previously suppressed bronchial asthma condition.

NURSING CONSIDERATIONS

BASELINE ASSESSMENT

Question for hypersensitivity to any corticosteroids.

INTERVENTION/EVALUATION

Teach proper use of nasal spray, oral inhaler. Instruct pt to clear nasal passages

M

before use. Contact physician if no improvement in symptoms, sneezing, nasal irritation occur. Assess lung sounds for wheezing, rales.

PATIENT/FAMILY TEACHING

• Do not change dose schedule or stop taking drug; must taper off gradually under medical supervision. **Nasal:** Contact physician if symptoms do not improve; sneezing, nasal irritation occur. • Clear nasal passages prior to use. **Inhalation:** Inhale rapidly, deeply; rinse mouth after inhalation. • Not indicated for acute asthma attacks. **Topical:** Do not cover affected area with bandage, dressing.

---

montelukast

mon-**tee**-loo-kast
(Apo-Montelukast ✦, <u>Singulair</u>)
Do not confuse Singulair with Sinequan.

◆CLASSIFICATION

PHARMACOTHERAPEUTIC: Leukotriene receptor inhibitor. **CLINICAL:** Antiasthmatic (see p. 78C).

ACTION

Binds to cysteinyl leukotriene receptors, inhibiting effects of leukotrienes on bronchial smooth muscle. **Therapeutic Effect:** Decreases bronchoconstriction, vascular permeability, mucosal edema, mucus production.

PHARMACOKINETICS

Route	Onset	Peak	Duration
PO	N/A	N/A	24 hrs
PO (chewable)	N/A	N/A	24 hrs

Rapidly absorbed from GI tract. Protein binding: 99%. Extensively metabolized in liver. Excreted almost exclusively in feces. **Half-life:** 2.7–5.5 hrs (slightly longer in elderly).

USES

Prophylaxis, chronic treatment of asthma. Prevention of exercise-induced bronchoconstriction. Treatment of seasonal allergic rhinitis (hay fever). Relief of perennial allergic rhinitis. **OFF-LABEL:** Acute asthma.

PRECAUTIONS

Contraindications: None known. **Cautions:** Systemic corticosteroid treatment reduction during montelukast therapy. Concomitant use of CYP3A4 inducers.

⌛ LIFESPAN CONSIDERATIONS

Pregnancy/Lactation: Unknown if distributed in breast milk. Use during pregnancy only if necessary. **Pregnancy Category B. Children/Elderly:** No age-related precautions noted in those older than 6 yrs or the elderly.

INTERACTIONS

DRUG: CYP3A4 inducers (e.g., carbamazepine, phenobarbital, rifampin) may decrease concentration/effect. **HERBAL: St. John's wort** may decrease concentration/effects. **FOOD:** None known. **LAB VALUES:** May increase serum AST, ALT, eosinophils.

AVAILABILITY (Rx)

Oral Granules: 4 mg per packet. **Tablets:** 10 mg. **Tablets (Chewable):** 4 mg, 5 mg.

ADMINISTRATION/HANDLING

PO

• When treating asthma, administer in evening without regard to meals. • When treating allergic rhinitis, may individualize administration times. • Granules may be given directly in mouth or mixed with carrots, rice, applesauce, ice cream, baby formula, or breast milk (do not add to any other liquid or food). • Give within 15 min of opening packet.

INDICATIONS/ROUTES/DOSAGE

Bronchial Asthma

PO: ADULTS, ELDERLY, CHILDREN 15 YRS AND OLDER: One 10-mg tablet a day, taken in the evening. **CHILDREN 6–14 YRS:** One 5-mg

---

M

chewable tablet a day, taken in the evening. **CHILDREN 2–5 YRS:** One 4-mg chewable tablet a day, taken in the evening. **CHILDREN 6–23 MOS:** 4 mg (oral granules) once daily in the evening.

Seasonal Allergic Rhinitis
PO: ADULTS, ELDERLY, CHILDREN 15 YRS AND OLDER: One 10-mg tablet, taken in the evening. **CHILDREN 6–14 YRS:** One 5-mg chewable tablet, taken in the evening. **CHILDREN 2–5 YRS:** One 4-mg chewable tablet, taken in the evening.

Perennial Allergic Rhinitis
PO: ADULTS, ELDERLY, CHILDREN 15 YRS AND OLDER: One 10-mg tablet, taken in the evening. **CHILDREN 6–14 YRS:** One 5-mg chewable tablet, taken in the evening. **CHILDREN 2–5 YRS:** One 4-mg chewable tablet, taken in the evening. **CHILDREN 6–23 MOS:** 4 mg oral granules, taken in the evening.

Exercise-Induced Bronchoconstriction Prevention
PO: ADULTS, ELDERLY, CHILDREN 15 YRS AND OLDER: 10 mg 2 or more hrs before exercise. No additional doses within 24 hrs. **CHILDREN 6–14 YRS:** 5 mg (chew tab) 2 or more hrs prior to exercise. No additional doses within 24 hrs.

SIDE EFFECTS

Adults, children 15 yrs and older: **Frequent (18%):** Headache. **Occasional (4%):** Influenza. **Rare (3%–2%):** Abdominal pain, cough, dyspepsia, dizziness, fatigue, dental pain. **Children 6–14 yrs: Rare (less than 2%):** Diarrhea, laryngitis, pharyngitis, nausea, otitis media, sinusitis, viral infection.

ADVERSE EFFECTS/ TOXIC REACTIONS

Suicidal ideation and behavior, depression has been noted.

NURSING CONSIDERATIONS

BASELINE ASSESSMENT

Chewable tablet contains phenylalanine (component of aspartame); parents of phenylketonuric pts should be informed. Assess lung sounds for wheezing. Assess for allergy symptoms.

INTERVENTION/EVALUATION

Monitor rate, depth, rhythm, type of respirations; quality/rate of pulse. Assess lung sounds for wheezing. Monitor for change in mood, behavior.

PATIENT/FAMILY TEACHING

• Increase fluid intake (decreases lung secretion viscosity). • Take as prescribed, even during symptom-free periods as well as during exacerbations of asthma. • Do not alter/stop other asthma medications. • Drug is not for treatment of acute asthma attacks. • Report increased use or frequency of short-acting bronchodilators, changes in behavior, suicidal ideation.

---

morphine

mor-feen
(Astramorph PF, <u>Avinza</u>, DepoDur, Duramorph, Infumorph, <u>Kadian</u>, M-Eslon ✦, MS Contin, MSIR ✦)

BLACK BOX ALERT Be alert for signs of abuse, misuse, diversion. ***Epidural:*** Monitor for delayed sedation. ***Sustained-release:*** Do not crush or chew. ***MS Contin:*** Use only in opioid-tolerant pts requiring over 400 mg/day. ***Kadian:*** Use only in opioid-tolerant pts. ***Avinza:*** Alcohol disrupts extended-release timing. ***Duramorph:*** Risk of severe and/or sustained cardiopulmonary depression. **Do not confuse Avinza with Evista or Invanz, morphine with hydromorphone, morphine sulfate with magnesium sulfate, MS Contin with Oxycontin. MSO₄ and MS are error-prone abbreviations.**

FIXED-COMBINATION(S)

Embeda: morphine/naloxone (an opioid antagonist): 20 mg/0.8 mg, 30 mg/1.2 mg, 50 mg/2 mg, 60 mg/2.4 mg, 80 mg/3.2 mg, 100 mg/4 mg.

◆CLASSIFICATION

PHARMACOTHERAPEUTIC: Narcotic agonist **(Schedule II). CLINICAL:** Opiate analgesic.

ACTION

Binds with opioid receptors within CNS. **Therapeutic Effect:** Alters pain perception, emotional response to pain.

PHARMACOKINETICS

Route	Onset	Peak	Duration
Oral solution	30 min	1 hr	3–5 hrs
Tablets	30 min	1 hr	3–5 hrs
Tablets (extended-release)	N/A	3–4 hrs	8–12 hrs
IV	Rapid	0.3 hr	3–5 hrs
IM	5–30 min	0.5–1 hr	3–5 hrs
Epidural	15–60 min	1 hr	12–20 hrs
Subcutaneous	10–30 min	1.1–5 hrs	3–5 hrs
Rectal	20–60 min	0.5–1 hr	3–7 hrs

Variably absorbed from GI tract. Readily absorbed after IM, subcutaneous administration. Protein binding: 20%–35%. Widely distributed. Metabolized in liver. Primarily excreted in urine. Removed by hemodialysis. **Half-life:** 2–4 hrs (increased in hepatic disease).

USES

Relief of moderate to severe, acute, or chronic pain; analgesia during labor. Drug of choice for pain due to MI, dyspnea from pulmonary edema not resulting from chemical respiratory irritant. **DepoDur:** Epidural (lumbar) single-dose management of surgical pain. **Infumorph:** Use in devices for managing intractable chronic pain. **Extended-release:** Use only when repeated doses for extended periods of time are required.

PRECAUTIONS

Contraindications: All Formulations: Acute or severe asthma, GI obstruction, paralytic ileus, severe hepatic/renal impairment, severe respiratory depression. **Sustained Release:** GI obstruction, acute postoperative pain. **Oral Solution:** HF due to lung disease; arrhythmias, head injury, seizures, acute alcoholism. **Injection:** Labor when premature birth expected. **Immediate Release** *(Tablets, Oral Solution):* Post biliary tract surgery, concurrent use of MAO inhibitors, general CNS depression. **Extreme Caution:** COPD, cor pulmonale, hypoxia, hypercapnia, preexisting respiratory depression, head injury, increased ICP, severe hypotension. **Cautions:** Biliary tract disease, pancreatitis, Addison's disease, hypothyroidism, urethral stricture, prostatic hyperplasia, debilitated pts, those with CNS depression, toxic psychosis, seizure disorders, alcoholism.

☒ LIFESPAN CONSIDERATIONS

Pregnancy/Lactation: Crosses placenta. Distributed in breast milk. May prolong labor if administered in latent phase of first stage of labor or before cervical dilation of 4–5 cm has occurred. Respiratory depression may occur in neonate if mother received opiates during labor. Regular use of opiates during pregnancy may produce withdrawal symptoms in neonate (irritability, excessive crying, tremors, hyperactive reflexes, fever, vomiting, diarrhea, yawning, sneezing, seizures). **Pregnancy Category C (D if used for prolonged periods or at high dosages at term). Children:** Paradoxical excitement may occur; those younger than 2 yrs are more susceptible to respiratory depressant effects. **Elderly:** Paradoxical excitement may occur. Age-related renal impairment may increase risk of urinary retention.

INTERACTIONS

DRUG: Alcohol, other CNS depressants may increase CNS effects, respiratory depression, hypotension. **MAOIs** may produce severe, sometimes fatal reaction (reduce dosage to ¼ of usual morphine dose). **HERBAL: Gotu kola, kava kava, St. John's wort, valerian** may increase CNS depression. **FOOD:**

None known. **LAB VALUES:** May increase serum amylase, lipase.

AVAILABILITY (Rx)

Injection, Liposomal Suspension (Depo-Dur): 10 mg/ml. **Injection, Solution:** 2 mg/ml, 4 mg/ml, 5 mg/ml, 10 mg/ml, 15 mg/ml, 25 mg/ml, 50 mg/ml. **Injection, Solution (Epidural, Intrathecal, IV Infusion) (Astramorph PF, Duramorph):** 0.5 mg/ml, 1 mg/ml. **Injection, Solution (Epidural or Intrathecal) (Infumorph):** 10 mg/ml, 25 mg/ml. **Injection, Solution Patient-Controlled Analgesia (PCA) Pump:** 1 mg/ml, 5 mg/ml. **Solution Oral:** 20 mg/ml, 10 mg/5 ml, 20 mg/5 ml. **Suppository:** 5 mg, 10 mg, 20 mg, 30 mg. **Tablets:** 15 mg, 30 mg.

Capsules, Extended-Release (Avinza): 30 mg, 45 mg, 60 mg, 75 mg, 90 mg, 120 mg. **Capsules, Sustained-Release (Kadian):** 10 mg, 20 mg, 30 mg, 50 mg, 60 mg, 80 mg, 100 mg, 200 mg. **Tablets, Extended-Release (MS Contin):** 15 mg, 30 mg, 60 mg, 100 mg, 200 mg.

ADMINISTRATION/HANDLING

 IV

Reconstitution • May give undiluted. • For IV injection, may dilute in Sterile Water for Injection or 0.9% NaCl to final concentration of 1–2 mg/ml. • For continuous IV infusion, dilute to concentration of 0.1–1 mg/ml in D_5W and give through controlled infusion device.
Rate of Administration • Always administer very slowly. Rapid IV increases risk of severe adverse reactions (apnea, chest wall rigidity, peripheral circulatory collapse, cardiac arrest, anaphylactoid effects).
Storage • Store at room temperature.

Epidural, Liposomal
• May give either diluted or undiluted. • Do not use an in-line filter. • Store solution in refrigerator; do not freeze. May store at room temperature for 7 days. • Following withdrawal from vial, use within 4 hrs. • Gently invert vial to resuspend drug; avoid aggressive agitation.

IM, Subcutaneous
• Administer slowly, rotating injection sites. • Pts with circulatory impairment experience higher risk of overdosage due to delayed absorption of repeated administration.

PO
• May give without regard to food. • Mix liquid form with fruit juice to improve taste. • Do not crush, break extended-release capsule, tablets. • **Avinza, Kadian:** May mix with applesauce immediately prior to administration.

Rectal
• If suppository is too soft, chill for 30 min in refrigerator or run cold water over foil wrapper. • Moisten suppository with cold water before inserting well into rectum.

IV INCOMPATIBILITIES

Amphotericin B complex (Abelcet, AmBisome, Amphotec), cefepime (Maxipime), doxorubicin (Doxil), phenytoin (Dilantin).

IV COMPATIBILITIES

Amiodarone (Cordarone), atropine, bumetanide (Bumex), bupivacaine (Marcaine, Sensorcaine), dexmedetomidine (Precedex), diltiazem (Cardizem), diphenhydramine (Benadryl), dobutamine (Dobutrex), dopamine (Intropin), glycopyrrolate (Robinul), heparin, hydroxyzine (Vistaril), lidocaine, lorazepam (Ativan), magnesium, midazolam (Versed), milrinone (Primacor), nitroglycerin, potassium, propofol (Diprivan).

INDICATIONS/ROUTES/DOSAGE

◀**ALERT**▶ Dosage should be titrated to desired effect.

Analgesia
PO *(Immediate-Release)*: **ADULTS, ELDERLY:** 10–30 mg q3–4h as needed. **CHILDREN:** 0.15–0.3 mg/kg q3–4h as needed.

◄ALERT► For the Avinza dosage below, be aware that this drug is to be administered once a day only.

◄ALERT► For the Kadian dosage information below, be aware that this drug is to be administered q12h or once a day.

◄ALERT► Be aware that pediatric dosages of extended-release preparations of Kadian and Avinza have not been established.

◄ALERT► For the MS Contin dosage information below, be aware that the daily dosage is divided and given q8h or q12h.

PO *(Extended-Release [Avinza])*: **ADULTS, ELDERLY:** Dosage requirement should be established using prompt-release formulations and is based on total daily dose. Avinza is given once a day only.

PO *(Extended-Release [Kadian])*: **ADULTS, ELDERLY:** Dosage requirement should be established using prompt-release formulations and is based on total daily dose. Dose is given once a day or divided and given q12h.

PO *(Extended-Release [MS Contin])*: **ADULTS, ELDERLY:** Dosage requirement should be established using prompt-release formulations and is based on total daily dose. Daily dose is divided and given q8h or q12h.

IV: ADULTS, ELDERLY: 2.5–5 mg q3–4h as needed. Note: Repeated doses (e.g., 1–2 mg) may be given more frequently (e.g., every hr) if needed. **CHILDREN:** 0.05–0.3 mg/kg q3–4h as needed. **NEONATES:** Initially, 0.05–0.1 mg/kg/dose q4–6h as needed.

IV Continuous Infusion: ADULTS, ELDERLY: 0.8–10 mg/hr. Range: Titrate up to 80 mg/hr. **CHILDREN:** Initially, 30 mcg/kg/hr. Titrate as needed to control pain. **NEONATES:** Initially, 0.01 mg/kg/hr (10 mcg/kg/hr). **Maximum:** 0.015–0.02 mg/kg/hr.

IM: ADULTS, ELDERLY: 5–10 mg q3–4h as needed. **CHILDREN:** 0.1–0.2 mg/kg q3–4h as needed.

Patient-Controlled Analgesia (PCA)
IV: ADULTS, ELDERLY: Usual concentration: 1 mg/ml. **Demand dose:** 1 mg (range: 0.5–2.5 mg). **Lockout interval:** 5–10 min.

SIDE EFFECTS

◄ALERT► Ambulatory pts, pts not in severe pain may experience nausea, vomiting more frequently than pts in supine position or who have severe pain. **Frequent:** Sedation, decreased B/P (including orthostatic hypotension), diaphoresis, facial flushing, constipation, dizziness, drowsiness, nausea, vomiting. **Occasional:** Allergic reaction (rash, pruritus), dyspnea, confusion, palpitations, tremors, urinary retention, abdominal cramps, vision changes, dry mouth, headache, decreased appetite, pain/burning at injection site. **Rare:** Paralytic ileus.

ADVERSE EFFECTS/ TOXIC REACTIONS

Overdose results in respiratory depression, skeletal muscle flaccidity, cold/clammy skin, cyanosis, extreme drowsiness progressing to seizures, stupor, coma. Tolerance to analgesic effect, physical dependence may occur with repeated use. Prolonged duration of action, cumulative effect may occur in those with hepatic/renal impairment. **Antidote:** Naloxone (see Appendix K for dosage).

NURSING CONSIDERATIONS

BASELINE ASSESSMENT

Pt should be in recumbent position before drug is given by parenteral route. Assess onset, type, location, duration of pain. Obtain vital signs before giving medication. If respirations are 12/min or less (20/min or less in children), withhold medication, contact physician. Effect of medication is reduced if full pain recurs before next dose.

INTERVENTION/EVALUATION

Monitor vital signs 5–10 min after IV administration, 15–30 min after subcutaneous, IM. Be alert for decreased respirations, B/P. Check for adequate voiding. Monitor daily pattern of bowel activity, stool consistency. Avoid constipation. Initiate deep breathing, coughing exercises, particularly in those with pulmonary impairment. Assess for clinical improvement, record onset of pain relief. Consult physician if pain relief is not adequate.

PATIENT/FAMILY TEACHING

• Discomfort may occur with injection. • Change positions slowly to avoid orthostatic hypotension. • Avoid tasks that require alertness, motor skills until response to drug is established. • Avoid alcohol, CNS depressants. • Tolerance, dependence may occur with prolonged use of high doses. • Report ineffective pain control, constipation, urinary retention.

---

moxifloxacin

mox-i-**flox**-a-sin
(Avelox, Avelox IV, Moxeza, Vigamox)
BLACK BOX ALERT May increase risk of tendonitis, tendon rupture (increased with concurrent corticosteroids, organ transplant recipients, those older than 60 yrs).
Do not confuse Avelox with Avonex.

◆CLASSIFICATION

PHARMACOTHERAPEUTIC: Fluoroquinolone. **CLINICAL:** Antibacterial, antibiotic (see p. 26C).

ACTION

Inhibits two enzymes, topoisomerase II and IV, in susceptible microorganisms. **Therapeutic Effect:** Interferes with bacterial DNA replication. Prevents/delays emergence of resistant organisms. Bactericidal.

PHARMACOKINETICS

Well absorbed from GI tract after PO administration. Protein binding: 50%. Widely distributed throughout body with tissue concentration often exceeding plasma concentration. Metabolized in liver. Primarily excreted in urine, with lesser amount in feces. **Half-life: PO:** 12 hrs; **IV:** 15 hrs.

USES

Treatment of susceptible infections due to *S. pneumoniae, S. pyogenes, S. aureus, H. influenzae, M. catarrhalis, K. pneumoniae, M. pneumoniae, C. pneumoniae* including acute bacterial exacerbation of chronic bronchitis, acute bacterial sinusitis, intra-abdominal infection, community-acquired pneumonia, uncomplicated skin/skin structure infections. **Ophthalmic:** Topical treatment of bacterial conjunctivitis due to susceptible strains of bacteria. **OFF-LABEL:** Legionella, pneumonia, tuberculosis (second-line therapy).

PRECAUTIONS

Contraindications: Hypersensitivity to quinolones. **Cautions:** Renal/hepatic impairment, bradycardia, acute myocardial ischemia, myasthenia gravis, diabetes, rheumatoid arthritis, seizures, pts with prolonged QT interval.

⌛ LIFESPAN CONSIDERATIONS

Pregnancy/Lactation: May be distributed in breast milk. May produce teratogenic effects. **Pregnancy Category C. Children:** Safety and efficacy not established. **Elderly:** No age-related precautions noted.

INTERACTIONS

DRUG: Antacids, iron preparations, sucralfate may decrease absorption. **NSAIDs** may increase risks of CNS stimulation/seizures. **HERBAL:** None significant. **FOOD:** None known. **LAB VALUES:** None known.

AVAILABILITY (Rx)

Injection Infusion (Avelox IV): 400 mg (250 ml). **Ophthalmic Solution (Moxeza, Vigamox):** 0.5%. **Tablets (Avelox):** 400 mg.

ADMINISTRATION/HANDLING

 IV

Reconstitution • Available in ready-to-use containers.
Rate of Administration • Give by IV infusion only. • Avoid rapid or bolus IV infusion. • Infuse over 60 min.
Storage • Store at room temperature. • Do not refrigerate.

PO

• Give without regard to meals. • Oral moxifloxacin should be administered 4 hrs before or 8 hrs after antacids, multivitamins, iron preparations, sucralfate, didanosine chewable/buffered tablets, pediatric powder for oral solution.

Ophthalmic

• Place gloved finger on lower eyelid and pull out until a pocket is formed between eye and lower lid. • Place prescribed number of drops into pocket. • Instruct pt to close eye gently (so medication will not be squeezed out of the sac) and to apply digital pressure to lacrimal sac at inner canthus for 1 min to minimize systemic absorption.

🔷 IV INCOMPATIBILITIES

Do not add or infuse other drugs simultaneously through the same IV line. Flush line before and after use if same IV line is used with other medications.

INDICATIONS/ROUTES/DOSAGE

Usual Dose
PO, IV: ADULTS, ELDERLY: 400 mg q24h.

Acute Bacterial Sinusitis
PO, IV: ADULTS, ELDERLY: 400 mg q24h for 10 days.

Acute Bacterial Exacerbation of Chronic Bronchitis
PO, IV: ADULTS, ELDERLY: 400 mg q24h for 5 days.

Community-Acquired Pneumonia
PO, IV: ADULTS, ELDERLY: 400 mg q24h for 7–14 days.

Intra-Abdominal Infection
PO, IV: ADULTS, ELDERLY: 400 mg q24h for 5–14 days.

Skin/Skin Structure Infection
PO, IV: ADULTS, ELDERLY: 400 mg once a day for 7–21 days.

Topical Treatment of Bacterial Conjunctivitis Due to Susceptible Strains of Bacteria
Ophthalmic: ADULTS, ELDERLY, CHILDREN 1 YR AND OLDER: (Vigamox): 1 drop 3 times a day for 7 days. **(Moxeza):** 1 drop 2 times a day for 7 days.

SIDE EFFECTS

Frequent (8%–6%): Nausea, diarrhea. **Occasional: PO, IV (3%–2%):** Dizziness, headache, abdominal pain, vomiting. **Ophthalmic (6%–1%):** Conjunctival irritation, reduced visual acuity, dry eye, keratitis, eye pain, ocular itching, swelling of tissue around cornea, eye discharge, fever, cough, pharyngitis, rash, rhinitis. **Rare (1%):** Change in sense of taste, dyspepsia (heartburn, epigastric pain, indigestion), photosensitivity.

ADVERSE EFFECTS/TOXIC REACTIONS

Pseudomembranous colitis (severe abdominal cramps/pain, severe watery diarrhea, fever) may occur. Superinfection (anal/genital pruritus, moderate to severe diarrhea, stomatitis) may occur.

NURSING CONSIDERATIONS

BASELINE ASSESSMENT

Question for history of hypersensitivity to moxifloxacin, quinolones.

INTERVENTION/EVALUATION

Monitor daily pattern of bowel activity, stool consistency. Assist with ambulation if dizziness occurs. Assess for headache, abdominal pain, vomiting, altered taste, dyspepsia (heartburn, indigestion). Monitor WBC, signs of infection.

PATIENT/FAMILY TEACHING

• May be taken without regard to food. • Drink plenty of fluids. • Avoid exposure to direct sunlight; may cause photosensitivity reaction. • Do not take antacids 4 hrs before or 8 hrs after dosing. • Take full course of therapy. • Report abdominal cramping/pain, persistent diarrhea.

---

mupirocin
[TOP 200]

mue-peer-oh-sin
(Bactroban, Bactroban Nasal)
Do not confuse Bactroban or Bactroban Nasal with bacitracin, baclofen, or Bactrim.

◆ CLASSIFICATION

PHARMACOTHERAPEUTIC: Anti-infective. **CLINICAL:** Topical antibiotic.

ACTION

Inhibits bacterial protein, RNA synthesis. Less effective on DNA synthesis. **Nasal:** Eradicates nasal colonization of methicillin-resistant *Staphylococcus aureus* (MRSA). **Therapeutic Effect:** Prevents bacterial growth, replication. Bacteriostatic.

PHARMACOKINETICS

Following topical administration, penetrates outer layer of skin (minimal through intact skin). Protein binding: 95%. Metabolized in liver. Excreted in urine. **Half-life:** 17–36 min.

USES

Ointment: Topical treatment of impetigo caused by *S. aureus*, *S. pyogenes*. **Cream:** Treatment of traumatic skin lesions due to *S. aureus*, *S. pyogenes*. **Intranasal ointment:** Eradication of *S. aureus* from nasal, perineal carriage sites. **OFF-LABEL:** Surgical prophylaxis to prevent wound infections (intranasal).

PRECAUTIONS

Contraindications: None known. **Cautions:** Renal impairment, burn pts.

⏳ LIFESPAN CONSIDERATIONS

Pregnancy/Lactation: Unknown if distributed in breast milk. Breast-feeding not recommended. **Pregnancy Category B. Children:** Safety and efficacy not established. **Elderly:** No age-related precautions noted.

INTERACTIONS

DRUG: None significant. **HERBAL:** None significant. **FOOD:** None known. **LAB VALUES:** None significant.

AVAILABILITY (Rx)

Cream, Topical (Bactroban): 2%. **Ointment, Intranasal (1-g single-use tube) (Bactroban Nasal):** 2%. **Ointment, Topical (Bactroban):** 2%.

ADMINISTRATION/HANDLING

Topical
Cream, Ointment • For topical use only. • May cover with gauze dressing. • Avoid contact with eyes.

Intranasal
• Apply ½ of the ointment from single-use tube into each nostril. • Avoid contact with eyes.

INDICATIONS/ROUTES/DOSAGE

Usual Topical Dosage
Topical Cream: ADULTS, ELDERLY, CHILDREN 3 MOS AND OLDER: Apply small amount 3 times a day for 10 days. **Topical Ointment: ADULTS, ELDERLY, CHILDREN 2 MOS AND OLDER:** Apply small amount 3 times a day for 5–14 days.

Usual Nasal Dosage
Intranasal: ADULTS, ELDERLY, CHILDREN 12 YRS AND OLDER: Apply small amount 2 times a day for 5–10 days.

SIDE EFFECTS

Frequent: Nasal (9%–3%): Headache, rhinitis, upper respiratory congestion,

---

 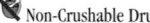

pharyngitis, altered taste. **Occasional: Nasal (2%):** Burning, stinging, cough. **Topical (2%–1%):** Pain, burning, stinging, pruritus. **Rare: Nasal (less than 1%):** Pruritus, diarrhea, dry mouth, epistaxis, nausea, rash. **Topical (less than 1%):** Rash, nausea, dry skin, contact dermatitis.

ADVERSE EFFECTS/ TOXIC REACTIONS

Superinfection may result in bacterial, fungal infections, esp. with prolonged, repeated therapy.

NURSING CONSIDERATIONS

BASELINE ASSESSMENT

Assess skin for type, extent of lesions.

INTERVENTION/EVALUATION

Monitor healing of skin lesions. In event of skin reaction, stop applications, cleanse area gently, notify physician.

PATIENT/FAMILY TEACHING

• For external use only. • Avoid contact with eyes. • Explain precautions to avoid spread of infection; teach how to apply medication. • Report skin reactions, irritation. • If no improvement is noted in 3–5 days, contact physician.

mycophenolate

mye-koe-**fen**-o-late
(Apo-Mycophenolate ✦, CellCept, Myfortic)

BLACK BOX ALERT Increased risk of congenital malformation, spontaneous abortion. Increased risk for development of lymphoma, skin malignancy. Increased susceptibility to infections.

◆ CLASSIFICATION

PHARMACOTHERAPEUTIC: Immunologic agent. **CLINICAL:** Immunosuppressant (see p. 123C).

ACTION

Suppresses immunologically-mediated inflammatory response by inhibiting inosine monophosphate dehydrogenase, an enzyme that deprives lymphocytes of nucleotides necessary for DNA, RNA synthesis, thus inhibiting proliferation of T and B lymphocytes. **Therapeutic Effect:** Prevents transplant rejection.

PHARMACOKINETICS

Rapidly, extensively absorbed after PO administration (food decreases drug plasma concentration but does not affect absorption). Protein binding: 97%. Completely hydrolyzed to active metabolite mycophenolic acid. Primarily excreted in urine. Not removed by hemodialysis. **Half-life:** 17.9 hrs.

USES

Should be used concurrently with cyclosporine and corticosteroids. **CellCept:** Prophylaxis of organ rejection in pts receiving allogeneic hepatic/renal/cardiac transplants. **Myfortic:** Renal transplants. **OFF-LABEL:** Treatment of hepatic transplant rejection, mild heart transplant rejection, moderate to severe psoriasis, proliferative lupus nephritis, myasthenia gravis, graft-vs-host disease.

PRECAUTIONS

Contraindications: Hypersensitivity to mycophenolic acid or polysorbate 80 (IV formulation). **Cautions:** Active severe GI disease, renal impairment, neutropenia, women of childbearing potential.

⧗ LIFESPAN CONSIDERATIONS

Pregnancy/Lactation: Unknown if drug crosses placenta or is distributed in breast milk. Breastfeeding not recommended. Increased risk of miscarriage, birth defects. **Pregnancy Category C. (Myfortic: Pregnancy Category D). Children:** Safety and efficacy not established. **Elderly:** Age-related renal impairment may require dosage adjustment.

INTERACTIONS

DRUG: May increase concentrations of **acyclovir, ganciclovir** in pts with renal impairment. **Antacids (aluminum- and magnesium-containing), cholestyramine** may decrease absorption. **Live virus vaccines** may potentiate virus replication, increase vaccine side effects, decrease pt's antibody response to vaccine. **Other immunosuppressants (e.g., cyclophosphamide, cyclosporine, tacrolimus)** may increase risk of infection, lymphomas. **Probenecid** may increase concentration. **HERBAL:** **Cat's claw, echinacea** may decrease effects (have immunostimulant properties). **FOOD:** **All foods** may decrease concentration. **LAB VALUES:** May increase serum cholesterol, alkaline phosphatase, creatinine, AST, ALT. May alter serum glucose, lipids, calcium, potassium, phosphate, uric acid.

AVAILABILITY (Rx)

Capsules (CellCept): 250 mg. **Injection, Powder for Reconstitution (CellCept):** 500 mg. **Oral Suspension (CellCept):** 200 mg/ml. **Tablets (CellCept):** 500 mg.

 Tablets (Delayed-Release [Myfortic]): 180 mg, 360 mg.

ADMINISTRATION/HANDLING

💧 **IV**

Reconstitution • Reconstitute each 500-mg vial with 14 ml D₅W. Gently agitate. • For 1-g dose, further dilute with 140 ml D₅W; for 1.5-g dose further dilute with 210 ml D₅W, providing a concentration of 6 mg/ml.
Rate of Administration • Infuse over at least 2 hrs. • Begin infusion within 4 hrs of reconstitution.
Storage • Store at room temperature. • IV infusion stable for 12 hrs at room temperature.

PO

• Give on empty stomach (1 hr before or 2 hrs after food). • Do not open capsules or crush, cut, or chew delayed-release tablets. Avoid inhalation of powder in capsules, direct contact of powder on skin/mucous membranes. If contact occurs, wash thoroughly, with soap, water. Rinse eyes profusely with plain water. • May store reconstituted suspension in refrigerator or at room temperature. • Suspension is stable for 60 days after reconstitution. • Suspension can be administered orally or via an NG tube (minimum size 8 French).

🞖 IV INCOMPATIBILITIES

Mycophenolate is compatible only with D₅W. Do not infuse concurrently with other drugs or IV solutions.

INDICATIONS/ROUTES/DOSAGE

Prevention of Renal Transplant Rejection
PO, IV *(Cellcept)*: **ADULTS, ELDERLY:** 1 g twice a day. **PO: CHILDREN** *(Cellcept Suspension)*: 600 mg/m²/dose twice a day. **Maximum:** 1 g twice a day.
PO *(Myfortic)*: **ADULTS, ELDERLY:** 720 mg twice a day. **CHILDREN 5–16 YRS:** 400 mg/m² twice a day. **Maximum:** 720 mg twice a day.

Prevention of Heart Transplant Rejection
PO, IV *(Cellcept)*: **ADULTS, ELDERLY:** 1.5 g twice a day.

Prevention of Hepatic Transplant Rejection
PO *(Cellcept)*: **ADULTS, ELDERLY:** 1.5 g twice a day.
IV *(Cellcept)*: **ADULTS, ELDERLY:** 1 g twice a day.

SIDE EFFECTS

Frequent (37%–20%): UTI, hypertension, peripheral edema, diarrhea, constipation, fever, headache, nausea. **Occasional (18%–10%):** Dyspepsia; dyspnea; cough; hematuria; asthenia (loss of strength, energy); vomiting; edema; tremors; abdominal, chest, back pain; oral candidiasis; acne. **Rare (9%–6%):** Insomnia, respiratory tract infection, rash, dizziness.

M

ADVERSE EFFECTS/ TOXIC REACTIONS

Significant anemia, leukopenia, thrombocytopenia, neutropenia, leukocytosis may occur, particularly in those undergoing renal transplant rejection. Sepsis, infection occur occasionally. GI tract hemorrhage occurs rarely. There is an increased risk of developing neoplasms. Immunosuppression results in increased susceptibility to infection.

NURSING CONSIDERATIONS

BASELINE ASSESSMENT

Women of childbearing potential should have a negative serum or urine pregnancy test within 1 wk before initiation of drug therapy. Assess medical history, esp. renal function, existence of active digestive system disease, drug history, esp. other immunosuppressants.

INTERVENTION/EVALUATION

CBC should be performed weekly during first mo of therapy, twice monthly during second and third mos of treatment, then monthly throughout the first yr. If rapid fall in WBC occurs, dosage should be reduced or discontinued. Assess particularly for delayed bone marrow suppression. Report any major change in assessment of pt.

PATIENT/FAMILY TEACHING

• Effective contraception should be used before, during, and for 6 wks after discontinuing therapy, even if pt has a history of infertility, other than hysterectomy. • Two forms of contraception must be used concurrently unless abstinence is absolute. • Report unusual bleeding/bruising, sore throat, mouth sores, abdominal pain, fever. • Laboratory followup while taking medication is important part of therapy. • Malignancies may occur.

M

nabumetone

na-**bue**-me-tone
(Apo-Nabumetone ✤, Novo-Nabumetone ✤, Relafen ✤)

BLACK BOX ALERT Increased risk of serious cardiovascular thrombotic events, including myocardial infarction, CVA. Increased risk of severe GI reactions, including ulceration, bleeding, perforation of stomach, intestines.

◆CLASSIFICATION

PHARMACOTHERAPEUTIC: NSAID. **CLINICAL:** Analgesic, anti-inflammatory (see p. 130C).

ACTION

Produces analgesic anti-inflammatory effects by inhibiting prostaglandin synthesis. **Therapeutic Effect:** Reduces inflammatory response, intensity of pain.

PHARMACOKINETICS

Readily absorbed from GI tract. Protein binding: 99%. Widely distributed. Metabolized in liver. Primarily excreted in urine. Not removed by hemodialysis. **Half-life:** 22–30 hrs.

USES

Acute, chronic treatment of osteoarthritis, rheumatoid arthritis (RA). **OFF-LABEL:** Moderate pain.

PRECAUTIONS

Contraindications: Perioperative pain in setting of CABG surgery, history of hypersensitivity to aspirin or NSAIDs. **Cautions:** Active peptic ulcer disease, chronic inflammation of GI tract, GI bleeding/ulceration, HF, fluid retention, hypertension, hepatic/renal impairment; concurrent use of anticoagulants, aspirin, or corticosteroids; asthma.

⊠ LIFESPAN CONSIDERATIONS

Pregnancy/Lactation: Distributed in low concentration in breast milk. Avoid use during last trimester (may adversely affect fetal cardiovascular system: premature closing of ductus arteriosus). **Pregnancy Category C (D if used in third trimester or near delivery). Children:** Safety and efficacy not established. **Elderly:** Age-related renal impairment may increase risk of hepatic/renal toxicity; reduced dosage recommended. More likely to have serious adverse effects with GI bleeding/ulceration.

INTERACTIONS

DRUG: May decrease effects of **antihypertensives, diuretics. Aspirin, other salicylates** may increase risk of GI side effects, bleeding. May increase effects of **heparin, oral anticoagulants, thrombolytics.** May increase concentration/risk of **lithium** toxicity. May increase risk of **methotrexate** toxicity. **HERBAL:** Cat's claw, dong quai, evening primrose, feverfew, garlic, ginger, ginkgo, ginseng, horse chestnut possess antiplatelet activity, may increase risk of bleeding. **FOOD:** None known. **LAB VALUES:** May increase urine protein levels, serum LDH, alkaline phosphatase, AST, ALT, BUN, creatinine, potassium. May decrease serum uric acid, Hgb, Hct, leukocytes, platelets.

AVAILABILITY (Rx)

Tablets (Relafen): 500 mg, 750 mg.

ADMINISTRATION/HANDLING

PO
• Give with food, milk, antacids to decrease GI irritation, increase absorption.

INDICATIONS/ROUTES/DOSAGE

Rheumatoid Arthritis (RA), Osteoarthritis
PO: ADULTS, ELDERLY: Initially, 1,000 mg as a single dose or in 2 divided doses. May increase up to 2,000 mg/day as a single dose or in 2 divided doses.

Dosage in Renal Impairment

Creatinine Clearance	Dosage
30–49 ml/min	Initially, 750 mg/day. **Maximum:** 1,500 mg/day
Less than 30 ml/min	Initially, 500 mg/day. **Maximum:** 1,000 mg/day

SIDE EFFECTS

Frequent (14%–12%): Diarrhea, abdominal cramps/pain, dyspepsia. **Occasional (9%–4%):** Nausea, constipation, flatulence, dizziness, headache. **Rare (3%–1%):** Vomiting, stomatitis, pruritus, rash, tinnitus, edema, fatigue, diaphoresis, insomnia, somnolence.

ADVERSE EFFECTS/ TOXIC REACTIONS

Overdose may result in acute hypotension, tachycardia. Rare reactions with long-term use include peptic ulcer, GI bleeding, gastritis, nephrotoxicity (dysuria, cystitis, hematuria, proteinuria, nephrotic syndrome), severe hepatic reactions (cholestasis, jaundice), severe hypersensitivity reactions (bronchospasm, angioedema).

NURSING CONSIDERATIONS

BASELINE ASSESSMENT

Assess onset, type, location, duration of pain/inflammation. Inspect appearance of affected joints for immobility, deformities, skin condition.

INTERVENTION/EVALUATION

Monitor renal function tests in pts with renal insufficiency. Assist with ambulation if drowsiness, dizziness occurs. Monitor for evidence of dyspepsia. Monitor daily pattern of bowel activity, stool consistency. Assess for therapeutic response: relief of pain, stiffness, swelling; increase in joint mobility; reduced joint tenderness; improved grip strength.

PATIENT/FAMILY TEACHING

• May cause serious GI bleeding with or without pain. • Avoid aspirin, alcohol.
• May take with food if GI upset occurs.
• Avoid tasks requiring mental alertness, motor skills until response to drug is established. • Report GI symptoms.

---

nadolol

na-**doe**-lol
(Apo-Nadol ✦, Corgard, Novo-Nadolol ✦)

BLACK BOX ALERT Severe angina exacerbation, MI, ventricular arrhythmias noted in angina pts after abrupt withdrawal.
Do not confuse Corgard with Coreg, or nadolol with labetolol or atenolol.

FIXED-COMBINATION(S)

Corzide: nadolol/bendroflumethiazide (a diuretic): 40 mg/5 mg, 80 mg/5 mg.

◆ CLASSIFICATION

PHARMACOTHERAPEUTIC: Beta-adrenergic blocker. **CLINICAL:** Antianginal, antihypertensive (see p. 73C).

ACTION

Blocks beta$_1$- and beta$_2$-adrenergenic receptors. Large doses increase airway resistance. **Therapeutic Effect:** Slows heart rate, decreases cardiac output, B/P. Decreases myocardial ischemia severity by decreasing oxygen requirements.

PHARMACOKINETICS

Variable absorption after PO administration. Protein binding: 28%–30%. Not metabolized. Excreted unchanged in feces. **Half-life:** 20–24 hrs.

USES

Management of mild to moderate hypertension; used alone or in combination with diuretics, esp. thiazide type. Management of chronic stable angina pectoris. Prophylaxis of migraine headaches. **OFF-LABEL:** Prophylaxis of variceal hemorrhage; management of thyrotoxicosis.

PRECAUTIONS

Contraindications: Bronchial asthma, cardiogenic shock, sinus node dysfunction, second- or third-degree heart block (except with functioning pacemaker), sinus bradycardia, uncontrolled cardiac failure. **Cautions:** Compensated HF, concurrent use of verapamil, digoxin, or diltiazem, diabetes, renal impairment, myasthenia gravis, peripheral vascular disease, psychiatric disease.

⧗ LIFESPAN CONSIDERATIONS

Pregnancy/Lactation: Crosses placenta; distributed in breast milk. **Pregnancy Category C (D if used in second or third trimester). Children:** Safety and efficacy not established. **Elderly:** No age-related precautions noted.

INTERACTIONS

DRUG: Digoxin may increase risk of bradycardia. May mask symptoms of hypoglycemia, prolong hypoglycemic effect of **insulin, oral hypoglycemics. HERBAL: Ephedra, garlic, ginseng, yohimbe** may worsen hypertension. **Licorice** may cause increased serum sodium, water retention, decreased serum potassium. **FOOD:** None known. **LAB VALUES:** May increase serum antinuclear antibody (ANA) titer, BUN, serum LDH, lipoprotein, alkaline phosphatase, bilirubin, potassium, uric acid, AST, ALT, triglycerides.

AVAILABILITY (Rx)

Tablets: 20 mg, 40 mg, 80 mg.

ADMINISTRATION/HANDLING

PO

• Give without regard to meals. • Tablets may be crushed.

INDICATIONS/ROUTES/DOSAGE

Hypertension, Angina

PO: ADULTS: Initially, 40 mg/day. May increase by 40–80 mg at 3- to 7-day intervals. **Maximum: (Hypertension)** 240–320 mg/day. **(Angina):** 160–240 mg. **ELDERLY:** Initially, 20 mg/day. May increase gradually. Range: 20–240 mg/day.

Dosage in Renal Impairment

Dosage is modified based on creatinine clearance.

Creatinine Clearance	Dosage
31–50 ml/min	q24–36 h
10–30 ml/min	q24–48 h
Less than 10 ml/min	q40–60 h

SIDE EFFECTS

Nadolol is generally well tolerated, with transient, mild side effects. **Occasional (6% or less):** Diminished sexual function, drowsiness, unusual fatigue/weakness, bradycardia, difficulty breathing, depression, cold hands/feet, diarrhea, constipation, anxiety, nasal congestion, nausea, vomiting, altered taste, dry eyes, pruritus.

ADVERSE EFFECTS/ TOXIC REACTIONS

Overdose may produce profound bradycardia, hypotension. Abrupt withdrawal may result in diaphoresis, palpitations, headache, tremors, exacerbation of angina, MI, ventricular arrhythmias. May precipitate HF, MI in pts with cardiac disease; thyroid storm in pts with thyrotoxicosis; peripheral ischemia in those with existing peripheral vascular disease. Hypoglycemia may occur in pts with previously controlled diabetes.

NURSING CONSIDERATIONS

BASELINE ASSESSMENT

Assess baseline renal/hepatic function tests. Assess B/P, apical pulse immediately before drug administration (if pulse is 60/min or less or systolic B/P is less than 90 mm Hg, withhold medication, contact physician). **Antianginal:** Record onset, type (sharp, dull, squeezing), radiation, location, intensity, duration of anginal pain; precipitating factors (exertion, emotional stress).

INTERVENTION/EVALUATION

Monitor B/P for hypotension, respiratory effort for dyspnea. Assess pulse for qual-

N

ity, irregular rate, bradycardia. Assess hands/feet for coldness, tingling, numbness. Assess for evidence of HF: dyspnea (particularly on exertion, lying down), night cough, peripheral edema, distended neck veins. Monitor I&O (increase in weight, decrease in urinary output may indicate HF).

PATIENT/FAMILY TEACHING

• Do not discontinue abruptly (may precipitate angina MI, ventricular arrhythmias). • Report difficulty breathing, night cough, swelling of arms/legs, slow pulse, dizziness, confusion, depression, rash, fever, sore throat, unusual bleeding/bruising. • Avoid tasks that require alertness, motor skills until response to drug is established. • Limit alcohol intake.

---

nafcillin

naf-**sill**-in

◆CLASSIFICATION

PHARMACOTHERAPEUTIC: Penicillinase-resistant penicillin. **CLINICAL:** Antibiotic (see p. 29C).

ACTION

Binds to bacterial membranes. **Therapeutic Effect:** Inhibits cell wall synthesis. Bactericidal.

USES

Treatment of respiratory tract, skin/skin structure infections, osteomyelitis, endocarditis, meningitis; perioperatively, esp. in cardiovascular, orthopedic procedures. Predominant treatment of infections caused by susceptible strains of staphylococci.

PRECAUTIONS

Contraindications: Hypersensitivity to any penicillin. **Cautions:** History of allergies, particularly cephalosporins, severe renal/hepatic impairment, asthma.

⧗ LIFESPAN CONSIDERATIONS

Pregnancy/Lactation: Readily crosses placenta; appears in cord blood, amniotic fluid. Distributed in breast milk. May lead to rash, diarrhea, candidiasis in neonate, infant. **Pregnancy Category B. Children:** Immature renal function in neonate may delay renal excretion. **Elderly:** Age-related renal impairment may require dosage adjustment.

INTERACTIONS

DRUG: High doses (2 g q4h) may decrease effects of **warfarin. HERBAL:** None significant. **FOOD:** None known. **LAB VALUES:** May cause false-positive Coombs' test.

AVAILABILITY (Rx)

Injection, Powder for Reconstitution: 1 g, 2 g. **Infusion (Premix):** 1 g/50 ml, 2g/100 ml.

ADMINISTRATION/HANDLING

◀**ALERT**▶ Space doses evenly around the clock.

 IV

Reconstitution • Reconstitute each vial with 10 ml Sterile Water for Injection or 0.9% NaCl. • For intermittent IV infusion (piggyback), further dilute with 50–100 ml 0.9% NaCl or D_5W to maximum concentration of 40 mg/ml.
Rate of Administration • Infuse over 30–60 min. • Because of potential for hypersensitivity/anaphylaxis, start initial dose at few drops per min, increase slowly to ordered rate; stay with pt first 10–15 min, then check q10min. • Limit IV therapy to less than 48 hrs, if possible. Stop infusion if pt complains of pain at IV site.
Storage *(IV infusion [piggyback])* • Stable for 24 hrs at room temperature, 96 hrs if refrigerated. • Discard if precipitate forms.

IM

• Reconstitute each 500 mg with 1.7 ml Sterile Water for Injection or 0.9% NaCl

to provide concentration of 250 mg/ml.
• Inject IM into large muscle mass.

▨ IV INCOMPATIBILITIES

Aztreonam (Azactam), diltiazem (Cardizem), droperidol (Inapsine), fentanyl, gentamicin, insulin, labetalol (Normodyne, Trandate), methylprednisolone (Solu-Medrol), midazolam (Versed), nalbuphine (Nubain), vancomycin (Vancocin), verapamil (Isoptin).

▨ IV COMPATIBILITIES

Acyclovir, famotidine (Pepcid), fluconazole (Diflucan), heparin, hydromorphone (Dilaudid), lidocaine, lipids, magnesium, morphine, potassium chloride, propofol (Diprivan).

INDICATIONS/ROUTES/DOSAGE

Usual Dosage
IV: ADULTS, ELDERLY: 0.5–2 g q4–6h. **CHILDREN:** 50–200 mg/kg/day in divided doses q4–6h. **Maximum:** 12 g/day. **NEONATES:** 25 mg/kg/dose in divided doses q6–12h.
IM: ADULTS, ELDERLY: 500 mg q4–6h. **CHILDREN:** 25 mg/kg twice daily.

SIDE EFFECTS

Frequent: Mild hypersensitivity reaction (fever, rash, pruritus), GI effects (nausea, vomiting, diarrhea). **Occasional:** Hypokalemia with high IV dosages, phlebitis, thrombophlebitis (common in elderly). **Rare:** Extravasation with IV administration.

ADVERSE EFFECTS/ TOXIC REACTIONS

Potentially fatal antibiotic-associated colitis, superinfections (abdominal cramps, severe watery diarrhea, fever) may result from altered bacterial balance in GI tract. Hematologic effects (esp. involving platelets, WBCs), severe hypersensitivity reactions, anaphylaxis occur rarely.

NURSING CONSIDERATIONS

BASELINE ASSESSMENT

Question for history of allergies, esp. penicillins, cephalosporins.

INTERVENTION/EVALUATION

Hold medication, promptly report rash (possible hypersensitivity), diarrhea (fever, abdominal pain, mucus/blood in stool may indicate antibiotic-associated colitis). Evaluate IV site frequently for phlebitis (heat, pain, red streaking over vein), infiltration (potential extravasation). Monitor periodic CBC, urinalysis, serum potassium, renal/hepatic function. Be alert for superinfection: fever, vomiting, diarrhea, anal/genital pruritus, oral mucosal changes (ulceration, pain, erythema).

PATIENT/FAMILY TEACHING

• Continue antibiotic for full length of treatment. • Doses should be evenly spaced. • Discomfort may occur with IM injection. • Report IV discomfort immediately. • Notify physician in event of diarrhea, rash, other new symptoms.

---

nalbuphine ^{HIGH ALERT}

nal-bue-feen

◆CLASSIFICATION

PHARMACOTHERAPEUTIC: Narcotic agonist, antagonist. **CLINICAL:** Opioid analgesic.

ACTION

Binds with opioid receptors within CNS. May displace opioid agonists, competitively inhibiting their action; may precipitate withdrawal symptoms. **Therapeutic Effect:** Alters pain perception, emotional response to pain.

PHARMACOKINETICS

Route	Onset	Peak	Duration
IV	2–3 min	2–3 min	3–4 hrs
IM	Less than 15 min	30 min	3–6 hrs
Subcutaneous	Less than 15 min	N/A	3–6 hrs

Well absorbed after IM, subcutaneous administration. Metabolized in liver. Primarily eliminated in feces by biliary secretion. **Half-life:** 3.5–5 hrs.

USES

Relief of moderate to severe pain, preop analgesia, obstetric analgesia, adjunct to anesthesia. **OFF-LABEL:** Opioid-induced pruritus.

PRECAUTIONS

Contraindications: None known. **Cautions:** Hepatic/renal impairment, respiratory depression, recent MI, recent biliary tract surgery, head trauma, increased intracranial pressure (ICP), pregnancy, pts suspected of being opioid dependent, obesity, thyroid dysfunction, prostatic hyperplasia, urinary stricture, adrenal insufficiency, cardiovascular disease.

⏳ LIFESPAN CONSIDERATIONS

Pregnancy/Lactation: Readily crosses placenta. Distributed in breast milk. Breastfeeding not recommended. May cause fetal, neonatal adverse effects during labor/delivery (e.g., fetal bradycardia). **Pregnancy Category B (D if used for prolonged periods or at high dosages at term). Children:** Paradoxical excitement may occur. Those younger than 2 yrs more susceptible to respiratory depression. **Elderly:** More susceptible to respiratory depression. Age-related renal impairment may increase risk of urinary retention.

INTERACTIONS

DRUG: Alcohol, other CNS depressants may increase CNS effects, respiratory depression, hypotension. **HERBAL: Gotu kola, kava kava, St. John's wort, valerian** may increase CNS depression. **FOOD:** None known. **LAB VALUES:** May increase serum amylase, lipase.

AVAILABILITY (Rx)

Injection Solution: 10 mg/ml, 20 mg/ml.

ADMINISTRATION/HANDLING

 IV

**Reconstitution • May give undiluted.
Rate of Administration •** For IV push, administer each 10 mg over 3–5 min. **Storage •** Store parenteral form at room temperature.

IM
• Rotate IM injection sites.

▦ IV INCOMPATIBILITIES

Amphotericin B complex (Abelcet, AmBisome, Amphotec), cefepime (Maxipime), ketorolac (Toradol), nafcillin (Nafcil), piperacillin and tazobactam (Zosyn).

▦ IV COMPATIBILITIES

Dexmedetomidine (Precedex), diphenhydramine (Benadryl), droperidol (Inapsine), glycopyrrolate (Robinul), hydroxyzine (Vistaril), lidocaine, midazolam (Versed), prochlorperazine (Compazine), propofol (Diprivan).

INDICATIONS/ROUTES/DOSAGE

Analgesia
IV, IM, Subcutaneous: ADULTS, ELDERLY: 10 mg q3–6h as needed. Do not exceed maximum single dose of 20 mg or daily dose of 160 mg. **CHILDREN 1 YR AND OLDER:** 0.1–0.2 mg/kg q3–4h as needed. **Maximum:** 20 mg/dose, 160 mg/day.

Supplement to Anesthesia
IV: ADULTS, ELDERLY: Induction: 0.3–3 mg/kg over 10–15 min. Maintenance: 0.25–0.5 mg/kg as needed.

SIDE EFFECTS

Frequent (36%): Sedation. **Occasional (9%–3%):** Diaphoresis, cold/clammy skin, nausea, vomiting, dizziness, vertigo, dry mouth, headache. **Rare (less than 1%):** Restlessness, emotional lability, paresthesia, flushing, paradoxical reaction.

ADVERSE EFFECTS/ TOXIC REACTIONS

Abrupt withdrawal after prolonged use may produce symptoms of narcotic withdrawal (abdominal cramping, rhinorrhea, lacrimation, anxiety, fever, piloerection [goose bumps]). Overdose results in severe respiratory depression, skeletal muscle flaccidity, cyanosis, extreme drowsiness progressing to seizures, stupor, coma. Tolerance to analgesic effect, physical dependence may occur with chronic use.

NURSING CONSIDERATIONS

BASELINE ASSESSMENT

Obtain vital signs before giving medication. If respirations are 12/min or less (20/min or less in children), withhold medication, contact physician. Assess onset, type, location, duration of pain. Effect of medication is reduced if full pain recurs before next dose. Low abuse potential.

INTERVENTION/EVALUATION

Monitor for change in respirations, B/P, rate/quality of pulse. Monitor daily pattern of bowel activity, stool consistency. Initiate deep breathing, coughing exercises, particularly in pts with pulmonary impairment. Assess for clinical improvement, record onset of relief of pain. Consult physician if pain relief is not adequate.

PATIENT/FAMILY TEACHING

• Avoid alcohol. • Avoid tasks that require alertness, motor skills until response to drug is established. • May cause dry mouth. • May be habit forming.

naloxone

nah-**lox**-own
Do not confuse naloxone
with Lanoxin or naltrexone.

FIXED-COMBINATION(S)

Embeda: naloxone/morphine (an opioid agonist): 0.8 mg/20 mg, 1.2 mg/30 mg, 2 mg/50 mg, 2.4 mg/60 mg, 3.2 mg/80 mg, 4 mg/100 mg. **Suboxone (sublingual film):** naloxone/buprenorphine (an analgesic): 0.5 mg/2 mg, 1 mg/4 mg, 2 mg/8 mg, 3 mg/12 mg.

◆CLASSIFICATION

PHARMACOTHERAPEUTIC: Narcotic antagonist. **CLINICAL:** Antidote.

ACTION

Displaces opioids at opioid-occupied receptor sites in CNS. **Therapeutic Effect:** Reverses opioid-induced sleep/sedation, increases respiratory rate, raises B/P to normal range.

PHARMACOKINETICS

Route	Onset	Peak	Duration
IV	1–2 min	N/A	20–60 min
IM	2–5 min	N/A	20–60 min
Subcutaneous	2–5 min	N/A	20–60 min

Well absorbed after IM, subcutaneous administration. Metabolized in liver. Primarily excreted in urine. **Half-life:** 60–100 min.

USES

Complete or partial reversal of opioid depression including respiratory depression. Diagnosis of suspected opioid tolerance or acute opioid overdose. Neonatal opiate depression. Coma of unknown origin. **OFF-LABEL:** Opioid-induced pruritus.

PRECAUTIONS

Contraindications: None known. **Cautions:** Chronic cardiac/pulmonary disease, coronary artery disease, pts suspected of being opioid dependent, postop pts (to avoid cardiovascular changes), history of seizures.

N

⏳ LIFESPAN CONSIDERATIONS

Pregnancy/Lactation: Unknown if drug crosses placenta or is distributed in breast milk. **Pregnancy Category B. Children/Elderly:** No age-related precautions noted.

INTERACTIONS

DRUG: None significant. **HERBAL:** None significant. **FOOD:** None known. **LAB VALUES:** None significant.

AVAILABILITY (Rx)

Injection Solution: 0.4 mg/ml, 1 mg/ml.

ADMINISTRATION/HANDLING
💧 IV

Reconstitution • May dilute 1 mg/ml with 50 ml Sterile Water for Injection to provide concentration of 0.02 mg/ml. • For continuous IV infusion, dilute each 2 mg of naloxone with 500 ml of D_5W or 0.9% NaCl, producing solution containing 0.004 mg/ml (4 mcg/ml).
Rate of Administration • May administer undiluted. • Give each 0.4 mg as IV push over 30 sec.
Storage • Store parenteral form at room temperature. • Use mixture within 24 hrs; discard unused solution. • Protect from light. • Stable in D_5W or 0.9% NaCl at 4 mcg/ml for 24 hrs.

IM

• Give deep IM in large muscle mass.

💊 IV INCOMPATIBILITY

Amphotericin B complex (Abelcet, AmBisome, Amphotec).

💊 IV COMPATIBILITIES

Heparin, ondansetron (Zofran), propofol (Diprivan).

INDICATIONS/ROUTES/DOSAGE

Opioid Overdose
IV, IM, Subcutaneous: ADULTS, ELDERLY: 2 mg q2–3min as needed. May repeat doses q20–60min. **CHILDREN 5 YRS AND OLDER, WEIGHING 20 KG OR MORE:** 2 mg/dose; if no response, may repeat q2–3min. May need to repeat doses q20–60min. **CHILDREN YOUNGER THAN 5 YRS, WEIGHING LESS THAN 20 KG:** 0.1 mg/kg (**maximum:** 2 mg); if no response, repeat q2–3min. May need to repeat doses q20–60min.

Reversal of Respiratory Depression With Therapeutic Opioid Dosing
IV, IM, Subcutaneous: ADULTS, ELDERLY: Initially, 0.04–0.4 mg. May repeat until desired response achieved. **CHILDREN:** 0.001–0.005 mg/kg. Dose may be repeated as needed.

Postanesthesia Narcotic Reversal
IV: ADULTS, ELDERLY: 0.1–0.2 mg q2–3min. **INFANTS, CHILDREN:** 0.01 mg/kg; may repeat q2–3min.

SIDE EFFECTS

None known; little or no pharmacologic effect in absence of narcotics.

ADVERSE EFFECTS/ TOXIC REACTIONS

Too-rapid reversal of narcotic-induced respiratory depression may result in agitation, nausea, vomiting, tremors, increased B/P, tachycardia. Excessive dosage in postop pts may produce significant reversal of analgesia, agitation, tremors. Hypotension or hypertension, ventricular tachycardia/fibrillation, pulmonary edema may occur in pts with cardiovascular disease.

NURSING CONSIDERATIONS

BASELINE ASSESSMENT

Maintain clear airway. Obtain weight of children to calculate drug dosage.

INTERVENTION/EVALUATION

Monitor vital signs, esp. rate, depth, rhythm of respiration, during and frequently following administration. Carefully observe pt after satisfactory response (duration of opiate may exceed duration of naloxone, resulting in recurrence of respiratory depression). Assess for increased pain with reversal of opiate.

naltrexone

nal-**trex**-own
(ReVia, Vivitrol)
BLACK BOX ALERT Can cause hepatic injury in excessive doses.
Do not confuse naltrexone with naloxone, or ReVia with Revatio or Revex.

◆CLASSIFICATION

PHARMACOTHERAPEUTIC: Opioid receptor antagonist. **CLINICAL:** Ethanol detoxification agent, antidote.

ACTION

Blocks effects of endogenous opioid peptides by competitively binding at opioid receptors. **Therapeutic Effect: Alcohol deterrent:** Decreases craving, drinking days, relapse rate. **Antidote:** Blocks physical dependence of morphine, heroin, other opioids.

PHARMACOKINETICS

Route	Onset	Peak	Duration
PO	N/A	N/A	24–72 hrs
IM	N/A	2 hrs	2–4 wks

Well absorbed following PO administration. Protein binding: 21%. Metabolized in liver. Reduction in first-pass hepatic metabolism when given by intramuscular route. Excreted primarily in urine; partial elimination in feces. **Half-life: PO:** 4 hrs; **IM:** 5–10 days.

USES

Vivitrol: Treatment of alcohol dependence in pts able to abstain from alcohol in outpatient setting prior to initiation of treatment. Prevention of relapse to opioid dependence following opioid detoxi-

fication. **ReVia:** Blocks effects of exogenously administered opioids.

PRECAUTIONS

Contraindications: Opioid dependence or current use of opioid analgesics, acute opioid withdrawal, failed naloxone challenge or positive urine screen for opioids, acute hepatitis, hepatic failure. **Cautions:** Active hepatic disease, history of suicide attempts, depression, history of bleeding disorders, concurrent anticoagulant therapy, renal impairment.

⌛ LIFESPAN CONSIDERATIONS

Pregnancy/Lactation: Unknown if drug crosses placenta or is distributed in breast milk. **Pregnancy Category C. Children:** Safety and efficacy not established in pts younger than 18 yrs. **Elderly:** No age-related precautions noted.

INTERACTIONS

DRUG: May decrease effects of **opioid analgesics. HERBAL:** None significant. **FOOD:** None known. **LAB VALUES:** May increase serum transaminase, AST, ALT.

AVAILABILITY (Rx)

Injection Suspension, Extended-Release Kit (Vivitrol): 380 mg/4 ml vial. **Tablets: (ReVia):** 50 mg.

ADMINISTRATION/HANDLING

◀**ALERT**▶ In pts with narcotic dependence, do not attempt treatment until pt has remained opioid free for 7–10 days. Test urine for opioids for verification. Pt should not be experiencing withdrawal symptoms.

IM
• Give in deep muscle mass of gluteal region, alternating buttocks. • Vivitrol must be suspended only in diluent supplied in kit.
Storage • Store entire diluent supplied in the kit. • All components (microspheres, diluent, preparation needle, administration needle with safety de-

vice) are required for preparation administration. Spare administration needle is provided in case of clogging.

PO
• Administer with food or antacids or after meals.

INDICATIONS/ROUTES/DOSAGE

Adjunct in Treatment of Alcohol Dependence, Prevention of Relapse to Opioid Dependence
IM: ADULTS, ELDERLY: (Vivitrol): 380 mg once every 4 wks or once/mo.

Block Effects of Opioids, Alcohol Dependence
PO: ADULTS, ELDERLY: Initially, 25 mg. Observe for 1 hr. If no withdrawal signs appear, give 50 mg on day 2. Maintenance regimen is flexible, variable, and individualized. May be given as 50 mg daily, 50 mg/day Monday thru Friday and 100 mg on Saturday, 100 mg every other day, or 150 mg every 3 days for 12 wks.

SIDE EFFECTS

Common: IM: (69%): Injection site reaction (induration, tenderness, pain, nodules, swelling, pruritus, ecchymosis). **Frequent: Alcohol Deterrent (33%–10%):** Nausea, headache, depression. **Narcotic Addiction (10%–5%):** Insomnia, anxiety, headache, low energy, abdominal cramps, nausea, vomiting, joint/muscle pain. **Occasional: Alcohol Deterrent (4%–2%):** Dizziness, anxiety, fatigue, insomnia, vomiting, suicidal ideation. **Narcotic Addiction (5% or less):** Irritability, increased energy, dizziness, anorexia, diarrhea, constipation, rash, chills, increased thirst.

ADVERSE EFFECTS/ TOXIC REACTIONS

Signs/symptoms of opioid withdrawal include stuffy/runny nose, tearing, yawning, diaphoresis, tremor, vomiting, piloerection (goose bumps), feeling of temperature change, arthralgia, myalgia, abdominal cramps, formication (feeling of skin crawling). Accidental naltrexone overdosage produces withdrawal symptoms within 5 min of ingestion, lasts up to 48 hrs. Symptoms present as confusion, visual hallucinations, drowsiness, significant vomiting, diarrhea. Hepatotoxicity may occur with large doses.

NURSING CONSIDERATIONS

BASELINE ASSESSMENT

Treatment should not be instituted unless pt is opioid free for 7–10 days, alcohol free for 3–5 days before therapy begins. Obtain medication history (esp. opioids), other medical conditions (esp. hepatitis, other hepatic disease). If opioid dependence suspected, a naloxone challenge test should be performed (naloxone administered to verify opioid dependence and eligibility for admission to opioid treatment program).

INTERVENTION/EVALUATION

Monitor for evidence of hepatotoxicity (abdominal pain that lasts longer than a few days, white bowel movements, dark urine, jaundice). Monitor serum AST, ALT, bilirubin.

PATIENT/FAMILY TEACHING

• If heroin, other opiates are self-administered, there will be no effect. However, any attempt to overcome naltrexone's prolonged 24- to 72-hr blockade of opioid effect by taking large amounts of opioids is dangerous and may result in coma, serious injury, fatal overdose. • Naltrexone blocks effects of opioid-containing medicine (cough/cold preparations, antidiarrheal preparations, opioid analgesics). • Report abdominal pain lasting longer than 3 days, white bowel movement, dark-colored urine, yellow eyes.

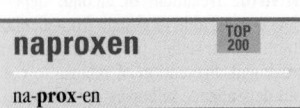

naproxen   TOP 200

na-**prox**-en

(Aleve, Anaprox, Anaprox DS, Apo-Naproxen ✦, EC-Naprosyn, Naprelan, Naprosyn, Pamprin)

BLACK BOX ALERT Increased risk of serious cardiovascular thrombotic events, including myocardial infarction, CVA. Increased risk of severe GI reactions, including ulceration, bleeding, perforation of stomach, intestines.

Do not confuse Aleve with Allese, or Anaprox with Anaspaz or Avapro.

FIXED-COMBINATION(S)

Prevacid NapraPac: naproxen/lansoprazole (proton pump inhibitor): 375 mg/15 mg, 500 mg/15 mg. **Treximet:** naproxen/sumatriptan (an antimigraine): 500 mg/85 mg. **Vimovo:** naproxen/esomeprazole (proton pump inhibitor): 375 mg/20 mg, 500 mg/20 mg.

◆CLASSIFICATION

PHARMACOTHERAPEUTIC: NSAID. **CLINICAL:** Analgesic, anti-inflammatory (see p. 130C).

ACTION

Produces analgesic, anti-inflammatory effects by inhibiting prostaglandin synthesis. **Therapeutic Effect:** Reduces inflammatory response, intensity of pain.

PHARMACOKINETICS

Route	Onset	Peak	Duration
PO (analgesic)	1 hr	2–4 hrs	7 hrs or less
PO (anti-inflammatory)	2 wks	2–4 wks	12 hrs

Completely absorbed from GI tract. Protein binding: 99%. Metabolized in liver. Primarily excreted in urine. Not removed by hemodialysis. **Half-life:** 13 hrs.

USES

Treatment of acute or long-term mild to moderate pain, primary dysmenorrhea, rheumatoid arthritis (RA), juvenile rheumatoid arthritis (JRA), osteoarthritis, ankylosing spondylitis, acute gouty arthritis, bursitis, tendonitis, fever. **OFF-LABEL:** Migraine prophylaxis.

PRECAUTIONS

Contraindications: Hypersensitivity to aspirin, naproxen, other NSAIDs. Perioperative pain in setting of CABG surgery. **Cautions:** GI/cardiac disease, renal/hepatic impairment, asthma, HF, concurrent use of anticoagulants, smoking, use of alcohol, elderly, debilitated.

⏳ LIFESPAN CONSIDERATIONS

Pregnancy/Lactation: Crosses placenta. Distributed in breast milk. Avoid use during third trimester (may adversely affect fetal cardiovascular system: premature closing of ductus arteriosus). **Pregnancy Category C (D if used in third trimester or near delivery). Children:** Safety and efficacy not established in those younger than 2 yrs. Children older than 2 yrs at increased risk for skin rash. **Elderly:** Age-related renal impairment may increase risk of hepatic/renal toxicity; reduced dosage recommended. More likely to have serious adverse effects with GI bleeding/ulceration.

INTERACTIONS

DRUG: May decrease effects of **antihypertensives, diuretics. Aspirin, other salicylates** may increase risk of GI side effects, bleeding. **Bone marrow depressants** may increase risk of hematologic reactions. May increase risk of bleeding with **heparin, oral anticoagulants, thrombolytics.** May increase concentration, risk of toxicity of **lithium.** May increase risk of **methotrexate** toxicity. **HERBAL:** Cat's claw, **dong quai, evening primrose, feverfew, garlic, ginger, ginkgo, ginseng, horse chestnut, red clover** possess antiplatelet activity, may increase risk of bleeding. **FOOD:** None known. **LAB VALUES:** May prolong bleeding time. May increase BUN, serum creatinine, ALT,

AST, alkaline phosphatase. May decrease Hgb, Hct, leukocytes, platelets, uric acid.

AVAILABILITY (Rx)

Gelcaps (Aleve [OTC]): 220 mg naproxen sodium (equivalent to 200 mg naproxen). **Oral Suspension (Naprosyn):** 125 mg/5 ml naproxen. **Tablets:** 220 mg naproxen sodium (equivalent to 200 mg naproxen) (Aleve [OTC]), 250 mg (Naprosyn), 275 mg naproxen sodium (equivalent to 250 mg naproxen) (Anaprox), 375 mg, 500 mg, 550 mg naproxen sodium (equivalent to 500 mg naproxen) (Anaprox DS).

✎ Tablets (Controlled-Release): 375 mg naproxen (EC-Naprosyn), 412.5 mg naproxen sodium (equivalent to 375 mg naproxen) (Naprelan), 500 mg naproxen (EC-Naprosyn), 550 mg naproxen sodium (equivalent to 500 mg naproxen) (Naprelan), 825 mg naproxen sodium (equivalent to 750 mg naproxen) (Naprelan).

ADMINISTRATION/HANDLING

PO
• Give controlled-release form whole. Do not break, crush, divide. • Scored tablets may be broken/crushed. • Best taken with food or milk (decreases GI irritation). • Shake suspension well.

INDICATIONS/ROUTES/DOSAGE

Note: Dosage expressed as naproxen base (200 mg naproxen base equivalent to 220 mg naproxen sodium).

Rheumatoid Arthritis (RA), Osteoarthritis, Ankylosing Spondylitis
PO: ADULTS, ELDERLY: 500–1,000 mg/day in 2 divided doses. May increase to 1,500 mg/day for limited time.

Acute Gouty Arthritis
PO: ADULTS, ELDERLY: Initially, 750 mg naproxen (825 mg naproxen sodium), then 250 mg naproxen (275 mg naproxen sodium) q8h until attack subsides. **Naprelan:** Initially, 1,000–1,500 mg, then 1,000 mg once daily until attack subsides.

Mild to Moderate Pain, Dysmenorrhea, Bursitis, Tendonitis
PO: ADULTS, ELDERLY: Initially, 500 mg naproxen (550 mg naproxen sodium), then 250 mg naproxen (275 mg naproxen sodium) q6–8h as needed. **Maximum:** 1.25 g/day naproxen (1.375 g/day naproxen sodium). **Naprelan:** 1,000 mg once daily.

Juvenile Rheumatoid Arthritis (JRA)
PO (Naproxen Only): **CHILDREN OLDER THAN 2 YRS:** 10 mg/kg/day in 2 divided doses. **Maximum:** 1,000 mg/day.

OTC Uses
PO: ADULTS 65 YRS AND YOUNGER, CHILDREN 12 YRS AND OLDER: 220 mg (200 mg naproxen sodium) q8–12h. May take 440 mg (400 mg naproxen sodium) as initial dose. **ADULTS OLDER THAN 65 YRS:** 220 mg (200 mg naproxen sodium) q12h.

Renal Impairment
Not recommended with creatinine clearance less than 30 ml/min.

SIDE EFFECTS

Frequent (9%–4%): Nausea, constipation, abdominal cramps/pain, heartburn, dizziness, headache, drowsiness. **Occasional (3%–1%):** Stomatitis, diarrhea, indigestion. **Rare (less than 1%):** Vomiting, confusion.

ADVERSE EFFECTS/ TOXIC REACTIONS

Rare reactions with long-term use include peptic ulcer, GI bleeding, gastritis, severe hepatic reactions (cholestasis, jaundice), nephrotoxicity (dysuria, hematuria, proteinuria, nephrotic syndrome), and severe hypersensitivity reaction (fever, chills, bronchospasm).

NURSING CONSIDERATIONS

BASELINE ASSESSMENT

Assess onset, type, location, duration of pain/inflammation. Inspect appearance of affected joints for immobility, deformities, skin condition.

INTERVENTION/EVALUATION

Assist with ambulation if dizziness occurs. Monitor CBC, serum renal/hepatic function tests, daily pattern of bowel activity, stool consistency. Evaluate for therapeutic response: relief of pain, stiffness, swelling; increased joint mobility; reduced joint tenderness; improved grip strength.

PATIENT/FAMILY TEACHING

• Avoid tasks that require alertness, motor skills until response to drug is established. • Take with food, milk. • Avoid aspirin, alcohol during therapy (increases risk of GI bleeding). • Report headache, rash, visual disturbances, weight gain, black or tarry stools, bleeding, persistent headache.

naratriptan

nar-a-**trip**-tan
(Amerge)
Do not confuse naratriptan with eletriptan or almotriptan, or Amerge with Altace or Amaryl.

◆CLASSIFICATION

PHARMACOTHERAPEUTIC: Serotonin receptor agonist. **CLINICAL:** Antimigraine (see p. 64C).

ACTION

Binds selectively to vascular receptors, producing vasoconstrictive effect on cranial blood vessels. **Therapeutic Effect:** Relieves migraine headache.

PHARMACOKINETICS

Well absorbed after PO administration. Protein binding: 28%–31%. Metabolized in liver. Eliminated primarily in urine and, to lesser extent, in feces. **Half-life:** 6 hrs (increased in hepatic/renal impairment).

USES

Treatment of acute migraine headache with or without aura in adults.

PRECAUTIONS

Contraindications: Basilar/hemiplegic migraine, cerebrovascular disease, peripheral vascular disease, coronary artery disease, ischemic heart disease (including angina pectoris, history of MI, silent ischemia, Prinzmetal's angina), severe hepatic impairment (Child-Pugh grade C), severe renal impairment (serum creatinine less than 15 ml/min), uncontrolled hypertension, use within 24 hrs of ergotamine-containing preparations or another serotonin receptor agonist, 5-HT agonist (e.g., sumatriptan), MAOI use within 14 days. **Cautions:** Mild to moderate renal/hepatic impairment, pt profile suggesting cardiovascular risks.

⏳ LIFESPAN CONSIDERATIONS

Pregnancy/Lactation: Unknown if drug is distributed in breast milk. **Pregnancy Category C. Children:** Safety and efficacy not established. **Elderly:** Not recommended in the elderly.

INTERACTIONS

DRUG: Ergotamine-containing medications may produce vasospastic reaction. **SSRIs** and **SNRIs (e.g., fluoxetine, fluvoxamine, paroxetine, sertraline)** may produce serotonin syndrome (e.g., hyperreflexia, incoordination, weakness). **HERBAL:** None significant. **FOOD:** None known. **LAB VALUES:** None significant.

AVAILABILITY (Rx)

🖤 **Tablets:** 1 mg, 2.5 mg.

ADMINISTRATION/HANDLING

PO
• Give without regard to food. • Do not break, crush, dissolve, or divide tablets. Swallow whole with water.

INDICATIONS/ROUTES/DOSAGE

Acute Migraine Attack
PO: ADULTS: 1 or 2.5 mg. If headache improves but then returns, dose may be repeated after 4 hrs. **Maximum:** 5 mg/24 hrs.

N

 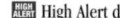

Dosage in Renal/Hepatic Impairment

Hepatic Failure	Creatinine Clearance	Dosage
Mild to moderate	15–39 ml/min	Initial, 1 mg. Max: 2.5/24 hrs
Severe	Less than 15 ml/min	Do not use

SIDE EFFECTS

Occasional (5%): Nausea. **Rare (2%):** Paresthesia, dizziness, fatigue, drowsiness, feeling of pressure in throat, neck, jaw.

ADVERSE EFFECTS/ TOXIC REACTIONS

Corneal opacities, other ocular defects may occur. Cardiac events (ischemia, coronary artery vasospasm, MI), noncardiac vasospasm-related reactions (hemorrhage, cerebrovascular accident [CVA]) occur rarely, particularly in pts with hypertension, diabetes, strong family history of coronary artery disease, obese pts, smokers, males older than 40 yrs, postmenopausal women.

NURSING CONSIDERATIONS

BASELINE ASSESSMENT

Question for history of peripheral vascular disease, renal/hepatic impairment, possibility of pregnancy. Question pt regarding possible precipitating symptoms, onset, location, duration of migraine.

INTERVENTION/EVALUATION

Assess for relief of migraine headache; potential for photophobia, phonophobia (sound sensitivity), nausea, vomiting.

PATIENT/FAMILY TEACHING

• Do not chew, crush, dissolve, or divide tablet; swallow whole with water. • May repeat dose after 4 hrs (maximum of 5 mg/24 hrs). • May cause dizziness, fatigue, drowsiness. • Avoid tasks that require alertness, motor skills until response to drug is established. • Report any chest pain, palpitations, tightness in throat, rash, hallucinations, anxiety, panic.

natalizumab

na-ta-**liz**-yoo-mab
(Tysabri)

BLACK BOX ALERT Restricted distribution program (TOUCH), given only to program-qualified/enrolled pts. Increased risk of leukoencephalopathy (progressive, often fatal viral brain infection).

◆CLASSIFICATION

PHARMACOTHERAPEUTIC: Monoclonal antibody. **CLINICAL:** Multiple sclerosis agent, immunologic agent.

ACTION

Binds to surface of leukocytes, inhibiting adhesion of leukocytes to vascular endothelial cells of GI tract, preventing migration of leukocytes across endothelium into inflamed parenchymal tissue. **Therapeutic Effect:** Inhibits inflammatory activity of activated immune cells, reduces clinical exacerbations of multiple sclerosis, Crohn's disease.

PHARMACOKINETICS

Steady state reached in approximately 16–24 wks. **Half-life:** 11 days.

USES

Treatment of relapsing forms of multiple sclerosis to reduce frequency of clinical exacerbations. Treatment of moderate to severe Crohn's disease in pts with inadequate response or unable to tolerate conventional Crohn's disease therapies.

PRECAUTIONS

Contraindications: Pts who have or have had progressive multifocal leukoencephalopathy (PML). **Cautions:** Chronic progressive multiple sclerosis, children younger than 18 yrs. Concomitant immunosuppressants (may increase risk of infection).

⌛ LIFESPAN CONSIDERATIONS

Pregnancy/Lactation: Unknown if drug crosses placenta or is distributed in breast milk. **Pregnancy Category C. Children:** Safety and efficacy not established in those younger than 18 yrs. **Elderly:** No age-related precautions noted.

INTERACTIONS

DRUG: Antineoplastics, immunomodulating agents, immunosuppresants may increase risk of PML. **HERBAL:** None significant. **FOOD:** None known. **LAB VALUES:** May increase basophils, lymphocytes, monocytes, eosinophils, red blood cells (usually reversible within 16 wks after last dose).

AVAILABILITY (Rx)

Injection Solution: 300 mg/15 ml concentrate.

ADMINISTRATION/HANDLING
 IV

Reconstitution • Withdraw 15 ml natalizumab from vial; inject concentrate into 100 ml 0.9% NaCl. • Invert solution to mix completely; do not shake. • Discard if solution is discolored or particulate forms.
Rate of Administration • Infuse over 1 hr. • Following completion of infusion, flush with 0.9% NaCl.
Storage • Refrigerate vials. • Do not shake, freeze. Protect from light. • After reconstitution, solution is stable for 8 hrs if refrigerated.

🔲 IV INCOMPATIBILITIES

Do not mix with any other medications or diluent other than 0.9% NaCl.

INDICATIONS/ROUTES/DOSAGE

Relapsed Multiple Sclerosis,
Crohn's Disease
IV Infusion: ADULTS 18 YRS AND OLDER, ELDERLY: 300 mg every 4 wks.

SIDE EFFECTS

Frequent (35%–15%): Headache, fatigue, depression, arthralgia. **Occasional (10%–5%):** Abdominal discomfort, rash, urinary urgency/frequency, irregular menstruation/dysmenorrhea, dermatitis. **Rare**

(4%–2%): Pruritus, chest discomfort, local bleeding, rigors, tremor, syncope.

ADVERSE EFFECTS/ TOXIC REACTIONS

UTI, lower respiratory tract infection, gastroenteritis, vaginitis, allergic reaction, tonsillitis, PMI.

NURSING CONSIDERATIONS

BASELINE ASSESSMENT

Obtain CBC, serum chemistries, hepatic function test. Assess home situation for support of therapy.

INTERVENTION/EVALUATION

Periodically monitor lab results. Assess for arthralgia, depression, urinary changes, menstrual irregularities. Assess skin for evidence of rash, pruritus, dermatitis. Monitor for signs/symptoms of UTI, respiratory infection.

---

nateglinide

na-**te**-glye-nide
(Starlix)

◆CLASSIFICATION

PHARMACOTHERAPEUTIC: Antihyperglycemic. **CLINICAL:** Antidiabetic agent (see p. 45C).

ACTION

Stimulates insulin release from beta cells of pancreas by depolarizing beta cells, leading to opening of calcium channels. Resulting calcium influx induces insulin secretion. **Therapeutic Effect:** Lowers serum glucose concentration.

PHARMACOKINETICS

Route	Onset	Peak	Duration
PO	20 min	1 hr	4 hrs

Rapidly absorbed from GI tract. Protein binding: 98%. Extensive metabolism in liver. Primarily excreted in urine; minimal elimination in feces. **Half-life:** 1.5 hrs.

USES

Treatment of type 2 diabetes mellitus in pts whose disease cannot be adequately controlled with diet and exercise; pts who have not been chronically treated with other antidiabetic agents. Used as monotherapy or in combination with metformin or a thiazolidinedione.

PRECAUTIONS

Contraindications: Diabetic ketoacidosis, type 1 diabetes mellitus. **Cautions:** Hepatic/renal impairment, adrenal/pituitary dysfunction.

⏳ LIFESPAN CONSIDERATIONS

Pregnancy/Lactation: Unknown if drug crosses placenta or is distributed in breast milk. **Pregnancy Category C. Children:** Safety and efficacy not established. **Elderly:** Increased susceptibility to hypoglycemia.

INTERACTIONS

DRUG: Beta-blockers may mask symptoms of hypoglycemia. **Beta-blockers, MAOIs, NSAIDs, salicylates** may increase hypoglycemic effect. **Corticosteroids, sympathomimetics, thiazide diuretics, thyroid medications** may decrease hypoglycemic effect. **HERBAL: Bilberry, garlic, ginger, ginseng** may increase hypoglycemic effect. **St. John's wort** may decrease concentration/effects. **FOOD:** None known. **LAB VALUES:** Decrease in serum glucose expected.

AVAILABILITY (Rx)

Tablets: 60 mg, 120 mg.

ADMINISTRATION/HANDLING

PO
• Ideally, give within 15 min of a meal, but may be given immediately before a meal to as long as 30 min before a meal.

INDICATIONS/ROUTES/DOSAGE

Diabetes Mellitus
PO: ADULTS, ELDERLY: 120 mg 3 times a day before meals. 60 mg 3 times a day may be given in pts close to HbA$_{1C}$ goal.

SIDE EFFECTS

Frequent (10%): Upper respiratory tract infection. **Occasional (4%–3%):** Back pain, flu symptoms, dizziness, arthropathy, diarrhea. **Rare (2% or less):** Bronchitis, cough.

ADVERSE EFFECTS/TOXIC REACTIONS

Hypoglycemia occurs in less than 2% of pts.

NURSING CONSIDERATIONS

BASELINE ASSESSMENT

Check fasting serum glucose, Hgb (A1c) periodically to determine minimum effective dose. Discuss lifestyle to determine extent of learning, emotional needs. Ensure follow-up instruction if pt, family do not thoroughly understand diabetes management, glucose-testing technique. At least 1 wk should elapse to assess response to drug before new dose adjustment is made.

INTERVENTION/EVALUATION

Monitor serum glucose, food intake. Assess for hypoglycemia (cool, wet skin, tremors, dizziness, anxiety, headache, tachycardia, numbness in mouth, hunger, diplopia), hyperglycemia (polyuria, polyphagia, polydipsia, nausea, vomiting, dim vision, fatigue, deep rapid breathing). Be alert to conditions that alter glucose requirements: fever, increased activity, stress, surgical procedures.

PATIENT/FAMILY TEACHING

• Diabetes mellitus requires lifelong control. • Prescribed diet, exercise are principal parts of treatment; do not skip, delay meals. • Continue to adhere to dietary instructions, regular exercise program, regular testing of serum glucose.

nebivolol

ne-**biv**-oh-lol
(Bystolic)
**Do not confuse nebivolol with
nadolol or atenolol.**

◆CLASSIFICATION

PHARMACOTHERAPEUTIC: Beta-adrenergic blocker. **CLINICAL:** Antihypertensive (see p. 73C).

ACTION

Predominantly blocks beta$_1$-adrenergic receptors. Large doses block both beta$_1$ and beta$_2$ receptors. **Therapeutic Effect:** Slows sinus heart rate, decreases myocardial contractility, B/P.

PHARMACOKINETICS

	Onset	Peak	Duration
PO	30 min	1.5–4 hrs	12 hrs

Completely absorbed from GI tract. Protein binding: 98%. Metabolized in liver. Excreted in feces (44%), urine (38%). **Half-life:** 12 hrs (increased in severe renal impairment).

USES

Management of hypertension. Used alone or in combination with other antihypertensives. **OFF-LABEL:** HF.

PRECAUTIONS

Contraindications: Severe bradycardia, overt cardiac failure, cardiogenic shock, heart block greater than first degree, severe hepatic impairment, sick sinus rhythm (unless pt has pacemaker). **Cautions:** Diabetes mellitus, acute exacerbation of coronary artery disease.

⧖ LIFESPAN CONSIDERATIONS

Pregnancy/Lactation: May cross placenta; appears to be distributed in breast milk. May produce low birthweight infants. **Pregnancy Category C (D** in second or third trimester). **Children:** Safety and efficacy not established. **Elderly:** No age-related precautions noted.

INTERACTIONS

DRUG: Diuretics, other hypotensives may increase hypotensive effect. **CYP2D6 inhibitors (e.g., fluoxetine, paroxetine)** may increase concentration/effect. **HERBAL: Ephedra, ginseng, yohimbe, ginger, licorice** may worsen hypertension. **Black cohosh, periwinkle** may increase antihypertensive effect. **FOOD:** None known. **LAB VALUES:** May increase BUN, serum uric acid, AST, ALT, bilirubin, triglycerides. May decrease platelet count, serum HDL.

AVAILABILITY (Rx)

▼ **Tablets:** 2.5 mg, 5 mg, 10 mg, 20 mg.

ADMINISTRATION/HANDLING

PO
• Give without regard to meals. • Do not break, crush, dissolve, or divide tablets.

INDICATIONS/ROUTES/DOSAGE

Hypertension
PO: ADULTS, ELDERLY: Initially, 5 mg once a day alone or in combination with other antihypertensives. May increase at 2-wk intervals to maximum 40 mg once a day.

Severe Renal Impairment (Creatinine Clearance Less Than 30 ml/min)
PO: ADULTS, ELDERLY: Initially, 2.5 mg once a day. Increase dose cautiously.

Moderate Hepatic Impairment
PO: ADULTS, ELDERLY: Initially, 2.5 mg once a day. Increase cautiously.

SIDE EFFECTS

Generally well tolerated, with mild and transient side effects. **Occasional (9%):** Headache. **Rare (2%–1%):** Fatigue, dizziness, diarrhea, nausea, insomnia, peripheral edema.

N

ADVERSE EFFECTS/ TOXIC REACTIONS

Large doses may produce bradycardia, dyspnea, rash. Acute pulmonary edema, renal failure, AV block reported. **Antidote:** Glucagon (see Appendix K for dosage).

NURSING CONSIDERATIONS

BASELINE ASSESSMENT

Assess baseline renal/hepatic function tests. Assess B/P, apical pulse immediately before drug administration (if pulse is 60/min or less, or systolic B/P is less than 90 mm Hg, withhold medication, contact physician).

INTERVENTION/EVALUATION

Measure B/P near end of dosing interval (determines whether B/P is controlled throughout day). Monitor B/P for hypotension. Assess pulse for quality, irregular rate, bradycardia. Question for evidence of headache.

PATIENT/FAMILY TEACHING

• Compliance with therapy regimen is essential to control hypertension. • Do not use nasal decongestants, OTC cold preparations (stimulants) without physician's approval. • Monitor B/P, pulse before taking medication. • Restrict salt, alcohol intake. • Do not chew, crush, dissolve, or divide tablets. Swallow whole.

---

nelarabine HIGH ALERT

nel-**ar**-a-bine
(Arranon, Atriance ✦)
BLACK BOX ALERT Dose-limiting neurotoxicity (confusion, severe drowsiness, seizures, ataxia, ascending neuropathy). Must be administered by certified chemotherapy personnel.

◆CLASSIFICATION

PHARMACOTHERAPEUTIC: DNA demethylation agent. **CLINICAL:** Antineoplastic; antimetabolite (see p. 89C).

ACTION

Incorporates into DNA, leading to inhibition of DNA synthesis. Exerts cytotoxic effect on rapidly dividing cells by causing demethylation of DNA. **Therapeutic Effect:** Produces cell death.

PHARMACOKINETICS

Rapidly eliminated from plasma. Widely distributed. Protein binding: less than 25%. Partially eliminated in urine. **Half-life:** 30 min.

USES

Treatment of T-cell acute lymphoblastic leukemia (ALL), T-cell lymphoblastic lymphoma in pts whose disease has not responded to or has relapsed following treatment with at least two chemotherapy regimens.

PRECAUTIONS

Contraindications: None known. **Cautions:** Bone marrow suppression, elevated uric acid, gout, history of uric acid stones, severe hepatic impairment, renal impairment.

▧ LIFESPAN CONSIDERATIONS

Pregnancy/Lactation: May cause developmental abnormalities of the fetus. Breastfeeding not recommended. **Pregnancy Category D. Children:** No age-related precautions noted. **Elderly:** Increased risk of neurologic toxicities.

INTERACTIONS

DRUG: Live virus vaccines may potentiate virus replication, increase vaccine side effects, decrease pt's antibody response to vaccine. **HERBAL: Echinacea** may decrease effects. **FOOD:** None known. **LAB VALUES:** May decrease Hgb, Hct, WBCs, RBCs, platelets, serum albumin, calcium, glucose, magnesium, potassium. May increase serum bilirubin, creatinine, AST.

AVAILABILITY (Rx)

Injection Solution: 250 mg (5 mg/ml) in 50-ml vials (Arranon).

ADMINISTRATION/HANDLING

 IV

Reconstitution • Do not dilute before administration. • Transfer appropriate dose into polyvinylchloride infusion bag or glass container before administration.
Rate of Administration • Administer as 2-hr infusion for adults, 1-hr infusion for pediatric pts.
Storage • Store vials at room temperature. • Solution should appear colorless, free of precipitate. Undiluted injection solution stable for 8 hrs in PVC infusion bag or glass container.

INDICATIONS/ROUTES/DOSAGE

T-Cell Leukemia, Lymphoma
IV: ADULTS, ELDERLY: 1,500 mg/m^2 infused over 2 hrs on days 1, 3, and 5 repeated q21days. **CHILDREN:** 650 mg/m^2 infused over 1 hr daily for 5 consecutive days repeated q21days.

SIDE EFFECTS

ADULTS
Frequent (50%–41%): Fatigue, nausea. **Occasional (25%–11%):** Cough, fever, drowsiness, vomiting, dyspnea, diarrhea, constipation, dizziness, asthenia (loss of strength, energy), peripheral edema, paresthesia, headache, peripheral neuropathy, myalgia, petechiae, generalized edema. **Rare (9%–4%):** Anorexia, abdominal pain, arthralgia, hypertension, tachycardia, confusion, rigors, stomatitis, back pain, epistaxis, insomnia, dehydration, extremity pain, depression, abdominal distention, blurred vision.

CHILDREN
Frequent (17%): Headache. **Occasional (10%–6%):** Vomiting, drowsiness, asthenia (loss of strength, energy), peripheral neuropathy. **Rare (4%–2%):** Paresthesia, tremor, ataxia.

ADVERSE EFFECTS/ TOXIC REACTIONS

Overdose may result in severe neurotoxicity, myelosuppression. Hematologic toxicity manifested as thrombocytopenia, neutropenia, anemia occurs in most cases. Pleural effusion occurs in 10% of pts, pneumonia in 8% of pts, seizures in 6% of pts.

NURSING CONSIDERATIONS

BASELINE ASSESSMENT

Give emotional support. Use strict asepsis, protect pt from infection. Hydration, urine alkalization, prophylaxis with allopurinol must be given to prevent hyperuricemia of tumor lysis syndrome. Perform blood counts as needed to monitor response and toxicity but esp. before each dosing cycle.

INTERVENTION/EVALUATION

Monitor for neurologic toxicity (severe drowsiness, confusion, seizure), hematologic toxicity (fever, sore throat, signs of local infections, unusual bruising/bleeding), symptoms of anemia (excessive fatigue, weakness). Assess response to medication; monitor and report nausea, vomiting, diarrhea. Avoid rectal temperatures, other traumas that may induce bleeding. Monitor renal/hepatic function.

PATIENT/FAMILY TEACHING

• Do not have immunizations without physician's approval (drug lowers resistance). • Avoid crowds, persons with known infections. • Report signs of infection at once (fever, flu-like symptoms). • Report persistent nausea/ vomiting. • Advise men to use barrier contraception while receiving treatment. • Measures should be taken to avoid pregnancy. • Report new or worsening symptoms of peripheral neuropathy.

---

nelfinavir

nel-**fin**-a-veer
(Viracept)
Do not confuse nelfinavir with nevirapine, or Viracept with Viramune.

N

◆CLASSIFICATION

PHARMACOTHERAPEUTIC: Protease inhibitor. **CLINICAL:** Antiviral (see pp. 70C, 120C).

ACTION

Inhibits activity of HIV-1 protease, the enzyme necessary for formation of infectious HIV. **Therapeutic Effect:** Formation of immature noninfectious viral particles rather than HIV replication.

PHARMACOKINETICS

Well absorbed after PO administration (absorption increased with food). Protein binding: 98%. Metabolized in liver. Eliminated primarily in feces. Unknown if removed by hemodialysis. **Half-life:** 3.5–5 hrs.

USES

Treatment of HIV infection in combination with at least two other antiretrovirals.

PRECAUTIONS

Contraindications: Concurrent administration with alfuzosin, amiodarone, ergot derivatives, lovastatin, midazolam (oral), pimozide, quinidine, rifampin, sildenafil (when used for pulmonary arterial hypertension), simvastatin, St. John's wort, triazolam. **Cautions:** Hepatic impairment.

⌛ LIFESPAN CONSIDERATIONS

Pregnancy/Lactation: Unknown if distributed in breast milk. **Pregnancy Category B. Children:** No age-related precautions noted in those older than 2 yrs. **Elderly:** No information available.

INTERACTIONS

DRUG: May increase toxicity of **colchicine. Anticonvulsants (e.g., carbamazepine, phenytoin)** may decrease concentration. May increase concentration of **fluticasone, immunosuppressants (e.g., cyclosporine, sirolimus, tacrolimus), saquinavir, trazodone,** lovastatin, atorvastatin. May decrease effects of **oral contraceptives. HERBAL: St. John's wort** may decrease concentration/effects. **FOOD: All foods** increase concentration. **LAB VALUES:** May decrease neutrophil.

AVAILABILITY (Rx)

Powder for Oral Suspension: 50 mg/g. **Tablets:** 250 mg, 625 mg.

ADMINISTRATION/HANDLING

PO
• Give with food (light meal, snack). • Tablets can be dissolved in water then mixed with milk or crushed and mixed with pudding. • Mix oral powder with small amount of water, milk, formula, soy formula, soy milk, dietary supplement. • Entire contents must be consumed in order to ingest full dose. • Do not mix with acidic food, orange juice, apple juice, applesauce (bitter taste), or with water in original oral powder container.

INDICATIONS/ROUTES/DOSAGE

HIV Infection
PO: ADULTS: 750 mg (three 250-mg tablets) 3 times a day or 1,250 mg (two 625-mg tablets) twice a day in combination with other antiretrovirals. **CHILDREN 2–13 YRS:** 45–55 mg/kg twice a day or 25–35 mg/kg 3 times a day. **Maximum:** 2,500 mg/day.

SIDE EFFECTS

Frequent (20%): Diarrhea. **Occasional (7%–3%):** Nausea, rash. **Rare (2%–1%):** Flatulence, asthenia (loss of strength, energy).

ADVERSE EFFECTS/ TOXIC REACTIONS

Diabetes mellitus, hyperglycemia occur rarely.

NURSING CONSIDERATIONS

BASELINE ASSESSMENT

Obtain baseline CBC, hepatic function tests for accurate baseline.

INTERVENTION/EVALUATION

Monitor daily pattern of bowel activity, stool consistency. Monitor hepatic enzyme studies for abnormalities. Be alert to development of opportunistic infections (fever, chills, cough, myalgia).

PATIENT/FAMILY TEACHING

• Take with food (optimizes absorption). • Take medication every day as prescribed. • Doses should be evenly spaced around the clock. • Do not alter dose, discontinue medication without informing physician. • Nelfinavir is not a cure for HIV infection nor does it reduce risk of transmission to others. • Illnesses, including opportunistic infections, may still occur.

neostigmine

nee-oh-**stig**-meen
(Prostigmin)
Do not confuse neostigmine or Prostigmin with physostigmine.

◆ CLASSIFICATION

PHARMACOTHERAPEUTIC: Cholinergic. **CLINICAL:** Antimyasthenic agent, antidote.

ACTION

Prevents destruction of acetylcholine by attaching to enzyme acetylcholinesterase, enhancing impulse transmission across myoneural junction. **Therapeutic Effect:** Improves intestinal/skeletal muscle tone; stimulates salivary, sweat gland secretions.

USES

Improvement of muscle strength in control of myasthenia gravis, diagnosis of myasthenia gravis, prevention/treatment of postop bladder distention, urinary retention; antidote for reversal of effects of nondepolarizing neuromuscular blocking agents after surgery.

PRECAUTIONS

Contraindications: GI/GU obstruction, history of hypersensitivity reaction to bromides. **Cautions:** Epilepsy, asthma, bradycardia, hyperthyroidism, arrhythmias, peptic ulcer. **Pregnancy Category C.**

INTERACTIONS

DRUG: Anticholinergics reverse, prevent effects. **Cholinesterase inhibitors** may increase risk of toxicity. Antagonizes effects of **neuromuscular blockers.** **HERBAL:** None significant. **FOOD:** None known. **LAB VALUES:** None significant.

AVAILABILITY (Rx)

Injection Solution (Prostigmin): 0.5 mg/ml, 1 mg/ml. **Tablets (Prostigmin):** 15 mg.

ADMINISTRATION/HANDLING

◀**ALERT**▶ Give 0.011 mg/kg atropine sulfate IV simultaneously with neostigmine or IM 30 min before administering neostigmine to prevent adverse effects.

PO
• May administer with or without food.

🔳 IV COMPATIBILITIES

Glycopyrrolate (Robinul), heparin, ondansetron (Zofran), potassium chloride, thiopental (Pentothal).

INDICATIONS/ROUTES/DOSAGE

Myasthenia Gravis
PO: ADULTS, ELDERLY: Initially, 15 mg 3–4 times a day. Gradually increase as necessary q1–2days. Maintenance: 150 mg/day (range of 15–375 mg). **CHILDREN:** 2 mg/kg/day or 60 mg/m²/day divided q3–4h, not to exceed 375 mg/day.
IV, IM, Subcutaneous: ADULTS: 0.5–2.5 mg q1–3h up to 10 mg/24 hrs. **CHILDREN:** 0.01–0.04 mg/kg q2–4h.

Diagnosis of Myasthenia Gravis
◀**ALERT**▶ Discontinue all cholinesterase medications at least 8 hrs before testing; atropine should be given IV immediately before or IM 30 min before neostigmine.

N

IM: ADULTS, ELDERLY: 0.02 mg/kg as single dose. CHILDREN: 0.025–0.04 mg/kg as a single dose.

Prevention of Postop Bladder Distention, Urinary Retention
IM, Subcutaneous: ADULTS, ELDERLY: 0.25 mg q4–6h for 2–3 days.

Treatment of Postop Bladder Distention, Urinary Retention
IM, Subcutaneous: ADULTS, ELDERLY: 0.5–1 mg q3h for 5 doses after bladder has been emptied.

Reversal of Neuromuscular Blockade After Surgery
IV: ADULTS, ELDERLY: 0.5–2.5 mg given slowly. CHILDREN: 0.025–0.08 mg/kg/dose. INFANTS: 0.025–0.1 mg/kg/dose.

Dosage in Renal Impairment

Creatinine Clearance	Dose
10–50 ml/min	50% of normal dose
Less than 10 ml/min	25% of normal dose

SIDE EFFECTS

Frequent: Muscarinic effects (diarrhea, diaphoresis, increased salivation, nausea, vomiting, abdominal cramps/pain). **Occasional:** Muscarinic effects (urinary urgency/frequency, increased bronchial secretions, miosis, lacrimation).

ADVERSE EFFECTS/ TOXIC REACTIONS

Overdose produces cholinergic crisis manifested as abdominal discomfort/cramps, nausea, vomiting, diarrhea, flushing, facial warmth, excessive salivation, diaphoresis, lacrimation, pallor, bradycardia, tachycardia, hypotension, bronchospasm, urinary urgency, blurred vision, miosis, fasciculation (involuntary muscular contractions visible under skin).

NURSING CONSIDERATIONS

BASELINE ASSESSMENT
Larger doses should be given at time of greatest fatigue. Avoid large doses in pts with megacolon, reduced GI motility.

INTERVENTION/EVALUATION
Monitor muscle strength, vital signs. Monitor for therapeutic response to medication (increased muscle strength, decreased fatigue, improved chewing, swallowing functions).

PATIENT/FAMILY TEACHING
• Report nausea, vomiting, diarrhea, diaphoresis, increased salivary secretions, palpitations, muscle weakness, severe abdominal pain, difficulty breathing.

nesiritide

ness-**ear**-i-tide
(Natrecor)

◆CLASSIFICATION
PHARMACOTHERAPEUTIC: Brain natriuretic peptide. **CLINICAL:** Endogenous hormone.

ACTION
Facilitates cardiovascular homeostasis, fluid status through counterregulation of renin-angiotensin-aldosterone system, stimulating cyclic guanosine monophosphate, thereby leading to smooth muscle cell relaxation. **Therapeutic Effect:** Promotes vasodilation, natriuresis, diuresis, correcting HF.

PHARMACOKINETICS

Route	Onset	Peak	Duration
IV	15 min	1 hr	Up to 4 hrs

Excreted primarily in heart by left ventricle. Metabolized by natriuretic neutral endopeptidase enzymes on vascular luminal surface. **Half-life:** 18–23 min.

USES

Treatment of acutely decompensated HF in pts who have dyspnea at rest or with minimal activity.

PRECAUTIONS

Contraindications: Cardiogenic shock, systolic B/P less than 100 mm Hg prior to therapy. **Cautions:** Significant valvular stenosis, restrictive/obstructive cardiomyopathy, constrictive pericarditis, pericardial tamponade, suspected low cardiac filling pressures, atrial/ventricular arrhythmias/conduction defects, renal insufficiency.

⌛ LIFESPAN CONSIDERATIONS

Pregnancy/Lactation: Unknown if drug crosses placenta or is distributed in breast milk. **Pregnancy Category C. Children:** Safety and efficacy not established. **Elderly:** No age-related precautions noted.

INTERACTIONS

DRUG: None significant. **HERBAL: Ephedra, ginger, ginseng, licorice** may increase B/P. **Black cohosh, goldenseal, hawthorne** may decrease B/P. **FOOD:** None known. **LAB VALUES:** May increase serum creatinine.

AVAILABILITY (Rx)

Injection, Powder for Reconstitution: 1.5 mg/5-ml vial.

ADMINISTRATION/HANDLING

◀**ALERT**▶ Do not mix with other injections, infusions. Do not give IM.

 IV

Reconstitution • Reconstitute one 1.5-mg vial with 5 ml D₅W or 0.9% NaCl, 0.2% NaCl, or any combination thereof. Swirl or rock gently, add to 250-ml bag D₅W or 0.9% NaCl, 0.2% NaCl, or any combination thereof, yielding a solution of 6 mcg/ml.
Rate of Administration • Give as IV bolus over approximately 60 sec initially, followed by continuous IV infusion.

Storage • Store vial at room temperature. Once reconstituted, vials are stable at 36°–77°F (2°–25°C) for up to 24 hrs. Use reconstituted solution within 24 hrs.

🚫 IV INCOMPATIBILITIES

Bumetanide (Bumex), enalapril (Vasotec), ethacrynic acid (Edecrin), furosemide (Lasix), heparin, hydralazine (Apresoline), insulin, sodium metabisulfite.

INDICATIONS/ROUTES/DOSAGE

Treatment of Acute HF
IV Bolus: ADULTS, ELDERLY: 2 mcg/kg followed by continuous IV infusion of 0.01 mcg/kg/min. At intervals of 3 hrs or longer, may be increased by 0.005 mcg/kg/min (preceded by bolus of 1 mcg/kg), up to maximum of 0.03 mcg/kg/min.

SIDE EFFECTS

Frequent (11%): Hypotension. **Occasional (8%–2%):** Headache, nausea, bradycardia. **Rare (1% or less):** Confusion, paresthesia, drowsiness, tremor.

ADVERSE EFFECTS/ TOXIC REACTIONS

Ventricular arrhythmias (ventricular tachycardia, atrial fibrillation, AV node conduction abnormalities), angina pectoris occur rarely.

NURSING CONSIDERATIONS

BASELINE ASSESSMENT

Obtain B/P immediately before each dose, in addition to regular monitoring (be alert to fluctuations).

INTERVENTION/EVALUATION

Monitor B/P, pulse rate for hypotension frequently during therapy. Hypotension is dose-limiting and dose-dependent. If excessive reduction in B/P occurs, place pt in supine position with legs elevated. With physician, establish parameters for adjusting rate, stopping infusion. Maintain accurate I&O; measure urinary output frequently. Immediately notify physician of decreased urinary output, cardiac

N

arrhythmias, significant decrease in B/P, heart rate.

PATIENT/FAMILY TEACHING
• Report chest pain, palpitations.

nevirapine

ne-**vye**-ra-peen
(Viramune, Viramune XR)

BLACK BOX ALERT Potentially severe, life-threatening dermatologic hypersensitivity, hepatic reactions may occur. Greatest risk occurs within first 6 wks of treatment.
Do not confuse nevirapine with nelfinavir, or Viramune with Viracept.

◆ CLASSIFICATION

PHARMACOTHERAPEUTIC: Non-nucleoside reverse transcriptase inhibitor. **CLINICAL:** Antiviral (see p. 119C).

ACTION

Binds directly to HIV-1 reverse transcriptase, changing shape of enzyme, blocking RNA-, DNA-dependent polymerase activity. **Therapeutic Effect:** Interferes with HIV replication, slowing progression of HIV infection.

PHARMACOKINETICS

Readily absorbed after PO administration. Protein binding: 60%. Widely distributed. Metabolized in liver. Excreted primarily in urine. **Half-life:** 45 hrs (single dose); 25–30 hrs (multiple doses).

USES

Used in combination with at least two other anti-retroviral agents for treatment of HIV-1 infected adults who have experienced clinical, immunologic deterioration.

PRECAUTIONS

Contraindications: Moderate to severe hepatic impairment, use in occupational or nonoccupational postexposure prophylaxis (PEP) regimens. **Cautions:** Elevated AST, ALT levels, history of chronic hepatitis (B or C), higher $CD4^+$ cell counts (greater risk of hepatic events), renal impairment.

⌛ LIFESPAN CONSIDERATIONS

Pregnancy/Lactation: Crosses placenta. Distributed in breast milk. Breastfeeding not recommended (possibility of HIV transmission). **Pregnancy Category C. Children:** Granulocytopenia occurs more frequently. **Elderly:** No information available.

INTERACTIONS

DRUG: May decrease concentrations of **ketoconazole, oral contraceptives, clarithromycin, protease inhibitors. Rifabutin, rifampin** may decrease concentration. **HERBAL: St. John's wort** may decrease concentration/effects. **FOOD:** None known. **LAB VALUES:** May increase serum bilirubin, alkaline phosphatase, GGT, AST, ALT. May decrease Hgb, neutrophil, platelet counts.

AVAILABILITY (Rx)

Oral Suspension: 50 mg/5 ml. **Tablets:** 200 mg.

🔖 **Tablets, Extended-Release:** 400 mg.

ADMINISTRATION/HANDLING
PO
• Give without regard to meals. May give with water, milk, or soda. • Shake suspension gently prior to administration. • Give extended-release tablets whole; do not break, crush, dissolve, or divide.

INDICATIONS/ROUTES/DOSAGE
HIV Infection
PO: ADULTS: 200 mg once daily for 14 days (to reduce risk of rash). Maintenance: 200 mg twice daily in combination with nucleoside analogues. **CHILDREN 8 YRS AND OLDER:** Initially, 120–150 mg/m²/dose (**maximum:** 200 mg) once daily for 14 days. Increase to 120–150 mg/m²/dose twice daily (if no rash).

CHILDREN 8 YRS OF AGE OR YOUNGER: 200 mg/m²/dose once daily for 14 days (**maximum:** 200 mg). Increase to 200 mg/m²/dose twice daily (if no rash).

Extended-Release Dosage
PO: ADULTS, ELDERLY: 400 mg once daily.

SIDE EFFECTS

Frequent (8%–3%): Rash, fever, headache, nausea, granulocytopenia (more common in children). **Occasional (2%–1%):** Stomatitis (burning, erythema, ulceration of oral mucosa; dysphagia). **Rare (less than 1%):** Paresthesia, myalgia, abdominal pain.

ADVERSE EFFECTS/ TOXIC REACTIONS

Skin reactions, hepatitis may become severe, life-threatening.

NURSING CONSIDERATIONS

BASELINE ASSESSMENT

Establish baseline lab values, esp. hepatic function tests, before initiating therapy and at intervals during therapy. Obtain full medication history (esp. use of oral contraceptives).

INTERVENTION/EVALUATION

Closely monitor for evidence of rash (usually appears on trunk, face, extremities; occurs within first 6 wks of drug initiation). Observe for rash accompanied by fever, blistering, oral lesions, conjunctivitis, swelling, muscle/joint aches, general malaise.

PATIENT/FAMILY TEACHING

• If therapy is missed for longer than 7 days, restart by using one 200-mg tablet daily for first 14 days, followed by one 200-mg tablet twice a day. • Continue therapy for full length of treatment. • Doses should be evenly spaced. • Swallow extended-release tablets whole; do not chew, crush, dissolve, or divide. • Nevirapine is not a cure for HIV infection, nor does it reduce risk of transmission to others. • Report any rash, yellowing of skin/eyes, nausea, loss of appetite.

niacin, nicotinic acid

`TOP 200`

nye-a-sin, nik-oh-**tin**-ik **as**-id
(Niacor, Niaspan, Slo-Niacin)
Do not confuse niacin, Niacor, or Niaspan with minocin or Nitro-Bid.

FIXED-COMBINATION(S)

Advicor: niacin/lovastatin (HMG-CoA reductase inhibitor [statin]): 500 mg/20 mg, 750 mg/20 mg, 1,000 mg/20 mg. **Simcor:** niacin/simvastatin (HMG-CoA reductase inhibitor [statin]): 500 mg/20 mg, 500 mg/40 mg, 750 mg/20 mg, 1,000 mg/20 mg, 1,000 mg/40 mg.

◆ CLASSIFICATION

CLINICAL: Antihyperlipidemic, water-soluble vitamin (see p. 58C).

ACTION

Component of two coenzymes needed for tissue respiration, lipid metabolism, glycogenolysis. Inhibits synthesis of very-low-density lipoproteins (VLDLs). **Therapeutic Effect:** Reduces total, LDL, VLDL cholesterol levels and triglyceride levels; increases HDL cholesterol concentration.

PHARMACOKINETICS

Readily absorbed from GI tract. Widely distributed. Protein binding: 20%. Metabolized in liver. Primarily excreted in urine. **Half-life:** 45 min.

USES

Treatment of dyslipidemias, lower risk of recurrent MI (pts with history of MI/hyperlipidemia, slow progression of CAD, treatment of hypertriglyceridemia in

N

✦ Canadian trade name   🚫 Non-Crushable Drug   🔺 High Alert drug pts at risk for pancreatitis, dietary supplement. **OFF-LABEL:** Treatment of pellagra.

PRECAUTIONS

Contraindications: Active peptic ulcer disease, arterial hemorrhaging, significant or unexplained persistent elevations in hepatic transaminases. **Cautions:** Diabetes mellitus, gallbladder disease, unstable angina, MI, renal impairment, heavy alcohol use, concomitant use of anticoagulants, gout, history of jaundice/hepatic disease.

⌛ LIFESPAN CONSIDERATIONS

Pregnancy/Lactation: Not recommended for use during pregnancy/lactation. Distributed in breast milk. **Pregnancy Category A (C if used at dosages above the recommended daily allowance). Children:** No age-related precautions noted. Not recommended in those younger than 2 yrs. **Elderly:** No age-related precautions noted.

INTERACTIONS

DRUG: Alcohol may increase risk of side effects. May increase effect of **antihypertensives. Lovastatin, pravastatin, simvastatin** may increase risk of acute renal failure, rhabdomyolysis. **Vasoactive drugs (e.g., calcium channel blockers, nitrates)** may increase hypotension. **HERBAL:** None significant. **FOOD:** None known. **LAB VALUES:** May increase serum uric acid, PT, amylase, bilirubin, fasting glucose, LDH, transaminase. May decrease platelets.

AVAILABILITY (OTC)

Tablets (Immediate-Release [Niacor]): 50 mg, 100 mg, 250 mg, 500 mg.
🔖 **Capsules (Extended-Release):** 250 mg, 400 mg, 500 mg. 🔖 **Tablets (Controlled-Release [Slo-Niacin]):** 250 mg, 500 mg, 750 mg. 🔖 **Tablets (Extended-Release [Niaspan]):** 500 mg, 750 mg, 1,000 mg.

ADMINISTRATION/HANDLING

PO
• For pts switching from immediate-release niacin to extended-release nia-

cin, initiate extended-release form with low doses and titrate to therapeutic response. • Give with food. • Give aspirin 30 min before taking extended-release niacin to minimize flushing. • Do not crush, break, or cut long-acting forms.

INDICATIONS/ROUTES/DOSAGE

Hyperlipidemia
PO (Immediate-Release): ADULTS, ELDERLY: Initially, 250 mg once a day (with evening meal). May increase dose q4–7days up to 1.5–2 g/day in 2–3 divided doses. After 2 mos may increase at 2- to 4-wk intervals to 3 g/day in 3 divided doses. **Maximum:** 6 g/day in 3 divided doses. Usual daily dose: 1.5–3 g/day.
PO (Controlled-Release): ADULTS, ELDERLY: Initially, 500 mg/day at bedtime for 4 wks, then 1 g at bedtime for 4 wks. May increase by 500 mg q4wks up to maximum of 2 g/day. Usual daily dose: 1–2 g/day.

SIDE EFFECTS

Frequent: Flushing (esp. face, neck) occurring within 20 min of drug administration and lasting for 30–60 min, GI upset, pruritus. **Occasional:** Dizziness, hypotension, headache, blurred vision, burning/tingling of skin, flatulence, nausea, vomiting, diarrhea. **Rare:** Hyperglycemia, glycosuria, rash, hyperpigmentation, dry skin.

ADVERSE EFFECTS/ TOXIC REACTIONS

Arrhythmias occur rarely.

NURSING CONSIDERATIONS

BASELINE ASSESSMENT
Obtain diet history, especially fat consumption. Question for history of hypersensitivity to niacin, tartrazine, aspirin. Assess serum baselines, cholesterol, triglyceride, glucose, hepatic function tests.

INTERVENTION/EVALUATION
Evaluate flushing, degree of GI discomfort. Check for headache, dizziness, blurred vision. Monitor daily pattern of

bowel activity, stool consistency. Monitor hepatic function, serum cholesterol, triglycerides. Check serum glucose carefully in pts on insulin, oral antihyperglycemics. Assess skin for rash, dryness. Monitor serum uric acid.

PATIENT/FAMILY TEACHING

• Transient flushing of the skin, sensation of warmth, pruritus, tingling may occur. • Notify physician if dizziness occurs (avoid sudden changes in posture). • Report nausea, vomiting, loss of appetite, yellowing of skin, dark urine, feeling of weakness. • If medically approved, take aspirin 30 min before taking extended-release niacin to minimize flushing. • Take at bedtime with low-fat snack. • Limit alcohol consumption.

---

*niCARdipine

nye-**kar**-di-peen
(Cardene IV, Cardene SR)
Do not confuse Cardene SR with Cardizem SR or codeine, or nicardipine with nifedipine or nimodipine.

◆CLASSIFICATION

PHARMACOTHERAPEUTIC: Calcium channel blocker. **CLINICAL:** Antianginal, antihypertensive (see p. 79C).

ACTION

Inhibits calcium ion movement across cell membranes, depressing contraction of cardiac, vascular smooth muscle. **Therapeutic Effect:** Increases heart rate, cardiac output. Decreases systemic vascular resistance, B/P.

PHARMACOKINETICS

Route	Onset	Peak	Duration
PO	0.5–2 hrs	—	8 hrs
IV	10 min	—	8 hrs or less

Rapidly, completely absorbed from GI tract. Protein binding: 95%. Metabolized in liver. Primarily excreted in urine. Not removed by hemodialysis. **Half-life:** 2–4 hrs.

USES

PO: Immediate-release: Treatment of chronic stable (effort-associated) angina, essential hypertension. **Sustained-release:** Treatment of essential hypertension. **Parenteral:** Short-term treatment of hypertension when oral therapy not feasible or desirable. **OFF-LABEL:** Subarachnoid hemorrhage with associated neurologic deficits, prevention of migraine headaches, HF, control blood pressure in acute ischemic stroke and intracranial hemorrhage, postoperative hypertension associated with carotid endarterectomy.

PRECAUTIONS

Contraindications: Advanced aortic stenosis. **Cautions:** Cardiac, renal, hepatic dysfunction; heart failure, hypertrophic cardiomyopathy, aortic stenosis, coronary artery disease, pheochromocytoma, portal hypertension.

⌛ LIFESPAN CONSIDERATIONS

Pregnancy/Lactation: Unknown if distributed in breast milk. **Pregnancy Category C. Children:** Safety and efficacy not established. **Elderly:** Age-related renal impairment may require dosage adjustment.

INTERACTIONS

DRUG: May increase concentration of **cyclosporine. HERBAL: Ephedra, ginger, ginseng, yohimbe** may increase hypertension. **Licorice** may cause retention of sodium, water; may increase loss of potassium. **St. John's wort** may decrease levels. **FOOD: Grapefruit products** may alter absorption. **LAB VALUES:** None significant.

AVAILABILITY (Rx)

Capsules: 20 mg, 30 mg. **Infusion, Ready to Use:** 20 mg/200 ml, 40 mg/200 ml.

N

Injection Solution (Cardene IV): 2.5 mg/ml (10-ml vial).

 Capsules (Sustained-Release [Cardene SR]): 30 mg, 45 mg, 60 mg.

ADMINISTRATION/HANDLING

IV

Reconstitution • Dilute 25-mg vial with 240 ml D₅W, 0.45% NaCl, or 0.9% NaCl to provide concentration of 0.1 mg/ml.

Rate of Administration • Give by slow IV infusion. • Change IV site q12h if administered peripherally.

Storage • Store at room temperature. • Diluted IV solution is stable for 24 hrs at room temperature.

PO

• Give without regard to food. • Do not break, crush, or divide capsules. Give whole.

🔲 IV INCOMPATIBILITIES

Ampicillin (Principen), ampicillin/sulbactam (Unasyn), cefepime (Maxipime), ceftazidime (Fortaz), furosemide (Lasix), heparin, sodium bicarbonate.

🔲 IV COMPATIBILITIES

Diltiazem (Cardizem), dobutamine (Dobutrex), dopamine (Intropin), epinephrine, hydromorphone (Dilaudid), labetalol (Trandate), lorazepam (Ativan), midazolam (Versed), milrinone (Primacor), morphine, nitroglycerin, norepinephrine (Levophed), potassium chloride.

INDICATIONS/ROUTES/DOSAGE

Chronic Stable Angina

PO: ADULTS, ELDERLY: Initially, 20 mg 3 times a day. Range: 20–40 mg 3 times a day (allow 3 days between dosage increases).

Essential Hypertension

PO: ADULTS, ELDERLY: Initially, 20 mg 3 times a day. Range: 20–40 mg 3 times a day (allow 3 days between dosage increases).

PO *(Sustained-Release):* **ADULTS, ELDERLY:** Initially, 30 mg twice a day. Range: 30–60 mg twice a day.

Short-Term Treatment of Hypertension (Parenteral Dosage as Substitute for Oral Nicardipine)

IV: ADULTS, ELDERLY: 0.5 mg/hr (for pt receiving 20 mg PO q8h), 1.2 mg/hr (for pt receiving 30 mg PO q8h), 2.2 mg/hr (for pt receiving 40 mg PO q8h).

Pts Not Already Receiving Nicardipine

IV: ADULTS, ELDERLY (GRADUAL B/P DECREASE): Initially, 5 mg/hr. May increase by 2.5 mg/hr q15min. After B/P goal is achieved, decrease rate to 3 mg/hr. **ADULTS, ELDERLY (RAPID B/P DECREASE):** Initially, 5 mg/hr. May increase by 2.5 mg/hr q5min. **Maximum:** 15 mg/hr until desired B/P attained. After B/P goal achieved, decrease rate to 3 mg/hr.

Changing From IV to Oral Antihypertensive Therapy

ADULTS, ELDERLY: Begin antihypertensives other than nicardipine when IV has been discontinued; for nicardipine, give first dose 1 hr before discontinuing IV.

Dosage in Hepatic Impairment

ADULTS, ELDERLY: Initially, give 20 mg twice a day, then titrate.

Dosage in Renal Impairment

ADULTS, ELDERLY: Initially, give 20 mg q8h (30 mg twice a day [sustained-release capsules]), then titrate.

SIDE EFFECTS

Frequent (10%–7%): Headache, facial flushing, peripheral edema, light-headedness, dizziness. **Occasional (6%–3%):** Asthenia (loss of strength, energy), palpitations, angina, tachycardia. **Rare (Less Than 2%):** Nausea, abdominal cramps, dyspepsia (heartburn, indigestion, epigastric pain), dry mouth, rash.

ADVERSE EFFECTS/ TOXIC REACTIONS

Overdose produces confusion, slurred speech, drowsiness, marked hypotension, bradycardia.

NURSING CONSIDERATIONS

BASELINE ASSESSMENT

Concurrent therapy of sublingual nitroglycerin may be used for relief of anginal pain. Record onset, type (sharp, dull, squeezing), radiation, location, intensity, duration of anginal pain, precipitating factors (exertion, emotional stress).

INTERVENTION/EVALUATION

Monitor B/P during and following IV infusion. Assess for peripheral edema behind medial malleolus. Assess skin for facial flushing, dermatitis, rash. Question for asthenia (loss of strength, energy), headache. Monitor serum hepatic enzyme results. Assess EKG, pulse for tachycardia.

PATIENT/FAMILY TEACHING

• May take without regard to food. • Sustained-release capsule taken whole; do not break, chew, crush, or divide. • Avoid alcohol, grapefruit juice, limit caffeine. • Inform physician if anginal pain not relieved or palpitations, shortness of breath, swelling, dizziness, constipation, nausea, hypotension occur. • Avoid tasks requiring motor skills, alertness until response to drug is established.

nicotine

nik-o-teen
(Commit, Habitrol ✤, NicoDerm ✤, NicoDerm CQ, Nicorette, Nicorette Plus ✤, Nicotrol ✤, Nicotrol Inhaler, Nicotrol NS, Thrive)
Do not confuse NicoDerm with Nitroderm.

◆CLASSIFICATION

PHARMACOTHERAPEUTIC: Cholinergic-receptor agonist. **CLINICAL:** Smoking deterrent (see p. 154C, 155C).

ACTION

Binds to acetylcholine receptors, producing both stimulating, depressant effects on peripheral, central nervous systems. **Therapeutic Effect:** Provides source of nicotine during nicotine withdrawal, reduces withdrawal symptoms.

PHARMACOKINETICS

Absorbed slowly after transdermal administration. Protein binding: 5%. Metabolized in liver. Excreted primarily in urine. **Half-life:** 4 hrs.

USES

Treatment to aid smoking cessation for relief of nicotine withdrawal symptoms. **OFF-LABEL: Transdermal:** Management of ulcerative colitis.

PRECAUTIONS

Contraindications: Smoking during immediate post-MI period, life-threatening arrhythmias, severe or worsening angina, active temporomandibular joint disease (gum), pregnancy. **Cautions:** Hyperthyroidism, pheochromocytoma, insulin-dependent diabetes mellitus, severe renal impairment, eczematous dermatitis, oral/pharyngeal inflammation, esophagitis, peptic ulcer (delays healing in peptic ulcer disease), coronary artery disease, recent MI, serious cardiac arrhythmias, vasospastic disease, angina, hypertension, hepatic impairment, oral inhaler/nasal spray, bronchospastic disease.

⧗ LIFESPAN CONSIDERATIONS

Pregnancy/Lactation: Distributed freely into breast milk. Use of cigarettes, nicotine gum associated with decrease in fetal breathing movements. **Pregnancy Category D. Children:** Not recommended in this pt population. **Elderly:** Age-related decrease

N

---

* "Tall Man" lettering   ✤ Canadian trade name   🖳 Non-Crushable Drug   🆖 High Alert drug

in cardiac function may require dosage adjustment.

INTERACTIONS

DRUG: Smoking cessation, decreased dosage of nicotine may alter effects of **tricyclic antidepressants, theophylline. HERBAL:** None significant. **FOOD:** None known. **LAB VALUES:** None significant.

AVAILABILITY (OTC)

Chewing Gum (Nicorette, Thrive): 2 mg, 4 mg. **Inhalation (Nicotrol Inhaler):** 10 mg cartridge. **Lozenges (Commit):** 2 mg, 4 mg. **Nasal Spray (Nicotrol NS):** 0.5 mg/spray. **Transdermal Patch (NicoDerm CQ):** 7 mg/24 hrs, 14 mg/24 hrs, 21 mg/24 hrs.

ADMINISTRATION/HANDLING

Gum
• Do not swallow. • Chew 1 piece when urge to smoke present. • Chew slowly and intermittently for 30 min. • Chew until distinctive nicotine taste (peppery) or slight tingling in mouth perceived, then stop; when tingling almost gone (about 1 min) repeat chewing procedure (this allows constant slow buccal absorption). • Too-rapid chewing may cause excessive release of nicotine, resulting in adverse effects similar to oversmoking (e.g., nausea, throat irritation).

Inhaler
• Insert cartridge into mouthpiece. • Puff on nicotine cartridge mouthpiece for 20 min.

Lozenge
• Do not chew or swallow. • Allow to dissolve slowly (20–30 min).

Transdermal
• Apply promptly upon removal from protective pouch (prevents evaporation, loss of nicotine). • Use only intact pouch. Do not cut patch. • Apply only once daily to hairless, clean, dry skin on upper body, outer arm. • Replace daily; rotate sites; do not use same site within 7 days; do not use same patch longer than 24 hrs. • Wash hands with water alone after applying patch (soap may increase nicotine absorption). • Discard used patch by folding patch in half (sticky side together), placing in pouch of new patch, and throwing away in such a way as to prevent child or pet accessibility. • Patch may contain conducting metal; remove prior to MRI.

INDICATIONS/ROUTES/DOSAGE

Smoking Cessation Aid to Relieve Nicotine Withdrawal Symptoms

PO *(Chewing Gum):* **ADULTS, ELDERLY:** Less than 25 cigarettes/day: Use 2 mg. 25 or more cigarettes/day: Use 4 mg. Chew 1 piece of gum when urge to smoke, up to 24/day. Use following schedule: wks 1–6: q1–2h (at least 9 pieces/day); wks 7–9: q2–4h; wks 10–12: q4–8h.

PO *(Lozenge):*
◄ALERT► For pts who smoke the first cigarette within 30 min of waking, administer the 4-mg lozenge; otherwise, administer the 2-mg lozenge.

ADULTS, ELDERLY: One 4-mg or 2-mg lozenge q1–2h for the first 6 wks (use at least 9 lozenges/day first 6 wks); 1 lozenge q2–4h for wks 7–9; and 1 lozenge q4–8h for wks 10–12. **Maximum:** 1 lozenge at a time, 5 lozenges/6 hrs, 20 lozenges/day.

Transdermal: ◄ALERT► Apply 1 new patch q24h. **ADULTS, ELDERLY WHO SMOKE 10 CIGARETTES OR MORE PER DAY:** Follow the guidelines below. **Step 1:** 21 mg/day for 6 wks. **Step 2:** 14 mg/day for 2 wks. **Step 3:** 7 mg/day for 2 wks. **ADULTS, ELDERLY WHO SMOKE LESS THAN 10 CIGARETTES PER DAY:** Follow the guidelines below. **Step 1:** 14 mg/day for 6 wks. **Step 2:** 7 mg/day for 2 wks.

Nasal: ADULTS, ELDERLY: Each dose (2 sprays, 1 spray in each nostril) = 1 mg nicotine. Initially, 1–2 doses/hr. **Maximum:** 5 doses/hr (10 sprays), 40 doses/day (80 sprays). Take at least 8 doses (16 sprays) per day.

Inhaler *(Nicotrol)*: **ADULTS, ELDERLY:**
Puff on nicotine cartridge mouthpiece for
about 20 min as needed.

SIDE EFFECTS

Frequent: All forms: Hiccups, nausea.
Gum: Mouth/throat soreness. **Transdermal:** Erythema, pruritus, burning at application site. **Occasional: All forms:** Eructation, GI upset, dry mouth, insomnia, diaphoresis, irritability. **Gum:** Hoarseness. **Inhaler:** Mouth/throat irritation, cough. **Rare: All forms:** Dizziness, myalgia, arthralgia.

ADVERSE EFFECTS/ TOXIC REACTIONS

Overdose produces palpitations, tachyarrhythmias, seizures, depression, confusion, diaphoresis, hypotension, rapid/weak pulse, dyspnea. Lethal dose for adults is 40–60 mg. Death results from respiratory paralysis.

NURSING CONSIDERATIONS

BASELINE ASSESSMENT

Screen, evaluate those with coronary heart disease (history of MI, angina pectoris), serious cardiac arrhythmias, Buerger's disease, Prinzmetal's variant angina.

INTERVENTION/EVALUATION

Monitor smoking habits, B/P, pulse, sleep pattern, skin for erythema, pruritus, burning at application site if transdermal system used.

PATIENT/FAMILY TEACHING

• Follow guidelines for proper application of transdermal system. • Chew gum slowly to avoid jaw ache, maximize benefit. • Report persistent rash, pruritus that occurs with patch. • Do not smoke while wearing patch.

---

*NIFEdipine

nye-**fed**-i-peen

(Adalat CC, Adalat XL ♣,
Afeditab CR, Apo-Nifed ♣, Nifediac
CC, Nifedical XL, Procardia,
Procardia XL)
**Do not confuse nifedipine with
nicardipine or nimodipine, or
Procardia XL with Cartia XT.**

◆CLASSIFICATION

PHARMACOTHERAPEUTIC: Calcium
channel blocker. **CLINICAL:** Antianginal, antihypertensive (see p. 63C, 80C).

ACTION

Inhibits calcium ion movement across
cell membranes, depressing contraction
of cardiac, vascular smooth muscle.
Therapeutic Effect: Increases heart
rate, cardiac output. Decreases systemic
vascular resistance, B/P.

PHARMACOKINETICS

Rapidly, completely absorbed from GI
tract. Protein binding: 92%–98%. Metabolized in liver. Primarily excreted in
urine. Not removed by hemodialysis.
Half-life: 2–5 hrs.

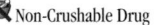

USES

Treatment of angina due to coronary artery spasm (Prinzmetal's variant angina),
chronic stable angina (effort-associated
angina). **Extended-release:** Treatment
of hypertension. **OFF-LABEL:** Treatment of
Raynaud's phenomenon, pulmonary hypertension, preterm labor, prevention/
treatment of high-altitude pulmonary
edema.

PRECAUTIONS

Contraindications: Cardiogenic shock,
concomitant administration with strong
CYP3A4 inducers (e.g., rifampin), acute
MI. **Immediate-Release:** Treatment of
urgent/emergent hypertension. **Cautions:**
Renal/hepatic impairment, obstructive
coronary disease, HF, severe aortic stenosis, severe left ventricular dysfunction,
hypertrophic cardiomyopathy, edema,
CYP3A4 inhibitors.

---

* "Tall Man" lettering ♣ Canadian trade name 🗲 Non-Crushable Drug 🔲 High Alert drug

⧗ LIFESPAN CONSIDERATIONS

Pregnancy/Lactation: Insignificant amount distributed in breast milk. **Pregnancy Category C. Children:** Safety and efficacy not established. **Elderly:** Age-related renal impairment may require dosage adjustment.

INTERACTIONS

DRUG: Strong CYP3A4 inducers (e.g., rifampin, phenobarbital, phenytoin, carbamazepine) may decrease concentration/effect. **CYP3A4 inhibitors (e.g., clarithromycin, ketoconazole)** may increase concentration. **Beta-blockers** may have additive effect. May increase **digoxin** concentration, risk of toxicity. **Hypokalemia-producing agents (e.g., furosemide, other diuretics)** may increase risk of arrhythmias. **HERBAL: Ephedra, garlic, ginseng, yohimbe** may increase hypertension. **Licorice** may cause retention of sodium, water; may increase loss of potassium. **St. John's wort** decreases concentration/effects. **FOOD: Grapefruit products** may increase risk for flushing headache, tachycardia, hypotension. **LAB VALUES:** May cause positive ANA, direct Coombs' test.

AVAILABILITY (Rx)

Capsules (Procardia): 10 mg, 20 mg.

▨ Tablets, Extended-Release: (Adalat CC, Afeditab CR, Procardia XL): 30 mg, 60 mg, 90 mg. (Nifediac CC, Nifedical XL): 30 mg, 60 mg.

ADMINISTRATION/HANDLING

PO

• Do not crush/break/cut extended-release tablets. • Give without regard to meals (Adalat CC, Nifediac CC should be taken on an empty stomach). • Grapefruit juice may alter absorption; avoid with all products.

Sublingual

• Capsules must be punctured, chewed, and/or squeezed to express liquid into mouth.

INDICATIONS/ROUTES/DOSAGE

Prinzmetal's Variant Angina, Chronic Stable (Effort-Associated) Angina
PO *(Immediate-Release)*: **ADULTS, ELDERLY:** Initially, 10 mg 3 times a day. Increase at 7- to 14-day intervals. Maintenance: 10 mg 3 times a day up to 30 mg 4 times a day. **Maximum:** 180 mg/day.
PO *(Extended-Release)*: **ADULTS, ELDERLY:** Initially, 30–60 mg/day. May increase at 7- to 14-day intervals. **Maximum:** 120–180 mg/day.

Hypertension
PO *(Extended-Release)*: **ADULTS, ELDERLY:** Initially, 30–60 mg/day. May increase at 7- to 14-day intervals. **Maximum:** 90–120 mg/day. **CHILDREN 1–17 YRS:** Initially, 0.25–0.5 mg/kg/day. **Maximum:** 3 mg/kg/day or 120 mg/day.

SIDE EFFECTS

Frequent (30%–11%): Peripheral edema, headache, flushed skin, dizziness. **Occasional (12%–6%):** Nausea, shakiness, muscle cramps/pain, drowsiness, palpitations, nasal congestion, cough, dyspnea, wheezing. **Rare (5%–3%):** Hypotension, rash, pruritus, urticaria, constipation, abdominal discomfort, flatulence, sexual dysfunction.

ADVERSE EFFECTS/ TOXIC REACTIONS

May precipitate HF, MI in pts with cardiac disease, peripheral ischemia. Overdose produces nausea, drowsiness, confusion, slurred speech. **Antidote:** Glucagon (see Appendix K for dosage).

NURSING CONSIDERATIONS

BASELINE ASSESSMENT

Concurrent therapy of sublingual nitroglycerin may be used for relief of anginal pain. Record onset, type (sharp, dull, squeezing), radiation, location, intensity, duration of anginal pain; precipitating factors (exertion, emotional stress). Check B/P for hypotension immediately before giving medication.

N

INTERVENTION/EVALUATION

Assist with ambulation if light-headedness, dizziness occurs. Assess for peripheral edema. Assess skin for flushing. Monitor serum hepatic enzymes. Observe for signs/symptoms of HF.

PATIENT/FAMILY TEACHING

• Go from lying to standing slowly. • Report palpitations, shortness of breath, pronounced dizziness, nausea, exacerbations of angina. • Avoid alcohol; concomitant grapefruit, grapefruit juice use.

---

nilotinib

HIGH ALERT

nye-**loe**-ti-nib
(Tasigna)

BLACK BOX ALERT Prolongs QT interval; sudden deaths reported. Do not use in pts with hypokalemia, hypomagnesemia, prolonged QT syndrome.

Do not confuse nilotinib with dasatinib, erlotinib, imatinib, nilutamide, sorafenib, sunitinib.

◆CLASSIFICATION

PHARMACOTHERAPEUTIC: Protein-tyrosine kinase inhibitor. **CLINICAL:** Antineoplastic (see p. 89C).

ACTION

Inhibits the Bcr-Abl tyrosine kinase, a translocation-created enzyme, created by the Philadelphia chromosome abnormality noted in chronic myelogenous leukemia (CML). **Therapeutic Effect:** Inhibits proliferation and tumor growth during two stages of CML: accelerated phase, chronic phase.

PHARMACOKINETICS

Well absorbed following PO administration. Protein binding: 98%. Metabolized in liver. Eliminated mainly in feces. Food increases concentration, and dose cannot be given less than 2 hrs before and less than 1 hr after food. **Half-life:** 17 hrs.

USES

Treatment of chronic phase and accelerated phase of chronic myelogenous leukemia (CML) in adult pts resistant or intolerant to prior therapy that included imatinib. Treatment of newly diagnosed Philadelphia chromosome positive chronic myeloid leukemia in chronic phase (Ph+ CML-CP). **OFF-LABEL:** Refractory gastrointestinal stromal tumor (GIST).

PRECAUTIONS

Contraindications: Hypokalemia, hypomagnesemia, long QT syndrome. **Cautions:** Myelosuppression, QT prolongation, history of pancreatitis, hepatic impairment, electrolyte abnormalities, pregnancy.

⧗ LIFESPAN CONSIDERATIONS

Pregnancy/Lactation: May cause fetal harm. Breastfeeding not recommended. **Pregnancy Category D. Children:** Safety and efficacy not established in those younger than 18 yrs. **Elderly:** No age-related precautions noted.

INTERACTIONS

DRUG: CYP3A4 inhibitors (e.g., clarithromycin, erythromycin, itraconazole, ketoconazole) increase concentration. **CYP3A4 inducers (e.g., carbamazepine, dexamethasone, phenobarbital, phenytoin, rifampicin)** decrease concentration. **QT-prolonging medications** may increase risk of prolonged QT interval. **HERBAL: St. John's wort** may decrease concentration. **FOOD: Grapefruit products** may increase risk for torsades de pointes, myelotoxicity. **LAB VALUES:** May decrease WBCs, platelets, serum magnesium, phosphorus, albumin, sodium. May increase serum glucose, lipase, bilirubin, ALT, AST. May alter serum potassium, alkaline phosphatase, creatinine.

N

AVAILABILITY (Rx)

Capsules: 150 mg, 200 mg.

ADMINISTRATION/HANDLING

PO

• Give at least 2 hrs before and 1 hr after ingestion of food. • Contents may be opened, mixed with applesauce and taken within 15 min. • Swallow capsules whole; do not crush. • Store at room temperature.

INDICATIONS/ROUTES/DOSAGE

Note: Dosage adjusted in hepatic impairment, hematologic toxicity, nonhematologic toxicity, QT prolongation (consult specific product labeling).

Chronic Myelogenous Leukemia (CML)
PO: ADULTS, ELDERLY: 400 mg twice daily every 12 hrs, without food.

Ph+ CML-CP
PO: ADULTS, ELDERLY: 300 mg twice daily.

SIDE EFFECTS

Frequent (33%–21%): Rash, nausea, headache, pruritus, fatigue, diarrhea, constipation, vomiting. **Occasional (18%–10%):** Arthralgia, cough, pharyngitis, asthenia (loss of strength, energy), fever, myalgia, abdominal pain, peripheral edema, weight gain, bone pain, muscle spasm, back pain. **Rare (9%–1%):** Anorexia, insomnia, dizziness, paresthesia, vertigo, palpitations, flushing, hypertension, flatulence, alopecia, night sweats.

ADVERSE EFFECTS/
TOXIC REACTIONS

Prolongation of QT interval producing ventricular tachycardia (torsades de pointes) may result in seizure, sudden death. Neutropenia, thrombocytopenia, anemia are expected response to drug. Respiratory toxicity manifested as dyspnea, pneumonia.

NURSING CONSIDERATIONS

BASELINE ASSESSMENT

Obtain CBC every 2 wks for the first 2 mos and then monthly thereafter. Hypokalemia or hypomagnesemia must be corrected prior to initiating therapy. Monitor hepatic function tests (AST, ALT, bilirubin, alkaline phosphatase) before treatment begins and monthly thereafter. Obtain baseline weight.

INTERVENTION/EVALUATION

Monitor serum electrolytes periodically during therapy, particularly potassium, magnesium, sodium, lipase. Monitor for unexpected weight gain. Offer antiemetics to control nausea, vomiting. Monitor daily pattern of bowel frequency, stool consistency. Monitor CBC for evidence of neutropenia, thrombocytopenia; assess hepatic function tests for hepatotoxicity. Monitor closely for QT-interval prolongation.

PATIENT/FAMILY TEACHING

• Avoid crowds, those with known infection. • Avoid contact with anyone who recently received live virus vaccine; do not receive vaccinations. • Do not ingest food less than 2 hours before and less than 1 hr after dose is taken. • Avoid grapefruit products.

---

nilutamide   `HIGH ALERT`

nye-**loo**-ta-myde
(Anandron ✲, Nilandron)

BLACK BOX ALERT Interstitial pneumonitis reported in 2% of pts manifested as progressive exertional dyspnea, cough, chest pain, fever.
Do not confuse nilutamide with nilotinib.

◆**CLASSIFICATION**

PHARMACOTHERAPEUTIC: Hormone.
CLINICAL: Antineoplastic (see p. 89C).

N

ACTION

Competitively inhibits androgen activity by binding to androgen receptors in target tissue. **Therapeutic Effect:** Decreases growth of abnormal prostate tissue.

PHARMACOKINETICS

Well absorbed following PO administration. Protein binding: 72%–85%. Metabolized in liver. Primarily excreted in urine. **Half-life:** 23–87 hrs.

USES

Treatment of metastatic prostatic carcinoma (stage D_2) in combination with surgical castration. For maximum benefit, begin on same day or day after surgical castration.

PRECAUTIONS

Contraindications: Severe hepatic impairment, severe respiratory insufficiency. **Cautions:** Hepatitis, marked increase in serum hepatic enzymes, alcoholism.

⌛ LIFESPAN CONSIDERATIONS

Pregnancy Category C. Children: Safety and efficacy not established. **Elderly:** No age-related precautions noted.

INTERACTIONS

DRUG: May increase effect of **warfarin.** May increase concentration, risk of toxicity with **fosphenytoin, phenytoin, theophylline. HERBAL: St. John's wort** may decrease concentration. **FOOD:** None known. **LAB VALUES:** May increase serum bilirubin, creatinine, AST, ALT, alkaline phosphatase, BUN, glucose. May decrease Hgb, WBC.

AVAILABILITY (Rx)

Tablets: 150 mg.

ADMINISTRATION/HANDLING

PO
• May give without regard to food.

INDICATIONS/ROUTES/DOSAGE

Prostatic Carcinoma
PO: ADULTS, ELDERLY: 300 mg once a day for 30 days, then 150 mg once a day.

Begin on day of, or day after, surgical castration.

SIDE EFFECTS

Frequent (28%): Skin flushing, hot flashes. **Occasional (10%–6%):** Nausea, dyspnea, constipation, dizziness, abnormal vision. **Rare (less than 6%):** Malaise, diarrhea, weight loss, dry mouth, paresthesia, pruritus, photophobia, rhinitis, decreased libido, diminished sexual function, gynecomastia, alcohol intolerance, increased B/P.

ADVERSE EFFECTS/ TOXIC REACTIONS

Interstitial pneumonitis occurs rarely.

NURSING CONSIDERATIONS

BASELINE ASSESSMENT

Obtain baseline chest X-ray, hepatic enzymes before beginning therapy.

INTERVENTION/EVALUATION

Monitor B/P periodically and hepatic function tests in long-term therapy.

PATIENT/FAMILY TEACHING

• Contact physician if any side effects occur at home, esp. signs of hepatic toxicity (jaundice, dark urine, fatigue, abdominal pain). • Tinted glasses may help improve night driving.

N

nimodipine

nye-**mode**-i-peen
(Nimotop, Nymalize)
BLACK BOX ALERT Severe cardiovascular events, including fatalities, have resulted when capsule contents have been withdrawn by syringe and administered by IV injection rather than nasogastric tube.

Do not confuse nimodipine with nicardipine or nifedipine.

 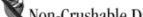

◆CLASSIFICATION

PHARMACOTHERAPEUTIC: Calcium channel blocker. **CLINICAL:** Cerebral vasospasm agent (see p. 80C).

ACTION

Inhibits movement of calcium ions across vascular smooth muscle cell membranes. Exerts greatest effect on cerebral arteries. **Therapeutic Effect:** Produces favorable effect on severity of neurologic deficits due to cerebral vasospasm. May prevent cerebral vasospasm.

PHARMACOKINETICS

Rapidly absorbed from GI tract. Protein binding: 95%. Metabolized in liver. Excreted in urine; eliminated in feces. Not removed by hemodialysis. **Half-life:** 1–2 hrs.

USES

Improvement of neurologic deficits due to cerebral vasospasm following subarachnoid hemorrhage from ruptured intracranial aneurysms.

PRECAUTIONS

Contraindications: None known. **Cautions:** Hepatic impairment, decreased GI motility, history of bowel obstruction, hypertrophic cardiomyopathy.

⌛ LIFESPAN CONSIDERATIONS

Pregnancy/Lactation: Unknown if drug crosses placenta or is distributed in breast milk. **Pregnancy Category C. Children:** Safety and efficacy not established. **Elderly:** Age-related renal impairment may require dosage adjustment. May experience greater hypotensive response, constipation.

INTERACTIONS

DRUG: Beta-blockers may have additive effect, increase depression of cardiac SA/AV conduction. May increase **digoxin** concentration. **Agents inducing hypokalemia** may increase risk of arrhythmias. **CYP3A4 inhibitors (e.g., erythromy-**cin, itraconazole, ketoconazole, protease inhibitors)** may inhibit metabolism. **CYP3A4 inducers (e.g., rifabutin, rifampin)** may increase metabolism. **HERBAL: Ephedra, garlic, ginseng, yohimbe** may increase hypertension. **Licorice** may cause retention of sodium, water; may increase loss of potassium. **St. John's wort** may decrease levels/effect. **FOOD: Grapefruit products** may increase concentration, risk of toxicity. **LAB VALUES:** None significant.

AVAILABILITY (Rx)

Solution, Oral (Nymalize): 60 mg/20 ml.
📦 **Capsules (Nimotop):** 30 mg.

ADMINISTRATION/HANDLING

PO
• If pt unable to swallow, place hole in both ends of capsule with 18-gauge needle to extract contents into syringe. • Empty into NG tube; flush tube with 30 ml water.

INDICATIONS/ROUTES/DOSAGE

Subarachnoid Hemorrhage
PO: ADULTS, ELDERLY: 60 mg q4h for 21 days. Begin within 96 hrs of subarachnoid hemorrhage.

Dosage in Hepatic Failure
PO: ADULTS, ELDERLY: 30 mg q4h.

SIDE EFFECTS

Occasional (6%–2%): Hypotension, peripheral edema, diarrhea, headache. **Rare (Less Than 2%):** Allergic reaction (rash, urticaria), tachycardia, flushing of skin.

ADVERSE EFFECTS/ TOXIC REACTIONS

Overdose produces nausea, weakness, dizziness, drowsiness, confusion, slurred speech.

NURSING CONSIDERATIONS

BASELINE ASSESSMENT

Assess LOC, neurologic response, initially and throughout therapy. Monitor baseline hepatic function tests. Assess B/P, apical pulse immediately before drug administration (if pulse is 60/min or less or systolic B/P is less than 90 mm Hg, withhold medication, contact physician).

INTERVENTION/EVALUATION

Monitor CNS response, heart rate, B/P for evidence of hypotension, signs/symptoms of HF. Monitor transcranial doppler results for evidence of vasospasm.

PATIENT/FAMILY TEACHING

• Do not chew, crush, dissolve, or divide capsules. • Report palpitations, shortness of breath, swelling, constipation, nausea, dizziness. Immediately report headache, blurry vision, confusion; may indicate vasospasm.

---

nitazoxanide

nye-ta-**zox**-a-nide
(Alinia)

◆CLASSIFICATION

PHARMACOTHERAPEUTIC: Antiparasitic. **CLINICAL:** Antiprotozoal agent.

ACTION

Interferes with body's reaction to pyruvate ferredoxin oxidoreductase, an enzyme essential for anaerobic energy metabolism. **Therapeutic Effect:** Produces antiprotozoal activity, reducing/terminating diarrheal episodes.

PHARMACOKINETICS

Rapidly hydrolyzed to active metabolite. Protein binding: 99%. Excreted in urine, bile, feces. **Half-life:** 2–4 hrs.

USES

Treatment of diarrhea caused by *Cryptosporidium parvum*, *Giardia lamblia* in children 12 mos and older, adults. **OFF-LABEL:** *C. difficile*-associated diarrhea.

PRECAUTIONS

Contraindications: None known. **Cautions:** Caution with use of suspension in diabetic pts (due to sucrose content), hepatic/biliary disease, renal impairment.

⧗ LIFESPAN CONSIDERATIONS

Pregnancy/Lactation: Unknown if distributed in breast milk. **Pregnancy Category B. Children:** Safety and efficacy not established in those younger than 1 yr (suspension) and younger than 12 yrs (tablet). **Elderly:** Not for use in this age group.

INTERACTIONS

DRUG: None significant. **HERBAL:** None significant. **FOOD:** None known. **LAB VALUES:** May increase serum creatinine, ALT.

AVAILABILITY (Rx)

Powder for Oral Suspension: 100 mg/5 ml. **Tablets:** 500 mg.

ADMINISTRATION/HANDLING

PO (Oral Suspension)
• Store unreconstituted powder at room temperature. • Reconstitute oral suspension with 48 ml water to provide concentration of 100 mg/5 ml. • Shake vigorously to suspend powder. • Reconstituted solution is stable for 7 days at room temperature. • Give with food.

PO (Tablets)
• Give with food.

INDICATIONS/ROUTES/DOSAGE

Diarrhea Caused by *C. Parvum*, *G. Lamblia*
PO: ADULTS, ELDERLY, CHILDREN 12 YRS AND OLDER: 500 mg q12h for 3 days. **CHILDREN 4–11 YRS:** 200 mg q12h for 3 days. **CHILDREN 1–3 YRS:** 100 mg q12h for 3 days.

SIDE EFFECTS

Occasional (8%): Abdominal pain. **Rare (2%–1%):** Diarrhea, vomiting, headache.

ADVERSE EFFECTS/ TOXIC REACTIONS

None known.

NURSING CONSIDERATIONS

BASELINE ASSESSMENT

Establish baseline B/P, weight, serum glucose, electrolytes. Assess for dehydration.

INTERVENTION/EVALUATION

Evaluate serum glucose in diabetics, electrolytes (therapy generally reduces abnormalities). Weigh pt daily. Encourage adequate fluid intake. Assess bowel sounds for peristalsis. Monitor daily pattern of bowel activity, stool consistency.

PATIENT/FAMILY TEACHING

• Parents of children with diabetes should be aware that the oral suspension contains 1.48 g of sucrose per 5 ml.
• Therapy should provide significant improvement of diarrhea.

nitrofurantoin

nye-troe-fue-**ran**-toyn
(Apo-Nitrofurantoin ❋, Furadantin, Macrobid, Macrodantin, Novo-Furantoin ❋)
Do not confuse Macrobid with MicroK or Nitro-Bid, or nitrofurantoin with Neurontin or nitroglycerin.

◆CLASSIFICATION

PHARMACOTHERAPEUTIC: Antibacterial. **CLINICAL:** Antibiotic, UTI prophylaxis.

ACTION

Inhibits synthesis of bacterial DNA, RNA, proteins, cell walls by altering, inactivating ribosomal proteins. **Therapeutic Effect:** Bacteriostatic (bactericidal at high concentrations).

PHARMACOKINETICS

Microcrystalline form rapidly, completely absorbed; macrocrystalline form more slowly absorbed. Food increases absorption. Protein binding: 60%. Primarily concentrated in urine, kidneys. Metabolized in most body tissues. Primarily excreted in urine. Removed by hemodialysis. **Half-life:** 20–60 min.

USES

Prevention/treatment of UTI caused by susceptible gram-negative, gram-positive organisms, including *E. coli, S. aureus, Enterococcus, Klebsiella, Enterobacter.*

PRECAUTIONS

Contraindications: Anuria, oliguria, substantial renal impairment (creatinine clearance less than 60 ml/min), infants younger than 1 mo due to risk of hemolytic anemia. Pregnancy at term, during labor, or delivery, or when onset of labor is imminent. **Cautions:** Renal impairment, diabetes mellitus, electrolyte imbalance, anemia, vitamin B deficiency, debilitated (greater risk of peripheral neuropathy), G6PD deficiency (greater risk of hemolytic anemia).

⌛ LIFESPAN CONSIDERATIONS

Pregnancy/Lactation: Readily crosses placenta. Distributed in breast milk. Contraindicated at term and during lactation when infant suspected of having G6PD deficiency. **Pregnancy Category B (contraindicated at term). Children:** No age-related precautions noted in pts older than 1 mo. **Elderly:** More likely to develop acute pneumonitis, peripheral neuropathy. Age-related renal impairment may require dosage adjustment.

INTERACTIONS

DRUG: Antacids containing magnesium trisilicate may decrease absorption. **Probenecid** may increase concentration, risk of toxicity. **HERBAL:** None significant. **FOOD:** None known. **LAB VALUES:** May increase serum ALT, AST, phosphorus. May decrease Hgb.

AVAILABILITY (Rx)

Capsules (Macrocrystalline, Monohydrate [Macrobid]): 100 mg. **Capsules (Macrocrystalline [Macrodantin]):** 25 mg, 50 mg,

100 mg. **Oral Suspension (Microcrystalline [Furadantin]):** 25 mg/5 ml.

ADMINISTRATION/HANDLING

PO

• Give with food, milk to enhance absorption, reduce GI upset. • May mix suspension with water, milk, fruit juice; shake well.

INDICATIONS/ROUTES/DOSAGE

UTI

PO *(Furadantin, Macrodantin)*: **ADULTS, ELDERLY:** 50–100 mg q6h. **Maximum:** 400 mg/day. **CHILDREN:** 5–7 mg/kg/day in divided doses q6h. **Maximum:** 400 mg/day.

PO *(Macrobid)*: **ADULTS, ELDERLY:** 100 mg twice daily.

Long-Term Prevention of UTI

PO: ADULTS, ELDERLY: 50–100 mg at bedtime. **CHILDREN:** 1–2 mg/kg/day as a single dose or 2 divided doses. **Maximum:** 100 mg/day.

Dosage in Renal Impairment

Contraindicated in pts with creatinine clearance less than 60 ml/min.

SIDE EFFECTS

Frequent: Anorexia, nausea, vomiting, dark urine. **Occasional:** Abdominal pain, diarrhea, rash, pruritus, urticaria, hypertension, headache, dizziness, drowsiness. **Rare:** Photosensitivity, transient alopecia, asthmatic exacerbation in those with history of asthma.

ADVERSE EFFECTS/ TOXIC REACTIONS

Superinfection, hepatotoxicity, peripheral neuropathy (may be irreversible), Stevens-Johnson syndrome, permanent pulmonary impairment, anaphylaxis occur rarely.

NURSING CONSIDERATIONS

BASELINE ASSESSMENT

Question for history of asthma. Evaluate lab test results for renal/hepatic baseline values.

INTERVENTION/EVALUATION

Monitor I&O, renal/hepatic function tests, CBC. Monitor daily pattern of bowel activity, stool consistency. Assess skin for rash, urticaria. Be alert for numbness/tingling, esp. of lower extremities (may signal onset of peripheral neuropathy). Observe for signs of hepatotoxicity (fever, rash, arthralgia, hepatomegaly). Perform respiratory assessment: auscultate lungs, check for cough, chest pain, difficulty breathing.

PATIENT/ FAMILY TEACHING

• Urine may become dark yellow/brown. • Take with food, milk for best results, reduce GI upset. • Complete full course of therapy. • Avoid sun, ultraviolet light; use sunscreen, wear protective clothing. • Notify physician if cough, fever, chest pain, difficulty breathing, numbness/tingling of fingers, toes occur. • Rare occurrence of alopecia is transient.

nitroglycerin

nye-troe-**glis**-er-in
(Minitran, Nitro-Bid, Nitro-Dur, Nitrolingual, Nitrostat, Nitro-Time, Trinipatch ✦)
Do not confuse Nitro-Bid with Macrobid or Nicobid, Nitro-Dur with Nicoderm, nitroglycerin with nitrofurantoin or nitroprusside, or Nitrostat with Nilstat or Nystatin.

◆CLASSIFICATION

PHARMACOTHERAPEUTIC: Nitrate. **CLINICAL:** Antianginal, antihypertensive, coronary vasodilator (see p. 128C).

ACTION

Dilates coronary arteries, improves collateral blood flow to ischemic areas within myocardium. IV form produces peripheral vasodilation. **Therapeutic Effect:** Decreases myocardial oxygen demand. Reduces left ventricular preload, afterload.

PHARMACOKINETICS

Route	Onset	Peak	Duration
Sublingual	1–3 min	4–8 min	30–60 min
Translingual spray	2 min	4–10 min	30–60 min
Buccal tablet	2–5 min	4–10 min	2 hrs
PO (extended-release)	20–45 min	45–120 min	4–8 hrs
Topical	15–60 min	30–120 min	2–12 hrs
Transdermal patch	40–60 min	60–180 min	18–24 hrs
IV	1–2 min	Immediate	3–5 min

Well absorbed after PO, sublingual, topical administration. Metabolized in liver, by enzymes in bloodstream. Protein binding: 60%. Excreted in urine. Not removed by hemodialysis. **Half-life:** 1–4 min.

USES

Lingual, sublingual, buccal dose used for acute relief of angina pectoris. Extended-release, topical forms used for prophylaxis, long-term angina management. IV form used in treatment of HF, acute MI, perioperative hypertension, induction of intraoperative hypotension. **OFF-LABEL:** Short-term management of pulmonary hypertension, esophageal spastic disorders, uterine relaxation.

PRECAUTIONS

Contraindications: Allergy to adhesives (transdermal); increased ICP; severe anemia; concurrent use of sildenafil, tadalafil, vardenafil (PDE5 inhibitors), right-sided MI (inferior wall). **IV:** Restrictive cardiomyopathy, pericardial tamponade, constrictive pericarditis. **Cautions:** Blood volume depletion, severe hypotension (systolic B/P less than 90 mm Hg), bradycardia (less than 50 beats/min).

⧗ LIFESPAN CONSIDERATIONS

Pregnancy/Lactation: Unknown if drug crosses placenta or is distributed in breast milk. **Pregnancy Category B. Children:** Safety and efficacy not established. **Elderly:** More susceptible to hypotensive effects. Age-related renal impairment may require dosage adjustment.

INTERACTIONS

DRUG: Alcohol, other antihypertensives, vasodilators may increase risk of orthostatic hypotension. Concurrent use of **sildenafil, tadalafil, vardenafil** (PDE5 inhibitors) produces significant hypotension. **HERBAL: Ephedra, ginger, ginseng, licorice** may increase hypertension. **Black cohosh, goldenseal, hawthorne** may cause hypotension. **FOOD:** None known. **LAB VALUES:** May increase serum methemoglobin, urine catecholamine concentrations.

AVAILABILITY (Rx)

Infusion, Pre-Mix: 25 mg/250 ml, 50 mg/500 ml (0.1 mg/ml), 50 mg/250 ml (0.2 mg/ml), 100 mg/250 ml. **Injection, Solution:** 5 mg/ml. **Ointment (Nitro-Bid):** 2%. **Translingual Spray (Nitrolingual):** 0.4 mg/spray. **Transdermal Patch (Minitran, Nitro-Dur):** 0.1 mg/hr, 0.2 mg/hr, 0.4 mg/hr, 0.6 mg/hr.

🖚 **Capsules, Extended-Release (Nitro-Time):** 2.5 mg, 6.5 mg, 9 mg. 🖚**Tablets, Sublingual (Nitrostat):** 0.4 mg.

ADMINISTRATION/HANDLING

◀**ALERT**▶   Cardioverter/defibrillator must not be discharged through paddle electrode overlying nitroglycerin (transdermal, ointment) system (may cause burns to pt or damage to paddle via arcing).

 IV

Reconstitution • Available in ready-to-use injectable containers. • Dilute vials in D₅W or 0.9% NaCl. Maximum concentration: 400 mcg/ml. • Use glass bottles.

Rate of Administration • Use microdrop or infusion pump.

Storage • Store at room temperature. • Reconstituted solutions stable for 48 hrs at room temperature or 7 days if refrigerated.

PO

• Do not cut, crush, split extended-release capsules. • Do not shake oral aerosol canister before lingual spraying.

Sublingual

• Instruct pt to not swallow. • Dissolve under tongue. • Administer while seated. • Slight burning sensation under tongue may be lessened by placing tablet in buccal pouch. • Keep sublingual tablets in original container.

Topical

• Spread thin layer on clean, dry, hairless skin of upper arm or body (not below knee or elbow), using applicator or dose-measuring papers. Do not use fingers; do not rub/massage into skin.

Transdermal

• Apply patch on clean, dry, hairless skin of upper arm or body (not below knee or elbow). • May keep patch on when bathing/showering. • Do not cut/trim to adjust dose.

🔲 IV INCOMPATIBILITIES

Alteplase (Activase), phenytoin (Dilantin).

🔲 IV COMPATIBILITIES

Amiodarone (Cordarone), dexmedetomidine (Precedex), diltiazem (Cardizem), dobutamine (Dobutrex), dopamine (Intropin), epinephrine, famotidine (Pepcid), fentanyl (Sublimaze), furosemide (Lasix), heparin, hydromorphone (Dilaudid), insulin, labetalol (Trandate), lidocaine, lipids, lorazepam (Ativan), midazolam (Versed), milrinone (Primacor), morphine, nicardipine (Cardene), nitroprusside (Nipride), norepinephrine (Levophed), propofol (Diprivan).

INDICATIONS/ROUTES/DOSAGE

Acute Treatment/Prophylaxis of Angina Pectoris

Translingual Spray: ADULTS, ELDERLY: 1–2 sprays onto or under tongue q3–5min until relief is noted (no more than 3 sprays in 15-min period).

Sublingual: ADULTS, ELDERLY: One tablet under tongue. If chest pain has not improved in 5 min, call 911. After the call, may take additional tablet. A third tablet may be taken 5 min after second dose (maximum of 3 tablets).

Long-Term Prophylaxis of Angina

PO (Extended-Release): ADULTS, ELDERLY: 2.5–6.5 mg 3–4 times a day. **Maximum:** 26 mg 4 times a day.

Topical: ADULTS, ELDERLY: Initially, ½ inch q6–8h during waking hours. Range: ½–2 inches q8h.

Transdermal Patch: ADULTS, ELDERLY: Initially, 0.2–0.4 mg/hr. **Maintenance:** 0.4–0.8 mg/hr. Consider patch on for 12–14 hrs, patch off for 10–12 hrs (prevents tolerance).

HF, Acute MI

IV: ADULTS, ELDERLY: Initially, 5 mcg/min via infusion pump. Increase in 5-mcg/min increments at 3- to 5-min intervals until B/P response is noted or until dosage reaches 20 mcg/min, then increase by 10–20 mcg/min q3–5min. Dosage may be further titrated according to clinical, therapeutic response up to 400 mcg/min. **CHILDREN:** Initially, 0.25–0.5 mcg/kg/min; titrate by 0.5–1 mcg/kg/min q3–5min up to 20 mcg/kg/min.

SIDE EFFECTS

Frequent: Headache (possibly severe; occurs mostly in early therapy, diminishes rapidly in intensity, usually disappears during continued treatment), transient flushing of face/neck, dizziness (esp. if pt is standing immobile or is in a warm environment), weakness, orthostatic hypotension. **Sublingual:** Burning, tingling sensation at oral point of dissolution. **Ointment:** Erythema, pruritus. **Occa-**

N

sional: GI upset. **Transdermal:** Contact dermatitis.

ADVERSE EFFECTS/ TOXIC REACTIONS

Discontinue drug if blurred vision, dry mouth occurs. Severe orthostatic hypotension may occur, manifested by syncope, pulselessness, cold/clammy skin, diaphoresis. Tolerance may occur with repeated, prolonged therapy; minor tolerance may occur with intermittent use of sublingual tablets. High doses tend to produce severe headache.

NURSING CONSIDERATIONS

BASELINE ASSESSMENT

Record onset, type (sharp, dull, squeezing), radiation, location, intensity, duration of anginal pain; precipitating factors (exertion, emotional stress). Assess B/P, apical pulse before administration and periodically following dose. Pt must have continuous EKG monitoring for IV administration. Rule out right-sided MI, if applicable (may precipitate life-threatening hypotension).

INTERVENTION/EVALUATION

Monitor B/P, heart rate. Assess for facial, neck flushing. Cardioverter/defibrillator must not be discharged through paddle electrode overlying nitroglycerin (transdermal, ointment) system (may cause burns to pt or damage to paddle via electrical arcing). Consider NS boluses for hypotension.

PATIENT/FAMILY TEACHING

• Go from lying to standing slowly. • Take oral form on empty stomach (however, if headache occurs during therapy, take medication with meals). • Use spray only when lying down. • Dissolve sublingual tablet under tongue; do not swallow. • Take at first sign of angina. • May take another dose q5min if needed up to a total of 3 doses. • If not relieved within 5 min, contact physician or immediately go to emergency room. • Do not change brands. • Keep container away from heat, moisture. • Do not inhale lingual aerosol but spray onto or under tongue (avoid swallowing after spray is administered). • Expel from mouth any remaining lingual, sublingual, intrabuccal tablet after pain is completely relieved. • Place transmucosal tablets under upper lip or buccal pouch (between cheek and gum); do not chew/swallow tablet. • Avoid alcohol (intensifies hypotensive effect). If alcohol is ingested soon after taking nitroglycerin, possible acute hypotensive episode (marked drop in B/P, vertigo, diaphoresis, pallor) may occur. • Do not use within 48 hrs of sildenafil, tadalafil, vardenafil (PDE$_5$ inhibitors). May cause acute hypotensive episode.

nitroprusside   HIGH ALERT

nye-troe-**prus**-ide
(Nipride ✦, Nitropress)
BLACK BOX ALERT Must dilute with D$_5$W. Can cause sharp decrease in B/P; may lead to irreversible ischemia, death. Unless used briefly or at low infusion rate (less than 2 mcg/kg/min), potentially lethal levels of cyanide may result. Do not use maximum dose for longer than 10 min.
Do not confuse nitroprusside with nitroglycerin or Nitrostat.

◆**CLASSIFICATION**

PHARMACOTHERAPEUTIC: Vasodilator. **CLINICAL:** Antihypertensive, vasodilator, antidote.

ACTION

Direct vasodilating action on arterial, venous smooth muscle. Decreases peripheral vascular resistance, preload, afterload; improves cardiac output. **Therapeutic Effect:** Dilates coronary arteries, decreases oxygen consumption, relieves persistent chest pain.

PHARMACOKINETICS

Route	Onset	Peak	Duration
IV	Less than 2 min	Dependent on infusion rate	1–10 min

Reacts with Hgb in erythrocytes, producing cyanmethemoglobin, cyanide ions. Primarily excreted in urine. **Half-life:** less than 10 min.

USES

Immediate reduction of B/P in hypertensive crisis. Produces controlled hypotension in surgical procedures to reduce bleeding. Treatment of acute HF.

PRECAUTIONS

Contraindications: Compensatory hypertension (AV shunt, coarctation of aorta), congenital (Leber's) optic atrophy, inadequate cerebral circulation, moribund pts, tobacco amblyopia (dim vision). **Cautions:** Severe hepatic/renal impairment, hypothyroidism, hyponatremia, elderly, increased intracranial pressure.

☒ LIFESPAN CONSIDERATIONS

Pregnancy/Lactation: Unknown if drug crosses placenta or is distributed in breast milk. **Pregnancy Category C. Children:** Safety and efficacy not established. **Elderly:** More sensitive to hypotensive effect. Age-related renal impairment may require dosage adjustment.

INTERACTIONS

DRUG: Antihypertensives may increase hypotensive effect. **HERBAL: Yohimbe** may decrease effects. **FOOD:** None known. **LAB VALUES:** None significant.

AVAILABILITY (Rx)

Injection Solution: 25 mg/ml.

ADMINISTRATION/HANDLING

IV

Reconstitution • Dilute with 250–1,000 ml D₅W to provide concentration of 200 mcg, 50 mcg/ml, respectively. **Maximum concentration:** 200 mg/250 ml. • Wrap infusion bottle in aluminum foil immediately after mixing.

Rate of Administration • Give by IV infusion only, using infusion rate chart provided by manufacturer or protocol. • Administer using IV infusion pump. • Be alert for extravasation (produces severe pain, sloughing).

Storage • Protect from light. • Solution should appear very faint brown. • Use only freshly prepared solution. Once prepared, do not keep or use longer than 24 hrs. • Deterioration evidenced by color change from brown to blue, green, dark red. • Discard unused portion.

☒ IV INCOMPATIBILITY

Insulin (regular).

☒ IV COMPATIBILITIES

Cisatracurium (Nimbex), dexmedetomidine (Precedex), diltiazem (Cardizem), dobutamine (Dobutrex), dopamine (Intropin), enalapril (Vasotec), heparin, labetalol (Normodyne, Trandate), lidocaine, midazolam (Versed), milrinone (Primacor), nitroglycerin, propofol (Diprivan).

INDICATIONS/ROUTES/DOSAGE

Usual Parenteral Dosage

IV Infusion: ADULTS, ELDERLY, CHILDREN: Initially, 0.3–0.5 mcg/kg/min. May increase by 0.5 mcg/kg/min to desired hemodynamic effect or appearance of headache, nausea. Usual dose: 3 mcg/kg/min. Doses greater than 4 mcg/kg/min rarely needed. **Maximum:** 10 mcg/kg/min (children: 8–10 mcg/kg/min).

SIDE EFFECTS

Occasional: Flushing of skin, pruritus, pain/redness at injection site.

ADVERSE EFFECTS/ TOXIC REACTIONS

Too-rapid IV infusion rate reduces B/P too quickly. Nausea, vomiting, diaphoresis, apprehension, headache, restless-

N

ness, muscle twitching, dizziness, palpitations, retrosternal pain, abdominal pain may occur. Symptoms disappear rapidly if rate of administration is slowed or temporarily discontinued. Overdose produces metabolic acidosis, tolerance to therapeutic effect.

NURSING CONSIDERATIONS

BASELINE ASSESSMENT

Check with physician for desired B/P parameters (B/P is normally maintained approximately 30%–40% below pretreatment levels). Medication should be discontinued if therapeutic response is not achieved within 10 min after IV infusion at 10 mcg/kg/min.

INTERVENTION/EVALUATION

Monitor EKG, B/P continuously. Monitor blood acid-base balance, electrolytes, laboratory results, I&O. Assess for metabolic acidosis (weakness, disorientation, headache, nausea, hyperventilation, vomiting). Assess for therapeutic response to medication. Monitor B/P for potential rebound hypertension after infusion is discontinued.

nizatidine

nye-**za**-ti-deen
(Apo-Nizatidine ✦, Axid,
Novo-Nizatidine ✦)
**Do not confuse Axid with
Ansaid.**

◆ CLASSIFICATION

PHARMACOTHERAPEUTIC: H_2 receptor antagonist. **CLINICAL:** Antiulcer, gastric acid secretion inhibitor (see p. 111C).

ACTION

Inhibits histamine action at histamine-2 (H_2) receptors of parietal cells. **Therapeutic Effect:** Inhibits basal/nocturnal gastric acid secretion.

PHARMACOKINETICS

Rapidly, well absorbed from GI tract. Protein binding: 35%. Metabolized in liver. Primarily excreted in urine. Not removed by hemodialysis. **Half-life:** 1–2 hrs (increased in renal impairment).

USES

Short-term treatment of active duodenal ulcer, active benign gastric ulcer. Prevention of duodenal ulcer recurrence. Treatment of gastroesophageal reflux disease (GERD), including erosive esophagitis. **OFF-LABEL:** Part of multidrug therapy for *H. pylori* eradication used to reduce risk of duodenal ulcer recurrence.

PRECAUTIONS

Contraindications: Hypersensitivity to other H_2 antagonists. **Cautions:** Renal impairment.

⧖ LIFESPAN CONSIDERATIONS

Pregnancy/Lactation: Unknown if drug crosses placenta or is distributed in breast milk. **Pregnancy Category B. Children:** Safety and efficacy not established in those younger than 12 yrs. **Elderly:** No age-related precautions noted.

INTERACTIONS

DRUG: None significant. **HERBAL:** None significant. **FOOD:** None known. **LAB VALUES:** Interferes with skin tests using allergen extracts. May increase serum alkaline phosphatase, AST, ALT.

AVAILABILITY (Rx)

Capsules (Axid): 150 mg, 300 mg. **Oral Solution (Axid):** 15 mg/ml.

ADMINISTRATION/HANDLING

PO

• Give without regard to meals. Best given after meals or at bedtime. • Do not administer within 1 hr of magnesium- or aluminum-containing antacids (decreases absorption). • May give immediately before eating for heartburn prevention.

INDICATIONS/ROUTES/DOSAGE

Active Duodenal Ulcer
PO: ADULTS, ELDERLY: 300 mg at bedtime or 150 mg twice daily.

Prevention of Duodenal Ulcer Recurrence
PO: ADULTS, ELDERLY: 150 mg at bedtime.

Gastroesophageal Reflux Disease (GERD)
PO: ADULTS, ELDERLY: 150 mg twice a day.

Active Benign Gastric Ulcer
PO: ADULTS, ELDERLY: 150 mg twice daily or 300 mg at bedtime.

Dosage in Renal Impairment
Dosage adjustment is based on creatinine clearance.

Creatinine Clearance	Active Ulcer	Maintenance Therapy
20–50 ml/min	150 mg at bedtime	150 mg every other day
Less than 20 ml/min	150 mg every other day	150 mg q3days

SIDE EFFECTS

Occasional (2%): Drowsiness, fatigue.
Rare (1%): Diaphoresis, rash.

ADVERSE EFFECTS/ TOXIC REACTIONS

Asymptomatic ventricular tachycardia, hyperuricemia not associated with gout, nephrolithiasis occur rarely.

NURSING CONSIDERATIONS

INTERVENTION/EVALUATION

Assess for abdominal pain, GI bleeding (overt blood in emesis/stool, tarry stools). Monitor liver function test (hepatocellular injury).

PATIENT/FAMILY TEACHING

• Avoid tasks that require alertness, motor skills until response to drug is established. • Avoid alcohol, aspirin, smoking, excessive amounts of caffeine. • Report symptoms of heartburn, acid indigestion, sour stomach persisting after 2 wks of continuous use of nizatidine.

---

norepinephrine

nor-ep-i-**nef**-rin
(Levophed)

BLACK BOX ALERT Extravasation may produce severe tissue necrosis, sloughing. Using fine hypodermic needle, liberally infiltrate area with 10–15 ml saline solution containing 5–10 mg phentolamine.
Do not confuse Levophed with Levaquin or levofloxacin, or norepinephrine with epinephrine.

◆CLASSIFICATION

PHARMACOTHERAPEUTIC: Sympathomimetic. **CLINICAL:** Vasopressor.

ACTION

Stimulates beta₁-adrenergic receptors, alpha-adrenergic receptors, increasing peripheral resistance. Enhances contractile myocardial force, increases cardiac output. Constricts resistance, capacitance vessels. **Therapeutic Effect:** Increases systemic B/P, coronary blood flow.

PHARMACOKINETICS

Route	Onset	Peak	Duration
IV	Rapid	1–2 min	N/A

Localized in sympathetic tissue. Metabolized in liver. Primarily excreted in urine.

USES

Severe hypotension, treatment of shock persisting after fluid volume replacement.

PRECAUTIONS

Contraindications: Hypovolemic states (unless as an emergency measure), mesenteric/peripheral vascular thrombosis,

---

profound hypoxia. **Cautions:** Occlusive vascular disease, those taking MAOIs.

⏳ LIFESPAN CONSIDERATIONS

Pregnancy/Lactation: Readily crosses placenta. May produce fetal anoxia due to uterine contraction, constriction of uterine blood vessels. **Pregnancy Category C. Children/Elderly:** No age-related precautions noted.

INTERACTIONS

DRUG: MAOIs, antidepressants (tricyclic) may prolong hypertension. **HERBAL:** None significant. **FOOD:** None known. **LAB VALUES:** None significant.

AVAILABILITY (Rx)

Injection Solution: 1 mg/ml.

ADMINISTRATION/HANDLING

◀ALERT▶ Blood, fluid volume depletion should be corrected before drug is administered.

🔋 **IV**

◀ALERT▶ Dilute only in dextrose-containing solutions (D$_5$W, D$_5$NS). Dextrose-containing fluids offer protection against significant loss of potency due to oxidation. Administration in saline solution only is not recommended.

Reconstitution • Add 4 ml (4 mg) to 250 ml D$_5$W (16 mcg/ml). **Maximum concentration:** 32 ml (32 mg) to 250 ml (128 mcg/ml).

Rate of Administration • Closely monitor IV infusion flow rate (use infusion pump). • Monitor B/P q2min during IV infusion until desired therapeutic response is achieved, then q5min during remaining IV infusion. • Never leave pt unattended. • Maintain B/P at 90–100 mm Hg in previously normotensive pts, and 30–40 mm Hg below preexisting B/P in previously hypertensive pts. • Reduce IV infusion gradually. Avoid abrupt withdrawal. • If using peripherally inserted catheter, it is imperative to check the IV site frequently for free flow and infused vein for blanching, hardness to vein, coldness, pallor to extremity. • If ex-

travasation occurs, area should be infiltrated with 10–15 ml sterile saline containing 5–10 mg phentolamine (does not alter pressor effects of norepinephrine).

Storage • Do not use if solution is brown or contains precipitate. • Store at room temperature.

🔲 IV INCOMPATIBILITIES

Pantoprazole (Protonix), regular insulin.

🔲 IV COMPATIBILITIES

Amiodarone (Cordarone), calcium gluconate, dexmedetomidine (Precedex), diltiazem (Cardizem), dobutamine (Dobutrex), dopamine (Intropin), epinephrine, esmolol (Brevibloc), fentanyl (Sublimaze), furosemide (Lasix), haloperidol (Haldol), heparin, hydromorphone (Dilaudid), labetalol (Trandate), lipids, lorazepam (Ativan), magnesium, midazolam (Versed), milrinone (Primacor), morphine, nicardipine (Cardene), nitroglycerin, potassium chloride, propofol (Diprivan).

INDICATIONS/ROUTES/DOSAGE

Acute Hypotension Unresponsive to Fluid Volume Replacement
IV INFUSION: ADULTS, ELDERLY: Initially, administer at 4–12 mcg/min. Adjust rate of flow to desired response. Average maintenance dose: 2–4 mcg/min. **Maximum:** 30 mcg/min. **CHILDREN:** Initially, 0.05–0.1 mcg/kg/min; titrate to desired effect. **Maximum:** 2 mcg/kg/min.

SIDE EFFECTS

Norepinephrine produces less pronounced, less frequent side effects than epinephrine. **Occasional (5%–3%):** Anxiety, bradycardia, palpitations. **Rare (2%–1%):** Nausea, anginal pain, shortness of breath, fever.

ADVERSE EFFECTS/ TOXIC REACTIONS

Extravasation may produce tissue necrosis, sloughing. Overdose manifested as severe hypertension with violent headache (may be first clinical sign of overdose), arrhythmias, photophobia, retrosternal or pharyngeal pain, pallor, diaphoresis, vomiting. Prolonged therapy may result in plasma volume depletion. Hypotension may recur if plasma volume is not maintained.

NURSING CONSIDERATIONS

BASELINE ASSESSMENT

Assess EKG, B/P continuously (be alert to precipitous B/P drop). Never leave pt alone during IV infusion. Be alert to pt complaint of headache.

INTERVENTION/EVALUATION

Monitor IV flow rate diligently. Assess for extravasation characterized by blanching of skin over vein, coolness (results from local vasoconstriction); color, temperature of IV site extremity (pallor, cyanosis, mottling). Assess nailbed capillary refill. Monitor I&O; measure output hourly, report urine output less than 30 ml/hr. Once B/P parameter has been reached, IV infusion should not be restarted unless systolic B/P falls below 90 mm Hg.

norfloxacin

nor-**flox**-a-sin
(Apo-Norflox ♣, Norfloxacine ♣,
Noroxin, Novo-Norfloxacin ♣,
PMS-Norfloxacin ♣)

BLACK BOX ALERT May increase risk of tendonitis, tendon rupture. **Do not confuse norfloxacin with Norflex, or Noroxin with Norflex or Neurontin.**

◆ CLASSIFICATION

PHARMACOTHERAPEUTIC: Quinolone. **CLINICAL:** Antibiotic (see p. 26C).

ACTION

Interferes with bacterial cell replication by inhibiting DNA-gyrase in susceptible microorganisms. **Therapeutic Effect:** Bactericidal.

USES

Treatment of susceptible infections due to *E. faecalis, E. coli, K. pneumoniae, P. mirabilis, P. aeruginosa, S. epidermidis, S. saprophyticus,* including UTIs, acute or chronic prostatitis.

PRECAUTIONS

Contraindications: Children younger than 18 yrs (increased risk of arthropathy), hypersensitivity to other quinolones. **Cautions:** Renal impairment, predisposition to seizures, diabetes.

⏳ LIFESPAN CONSIDERATIONS

Pregnancy/Lactation: Unknown if drug crosses placenta or is distributed in breast milk. **Pregnancy Category C. Children:** Safety and efficacy not established. **Elderly:** Age-related renal impairment may require dosage adjustment.

INTERACTIONS

DRUG: Antacids, sucralfate, didanosine may decrease absorption. May increase effects of **oral anticoagulants.** May increase concentration of **cyclosporine.** Decreases clearance of **theophylline,** may increase concentration, risk of toxicity. **HERBAL: Dong quai, St. John's wort** may increase risk of photosensitization. **FOOD:** None known. **LAB VALUES:** May increase serum alkaline phosphatase, LDH, AST, ALT, amylase.

AVAILABILITY (Rx)

Tablets: 400 mg.

ADMINISTRATION/HANDLING

PO
• Give 1 hr before or 2 hrs after meals with 8 oz of water. • Encourage additional glasses of water between meals. • Do not administer antacids with or within 2 hrs of norfloxacin dose. • Encourage cranberry juice, citrus fruits (to acidify urine).

INDICATIONS/ROUTES/DOSAGE

UTI
PO: ADULTS, ELDERLY: 400 mg twice daily for 3–21 days.

N

♣ Canadian trade name   🍶 Non-Crushable Drug   **HIGH ALERT** High Alert drug

Prostatitis
PO: ADULTS: 400 mg twice daily for 4–6 wks.

Dosage in Renal Impairment
Dosage and frequency are modified based on creatinine clearance.

Creatinine Clearance	Dosage
30 ml/min or higher	400 mg twice daily
Less than 30 ml/min	400 mg once daily

SIDE EFFECTS

Frequent: Nausea, headache, dizziness. **Rare:** Vomiting, diarrhea, dry mouth, bitter taste, anxiety, drowsiness, insomnia, photosensitivity, tinnitus, crystalluria, rash, fever, seizures.

ADVERSE EFFECTS/ TOXIC REACTIONS

Superinfection, anaphylaxis, Stevens-Johnson syndrome, arthropathy occur rarely. Hypersensitivity reactions, including photosensitivity, rash, pruritus, blisters, edema, burning skin, may be noted.

NURSING CONSIDERATIONS

BASELINE ASSESSMENT
Question for history of hypersensitivity to norfloxacin, quinolones.

INTERVENTION/EVALUATION
Assess for nausea, headache, dizziness. Evaluate food tolerance. Assess for chest, joint pain (arthropathy).

PATIENT/FAMILY TEACHING
• Take 1 hr before or 2 hrs after meals. • Complete full course of therapy. • Take with 8 oz of water; drink several glasses of water between meals. • May cause dizziness, drowsiness. • Do not take antacids with or within 2 hrs of norfloxacin dose (reduces or destroys effectiveness).

nortriptyline

nor-**trip**-ti-leen
(Apo-Nortriptyline ♣, Aventyl ♣, Norventyl ♣, Pamelor)

BLACK BOX ALERT Increased risk of suicidal thinking and behavior in children, adolescents, young adults 18–24 yrs with major depressive disorder, other psychiatric disorders.
Do not confuse Aventyl with Bentyl, or nortriptyline with amitriptyline, desipramine, or Norpramin.

◆CLASSIFICATION

PHARMACOTHERAPEUTIC: Tricyclic compound. **CLINICAL:** Antidepressant (see pp. 39C, 155C).

ACTION

Blocks reuptake of neurotransmitters (norepinephrine, serotonin) at neuronal presynaptic membranes, increasing their availability at postsynaptic receptor sites. **Therapeutic Effect:** Relieves depression, anxiety disorders, nocturnal enuresis.

USES

Treatment of various forms of depression, often in conjunction with psychotherapy. Treatment of nocturnal enuresis. **OFF-LABEL:** Treatment of neurogenic pain, anxiety disorders, ADHD, adjunctive therapy for smoking cessation.

PRECAUTIONS

Contraindications: Acute recovery period after MI, MAOI use within 14 days. **Cautions:** Prostatic hyperplasia, history of urinary retention/obstruction, glaucoma, diabetes mellitus, history of seizures, hyperthyroidism, cardiac/hepatic/renal disease, psychosis, increased intraocular pressure, pts at high risk for suicide. **Pregnancy Category C.**

INTERACTIONS

DRUG: Alcohol, other CNS depressants may increase CNS effects, respiratory depression, hypotensive effects. **Cimetidine** may increase concentration, risk of toxicity. **MAOIs** may increase risk of neuroleptic malignant syndrome, seizures, hyperpyrexia, hypertensive crisis. **HERBAL: Gotu kola, kava kava, St. John's wort, valerian** may increase CNS depression and risk of serotonin syndrome. **FOOD:** None known. **LAB VALUES:** May alter serum glucose, EKG readings. **Therapeutic peak serum level:** 6–10 mcg/ml; **therapeutic trough serum level:** 0.5–2 mcg/ml. **Toxic peak serum level:** greater than 12 mcg/ml; **toxic trough serum level:** greater than 2 mcg/ml.

AVAILABILITY (Rx)

Capsules (Pamelor): 10 mg, 25 mg, 50 mg, 75 mg. **Oral Solution (Pamelor):** 10 mg/5 ml.

ADMINISTRATION/HANDLING

◄**ALERT**► At least 14 days must elapse between use of MAOIs and nortriptyline.

PO
• Give with food, milk if GI distress occurs.
• Dilute oral solution in water, milk, or fruit juice. Give immediately. (Do not mix with grape juice/carbonated beverages.)

INDICATIONS/ROUTES/DOSAGE

Depression
PO: ADULTS: 25 mg 3–4 times a day up to 150 mg/day. **ELDERLY:** Initially, 10–25 mg at bedtime. May increase by 25 mg every 3–7 days. **Maximum:** 150 mg/day. **CHILDREN 12 YRS AND OLDER:** 1–3 mg/kg/day or 30–50 mg/day in 3–4 divided doses. **Maximum:** 150 mg/day. **CHILDREN 6–11 YRS:** 1–3 mg/kg/day or 10–20 mg/day in 3–4 divided doses.

Enuresis
PO: CHILDREN 12 YRS AND OLDER: 25–35 mg/day. **CHILDREN 8–11 YRS:** 10–20 mg/day. **CHILDREN 6–7 YRS:** 10 mg/day.

SIDE EFFECTS

Frequent: Drowsiness, fatigue, dry mouth, blurred vision, constipation, delayed micturition, orthostatic hypotension, diaphoresis, impaired concentration, increased appetite, urinary retention. **Occasional:** GI disturbances (nausea, GI distress, metallic taste), photosensitivity. **Rare:** Paradoxical reactions (agitation, restlessness, nightmares, insomnia), extrapyramidal symptoms (particularly fine hand tremor).

ADVERSE EFFECTS/ TOXIC REACTIONS

High dosage may produce cardiovascular effects (severe orthostatic hypotension, dizziness, tachycardia, palpitations, arrhythmias), altered temperature regulation (hyperpyrexia, hypothermia). Abrupt discontinuation from prolonged therapy may produce headache, malaise, nausea, vomiting, vivid dreams.

NURSING CONSIDERATIONS

BASELINE ASSESSMENT

Assess for suicidal ideation/tendencies, behavior, thought content, appearance. Obtain baseline glucose, cholesterol levels. For pts on long-term therapy, hepatic/renal function tests, blood counts should be performed periodically.

INTERVENTION/EVALUATION

Supervise suicidal-risk pt closely during early therapy (as depression lessens, energy level improves, increasing suicide potential). Assess appearance, behavior, speech pattern, level of interest, mood. Monitor daily pattern of bowel activity, stool consistency. Avoid constipation with increased fluids, bulky foods. Monitor B/P, pulse for hypotension, arrhythmias, weight. Assess for urinary retention, including output estimate, bladder palpation if indicated. Therapeutic peak serum level: 6–10 mcg/ml; trough serum level: 0.5–2 mcg/ml. Toxic peak serum level: greater than 12 mcg/ml; toxic trough: greater than 2 mcg/ml.

N

PATIENT/FAMILY TEACHING

• Change positions slowly to avoid hypotensive effect. • Tolerance to postural hypotension, sedative, anticholinergic effects usually develops during early therapy. • Avoid alcohol. • Avoid tasks that require alertness, motor skills until response to drug is established. • Therapeutic effect may be noted in 2 wks or longer. • Photosensitivity to sun may occur. • Use sunscreen, protective clothing. • Dry mouth may be relieved by sugarless gum, sips of water. • Report visual disturbances, worsening depression, suicidal ideation, unusual changes in behavior (esp. at initiation of therapy or with changes in dosage). • Do not abruptly discontinue medication.

nystatin

nye-**stat**-in
(Candistatin ✤, Nystop, Pedi-Dri)
Do not confuse nystatin with atorvastatin, fluvastatin, lovastatin, Nitrostat, pitavastatin, pravastatin, rosuvastatin, or simvastatin.

FIXED-COMBINATION(S)

Mycolog, Myco-Triacet: nystatin/triamcinolone (a steroid): 100,000 units/0.1%.

◆ CLASSIFICATION

PHARMACOTHERAPEUTIC: Polyene antifungal antibiotic. **CLINICAL:** Antifungal (see p. 50C).

ACTION

Binds to sterols in cell membrane, increasing fungal cell membrane permeability, permitting loss of potassium, other cellular components. **Therapeutic Effect:** Fungistatic.

PHARMACOKINETICS

PO: Poorly absorbed from GI tract. Eliminated unchanged in feces. **Topical:** Not absorbed systemically from intact skin.

USES

Treatment of cutaneous, intestinal, oral cavity, infections caused by *Candida* spp.

PRECAUTIONS

Contraindications: None known. **Cautions:** None known.

⧖ LIFESPAN CONSIDERATIONS

Pregnancy/Lactation: Unknown if distributed in breast milk. Vaginal applicators may be contraindicated, requiring manual insertion of tablets during pregnancy. **Pregnancy Category B (C: oral). Children:** No age-related precautions noted for suspension, topical use. Lozenges not recommended in those younger than 5 yrs. **Elderly:** No age-related precautions noted.

INTERACTIONS

DRUG: None significant. **HERBAL:** None significant. **FOOD:** None known. **LAB VALUES:** None significant.

AVAILABILITY (Rx)

Cream: 100,000 units/g. **Ointment:** 100,000 units/g. **Oral Suspension:** 100,000 units/ml. **Tablets:** 500,000 units. **Topical Powder (Nystop, Pedi-Dri):** 100,000 units/g.

ADMINISTRATION/HANDLING

PO
• Shake suspension well before administration. • Place and hold suspension in mouth or swish throughout mouth as long as possible before swallowing. • For neonates and infants, paint into recesses of the mouth.

INDICATIONS/ROUTES/DOSAGE

Intestinal Infection
PO: ADULTS, ELDERLY: 500,000–1,000,000 units q8h.

Oral Candidiasis
PO: ADULTS, ELDERLY, CHILDREN: 400,000–600,000 units 4 times a day. **INFANTS:** 200,000 units 4 times a day. **PREMATURE INFANTS:** 100,000 units 4 times a day.

Cutaneous Candidal Infections
Topical: ADULTS, ELDERLY, CHILDREN: Apply 2–3 times a day.

SIDE EFFECTS

Occasional: **PO:** None known. **Topical:** Skin irritation. **Vaginal:** Vaginal irritation.

ADVERSE EFFECTS/ TOXIC REACTIONS

High dosages of oral form may produce nausea, vomiting, diarrhea, GI distress.

NURSING CONSIDERATIONS

BASELINE ASSESSMENT

Confirm that cultures, histologic tests were obtained for accurate diagnosis. Inspect oral mucous membranes.

INTERVENTION/EVALUATION

Assess for increased skin irritation with topical, increased vaginal discharge with vaginal application.

PATIENT/FAMILY TEACHING

• Do not miss doses; complete full length of treatment (continue vaginal use during menses). • Notify physician if nausea, vomiting, diarrhea, stomach pain develops. • **Vaginal:** Insert high in vagina. • Check with physician regarding douching, sexual intercourse. • **Topical:** Rub well into affected areas. • Avoid contact with eyes. • Use cream (sparingly) or powder on erythematous areas. • Keep areas clean, dry; wear light clothing for ventilation. • Separate personal items in contact with affected areas.

N

obinutuzumab

oh-bi-nue-**tooz**-ue-mab
(Gazyva)

BLACK BOX ALERT Hepatitis B reactivation resulting in hepatic failure, fulminant hepatitis, and death have occurred. Screen all pt for hepatitis B infection before initiating treatment. Progressive multifocal leukoencephalopathy (PML) including fatal PML reported.

◆CLASSIFICATION

PHARMACOTHERAPEUTIC: Monoclonal antibody. **CLINICAL:** Antineoplastic.

ACTION

Targets CD20 antigen expressed on surface of B lymphocytes. Mediates B-cell lysis, cellular cytotoxicity, and antibody-dependant cellular phagocytosis (macrophage ingestion). **Therapeutic Effect:** Inhibits tumor cell growth and proliferation in chronic lymphocytic leukemia.

PHARMACOKINETICS

Metabolism and elimination not specified. **Half-life:** 28 days.

USES

Treatment of previously untreated chronic lymphocytic leukemia (CLL), in combination with chlorambucil.

PRECAUTIONS

Contraindications: None known. **Cautions:** History of anemia, leukopenia, neutropenia, thrombocytopenia; asthma, COPD, electrolyte imbalance, GI bleeding, gout, elderly, renal/hepatic impairment. Avoid use of live virus vaccines.

☒ LIFESPAN CONSIDERATIONS

Pregnancy/Lactation: Unknown if distributed in breast milk. Must either discontinue drug or discontinue breastfeeding. **Pregnancy Category C. Children:** Safety and efficacy not established. **El-**

derly: May have increased risk of adverse reactions.

INTERACTIONS

DRUG: ACE inhibitors, angiotensin receptor blockers, beta blockers may increase risk of hypotension. **HERBAL:** None significant. **FOOD:** None known. **LAB VALUES:** May increase serum alkaline phosphatase, AST, ALT, bilirubin, creatinine, uric acid. May decrease serum albumin, Hgb, Hct, lymphocytes, neutrophils, platelets, potassium, sodium.

AVAILABILITY (Rx)

Solution, Injection: 1,000 mg/40 ml (25 mg/ml) single-use vial.

ADMINISTRATION/HANDLING

◀ALERT▶ Administer via dedicated line. Do not administer IV push or bolus. Withhold hypertensive medications at least 12 hrs before and 1 hr after administration. Do not mix with dextrose-containing fluids.

IV

Reconstitution • Visually inspect for particulate matter or discoloration. • For 100-mg dose: withdraw 4 ml solution from vial and dilute only 4 ml (100 mg) in 100 ml 0.9% NaCl for immediate administration. Dilute remaining 36 ml (900 mg) into 250 ml 0.9% NaCl at same time and refrigerate for up to 24 hrs for cycle 1: day 2. For remaining infusions (Day 8 and 15 of cycle 1), and day 1 of cycles 2–6, dilute 40 ml (1,000 mg) solution in 250 ml NaCl infusion bag. • Gently mix by inversion. • Do not shake. **Rate of Administration** • **Day 1 of Cycle 1 (100 mg):** Infuse over 4 hrs (25 mg/hr). • Do not increase infusion rate. • **Day 2 of Cycle 1 (900 mg):** Infuse at 50 mg/hr. • May increase by 50mg/hr every 30 min to maximum rate of 400 mg/hr. • **Day 8 and Day 15 of Cycle 1, and Day 1 of Cycles 2–6 (1,000 mg):** Start at 100 mg/hr. May increase by 100 mg/hr every 30 min to maximum rate of 400 mg/hr. • Increase rate based on tolerability.

Storage • Solution should appear clear, colorless to slightly brown. • May refrigerate diluted solution up to 24 hrs.

INDICATIONS/ROUTES/DOSAGE

Chronic Lymphocytic Leukemia (CLL)

◀ALERT▶ Premedicate with glucocorticoid, acetaminophen, and antihistamine to decrease severity of infusion reaction. Consider premedication with antihyperuricemics (allopurinol) 12–24 hrs for pts with high tumor burden or high circulating absolute lymphocyte count greater than 25×10^9/L. Recommend antimicrobial prophylaxis throughout treatment for pts with neutropenia.

IV: ADULTS/ELDERLY: Six treatment cycles of 28 day cycle. **Day 1 of Cycle 1:** 100 mg. **Day 2 of Cycle 1:** 900 mg. **Day 8 and Day 15 of Cycle 1 and Day 1 of Cycles 2–6:** 1,000 mg. Discontinue treatment if any severe to life-threatening infusion reactions occur.

SIDE EFFECTS

Frequent (69%): Infusion reactions (pruritis, flushing, urticaria). **Occasional (10%):** Pyrexia, cough.

ADVERSE EFFECTS/ TOXIC REACTIONS

Thrombocytopenia, neutropenia, leukopenia, lymphopenia (47%–80% of pts) is an expected response to therapy, but more severe reactions including bone marrow failure, febrile neutropenia, opportunistic infection may result in life-threatening events. Hepatitis B reactivation may occur. Infusion reactions including hypotension, tachycardia, dyspnea, bronchospasm, wheezing, laryngeal edema, nausea, vomiting, flushing, pyrexia may occur during infusion. Tumor lysis syndrome may present as acute renal failure, hypocalcemia, hyperuricemia, hyperphosphatemia within 12–24 hrs of infusion. Immunogenicity (autoantibodies) occurred in 13% of pts. Progressive multifocal leukoencephalopathy (PML) occurred rarely and may include weakness, paralysis, vision loss, aphasia, cognition impairment.

NURSING CONSIDERATIONS

BASELINE ASSESSMENT

Obtain baseline CBC, serum chemistries, ionized calcium, phosphate, uric acid; vital signs. Screen for history of anemia, asthma, arrhythmias, COPD, diabetes mellitus, GI bleeding, hypertension, hepatitis B infection, hepatic/renal impairment, peripheral edema. Receive full medication history esp. hypertension, anticoagulant medications. Perform baseline visual acuity.

INTERVENTION/EVALUATION

Monitor CBC, serum electrolytes, hepatic function test, vital signs. Monitor all pts for cardiovascular alterations, respiratory distress. If respiratory reactions occur, consider administration of oxygen, epinephrine, albuterol treatments. Locate rapid-sequence intubation kit if respiratory compromise occurs. Monitor strict I&O, hydration status. If PML suspected, consult neurologist for proper management. Obtain EKG for palpitations, severe hypokalemia, hyponatremia.

PATIENT/FAMILY TEACHING

• Blood levels will be routinely monitored. • Avoid pregnancy. • Report any yellowing of skin or eyes, abdominal pain, bruising, black/tarry stools, amber or bloody urine. • Fever, cough, burning with urination, body aches, chills may indicate acute infection. • Avoid alcohol. • Immediately report difficult breathing, severe coughing, chest tightness, wheezing. • Paralysis, vision changes, impaired speech, altered mental status may indicate life-threatening neurologic event.

octreotide

ock-**tree**-oh-tide
(Sandostatin, Sandostatin LAR)

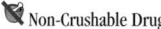

Do not confuse Sandostatin with Sandimmune, Sandostatin LAR, sargramostim, or simvastatin.

◆CLASSIFICATION

PHARMACOTHERAPEUTIC: Somatostatin analogue. **CLINICAL:** Secretory inhibitory, growth hormone suppressant.

ACTION

Suppresses secretion of serotonin, gastroenteropancreatic peptides. Enhances fluid/electrolyte absorption from GI tract. **Therapeutic Effect:** Prolongs intestinal transit time.

PHARMACOKINETICS

Route	Onset	Peak	Duration
Subcutaneous	N/A	N/A	Up to 12 hrs

Rapidly, completely absorbed from injection site. Protein binding: 65%. Metabolized in liver. Excreted in urine. Removed by hemodialysis. **Half-life:** 1.7–1.9 hrs.

USES

Controls diarrhea and flushing in pts with metastatic carcinoid tumors, treatment of watery diarrhea associated with vasoactive intestinal peptic-secreting tumors (VIPomas), acromegaly. **OFF-LABEL:** Control of bleeding esophageal varices, treatment of AIDS-associated secretory diarrhea, chemotherapy-induced diarrhea, insulinomas, small-bowel fistulas, Zollinger-Ellison syndrome, Cushing's syndrome, hypothalamic obesity, malignant bowel obstruction, postgastrectomy dumping syndrome.

PRECAUTIONS

Contraindications: None known. **Cautions:** Diabetic pts with gastroparesis, renal failure, hepatic impairment, HF, concomitant medications altering heart rate or rhythm.

⧗ LIFESPAN CONSIDERATIONS

Pregnancy/Lactation: Unknown if distributed in breast milk. **Pregnancy Cate-**gory B. **Children:** Safety and efficacy not established. **Elderly:** No age-related precautions noted.

INTERACTIONS

DRUG: May decrease effectiveness of **cyclosporine. Glucagon, growth hormone, insulin, oral antidiabetics** may alter glucose concentrations. **HERBAL:** Avoid herbs that have hypoglycemic activity (e.g., **garlic, ginger, ginseng**). **FOOD:** None known. **LAB VALUES:** May decrease serum thyroxine (T_4). May increase serum alkaline phosphatase, ALT, AST, GGT.

AVAILABILITY (Rx)

Injection Solution (Sandostatin): 0.05 mg/ml, 0.1 mg/ml, 0.2 mg/ml, 0.5 mg/ml, 1 mg/ml. **Injection Suspension (Sandostatin LAR):** 10-mg, 20-mg, 30-mg vials.

ADMINISTRATION/HANDLING

◀**ALERT**▶ Sandostatin may be given IV, IM, subcutaneous. Sandostatin LAR Depot may be given only IM.

IM
• Give immediately after mixing. • Administer deep IM in large muscle mass at 4-wk intervals. • Avoid deltoid injections.

Subcutaneous
• Do not use if discolored or particulates form. • Avoid multiple injections at same site within short periods.

 IV
• Dilute in 50–100 ml 0.9% NaCl or D_5W and infuse over 15–30 min. In emergency, may give IV push over 3 min.

INDICATIONS/ROUTES/DOSAGE

Diarrhea
IV *(Sandostatin)*: **ADULTS, ELDERLY:** Initially, 50–100 mcg q8h. May increase by 100 mcg/dose q48h. **Maximum:** 500 mcg q8h.

IV, Subcutaneous *(Sandostatin)*: 1–10 mcg/kg q12h.

Carcinoid Tumor
IV, Subcutaneous *(Sandostatin)*: **ADULTS, ELDERLY:** Initial 2 wks, 100–600 mcg/day in 2–4 divided doses. Range: 50–750 mcg.
IM *(Sandostatin Lar)*: **ADULTS, ELDERLY:** Must be stabilized on subcutaneous octreotide for at least 2 wks. 20 mg q4wks.

Vasoactive Intestinal Peptic-Secreting Tumor (VIPoma)
IV, Subcutaneous *(Sandostatin)*: **ADULTS, ELDERLY:** Initial 2 wks, 200–300 mcg/day in 2–4 divided doses. **Range:** 150–750 mcg.
IM *(Sandostatin Lar)*: **ADULTS, ELDERLY:** Must be stabilized on subcutaneous octreotide for at least 2 wks. 20 mg q4wks.

Esophageal Varices
IV *(Sandostatin)*: **ADULTS, ELDERLY:** Bolus of 25–100 mcg followed by IV infusion of 25–50 mcg/hr for 2–5 days.

Acromegaly
IV, Subcutaneous *(Sandostatin)*: **ADULTS, ELDERLY:** 50 mcg 3 times a day. Increase as needed. **Range:** 300–1,500 mcg/day.
IM *(Sandostatin Lar)*: **ADULTS, ELDERLY:** Must be stabilized on subcutaneous octreotide for at least 2 wks. 20 mg q4wks for 3 mos. **Maximum:** 40 mg q4wks.

SIDE EFFECTS

Frequent (10%–6%; 58%–30% in Acromegaly Pts): Diarrhea, nausea, abdominal discomfort, headache, injection site pain. **Occasional (5%–1%):** Vomiting, flatulence, constipation, alopecia, facial flushing, pruritus, dizziness, fatigue, arrhythmias, ecchymosis, blurred vision. **Rare (Less Than 1%):** Depression, diminished libido, vertigo, palpitations, dyspnea.

ADVERSE EFFECTS/ TOXIC REACTIONS

Increased risk of cholelithiasis. Prolonged high-dose therapy may produce hypothyroidism. GI bleeding, hepatitis, seizures occur rarely.

NURSING CONSIDERATIONS

BASELINE ASSESSMENT
Establish baseline B/P, weight, thyroid function, serum glucose, electrolytes.

INTERVENTION/EVALUATION
Monitor serum glucose, thyroid function tests; fluid, electrolyte balance; fecal fat. In acromegaly, monitor growth hormone levels. Weigh every 2–3 days, report over 5-lb gain per wk. Monitor B/P, pulse, respirations periodically during treatment. Be alert for decreased urinary output, peripheral edema (esp. ankles). Monitor daily pattern of bowel activity, stool consistency.

PATIENT/FAMILY TEACHING
• Therapy should provide significant improvement of severe, watery diarrhea.

---

ocular lubricant

ock-yoo-lar **lube**-ri-cant
(Hypotears, Lacrilube, Tears Naturale)

◆CLASSIFICATION
PHARMACOTHERAPEUTIC: Topical ophthalmic. **CLINICAL:** Lubricant, toner, buffer, viscosity agent.

ACTION

Forms an occlusive film on eye surface. **Therapeutic Effect:** Lubricates/protects eye from drying.

USES

Protection/lubrication of eye in exposure keratitis, decreased corneal sensitivity, recurrent corneal erosions, keratitis sicca (particularly for nighttime use), after removal of foreign body, during and following surgery.

PRECAUTIONS

Contraindications: None known. **Cautions:** None known. **Pregnancy Category Unknown.**

INTERACTIONS

DRUG: None significant. **HERBAL:** None significant. **FOOD:** None known. **LAB VALUES:** None significant.

AVAILABILITY (OTC)

Ophthalmic Ointment. Solution.

ADMINISTRATION/HANDLING

Ophthalmic
• Do not use with contact lenses. • Place gloved finger on lower eyelid and pull out until a pocket is formed between eye and lower lid. • Place prescribed number of drops (¼–½ inch of ointment) into pocket. • Instruct pt to close eye gently (so medication will not be squeezed out of the sac).

Solution
• Instruct pt to apply digital pressure to lacrimal sac at inner canthus for 1 min to minimize systemic absorption.

Ointment
• Instruct pt to roll eyeball to increase contact area of drug to eye.

INDICATIONS/ROUTES/DOSAGE

Usual Ophthalmic Dosage
Ophthalmic: ADULTS, ELDERLY: Small amount in conjunctival sac as needed.

SIDE EFFECTS

Frequent: Temporary blurred vision after administration, esp. with ointment.

ADVERSE EFFECTS/ TOXIC REACTIONS

None known.

NURSING CONSIDERATIONS

PATIENT/FAMILY TEACHING
• Do not use with contact lenses. • Do not touch tip of tube or dropper to any surface (may contaminate). • Temporary blurred vision will occur, esp. with administration of ointment. • Avoid activities requiring visual acuity until blurring clears. • Report eye pain, change of vision, worsening of condition or if condition is unchanged after 72 hrs.

ofatumumab

oh-fa-**tue**-mue-mab
(Arzerra)
Do not confuse ofatumumab with omalizumab.

◆CLASSIFICATION

PHARMACOTHERAPEUTIC: Monoclonal antibody. **CLINICAL:** Antineoplastic.

ACTION

Binds to CD20 molecule, the antigen on surface of B-cell lymphocytes; inhibits early-stage B-lymphocyte activation. **Therapeutic Effect:** Controls tumor growth, triggers cell death.

PHARMACOKINETICS

Eliminated through both a target-independent route and a B-cell–mediated route. Due to depletion of B cells, clearance is decreased substantially after subsequent infusions compared to first infusion. **Half-life:** 12–16 days.

USES

Treatment of chronic lymphocytic leukemia (CLL).

PRECAUTIONS

Contraindications: None known. **Cautions:** Carriers of hepatitis B virus.

⌛ LIFESPAN CONSIDERATIONS

Pregnancy/Lactation: Unknown if distributed in breast milk. **Pregnancy Category C. Children:** Safety and efficacy not established. **Elderly:** No age-related precautions noted.

INTERACTIONS

DRUG: **Bone marrow depressants** may increase myelosuppression. **Live virus vaccines** may potentiate virus replication, increase vaccine side effects, decrease pt's antibody response to vaccine. **HERBAL:** **Echinacea** may decrease concentration/effects. **FOOD:** None known. **LAB VALUES:** May decrease WBC count, platelets.

AVAILABILITY (Rx)

Solution for Injection: 100 mg/5 ml single-use vial.

ADMINSTRATION/HANDLING

 IV

◄**ALERT**► Do not give by IV push or bolus. Use in-line filter supplied with product.

Reconstitution • **300-mg dose:** Withdraw and discard 15 ml from 1,000 ml 0.9% NaCl. • Withdraw 5 ml from each of 3 vials and add to bag. • Gently invert. • **2,000-mg dose:** Withdraw and discard 100 ml from 1,000 ml 0.9% NaCl. • Withdraw 5 ml from each of 2 vials and add to bag. • Gently invert.

Rate of Administration • **Dose 1:** Initiate infusion at rate of 3.6 mg/hr (12 ml/hr). • **Dose 2:** Initiate infusion at rate of 24 mg/hr (12 ml/hr). • **Dose 3–12:** Initiate infusion at rate of 50 mg/hr (25 ml/hr). • If no infusion toxicity, rate of infusion may be increased every 30 min, using following table:

Interval After Start of Infusion (min)	Dose 1 (ml/hr)	Dose 2 (ml/hr)	Doses 3–12 (ml/hr)
0–30	12	12	25
31–60	25	25	50
61–90	50	50	100
91–120	100	100	200
Over 120	200	200	400

Storage • Refrigerate vials. • After dilution, solution should be used within first 12 hrs; discard preparation after 24 hrs. • Discard if discoloration is present, but solution may contain visible, translucent-to-white particulates (will be removed by in-line filter).

🔲 IV COMPATIBILITY

Prepare all doses with 0.9% NaCl. Do not mix with dextrose solutions or any other medications.

INDICATIONS/ROUTES/DOSAGE

◄**ALERT**► Premedicate 30 min to 2 hrs before each infusion with acetaminophen, an antihistamine, and a corticosteroid as prophylaxis for infusion reaction. Flush IV line with 0.9% NaCl before and after each dose.

Chronic Lymphocytic Leukemia
IV Infusion: ADULTS, ELDERLY: Recommended dosage is 12 doses given on the following schedule: 300 mg initial dose (dose 1), followed 1 wk later by 2,000 mg weekly for 7 doses (doses 2–8), followed 4 wks later by 2,000 mg every 4 wks for 4 doses (doses 9–12).

SIDE EFFECTS

Frequent (20%–14%): Fever, cough, diarrhea, fatigue, rash. **Occasional (13%–5%):** Nausea, bronchitis, peripheral edema, nasopharyngitis, urticaria, insomnia, headache, sinusitis, muscle spasm, hypertension.

ADVERSE EFFECTS/ TOXIC REACTIONS

Most common serious adverse reactions were bacterial, viral, fungal infections (including pneumonia and sepsis), septic shock, neutropenia, thrombocytopenia. Infusion reactions occur more frequently with first 2 infusions. Severe infusion reactions manifested as angioedema, bronchospasm, dyspnea, fever, chills, back pain, hypotension. Progressive multifocal leukoencephalopathy may occur. Small bowel obstruction has been noted.

NURSING CONSIDERATIONS

BASELINE ASSESSMENT

Screen pts at high risk of hepatitis B virus. Assess baseline CBC prior to therapy.

INTERVENTION/EVALUATION

Monitor CBC for evidence of myelosuppression during therapy, and increase frequency of monitoring in pts who develop grade 3 or 4 cytopenia. Monitor for blood dyscrasias (fever, sore throat, signs of local infection, unusual bruising/bleeding from any site), symptoms of anemia (excessive fatigue, weakness). Closely monitor for infusion reactions.

PATIENT/FAMILY TEACHING

• Do not have immunizations without physician's approval (lowers body's resistance). • Avoid contact with those who have recently received live virus vaccine. • Avoid crowds, those with infection. • Promptly report fever, sore throat, signs of infection. • Report symptoms of infusion reactions (e.g., fever, chills, breathing problems, rash); bleeding, bruising, petechiae, worsening weakness or fatigue; new neurologic symptoms (e.g., confusion, loss of balance, vision problems); symptoms of hepatitis (e.g., fatigue, yellow discoloration of skin/eyes); worsening abdominal pain, nausea.

ofloxacin

o-**flox**-a-sin
(Apo-Oflox ✦, Floxin Otic,
Novo-Ofloxacin ✦, Ocuflox)

BLACK BOX ALERT May increase risk of tendonitis, tendon rupture. **Do not confuse Ocuflox with Ocufen.**

◆ CLASSIFICATION

PHARMACOTHERAPEUTIC: Fluoroquinolone. **CLINICAL:** Antibiotic (see p. 26C).

ACTION

Interferes with bacterial cell replication, repair by inhibiting DNA-gyrase in susceptible microorganisms. **Therapeutic Effect:** Bactericidal.

PHARMACOKINETICS

Rapidly, well absorbed from GI tract. Protein binding: 20%–25%. Widely distributed (including CSF). Metabolized in liver. Primarily excreted in urine. Removed by hemodialysis. **Half-life:** 4.7–7 hrs (increased in renal impairment, cirrhosis, elderly).

USES

Treatment of susceptible infections due to *S. pneumoniae, S. aureus, S. pyogenes, H. influenzae, P. mirabilis, N. gonorrhoeae, C. trachomatis, E. coli, K. pneumoniae, P. aeruginosa,* including infections of urinary tract, lower respiratory tract, skin/skin structure; sexually transmitted diseases, prostatitis due to *E. coli,* pelvic inflammatory disease (PID). **Ophthalmic:** Bacterial conjunctivitis, corneal ulcers. **Otic:** Otitis externa, acute or chronic otitis media. **OFF-LABEL: Oral:** Epididymitis, leprosy, traveler's diarrhea.

PRECAUTIONS

Contraindications: Hypersensitivity to any quinolones. **Otic:** Viral infection of external ear canal. **Cautions:** Renal impairment, CNS disorders, seizures, severe cerebral arteriosclerosis, prolongation of QT interval, bradycardia, cardiomyopathy, hypokalemia, hypomagnesemia, rheumatoid arthritis.

⌛ LIFESPAN CONSIDERATIONS

Pregnancy/Lactation: Distributed in breast milk; potentially serious adverse reactions in breastfeeding infants. Risk of arthropathy to fetus. **Pregnancy Category C. Children:** Safety and efficacy not established (otic not established in those younger than 1 yr). **Elderly:** No age-related precautions for otic. Age-related renal impairment may require dosage adjustment for oral administration.

INTERACTIONS

DRUG: Antacids, sucralfate may decrease absorption, effect. **NSAIDs** may increase risk of CNS stimulation, seizures. May increase **theophylline** concentration, risk of toxicity. **HERBAL: Dong quai, St. John's wort** may increase photosensitization. **FOOD:** None known. **LAB VALUES:** May increase ALT, AST, alkaline phosphatase, amylase, LDH.

AVAILABILITY (Rx)

Ophthalmic Solution (Ocuflox): 0.3%. **Otic Solution (Floxin Otic):** 0.3%. **Tablets:** 200 mg, 300 mg, 400 mg.

ADMINISTRATION/HANDLING

PO

• Do not give with food; preferred dosing time is 1 hr before or 2 hrs following meals. • Do not administer antacids (aluminum, magnesium) or iron/zinc-containing products within 2 hrs of ofloxacin. • Encourage cranberry juice, citrus fruits (to acidify urine). • Give with 8 oz of water; encourage fluid intake.

Ophthalmic

• Place gloved finger on lower eyelid and pull out until a pocket is formed between eye and lower lid. Place prescribed number of drops into pocket. Instruct pt to close eye gently (so medication will not be squeezed out of the sac) and apply digital pressure to lacrimal sac at inner canthus for 1 min to minimize systemic absorption.

Otic

• Instruct pt to lie down with head turned so affected ear is upright. • Instill toward canal wall, not directly on eardrum. • Pull auricle down and posterior in children; up and posterior in adults.

INDICATIONS/ROUTES/DOSAGE

Usual Dosage Range
PO: ADULTS, ELDERLY: 200–400 mg q12h.
Ophthalmic: ADULTS, ELDERLY, CHILDREN 1 YR AND OLDER: 1–2 drops q30min to 4 hrs initially, decreasing to q4–6h.
Otic: ADULTS, ELDERLY, CHILDREN OLDER THAN 12 YRS: 10 drops 1–2 times/day. **CHILDREN 6 MOS–12 YRS:** 5 drops once daily.

UTI
PO: ADULTS: 200 mg q12h for 3–10 days.

Pelvic Inflammatory Disease (PID)
PO: ADULTS: 400 mg q12h for 10–14 days.

Lower Respiratory Tract, Skin/Skin Structure Infection
PO: ADULTS: 400 mg q12h for 10 days.

Prostatitis, Sexually Transmitted Disease (Cervicitis, Urethritis)
PO: ADULTS: 400 mg once, then 300 mg q12h for 10 days.

Usual Elderly Dosage
PO: ELDERLY: 200–400 mg q12–24h for 7 days up to 6 wks.

Bacterial Conjunctivitis
Ophthalmic: ADULTS, ELDERLY: 1–2 drops q2–4h for 2 days, then 4 times a day for 5 days.

Corneal Ulcer
Ophthalmic: ADULTS: 1–2 drops q30min while awake and q4–6h at night for 2 days, then q60min while awake for 5–7 days, then 4 times a day until clinical cure achieved.

O

Acute Otitis Media
Otic: CHILDREN 1–12 YRS: 5 drops into affected ear twice a day for 10 days.

Otitis Externa
Otic: ADULTS, ELDERLY, CHILDREN 12 YRS AND OLDER: 10 drops into affected ear once daily for 7 days. **CHILDREN 6 MOS–11 YRS:** 5 drops into affected ear once daily for 7 days.

Dosage in Renal Impairment
After normal initial dose, dosage and frequency are based on creatinine clearance.

Creatinine Clearance	Adjusted Dose	Dosage Interval
Greater than 50 ml/min	None	q12h
20–50 ml/min	None	q24h
Less than 20 ml/min	Half	q24h

SIDE EFFECTS

Frequent (10%–7%): Nausea, headache, insomnia. **Occasional (5%–3%):** Abdominal pain, diarrhea, vomiting, dry mouth, flatulence, dizziness, fatigue, drowsiness, rash, pruritus, fever. **Rare (Less Than 1%):** Constipation, paresthesia.

ADVERSE EFFECTS/ TOXIC REACTIONS

Antibiotic-associated colitis, other superinfections (abdominal cramps, severe watery diarrhea, fever) may occur from altered bacterial balance in GI tract. Hypersensitivity reaction (evidenced by rash, pruritus, blisters, edema, photosensitivity) occurs rarely. Arthropathy (swelling, pain, clubbing of fingers/toes, degeneration of stress-bearing portion of joint) may occur in children.

NURSING CONSIDERATIONS

BASELINE ASSESSMENT
Question for history of hypersensitivity to ofloxacin, other quinolones.

INTERVENTION/EVALUATION
Monitor signs/symptoms of infection, altered mental status. Monitor renal/hepatic

function, WBC. Assess skin, discontinue medication at first sign of rash, other allergic reaction. Monitor daily pattern of bowel activity, stool consistency. Assess for insomnia. Check for dizziness, headache, visual difficulties, tremors; provide assistance with ambulation as needed. Be alert for superinfection: fever, vomiting, diarrhea, anal/genital pruritus, oral mucosal changes (ulceration, pain, erythema).

PATIENT/FAMILY TEACHING
• Do not take antacids within 2 hrs before or 2 hrs after taking ofloxacin. • Best taken 1 hr before or 2 hrs after meals. • May cause insomnia, headache, drowsiness, dizziness. • Avoid tasks requiring alertness, motor skills until response to drug is established. • Report tendon pain/ swelling, persistent diarrhea.

olanzapine   TOP 200

oh-**lan**-za-peen
(Apo-Olanzapine ♦, Zyprexa, Zyprexa Intramuscular, Zyprexa Relprevv, Zyprexa Zydis)

BLACK BOX ALERT Elderly pts with dementia-related psychosis are at increased risk for mortality due to cerebrovascular events.
Do not confuse olanzapine with olsalazine or quetiapine, or Zyprexa with Celexa or Zyrtec.

FIXED-COMBINATION(S)

Symbyax: olanzapine/fluoxetine (an antidepressant): 6 mg/25 mg, 6 mg/ 50 mg, 12 mg/25 mg, 12 mg/50 mg.

◆CLASSIFICATION

PHARMACOTHERAPEUTIC: Dibenzazepine derivative. **CLINICAL:** Antipsychotic (see p. 67C).

ACTION

Antagonizes alpha$_1$-adrenergic, dopamine, histamine, muscarinic, serotonin receptors. Produces anticholinergic, histaminic, CNS depressant effects. **Therapeutic Effect:** Diminishes psychotic symptoms.

PHARMACOKINETICS

Well absorbed after PO administration. Rapid absorption following IM administration. Protein binding: 93%. Widely distributed. Excreted in urine (57%), feces (30%). Not removed by dialysis. **Half-life:** 21–54 hrs.

USES

PO: Management of manifestations of schizophrenia. Treatment of acute mania associated with bipolar disorder. In combination with fluoxetine: treatment of depressive episodes associated with bipolar I disorder and treatment of treatment-resistant bipolar depression. **IM: Zyprexa Intramuscular:** Controls agitation in schizophrenia and bipolar mania. **Relprevv:** Long acting antipsychotic for IM injection for treatment of schizophrenia. **OFF-LABEL:** Psychosis/schizophrenia in children, chronic pain, prevention of chemotherapy-induced nausea/vomiting, psychosis/agitation related to Alzheimer's dementia.

PRECAUTIONS

Contraindications: None known. **Cautions:** Benign prostatic hyperplasia, suicidal pts, decrease GI motility, paralytic ileus, urinary retention, glaucoma, myasthenia gravis, breast cancer or history of breast cancer, hepatic impairment, elderly, concurrent use of potentially hepatotoxic drugs, dose escalation, known cardiovascular disease (history of MI, ischemia, heart failure, conduction abnormalities), cerebrovascular disease, conditions predisposing pts to hypotension (dehydration, hypovolemia, hypertensive medications), history of seizures, conditions lowering seizure threshold (e.g., Alzheimer's dementia), those at risk for aspiration pneumonia, pts with diabetes, pts at risk for suicide.

⌛ LIFESPAN CONSIDERATIONS

Pregnancy/Lactation: Unknown if drug crosses placenta or is distributed in breast milk. **Pregnancy Category C. Children:** Safety and efficacy not established. **Elderly:** No age-related precautions noted.

INTERACTIONS

DRUG: Alcohol, CNS depressants may increase CNS depressant effects. **Anticholinergics** may increase anticholinergic effects. **Hepatotoxic medications** may increase hepatic function test levels. **HERBAL: Dong quai, St. John's wort** may increase photosensitization. **Gotu kola, kava kava, St. John's wort, valerian** may increase CNS depression. **FOOD:** None known. **LAB VALUES:** May increase serum GGT, cholesterol, prolactin, AST, ALT.

AVAILABILITY (Rx)

Injection, Powder for Reconstitution (Zyprexa Intramuscular): 10 mg. **Suspension for IM Injection (Relprevv):** 210 mg, 300 mg, 405 mg. **Tablets (Zyprexa):** 2.5 mg, 5 mg, 7.5 mg, 10 mg, 15 mg, 20 mg. **Tablets (Orally Disintegrating [Zyprexa Zydis]):** 5 mg, 10 mg, 15 mg, 20 mg.

ADMINISTRATION/HANDLING

PO
• Give without regard to meals.

Orally Disintegrating
• Remove by peeling back foil (do not push through foil). • Place in mouth immediately. • Tablet dissolves rapidly with saliva and may be swallowed with or without liquid.

IM (Zyprexa Intramuscular)
• Reconstitute 10-mg vial with 2.1 ml Sterile Water for Injection to provide concentration of 5 mg/ml. • Use within 1 hr following reconstitution. • Discard unused portion.

IM (Relprevv)
• Dilute to final concentration of 150 mg/ml. • Shake vigorously to mix.

• Store at room temperature for up to 24 hrs.

INDICATIONS/ROUTES/DOSAGE

Schizophrenia

PO: ADULTS: Initially, 5–10 mg once daily. May increase to 10 mg/day within 5–7 days. If further adjustments are indicated, may increase by 5 mg/day at 7-day intervals. **Maximum**: 20 mg/day. **ELDERLY**: Initially, 2.5 mg/day. May increase as indicated. Range: 2.5–10 mg/day. **CHILDREN**: Initially, 2.5–5 mg/day. Titrate in 2.5- or 5-mg increments at weekly intervals. **Maximum**: 20 mg/day.

IM (Short-Acting [Zyprexa Intramuscular]): **ADULTS**: 10 mg. May repeat after 2–4 hrs. **Maximum**: 30 mg/day.

IM (Long-Acting [Relprevv]): **ADULTS, ESTABLISHED ON 10 MG/DAY ORALLY**: 210 mg q2wks for 4 doses or 405 mg q4wks for 2 doses. Maintenance: 150 mg q2wks or 300 mg q4wks. **ESTABLISHED ON 15 MG/DAY ORALLY**: 300 mg q2wks for 4 doses. Maintenance: 210 mg q2wks or 405 mg q4wks. **ESTABLISHED ON 20 MG/DAY ORALLY**: 300 mg q2wks.

Depression Associated with Bipolar Disorder (with fluoxetine)

PO: ADULTS: Initially, 5 mg in evening. Range: 5–12.5 mg/day.

Bipolar Mania

PO: ADULTS: Initially, 10–15 mg/day. May increase by 5 mg/day at intervals of at least 24 hrs. **Maximum**: 20 mg/day. **CHILDREN**: Initially, 2.5–5 mg/day. Titrate as necessary up to 20 mg/day.

Dosage for Elderly, Debilitated Pts, Those Predisposed to Hypotensive Reactions
Initial dosage: 5 mg/day.

Control of Agitation

IM: ADULTS, ELDERLY: 2.5–10 mg. May repeat 2 hrs after first dose and 4 hrs after 2nd dose. **Maximum**: 30 mg/day.

SIDE EFFECTS

Frequent (26%–10%): Drowsiness, agitation, insomnia, headache, nervousness, hostility, dizziness, rhinitis. **Occasional (9%–5%)**: Anxiety, constipation, nonaggressive atypical behavior, dry mouth, weight gain, orthostatic hypotension, fever, arthralgia, restlessness, cough, pharyngitis, visual changes (dim vision). **Rare**: Tachycardia; back, chest, abdominal, or extremity pain; tremor.

ADVERSE EFFECTS/TOXIC REACTIONS

Rare reactions include seizures, neuroleptic malignant syndrome, a potentially fatal syndrome characterized by hyperpyrexia, muscle rigidity, irregular pulse or B/P, tachycardia, diaphoresis, cardiac arrhythmias. Extrapyramidal symptoms (EPS), dysphagia may occur. Overdose (300 mg) produces drowsiness, slurred speech.

NURSING CONSIDERATIONS

BASELINE ASSESSMENT

Obtain baseline hepatic function tests, glucose, weight, lipid profile before initiating treatment. Assess behavior, appearance, emotional status, response to environment, speech pattern, thought content.

INTERVENTION/EVALUATION

Monitor B/P, glucose, lipids, hepatic function tests. Assess for tremors, changes in gait, abnormal muscular movements, behavior. Supervise suicidal-risk pt closely during early therapy (as depression lessens, energy level improves, increasing suicide potential). Assess for therapeutic response (interest in surroundings, improvement in self-care, increased ability to concentrate, relaxed facial expression). Assist with ambulation if dizziness occurs. Assess sleep pattern. Notify physician if extrapyramidal symptoms (EPS) occur.

PATIENT/FAMILY TEACHING

• Avoid dehydration, particularly during exercise, exposure to extreme heat, concurrent use of medication causing dry mouth, other drying effects. • Sugarless gum, sips of water may relieve dry mouth. • Report if suspected pregnancy. • Take medication as prescribed; do not stop taking or increase dosage. • Rise slowly from sitting/lying position. • Avoid alcohol. • Avoid tasks that require alertness, motor skills until response to drug is established. • Monitor diet, exercise program to prevent weight gain.

---

olmesartan

TOP 200

ol-me-**sar**-tan
(Benicar, Olmetec ♦)

BLACK BOX ALERT May cause fetal injury, mortality if used during second or third trimester of pregnancy.
Do not confuse Benicar with Mevacor.

FIXED-COMBINATION(S)

Azor: olmesartan/amlodipine (calcium channel blocker): 20 mg/5 mg, 40 mg/5 mg, 20 mg/10 mg, 40 mg/10 mg. **Benicar HCT:** olmesartan/hydrochlorothiazide (a diuretic): 20 mg/12.5 mg, 40 mg/12.5 mg, 40 mg/25 mg. **Tribenzor:** olmesartan/hydrochlorothiazide/amlodipine: 20 mg/12.5 mg/5 mg, 40 mg/12.5 mg/5 mg, 40 mg/25 mg/5 mg, 40 mg/12.5 mg/10 mg, 40 mg/25 mg/10 mg.

◆CLASSIFICATION

PHARMACOTHERAPEUTIC: Angiotensin II receptor antagonist. **CLINICAL:** Antihypertensive (see pp. 11C, 62C).

ACTION

Blocks vasoconstrictor, aldosterone-secreting effects of angiotensin II by inhibiting binding of angiotensin II to AT_1 receptors in vascular smooth muscle. **Therapeutic Effect:** Causes vasodilation, decreases peripheral resistance, decreases B/P.

PHARMACOKINETICS

Moderately absorbed after PO administration. Hydrolyzed in GI tract to olmesartan. Protein binding: 99%. Eliminated in urine (35%–50%), remainder in feces. Not removed by hemodialysis. **Half-life:** 13 hrs.

USES

Treatment of hypertension alone or in combination with other antihypertensives.

PRECAUTIONS

Contraindications: Concomitant use with aliskiren in pts with diabetes. **Cautions:** Renal impairment, unstented unilateral or bilateral renal arterial stenosis, significant aortic/mitral stenosis.

⌛ LIFESPAN CONSIDERATIONS

Pregnancy/Lactation: Unknown if distributed in breast milk. **Pregnancy Category C (D if used in second or third trimester). Children:** Safety and efficacy not established. **Elderly:** No age-related precautions noted.

INTERACTIONS

DRUG: NSAIDs may decrease antihypertensive effect. **HERBAL: Ephedra, ginseng, yohimbe** may worsen hypertension. **Garlic** may increase antihypertensive effect. **FOOD:** None known. **LAB VALUES:** May slightly decrease Hgb, Hct. May increase serum BUN, creatinine, bilirubin, hepatic enzymes.

AVAILABILITY (Rx)

Tablets: 5 mg, 20 mg, 40 mg.

ADMINISTRATION/HANDLING

PO
• Give without regard to meals.

INDICATIONS/ROUTES/DOSAGE

Hypertension
PO: ADULTS, ELDERLY: Initially, 20 mg/day. May increase to 40 mg/day after 2 wks.

O

Lower initial dose may be necessary in pts receiving volume-depleting medications (e.g., diuretics). **CHILDREN 6–16 YRS, WEIGHING 20 TO LESS THAN 35 KG:** Initially, 10 mg once daily. **Range:** 10–20 mg once daily. **WEIGHING 35 KG OR GREATER:** Initially, 20 mg once daily. **Range:** 20–40 mg once daily.

SIDE EFFECTS

Occasional (3%): Dizziness. **Rare (less than 2%):** Headache, diarrhea, upper respiratory tract infection.

ADVERSE EFFECTS/ TOXIC REACTIONS

Overdosage may manifest as hypotension, tachycardia. Bradycardia occurs less often. Rare cases of rhabdomyolysis have been reported.

NURSING CONSIDERATIONS

BASELINE ASSESSMENT

Obtain B/P, apical pulse immediately before each dose in addition to regular monitoring (be alert to fluctuations). If excessive reduction in B/P occurs, place pt in supine position, feet slightly elevated. Question for possibility of pregnancy (see Pregnancy Category). Assess medication history (esp. diuretics).

INTERVENTION/EVALUATION

Maintain hydration (offer fluids frequently). Assess for evidence of upper respiratory infection. Assist with ambulation if dizziness occurs. Monitor serum potassium level. Assess B/P for hypertension, hypotension.

PATIENT/FAMILY TEACHING

• Avoid pregnancy. • Avoid tasks that require alertness, motor skills until response to drug is established (possible dizziness effect). • Report any signs of infection (sore throat, fever). • Therapy requires lifelong control, diet, exercise. • Maintain adequate hydration.

olsalazine

ol-**sal**-a-zeen
(Dipentum)
Do not confuse Dipentum with Dilantin, or olsalazine with olanzapine.

◆CLASSIFICATION

PHARMACOTHERAPEUTIC: Salicylic acid derivative. **CLINICAL:** Anti-inflammatory.

ACTION

Converted to mesalamine in colon by bacterial action. Blocks prostaglandin production in bowel mucosa. **Therapeutic Effect:** Reduces colonic inflammation.

PHARMACOKINETICS

Small amount absorbed. Protein binding: 99%. Metabolized by bacteria in colon. Minimal elimination in urine, feces. **Half-life:** 0.9 hr.

USES

Maintenance of remission of ulcerative colitis in pts intolerant of sulfasalazine medication.

PRECAUTIONS

Contraindications: History of hypersensitivity to salicylates. **Cautions:** Renal/hepatic impairment, elderly, severe allergies, asthma.

⧖ LIFESPAN CONSIDERATIONS

Pregnancy/Lactation: Crosses placenta; distributed in breast milk. **Pregnancy Category C. Children:** Safety and efficacy not established. **Elderly:** Age-related renal impairment may require dosage adjustment.

INTERACTIONS

DRUG: May increase risk of bleeding with **warfarin, heparin.** May increase risk of myelosuppression with **mercapto-**

purine, **thioguanine. HERBAL:** None significant. **FOOD:** None known. **LAB VALUES:** May increase serum AST, ALT.

AVAILABILITY (Rx)

Capsules: 250 mg.

ADMINISTRATION/HANDLING

PO
• Give with food.

INDICATIONS/ROUTES/DOSAGE

Maintenance of Controlled Ulcerative Colitis
PO: ADULTS, ELDERLY: 1 g/day in 2 divided doses, preferably q12h.

SIDE EFFECTS

Frequent (10%–5%): Headache, diarrhea, abdominal pain/cramps, nausea. **Occasional (4%–2%):** Depression, fatigue, dyspepsia, upper respiratory tract infection, decreased appetite, rash, pruritus, arthralgia. **Rare (1%):** Dizziness, vomiting, stomatitis.

ADVERSE EFFECTS/ TOXIC REACTIONS

Sulfite sensitivity may occur in susceptible pts (manifested as cramping, headache, diarrhea, fever, rash, urticaria, pruritus, wheezing). Discontinue drug immediately. Excessive diarrhea associated with extreme fatigue is rarely noted.

NURSING CONSIDERATIONS

INTERVENTION/EVALUATION

Encourage adequate fluid intake. Assess bowel sounds for peristalsis. Monitor daily pattern of bowel activity, stool consistency; record time of evacuation. Assess for abdominal disturbances. Assess skin for rash, urticaria. Medication should be discontinued if rash, fever, cramping, diarrhea occur.

PATIENT/FAMILY TEACHING

• Report if diarrhea, cramping continues or worsens or if rash, fever, pruritus occur.

omacetaxine

oh-ma-set-**ax**-een
(Synribo)

◆CLASSIFICATION

PHARMACOTHERAPEUTIC: Protein synthesis inhibitor. **CLINICAL:** Antineoplastic.

ACTION

Inhibits protein synthesis of Bcr-Abl tyrosine kinase, a translocation-created enzyme, created by the Philadelphia chromosome abnormality noted in chronic myeloid leukemia (CML). **Therapeutic Effect:** Inhibits tumor proliferation and growth during accelerated and chronic stages of CML.

PHARMACOKINETICS

Rapidly absorbed following subcutaneous administration. Maximum concentration: 30 min. Protein binding: Less than 50%. Hydrolyzed via plasma esterases. **Half-life:** 6 hrs.

USES

Treatment of adult pts with chronic or accelerated phase chronic myeloid leukemia (CML) with resistance and/or intolerance to two or more tyrosine kinase inhibitors.

PRECAUTIONS

Contraindications: None known. **Cautions:** Glucose intolerance, poorly controlled diabetes, recent GI bleeding.

⧖ LIFESPAN CONSIDERATIONS

Pregnancy/Lactation: May cause fetal harm. Not recommended in nursing mothers. Unknown if distributed in breast milk. **Pregnancy Category D. Children:** Safety and efficacy not established. **Elderly:** Increased risk for toxicity (e.g., hematologic).

INTERACTIONS

DRUG: NSAIDs, anticoagulants, antiplatelets may increase risk for bleeding. **HERBAL:** None significant. **FOOD:** None known. **LAB VALUES:** May decrease platelets, Hgb, Hct, leukocytes, lymphocytes. May increase serum ALT.

AVAILABILITY (Rx)

Injection, Powder for Reconstitution: 3.5-mg vial.

ADMINISTRATION/HANDLING

◀**ALERT**▶ Must be administered by health care workers trained in proper chemotherapy handling and disposal procedures.

Subcutaneous

Reconstitution • Reconstitute with 1 ml 0.9% NaCl. • Gently swirl until powder is completely dissolved. • Inspect vial for particular matter or discoloration. • Reconstituted vial will provide a concentration of 3.5 mg/ml. • Avoid contact with skin.
Storage • Solution should appear clear. • May store solution at room temperature for up to 12 hrs or may refrigerate up to 24 hrs. • Discard unused solution.

INDICATIONS/ROUTES/DOSAGE

Chronic or Accelerated Myeloid Leukemia

Subcutaneous: ADULTS, ELDERLY: Induction dose: 1.25 mg/m^2 twice daily for 14 consecutive days every 28 days, over 28-day cycle. Continue induction dose until hematologic response achieved. **Maintenance dose:** 1.25 mg/m^2 twice daily for 7 consecutive days every 28 days over 28-day cycle.

Dosage Modification

Hematologic Toxicity: If neutrophils less than 0.5/mm^3 or platelet less than 50,000/mm^3, interrupt therapy. Restart when neutrophil count greater than or equal to 1.0/mm^3 or platelet count greater than or equal to 50,000/mm^3 and reduce number of dosing days by 2. **Nonhematologic Toxicity:** Interrupt therapy until toxicity/adverse effects resolved. Continue indefinitely until pt no longer benefits from therapy.

SIDE EFFECTS

Chronic Phase
Frequent (45%–25%): Diarrhea, nausea, fatigue, pyrexia, asthenia (loss of strength, energy). **Occasional (20%–11%):** Headache, arthralgia, cough, epistaxis, alopecia, constipation, abdominal pain, peripheral edema, vomiting, back pain, insomnia, rash.

Accelerated Phase
Occasional (19%–7%): Diarrhea, nausea, fatigue, pyrexia, asthenia, vomiting, cough, abdominal pain, chills, anorexia, headache. **Rare (7% or Less):** Dyspnea, epistaxis.

ADVERSE EFFECTS/ TOXIC REACTIONS

Thrombocytopenia, neutropenia, leukopenia, lymphopenia, or myelosuppression is an expected response to therapy, but more severe reactions including bone marrow failure, febrile neutropenia may result in life-threatening events. Pts with neutropenia are at increased risk for infection. Thrombocytopenia may increase risk for intracranial hemorrhage, GI bleeding. Avoid anticoagulants, antiplatelets, NSAIDs if platelet count less than 50,000/mm^3. Hyperglycemic events including hyperglycemic hyperosmolar nonketotic syndrome (HHNK) may occur. Pts with uncontrolled diabetes are at increased risk for hyperglycemic emergency.

NURSING CONSIDERATIONS

BASELINE ASSESSMENT

Obtain baseline serum chemistries, CBC; PT/INR if on anticoagulants. Question for possibility of pregnancy, current breast-feeding status. Obtain negative urine pregnancy before initiating treatment. Obtain full medication history including vitamins, supplements, herbal products, anticoagulants. Question for history of diabetes mellitus, GI bleeding.

INTERVENTION/EVALUATION

Monitor CBC weekly, then every 2 wks during maintenance phase. Obtain frequent blood glucose levels, especially in diabetic pts. Do not initiate therapy until negative urine pregnancy confirmed. Monitor hepatic function panel if hepatic impairment suspected. If drug exposure occurs, immediately wash affected area with soap and water. Consider isolation protocol if pt develops neutropenia.

PATIENT/FAMILY TEACHING

• May cause male infertility. • Serum lab studies will be routinely monitored. • Notify physician if pregnant or planning to become pregnant. • Use barrier methods during sexual activity. • Strictly avoid pregnancy. • Immediately report yellowing of skin or eyes, abdominal pain, bruising, black/tarry stools, dark urine, dehydration, GI bleeding, nausea, vomiting, rash. • Report fever, cough, night sweats, flu-like symptoms, skin changes. • Avoid tasks that require alertness, motor skills until response to drug is established. • Shortness of breath, pale skin, weakness may indicate bleeding or severe myelosuppression.

---

omalizumab ^{TOP 200}

oh-ma-**liz**-ue-mab
(Xolair)

BLACK BOX ALERT Anaphylaxis (severe bronchospasm, hypotension, angioedema, syncope, urticaria) has occurred after first dose, and in some cases, after 1 yr of regular treatment.
Do not confuse omalizumab with ofatumumab.

◆ CLASSIFICATION

PHARMACOTHERAPEUTIC: Monoclonal antibody. **CLINICAL:** Antiasthmatic.

ACTION

Selectively binds to human immunoglobulin E (IgE). Inhibits binding of IgE on surface of mast cells, basophiles. **Thera-**peutic Effect: Prevents/reduces number of asthmatic attacks.

PHARMACOKINETICS

Absorbed slowly after subcutaneous administration, with peak concentration in 7–8 days. Excreted primarily via hepatic degradation. **Half-life:** 26 days.

USES

Treatment of moderate to severe persistent asthma in pts reactive to perennial allergens and inadequately controlled asthma symptoms with inhaled corticosteroids.

PRECAUTIONS

Contraindications: Acute bronchospasm, status asthmaticus. **Cautions:** Pts at risk for parasitic infections.

⌛ LIFESPAN CONSIDERATIONS

Pregnancy/Lactation: Because IgE is present in breast milk, omalizumab is expected to be present in breast milk. Use only if clearly needed. **Pregnancy Category B. Children:** Safety and efficacy not established in those younger than 12 yrs. **Elderly:** No age-related precautions noted.

INTERACTIONS

DRUG: None significant. **HERBAL: Echinacea** may decrease effects. **FOOD:** None known. **LAB VALUES:** May increase serum IgE levels.

AVAILABILITY (Rx)

Injection, Powder for Reconstitution: 150 mg/1.2 ml after reconstitution.

ADMINISTRATION/HANDLING

Subcutaneous
Reconstitution • Use only Sterile Water for Injection to prepare for subcutaneous administration. • Medication takes 15–20 min to dissolve. • Draw 1.4 ml Sterile Water for Injection into 3-ml syringe with 1-inch, 18-gauge needle; inject contents into powdered vial. • Swirl vial for approximately 1 min (do not shake) and

 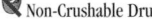

again swirl vial for 5–10 sec every 5 min until no gel-like particles appear in the solution. • Do not use if contents do not dissolve completely within 40 min. • Invert vial for 15 sec (allows solution to drain toward the stopper). • Using new 3-ml syringe with 1-inch 18-gauge needle, obtain required 1.2-ml dose, replace 18-gauge needle with 25-gauge needle for subcutaneous administration.

Rate of Administration • Subcutaneous administration may take 5–10 sec to administer due to its viscosity.

Storage • Use only clear or slightly opalescent solution; solution is slightly viscous. • Refrigerate. • Reconstituted solution is stable for 8 hrs if refrigerated or within 4 hrs of reconstitution when stored at room temperature.

INDICATIONS/ROUTES/DOSAGE

◄ALERT► Dosage and frequency of administration is based upon total IgE levels and body weight (see table). IgE levels should be measured prior to initiating treatment and not during treatment. Pts should be observed a minimum of 2 hrs following each omalizumab treatment.

Asthma

Subcutaneous: ADULTS, ELDERLY, CHILDREN 12 YRS AND OLDER: 150–375 mg every 2 or 4 wks; dose and dosing frequency are individualized based on body weight and pretreatment IgE level (as shown below). (Consult specific product labeling.)

SIDE EFFECTS

Frequent (45%–11%): Injection site ecchymosis, redness, warmth, stinging, urticaria, viral infection, sinusitis, headache, pharyngitis. **Occasional (8%–3%):** Arthralgia, leg pain, fatigue, dizziness. **Rare (2%):** Arm pain, earache, dermatitis, pruritus.

ADVERSE EFFECTS/ TOXIC REACTIONS

Anaphylaxis, occurring within 2 hrs of first dose or subsequent doses, occurs in 0.1% of pts. Malignant neoplasms occur in 0.5% of pts.

NURSING CONSIDERATIONS

BASELINE ASSESSMENT

Obtain baseline serum total IgE level before initiation of treatment (dosage is based on

4-Wk Dosing Table

Pretreatment Serum IgE Levels (units/ml)	Weight 30–60 kg	Weight 61–70 kg	Weight 71–90 kg	Weight 91–150 kg
30–100	150 mg	150 mg	150 mg	300 mg
101–200	300 mg	300 mg	300 mg	See next table
201–300	300 mg	See next table	See next table	See next table

2-Wk Dosing Table

Pretreatment Serum IgE Levels (units/ml)	Weight 30–60 kg	Weight 61–70 kg	Weight 71–90 kg	Weight 91–150 kg
101–200	See preceding table	See preceding table	See preceding table	225 mg
201–300	See preceding table	225 mg	225 mg	300 mg
301–400	225 mg	225 mg	300 mg	Do not dose
401–500	300 mg	300 mg	375 mg	Do not dose
501–600	300 mg	375 mg	Do not dose	Do not dose
601–700	375 mg	Do not dose	Do not dose	Do not dose

pretreatment levels). Drug is not for treatment of acute exacerbations of asthma, acute bronchospasm, status asthmaticus.

INTERVENTION/EVALUATION

Monitor rate, depth, rhythm, type of respirations, quality/rate of pulse. Assess lung sounds for rhonchi, wheezing, rales. Observe lips, fingernails for cyanosis (blue/dusky color in light-skinned pts, gray in dark-skinned pts).

PATIENT/FAMILY TEACHING

• Increase fluid intake (decreases viscosity of pulmonary secretions). • Do not alter/stop other asthma medications. • Report allergic reactions (e.g., breathing difficulty, swelling of throat/tongue).

---

omega-3 acid ethyl esters   TOP 200

oh-**may**-ga 3 **as**-id **eth**-il **es**-ters (Lovaza)
Do not confuse Lovaza with lorazepam.

◆ CLASSIFICATION

PHARMACOTHERAPEUTIC: Omega-3 fatty acid. **CLINICAL:** Antihypertriglyceride agent (see p. 59C).

ACTION

Inhibits esterification of fatty acids, prevents hepatic enzymes from catalyzing final step of triglyceride synthesis. **Therapeutic Effect:** Reduces serum triglyceride levels.

PHARMACOKINETICS

Well absorbed following PO administration. Incorporated into phospholipids. **Half-life:** N/A.

USES

Adjunct to diet to reduce very high (500 mg/dl or higher) serum triglyceride levels in adult pts. **OFF-LABEL:** Treatment of IgA nephropathy.

PRECAUTIONS

Contraindications: None known. **Cautions:** Known sensitivity, allergy to fish.

⧗ LIFESPAN CONSIDERATIONS

Pregnancy/Lactation: Unknown if distributed in breast milk. **Pregnancy Category C. Children:** Safety and efficacy not established in those younger than 18 yrs. **Elderly:** No age-related precautions noted.

INTERACTIONS

DRUG: May increase bleeding time with **anticoagulants. HERBAL:** None significant. **FOOD:** None known. **LAB VALUES:** May increase serum ALT, LDL.

AVAILABILITY (Rx)

Capsules, Soft Gelatin (Oil-Filled): 1 g.

ADMINISTRATION/HANDLING

PO
• Give without regard to meals.

INDICATIONS/ROUTES/DOSAGE

◄ **ALERT** ► Before initiating therapy, pt should be on standard cholesterol-lowering diet for minimum of 3–6 mos. Continue diet throughout therapy.

Usual Dosage
PO: ADULTS, ELDERLY: 4 g/day, given as a single dose (4 capsules), or 2 capsules twice daily.

SIDE EFFECTS

Occasional (5%–3%): Eructation, altered taste, dyspepsia. **Rare (2%–1%):** Rash, back pain.

ADVERSE EFFECTS/ TOXIC REACTIONS

None known.

NURSING CONSIDERATIONS

BASELINE ASSESSMENT

Assess baseline serum triglyceride level, hepatic function tests. Obtain diet history, esp. fat consumption.

INTERVENTION/EVALUATION

Monitor serum triglyceride levels for therapeutic response. Monitor serum ALT, LDL periodically during therapy. Discontinue therapy if no response after 2 mos of treatment.

PATIENT/FAMILY TEACHING

• Continue to adhere to lipid-lowering diet (important part of treatment). • Periodic lab tests are essential part of therapy to determine drug effectiveness.

omeprazole

oh-**mep**-ra-zole
(Apo-Omeprazole ❖, Losec ✚, Prilosec, Prilosec OTC)
Do not confuse omeprazole with aripiprazole, pantoprazole or esomeprazole, or Prilosec with Plendil, Prevacid, Prinivil, or Prozac.

FIXED-COMBINATION(S)

Zegerid: omeprazole/sodium bicarbonate (an antacid): 20 mg/1,100 mg, 40 mg/1,100 mg. **Zegerid Powder:** 20 mg/1,680 mg, 40 mg/1,680 mg.

◆CLASSIFICATION

PHARMACOTHERAPEUTIC: Benzimidazole. **CLINICAL:** Proton pump inhibitor (see p. 147C).

ACTION

Converted to active metabolites that irreversibly bind to, inhibit hydrogen-potassium adenosine triphosphatase, an enzyme on the surface of gastric parietal cells. Inhibits hydrogen ion transport into gastric lumen. **Therapeutic Effect:** Increases gastric pH, reduces gastric acid production.

PHARMACOKINETICS

Route	Onset	Peak	Duration
PO	1 hr	2 hrs	72 hrs

Rapidly absorbed from GI tract. Protein binding: 95%. Primarily distributed into gastric parietal cells. Metabolized in liver. Primarily excreted in urine. Unknown if removed by hemodialysis. **Half-life:** 0.5–1 hr (increased in hepatic impairment).

USES

Short-term treatment (4–8 wks) of erosive esophagitis (diagnosed by endoscopy), symptomatic gastroesophageal reflux disease (GERD) poorly responsive to other treatment. *H. pylori*–associated duodenal ulcer (with amoxicillin and clarithromycin). Long-term treatment of pathologic hypersecretory conditions, treatment of active duodenal ulcer or active benign gastric ulcer. Maintenance healing of erosive esophagitis. **OTC, short-term:** Treatment of frequent, uncomplicated heartburn occurring 2 or more days/wk. **OFF-LABEL:** Prevention/treatment of NSAID-induced ulcers, stress ulcer prophylaxis in critically ill pts.

PRECAUTIONS

Contraindications: None known. **Cautions:** May increase risk of fractures, gastrointestinal infections. Hepatic impairment, pts of Asian descent.

⌛ LIFESPAN CONSIDERATIONS

Pregnancy/Lactation: Unknown if drug crosses placenta or is distributed in breast milk. **Pregnancy Category C. Children:** Safety and efficacy not established. **Elderly:** No age-related precautions noted.

INTERACTIONS

DRUG: May decrease concentration/effects of **atazanavir, clopidogrel.** May increase concentration/effects of **diazepam, oral anticoagulants, phenytoin. HERBAL:** St. John's wort may decrease concentration/effects. **FOOD:** None known. **LAB VALUES:** May increase serum alkaline phosphatase, AST, ALT.

AVAILABILITY (Rx)

Granules for Oral Suspension: 2.5 mg/packet, 10 mg/packet. **Powder for Oral Suspension:** 2 mg/ml.

Capsules (Delayed-Release [Prilosec]): 10 mg, 20 mg, 40 mg. **Tablets (Delayed-Release [Prilosec OTC]):** 20 mg.

ADMINISTRATION/HANDLING

PO

• Give before meals (breakfast preferred). • Give whole. Do not break, crush, dissolve, or divide delayed-release forms. • May open capsule, mix with applesauce and give immediately.

PO (Suspension)

• Following reconstitution, allow to thicken (2–3 min). • Administer within 30 min.

INDICATIONS/ROUTES/DOSAGE

Erosive Esophagitis, Poorly Responsive Gastroesophageal Reflux Disease (GERD), Active Duodenal Ulcer, Prevention/Treatment of NSAID-Induced Ulcers
PO: ADULTS, ELDERLY: 20 mg/day.

Maintenance Healing of Erosive Esophagitis
PO: ADULTS, ELDERLY: 20 mg/day for up to 12 mos.

Pathologic Hypersecretory Conditions
PO: ADULTS, ELDERLY: Initially, 60 mg/day up to 120 mg 3 times a day.

H. Pylori **Duodenal Ulcer**
PO: ADULTS, ELDERLY: 20 mg once daily or 40 mg/day as a single or in 2 divided doses in combination therapy with antibiotics. Dose varies with regimen used.

Gastric Ulcer
PO: ADULTS, ELDERLY: 40 mg/day for 4–8 wks.

OTC Use (Frequent Heartburn)
PO: ADULTS, ELDERLY: 20 mg/day for 14 days. May repeat after 4 mos if needed.

Usual Pediatric Dosage
CHILDREN 1–16 YRS, WEIGHT 20 KG OR MORE: 20 mg/day. **CHILDREN OLDER THAN 2 YRS, WEIGHT 10–19 KG:** 10 mg/day. **WEIGHT 5–9 KG:** 5 mg/day.

SIDE EFFECTS

Frequent (7%): Headache. **Occasional (3%–2%):** Diarrhea, abdominal pain, nausea. **Rare (2%):** Dizziness, asthenia (loss of strength, energy), vomiting, constipation, upper respiratory tract infection, back pain, rash, cough.

ADVERSE EFFECTS/TOXIC REACTIONS

Pancreatitis, hepatotoxicity, interstitial nephritis occur rarely.

NURSING CONSIDERATIONS

INTERVENTION/EVALUATION

Evaluate for therapeutic response (relief of GI symptoms). Question if GI discomfort, nausea, diarrhea occurs.

PATIENT/FAMILY TEACHING

• Report headache, onset of black, tarry stools, diarrhea, abdominal pain. • Avoid alcohol. • Swallow capsules whole; do not chew, crush, dissolve, or divide. • Take before eating.

ondansetron

on-**dan**-se-tron
(Apo-Ondansetron ✤, Zofran, Zofran ODT, Zuplenz)
Do not confuse ondansetron with dolasetron, granisetron, or palonosetron, or Zofran with Zantac or Zosyn.

◆CLASSIFICATION

PHARMACOTHERAPEUTIC: Selective serotonin and 5-HT$_3$ receptor antagonist. **CLINICAL:** Antinausea, antiemetic.

ACTION

Blocks serotonin, both peripherally on vagal nerve terminals and centrally in chemoreceptor trigger zone. **Therapeutic Effect:** Prevents nausea/vomiting.

PHARMACOKINETICS

Readily absorbed from GI tract. Protein binding: 70%–76%. Metabolized in liver. Primarily excreted in urine. Unknown if removed by hemodialysis. **Half-life:** 3–6 hrs (increased in hepatic impairment).

USES

Prevention/treatment of nausea/vomiting due to cancer chemotherapy (including high-dose cisplatin). Prevention and treatment of postop nausea, vomiting. Prevention of radiation-induced nausea, vomiting. **OFF-LABEL:** Breakthrough treatment of nausea and vomiting associated with chemotherapy, hyperemesis gravidarum.

PRECAUTIONS

Contraindications: Use of apomorphine. **Cautions:** Mild to moderate hepatic impairment, pts at risk for QT prolongation or ventricular arrhythmia (congenital long QT prolongation, medications prolonging QT interval, electrolyte abnormalities).

⧗ LIFESPAN CONSIDERATIONS

Pregnancy/Lactation: Unknown if drug crosses placenta or is distributed in breast milk. **Pregnancy Category B. Children:** Safety and efficacy not established. **Elderly:** No age-related precautions noted.

INTERACTIONS

DRUG: Apomorphine may cause profound hypotension, altered LOC. **HERBAL: St. John's wort** may decrease concentration. **FOOD:** None known. **LAB VALUES:** May transiently increase serum bilirubin, AST, ALT.

AVAILABILITY (Rx)

Injection (Premix): 32 mg/50 ml. **Injection Solution (Zofran):** 2 mg/ml. **Oral Soluble Film (Zuplenz):** 4 mg, 8 mg. **Oral Solution** (Zofran): 4 mg/5 ml. **Tablets (Zofran):** 4 mg, 8 mg. **Tablets (Orally Disintegrating [Zofran ODT]):** 4 mg, 8 mg.

ADMINISTRATION/HANDLING

 IV

Reconstitution • May give undiluted. • For IV infusion, dilute with 50 ml D_5W or 0.9% NaCl before administration.
Rate of Administration • Give IV push over 2–5 min. • Give IV infusion over 15–30 min.
Storage • Store at room temperature. • Stable for 48 hrs at room temperature following dilution.

IM
• Inject undiluted into large muscle mass.

PO
• Give without regard to food.

Orally Disintegrating Tablets
• Do not remove from blister until needed. • Peel backing off; do not push through. • Place tablet on tongue; allow to dissolve. • Swallow with saliva.

Oral Soluble Film
• Keep film in pouch until ready to use. • Remove film strip from pouch and place on top of tongue, allow to dissolve. • Swallow after film dissolves. Do not chew or swallow film whole. • If using more than one, each should be allowed to dissolve before administering the next one.

▦ IV INCOMPATIBILITIES

Acyclovir (Zovirax), allopurinol (Aloprim), amphotericin B (Fungizone), amphotericin B complex (Abelcet, AmBisome, Amphotec), ampicillin (Polycillin), ampicillin and sulbactam (Unasyn), cefepime (Maxipime), 5-fluorouracil, lorazepam (Ativan), meropenem (Merrem IV), methylprednisolone (Solu-Medrol).

▦ IV COMPATIBILITIES

Carboplatin (Paraplatin), cisplatin (Platinol), cyclophosphamide (Cytoxan), cytarabine (Cytosar), dacarbazine (DTIC-Dome), daunorubicin (Cerubidine), dexmedetomidine (Precedex), dexamethasone (Decadron), diphenhydramine (Benadryl), docetaxel (Taxotere), dopamine (Intropin), etoposide (VePesid), gemcitabine (Gemzar), heparin, hydromorphone (Dilaudid), ifosfamide (Ifex), magnesium, mannitol, mesna (Mesnex), methotrexate, metoclopramide (Reglan), mitomycin (Mutamycin), mitoxantrone (Novantrone), morphine, paclitaxel (Taxol), potassium chloride, teniposide (Vumon), topotecan (Hycamtin), vinblastine (Velban), vincristine (Oncovin), vinorelbine (Navelbine).

INDICATIONS/ROUTES/DOSAGE

Chemotherapy-Induced Nausea/Vomiting

IV: ADULTS, ELDERLY: 0.15 mg/kg 3 times a day beginning 30 min before chemotherapy, followed by subsequent doses 4 and 8 hrs after the first dose. **CHILDREN 6 MOS AND OLDER:** 0.15 mg/kg 3 times a day beginning 30 min before chemotherapy and again 4 and 8 hrs after first dose.

PO: ADULTS, ELDERLY, CHILDREN 12 YRS AND OLDER: (highly emetogenic) 24 mg 30 min before start of chemotherapy, (moderately emetogenic) 8 mg q12h beginning 30 min before chemotherapy and continuing for 1–2 days after completion of chemotherapy. **Zuplenz:** 8 mg 30 min before chemotherapy, followed by 8 mg 8 hrs later, then continue q12h for 1–2 days after completion of chemotherapy. **CHILDREN 4–11 YRS:** 4 mg 30 min before chemotherapy, repeat 4 and 8 hrs after initial dose then q8h for 1–2 days after chemotherapy completed.

Prevention of Postop Nausea/Vomiting

IV, IM: ADULTS, ELDERLY, CHILDREN OLDER THAN 12 YRS: 4 mg as a single dose. **CHILDREN 1 MO–12 YRS, WEIGHING MORE THAN 40 KG:** 4 mg as a single dose. **CHILDREN 1 MO–12 YRS, WEIGHING 40 KG AND LESS:** 0.1 mg/kg as a single dose. **PO: ADULTS, ELDERLY:** 16 mg 1 hr before induction of anesthesia.

Prevention of Radiation-Induced Nausea/Vomiting

PO: ADULTS, ELDERLY: (total body irradiation) 8 mg 1–2 hrs daily before each fraction of radiotherapy, (single high-dose radiotherapy to abdomen) 8 mg 1–2 hrs before irradiation, then 8 mg q8h after first dose for 1–2 days after completion of radiotherapy, (daily fractionated radiotherapy to abdomen) 8 mg 1–2 hrs before irradiation, then 8 mg 8 hrs after first dose for each day of radiotherapy. **Zuplenz:** 8 mg q8h.

Dosage in Hepatic Impairment

Severe Impairment: ADULTS, ELDERLY: Maximum daily dose: 8 mg.

SIDE EFFECTS

Frequent (13%–5%): Anxiety, dizziness, drowsiness, headache, fatigue, constipation, diarrhea, hypoxia, urinary retention. **Occasional (4%–2%):** Abdominal pain, xerostomia, fever, feeling of cold, redness/pain at injection site, paresthesia, asthenia (loss of strength, energy). **Rare (1%):** Hypersensitivity reaction (rash, pruritus), blurred vision.

ADVERSE EFFECTS/TOXIC REACTIONS

Hypertension, acute renal failure, GI bleeding, respiratory depression, coma, extrapyramidal effects occur rarely.

NURSING CONSIDERATIONS

BASELINE ASSESSMENT

Assess degree of nausea, vomiting. Assess for dehydration if excessive vomiting occurs (poor skin turgor, dry mucous membranes, longitudinal furrows in tongue). Provide emotional support.

INTERVENTION/EVALUATION

Monitor EKG in pts with electrolyte abnormalities (e.g., hypokalemia, hypomagnesemia), HF, bradyarrhythmias, concurrent use of other medications that may cause QT prolongation. Assess bowel sounds for peristalsis. Provide

O

supportive measures. Assess mental status. Monitor daily pattern of bowel activity, stool consistency. Record time of evacuation.

PATIENT/FAMILY TEACHING
• Relief from nausea/vomiting generally occurs shortly after drug administration. • Avoid alcohol, barbiturates. • Report persistent vomiting. • Avoid tasks that require alertness, motor skills until response to drug is established (may cause drowsiness, dizziness).

oprelvekin (interleukin-2, IL-2)

oh-**prel**-vee-kin
(Neumega)

BLACK BOX ALERT Allergic or hypersensitivity reactions, including anaphylaxis, have occurred.
Do not confuse Neumega with Neulasta or Neupogen, or oprelvekin with aldesleukin or Proleukin.

◆**CLASSIFICATION**
PHARMACOTHERAPEUTIC: Hematopoietic. **CLINICAL:** Platelet growth factor.

ACTION
Stimulates production of blood platelets, essential to blood-clotting process. **Therapeutic Effect:** Increases platelet production.

PHARMACOKINETICS
Renal elimination as metabolite. **Half-life:** 5–8 hrs.

USES
Prevents severe thrombocytopenia, reduces need for platelet transfusions following myelosuppressive chemotherapy in pts with nonmyeloid malignancies.

PRECAUTIONS
Contraindications: None known. **Cautions:** HF, left ventricular dysfunction, hypertension, cardiac arrhythmias, conduction defect, respiratory disease, history of thromboembolic disease, renal/hepatic impairment.

⏳ LIFESPAN CONSIDERATIONS
Pregnancy/Lactation: Unknown if drug crosses placenta or is distributed in breast milk. **Pregnancy Category C. Children:** Safety and efficacy not established. **Elderly:** No age-related precautions noted.

INTERACTIONS
DRUG: None significant. **HERBAL:** None significant. **FOOD:** None known. **LAB VALUES:** May decrease Hgb, Hct, usually within 3–5 days of initiation of therapy; reverses approximately 1 wk after discontinuation of therapy.

AVAILABILITY (Rx)
Injection, Powder for Reconstitution: 5 mg.

ADMINISTRATION/HANDLING
Subcutaneous
Reconstitution • Add 1 ml Sterile Water for Injection directed at side of vial; swirl contents gently (avoid excessive agitation) to provide concentration of 5 mg/ml oprelvekin. • Discard unused portion.
Storage • Store in refrigerator. Once reconstituted, use within 3 hrs. • Give single injection in abdomen, thigh, hip, upper arm.

INDICATIONS/ROUTES/DOSAGE
◀ALERT▶ Give first dose 6–24 hrs after end of chemotherapy and stop at least 48 hrs before starting next cycle of chemotherapy.

Prevention of Thrombocytopenia
Subcutaneous: **ADULTS:** 50 mcg/kg once daily. **CHILDREN:** 25–50 mcg/kg once daily. Continue for 10–21 days or until platelet count reaches 50,000 cells/mm^3 after its nadir.

Dosage in Renal Impairment
ADULTS WITH CREATININE CLEARANCE LESS THAN 30 ML/MIN: 25 mcg once daily.

SIDE EFFECTS

Frequent (77%–19%): Nausea/vomiting, fluid retention, neutropenic fever, diarrhea, rhinitis, headache, dizziness, fever, insomnia, cough, rash, pharyngitis, tachycardia, vasodilation.

ADVERSE EFFECTS/ TOXIC REACTIONS

Transient atrial fibrillation/flutter occurs in 10% of pts (may be due to increased plasma volume; oprelvekin is not directly arrhythmogenic). Arrhythmias usually are brief in duration and spontaneously convert to normal sinus rhythm. Papilledema may occur in children.

NURSING CONSIDERATIONS

BASELINE ASSESSMENT
Obtain CBC before chemotherapy and at regular intervals thereafter.

INTERVENTION/EVALUATION
Monitor platelet count periodically to assess therapeutic duration of therapy. Dosing should continue until postnadir platelet count is more than 50,000 cells/mcl. Treatment should be stopped longer than 2 days before starting next round of chemotherapy. Closely monitor fluid and electrolyte status, esp. in pts receiving diuretic therapy. Assess for fluid retention (peripheral edema, dyspnea on exertion, generally occurs during first wk of therapy and continues for duration of treatment).

PATIENT/FAMILY TEACHING
• Report swelling in arms or legs, shortness of breath, irregular heartbeat, hypersensitivity reaction.

orlistat

or-lye-stat
(Alli, Xenical)
Do not confuse Xenical with Xeloda.

◆CLASSIFICATION

PHARMACOTHERAPEUTIC: Gastric/pancreatic lipase inhibitor. CLINICAL: Obesity management agent (see p. 138C).

ACTION

Inhibits absorption of dietary fats by inactivating gastric, pancreatic enzymes. **Therapeutic Effect:** Resulting caloric deficit may have positive effects on weight control.

PHARMACOKINETICS

Minimal absorption after administration. Protein binding: 99%. Metabolized within GI wall. Primarily eliminated in feces. Unknown if removed by hemodialysis. **Half-life:** 1–2 hrs.

USES

Management of obesity, including weight loss/maintenance, when used in conjunction with reduced-calorie diet. Reduces risk of weight regain after previous weight loss. Indicated for pts with initial BMI of 30 kg/m^2 or greater or 27 kg/m^2 or greater with other risk factors (e.g., diabetes, dyslipidemia, hypertension).

PRECAUTIONS

Contraindications: Cholestasis, chronic malabsorption syndrome, pregnancy. Cautions: History of hyperoxaluria or calcium oxalate nephrolithiasis.

⧗ LIFESPAN CONSIDERATIONS

Pregnancy/Lactation: Unknown if distributed in breast milk. Not recommended during pregnancy. Breastfeeding not recommended. **Pregnancy Category B. Children:** Safety and efficacy not established.

O

◆ Canadian trade name   🗡 Non-Crushable Drug   HIGH ALERT High Alert drug

Elderly: No age-related precautions noted.

INTERACTIONS

DRUG: May decrease concentration/effects of **cyclosporine, levothyroxine.** May reduce absorption of **vitamin E.** May alter effect of **warfarin** by altering vitamin K level. **HERBAL:** None significant. **FOOD:** None known. **LAB VALUES:** May decrease serum glucose, cholesterol, LDL.

AVAILABILITY (Rx)

Capsules (Alli): 60 mg. **(Xenical):** 120 mg.

ADMINISTRATION/HANDLING

PO
• Multivitamin supplements containing fat-soluble vitamins should be taken once daily at least 2 hrs before or after taking orlistat. • Distribute daily fat intake over 3 main meals (GI effects may increase when taken with any 1 meal very high in fat). Administer during or up to 1 hr after each meal containing fat.

INDICATIONS/ROUTES/DOSAGE

Weight Reduction
PO: ADULTS, ELDERLY, CHILDREN 12–16 YRS: (XENICAL): 120 mg 3 times a day. **(ALLI):** 60 mg 3 times a day with each main meal containing fat (do not take if meal is occasionally missed or contains no fat).

SIDE EFFECTS

Frequent (30%–20%): Headache, abdominal discomfort, flatulence, fecal urgency, fatty/oily stool. **Occasional (14%–5%):** Back pain, menstrual irregularity, nausea, fatigue, diarrhea, dizziness. **Rare (Less Than 4%):** Anxiety, rash, myalgia, dry skin, vomiting.

ADVERSE EFFECTS/ TOXIC REACTIONS

Hypersensitivity reaction occurs rarely.

NURSING CONSIDERATIONS

BASELINE ASSESSMENT
Obtain baseline laboratory tests. Obtain pt weight.

INTERVENTION/EVALUATION
Monitor serum cholesterol, LDL, glucose, changes in coagulation parameters. Monitor weight weekly.

PATIENT/FAMILY TEACHING
• Maintain nutritionally balanced, reduced-calorie diet. • Daily intake of fat, carbohydrates, protein to be distributed over 3 main meals.

---

oseltamivir

oh-sel-**tam**-i-veer
(Tamiflu)
Do not confuse Tamiflu with Thera-flu.

◆CLASSIFICATION

PHARMACOTHERAPEUTIC: Neuraminidase inhibitor. **CLINICAL:** Antiviral (see p. 70C).

ACTION

Selective inhibitor of influenza virus neuraminidase, an enzyme essential for viral replication. Acts against influenza A and B viruses. **Therapeutic Effect:** Suppresses spread of infection within respiratory system, reduces duration of clinical symptoms.

PHARMACOKINETICS

Readily absorbed after PO administration. Protein binding: 3%. Extensively converted to active drug in liver. Primarily excreted in urine. **Half-life:** 6–10 hrs.

USES

Symptomatic treatment of uncomplicated acute illness caused by influenza A or B virus in adults and children 1 yr and older who are symptomatic no longer than 2 days. Prevention of influenza in adults, children 1 yr and older.

PRECAUTIONS

Contraindications: None known. **Cautions:** Renal impairment.

⌛ LIFESPAN CONSIDERATIONS

Pregnancy/Lactation: Unknown if distributed in breast milk. **Pregnancy Category C. Children:** Safety and efficacy not established in those younger than 1 yr. **Elderly:** No age-related precautions noted.

INTERACTIONS

DRUG: Live attenuated influenza virus vaccine intranasal may interfere with effect. **HERBAL:** None significant. **FOOD:** None known. **LAB VALUES:** None significant.

AVAILABILITY (Rx)

Capsules: 30 mg, 45 mg, 75 mg. **Powder for Oral Suspension:** 6 mg/ml.

ADMINISTRATION/HANDLING

PO

• Give without regard to food. • May open capsules and mix with sweetened liquid. • Oral suspension stable for 10 days following reconstitution.

INDICATIONS/ROUTES/DOSAGE

Treatment of Influenza

Note: Hospitalized pts may require longer treatment course.

PO: ADULTS, ELDERLY, CHILDREN 13 YRS AND OLDER: 75 mg twice daily for 5 days. **CHILDREN 1–12 YRS, WEIGHING MORE THAN 40 KG:** 75 mg twice daily for 5 days. **CHILDREN 1–12 YRS, WEIGHING 24–40 KG:** 60 mg twice daily for 5 days. **CHILDREN 1–12 YRS, WEIGHING 15–23 KG:** 45 mg twice daily for 5 days. **CHILDREN 1–12 YRS, WEIGHING LESS THAN 15 KG:** 30 mg twice daily for 5 days. **CHILDREN 2 WKS TO YOUNGER THAN 1 YR:** 3 mg/kg twice daily for 5 days.

Prevention of Influenza

PO: ADULTS, ELDERLY, CHILDREN 13 YRS AND OLDER: 75 mg once daily. **CHILDREN 1–12 YRS, WEIGHING MORE THAN 40 KG:** 75 mg once daily. **WEIGHING 24–40 KG:** 60 mg once daily. **WEIGHING 15–23 KG:** 45 mg once daily. **WEIGHING LESS THAN 15 KG:** 30 mg once daily.

Dosage in Renal Impairment

Creatinine clearance 10–30 ml/min: Treatment: 75 mg/day. Prevention: 75 mg every other day or 30 mg daily.

SIDE EFFECTS

Frequent (10%–7%): Nausea, vomiting, diarrhea. **Rare (2%–1%):** Abdominal pain, bronchitis, dizziness, headache, cough, insomnia, fatigue, vertigo.

ADVERSE EFFECTS/ TOXIC REACTIONS

Colitis, pneumonia, tympanic membrane disorder, fever occur rarely.

NURSING CONSIDERATIONS

BASELINE ASSESSMENT

Obtain baseline laboratory tests as indicated. Confirm presence of influenza A or B virus.

INTERVENTION/EVALUATION

Monitor serum glucose, renal function in pts with influenza symptoms, diabetes.

PATIENT/FAMILY TEACHING

• Begin as soon as possible from first appearance of flu symptoms. • Avoid contact with those who are at high risk for influenza. • Not a substitute for flu shot.

O

ospemifene

os-**pem**-i-feen
(Osphena)

BLACK BOX ALERT Increased risk of endometrial cancer in women with a uterus who use unopposed estrogens. Supplemental progestin with estrogen therapy may reduce risk of endometrial hyperplasia. Use adequate diagnostic measures such as uterine sampling to rule out malignancy if abnormal bleeding occurs. May increase risk of stroke, deep vein thrombosis (DVT), hemorrhagic or thrombotic stroke.

✦ Canadian trade name   🗲 Non-Crushable Drug   **HIGH ALERT** High Alert drug

◆CLASSIFICATION

PHARMACOTHERAPEUTIC: Estrogen agonist/antagonist. **CLINICAL:** Hormonal modulator.

ACTION

Activates or blocks estrogenic pathway in differential tissues by binding to estrogen receptors. Alters vaginal epithelium. **Therapeutic Effect:** Alleviates painful intercourse in postmenopausal women.

PHARMACOKINETICS

Readily absorbed following PO administration. Metabolized in liver. Protein binding: 99%. Peak plasma concentration: 2 hrs. Excreted in feces (75%), urine (7%). **Half-life:** 26 hrs.

USES

Treatment of moderate to severe dyspareunia, a symptom of vulvar and vaginal atrophy, due to menopause.

PRECAUTIONS

Contraindications: Pregnancy (Pregnancy Category X) or women who may become pregnant, known or suspected estrogen-dependant neoplasia, breast cancer, undiagnosed abnormal genital bleeding, history of DVT, stroke, myocardial infarction. **Cautions:** Arterial vascular disease, breast cancer (known or suspected history), cardiovascular disease, diabetes mellitus, hypercholesterolemia, hypertension, obesity, smoking, surgery or immobilization, systemic lupus erythematosus, severe hepatic impairment.

⧖ LIFESPAN CONSIDERATIONS

Pregnancy/Lactation: Therapy contraindicated in pregnant women or those who may become pregnant. May cause fetal harm. Unknown if distributed in breast milk. **Pregnancy Category X. Children:** Not indicated in children. **Elderly:** No age-related precautions noted.

INTERACTIONS

DRUG: CYP3A4 inhibitors (e.g., fluconazole, ketoconazole) may increase concentration/effect. **CYP3A4 inducers (e.g., rifampin)** may decrease concentration/effect. **HERBAL:** None significant. **FOOD:** None known. **LAB VALUES:** None known.

AVAILABILITY (Rx)

Tablets: 60 mg.

ADMINISTRATION/HANDLING

PO
• Give with a meal or food.

INDICATIONS/ROUTES/DOSAGE

Dyspareunia
PO: ADULTS/ELDERLY: 60 mg once daily with food.

SIDE EFFECTS

Occasional (7%–4%): Flushing, benign vaginal discharge, muscle spasm. **Rare (Less than 2%):** Hyperhidrosis.

ADVERSE EFFECTS/ TOXIC REACTIONS

Increased risk of arterial/venous occlusive disease (DVT, MI, stroke). May increase risk of cardiovascular disease, malignant neoplasms (endometrial cancer), uterine polyps.

NURSING CONSIDERATIONS

BASELINE ASSESSMENT

Obtain baseline vital signs. Question history of DVT, MI, stroke; breast cancer, diabetes mellitus, hypertension, smoking history. Receive full medication history.

INTERVENTION/EVALUATION

Monitor for signs and symptoms of DVT (extremity pain, swelling), myocardial infarction (chest pain, sweating, left arm numbness, jaw pain), stroke (aphasia, hemiparesis, altered mental status, homonymous hemianopsia [blindness of one half of vision on same side of both eyes]). Monitor for abnormal bleeding.

Recommend pelvic exam, breast exam, mammogram every year.

PATIENT/FAMILY TEACHING

• There is an increased risk of uterine cancer. • Report signs of blood clots in extremities (leg pain, swelling of lower extremity), chest pains, difficulty speaking, one-sided paralysis, abnormal vaginal bleeding. • Report any planned surgery or bed rest. • Take with food. • Hot flashes are common. • Speak with gynecologist about routine breast and uterine exams. • If yeast infection occurs, do not take fluconazole. • Conduct routine breast exams, esp. with breast cancer history.

---

oxaliplatin

TOP 200   HIGH ALERT

ox-**al**-i-**pla**-tin
(Eloxatin)

BLACK BOX ALERT Anaphylactic-like reaction may occur within minutes of administration; may be controlled with epinephrine, corticosteroids, antihistamines.
Do not confuse oxaliplatin with Aloxi, carboplatin, or cisplatin.

◆**CLASSIFICATION**

PHARMACOTHERAPEUTIC: Platinum-containing complex. **CLINICAL:** Antineoplastic (see p. 89C).

ACTION

Inhibits DNA replication by cross-linking with DNA strands. Cell cycle–phase nonspecific. **Therapeutic Effect:** Prevents cell division.

PHARMACOKINETICS

Rapidly distributed. Protein binding: 90%. Undergoes rapid, extensive nonenzymatic biotransformation. Excreted in urine. **Half-life:** 391 hrs.

USES

Combination treatment of metastatic carcinoma of colon, rectum with 5-fluoroura-

cil (5-FU)/leucovorin in pts whose disease has recurred or progressed during or within 6 mos of completion of first-line therapy with bolus 5-FU/leucovorin and irinotecan. **OFF-LABEL:** Treatment of ovarian cancer, pancreatic cancer, hepatobiliary cancer, testicular cancer, esophageal cancer, gastric cancer, non-Hodgkin's lymphoma.

PRECAUTIONS

Contraindications: History of allergy to other platinum compounds. **Cautions:** Previous therapy with other antineoplastic agents; radiation, renal impairment, infection, pregnancy, immunosuppression, presence or history of peripheral neuropathy, elderly.

⌛ LIFESPAN CONSIDERATIONS

Pregnancy/Lactation: If possible, avoid use during pregnancy, esp. first trimester. May cause fetal harm. Breastfeeding not recommended. **Pregnancy Category D. Children:** Safety and efficacy not established. **Elderly:** Increased incidence of diarrhea, dehydration, hypokalemia, fatigue.

INTERACTIONS

DRUG: Bone marrow depressants may increase myelosuppression, GI effects. **Live virus vaccines** may potentiate virus replication, increase vaccine side effects, decrease pt's antibody response to vaccine. **Nephrotic medications** may increase concentration. **HERBAL: Echinacea** may decrease effects. **FOOD:** None known. **LAB VALUES:** May increase serum creatinine, bilirubin, AST, ALT.

AVAILABILITY (Rx)

Injection, Solution: 5 mg/ml (10-ml, 20-ml, 40-ml vials).

ADMINISTRATION/HANDLING

◄**ALERT**► Wear protective gloves during handling of oxaliplatin. If solution comes in contact with skin, wash skin immediately with soap, water. Do not use aluminum needles or administration sets that may

O

---

come in contact with drug; may cause degradation of platinum compounds. ◄ALERT► Pt should avoid ice, drinking cold beverages, touching cold objects during infusion and for 5 days thereafter (can exacerbate acute neuropathy).

 IV

Reconstitution • Dilute with 250–500 ml D₅W (never dilute with sodium chloride solution or other chloride-containing solutions) to final concentration of 0.2–0.6 mg/ml.
Rate of Administration • Infuse over 2–6 hrs.
Storage • Do not freeze. • Protect from light. • Store vials at room temperature. • After dilution, solution is stable for 6 hrs at room temperature, 24 hrs if refrigerated.

▦ IV INCOMPATIBILITIES

Do not infuse oxaliplatin with alkaline medications.

▦ IV COMPATIBILITIES

Dexamethasone, diphenhydramine (Benadryl), granisetron (Kytril), ondansetron (Zofran), palonosetron (Aloxi).

INDICATIONS/ROUTES/DOSAGE

Refer to individual protocols.
◄ALERT►Pretreat pt with antiemetics. Repeat courses should not be given more frequently than every 2 wks.

Colorectal Cancer
IV: ADULTS: Day 1: Oxaliplatin 85 mg/m² in 250–500 ml D₅W and leucovorin 200 mg/m², given simultaneously over more than 2 hrs in separate bags using a Y-line, followed by 5-FU 400 mg/m² IV bolus given over 2–4 min, followed by 5-FU 600 mg/m² in 500 ml D₅W as a 22-hr continuous IV infusion. **Day 2:** Leucovorin 200 mg/m² IV infusion given over more than 2 hrs, followed by 5-FU 400 mg/m² IV bolus given over 2–4 min, followed by 5-FU 600 mg/m² in 500 ml D₅W as a 22-hr continuous IV infusion. Repeat cycle every 2 wks for total of 6 mos. Prior

to subsequent therapy cycles, evaluate pt for clinical toxicities and laboratory tests.

Ovarian Cancer (Off-Label Use)
IV: ADULTS: Oxaliplatin 130 mg/m² q3wks. Prior to subsequent therapy cycles, evaluate pt for clinical toxicities and laboratory tests.

SIDE EFFECTS

Frequent (76%–20%): Peripheral/sensory neuropathy (usually occurs in hands, feet, perioral area, throat but may present as: jaw spasm, abnormal tongue sensation, eye pain, chest pressure, difficulty walking, swallowing, writing), nausea, fatigue, diarrhea, vomiting, constipation, abdominal pain, fever, anorexia. **Occasional (14%–10%):** Stomatitis, earache, insomnia, cough, difficulty breathing, backache, edema. **Rare (7%–3%):** Dyspepsia, dizziness, rhinitis, flushing, alopecia.

ADVERSE EFFECTS/ TOXIC REACTIONS

Peripheral/sensory neuropathy can occur without any prior event by drinking or holding a glass of cold liquid during IV infusion. Pulmonary fibrosis (characterized as nonproductive cough, dyspnea, crackles, radiologic pulmonary infiltrates) may warrant drug discontinuation. Hypersensitivity reaction (rash, urticaria, pruritus) occurs rarely.

NURSING CONSIDERATIONS

BASELINE ASSESSMENT
Obtain baseline renal function, WBC, platelet count.

INTERVENTION/EVALUATION
Monitor for decrease in WBC, platelets (myelosuppression is minimal). Monitor for diarrhea, GI bleeding (bright red, tarry stool), signs of neuropathy. Pt should avoid ice or drinking, holding glass of cold liquid during IV infusion and for 5 days following completion of infusion; may precipitate/exacerbate neurotoxicity (occurs within hrs or 1–2 days of dosing, lasts up

to 14 days). Maintain strict I&O. Assess oral mucosa for stomatitis.

PATIENT/FAMILY TEACHING
• Promptly report fever, sore throat, signs of local infection, unusual bruising/ bleeding from any site, persistent diarrhea, difficulty breathing. • Do not have immunizations without physician's approval (drug lowers resistance). • Avoid contact with those who have recently taken oral polio vaccine. • Avoid cold drinks, ice, cold objects (may produce neuropathy).

oxaprozin

ox-a-**pro**-zin
(Apo-Oxaprozin ✤, Daypro)

BLACK BOX ALERT Increased risk of serious cardiovascular thrombotic events, including myocardial infarction, CVA, new onset or worsening of preexisting hypertension. Increased risk of severe GI reactions, including ulceration, bleeding, perforation of stomach, intestines.
Do not confuse oxaprozin with oxazepam.

◆CLASSIFICATION
PHARMACOTHERAPEUTIC: NSAID. **CLINICAL:** Analgesic, anti-inflammatory (see p. 130C).

ACTION
Produces analgesic, anti-inflammatory effects by inhibiting prostaglandin synthesis. **Therapeutic Effect:** Reduces inflammatory response, intensity of pain.

PHARMACOKINETICS
Well absorbed from GI tract. Protein binding: 99%. Widely distributed. Metabolized in liver. Primarily excreted in urine; partially eliminated in feces. Not removed by hemodialysis. **Half-life:** 42–50 hrs.

USES
Acute, chronic treatment of osteoarthritis, juvenile rheumatoid arthritis (JRA), rheumatoid arthritis (RA).

PRECAUTIONS
Contraindications: History of hypersensitivity to aspirin, NSAIDs. Perioperative pain in the setting of CABG surgery. **Cautions:** Renal/hepatic impairment, asthma, history of GI tract disease, predisposition to fluid retention, HF, dehydration, coagulation disorders, concomitant anticoagulant therapy.

⧗ LIFESPAN CONSIDERATIONS
Pregnancy/Lactation: Unknown if drug is distributed in breast milk. Avoid use during third trimester (may adversely affect fetal cardiovascular system: premature closure of ductus arteriosus). **Pregnancy Category C (D if used in third trimester or near delivery). Children:** Safety and efficacy not established. **Elderly:** Age-related renal impairment may increase risk of hepatic/renal toxicity; decreased dosage recommended. GI bleeding/ulceration more likely to cause serious adverse effects.

INTERACTIONS
DRUG: May decrease effects of **antihypertensives, diuretics. Aspirin, other salicylates** may increase risk of GI side effects, bleeding. May increase risk of bleeding with **heparin, oral anticoagulants, thrombolytics.** May increase concentration, risk of toxicity of **lithium, methotrexate. HERBAL: Cat's claw, dong quai, evening primrose, feverfew, garlic, ginger, ginkgo, ginseng, horse chestnut, red clover** possess antiplatelet activity, may increase risk of bleeding. **FOOD:** None known. **LAB VALUES:** May increase serum BUN, creatinine, AST, ALT, potassium, LDH, alkaline phosphatase. May decrease Hgb, Hct.

AVAILABILITY (Rx)
Tablets: 600 mg.

 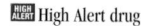

ADMINISTRATION/HANDLING

PO
• May give with food, milk, antacids if GI distress occurs.

INDICATIONS/ROUTES/DOSAGE

Osteoarthritis
PO: ADULTS, ELDERLY: 600–1,200 mg once a day (600 mg in pts with low body weight or mild disease).

Rheumatoid Arthritis (RA)
PO: ADULTS, ELDERLY: 1,200 mg once daily. **Range:** 600–1,800 mg/day. **Maximum dose: WEIGHT GREATER THAN 50 KG:** 1,800 mg; **WEIGHT 50 KG OR LESS:** 1,200 mg.

Juvenile Rheumatoid Arthritis (JRA)
PO: CHILDREN 6–16 YRS OF AGE WEIGHING MORE THAN 54 KG: 1,200 mg/day. **CHILDREN WEIGHING 32–54 KG:** 900 mg/day. **CHILDREN WEIGHING 22–31 KG:** 600 mg/day.

Dosage in Renal Impairment
ADULTS, ELDERLY PTS WITH RENAL IMPAIRMENT: Recommended initial dose is 600 mg/day; may be increased up to 1,200 mg/day.

SIDE EFFECTS

Occasional (9%–3%): Nausea, diarrhea, constipation, dyspepsia (heartburn, indigestion, epigastric pain), edema. **Rare (Less Than 3%):** Vomiting, abdominal cramps/pain, flatulence, anorexia, confusion, tinnitus, insomnia, drowsiness.

ADVERSE EFFECTS/ TOXIC REACTIONS

Hypertension, acute renal failure, respiratory depression, GI bleeding, coma occur rarely.

NURSING CONSIDERATIONS

BASELINE ASSESSMENT
Assess onset, type, location, duration of pain/inflammation.

INTERVENTION/EVALUATION
Observe for weight gain, edema, bleeding, ecchymoses, mental confusion. Monitor renal/hepatic function tests. Assess for therapeutic response: relief of pain, stiffness, swelling; increased joint mobility; reduced joint tenderness; improved grip strength.

PATIENT/FAMILY TEACHING
• Avoid aspirin, alcohol during therapy (increases risk of GI bleeding). • If gastric upset occurs, take with food, milk, antacids. • Report persistent GI effects. • Report blood in stool, weight gain, persistent abdominal pain. • Avoid tasks that require alertness, motor skills until response to drug is established.

oxcarbazepine

ox-kar-**baz**-e-peen
(Apo-Oxcarbazepine ❖, Oxtellar XR, <u>Trileptal</u>)
Do not confuse oxcarbazepine with carbamazepine, or Trileptal with TriLipix.

◆CLASSIFICATION

PHARMACOTHERAPEUTIC: Carboxamide derivative, anticonvulsant. **CLINICAL:** Anticonvulsant (see p. 36C).

ACTION

Blocks sodium channels, stabilizing hyperexcited neural membranes, inhibiting repetitive neuronal firing, diminishing synaptic impulses. **Therapeutic Effect:** Prevents seizures.

PHARMACOKINETICS

Completely absorbed from GI tract. Metabolized in liver. Protein binding: 40%. Primarily excreted in urine. **Half-life:** 2 hrs; metabolite, 6–10 hrs.

USES

Trileptal: Monotherapy, adjunctive therapy in adults, children 4 yrs and older for treatment of partial seizures. Adjunctive therapy in children 2 yrs and older for partial seizures. **Oxtellar XR:** Adjunctive therapy in treatment of partial seizures. **OFF-LABEL:** Treatment of neuropathic pain, bipolar disorder.

PRECAUTIONS

Contraindications: None known. **Cautions:** Renal impairment, sensitivity to carbamazepine, pts at increased risk for suicide.

⚖ LIFESPAN CONSIDERATIONS

Pregnancy/Lactation: Crosses placenta. Distributed in breast milk. **Pregnancy Category C. Children:** No age-related precautions in those older than 4 yrs. **Elderly:** Age-related renal impairment may require dosage adjustment.

INTERACTIONS

DRUG: **Alcohol, CNS depressants** may have additive sedative effect. May decrease effectiveness of **felodipine, oral contraceptives, verapamil.** May increase concentration, risk of toxicity of **phenobarbital, phenytoin. HERBAL: Gotu kola, kava kava, St. John's wort, valerian** may increase CNS depression. **Evening primrose** may decrease seizure threshold. **St. John's wort** may decrease concentration. **FOOD:** None known. **LAB VALUES:** May increase serum alkaline phosphatase, AST, ALT. May decrease serum sodium.

AVAILABILITY (Rx)

Oral Suspension (Trileptal): 300 mg/5 ml. **Tablets (Trileptal):** 150 mg, 300 mg, 600 mg.

🜆 **Tablets, Extended-Release (Oxtellar XR):** 150 mg, 300 mg, 600 mg.

ADMINISTRATION/HANDLING

PO

• Give without regard to food. Do not crush, cut, or break extended-release tablets. Swallow whole.

INDICATIONS/ROUTES/DOSAGE

Adjunctive Treatment of Seizures
PO: ADULTS, ELDERLY: (Immediate-Release): Initially, 600 mg/day in 2 divided doses. May increase by up to 600 mg/day at weekly intervals. **Maximum:** 2,400 mg/day. **Usual maintenance dose:** 600 mg twice daily. **CHILDREN 4–16 YRS:** Initially, 8–10 mg/kg in 2 divided doses. **Maximum:** 600 mg/day. Increase dose slowly over 2 wks. **Maintenance (based on weight): CHILDREN WEIGHING MORE THAN 39 KG:** 1,800 mg/day in 2 divided doses; **CHILDREN WEIGHING 29.1–39 KG:** 1,200 mg/day in 2 divided doses; **CHILDREN WEIGHING 20–29 KG:** 900 mg/day in 2 divided doses. **CHILDREN 2–3 YRS:** Initially, 8–10 mg/kg/day in 2 divided doses. **Maximum:** 600 mg/day in 2 divided doses. Increase dose slowly over 2 wks up to a **maximum** of 60 mg/kg/day in 2 divided doses. **(Extended-Release):** **ADULTS:** Initially, 600 mg once daily. May increase by 600 mg/day at weekly intervals. **Range:** 1,200–2,400 mg/day. **ELDERLY:** Initially, 300–450 mg/day. May increase by 300–450 mg/day at weekly intervals. **Range:** Up to 2,400 mg/day.

Conversion to Monotherapy
PO: ADULTS, ELDERLY: (Immediate-Release): 600 mg/day in 2 divided doses (while decreasing concomitant anticonvulsant over 3–6 wks). May increase by 600 mg/day at weekly intervals up to 2,400 mg/day. **CHILDREN 4–16 YRS:** Initially, 8–10 mg/kg/day in 2 divided doses with simultaneous initial reduction of dose of concomitant antiepileptic over 3–6 wks. May increase by maximum of 10 mg/kg/day at weekly intervals (see below for recommended daily dose by weight).

Initiation of Monotherapy
PO: ADULTS, ELDERLY: (Immediate-Release): 600 mg/day in 2 divided doses. May increase by 300 mg/day every 3 days up to 1,200 mg/day. **CHILDREN 4–16 YRS:** Initially, 8–10 mg/kg/day in 2 divided doses. Increase at 3-day intervals by 5 mg/kg/day to achieve maintenance dose by weight as follows:

Weight	Dosage
70+ kg	1,500–2,100 mg/day
60–69 kg	1,200–2,100 mg/day
50–59 kg	1,200–1,800 mg/day

O

Weight	Dosage
41–49 kg	1,200–1,500 mg/day
35–40 kg	900–1,500 mg/day
25–34 kg	900–1,200 mg/day
20–24 kg	600–900 mg/day

Dosage in Renal Impairment
Creatinine clearance less than 30 ml/min: Give 50% of normal starting dose, then titrate slowly to desired dose.

SIDE EFFECTS

Frequent (22%–13%): Dizziness, nausea, headache. **Occasional (7%–5%):** Vomiting, diarrhea, ataxia (muscular incoordination), nervousness, dyspepsia (heartburn, indigestion, epigastric pain), constipation. **Rare (4%):** Tremor, rash, back pain, epistaxis, sinusitis, diplopia.

ADVERSE EFFECTS/ TOXIC REACTIONS

Clinically significant hyponatremia may occur, manifested as leg cramping, hypotension, cold/clammy skin, increased pulse rate, headache, nausea, vomiting, diarrhea. Suicidal ideation occurs rarely.

NURSING CONSIDERATIONS

BASELINE ASSESSMENT

Review history of seizure disorder (type, onset, intensity, frequency, duration, LOC), drug history (esp. other anticonvulsants). Provide safety precautions; quiet, dark environment.

INTERVENTION/EVALUATION

Assist with ambulation if dizziness, ataxia occur. Assess for visual abnormalities, headache. Monitor serum sodium. Assess for signs of hyponatremia (nausea, malaise, headache, lethargy, confusion). Assess for clinical improvement (decrease in intensity, frequency of seizures). Monitor for worsening depression, suicidal ideation.

PATIENT/FAMILY TEACHING

• Do not abruptly stop taking medication (may increase seizure activity). • Inform physician if rash, nausea, headache, dizziness occurs. • May need periodic blood tests. • Avoid tasks that require alertness, motor skills until response to drug is established. • Avoid alcohol. • May decrease effectiveness of oral contraceptives.

oxybutynin

ox-i-**bue**-ti-nin
(Apo-Oxybutynin ✤, <u>Ditropan XL</u>, Gelnique, Novo-Oxybutynin ✤, Oxytrol)
Do not confuse Ditropan with Detrol, diazepam, or Diprivan, or oxybutynin with OxyContin.

◆CLASSIFICATION

PHARMACOTHERAPEUTIC: Anticholinergic. **CLINICAL:** Antispasmodic.

ACTION

Exerts antispasmodic (papaverine-like), antimuscarinic (atropine-like) action on detrusor smooth muscle of bladder. **Therapeutic Effect:** Increases bladder capacity, delays desire to void.

PHARMACOKINETICS

Route	Onset	Peak	Duration
PO	0.5–1 hr	3–6 hrs	6–10 hrs

Rapidly, well absorbed from GI tract. Metabolized in liver. Primarily excreted in urine. Unknown if removed by hemodialysis. **Half-life:** 1–2.3 hrs; metabolite, 7–8 hrs.

USES

Relief of symptoms (urgency, incontinence, frequency, nocturia, urge incontinence) associated with uninhibited neurogenic bladder, reflex neurogenic bladder. Extended-release also indicated for treatment of symptoms associated with detrusor overactivity due to neurologic disorder.

PRECAUTIONS

Contraindications: Partial or complete GI/GU obstruction, with or at risk for uncontrolled narrow-angle glaucoma, toxic megacolon. **Cautions:** Renal/hepatic impairment, cardiovascular disease, hyperthyroidism, reflux esophagitis, hypertension, prostatic hypertrophy, neuropathy, myasthenia gravis, ulcerative colitis, intestinal atony.

⧖ LIFESPAN CONSIDERATIONS

Pregnancy/Lactation: Unknown if drug crosses placenta or is distributed in breast milk. **Pregnancy Category B. Children:** No age-related precautions noted in those older than 5 yrs. **Elderly:** May be more sensitive to anticholinergic effects (e.g., dry mouth, urinary retention).

INTERACTIONS

DRUG: Medications with anticholinergic action (e.g., antihistamines) may increase anticholinergic effects. **Clarithromycin, erythromycin, itraconazole, ketoconazole** may alter pharmacokinetic parameters. **HERBAL:** None significant. **FOOD:** None known. **LAB VALUES:** None significant.

AVAILABILITY (Rx)

Syrup: 5 mg/5 ml. **Tablets:** 5 mg. **Topical Gel (Gelnique):** 100 mg/unit dose sachet. **(3% Gel):** 30 mg/ml. **Transdermal (Oxytrol):** 3.9 mg.

🦉 Tablets (Extended-Release [Ditropan XL]): 5 mg, 10 mg, 15 mg.

ADMINISTRATION/HANDLING

PO
• Give without regard to meals. • Extended-release tablet must be swallowed whole; do not crush, divide, cut.

Transdermal
• Apply patch to dry, intact skin on abdomen, hip, buttock. • Use new application site for each new patch; avoid reapplication to same site within 7 days.

Topical Gel
• **(Gelnique):** Apply contents of 1 sachet once daily to dry, intact skin on abdomen, upper arms/shoulders, or thighs. • Do not bathe/shower until 1 hr after gel is applied. • **(3% Gel):** Apply 3 ml to thigh, upper arm, or shoulder.

INDICATIONS/ROUTES/DOSAGE

Neurogenic Bladder
PO: ADULTS: 5 mg 2–3 times a day. May increase 5 mg 4 times a day. **ELDERLY:** 2.5–5 mg 2–3 times a day. **CHILDREN OLDER THAN 5 YRS:** 5 mg twice a day. May increase 5 mg 3 times a day. **CHILDREN 1–5 YRS:** 0.2 mg/kg/dose 2–4 times a day. **PO (Extended-Release): ADULTS, ELDERLY:** 5–10 mg/day. May increase 30 mg/day. **CHILDREN 6 YRS AND OLDER:** Initially, 5–10 mg once a day. May increase in 5–10 mg increments. **Maximum:** 20 mg/day.
Transdermal: ADULTS: 3.9 mg applied twice a wk. Apply every 3–4 days.
Topical Gel: ADULTS, ELDERLY: 100 mg once daily.
Gel 3%: Apply 3 ml (84 mg) once daily.

SIDE EFFECTS

Frequent: Constipation, dry mouth, drowsiness, decreased perspiration. **Occasional:** Decreased lacrimation/salivation, impotence, urinary hesitancy/retention, suppressed lactation, blurred vision, mydriasis, nausea/vomiting, insomnia.

ADVERSE EFFECTS/TOXIC REACTIONS

Overdose produces CNS excitation (nervousness, restlessness, hallucinations, irritability), hypotension/hypertension, confusion, tachycardia, facial flushing, respiratory depression.

NURSING CONSIDERATIONS

BASELINE ASSESSMENT

Assess dysuria, urgency, frequency, incontinence.

INTERVENTION/EVALUATION

Monitor for symptomatic relief. Monitor I&O; palpate bladder for urine retention. Monitor daily pattern of bowel activity, stool consistency.

PATIENT/FAMILY TEACHING

• Avoid alcohol. • May cause dry mouth (sugarless candy/gum may reduce effect). • Avoid tasks that require alertness, motor skills until response to drug is established (may cause drowsiness). • Avoid strenuous activity in warm environment.

---

oxycodone

ox-ee-**koe**-done
(Oxecta, <u>OxyContin</u>, OxyIR ✦,
Roxicodone, Supeudol ✦)

BLACK BOX ALERT OxyContin **(controlled-release):** Not intended as an "as needed" analgesic or for immediate postop pain control. Extended-release should not be crushed, broken, or chewed (otherwise leads to rapid release and absorption of potentially fatal dose). Be alert to signs of abuse, misuse, and diversion. CYP3A4 inhibitors or inducers can affect oxycodone levels. **Do not confuse oxycodone with hydrocodone, oxybutynin, or oxymorphone, OxyContin with MS Contin or oxybutynin, or Roxicodone with Roxanol.**

FIXED-COMBINATION(S)

Combunox: oxycodone/ibuprofen (an NSAID): 5 mg/400 mg. **Endocet:** oxycodone/acetaminophen (a non-narcotic analgesic): 5 mg/325 mg, 7.5 mg/325 mg, 7.5 mg/500 mg, 10 mg/325 mg, 10 mg/650 mg. **Magnacet:** oxycodone/acetaminophen (a non-narcotic analgesic): 2.5 mg/400 mg, 7.5 mg/400 mg, 10 mg/400 mg. **Percocet:** oxycodone/acetaminophen: 2.5 mg/325 mg, 5 mg/325 mg, 5 mg/500 mg, 7.5 mg/325 mg, 7.5 mg/500 mg, 10 mg/325 mg, 10 mg/650 mg. **Percocet, Roxicet, Ty-**lox: oxycodone/acetaminophen (a non-narcotic analgesic): 5 mg/500 mg. **Percodan:** oxycodone/aspirin (a non-narcotic analgesic): 2.25 mg/325 mg, 4.5 mg/325 mg.

◆CLASSIFICATION

PHARMACOTHERAPEUTIC: Opioid analgesic **(Schedule II). CLINICAL:** Narcotic analgesic.

ACTION

Binds with opioid receptors within CNS. **Therapeutic Effect:** Alters perception of and emotional response to pain.

PHARMACOKINETICS

Route	Onset	Peak	Duration
PO (immediate-release)	10–15 min	0.5–1 hr	3–6 hrs
PO (controlled-release)	10–15 min	0.5–1 hr	Up to 12 hrs

Moderately absorbed from GI tract. Protein binding: 38%–45%. Widely distributed. Metabolized in liver. Excreted in urine. Unknown if removed by hemodialysis. **Half-life:** 2–3 hrs (5 hrs controlled-release).

USES

Relief of moderate to severe pain (usually in combination with nonopioid analgesics).

PRECAUTIONS

Contraindications: Acute or severe bronchial asthma, hypercarbia, paralytic ileus, significant respiratory depression. **Extreme Caution:** CNS depression, anoxia, hypercapnia, respiratory depression, seizures, acute alcoholism, shock, untreated myxedema, respiratory dysfunction. **Cautions:** Elevated ICP, hepatic impairment, coma, debilitated pts, head injury, biliary tract disease, toxic psychosis, acute abdominal conditions, hypothyroidism, prostatic hypertrophy, Addison's disease, urethral stricture, COPD, history of substance abuse.

LIFESPAN CONSIDERATIONS

Pregnancy/Lactation: Readily crosses placenta. Distributed in breast milk. Respiratory depression may occur in neonate if mother received opiates during labor. Regular use of opiates during pregnancy may produce withdrawal symptoms in neonate (irritability, excessive crying, tremors, hyperactive reflexes, fever, vomiting, diarrhea, yawning, sneezing, seizures). **Pregnancy Category B (D if used for prolonged periods or at high dosages at term). Children:** Paradoxical excitement may occur. Pts younger than 2 yrs are more susceptible to respiratory depressant effects. **Elderly:** Age-related renal impairment may increase risk of urinary retention. May be more susceptible to respiratory depressant effects.

INTERACTIONS

DRUG: Alcohol, other CNS depressants may increase CNS effects, respiratory depression, hypotension. **CYP3A4 inhibitors (clarithromycin, ketoconazole)** may increase concentration, toxicity. **CYP3A4 inducers (carbamazepine, rifampin)** may decrease concentration/effects. **MAOIs** may produce severe, sometimes fatal reaction (administer ¼ of usual oxycodone dose). **HERBAL: Gotu kola, kava kava, St. John's wort, valerian** may increase CNS depression. **FOOD: Grapefruit products** may increase potential for respiratory depression. **LAB VALUES:** May increase serum amylase, lipase.

AVAILABILITY (Rx)

Note: New formulation of controlled-release intended to prevent medication from being cut, broken, chewed, crushed, or dissolved to reduce risk of overdose due to tampering, snorting, or injection. **Capsules (Immediate-Release):** 5 mg. **Oral Concentrate:** 20 mg/ml. **Oral Solution (Roxicodone):** 5 mg/5 ml. **Tablets (Oxecta, Roxicodone):** 5 mg, 7.5 mg, 10 mg, 15 mg, 20 mg, 30 mg.

Tablets (Controlled-Release [Oxycontin]): 10 mg, 15 mg, 20 mg, 30 mg, 40 mg, 60 mg, 80 mg.

ADMINISTRATION/HANDLING

PO

• Give without regard to meals. • Tablets may be crushed. • **Controlled-release:** Swallow whole; do not break, crush, dissolve, or divide.

INDICATIONS/ROUTES/DOSAGE

Note: All doses should be titrated to desired effect.

Analgesia
PO (Immediate-Release): ADULTS, ELDERLY: Initially, 5–15 mg q4–6h as needed. Range: 5–20 mg/dose. **CHILDREN, 6–18 YRS:** 0.1–0.2 mg/kg/dose q4–6h as needed. **Maximum dose:** 10 mg for moderate pain, 20 mg for severe pain.

Opioid Naive
PO (Controlled-Release): ADULTS, ELDERLY: Initially, 10 mg q12h.
◄**ALERT**► To convert from other opioids or nonopioid analgesics to oxycodone controlled-release, refer to OxyContin package insert. Dosages are reduced in pts with severe hepatic disease.

SIDE EFFECTS

◄**ALERT**► Effects are dependent on dosage amount. Ambulatory pts, those not in severe pain may experience dizziness, nausea, vomiting, hypotension more frequently than those in supine position or having severe pain. **Frequent:** Drowsiness, dizziness, hypotension (including orthostatic hypotension), anorexia. **Occasional:** Confusion, diaphoresis, facial flushing, urinary retention, constipation, dry mouth, nausea, vomiting, headache. **Rare:** Allergic reaction, depression, paradoxical CNS hyperactivity, nervousness in children, paradoxical excitement, restlessness in elderly, debilitated pts.

O

ADVERSE EFFECTS/ TOXIC REACTIONS

Overdose results in respiratory depression, skeletal muscle flaccidity, cold/ clammy skin, cyanosis, extreme drowsiness progressing to seizures, stupor, coma. Hepatotoxicity may occur with overdose of acetaminophen component of fixed-combination product. Tolerance to analgesic effect, physical dependence may occur with repeated use. **Antidote:** Naloxone (see Appendix K for dosage).

NURSING CONSIDERATIONS

BASELINE ASSESSMENT

Assess onset, type, location, duration of pain. Effect of medication is reduced if full pain recurs before next dose. Obtain vital signs before giving medication. If respirations are 12/min or less (20/min or less in children), withhold medication, contact physician.

INTERVENTION/EVALUATION

Palpate bladder for urinary retention. Monitor daily pattern of bowel activity, stool consistency. Initiate deep breathing, coughing exercises, esp. in pts with pulmonary impairment. Monitor pain relief, respiratory rate, mental status, B/P, LOC.

PATIENT/FAMILY TEACHING

• May cause dry mouth, drowsiness. • Avoid tasks that require alertness, motor skills until response to drug is established. • Avoid alcohol. • May be habit forming. • Do not chew, crush, dissolve or divide controlled-release tablets. • Report severe constipation, absence of pain relief.

---

oxymorphone

ox-ee-**mor**-fone
(Opana, Opana ER)
BLACK BOX ALERT Has abuse liability. Concern about increased risk of abuse, misuse, or diversion.
Do not confuse oxymorphone with oxycodone.

♦ CLASSIFICATION

PHARMACOTHERAPEUTIC: Opioid agonist **(Schedule II). CLINICAL:** Narcotic analgesic, antianxiety, preop anesthetic.

ACTION

Binds to opiate receptor sites within CNS. **Therapeutic Effect:** Reduces intensity of pain stimuli, alters pain perception, emotional response to pain. Parenterally, 1 mg oxymorphone equivalent to 10 mg morphine.

PHARMACOKINETICS

Route	Onset	Peak	Duration
Parenteral	5–10 min	N/A	3–6 hrs

Well absorbed. Protein binding: 10%. Widely distributed. Metabolized in liver. Excreted in urine. **Half-life:** 7–9 hrs; **extended-release:** 9–11 hrs.

USES

Injection: Relief of moderate to severe pain. **PO (Immediate-release):** Relief of moderate to severe acute pain. **(Extended-release):** Relief of moderate to severe pain in pts requiring continuous treatment for extended period of time.

PRECAUTIONS

Contraindications: Hypersensitivity to morphine, acute asthma attack, severe respiratory depression, paralytic ileus, pulmonary edema secondary to chemical respiratory irritants, moderate to severe hepatic function impairment, hypercarbia. **Extreme Cautions:** Anoxia, hypercapnia, seizures, acute alcoholism, shock, untreated myxedema. **Cautions:** Hypothyroidism, prostatic hypertrophy, Addison's disease, urethral stricture, prostatic hyperplasia, toxic psychosis, renal impairment, COPD, biliary tract disease, acute pancreatitis, head injury, increased ICP, morbid obesity, mild hepatic dysfunction, history of substance abuse.

LIFESPAN CONSIDERATIONS

Pregnancy/Lactation: Unknown if distributed in breast milk. May prolong labor if administered in latent phase of first stage of labor or before cervical dilation of 4–5 cm has occurred. Respiratory depression may occur in neonate if mother received opiates during labor. Regular use of opiates during pregnancy may produce withdrawal symptoms in the neonate (irritability, excessive crying, tremors, hyperactive reflexes, fever, vomiting, diarrhea, yawning, sneezing, seizures). **Pregnancy Category C. (Category D if used for prolonged periods or high doses at term.) Children:** Safety and efficacy not established in those younger than 18 yrs. **Elderly:** May be more susceptible to respiratory depression, may cause paradoxical excitement. Age-related hepatic impairment, debilitation may require dosage adjustment.

INTERACTIONS

DRUG: Alcohol, other CNS depressants may increase CNS effects, respiratory depression, hypotension. **Anticholinergics** may increase risk of urinary retention, severe constipation (may lead to paralytic ileus). **Propofol** increases risk of bradycardia. Decreased effect when given concurrently with **phenothiazines. HERBAL: Gotu kola, kava kava, St. John's wort, valerian** may produce CNS depressant effects. **FOOD:** None known. **LAB VALUES:** May increase serum amylase, lipase.

AVAILABILITY (Rx)

Injection: 1 mg/ml. **Tablets:** 5 mg, 10 mg.

Tablets (Extended-Release): 5 mg, 7.5 mg, 10 mg, 15 mg, 20 mg, 30 mg, 40 mg.

ADMINISTRATION/HANDLING

IV

Rate of Administration • Administer IV push very slowly. • Rapid IV increases risk of severe adverse reactions (chest wall rigidity, apnea, peripheral circulatory collapse, anaphylactoid effects, cardiac arrest).

IM/Subcutaneous

• Inject deep IM, preferably in upper, outer quadrant of buttock. • Use short 30-gauge needle for subcutaneous injection. • Administer slowly, rotating injection sites. • Pts with circulatory impairment experience higher risk of overdosage due to delayed absorption of repeated administration.

Storage • Store parenteral form at room temperature. Refrigerate suppository form. • Discard parenteral form if discolored or particulate forms.

PO

• Give 1 hr before or 2 hrs after meals. • Do not cut, break, crush extended-release tablet.

IV COMPATIBILITIES

Glycopyrrolate, hydroxyzine, ranitidine.

INDICATIONS/ROUTES/DOSAGE

Analgesia

IV: ADULTS 18 YRS AND OLDER, ELDERLY: Initially, 0.5 mg. Dose may be cautiously increased until satisfactory response is achieved.

ALERT IM preferred over subcutaneous route (subcutaneous rate of absorption is less reliable).

IM/Subcutaneous: ADULTS 18 YRS AND OLDER, ELDERLY: Initially, 1–1.5 mg every 4–6 hrs as needed.

PO: ADULTS, ELDERLY: (IMMEDIATE-RELEASE): 5–10 mg q4–6h. **(EXTENDED-RELEASE):** Initially, 5 mg q12h. May increase by 5–10 mg q12h every 3–7 days.

Analgesia during Labor

IM/Subcutaneous: ADULTS 18 YRS AND OLDER, ELDERLY: 0.5–1 mg.

SIDE EFFECTS

Note: Effects are dependent on dosage amount, route of administration. Ambulatory pts, those not in severe pain may experience dizziness, nausea, vomiting, hypotension more frequently than those

in supine position or having severe pain. **Frequent (10% or higher):** Drowsiness, hypotension, dizziness, nausea, vomiting, constipation, weakness. **Occasional (9%–2%):** Nervousness, headache, restlessness, malaise, confusion, anorexia, abdominal cramps, dry mouth, decreased urinary output, ureteral spasm, pain at injection site. **Rare (1% or less):** Depression, paradoxical CNS stimulation, hallucinations, rash, urticaria.

ADVERSE EFFECTS/ TOXIC REACTIONS

Overdose results in respiratory depression, skeletal muscle flaccidity, cold/clammy skin, cyanosis, extreme drowsiness progressing to convulsions, stupor, coma. Tolerance to analgesic effect, physical dependence may occur with repeated use. Prolonged duration of action, cumulative effect may occur in those with hepatic/renal impairment.

NURSING CONSIDERATIONS

BASELINE ASSESSMENT

Assess onset, type, location, duration of pain. Obtain vital signs before giving medication. If respirations are 12/min or lower, withhold medication, contact physician. Effect of medication is reduced if full pain recurs before next dose.

INTERVENTION/EVALUATION

Monitor vital signs 5–10 min after IV administration, 15–30 min after subcutaneous, IM. Be alert for decreased respirations, B/P. To prevent pain cycles, instruct pt to request pain medication as soon as discomfort begins. Assess for clinical improvement, record onset of pain relief. Consult physician if pain relief is not adequate.

PATIENT/FAMILY TEACHING

• Discomfort may occur with injection. • Change positions slowly to avoid postural hypotension. • Avoid tasks that require alertness, motor skills until response to drug is established. • Avoid

alcohol. • Tolerance/dependence may occur with prolonged use of high doses.

oxytocin

ox-ee-**toe**-sin
(Pitocin, Syntocinon ✤)

BLACK BOX ALERT Not to be given for elective labor induction, but when medically indicated.
Do not confuse Pitocin with Pitressin.

◆CLASSIFICATION

PHARMACOTHERAPEUTIC: Uterine smooth muscle stimulant. **CLINICAL:** Oxytocic agent.

ACTION

Affects uterine myofibril activity, stimulates mammary smooth muscle. **Therapeutic Effect:** Contracts uterine smooth muscle. Enhances lactation.

PHARMACOKINETICS

Route	Onset	Peak	Duration
IV	Immediate	N/A	1 hr
IM	3–5 min	N/A	2–3 hrs

Rapidly absorbed through nasal mucous membranes. Protein binding: 30%. Distributed in extracellular fluid. Metabolized in liver, kidney. Primarily excreted in urine. Half-life: 1–6 min.

USES

Induction of labor at term, control of postpartum bleeding. Adjunct in management of abortion.

PRECAUTIONS

Contraindications: Adequate uterine activity that fails to progress, cephalopelvic disproportion, fetal distress without imminent delivery, grand multiparity, hyperactive or hypertonic uterus, obstetric emergencies that favor surgical intervention, prematurity, unengaged fetal head, unfavorable fetal position/presentation, when vaginal delivery is contraindicated, (e.g., active genital herpes infection, invasive cervical cancer, placenta previa, cord presentation). **Cautions:** Induction of labor should be for medical, not elective, reasons.

⧗ LIFESPAN CONSIDERATIONS

Pregnancy/Lactation: Used as indicated, not expected to present risk of fetal abnormalities. Small amounts in breast milk. Breast-feeding not recommended. **Pregnancy Category X. Children/Elderly:** Not used in these pt populations.

INTERACTIONS

DRUG: Caudal block anesthetics, vasopressors may increase pressor effects. **Other oxytocics** may cause cervical lacerations, uterine hypertonus, uterine rupture. **HERBAL:** None significant. **FOOD:** None known. **LAB VALUES:** None significant.

AVAILABILITY (Rx)

Injection (Pitocin): 10 units/ml.

ADMINISTRATION/HANDLING
🖢 IV

Reconstitution • Dilute 10–40 units (1–4 ml) in 1,000 ml of 0.9% NaCl, lactated Ringer's, or D₅W to provide concentration of 10–40 milliunits/ml solution.
Rate of Administration • Give by IV infusion (use infusion device to carefully control rate of flow as ordered by physician).
Storage • Store at room temperature.

🗎 IV INCOMPATIBILITIES

No known incompatibilities via Y-site administration.

🗎 IV COMPATIBILITIES

Heparin, insulin (regular), multivitamins, potassium chloride, zidovudine.

INDICATIONS/ROUTES/DOSAGE

Induction or Stimulation of Labor
IV: ADULTS: 0.5–1 milliunit/min. May gradually increase in increments of 1–2 milliunits/min. Rates of 9–10 milliunits/min are rarely required.

Abortion
IV: ADULTS: 10–20 milliunits/min. **Maximum:** 30 units/12-hr dose.

Control of Postpartum Bleeding
IV Infusion: ADULTS: 10–40 units in 1,000 ml IV fluid at rate sufficient to control uterine atony.
IM: ADULTS: 10 units (total dose) after delivery.

SIDE EFFECTS

Occasional: Tachycardia, premature ventricular contractions, hypotension, nausea, vomiting. **Rare: Nasal:** Lacrimation/tearing, nasal irritation, rhinorrhea, unexpected uterine bleeding/contractions.

ADVERSE EFFECTS/ TOXIC REACTIONS

Hypertonicity may occur with tearing of uterus, increased bleeding, abruptio placentae (i.e., placental abruption), cervical/vaginal lacerations. **Fetal:** Bradycardia, CNS/brain damage, trauma due to rapid propulsion, low Apgar score at 5 min, retinal hemorrhage occur rarely. Prolonged IV infusion of oxytocin with excessive fluid volume has caused severe water intoxication with seizures, coma, death.

NURSING CONSIDERATIONS

BASELINE ASSESSMENT

Assess baselines for vital signs, B/P, fetal heart rate. Determine frequency, duration, strength of contractions.

INTERVENTION/EVALUATION

Monitor B/P, pulse, respirations, fetal heart rate, intrauterine pressure, contractions (duration, strength, frequency) q15min. Notify physician of contractions that last longer than 1 min, occur more frequently than every 2 min, or stop. Maintain careful I&O; be alert to potential water intoxication. Check for blood loss.

PATIENT/FAMILY TEACHING

• Keep pt, family informed of labor progress.

O

 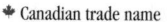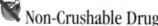

paclitaxel

pak-li-**tak**-sel
(Abraxane, Apo-Paclitaxel ❖)

BLACK BOX ALERT Myelosuppression is major dose-limiting toxicity. Must be administered by certified chemotherapy personnel. Severe hypersensitivity reactions reported. **Do not confuse paclitaxel with docetaxel, paroxetine, or Paxil.**

◆ CLASSIFICATION

PHARMACOTHERAPEUTIC: Taxoid, antimitotic agent. **CLINICAL:** Antineoplastic (see p. 89C).

ACTION

Promotes the polymerization of tubulin, disrupting normal microtubule dynamics required for cell division in late G_2, M phases of cell cycle. **Therapeutic Effect:** Inhibits cellular mitosis, replication.

PHARMACOKINETICS

Does not readily cross blood-brain barrier. Protein binding: 89%–98%. Metabolized in liver. Eliminated by bile. Not removed by hemodialysis. **Half-life:** 3-hr infusion: 13.1–20.2 hrs; 24-hr infusion: 15.7–52.7 hrs.

USES

First-line treatment of advanced ovarian cancer, treatment of metastatic ovarian cancer following failure of first-line or subsequent chemotherapy. Treatment of breast cancer, AIDS-related Kaposi's sarcoma, non–small-cell lung cancer (NSCLC). **Abraxane:** Treatment of breast cancer after failure of combination chemotherapy or relapse within 6 mos of adjuvant chemotherapy. First-line treatment of metastatic adenocarcinoma of pancreas. Treatment of locally advanced or metastatic non–small-cell lung cancer (NSCLC). **OFF-LABEL:** Bladder, cervical, small-cell lung, head and neck cancers. Treatment of adenocarcinoma.

PRECAUTIONS

Contraindications: Hypersensitivity to drugs developed with Cremophor EL (polyoxyethylated castor oil). **Cautions:** Hepatic impairment, severe neutropenia, peripheral neuropathy. Baseline neutropenia (neutrophil count 1,500 cells/mm^3 or less), 1,000 cells/mm^3 or less when treating AIDS-related Kaposi's sarcoma.

⧖ LIFESPAN CONSIDERATIONS

Pregnancy/Lactation: May cause fetal harm. Unknown if distributed in breast milk. Avoid use in pregnancy. **Pregnancy Category D. Children:** Safety and efficacy not established. **Elderly:** No age-related precautions noted.

INTERACTIONS

DRUG: CYP3A4, CYP2C8 inhibitors (e.g., ritonavir, clarithromycin, ketoconazole) may increase concentration/effects. **CYP3A4, CYP2C8 inducers (e.g., rifampin, carbamazepine)** may decrease effects. **Bone marrow depressants** may increase myelosuppression. **Live virus vaccines** may potentiate virus replication, increase vaccine side effects, decrease pt's antibody response to vaccine. **HERBAL:** Avoid **black cohosh, dong quai** in estrogen-dependent tumors. **Gotu kola, kava kava, St. John's wort, valerian** may increase CNS depression. **St. John's wort** may decrease levels. **FOOD:** None known. **LAB VALUES:** May elevate serum alkaline phosphatase, bilirubin, AST, ALT, triglycerides.

AVAILABILITY (Rx)

Injection, Powder for Reconstitution (Abraxane): 100-mg vial. **Injection Solution:** 6 mg/ml.

ADMINISTRATION/HANDLING

 IV

◀ALERT▶ Wear gloves during handling; if contact with skin occurs, wash hands thoroughly with soap, water. If contact with mucous membranes occurs, flush with water.

Paclitaxel
Reconstitution • Dilute with 250–1,000 ml 0.9% NaCl, D₅W to final concentration of 0.3–1.2 mg/ml.
Rate of Administration • Administer at rate as ordered by physician (over 1–24 hrs) through in-line filter not greater than 0.22 microns. • Monitor vital signs during infusion, esp. during first hour. • Discontinue administration if severe hypersensitivity reaction occurs.
Storage • Store unopened vials at room temperature. • Reconstituted solution is stable at room temperature for 72 hrs. • Store diluted solutions in bottles or plastic bags. Administer through polyethylene-lined administration sets (avoid plasticized PVC equipment or devices).

Abraxane (Paclitaxel—Protein Bound)
Reconstitution • Reconstitute each vial with 20 ml 0.9% NaCl to provide concentration of 5 mg/ml. • Slowly inject onto inside wall of vial; gently swirl over 2 min to avoid foaming. • Inject appropriate amount into empty PVC-type bag.
Rate of Administration • Infuse over 30 min. Do not use in-line filter.
Storage • Store unopened vials at room temperature • Once reconstituted, use immediately but may refrigerate for up to 8 hrs.

⊞ IV INCOMPATIBILITIES

◀ALERT▶ IV compatibility: Data for Abraxane not known; avoid mixing with other medication. Amphotericin B complex (Abelcet, AmBisome, Amphotec), doxorubicin liposomal (Doxil), hydroxyzine (Vistaril), methylprednisolone (Solu-Medrol), mitoxantrone (Novantrone).

⊞ IV COMPATIBILITIES

Carboplatin (Paraplatin), cisplatin (Platinol AQ), cyclophosphamide (Cytoxan), cytarabine (Cytosar), dacarbazine (DTIC-Dome), dexamethasone (Decadron), diphenhydramine (Benadryl), doxorubicin (Adriamycin), etoposide (VePesid), gemcitabine (Gemzar), granisetron (Kytril), hydromorphone (Dilaudid), lipids, magnesium sulfate, mannitol, methotrexate, morphine, ondansetron (Zofran), potassium chloride, vinblastine (Velban), vincristine (Oncovin).

INDICATIONS/ROUTES/DOSAGE

Note: Premedication with dexamethasone, diphenhydramine, and cimetidine, famotidine, or ranitidine recommended. Refer to individual protocols.

Paclitaxel
Ovarian Cancer
IV: ADULTS: 135–175 mg/m²/dose over 3 hrs q3wks, 135 mg/m² over 24 hrs q3wks, or 50–80 mg/m² over 1–3 hrs weekly.

Breast Cancer
IV: ADULTS, ELDERLY: 175–250 mg/m² over 3 hrs q3wks or 50–80 mg/m² over 1–3 hrs weekly.

Non-Small-Cell Lung Cancer
IV: ADULTS, ELDERLY: 135 mg/m² over 24 hrs.

Kaposi's Sarcoma
IV: ADULTS, ELDERLY: 135 mg/m²/dose over 3 hrs q3wks or 100 mg/m²/dose over 3 hrs q2wks.

Dosage in Hepatic Impairment

Transaminase Level	Bilirubin	Dose
24-HR INFUSION		
Less than 2 times ULN	1.5 mg/dl or less	135 mg/m²
2 to less than 10 times ULN	1.5 mg/dl or less	100 mg/m²
Less than 10 times ULN	1.6–7.5 mg/dl or less	50 mg/m²
3-HR INFUSION		
Less than 10 times ULN	1.25 mg/dl or less	175 mg/m²
Less than 10 times ULN	1.26–2 times ULN	135 mg/m²
Less than 10 times ULN	2.01–5 times ULN	90 mg/m²
10 times ULN or greater	Greater than 5 times ULN	Avoid use

ULN: upper limit of normal

P

Abraxane
Breast Cancer
IV Infusion: ADULTS, ELDERLY: 260 mg/m^2 q3wks. For pts who experience severe neutropenia (neutrophils less than 500 cells/mm^3 for a wk or longer) or severe sensory neuropathy, reduce dosage to 220 mg/m^2 for subsequent courses. For recurrence of severe neutropenia or severe sensory neuropathy, reduce dosage to 180 mg/m^2 q3wks for subsequent courses. For grade 3 sensory neuropathy, hold until resolution to grade 1 or 2, followed by reduced dose for subsequent courses. Dosage of Abraxane for bilirubin greater than 1.5 mg/dl is not known.

NSCLC
IV: ADULTS, ELDERLY: 100 mg/m^2 on days 1, 8, 15 of each 21-day cycle (in combination with carboplatin).

Adenocarcinoma of Pancreas (in combination with gemcitabine)
IV: ADULTS, ELDERLY: 125 mg/m^2 on days 1, 8, 15 of each 28-day cycle.

SIDE EFFECTS

Expected (90%–70%): Diarrhea, alopecia, nausea, vomiting. **Frequent (48%–46%):** Myalgia, arthralgia, peripheral neuropathy. **Occasional (20%–13%):** Mucositis, hypotension during infusion, pain/redness at injection site. **Rare (3%):** Bradycardia.

ADVERSE EFFECTS/ TOXIC REACTIONS

Neutropenic nadir occurs at median of 11 days. Anemia, leukopenia occur commonly; thrombocytopenia occurs occasionally. Severe hypersensitivity reaction (dyspnea, severe hypotension, angioedema, generalized urticaria) occurs rarely.

NURSING CONSIDERATIONS

BASELINE ASSESSMENT

Offer emotional support. Use strict asepsis, protect pt from infection. Check blood counts, particularly neutrophil, platelet count, before each course of therapy or as clinically indicated.

INTERVENTION/EVALUATION

Monitor CBC, hepatic function tests, vital signs. Monitor for hematologic toxicity (fever, sore throat, signs of local infections, unusual bleeding/bruising), symptoms of anemia (excessive fatigue, weakness). Assess response to medication. Monitor, report diarrhea. Avoid IM injections, rectal temperatures, other traumas that may induce bleeding. Hold pressure to injection sites for full 5 min.

PATIENT/FAMILY TEACHING

• Hair loss is reversible, but new hair may have different color, texture. • Do not have immunizations without physician's approval (drug lowers resistance). • Avoid crowds, persons with known infections. • Report signs of infection at once (fever, flu-like symptoms). • Report persistent nausea/vomiting. • Be alert for signs of peripheral neuropathy. • Avoid pregnancy. • Avoid tasks that may require alertness, motor skills until response to drug is established.

palifermin

pal-ee-**fer**-min
(Kepivance)

◆CLASSIFICATION

PHARMACOTHERAPEUTIC: Keratinocyte growth factor. **CLINICAL:** Antineoplastic adjunct.

ACTION

Binds to keratinocyte growth factor receptor, present on epithelial cells of buccal mucosa, tongue, resulting in proliferation, differentiation, migration of epithelial cells. **Therapeutic Effect:** Reduces incidence, duration of severe oral mucositis.

PHARMACOKINETICS

Clearance is higher in pts with cancer compared to healthy subjects. **Half-life:** 4.5 hrs.

USES

Reduces incidence, duration, severity of severe stomatitis in pts with hematologic malignancies receiving myelotoxic therapy requiring hematopoietic stem cell support.

PRECAUTIONS

Contraindications: (Canada) Pts allergic to *Escherichia coli*–derived proteins. **Cautions:** None known.

⌛ LIFESPAN CONSIDERATIONS

Pregnancy/Lactation: Unknown if drug crosses placenta or is excreted in breast milk. Use only if potential benefit justifies fetal risk. **Pregnancy Category C. Children:** Safety and efficacy not established. **Elderly:** No age-related precautions noted.

INTERACTIONS

DRUG: Binds to **heparin, low molecular weight heparins (e.g., enoxaparin),** decreasing effectiveness. Administration during or within 24 hrs before or after **myelotoxic chemotherapy** results in increased severity, duration of oral mucositis. **HERBAL:** None significant. **FOOD:** None known. **LAB VALUES:** May elevate serum lipase, amylase.

AVAILABILITY (Rx)

Injection, Powder for Reconstitution: 6.25-mg vials.

ADMINISTRATION/HANDLING
 IV

Reconstitution • Reconstitute only with 1.2 ml Sterile Water for Injection, using aseptic technique. • Swirl gently to dissolve. Dissolution takes less than 3 min. Do not shake/agitate solution. • Yields final concentration of 5 mg/ml.

Rate of Administration • If heparin is being used to maintain an IV line, use 0.9% NaCl to rinse IV line before and af-

ter palifermin administration. • Administer by IV bolus injection.

Storage • Store intact vials in refrigerator. • If reconstituted solution is not used immediately, may be refrigerated for up to 24 hrs. • Before administration, may be warmed to room temperature for up to 1 hr. • Discard if left at room temperature for more than 1 hr, if discolored or particulate forms. • Protect from light.

INDICATIONS/ROUTES/DOSAGE

Mucositis (Premyelotoxic Therapy)
IV: ADULTS, ELDERLY: 60 mcg/kg/day for 3 consecutive days, with 3rd dose 24–48 hrs before chemotherapy.

Mucositis (Postmyelotoxic Therapy)
IV: ADULTS, ELDERLY: Last 3 doses of 60 mcg/kg/day should be administered after myelotoxic therapy; first of these doses should be administered after, but on the same day of, hematopoietic stem cell infusion and at least 4 days after most recent administration of palifermin.

SIDE EFFECTS

Frequent (62%–28%): Rash, fever, pruritus, erythema, edema. **Occasional (17%–10%):** Mouth/tongue thickness/discoloration, altered taste, dysesthesia manifested as hyperesthesia, hypoesthesia, paresthesia, arthralgia.

ADVERSE EFFECTS/ TOXIC REACTIONS

Transient hypertension occurs occasionally.

NURSING CONSIDERATIONS

BASELINE ASSESSMENT

Assess oral mucous membranes for degree of stomatitis (erythema, white patches, ulceration, bleeding). Offer emotional support.

INTERVENTION/EVALUATION

Assess for oral inflammation, difficulty swallowing, mucosal bleeding. Offer sponge sticks to wash mouth with water. Monitor pt's pain level; medicate as necessary for improved pain control.

PATIENT/FAMILY TEACHING

• Consume bland meals; avoid eating any spicy food. • Rinse mouth often with water; avoid hot, cold liquids. • Take measures to prevent pregnancy.

---

paliperidone

TOP 200

pal-ee-**per**-i-done
(Invega, Invega Sustenna)

BLACK BOX ALERT Elderly pts with dementia-related psychosis are at increased risk for mortality due to cerebrovascular events.

◆CLASSIFICATION

PHARMACOTHERAPEUTIC: Benzisoxazole derivative. **CLINICAL:** Antipsychotic (see p. 67C).

ACTION

Exact mechanism of action is unknown, but may antagonize dopamine and serotonin receptors. **Therapeutic Effect:** Suppresses behavioral response in psychosis.

PHARMACOKINETICS

Absorbed from GI tract. Metabolized in liver. Primarily excreted in urine. **Half-life:** 23 hrs.

USES

Oral: Treatment of acute (short-term) and long-term maintenance of schizophrenia. Acute treatment of schizoaffective disorder as monotherapy or as adjunct to mood stabilizers and/or antidepressants. **Injection:** Acute and maintenance treatment of schizophrenia. **OFF-LABEL:** Psychosis/agitation related to Alzheimer's dementia.

PRECAUTIONS

Contraindications: Sensitivity to risperidone. **Cautions:** History of cardiac arrhythmias, renal impairment, diabetes mellitus, HF, active seizures or predisposition to seizures, history of seizures, cardiovascular disease, congenital long QT syndrome, concomitant use with other medications that prolong QT interval (e.g., amiodarone, quinidine), pts at risk for aspiration pneumonia. May increase risk of stroke in pts with dementia-related psychosis. CNS depression, medications for hypertension, hypovolemia, high risk for suicide. Pts with breast cancer, other prolactin-dependent tumors, children, adolescents.

⏳ LIFESPAN CONSIDERATIONS

Pregnancy/Lactation: Unknown if drug crosses placenta or is distributed in breast milk. **Pregnancy Category C. Children:** Safety and efficacy not established. **Elderly:** Potential for orthostatic hypotension. Age-related renal impairment may require dosage adjustment.

INTERACTIONS

DRUG: May decrease effects of **dopamine agonists, levodopa. Alcohol, CNS depressants** may increase CNS depression. **HERBAL:** None significant. **FOOD:** None known. **LAB VALUES:** May increase serum creatine phosphatase, uric acid, triglycerides, AST, ALT, prolactin. May decrease serum potassium, sodium, protein, glucose. May cause EKG changes (including prolonged QT interval).

AVAILABILITY (Rx)

Injection Suspension: 39 mg/0.25 ml, 78 mg/0.5 ml, 117 mg/0.75 ml, 156 mg/ml, 234 mg/1.5 ml.

🖋 **Tablets, Extended-Release:** 1.5 mg, 3 mg, 6 mg, 9 mg, 12 mg.

ADMINISTRATION/HANDLING

PO
• May give without regard to food. • Do not break, crush, dissolve, or divide extended-release tablets.

IM
• Administer 2 initial injections in deltoid muscle (helps attain therapeutic

concentration rapidly). • Maintenance doses may be given in gluteal or deltoid muscle.

INDICATIONS/ROUTES/DOSAGE

Treatment of Schizophrenia
PO: ADULTS, ELDERLY: Initially, 6 mg once daily in the morning. May increase dose in increments of 3 mg/day at intervals of more than 5 days. Range: 3–12 mg/day. **ADOLESCENTS (51 KG OR GREATER):** Initially, 3 mg once daily. Range: 3–12 mg/day. **(50 KG OR LESS):** Initially, 3 mg once daily. Range: 3–6 mg/day.
IM: ADULTS, ELDERLY: 234 mg on day 1 followed by 156 mg 1 wk later (second dose may be given 4 days before or after the weekly time point). Maintenance: Initially, 117 mg monthly. Range: 39–234 mg.

Schizoaffective Disorder
PO: ADULTS, ELDERLY: 6 mg once daily in the morning. May increase in increments of 3 mg/day at intervals of more than 4 days. Range: 3–12 mg/day.

Dosage in Renal Impairment

Creatinine Clearance	Oral Dosage	IM Dosage
50–80 ml/min	6 mg/day maximum	156 mg on day 1, then 117 mg 1 wk later Maintenance: 78 mg once monthly
10–49 ml/min	3 mg/day maximum	Not recommended

SIDE EFFECTS

Occasional (14%–4%): Tachycardia, headache, drowsiness, akathisia (motor restlessness), anxiety, dizziness, dyspepsia, nausea.

ADVERSE EFFECTS/TOXIC REACTIONS

Neuroleptic malignant syndrome (NMS), hyperpyrexia, muscle rigidity, change in mental status, unstable pulse or B/P, tachycardia, diaphoresis, cardiac arrhythmias, rhabdomyolysis, acute renal failure, tardive dyskinesia (protrusion of tongue, puffing of cheeks, chewing/puckering of mouth) may occur rarely.

NURSING CONSIDERATIONS

BASELINE ASSESSMENT
Obtain baseline renal function test. Assess behavior, appearance, emotional status, response to environment, speech pattern, thought content.

INTERVENTION/EVALUATION
Monitor B/P, heart rate, weight, renal function tests, EKG. Monitor for fine tongue movement (may be first sign of tardive dyskinesia). Supervise suicidal-risk pt closely during early therapy (as depression lessons, energy level improves, increasing suicide potential). Assess for therapeutic response (greater interest in surroundings, improved self-care, increased ability to concentrate, relaxed facial expression). Monitor for potential neuroleptic malignant syndrome (fever, muscle rigidity, unstable B/P or pulse, altered mental status).

PATIENT/FAMILY TEACHING
• Avoid tasks that may require alertness, motor skills until response to drug is established. • Use caution when changing position from lying or sitting to standing. • Report trembling in fingers, altered gait, unusual muscle/skeletal movements, palpitations, severe dizziness, fainting, swelling/pain in breasts, visual changes, rash, difficulty in breathing.

palivizumab
pal-i-**viz**-ue-mab
(Synagis)
Do not confuse Synagis with Synalgos-DC.

◆CLASSIFICATION

PHARMACOTHERAPEUTIC: Monoclonal antibody. **CLINICAL:** Antiviral.

ACTION

Exhibits neutralizing activity against respiratory syncytial virus (RSV) in infants. **Therapeutic Effect:** Inhibits RSV replication in lower respiratory tract of children.

USES

Prevention of serious lower respiratory tract disease caused by RSV in pediatric pts younger than 2 yrs at high risk for RSV disease (e.g., hemodynamically significant congenital heart disease).

PRECAUTIONS

Contraindications: None known. **Cautions:** Thrombocytopenia, any coagulation disorder after mild hypersensitivity reaction to palivizumab. Not to be used for treatment of established RSV disease. **Pregnancy Category C.**

INTERACTIONS

DRUG: None significant. **HERBAL:** None significant. **FOOD:** None known. **LAB VALUES:** May increase serum AST.

AVAILABILITY (Rx)

Injection Solution: 100 mg/ml.

ADMINISTRATION/HANDLING

IM
• Refrigerate vials. • Give undiluted in anterolateral aspect of thigh.

INDICATIONS/ROUTES/DOSAGE

Prevention of Respiratory Syncytial Virus (RSV)
IM: CHILDREN: 15 mg/kg once/mo during RSV season. (First dose prior to commencement of RSV season.)

SIDE EFFECTS

Frequent (49%–22%): Upper respiratory tract infection, otitis media, rhinitis, rash. **Occasional (10%–2%):** Pain, pharyngitis.

Rare (Less Than 2%): Cough, diarrhea, vomiting, injection site reaction.

ADVERSE EFFECTS/ TOXIC REACTIONS

Anaphylaxis, severe acute hypersensitivity reaction occur very rarely.

NURSING CONSIDERATIONS

BASELINE ASSESSMENT
Assess for sensitivity to palivizumab.

INTERVENTION/EVALUATION
Monitor potential side effects, esp. otitis media, rhinitis, skin rash, upper respiratory tract infection.

PATIENT/FAMILY TEACHING
• Discuss the purpose, potential side effects of medication with family.

palonosetron

pal-oh-**noe**-se-tron
(Aloxi)
Do not confuse Aloxi with Eloxatin or oxaliplatin, or palonosetron with dolasetron, granisetron, or ondansetron.

◆CLASSIFICATION

PHARMACOTHERAPEUTIC: 5-HT$_3$ receptor antagonist. **CLINICAL:** Antiemetic.

ACTION

Acts centrally in chemoreceptor trigger zone, peripherally at vagal nerve terminals. **Therapeutic Effect:** Prevents nausea/ vomiting associated with chemotherapy.

PHARMACOKINETICS

Protein binding: 52%. Metabolized in liver. Eliminated in urine. **Half-life:** 40 hrs.

USES

Prevention of acute and delayed nausea/ vomiting associated with initial/repeated courses of moderately or highly emetogenic chemotherapy. Prevention of postop nausea/vomiting for up to 24 hrs following surgery.

PRECAUTIONS

Contraindications: None known. **Cautions:** History of cardiovascular disease; congenital long QT syndrome, risk factors for QT prolongation (hypokalemia, hypomagnesemia), medications that prolong QT interval or reduce potassium/magnesium levels, pts at risk for ventricular arrhythmias.

⚖ LIFESPAN CONSIDERATIONS

Pregnancy/Lactation: Unknown if distributed in breast milk. **Pregnancy Category B. Children:** Safety and efficacy not established. **Elderly:** No age-related precautions noted.

INTERACTIONS

DRUG: None significant. **HERBAL:** None significant. **FOOD:** None known. **LAB VALUES:** May transiently increase serum bilirubin, AST, ALT.

AVAILABILITY (Rx)

Injection Solution: 0.05 mg/ml.

ADMINISTRATION/HANDLING
 IV

Reconstitution • Give undiluted as IV push.
Rate of Administration • Give IV push over 30 sec. • Flush infusion line with 0.9% NaCl before and following administration.
Storage • Store at room temperature. Solution should appear colorless, clear. Discard if cloudy precipitate forms.

▦ IV COMPATIBILITIES

Famotidine (Pepcid), lorazepam (Ativan), midazolam (Versed), potassium chloride.

INDICATIONS/ROUTES/DOSAGE

Chemotherapy-Induced Nausea/Vomiting
IV: ADULTS, ELDERLY: 0.25 mg as single dose 30 min before starting chemotherapy.

Postop Nausea/Vomiting
IV: ADULTS, ELDERLY: 0.075 mg over 10 sec immediately before induction of anesthesia.

SIDE EFFECTS

Occasional (9%–5%): Headache, constipation. **Rare (Less Than 1%):** Diarrhea, dizziness, fatigue, abdominal pain, insomnia.

ADVERSE EFFECTS/ TOXIC REACTIONS

Overdose may produce combination of CNS stimulation, depressant effects.

NURSING CONSIDERATIONS

BASELINE ASSESSMENT

Assess for signs of dehydration due to excessive vomiting (poor skin turgor, dry mucous membranes, longitudinal furrows in tongue). Provide emotional support.

INTERVENTION/EVALUATION

Monitor pt for signs of dehydration. Provide supportive measures. Assess mental status. Monitor daily pattern of bowel activity, stool consistency. Record time of evacuation.

PATIENT/FAMILY TEACHING

• Relief from nausea/vomiting generally occurs shortly after drug administration. • Avoid alcohol, barbiturates. • Report persistent vomiting.

pamidronate

pam-i-**droe**-nate
(Aredia)
Do not confuse Aredia with Adriamycin, or pamidronate with alendronate, ibandronate, or risedronate.

◆CLASSIFICATION

PHARMACOTHERAPEUTIC: Bisphosphonate. **CLINICAL:** Hypocalcemic.

P

 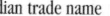

ACTION

Binds to bone, inhibits osteoclast-mediated calcium resorption. **Therapeutic Effect:** Lowers serum calcium concentration.

PHARMACOKINETICS

Route	Onset	Peak	Duration
IV	24–48 hrs	3–7 days	N/A

After IV administration, rapidly absorbed by bone. Slowly excreted unchanged in urine. Unknown if removed by hemodialysis. **Half-life:** 21–35 hrs.

USES

Treatment of moderate to severe hypercalcemia associated with malignancy (with/without bone metastases). Treatment of moderate to severe Paget's disease, osteolytic bone lesions of multiple myeloma, breast cancer. **OFF-LABEL:** Inhibits bone resorption in osteogenesis imperfecta, treatment of bone metastases of thyroid cancer, prevention of bone loss associated with androgen deprivation treatment in prostate cancer.

PRECAUTIONS

Contraindications: Hypersensitivity to other bisphosphonates (e.g., etidronate, tiludronate, risedronate, alendronate). **Cautions:** Renal impairment, concurrent use with other nephrotoxic medications, history of thyroid surgery.

⧗ LIFESPAN CONSIDERATIONS

Pregnancy/Lactation: No adequate, well-controlled studies in pregnant women; unknown if fetal harm can occur. Unknown if distributed in breast milk. **Pregnancy Category D. Children:** Safety and efficacy not established. **Elderly:** May become overhydrated. Careful monitoring of fluid and electrolytes indicated; recommend dilution in smaller volume.

INTERACTIONS

DRUG: Nephrotoxic medications may increase potential for nephrotoxicity. **HERBAL:** None significant. **FOOD:** None known. **LAB VALUES:** None significant.

AVAILABILITY (Rx)

Injection, Powder for Reconstitution: 30 mg, 90 mg. **Injection Solution:** 3 mg/ml, 6 mg/ml, 9 mg/ml.

ADMINISTRATION/HANDLING

 IV

Reconstitution • Reconstitute each vial with 10 ml Sterile Water for Injection to provide concentration of 3 mg/ml or 9 mg/ml. • Allow drug to dissolve before withdrawing. • Further dilute with 250–1,000 ml sterile 0.45% or 0.9% NaCl or D₅W (1,000 ml for hypercalcemia of malignancy, 500 ml for Paget's disease, multiple myeloma, 250 ml for breast cancer).

Rate of Administration • Adequate hydration is essential in conjunction with pamidronate therapy (avoid overhydration in pts with potential for cardiac failure). • Administer as IV infusion over 2–24 hrs for treatment of hypercalcemia; over 2–4 hrs for other indications.

Storage • Store parenteral form at room temperature. • Reconstituted vial is stable for 24 hrs if refrigerated; IV solution is stable for 24 hrs after dilution.

▣ IV INCOMPATIBILITIES

Calcium-containing IV fluids.

INDICATIONS/ROUTES/DOSAGE

Hypercalcemia
IV Infusion: ADULTS, ELDERLY: Moderate hypercalcemia (corrected serum calcium level 12–13.5 mg/dl): 60–90 mg. **Severe hypercalcemia (corrected serum calcium level greater than 13.5 mg/dl):** 90 mg.

Paget's Disease
IV Infusion: ADULTS, ELDERLY: 30 mg/day over 4 hrs for 3 consecutive days.

Osteolytic Bone Lesion (Multiple Myeloma)
IV Infusion: ADULTS, ELDERLY: 90 mg over 4 hrs once q mo.

Osteolytic Bone Lesion (Breast Cancer)
IV Infusion: ADULTS, ELDERLY: 90 mg over 2 hrs q3–4wks.

SIDE EFFECTS

Frequent (Greater Than 10%): Temperature elevation (at least 1°C) 24–48 hrs after administration (27%); erythema, swelling, induration, pain at catheter site in pts receiving 90 mg (18%); anorexia, nausea, fatigue. **Occasional (10%–1%):** Constipation, rhinitis.

ADVERSE EFFECTS/ TOXIC REACTIONS

Hypophosphatemia, hypokalemia, hypomagnesemia, hypocalcemia occur more frequently with higher dosages. Anemia, hypertension, tachycardia, atrial fibrillation, drowsiness occur more frequently with 90-mg doses. GI hemorrhage occurs rarely.

NURSING CONSIDERATIONS

BASELINE ASSESSMENT

Obtain corrected serum calcium level, ionized calcium level prior to therapy. Determine hydration status.

INTERVENTION/EVALUATION

Monitor serum calcium, ionized calcium level, potassium, magnesium, creatinine, CBC. Provide adequate hydration; assess overhydration. Monitor I&O carefully; assess lungs for rales, dependent body parts for edema. Monitor B/P, temperature, pulse. Assess catheter site for redness, swelling, pain. Monitor food intake, daily pattern of bowel activity, stool consistency. Be alert for potential GI hemorrhage with 90-mg dosage.

pancrelipase

pan-kree-**lye**-pace
(Creon, Pancreaze, Zenpep, Pertyze, Ultresa, Viokace)

◆CLASSIFICATION

PHARMACOTHERAPEUTIC: Digestive enzyme. **CLINICAL:** Pancreatic enzyme replenisher.

ACTION

Replaces endogenous pancreatic enzymes. **Therapeutic Effect:** Assists in digestion of protein, starch, fats.

USES

Creon, Pancreaze, Pertyze, Ultresa Zenpep: Treatment of exocrine pancreatic insufficiency (EPI) due to cystic fibrosis or other conditions. **Creon:** Chronic pancreatitis, pancreatectomy. **Viokace: (with a proton pump inhibitor):** Chronic pancreatitis, pancreatectomy.

PRECAUTIONS

Contraindications: None known. **Cautions:** Gout, hyperuricemia, renal impairment, hypersensitivity to pork proteins. **Pregnancy Category C.**

INTERACTIONS

DRUG: May decrease absorption of **iron supplements. HERBAL:** None significant. **FOOD:** None known. **LAB VALUES:** May increase serum uric acid.

AVAILABILITY (Rx)

Capsules, Delayed-Release: (Creon): 3,000 units lipase; 9,500 units protease; 15,000 units amylase. 6,000 units lipase; 19,000 units protease; 30,000 units amylase. 12,000 units lipase; 38,000 units protease; 60,000 units amylase. 24,000 units lipase; 76,000 units protease; 120,000 units amylase. **(Pancreaze):** 4,200 units lipase; 10,000 units protease; 17,500 units amylase; 10,500 units lipase; 25,000 units protease; 43,750 units amylase; 16,800 units lipase; 40,000 units protease; 70,000 units amylase; 21,000 units lipase; 37,000 units protease; 61,000 units amylase. **(Zenpep):** 3,000 units lipase; 10,000 units protease; 16,000 units amylase; 5,000 units lipase; 17,000 units protease; 27,000 units amy-

P

lase. 10,000 units lipase; 34,000 units protease; 55,000 units amylase. 15,000 units lipase; 51,000 units protease; 82,000 units amylase. 20,000 units lipase; 68,000 units protease; 109,000 units amylase. 25,000 units lipase; 85,000 units protease; 136,000 units amylase. **Pertyze:** 8,000 units lipase; 28,750 units protease; 30,250 units amylase. 16,000 units lipase; 57,500 units protease; 60,500 units amylase. **Ultresa:** 13,800 units lipase; 27,600 units protease; 27,600 units amylase. 20,700 units lipase; 41,400 units protease; 41,400 units amylase. 23,000 units lipase; 46,000 units protease; 46,000 units amylase. ✎ **Tablets, Viokace:** 10,440 units lipase; 39,150 units protease; 39,150 units amylase. 20,880 units lipase; 78,300 units protease; 78,300 units amylase.

ADMINISTRATION/HANDLING

PO

• Give capsules whole with generous amount of liquid. • If pt unable to swallow intact capsule, contents may be given without crushing/chewing, followed by fluid. Contents may be sprinkled on soft acidic food such as applesauce. • Swallow immediately after mixing. Give tablets whole, do not break, crush, dissolve, or divide. • **Viokace:** must be given with a proton pump inhibitor.

INDICATIONS/ROUTES/DOSAGE

◄ALERT► Dosage expressed as lipase units/kg. Individualize dose based on clinical symptoms, degree of steatorrhea, fat content in diet.

Pancreatic Insufficiency (Due to Conditions Such As Cystic Fibrosis)
PO: ADULTS, ELDERLY, CHILDREN 4 YRS AND OLDER: Initially, 500 units/kg lipase/kg/meal up to 2,500 units lipase/kg/meal (or less than or equal to 10,000 lipase units/kg/day) or less than 4,000 units/g of fat ingested/day. **CHILDREN OLDER THAN 12 MOS AND YOUNGER THAN 4 YRS:** Initially, 1,000 units lipase/kg/meal up to 2,500 units lipase/kg/meal (or less than or equal to 10,000 lipase units/kg/day) or less than 4,000 lipase units/g of fat ingested/day. **INFANTS UP TO 12 MOS:** 2,000–4,000 units lipase per 120 ml of formula or per breastfeeding. Do not mix Creon or Zenpep capsule contents directly into formula or breast milk prior to administration.

Pancreatic Insufficiency (Due to Chronic Pancreatitis or Pancreatectomy)
PO: ADULTS, ELDERLY: (Cream): 72,000 units/meal, while consuming 100 g or more of fat daily. **(Viokace):** 500 units/kg/meal. **Range:** 500–2,500 units/kg/meal.

SIDE EFFECTS

Rare: Allergic reaction, mouth irritation, shortness of breath, wheezing.

ADVERSE EFFECTS/ TOXIC REACTIONS

Excessive dosage may produce nausea, cramping, diarrhea. Hyperuricosuria, hyperuricemia reported with extremely high dosages.

NURSING CONSIDERATIONS

INTERVENTION/EVALUATION

Question for therapeutic relief from GI symptoms. Do not change brands without consulting physician.

PATIENT/FAMILY TEACHING

• Do not chew capsules. • Instruct pts with trouble swallowing to open capsules, spread contents over applesauce, mashed fruit, rice cereal or follow with glass of water or juice to ensure swallowing. • Do not break, crush, dissolve, or divide tablets. Swallow whole.

panitumumab

pan-i-**toom**-ue-mab
(Vectibix)
BLACK BOX ALERT 90% of pts experience dermatologic toxicities (der-

matitis acneiform, pruritus, erythema, rash, skin exfoliation, skin fissures, abscess). Potential for severe infusion reaction (anaphylaxis, bronchospasm, fever, chills, hypotension) (fatal reactions have occurred).

◆ CLASSIFICATION

PHARMACOTHERAPEUTIC: Monoclonal antibody. **CLINICAL:** Antineoplastic (see p. 89C).

ACTION

Binds specifically to epidermal growth factor receptor (EGFR) and competitively inhibits binding of epidermal growth factor. **Therapeutic Effect:** Prevents cell growth, proliferation, transformation, survival.

PHARMACOKINETICS

Clearance varies by body weight, gender, tumor burden. **Half-life:** 3–10 days.

USES

Monotherapy in metastatic colorectal carcinoma with disease progression on or following fluoropyrimidine-, oxaliplatin-, or irinotecan-based regimens.

PRECAUTIONS

Contraindications: None known. **Cautions:** Interstitial pneumonitis, pulmonary fibrosis, pulmonary infiltrates.

⌛ LIFESPAN CONSIDERATIONS

Pregnancy/Lactation: Teratogenic. Potential for fertility impairment. May decrease fetal body weight; increase risk of skeletal fetal abnormalities. Breastfeeding not recommended. **Pregnancy Category C. Children:** Safety and efficacy not established. **Elderly:** No age-related precautions noted.

INTERACTIONS

DRUG: None significant. **HERBAL:** None significant. **FOOD:** None known. **LAB VALUES:** May decrease serum magnesium, calcium.

AVAILABILITY (Rx)

Injection Solution: 20 mg/ml vial (5-ml, 20-ml vials).

ADMINISTRATION/HANDLING
 IV

◀**ALERT**▶ Do not give by IV push or bolus. Use low protein-binding 0.2- or 0.22-micron in-line filter. Flush IV line before and after chemotherapy administration with 0.9% NaCl.

Reconstitution • Dilute in 100–150 ml 0.9% NaCl to provide concentration of 10 mg/ml or less. • Do not shake solution. Invert gently to mix. • Discard any unused portion.

Rate of Administration • Give as IV infusion over 60 min. • Infuse doses greater than 1,000 mg over 90 min.

Storage • Refrigerate vials. • After dilution, solution may be stored for up to 6 hrs at room temperature, up to 24 hrs if refrigerated. • Discard if discolored but solution may contain visible, translucent-to-white particulates (will be removed by in-line filter).

🔳 IV INCOMPATIBILITY

Do not mix with dextrose solutions or any other medications.

INDICATIONS/ROUTES/DOSAGE

◀**ALERT**▶ Stop infusion immediately in pts experiencing severe infusion reactions.

Metastatic Colorectal Carcinoma
IV Infusion: ADULTS, ELDERLY: 6 mg/kg given over 60 min once every 14 days. Doses greater than 1,000 mg should be infused over 90 min.

SIDE EFFECTS

Common (65%–57%): Erythema, acneiform dermatitis, pruritus. **Frequent (26%–20%):** Fatigue, abdominal pain, skin exfoliation, paronychia (inflammation involving folds of tissue surrounding fingernail), nausea, rash, diarrhea, constipation, skin fissures. **Occasional (19%–10%):** Vomiting, acne,

P

cough, peripheral edema, dry skin. **Rare (7%–2%):** Stomatitis, mucosal inflammation, eyelash growth, conjunctivitis, increased lacrimation.

ADVERSE EFFECTS/TOXIC REACTIONS

Pulmonary fibrosis, severe dermatologic toxicity (complicated by infectious sequelae), sepsis occur rarely. Severe infusion reactions manifested as bronchospasm, fever, chills, hypotension occur rarely. Hypomagnesemia occurs in 39% of pts.

NURSING CONSIDERATIONS

BASELINE ASSESSMENT

Assess baseline serum magnesium, calcium prior to therapy, periodically during therapy, and for 8 wks after completion of therapy.

INTERVENTION/EVALUATION

Assess for skin, ocular, mucosal toxicity; report effects. Median time to development of skin/ocular toxicity is 14–15 days; resolution after last dosing is 84 days. Monitor serum electrolytes for hypomagnesemia, hypocalcemia. Offer antiemetic if nausea/vomiting occurs. Monitor daily pattern of bowel activity, stool consistency.

PATIENT/FAMILY TEACHING

• Do not have immunizations without physician's approval (drug lowers resistance). • Avoid contact with those who have recently received a live virus vaccine. • Avoid crowds, those with infection. • There is a potential risk for development of fetal abnormalities if pregnancy occurs; take measures to prevent pregnancy.

---

pantoprazole

pan-**toe**-pra-zole
(Apo-Pantoprazole ✦, <u>Protonix</u>, <u>Protonix IV</u>)

Do not confuse pantoprazole with aripiprazole.

◆ CLASSIFICATION

PHARMACOTHERAPEUTIC: Benzimidazole. **CLINICAL:** Proton pump inhibitor (see p. 147C).

ACTION

Irreversibly binds to, inhibits hydrogen-potassium adenosine triphosphate, an enzyme on surface of gastric parietal cells. Inhibits hydrogen ion transport into gastric lumen. **Therapeutic Effect:** Increases gastric pH, reduces gastric acid production.

PHARMACOKINETICS

Route	Onset	Peak	Duration
PO	N/A	N/A	24 hrs

Well absorbed from GI tract. Protein binding: 98% (primarily albumin). Primarily distributed into gastric parietal cells. Metabolized in liver. Primarily excreted in urine. Not removed by hemodialysis. **Half-life:** 1 hr.

USES

PO: Treatment, maintenance of healing of erosive esophagitis associated with gastroesophageal reflux disease (GERD). Reduction of relapse rate of heartburn symptoms in GERD. Treatment of hypersecretory conditions including Zollinger-Ellison syndrome. **IV:** Short-term treatment of erosive esophagitis associated with GERD, treatment of hypersecretory conditions. **OFF-LABEL:** Peptic ulcer disease, active ulcer bleeding (injection), adjunct in treatment of *H. pylori,* stress ulcer prophylaxis in critically ill pts.

PRECAUTIONS

Contraindications: Hypersensitivity to proton pump inhibitors (e.g., omeprazole). **Cautions:** May increase risk of fractures, GI infections.

⧗ LIFESPAN CONSIDERATIONS

Pregnancy/Lactation: Unknown if drug crosses placenta or is distributed in breast milk. **Pregnancy Category B. Children:** Safety and efficacy not established. **Elderly:** No age-related precautions noted.

INTERACTIONS

DRUG: May increase effects of **warfarin.** May decrease effects of **clopidogrel, atazanavir. HERBAL:** None significant. **FOOD:** None known. **LAB VALUES:** May increase serum creatinine, cholesterol, uric acid, glucose, lipoprotein, ALT.

AVAILABILITY (Rx)

Granules for Suspension: 40 mg/packet. **Injection, Powder for Reconstitution (Protonix IV):** 40 mg.

🔰 **Tablets (Delayed-Release [Protonix]):** 20 mg, 40 mg.

ADMINISTRATION/HANDLING
 IV

Reconstitution • Mix 40-mg vial with 10 ml 0.9% NaCl injection. **•** May be further diluted with 100 ml D₅W, 0.9% NaCl, or lactated Ringer's.
Rate of Administration • Infuse 10 ml solution over at least 2 min. **•** Infuse 100 ml solution over at least 15 min.
Storage • Store undiluted vials at room temperature. **•** Once diluted with 10 ml 0.9% NaCl, stable for 96 hrs at room temperature; when further diluted with 100 ml, stable for 24 hrs at room temperature.

PO
• May be given without regard to food. Best given before breakfast. **•** Do not break, crush, dissolve, or divide tablets; give whole. **•** Administer oral suspension only in apple juice or applesauce. Best taken 30 min before a meal.

🔲 IV COMPATIBILITIES

Dopamine, epinephrine, furosemide (Lasix), insulin (regular), potassium chloride, vasopressin.

🔲 IV INCOMPATIBILITIES

Dobutamine.

INDICATIONS/ROUTES/DOSAGE

Erosive Esophagitis
PO: ADULTS, ELDERLY: 40 mg/day for up to 8 wks. If not healed after 8 wks, may continue an additional 8 wks. **CHILDREN 5 YRS AND OLDER:** 20–40 mg/day.
IV: ADULTS, ELDERLY: 40 mg/day for 7–10 days.

Maintenance of Healing of Erosive Esophagitis
PO: ADULTS, ELDERLY: 40 mg once daily.

Hypersecretory Conditions
PO: ADULTS, ELDERLY: Initially, 40 mg twice a day. May increase to 240 mg/day.
IV: ADULTS, ELDERLY: 80 mg twice a day. May increase to 80 mg q8h.

Peptic Ulcer Bleed (Unlabeled)
IV: ADULTS, ELDERLY: 80 mg followed by 8 mg/hr infusion for 72 hrs.

SIDE EFFECTS

Rare (less than 2%): Diarrhea, headache, dizziness, pruritus, rash.

ADVERSE EFFECTS/ TOXIC REACTIONS

Hyperglycemia occurs rarely.

NURSING CONSIDERATIONS

BASELINE ASSESSMENT
Obtain baseline lab values, including serum creatinine, cholesterol.

INTERVENTION/EVALUATION
Evaluate for therapeutic response (relief of GI symptoms). Question if GI discomfort, nausea occur.

PATIENT/FAMILY TEACHING
• Report headache, onset of black, tarry stools, diarrhea. **•** Avoid alcohol. **•** Swallow tablets whole; do not chew, crush, dissolve, or divide. **•** Best if given before breakfast. May give without regard to food.

P

---

paroxetine `TOP 200`

par-**ox**-e-teen
(Apo-Paroxetine ✦, Brisdelle, Novo-Paroxetine ✦, Paxil, Paxil CR, Pexeva)

BLACK BOX ALERT Increased risk of suicidal thinking and behavior in children, adolescents, young adults 18–24 yrs with major depressive disorder, other psychiatric disorders.
Do not confuse paroxetine with piroxicam, fluoxetine or pyridoxine, or Paxil with Doxil, Plavix, Prozac, or Taxol.

◆CLASSIFICATION

PHARMACOTHERAPEUTIC: Serotonin uptake inhibitor. **CLINICAL:** Antidepressant, antiobsessive-compulsive, antianxiety (see pp. 15C, 40C).

ACTION

Selectively blocks uptake of neurotransmitter serotonin at CNS neuronal presynaptic membranes, increasing its availability at postsynaptic receptor sites. **Therapeutic Effect:** Relieves depression, reduces obsessive-compulsive behavior, decreases anxiety.

PHARMACOKINETICS

Well absorbed from GI tract. Protein binding: 95%. Widely distributed. Metabolized in liver. Excreted in urine. Not removed by hemodialysis. **Half-life:** 24 hrs.

USES

Treatment of major depressive disorder (MDD). Treatment of panic disorder, obsessive-compulsive disorder (OCD). Treatment of social anxiety disorder (SAD), generalized anxiety disorder (GAD), premenstrual dysphoric disorder (PMDD), post-traumatic stress disorder (PTSD). **(Brisdelle):** Treatment of moderate to severe vasomotor symptoms associated with menopause. **OFF-LABEL:** Eating disorders, impulse disorders, menopause symptoms, premenstrual disorders, treatment of depression and OCD in children, mild dementia-associated agitation in nonpsychotic pts.

PRECAUTIONS

Contraindications: Use of MAOIs with or within 14 days, concurrent use of reversible MAOIs (e.g., linezolid) or thioridazine. **Cautions:** History of seizures, mania, renal/hepatic impairment, cardiac disease, pts with suicidal tendencies, impaired platelet aggregation. Concurrent use of aspirin or NSAIDs, children, breastfeeding, those who are volume depleted or using diuretics.

⧖ LIFESPAN CONSIDERATIONS

Pregnancy/Lactation: May impair reproductive function. Not distributed in breast milk. May increase risk of congenital malformations. **Pregnancy Category D. Children:** Safety and efficacy not established. **Elderly:** Age-related renal impairment may require dosage adjustment.

INTERACTIONS

DRUG: May increase concentration, risk of toxicity of **tricyclic antidepressants. Triptans, lithium, tramadol** may increase risk of serotonin syndrome. **Aspirin, NSAIDs, warfarin** may increase risk of bleeding. **MAOIs** may cause confusion, agitation, severe seizures; increase risk of serotonin syndrome, hypertensive crises. **Thioridazine** may prolong QT interval. **HERBAL: Kava kava, St. John's wort, valerian** may increase CNS depression, risk of serotonin syndrome. **FOOD:** None known. **LAB VALUES:** May decrease Hgb, Hct, WBC count.

AVAILABILITY (Rx)

Capsules (Brisdelle): 7.5 mg. **Oral Suspension (Paxil):** 10 mg/5 ml. **Tablets (Paxil, Pexeva):** 10 mg, 20 mg, 30 mg, 40 mg.
✦ **Tablets (Controlled-Release [Paxil CR]):** 12.5 mg, 25 mg, 37.5 mg.

ADMINISTRATION/HANDLING

PO

• May give without regard to food. • Give with food, milk if GI distress occurs. • Scored tablet may be crushed. • Do not crush, break, dissolve, or divide controlled-release tablets.

INDICATIONS/ROUTES/DOSAGE

Depression

PO: ADULTS: Initially, 20 mg/day. May increase by 10 mg/day at intervals of more than 1 wk. **Maximum:** 50 mg/day.
PO (Controlled-Release): ADULTS: Initially, 25 mg/day. May increase by 12.5 mg/day at intervals of more than 1 wk. **Maximum:** 62.5 mg/day.

Generalized Anxiety Disorder (GAD)

PO: ADULTS: Initially, 20 mg/day. May increase by 10 mg/day at intervals of more than 1 wk. **Range:** 20–50 mg/day.

Obsessive-Compulsive Disorder (OCD)

PO: ADULTS: Initially, 20 mg/day. May increase by 10 mg/day at intervals of more than 1 wk. **Range:** 20–60 mg/day.

Panic Disorder

PO: ADULTS: Initially, 10–20 mg/day. May increase by 10 mg/day at intervals of more than 1 wk. **Range:** 10–60 mg/day.
PO (Controlled-Release): ADULTS, ELDERLY: Initially, 12.5 mg once daily. May increase by 12.5 mg/day at weekly intervals. **Maximum:** 75 mg/day.

Social Anxiety Disorder (SAD)

PO: ADULTS: Initially 20 mg/day. **Range:** 20–60 mg/day.
PO (Controlled-Release): ADULTS, ELDERLY: Initially, 12.5 mg once daily. May increase by 12.5 mg/day at weekly intervals. **Maximum:** 37.5 mg/day.

Post-Traumatic Stress Disorder (PTSD)

PO: ADULTS: Initially, 20 mg/day. May increase by 10 mg/day at intervals of more than 1 wk. **Range:** 20–50 mg/day.

Premenstrual Dysphoric Disorder (PMDD)

PO (Controlled-Release): ADULTS: Initially, 12.5 mg/day. May increase by 12.5 mg at weekly intervals. **Maximum:** 25 mg/day.

Vasomotor Symptoms

PO: ADULTS: 7.5 mg once daily at bedtime.

Usual Elderly Dosage

PO: Initially, 10 mg/day. May increase by 10 mg/day at intervals of more than 1 wk. **Maximum:** 40 mg/day.
PO (Controlled-Release): Initially, 12.5 mg/day. May increase by 12.5 mg/day at intervals of more than 1 wk. **Maximum:** 50 mg/day.

Dosage Renal/Hepatic Impairment

Creatinine clearance less than 30 ml/min, severe hepatic impairment. **Immediate-Release:** Initially, 10 mg/day. May increase by 10 mg/dose at weekly intervals. **Maximum:** 40 mg/day. **Extended-Release:** Initially, 12.5 mg/day. May increase by 12.5/day at weekly intervals. **Maximum:** 50 mg/day.

SIDE EFFECTS

Frequent (26%–8%): Nausea, drowsiness, headache, dry mouth, asthenia (loss of strength, energy), constipation, dizziness, insomnia, diarrhea, diaphoresis, tremor. **Occasional (6%–3%):** Decreased appetite, respiratory disturbance (e.g., increased cough), anxiety, flatulence, paresthesia, yawning, decreased libido, sexual dysfunction, abdominal discomfort. **Rare:** Palpitations, vomiting, blurred vision, altered taste, confusion.

ADVERSE EFFECTS/TOXIC REACTIONS

Hyponatremia, seizures have been reported. Serotonin syndrome (agitation, confusion, diaphoresis, hallucinations, hyperreflexia) occurs rarely.

P

❦ Canadian trade name   🔪 Non-Crushable Drug   🔲 High Alert drug

NURSING CONSIDERATIONS

BASELINE ASSESSMENT

Assess appearance, behavior, speech pattern, level of interest, mood.

INTERVENTION/EVALUATION

For pts on long-term therapy, hepatic/renal function tests, blood counts should be performed periodically. Assess mental status for depression, suicidal ideation (esp. at beginning of therapy or change in dosage), anxiety, social functioning, panic attacks. Assess appearance, behavior, speech pattern, level of interest, mood.

PATIENT/FAMILY TEACHING

• May cause dry mouth. • Avoid alcohol, St. John's wort. • Therapeutic effect may be noted within 1–4 wks. • Do not abruptly discontinue medication. • Avoid tasks that require alertness, motor skills until response to drug is established. • May impair reproductive function. • Inform physician of intention for pregnancy or if pregnancy occurs. • Report worsening depression, suicidal ideation, unusual changes in behavior.

pazopanib

paz-**oh**-pa-nib
(Votrient)
BLACK BOX ALERT Severe, fatal hepatotoxicity has been observed.

◆CLASSIFICATION

PHARMACOTHERAPEUTIC: Tyrosine kinase inhibitor. **CLINICAL:** Antineoplastic.

ACTION

Interferes with proliferation of tumor vasculature, preventing tumor growth. **Therapeutic Effect:** Inhibits angiogenesis, blocks tumor growth.

PHARMACOKINETICS

Peak concentration occurs 2–4 hrs following oral administration. Metabolized in liver. Protein binding: greater than 99%. Eliminated primarily in feces, with a lesser amount excreted in urine. **Half-life:** 31 hrs.

USES

Treatment of advanced renal cell carcinoma, advanced soft-tissue sarcoma (in pts previously treated with chemotherapy). **OFF-LABEL:** Advanced thyroid cancer.

PRECAUTIONS

Contraindications: None known. **Cautions:** Avoid use of strong CYP3A4 inhibitors (e.g., clarithromycin, ketoconazole, ritonavir) or inducers (carbamazepine, dexamethasone, phenobarbital, phenytoin, rifabutin, rifampin), and grapefruit products. Cautious use in pts with increased risk or history of arterial thrombotic events (e.g., angina, MI, ischemic stroke), QT prolongation, hypertension, severe hepatic impairment, concomitant use of medications that may prolong QT interval, history of hemoptysis, cerebral hemorrhage or significant GI hemorrhage.

⧖ LIFESPAN CONSIDERATIONS

Pregnancy/Lactation: May cause fetal harm. Unknown if distributed in breast milk. **Pregnancy Category D. Children:** Safety and efficacy not established in those younger than 18 yrs. **Elderly:** No age-related precautions noted.

INTERACTIONS

DRUG: Concurrent use of **CYP3A4 inhibitors** (e.g., **clarithromycin, ketoconazole, ritonavir**) may increase concentration. Concomitant use of **CYP3A4 inducers** (e.g., **carbamazepine, dexamethasone, phenobarbital, phenytoin, rifabutin, rifampin**) may decrease concentration. **Simvastatin** may increase incidence of serum ALT elevations. **HERBAL:** **St. John's wort** decreases concentration. **FOOD:** **Food** may increase con-

P

centration. Give 1 hr before or 2 hrs after meals. **Grapefruit products** may increase concentration, potential for torsades, myelotoxicity. **LAB VALUES:** May decrease serum phosphorus, sodium, magnesium, glucose, WBC count. May increase serum ALT, AST.

AVAILABILITY (Rx)

 Tablets: 200 mg.

ADMINISTRATION/HANDLING

PO

• Give at least 1 hr before or 2 hrs after ingestion of food. • Give tablets whole; do not break, crush, dissolve, or divide.

INDICATIONS/ROUTES/DOSAGE

Renal Cell Carcinoma, Soft-Tissue Sarcoma

PO: ADULTS, ELDERLY: 800 mg once daily. Initial dose reduction should be 400 mg with additional increases/decreases in 200-mg steps based on individual tolerability. Initial dose of 400 mg/day with concomitant strong CYP3A4 inhibitors.

Dosage in Hepatic Impairment

Reduce dose to 200 mg/day for moderate hepatic impairment. Not recommended in pts with severe hepatic impairment.

SIDE EFFECTS

Frequent (52%–19%): Diarrhea, hypertension, hair color changes, nausea, fatigue, anorexia, vomiting. **Occasional (14%–10%):** Asthenia (loss of strength, energy), abdominal pain, headache. **Rare (Less Than 10%):** Alopecia, chest pain, altered taste, dyspepsia, proteinuria, rash, decreased weight.

ADVERSE EFFECTS/ TOXIC REACTIONS

Hepatotoxicity, manifested as increase in serum bilirubin, ALT, AST, has been observed and may be fatal. Hemorrhagic events (hematuria, epistaxis, hemoptysis, GI bleeding or perforation, intracranial hemorrhage) have been noted and may be fatal. Hypertension (B/P greater than 150/100 mm Hg) is common (47%), usually occurring early in the first 18 wks of treatment. Hypothyroidism has been reported occasionally. Arterial thrombotic events (MI, CVA), QT prolongation, torsade de pointes have been seen rarely.

NURSING CONSIDERATIONS

BASELINE ASSESSMENT

Assess medical history, esp. hepatic function abnormalities. Obtain baseline EKG, CBC, serum chemistries, hepatic function tests (ALT, AST, bilirubin).

INTERVENTION/EVALUATION

Monitor B/P, serum hepatic function tests periodically for elevations. Monitor CBC, serum chemistries for changes from baseline. Observe for signs of hepatotoxicity (jaundice, dark-colored urine, unusual fatigue, right upper quadrant abdominal pain). Observe EKG for QT-interval prolongation. Monitor for evidence of bleeding, hemorrhage. Monitor daily pattern of bowel activity, stool consistency.

PATIENT/FAMILY TEACHING

• Avoid crowds, those with known infection. • Avoid contact with anyone who recently received live virus vaccine; do not receive vaccinations. • Swallow tablets whole; do not chew, crush, dissolve, or divide. • No food should be taken at least 1 hr before and 2 hrs after dose is taken. • Avoid grapefruit products. • Report diarrhea, abdominal pain, yellowing of skin or sclera, discolored urine, fatigue.

pegaspargase

peg-ah-**spar**-jase
(Oncaspar)
Do not confuse pegaspargase with asparaginase.

P

♣ Canadian trade name   🔖 Non-Crushable Drug   ⬛ **HIGH ALERT** High Alert drug

◆CLASSIFICATION

PHARMACOTHERAPEUTIC: Enzyme, immunomodulator. **CLINICAL:** Antineoplastic (see p. 89C).

ACTION

Inhibits protein synthesis by deaminating asparagine in plasma and extracellular fluid. **Therapeutic Effect:** Deprives tumor cells of amino acids necessary for protein synthesis, thereby inhibiting tumor cell growth.

PHARMACOKINETICS

Slowly absorbed following IM administration. Primarily excreted in urine elimination. **Half-life:** 6 days.

USES

Treatment of acute lymphoblastic leukemia (ALL).

PRECAUTIONS

Contraindications: Hypersensitivity reaction to pegaspargase, history of hemorrhage, pancreatitis, or thrombosis with L-asparaginase therapy. **Cautions:** Pts with diabetes mellitus, underlying coagulopathy, hepatic impairment, or concurrent hepatotoxic medications.

⧖ LIFESPAN CONSIDERATIONS

Pregnancy/Lactation: Unknown if distributed in breast milk. Must either discontinue drug or discontinue breastfeeding. **Pregnancy Category C. Children:** Safety and efficacy not established. **Elderly:** No age-related precautions noted.

INTERACTIONS

DRUG: Anticoagulants, antiplatelets, NSAIDs may increase risk of coagulopathy, bleeding. **HERBAL: Echinacea** may decrease concentration/effects. **FOOD:** None known. **LAB VALUES:** May increase serum AST, ALT, bilirubin, glucose.

AVAILABILITY (Rx)

Injection Solution: 3,750 international units/5 ml (750 international unit/ml).

ADMINISTRATION/HANDLING

Note: Refrigerate unused vial.

IM
• Visually inspect for particulate matter.
• Do not inject volume greater than 2 ml for single injection site. • Use multiple sites if injecting more than 2 ml of volume.

 IV

Reconstitution • Withdraw appropriate volume and dilute in 100 ml bag of NaCl or D_5 Sterile Water for Injection. • Gently mix bag by inversion. • Do not shake or agitate.
Rate of Administration • Infuse over 1–2 hrs.
Storage • Solution should appear clear, colorless. • May refrigerate diluted solution up to 48 hrs. • Protect infusion bag from direct sunlight.

▦ IV INCOMPATIBILITIES

Do not mix with other intravenous medications.

INDICATIONS/ROUTES/DOSAGE

Acute Lymphoblastic Leukemia (ALL)
IM/IV: ADULTS/ELDERLY: 2,500 international units every 14 days (of 28-day cycle).

SIDE EFFECTS

Occasional: Nausea, headache.

ADVERSE EFFECTS/ TOXIC REACTIONS

Hypersensitivity reactions including anaphylactic reaction may include angioedema, dyspnea, flushing, hypotension, laryngeal edema, urticaria, wheezing. Central nervous system thrombosis including acute CVA occurred in 3% of pts. Pancreatitis (autodigestion of pancreas) may result in septic shock, acute respiratory distress syndrome (ARDS), hypotension, or death. Coagulopathy may increase risk of fatal bleeding. Immunogenicity (autoantibody formation) reported in 2%–10% of pts.

NURSING CONSIDERATIONS

BASELINE ASSESSMENT

Obtain baseline serum chemistries, PT/INR, capillary blood glucose. Question history of hepatic impairment, pancreatitis, prior hypersensitivity, DVT, MI, stroke. Receive full medication history.

INTERVENTION/EVALUATION

Monitor serum hepatic function tests, capillary blood glucose, PT/INR regularly. Monitor pt for hypersensitivity reaction for at least 1 hr after administration. If anaphylactic reaction occurs, consider treatment with antihistamine, intravenous steroids, racemic epinephrine; locate rapid sequence intubation kit. If pancreatitis suspected (abdominal pain, Grey Turner's sign, intractable vomiting), contact physician to obtain serum chemistries, amylase and lipase levels, possible radiologic testing. Immediately report dyspnea, chest pain, hypoxia, unilateral peripheral edema/pain (may indicate thromboembolic event).

PATIENT/FAMILY TEACHING

• Treatment may induce allergic reaction (difficulty breathing, itching, wheezing, rash, dizziness). • Increased urination, thirst, confusion, dehydration, fruity breath may indicate elevated blood sugar levels. • Immediately report flank bruising, vomiting, abdominal pain (may indicate pancreatitis). • Report difficulty breathing, chest pain, extremity pain swelling. • Report abdominal pain, yellowing of skin or eyes, dark-amber urine, clay-colored stools, fatigue, loss of appetite; may indicate liver problems.

---

pegfilgrastim   `TOP 200`

peg-fil-**gras**-tim
(Neulasta)
Do not confuse Neulasta with Lunesta, Neumega, or Neupogen.

◆ CLASSIFICATION

PHARMACOTHERAPEUTIC: Colony-stimulating factor. **CLINICAL:** Hematopoietic, antineutropenic.

ACTION

Regulates production of neutrophils within bone marrow. A glycoprotein, primarily affects neutrophil progenitor proliferation, differentiation, selected end-cell functional activation. **Therapeutic Effect:** Increases phagocytic ability, antibody-dependent destruction; decreases incidence of infection.

PHARMACOKINETICS

Readily absorbed after subcutaneous administration. **Half-life:** 15–80 hrs.

USES

Decreases incidence of infection manifested by febrile neutropenia in cancer pts receiving moderately myelosuppressive chemotherapy. Stimulates granulocyte production in pts receiving myelosuppressive chemotherapy.

PRECAUTIONS

Contraindications: Hypersensitivity to filgrastim. Do not administer within 14 days before and 24 hrs after cytotoxic chemotherapy. **Cautions:** Any malignancy with myeloid characteristics, gout, psoriasis, sickle cell, or respiratory disease. The 6-mg fixed dose not to be used in infants, children, or adolescents weighing less than 45 kg.

⊠ LIFESPAN CONSIDERATIONS

Pregnancy/Lactation: Unknown if drug crosses placenta or is distributed in breast milk. **Pregnancy Category C. Children:** Safety and efficacy not established in children younger than 12 yrs of age. **Elderly:** No age-related precautions noted.

INTERACTIONS

DRUG: None significant. **HERBAL:** None significant. **FOOD:** None known. **LAB VALUES:** May increase serum LDH, alkaline phosphatase, uric acid.

AVAILABILITY (Rx)

Injection Solution: 6 mg/0.6 ml syringe.

ADMINISTRATION/HANDLING

Subcutaneous

Storage • Store in refrigerator. Warm to room temperature prior to administering injection. Discard if left at room temperature for more than 48 hrs. • Protect from light. • Avoid freezing; but if accidentally frozen, may allow to thaw in refrigerator before administration. Discard if freezing takes place a second time. • Discard if discolored or precipitate forms.

INDICATIONS/ROUTES/DOSAGE

Myelosuppression

Subcutaneous: ADULTS, ELDERLY, CHILDREN 12–17 YRS, WEIGHING MORE THAN 45 KG: Give as single 6-mg injection once per chemotherapy cycle beginning 24–72 hrs after completion of chemotherapy. **◀ALERT▶** Do not administer between 14 days before and 24 hrs after cytotoxic chemotherapy. Do not use in infants, children, adolescents weighing less than 45 kg.

SIDE EFFECTS

Frequent (72%–15%): Bone pain, nausea, fatigue, alopecia, diarrhea, vomiting, constipation, anorexia, abdominal pain, arthralgia, generalized weakness, peripheral edema, dizziness, stomatitis, mucositis, neutropenic fever.

ADVERSE EFFECTS/ TOXIC REACTIONS

Allergic reactions (anaphylaxis, rash, urticaria) occur rarely. Cytopenia resulting from antibody response to growth factors occurs rarely. Splenomegaly occurs rarely. Adult respiratory distress syndrome (ARDS) may occur in septic pts.

NURSING CONSIDERATIONS

BASELINE ASSESSMENT

CBC should be obtained before initiating therapy and routinely thereafter.

INTERVENTION/EVALUATION

Monitor for allergic reactions. Assess for peripheral edema, particularly behind medial malleolus (usually first area showing peripheral edema). Assess mucous membranes for evidence of stomatitis, mucositis (red mucous membranes, white patches, extreme mouth soreness). Assess muscle strength. Monitor daily pattern of bowel activity, stool consistency. Adult respiratory distress syndrome (ARDS) may occur in septic pts.

PATIENT/FAMILY TEACHING

• Inform pt of possible side effects, signs/ symptoms of allergic reaction. • Counsel pt on importance of compliance with pegfilgrastim treatment, including regular monitoring of blood counts. • Report unusual fever or chills, severe bone pain, chest pain or palpitations.

peginterferon alfa-2a

peg-in-ter-**feer**-on
(Pegasys)
BLACK BOX ALERT Can cause or aggravate fatal or life-threatening autoimmune, neuropsychiatric (depression, suicidal ideation/behaviors), ischemic, including worsening hepatic function, and infectious disorders. Combination with ribavirin can cause fetal mortality, birth defects, hemolytic anemia. May be carcinogenic.
Do not confuse peginterferon alfa-2a with interferon alfa-2b, interferon alfa-n3, or peginterferon alfa-2b.

◆CLASSIFICATION

PHARMACOTHERAPEUTIC: Immunomodulator. **CLINICAL:** Immunologic agent.

ACTION

Binds to specific membrane receptors on virus-infected cell surface, inhibiting viral replication. Suppresses cell proliferation, producing reversible decreases in leukocyte, platelet counts. **Therapeutic Effect:** Inhibits viral hepatitis.

PHARMACOKINETICS

Readily absorbed after subcutaneous administration. Excreted by kidneys. **Half-life:** 50–140 hrs.

USES

Treatment of chronic hepatitis C (CHC) alone or in combination with ribavirin (unless contraindicated or significant intolerance to ribavirin) in pts 5 yrs or older who have compensated hepatic disease. Treatment of adults coinfected with CHC and clinically stable HIV disease. Treatment of chronic hepatitis B with compensated hepatic disease and evidence of viral replication and hepatic inflammation.

PRECAUTIONS

Contraindications: Autoimmune hepatitis, decompensated hepatic disease with cirrhosis, or pts co-infected with HIV, infants, neonates. **Extreme Caution:** History of neuropsychiatric disorders, depression. **Cautions:** Renal impairment (creatinine clearance less than 30 ml/min), elderly, pulmonary disorders, compromised CNS function, cardiac diseases, autoimmune disorders, endocrine abnormalities (e.g., diabetes, thyroid disorders), colitis, ophthalmologic disorders, myelosuppression.

⧗ LIFESPAN CONSIDERATIONS

Pregnancy/Lactation: May have abortifacient potential. Unknown if distributed in breast milk. **Pregnancy Category C (X when used with ribavirin). Children:** Safety and efficacy not established in those younger than 18 yrs. **Elderly:** CNS, cardiac, systemic effects may be more severe in the elderly, particularly in those with renal impairment.

INTERACTIONS

DRUG: Didanosine may cause hepatic failure, peripheral neuropathy, pancreatitis, lactic acidosis. May increase concentration, risk of toxicity of **methadone, theophylline.** Concurrent use of **ribavirin** may increase risk of hemolytic anemia. **HERBAL:** None significant. **FOOD:** None known. **LAB VALUES:** May increase serum ALT. May decrease absolute neutrophil, platelet.

AVAILABILITY (Rx)

Injection, Prefilled Syringe: 135 mcg/0.5 ml, 180 mcg/0.5 ml. **Injection Solution:** 180 mcg/ml.

ADMINISTRATION/HANDLING

Subcutaneous
• Refrigerate. • Vials are for single use only; discard unused portion. • Give subcutaneously in abdomen, thigh.

INDICATIONS/ROUTES/DOSAGE

Hepatitis C, Hepatitis B
Subcutaneous: ADULTS 18 YRS AND OLDER, ELDERLY: 180 mcg injected in abdomen or thigh once weekly (duration of therapy based on genotype).

Dosage in Renal Impairment
For pts who require hemodialysis or creatinine clearance less than 30 ml/min, dosage is 135 mg injected in abdomen or thigh once weekly.

Dosage in Hepatic Impairment
For pts with progressive ALT increases above baseline values, dosage is 135 mcg injected in abdomen or thigh once weekly.

SIDE EFFECTS

Frequent (54%): Headache. **Occasional (23%–13%):** Alopecia, nausea, insomnia, anorexia, dizziness, diarrhea, abdominal pain, flu-like symptoms, psychiatric reactions (depression, irritability, anxiety), injection site reaction. **Rare (8%–5%):** Impaired concentration, diaphoresis, dry mouth, nausea, vomiting.

P

✦ Canadian trade name   🦺 Non-Crushable Drug   🔺 High Alert drug

ADVERSE EFFECTS/ TOXIC REACTIONS

Serious, acute hypersensitivity reactions (urticaria, angioedema, bronchoconstriction, anaphylaxis), pancreatitis, colitis, endocrine disorders (diabetes mellitus, hyperthyroidism, hypothyroidism), ophthalmologic disorders, pulmonary abnormalities occur rarely.

NURSING CONSIDERATIONS

BASELINE ASSESSMENT

CBC, blood chemistry, urinalysis, renal/ hepatic function tests, EKG should be performed before initial therapy and routinely thereafter. Pts with diabetes, hypertension should have ophthalmologic exam before treatment begins.

INTERVENTION/EVALUATION

Monitor for evidence of depression. Offer emotional support. Monitor for abdominal pain, bloody diarrhea as evidence of colitis. Assess for pulmonary impairment. Monitor chest X-ray for pulmonary infiltrates. Encourage ample fluid intake, particularly during early therapy. Assess serum hepatitis C virus RNA levels after 24 wks of treatment.

PATIENT/FAMILY TEACHING

• Clinical response occurs in 1–3 mos. • Flu-like symptoms tend to diminish with continued therapy. • Immediately report symptoms of depression, suicidal ideation. • Avoid tasks requiring alertness, motor skills until response to drug is established. • Avoid alcohol.

peginterferon alfa-2b

peg-in-ter-**feer**-on
(PEG-Intron, PEG-Intron RediPen, Sylatron)

BLACK BOX ALERT Can cause or aggravate fatal or life-threatening autoimmune, neuropsychiatric (depression, suicidal ideation/behaviors), ischemic, including worsening hepatic function, and infectious disorders. Combination with ribavirin can cause fetal mortality, birth defects, hemolytic anemia. May be carcinogenic.

Do not confuse peginterferon alfa-2b with interferon alfa-2b, interferon alfa-n3, or peginterferon alfa-2a.

◆CLASSIFICATION

PHARMACOTHERAPEUTIC: Immunomodulator. **CLINICAL:** Immunologic agent.

ACTION

Inhibits viral replication in virus-infected cells, suppresses cell proliferation, increases phagocytic action of macrophages, augments specific cytotoxicity of lymphocytes for target cells. **Therapeutic Effect:** Inhibits viral hepatitis.

PHARMACOKINETICS

Bioavailability is increased after multiple weekly doses. Excreted in urine. **Half-life:** 22–60 hrs.

USES

PEG-Intron: As monotherapy or in combination with ribavirin for treatment of chronic hepatitis C in pts not previously treated with interferon alfa who have compensated hepatic disease and are older than 18 yrs. **Sylatron:** Treatment of melanoma or gross nodal involvement within 84 days of definitive surgical resection including complete lymphadenectomy.

PRECAUTIONS

Contraindications: Autoimmune hepatitis, decompensated hepatic disease with cirrhosis. Hypersensitivity to interferon alfa-2b, other alfa interferons. **Cautions:** Renal impairment (creatinine clearance less than 50 ml/min), elderly, pulmonary disorders, history of psychiatric disorders, compromised CNS function, cardiac diseases, autoimmune disorders, endocrine disorders (diabetes, hyperthyroidism, hypothyroidism), ophthalmologic disorders, myelosuppression.

⌛ LIFESPAN CONSIDERATIONS

Pregnancy/Lactation: May have abortifacient potential. Unknown if distributed in breast milk. **Pregnancy Category C (X when used with ribavirin). Children:** Safety and efficacy not established in those younger than 18 yrs. **Elderly:** CNS, cardiac, systemic effects may be more severe in the elderly, particularly in those with renal impairment.

INTERACTIONS

DRUG: None significant. **HERBAL:** None significant. **FOOD:** None known. **LAB VALUES:** May increase serum ALT. May decrease neutrophil, platelet counts.

AVAILABILITY (Rx)

Injection, Powder for Reconstitution: (PEG-Intron): 50 mcg, 80 mcg, 120 mcg, 150 mcg. **(Sylatron):** 296 mcg, 444 mcg, 888 mcg. **Prefilled Syringe (RediPen):** 50 mcg, 80 mcg, 120 mcg, 150 mcg.

ADMINISTRATION/HANDLING

Subcutaneous

Reconstitution • To reconstitute, add 0.7 ml Sterile Water for Injection (supplied) to vial. • Gently swirl. Use immediately. Reconstituted solution may be refrigerated for up to 24 hrs before use. • Prefilled Syringe (RediPen): Hold cartridge upright, press two halves together until "click" is heard. • Gently invert to mix.

Storage • Store at room temperature. • Refrigerate RediPen. Once reconstituted, both products stable for 24 hrs if refrigerated.

INDICATIONS/ROUTES/DOSAGE

Melanoma

Subcutaneous: ADULTS, ELDERLY: (Sylatron): 6 mcg/kg/wk for 8 doses, then 3 mcg/kg/wk for up to 5 yrs.

Chronic Hepatitis C, Monotherapy
Subcutaneous: ADULTS 18 YRS AND OLDER, ELDERLY: (PEG-Intron): Initially,

1 mcg/kg/wk. Administer appropriate dosage (see chart below) once weekly for 1 yr on same day each wk.

Weight (kg)	mcg*
45 or less	40
46–56	50
57–72	64
73–88	80
89–106	96
107–136	120
137–160	150

*Of peginterferon alfa-2b to administer.

Chronic Hepatitis C with Ribavirin
Subcutaneous: COMBINATION THERAPY WITH RIBAVIRIN: ADULTS, ELDERLY: Initially, 1.5 mcg/kg/wk. **CHILDREN 3 YRS AND OLDER:** 60 mcg/m^2 once weekly.

Weight	Dosage
Less than 40 kg	50 mcg
40–50 kg	64 mcg
51–60 kg	80 mcg
61–75 kg	96 mcg
76–85 kg	120 mcg
86–105 kg	150 mcg
Greater than 105 kg	1.5 mcg/kg/wk

◀ALERT▶ Do not use in pts with creatinine clearance less than 50 ml/min. Dosage adjustments needed for hematologic toxicity (hemoglobin, WBCs, neutrophils, platelets) and depression.

SIDE EFFECTS

Frequent (50%–47%): Flu-like symptoms; inflammation, bruising, pruritus, irritation at injection site. **Occasional (29%–18%):** Psychiatric reactions (depression, anxiety, emotional lability, irritability), insomnia, alopecia, diarrhea. **Rare:** Rash, diaphoresis, dry skin, dizziness, flushing, vomiting, dyspepsia.

ADVERSE EFFECTS/ TOXIC REACTIONS

Serious, acute hypersensitivity reactions (urticaria, angioedema, bronchoconstriction, anaphylaxis), pulmonary disorders, endocrine disorders (diabetes mellitus,

P

hypothyroidism, hyperthyroidism) pancreatitis occur rarely. Ulcerative colitis may occur within 12 wks of starting treatment.

NURSING CONSIDERATIONS

BASELINE ASSESSMENT

CBC, blood chemistry, urinalysis, renal/hepatic function tests, EKG should be performed before initial therapy and routinely thereafter. Pts with diabetes, hypertension should have ophthalmologic exam before treatment begins.

INTERVENTION/EVALUATION

Monitor for abdominal pain, bloody diarrhea as evidence of colitis. Assess for pulmonary impairment. Monitor chest X-ray for pulmonary infiltrates. Encourage adequate fluid intake, particularly during early therapy. Assess serum hepatitis C virus RNA levels after 24 wks of treatment. Monitor for depression, suicidal ideation.

PATIENT/FAMILY TEACHING

• Maintain adequate hydration. • Avoid alcohol. • May experience flu-like syndrome (nausea, body aches, headache). • Report persistent abdominal pain, bloody diarrhea, fever, signs of depression, suicidal ideation, or infection, unusual bruising/bleeding.

pegloticase

peg-**loe**-ti-kase
(Krystexxa)

BLACK BOX ALERT Severe infusion reactions, anaphylaxis (bronchospasm, stridor, urticaria, hypotension, dyspnea, flushing, circumoral swelling) have occurred, especially within 2 hrs of first infusion. Premedicate pt with corticosteroids, antihistamines. Should be administered in health care setting by health care providers prepared to manage infusion reactions.

Do not confuse pegloticase with Activase, cholinesterase, or pegaspargase.

♦CLASSIFICATION

PHARMACOTHERAPEUTIC: Uric acid enzyme. **CLINICAL:** Antigout agent.

ACTION

Decreases uric acid production by catalyzing oxidation of uric acid to allantoin, lowering serum uric acid. **Therapeutic Effect:** Lowers serum uric acid concentration.

PHARMACOKINETICS

Catalyzes oxidation of uric acid to allantoin, an inert and water-soluble purine metabolite. Readily eliminated, primarily by renal excretion. **Half-life:** 14.5 days.

USES

Treatment of chronic gout in adult pts refractory to conventional therapy. Not recommended for treatment of asymptomatic hyperuricemia.

PRECAUTIONS

Contraindications: Glucose-6-phosphate dehydrogenase (G6PD) deficiency due to hemodialysis, methemoglobinemia. **Cautions:** History of HF, elderly, debilitated.

☒ LIFESPAN CONSIDERATIONS

Pregnancy/Lactation: Unknown if drug crosses placenta or is distributed in breast milk. **Pregnancy Category C. Children:** Safety and efficacy not established in those younger than 18 yrs. **Elderly:** No age-related precautions noted.

INTERACTIONS

DRUG: None significant. **HERBAL:** None significant. **FOOD:** None known. **LAB VALUES:** Decreases serum uric acid (expected).

AVAILABILITY (Rx)

Injection Solution: 2-ml (8 mg/ml) single-use vials.

ADMINISTRATION/HANDLING

🖐 IV

Reconstitution • Withdraw 1 ml from single-use vial and inject into 250 ml

0.9% NaCl or 0.45% NaCl. • Invert infusion bag a number of times to ensure thorough mixing; do not shake.

Rate of Administration • Infuse slowly over no less than 120 min.

Storage • Store in refrigerator. • Solution should appear clear; discard if particulate is present. • Allow diluted solution to reach room temperature prior to infusion. • Following dilution, solution remains stable for 4 hrs if refrigerated or at room temperature.

INDICATIONS/ROUTES/DOSAGE

◄**ALERT**► Give by IV infusion; do not give as IV push or IV bolus. Pt to be pretreated with corticosteroids, antihistamines to reduce risk of infusion reaction, anaphylaxis.

Gout
IV Infusion: ADULTS, ELDERLY: 8 mg every 2 wks.

SIDE EFFECTS

Occasional (12%–9%): Nausea, ecchymosis at IV site, nasopharyngitis. **Rare (6%–5%):** Constipation, vomiting.

ADVERSE EFFECTS/ TOXIC REACTIONS

Exacerbation of HF has been noted. Infusion-related reaction (urticaria, dyspnea, chest discomfort, chest pain, erythema, pruritus) occurs in 26% of pts; anaphylaxis occurs in 7% of pts. Increase in gout flares is frequently noted upon initiation of antihyperuricemic therapy due to changing serum uric acid levels.

NURSING CONSIDERATIONS

BASELINE ASSESSMENT

If gout flare occurs during treatment, prophylaxis with an NSAID or colchicine is recommended. Pts at higher risk for G6PD deficiency (e.g., those of African or Mediterranean ancestry) should be screened for G6PD deficiency before starting therapy. Obtain serum uric acid levels prior to each infusion. If levels reach greater than 6 mg/dl, particularly when 2 consecutive levels greater than 6 mg/dl are observed, treatment should be discontinued.

INTERVENTION/EVALUATION

Monitor closely for infusion reaction during therapy and for 2 hrs post treatment. If infusion reaction occurs during administration, infusion may be slowed, or stopped and restarted at slower rate. If severe infusion reaction occurs, discontinue infusion and institute treatment as needed. Assess for therapeutic response (reduced joint tenderness, swelling, redness, limitation of motion).

PATIENT/FAMILY TEACHING

• Educate pts on the most common signs and symptoms of infusion reaction (rash, redness of skin, difficulty breathing, flushing, chest discomfort, chest pain). • Advise pts to seek medical care immediately if they experience any symptoms of allergic reaction during or at any time after infusion.

pegvisomant

peg-**vie**-soe-mant
(Somavert)
Do not confuse Somavert with somatrem or somatropin.

◆**CLASSIFICATION**

PHARMACOTHERAPEUTIC: Protein analog of human growth hormone. **CLINICAL:** Acromegaly agent.

ACTION

Selectively binds to growth hormone receptors on cell surfaces, blocking binding of endogenous growth hormones, interfering with growth hormone signal transduction. **Therapeutic Effect:** Decreases serum concentrations of insulin-like growth factor 1 (IGF-1) serum protein, normalizing serum IGF-1 levels.

P

PHARMACOKINETICS

Not distributed extensively into tissues after subcutaneous administration. Less than 1% excreted in urine. **Half-life:** 6 days.

USES

Treatment of acromegaly in pts with inadequate response to surgery, radiation, other medical therapies or pts for whom these therapies are inappropriate.

PRECAUTIONS

Contraindications: None known. **Cautions:** Elderly, diabetes mellitus.

⏳ LIFESPAN CONSIDERATIONS

Pregnancy/Lactation: Unknown if distributed in breast milk. **Pregnancy Category B. Children:** Safety and efficacy not established. **Elderly:** Initiation of treatment should begin at low end of dosage range.

INTERACTIONS

DRUG: May enhance effects of **insulin, oral antidiabetics** (may result in hypoglycemia); dosage should be decreased when initiating therapy. **Opioids** may decrease serum concentration. **HERBAL:** None significant. **FOOD:** None known. **LAB VALUES:** May increase serum alkaline phosphatase, total bilirubin, AST, ALT. Interferes with measurement of serum growth hormone concentration. Glucose tolerance test results may be elevated.

AVAILABILITY (Rx)

Injection, Powder for Reconstitution: 10-mg, 15-mg, 20-mg vials.

ADMINISTRATION/HANDLING

Subcutaneous

Reconstitution • Withdraw 1 ml Sterile Water for Injection, inject into vial of pegvisomant, aiming stream against glass wall. • Roll to dissolve powder (do not shake).

Rate of Administration • Administer subcutaneously only 1 dose from each vial. **Storage** • Refrigerate unreconstituted vials. • Administer within 6 hrs following reconstitution. • Solution should appear clear after reconstitution. Discard if cloudy or particulate forms.

INDICATIONS/ROUTES/DOSAGE

Acromegaly

Subcutaneous: ADULTS, ELDERLY: Initially, 40 mg, as a loading dose, then 10 mg daily. Adjust dosage in 5-mg increments in 4–6 wk intervals if serum IGF-1 level is still elevated, or in 5-mg decrements if IGF-1 level has decreased below the normal range. **Maximum maintenance dose:** 30 mg daily.

Dosage in Hepatic Impairment

Baseline Hepatic Function Tests Greater Than 3 Times Upper Limit of Normal (ULN): Do not initiate without comprehensive workup to determine cause.

Hepatic Function Tests 3–5 Times ULN: Continue treatment but monitor for hepatitis, hepatic injury.

Hepatic Function Tests 5 Times or Greater or Serum Transaminase Greater Than 3 Times ULN Associated With Any Increase in Total Bilirubin: Discontinue immediately and perform comprehensive hepatic workup.

SIDE EFFECTS

Frequent (23%): Infection (cold symptoms, upper respiratory tract infection, blister, ear infection). **Occasional (8%–5%):** Back pain, dizziness, injection site reaction, peripheral edema, sinusitis, nausea. **Rare (Less Than 4%):** Diarrhea, paresthesia.

ADVERSE EFFECTS/ TOXIC REACTIONS

May produce marked elevation of hepatic enzymes (transaminase). Substantial weight gain occurs rarely.

NURSING CONSIDERATIONS

BASELINE ASSESSMENT

Obtain baseline IGF-1 serum tests, hepatic function tests.

INTERVENTION/EVALUATION

Monitor hepatic function tests. Monitor all pts with tumors that secrete growth hormone with periodic imaging scans of sella turcica for progressive tumor growth. Monitor diabetic pts for hypoglycemia. Obtain IGF-1 serum concentrations 4–6 wks after therapy begins and periodically thereafter; dosage adjustment based on results; dosage adjustment should not be based on growth hormone assays.

PATIENT/FAMILY TEACHING

• Routine monitoring of liver function is essential during treatment. • Report abdominal pain, discolored urine, jaundice (yellowing of eyes, skin).

---

pemetrexed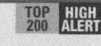

pem-e-**trex**-ed
(<u>Alimta</u>)
Do not confuse pemetrexed with methotrexate or pralatrexate.

◆CLASSIFICATION

PHARMACOTHERAPEUTIC: Antimetabolite. **CLINICAL:** Antineoplastic (see p. 87C).

ACTION

Disrupts folate-dependent enzymes essential for cell replication. **Therapeutic Effect:** Inhibits growth of mesothelioma cell lines.

PHARMACOKINETICS

Protein binding: 81%. Not metabolized. Excreted in urine. **Half-life:** 3.5 hrs.

USES

Combination chemotherapy with cisplatin for treatment of unresectable malignant pleural mesothelioma. Single agent treatment of locally advanced or metastatic non–small-cell lung cancer (NSCLC) after prior chemotherapy. Initial treatment of NSCLC in combination with cisplatin. Maintenance treatment of NSCLC in pts whose disease has not progressed following 4 cycles of platinum-based first-line chemotherapy. **OFF-LABEL:** Treatment of bladder, cervical, ovarian cancer; malignant pleural mesothelioma.

PRECAUTIONS

Contraindications: None known. **Cautions:** Hepatic/renal impairment. Concurrent nephrotoxins. Not indicated for squamous cell NSCLC.

⚖ LIFESPAN CONSIDERATIONS

Pregnancy/Lactation: Unknown if drug crosses placenta or is distributed in breast milk. Breastfeeding not recommended. May cause fetal harm. Not recommended during pregnancy. **Pregnancy Category D. Children:** Safety and efficacy not established in those younger than 18 yrs. **Elderly:** Higher incidence of fatigue, leukopenia, neutropenia, thrombocytopenia in those 65 yrs and older.

INTERACTIONS

DRUG: NSAIDs may increase concentration/effects. **Bone marrow depressants** may increase risk of myelosuppression. **Live virus vaccines** may potentiate virus replication, increase vaccine side effects, decrease pt's antibody response to vaccine. **HERBAL: Echinacea** may decrease effects. **FOOD:** None known. **LAB VALUES:** May increase serum ALT, AST, creatinine.

AVAILABILITY (Rx)

Injection, Powder for Reconstitution: 100 mg; 500 mg.

ADMINISTRATION/HANDLING

 IV Infusion

Reconstitution • Dilute 500-mg vial with 20 ml (4.2 ml to 100-mg vial) 0.9% NaCl to provide concentration of 25 mg/ml. • Gen-

P

tly swirl each vial until powder is completely dissolved. • Solution appears clear and ranges in color from colorless to yellow or green-yellow. • Further dilute reconstituted solution with 100 ml 0.9% NaCl.

Rate of Administration • Infuse over 10 min.

Storage • Store at room temperature. • Diluted solution is stable for up to 24 hrs at room temperature or if refrigerated.

🏵 IV INCOMPATIBILITIES

Use only 0.9% NaCl to reconstitute; flush line prior to and following infusion. Do not add any other medications to IV line.

INDICATIONS/ROUTES/DOSAGE

Refer to individual protocols.

◀ALERT▶ Pretreatment with dexamethasone (or equivalent) will reduce risk, severity of cutaneous reaction; treatment with folic acid and vitamin B_{12} beginning 1 wk before treatment and continuing for 21 days after last pemetrexed dose will reduce risk of side effects. Do not begin new treatment cycles unless ANC 1,500/mm^3 or greater, platelets 100,000/mm^3 or greater, and CrCl 45 ml/min or greater.

Malignant Pleural Mesothelioma
IV: ADULTS, ELDERLY: 500 mg/m^2 q3wks in combination with cisplatin 75 mg/m^2.

Non–Small-Cell Lung Cancer (NSCLC)
IV: ADULTS, ELDERLY: Initial treatment 500 mg/m^2 q3wks (in combination with cisplatin). Maintenance or second-line treatment: 500 mg/m^2 on day 1 of each 21-day cycle (as single agent).

Dosage in Hepatic Impairment
Grade 3 *(5.1–20 Times Upper Level Normal)* or Grade 4 *(Greater Than 20 Times Upper Level Normal)*: 75% of previous dose.

SIDE EFFECTS

Frequent (12%–10%): Fatigue, nausea, vomiting, rash, desquamation. **Occasional (8%–4%):** Stomatitis, pharyngitis, diarrhea,

anorexia, hypertension, chest pain. **Rare (Less Than 3%):** Constipation, depression, dysphagia.

ADVERSE EFFECTS/ TOXIC REACTIONS

Myelosuppression, characterized as grade 1–4 neutropenia, thrombocytopenia, anemia, has been noted.

NURSING CONSIDERATIONS

BASELINE ASSESSMENT

Question for possibility of pregnancy before initiating therapy (Pregnancy Category D). Obtain CBC, serum chemistry tests before therapy and at regular intervals throughout therapy.

INTERVENTION/EVALUATION

Monitor Hgb, Hct, WBC, platelet count, renal/hepatic function. Monitor for hematologic toxicity (fever, sore throat, signs of local infection, unusual bruising/bleeding from any site), symptoms of anemia (excessive fatigue, weakness). Assess skin for evidence of dermatologic toxicity. Keep pt well hydrated, urine alkaline. Monitor WBC count for nadir, recovery.

PATIENT/FAMILY TEACHING

• Maintain strict oral hygiene. • Do not have immunizations without physician's approval (drug lowers resistance). • Avoid crowds, those with infection. • Use contraceptive measures during therapy. • Promptly report fever, sore throat, signs of local infection, unusual bruising/bleeding from any site. • Do not breastfeed.

penicillamine

pen-i-**sil**-a-meen
(Cuprimine, Depen)

BLACK BOX ALERT Pt must remain under close medical supervision for signs of toxicity (fever, sore throat, chills, ecchymosis, bleeding). **Do not confuse penicillamine with penicillin.**

◆ CLASSIFICATION

PHARMACOTHERAPEUTIC: Heavy metal antagonist. **CLINICAL:** Chelating agent, anti-inflammatory.

ACTION

Chelates with lead, copper, mercury, iron to form soluble complexes; depresses circulating IgM rheumatoid factor levels; depresses T-cell activity; combines with cystine to form more soluble compound. **Therapeutic Effect:** Promotes excretion of heavy metals, acts as anti-inflammatory drug, prevents renal calculi (may dissolve existing stones).

USES

Treatment of Wilson's disease, cystinuria. Treatment of severe active rheumatoid arthritis (RA) not controlled with conventional therapy. **OFF-LABEL:** Treatment of lead poisoning.

PRECAUTIONS

Contraindications: History of penicillamine-related aplastic anemia or agranulocytosis, rheumatoid arthritis with renal insufficiency, pregnancy (except for treatment of Wilson's disease), breastfeeding. **Cautions:** Elderly, debilitated, concurrent hematopoietic depressant medications (e.g., immunosuppressants), renal impairment.

⌛ LIFESPAN CONSIDERATIONS

Pregnancy/Lactation: Contraindicated in pregnancy. Teratogenic; may cause fetal death. **Pregnancy Category D. Children:** Efficacy not established. **Elderly:** Age-related renal/hepatic impairment may require dosage adjustment.

INTERACTIONS

DRUG: Iron supplements may decrease absorption. May decrease levels of **di-goxin. Bone marrow depressants, gold compounds, immunosuppressants** may increase risk of adverse hematologic, renal effects. **HERBAL:** None significant. **FOOD: All foods** may decrease absorption. **LAB VALUES:** None significant.

AVAILABILITY (Rx)

Capsules (Cuprimine): 250 mg. **Tablets (Depen):** 250 mg.

ADMINISTRATION/HANDLING

PO

• Administer 1 hr before or 2 hrs after meals, milk, other medication. • Contents of capsule may be mixed with fruit juice or pureed fruit. • For cystinuria, drink copious amounts of water.

INDICATIONS/ROUTES/DOSAGE

Rheumatoid Arthritis (RA)
◄**ALERT**► Avoid use in pts with creatinine clearance 50 ml/min or less.
PO: ADULTS, ELDERLY: 125–250 mg/day. **Maximum (adults):** May increase at 1- to 3-mo intervals up to 1–1.5 g/day. **Maximum (elderly):** 750 mg/day.
◄**ALERT**► Dose more than 500 mg/day should be in divided doses.
CHILDREN YOUNGER THAN 12 YRS: Initially, 3 mg/kg/day (**maximum:** 250 mg) for 3 mos, then 6 mg/kg/day (**maximum:** 500 mg) in 2 divided doses for 3 mos. **Maximum:** 10 mg/kg/day (750 mg/day) in 3–4 divided doses.

Wilson's Disease
PO: ADULTS, CHILDREN 12 YRS AND OLDER: 750–1,500 mg/day in 4 divided doses. **Maximum:** 2 g/day. **ELDERLY:** 750 mg/day in 3–4 divided doses. **CHILDREN YOUNGER THAN 12 YRS:** 20 mg/kg/day in 2–4 doses. **Maximum:** 1 g/day.
◄**ALERT**► Dose that results in initial 24-hr urinary copper excretion greater than 2 mg/day should continue for 3 mos. Maintenance dose: less than 10 mcg serum-free copper/dl.

P

Cystinuria
PO: ADULTS, ELDERLY: Initially, 2 g/day in divided doses q6h. Range: 1–4 g/day. **CHILDREN:** 30 mg/kg/day in 4 divided doses. **Maximum:** 4 g/day.

◀ **ALERT** ▶ Titrate to maintain urinary cystine excretion at 100–200 mg/day.

SIDE EFFECTS

Frequent: Rash (pruritic, erythematous, maculopapular, morbilliform), reduced/altered sense of taste (hypogeusia), GI disturbances (anorexia, epigastric pain, nausea, vomiting, diarrhea), oral ulcers, glossitis. **Occasional:** Proteinuria, hematuria, hot flashes, drug-induced hyperthermia (drug fever). **Rare:** Alopecia, tinnitus, pemphigoid rash (water blisters).

ADVERSE EFFECTS/TOXIC REACTIONS

Aplastic anemia, agranulocytosis, thrombocytopenia, leukopenia, myasthenia gravis, bronchiolitis, erythematous-like syndrome, evening hypoglycemia, skin friability at sites of pressure/trauma producing extravasation or white papules at venipuncture, surgical sites were reported. Iron deficiency may develop, particularly in children, menstruating women.

NURSING CONSIDERATIONS

BASELINE ASSESSMENT

CBC with differential should be performed before beginning therapy, q2wks thereafter for first 6 mos, then monthly during therapy. Hepatic function tests (GGT, AST, ALT, LDH), CT scan for renal stones may also be ordered by physician. A 2-hr interval is necessary between iron and penicillamine therapy. In event of upcoming surgery, dosage should be reduced to 250 mg/day until wound healing is complete.

INTERVENTION/EVALUATION

Encourage copious amounts of water in pts with cystinuria. Monitor WBC, differ-

ential, platelet count. If WBC less than 3,500, neutrophils less than 2,000/mm^3, monocytes more than 500/mm^3, or platelet counts less than 100,000, or if progressive fall in platelet count or WBC in 3 successive determinations noted, inform physician (drug withdrawal necessary). Assess for evidence of hematuria. Monitor urinalysis for hematuria, proteinuria (if proteinuria exceeds 1 g/24 hrs, inform physician).

PATIENT/FAMILY TEACHING

• Promptly report any possibilities of pregnancy. • Report fever, sore throat, chills, bruising, bleeding, difficulty breathing on exertion, unexplained cough or wheezing. • Take medication 1 hr before or 2 hrs after meals or at least 1 hr before or after any other drug, food, or milk.

penicillin G benzathine

pen-i-**sill**-in G **benz**-ah-theen
(Bicillin LA)
Do not confuse penicillin G benzathine with penicillin G potassium.

FIXED-COMBINATION(S)

Bicillin CR: penicillin G benzathine/penicillin procaine: 600,000 units benzathine/600,000 units procaine.

◆CLASSIFICATION

PHARMACOTHERAPEUTIC: Penicillin.
CLINICAL: Antibiotic (see p. 28C).

ACTION

Inhibits bacterial cell wall synthesis by binding to one or more of the penicillin-binding proteins of bacteria. **Therapeutic Effect:** Bactericidal.

USES

Treatment of mild to moderate severe infections caused by organisms suscepti-

P

ble to low concentrations of penicillin including streptococcal (group A) upper respiratory infections, syphilis. Prophylaxis of infections caused by susceptible organisms (e.g., rheumatic fever prophylaxis).

PRECAUTIONS

Contraindications: Hypersensitivity to any penicillin. **Cautions:** Renal/cardiac impairment, seizure disorder, hypersensitivity to cephalosporins, history of significant allergies and/or asthma.

⧖ LIFESPAN CONSIDERATIONS

Pregnancy/Lactation: Readily crosses placenta; distributed in breast milk. **Pregnancy Category B. Children:** May delay renal excretion in neonates, young infants. **Elderly:** Age-related renal impairment may require dosage adjustment.

INTERACTIONS

DRUG: Probenecid increases concentration. **HERBAL:** None significant. **FOOD:** None known. **LAB VALUES:** May cause positive Coombs' test. May increase serum ALT, AST, alkaline phosphatase, LDH. May decrease WBC count.

AVAILABILITY (Rx)

Injection (Prefilled Syringe [Bicillin LA]): 600,000 units/ml.

ADMINISTRATION/HANDLING

◀ALERT▶ Do not give IV, intra-arterially, subcutaneously (may cause thrombosis, severe neurovascular damage, cardiac arrest, death).

IM
• Store in refrigerator. Do not freeze.
• Administer undiluted by deep IM injection.

INDICATIONS/ROUTES/DOSAGE

Usual Dosage Range
IM: ADULTS, ELDERLY: 1.2–2.4 million units as single dose. **CHILDREN:** 25,000–50,000 units/kg as single dose. **Maximum:** 2.4 million units.

SIDE EFFECTS

Occasional: Lethargy, fever, dizziness, rash, pain at injection site. **Rare:** Seizures, interstitial nephritis.

ADVERSE EFFECTS/ TOXIC REACTIONS

Hypersensitivity reactions, ranging from chills, fever, rash to anaphylaxis, may occur.

NURSING CONSIDERATIONS

BASELINE ASSESSMENT
Question for history of allergies, particularly penicillins, cephalosporins.

INTERVENTION/EVALUATION
Monitor CBC, urinalysis, renal function tests.

penicillin G potassium

pen-i-**sil**-in G po-**tas**-ee-um
(Crystapen ♣, Pfizerpen)
Do not confuse penicillin with penicillamine.

◆**CLASSIFICATION**

PHARMACOTHERAPEUTIC: Penicillin. **CLINICAL:** Antibiotic (see p. 28C).

ACTION

Inhibits bacterial cell wall synthesis by binding to one or more of the penicillin-binding proteins of bacteria. **Therapeutic Effect:** Bactericidal.

PHARMACOKINETICS

Protein binding: 60%. Widely distributed (poor CNS penetration). Metabolized in liver. Primarily excreted in urine. **Half-life:** 0.5–1 hr (increased in renal impairment).

USES

Treatment of susceptible infections including sepsis, meningitis, endocarditis, pneumonia. Active against gram-positive organisms (except *S. aureus*), some gram-negative organisms (e.g., *N. gonorrhoeae*), and some anaerobes and spirochetes.

PRECAUTIONS

Contraindications: Hypersensitivity to any penicillin. **Cautions:** Renal/hepatic impairment, seizure disorder, hypersensitivity to cephalosporins.

⧗ LIFESPAN CONSIDERATIONS

Pregnancy/Lactation: Readily crosses placenta; distributed in breast milk. **Pregnancy Category B. Children:** May delay renal excretion in neonates, young infants. **Elderly:** Age-related renal impairment may require dosage adjustment.

INTERACTIONS

DRUG: Probenecid increases concentration. **HERBAL:** None significant. **FOOD: Food, milk** decrease absorption. **LAB VALUES:** May cause positive Coombs' test. May increase serum ALT, AST, alkaline phosphatase, LDH. May decrease WBC count.

AVAILABILITY (Rx)

Infusion (Premix): 1 million units/50 ml, 2 million units/50 ml, 3 million units/50 ml. **Injection, Powder for Reconstitution:** 5 million units.

ADMINISTRATION/HANDLING
 IV

Reconstitution • Follow dilution guide per manufacturer. • After reconstitution, further dilute with 50–100 ml D₅W or 0.9% NaCl for final concentration of 100,000–500,000 units/ml (50,000 units/ml for infants, neonates).
Rate of Administration • Infuse over 15–60 min (15–30 min for infants, neonates).
Storage • Reconstituted solution is stable for 7 days if refrigerated.

▦ IV INCOMPATIBILITIES

Dopamine (Intropin), sodium bicarbonate.

▦ IV COMPATIBILITIES

Amiodarone (Cordarone), calcium gluconate, diltiazem (Cardizem), heparin, magnesium sulfate, potassium chloride.

INDICATIONS/ROUTES/DOSAGE
Usual Dosage
IV, IM: ADULTS, ELDERLY: 2–30 million units/day in divided doses q4–6h. **CHILDREN:** 100,000–400,000 units/kg/day in divided doses q4–6h. **NEONATES:** 25,000–50,000 units/kg/dose q8–12h.

Dosage in Renal Impairment
Dosage interval is modified based on creatinine clearance.

Creatinine Clearance (CrCl)	Dosage
Uremic pts with CrCl greater than 10 ml/min	Full loading dose, then 1/2 loading dose q4–5h
Less than 10 ml/min	Full loading dose, then 1/2 loading dose q8–10h
Hemodialysis:	50%–100% normal dose q8–12h
Continuous renal replacement therapy	
Continuous venovenous hemofiltration:	Loading dose 4 million units, then 2 million units q4–6h
Continuous venovenous hemodialysis:	Loading dose 4 million units, then 2–3 million units q4–6h
Continuous venovenous hemodiafiltration:	Loading dose 4 million units, then 2–4 million units q4–6h

SIDE EFFECTS

Occasional: Lethargy, fever, dizziness, rash, electrolyte imbalance, diarrhea, thrombophlebitis. **Rare:** Seizures, interstitial nephritis.

ADVERSE EFFECTS/ TOXIC REACTIONS

Hypersensitivity reactions ranging from rash, fever, chills to anaphylaxis occur occasionally.

NURSING CONSIDERATIONS

BASELINE ASSESSMENT

Question for history of allergies, particularly penicillins, cephalosporins.

INTERVENTION/EVALUATION

Promptly report rash (hypersensitivity), diarrhea (with fever, abdominal pain, mucus, or blood in stool, may indicate antibiotic-associated colitis). Monitor I&O, urinalysis electrolytes, renal function tests for nephrotoxicity.

penicillin V potassium

TOP 200

pen-i-**sil**-in V po-**tas**-ee-um
(Apo-Pen-VK ♣, Novo-Pen-VK ♣,
NuPen VK ♣)

◆CLASSIFICATION

PHARMACOTHERAPEUTIC: Penicillin.
CLINICAL: Antibiotic (see p. 29C).

ACTION

Inhibits cell wall synthesis by binding to bacterial cell membranes. **Therapeutic Effect:** Bactericidal.

PHARMACOKINETICS

Moderately absorbed from GI tract. Protein binding: 80%. Widely distributed. Metabolized in liver. Primarily excreted in urine. **Half-life:** 1 hr (increased in renal impairment).

USES

Treatment of mild to moderate infections of respiratory tract, skin/skin structure, otitis media, necrotizing ulcerative gingivitis; prophylaxis for rheumatic fever, dental procedures.

PRECAUTIONS

Contraindications: Hypersensitivity to any penicillin. **Cautions:** Renal impairment, history of allergies (particularly cephalosporins), history of seizures.

⌛ LIFESPAN CONSIDERATIONS

Pregnancy/Lactation: Readily crosses placenta; appears in cord blood, amniotic fluid. Distributed in breast milk in low concentrations. May lead to allergic sensitization, diarrhea, candidiasis, skin rash in infant. **Pregnancy Category B. Children:** Use caution in neonates and young infants (may delay renal elimination). **Elderly:** Age-related renal impairment may require dosage adjustment.

INTERACTIONS

DRUG: ACE inhibitors, potassium-sparing diuretics, potassium supplements may increase risk of hyperkalemia. May increase **methotrexate** concentration, toxicity. **Probenecid** may increase concentration, risk of toxicity. **HERBAL:** None significant. **FOOD:** None known. **LAB VALUES:** May cause positive Coombs' test. May increase serum ALT, AST, alkaline phosphatase, LDH. May decrease WBC count.

AVAILABILITY (Rx)

Powder for Oral Solution: 125 mg/5 ml, 250 mg/5 ml. **Tablets:** 250 mg, 500 mg.

ADMINISTRATION/HANDLING

PO
• Give on empty stomach 1 hr before or 2 hrs after meals (increases absorption).
• After reconstitution, oral solution is stable for 14 days if refrigerated. • Space doses evenly around the clock.

INDICATIONS/ROUTES/DOSAGE

Usual Dosage
PO: ADULTS, ELDERLY, CHILDREN 12 YRS AND OLDER: 125–500 mg q6–8h. **CHILDREN YOUNGER THAN 12 YRS:** 25–50 mg/kg/day in divided doses q6–8h. **Maximum:** 3 g/day.

Prophylaxis of Pneumococcal Infections, Recurrent Rheumatic Fever
PO: ADULTS, ELDERLY, CHILDREN 5 YRS AND OLDER: 250 mg twice a day. **CHILDREN YOUNGER THAN 5 YRS:** 125 mg twice a day.

P

♣ Canadian trade name   🗡 Non-Crushable Drug   🔴 High Alert drug

Dosage in Renal Impairment
Creatinine clearance less than 10 ml/min: 250 mg q6h.

SIDE EFFECTS

Frequent: Mild hypersensitivity reaction (chills, fever, rash), nausea, vomiting, diarrhea. **Rare:** Bleeding, allergic reaction.

ADVERSE EFFECTS/ TOXIC REACTIONS

Severe hypersensitivity reactions, including anaphylaxis, may occur. Nephrotoxicity, antibiotic-associated colitis, other superinfections (abdominal cramps, severe watery diarrhea, fever) may result from high dosages, prolonged therapy.

NURSING CONSIDERATIONS

BASELINE ASSESSMENT

Question for history of allergies, particularly penicillins, cephalosporins.

INTERVENTION/EVALUATION

Hold medication, promptly report rash (hypersensitivity), diarrhea (with fever, abdominal pain, mucus or blood in stool may indicate antibiotic-associated colitis). Be alert for superinfection: fever, vomiting, diarrhea, anal/genital pruritus, oral mucosal change (ulceration, pain, erythema). Review Hgb levels; check for bleeding (overt/occult bleeding, ecchymosis, swelling of tissue). Monitor I&O, urinalysis, renal function tests for nephrotoxicity.

PATIENT/FAMILY TEACHING

• Continue antibiotic for full length of treatment. • Space doses evenly. • Notify physician immediately if rash, diarrhea, bleeding, bruising, other new symptoms occur.

pentamidine

pen-**tam**-i-deen
(NebuPent, Pentam-300)

◆ CLASSIFICATION

PHARMACOTHERAPEUTIC: Antiinfective. **CLINICAL:** Antiprotozoal, antifungal agent.

ACTION

Interferes with nuclear metabolism, incorporation of nucleotides, inhibiting DNA, RNA, phospholipid, protein synthesis. **Therapeutic Effect:** Produces antibacterial, antiprotozoal effects.

PHARMACOKINETICS

Well absorbed after IM administration; minimally absorbed after inhalation. Widely distributed. Primarily excreted in urine. Minimally removed by hemodialysis. **Half-life:** 6.4–9.4 hrs (increased in renal impairment).

USES

IM/IV: Treatment of pneumonia caused by *Pneumocystis jiroveci* (PCP). **Inhalation:** Prevention of PCP in high-risk HIV-infected pts either with history of PCP or with a CD4+ count 200/mm³ or less. **OFF-LABEL:** Treatment of African trypanosomiasis, cutaneous/visceral leishmaniasis. Prevention of PCP in non–HIV-infected pts.

PRECAUTIONS

Contraindications: None known. **Cautions:** Diabetes mellitus, hepatic impairment, hypertension/hypotension, anemia, thrombocytopenia, preexisting cardiac disease, hypocalcemia, prolonged QT interval, ventricular tachycardia, severe renal impairment, asthma, history of seizures or hematologic disorders.

⧗ LIFESPAN CONSIDERATIONS

Pregnancy/Lactation: Unknown if drug crosses placenta or is distributed in breast milk. **Pregnancy Category C. Children:** No age-related precautions noted. **Elderly:** No age-related information available.

INTERACTIONS

DRUG: Nephrotoxic medications may increase risk of nephrotoxicity. **HERBAL:**

None significant. **FOOD**: None known. **LAB VALUES**: May increase serum alkaline phosphatase, bilirubin, BUN, creatinine, AST, ALT. May decrease serum calcium, magnesium. May alter serum glucose.

AVAILABILITY (Rx)

Injection, Powder for Reconstitution (Pentam-300): 300 mg. **Powder for Nebulization (NebuPent)**: 300 mg.

ADMINISTRATION/HANDLING

◀ **ALERT** ▶ Pt must be in supine position during IM, IV administration, with frequent B/P checks until stable (potential for life-threatening hypotensive reaction). Have resuscitative equipment immediately available.

 IV

Reconstitution • For intermittent IV infusion (piggyback), reconstitute each vial with 3–5 ml D_5W or Sterile Water for Injection. • Withdraw desired dose; further dilute with 50–250 ml D_5W to concentration not to exceed 6 mg/ml.
Rate of Administration • Infuse over 60–120 min. • Do not give by IV injection or rapid IV infusion (increases potential for severe hypotension).
Storage • Store vials at room temperature. • After reconstitution, IV solution is stable for 48 hrs at room temperature (24 hrs if reconstituted with D_5W). • Discard unused portion.

IM

• Reconstitute 300-mg vial with 3 ml Sterile Water for Injection to provide concentration of 100 mg/ml. • Administer deep IM.

Aerosol (Nebulizer)

• Aerosol stable for 48 hrs at room temperature. • Reconstitute 300-mg vial with 6 ml Sterile Water for Injection. Avoid NaCl (may cause precipitate). • Do not mix with other medication in nebulizer reservoir.

🔲 IV INCOMPATIBILITIES

Cefazolin (Ancef), cefotaxime (Claforan), ceftazidime (Fortaz), ceftriaxone (Rocephin), fluconazole (Diflucan), foscarnet (Foscavir), interleukin (Proleukin).

🔲 IV COMPATIBILITIES

Diltiazem (Cardizem), total parenteral nutrition (TPN), zidovudine (Retrovir).

INDICATIONS/ROUTES/DOSAGE

Treatment of *Pneumocystis Jiroveci* Pneumonia (PCP)
IV, IM: ADULTS, ELDERLY, CHILDREN OLDER THAN 4 MOS: 4 mg/kg/day once daily for 14–21 days.

Prevention of PCP
Inhalation: ADULTS, ELDERLY, CHILDREN 5 YRS AND OLDER: 300 mg once q4wks.

SIDE EFFECTS

Frequent: Injection (Greater Than 10%): Abscess, pain at injection site. **Inhalation (Greater Than 5%):** Fatigue, metallic taste, shortness of breath, decreased appetite, dizziness, rash, cough, nausea, vomiting, chills. **Occasional: Injection (10%–1%):** Nausea, decreased appetite, hypotension, fever, rash, altered taste, confusion. **Inhalation (5%–1%):** Diarrhea, headache, anemia, muscle pain. **Rare: Injection (less than 1%):** Neuralgia, thrombocytopenia, phlebitis, dizziness.

ADVERSE EFFECTS/ TOXIC REACTIONS

Life-threatening/fatal hypotension, arrhythmias, hypoglycemia, leukopenia, nephrotoxicity, renal failure, anaphylactic shock, Stevens-Johnson syndrome, toxic epidural necrolysis occur rarely. Hyperglycemia, insulin-dependent diabetes mellitus (often permanent) may occur even mos after therapy has stopped.

NURSING CONSIDERATIONS

BASELINE ASSESSMENT

Avoid concurrent use of nephrotoxic drugs. Establish baseline for B/P, serum

P

 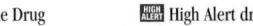

glucose. Obtain specimens for diagnostic tests before giving first dose.

INTERVENTION/EVALUATION

Monitor B/P during administration until stable for both IM and IV administration (pt should remain supine). Check serum glucose levels; observe for clinical signs of hypoglycemia (diaphoresis, anxiety, tremor, tachycardia, palpitations, dizziness, headache, numbness of lips, double vision, incoordination), hyperglycemia (polyuria, polyphagia, polydipsia, malaise, visual changes, abdominal pain, headache, nausea/vomiting). Evaluate IM sites for pain, redness, induration; IV sites for phlebitis (heat, pain, red streaking over vein). Monitor renal, hepatic, hematology test results. Assess skin for rash. Evaluate equilibrium during ambulation. Be alert for respiratory difficulty when administering by inhalation route.

PATIENT/FAMILY TEACHING

• Remain flat in bed during administration of medication; get up slowly with assistance only when B/P stable. • Immediately report profuse sweating, shakiness, dizziness, palpitations. • Drowsiness, increased urination, thirst, anorexia may develop in mos following therapy. • Maintain adequate fluid intake. • Report fever, cough, shortness of breath. • Avoid alcohol.

---

perampanel

per-**am**-pa-nel
(Fycompa)

BLACK BOX ALERT Risk for serious neuropsychiatric events, including irritability, aggression, anger, anxiety, paranoia, euphoric mood, agitation, mental status changes. Some of these events reported as serious and life-threatening. Violent thoughts or threatening behavior were also observed. Immediately report any changes in mood or behavior that are not typical for the patient are observed. Health care professionals should closely monitor patients during titration period when higher doses are used.

◆CLASSIFICATION

PHARMACOTHERAPEUTIC: Noncompetitive AMPA glutamate receptive antagonist. **CLINICAL:** Anticonvulsant.

ACTION

Non-competitive antagonist of AMPA glutamate receptors, a primary excitatory neurotransmitter on post-synaptic neurons. **Therapeutic Effect:** Reduces neuronal over excitation.

PHARMACOKINETICS

Rapidly, completely absorbed. Peak concentration: 0.5–2.5 hrs. Protein binding: 95%–96%. Steady-state levels reached in 2–3 wks. Metabolized via oxidation/glucuronidation. Excreted in feces (48%), urine (22%). **Half-life:** 105 hrs.

USES

Adjunctive treatment of partial-onset seizures with or without secondary generalized seizures in pts with epilepsy age 12 yrs and older.

PRECAUTIONS

Contraindications: None known. **Cautions:** Hepatic/renal impairment, elderly (increased falls, dizziness, gait disturbances), severe renal/hepatic impairment, concurrent use of CNS depressants, pts at risk for suicidal behavior.

⚕ LIFESPAN CONSIDERATIONS

Pregnancy/Lactation: Unknown if distributed in breast milk. Use caution when breastfeeding. **Pregnancy Category C. Children:** Safety and efficacy not established in children less than 12 yrs. **Elderly:** Owing to greater likelihood for adverse reactions in the elderly, dosing titration should proceed very slowly.

INTERACTIONS

DRUG: **CYP450 inducers (e.g., carbamazepine, oxcarbazepine, phenytoin)** may decrease concentration/effects. May decrease effectiveness of **hormonal contraceptives containing levonorgestrel. Alcohol, other CNS depressants** may increase CNS depression. **HERBAL: St. John's wort, kava kava, valerian** may increase CNS depression. **Evening primrose** may decrease seizure threshold. **FOOD:** None known. **LAB VALUES:** None significant.

AVAILABILITY (Rx)

Tablets, Film-Coated: 2 mg, 4 mg, 6 mg, 8 mg, 10 mg, 12 mg.

ADMINISTRATION/HANDLING

PO
• Give at bedtime. • Give tablet whole; do not break, crush, dissolve, or divide tablet.

INDICATIONS/ROUTES/DOSAGE

◄ALERT► Initial starting dose should be increased when enzyme-inducing anticonvulsants are given concurrently. Individual dosing based on clinical response, tolerability. Do not use in severe hepatic/renal impairment, pts on hemodialysis.

Partial-Onset Seizures in Absence of an Enzyme-Inducing Anticonvulsant
PO: ADULTS, ELDERLY, CHILDREN 13 YRS AND OLDER: Initially, 2 mg once daily at bedtime. May titrate in 2-mg increments at weekly intervals (in elderly, no more frequently than every 2 wks). **Recommended dose:** 8–12 mg/day at bedtime.

Partial-Onset Seizures (Concurrently Taking an Enzyme-Inducing Anticonvulsant)
PO: ADULTS, ELDERLY, CHILDREN 13 YRS AND OLDER: Initially, 4 mg once daily at bedtime. May titrate in 2-mg increments at weekly intervals (in elderly, no more frequently than every 2 wks). **Recom-**

mended dose: 8–12 mg/day at bedtime.

Mild to Moderate Hepatic Impairment
PO: ADULTS, ELDERLY, CHILDREN 13 YRS AND OLDER: 2 mg once daily with weekly increase of 2 mg daily every 2 wks until target dose is achieved. **Maximum (mild hepatic impairment):** 6 mg. **Maximum (moderate hepatic impairment):** 4 mg.

SIDE EFFECTS

Frequent (32%–11%): Dizziness, sleepiness, headache. **Occasional (8%–3%):** Fatigue, irritability, nausea, balance disorder, weight gain, gait disturbance, vertigo, blurred vision, vomiting, arthralgia, anxiety. **Rare (2%–1%):** Constipation, back pain, extremity pain, asthenia (lack of strength, energy), oropharyngeal pain, aggression.

ADVERSE EFFECTS/ TOXIC REACTIONS

Irritability, aggression, anger, anxiety, affect lability, agitation occurred rarely (2%). Increased risk for seizures when anticonvulsants are withdrawn abruptly.

NURSING CONSIDERATIONS

BASELINE ASSESSMENT

Review history of seizure disorder (intensity, frequency, duration, LOC). Initiate seizure precautions. Obtain medication history (esp. use of other anticonvulsant therapy; dosage based on concurrent seizure medication). Observe clinically. Assist with ambulation until response to drug is established (32% experience dizziness).

INTERVENTION/EVALUATION

Assess mental status, cognitive abilities, behavioral changes. Monitor for clinical response, tolerability to medication, dosing level during treatment and for at least 1 mo after last therapy dose. Report persistent, severe, or worsening psychiatric symptoms or behaviors. Assess for clinical improvement (decrease in intensity, frequency of seizures).

PATIENT/FAMILY TEACHING

• Avoid alcohol (greater risk for adverse effects). • The combination of alcohol and perampanel may significantly worsen mood, increase anger. • Counsel pts, families, and caregivers of need to monitor for emergence of anger, aggression, hostility, unusual changes in mental status. • Avoid tasks that require alertness, motor skills until response to drug is established (greater risk for dizziness, sleepiness).

---

pertuzumab

per-**tue**-zue-mab
(Perjeta)

BLACK BOX ALERT Can result in embryo-fetal death, birth defects. Pts must be made aware of danger to fetus, need for effective contraception.

◆CLASSIFICATION

PHARMACOTHERAPEUTIC: *HER2* receptor antagonist. **CLINICAL:** Antineoplastic (see p. 89C).

ACTION

Targets human epidermal growth factor 2 (*HER2*), blocking ligand-initiated intercellular signaling, which can result in cell growth arrest and cell death. **Therapeutic Effect:** Inhibits proliferation of human tumor cells.

PHARMACOKINETICS

Peak plasma concentration reached after first maintenance dose. **Half-life:** 18 days.

USES

Used in combination with trastuzumab and docetaxel for treatment of pts with *HER2*-positive metastatic breast cancer who have not received prior anti-*HER2* therapy or chemotherapy for metastatic disease. Neoadjuvant treatment of pts with *HER2*-positive, locally advanced inflammatory, or early-stage breast cancer.

PRECAUTIONS

Contraindications: None known. **Cautions:** Conditions that may impair left ventricular function (e.g., uncontrolled hypertension, recent MI, severe cardiac arrhythmia), history of sensitivity to medication, history of infusion-related reaction.

⌛ LIFESPAN CONSIDERATIONS

Pregnancy/Lactation: May cause embryo-fetal harm. Must use effective contraception in addition to barrier methods. Unknown if distributed in breast milk. **Pregnancy Category D. Children:** Safety and efficacy not established. **Elderly:** No age-related precautions noted.

INTERACTIONS

DRUG: None significant. **HERBAL:** None significant. **FOOD:** None known. **LAB VALUES:** None known.

AVAILABILITY (Rx)

Injection Solution: 420 mg/14 ml (30 mg/ml) vial.

ADMINISTRATION/HANDLING
🖉 IV

Reconstitution • Withdraw ordered volume of solution from vial. • Dilute into 250 ml 0.9% NaCl only (do not use D₅W). • Gently invert solution (do not shake). • Once diluted, use immediately or refrigerate for up to 24 hrs.
Rate of Administration • Initial dose to be infused over 60 min. • Subsequent doses may be infused over 30–60 min.
Storage • Refrigerate vials. Store vials in outside cartons (protects from light). • Do not use if solution appears cloudy or contains particulate.

▦ IV INCOMPATIBILITIES

Do not mix with any other medications.

INDICATIONS/ROUTES/DOSAGE

◄ALERT► Give as an IV infusion only. Do not give by IV push or bolus. If diluted solution is not used immediately, may refrigerate for up to 24 hrs.

Breast Carcinoma
IV Infusion: ADULTS/ELDERLY: Initially, 840 mg given over 60 min, followed every 3 wks thereafter by 420 mg given as a 30–60 min infusion.

Concurrent Dose With Trastuzumab
IV Infusion: ADULTS/ELDERLY: Initially, trastuzumab is given at 8 mg/kg over 90 min, followed every 3 wks thereafter by 6 mg/kg given as a 30- to 90-min infusion.

Concurrent Dose With Docetaxel
IV Infusion: ADULTS/ELDERLY: Initially, docetaxel is given at 75 mg/m². Dose may be escalated to 100 mg/m² every 3 wks if initial dose is well tolerated.

SIDE EFFECTS

Frequent (67%–21%): Diarrhea, alopecia, nausea, fatigue, rash, peripheral neuropathy, anorexia, asthenia (loss of strength, energy), mucosal inflammation, vomiting, peripheral edema, myalgia, nail disorder, headache. **Occasional (19%–12%):** Stomatitis, pyrexia, dysgeusia (abnormal taste sensation), arthralgia, constipation, increased lacrimation, pruritus, insomnia, dizziness. **Rare (10%–7%):** Nasopharyngitis, dry skin, paronychia (inflammation of folds around skin of nails).

ADVERSE EFFECTS/ TOXIC REACTIONS

Neutropenia occurs in 53% of pts, anemia occurs in 23%, and leukopenia occurs in 18%. Upper respiratory tract infection occurs in 17% of pts. Dyspnea, febrile neutropenia occurs in 14% of pts. Pleural effusion occurs in 5%, left ventricular dysfunction occurs in 4%.

NURSING CONSIDERATIONS

BASELINE ASSESSMENT

Negative pregnancy test must be confirmed before initiating treatment (Pregnancy Category D). Obtain *HER2* testing by an FDA-approved laboratory. Assess daily serum blood chemistries, CBC.

INTERVENTION/EVALUATION

Monitor daily ANC. Monitor left ventricular ejection fraction (LVEF) and withhold dosing if ordered. Assess skin, IV site for infusion-associated reactions, hypersensitivity reactions, anaphylaxis. If a significant infusion-associated reaction occurs, slow or interrupt infusion and administer appropriate medical treatment. If a reaction is noted, the most common is pyrexia. Chills, fatigue, headache, asthenia, or vomiting usually occurs during the infusion or on the same day as the infusion. Observe pt closely for 60 min after the first infusion and for 30 min after subsequent infusions. Offer antiemetics if nausea occurs.

PATIENT/FAMILY TEACHING

• Avoid pregnancy. • Use effective contraceptive measures, including barrier precautions during treatment and for 6 mos after treatment in women of childbearing potential. • If pregnancy occurs, inform physician immediately. • Do not breastfeed. • Alopecia is reversible, but new hair growth may have different color, texture.

phenazopyridine

fen-**ay**-zoe-**pir**-i-deen
(Azo-Gesic, Azo-Standard, Phenazo ✤, Pyridium, Uristat)
Do not confuse phenazopyridine with pyridoxine, or Pyridium with Dyrenium or Perdiem.

P

 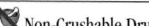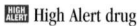

◆CLASSIFICATION

PHARMACOTHERAPEUTIC: Interstitial cystitis agent. **CLINICAL:** Urinary tract analgesic.

ACTION

Exerts topical analgesic effect on urinary tract mucosa. **Therapeutic Effect:** Relieves urinary pain, burning, urgency, frequency.

PHARMACOKINETICS

Well absorbed from GI tract. Partially metabolized in liver. Primarily excreted in urine. **Half-life:** Unknown.

USES

Symptomatic relief of pain, burning, urgency, frequency resulting from lower urinary tract mucosa irritation (may be caused by infection, trauma, surgery).

PRECAUTIONS

Contraindications: Hepatic impairment, renal impairment (creatinine clearance less than 50 ml/min). **Cautions:** Renal impairment (creatinine clearance 50–80 ml/min).

☒ LIFESPAN CONSIDERATIONS

Pregnancy/Lactation: Unknown if drug crosses placenta or is distributed in breast milk. **Pregnancy Category B. Children:** No age-related precautions noted in those older than 6 yrs. **Elderly:** Age-related renal impairment may increase toxicity.

INTERACTIONS

DRUG: None significant. **HERBAL:** None significant. **FOOD:** None known. **LAB VALUES:** May interfere with urinalysis tests based on color reactions (e.g., urinary glucose, ketones, protein, 17-ketosteroids).

AVAILABILITY (Rx)

Tablets: (Azo-Gesic, Azo-Standard, Uristat): 95 mg. **(Pyridium):** 100 mg, 200 mg.

ADMINISTRATION/HANDLING

PO
• Give with meals.

INDICATIONS/ROUTES/DOSAGE

Urinary Analgesic
PO: ADULTS: 95–200 mg 3–4 times/day for 2 days. **CHILDREN 6 YRS AND OLDER:** 12 mg/kg/day in 3 divided doses for 2 days.

Dosage in Renal Impairment
Dosage interval is modified based on creatinine clearance.

Creatinine Clearance	Dosage
50–80 ml/min	Usual dose q8–16h
Less than 50 ml/min	Avoid use

SIDE EFFECTS

Occasional: Headache, GI disturbance, rash, pruritus.

ADVERSE EFFECTS/ TOXIC REACTIONS

Overdose in pts with renal impairment, severe hypersensitivity may lead to hemolytic anemia, nephrotoxicity, hepatotoxicity. Methemoglobinemia generally occurs as result of massive, acute overdose.

NURSING CONSIDERATIONS

BASELINE ASSESSMENT

Assess pt for dysuria, urinary urgency or frequency.

INTERVENTION/EVALUATION

Monitor for therapeutic response: relief of dysuria (pain, burning), urgency, frequency of urination.

PATIENT/FAMILY TEACHING

• Reddish orange discoloration of urine should be expected. • May stain fabric. • Take with meals (reduces possibility of GI upset).

phenelzine

fen-el-zeen
(Nardil)

BLACK BOX ALERT Increased risk of suicidal ideation and behavior in children, adolescents, young adults 18–24 yrs with major depressive disorder, other psychiatric disorders.

Do not confuse phenelzine with phenytoin.

◆CLASSIFICATION

PHARMACOTHERAPEUTIC: MAOI. **CLINICAL:** Antidepressant (see p. 39C).

ACTION

Inhibits activity of the enzyme monoamine oxidase at CNS storage sites, leading to increased levels of epinephrine, norepinephrine, serotonin, dopamine at neuronal receptor sites. **Therapeutic Effect:** Relieves depression.

USES

Treatment of depression refractory to other antidepressants, electroconvulsive therapy.

PRECAUTIONS

Contraindications: HF, hepatic/renal impairment, pheochromocytoma. Concurrent use of sympathomimetics, CNS depressants, foods high in tyramine content, cyclobenzaprine, dextromethorphan, meperidine, bupropion, buspirone. **Cautions:** Cardiac arrhythmias, severe/frequent headaches, hypertension, cardiovascular/cerebrovascular disease, suicidal tendencies, glaucoma, hyperthyroidism, seizure disorder. Do not use with other MAOIs/antidepressants, within 5 wks of fluoxetine, 2 wks with other antidepressants.

⌛ LIFESPAN CONSIDERATIONS

Pregnancy/Lactation: Crosses placenta. Minimally distributed in breast milk. **Pregnancy Category C. Children:** Not recommended for children (increased risk of suicidal ideation). **Elderly:** Increased risk of drug toxicity may require dosage adjustment.

INTERACTIONS

DRUG: Fluoxetine, trazodone, paroxetine, citalopram, venlafaxine, tricyclic antidepressants may cause serotonin syndrome. **HERBAL: Valerian, St. John's wort, SAMe, kava kava** may increase risk of serotonin syndrome. **FOOD: Caffeine, chocolate, tyramine-containing foods** may cause sudden, severe hypertension. **LAB VALUES:** None significant.

AVAILABILITY (Rx)

Tablets: 15 mg.

ADMINISTRATION/HANDLING

PO
• Store tablets at room temperature.
• Give with food, milk if GI distress occurs. • Tablets may be crushed.

INDICATIONS/ROUTES/DOSAGE

Depression
PO: ADULTS: 15 mg 3 times daily. May increase to 60–90 mg/day. **ELDERLY:** Initially, 7.5 mg/day. May increase by 7.5–15 mg/day q3–4days up to 60 mg/day in 3–4 divided doses.

SIDE EFFECTS

Frequent: Orthostatic hypotension, restlessness, GI upset, insomnia, dizziness, headache, lethargy, asthenia (loss of strength, energy), dry mouth, peripheral edema. **Occasional:** Flushing, diaphoresis, rash, urinary frequency, increased appetite, transient impotence. **Rare:** Visual disturbances.

ADVERSE EFFECTS/ TOXIC REACTIONS

Hypertensive crisis occurs rarely, marked by severe hypertension, occipital headache radiating frontally, neck stiffness/soreness, nausea, vomiting, diaphoresis, fever, chills, clammy skin, dilated pupils,

P

palpitations, tachycardia or bradycardia, constricting chest pain. **Antidote for hypertensive crisis:** 5–10 mg phentolamine IV.

NURSING CONSIDERATIONS

BASELINE ASSESSMENT

Assess appearance, behavior, speech pattern, level of interest, mood.

INTERVENTION/EVALUATION

Periodic hepatic function tests should be performed for pts requiring high dosage who are undergoing prolonged therapy. Assess appearance, behavior, speech pattern, level of interest, mood. Monitor for suicidal ideation, worsening depression. Monitor for occipital headache radiating frontally and/or neck stiffness/soreness (may be first signal of impending hypertensive crisis). Monitor B/P, heart rate, diet, weight.

PATIENT/FAMILY TEACHING

• Notify physician if depression worsens, suicidal ideation, or unusual changes in behavior occur. • Antidepressant relief may be noted during first wk of therapy; maximum benefit noted in 2–6 wks. • Report headache, neck stiffness/soreness immediately. • Avoid foods that require bacteria/molds for their preparation/preservation or those that contain tyramine (e.g., cheese, sour cream, beer, wine, yeast extracts, yogurt, papaya, meat tenderizers), excessive amounts of caffeine (coffee, tea, chocolate), OTC preparations for hay fever, colds, weight reduction.

phenobarbital

fee-noe-**bar**-bi-tal
(Luminal)
Do not confuse phenobarbital with Phenergan or phenytoin.

FIXED-COMBINATION(S)

Bellergal-S: phenobarbital/ergotamine/belladonna (an anticholinergic): 40 mg/0.6 mg/0.2 mg. **Dilantin with PB:** phenobarbital/phenytoin (an anticonvulsant): 15 mg/100 mg, 30 mg/100 mg. **Donnatal:** phenobarbital/atropine (an anticholinergic)/hyoscyamine (an anticholinergic)/scopolamine (an anticholinergic): 16.2 mg/0.0194 mg/0.1037 mg/0.0065 mg.

◆CLASSIFICATION

PHARMACOTHERAPEUTIC: Barbiturate **(Schedule IV). CLINICAL:** Anticonvulsant, hypnotic (see p. 36C).

ACTION

Enhances activity of gamma-aminobutyric acid (GABA) by binding to GABA receptor complex. **Therapeutic Effect:** Depresses CNS activity.

PHARMACOKINETICS

Route	Onset	Peak	Duration
PO	20–60 min	N/A	6–10 hrs
IV	5 min	30 min	4–10 hrs

Well absorbed after PO, parenteral administration. Protein binding: 20%–45%. Rapidly and widely distributed. Metabolized in liver. Primarily excreted in urine. Removed by hemodialysis. **Half-life:** 53–140 hrs.

USES

Management of generalized tonic-clonic (grand mal) seizures, partial seizures, control of acute seizure episodes (status epilepticus, eclampsia, febrile seizures). **OFF-LABEL:** Prevention/treatment of neonatal hyperbilirubinemia and lowering of bilirubin in chronic cholestasis; neonatal seizures.

PRECAUTIONS

Contraindications: Hypersensitivity to other barbiturates, porphyria, preexisting CNS depression, severe uncontrolled pain, severe respiratory disease with dyspnea or

P

obstruction, use in nephritic pts. **Cautions:** Renal/hepatic impairment, acute/chronic pain, depression, suicidal tendencies, history of drug abuse.

⧗ LIFESPAN CONSIDERATIONS

Pregnancy/Lactation: Readily crosses placenta. Distributed in breast milk. Produces respiratory depression in neonates during labor. May cause postpartum hemorrhage, hemorrhagic disease in newborn. Withdrawal symptoms may appear in neonates born to women receiving barbiturates during last trimester of pregnancy. Lowers serum bilirubin in neonates. **Pregnancy Category D. Children:** May cause paradoxical excitement. **Elderly:** May exhibit excitement, confusion, mental depression.

INTERACTIONS

DRUG: Alcohol, other CNS depressants may increase effects. May decrease effects of **warfarin, oral contraceptives. Valproic acid** may increase concentration, risk of toxicity. **HERBAL: Evening primrose** may decrease seizure threshold. **Gotu kola, kava kava, St. John's wort, valerian** may increase CNS depression. **FOOD:** None known. **LAB VALUES:** May decrease serum bilirubin. **Therapeutic serum level:** 10–40 mcg/ml; **toxic serum level:** greater than 40 mcg/ml.

AVAILABILITY (Rx)

Elixir: 20 mg/5 ml. **Injection, Solution:** 65 mg/ml, 130 mg/ml. **Tablets:** 15 mg, 16.2 mg, 30 mg, 32.4 mg, 60 mg, 100 mg.

ADMINISTRATION/HANDLING
 IV

Reconstitution • May give undiluted or may dilute with NaCl, D₅W, lactated Ringer's.
Rate of Administration • Adequately hydrate pt before and immediately after drug therapy (decreases risk of adverse renal effects). • Do not inject IV faster than 1 mg/kg/min and maximum of 30

mg/min for children and 60 mg/min for adults. Too-rapid IV may produce severe hypotension, marked respiratory depression. • Inadvertent intra-arterial injection may result in arterial spasm with severe pain, tissue necrosis. Extravasation in subcutaneous tissue may produce redness, tenderness, tissue necrosis. If this occurs, treat with 0.5% procaine solution into affected area, apply moist heat.
Storage • Store vials at room temperature.

IM
• Do not inject more than 5 ml in any one IM injection site (produces tissue irritation). • Inject deep IM into large muscle mass.

PO
• Give without regard to meals. • Tablets may be crushed. • Elixir may be mixed with water, milk, fruit juice.

▨ IV INCOMPATIBILITIES
Amphotericin B complex (Abelcet, AmBisome, Amphotec).

▨ IV COMPATIBILITIES
Calcium gluconate, enalapril (Vasotec), fosphenytoin (Cerebyx), propofol (Diprivan).

INDICATIONS/ROUTES/DOSAGE
Status Epilepticus
IV: ADULTS, ELDERLY: 10–20 mg/kg. May repeat dose in 20-min intervals. **Maximum total dose:** 30 mg/kg. **CHILDREN, INFANTS:** 15–20 mg/kg (**maximum:** 1,000 mg). May repeat q15–30min until seizures controlled or total dose of 40 mg/kg administered.

Seizure Control
PO, IV: ADULTS, ELDERLY, CHILDREN OLDER THAN 12 YRS: 1–3 mg/kg/day or 50–100 mg 2–3 times daily. **CHILDREN 6–12 YRS:** 4–6 mg/kg/day. **CHILDREN 1–5 YRS:** 6–8 mg/kg/day. **CHILDREN YOUNGER THAN 1 YR:** 5–8 mg/kg/day in 1–2 divided doses.

NEONATES: 3–4 mg/kg/day given once daily.

SIDE EFFECTS

Occasional (3%–1%): Drowsiness. **Rare (less than 1%):** Confusion, paradoxical CNS reactions (hyperactivity, anxiety in children; excitement, restlessness in elderly, generally noted during first 2 wks of therapy, particularly in presence of uncontrolled pain).

ADVERSE EFFECTS/ TOXIC REACTIONS

Abrupt withdrawal after prolonged therapy may produce increased dreaming, nightmares, insomnia, tremor, diaphoresis, vomiting, hallucinations, delirium, seizures, status epilepticus. Skin eruptions appear as hypersensitivity reaction. Blood dyscrasias, hepatic disease, hypocalcemia occur rarely. Overdose produces cold/clammy skin, hypothermia, severe CNS depression, cyanosis, tachycardia, Cheyne-Stokes respirations. Toxicity may result in severe renal impairment.

NURSING CONSIDERATIONS

BASELINE ASSESSMENT

Assess B/P, pulse, respirations immediately before administration. **Hypnotic:** Raise bed rails, provide environment conducive to sleep (back rub, quiet environment, low lighting). **Seizures:** Review history of seizure disorder (length, presence of auras, LOC). Observe frequently for recurrence of seizure activity. Initiate seizure precautions.

INTERVENTION/EVALUATION

Monitor CNS status, seizure activity, hepatic/renal function, respiratory rate, heart rate, B/P. Monitor for therapeutic serum level. **Therapeutic serum level:** 10–40 mcg/ml; **toxic serum level:** greater than 40 mcg/ml.

PATIENT/FAMILY TEACHING

• Avoid alcohol, limit caffeine. • May be habit forming. • Do not discontinue abruptly. • May cause dizziness/drowsiness; avoid tasks that require alertness, motor skills until response to drug is established.

phentolamine

fen-**tol**-a-meen
(OraVerse, Regitine ✦, Rogitine ✦)
Do not confuse phentolamine with Ventolin.

◆CLASSIFICATION

PHARMACOTHERAPEUTIC: Alpha-adrenergic blocking agent. **CLINICAL:** Antihypertensive agent.

ACTION

Blocks presynaptic (alpha$_2$), postsynaptic (alpha$_1$) adrenergic receptors, acting on arterial tree, venous bed. **Therapeutic Effect:** Decreases total peripheral resistance, diminishes venous return to heart.

PHARMACOKINETICS

Route	Onset	Peak	Duration
IM	15–20 min	20 min	30–45 min
IV	Immediate	2 min	15–30 min

Metabolized in liver. Excreted in urine. **Half-life:** 19 min.

USES

Diagnosis of pheochromocytoma. Control/prevention of hypertensive episodes in pts with pheochromocytoma immediately before, during surgical excision. Prevention/treatment of dermal necrosis, sloughing after IV administration of alpha-adrenergic drugs (e.g., norepinephrine/dopamine). **OFF-LABEL:** Pralidoxime-induced hypertension.

PRECAUTIONS

Contraindications: Renal impairment; coronary or cerebral arteriosclerosis; concurrent use of sildenafil, tadalafil, or vardenafil. **Cautions:** Gastritis, peptic ulcer, history of arrhythmias, MI.

⧗ LIFESPAN CONSIDERATIONS

Pregnancy/Lactation: Unknown if drug crosses placenta or is distributed in breast milk. **Pregnancy Category C. Children:** Safety and efficacy not established. **Elderly:** No age-related precautions noted.

INTERACTIONS

DRUG: None significant. **HERBAL: Yohimbe** may decrease effects. **FOOD:** None known. **LAB VALUES:** None significant.

AVAILABILITY (Rx)

Injection, Powder for Reconstitution: 5-mg vials. **Injection Solution (OraVerse):** 0.4 mg/1.7 ml.

ADMINISTRATION/HANDLING

◄**ALERT**► Maintain pt in supine position (preferably in quiet, darkened room) during pheochromocytoma testing. Decrease in B/P generally noted in less than 2 min.

 IV

Reconstitution • Reconstitute 5-mg vial with 1 ml Sterile Water for Injection to provide concentration of 5 mg/ml.
Rate of Administration • Pheochromocytoma: Inject each 5 mg over 1 min. Monitor B/P immediately after injection, q30sec for 3 min, then q60sec for 7 min.
Storage • Store vials at room temperature. • After reconstitution, stable for 48 hrs at room temperature or 1 wk if refrigerated.

⊞ IV INCOMPATIBILITIES

None known.

⊞ IV COMPATIBILITIES

Amiodarone (Cordarone), dobutamine (Dobutrex), verapamil (Calan), papaverine.

INDICATIONS/ROUTES/DOSAGE

Diagnosis of Pheochromocytoma
IM, IV: ADULTS, ELDERLY: 5 mg. **CHILDREN:** 0.05–0.1 mg/kg/dose. **Maximum:** 5 mg.

Control/Prevention of Hypertension in Pheochromocytoma
IV: ADULTS, ELDERLY: 5 mg 1–2 hrs before surgery. May repeat q2–4h. **CHILDREN:** 0.05–0.1 mg/kg/dose 1–2 hrs before surgery. May repeat q2–4h. **Maximum single dose:** 5 mg.

Prevention/Treatment of Tissue Necrosis/Sloughing
ADULTS, ELDERLY: Infiltrate area with 1 ml of solution (reconstituted by diluting 5–10 mg in 0.9% NaCl) within 12 hrs of extravasation. Infiltrate with multiple small injections using only 27- or 30-gauge needles; change needles between each skin entry. **CHILDREN:** 0.1–0.2 mg/kg diluted in 10 ml 0.9% NaCl infiltrated into area of extravasation within 12 hrs. If dose is effective, normal skin color should return within 1 hr. **Maximum:** 0.1–0.2 mg/kg or 5 mg total.

SIDE EFFECTS

Occasional (3%–2%): Weakness, dizziness, flushing, nausea, vomiting, diarrhea, orthostatic hypotension.

ADVERSE EFFECTS/TOXIC REACTIONS

Tachycardia, arrhythmias, acute/prolonged hypotension may occur. Do not use epinephrine (will produce further drop in B/P).

NURSING CONSIDERATIONS

BASELINE ASSESSMENT

Positive pheochromocytoma test indicated by decrease in B/P greater than 35 mm Hg systolic, greater than 25 mm Hg diastolic pressure. Negative test indicated by no change in B/P or elevation of B/P. B/P generally returns to baseline within 15–30 min following administration.

INTERVENTION/EVALUATION

Monitor B/P, heart rate. Assess for orthostatic hypotension. Monitor for extravasation (skin color streaking).

P

phenylephrine

fen-il-**ef**-rin
(AK-Dilate, Mydfrin, Neo-Synephrine,
Sudafed PE)

BLACK BOX ALERT Intravenous use
should be administered by adequately trained individuals familiar
with its use.
**Do not confuse Mydrin with
Midrin, or Sudafed PE with
Sudafed.**

◆CLASSIFICATION

PHARMACOTHERAPEUTIC: Sympathomimetic, alpha-receptor stimulant.
CLINICAL: Nasal decongestant, mydri-
atic, vasopressor (see p. 4C).

ACTION

Acts on alpha-adrenergic receptors of vascular smooth muscle. Causes vasoconstriction of arterioles of nasal mucosa/conjunc-
tiva, activates dilator muscle of pupil,
causing contraction, producing systemic
arterial vasoconstriction. **Therapeutic Effect:** Decreases mucosal blood flow, relieves congestion. Increases B/P.

PHARMACOKINETICS

Route	Onset	Peak	Duration
IV	Immediate	N/A	15–20 min
IM	10–15 min	N/A	0.5–2 hrs
Subcuta-neous	10–15 min	N/A	1 hr

Minimal absorption after intranasal, ophthalmic administration. Metabolized in
liver, GI tract. Primarily excreted in
urine. **Half-life:** 2.5 hrs.

USES

Nasal decongestant: Topical application
to nasal mucosa reduces nasal secretion,
promoting drainage of sinus secretions.
Ophthalmic: Topical application to conjunctiva relieves congestion, itching, minor
irritation; whitens sclera of eye. **Parenteral:** Vascular failure in shock, supraventricular tachycardia, hypotension.

PRECAUTIONS

Contraindications: (Systemic): Acute pancreatitis, heart disease, hepatitis, narrow-
angle glaucoma, pheochromocytoma, severe hypertension, thrombosis, asthma,
ventricular tachycardia, MAOIs within 2
wks. **(Ophthalmic):** Severe hypertension,
ventricular tachycardia, narrow-angle
glaucoma. **Cautions:** Hyperthyroidism, bradycardia, partial heart block, severe arteriosclerosis, myocardial disease.

⌛ LIFESPAN CONSIDERATIONS

Pregnancy/Lactation: Crosses placenta. Distributed in breast milk. **Pregnancy Category C. Children:** May exhibit
increased absorption, toxicity with nasal
preparation. No age-related precautions
noted with systemic use. **Elderly:** More
likely to experience adverse effects.

INTERACTIONS

DRUG: MAOIs may increase vasopressor
effects. **Tricyclic antidepressants** may
increase cardiovascular effects. **HERBAL:
Ephedra, yohimbe** may increase CNS
stimulation. **FOOD:** None known. **LAB
VALUES:** None significant.

AVAILABILITY (OTC)

Injection, Solution: 1% (10 mg/ml). **Solution, Nasal Drops (Neo-Synephrine):**
0.125%, 0.25%. **Solution, Nasal Spray
(Neo-Synephrine):** 0.25%, 0.5%, 1%. **Solution, Ophthalmic (AK-Dilate, Mydfrin, Neo-
Synephrine):** 0.12%, 2.5%, 10%. **Tablets
(Sudafed PE):** 10 mg.

ADMINISTRATION/HANDLING
IV

Reconstitution • For IV push, dilute
1 ml of 10 mg/ml solution with 9 ml Sterile
Water for Injection to provide concentration of 1 mg/ml. • For IV infusion, dilute
with 0.9% NaCl or D₅W. Usual concentration: 20–60 mcg/ml.
Rate of Administration • For IV push,
give over 20–30 sec. • For IV infusion,
titrate dose to maintain systolic B/P
greater than 90 mm Hg.

Storage • Store vials at room temperature.

Nasal
• Instruct pt to blow nose prior to administering medication. • With head tilted back, apply drops in 1 nostril. Wait 5 min before applying drops in other nostril. • Sprays should be administered into each nostril with head erect. • Pt should sniff briskly while squeezing container, then wait 3–5 min before blowing nose gently. • Rinse tip of spray bottle.

Ophthalmic
• Instruct pt to tilt head backward, look up. • Gently pull lower lid down to form pouch, then instill medication. • Do not touch tip of applicator to lids or any surface. • When lower lid is released, have pt keep eye open without blinking for at least 30 sec. • Apply gentle finger pressure to lacrimal sac (bridge of nose, inside corner of eye) for 1–2 min. • Remove excess solution around eye with tissue. • Wash hands immediately to remove medication on hands.

▧ IV INCOMPATIBILITY
Furosemide (Lasix).

▧ IV COMPATIBILITIES
Amiodarone (Cordarone), dexmedetomidine (Precedex), dobutamine (Dobutrex), lidocaine, potassium chloride, propofol (Diprivan), vasopressin.

INDICATIONS/ROUTES/DOSAGE
Nasal Decongestant
◀ALERT▶ Do not use for more than 3 days.
Intranasal: ADULTS, ELDERLY, CHILDREN 12 YRS AND OLDER: 1–2 drops or 1–2 sprays of 0.25%–0.5% solution into each nostril q4h as needed. **CHILDREN 6–11 YRS:** 1–2 drops or 1–2 sprays of 0.25% solution into each nostril q4h as needed. **CHILDREN 2–5 YRS:** 1 drop of 0.125% solution (dilute 0.5% solution with 0.9%

NaCl to achieve 0.125%) in each nostril. Repeat q2–4h as needed.
PO: ADULTS, ELDERLY, CHILDREN 13 YRS AND OLDER: 10 mg q4h as needed for up to 7 days. **CHILDREN 6–11 YRS:** 5 mg q4h as needed for up to 7 days. **CHILDREN 4–5 YRS:** 2.5 mg q4h as needed for up to 7 days.

Conjunctival Congestion, Itching, Minor Irritation
Ophthalmic: ADULTS, ELDERLY, CHILDREN 12 YRS AND OLDER: 1–2 drops of 0.12% solution q3–4h.

Hypotension, Shock
IV Bolus: ADULTS, ELDERLY: 0.1–0.5 mg/dose q10–15min as needed. **CHILDREN:** 5–20 mcg/kg/dose q10–15min as needed.
IV Infusion: ADULTS, ELDERLY: 100–180 mcg/min or 0.5 mcg/kg/min. Titrate to desired response. When B/P is stabilized, maintenance rate: 0.4–9.1 mcg/kg/min. **CHILDREN:** 0.1–0.5 mcg/kg/min. Titrate to desired effect.

SIDE EFFECTS
Frequent: Nasal: Rebound nasal congestion due to overuse, esp. when used longer than 3 days. **Occasional:** Mild CNS stimulation (restlessness, nervousness, tremors, headache, insomnia, particularly in those hypersensitive to sympathomimetics, such as elderly pts). **Nasal:** Stinging, burning, drying of nasal mucosa. **Ophthalmic:** Transient burning/stinging, brow ache, blurred vision.

ADVERSE EFFECTS/TOXIC REACTIONS
Large doses may produce tachycardia, palpitations (particularly in those with cardiac disease), dizziness, nausea, vomiting. Overdose in those older than 60 yrs may result in hallucinations, CNS depression, seizures. Prolonged nasal use may produce chronic swelling of nasal mucosa, rhinitis. If phenylephrine 10% ophthalmic is instilled into denuded/damaged corneal epithelium, corneal clouding may result.

P

✤ Canadian trade name   ▨ Non-Crushable Drug   ▧ High Alert drug

NURSING CONSIDERATIONS

BASELINE ASSESSMENT

Obtain baseline symptomology, vital signs.

INTERVENTION/EVALUATION

Monitor B/P, heart rate. For severe hypotension or shock states, monitor central venous pressure.

PATIENT/FAMILY TEACHING

• Discontinue drug if adverse reactions occur. • Do not use for nasal decongestion for longer than 5 days (rebound congestion). • Discontinue drug if insomnia, dizziness, weakness, tremor, palpitations occur. • **Nasal:** Stinging/burning of nasal mucosa may occur. • **Ophthalmic:** Blurring of vision with eye instillation generally subsides with continued therapy. • Discontinue medication if redness/swelling of eyelids, itching occurs.

---

phenytoin

fen-i-toyn
(Dilantin, Novo-Phenytoin ✦, Phenytek)
BLACK BOX ALERT Do not exceed IV rate of 50 mg/min in adults and 1–3 mg/kg/min in neonates.
Do not confuse Dilantin with Dilaudid or diltiazem, or phenytoin with phenelzine or fosphenytoin.

◆ CLASSIFICATION

PHARMACOTHERAPEUTIC: Hydantoin. **CLINICAL:** Anticonvulsant, antiarrhythmic (see p. 37C).

ACTION

Anticonvulsant: Stabilizes neuronal membranes in motor cortex. **Therapeutic Effect:** Limits spread of seizure activity. Stabilizes threshold against hyperexcitability. Decreases post-tetanic potentiation, repetitive discharge.

PHARMACOKINETICS

Slowly, variably absorbed after PO administration. Protein binding: 90%–95%. Widely distributed. Metabolized in liver. Primarily excreted in urine. Not removed by hemodialysis. **Half-life:** 7–42 hrs.

USES

PO: Management of generalized tonic-clonic seizures (grand mal), complex partial seizures, status epilepticus. Prevention of seizures following head trauma/neurosurgery. **IV:** Management of status epilepticus, prevention and treatment of seizures occurring during neurosurgery. **OFF-LABEL:** Simple partial seizures, ventricular arrhythmias, prevention of early post-traumatic seizures following traumatic brain injury.

PRECAUTIONS

Contraindications: Hypersensitivity to hydantoins, concurrent use of delavirdine, IV (additional), second- and third-degree AV block, sinoatrial block, sinus bradycardia, Adams-Stokes syndrome. **Cautions:** Porphyria, renal/hepatic impairment, those at increased risk of suicidal behavior/thoughts, elderly/debilitated pts, low serum albumin, underlying cardiac disease.

⌛ LIFESPAN CONSIDERATIONS

Pregnancy/Lactation: Crosses placenta; distributed in small amount in breast milk. Fetal hydantoin syndrome (craniofacial abnormalities, nail/digital hypoplasia, prenatal growth deficiency) has been reported. Increased frequency of seizures in pregnant women due to altered absorption of metabolism of phenytoin. May increase risk of hemorrhage in neonate, maternal bleeding during delivery. **Pregnancy Category D. Children:** More susceptible to gingival hyperplasia, coarsening of facial hair; excess body hair. **Elderly:** No age-related precautions noted but lower dosages recommended.

INTERACTIONS

DRUG: Alcohol, other CNS depressants may increase CNS depression. **Amiodarone, cimetidine, disulfiram, fluoxetine, isoniazid, sulfonamides** may increase concentration/effects, risk of toxicity. **Calcium-containing antacids** may decrease absorption. May decrease effects of **glucocorticoids, anticoagulants, oral contraceptives. Lidocaine, propranolol** may increase cardiac depressant effects. **Valproic acid** may decrease metabolism, increase concentration. May increase metabolism, decrease effect of **xanthines. HERBAL: Evening primrose** may decrease seizure threshold. **Gotu kola, kava kava, St. John's wort, valerian** may increase CNS depression. **FOOD:** None known. **LAB VALUES:** May increase serum glucose, GGT, alkaline phosphatase. **Therapeutic serum level:** 10–20 mcg/ml; **toxic serum level:** greater than 20 mcg/ml.

AVAILABILITY (Rx)

Capsules, Extended-Release (Dilantin): 30 mg, 100 mg. **(Phenytek):** 200 mg, 300 mg. **Injection, Solution (Dilantin):** 50 mg/ml. **Suspension, Oral (Dilantin):** 100 mg/4 ml, 125 mg/5 ml. **Tablets, Chewable (Dilantin):** 50 mg.

ADMINISTRATION/HANDLING

IV

◀**ALERT**▶ Give by IV push or IV piggyback. IV push very painful (chemical irritation of vein due to alkalinity of solution). To minimize effect, flush vein with sterile saline solution through same IV needle and catheter after each IV push.

Reconstitution • May give undiluted or may dilute with 0.9% NaCl to a concentration of 1–10 mg/ml.

Rate of Administration • Administer 50 mg over 2–3 min for elderly. In neonates, administer at rate not exceeding 1–3 mg/kg/min. • Severe hypotension, cardiovascular collapse occur if rate of IV injection exceeds 50

mg/min for adults. • IV toxicity characterized by CNS depression, cardiovascular collapse.

Storage • Precipitate may form if parenteral form is refrigerated (will dissolve at room temperature). • Slight yellow discoloration of parenteral form does not affect potency, but do not use if solution is cloudy or precipitate forms. Discard if not used within 4 hrs of preparation.

PO

• Give with food if GI distress occurs. • Tablets may be chewed. • Shake oral suspension well before using. • Separate administration of phenytoin with antacids or tube feeding by 2 hrs.

IV INCOMPATIBILITIES

Diltiazem (Cardizem), dobutamine (Dobutrex), enalapril (Vasotec), heparin, hydromorphone (Dilaudid), insulin, lidocaine, morphine, nitroglycerin, norepinephrine (Levophed), potassium chloride, propofol (Diprivan).

INDICATIONS/ROUTES/DOSAGE

Status Epilepticus
IV: ADULTS, ELDERLY, CHILDREN, NEONATES: Loading dose: 15–20 mg/kg. **Maintenance dose for adults and elderly:** IV/PO: 100 mg q6–8h. Range: 300–600 mg/day. **Maintenance dose for infants/children:** 5 mg/kg/day in 2–3 divided doses. **NEONATES:** Range: 4–8 mg/kg/day. **Maximum:** 300 mg/day.

Seizure Control
PO: ADULTS, ELDERLY, CHILDREN: Loading dose: 15–20 mg/kg in 3 divided doses 2–4 hrs apart. Maintenance dose: Same as for status epilepticus.

SIDE EFFECTS

Frequent: Drowsiness, lethargy, confusion, slurred speech, irritability, gingival hyperplasia, hypersensitivity reaction (fever, rash, lymphadenopathy), constipation, dizziness, nausea. **Occasional:** Headache, hirsutism, coarsening of facial features, insomnia, muscle twitching.

ADVERSE EFFECTS/ TOXIC REACTIONS

Abrupt withdrawal may precipitate status epilepticus. Blood dyscrasias, lymphadenopathy, osteomalacia (due to interference of vitamin D metabolism) may occur. Toxic phenytoin blood concentration (25 mcg/ml or more) may produce ataxia (muscular incoordination), nystagmus (rhythmic oscillation of eyes), diplopia. As level increases, extreme lethargy to comatose state occurs.

NURSING CONSIDERATIONS

BASELINE ASSESSMENT

Anticonvulsant: Review history of seizure disorder (intensity, frequency, duration, LOC). Initiate seizure precautions. Hepatic function tests, CBC should be performed before beginning therapy and periodically during therapy. Repeat CBC 2 wks following initiation of therapy and 2 wks following administration of maintenance dose.

INTERVENTION/EVALUATION

Observe frequently for recurrence of seizure activity. Assess for clinical improvement (decrease in intensity/frequency of seizures). Monitor for signs/symptoms of depression, suicidal tendencies, unusual behavior. Monitor CBC with differential, hepatic/renal function tests, B/P (with IV use). Assist with ambulation if drowsiness, lethargy occurs. Monitor for therapeutic serum level (10–20 mcg/ml). **Therapeutic serum level:** 10–20 mcg/ml; **toxic serum level:** greater than 20 mcg/ml.

PATIENT/FAMILY TEACHING

• Pain may occur with IV injection. • To prevent gingival hyperplasia (bleeding, tenderness, swelling of gums), maintain good oral hygiene, gum massage, regular dental visits. • Blood counts should be performed every mo for 1 yr after maintenance dose is established and q3mos thereafter. • Report sore throat, fever, glandular swelling, skin reaction (hema-

tologic toxicity). • Drowsiness usually diminishes with continued therapy. • Avoid tasks that require alertness, motor skills until response to drug is established. • Do not abruptly withdraw medication after long-term use (may precipitate seizures). • Strict maintenance of drug therapy is essential for seizure control, arrhythmias. • Avoid alcohol. • Report any unusual changes in behavior.

phosphates potassium sodium

fos-fates

◆CLASSIFICATION

PHARMACOTHERAPEUTIC: Electrolyte supplement. **CLINICAL:** Mineral.

ACTION

Active in bone deposition, calcium metabolism, utilization of B complex vitamins. Acts as buffers in maintaining acid-base balance. Exerts osmotic effect in small intestine. **Therapeutic Effect:** Corrects hypophosphatemia, acidifies urine, prevents calcium deposits in urinary tract, promotes peristalsis in GI tract.

PHARMACOKINETICS

Poorly absorbed after PO administration. PO form excreted in feces; IV form excreted in urine.

USES

Prevention and treatment of hypophosphatemia.

PRECAUTIONS

Contraindications: Hyperkalemia, hypernatremia, hyperphosphatemia, hypocalcemia, hypomagnesemia, severe renal impairment. **Cautions:** Renal impairment, concomitant use of potassium-sparing drugs, acid-base alteration, digitalized pts.

⚥ LIFESPAN CONSIDERATIONS

Pregnancy/Lactation: Unknown if drug crosses placenta or is distributed in breast milk. **Pregnancy Category C. Children:** Increased risk of dehydration in those younger than 12 yrs. **Elderly:** No age-related precautions noted.

INTERACTIONS

DRUG: ACE inhibitors, NSAIDs, potassium-containing medications, potassium-sparing diuretics, salt substitutes containing potassium phosphate may increase serum potassium. **Antacids** may decrease absorption. **Calcium-containing medications** may increase risk of calcium deposition in soft tissues, decrease phosphate absorption. **HERBAL:** None significant. **FOOD:** None known. **LAB VALUES:** None significant.

AVAILABILITY (Rx)

Injection Solution (Potassium Phosphate): 3 mmol phosphate and 4.4 mEq potassium per ml. **Injection Solution (Sodium Phosphate):** 3 mmol phosphate and 4 mEq sodium per ml.

ADMINISTRATION/HANDLING

 IV

Reconstitution • Must be diluted. Soluble in all commonly used IV solutions. **Rate of Administration •** Infuse over minimum of 4 hrs (usually over 6 hrs). Maximum rate: 0.06 mmol/kg/hr. **Storage •** Store at room temperature.

🜄 IV INCOMPATIBILITY

Amiodarone, dobutamine (Dobutrex), pantoprazole (Protonix).

🜄 IV COMPATIBILITIES

Diltiazem (Cardizem), enalapril (Vasotec), famotidine (Pepcid), metoclopramide (Reglan), nicardipine (Cardene).

INDICATIONS/ROUTES/DOSAGE

Hypophosphatemia
Potassium/Sodium Phosphate: (Phosphate level 2.3–3 mg/dL): 0.16–0.32 mmol/kg over 4–6 hr. (Phosphate level 1.6–22 mg/dL): 0.32–0.64 mmol/kg over 4–6 hr. (Phosphate level <1.5 mg/dL): 0.64–1 mmol/kg over 8–12 hr.

SIDE EFFECTS

Frequent: Mild laxative effect (in first few days of therapy). **Occasional:** Diarrhea, nausea, abdominal pain, vomiting. **Rare:** Headache, dizziness, confusion, heaviness of lower extremities, fatigue, muscle cramps, paresthesia, peripheral edema, arrhythmias, weight gain, thirst.

ADVERSE EFFECTS/ TOXIC REACTIONS

Hyperphosphatemia may produce extraskeletal calcification.

NURSING CONSIDERATIONS

INTERVENTION/EVALUATION

Routinely monitor serum calcium, phosphorus, potassium, sodium, AST, ALT, alkaline phosphatase, bilirubin.

PATIENT/FAMILY TEACHING

• Report diarrhea, nausea, vomiting.

---

pimecrolimus

pim-e-**kroe**-li-mus
(Elidel)

BLACK BOX ALERT Rare cases of lymphoma, skin malignancy have occurred. Use only for short-term, intermittent treatment using minimum amount needed. Not recommended in children younger than 2 yrs.

Do not confuse Elidel with Elavil, or pimecrolimus with tacrolimus.

◆CLASSIFICATION

PHARMACOTHERAPEUTIC: Immunomodulator. **CLINICAL:** Anti-inflammatory.

ACTION

Inhibits release of cytokine, an enzyme that produces an inflammatory reaction. **Therapeutic Effect:** Produces anti-inflammatory activity.

USES

Treatment of mild to moderate atopic dermatitis (eczema).

PRECAUTIONS

Contraindications: Active cutaneous viral infection, application on malignant or premalignant skin conditions. **Cautions:** Immunocompromised pts.

⌛ LIFESPAN CONSIDERATIONS

Pregnancy/Lactation: Embryotoxic. Unknown if distributed in breast milk. **Pregnancy Category C. Children:** May be used in those 2 yrs and older. **Elderly:** No age-related precautions noted.

INTERACTIONS

DRUG: None significant. **HERBAL:** None significant. **FOOD:** None known. **LAB VALUES:** None significant.

AVAILABILITY (Rx)

Topical: 1% cream.

INDICATIONS/ROUTES/DOSAGE

Atopic Dermatitis (Eczema)
Topical: ADULTS, ELDERLY, CHILDREN 2–17 YRS: Apply to affected area twice daily. Rub in gently, completely. Reevaluate if symptoms persist for more than 6 wks.

SIDE EFFECTS

Rare: Transient sensation of burning/feeling of heat at application site.

ADVERSE EFFECTS/TOXIC REACTIONS

Lymphadenopathy, phototoxicity occur rarely.

NURSING CONSIDERATIONS

PATIENT/FAMILY TEACHING

• Wash hands after application. • May cause mild to moderate feeling of warmth, sensation of burning at application site. • Inform physician if application site reaction is severe or lasts for longer than 1 wk. • Avoid exposure to sunlight, artificial sunlight, tanning beds. • Report if no improvement in atopic dermatitis is seen following 6 wks of treatment or if condition worsens.

---

pioglitazone

pie-oh-**glit**-a-zone
(<u>Actos</u>, Apo-Pioglitazone ✦,
Novo-Pioglitazone ✦)
BLACK BOX ALERT May cause or exacerbate HF.
Do not confuse Actos with Actidose or Actonel.

FIXED-COMBINATION(S)

Actoplus Met: pioglitazone/metformin (an antidiabetic): 15 mg/500 mg, 15 mg/850 mg. **Duetact:** pioglitazone/glimepiride (an antidiabetic): 30 mg/2 mg, 30 mg/4 mg. **Oseni:** pioglitazone/alogliptin (an antidiabetic): 15 mg/25 mg, 30 mg/25 mg, 45 mg/25 mg, 15 mg/12.5 mg, 30 mg/12.5 mg, 45 mg/12.5 mg.

◆CLASSIFICATION

PHARMACOTHERAPEUTIC: Thiazolidinedione antidiabetic. **CLINICAL:** Antidiabetic agent (see p. 45C).

ACTION

Improves target-cell response to insulin without increasing pancreatic insulin secretion. Decreases hepatic glucose output, increases insulin-dependent glucose utilization in skeletal muscle. **Therapeutic Effect:** Lowers serum glucose concentration.

PHARMACOKINETICS

Rapidly absorbed. Protein binding: 99%. Metabolized in liver. Excreted in urine. Unknown if removed by hemodialysis. **Half-life:** 16–24 hrs.

USES

Adjunct to diet and exercise to lower serum glucose in those with type 2 non–insulin-dependent diabetes mellitus (NIDDM). Used as monotherapy or combination therapy.

PRECAUTIONS

Contraindications: NYHA class III/IV heart failure (at initiation of therapy). **Cautions:** Hepatic impairment, active liver disease, anemia. For premenopausal, anovulatory women may result in ovulation resumption, increase risk of pregnancy.

⌛ LIFESPAN CONSIDERATIONS

Pregnancy/Lactation: Unknown if drug crosses placenta or is distributed in breast milk. Not recommended in pregnant or breastfeeding women. **Pregnancy Category C. Children:** Safety and efficacy not established. **Elderly:** No age-related precautions noted.

INTERACTIONS

DRUG: CYP2C8 inhibitors (e.g., gemfibrozil) may increase concentration/effects. **CYP2C8 inducers (e.g., rifampin)** may decrease concentration. **HERBAL: Garlic, ginger, ginseng** may cause hypoglycemia. **FOOD:** None known. **LAB VALUES:** May increase serum creatine kinase (CK). May decrease Hgb (by 2%–4%). May increase serum alkaline phosphatase, bilirubin, ALT. Less than 1% of pts experience ALT values 3 times the normal level.

AVAILABILITY (Rx)

Tablets: 15 mg, 30 mg, 45 mg.

ADMINISTRATION/HANDLING

PO
• Give without regard to meals.

INDICATIONS/ROUTES/DOSAGE

Diabetes Mellitus
PO: ADULTS, ELDERLY: 15–30 mg once daily.

Dosage Adjustment in HF
Note: Not recommended in pts with symptomatic heart failure.
PO: ADULTS, ELDERLY: 15 mg once a day.

SIDE EFFECTS

Frequent (13%–9%): Headache, upper respiratory tract infection. **Occasional (6%–5%):** Sinusitis, myalgia, pharyngitis, aggravated diabetes mellitus.

ADVERSE EFFECTS/TOXIC REACTIONS

Hepatotoxicity occurs rarely. May cause/worsen macular edema. Increased risk of HF. May increase risk of fractures. Pts with ischemic heart disease are at high risk of MI.

NURSING CONSIDERATIONS

BASELINE ASSESSMENT

Obtain baseline chemistries, esp. hepatic function test, before initiating therapy and periodically thereafter.

INTERVENTION/EVALUATION

Monitor serum glucose, Hgb A1c, hepatic function tests. Assess for hypoglycemia (cool/wet skin, tremors, dizziness, anxiety, headache, tachycardia, numbness in mouth, hunger, diplopia), hyperglycemia (polyuria, polyphagia, polydipsia, nausea, vomiting, dim vision, fatigue, deep rapid breathing). Be alert to conditions that alter serum glucose requirements: fever, increased activity, trauma, stress, surgical procedures. Monitor for signs/symptoms of HF.

PATIENT/FAMILY TEACHING

• Be alert for signs/symptoms of hypoglycemia and take measures to manage it. • Avoid alcohol. • Inform physician of chest pain, palpitations, abdominal pain, fever, rash, hypoglyce-

P

mic reactions, yellowing of skin/eyes, dark urine, light stool, nausea, vomiting. • Report any change in vision. • Report rapid weight gain, edema, difficulty breathing. • Ensure follow-up instruction if pt, family do not thoroughly understand diabetes management, glucose-testing technique.

piperacillin sodium/tazobactam sodium

TOP 200

pye-per-a-**sil**-in/tay-zoe-**bak**-tam (Tazocin ✦, Zosyn).
Do not confuse Zosyn with Zofran or Zyvox.

◆ CLASSIFICATION

PHARMACOTHERAPEUTIC: Penicillin.
CLINICAL: Antibiotic (see p. 30C).

ACTION

Piperacillin: Inhibits cell wall synthesis by binding to bacterial cell membranes. **Therapeutic Effect:** Bactericidal. **Tazobactam:** Inactivates bacterial beta-lactamase. **Therapeutic Effect:** Protects piperacillin from enzymatic degradation, extends its spectrum of activity, prevents bacterial overgrowth.

PHARMACOKINETICS

Protein binding: 16%–30%. Widely distributed. Primarily excreted unchanged in urine. Removed by hemodialysis. **Half-life:** 0.7–1.2 hrs (increased in hepatic cirrhosis, renal impairment).

USES

Treatment of appendicitis (complicated by rupture, abscess), peritonitis, uncomplicated and complicated skin/skin structure infections, including cellulitis, cutaneous abscesses, ischemic/diabetic foot infections, postpartum endometritis, pelvic inflammatory disease (PID), community-acquired pneumonia (moderate severity only), moderate to severe nosocomial pneumonia. Tazobactam expands, piperacillin activity to include beta-lactamase-producing strains of *S. aureus, H. influenzae, Bacteroides.* **OFF-LABEL:** Treatment of UTI, bone and joint infections, septicemia, endocarditis, cystic fibrosis exacerbations.

PRECAUTIONS

Contraindications: Hypersensitivity to any penicillin. **Cautions:** History of allergies (esp. cephalosporins, other drugs), renal impairment, preexisting seizure disorder.

⌛ LIFESPAN CONSIDERATIONS

Pregnancy/Lactation: Readily crosses placenta; appears in cord blood, amniotic fluid. Distributed in breast milk in low concentrations. May lead to allergic sensitization, diarrhea, candidiasis, skin rash in infant. **Pregnancy Category B. Children:** Dosage not established for those younger than 12 yrs. **Elderly:** Age-related renal impairment may require dosage adjustment.

INTERACTIONS

DRUG: Concurrent use of **aminoglycosides** may cause mutual inactivation (must give at least 1 hr apart). May increase concentration, toxicity of **methotrexate. Probenecid** may increase concentration, risk of toxicity. High-dose piperacillin may increase risk of bleeding with **heparin, NSAIDs, platelet inhibitors, thrombolytic agents, warfarin. HERBAL:** None significant. **FOOD:** None known. **LAB VALUES:** May increase serum sodium, alkaline phosphatase, bilirubin, LDH, AST, ALT, BUN, creatinine, PT, PTT. May decrease serum potassium. May cause positive Coombs' test.

AVAILABILITY (Rx)

◀**ALERT**▶ Piperacillin/tazobactam is a combination product in an 8:1 ratio of piperacillin to tazobactam. **Injection Powder:** 2.25 g, 3.375 g, 4.5 g. **Premix Ready to Use:** 2.25 g (50 ml), 3.375 g (50 ml), 4.5 g (100 ml).

P

ADMINISTRATION/HANDLING

IV

Reconstitution • Reconstitute each 1 g with 5 ml D_5W or 0.9% NaCl. Shake vigorously to dissolve. • Further dilute with at least 50 ml D_5W or 0.9% NaCl.
Rate of Administration • Infuse over 30 min. Expanded infusion over 3–4 hrs.
Storage • Reconstituted vial is stable for 24 hrs at room temperature or 48 hrs if refrigerated. • After further dilution, stable for 24 hrs at room temperature or 7 days if refrigerated.

IV INCOMPATIBILITIES

Amphotericin B (Fungizone), amphotericin B complex (Abelcet, AmBisome, Amphotec), famotidine (Pepcid), haloperidol (Haldol), hydroxyzine (Vistaril), vancomycin (Vancocin).

IV COMPATIBILITIES

Bumetanide (Bumex), calcium gluconate, dexmedetomidine (Precedex), diphenhydramine (Benadryl), dopamine (Intropin), enalapril (Vasotec), furosemide (Lasix), granisetron (Kytril), heparin, hydrocortisone (Solu-Cortef), hydromorphone (Dilaudid), lorazepam (Ativan), magnesium sulfate, methylprednisolone (Solu-Medrol), metoclopramide (Reglan), morphine, ondansetron (Zofran), potassium chloride.

INDICATIONS/ROUTES/DOSAGE

Severe Infections
IV: **ADULTS, ELDERLY, CHILDREN 12 YRS AND OLDER:** 4.5 g q6–8h or 3.375 g q6h. **Maximum:** 18 g daily. **CHILDREN 9 MOS AND OLDER AND 40 KG OR LESS:** 100 mg piperacillin component/kg/dose q8h. **CHILDREN 2–8 MOS:** 80 mg piperacillin component/kg/dose q8h. **NEONATES:** 75 mg piperacillin component/kg/dose q6–12h.

Dosage in Renal Impairment
Dosage and frequency are modified based on creatinine clearance.

Creatinine Clearance	Dosage
20–40 ml/min	2.25 g q6h (3.375 g q6h for nosocomial pneumonia)
Less than 20 ml/min	2.25 g q8h (2.25 g q6h for nosocomial pneumonia)

Dosage for Hemodialysis
IV: **ADULTS, ELDERLY:** 2.25 g q8–12h with additional dose of 0.75 g after each dialysis session.

Dosage for CRRT

CVVH	2.25–3.375 g q6–8h
CVVHD	2.25–3.375 g q6h
CVVHDF	3.375 g q6h

SIDE EFFECTS

Frequent: Diarrhea, headache, constipation, nausea, insomnia, rash. **Occasional:** Vomiting, dyspepsia (heartburn, indigestion, epigastric pain), pruritus, fever, agitation, candidiasis, dizziness, abdominal pain, edema, anxiety, dyspnea, rhinitis.

ADVERSE EFFECTS/ TOXIC REACTIONS

Antibiotic-associated colitis, other superinfections (abdominal cramps, severe watery diarrhea, fever) may result from altered bacterial balance in GI tract. Overdose, more often with renal impairment, may produce seizures, neurologic reactions. Severe hypersensitivity reactions, including anaphylaxis, occur rarely.

NURSING CONSIDERATIONS

BASELINE ASSESSMENT
Question for history of allergies, esp. to penicillins, cephalosporins.

INTERVENTION/EVALUATION
Monitor daily pattern of bowel activity, stool consistency; mild GI effects may be tolerable, but increasing severity may indicate onset of antibiotic-associated coli-

P

tis. Be alert for superinfection: fever, vomiting, diarrhea, anal/genital pruritus, oral mucosal changes (ulceration, pain, erythema). Monitor I&O, urinalysis. Monitor serum electrolytes, esp. potassium, renal function tests.

piroxicam

peer-**ox**-i-kam
(Apo-Piroxicam ✦, Feldene, Novo-Pirocam ✦)

BLACK BOX ALERT May increase risk of serious, potentially fatal cardiovascular thrombotic events, MI, stroke. Increased risk of serious GI events (bleeding, ulceration, perforation).

Do not confuse Feldene with fluoxetine, or piroxicam with paroxetine.

◆CLASSIFICATION

PHARMACOTHERAPEUTIC: NSAID.
CLINICAL: Anti-inflammatory, analgesic (see p. 130C).

ACTION

Produces analgesic, anti-inflammatory effects by inhibiting prostaglandin synthesis. **Therapeutic Effect:** Reduces inflammatory response, intensity of pain.

PHARMACOKINETICS

Route	Onset	Peak	Duration
PO	1 hr	3–5 hrs	—

Well absorbed following PO administration. Protein binding: 99%. Metabolized in liver. Primarily excreted in urine; small amount eliminated in feces. **Half-life:** 50 hrs.

USES

Symptomatic treatment of acute or chronic rheumatoid arthritis (RA), osteoarthritis.

PRECAUTIONS

Contraindications: Perioperative pain in setting of CABG surgery, history of hypersensitivity to aspirin/NSAIDs, active GI bleeding. **Cautions:** Advanced renal disease, hepatic impairment, asthma, coagulation disorders, concomitant use of anticoagulants, poor CYP2C9 metabolizers.

⧖ LIFESPAN CONSIDERATIONS

Pregnancy/Lactation: Crosses placenta; distributed in breast milk. Avoid use during third trimester (may adversely affect fetal cardiovascular system: premature closing of ductus arteriosus). **Pregnancy Category C (D if used in third trimester or near delivery). Children:** Safety and efficacy not established. **Elderly:** Age-related renal impairment may increase risk of hepatotoxicity, renal toxicity; reduced dosage recommended. More likely to have serious adverse effects with GI bleeding/ulceration.

INTERACTIONS

DRUG: May decrease effects of **antihypertensives, diuretics. Aspirin, other salicylates** may increase risk of GI side effects, bleeding. May increase effects of **heparin, oral anticoagulants, thrombolytics.** May increase concentration, risk of toxicity of **lithium, methotrexate. HERBAL: Cat's claw, dong quai, evening primrose, feverfew, garlic, ginger, ginkgo, ginseng, horse chestnut, red clover** possess antiplatelet activity, may increase risk of bleeding. **St. John's wort** may increase risk of phototoxicity. **FOOD:** None known. **LAB VALUES:** May increase BUN, serum creatinine, LDH, alkaline phosphatase, AST, ALT. May decrease serum uric acid, Hgb, Hct, platelets, leukocytes.

AVAILABILITY (Rx)

🖤 **Capsules:** 10 mg, 20 mg.

ADMINISTRATION/HANDLING

PO
• Do not crush/break capsules. • May give with food, milk, antacids if GI distress occurs.

INDICATIONS/ROUTES/DOSAGE

Rheumatoid Arthritis (RA), Osteoarthritis
PO: ADULTS, ELDERLY: Initially, 10–20 mg/
day as a single dose or in divided doses.
Some pts may require up to 30–40 mg/
day. **CHILDREN:** 0.2–0.4 mg/kg/day. **Maximum:** 15 mg/day.

SIDE EFFECTS

Frequent (9%–4%): Dyspepsia (heartburn,
indigestion, epigastric pain), nausea, dizziness. **Occasional (3%–1%):** Diarrhea,
constipation, abdominal cramps/pain,
flatulence, stomatitis. **Rare (less than 1%):**
Hypertension, urticaria, dysuria, ecchymosis, blurred vision, insomnia, photo-toxicity.

ADVERSE EFFECTS/ TOXIC REACTIONS

Peptic ulcer, GI bleeding, gastritis, severe
hepatic reaction (cholestasis, jaundice)
occur rarely. Nephrotoxicity (dysuria,
hematuria, proteinuria, nephrotic syndrome), hematologic toxicity (anemia,
leukopenia, eosinophilia, thrombocytopenia), severe hypersensitivity reaction
(fever, chills, bronchospasm) occur
rarely with long-term treatment.

NURSING CONSIDERATIONS

BASELINE ASSESSMENT

Assess onset, type, location, duration of
pain/inflammation. Inspect appearance
of affected joints for immobility, deformities, skin condition.

INTERVENTION/EVALUATION

Monitor daily pattern of bowel activity,
stool consistency. Monitor for evidence of
nausea, GI distress. Assess for therapeutic
response: relief of pain, stiffness, swelling;
increased joint mobility; reduced joint
tenderness; improved grip strength. Monitor CBC, renal/hepatic function tests.

PATIENT/FAMILY TEACHING

• Avoid aspirin, alcohol during therapy
(increases risk of GI bleeding). • If GI
upset occurs, take with food, milk, antacids. • Avoid tasks that require alertness
until response to drug is established.

pitavastatin

pit-a-va-**stat**-in
(Livalo)
**Do not confuse pitavastatin with
atorvastatin, lovastatin, pravastatin, or simvastatin.**

◆CLASSIFICATION

PHARMACOTHERAPEUTIC: HMG-CoA
reductase inhibitor. **CLINICAL:** Antihyperlipidemic (see p. 58C).

ACTION

Interferes with cholesterol biosynthesis
by inhibiting conversion of HMG-CoA reductase to a precursor to cholesterol.
Therapeutic Effect: Lowers total cholesterol, LDL cholesterol, apolipoprotein
B (Apo B), plasma triglycerides; increases HDL cholesterol.

PHARMACOKINETICS

Poorly absorbed from GI tract. Protein
binding: greater than 99%. Metabolized
in liver. Primarily excreted in feces via
biliary system. **Half-life:** 12 hrs.

USES

Reduces elevated total cholesterol, low-density lipoproteins (LDLs), apolipoprotein B, triglycerides; increases low
high-density lipoproteins (HDLs) in primary hyperlipidemia and mixed dyslipidemia.

PRECAUTIONS

Contraindications: Active hepatic disease
persistent or unexplained elevations of
hepatic function tests; concurrent cyclosporine use, pregnancy, breastfeeding.
Cautions: History of hepatic disease, substantial alcohol consumption, moderate
renal impairment. Withholding/discontinuing pitavastatin may be necessary

P

when pt at risk for renal failure. Pts at risk for myopathy: advanced age, renal impairment, inadequately treated hypothyroidism.

⌛ LIFESPAN CONSIDERATIONS

Pregnancy/Lactation: Contraindicated in pregnancy (suppression of cholesterol biosynthesis may cause fetal toxicity) and lactation. Unknown if drug is distributed in breast milk (risk of serious adverse reactions in nursing infants). **Pregnancy Category X. Children:** Safety and efficacy not established in those younger than 18 yrs. **Elderly:** No age-related precautions noted.

INTERACTIONS:

DRUG: Increased risk of rhabdomyolysis, acute renal failure with **gemfibrozil, niacin, other fibrates. Cyclosporine, erythromycin, rifampin** significantly increase serum pitavastatin levels. **HERBAL:** None significant. **FOOD:** None known. **LAB VALUES:** May increase serum creatine kinase (CPK), AST, ALT concentrations.

AVAILABILITY (Rx)

Tablets: 1 mg, 2 mg, 4 mg.

ADMINISTRATION/HANDLING

PO
• Give without regard to meals or time of day.

INDICATIONS/ROUTES/DOSAGE

◄**ALERT**► Before initiating therapy, pt should be on standard cholesterol-lowering diet for minimum of 3–6 mos. Continue diet throughout pitavastatin therapy.

Usual Dosage
PO: ADULTS: Initially, 2 mg/day. **Maximum:** 4 mg/day. **Range:** 1–4 mg/day. **Dosage with erythromycin:** 1 mg/day; with rifampin: 2 mg/day.

Dosage in Renal Impairment
CrCl 15–59 or end-stage renal disease in pts on hemodialysis: Initially, 1 mg/day. **Maximum:** 2 mg/day. **Severe**

renal disease not on hemodialysis: Not recommended.

SIDE EFFECTS

Generally well tolerated. Side effects usually mild and transient. **Rare (Less Than 4%):** Myalgia, constipation/diarrhea, back/extremity pain, arthralgia, headache, nasopharyngitis.

ADVERSE EFFECTS/TOXIC REACTIONS

Hypersensitivity (rash, pruritus, urticaria) occurs rarely.

NURSING CONSIDERATIONS

BASELINE ASSESSMENT

Question for possibility of pregnancy before initiating therapy (Pregnancy Category X). Assess baseline lab results: cholesterol, triglycerides, hepatic function tests.

INTERVENTION/EVALUATION

Monitor cholesterol and triglyceride levels. Monitor hepatic function tests. Monitor daily pattern of bowel activity, stool consistency. Check for myalgia, arthralgia, headache. Assess for rash, pruritus. Be alert for malaise, muscle cramping/weakness.

PATIENT/FAMILY TEACHING

• Follow special diet (important part of treatment). • Periodic lab tests are essential part of therapy. • Report promptly any muscle pain/weakness. • Use nonhormonal contraception.

plerixafor

pler-**ix**-a-for
(Mozobil)

◆CLASSIFICATION

PHARMACOTHERAPEUTIC: Chemokine receptor inhibitor. **CLINICAL:** Hematopoietic stem cell mobilizer.

P

ACTION

Immobilizes hematopoietic stem cells in bone marrow. Once in the marrow, acts to help anchor these cells to marrow matrix through induction of adhesion molecules. **Therapeutic Effect:** Results in leukocytosis, elevation in circulating hematopoietic progenitor cells in peripheral blood system.

PHARMACOKINETICS

Readily absorbed after subcutaneous administration. Generally confines to extravascular fluid space. Protein binding: 58%. Peak plasma concentration: 30–60 min. Eliminated in urine. Clearance reduced with renal impairment. **Half-life:** 3–5 hrs.

USES

Indicated in combination with granulocyte colony-stimulating factor (G-CSF) to mobilize stem cells to peripheral blood for collection and transplantation in pts with non-Hodgkin's lymphoma and multiple myeloma.

PRECAUTIONS

Contraindications: None known. **Cautions:** Avoid use in leukemic pts, in pts with neutrophil count greater than 50,000/mm^3, those with renal impairment.

⧗ LIFESPAN CONSIDERATIONS

Pregnancy/Lactation: Potential for teratogenic effects. May cause fetal harm. **Pregnancy Category D. Children:** Safety and efficacy not established. **Elderly:** Age-related renal impairment may require dosage adjustment.

INTERACTIONS

DRUG: None significant. **HERBAL:** None significant. **FOOD:** None known. **LAB VALUES:** May increase WBC count. May decrease platelet count.

AVAILABILITY (Rx)

Injection Solution: 20 mg/ml (1.2-ml vial).

ADMINISTRATION/HANDLING

Subcutaneous
• Aspirate syringe before injection (avoid intra-arterial administration).
Storage • Store at room temperature.
• Discard if particulate matter is present or if solution is discolored. • Use single-dose vial; discard unused drug.

INDICATIONS/ROUTES/DOSAGE

◀**ALERT**▶ Begin therapy after pt has received daily morning doses of G-CSF, 10 mcg/kg once daily for 4 days prior to the first evening dose of plerixafor and approximately 11 hrs prior to initiation of apheresis for up to 4 consecutive days.

Daily Dosage
Subcutaneous: ADULTS, ELDERLY: 0.24 mg/kg using following formula: 0.012 × pt's actual body weight (in kg) = volume to be administered (in ml). **Maximum:** 40 mg/day.

Moderate to Severe Renal Impairment (Creatinine Clearance Equal to or Less Than 50 ml/min):
Subcutaneous: ADULTS, ELDERLY: Decrease dose by one-third to 0.16 mg/kg, not to exceed 27 mg/day.

SIDE EFFECTS

Frequent (37%–22%): Diarrhea, nausea, injection site irritation, fatigue, headache. **Occasional (13%–7%):** Arthralgia, dizziness, vomiting, insomnia, flatulence.

ADVERSE EFFECTS/TOXIC REACTIONS

Thrombocytopenia may occur. Dyspnea, hypoxia, vasovagal reaction, periorbital edema, urticaria have been noted; may resolve spontaneously, generally responds to antihistamines, corticosteroids.

NURSING CONSIDERATIONS

BASELINE ASSESSMENT
Obtain baseline CBC.

P

INTERVENTION/EVALUATION

Monitor WBC, platelet count. Assess for potential systemic reaction (periorbital edema, dyspnea, urticaria), orthostatic hypotension during or shortly after injection. Advise female pt with reproductive potential to use effective contraceptive method (Pregnancy Category D).

PATIENT/FAMILY TEACHING

• Manage gastrointestinal disorders; report severe diarrhea, nausea, vomiting. • Report upper quadrant pain or scapular/shoulder pain.

---

polyethylene glycol

TOP 200

polyethylene glycol-electrolyte solution (PEG-ES) (CoLyte, GoLYTELY)

poly-**eth**-ah-leen **glye**-col
(CoLyte, GoLYTELY, Klean-Prep ✷,
MiraLax, NuLytely, Peglyte ✷, TriLyte)
Do not confuse MiraLax with Mirapex.

◆ CLASSIFICATION

PHARMACOTHERAPEUTIC: Laxative.
CLINICAL: Bowel evacuant (see p. 126C).

ACTION

Osmotic effect. **Therapeutic Effect:** Induces diarrhea, cleanses bowel without depleting electrolytes.

PHARMACOKINETICS

Route	Onset	Peak	Duration
PO (bowel cleansing)	1–2 hrs	N/A	N/A
PO (constipation)	2–4 days	N/A	N/A

USES

Polyethylene glycol-electrolyte solution: Bowel cleansing before GI examination, colon surgery. **Polyethylene glycol:** Treatment of occasional constipation.

PRECAUTIONS

Contraindications: Bowel perforation, gastric retention, GI obstruction, megacolon, toxic colitis, toxic ileus. **Cautions: (Propylene glycol):** Renal impairment. **(Propylene glycol–electrolyte solution):** Ulcerative colitis, medications altering electrolytes, hyponatremia, cardiac arrhythmias, impaired gag reflex.

⌛ LIFESPAN CONSIDERATIONS

Pregnancy/Lactation: Unknown if drug crosses placenta or is distributed in breast milk. **Pregnancy Category C. Children/Elderly:** No age-related precautions noted.

INTERACTIONS

DRUG: May decrease absorption of **oral medications** if given within 1 hr (may be flushed from GI tract). **HERBAL:** None significant. **FOOD:** None known. **LAB VALUES:** None significant.

AVAILABILITY (Rx)

Powder for Oral Solution: Propylene glycol (Miralax): 17 g/dose. **Propylene glycol–electrolyte solution (CoLyte, GoLYTELY):** See individual product for specific ingredients.

ADMINISTRATION/HANDLING

PO

Polyethylene glycol-electrolyte solution

• Refrigerate reconstituted solutions; use within 48 hrs. • May use tap water to prepare solution. Shake vigorously for several min to ensure complete dissolution of powder. • Fasting should occur for more than 3 hrs prior to ingestion of solution (always avoid solid food less than 2 hrs prior to administration). • Only clear liquids permitted after administration. • May give via NG tube. • Rapid drinking preferred. Chilled solution is more palatable.

Polyethylene glycol
• Add to 4- to 8-oz beverage.

INDICATIONS/ROUTES/DOSAGE

Bowel Evacuant
PO: ADULTS, ELDERLY: Before GI examination: 240 ml (8 oz) q10min until 4 liters consumed or rectal effluent clear. NG tube: 20–30 ml/min until 4 liters given. **CHILDREN 6 MOS AND OLDER:** 25–40 ml/kg/hr until rectal effluent clear. **Maximum:** 4 L.

Constipation
PO (Miralax): ADULTS: 17 g or 1 heaping tbsp a day. **CHILDREN 6 MOS AND OLDER:** 0.5–1.5 g/kg/day. **Maximum:** 17 g/day.

SIDE EFFECTS

Frequent (50%): Some degree of abdominal fullness, nausea, bloating. **Occasional (10%–1%):** Abdominal cramping, vomiting, anal irritation. **Rare (less than 1%):** Urticaria, rhinorrhea, dermatitis.

ADVERSE EFFECTS/ TOXIC REACTIONS

None known.

NURSING CONSIDERATIONS

BASELINE ASSESSMENT

Do not give oral medication within 1 hr of start of therapy (may not adequately be absorbed before GI cleansing).

INTERVENTION/EVALUATION

Assess bowel sounds for peristalsis. Monitor daily pattern of bowel activity, stool consistency; record time of evacuation. Assess for abdominal disturbances. Monitor serum electrolytes, BUN, glucose, urine osmolality.

PATIENT/FAMILY TEACHING

• May take 2–4 days to produce a bowel movement. • Report unusual cramps, bloating, diarrhea.

pomalidomide

poe-ma-**lid**-oh-mide
(Pomalyst)

BLACK BOX ALERT May cause life-threatening birth defects. Pregnancy contraindicated. Exclude pregnancy before initiating treatment. Females of reproductive potential must use two reliable forms of contraception or continuously abstain during treatment and for 4 wks after treatment. Deep vein thrombosis and pulmonary embolism may occur. Consider venous thromboembolism (VTE) prophylaxis during treatment. Treatment only available through restricted program under the Risk Evaluation and Mitigation Strategy (REMS) named POMALYST REMS PROGRAM.

◆CLASSIFICATION

PHARMACOTHERAPEUTIC: Thalidomide analogue. **CLINICAL:** Antineoplastic.

ACTION

Inhibits tumor cell proliferation and induces apoptosis (cell death) of hematopoietic cells. Enhances T-cell– and natural killer (NK) cell–mediated immunity. Inhibits proinflammatory cytokines. **Therapeutic Effect:** Inhibits tumor cell growth and metastasis. Promotes tumor cell death.

PHARMACOKINETICS

Readily absorbed following PO administration. Metabolized in liver. Protein binding: 12%–44%. Peak plasma concentration: 2–3 hrs. Eliminated in urine (73%), feces (15%). **Half-life:** 8–10 hrs.

USES

Treatment of multiple myeloma in pts who have received at least two prior therapies including lenalidomide and bortezomib and have demonstrated disease progression on or within 60 days of completion of the last therapy.

P

PRECAUTIONS

◄ **ALERT** ► Do not donate blood products.

Contraindications: Pregnancy (Category X). **Cautions:** Anemia, HF, hepatic/renal impairment, smoking, or prior history of CVA, MI, DVT, PE, breastfeeding.

⌛ LIFESPAN CONSIDERATIONS

Pregnancy/Lactation: Pregnancy/breastfeeding contraindicated. May cause fetal harm. Unknown if distributed in breast milk. Do not breastfeed. Must verify negative pregnancy status before initiation. Must use two reliable forms of birth control (intrauterine device [IUD], tubal ligation) plus barrier methods. Avoid pregnancy for at least 4 wks after discontinuation.

Males: Must use condoms during treatment and up to 1 mo after treatment, despite prior history of vasectomy. Do not donate sperm. **Pregnancy Category X. Children:** Safety and efficacy not established. **Elderly:** May have increased risk of serious adverse effects, renal failure, electrolyte imbalance.

INTERACTIONS

DRUG: CYP3A4, P-glycoprotein inhibitors (e.g., erythromycin, ketoconazole) may increase concentration/effect. **CYP3A4, P-glycoprotein inducers (e.g., carbamazepine, rifampin)** may decrease concentration/effect. **HERBAL:** None significant. **FOOD:** Meals may reduce absorption/concentration. **LAB VALUES:** May decrease Hgb, Hct, neutrophils, platelets, leukocytes, lymphocytes, serum calcium, potassium, sodium. May increase serum calcium, creatinine, glucose.

AVAILABILITY (Rx)

🗊 **Capsules:** 1 mg, 2 mg, 3 mg, 4 mg.

ADMINISTRATION/HANDLING

PO

• Do not break, crush, dissolve, or open capsule. • Give on empty stomach; must administer at least 2 hrs before or 2 hrs after meal.

INDICATIONS/ROUTES/DOSAGE

Multiple Myeloma
PO: ADULTS/ELDERLY: 4 mg once daily on days 1–21 of 28-day cycle.

Dose Modification
Neutropenia
Absolute Neutrophil Count (ANC) Less Than 500 mm^3 or Febrile Neutropenia: Interrupt treatment until ANC is greater than 500 mm^3, then reduce dose to 3 mg once daily. **Any Subsequent Drop of ANC Less Than 500 mm^3 After Prior Reduction:** Interrupt treatment until ANC is greater than 500 mm^3, then reduce dose at 1 mg less than previous dose. Discontinue if 1-mg dose is intolerable.
Thrombocytopenia
Platelet Count Less Than 25,000 mm^3: Interrupt treatment until platelet count greater than 50,000 mm^3, then reduce dose to 3 mg once daily. **Any Subsequent Platelet Drop to Less Than 25,000 mm^3:** Interrupt treatment until platelet count greater than 50,000 mm^3, then reduce dose at 1 mg less than previous dose. Discontinue if 1-mg dose is intolerable.

SIDE EFFECTS

Frequent (55%–22%): Fatigue, constipation, nausea, diarrhea, dyspnea, back pain, peripheral edema, musculoskeletal chest pain, anorexia, rash. **Occasional (20%–7%):** Dizziness, pyrexia, muscle spasms, arthralgia, pruritus, vomiting, cough, weight loss, headache, bone pain, muscular weakness, anxiety, musculoskeletal pain, peripheral neuropathy, chills, dry skin, tremor, insomnia. **Rare (6%–1%):** Hyperhidrosis, extremity pain, back pain, night sweats, constipation.

ADVERSE EFFECTS/ TOXIC REACTIONS

Neutropenia, leukopenia, thrombocytopenia is an expected outcome of therapy; may increase risk of infection such as pneumonia, upper respiratory tract infection, UTI. Neurologic events such as acute confusion, dizziness reported. Peripheral neuropathy occurred in 18% of pts. Venous thromboembolism including DVT, PE occurred in 3% of pts. Epistaxis (nosebleed) occurred in 15% of pts. Increased risk of secondary malignancies reported. Acute renal failure reported in 16% of pts. Additional adverse events may include interstitial lung disease (ILD), neutropenic sepsis, *Pneumocystis jiroveci* pneumonia, respiratory syncytial virus infection, urinary retention, vertigo.

NURSING CONSIDERATIONS

BASELINE ASSESSMENT

Obtain baseline vital signs, CBC with differential, serum chemistries, esp. magnesium, phosphate, ionized calcium, PT/INR, urinalysis. Confirm negative pregnancy status 10–14 days before and 24 hrs before starting treatment. Receive full medication history. Obtain baseline neurologic exam. Question history of diabetes mellitus, electrolyte imbalance, hepatic/renal impairment, pulmonary disease, thromboembolism, smoking.

INTERVENTION/EVALUATION

Monitor CBC, serum chemistries, PT/INR. Offer antiemetics for nausea, vomiting. Monitor pregnancy status every mo during treatment and for at least 4 mos after discontinuation. Obtain EKG for palpitation, chest pain, hypokalemia, hyperkalemia, hypocalcemia, bradycardia, ventricular arrhythmias. Immediately report dyspnea, chest pain, hypoxia, unilateral peripheral edema/pain (may indicate thromboembolic event). Consider sequential compression device (SCD) for immobilized pts. Perform routine neurologic assessments to screen for confusion, delirium. Monitor urine output, frequency.

PATIENT/FAMILY TEACHING

• Blood levels will be routinely monitored.• May cause birth defects or miscarriage. Do not breastfeed. Consult with gynecologist for appropriate birth control methods. Female pts must use contraception during treatment and for at least 1 mo after treatment. Immediately report suspected pregnancy. Male pts must use condoms with spermicide during sexual activity, despite history of vasectomy.• Do not donate blood.• Swallow capsules whole; do not break, chew, crush, or open.• Go from lying to standing slowly (prevents postural hypotension, dizziness). Avoid tasks that require alertness, motor skills until response to drug is established.• Do not smoke.• Do not eat 2 hrs before or 2 hrs after dose. • Avoid alcohol.• Report difficulty breathing, chest pain, extremity pain swelling, confusion.

poractant alfa

pore-**ack**-tant
(Curosurf)

◆CLASSIFICATION

PHARMACOTHERAPEUTIC: Natural porcine lung extract. **CLINICAL:** Pulmonary surfactant.

ACTION

Reduces alveolar surface tension during ventilation; stabilizes alveoli against collapse that may occur at resting transpulmonary pressures. **Therapeutic Effect:** Improves lung compliance, respiratory gas exchange.

USES

Rescue treatment for respiratory distress syndrome (RDS), hyaline membrane disease in premature infants.

PRECAUTIONS

Contraindications: None known. **Cautions:** Pts at risk for circulatory overload. Acidosis, hypotension, anemia, hypoglycemia, hypothermia should be corrected prior to administration.

P

⌛ LIFESPAN CONSIDERATIONS

Pregnancy/Lactation: Neonate: No age-related precautions noted for neonates.

INTERACTIONS

DRUG: None significant. **HERBAL:** None significant. **FOOD:** None known. **LAB VALUES:** None significant.

AVAILABILITY (Rx)

Intratracheal Suspension: 80 mg/ml (1.5 ml, 3 ml), 1.5 ml (120 mg), 3 ml (240 mg).

ADMINISTRATION/HANDLING

Intratracheal

Administration • Attach syringe to catheter and instill through catheter inserted into infant's endotracheal tube. • Monitor for bradycardia, decreased O_2 saturation during administration. • Stop dosing procedure if these effects occur; begin appropriate measures before reinstituting therapy.
Storage • Refrigerate vials. • Warm by standing vial at room temperature for 20 min or warm in hand 8 min. • To obtain uniform suspension, turn upside down gently, swirl vial (do not shake). • After warming, may return to refrigerator one time only. • Withdraw entire contents of vial into 3- or 5-ml plastic syringe through large-gauge needle (20 gauge or larger).

INDICATIONS/ROUTE/DOSAGE

Respiratory Distress Syndrome (RDS)
Intratracheal: INFANTS: Initially, 2.5 ml/kg of birth weight. May give up to 2 subsequent doses of 1.25 ml/kg of birth weight at 12-hr intervals. **Maximum:** 5 ml/kg (total dose).

SIDE EFFECTS

Frequent: Transient bradycardia, oxygen (O_2) desaturation, increased carbon dioxide (CO_2) retention. **Occasional:** Endotracheal tube reflux. **Rare:** Hypotension, hypertension, apnea, pallor, vasoconstriction.

ADVERSE EFFECTS/ TOXIC REACTIONS

None known.

NURSING CONSIDERATIONS

BASELINE ASSESSMENT

Immediately before administration, change ventilator setting to 40–60 breaths/min, inspiratory time 0.5 sec, supplemental O_2 sufficient to maintain SaO_2 over 92%. Drug must be administered in highly supervised setting. Clinicians caring for neonate must be experienced with intubation, ventilator management. Offer emotional support to parents.

INTERVENTION/EVALUATION

Monitor infant with arterial or transcutaneous measurement of systemic O_2 and CO_2. Assess lung sounds for rales, moist breath sounds. Monitor heart rate.

posaconazole

poe-sa-**kon**-a-zole
(Noxafil, Posanol ✹)
Do not confuse Noxafil with minoxidil.

◆CLASSIFICATION

PHARMACOTHERAPEUTIC: Azole derivative. **CLINICAL:** Antifungal (see p. 48C).

ACTION

Inhibits synthesis of ergosterol, a vital component of fungal cell wall formation. **Therapeutic Effect:** Damages fungal cell wall membrane, altering its function.

PHARMACOKINETICS

Moderately absorbed following PO administration. Absorption increased if drug is taken with food. Widely distributed. Protein binding: 98%. Not significantly metabolized. Primarily excreted in feces. **Half-life:** 20–66 hrs.

USES

Prophylaxis of invasive *Aspergillus* and *Candida* infections in pts 13 yrs and older who are at high risk for developing these infections due to severely immunocompromised conditions. Treatment of oropharyngeal candidiasis. **OFF-LABEL:** Salvage therapy of refractory invasive fungal infections, mucomycosis, pulmonary infections.

PRECAUTIONS

Contraindications: Coadministration with pimozide, quinidine, HMG-CoA reductase inhibitors metabolized by CYP3A4 (e.g., atorvastatin, simvastatin), sirolimus, ergot alkaloids (may cause QT prolongation, torsade de pointes). **Cautions:** Renal/hepatic impairment, hypersensitivity to other azole antifungal agents, pts at increased risk of arrhythmias. Concomitant administration of medications that prolong QT interval.

⧗ LIFESPAN CONSIDERATIONS

Pregnancy/Lactation: May cause fetal harm. Breastfeeding not recommended. **Pregnancy Category C. Children:** Safety and efficacy not established in those younger than 13 yrs. **Elderly:** No age-related precautions noted.

INTERACTIONS

DRUG: May increase concentrations of **atorvastatin, cyclosporine, ergot alkaloids, felodipine, midazolam, phenytoin, pimozide, quinidine, rifabutin, simvastatin, sirolimus, tacrolimus, vinblastine, vincristine. Cimetidine, phenytoin** may decrease concentration. **HERBAL:** None significant. **FOOD:** Concentration higher when given with **food or nutritional supplements. Grapefruit products** may decrease concentration/effects. **LAB VALUES:** May decrease WBC, RBC, Hgb, Hct, platelets, serum calcium, potassium, magnesium. May increase serum glucose, bilirubin, ALT, AST, alkaline phosphatase.

AVAILABILITY (Rx)

Oral Suspension: 40 mg/ml. **Tablets (Delayed-Release):** 100 mg.

ADMINISTRATION/HANDLING

PO

• Administer with or within 20 min of full meal, liquid nutritional supplement, or acidic carbonated beverage (e.g., ginger ale) (enhances absorption). • Store oral suspension at room temperature. • Shake suspension well before use.

INDICATIONS/ROUTES/DOSAGE

Prophylaxis of Invasive *Aspergillus* and *Candida*
PO: ADULTS, ELDERLY, CHILDREN 13 YRS AND OLDER: 200 mg (5 ml) 3 times daily, given with full meal or liquid nutritional supplement. **(DELAYED-RELEASE):** 300 mg twice a day on first day, then 300 mg once daily.

Oropharyngeal Candidiasis
PO: ADULTS, ELDERLY, CHILDREN 13 YRS AND OLDER: 100 mg twice daily for 1 day, then 100 mg once daily for 13 days.

Refractory Oropharyngeal Candidiasis
PO: ADULTS, ELDERLY: 400 mg twice daily.

SIDE EFFECTS

Common (42%–24%): Diarrhea, nausea, vomiting, headache, abdominal pain, cough. **Frequent (20%–15%):** Constipation, rigors, rash, hypertension, fatigue, insomnia, mucositis, musculoskeletal pain, edema of lower extremities, herpes simplex, anorexia. **Occasional (14%–8%):** Hypotension, epistaxis, tachycardia, pharyngitis, dizziness, pruritus, arthralgia, dyspepsia (heartburn, indigestion, epigastric pain), back pain, generalized edema, weakness.

ADVERSE EFFECTS/ TOXIC REACTIONS

Bacteremia occurs in 18% of pts; upper respiratory tract infection occurs in 7%. Allergic/hypersensitivity reactions, QT prolongation, hemolytic uremic syndrome, thrombotic thrombocytopenic purpura, pulmonary embolus have been reported.

P

NURSING CONSIDERATIONS

BASELINE ASSESSMENT

Obtain baselines for CBC, hepatic function test, serum chemistries prior to therapy.

INTERVENTION/EVALUATION

Monitor hepatic function tests periodically. Monitor daily pattern of bowel activity, stool consistency. Obtain order for antiemetic if excessive vomiting occurs. Monitor B/P for hypertension, hypotension. Assess for lower extremity edema (first sign of edema appears behind medial malleolus).

PATIENT/FAMILY TEACHING

• Take each dose with full meal or liquid nutritional supplement. • Report severe diarrhea, vomiting, chest pain, yellowing of skin/eyes. • Maintain strict oral hygiene.

---

potassium acetate

potassium bicarbonate/citrate

(Effer-K, <u>Klor-Con EF</u>)

potassium chloride

(Apo-K ✷, Kaon-Cl, Klor-Con, <u>Klor-Con M10</u>, <u>Klor-Con M20</u>, Micro-K)

potassium gluconate

poe-**tass**-ee-um
Do not confuse Micro-K with Macrobid or Micronase.

◆CLASSIFICATION

PHARMACOTHERAPEUTIC: Electrolyte. **CLINICAL:** Potassium replenisher.

ACTION

Necessary for multiple cellular metabolic processes. Primary action is intracellular. **Therapeutic Effect:** Required for nerve impulse conduction, contraction of cardiac, skeletal, smooth muscle; maintains normal renal function, acid-base balance.

PHARMACOKINETICS

Well absorbed from GI tract. Enters cells by active transport from extracellular fluid. Primarily excreted in urine.

USES

Potassium acetate, potassium bicarbonate/citrate: Treatment, prevention of hypokalemia when necessary to avoid chloride or acid/base imbalance (requires bicarbonate). **Potassium chloride, potassium gluconate:** Treatment, prevention of hypokalemia.

PRECAUTIONS

Contraindications: Severe renal impairment, untreated Addison's disease, heat cramps, hyperkalemia, severe tissue trauma. **Cautions:** Cardiac disease, concurrent use of potassium-sparing medications, renal impairment.

⧖ LIFESPAN CONSIDERATIONS

Pregnancy/Lactation: Unknown if drug crosses placenta or is distributed in breast milk. **Pregnancy Category C. Children:** No age-related precautions noted. **Elderly:** May be at increased risk for hyperkalemia. Age-related ability to excrete potassium is reduced.

INTERACTIONS

DRUG: Angiotensin-converting enzyme (ACE) inhibitors, potassium-containing medications, potassium-sparing diuretics, salt substitutes may increase serum potassium concentration. **HERBAL:** None significant. **FOOD:** None known. **LAB VALUES:** None known.

AVAILABILITY (Rx)

POTASSIUM ACETATE
Injection, Solution: 2 mEq/ml.
POTASSIUM BICARBONATE
AND POTASSIUM CITRATE
Tablets for Solution: (**Effer-K**): 10 mEq,
20 mEq, 25 mEq. (**Klor-Con EF**): 25
mEq.
POTASSIUM CHLORIDE
Injection, Solution: 2 mEq/ml. Oral Solution: 20 mEq/15 ml, 40 mEq/15 ml.
Powder for Oral Solution: 20 mEq/packet,
25 mEq/packet.

Capsules, Extended-Release (Micro-K):
8 mEq, 10 mEq. Tablets, Extended-Release: 8 mEq, 10 mEq, 15 mEq, 20 mEq.
POTASSIUM GLUCONATE
Tablets (Glu-K): 550 mg, 595 mg.

ADMINISTRATION/HANDLING
IV

Reconstitution • For IV infusion only,
must dilute before administration, mix
well, infuse slowly. • Avoid adding potassium to hanging IV.
Rate of Administration • Routinely,
give at concentration of no more than
40 mEq/L, no faster than 10 mEq/hr for
peripheral infusion, 40 mEq/hr for central infusion. • Check IV site closely
during infusion for evidence of phlebitis
(heat, pain, red streaking of skin over
vein, hardness to vein), extravasation
(swelling, pain, cool skin, little/no blood
return).
Storage • Store at room temperature.

PO

• Take with or after meals, with full glass
of water (decreases GI upset). • Liquids,
powder, effervescent tablets: Mix, dissolve with juice, water before administering. • Do not break, crush, or divide
tablets; give whole.

IV INCOMPATIBILITIES

Amphotericin B complex (Abelcet, AmBisome, Amphotec), phenytoin (Dilantin).

IV COMPATIBILITIES

Amiodarone (Cordarone), atropine, aztreonam (Azactam), calcium gluconate,
cefepime (Maxipime), ciprofloxacin
(Cipro), clindamycin (Cleocin), dexamethasone (Decadron), dexmedetomidine
(Precedex), digoxin (Lanoxin), diltiazem
(Cardizem), diphenhydramine (Benadryl), dobutamine (Dobutrex), dopamine
(Intropin), enalapril (Vasotec), famotidine
(Pepcid), fluconazole (Diflucan), furosemide (Lasix), granisetron (Kytril), heparin, hydrocortisone (Solu-Cortef), insulin,
lidocaine, lorazepam (Ativan), magnesium
sulfate, methylprednisolone (Solu-Medrol), metoclopramide (Reglan), midazolam (Versed), milrinone (Primacor),
morphine, norepinephrine (Levophed),
ondansetron (Zofran), oxytocin (Pitocin),
piperacillin and tazobactam (Zosyn), procainamide (Pronestyl), propofol (Diprivan), propranolol (Inderal).

INDICATIONS/ROUTES/DOSAGE

Prevention of Hypokalemia with Diuretic Therapy
PO: ADULTS, ELDERLY: 20–40 mEq/day in
1–2 divided doses. CHILDREN: 1–2 mEq/
kg/day in 1–2 divided doses.

Treatment of Hypokalemia
PO: ADULTS, ELDERLY: 40–100 mEq/day
in divided doses (generally limit amount
per dose to 40 mEq); further doses
based on laboratory values. CHILDREN:
Initially, 1–2 mEq/kg; further doses
based on laboratory values.
IV: ADULTS, ELDERLY: 5–10 mEq/hr. **Maximum:** 400 mEq/day. CHILDREN: 0.5–1
mEq/kg per dose. **Maximum dose:** 40
mEq per dose to infuse at 0.3–0.5 mEq/
kg/hr. **Maximum rate:** 1 mEq/kg/hr.

SIDE EFFECTS

Occasional: Nausea, vomiting, diarrhea,
flatulence, abdominal discomfort with distention, phlebitis with IV administration
(particularly when potassium concentration of greater than 40 mEq/L is infused).
Rare: Rash.

♣ Canadian trade name   Non-Crushable Drug   High Alert drug

ADVERSE EFFECTS/ TOXIC REACTIONS

Hyperkalemia (more common in elderly, pts with renal impairment) manifested as paresthesia, feeling of heaviness in lower extremities, cold skin, grayish pallor, hypotension, confusion, irritability, flaccid paralysis, cardiac arrhythmias.

NURSING CONSIDERATIONS

BASELINE ASSESSMENT

Assess for hypokalemia (weakness, fatigue, polyuria, polydipsia). PO should be given with food or after meals with full glass of water, fruit juice (minimizes GI irritation).

INTERVENTION/EVALUATION

Monitor serum potassium (particularly in renal impairment). If GI disturbance is noted, dilute preparation further or give with meals. Be alert to decreased urinary output (may be indication of renal insufficiency). Monitor daily pattern of bowel activity, stool consistency. Assess I&O diligently during diuresis, IV site for extravasation, phlebitis. Be alert to evidence of hyperkalemia (skin pallor/coldness, complaints of paresthesia, feeling of heaviness of lower extremities).

PATIENT/FAMILY TEACHING

• Foods rich in potassium include beef, veal, ham, chicken, turkey, fish, milk, bananas, dates, prunes, raisins, avocados, watermelon, cantaloupe, apricots, molasses, beans, yams, broccoli, Brussels sprouts, lentils, potatoes, spinach.
• Report paresthesia, feeling of heaviness of lower extremities, tarry or bloody stools, weakness, unusual fatigue.

pralatrexate

pral-a-**trex**-ate
(Folotyn)
Do not confuse Folotyn with Focalin, or pralatrexate with methotrexate or pemetrexed.

◆CLASSIFICATION

PHARMACOTHERAPEUTIC: Antimetabolite. **CLINICAL:** Antineoplastic.

ACTION

Folate analogue metabolic inhibitor that competes with enzymes necessary for tumor cell reproduction. **Therapeutic Effect:** Inhibits tumor growth.

PHARMACOKINETICS

Protein binding: 67%. Partially excreted in urine. **Half-life:** 12–18 hrs.

USES

Treatment of relapsed or refractory peripheral T-cell lymphoma (PTCL). **OFF-LABEL:** Treatment of relapsed/refractory cutaneous T-cell lymphoma.

PRECAUTIONS

Contraindications: None known. **Cautions:** Moderate to severe renal impairment, hepatic impairment.

⧖ LIFESPAN CONSIDERATIONS

Pregnancy/Lactation: May cause fetal harm. Unknown if drug is distributed in breast milk. **Pregnancy Category D. Children:** Safety and efficacy not established. **Elderly:** No age-related precautions noted.

INTERACTIONS

DRUG: NSAIDs, probenecid, trimethoprim/sulfamethoxazole may delay clearance, increase concentration. **HERBAL: Echinacea** may decrease concentration/effects. **FOOD:** None known. **LAB VALUES:** May decrease RBC, WBC, Hgb, Hct, serum potassium, platelet count. May increase serum ALT, AST.

AVAILABILITY (Rx)

Injection Solution: 20 mg/ml.

ADMINISTRATION/HANDLING

◀**ALERT**▶ May be carcinogenic, mutagenic, teratogenic. Handle with extreme care during preparation/administration.

P

Wear gloves when preparing solution. If powder or solution comes in contact with skin, wash immediately, thoroughly with soap, water.

◄ ALERT ► Pt should begin taking oral folic acid (1 mg) daily starting 10 days prior to first IV pralatrexate dose and continue for 30 days after last dose. Pt should also receive vitamin B$_{12}$ (1 mg) IM injection no more than 10 wks prior to first IV pralatrexate dose and every 8–10 wks thereafter.

 IV

Reconstitution • Withdraw calculated dose into syringe for immediate use. • Intended for single use only. • Do not dilute.

Rate of Administration • Administer as IV push over 3–5 min into IV infusion of 0.9% NaCl.

Storage • Refrigerate vials until use, protect from light. Stable at room temperature for 72 hrs. • Discard vial if solution is discolored (solution should appear clear to yellow) or particulate matter is present.

▩ IV INCOMPATIBILITY

Do not mix with any other medication.

INDICATIONS/ROUTES/DOSAGE

◄ ALERT ► Prior to any dose, mucositis should be no higher than grade 1, platelets 100,000/mm^3 or greater for first dose and 50,000/mm^3 or greater for subsequent doses, and absolute neutrophil count (ANC) 1,000/mm^3 or greater.

Refractory/Relapsed Peripheral T-Cell Lymphoma
IV: ADULTS, ELDERLY: 30 mg/m^2 administered once weekly for 6 wks in 7-wk cycles. Dose may be decreased to 20 mg/m^2 to manage adverse reactions.

SIDE EFFECTS

Common (70%–36%): Mucositis, nausea, fatigue. **Frequent (34%–10%):** Constipation/diarrhea, pyrexia, edema, cough, epistaxis, vomiting, dyspnea, anorexia,

rash, throat/abdominal/back pain, night sweats, asthenia (loss of strength, energy), tachycardia, upper respiratory infection.

ADVERSE EFFECTS/ TOXIC REACTIONS

Hematologic toxicity, resulting from blood dyscrasias, may manifest as thrombocytopenia (41%), anemia (34%), neutropenia (24%), leukopenia (11%). High potential for development of mucositis (70%). Mucositis is less severe when folic acid, vitamin B$_{12}$ therapy is ongoing. Sepsis, pyrexia, febrile neutropenia, dehydration have occurred. Overdosage requires general supportive care. Prompt administration of leucovorin should be considered in case of overdose, based on mechanism of action of pralatrexate.

NURSING CONSIDERATIONS

BASELINE ASSESSMENT

Question for possibility of pregnancy before initiating therapy (Pregnancy Category D). Assess baseline vital signs, temperature. Evaluate baseline CBC with differential, hepatic/renal function, serum potassium level. Antiemetics before and during therapy may alleviate nausea/vomiting. Initiate folic acid, vitamin B$_{12}$ administration prior to and throughout therapy.

INTERVENTION/EVALUATION

Prior to any dose: mucositis should be grade 1 or less. Platelet count 100,000 or greater for 1st dose (50,000 or greater for all subsequent doses). Absolute neutrophil count (ANC) 1,000 or greater. Assess for signs of mucositis (oropharyngeal ulcers, oral/throat pain, local infection). Monitor for signs of hematologic toxicity, sepsis (fever, signs of local infection, altered CBC results). Monitor hepatic/renal function. Monitor for hypokalemia (muscle cramps, weakness, EKG changes).

PATIENT/FAMILY TEACHING

• Explain importance of folic acid, vitamin B$_{12}$ therapy to reduce adverse ef-

P

 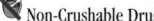

fects. • Maintain fastidious oral hygiene. • Do not have immunizations without physician's approval (drug lowers body's resistance). • Avoid crowds, those with infection. • Promptly report fever, sore throat, signs of local infection, unusual bruising/bleeding from any site. • Use nonhormonal contraception. • Report persistent nausea/vomiting.

pramipexole

pram-i-**pex**-ole
(Apo-Pramipexole ❋, <u>Mirapex</u>, Mirapex ER)
Do not confuse Mirapex with Mifeprex or MiraLax.

◆CLASSIFICATION

PHARMACOTHERAPEUTIC: Dopamine receptor agonist. **CLINICAL:** Antiparkinson agent (see p. 145C).

ACTION

Stimulates dopamine receptors in striatum. **Therapeutic Effect:** Relieves signs/symptoms of Parkinson's disease.

PHARMACOKINETICS

Rapidly, extensively absorbed after PO administration. Protein binding: 15%. Widely distributed. Steady-state concentrations achieved within 2 days. Primarily eliminated in urine. Not removed by hemodialysis. **Half-life:** 8 hrs (12 hrs in pts older than 65 yrs).

USES

Mirapex: Treatment of signs/symptoms of idiopathic Parkinson's disease, restless legs syndrome. **Mirapex ER:** Treatment of Parkinson's disease. **OFF-LABEL:** Depression (due to bipolar disorder), fibromyalgia.

PRECAUTIONS

Contraindications: None known. **Cautions:** History of orthostatic hypotension,

syncope, hallucinations, renal impairment, concomitant use of CNS depressants, preexisting dyskinesia, elderly.

⌛ LIFESPAN CONSIDERATIONS

Pregnancy/Lactation: Unknown if drug is distributed in breast milk. **Pregnancy Category C. Children:** Safety and efficacy not established. **Elderly:** Increased risk of hallucinations.

INTERACTIONS

DRUG: May increase plasma concentrations of **carbidopa, levodopa. HERBAL: Gotu kola, kava kava, St. John's wort, SAMe, valerian** may increase CNS depression, risk of serotonin syndrome. **FOOD: All foods** delay peak drug plasma levels by 1 hr (extent of absorption not affected). **LAB VALUES:** None significant.

AVAILABILITY (Rx)

Tablets: 0.125 mg, 0.25 mg, 0.5 mg, 0.75 mg, 1 mg, 1.5 mg.

Tablets (Extended-Release [Mirapex ER]): 0.375 mg, 0.75 mg, 1.5 mg, 2.25 mg, 3 mg, 3.75 mg, 4.5 mg.

ADMINISTRATION/HANDLING

PO (Mirapex)
• Give without regard to food.

PO (Mirapex ER)
• Give once daily, without regard to food.
• Give whole; do not break, crush, dissolve, or divide tablets.

INDICATIONS/ROUTES/DOSAGE

Parkinson's Disease (Mirapex)
PO: ADULTS, ELDERLY: Initially, 0.375 mg/day in 3 divided doses. Increase dosage by 0.125–0.25 mg/dose no more frequently than every 5–7 days. **Maintenance:** 0.5–1.5 mg/day in 3 equally divided doses.

Parkinson's Disease (Mirapex ER)
Initially, 0.375 mg once daily. May increase to 0.75 mg, then by 0.75-mg in-

crements no more frequently than 5–7 days. **Maximum:** 4.5 mg once daily. Note: May switch overnight from immediate-release to extended-release at same daily dose.

Dosage in Renal Impairment

Dosage and frequency are modified based on creatinine clearance.

Mirapex

Creatinine	Dosage	
Clearance	Initial	Maximum
30–50 ml/min	0.125 mg twice daily	0.75 mg 3 times/day
15–29 ml/min	0.125 mg once daily	1.5 mg once daily

Mirapex ER
Creatinine Clearance 30–50 ml/min: Initially, 0.375 mg q every other day. May increase to 0.375 mg daily after 1 wk, then 0.375 mg/dose not more frequently than q7days. **Maximum:** 2.25 mg/day.

Restless Legs Syndrome
PO: ADULTS, ELDERLY: Initially, 0.125 mg once daily 2–3 hrs before bedtime. May increase to 0.25 mg after 4–7 days, then to 0.5 mg after 4–7 days (interval is 14 days in pts with renal impairment). **Maximum:** 0.5 mg/day.

SIDE EFFECTS

Frequent: Early Parkinson's disease (28%–10%): Nausea, asthenia (loss of strength, energy), dizziness, drowsiness, insomnia, constipation. **Advanced Parkinson's disease (53%–17%):** Orthostatic hypotension, extrapyramidal reactions, insomnia, dizziness, hallucinations. **Occasional: Early Parkinson's disease (5%–2%):** Edema, malaise, confusion, amnesia, akathisia, anorexia, dysphagia, peripheral edema, vision changes, impotence. **Advanced Parkinson's disease (10%–7%):** Asthenia (loss of strength, energy), drowsiness, confusion, consti-

pation, abnormal gait, dry mouth. **Rare: Advanced Parkinson's disease (6%–2%):** General edema, malaise, angina, amnesia, tremor, urinary frequency/incontinence, dyspnea, rhinitis, vision changes. **Restless legs syndrome: Frequent (16%):** Headache, nausea. **Occasional (13%–9%):** Insomnia, fatigue. **Rare (6%–3%):** Drowsiness, constipation, diarrhea, dry mouth.

ADVERSE EFFECTS/ TOXIC REACTIONS

Vascular disease, atrial fibrillation, arrhythmias, pulmonary embolism, impulsive/compulsive behavior (pathological gambling, hypersexuality, binge eating) have been reported.

NURSING CONSIDERATIONS

BASELINE ASSESSMENT

Parkinson's disease: Assess for tremor, muscle weakness and rigidity, ataxia. **Restless legs syndrome:** Assess frequency of symptoms, sleep pattern.

INTERVENTION/EVALUATION

Instruct pt to rise from lying to sitting or sitting to standing position slowly to prevent risk of postural hypotension. Assess for clinical improvement. Assist with ambulation if dizziness occurs. Assess for constipation; encourage fiber, fluids, exercise.

PATIENT/FAMILY TEACHING

• Inform pt that hallucinations may occur, esp. in the elderly. • Go from lying to standing slowly. • Avoid tasks that require alertness, motor skills until response to drug is established. • If nausea occurs, take medication with food. • Avoid abrupt withdrawal. • Avoid alcohol. • Report new or increased impulsive/compulsive behaviors (gambling, sexual urges, compulsive eating or buying).

P

pramlintide

pram-lin-tide
(SymlinPen 60, SymlinPen 120)

BLACK BOX ALERT Increased risk of severe hypoglycemia; usually occurs within 3 hrs of injection.

◆ CLASSIFICATION

PHARMACOTHERAPEUTIC: Antihyperglycemic. **CLINICAL:** Antidiabetic agent (see p. 45C).

ACTION

Cosecreted with insulin by pancreatic beta cells, reduces postprandial glucose increases by slowing gastric emptying time, reducing postprandial glucagon secretion, reducing caloric intake through centrally mediated appetite suppression. **Therapeutic Effect:** Improves glycemic control by reducing postprandial glucose concentrations in pts with type 1, type 2 diabetes mellitus.

PHARMACOKINETICS

	Onset	Peak	Duration
Subcuta-neous	NA	20 min	3 hrs

Metabolized primarily by kidneys. Protein binding: 60%. Excreted in urine. **Half-life:** 48 min.

USES

Adjunctive treatment with mealtime insulin in type 1, type 2 diabetes mellitus pts who have failed to achieve desired glucose control despite optimal insulin therapy, with/without concurrent sulfonylurea and/or metformin in type 2 diabetes mellitus.

PRECAUTIONS

Contraindications: Diagnosed gastroparesis, presence of hypoglycemia or recurrent severe hypoglycemic episodes in the past 6 mos. **Cautions:** Coadministration with insulin may induce severe hypoglycemia (usually within 3 hrs following administration); concurrent use of other glucose-lowering agents may increase risk of hypoglycemia. History of nausea, visual or dexterity impairment, poor compliance with insulin monitoring or current insulin therapy, pts with hemoglobin A_{1c} greater than 9%, pts with conditions or taking concurrent medications likely to impair gastric motility (e.g., anticholinergics), pts requiring medication to stimulate gastric emptying.

LIFESPAN CONSIDERATIONS

Pregnancy/Lactation: Unknown if distributed in breast milk. **Pregnancy Category C. Children:** Safety and efficacy not established. **Elderly:** No age-related precautions noted.

INTERACTIONS

DRUG: Anticholinergics may cause additive impairment of gastric motility. **HERBAL: Garlic** may increase hypoglycemia. **FOOD: Ethanol** may increase risk of hypoglycemia. **LAB VALUES:** None significant.

AVAILABILITY (Rx)

Injection, Solution (SymlinPen 120): Delivers fixed doses of 120 mcg. **(SymlinPen 60):** Delivers fixed doses of 60 mcg.

ADMINISTRATION/HANDLING

Subcutaneous
• Administer immediately before each major meal (350 or more kcal or containing 30 g or more carbohydrate). • Give in abdomen or thigh; do not give in arm (variable absorption). • Injection site should be distinct from insulin injection site. • Rotation of injection sites is essential. • Use U-100 insulin syringe for accuracy. • Always give pramlintide and insulin as separate injections.
Storage • Store unopened vials in refrigerator. • Discard if freezing occurs. • Vials that have been opened (punctured) may be stored in refrigerator or kept at room temperature for up to 30 days.

P

INDICATIONS/ROUTES/DOSAGE

◄ALERT► Initially, current insulin dosage in all pts with type 1, type 2 diabetes mellitus should be reduced by 50%. This includes preprandial, rapid-acting, short-acting, fixed-mixed insulins.

Type 1 Diabetes Mellitus
Subcutaneous: ADULTS, ELDERLY: Initially, 15 mcg immediately before major meal. Titrate in 15-mcg increments every 3 days (if no significant nausea occurs) to target dose of 30–60 mcg.

Type 2 Diabetes Mellitus
Subcutaneous: ADULTS, ELDERLY: Initially, 60 mcg immediately before major meal. After 3–7 days, increase to 120 mcg if no significant nausea occurs (if nausea occurs at 120 mcg dose, reduce to 60 mcg).

SIDE EFFECTS

TYPE 1 DIABETES MELLITUS
Frequent (48%): Nausea. Occasional (17%–11%): Anorexia, vomiting. Rare (7%–5%): Fatigue, arthralgia, allergic reaction, dizziness.
TYPE 2 DIABETES MELLITUS
Frequent (28%): Nausea. Occasional (13%–8%): Headache, anorexia, vomiting, abdominal pain. Rare (7%–5%): Fatigue, dizziness, cough, pharyngitis.

ADVERSE EFFECTS/ TOXIC REACTIONS

Overdose produces severe nausea, vomiting, diarrhea, vasodilation, dizziness. No hypoglycemia was reported. Increased risk of severe hypoglycemia when given concurrently with nontitrated insulin.

NURSING CONSIDERATIONS

BASELINE ASSESSMENT

Check serum glucose concentration before administration, both before and after meals and at bedtime. Discuss lifestyle to determine extent of learning, emotional needs. Ensure follow-up instruction if pt, family does not thoroughly understand diabetes management, glucose testing technique.

INTERVENTION/EVALUATION

Risk for hypoglycemia occurs within first 3 hrs following drug administration if given concurrently with insulin. Assess for hypoglycemia (diaphoresis, tremors, dizziness, anxiety, headache, tachycardia, numbness in mouth, hunger, diplopia, difficulty concentrating). Be alert to conditions that alter glucose requirements (fever, increased activity, stress, surgical procedures).

PATIENT/FAMILY TEACHING

• Diabetes mellitus requires lifelong control. • Prescribed diet, exercise are principal parts of treatment; do not skip/delay meals. • Continue to adhere to dietary instructions, regular exercise program, regular testing of serum glucose. • When taking combination drug therapy, have source of glucose available to treat symptoms of low blood sugar.

---

prasugrel

pra-soo-grel
(Effient)
BLACK BOX ALERT Serious, sometimes fatal, hemorrhage may occur. **Do not confuse Effient with Effexor, or prasugrel with praziquantel.**

◆CLASSIFICATION

PHARMACOTHERAPEUTIC: Thienopyridine derivative inhibitor. **CLINICAL:** Antiplatelet agent (see p. 34C).

ACTION

Inhibits binding of the enzyme adenosine phosphate (ADP) to its platelet receptor and subsequent ADP-mediated activation of a glycoprotein complex. **Therapeutic Effect:** Inhibits platelet aggregation.

PHARMACOKINETICS

Rapidly absorbed, with peak concentration occurring 30 min following adminis-

P

 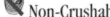

tration. Metabolized in liver. Protein binding: 98%. Eliminated in urine (68%), feces (27%). **Half-life:** 7 hrs.

USES

Reduction of thrombotic cardiovascular events (MI, CVA, stent thrombosis) in pts with acute coronary syndrome (unstable angina, non–ST-segment elevation MI, ST-segment MI) who are to be managed with percutaneous coronary intervention (PCI). **OFF-LABEL:** Initial treatment of unstable angina, STEMI in pts undergoing PCI with allergy or major GI intolerance to aspirin.

PRECAUTIONS

Contraindications: Active bleeding, prior transient ischemic attack (TIA), CVA. **Cautions:** Pts who undergo coronary artery bypass graft (CABG) after receiving prasugrel, pts at risk for bleeding (age 75 yrs or older, body weight less than 60 kg, recent trauma/surgery, recent GI bleeding or active peptic ulcer disease, severe hepatic impairment).

⧗ LIFESPAN CONSIDERATIONS

Pregnancy/Lactation: Unknown if drug crosses placenta or is distributed in breast milk. **Pregnancy Category B. Children:** Safety and efficacy not established. **Elderly:** May have increased risk for intracranial hemorrhage; caution advised in pts 75 yrs and older.

INTERACTIONS

DRUG: Aspirin, NSAIDs, warfarin may increase risk of bleeding. **HERBAL:** Cat's claw, dong quai, evening primrose, feverfew, garlic, ginger, ginseng, green tea, horse chestnut, red clover may have additive platelet effects. Ginkgo biloba may increase risk of bleeding. **FOOD:** None known. **LAB VALUES:** May decrease Hgb, Hct, WBC, platelet count. May increase bleeding time, serum cholesterol, AST, ALT.

AVAILABILITY (Rx)

▧ **Tablets:** 5 mg, 10 mg.

ADMINISTRATION/HANDLING

PO
• Give without regard to food. • Do not crush tablet.

INDICATIONS/ROUTES/DOSAGE

Acute Coronary Syndrome
◀**ALERT**▶ Consider 5 mg once daily for pts weighing less than 60 kg.
PO: ADULTS, ELDERLY: Initially, 60-mg loading dose, then 10 mg once daily (in combination with aspirin).

SIDE EFFECTS

Occasional (8%–4%): Hypertension, headache, back pain, dyspnea, nausea, dizziness. **Rare (Less Than 4%):** Cough, hypotension, fatigue, noncardiac chest pain, bradycardia, rash, pyrexia, peripheral edema, extremity pain, minor bleeding, diarrhea.

ADVERSE EFFECTS/ TOXIC REACTIONS

Major bleeding (intracranial hemorrhage, epistaxis, GI bleeding, hemoptysis, subcutaneous hematoma, postprocedural hemorrhage, retroperitoneal hemorrhage, retinal hemorrhage) has been reported. Severe thrombocytopenia, anemia, abnormal hepatic function, anaphylactic reaction, angioedema, atrial fibrillation occur rarely. Overdosage may require platelet transfusion to restore clotting ability.

NURSING CONSIDERATIONS

BASELINE ASSESSMENT

Obtain baseline vital signs, CBC, EKG, hepatic function tests.

INTERVENTION/EVALUATION

Monitor vital signs for changes in B/P, pulse. Assess for signs of unusual bleeding or hemorrhage, pain. Monitor platelet count, hepatic function tests, EKG for changes from baseline.

PATIENT/FAMILY TEACHING

• It may take longer to stop minor bleeding during drug therapy. Report unusual bleeding/bruising, blood noted in stool or urine, chest/back pain, extremity pain. • Monitor for dyspnea. • Report fever, weakness, extreme skin paleness, purple skin patches, yellowing of skin or eyes, changes in mental status. • Do not discontinue drug therapy without physician approval. • Inform physicians, dentists before undergoing any invasive procedure or surgery.

---

pravastatin
TOP 200

pra-va-sta-tin
(Apo-Pravastatin ✦, Novo-Pravastatin ✦, Pravachol)
Do not confuse pravastatin with atorvastatin, lovastatin, nystatin, pitavastatin, or simvastatin, or Pravachol with Prevacid, Prinivil, or propranolol.

FIXED-COMBINATION(S)

Pravigard: pravastatin/aspirin (anticoagulant): 20 mg/81 mg, 40 mg/81 mg, 80 mg/81 mg, 20 mg/325 mg, 40 mg/325 mg, 80 mg/325 mg.

◆CLASSIFICATION

PHARMACOTHERAPEUTIC: Hydroxymethylglutaryl CoA (HMG-CoA) reductase inhibitor. **CLINICAL:** Antihyperlipidemic (see p. 59C).

ACTION

Interferes with cholesterol biosynthesis by preventing conversion of HMG-CoA reductase to mevalonate, a precursor to cholesterol. **Therapeutic Effect:** Lowers LDL, VLDL cholesterol, plasma triglycerides; increases HDL.

PHARMACOKINETICS

Rapidly absorbed from GI tract. Protein binding: 50%. Metabolized in liver. Primarily excreted in feces via biliary system. Not removed by hemodialysis. **Half-life:** 2–3 hrs.

USES

Treatment of primary hyperlipidemias and mixed dyslipidemias to reduce total cholesterol, LDL cholesterol, apolipoprotein B, triglycerides; increase HDL cholesterol. Reduces risk of MI, revascularization, and mortality in hypercholesterolemia without clinically evident CHD. Reduces mortality risk in pts with CHD. Reduces elevated triglycerides in hypertriglyceridemia. Treatment of heterozygous familial hypercholesterolemia in pediatric pts 8–18 yrs.

PRECAUTIONS

Contraindications: Active hepatic disease or unexplained, persistent elevations of hepatic function test results. Pregnancy, nursing mothers. **Cautions:** History of hepatic disease, substantial alcohol consumption. Withholding/discontinuing pravastatin may be necessary when pt is at risk for renal failure secondary to rhabdomyolysis.

⊠ LIFESPAN CONSIDERATIONS

Pregnancy/Lactation: Contraindicated in pregnancy (suppression of cholesterol biosynthesis may cause fetal toxicity) and lactation. Unknown if drug is distributed in breast milk, but there is risk of serious adverse reactions in breastfeeding infants. **Pregnancy Category X. Children:** Safety and efficacy not established. **Elderly:** No age-related precautions noted.

INTERACTIONS

DRUG: Cyclosporine, clarithromycin, colchicine, erythromycin, gemfibrozil, immunosuppressants, niacin increase risk of myopathy, rhabdomyolysis. **HERBAL: St. John's wort** may decrease concentration. **FOOD: Red yeast rice** contains 2.4 mg **lovastatin** per 600 mg rice. **LAB VALUES:** May increase serum creatine kinase (CK), transaminase.

P

✦ Canadian trade name   🦃 Non-Crushable Drug   **HIGH ALERT** High Alert drug

AVAILABILITY (Rx)

Tablets: 10 mg, 20 mg, 40 mg, 80 mg.

ADMINISTRATION/HANDLING

PO

• Give without regard to meals.

INDICATIONS/ROUTES/DOSAGE

◄**ALERT**► Prior to initiating therapy, pt should be on standard cholesterol-lowering diet for 3–6 mos. Low-cholesterol diet should be continued throughout pravastatin therapy.

Usual Dosage
PO: ADULTS, ELDERLY: Initially, 40 mg/day. Titrate to desired response. **Range:** 10–80 mg/day. **CHILDREN 14–18 YRS:** 40 mg/day. **CHILDREN 8–13 YRS:** 20 mg/day.

Dosage in Renal Impairment
For adults, give 10 mg/day initially. Titrate to desired response.

Dosage with Clarithromycin
Maximum: 40 mg/day.

Dosage with Cyclosporine
ADULTS, ELDERLY: Initially, 10 mg/day. **Maximum:** 20 mg/day.

SIDE EFFECTS

Pravastatin is generally well tolerated. Side effects are usually mild and transient. **Occasional (7%–4%):** Nausea, vomiting, diarrhea, constipation, abdominal pain, headache, rhinitis, rash, pruritus. **Rare (3%–2%):** Heartburn, myalgia, dizziness, cough, fatigue, flu-like symptoms, depression, photosensitivity.

ADVERSE EFFECTS/
TOXIC REACTIONS

Potential for malignancy, cataracts. Hypersensitivity, myopathy occur rarely. Rhabdomyolysis has been reported.

NURSING CONSIDERATIONS

BASELINE ASSESSMENT

Obtain dietary history, esp. fat consumption. Question for possibility of pregnancy before initiating therapy (Pregnancy Category X). Assess baseline serum lab results (cholesterol, triglycerides, hepatic function tests).

INTERVENTION/EVALUATION

Monitor serum cholesterol, triglyceride lab results for therapeutic response. Monitor hepatic function tests, CPK. Monitor daily pattern of bowel activity, stool consistency. Check for headache, dizziness (provide assistance as needed). Assess for rash, pruritus. Be alert for malaise, muscle cramping/weakness; if accompanied by fever, may require discontinuation of medication.

PATIENT/FAMILY TEACHING

• Follow special diet (important part of treatment). • Periodic lab tests are essential part of therapy. • Report promptly any muscle pain/weakness, esp. if accompanied by fever, malaise. • Avoid tasks that require alertness, motor skills until response to drug is established (potential for dizziness). • Use nonhormonal contraception. • Avoid direct exposure to sunlight.

prazosin

praz-oh-sin
(Apo-Prazo ✦, Minipress, Novo-Prazin ✦)
Do not confuse prazosin with prednisone.

◆ **CLASSIFICATION**

PHARMACOTHERAPEUTIC: Alpha-adrenergic blocker. **CLINICAL:** Antihypertensive, antidote, vasodilator (see p. 61C).

ACTION

Selectively blocks alpha₁-adrenergic receptors, decreasing peripheral vascular resistance. **Therapeutic Effect:** Produces vasodilation of veins, arterioles; decreases total peripheral resistance; relaxes smooth muscle in bladder neck, prostate.

PHARMACOKINETICS

Route	Onset	Peak	Duration
PO (B/P reduction)	2 hrs	2–4 hrs	10–24 hrs

Well absorbed following PO administration. Protein binding: 92%–97%. Metabolized in liver. Primarily excreted in feces. **Half-life:** 2–4 hrs.

USES

Treatment of mild to moderate hypertension. Used alone or in combination with other antihypertensives. **OFF-LABEL:** Treatment of benign prostate hyperplasia, Raynaud's phenomenon, post-traumatic stress disorder with related nightmares and sleep disruption.

PRECAUTIONS

Contraindications: Hypersensitivity to quinazolines. **Cautions:** Chronic renal failure, hepatic impairment.

⧗ LIFESPAN CONSIDERATIONS

Pregnancy/Lactation: Unknown if drug crosses placenta; is distributed in breast milk. **Pregnancy Category C. Children:** Safety and efficacy not established. **Elderly:** May be more sensitive to hypotensive effects.

INTERACTIONS

DRUG: Antihypertensives, diuretics, hypotension-producing medications may increase hypotensive effects. **HERBAL: Ephedra, ginseng, yohimbe, saw palmetto, garlic** may increase antihypertensive effect. **Licorice** causes sodium and water retention, potassium loss. **FOOD:** None known. **LAB VALUES:** None significant.

AVAILABILITY (Rx)

Capsules: 1 mg, 2 mg, 5 mg.

ADMINISTRATION/HANDLING

PO
• Give without regard to food. • Administer first dose at bedtime (minimizes risk of fainting due to "first-dose syncope").

INDICATIONS/ROUTES/DOSAGE

Hypertension
PO: ADULTS, ELDERLY: Initially, 1 mg 2–3 times a day. **Maintenance:** 2–20 mg/day in divided doses. **Maximum:** 20 mg/day. **CHILDREN:** Initially, 0.05–0.1 mg/kg/day in 3 divided doses. **Maximum:** 0.5 mg/kg/day or 20 mg.

SIDE EFFECTS

Frequent (10%–7%): Dizziness, drowsiness, headache, asthenia (loss of strength, energy). **Occasional (5%–4%):** Palpitations, nausea, dry mouth, nervousness. **Rare (Less Than 1%):** Angina, urinary urgency.

ADVERSE EFFECTS/ TOXIC REACTIONS

First-dose syncope (hypotension with sudden loss of consciousness) may occur 30–90 min following initial dose of more than 2 mg, too-rapid increase in dosage, addition of another antihypertensive agent to therapy. May be preceded by tachycardia (pulse rate of 120–160 beats/min).

NURSING CONSIDERATIONS

BASELINE ASSESSMENT

Give first dose at bedtime. If initial dose is given during daytime, pt must remain recumbent for 3–4 hrs. Assess B/P, pulse immediately before each dose and q15–30min until stabilized (be alert to B/P fluctuations).

INTERVENTION/EVALUATION

Monitor B/P, pulse diligently (first-dose syncope may be preceded by tachycardia). Monitor daily pattern of bowel ac-

P

tivity, stool consistency. Assist with ambulation if dizziness occurs.

PATIENT/FAMILY TEACHING

• Avoid tasks that require alertness, motor skills until response to drug is established. • Use caution when rising from sitting or lying position. • Report continued dizziness, palpitations.

---

*prednisoLONE

pred-**niss**-oh-lone
(Millipred, Novo-Prednisolone ❖, Omnipred, Orapred, Orapred ODT, Pediapred, Pred Forte, Pred Mild, Prelone, Veripred)
Do not confuse Pediapred with Pediazole, prednisolone with prednisone or primidone, or Prelone with Prozac.

FIXED-COMBINATION(S)

Blephamide: prednisolone/sulfacetamide (an anti-infective): 0.2%/10%. **Vasocidin:** prednisolone/sulfacetamide: 0.25%/10%.

◆CLASSIFICATION

PHARMACOTHERAPEUTIC: Adrenal corticosteroid. **CLINICAL:** Glucocorticoid (see pp. 100C, 141C).

ACTION

Inhibits accumulation of inflammatory cells at inflammation sites, phagocytosis, lysosomal enzyme release/synthesis, release of mediators of inflammation. **Therapeutic Effect:** Prevents/suppresses cell-mediated immune reactions. Decreases/prevents tissue response to inflammatory process.

PHARMACOKINETICS

Protein binding: 65%–91%. Metabolized in liver. Excreted in urine. **Half-life:** 3.6 hrs.

USES

Systemic: Endocrine, rheumatic, hematologic disorders; collagen, respiratory, neoplastic, GI diseases; allergic states; acute or chronic solid organ rejection. **Ophthalmic:** Treatment of conjunctivitis, corneal injury (from chemical/thermal burns, foreign body).

PRECAUTIONS

Contraindications: Acute superficial herpes simplex keratitis, systemic fungal infections, varicella, live or attenuated virus vaccines. **Cautions:** Hyperthyroidism, cirrhosis, ocular herpes simplex, respiratory tuberculosis, untreated systemic infections, renal/hepatic impairment, diabetes, cataracts, glaucoma, history of seizure disorder, peptic ulcer disease, osteoporosis, myasthenia gravis, hypertension, HF, ulcerative colitis, thromboembolic disorders.

⧗ LIFESPAN CONSIDERATIONS

Pregnancy/Lactation: Crosses placenta. Distributed in breast milk. Fetal cleft palate often occurs with chronic, first-trimester use. Breastfeeding not recommended. **Pregnancy Category C (D if used in first trimester). Children:** Prolonged treatment or high dosages may decrease short-term growth rate, cortisol secretion. **Elderly:** May be more susceptible to developing hypertension or osteoporosis.

INTERACTIONS

DRUG: **Hepatic enzyme inducers (e.g., phenobarbital, phenytoin, rifampin)** may decrease effects. **Live virus vaccines** increase vaccine side effects, potentiate virus replication, decrease pt's antibody response to vaccine. **HERBAL:** **St. John's wort** may decrease concentration. **Cat's claw, echinacea** have immunostimulant properties. **Echinacea** may decrease levels/effects. **FOOD:** None known. **LAB VALUES:** May increase serum glucose, lipids, sodium, uric acid. May decrease serum calcium, WBC, hypothalamic pituitary adrenal (HPA) axis function, potassium.

AVAILABILITY (Rx)

Solution, Ophthalmic: 1%. Solution, Oral (Orapred): 15 mg/5 ml. (Pediapred): 5 mg/5 ml. (Millipred): 10 mg/5 ml. (Veripred): 20 mg/5 ml. Suspension, Ophthalmic (Pred Forte): 1%; (Pred Mild): 0.12%. Syrup (Prelone): 5 mg/5 ml, 15 mg/5 ml. Tablets: 5 mg.

🏷 Tablets, Orally Disintegrating: 10 mg, 15 mg, 30 mg.

ADMINISTRATION/HANDLING

PO
• Give with food or fluids.

Orally Disintegrating Tablets
• Do not cut, split, break, or use partial tablets. • Remove from blister just prior to giving, place on tongue. • Pt may swallow whole or allow to dissolve in mouth with/without water.

Ophthalmic
• For ophthalmic solution, shake well before using. • Instill drops into conjunctival sac, as prescribed. • Avoid touching applicator tip to conjunctiva to avoid contamination.

INDICATIONS/ROUTES/DOSAGE

Usual Dosage
PO: ADULTS, ELDERLY: 5–60 mg/day in divided doses. **CHILDREN:** 0.1–2 mg/kg/day in 1–4 divided doses.

Treatment of Conjunctivitis, Corneal Injury
Ophthalmic: ADULTS, ELDERLY, CHILDREN: 1–2 drops every hr during day and q2h during night. After response, decrease dosage to 1 drop q4h, then 1 drop 3–4 times a day.

SIDE EFFECTS

Frequent: Insomnia, heartburn, nervousness, abdominal distention, diaphoresis, acne, mood swings, increased appetite, facial flushing, delayed wound healing, increased susceptibility to infection, diarrhea, constipation. **Occasional:** Headache, edema, change in skin color, frequent urination. **Rare:** Tachycardia, allergic reaction (rash, urticaria), psychological changes, hallucinations, depression. **Ophthalmic:** Stinging/burning, posterior subcapsular cataracts.

ADVERSE EFFECTS/ TOXIC REACTIONS

LONG-TERM THERAPY: Hypocalcemia, hypokalemia, muscle wasting (esp. arms, legs) osteoporosis, spontaneous fractures, amenorrhea, cataracts, glaucoma, peptic ulcer, HF. **ABRUPT WITHDRAWAL FOLLOWING LONG-TERM THERAPY:** Anorexia, nausea, fever, headache, severe/sudden joint pain, rebound inflammation, fatigue, weakness, lethargy, dizziness, orthostatic hypotension. Sudden discontinuance may be fatal.

NURSING CONSIDERATIONS

BASELINE ASSESSMENT

Obtain baselines for height, weight, B/P, serum glucose, electrolytes. Check results of initial tests (tuberculosis [TB] skin test, X-rays, EKG). Never give live virus vaccine (e.g., smallpox).

INTERVENTION/EVALUATION

Monitor B/P, weight, serum electrolytes, glucose, results of bone mineral density test, height, weight in children. Be alert to infection (sore throat, fever, vague symptoms); assess oral cavity daily for signs of candida infection (white patches, painful tongue/mucous membranes).

PATIENT/FAMILY TEACHING

• Report fever, sore throat, muscle aches, sudden weight gain, swelling, loss of appetite, fatigue. • Avoid alcohol, limit caffeine. • Do not abruptly discontinue without physician's approval. • Avoid exposure to chickenpox, measles.

P

---

*predniSONE

pred-ni-sone
(Apo-Prednisone ✤, Novo-Predni-sone ✤, Prednisone Intensol, Rayos, Winpred ✤)
Do not confuse prednisone with methylprednisolone, prazosin, prednisolone, Prilosec, primidone, or promethazine.

◆CLASSIFICATION

PHARMACOTHERAPEUTIC: Adrenal corticosteroid. **CLINICAL:** Glucocorticoid (see p. 100C).

ACTION

Inhibits accumulation of inflammatory cells at inflammation sites, phagocytosis, lysosomal enzyme release/synthesis, release of mediators of inflammation. **Therapeutic Effect:** Prevents/suppresses cell-mediated immune reactions. Decreases/prevents tissue response to inflammatory process.

PHARMACOKINETICS

Well absorbed from GI tract. Protein binding: 70%–90%. Widely distributed. Metabolized in liver, converted to prednisolone. Primarily excreted in urine. Not removed by hemodialysis. **Half-life:** 2.5–3.5 hrs.

USES

Substitution therapy in deficiency states: Acute or chronic adrenal insufficiency, congenital adrenal hyperplasia, adrenal insufficiency secondary to pituitary insufficiency. **Nonendocrine disorders:** Arthritis; rheumatic carditis; allergic, collagen, intestinal tract, multiple sclerosis exacerbations; liver, ocular, renal, skin diseases; bronchial asthma; cerebral edema; malignancies. **OFF-LABEL:** Prevention of postherpetic neuralgia, relief of acute pain in pts with herpes zoster, autoimmune hepatitis.

PRECAUTIONS

Contraindications: Acute superficial herpes simplex keratitis, systemic fungal infections, varicella, administration of live or attenuated virus vaccines. **Cautions:** Hyperthyroidism, cirrhosis, ocular herpes simplex, respiratory tuberculosis, untreated systemic infections, renal/hepatic impairment; following acute MI, diabetes, cataracts, glaucoma, seizures, peptic ulcer disease, osteoporosis, myasthenia gravis, hypertension, HF, ulcerative colitis, thromboembolic disorders.

⏳ LIFESPAN CONSIDERATIONS

Pregnancy/Lactation: Crosses placenta. Distributed in breast milk. Fetal cleft palate often occurs with chronic, first trimester use. Breastfeeding not recommended. **Pregnancy Category C (D if used in first trimester). Children:** Prolonged treatment or high dosages may decrease short-term growth rate, cortisol secretion. **Elderly:** May be more susceptible to developing hypertension or osteoporosis.

INTERACTIONS

DRUG: Hepatic enzyme inducers (e.g., phenobarbital, phenytoin, rifampin) may decrease effects. **Live virus vaccines** may increase vaccine side effects, potentiate virus replication, decrease pt's antibody response to vaccine. **HERBAL: St. John's wort** may decrease concentration. **Cat's claw, echinacea** have immunostimulant properties. **FOOD:** None known. **LAB VALUES:** May increase serum glucose, lipids, sodium, uric acid. May decrease serum calcium, potassium, WBC, hypothalamic pituitary adrenal (HPA) axis function.

AVAILABILITY (Rx)

Solution, Oral: 1 mg/ml. **Solution, Oral Concentrate (Prednisone Intensol):** 5 mg/ml. **Tablets:** 1 mg, 2.5 mg, 5 mg, 10 mg, 20 mg, 50 mg.

 Tablet: (Delayed-Release [Rayos]): 1 mg, 2 mg, 5 mg.

ADMINISTRATION/HANDLING

PO

• Give with food or fluids. • Give single doses before 9 AM, multiple doses at evenly spaced intervals. • Give delayed-release tablet whole. • Do not break, crush, dissolve, or divide.

INDICATIONS/ROUTES/DOSAGE

Note: Dose dependent upon condition treated, pt response rather than by rigid adherence to age, weight, or body surface area.

Usual Dosage

PO: ADULTS, ELDERLY: 5–60 mg/day in divided doses. **CHILDREN:** 0.05–2 mg/kg/day in 1–4 divided doses.

SIDE EFFECTS

Frequent: Insomnia, heartburn, nervousness, abdominal distention, diaphoresis, acne, mood swings, increased appetite, facial flushing, delayed wound healing, increased susceptibility to infection, diarrhea, constipation. **Occasional:** Headache, edema, change in skin color, frequent urination. **Rare:** Tachycardia, allergic reaction (rash, urticaria), psychological changes, hallucinations, depression.

ADVERSE EFFECTS/ TOXIC REACTIONS

LONG-TERM THERAPY: Muscle wasting (esp. in arms, legs), osteoporosis, spontaneous fractures, amenorrhea, cataracts, glaucoma, peptic ulcer, HF. **ABRUPT WITHDRAWAL FOLLOWING LONG-TERM THERAPY:** Anorexia, nausea, fever, headache, rebound inflammation, fatigue, weakness, lethargy, dizziness, orthostatic hypotension. Sudden discontinuance may be fatal.

NURSING CONSIDERATIONS

BASELINE ASSESSMENT

Obtain baselines for height, weight, B/P, serum glucose, electrolytes. Check results of initial tests (tuberculosis [TB] skin test, X-rays, EKG). Never give live virus vaccine (e.g., smallpox).

INTERVENTION/EVALUATION

Monitor B/P, serum electrolytes, glucose, results of bone mineral density test, height, weight in children. Be alert to infection (sore throat, fever, vague symptoms); assess oral cavity daily for signs of candida infection (white patches, painful tongue/mucous membranes).

PATIENT/FAMILY TEACHING

• Report fever, sore throat, muscle aches, sudden weight gain, swelling, loss of appetite, or fatigue. • Avoid alcohol, minimize use of caffeine. • Do not abruptly discontinue without physician's approval. • Avoid exposure to chickenpox, measles.

pregabalin TOP 200

pre-**gab**-a-lin
(Lyrica)

◆CLASSIFICATION

CLINICAL: Anticonvulsant, antineuralgic, analgesic **(Schedule V)** (see p. 37C).

ACTION

Binds to calcium channel sites in CNS tissue, inhibiting excitatory neurotransmitter release. Exerts antinociceptive, anticonvulsant activity. **Therapeutic Effect:** Decreases symptoms of painful peripheral neuropathy; decreases frequency of partial seizures.

PHARMACOKINETICS

Well absorbed following PO administration. Eliminated in urine unchanged. **Half-life:** 6 hrs.

USES

Adjunctive therapy in treatment of partial-onset seizures. Management of neuropathic pain associated with dia-

P

 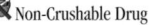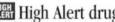

betic peripheral neuropathy or spinal cord injury. Management of postherpetic neuralgia. Management of fibromyalgia.

PRECAUTIONS

Contraindications: None known. **Cautions:** HF, renal impairment, cardiovascular disease, diabetes, history of angioedema, pts at high risk for suicide.

⧗ LIFESPAN CONSIDERATIONS

Pregnancy/Lactation: Increased risk of fetal skeletal abnormalities. Unknown if distributed in breast milk. **Pregnancy Category C. Children:** Safety and efficacy not established. **Elderly:** Age-related renal impairment may require dosage adjustment.

INTERACTIONS

DRUG: Alcohol, barbiturates, narcotic analgesics, other sedative agents may increase sedative effect. **HERBAL: Gotu kola, kava kava, St. John's wort, valerian** may increase CNS depression. **FOOD:** None known. **LAB VALUES:** May increase CPK. May cause mild PR interval prolongation. May decrease platelet count.

AVAILABILITY (Rx)

Solution, Oral: 20 mg/ml.

🍶 **Capsules (Lyrica):** 25 mg, 50 mg, 75 mg, 100 mg, 150 mg, 200 mg, 225 mg, 300 mg.

ADMINISTRATION/HANDLING

• Give without regard to food. • Do not open/crush capsule.

INDICATIONS/ROUTES/DOSAGE

Partial-Onset Seizures
PO: ADULTS, ELDERLY: Initially, 75 mg twice a day or 50 mg 3 times a day. May increase dose based on tolerability/effect. **Maximum:** 600 mg/day.

Neuropathic Pain
PO: ADULTS, ELDERLY: Initially, 50 mg 3 times a day. **Maximum:** 300 mg/day, in-

creased dose based on efficacy and tolerability.

Postherpetic Neuralgia, Neuropathic Pain Associated with Spinal Cord Injury
PO: ADULTS, ELDERLY: Initially, 75 mg twice a day or 50 mg 3 times a day. May increase to 300 mg/day within 1 wk. May further increase to 600 mg/day after 2–4 wks. **Maximum:** 600 mg/day.

Fibromyalgia
PO: ADULTS, ELDERLY: Initially, 75 mg twice a day. May increase to 150 mg twice a day within 1 wk. **Maximum:** 225 mg twice a day.

Dosage in Renal Impairment

Creatinine Clearance	Daily Dosage
30–60 ml/min	75–300 mg in 2–3 divided doses
15–29 ml/min	25–150 mg in 1 or 2 doses
Less than 15 ml/min	25–75 mg once daily

Dosage for Hemodialysis
◀ **ALERT** ▶ Take supplemental dose immediately following dialysis.

Daily Dosage	Supplemental Dosage
25 mg	Single dose of 25 mg or 50 mg
25–50 mg	Single dose of 50 mg or 75 mg
75 mg	Single dose of 100 mg or 150 mg

SIDE EFFECTS

Frequent (32%–12%): Dizziness, drowsiness, ataxia, peripheral edema. **Occasional (12%–5%):** Weight gain, blurred vision, diplopia, difficulty with concentration, attention, cognition; tremor, dry mouth, headache, constipation, asthenia (loss of strength, energy). **Rare (4%–2%):** Abnormal gait, confusion, incoordination, twitching, flatulence, vomiting, edema, myopathy.

underlined – top prescribed drug

ADVERSE EFFECTS/ TOXIC REACTIONS

Abrupt withdrawal increases risk of seizure frequency in pts with seizure disorders; withdraw gradually over a minimum of 1 wk.

BASELINE ASSESSMENT

Seizure: Review history of seizure disorder (type, onset, intensity, frequency, duration, LOC). **Pain:** Assess onset, type, location, and duration of pain.

INTERVENTION/EVALUATION

Provide safety measures as needed. Assess for seizure activity. Assess for clinical improvement; record onset of relief of pain. Assess for evidence of peripheral edema behind medial malleolus (usually first area of edema). Question for changes in visual acuity.

PATIENT/FAMILY TEACHING

• Do not abruptly stop taking drug because seizure frequency may be increased. • Do not drive, operate machinery, perform activities requiring mental acuity due to potential dizziness, drowsiness, ataxia. • Avoid alcohol. • Carry identification card, bracelet to note anticonvulsant therapy.

primidone

prim-i-done
(Apo-Primidone ✤, Mysoline)
**Do not confuse primidone with
prednisone or pyridoxine.**

◆CLASSIFICATION

PHARMACOTHERAPEUTIC: Barbiturate. **CLINICAL:** Anticonvulsant (see p. 37C).

ACTION

Decreases motor activity from electrical/chemical stimulation, stabilizes seizure threshold against hyperexcitability. **Therapeutic Effect:** Reduces seizure activity.

PHARMACOKINETICS

Rapidly, usually completely absorbed following PO administration. Protein binding: 99%. Extensively metabolized in liver to phenobarbital and phenylethylmalonamide (PEMA). Minimal excretion in urine. **Half-life:** 10–12 hrs.

USES

Management of partial seizures with complex symptomatology (psychomotor seizures), generalized tonic-clonic (grand mal) seizures, focal seizures. **OFF-LABEL:** Treatment of essential tremor (familial tremor).

PRECAUTIONS

Contraindications: Hypersensitivity to phenobarbital, porphyria. **Cautions:** Renal/hepatic impairment, pulmonary insufficiency, elderly, debilitated, children, hypoadrenalism, pts at risk for suicidal thoughts/behavior, depression.

⌛ LIFESPAN CONSIDERATIONS

Pregnancy/Lactation: Crosses placenta; distributed in breast milk. **Pregnancy Category D. Children, Elderly:** May produce paradoxical excitement, restlessness.

INTERACTIONS

DRUG: Alcohol, other CNS depressants may increase effects. **Valproic acid** increases concentration, risk of toxicity. **HERBAL: Evening primrose** may decrease seizure threshold. **Gotu kola, kava kava, St. John's wort, valerian** may increase CNS depression. **FOOD:** None known. **LAB VALUES:** May decrease serum bilirubin. **Therapeutic serum level:** 4–12 mcg/ml; **toxic serum level:** greater than 12 mcg/ml.

AVAILABILITY (Rx)

Tablets: 50 mg, 250 mg.

 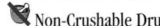

ADMINISTRATION/HANDLING

PO

• Give with food to minimize GI effects.

INDICATIONS/ROUTES/DOSAGE

Seizure Control

PO: ADULTS, ELDERLY, CHILDREN 8 YRS AND OLDER: Initially, 100–125 mg/day at bedtime for days 1–3. **Days 4–6:** 100–125 mg twice daily. **Days 7–9:** 100–125 mg 3 times/day. **Usual dose:** 750–1,500 mg/day. **Maximum:** 2 g/day. **CHILDREN YOUNGER THAN 8 YRS:** Initially, 50 mg/day at bedtime for days 1–3. **Days 4–6:** 50 mg twice daily. **Days 7–9:** 100 mg twice daily. **Usual dose:** 10–25 mg/kg/day (375–750 mg) in 3–4 divided doses. **NEONATES:** 12–20 mg/kg/day in divided doses 2–4 times a day.

Dosage Interval in Renal Impairment

Creatine Clearance	Interval
50 ml/min or greater	q12h
10–49 ml/min	q12–24h
Less than 10 ml/min	q24h

SIDE EFFECTS

Frequent: Ataxia, dizziness. **Occasional:** Anorexia, drowsiness, altered mental status, nausea, vomiting, paradoxical excitement. **Rare:** Rash.

ADVERSE EFFECTS/ TOXIC REACTIONS

Abrupt withdrawal after prolonged therapy may produce effects ranging from markedly increased dreaming, nightmares, insomnia, tremor, diaphoresis, vomiting to hallucinations, delirium, seizures, status epilepticus. Skin eruptions may appear as hypersensitivity reaction. Blood dyscrasias, hepatic disease, hypocalcemia occur rarely. Overdose produces cold/clammy skin, hypothermia, severe CNS depression, followed by high fever, coma.

NURSING CONSIDERATIONS

BASELINE ASSESSMENT

Review history of seizure disorder (intensity, frequency, duration, LOC). Observe frequently for recurrence of seizure activity. Initiate seizure precautions.

INTERVENTION/EVALUATION

Monitor for changes in behavior, depression, suicidal ideation. Monitor serum primidone concentrations, CBC; neurologic status (frequency, duration, severity of seizures). Monitor for **therapeutic serum level:** 4–12 mcg/ml; **toxic serum level:** more than 12 mcg/ml.

PATIENT/FAMILY TEACHING

• Do not abruptly discontinue medication after long-term use (may precipitate seizures). • Strict maintenance of drug therapy is essential for seizure control. • Avoid tasks that require alertness, motor skills until response to drug is established. • Drowsiness usually disappears during continued therapy. • If dizziness occurs, change positions slowly from recumbent to sitting position before standing. • Avoid alcohol. • Report depression, thoughts of suicide, unusual changes in behavior.

probenecid

pro-**ben**-e-sid
(Benuryl ✦)
Do not confuse probenecid with procainamide or Procanbid.

FIXED-COMBINATION(S)

Probenecid/colchicine (an antigout agent): 500 mg/0.5 mg.

◆CLASSIFICATION

PHARMACOTHERAPEUTIC: Uricosuric. **CLINICAL:** Antigout agent.

ACTION

Competitively inhibits reabsorption of uric acid at proximal convoluted tubule.

Inhibits renal tubular secretion of weak organic acids (e.g., penicillins). **Therapeutic Effect:** Promotes uric acid excretion, reduces serum uric acid level, increases plasma levels of penicillins, cephalosporins.

PHARMACOKINETICS

Rapidly absorbed following PO administration. Metabolized in liver. Excreted in urine. Excretion is dependent upon urinary pH, is increased in alkaline urine. **Half-life:** 6–12 hrs.

USES

Treatment of hyperuricemia associated with gout, gouty arthritis. Adjunctive therapy with penicillins, cephalosporins to elevate/prolong antibiotic plasma levels. **OFF-LABEL:** Prolongation/elevation of beta-lactam plasma levels.

PRECAUTIONS

Contraindications: Blood dyscrasias, children younger than 2 yrs, concurrent high-dose aspirin therapy, uric acid calculi. **Cautions:** Peptic ulcer, hematuria, renal colic, severe renal impairment (creatinine clearance less than 30 ml/min), pts with G6PD deficiency.

⌛ LIFESPAN CONSIDERATIONS

Pregnancy/Lactation: Unknown if drug crosses placenta or is distributed in breast milk. **Pregnancy Category C. Children:** Safety and efficacy not established in those younger than 2 yrs. **Elderly:** No age-related precautions noted.

INTERACTIONS

DRUG: Increases effect, toxicity of **methotrexate.** Increases concentration of **cephalosporins, ketorolac, NSAIDs, penicillins.** **HERBAL:** None significant. **FOOD:** None known. **LAB VALUES:** May inhibit renal excretion of serum PSP (phenolsulfonphthalein), 17-ketosteroids, BSP (sulfobromophthalein).

AVAILABILITY (Rx)

Tablets: 500 mg.

ADMINISTRATION/HANDLING

PO
• Give with or immediately after meals, milk. • Instruct pt to drink at least 6–8 glasses (8 oz) of water/day (prevents kidney stone development).

INDICATIONS/ROUTES/DOSAGE

Gout
PO: ADULTS, ELDERLY: Initially, 250 mg twice daily for 1 wk, then 500 mg twice daily. May increase by 500 mg q4wks. **Maximum:** 2 g/day. Maintenance: Dosage that maintains normal uric acid level.

Adjunct to Penicillin, Cephalosporin Therapy
PO: ADULTS, ELDERLY, CHILDREN OLDER THAN 14 YRS: 500 mg 4 times/day. **CHILDREN 2–14 YRS:** Initially, 25 mg/kg. **Maintenance:** 40 mg/kg/day in 4 divided doses. **Maximum:** 500-mg dose.

Dosage in Renal Impairment
Creatinine clearance less than 30 ml/min: Avoid use.

SIDE EFFECTS

Frequent (10%–6%): Headache, anorexia, nausea, vomiting. **Occasional (5%–1%):** Lower back or side pain, rash, urticaria, pruritus, dizziness, flushed face, urinary urgency, gingivitis.

ADVERSE EFFECTS/ TOXIC REACTIONS

Severe hypersensitivity reactions, including anaphylaxis, occur rarely (usually within few hrs after administration following previous use); discontinue drug immediately, contact physician. Pruritic maculopapular rash should be considered a toxic reaction. May be accompanied by malaise, fever, chills, arthralgia, nausea, vomiting, leukopenia, aplastic anemia.

NURSING CONSIDERATIONS

BASELINE ASSESSMENT

Do not initiate therapy until acute gouty attack has subsided. Question for hyper-

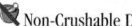 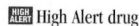

sensitivity to probenecid or if taking penicillin, cephalosporin antibiotics.

INTERVENTION/EVALUATION

If exacerbation of gout recurs after therapy, use other agents for gout. Discontinue medication immediately if rash, other evidence of allergic reaction appears. Encourage high fluid intake (3,000 ml/day). Monitor I&O (output should be at least 2,000 ml/day). Assess CBC, serum uric acid levels. Assess urine for cloudiness, unusual color, odor. Assess for therapeutic response (reduced joint tenderness, swelling, redness, limitation of motion).

PATIENT/FAMILY TEACHING

• Drink plenty of fluids to decrease risk of uric acid kidney stones. • Avoid alcohol, large doses of aspirin, other salicylates. • Consume low-purine food (reduce/omit meat, fowl, fish; use eggs, cheese, vegetables). • May take over 1 wk for full therapeutic effect. • Drink 6–8 glasses (8 oz) of fluid daily while on medication.

---

procainamide HIGH ALERT

proe-**kane**-a-mide
(Apo-Procainamide ❖,
Procan-SR ❖)

BLACK BOX ALERT Prolonged use results in positive ANA tests in 50% of pts, may lead to lupus erythematosus-like syndrome. Agranulocytosis, neutropenia, hypoplastic anemia, thrombocytopenia reported; 20%–25% mortality with agranulocytosis.

◆CLASSIFICATION

PHARMACOTHERAPEUTIC: Class 1 antiarrhythmic. **CLINICAL:** Antiarrhythmic (see p. 16C).

ACTION

Increases electrical stimulation threshold of ventricles, His-Purkinje system. Decreases myocardial excitability, conduction velocity; depresses myocardial contractility. Exerts direct cardiac effects. **Therapeutic Effect:** Suppresses arrhythmias.

PHARMACOKINETICS

Rapidly, completely absorbed from GI tract. Protein binding: 15%–20%. Widely distributed. Metabolized in liver. Primarily excreted in urine. Removed by hemodialysis. **Half-life:** 2.5–4.5 hrs; metabolite, 6–8 hrs.

USES

IV: Treatment of life-threatening ventricular arrhythmias. **OFF-LABEL:** Paroxysmal supraventricular tachycardia (PSVT); prevention of ventricular tachycardia, symptomatic premature ventricular contractions (PVCs).

PRECAUTIONS

Contraindications: Complete heart block, second-degree heart block without a functional pacemaker, systemic lupus erythematosus, torsade de pointes. **Cautions:** Marked AV conduction disturbances, bundle-branch block, severe digoxin toxicity, HF, supraventricular tachyarrhythmias, renal/hepatic impairment, preexisting QT prolongation, myasthenia gravis.

⏳ LIFESPAN CONSIDERATIONS

Pregnancy/Lactation: Crosses placenta. Unknown if distributed in breast milk. **Pregnancy Category C. Children:** No age-related precautions noted. **Elderly:** More susceptible to hypotensive effect. Age-related renal impairment may require dosage adjustment.

INTERACTIONS

DRUG: May increase effects of **neuromuscular blockers. Other antiarrhythmics** may increase cardiac effects. **HERBAL: Ephedra** may worsen arrhythmias. **FOOD:** None known. **LAB VALUES:** May cause EKG changes, positive ANA titers, Coombs' test. May increase serum alkaline phosphatase, bilirubin, AST, ALT, LDH. **Therapeutic serum level:** 4–8 mcg/ml; **toxic serum level:** greater than 10 mcg/ml.

AVAILABILITY (Rx)

Injection Solution: 100 mg/ml, 500 mg/ml.

ADMINISTRATION/HANDLING

 IV, IM

◀ **ALERT** ▶ May give by IM injection, IV push, IV infusion.

Reconstitution • For IV push, dilute with 5–10 ml D₅W. Maximum concentration: 20 mg/ml. • For initial loading infusion, add 1 g to 50 ml D₅W to provide concentration of 20 mg/ml. • For IV infusion, add 1 g to 250–500 ml D₅W to provide concentration of 2–4 mg/ml. Maximum concentration: 4 g/250 ml.

Rate of Administration • For IV push, with pt in supine position, administer at rate not exceeding 25–50 mg/min. • For initial loading infusion, infuse 1 ml/min for up to 25–30 min. • For IV infusion, infuse at 1–3 ml/min. • Check B/P q5–10min during infusion. If fall in B/P exceeds 15 mm Hg, discontinue drug, contact physician. Notify physician of any significant interval changes. • B/P, EKG should be monitored continuously during IV administration and rate of infusion adjusted to eliminate arrhythmias.

Storage • Solution appears clear, colorless to light yellow. • Discard if solution darkens or is discolored or if precipitate forms. • When diluted with 0.9% NaCl or D₅W, solution is stable for 24 hrs at room temperature, for 7 days if refrigerated.

IV INCOMPATIBILITY

Milrinone (Primacor).

IV COMPATIBILITIES

Amiodarone (Cordarone), dobutamine (Dobutrex), heparin, lidocaine, potassium chloride.

INDICATIONS/ROUTES/DOSAGE

Management of Arrhythmias

IV: ADULTS, ELDERLY: Loading dose: 15–18 mg/kg given as slow infusion over 25–30 min. **Maintenance infusion:** 1–4 mg/min. **CHILDREN:** Loading dose: 3–6 mg/kg over 5 min (**maximum:** 100 mg). May repeat q5–10min to maximum total dose of 15 mg/kg. **Maintenance dose:** 20–80 mcg/kg/min. **Maximum:** 2 g/day.

SIDE EFFECTS

Frequent: Transient, but at times, marked hypotension. **Rare:** Confusion, mental depression, psychosis.

ADVERSE EFFECTS/ TOXIC REACTIONS

Paradoxical, extremely rapid ventricular rate may occur during treatment of atrial fibrillation/flutter. Systemic lupus erythematosus-like syndrome (fever, myalgia, pleuritic chest pain) may occur with prolonged therapy. Cardiotoxic effects occur most commonly with IV administration and appear as conduction changes (50% widening of QRS complex, frequent ventricular premature contractions, ventricular tachycardia, complete AV block). Prolonged PR and QT intervals, flattened T waves occur less frequently.

NURSING CONSIDERATIONS

BASELINE ASSESSMENT

Check B/P, pulse for 1 full min (unless pt is on continuous monitor) before giving medication.

INTERVENTION/EVALUATION

Check B/P q5–10 min during infusion. If fall in B/P exceeds 15 mm/Hg, discontinue drug, contact physician. Monitor EKG for cardiac changes, particularly widening of QRS, prolongation of PR and QT intervals. Assess pulse for strength/weakness, irregular rate. Monitor I&O, serum electrolyte levels (potassium, chloride, sodium). Assess for complaints of GI upset, headache, arthralgia. Monitor daily pattern of bowel activity, stool consistency. Assess for dizziness. Assess skin for evidence of hypersensitivity reaction (esp. in pts on high-dose therapy). Monitor for therapeutic serum level. **Therapeutic serum level:** 4–8 mcg/ml; **toxic serum level:** greater than 10 mcg/ml.

P

procarbazine HIGH ALERT

proe-**kar**-ba-zeen
(Matulane, Natulan ✱)
BLACK BOX ALERT Must be administered by personnel trained in administration/handling of chemotherapeutic agents.
Do not confuse procarbazine with dacarbazine.

◆CLASSIFICATION

PHARMACOTHERAPEUTIC: Methylhydrazine derivative. **CLINICAL:** Antineoplastic (see p. 90C).

ACTION

Inhibits DNA, RNA, protein synthesis. May directly damage DNA. Cell cycle–phase specific for S phase of cell division. **Therapeutic Effect:** Causes cell death.

PHARMACOKINETICS

Rapidly, completely absorbed from GI tract. Crosses blood-brain barrier. Metabolized primarily in liver, kidneys. Excreted in urine, feces. **Half-life:** 1 hr.

USES

Treatment of Hodgkin's disease. **OFF-LABEL:** Non-Hodgkin's lymphoma, primary brain tumors.

PRECAUTIONS

Contraindications: Preexisting bone marrow aplasia, alcohol ingestion, pregnancy. **Cautions:** Renal/hepatic impairment.

⌛ LIFESPAN CONSIDERATIONS

Pregnancy/Lactation: Unknown if distributed in breast milk. May cause fetal harm. **Pregnancy Category D. Children:** Safety and efficacy not established. **Elderly:** Age-related renal impairment may require dosage adjustment.

INTERACTIONS

DRUG: Alcohol may cause disulfiram-like reaction. May increase anticho-linergic effects of **anticholinergics, antihistamines. Bone marrow depressants** may increase myelosuppression. **CNS depressants** may increase CNS depression. **Tricyclic antidepressants** may increase anticholinergic effects; may cause seizures, hyperpyretic crisis. **Live virus vaccines** may potentiate virus replication, increase vaccine side effects, decrease pt's antibody response to vaccine. **HERBAL: Echinacea** may decrease levels/effects. **FOOD: Caffeine** may increase B/P. **Foods containing tyramine** may cause clinically severe (possibly life-threatening) hypertension. **LAB VALUES:** None significant.

AVAILABILITY (Rx)

Capsules: 50 mg.

ADMINISTRATION/HANDLING

PO
• Administer with food or immediately after meals.

INDICATIONS/ROUTES/DOSAGE

◄**ALERT**► Base dosage on ideal body weight.

Advanced Hodgkin's Disease
PO: ADULTS, ELDERLY: Initially, 2–4 mg/kg/day as single dose or in divided doses for 1 wk, then 4–6 mg/kg/day. Maintenance: 1–2 mg/kg/day. **CHILDREN:** 100 mg/m^2/day for 14 days of a 28-day cycle and repeated q4wks. Continue until maximum response occurs, leukocyte count falls below 4,000/mm^3, or platelet count falls below 100,000/mm^3.

SIDE EFFECTS

Frequent: Severe nausea, vomiting, respiratory disorders (cough, effusion), myalgia, arthralgia, drowsiness, nervousness, insomnia, nightmares, diaphoresis, hallucinations, seizures. **Occasional:** Hoarseness, tachycardia, nystagmus, retinal hemorrhage, photophobia, photosensitivity, urinary frequency, nocturia, hypotension, diarrhea, stomatitis, paresthesia, unsteadi-

P

ness, confusion, decreased reflexes, foot drop. **Rare:** Hypersensitivity reaction (dermatitis, pruritus, rash, urticaria), hyperpigmentation, alopecia.

ADVERSE EFFECTS/ TOXIC REACTIONS

Major toxic effects are myelosuppression manifested as hematologic toxicity (principally leukopenia, thrombocytopenia, anemia), hepatotoxicity manifested as jaundice, ascites. UTIs secondary to leukopenia may occur.

NURSING CONSIDERATIONS

BASELINE ASSESSMENT

Obtain bone marrow tests, CBC, renal function test, hepatic function results before therapy and periodically thereafter. Therapy should be interrupted if WBC falls below 4,000/mm³ or platelet count falls below 100,000/mm³.

INTERVENTION/EVALUATION

Monitor hematologic status, renal/hepatic function studies. Assess for stomatitis. Monitor for hematologic toxicity (fever, sore throat, signs of local infection, unusual bruising/bleeding from any site), symptoms of anemia (excessive fatigue, weakness).

PATIENT/FAMILY TEACHING

• Report fever, sore throat, bleeding, bruising. • Avoid alcohol (may cause disulfiram reaction: nausea, vomiting, headache, sedation, visual disturbances). • Avoid tyramine-containing foods.

prochlorperazine

proe-klor-**per**-a-zeen
(Apo-Prochlorperazine ✤, Compro)
BLACK BOX ALERT Increased risk for death in elderly with dementia-related psychosis.
Do not confuse prochlorperazine with chlorpromazine.

◆CLASSIFICATION

PHARMACOTHERAPEUTIC: Phenothiazine. **CLINICAL:** Antiemetic, antipsychotic.

ACTION

Acts centrally to inhibit/block dopamine receptors in chemoreceptor trigger zone, peripherally to block vagus nerve in GI tract. **Therapeutic Effect:** Relieves nausea/vomiting, improves psychosis.

PHARMACOKINETICS

Route	Onset*	Peak	Duration
PO	30–40 min	N/A	3–4 hrs
IM	10–20 min	N/A	4–6 hrs
Rectal	60 min	N/A	12 hrs

*As an antiemetic.

Variably absorbed after PO administration. Widely distributed. Metabolized in liver, GI mucosa. Primarily excreted in urine. Unknown if removed by hemodialysis. **Half-life: PO:** 3–5 hrs, **IV:** 7 hrs.

USES

Management of nausea/vomiting. Treatment of acute or chronic psychosis. **OFF-LABEL:** Behavior syndromes in dementia, psychosis/agitation related to Alzheimer's dementia.

PRECAUTIONS

Contraindications: Narrow-angle glaucoma, severe CNS depression, coma, children younger than 2 yrs or less than 9 kg; severe cardiac/hepatic impairment, pediatric surgery. **Cautions:** History of seizures, Parkinson's disease, elderly, pts at risk for pneumonia, severe renal impairment, decreased GI motility, urinary retention, visual problems, paralytic ileus, myasthenia gravis, cerebrovascular/cardiovascular disease.

⌛ LIFESPAN CONSIDERATIONS

Pregnancy/Lactation: Crosses placenta. Distributed in breast milk. **Pregnancy Category C. Children:** Safety and efficacy not established in those weighing

P

less than 9 kg or younger than 2 yrs. **Elderly:** More susceptible to orthostatic hypotension, anticholinergic effects (e.g., dry mouth), sedation, extrapyramidal symptoms (EPS); lower dosage recommended.

INTERACTIONS

DRUG: Alcohol, other CNS depressants may increase CNS, respiratory depression, hypotensive effects. **Extrapyramidal symptom (EPS)–producing medications** may increase EPS. **Lithium** may decrease absorption, produce adverse neurologic effects. **MAOIs, tricyclic antidepressants** may increase anticholinergic, sedative effects. **HERBAL: Dong quai, St. John's wort** may increase photosensitization. **Gotu kola, kava kava, St. John's wort, valerian** may increase CNS depression. **FOOD:** None known. **LAB VALUES:** None significant.

AVAILABILITY (Rx)

Injection Solution: 5 mg/ml. **Suppositories (Compro):** 25 mg. **Tablets:** 5 mg, 10 mg.

ADMINISTRATION/HANDLING

 IV

Rate of Administration • May give by IV push slowly. Maximum rate: 5 mg/min. **Storage** • Store at room temperature. • Protect from light. • Clear or slightly yellow solutions may be used.

IM
• Inject deep IM into outer quadrant of buttocks.

PO
• Should be administered with food or water.

Rectal
• Moisten suppository with cold water before inserting well into rectum.

▣ IV INCOMPATIBILITIES

Furosemide (Lasix), hydrocortisone, hydromorphone (Dilaudid), midazolam (Versed).

▣ IV COMPATIBILITIES

Calcium gluconate, dexmedetomidine (Precedex), diphenhydramine (Benadryl), fentanyl, heparin, metoclopramide (Reglan), morphine, potassium chloride, promethazine (Phenergan), propofol (Diprivan).

INDICATIONS/ROUTES/DOSAGE

Nausea/Vomiting
PO: ADULTS, ELDERLY: 5–10 mg 3–4 times a day. **CHILDREN: GREATER THAN 39 KG:** 5–10 mg q6–8h. **Maximum:** 40 mg/day. **18 KG TO 39KG:** 2.5 mg q8h or 5 mg q12h. **Maximum:** 15 mg/day. **13 KG TO 18 KG:** 2.5 mg q8–12h. **Maximum:** 10 mg/day. **9–13 KG:** 2.5 mg q12–24h. **Maximum:** 7.5 mg/day.
IV: ADULTS, ELDERLY: 2.5–10 mg. May repeat q3–4h. **Maximum:** 10 mg/dose or 40 mg/day. **CHILDREN:** 0.1–0.15 mg/kg/dose q8–12h. **Maximum:** 40 mg/day.
IM: ADULTS, ELDERLY: 5–10 mg q3–4h. **CHILDREN:** 0.1–0.15 mg/kg/dose q8–12h. **Maximum:** 40 mg/day.
Rectal: ADULTS, ELDERLY: 25 mg twice a day.

Psychosis
PO: ADULTS, ELDERLY: 5–10 mg 3–4 times a day. **Maximum:** 150 mg/day. **CHILDREN 2–12 YRS:** 2.5 mg 2–3 times a day. **Maximum daily dose:** 25 mg for children 6–12 yrs; 20 mg for children 2–5 yrs.
IM: ADULTS, ELDERLY: 10–20 mg q4h. **CHILDREN:** 0.13 mg/kg/dose.

SIDE EFFECTS

Frequent: Drowsiness, hypotension, dizziness, fainting (commonly occurring after first dose, occasionally after subsequent doses, rarely with oral form). **Occasional:** Dry mouth, blurred vision, lethargy, constipation, diarrhea, myalgia, nasal congestion, peripheral edema, urinary retention.

ADVERSE EFFECTS/ TOXIC REACTIONS

Extrapyramidal symptoms (EPS) appear dose related and are divided into three categories: akathisia (e.g., inability to sit still, tapping of feet), parkinsonian symptoms (mask-like face, tremors, shuffling gait, hypersalivation), acute dystonias (torticollis [neck muscle spasm], opisthotonos [rigidity of back muscles], oculogyric crisis [rolling back of eyes]). Dystonic reaction may produce diaphoresis, pallor. Tardive dyskinesia (tongue protrusion, puffing of cheeks, puckering of mouth) occurs rarely and may be irreversible. Abrupt withdrawal after long-term therapy may precipitate nausea, vomiting, gastritis, dizziness, tremors. Blood dyscrasias, particularly agranulocytosis, mild leukopenia, may occur. May lower seizure threshold.

NURSING CONSIDERATIONS

BASELINE ASSESSMENT

Avoid skin contact with solution (contact dermatitis). **Antiemetic:** Assess for dehydration (poor skin turgor, dry mucous membranes, longitudinal furrows in tongue). **Antipsychotic:** Assess behavior, appearance, emotional status, response to environment, speech pattern, thought content.

INTERVENTION/EVALUATION

Monitor B/P for hypotension. Assess for EPS. Monitor WBC, differential count for blood dyscrasias. Monitor for fine tongue movement (may be early sign of tardive dyskinesia). Supervise suicidal-risk pt closely during early therapy (as depression lessens, energy level improves, increasing suicide potential). Assess for therapeutic response (interest in surroundings, improvement in self-care, increased ability to concentrate, relaxed facial expression or relief of nausea, vomiting).

PATIENT/FAMILY TEACHING

• Limit caffeine. • Avoid alcohol. • Avoid tasks requiring alertness, motor skills until response to drug is established (may cause drowsiness, impairment).

---

progesterone

pro-**jes**-te-rone
(Crinone, Endometrin Vaginal Insert, Prochieve, Prometrium)
BLACK BOX ALERT Not indicated to prevent coronary heart disease. Risk of dementia may be increased in postmenopausal women.

◆CLASSIFICATION

PHARMACOTHERAPEUTIC: Progestin.
CLINICAL: Hormone.

ACTION

Promotes mammary gland development, relaxes uterine smooth muscle. **Therapeutic Effect:** Decreases abnormal uterine bleeding; transforms endometrium from proliferative to secretory in estrogen-primed endometrium.

PHARMACOKINETICS

Protein binding: 96%–99%. Metabolized in liver. Excreted in bile, urine. **Half-life (vaginal gel):** 5–20 min.

USES

PO: Prevent endometrial hyperplasia, secondary amenorrhea. **IM:** Amenorrhea, abnormal uterine bleeding due to hormonal imbalance. **Vaginal gel:** Treatment of infertility, secondary amenorrhea. **Vaginal insert:** Treatment of infertility. **OFF-LABEL:** Reduce risk of recurrent spontaneous preterm birth.

PRECAUTIONS

Contraindications: History of or suspected carcinoma of breast, active breast cancer; thromboembolic disorders, thrombophlebitis, missed abortion or ectopic pregnancy, severe hepatic dysfunction, undiagnosed abnormal vaginal bleeding, use as a pregnancy test. **Cautions:** Diabetes, conditions aggravated by fluid retention (e.g., asthma, epilepsy, migraine, cardiac/renal dysfunction), history of mental depression.

⧗ LIFESPAN CONSIDERATIONS

Pregnancy/Lactation: Distributed in breast milk. Avoid use during pregnancy. **Pregnancy Category B (Prometrium).** None established for vaginal gel, vaginal insert, or injection. **Children:** Safety and efficacy not established. **Elderly:** No age-related precautions noted.

INTERACTIONS

DRUG: CYP3A4 inducers (e.g., **carbamazepine, phenobarbital, phenytoin, rifampin**) may decrease effects of progesterone. **HERBAL: St. John's wort** may decrease effect. **FOOD:** None known. **LAB VALUES:** May alter HDL, cholesterol, triglycerides, LDL. May increase hepatic function values.

AVAILABILITY (Rx)

Capsules (Prometrium): 100 mg, 200 mg. **Injection Oil:** 50 mg/ml. **Vaginal Gel (Crinone, Prochieve):** 4% (45 mg/dose), 8% (90 mg/dose). **Vaginal Insert (Endometrin Vaginal Insert):** 25 mg, 50 mg, 100 mg, 200 mg, 400 mg.

ADMINISTRATION/HANDLING

IM

• Store at room temperature. • Administer only deep IM in large muscle mass.

PO

• If given in morning, administer 2 hrs after breakfast with full glass of water.

Vaginal Gel

• Remove applicator from sealed wrapper. Do not remove twist-off tab at this time. • Hold applicator by thick end. Shake down several times (like a thermometer) to ensure contents are at thin end. • Hold applicator by flat section of thick end and twist off tab at other end. Do not squeeze thick end while twisting tab (could force some gel to be released before insertion). • Insert applicator into vagina either in sitting position or lying on back with knees bent. • Insert thin end well into vagina. • Squeeze thick end of applicator to deposit gel. • Remove applicator, discard.

INDICATIONS/ROUTES/DOSAGE

Amenorrhea

PO: ADULTS: 400 mg daily in evening for 10 days.

IM: ADULTS: 5–10 mg for 6–8 days. Withdrawal bleeding expected in 48–72 hrs if ovarian activity produced proliferative endometrium.

Vaginal: ADULTS: Apply 45 mg (4% gel) every other day for 6 or fewer doses.

Abnormal Uterine Bleeding

IM: ADULTS: 5–10 mg/day for 6 days. When estrogen given concomitantly, begin progesterone after 2 wks of estrogen therapy; discontinue when menstruation begins.

Prevention of Endometrial Hyperplasia

PO: ADULTS: 200 mg in evening for 12 days per 28-day cycle, in combination with daily conjugated estrogen.

Infertility

Vaginal: ADULTS: 90 mg (8% gel) once a day (twice a day in women with partial or complete ovarian failure). If pregnancy occurs, may continue up to 10–12 wks.

Support of Embryo/Early Pregnancy

Vaginal Insert: 100 mg 2–3 times a day for up to 10 wks.

SIDE EFFECTS

Frequent: Breakthrough bleeding/spotting at beginning of therapy, amenorrhea, change in menstrual flow, breast tenderness. **Gel:** Drowsiness. **Occasional:** Edema, weight gain/loss, rash, pruritus, photosensitivity, skin pigmentation. **Rare:** Pain/swelling at injection site, acne, depression, alopecia, hirsutism.

ADVERSE EFFECTS/
TOXIC REACTIONS

Thrombophlebitis, cerebrovascular disorders, retinal thrombosis, pulmonary embolism occur rarely.

NURSING CONSIDERATIONS

BASELINE ASSESSMENT

Question for possibility of pregnancy, hypersensitivity to progestins before initiating therapy. Obtain baseline weight, serum glucose level, B/P.

INTERVENTION/EVALUATION

Check weight daily; report weekly gain over 5 lbs. Assess skin for rash, urticaria. Immediately report development of chest pain, sudden shortness of breath, sudden decrease in vision, migraine headache, pain (esp. with swelling, warmth, redness) in calves, numbness of arm/leg (thrombotic disorders). Check B/P periodically. Note progesterone therapy on pathology specimens.

PATIENT/FAMILY TEACHING

• Use sunscreen, protective clothing to protect from sunlight, ultraviolet light until tolerance determined. • Report abnormal vaginal bleeding, other related symptoms. • Stop taking medication, contact physician at once if pregnancy suspected. • If using vaginal gel, avoid tasks that require alertness, motor skills until response to drug is established.

---

promethazine

proe-**meth**-a-zeen
(Phenadoz, <u>Phenergan</u>, Promethegan)

BLACK BOX ALERT Fatalities due to respiratory depression reported in children 2 yrs and younger. Severe tissue injury, including gangrene, may occur with intravenous injection (preferred route is deep intramuscular). Be alert for signs and symptoms of tissue injury including

burning or pain at injection site, phlebitis, swelling, blistering. Risk reduced by diluting promethazine with 10–20 ml 0.9% NaCl or diluting in a minibag (piggyback); administer slowly over 10–15 min; use large veins or central venous site (no hand or wrist veins).

Do not confuse Phenergan with phenelzine, or promethazine with chlorpromazine or prednisone.

FIXED-COMBINATION(S)

Phenergan with codeine: promethazine/codeine (a cough suppressant): 6.25 mg/10 mg/5 ml. **Phenergan VC:** promethazine/phenylephrine (a vasoconstrictor): 6.25 mg/5 mg/5 ml. **Phenergan VC with codeine:** promethazine/phenylephrine/codeine: 6.25 mg/5 mg/10 mg/5 ml.

◆CLASSIFICATION

PHARMACOTHERAPEUTIC: Phenothiazine. **CLINICAL:** Antihistamine, antiemetic, sedative-hypnotic (see p. 55C).

ACTION

Antihistamine: Inhibits histamine at histamine receptor sites. **Antiemetic:** Diminishes vestibular stimulation, depresses labyrinthine function, acts on chemoreceptor trigger zone. **Sedative-hypnotic:** Produces CNS depression by decreasing stimulation to brain stem reticular formation. **Therapeutic Effect:** Prevents allergic responses mediated by histamine (urticaria, pruritus). Prevents, relieves nausea/vomiting. Produces mild sedative effect.

PHARMACOKINETICS

Route	Onset	Peak	Duration
PO	20 min	N/A	2–8 hrs
IV	3–5 min	N/A	2–8 hrs
IM	20 min	N/A	2–8 hrs
Rectal	20 min	N/A	2–8 hrs

Well absorbed from GI tract after IM administration. Protein binding: 83%.

P

Widely distributed. Metabolized in liver. Primarily excreted in urine. Not removed by hemodialysis. **Half-life:** 9–16 hrs.

USES

Treatment of allergic conditions, motion sickness, nausea, vomiting. May be used as mild sedative. Adjunct to postoperative analgesia.

PRECAUTIONS

Contraindications: Children 2 yrs and younger (may cause fatal respiratory depression), hypersensitivity to phenothiazines, severe CNS depression, coma, treatment of lower respiratory tract symptoms including asthma. **Cautions:** Cardiovascular/hepatic impairment, narrow-angle glaucoma, prostatic hypertrophy, GI/GU obstruction, bone marrow depression, asthma, peptic ulcer, history of seizures, sleep apnea, pts suspected of Reye's syndrome.

⌛ LIFESPAN CONSIDERATIONS

Pregnancy/Lactation: Readily crosses placenta. Unknown if drug is distributed in breast milk. May inhibit platelet aggregation in neonates if taken within 2 wks of birth. May produce jaundice, extrapyramidal symptoms (EPS) in neonates if taken during pregnancy. **Pregnancy Category** C. **Children:** May experience increased excitement. Not recommended for those younger than 2 yrs. **Elderly:** More sensitive to dizziness, sedation, confusion, hypotension, hyperexcitability, anticholinergic effects (e.g., dry mouth).

INTERACTIONS

DRUG: Alcohol, CNS depressants may increase CNS depressant effects. **Anticholinergics** may increase anticholinergic effects. **MAOIs** may prolong, intensify anticholinergic, CNS depressant effects. **HERBAL: Gotu kola, kava kava, St. John's wort, valerian** may increase CNS depression. **FOOD:** None known. **LAB VALUES:** May suppress wheal/flare reactions to antigen skin testing unless discontinued 4 days before testing.

AVAILABILITY (Rx)

Injection Solution (Phenergan): 25 mg/ml, 50 mg/ml. **Suppositories (Phenadoz, Phenergan, Promethegan):** 12.5 mg, 25 mg, 50 mg. **Syrup (Phenergan):** 6.25 mg/5 ml. **Tablets (Phenergan):** 12.5 mg, 25 mg, 50 mg.

ADMINISTRATION/HANDLING

◀**ALERT**▶ IM is preferred route; avoid IV if possible. Significant tissue necrosis may occur if given subcutaneously. Inadvertent intra-arterial injection may produce severe arteriospasm, resulting in severe circulation impairment.

 IV

Reconstitution • Dilute with 10–20 ml 0.9% NaCl or prepare minibag.
Rate of Administration • Administer slowly over 10–15 min. • Use large vein or central venous site (no hand or wrist veins). • Too-rapid rate of infusion may result in transient fall in B/P, producing orthostatic hypotension, reflex tachycardia, serious tissue injury.
Storage • Store at room temperature.

IM
• Inject deep IM.

PO
• Give with food or fluids to reduce GI distress. • Scored tablets may be crushed.

Rectal
• Refrigerate suppository. • Moisten suppository with cold water before inserting well into rectum.

▦ IV INCOMPATIBILITIES

Allopurinol (Aloprim), amphotericin B complex (Abelcet, AmBisome, Amphotec), heparin, ketorolac (Toradol), nalbuphine (Nubain), piperacillin and tazobactam (Zosyn).

▦ IV COMPATIBILITIES

Dexmedetomidine (Precedex), diphenhydramine (Benadryl), hydromorphone (Dilaudid), midazolam (Versed), morphine.

INDICATIONS/ROUTES/DOSAGE

◄ALERT► Contraindicated in children 2 yrs and younger.

Allergic Symptoms
PO: ADULTS, ELDERLY: 6.25–12.5 mg 3 times a day plus 25 mg at bedtime. **CHILDREN:** 0.1 mg/kg/dose (**Maximum:** 12.5 mg) 4 times a day plus 0.5 mg/kg/dose (**Maximum:** 25 mg) at bedtime.
IV, IM: ADULTS, ELDERLY: 25 mg. May repeat in 2 hrs.

Motion Sickness
PO: ADULTS, ELDERLY: 25 mg 30–60 min before departure; may repeat in 8–12 hrs, then every morning on rising and before evening meal. **CHILDREN:** 0.5 mg/kg 30–60 min before departure; may repeat in 8–12 hrs, then every morning on rising and before evening meal. **Maximum:** 25 mg twice a day.

Prevention of Nausea/Vomiting
PO, IV, IM, Rectal: ADULTS, ELDERLY: 12.5–25 mg q4–6h as needed. **CHILDREN:** 0.25–1 mg/kg q4–6h as needed. **Maximum:** 25 mg/dose.

Preop/Postop Sedation, Adjunct to Analgesics
IV, IM: ADULTS, ELDERLY: 25–50 mg. **CHILDREN:** 1.1 mg/kg not to exceed 1/2 suggested adult dose.

Sedative
PO, IV, IM, Rectal: ADULTS, ELDERLY: 12.5–50 mg/dose. May repeat q4–6h as needed. **CHILDREN:** 0.5–1 mg/kg/dose q6h as needed. **Maximum:** 50 mg/dose.

SIDE EFFECTS

Frequent: Drowsiness, dry mouth, nose, throat; urinary retention, thickening of bronchial secretions. **Occasional:** Epigastric distress, flushing, visual disturbances, hearing disturbances, wheezing, paresthesia, diaphoresis, chills, disorientation, hypotension, confusion, syncope in elderly. **Rare:** Dizziness, urticaria, photosensitivity, nightmares.

ADVERSE EFFECTS/ TOXIC REACTIONS

Paradoxical reaction (particularly in children) manifested as excitation, anxiety, tremor, hyperactive reflexes, seizures. Long-term therapy may produce extrapyramidal symptoms (EPS) noted as dystonia (abnormal movements), pronounced motor restlessness (most frequently in children), parkinsonism (esp. noted in elderly). Blood dyscrasias, particularly agranulocytosis, occur rarely.

NURSING CONSIDERATIONS

BASELINE ASSESSMENT

Assess allergy symptoms. Assess B/P, pulse for bradycardia, tachycardia if pt is given parenteral form. If used as antiemetic, assess for dehydration (poor skin turgor, dry mucous membranes, longitudinal furrows in tongue). Assess LOC.

INTERVENTION/EVALUATION

Monitor serum electrolytes in pts with severe vomiting. Assist with ambulation if drowsiness, dizziness occurs. Monitor for relief of nausea, vomiting, allergic symptoms.

PATIENT/FAMILY TEACHING

• Drowsiness, dry mouth may be expected response to drug. • Avoid tasks that require alertness, motor skills until response to drug is established. • Sugarless gum, sips of water may relieve dry mouth. • Coffee, tea may help reduce drowsiness. • Report visual disturbances, involuntary movements, restlessness. • Avoid alcohol, other CNS depressants. • Avoid prolonged exposure to sunlight.

P

propafenone

proe-**pa**-fen-own
(Rythmol, Rythmol SR)
BLACK BOX ALERT Mortality or non-fatal cardiac arrest rate (7.7%) in

asymptomatic non–life-threatening ventricular arrhythmia pts with recent MI (more than 6 days but less than 2 years prior) reported.

◆ **CLASSIFICATION**

PHARMACOTHERAPEUTIC: Class 1c antiarrhythmic. **CLINICAL:** Antiarrhythmic (see p. 17C).

ACTION

Decreases fast sodium current in Purkinje/myocardial cells. Decreases excitability, automaticity; prolongs conduction velocity, refractory period. **Therapeutic Effect:** Suppresses arrhythmias.

PHARMACOKINETICS

Nearly completely absorbed following PO administration. Protein binding: 85%–97%. Metabolized in liver. Primarily excreted in feces. **Half-life:** 2–10 hrs.

USES

Treatment of life-threatening ventricular arrhythmias (e.g., sustained ventricular tachycardias). Treatment of paroxysmal atrial fibrillation/flutter (PAF) or paroxysmal supraventricular tachycardia (PSVT) in pts with disabling symptoms and without structural heart disease. **Rythmol SR:** Maintenance of normal sinus rhythm in pts with symptomatic atrial fibrillation. **OFF-LABEL:** Treatment following cardioversion of recent-onset atrial fibrillation; supraventricular tachycardia in pts with Wolff-Parkinson-White syndrome.

PRECAUTIONS

Contraindications: Bradycardia, bronchospastic disorders, cardiogenic shock, electrolyte imbalance, sinoatrial, AV, intraventricular impulse generation or conduction disorders (e.g., sick sinus syndrome, AV block) without pacemaker, uncontrolled HF, hypotension, concurrent use with ritonavir. **Cautions:** Renal/hepatic impairment, myasthenia gravis, concurrent use of other medications that prolong QT interval.

⏳ LIFESPAN CONSIDERATIONS

Pregnancy/Lactation: Unknown if drug crosses placenta or is distributed in breast milk. **Pregnancy Category C. Children:** Safety and efficacy not established. **Elderly:** No age-related precautions noted.

INTERACTIONS

DRUG: Amiodarone may affect conduction, repolarization. May increase **digoxin** concentration. May increase effects of **warfarin. CYP3A4 inhibitors (e.g., ketoconazole, erythromycin)** may increase concentration/toxicity. **HERBAL: St. John's wort** may decrease concentration/effect. **Ephedra** may worsen arrhythmias. **FOOD: Grapefruit products** may increase concentration. **LAB VALUES:** May cause EKG changes (e.g., QRS widening, PR interval prolongation), positive ANA titers.

AVAILABILITY (Rx)

Tablets (Rythmol): 150 mg, 225 mg, 300 mg.

🔖 Capsules (Extended-Release [Rythmol SR]): 225 mg, 325 mg, 425 mg.

ADMINISTRATION/HANDLING

PO
• May take without regard to meals.
• Give whole; do not break, crush, divide, or open capsules.

INDICATIONS/ROUTES/DOSAGE

Ventricular Arrhythmias, PAT, PSVT
PO: ADULTS, ELDERLY: Initially, 150 mg q8h. May increase at 3- to 4-day intervals to 225 mg q8h, then to 300 mg q8h. **Maximum:** 900 mg/day.

Atrial Fibrillation (Prevention of Recurrence)
PO *(Extended-Release)***: ADULTS, ELDERLY:** Initially, 225 mg q12h. May increase at 5-day intervals. **Maximum:** 425 mg q12h.

Dosage in Hepatic Impairment
Reduce dose by 70%–80% (immediate-release).

SIDE EFFECTS

Frequent (13%–7%): Dizziness, nausea, vomiting, altered taste, constipation. **Occasional (6%–3%):** Headache, dyspnea, blurred vision, dyspepsia (heartburn, indigestion, epigastric pain). **Rare (Less Than 2%):** Rash, weakness, dry mouth, diarrhea, edema, hot flashes.

ADVERSE EFFECTS/ TOXIC REACTIONS

May produce, worsen arrhythmias. Overdose may produce hypotension, drowsiness, bradycardia, atrioventricular conduction disturbances.

NURSING CONSIDERATIONS

BASELINE ASSESSMENT

Correct electrolyte imbalance before administering medication. Obtain baseline EKG. Screen for cardiac contraindications.

INTERVENTION/EVALUATION

Assess pulse for quality, rhythm, rate. Monitor EKG for cardiac performance or changes, particularly widening of QRS, prolongation of PR interval. Question for visual disturbances, headache, GI upset. Monitor fluid, serum electrolyte levels. Monitor daily pattern of bowel activity, stool consistency. Assess for dizziness, unsteadiness. Monitor hepatic enzymes results. Monitor for therapeutic serum level (0.06–1 mcg/ml).

PATIENT/FAMILY TEACHING

• Compliance with therapy regimen is essential to control arrhythmias. • Altered taste sensation may occur. • Report headache, blurred vision. • Avoid tasks that require alertness, motor skills until response to drug is established. • Report chest pain, difficulty breathing, palpitations.

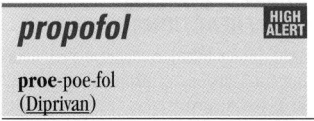

propofol **HIGH ALERT**

proe-poe-fol
(Diprivan)

Do not confuse Diprivan with Diflucan or Ditropan, or propofol with fospropofol.

◆ CLASSIFICATION

PHARMACOTHERAPEUTIC: Rapid-acting general anesthetic. **CLINICAL:** Sedative-hypnotic (see p. 6C).

ACTION

Inhibits sympathetic vasoconstrictor nerve activity; decreases vascular resistance. **Therapeutic Effect:** Produces hypnosis rapidly.

PHARMACOKINETICS

Route	Onset	Peak	Duration
IV	40 sec	N/A	3–10 min

Rapidly, extensively distributed. Protein binding: 97%–99%. Metabolized in liver. Primarily excreted in urine. Unknown if removed by hemodialysis. Rapid awakening can occur 10–15 min after discontinuation. **Half-life:** 3–12 hrs.

USES

Induction/maintenance of anesthesia. Continuous sedation in intubated and respiratory controlled adult pts in ICU. **OFF-LABEL:** Postop antiemetic, refractory delirium tremens.

PRECAUTIONS

Contraindications: Hypersensitivity to eggs, egg products, soybean or soy products. **Cautions:** Hemodynamically unstable pts, hypovolemia, severe cardiac/respiratory disease, elevated ICP, impaired cerebral circulation, preexisting pancreatitis, hyperlipidemia, history of epilepsy, seizure disorder.

⌛ LIFESPAN CONSIDERATIONS

Pregnancy/Lactation: Unknown if drug crosses placenta. Distributed in breast milk. Not recommended for obstetrics, breastfeeding mothers. **Pregnancy Category B. Children:** Safety and

P

✤ Canadian trade name   🥄 Non-Crushable Drug   **HIGH ALERT** High Alert drug efficacy not established. FDA approved for use in those 2 mos and older. **Elderly:** No age-related precautions noted; lower dosages recommended.

INTERACTIONS

DRUG: Alcohol, CNS depressants may increase CNS, respiratory depression, hypotensive effects. **Antihypertensive medications** may increase hypotensive effects. **HERBAL:** None significant. **FOOD:** None known. **LAB VALUES:** None significant.

AVAILABILITY (Rx)

Injection Emulsion: 10 mg/ml.

ADMINISTRATION/HANDLING
🔲 IV

◀ALERT▶ Do not give through same IV line with blood or plasma.

Reconstitution • May give undiluted, or dilute only with D₅W. • Do not dilute to concentration less than 2 mg/ml (4 ml D₅W to 1 ml propofol yields 2 mg/ml).
Rate of Administration • Too-rapid IV administration may produce marked severe hypotension, respiratory depression, irregular muscular movements. • Observe for signs of extravasation (pain, discolored skin patches, white or blue color to peripheral IV site area, delayed onset of drug action).
Storage • Store at room temperature. • Discard unused portions. • Do not use if emulsion separates. • Shake well before using.

🔲 IV INCOMPATIBILITIES

Amikacin (Amikin), amphotericin B complex (Abelcet, AmBisome, Amphotec), bretylium (Bretylol), calcium chloride, ciprofloxacin (Cipro), diazepam (Valium), digoxin (Lanoxin), doxorubicin (Adriamycin), gentamicin (Garamycin), methylprednisolone (Solu-Medrol), minocycline (Minocin), phenytoin (Dilantin), tobramycin (Nebcin), verapamil (Isoptin).

🔲 IV COMPATIBILITIES

Acyclovir (Zovirax), bumetanide (Bumex), calcium gluconate, ceftazidime (Fortaz), dexmedetomidine (Precedex), dobutamine (Dobutrex), dopamine (Intropin), enalapril (Vasotec), fentanyl, heparin, insulin, labetalol (Normodyne, Trandate), lidocaine, lorazepam (Ativan), magnesium, milrinone (Primacor), nitroglycerin, norepinephrine (Levophed), potassium chloride, vancomycin (Vancocin).

INDICATIONS/ROUTES/DOSAGE

Anesthesia
IV: ADULTS, ELDERLY: Induction, 20–40 mg every 10 sec until induction onset, then infusion of 50–200 mcg/kg/min with 20–50 mg bolus as needed. **CHILDREN 3–16 YRS:** Induction, 2.5–3.5 mg/kg over 20–30 sec, then infusion of 125–300 mcg/kg/min.

Sedation in ICU
IV: ADULTS, ELDERLY: Initially, 5 mcg/kg/min (0.3 mg/kg/hr) for 5 min, then titrate to 5–80 mcg/kg/min (0.3–4.8 mg/kg/hr) in 5–10 mcg/kg/min (0.3–0.6 mg/kg/hr) increments allowing minimum of 5 min between dose adjustments. Usual maintenance: 5–50 mcg/kg/min (0.3–3 mg/kg/hr).

SIDE EFFECTS

Frequent: Involuntary muscle movements, apnea (common during induction; often lasts longer than 60 sec), hypotension, nausea, vomiting, IV site burning/stinging. **Occasional:** Twitching, thrashing, headache, dizziness, bradycardia, hypertension, fever, abdominal cramps, paresthesia, coldness, cough, hiccups, facial flushing, green-tinted urine. **Rare:** Rash, dry mouth, agitation, confusion, myalgia, thrombophlebitis.

ADVERSE EFFECTS/
TOXIC REACTIONS

Continuous infusion or repeated intermittent infusions of propofol may result in extreme drowsiness, respiratory depression, circulatory depression. Too-rapid IV administration may produce severe hypotension, respiratory depression, involuntary muscle movements. Pt may experience acute allergic reaction, characterized by abdominal pain, anxiety, restlessness, dyspnea, erythema, hypotension, pruritus, rhinitis, urticaria.

NURSING CONSIDERATIONS

BASELINE ASSESSMENT

Resuscitative equipment, suction, O_2 must be available. Obtain vital signs before administration.

INTERVENTION/EVALUATION

Observe pt for signs of wakefulness, agitation. Monitor respiratory rate, B/P, heart rate, O_2 saturation, ABGs, depth of sedation, serum lipid, triglycerides (if used longer than 24 hrs). May change urine color to green.

---

propranolol

proe-**pran**-oh-lol
(Apo-Propranolol ✦, Inderal LA, InnoPran XL, Novo-Pranol ✦)
BLACK BOX ALERT Severe angina exacerbation, MI, ventricular arrhythmias may occur in angina pts after abrupt discontinuation; must taper gradually over 1–2 wks.
Do not confuse Inderal LA with Adderall, Imdur, Isordil, or Toradol, or propranolol with Pravachol.

FIXED-COMBINATION(S)

Inderide: propranolol/hydrochlorothiazide (a diuretic): 40 mg/25 mg, 80 mg/25 mg. **Inderide LA:** propranolol/hydrochlorothiazide (a diuretic): 80 mg/50 mg, 120 mg/50 mg, 160 mg/50 mg.

◆CLASSIFICATION

PHARMACOTHERAPEUTIC: Beta-adrenergic blocker. **CLINICAL:** Antihypertensive, antianginal, antiarrhythmic, antimigraine (see pp. 18C, 74C).

ACTION

Blocks beta$_1$-, beta$_2$-adrenergic receptors. Decreases oxygen requirements. Slows AV conduction, increases refractory period in AV node. Large doses increase airway resistance. **Therapeutic Effect:** Slows heart rate; decreases cardiac output, B/P, myocardial ischemia severity. Exhibits antiarrhythmic activity.

PHARMACOKINETICS

Route	Onset	Peak	Duration
PO	1–2 hrs	N/A	6 hrs

Well absorbed from GI tract. Protein binding: 93%. Widely distributed. Metabolized in liver. Primarily excreted in urine. Not removed by hemodialysis. **Half-life:** 4–6 hrs.

USES

Treatment of angina pectoris, arrhythmias, essential tremors, hypertension, hypertrophic subaortic stenosis, migraine headache, pheochromocytoma, prevention of MI. **OFF-LABEL:** Treatment adjunct for anxiety, tremor due to Parkinson's disease, alcohol withdrawal, aggressive behavior, schizophrenia, antipsychotic-induced akathisia, variceal hemorrhage, acute panic.

PRECAUTIONS

Contraindications: Asthma, bradycardia, cardiogenic shock, COPD, heart block greater than first-degree (unless pt has functional pacemaker), Raynaud's syndrome, uncompensated HF. **Cautions:** Diabetes, renal/hepatic impairment, peripheral vascular disease, skeletal muscle disease, concurrent use of calcium blockers when using IV form.

⌛ LIFESPAN CONSIDERATIONS

Pregnancy/Lactation: Crosses placenta. Distributed in breast milk. Avoid use during first trimester. May produce

P

---

low birth-weight infants, bradycardia, apnea, hypoglycemia, hypothermia during delivery. **Pregnancy Category C (D if used in second or third trimester).** **Children:** No age-related precautions noted. **Elderly:** Age-related peripheral vascular disease may increase susceptibility to decreased peripheral circulation.

INTERACTIONS

DRUG: Diuretics, other antihypertensives may increase hypotensive effect. May mask symptoms of hypoglycemia, prolong hypoglycemic effect of **insulin, oral hypoglycemics. Digoxin** may increase risk for bradycardia. **NSAIDs** may decrease antihypertensive effect. **HERBAL: Ephedra, ginger, licorice, ginseng, yohimbe** may worsen hypertension. **Licorice** may increase water retention. **Garlic, periwinkle** has antihypertensive effects. **FOOD:** None known. **LAB VALUES:** May increase serum antinuclear antibody (ANA) titer, BUN, serum LDH, lipoprotein, alkaline phosphatase, potassium, uric acid, AST, ALT, triglycerides.

AVAILABILITY (Rx)

Injection Solution: 1 mg/ml. **Oral Solution:** 20 mg/5 ml, 40 mg/5 ml. **Tablets:** 10 mg, 20 mg, 40 mg, 60 mg, 80 mg.

 Capsules (Extended-Release [Inno-Pran XL]): 80 mg, 120 mg. **Capsules (Sustained-Release [Inderal LA]):** 60 mg, 80 mg, 120 mg, 160 mg.

ADMINISTRATION/HANDLING

IV

Reconstitution • Give undiluted for IV push. • For IV infusion, may dilute each 1 mg in 10 ml D_5W.
Rate of Administration • Do not exceed 1 mg/min injection rate. • For IV infusion, give over 30 min.
Storage • Store at room temperature. • Once diluted, stable for 24 hrs at room temperature.

PO

• May crush scored tablets. • Do not crush extended- or sustained-release capsules. • Give immediate-release tablets on empty stomach. • Give extended-release, sustained-release without regard to food.

IV INCOMPATIBILITY

Amphotericin B complex (Abelcet, AmBisome, Amphotec).

IV COMPATIBILITIES

Alteplase (Activase), heparin, milrinone (Primacor), potassium chloride, propofol (Diprivan).

INDICATIONS/ROUTES/DOSAGE

Hypertension

PO: ADULTS, ELDERLY: Initially, 40 mg twice daily. May increase dose q3–7days. **Maximum:** 640 mg/day. **CHILDREN:** Initially, 0.5–1 mg/kg/day in divided doses q6–12h. May increase at 3- to 5-day intervals. Usual dose: 1–5 mg/kg/day. **Maximum:** 16 mg/kg/day.
PO (Long-Acting): (Inderal LA): Initially, 80 mg once daily. **Usual maintenance:** 120–160 mg/day.
(Innopran XL): Initially, 80 mg at bedtime. **Maximum:** 120 mg.

Angina

PO: ADULTS, ELDERLY: 80–320 mg/day in 2–4 divided doses.
PO (Long-Acting): Initially, 80 mg/day. **Maximum:** 320 mg/day.

Arrhythmia

IV: ADULTS, ELDERLY: 1–3 mg. Repeat q5min up to total of 5 mg. **CHILDREN:** 0.01–0.1 mg/kg. **Maximum:** Infants, 1 mg; children, 3 mg.
PO: ADULTS, ELDERLY: Initially, 10–30 mg q6–8h. May gradually increase dose. Range: 40–320 mg/day. **CHILDREN:** Initially, 0.5–1 mg/kg/day in divided doses q6–8h. May increase q3days. Usual dosage: 2–6 mg/kg/day. **Maximum:** 16 mg/kg/day or 60 mg/day.

Hypertrophic Subaortic Stenosis
PO: ADULTS, ELDERLY: 20–40 mg 3–4 times/day or 80–160 mg once daily as extended-release capsule.

Adjunct to Alpha-Blocking Agents to Treat Pheochromocytoma
PO: ADULTS, ELDERLY: 30–60 mg/day in divided doses.

Migraine Headache
PO: ADULTS, ELDERLY: 80 mg/day in divided doses or 80 mg once daily as extended-release capsule. Increase up to 160–240 mg/day in divided doses. **CHILDREN WEIGHING 35 KG OR LESS:** 10–20 mg 3 times a day. **CHILDREN WEIGHING OVER 35 KG:** 20–40 mg 3 times a day.
Extended-Release *(Inderal LA):* **ADULTS, ELDERLY:** Initially, 80 mg daily. **Effective range:** 160–240 mg/day.

Reduction of Cardiovascular Mortality, Reinfarction in Pts With Previous MI
PO: ADULTS, ELDERLY: Initially, 40 mg 3 times/day. Range: 180–240 mg/day in 3–4 divided doses.

Essential Tremor
PO: ADULTS, ELDERLY: Initially, 40 mg twice daily increased up to 120–320 mg/day in 3 divided doses.

SIDE EFFECTS

Frequent: Diminished sexual function, drowsiness, difficulty sleeping, unusual fatigue/weakness. **Occasional:** Bradycardia, depression, sensation of coldness in extremities, diarrhea, constipation, anxiety, nasal congestion, nausea, vomiting. **Rare:** Altered taste, dry eyes, pruritus, paresthesia.

ADVERSE EFFECTS/ TOXIC REACTIONS

Overdose may produce profound bradycardia, hypotension. Abrupt withdrawal may result in diaphoresis, palpitations, headache, tremulousness. May precipitate HF, MI in pts with cardiac disease; thyroid storm in pts with thyrotoxicosis; peripheral ischemia in those with existing peripheral vascular disease. Hypoglycemia may occur in pts with previously controlled diabetes. **Antidote:** Glucagon (see Appendix K for dosage).

NURSING CONSIDERATIONS

BASELINE ASSESSMENT

Assess baseline renal/hepatic function tests. Assess B/P, apical pulse immediately before administering drug (if pulse is 60/min or less or systolic B/P is less than 90 mm Hg, withhold medication, contact physician). **Angina:** Record onset, quality, radiation, location, intensity, duration of anginal pain, precipitating factors (exertion, emotional stress).

INTERVENTION/EVALUATION

Assess pulse for quality, irregular rate, bradycardia. Monitor EKG for cardiac arrhythmias. Assess fingers for color, numbness (Raynaud's). Assess for evidence of HF (dyspnea [particularly on exertion or lying down], night cough, peripheral edema, distended neck veins). Monitor I&O (increase in weight, decrease in urinary output may indicate HF). Assess for rash, fatigue, behavioral changes. Therapeutic response time ranges from a few days to several wks. Measure B/P near end of dosing interval (determines if B/P is controlled throughout day).

PATIENT/FAMILY TEACHING

• Do not abruptly discontinue medication. • Compliance with therapy regimen is essential to control hypertension, arrhythmia, anginal pain. • To avoid hypotensive effect, rise slowly from lying to sitting position. • Avoid tasks that require alertness, motor skills until response to drug is established. • Report excessively slow pulse rate (less than 50 beats/min), peripheral numbness, dizziness. • Do not use nasal decongestants, OTC cold preparations (stimulants) without physician approval. • Restrict salt, alcohol intake.

P

✤ Canadian trade name 🦃 Non-Crushable Drug 🔲 High Alert drug

propylthiouracil

proe-pil-**thye**-oh-**ure**-a-sil
(Propyl-Thyracil ✦)

BLACK BOX ALERT May cause severe hepatic injury, acute hepatic failure, death.

Do not confuse propylthiouracil with purinethol.

◆ CLASSIFICATION

PHARMACOTHERAPEUTIC: Thiourea derivative. **CLINICAL:** Antithyroid agent.

ACTION

Blocks oxidation of iodine in thyroid gland, blocks synthesis of thyroxine, triiodothyronine. **Therapeutic Effect:** Inhibits synthesis of thyroid hormone.

PHARMACOKINETICS

Readily absorbed from GI tract. Protein binding: 80%. Metabolized in liver. Excreted in urine. **Half-life:** 1.5–5 hrs.

USES

Palliative treatment of hyperthyroidism; adjunct to ameliorate hyperthyroidism in preparation for surgical treatment, radioactive iodine therapy. **OFF-LABEL:** Management of thyrotoxic crises, Graves' disease, thyroid storm.

PRECAUTIONS

Contraindications: None known. **Cautions:** In combination with other agranulocytosis-inducing drugs. **Pregnancy Category D.**

INTERACTIONS

DRUG: May increase concentration of **digoxin** (as pt becomes euthyroid). May increase effect of **oral anticoagulants.** **HERBAL:** None significant. **FOOD:** None known. **LAB VALUES:** May increase LDH, serum alkaline phosphatase, bilirubin, AST, ALT, prothrombin time.

AVAILABILITY (Rx)

Tablets: 50 mg.

ADMINISTRATION/HANDLING

PO
• Give with food.

INDICATIONS/ROUTES/DOSAGE

Hyperthyroidism
PO: ADULTS, ELDERLY: Initially, 300–400 mg/day (**ELDERLY:** 150–300 mg/day) in divided doses q8h. **Maintenance:** 100–150 mg/day in divided doses q8–12h. **CHILDREN:** Initially, 5–7 mg/kg/day in divided doses q8h. **Maintenance:** 33%–66% of initial dose in divided doses q8–12h. **NEONATES:** Initially, 5 mg/kg/day in divided doses q8h. May increase in 36–48 hrs by 50% if no response. Range: 5–10 mg/kg/day in divided doses q8h.

SIDE EFFECTS

Frequent: Urticaria, rash, pruritus, nausea, skin pigmentation, hair loss, headache, paresthesia. **Occasional:** Drowsiness, lymphadenopathy, vertigo. **Rare:** Drug fever, lupus-like syndrome.

ADVERSE EFFECTS/ TOXIC REACTIONS

Agranulocytosis (may occur as long as 4 mos after therapy), pancytopenia, fatal hepatitis have occurred.

NURSING CONSIDERATIONS

BASELINE ASSESSMENT

Obtain baseline weight, pulse.

INTERVENTION/EVALUATION

Monitor pulse, weight daily. Check for skin eruptions, pruritus, swollen lymph glands. Be alert for signs, symptoms of hepatic injury, hepatitis (nausea, vomiting, drowsiness, jaundice). Monitor hematology results for bone marrow suppression; observe for signs of infection, bleeding.

PATIENT/FAMILY TEACHING

• Space doses evenly around the clock. • Take resting pulse daily. • Report pulse rate less than 60 beats/min. • Seafood, iodine products may be restricted. • Report fever, sore throat, yellowing of skin/

eyes, unusual bleeding/bruising immediately. • Report sudden or continuous weight gain, cold intolerance, depression.

---

protamine

proe-ta-meen
(Protamine ✤, Protamine sulfate)
BLACK BOX ALERT May cause severe hypotension, cardiovascular collapse, noncardiogenic pulmonary edema, pulmonary hypertension.
Do not confuse protamine with ProAmatine or Protonix.

◆CLASSIFICATION

PHARMACOTHERAPEUTIC: Protein. **CLINICAL:** Heparin antagonist, antidote.

ACTION

Combines with heparin to form stable salt. **Therapeutic Effect:** Reduces anticoagulant activity of heparin.

PHARMACOKINETICS

Metabolized by fibrinolysin. **Half-life:** 7.4 min. Heparin neutralized in 5 min.

USES

Treatment of severe heparin overdose (causing hemorrhage). Neutralizes effects of heparin administered during extracorporeal circulation. **OFF-LABEL:** Treatment of low molecular weight heparin toxicity.

PRECAUTIONS

Contraindications: None known. **Cautions:** History of allergy to fish, seafood; vasectomized/infertile men; those on isophane (NPH) insulin, previous protamine therapy (propensity to hypersensitivity reaction).

⧖ LIFESPAN CONSIDERATIONS

Pregnancy/Lactation: Unknown if drug crosses placenta or is distributed in breast milk. **Pregnancy Category C. Children:** Safety and efficacy not established. **Elderly:** No age-related precautions noted.

INTERACTIONS

DRUG: None significant. **HERBAL:** None significant. **FOOD:** None known. **LAB VALUES:** None significant.

AVAILABILITY (Rx)

Injection Solution: 10 mg/ml.

ADMINISTRATION/HANDLING
🖳 IV

Rate of Administration • May give undiluted over 10 min. Do not exceed 5 mg/min (50 mg in any 10-min period). **Storage** • Store vials at room temperature.

INDICATIONS/ROUTES/DOSAGE

Heparin Overdose (Antidote, Treatment)
IV: ADULTS, ELDERLY: 1–1.5 mg protamine neutralizes 100 units heparin. Heparin disappears rapidly from circulation, reducing dosage demand for protamine as time elapses.

SIDE EFFECTS

Frequent: Decreased B/P, dyspnea. **Occasional:** Hypersensitivity reaction (urticaria, angioedema); nausea/vomiting, which generally occur in those sensitive to fish/seafood, vasectomized men, infertile men, those on isophane (NPH) insulin, those previously on protamine therapy. **Rare:** Back pain.

ADVERSE EFFECTS/ TOXIC REACTIONS

Too-rapid IV administration may produce acute hypotension, bradycardia, pulmonary hypertension, dyspnea, transient flushing, feeling of warmth. Heparin rebound may occur several hrs after heparin has been neutralized by protamine (usually evident 8–9 hrs after protamine administration). Heparin rebound occurs most often after arterial/cardiac surgery.

P

NURSING CONSIDERATIONS

BASELINE ASSESSMENT
Check PT, aPTT, Hct; assess for bleeding.

INTERVENTION/EVALUATION
Monitor coagulation tests, aPTT or ACT, B/P, cardiac function.

prothrombin complex concentrate (human)

pro-**throm**-bin
(Kcentra)

BLACK BOX ALERT Pts treated with vitamin K antagonists (VKA) have underlying disease states that predispose them to thromboembolic events. Benefits of VKA reversal must outweigh risks of thromboembolic events. Consider resumption of anticoagulant therapy after acute bleeding resolves. Both fatal and nonfatal arterial/venous thromboembolic events were reported. Not studied in pts with cerebral vascular accident (CVA), disseminated intravascular coagulation (DIC), myocardial infarction (MI), transient ischemic attack (TIA), or severe peripheral vascular disease (PVD) within prior 3 mos. Monitor for thromboembolic events during therapy.

◆CLASSIFICATION

PHARMACOTHERAPEUTIC: Coagulant. **CLINICAL:** Hemostatic.

ACTION

Replaces vitamin K–dependent clotting factors, essential for blood coagulation. Activates coagulation cascade of procoagulant reactions. **Therapeutic Effect:** Antagonizes warfarin-like medications; produces hemostatis; corrects international normalized ratio (INR) levels.

PHARMACOKINETICS

Extensively distributed in plasma. Peak plasma concentration: rapid/immediate. No physiologic system of elimination. **Half-life:** 4–60 hrs (varied among numerous clotting factors).

USES

Urgent reversal of acquired coagulation factor deficiency induced by VKA (e.g., warfarin) therapy in adult pts with acute major bleeding.
◀ALERT▶ Not indicated for urgent reversal of VKA anticoagulation in pts without acute major bleeding. Administer vitamin K concurrently to maintain factor levels once drug effects have diminished.

PRECAUTIONS

Contraindications: Hypersensitivity reaction to: drug class, antithrombin III, factors II, VII, IX, X, protein C and S, heparin, human albumin. History of DIC, heparin-induced thrombocytopenia. **Cautions:** History of CVA, DVT, HF, MI, PE, hypertension, peripheral edema, peripheral vascular disease, unstable angina, transient ischemic attack (TIA), disseminated intravascular coagulation (DIC).

⌛ LIFESPAN CONSIDERATIONS

Pregnancy/Lactation: Unknown if distributed in breast milk. **Pregnancy Category C. Children:** Safety and efficacy not established. **Elderly:** No age-related precautions noted.

INTERACTIONS

DRUG: None known. **HERBAL:** None significant. **FOOD:** None known. **LAB VALUES:** May decrease serum potassium.

AVAILABILITY (Rx)

Lyophilized Powder for Reconstitution (Units Defined by Factor IX Content): 500 units/vial (range 400–620 units), 1,000 units/vial (range 800–1,200 units).

ADMINISTRATION/HANDLING

 IV

Reconstitution • Verify all components are present in administration kit: 500-unit or 1,000-unit single-use vial, 20-ml or 40-ml vial of Sterile Water for Injection, Mix-2Vial filter transfer set, alcohol swab. • Use proper aseptic technique. • Ensure vial is at room temperature. • Remove flip caps from drug vial and diluent. • Wipe stoppers with alcohol and allow to dry. • Open Mix2Vial transfer set package by peeling away lid. • Leave Mix2Vial set in clear package. • Place Mix2Vial set on flat surface and grip Mix2Vial transfer set with clear package intact. • Push plastic spike at the blue end of Mix2Vial transfer set firmly through center of diluent vial stopper. • Carefully remove clear package from Mix2Vial transfer set by only pulling up clear package; do not touch/grab Mix-2Vial transfer set itself to ensure aseptic technique. • With Kcentra vial placed firmly on flat surface, invert diluent vial (with Mix2Vial transfer set attached) and push plastic spike of transparent adapter firmly through center of Kcentra vial stopper. • Diluent will automatically transfer. • Gently swirl until fully dissolved. • Separate diluent vial by gently unscrewing set into two pieces. • Draw air into empty, sterile syringe. • While Kcentra bottle is upright, screw syringe into Mix2Vial transfer set and inject air. • While keeping plunger pressed, invert system and draw solution into syringe slowly • Once transferred, unscrew syringe from Mix2Vial transfer set and administer • If pt is to receive more than one vial, may pool contents of multiple vials. • Enter product lot number in medical record.

Rate of Administration • Do not allow blood to enter syringe during administration (may cause fibrin clot formation). • Infuse at 0.12 ml/kg/min (~3 units/kg/min). • May titrate to maximum rate of 8.4 ml/min (~210 unit/min).

Storage • Reconstituted solution should appear clear, colorless to slightly opalescent and free of visible particles. • May re-frigerate reconstituted solution for up to 4 hrs. • Store unused vial at room temperature until time of use (may also refrigerate). • Do not freeze. • Protect from light.

IV INCOMPATIBILITIES

Infuse via dedicated line. Do not mix with other medications.

INDICATIONS/ROUTES/DOSAGE

Acute Major Bleeding with Concurrent Use of Vitamin K Antagonist
Contains factors II, VII, IX, X, antithrombotic proteins C and S. Vial potency defined by factor IX content (in units).
IV: ADULTS/ELDERLY: INR 2–3.9: 25 units/kg. **Maximum:** 2,500 units. **INR 4–5.9:** 35 unit/kg. **Maximum:** 3,500 units.
INR GREATER THAN 6: 50 units/kg. **Maximum:** 5,000 units. Repeat dosing not recommended.

SIDE EFFECTS

Occasional (8%–3%): Headache, hypotension, nausea, vomiting, arthralgia, hypertension, tachycardia. **Rare (2%–1%):** Constipation, hypokalemia, insomnia.

ADVERSE EFFECTS/ TOXIC REACTIONS

Hypersensitivity reactions including angioedema, anxiety, bronchospasm, dyspnea, flushing, hypotension, pulmonary edema, tachycardia, urticaria, wheezing was reported. Fatal and nonfatal thromboembolic events (CVA, DVT, MI, PE) reported in 9% of pts. Due to human blood component, drug may carry risk of infectious diseases transmission such as Creutzfeldt-Jakob disease; hepatitis A, B, C; or HIV. Hemodynamic/cardiac instability including angina, HF, hypoxia, hypotension, orthostatic hypotension, fluid overload have occurred. Coagulopathy-related intracranial hemorrhage, altered mental status was reported.

NURSING CONSIDERATIONS

BASELINE ASSESSMENT

Obtain baseline vital signs, CBC, serum chemistries, PT/INR, APTT. Question his-

P

tory of DIC, heparin-induced thrombocytopenia, CVA, DVT, MI, PE. Question any personal or religious objections to blood products. Ensure patency of IV access.

INTERVENTION/EVALUATION

Monitor CBC, serum electrolytes. Monitor PT/INR post infusion and as indicated. Monitor pt for hypersensitivity reactions. If anaphylactic reactions occur, consider treatment with antihistamine, intravenous steroids, racemic epinephrine; locate rapid sequence intubation kit. Monitor for signs and symptoms of DVT (extremity pain, swelling), MI (chest pain, sweating, left arm numbness, jaw pain), CVA (aphasia, hemiparesis, altered mental status, homonymous hemianopsia [blindness of one half of vision on same side of both eyes]).

PATIENT/FAMILY TEACHING

• Treatment may cause allergic reactions (difficulty breathing, dizziness, itching, rash, tongue swelling, wheezing). • Report signs of blood clots in extremities (extremity pain, swelling), heart attack (chest pain, left arm pain, sweating, nausea), stroke (confusion, difficulty speaking, one-sided paralysis, partial blindness). • Drug is a blood component and may carry risk of viral infection/transmission.

---

pseudoephedrine

soo-doe-e-**fed**-rin
(Balminil Decongestant ✦, Nexafed, PMS-Pseudoephedrine ✦, Robidrine ✦, Sudafed, Sudafed 12 Hour, Sudafed 24 Hour, Sudafed Children's)

FIXED-COMBINATION(S)

Advil Cold, Motrin Cold: pseudoephedrine/ibuprofen (an NSAID): 30 mg/200 mg, 15 mg/100 mg per 5 ml. **Allegra-D:** pseudoephedrine/fexofenadine (an antihistamine): 120 mg/60 mg. **Allegra-D 24 Hour:** pseudoephedrine/fexofenadine: 240 mg/180

mg. **Claritin-D:** pseudoephedrine/loratadine (an antihistamine): 120 mg/5 mg, 240 mg/10 mg. **Clarinex-D 24-Hour:** pseudoephedrine/desloratadine (an antihistamine): 240 mg/5 mg. **Clarinex-D 12-Hour:** pseudoephedrine/desloratadine: 120 mg/2.5 mg. **Rezira:** pseudoephedrine/hydrocodone (an opioid analgesic): 60 mg/5 mg per 5 ml. **Zyrtec-D:** pseudoephedrine/cetirizine (an antihistamine): 120 mg/5 mg.

◆CLASSIFICATION

PHARMACOTHERAPEUTIC: Sympathomimetic. **CLINICAL:** Nasal decongestant.

ACTION

Directly stimulates alpha-adrenergic, beta-adrenergic receptors. **Therapeutic Effect:** Produces vasoconstriction of respiratory tract mucosa; shrinks nasal mucous membranes; reduces edema, nasal congestion.

PHARMACOKINETICS

Route	Onset	Peak	Duration
PO (tablets, syrup)	15–30 min	30–60 min	4–6 hrs
PO (extended-release)	N/A	N/A	8–12 hrs

Well absorbed from GI tract. Partially metabolized in liver. Primarily excreted in urine. Not removed by hemodialysis. **Half-life:** 9–16 hrs.

USES

Temporary relief of nasal congestion due to common cold, upper respiratory allergies, sinusitis. Enhances nasal, sinus drainage.

PRECAUTIONS

Contraindications: Coronary artery disease, severe hypertension, use of MAOIs within 14 days. **Extended-release:** Children younger than 12 yrs. **Cautions:** Elderly, hyperthyroidism, diabetes, ischemic heart disease, prostatic hypertrophy, mild-to-moderate hypertension, arrhythmias, renal impairment, seizure disorder.

⌛ LIFESPAN CONSIDERATIONS

Pregnancy/Lactation: Crosses placenta. Distributed in breast milk. **Pregnancy Category C. Children:** Safety and efficacy not established in pts younger than 2 yrs. **Elderly:** Age-related prostatic hypertrophy may require dosage adjustment.

INTERACTIONS

DRUG: May decrease effects of **antihypertensives, beta-blockers, diuretics. HERBAL: Ephedra, yohimbe** may cause hypertension. **FOOD:** None known. **LAB VALUES:** None significant.

AVAILABILITY (OTC)

Liquid (Sudafed Children's): 15 mg/5 ml, 30 mg/5 ml. **Syrup:** 30 mg/5 ml. **Tablets: (Sudafed):** 30 mg, 60 mg. **(Nexafed):** 30 mg.
 Caplets, Extended-Release: (Sudafed 12 Hour): 120 mg. **Tablets, Extended-Release: (Sudafed 24 Hour):** 240 mg.

◄ALERT► Pseudoephedrine is key ingredient in synthesizing methamphetamine. Many pharmacies have moved pseudoephedrine behind the counter due to concerns about its purchase and theft for purposes of methamphetamine manufacture.

ADMINISTRATION/HANDLING

PO
• Administer with water or milk to decrease GI upset. • Do not break, crush, or divide extended-release forms; give whole.

INDICATIONS/ROUTES/DOSAGE

Decongestant
PO: ADULTS, ELDERLY, CHILDREN 12 YRS AND OLDER: 30–60 mg q4–6h. **Maximum:** 240 mg/day. **CHILDREN 6–11 YRS:** 30 mg q4–6h. **Maximum:** 120 mg/day. **CHILDREN 4–5 YRS:** 15 mg q4–6h. **Maximum:** 60 mg/day. **CHILDREN YOUNGER THAN 4 YRS:** 1 mg/kg/dose q6h. **Maximum single dose:** 15 mg.

PO *(Extended-Release)*: ADULTS, CHILDREN 12 YRS AND OLDER: 120 mg q12h or 240 mg once daily.

SIDE EFFECTS

Occasional (10%–5%): Nervousness, restlessness, insomnia, tremor, headache. **Rare (4%–1%):** Diaphoresis, weakness.

ADVERSE EFFECTS/ TOXIC REACTIONS

Large doses may produce tachycardia, palpitations (particularly in pts with cardiac disease), light-headedness, nausea, vomiting. Overdose in those older than 60 yrs may result in hallucinations, CNS depression, seizures.

NURSING CONSIDERATIONS

PATIENT/FAMILY TEACHING
• Discontinue drug if adverse reactions occur. • Report insomnia, dizziness, tremors, tachycardia, palpitations.

psyllium

sil-ee-yum
(Fiberall, Hydrocil, Konsyl, Metamucil)
Do not confuse Fiberall with Feverall.

P

◆CLASSIFICATION

PHARMACOTHERAPEUTIC: Bulk-forming laxative (see p. 125C).

ACTION

Dissolves and swells in water providing increased bulk, moisture content in stool. **Therapeutic Effect:** Promotes peristalsis, bowel motility.

PHARMACOKINETICS

Route	Onset	Peak	Duration
PO	12–24 hrs	2–3 days	N/A

Acts in small, large intestines.

 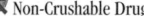

USES

Treatment of occasional constipation, constipation associated with rectal disorders. Dietary fiber supplement. Reduce risk of CHD. **OFF-LABEL:** Diarrhea, chronic constipation, inflammatory bowel disease, colon cancer, diabetes.

PRECAUTIONS

Contraindications: Fecal impaction, GI obstruction, undiagnosed abdominal pain. **Cautions:** Esophageal strictures, ulcers, stenosis, intestinal adhesions, difficulty swallowing, management of irritable bowel syndrome (IBS).

⌛ LIFESPAN CONSIDERATIONS

Pregnancy/Lactation: Safe for use in pregnancy. **Pregnancy Category B. Children:** Safety and efficacy not established in those younger than 6 yrs. **Elderly:** No age-related precautions noted.

INTERACTIONS

DRUG: None significant. **HERBAL:** None significant. **FOOD:** None known. **LAB VALUES:** May increase serum glucose. May decrease serum potassium.

AVAILABILITY (OTC)

Capsules (Konsyl, Metamucil): 500 mg. **Powder (Fiberall, Hydrocil, Konsyl, Metamucil):** 4.1 g/5 ml. **Wafer (Metamucil):** 3.4 g/dose.

ADMINISTRATION/HANDLING

PO

• Administer at least 2 hrs before or after other medication. • All doses should be followed with 8 oz liquid. • Drink 6–8 glasses of water/day (aids stool softening). • Do not swallow in dry form; mix with at least 1 full glass (8 oz) of liquid.

INDICATIONS/ROUTES/DOSAGE

Constipation, Irritable Bowel Syndrome (IBS)
Refer to specific dosing guidelines on product labeling.
PO: ADULTS, ELDERLY: (2.5–30 g/day in divided doses) 2–5 capsules/dose up to 3 times daily. 1 rounded tsp or 1 tbsp of powder up to 3 times daily. 2 wafers up to 3 times daily. **CHILDREN 6–11 YRS:** (1.25–15 g/day in divided doses). Approximately ½ adult dose up to 3 times daily.

CHD
PO: ADULTS, ELDERLY: 7 g or more daily.

SIDE EFFECTS

Rare: Some degree of abdominal discomfort, nausea, mild abdominal cramps, griping, faintness.

ADVERSE EFFECTS/ TOXIC REACTIONS

Esophageal/bowel obstruction may occur if administered with insufficient liquid (less than 250 ml).

NURSING CONSIDERATIONS

INTERVENTION/EVALUATION

Encourage adequate fluid intake. Assess bowel sounds for peristalsis. Monitor daily pattern of bowel activity, stool consistency. Monitor serum electrolytes in pts exposed to prolonged, frequent, excessive use of medication.

PATIENT/FAMILY TEACHING

• Take each dose with full glass (250 ml) of water. • Inadequate fluid intake may cause GI obstruction. • Institute measures to promote defecation (increase fluid intake, exercise, high-fiber diet).

pyrazinamide

peer-a-**zin**-a-mide
(Tebrazid ✱)

FIXED-COMBINATION(S)

Rifater: pyrazinamide/isoniazid/rifampin (an antitubercular): 300 mg/50 mg/120 mg.

◆CLASSIFICATION

PHARMACOTHERAPEUTIC: Synthetic pyrazine analogue. **CLINICAL:** Antitubercular.

ACTION

May disrupt mycobacterium tuberculosis membrane transport. **Therapeutic Effect:** Bacteriostatic or bactericidal, depending on drug concentration at infection site, susceptibility of infecting bacteria.

PHARMACOKINETICS

Well absorbed from GI tract. Protein binding: 5%–10%. Widely distributed. Metabolized in liver. Excreted in urine. **Half-life:** 9–10 hrs.

USES

Treatment of clinical tuberculosis in conjunction with other antitubercular agents.

PRECAUTIONS

Contraindications: Acute gout, severe hepatic dysfunction. **Cautions:** Diabetes mellitus, porphyria, renal impairment, history of gout, children (safety not established), history of alcoholism, concurrent medication associated with hepatotoxicity.

⌛ LIFESPAN CONSIDERATIONS

Pregnancy/Lactation: Unknown if drug crosses placenta or is distributed in breast milk. **Pregnancy Category C. Children:** Safety and efficacy not established. **Elderly:** No age-related precautions noted.

INTERACTIONS

DRUG: None significant. **HERBAL:** None significant. **FOOD:** None known. **LAB VALUES:** May increase serum AST, ALT, uric acid.

AVAILABILITY (Rx)

Tablets: 500 mg.

INDICATIONS/ROUTES/DOSAGE

Tuberculosis (in Combination With Other Antituberculars)
PO: ADULTS: Based on lean body weight. **40–55 KG:** 1,000 mg daily; **56–75 KG:** 1,500 mg daily; **76–90 KG:** 2,000 mg (**maximum dose** regardless of weight). **CHILDREN:** 15–30 mg/kg/day in 1 or 2 doses. **Maximum:** 2 g/day.

Dosage in Renal/Hepatic Impairment
Creatinine clearance less than 30 ml/min or receiving HD: 25–35 mg/kg/dose 3 times/wk (give after dialysis).

SIDE EFFECTS

Frequent: Arthralgia, myalgia (usually mild, self-limited). **Rare:** Hypersensitivity reaction (rash, pruritus, urticaria), photosensitivity, gouty arthritis.

ADVERSE EFFECTS/ TOXIC REACTIONS

Hepatotoxicity, gouty arthritis, thrombocytopenia, anemia occur rarely.

NURSING CONSIDERATIONS

BASELINE ASSESSMENT

Question for hypersensitivity to pyrazinamide, isoniazid, ethionamide, niacin. Ensure collection of specimens for culture, sensitivity. Evaluate results of initial CBC, hepatic function tests, serum uric acid levels.

INTERVENTION/EVALUATION

Monitor hepatic function test results; be alert for hepatic reactions: jaundice, malaise, fever, abdominal (RUQ) tenderness, anorexia, nausea, vomiting (stop drug, notify physician promptly). Check serum uric acid levels; assess for hot, painful, swollen joints, esp. big toe, ankle, knee (gout). Evaluate serum blood glucose levels, diabetic status carefully (pyrazinamide makes management difficult). Assess for rash, skin eruptions. Monitor CBC for thrombocytopenia, anemia.

PATIENT/FAMILY TEACHING

• Do not skip doses; complete full length of therapy (may be mos or yrs). • Office visits, lab tests are essential part of treatment. • Take with food to reduce GI upset. • Avoid excessive exposure to sun, ultra-

P

violet light until photosensitivity is determined. • Report any new symptom, immediately for jaundice (yellowing sclera of eyes/skin); unusual fatigue; fever; loss of appetite; hot, painful, swollen joints.

---

pyridostigmine

peer-id-oh-**stig**-meen
(Mestinon, Mestinon SR ✦,
Mestinon Timespan, Regonol)
Do not confuse pyridostigmine with physostigmine, or Regonol with Reglan or Renagel.

◆CLASSIFICATION

PHARMACOTHERAPEUTIC: Anticholinesterase. **CLINICAL:** Cholinergic muscle stimulant.

ACTION

Prevents destruction of acetylcholine by inhibiting the enzyme acetylcholinesterase, enhancing impulse transmission across myoneural junction. **Therapeutic Effect:** Produces miosis; increases intestinal, skeletal muscle tone; stimulates salivary, sweat gland secretions.

PHARMACOKINETICS

Poorly absorbed from GI tract. Metabolized in liver. Excreted primarily unchanged in urine. **Half-life:** 1–2 hrs.

USES

Improvement of muscle strength in control of myasthenia gravis, reversal of effects of nondepolarizing neuromuscular blocking agents after surgery.

PRECAUTIONS

Contraindications: Mechanical GI/urinary tract obstruction, hypersensitivity to anticholinesterase agents. **Cautions:** Bronchial asthma, bradycardia, epilepsy, recent coronary occlusion, vagotonia, hyperthyroidism, cardiac arrhythmias, peptic ulcer, renal impairment.

⌛ LIFESPAN CONSIDERATIONS

Pregnancy/Lactation: Unknown if drug crosses placenta or is distributed in breast milk. **Pregnancy Category B. Children:** Safety and efficacy not established. **Elderly:** No age-related precautions noted.

INTERACTIONS

DRUG: Antagonizes effects of **neuromuscular blockers. Anticholinergics** prevent, reverse effects. **Cholinesterase inhibitors** may increase risk of toxicity. **HERBAL:** None significant. **FOOD:** None known. **LAB VALUES:** None significant.

AVAILABILITY (Rx)

Injection Solution (Regonol): 5 mg/ml. **Syrup (Mestinon):** 60 mg/5 ml. **Tablets (Mestinon):** 60 mg.

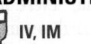 **Tablets (Extended-Release [Mestinon Timespan]):** 180 mg.

ADMINISTRATION/HANDLING
💉 IV, IM

• Give large parenteral doses concurrently with 0.6–1.2 mg atropine sulfate IV to minimize side effects.

PO

• Give with food, milk. • Tablets may be crushed. Instruct pt to not chew, crush extended-release tablets (may be broken). • Give larger dose at times of increased fatigue (e.g., for those with difficulty in chewing, 30–45 min before meals).

🗒 IV INCOMPATIBILITIES

Do not mix with any other medications.

INDICATIONS/ROUTES/DOSAGE
Myasthenia Gravis
PO: ADULTS, ELDERLY: Initially, 60 mg 3 times a day. Dosage increased at 48-hr intervals. **Maintenance:** 60 mg–1.5 g a day divided into 5–6 doses/day. **CHILDREN:** 7 mg/kg/24 hr divided into 5–6 doses.

PO *(Extended-Release)*: **ADULTS, ELDERLY:** 180–540 mg 1–2 times a day with at least a 6-hr interval between doses.
IV, IM: ADULTS, ELDERLY: 2 mg or 1/30th of oral dose q2–3h. **CHILDREN:** 0.05–0.15 mg/kg/dose. **Maximum single dose:** 10 mg.

SIDE EFFECTS

Frequent: Miosis, increased GI/skeletal muscle tone, bradycardia, constriction of bronchi/ureters, diaphoresis, increased salivation. **Occasional:** Headache, rash, temporary decrease in diastolic B/P with mild reflex tachycardia, short periods of atrial fibrillation (in hyperthyroid pts), marked drop in B/P (in hypertensive pts).

ADVERSE EFFECTS/ TOXIC REACTIONS

Overdose may produce cholinergic crisis, manifested as increasingly severe descending muscle weakness (appears first in muscles involving chewing, swallowing, followed by muscle weakness of shoulder girdle, upper extremities), respiratory muscle paralysis, followed by pelvis girdle/leg muscle paralysis. Requires withdrawal of all cholinergic drugs and immediate use of 1–4 mg atropine sulfate IV for adults, 0.01 mg/kg for infants and children younger than 12 yrs.

NURSING CONSIDERATIONS

BASELINE ASSESSMENT

Larger doses should be given at time of greatest fatigue. Assess muscle strength before testing for diagnosis of myasthenia gravis and following drug administration. Avoid large doses in pts with megacolon, reduced GI motility.

INTERVENTION/EVALUATION

Have facial tissues readily available at pt's bedside. Monitor respirations closely during myasthenia gravis testing or if dosage is increased. Assess diligently for cholinergic reaction, bradycardia in myasthenic pt in crisis. Coordinate dosage time with periods of fatigue and increased/decreased muscle strength. Monitor for therapeutic response to medication (increased muscle strength, decreased fatigue, improved chewing/swallowing functions).

PATIENT/FAMILY TEACHING

• Report nausea, vomiting, diarrhea, diaphoresis, profuse salivary secretions, palpitations, muscle weakness, severe abdominal pain, difficulty breathing.

pyridoxine (vitamin B$_6$)

peer-i-**dox**-een
(Aminoxin, Pyri-500)
Do not confuse pyridoxine with paroxetine, pralidoxime, or Pyridium.

◆CLASSIFICATION

PHARMACOTHERAPEUTIC: Coenzyme.
CLINICAL: Vitamin (B$_6$) (see p. 158C).

ACTION

Coenzyme for various metabolic functions, including metabolism of proteins, carbohydrates, fats. Aids in breakdown of glycogen and in synthesis of gamma-aminobutyric acid (GABA) in CNS. **Therapeutic Effect:** Prevents pyridoxine deficiency. Increases excretion of certain drugs (e.g., isoniazid) that are pyridoxine antagonists.

PHARMACOKINETICS

Readily absorbed, primarily in jejunum. Stored in liver, muscle, brain. Metabolized in liver. Primarily excreted in urine. Removed by hemodialysis. **Half-life:** 15–20 days.

USES

Prevention/treatment of vitamin B$_6$ deficiency. **OFF-LABEL:** Pyridoxine-dependent seizures in infants, drug-induced neuritis (e.g., associated with isoniazid). Treatment of peripheral neuropathy associ-

P

ated with isoniazid; nausea and vomiting of pregnancy.

PRECAUTIONS

Contraindications: None known. **Cautions:** Impaired renal function, neonates.

⌛ LIFESPAN CONSIDERATIONS

Pregnancy/Lactation: Crosses placenta. Distributed in breast milk. High dosages in utero may produce seizures in neonates. **Pregnancy Category A. Children/Elderly:** No age-related precautions noted.

INTERACTIONS

DRUG: Decreases effects of **levodopa. HERBAL:** None significant. **FOOD:** None known. **LAB VALUES:** None significant.

AVAILABILITY (OTC)

Capsules: 50 mg, 250 mg. **Injection Solution (Vitamin B₆):** 100 mg/ml. **Tablets:** 25 mg, 50 mg, 100 mg, 250 mg, 500 mg. **Tablet, Sustained-Release (Pyri-500):** 500 mg.

ADMINISTRATION/HANDLING

◄ **ALERT** ► Give PO unless nausea, vomiting, malabsorption occurs. Avoid IV use in cardiac pts.

 IV

• Give undiluted or may be added to IV solutions and given as infusion.

PO
• Give without regard to food.

▦ IV INCOMPATIBILITIES

Do not mix with any other medications.

INDICATIONS/ROUTES/DOSAGE

Pyridoxine Deficiency
PO/IM/IV: ADULTS, ELDERLY: 10–20 mg/day for 3 wks. **CHILDREN:** Initially, 5–25 mg/day for 3 wks, then 1.5–2.5 mg/day in multivitamin product.

SIDE EFFECTS

Occasional: Stinging at IM injection site. **Rare:** Headache, nausea, drowsiness, sensory neuropathy (paresthesia, unstable gait, clumsiness of hands) with high doses.

ADVERSE EFFECTS/ TOXIC REACTIONS

Long-term megadoses (2–6 g for longer than 2 mos) may produce sensory neuropathy (reduced deep tendon reflexes, profound impairment of sense of position in distal limbs, gradual sensory ataxia). Toxic symptoms subside when drug is discontinued. Seizures have occurred after IV megadoses.

NURSING CONSIDERATIONS

INTERVENTION/EVALUATION

Observe for improvement of deficiency symptoms, glossitis. Evaluate for nutritional adequacy.

PATIENT/FAMILY TEACHING

• Discomfort may occur with IM injection.
• Consume foods rich in pyridoxine (legumes, soybeans, eggs, sunflower seeds, hazelnuts, organ meats, tuna, shrimp, carrots, avocados, bananas, wheat germ, bran).

P

quetiapine

kwet-**eye**-a-peen
(Apo-Quetiapine ✤, <u>Seroquel</u>,
Seroquel XR)

BLACK BOX ALERT Increased risk of suicidal ideation and behavior in children, adolescents, young adults 18–24 yrs with major depressive disorder, other psychiatric disorders. Elderly with dementia-related psychosis are at increased risk for death.

Do not confuse quetiapine with olanzapine, or Seroquel with Sinequan.

◆CLASSIFICATION

PHARMACOTHERAPEUTIC: Dibenzapine derivative. **CLINICAL:** Antipsychotic (see p. 67C).

ACTION

Antagonizes dopamine, serotonin, histamine, alpha₁-adrenergic receptors. **Therapeutic Effect:** Diminishes psychotic disorders. Produces moderate sedation, few extrapyramidal effects. No anticholinergic effects.

PHARMACOKINETICS

Rapidly, well absorbed after PO administration. Protein binding: 83%. Widely distributed in tissues; CNS concentration exceeds plasma concentration. Metabolized in liver. Primarily excreted in urine. **Half-life:** 6 hrs.

USES

Treatment of schizophrenia. Treatment of acute manic episodes with bipolar disorder (alone or in combination with lithium or valproate). Maintenance treatment of bipolar disorder. Treatment of acute depressive episodes associated with bipolar disorder. Adjunctive treatment in major depressive disorder (MDD). **OFF-LABEL:** Autism, delirium in critically ill pts, psychosis/agitation related to Alzheimer's dementia.

PRECAUTIONS

Contraindications: None known. **Cautions:** Renal impairment, preexisting abnormal lipid profile, those at risk for aspiration pneumonia, cardiovascular disease (e.g., HF, history of MI), cerebrovascular disease, hepatic impairment, dehydration, hypovolemia, history of drug abuse/dependence, seizures, hypothyroidism, pts at risk for suicide, Parkinson's disease, decreased GI motility, urinary retention, narrow-angle glaucoma, diabetes, visual problems.

⌛ LIFESPAN CONSIDERATIONS

Pregnancy/Lactation: Unknown if drug is distributed in breast milk. Not recommended for breast-feeding mothers. **Pregnancy Category C. Children:** Safety and efficacy not established. **Elderly:** No age-related precautions noted, but lower initial and target dosages may be necessary.

INTERACTIONS

DRUG: Medications prolonging QT interval (e.g., amiodarone) may increase risk of QT prolongation. **Alcohol, other CNS depressants** may increase CNS depression. May increase hypotensive effects of **antihypertensives. Hepatic enzyme inducers (e.g., phenytoin)** may increase clearance. **CYP3A4 inhibitors (e.g., clarithromycin, erythromycin, fluconazole, itraconazole)** may increase effects. **HERBAL: St. John's wort** may decrease concentration. **Gotu kola, kava kava, St. John's wort, valerian** may increase CNS depression. **FOOD:** None known. **LAB VALUES:** May decrease total free thyroxine (T₄) serum levels. May increase serum cholesterol, triglycerides, AST, ALT, WBC, GGT. May produce false-positive pregnancy test result.

AVAILABILITY (Rx)

Tablets: 25 mg, 50 mg, 100 mg, 200 mg, 300 mg, 400 mg.

🥄 **Tablets, Extended-Release:** 50 mg, 150 mg, 200 mg, 300 mg, 400 mg.

Q

ADMINISTRATION/HANDLING

PO

• Give immediate-release tablets without regard to food. • Do not break, crush, dissolve, or divide extended-release tablets. • Extended-release tablets should be given without regard to food or with a light meal in evening.

INDICATIONS/ROUTES/DOSAGE

Note: When restarting pts who have been off quetiapine for less than 1 wk, titration is not required and maintenance dose can be reinstituted. • When restarting pts who have been off quetiapine for longer than 1 wk, follow initial titration schedule.

Psychotic Disorders, Schizophrenia

PO: ADULTS, ELDERLY: Initially, 25 mg twice a day, then 25–50 mg 2–3 times a day on the second and third days, up to 300–400 mg/day in divided doses 2–3 times a day by the fourth day. Further adjustments of 25–50 mg twice a day may be made at intervals of 2 days or longer. Maintenance: 300–800 mg/day (adults); 50–200 mg/day (elderly). **CHILDREN 13 YRS AND OLDER:** Initially, 25 mg twice daily on day 1, 50 mg twice daily on day 2, then increase by 100 mg/day to target dose of 400 mg/day on day 5. **Seroquel XR:** Initially, 300 mg/day in evening. May increase at intervals as short as 1 day up to 300 mg/day. Range: 400–800 mg/day.

Mania in Bipolar Disorder

PO: ADULTS, ELDERLY: Initially, 50 mg twice a day for 1 day. May increase in increments of 100 mg/day to 200 mg twice a day on day 4. May increase in increments of 200 mg/day to 800 mg/day on day 6. Range: 400–800 mg/day. **CHILDREN 10 YRS AND OLDER:** 25 mg twice daily on day 1, 50 mg twice daily on day 2, then increase by 100 mg/day until target dose of 400 mg/day reached on day 5. May increase up to 600 mg/day. Range: 400–600 mg/day. **Seroquel XR:** Initially, 300 mg on day 1 in the evening; 600 mg on day 2 and adjust between 400–800 mg/day thereafter.

Depression in Bipolar Disorder

PO: ADULTS, ELDERLY: Initially, 50 mg/day on day 1, increase to 100 mg/day on day 2, then increase by 100 mg/day up to target dose of 300 mg/day. **Seroquel XR:** Initially, 50 mg on day 1 in the evening, 100 mg on day 2, 200 mg on day 3, 300 mg on day 4 and thereafter.

Adjunctive Therapy in MDD

PO: ADULTS, ELDERLY: (SEROQUEL XR): Initially, 50 mg on days 1 and 2; then 150 mg on days 3 and 4; then 150–300 mg/day thereafter.

Dosage in Hepatic Impairment

Immediate-Release: Initially, 25 mg/day. Increase by 25–50 mg/day to effective dose.
Extended-Release: Initially, 50 mg/day, increase by 50 mg/day until effective dose.

SIDE EFFECTS

Frequent (19%–10%): Headache, drowsiness, dizziness. **Occasional (9%–3%):** Constipation, orthostatic hypotension, tachycardia, dry mouth, dyspepsia (heartburn, indigestion, epigastric pain), rash, asthenia (loss of strength, energy), abdominal pain, rhinitis. **Rare (2%):** Back pain, fever, weight gain.

ADVERSE EFFECTS/TOXIC REACTIONS

Overdose may produce heart block, hypotension, hypokalemia, tachycardia.

NURSING CONSIDERATIONS

BASELINE ASSESSMENT

Assess behavior, appearance, emotional status, response to environment, speech pattern, thought content. Obtain baseline CBC, hepatic enzyme levels before initiating treatment and periodically thereafter.

INTERVENTION/EVALUATION

Monitor mental status, onset of extrapyramidal symptoms. Assist with ambulation if dizziness occurs. Supervise suicidal-risk pt closely during early therapy (as psychosis, depression lessens, energy level improves, increasing suicide potential). Monitor B/P for hypotension, lipid profile, blood glucose, CBC, or worsening depression, unusual behavior. Assess pulse for tachycardia (esp. with rapid increase in dosage). Assess bowel activity for evidence of constipation. Assess for therapeutic response (improved thought content, increased ability to concentrate, improvement in self-care). Eye exam to detect cataract formation should be obtained q6mos during treatment.

PATIENT/ FAMILY TEACHING

• Avoid exposure to extreme heat. • Drink fluids often, esp. during physical activity. • Take medication as ordered; do not stop taking or increase dosage. • Drowsiness generally subsides during continued therapy. • Avoid tasks that require alertness, motor skills until response to drug is established. • Avoid alcohol. • Change positions slowly to reduce hypotensive effect. • Report suicidal ideation, unusual changes in behavior.

---

quinapril   _{TOP 200}

kwin-a-pril
(Accupril)

BLACK BOX ALERT May cause fetal injury, mortality if used during second or third trimester of pregnancy. **Do not confuse Accupril with Accolate, Accutane, Aciphex, or Monopril.**

FIXED-COMBINATION(S)

Accuretic: quinapril/hydrochlorothiazide (a diuretic): 10 mg/12.5 mg, 20 mg/12.5 mg, 20 mg/25 mg.

◆CLASSIFICATION

PHARMACOTHERAPEUTIC: Angiotensin-converting enzyme (ACE) inhibitor. **CLINICAL:** Antihypertensive (see p. 9C, 61C).

ACTION

Suppresses renin-angiotensin-aldosterone system, preventing conversion of angiotensin I to angiotensin II, a potent vasoconstrictor; may inhibit angiotensin II at local vascular renal sites. **Therapeutic Effect:** Reduces peripheral arterial resistance, B/P, pulmonary capillary wedge pressure; improves cardiac output.

PHARMACOKINETICS

Route	Onset	Peak	Duration
PO	1 hr	N/A	24 hrs

Readily absorbed from GI tract. Protein binding: 97%. Rapidly hydrolyzed to active metabolite. Primarily excreted in urine. Minimal removal by hemodialysis. **Half-life:** 1–2 hrs; metabolite, 3 hrs (increased in renal impairment).

USES

Treatment of hypertension. Used alone or in combination with other antihypertensives. Adjunctive therapy in management of heart failure. **OFF-LABEL:** Treatment of pediatric hypertension, treatment of left ventricular dysfunction following MI. Delays progression of nephropathy and reduces risk of cardiovascular events in hypertensive pts with diabetes.

PRECAUTIONS

Contraindications: History of angioedema from previous treatment with ACE inhibitors, concomitant use with aliskiren in pts with diabetes. **Cautions:** Renal impairment, hypertrophic cardiomyopathy, major surgery, HF, collagen vascular disease, hypovolemia, bilateral renal artery stenosis, hyperkalemia, severe aortic stenosis.

⏳ LIFESPAN CONSIDERATIONS

Pregnancy/Lactation: Crosses placenta. Unknown if distributed in breast milk. May cause fetal, neonatal mortality or morbidity. **Pregnancy Category C (D if used in second or third trimester). Children:** Safety and efficacy not established.

Elderly: May be more sensitive to hypotensive effects.

INTERACTIONS

DRUG: Alcohol, antihypertensives, diuretics may increase effects. May increase concentration, risk of toxicity of **lithium. NSAIDs** may decrease effects. **Potassium-sparing diuretics, potassium supplements** may cause hyperkalemia. **HERBAL: Black cohosh, periwinkle** may increase antihypertensive effect. **Ginseng, yohimbe, licorice** may worsen hypertension. **FOOD:** None known. **LAB VALUES:** May increase BUN, serum alkaline phosphatase, bilirubin, creatinine, potassium, AST, ALT. May decrease serum sodium. May cause positive antinuclear antibody (ANA) titer.

AVAILABILITY (Rx)

Tablets: 5 mg, 10 mg, 20 mg, 40 mg.

ADMINISTRATION/HANDLING

PO
• Give without regard to food. • Tablets may be crushed.

INDICATIONS/ROUTES/DOSAGE

Hypertension (Monotherapy)
PO: ADULTS: Initially, 10–20 mg/day. May adjust dosage at intervals of at least 2 wks or longer. Maintenance: 10–40 mg/day as single dose or 2 divided doses. **Maximum:** 40 mg/day. **ELDERLY:** Initially, 2.5–5 mg/day. May increase by 2.5–5 mg q1–2wks. **CHILDREN:** Initially, 5–10 mg once daily. **Maximum:** 80 mg/day.

Hypertension (Combination Diuretic Therapy)
PO: ADULTS: Initially, 5 mg/day titrated to pt's needs. **ELDERLY:** Initially, 2.5–5 mg/day. May increase by 2.5–5 mg q1–2wks.

Adjunct to Manage Heart Failure
PO: ADULTS, ELDERLY: Initially, 5 mg once or twice a day. Titrate at weekly intervals. Range: 20–40 mg/day.

Dosage in Renal Impairment
Dosage is titrated to pt's needs after the following initial doses:

Hypertension

Creatinine Clearance	Initial Dose
More than 60 ml/min	10 mg
30–60 ml/min	5 mg
10–29 ml/min	2.5 mg

HF

Creatinine Clearance	Initial Dose
Greater than 30 ml/min	5 mg
10–30 ml/min	2.5 mg

SIDE EFFECTS

Frequent (7%–5%): Headache, dizziness. **Occasional (4%–2%):** Fatigue, vomiting, nausea, hypotension, chest pain, cough, syncope. **Rare (less than 2%):** Diarrhea, cough, dyspnea, rash, palpitations, impotence, insomnia, drowsiness, malaise.

ADVERSE EFFECTS/ TOXIC REACTIONS

Excessive hypotension ("first-dose syncope") may occur in pts with HF, those who are severely salt/volume depleted. Angioedema, hyperkalemia occur rarely. Agranulocytosis, neutropenia may be noted in those with collagen vascular disease (scleroderma, systemic lupus erythematosus), renal impairment. Nephrotic syndrome may be noted in those with history of renal disease.

NURSING CONSIDERATIONS

BASELINE ASSESSMENT

Obtain B/P immediately before each dose in addition to regular monitoring (be alert to fluctuations). If excessive reduction in B/P occurs, place pt in supine position with legs slightly elevated. Renal function tests should be performed before beginning therapy. In pts with prior renal disease, urine test for protein by dipstick method should be made with first urine of day before beginning ther-

Q

apy and periodically thereafter. In pts with renal impairment, autoimmune disease, or taking drugs that affect leukocytes or immune response, CBC, differential count should be performed before beginning therapy and q2wks for 3 mos, then periodically thereafter.

INTERVENTION/EVALUATION

Monitor B/P, renal function, serum potassium, WBC. Assist with ambulation if dizziness occurs. Question for evidence of headache. Noncola carbonated beverage, unsalted crackers, dry toast may relieve nausea.

PATIENT/ FAMILY TEACHING

• Go from lying to standing slowly. • Full therapeutic effect may take 1–2 wks. • Report any sign of infection (sore throat, fever). • Skipping doses or voluntarily discontinuing drug may produce severe rebound hypertension. • Avoid tasks that require alertness, motor skills until response to drug is established. • Avoid alcohol.

---

quinupristin-dalfopristin

kwi-**nyoo**-pris-tin **dal**-foe-pris-tin (Synercid)

◆CLASSIFICATION

PHARMACOTHERAPEUTIC: Streptogramin. **CLINICAL:** Antimicrobial.

ACTION

Two chemically distinct compounds that, when given together, bind to different sites on bacterial ribosomes, inhibiting protein synthesis. **Therapeutic Effect:** Bactericidal.

PHARMACOKINETICS

After IV administration, both are extensively metabolized in liver, with dalfopris-

tin to active metabolite. Protein binding: quinupristin, 23%–32%; dalfopristin, 50%–56%. Primarily eliminated in feces. **Half-life:** quinupristin, 0.85 hr; dalfopristin, 0.7 hr.

USES

Complicated skin/skin structure infections caused by *S. aureus, S. pyogenes.* **OFF-LABEL:** Treatment of serious or life-threatening infections caused by vancomycin-resistant *Enterococcus faecium* (VRE).

PRECAUTIONS

Contraindications: Hypersensitivity to pristinamycin, virginiamycin. **Cautions:** Hepatic/renal dysfunction.

⧗ LIFESPAN CONSIDERATIONS

Pregnancy/Lactation: Unknown if drug crosses placenta or is distributed in breast milk. **Pregnancy Category B. Children:** Safety and efficacy not established. **Elderly:** No age-related precautions noted.

INTERACTIONS

DRUG: May increase concentration, risk of toxicity of **cyclosporine.** **HERBAL:** None significant. **FOOD:** None known. **LAB VALUES:** May increase serum bilirubin, creatinine, LDH, AST, ALT, BUN, alkaline phosphatase, glucose. May decrease Hgb, Hct; alter platelets.

AVAILABILITY (Rx)

Injection, Powder for Reconstitution: 500-mg vial (150 mg quinupristin/350 mg dalfopristin).

ADMINISTRATION/HANDLING
 IV

Reconstitution • Reconstitute vial by slowly adding 5 ml D_5W or Sterile Water for Injection to make 100 mg/ml solution. • Gently swirl vial contents to minimize foaming. • Further dilute with D_5W to final concentration of 2 mg/ml (5 mg/ml using central line).

Q

Rate of Administration • Infuse over 60 min. • After infusion, flush line with D_5W to minimize vein irritation. Do not flush with 0.9% NaCl (incompatible).

Storage • Refrigerate unopened vials. • Reconstituted vials are stable for 1 hr at room temperature. Diluted infusion bag is stable for 5 hrs at room temperature or 54 hrs if refrigerated.

🔹 IV INCOMPATIBILITIES

Sodium chloride.

🔹 IV COMPATIBILITIES

Aztreonam (Azactam), ciprofloxacin (Cipro), fluconazole (Diflucan), haloperidol (Haldol), metoclopramide (Reglan), potassium chloride.

INDICATIONS/ROUTES/DOSAGE

Infections Due to Vancomycin-Resistant *Enterococcus Faecium* (VRE)
IV: **ADULTS, ELDERLY:** 7.5 mg/kg/dose q8h.

Skin/Skin Structure Infections
IV: **ADULTS, ELDERLY:** 7.5 mg/kg/dose q12h.

SIDE EFFECTS

Frequent: Mild erythema, pruritus, pain/burning at infusion site (with doses greater than 7 mg/kg). **Occasional:** Headache, diarrhea. **Rare:** Vomiting, arthralgia, myalgia.

ADVERSE EFFECTS/ TOXIC REACTIONS

Antibiotic-associated colitis, other superinfections (abdominal cramps, severe watery diarrhea, fever) may result from altered bacterial balance. Hepatic function abnormalities, severe venous pain, inflammation may occur.

NURSING CONSIDERATIONS

BASELINE ASSESSMENT

Assess temperature, B/P, respiratory rate, pulse. Obtain baseline hepatic function tests, BUN, CBC, urinalysis.

INTERVENTION/EVALUATION

Monitor CBC, hepatic function tests. Observe infusion site for redness, vein irritation. Hold medication, promptly inform physician of diarrhea (with fever, abdominal pain, mucus/blood in stool may indicate antibiotic-associated colitis). Evaluate IV site for erythema, pruritus, pain, burning. Be alert for superinfection: fever, vomiting, diarrhea, anal/genital pruritus, oral mucosal changes (ulceration, pain, erythema).

Q

rabeprazole

TOP 200

rah-**bep**-rah-zole
(<u>Aciphex</u>, Apo-Rabeprazole)
Do not confuse Aciphex with Accupril or Aricept, or rabeprazole with aripiprazole, lansoprazole, omeprazole, or raloxifene.

◆ CLASSIFICATION

PHARMACOTHERAPEUTIC: Proton pump inhibitor. **CLINICAL:** Gastric acid inhibitor (see p. 147C).

ACTION

Converts to active metabolites that irreversibly bind to, inhibit hydrogen-potassium adenosine triphosphate, an enzyme on surface of gastric parietal cells. Actively secretes hydrogen ions for potassium ions, resulting in accumulation of hydrogen ions in gastric lumen. **Therapeutic Effect:** Increases gastric pH, reducing gastric acid production.

PHARMACOKINETICS

Rapidly absorbed from GI tract after passing through stomach relatively intact as delayed-release tablet. Protein binding: 96%. Metabolized in liver. Primarily excreted in urine. Unknown if removed by hemodialysis. **Half-life:** 1–2 hrs (increased with hepatic impairment).

USES

Short-term treatment (4–8 wks), maintenance of erosive or ulcerative gastro-esophageal reflux disease (GERD). Treatment of daytime/nighttime heartburn, other symptoms of GERD. Short-term treatment (4 wks or less) in healing, symptomatic relief of duodenal ulcers. Long-term treatment of pathologic hypersecretory conditions, including Zollinger-Ellison syndrome. Treatment of *H. pylori* (in combination with other medication). Sprinkle dose form approved for treatment of GERD in children 1–11 yrs. **OFF-LABEL:** Maintenance of healing and prevention of relapse of duodenal ulcers. Treatment of NSAID-induced ulcers.

PRECAUTIONS

Contraindications: Hypersensitivity to proton pump inhibitors (e.g., omeprazole). **Cautions:** Severe hepatic impairment. May increase risk of fractures, GI infections.

⌛ LIFESPAN CONSIDERATIONS

Pregnancy/Lactation: Unknown if drug crosses placenta or is distributed in breast milk. **Pregnancy Category B. Children:** Safety and efficacy not established. **Elderly:** No age-related precautions noted.

INTERACTIONS

DRUG: May increase concentration/effects of **cyclosporine, warfarin.** May decrease concentration of **ketoconazole, clopidogrel, atazanavir. HERBAL: St. John's wort** may decrease concentration/effects. **FOOD:** None known. **LAB VALUES:** May increase serum AST, ALT, thyroid stimulating hormone (TSH).

AVAILABILITY (Rx)

🐦 **Tablets (Delayed-Release):** 10 mg, 20 mg.

ADMINISTRATION/HANDLING

PO
• May give without regard to meals; best taken before breakfast. • Do not crush, break, split tablet; give whole.

INDICATIONS/ROUTES/DOSAGE

Gastroesophageal Reflux Disease (GERD)
PO: ADULTS, ELDERLY: 20 mg/day for 4–8 wks. Maintenance: 20 mg/day.

Short-Term Treatment of GERD
PO: CHILDREN 12 YRS AND OLDER: 20 mg/day for up to 8 wks. **CHILDREN, 1–11 YRS (15 KG OR GREATER):** 10 mg once a day. **(LESS THAN 15 KG):** 5 mg once daily; may increase to 10 mg once daily.

R

Duodenal Ulcer
PO: ADULTS, ELDERLY: 20 mg/day after morning meal for 4 wks.

Pathologic Hypersecretory Conditions
PO: ADULTS, ELDERLY: Initially, 60 mg once a day. May increase to 60 mg twice a day.

H. Pylori Infection
PO: ADULTS, ELDERLY: 20 mg twice a day for 10–14 days (given with amoxicillin 1,000 mg and clarithromycin 500 mg).

SIDE EFFECTS

Rare (less than 2%): Headache, nausea, dizziness, rash, diarrhea, malaise.

ADVERSE EFFECTS/ TOXIC REACTIONS

Hyperglycemia, hypokalemia, hyponatremia, hyperlipemia occur rarely.

NURSING CONSIDERATIONS

BASELINE ASSESSMENT
Obtain baseline lab values, esp. serum chemistries.

INTERVENTION/EVALUATION
Monitor ongoing laboratory results. Evaluate for therapeutic response (relief of GI symptoms). Question if GI discomfort, nausea, diarrhea, headache occurs. Assess skin for evidence of rash. Observe for evidence of dizziness; utilize appropriate safety precautions.

PATIENT/FAMILY TEACHING
• Swallow tablets whole; do not chew, split, crush tablets. • Report headache.

---

raloxifene

TOP
200

ra-**lox**-i-feen
(Evista, Apo-Raloxifene ✦, Novo-Raloxifene ✦)

BLACK BOX ALERT Increases risk of deep vein thrombosis, pulmonary embolism. Women with coronary heart disease or pts at risk for coronary events are at increased risk for death due to stroke.
Do not confuse Evista with Avinza.

◆CLASSIFICATION

PHARMACOTHERAPEUTIC: Selective estrogen receptor modulator. **CLINICAL:** Osteoporosis preventive (see p. 143C).

ACTION

Selective estrogen receptor modulator that binds to estrogen receptors, increasing bone mineral density. **Therapeutic Effect:** Reduces bone resorption, decreases bone turnover, prevents bone loss.

PHARMACOKINETICS

Rapidly absorbed after PO administration. Protein binding: 95%. Metabolized in liver. Excreted mainly in feces and, to a lesser extent, in urine. Unknown if removed by hemodialysis. **Half-life:** 27.7–32.5 hrs.

USES

Prevention/treatment of osteoporosis in postmenopausal women. Reduces risk of invasive breast cancer in postmenopausal women with osteoporosis and postmenopausal women at high risk for invasive breast cancer.

PRECAUTIONS

Contraindications: Active or history of venous thromboembolic events, such as deep vein thrombosis (DVT), pulmonary embolism, retinal vein thrombosis; women who are or may become pregnant, or are breastfeeding. **Cautions:** Cardiovascular disease, renal/hepatic impairment, risk for venous thromboembolism, unexplained uterine bleeding, elevated triglycerides in response to oral estrogen therapy.

⌛ LIFESPAN CONSIDERATIONS

Pregnancy/Lactation: Unknown if distributed in breast milk. Not recommended for breastfeeding mothers. **Pregnancy Category X. Children:** Not used in this population. **Elderly:** No age-related precautions noted.

INTERACTIONS

DRUG: Cholestyramine reduces peak levels, extent of absorption. Do not use concurrently with **hormone replacement therapy, systemic estrogen.** May decrease effect of **warfarin** (decreases INR). **HERBAL:** None significant. **FOOD:** None known. **LAB VALUES:** May lower serum total cholesterol, LDL. May decrease platelet count, serum inorganic phosphate, albumin, calcium, protein.

AVAILABILITY (Rx)

Tablets: 60 mg.

ADMINISTRATION/HANDLING

PO

• Give without regard to meals.

INDICATIONS/ROUTES/DOSAGE

Prophylaxis/Treatment of Osteoporosis, Breast Cancer Risk Reduction
PO: ADULTS, ELDERLY: 60 mg a day.

SIDE EFFECTS

Frequent (25%–10%): Hot flashes, flu-like symptoms, arthralgia, sinusitis. **Occasional (9%–5%):** Weight gain, nausea, myalgia, pharyngitis, cough, dyspepsia, leg cramps, rash, depression. **Rare (4%–3%):** Vaginitis, UTI, peripheral edema, flatulence, vomiting, fever, migraine, diaphoresis.

ADVERSE EFFECTS/ TOXIC REACTIONS

Pneumonia, gastroenteritis, chest pain, vaginal bleeding, breast pain occur rarely.

NURSING CONSIDERATIONS

BASELINE ASSESSMENT

Question for possibility of pregnancy (Pregnancy Category X). Drug should be discontinued 72 hrs before and during prolonged immobilization (postop recovery, prolonged bed rest). Therapy may be resumed only after pt is fully ambulatory. Determine serum total, LDL cholesterol before therapy and routinely thereafter.

INTERVENTION/EVALUATION

Monitor serum total, LDL cholesterol, total calcium, inorganic phosphate, total protein, albumin, bone mineral density, platelet count.

PATIENT/FAMILY TEACHING

• Avoid prolonged restriction of movement during travel (increased risk of venous thromboembolic events). • Take supplemental calcium, vitamin D if daily dietary intake is inadequate. • Engage in regular weight-bearing exercise. • Modify, discontinue habits of cigarette smoking, alcohol consumption.

raltegravir
TOP 200

ral-**teg**-ra-veer
(Isentress)

◆CLASSIFICATION

PHARMACOTHERAPEUTIC: Integrase inhibitor. **CLINICAL:** Antiviral (see p. 70C, 121C).

ACTION

Inhibits activity of HIV-1 integrase, an enzyme required for viral replication. **Therapeutic Effect:** Prevents integration and replication of viral HIV-1.

PHARMACOKINETICS

Variably absorbed following PO administration. Protein binding: 83%. Metabo-

R

lized in liver, primarily hepatic glucuronidation mediated by UGT1A1. Eliminated mainly in feces (51%), urine (32%). **Half-life:** 9 hrs.

USES

Treatment of HIV-1 infection in adults and children 2 yrs and older and weighing at least 10 kg. Used in combination with at least two other antiretroviral agents.

PRECAUTIONS

Contraindications: None known. **Cautions:** Elderly, pts at increased risk for myopathy, rhabdomyolysis, medications that induce (e.g., rifampin) or inhibit (e.g., atazanavir) UGT1A1 glucouronidation.

⧗ LIFESPAN CONSIDERATIONS

Pregnancy/Lactation: May cross placenta. Breastfeeding not recommended. **Pregnancy Category C. Children:** Safety and efficacy not established in those younger than 16 yrs. **Elderly:** Age-related hepatic, renal, cardiac impairment requires strict monitoring.

INTERACTIONS

DRUG: Proton pump inhibitors may increase concentration. **HERBAL: St. John's wort** may decrease concentration/effects. **FOOD:** None known. **LAB VALUES:** May increase serum glucose, bilirubin, aminotransferase, alkaline phosphatase, amylase, lipase, creatine kinase. May decrease lymphocytes/neutrophil count (ANC), Hgb, platelets.

AVAILABILITY (Rx)

Tablets, Chewable: 25 mg, 100 mg.

⧉ Tablets, Film-Coated: 400 mg.

ADMINISTRATION/HANDLING

PO

• Give without regard to food. • Do not break, crush, or divide film-coated tablets. • Chewable tablets may be chewed or taken whole.

INDICATIONS/ROUTES/DOSAGE

HIV Infection

PO: ADULTS, ELDERLY, CHILDREN 12 YRS AND OLDER: 400 mg twice a day. Dosage increased to 800 mg twice a day when given with rifampin. **CHILDREN 2–11 YRS (CHEWABLE TABLETS): 40 KG OR GREATER:** 300 mg twice daily. **28–39 KG:** 200 mg twice daily. **20–27 KG:** 150 mg twice daily. **14–19 KG:** 100 mg twice daily. **10–13 KG:** 75 mg twice daily. **Note:** Children 6–11 yrs and greater than 25 kg may use adult dosing.

SIDE EFFECTS

Frequent (17%–10%): Diarrhea, nausea, headache. **Occasional (5%):** Fever. **Rare (2%–1%):** Vomiting, abdominal pain, fatigue, dizziness.

ADVERSE EFFECTS/TOXIC REACTIONS

Hypersensitivity, anemia, neutropenia, MI, gastritis, hepatitis, herpes simplex, toxic nephropathy, renal failure, chronic renal failure, renal tubular necrosis occur rarely.

NURSING CONSIDERATIONS

BASELINE ASSESSMENT

Obtain baseline laboratory testing before beginning therapy and at periodic intervals during therapy. Offer emotional support. Obtain medication history.

INTERVENTION/EVALUATION

Closely monitor for evidence of GI discomfort. Monitor daily pattern of bowel activity, stool consistency. Monitor serum chemistry tests for marked laboratory abnormalities. Assess for opportunistic infections: onset of fever, cough, other respiratory symptoms.

PATIENT/FAMILY TEACHING

• Report fever, abdominal pain, yellowing of skin/eyes, dark urine. • Avoid tasks that require alertness, motor skills until response to drug is established. • Raltegravir is not a cure for HIV infection, nor does it reduce risk of transmission to others.

R

• Pt may continue to experience illnesses, including opportunistic infections.

ramelteon

ra-**mel**-tee-on
(Rozerem)
Do not confuse ramelteon with Remeron, or Rozerem with Razadyne or Remeron.

◆CLASSIFICATION

PHARMACOTHERAPEUTIC: Melatonin receptor agonist. **CLINICAL:** Hypnotic (see p. 149C).

ACTION

Selectively targets melatonin receptors thought to be involved in maintenance of circadian rhythm underlying normal sleep-wake cycle. **Therapeutic Effect:** Prevents insomnia characterized by difficulty with sleep onset.

PHARMACOKINETICS

Rapidly absorbed following PO administration. Protein binding: 82%. Substantial tissue distribution. Metabolized in liver. Excreted in urine (84%), feces (4%). **Half-life:** 2–5 hrs.

USES

Treatment of insomnia in pts who experience difficulty with sleep onset.

PRECAUTIONS

Contraindications: Concurrent fluvoxamine therapy, history of angioedema with previous ramelteon therapy. **Cautions:** Clinical depression, other psychiatric conditions, alcohol consumption, other CNS depressants, moderate to severe hepatic impairment, severe sleep apnea, COPD.

⌛ LIFESPAN CONSIDERATIONS

Pregnancy/Lactation: Unknown if distributed in breast milk. Breastfeeding not recommended. **Pregnancy Category C. Children:** Safety and efficacy not established. **Elderly:** Age-related hepatic impairment may require dosage adjustment.

INTERACTIONS

DRUG: Concurrent use with **alcohol** may produce additive effect. **Fluconazole, ketoconazole** may increase serum concentration/effects. **Donepezil, doxepin, fluvoxamine** may cause marked increase in serum level, toxicity. **Rifampin** may decrease serum level, effects. **HERBAL: Gotu kola, kava kava, St. John's wort, valerian** may increase CNS depression. **FOOD:** Onset of action may be reduced if taken with or immediately after a **high-fat meal. LAB VALUES:** May decrease serum cortisol.

AVAILABILITY (Rx)

🔖 **Tablets, Film-Coated:** 8 mg (Rozerem).

ADMINISTRATION/HANDLING

PO
• Administer within 30 min before bedtime. • Do not give with, or immediately following, a high-fat meal. • Do not break, crush, dissolve, or divide tablet.

INDICATIONS/ROUTES/DOSAGE

Insomnia
PO: ADULTS, ELDERLY: 8 mg 30 min before bedtime.

SIDE EFFECTS

Frequent (7%–5%): Headache, dizziness, drowsiness (expected effect). **Occasional (4%–3%):** Fatigue, nausea, exacerbated insomnia. **Rare (2%):** Diarrhea, myalgia, depression, altered taste, arthralgia.

ADVERSE EFFECTS/ TOXIC REACTIONS

May affect reproductive hormones in adults (decreased testosterone levels, increased prolactin levels), resulting in unexplained amenorrhea, galactorrhea, decreased libido, impaired fertility.

R

✦ Canadian trade name   🔖 Non-Crushable Drug   🟥 High Alert drug

NURSING CONSIDERATIONS

BASELINE ASSESSMENT

Assess B/P, pulse, respirations. Raise bed rails, provide call light. Provide environment conducive to sleep (quiet environment, low/no lighting, TV off).

INTERVENTION/EVALUATION

Assess sleep pattern of pt. Evaluate for therapeutic response: rapid induction of sleep onset, decrease in number of nocturnal awakenings.

PATIENT/FAMILY TEACHING

• Take within 30 min before going to bed; confine activities to those necessary to prepare for bed. • Avoid tasks that require alertness, motor skills until response to drug is established. • Avoid alcohol. • Do not take medication with or immediately after a high-fat meal.

---

ramipril

TOP 200

ram-i-pril
(<u>Altace</u>, Apo-Ramipril)

BLACK BOX ALERT May cause fetal injury, mortality if used during second or third trimester of pregnancy. **Do not confuse Altace with alteplase, Amaryl, or Artane, or ramipril with enalapril or Monopril.**

◆CLASSIFICATION

PHARMACOTHERAPEUTIC: Renin-angiotensin system antagonist. **CLINICAL:** Antihypertensive (see pp. 10C, 61C).

ACTION

Suppresses renin-angiotensin-aldosterone system. Decreases plasma angiotensin II, increases plasma renin activity, decreases aldosterone secretion. **Therapeutic Effect:** Reduces peripheral arterial resistance, decreasing B/P.

PHARMACOKINETICS

Route	Onset	Peak	Duration
PO	1–2 hrs	3–6 hrs	24 hrs

Well absorbed from GI tract. Protein binding: 73%. Metabolized in liver. Primarily excreted in urine. Not removed by hemodialysis. **Half-life:** 5.1 hrs.

USES

Treatment of hypertension. Used alone or in combination with other antihypertensives. Treatment of left ventricular dysfunction following MI. Reduce risk of heart attack, stroke in pts at increased risk for these events. **OFF-LABEL:** HF. Delay progression of nephropathy, reduce risks of cardiovascular events in hypertensive pts with type 1 or type 2 diabetes.

PRECAUTIONS

Contraindications: Hypersensitivity to ACE inhibitors. History of ACE-inhibitor induced angioedema, concomitant use with aliskiren in pts with diabetes. **Cautions:** Renal impairment, collagen vascular disease, hyperkalemia, hypertrophic cardiomyopathy with outflow tract obstruction; unstented unilateral, bilateral renal artery stenosis; severe aortic stenosis; before, during, or immediately after major surgery.

⧗ LIFESPAN CONSIDERATIONS

Pregnancy/Lactation: Crosses placenta. Distributed in breast milk. May cause fetal or neonatal mortality or morbidity. **Pregnancy Category C (D if used in second or third trimester). Children:** Safety and efficacy not established. **Elderly:** May be more sensitive to hypotensive effects.

INTERACTIONS

DRUG: Alcohol, antihypertensives, diuretics may increase effects. May increase **lithium** concentration, risk of toxicity. **NSAIDs** may decrease effects. **Potassium-sparing diuretics, potas-**

sium supplements may cause hyperkalemia. **HERBAL: Black cohosh, periwinkle** may increase antihypertensive effect. **Ginseng, ginger, licorice, yohimbe** may worsen hypertension. **FOOD:** None known. **LAB VALUES:** May increase BUN, serum alkaline phosphatase, bilirubin, creatinine, potassium, AST, ALT. May decrease serum sodium. May cause positive antinuclear antibody (ANA) titer.

AVAILABILITY (Rx)

Capsules: 1.25 mg, 2.5 mg, 5 mg, 10 mg.

ADMINISTRATION/HANDLING

PO
• Give without regard to food. • May mix with water, apple juice/sauce.

INDICATIONS/ROUTES/DOSAGE

Hypertension (Monotherapy)
PO: ADULTS, ELDERLY: Initially, 2.5 mg/day. **Maintenance:** 2.5–20 mg/day as single dose or in 2 divided doses.

Hypertension (in Combination with Other Antihypertensives)
PO: ADULTS, ELDERLY: Initially, 1.25 mg/day titrated to pt's needs.

Left Ventricular Dysfunction Following MI
PO: ADULTS, ELDERLY: Initially, 1.25–2.5 mg twice a day. **Maximum:** 5 mg twice a day.

Risk Reduction for MI/Stroke
PO: ADULTS, ELDERLY: Initially, 2.5 mg/day for 7 days, then 5 mg/day for 21 days, then 10 mg/day as a single dose or in divided doses.

Dosage in Renal Impairment
Creatinine Clearance Equal To or Less Than 40 ml/min: 25% of normal dose.

Renal Failure and Hypertension
Initially, 1.25 mg/day titrated upward. **Maximum:** 5 mg/day.
HF: Initially, 1.25 mg/day, titrated up to 2.5 mg twice a day.

SIDE EFFECTS

Frequent (12%–5%): Cough, headache. **Occasional (4%–2%):** Dizziness, fatigue, nausea, asthenia (loss of strength, energy). **Rare (less than 2%):** Palpitations, insomnia, nervousness, malaise, abdominal pain, myalgia.

ADVERSE EFFECTS/ TOXIC REACTIONS

Excessive hypotension ("first-dose syncope") may occur in pts with HF, severely salt or volume depleted. Angioedema, hyperkalemia occur rarely. Agranulocytosis, neutropenia may be noted in pts with collagen vascular disease (scleroderma, systemic lupus erythematosus), renal impairment. Nephrotic syndrome may be noted in those with history of renal disease.

NURSING CONSIDERATIONS

BASELINE ASSESSMENT

Obtain B/P immediately before each dose, in addition to regular monitoring (be alert to fluctuations). If excessive reduction in B/P occurs, place pt in supine position with legs elevated. Renal function tests should be performed before beginning therapy. In pts with prior renal disease, urine test for protein (by dipstick method) should be made with first urine of day before beginning therapy and periodically thereafter. In pts with renal impairment, autoimmune disease, or taking drugs that affect leukocytes or immune response, CBC, differential count should be performed before beginning therapy and q2wks for 3 mos periodically thereafter.

INTERVENTION/EVALUATION

Monitor B/P, renal function, serum potassium, WBC. Assess for cough (frequent effect). Assist with ambulation if dizziness occurs. Assess lung sounds for rales, wheezing in pts with HF. Monitor urinalysis for proteinuria. Monitor serum potassium in those on concurrent diuretic therapy.

R

PATIENT/FAMILY TEACHING

• Do not discontinue medication without physician's approval. • Rise slowly from sitting/lying position to reduce hypotensive effect. • Report palpitations, cough, chest pain. • Dizziness may occur in first few days. • Avoid tasks that require alertness, motor skills until response to drug is established. • Avoid alcohol.

ranitidine

 TOP 200

ra-**nit**-i-deen
(Apo-Ranitidine ✦, Zantac, Zantac-75, Zantac-150, Zantac EFFERdose)
Do not confuse ranitidine with amantadine or rimantadine, or Zantac with Xanax, Ziac, Zofran, or Zyrtec.

◆CLASSIFICATION

PHARMACOTHERAPEUTIC: Histamine H_2 receptor antagonist. **CLINICAL:** Antiulcer (see p. 111C).

ACTION

Inhibits histamine action at histamine 2 receptors of gastric parietal cells. **Therapeutic Effect:** Inhibits gastric acid secretion (fasting, nocturnal, when stimulated by food, caffeine, insulin). Reduces volume, hydrogen ion concentration of gastric juice.

PHARMACOKINETICS

Rapidly absorbed from GI tract. Protein binding: 15%. Widely distributed. Metabolized in liver. Primarily excreted in urine. Not removed by hemodialysis. **Half-life: PO:** 2.5 hrs; **IV:** 2–2.5 hrs (increased with renal impairment).

USES

Short-term treatment of active duodenal ulcer. Prevention of duodenal ulcer recurrence. Treatment of active benign gastric ulcer, pathologic GI hypersecretory conditions, acute gastroesophageal reflux disease (GERD), including erosive esophagitis. Maintenance of healed erosive esophagitis. Part of regimen for *H. pylori* eradication to reduce risk of duodenal ulcer recurrence. **OTC:** Relieve heartburn, acid indigestion, sour stomach. **OFF-LABEL:** Prevention of aspiration pneumonia, treatment of recurrent postop ulcer, upper GI bleeding, prevention of acid aspiration pneumonitis during surgery, prevention of stress-induced ulcers.

PRECAUTIONS

Contraindications: None known. **Cautions:** Renal/hepatic impairment, elderly, history of acute porphyria.

⏳ LIFESPAN CONSIDERATIONS

Pregnancy/Lactation: Unknown if drug crosses placenta or is distributed in breast milk. **Pregnancy Category B. Children:** No age-related precautions noted. **Elderly:** Confusion more likely with hepatic/renal impairment.

INTERACTIONS

DRUG: Magnesium or aluminum antacids may decrease absorption. May decrease absorption of **atazanavir, itraconazole, ketoconazole. HERBAL:** None significant. **FOOD:** None known. **LAB VALUES:** Interferes with skin tests using allergen extracts. May increase serum AST, ALT, gamma-glutamyl transpeptidase, creatinine.

AVAILABILITY (Rx)

Capsules (Zantac): 150 mg, 300 mg. **Injection Solution (Zantac):** 25 mg/ml. **Syrup (Zantac):** 15 mg/ml. **Tablets (Zantac):** 75 mg, 150 mg, 300 mg. **Tablet for Solution (Zantac EFFERdose):** 25 mg.

ADMINISTRATION/HANDLING
💉 IV

Reconstitution • For IV push, dilute each 50 mg with 20 ml 0.9% NaCl, D_5W. • For intermittent IV infusion (piggyback), dilute each 50 mg with 0.9% NaCl, D$_5$W to a maximum concentration of 0.5 mg/ml. • For IV infusion, dilute with 0.9% NaCl, D$_5$W to a maximum concentration of 2.5 mg/ml.

Rate of Administration • Administer IV push over minimum of 5 min (prevents arrhythmias, hypotension). • Infuse IV piggyback over 15–20 min. • Infuse IV infusion over 24 hrs.

Storage • IV solutions appear clear, colorless to yellow (slight darkening does not affect potency). • IV infusion (piggyback) is stable for 48 hrs at room temperature (discard if discolored or precipitate forms).

IM

• May be given undiluted. • Give deep IM into large muscle mass.

PO

• Give without regard to meals (best given with meals or at bedtime). • Do not administer within 1 hr of magnesium- or aluminum-containing antacids (decreases absorption). • **EFFERdose:** Instruct pt to not chew; swallow whole or dissolve on tongue.

▓ IV INCOMPATIBILITY

Amphotericin B complex (Abelcet, AmBisome, Amphotec).

▓ IV COMPATIBILITIES

Dexmedetomidine (Precedex), diltiazem (Cardizem), dobutamine (Dobutrex), dopamine (Intropin), heparin, hydromorphone (Dilaudid), insulin, lidocaine, lorazepam (Ativan), morphine, norepinephrine (Levophed), potassium chloride, propofol (Diprivan).

INDICATIONS/ROUTES/DOSAGE

Duodenal Ulcer, Gastric Ulcer
PO: ADULTS, ELDERLY: (Treatment): 150 mg twice daily or 300 mg once daily. **(Maintenance):** 150 mg once daily at bedtime. **CHILDREN 1 MO TO 16 YRS: (Treatment):** 4–8 mg/kg/day in 2 divided doses. **Maximum:** 300 mg.

(Maintenance): 2–4 mg/kg/day once daily. **Maximum:** 150 mg.

H. Pylori
PO: ADULTS, ELDERLY: 150 mg twice daily (in combination therapy).

Hypersecretory Conditions
PO: ADULTS, ELDERLY: 150 mg twice daily up to 6 g/day. **IV Infusion:** Initially, 1 mg/kg/hr. May increase by 0.5 mg/kg/hr up to 2.5 mg/kg/hr.

GERD
PO: ADULTS, ELDERLY: 150 mg twice daily. **CHILDREN 1 MO TO 16 YRS:** 5–10 mg/kg/day in 2 divided doses. **Maximum:** 300 mg/day.

Erosive Esophagitis
PO: ADULTS, ELDERLY: (Treatment): 150 mg four times/day. **(Maintenance):** 150 mg twice daily. **CHILDREN 1 MO TO 16 YRS: (Treatment):** 5–10 mg/kg/day in 2 divided doses. **Maximum:** 600 mg/day.

Prevention of Heartburn
PO: ADULTS, ELDERLY, CHILDREN 12 YRS AND OLDER: 75 mg 30–60 min before eating or drinking beverages that cause heartburn. **Maximum:** 150 mg/24 hrs for 14 days.

Usual Parenteral Dosage
IV Infusion: ADULTS, ELDERLY: 6.25 mg/hr. **CHILDREN:** 1 mg/kg for one dose then 0.08–0.17 mg/kg/hr (2–4 mg/kg/day).

Usual Neonatal Dosage
PO: NEONATES: 2 mg/kg/day in divided doses q12h.
IV: NEONATES: Initially, 1.5 mg/kg/dose, then 1.5–2 mg/kg/day in divided doses q12h.
IV Infusion: NEONATES: Loading dose: 1.5 mg/kg, then 1–2 mg/kg/day.

Dosage in Renal Impairment
Creatinine clearance less than 50 ml/min: Give 150 mg PO q24h or 50 mg IV or IM q18–24h.

R

SIDE EFFECTS

Occasional (2%): Diarrhea. **Rare (1%):** Constipation, headache (may be severe).

ADVERSE EFFECTS/ TOXIC REACTIONS

Reversible hepatitis, blood dyscrasias occur rarely.

NURSING CONSIDERATIONS

BASELINE ASSESSMENT

Obtain history of epigastric/abdominal pain. Obtain baseline hepatic/renal function tests.

INTERVENTION/EVALUATION

Monitor serum AST, ALT levels, BUN, creatinine. Assess mental status in elderly. Question present abdominal pain, GI distress.

PATIENT/FAMILY TEACHING

• Smoking decreases effectiveness of medication. • Do not take medicine within 1 hr of magnesium- or aluminum-containing antacids. • Transient burning/pruritus may occur with IV administration. • Report headache. • Avoid alcohol, aspirin.

---

ranolazine

rah-**noe**-la-zeen
(Ranexa)
Do not confuse Ranexa with Celexa.

◆CLASSIFICATION

PHARMACOTHERAPEUTIC: Sodium current inhibitor. **CLINICAL:** Antianginal, anti-ischemic.

ACTION

Thought to elicit changes in cardiac metabolism. Does not reduce heart rate, B/P. **Therapeutic Effect:** Exerts antianginal, anti-ischemic effects on cardiac tissue.

PHARMACOKINETICS

Absorption highly variable. Peak plasma concentration: 2–5 hrs. Rapidly, extensively metabolized in intestine, liver. Protein binding: 62%. Eliminated in urine (75%), feces (25%). **Half-life:** 7 hrs.

USES

Treatment of chronic angina.

PRECAUTIONS

Contraindications: Hepatic cirrhosis, concurrent use of potent **CYP3A inhibitors (rifampin, carbamazepine)** or **inducers (ketoconazole, itraconazole, fluconazole, clarithromycin, erythromycin).** **Cautions:** Renal/hepatic impairment. Preexisting QT prolongation, concurrent use with medications known to cause QT interval prolongation, pts 75 yrs of age or older, history of malignant neoplasms or adenomatous polyps.

⌛ LIFESPAN CONSIDERATIONS

Pregnancy/Lactation: Unknown if drug crosses placenta or is distributed in breast milk. **Pregnancy Category C. Children:** Safety and efficacy not established. **Elderly:** No age-related precautions noted.

INTERACTIONS

DRUG: See contraindications. **Diltiazem, verapamil** may increase serum concentration. May increase concentration of **cyclosporine, digoxin, simvastatin, sirolimus, tacrolimus. Antiarrhythmic agents, dofetilide, quinidine, sotalol, thioridazine, ziprasidone** may increase risk of QT prolongation. **HERBAL: St. John's wort** may decrease concentration/effects. **FOOD: Grapefruit products** may increase plasma concentration, risk of QT prolongation. **LAB VALUES:** May slightly elevate BUN, serum creatinine.

AVAILABILITY (Rx)

🏷 **Tablets (Extended-Release):** 500 mg, 1,000 mg.

ADMINISTRATION/HANDLING

PO

• May give without regard to food. • Do not break, crush, dissolve, or divide extended-release tablets.

INDICATIONS/ROUTES/DOSAGE

Chronic Angina

PO: ADULTS, ELDERLY: Initially, 500 mg twice daily. May increase to 1,000 mg twice daily, based on clinical response. Dose should not exceed 500 mg twice daily when used concurrently with moderate CYP3A inhibitors (e.g., diltiazem, verapamil).

SIDE EFFECTS

Occasional (6%–4%): Dizziness, headache, constipation, nausea. **Rare (2%–1%):** Peripheral edema, abdominal pain, dry mouth, vomiting, tinnitus, vertigo, palpitations.

ADVERSE EFFECTS/
TOXIC REACTIONS

Overdose manifested as confusion, diplopia, dizziness, paresthesia, syncope.

NURSING CONSIDERATIONS

BASELINE ASSESSMENT

Record onset, type (sharp, dull, squeezing), radiation, location, intensity, duration of anginal pain, precipitating factors (exertion, emotional stress). Obtain baseline EKG.

INTERVENTION/EVALUATION

Assist with ambulation if dizziness occurs. Give with food if nausea occurs. Monitor daily pattern of bowel activity, stool consistency. Assess for relief of anginal pain. Monitor EKG, pulse for irregularities.

PATIENT/FAMILY TEACHING

• Avoid grapefruit products. • Do not chew, crush, dissolve, or divide extended-release tablets. • Avoid tasks requiring alertness, motor skills until response to drug is established.

---

rasagiline

ra-**sa**-ji-leen
(Azilect)
Do not confuse Azilect with Aricept.

◆CLASSIFICATION

PHARMACOTHERAPEUTIC: MAOI.
CLINICAL: Antiparkinson agent (see p. 146C).

ACTION

Inhibits monoamine oxidase, an enzyme that plays a major role in catabolism of dopamine. Inhibition of dopamine depletion reduces symptomatic motor deficits of Parkinson's disease. **Therapeutic Effect:** Reduces symptoms of Parkinson's disease, appears to delay disease progression.

PHARMACOKINETICS

Rapidly absorbed following PO administration. Protein binding: 88%–94%. Metabolized in liver. Eliminated in urine (62%), feces (7%). **Half-life:** 1.3–3 hrs.

USES

Treatment of signs/symptoms of Parkinson's disease as initial monotherapy or as adjunct therapy to levodopa.

PRECAUTIONS

Contraindications: Concurrent use with meperidine, methadone, tramadol, dextromethorphan, St. John's wort, other MAOIs (selective or nonselective), cyclobenzaprine. **Cautions:** Hepatic impairment; cardiovascular, cerebrovascular disease, pts with hypotension. Avoid foods high in tyramine.

⧗ LIFESPAN CONSIDERATIONS

Pregnancy/Lactation: Unknown if distributed in breast milk. **Pregnancy Category C. Children:** Safety and efficacy not established. **Elderly:** No age-related precautions noted.

R

INTERACTIONS

DRUG: Amphetamines, other MAOIs (phenelzine, tranylcypromine), sympathomimetics (dopamine, metaraminol, phenylephrine, pseudoephedrine) may cause hypertensive crisis. **Anorexiants (dexfenfluramine, fenfluramine, sibutramine), CNS stimulants (methylphenidate), cyclobenzaprine, dextromethorphan, meperidine, methadone, mirtazapine, serotonin or norepinephrine reuptake inhibitors, sibutramine, tramadol, trazodone, tricyclic antidepressants, venlafaxine** may cause serotonin syndrome. May increase risk of **atomoxetine, bupropion** toxicity. **Ciprofloxacin, entacapone, tolcapone** may increase concentration (reduced dosage recommended). **Levodopa** may cause hypertensive/hypotensive reaction. **HERBAL: Kava kava, SAMe, St. John's wort, valerian** may increase risk of serotonin syndrome, excessive sedation. **FOOD: Caffeine, foods/beverages containing tyramine** may result in hypertensive reaction, hypertensive crisis. **LAB VALUES:** May increase serum alkaline phosphatase, bilirubin, ALT, AST. May cause leukopenia.

AVAILABILITY (Rx)

Tablets: 0.5 mg, 1 mg.

ADMINISTRATION/HANDLING

PO
• Give without regard to food. • Avoid food, beverages containing tyramine (cheese, sour cream, yogurt, pickled herring, liver, canned figs, raisins, bananas, avocados, soy sauce, broad beans, yeast extracts, meats prepared with tenderizers, red wine, beer).

INDICATIONS/ROUTES/DOSAGE

◀**ALERT**▶ When used in combination with levodopa, dosage reduction of levodopa should be considered.

Parkinson's Disease
PO: ADULTS, ELDERLY, MONOTHERAPY: 1 mg once daily.

PO: ADULTS, ELDERLY, ADJUNCTIVE THERAPY WITH LEVODOPA: Initially, 0.5 mg once daily. If therapeutic response is not achieved, dose may be increased to 1 mg once daily.

Mild Hepatic Impairment, Concurrent Use of Ciprofloxacin, Other CYP1A2 Inhibitors
PO: ADULTS, ELDERLY: 0.5 mg once daily.

SIDE EFFECTS

Frequent (14%–12%): Headache, nausea. **Occasional (9%–5%):** Orthostatic hypotension, weight loss, dyspepsia (heartburn, indigestion, epigastric pain), dry mouth, arthralgia, depression, hallucinations, constipation. **Rare (4%–2%):** Fever, vertigo, ecchymosis, rhinitis, neck pain, arthritis, paresthesia.

ADVERSE EFFECTS/ TOXIC REACTIONS

Increase in dyskinesia (impaired voluntary movement), dystonia (impaired muscular tone) occur in 18% of pts, angina occurs in 9%. Gastroenteritis, conjunctivitis occur rarely (3%).

NURSING CONSIDERATIONS

BASELINE ASSESSMENT
Obtain baseline hepatic enzyme levels, blood pressure.

INTERVENTION/EVALUATION
Give with food if nausea occurs. Monitor B/P. Instruct pt to rise from lying to sitting or sitting to standing position slowly to prevent orthostatic hypotension. Assess for clinical reversal of symptoms (improvement of tremor of head/hands at rest, mask-like facial expression, shuffling gait, muscular rigidity). If hallucinations or dyskinesia occur, symptoms may be eliminated if levodopa dosage is reduced. Hallucinations generally are accompanied by confusion and, to a lesser extent, insomnia.

PATIENT/FAMILY TEACHING
• Orthostatic hypotension may occur more frequently during initial therapy.

• Avoid tasks that require alertness, motor skills until response to drug is established. • Hallucinations may occur (more so in the elderly with Parkinson's disease), typically within first 2 wks of therapy. • Avoid foods that contain tyramine (cheese, sour cream, beer, wine, pickled herring, liver, figs, raisins, bananas, avocados, soy sauce, yeast extracts, yogurt, papaya, broad beans, meat tenderizers), excessive amounts of caffeine (coffee, tea, chocolate), OTC preparations for hay fever, colds, weight reduction (may produce significant rise in B/P).

rasburicase

ras-**bur**-i-kase
(Elitek, Fasturtec ✦)

BLACK BOX ALERT Severe hypersensitivity reactions including anaphylaxis reported. May cause severe hemolysis in pts with glucose-6-phosphate dehydrogenase (G6PD) deficiency. Screen pts at high risk for G6PD (African or Mediterranean descent) prior to therapy. Methemoglobinemia has been reported. Blood samples left at room temperature may interfere with uric acid measurements. Must collect blood samples in prechilled tubes containing heparin and immediately immerse in ice water bath. Assay plasma samples within 4 hrs of collection. Elitek enzymatically degrades uric acid in blood samples left at room temperature.

◆CLASSIFICATION

PHARMACOTHERAPEUTIC: Urate-oxidase inhibitor. **CLINICAL:** Antihyperuricemic.

ACTION

Catalyzes enzymatic oxidation of poorly soluble uric acid into soluble, inactive metabolites by converting uric acid into allantoin. Does not inhibit formation of uric acid. **Therapeutic Effect:** Decreases uric acid levels.

PHARMACOKINETICS

Half-life: 16–23 hrs.

USES

Initial management of uric acid levels in pts with leukemia, lymphoma, and solid tumor malignancies who are receiving chemotherapy expected to result in tumor lysis and subsequent elevation of plasma uric acid.

PRECAUTIONS

Contraindications: Prior drug reaction including hypersensitivity reactions, hemolysis, methemoglobinemia, G6PD deficiency. **Cautions:** Pts at high risk for G6PD deficiency (e.g., African, Mediterranean, or Southeast Asian descent).

⧖ LIFESPAN CONSIDERATIONS

Pregnancy/Lactation: Unknown if distributed in breast milk. Unknown if it crosses placenta. May cause fetal harm. **Pregnancy Category C. Children/Elderly:** No age-related precautions noted.

INTERACTIONS

DRUG: None significant. **HERBAL:** None significant. **FOOD:** None known. **LAB VALUES:** May increase serum bilirubin, ALT. May decrease serum phosphate.

AVAILABILITY (Rx)

Injection, Powder for Reconstitution: 1.5 mg/vial, 7.5 mg/vial.

ADMINISTRATION/HANDLING
 IV

Reconstitution • Must use diluent provided in carton. • Reconstitute 1.5-mg vial with 1 ml of diluent or 7.5-mg vial with 5 ml of diluent to provide concentration of 1.5 mg/ml. • Gently swirl to mix. Do not shake. • Inspect for particulate matter or discoloration. • Inject calculated dose into appropriate volume of 0.9% NaCl to achieve a final volume of 100 ml.
Rate of Administration • Infuse over 30 min. • Do not use filter during reconstitution or infusion.

R

Storage • Refrigerate solution until time of use. • Discard after 24 hrs following reconstitution.

🏵 IV INCOMPATIBILITIES

Do not mix with other IV medications.

INDICATIONS/ROUTES/DOSAGE

Management of Hyperuricemia
IV: ADULTS/CHILDREN: 0.2 mg/kg daily up to 5 days.

SIDE EFFECTS

Frequent (50%–46%): Vomiting, fever. **Occasional (27%–13%):** Nausea, headache, abdominal pain, constipation, diarrhea, mucositis, rash.

ADVERSE EFFECTS/ TOXIC REACTIONS

Hypersensitivity reactions occurred in 4.3% of pts including injection irritation, peripheral edema, urticaria, pruritus. Anaphylaxis, hemolysis, methemoglobinemia occurred in less than 1%. Pulmonary hemorrhage, respiratory failure, supraventricular arrhythmias, ischemic coronary artery disorders, sepsis, abdominal, gastrointestinal infections occurred in greater than 2% of pts. Clinical tumor lysis syndrome (TLS), manifested by hyperuricemia, hyperkalemia, hyperphosphatemia, seizure, increased serum creatinine, renal failure reported in 3% of pts. Anti-rasburicase antibodies reported.

NURSING CONSIDERATIONS

BASELINE ASSESSMENT

Obtain CBC, serum chemistries, hepatic function test, serum phosphate, uric acid level; urine pregnancy if applicable. Question for history of prior hypersensitivity reactions. Assess G6PD deficiency risk in potential candidates.

INTERVENTION/EVALUATION

Offer antiemetics to control nausea, vomiting. Monitor CBC, serum chemistries, hepatic function test, serum phosphate. If hypersensitivity reaction occurs, stop infusion and immediately notify physician. Screen for clinical tumor lysis syndrome, hemolysis, methemoglobinemia. Follow strict procedure when collecting uric acid levels. Obtain EKG for chest pain/ tightness, hyperkalemia, dyspnea. Assess skin for rash.

PATIENT/FAMILY TEACHING

• Report any allergic reaction, bronchospasm, chest pain or tightness, cough, difficulty breathing, dizziness, fainting, rash or itching.

regorafenib

re-goe-**raf**-e-nib
(Stivarga)
BLACK BOX ALERT Severe, sometimes fatal, hepatotoxicity reported. Monitor hepatic function prior to and during treatment. Interrupt, reduce, or discontinue therapy if hepatotoxicity or hepatocellular necrosis occurs.

◆CLASSIFICATION

PHARMACOTHERAPEUTIC: Multikinase inhibitor. **CLINICAL:** Antineoplastic.

ACTION

Inhibits tyrosine kinase activity involved with tumor angiogenesis, oncogenesis, and maintenance of tumor microenviroment. **Therapeutic Effect:** Inhibits colorectal tumor cell growth and metastasis.

PHARMACOKINETICS

Readily absorbed following PO administration. Metabolized in liver. Protein binding: 99.5%. Peak plasma concentration: 4 hrs. Excreted in feces (71%), urine (19%). **Half-life:** 28 hrs (Range: 14–58 hrs).

USES

Treatment of metastatic colorectal cancer in pts who have been previously treated with fluoropyrimidine/oxaliplatin/irinotecan-based chemotherapy, anti-VEGF or anti-EGFR therapy. Metastatic GI stromal tumor previously treated with imatinib and sunitinib.

PRECAUTIONS

Contraindications: None known. **Cautions:** Mild to moderate hepatic impairment (not recommended with severe hepatic impairment), hypertension (not recommended with severe or uncontrolled hypertension), recent surgical/dental procedures, chronic open wounds/ulcers, hemoptysis, concomitant warfarin therapy, cardiovascular disease, recent MI.

⧗ LIFESPAN CONSIDERATIONS

Pregnancy/Lactation: May cause fetal harm. Not recommended in nursing mothers. Unknown if distributed in breast milk. Contraception recommended during treatment and up to 2 mos after discontinuation of therapy. **Pregnancy Category D. Children:** Safety and efficacy not established in pts younger than 18 years old. **Elderly:** No age-related precautions noted.

INTERACTIONS

DRUG: Strong **CYP3A4 inducers (e.g., carbamazepine, phenytoin)** may decrease concentration/effects. Strong **CYP3A4 inhibitors (e.g., clurithromycin, ketoconazole)** may increase concentration/effects. **HERBAL: St. John's wort** may decrease concentration/effects. **FOOD: Grapefruit products** may increase concentration/effects. **High-fat meal** may increase absorption/concentration. **LAB VALUES:** May decrease lymphocytes, neutrophils, platelets, serum calcium, phosphorus, potassium, sodium. May increase serum bilirubin, AST, ALT, lipase, amylase, INR, urine protein.

AVAILABILITY (Rx)

⧗ **Tablets:** 40 mg.

ADMINISTRATION/HANDLING

PO

• Take at same time each day with low-fat (less than 30%) breakfast. • Give whole; do not break, crush, dissolve, or divide tablet.

INDICATIONS/ROUTES/DOSAGE

Metastatic Colorectal Cancer, GI Stromal Tumor

PO: ADULTS/ELDERLY: 160 mg once daily for first 21 days, of each 28-day cycle.

Dosage Modification

Symptomatic Hypertension, Toxic Skin Reactions, Severe Side Effects (Grades 3–4)

PO: ADULTS/ELDERLY: Reduce dose to 120 mg once daily. If recovery does not occur within 7 days (despite dose reduction), interrupt treatment for minimum of 7 days and reassess. If recovery does not occur after interruption, reduce dose to 80 mg once daily. Discontinue for intolerance of 80-mg dose, hepatic function tests greater than 20 times upper limit of normal, recovery failure of grades 3–4 side effects, toxic skin reaction.

SIDE EFFECTS

Frequent (64%–26%): Asthenia/fatigue, anorexia, diarrhea, mucositis, weight loss, hypertension, dysphonia, generalized pain, fever, rash. **Occasional (10%–5%):** Headache, alopecia, dysgeusia, musculoskeletal stiffness, dry mouth. **Rare (2% or Less):** Tremor, gastric reflux.

ADVERSE EFFECTS/ TOXIC REACTIONS

May cause GI perforation, GI fistula formation. Hemorrhaging of respiratory, GI, genitourinary tracts reported in 21% of pts. Hypertension (30% of pts) may lead to hypertensive crisis. May cause ineffective wound healing or wound dehiscence requiring medical intervention. Palmarplantar erythrodysesthesia syndrome (PPES), a chemotherapy-induced skin condition that presents with redness, swelling, numbness, skin sloughing of

R

hands, feet (45% of pts). Reversible posterior leukoencephalopathy syndrome (RPLS) reported in less than 1% of pts. May induce cardiac ischemia and/or MI. Severe, sometimes fatal, hepatotoxicity including hepatocellular necrosis reported in less than 1%. Various, unspecified infections reported in 31% of pts (most likely due to neutropenia).

NURSING CONSIDERATIONS

BASELINE ASSESSMENT

Obtain baseline vital signs, CBC with differential, serum chemistries also including magnesium, phosphate, ionized calcium, urinalysis, urine pregnancy, urine protein, hepatic/renal function test, amylase, lipase, PT/INR. Assess recent surgical/dental procedures. Question possibility of pregnancy, current breast-feeding status. Obtain full medication history including vitamins, supplements, herbal products. Question for history of hypertension, hepatic impairment, cardiovascular disease. Assess skin for open/unhealed wounds.

INTERVENTION/EVALUATION

Monitor CBC, electrolytes, urinalysis. Monitor hepatic function tests q2wks for 2 mos, then monthly; or every week if elevated hepatic function tests occur. Persistent diastolic hypertension may indicate hypertensive emergency. Obtain EKG for palpitation, chest pain, hypokalemia, hyperkalemia, hypocalcemia, bradycardia, ventricular arrhythmias. Reverse Posterior Leukoencephalopathy Syndrome (RPLS) should be considered in pts with seizure, headache, visual disturbances, altered mental status, malignant hypertension. Assess hydration status. Encourage PO intake. Immediately report any hemorrhaging, bloody stools, hematuria, abdominal pain, hemoptysis (may indicate GI perforation/fistula formation).

PATIENT/FAMILY TEACHING

• Blood levels will be routinely monitored.
• Avoid pregnancy. Contraception should be practiced during treatment and up to 2 mos after discontinuation. • Report any yellowing of skin or eyes, abdominal pain, bruising, black/tarry stools, dark urine, decreased urine output, skin changes. • Neurological changes including confusion, seizures, vision loss, high blood pressure crisis may indicate RPLS. • Do no take herbal products. • Contact doctor before any planned surgical/dental procedures. • Do not ingest grapefruit products. • Take with low-fat food only. • Drink liquids often if diarrhea occurs (may lead to dehydration). • Immediately report bleeding of any kind. • Swallow tablet whole; do not chew, crush, dissolve, or divide.

---

repaglinide

re-**pag**-li-nide
(GlucoNorm ✦, Prandin)
Do not confuse Prandin with Avandia.

FIXED-COMBINATION(S)

Prandimet: repaglinide/metformin (an antidiabetic): 1 mg/500 mg, 2 mg/500 mg.

◆CLASSIFICATION

PHARMACOTHERAPEUTIC: Antihyperglycemic. **CLINICAL:** Antidiabetic agent (see p. 45C).

ACTION

Stimulates release of insulin from beta cells of pancreas by depolarizing beta cells, leading to opening of calcium channels. Resulting calcium influx induces insulin secretion. **Therapeutic Effect:** Lowers serum glucose concentration.

PHARMACOKINETICS

Rapidly, completely absorbed from GI tract. Protein binding: 98%. Metabolized in liver. Excreted in feces (90%), urine (8%). Unknown if removed by hemodialysis. **Half-life:** 1 hr.

USES

Adjunct to diet and exercise to lower serum glucose in pts with type 2 diabetes mellitus. Used as monotherapy or in combination with metformin, pioglitazone, rosiglitazone.

PRECAUTIONS

Contraindications: Diabetic ketoacidosis, type 1 diabetes mellitus, concurrent gemfibrozil therapy. **Cautions:** Hepatic/renal impairment, elderly, malnourished, adrenal/pituitary dysfunction.

⌛ LIFESPAN CONSIDERATIONS

Pregnancy/Lactation: Unknown if drug is distributed in breast milk. **Pregnancy Category C. Children:** Safety and efficacy not established. **Elderly:** No age-related precautions noted, but hypoglycemia may be more difficult to recognize.

INTERACTIONS

DRUG: CYP3A4 inhibitors (e.g., ketoconazole, erythromycin), CYP2C8 inhibitors (e.g., gemfibrozil) may increase concentration/toxicity. **CYP3A4 inducers (e.g., carbamazepine, rifampin)** may decrease effects. **Beta blockers, NSAIDs** may increase hypoglycemic effect. **HERBAL: St. John's wort** may decrease concentration. **Garlic, ginger, ginseng** may cause hypoglycemia. **FOOD: Food** decreases concentration. **LAB VALUES:** Serum alkaline phosphatase, ALT, AST may be elevated.

AVAILABILITY (Rx)

Tablets: 0.5 mg, 1 mg, 2 mg.

ADMINISTRATION/HANDLING

PO
• Ideally, give within 15 min of a meal but may be given immediately before a meal to as long as 30 min before a meal.

INDICATIONS/ROUTES/DOSAGE

Diabetes Mellitus
PO: ADULTS, ELDERLY: 0.5–4 mg 2–4 times daily. **Maximum:** 16 mg/day.

Dosage in Renal Impairment
Creatinine clearance 20–40 ml/min: Initially, 0.5 mg with meals, titrate carefully.

SIDE EFFECTS

Frequent (10%–6%): Upper respiratory tract infection, headache, rhinitis, bronchitis, back pain. **Occasional (5%–3%):** Diarrhea, dyspepsia (heartburn, indigestion, epigastric pain), sinusitis, nausea, arthralgia, UTI. **Rare (2%):** Constipation, vomiting, paresthesia, allergy.

ADVERSE EFFECTS/TOXIC REACTIONS

Hypoglycemia occurs in 16% of pts. Chest pain occurs rarely.

NURSING CONSIDERATIONS

BASELINE ASSESSMENT

Check fasting serum glucose, glycosylated Hgb A1c levels periodically to determine minimum effective dose.

INTERVENTION/EVALUATION

Monitor fasting serum glucose, glycosylated Hgb A1c levels, food intake. Assess for hypoglycemia (cool/wet skin, tremors, dizziness, anxiety, headache, tachycardia, numbness in mouth, hunger, diplopia), hyperglycemia (polyuria, polyphagia, polydipsia, nausea, vomiting, dim vision, fatigue, deep or rapid breathing). Be alert to conditions that alter glucose requirements (fever, increased activity/stress, surgical procedures). Ensure follow-up instruction if pt, family do not thoroughly understand diabetes management, glucose-testing technique. At least 1 wk should elapse to assess response to drug before new dosage adjustment is made.

PATIENT/FAMILY TEACHING

• Diabetes mellitus requires lifelong control. • Prescribed diet, exercise is principal part of treatment; do not skip, delay meals. • Continue to adhere to dietary instructions, regular exercise program, regular testing of urine or serum glucose. • When taking combination drug

R

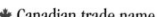

therapy with a sulfonylurea or insulin, have source of glucose available to treat symptoms of low blood sugar.

reteplase **HIGH ALERT**

reh-te-plase
(Retavase)
Do not confuse reteplase or Retavase with Restasis.

◆ CLASSIFICATION

PHARMACOTHERAPEUTIC: Tissue plasminogen activator. **CLINICAL:** Thrombolytic (see p. 34C).

ACTION

Activates fibrinolytic system by directly cleaving plasminogen to generate plasmin, an enzyme that degrades fibrin clot within a thrombus. **Therapeutic Effect:** Exerts thrombolytic action.

PHARMACOKINETICS

Rapidly cleared from plasma. Onset: 30–90 min. Eliminated primarily by liver, kidney. **Half-life:** 13–16 min.

USES

Management of acute myocardial infarction (AMI), improvement of ventricular function following AMI, reduction of incidence of HF, reduction of mortality associated with AMI.

PRECAUTIONS

Contraindications: Active internal bleeding, AV malformation/aneurysm, bleeding diathesis, history of CVA, intracranial neoplasm, recent intracranial/intraspinal surgery or trauma, severe uncontrolled hypertension. **Cautions:** Recent major surgery (coronary artery bypass graft, OB delivery, organ biopsy), cerebrovascular disease, recent GI/GU bleeding, hypertension, mitral stenosis with atrial fibrillation, acute pericarditis, bacterial endocarditis, hepatic/renal impairment, diabetic retinopathy, ophthalmic hemorrhage, septic thrombophlebitis, occluded AV cannula at infected site, advanced age (75 yrs of age or older), pts receiving oral anticoagulants.

⌛ LIFESPAN CONSIDERATIONS

Pregnancy/Lactation: Unknown if drug is distributed in breast milk. **Pregnancy Category C. Children:** Safety and efficacy not established. **Elderly:** More susceptible to bleeding; caution advised.

INTERACTIONS

DRUG: Heparin, platelet aggregation antagonists (e.g., abciximab, aspirin, dipyridamole), warfarin increase risk of bleeding. **HERBAL:** Cat's claw, dong quai, evening primrose, feverfew, garlic, ginger, ginkgo, ginseng, red clover possess antiplatelet action, may increase bleeding. **FOOD:** None known. **LAB VALUES:** May decrease serum fibringen, plasminogen.

AVAILABILITY (Rx)

Injection, Powder for Reconstitution: 10.4 units (18.1 mg) (packaged with Sterile Water for Injection).

ADMINISTRATION/HANDLING
 IV

Reconstitution • Reconstitute only with Sterile Water for Injection immediately before use. Use diluent, syringe, needle, dispensing pin provided with each kit. • Reconstituted solution contains 1 unit/ml. • Do not shake. • Slight foaming may occur; let stand for a few minutes to allow bubbles to dissipate.
Rate of Administration • Give through dedicated IV line. • Administer each IV bolus over 2-min period. • Give second bolus 30 min after first bolus injection. • Do not add other medications to bolus injection solution. • Do not give second bolus if serious bleeding occurs after first IV bolus is given.
Storage • Use within 4 hrs of reconstitution. • Discard any unused portion.

IV INCOMPATIBILITIES

Do not mix with other medications.

INDICATIONS/ROUTES/DOSAGE

Acute MI, HF
IV Bolus: ADULTS, ELDERLY: 10 units over 2 min; repeat in 30 min.

SIDE EFFECTS

Frequent: Bleeding at superficial sites, such as venous injection sites, catheter insertion sites, venous cutdowns, arterial punctures, sites of recent surgical procedures, gingival bleeding.

ADVERSE EFFECTS/ TOXIC REACTIONS

Bleeding at internal sites (intracranial, retroperitoneal, GI, GU, respiratory) occurs occasionally. Lysis of coronary thrombi may produce atrial or ventricular arrhythmias, stroke.

NURSING CONSIDERATIONS

BASELINE ASSESSMENT

Obtain baseline B/P, apical pulse. Evaluate 12-lead EKG, CPK, CPK-MB, serum electrolytes. Assess Hct, platelet count, thrombin time (TT), aPTT, PT, serum plasminogen, fibrinogen levels before therapy is instituted. Type, hold blood.

INTERVENTION/EVALUATION

Carefully monitor all needle puncture sites, catheter insertion sites for bleeding. Observe continuous cardiac monitoring for arrhythmias; monitoring B/P, pulse, respiration is essential until pt is stable. Check peripheral pulses, lung sounds. Monitor for chest pain relief; notify physician of continuation/recurrence of chest pain (note location, type, intensity). Avoid any trauma that may increase risk of bleeding (injections, shaving).

Rho (D) immune globulin

row D im-**myoon glob**-yoo-lin (Hyper-RHO S/D Full Dose, Hyper-RHO S/D Mini Dose, MICRhoGAM UF Plus, RhoGAM UF Plus, Rhophylac, WinRho SDF)

BLACK BOX ALERT May cause intravascular hemolysis in pts treated for idiopathic thrombocytopenic purpura (ITP).

◆CLASSIFICATION

CLINICAL: Immune globulin.

ACTION

Suppresses active antibody response, formation of anti-Rho(D) in Rho(D)-negative women exposed to Rho-positive blood from pregnancy with Rho(D)-positive fetus or transfusion with Rho(D)-positive blood. Injection of Rho(D) immune globulin into Rh-positive pt with ITP coats pt's own D-positive RBCs with antibody; as RBCs are cleared by spleen, they saturate capacity of spleen to clear antibody-coated cells. **Therapeutic Effect:** Prevents antibody response, hemolytic disease of newborn in women who previously conceived Rho(D)-positive fetus. Prevents Rho(D) sensitization in pts who have received Rho(D)-positive blood. Decreases bleeding in pts with ITP.

PHARMACOKINETICS

	Onset	Peak	Duration
ITP (increase platelets)	1–2 days	7–14 days	30 days

Half-life: 21–30 days.

USES

Suppression of Rh isoimmunization: Used in situations when an Rho(D)-negative individual is exposed to Rho(D)-positive blood: delivery of an Rho(D)-positive infant, abortion, amniocentesis, chorionic villus

R

sampling, ruptured tubal pregnancy, abdominal pregnancy, transplacental hemorrhage. Used when the mother is Rh₀(D) negative, the father is either Rh₀(D) positive or Rh₀(D) unknown, the baby is either Rh₀(D) positive or Rh₀(D) unknown. **Transfusion:** Suppression of Rh isoimmunization in Rh₀(D)-negative female children and female adults in their childbearing years transfused with Rh₀(D) antigen-positive RBCs or blood components containing Rh₀(D) antigen-positive RBCs. **Treatment of ITP:** Children with acute or chronic ITP, adults with chronic ITP, children and adults with ITP secondary to HIV infection.

PRECAUTIONS

Contraindications: Hypersensitivity to any component, IgA deficiency, mothers whose Rh group or immune status is uncertain, prior sensitization to Rh₀(D), Rh₀(D)-positive mother or pregnant woman, transfusion of Rh₀(D)-positive blood in previous 3 mos. **Cautions:** Thrombocytopenia, bleeding disorders. Hgb less than 8 g/dl.

⏳ LIFESPAN CONSIDERATIONS

Pregnancy/Lactation: Does not appear to harm fetus. **Pregnancy Category C. Children/Elderly:** No age-related precautions noted.

INTERACTIONS

DRUG: May interfere with pt's immune response to **live virus vaccines. HERBAL:** None significant. **FOOD:** None known. **LAB VALUES:** None significant.

AVAILABILITY (Rx)

Injection Solution: (Hyper-RHO): 50 mcg, 300 mcg. (MICRhoGAM UF Plus): 50 mcg. (RhoGAM UF Plus): 300 mcg. (Rhophylac): 300 mcg/2 ml. (WinRho SDF): 120 mcg/0.5 ml, 300 mcg/1.3 ml, 500 mcg/2.2 ml, 1,000 mcg/4.4 ml, 3,000 mcg/13 ml.

ADMINISTRATION/HANDLING

IM
• Administer into deltoid muscle of upper arm, anterolateral aspect of upper thigh.

INDICATIONS/ROUTES/DOSAGE

Idiopathic Thrombocytopenic Purpura (ITP)
IV (WinRho SDF): ADULTS, ELDERLY, CHILDREN: Initially, 50 mcg/kg as single dose (reduce to 25–40 mcg/kg if Hgb is less than 10 g/dl). **Maintenance:** 25–60 mcg/kg based on platelet count and Hgb level. **(Rhophylac):** 50 mcg/kg.

Suppression of Active Antibody Response in Pregnancy
IM (Hyper-RHO Full Dose, RhoGAM UF Plus): ADULTS: 300 mcg preferably within 72 hrs of delivery.
IV, IM (WinRho SDF): ADULTS: 300 mcg at 28 wks' gestation. After delivery: 120 mcg preferably within 72 hrs.

Suppression of Active Antibody Response in Threatened Abortion
IM (Hyper-RHO Full Dose, RhoGAM UF Plus): ADULTS: 300 mcg as soon as possible.

Suppression of Active Antibody Response in Abortion, Miscarriage, Termination of Ectopic Pregnancy
IM (Hyper-RHO, RhoGAM UF Plus): ADULTS: 300 mcg if more than 13 wks' gestation, 50 mcg if less than 13 wks' gestation.
IV, IM (WinRho SDF): ADULTS: 120 mcg after 34 wks' gestation.

Transfusion Incompatibility
◀**ALERT**▶ Must give within 72 hrs after exposure to incompatible blood transfusion, massive fetal hemorrhage. Dose is calculated based on exposure to Rh₀(D)-positive whole blood or red blood cells.
IV: ADULTS: 3,000 units (600 mcg) q8h until total dose given.
IM: ADULTS: 6,000 units (1,200 mcg) q12h until total dose given.

SIDE EFFECTS

Hypotension, pallor, vasodilation (IV formulation), fever, headache, chills, dizziness, drowsiness, lethargy, rash, pruritus, abdominal pain, diarrhea, discomfort/swelling at injection site, back pain, myalgia, arthralgia, asthenia (loss of strength, energy).

ADVERSE EFFECTS/ TOXIC REACTIONS

Acute renal failure occurs rarely.

NURSING CONSIDERATIONS

BASELINE ASSESSMENT

Determine existence of bleeding disorders. Assess pt's Hgb level; give drug cautiously to pts with Hgb level less than 8 g/dl.

INTERVENTION/EVALUATION

Monitor CBC (esp. Hgb, platelet count), BUN, serum creatinine, reticulocyte count, urinalysis results. Assess for signs/symptoms of hemolysis.

PATIENT/FAMILY TEACHING

• IM injection may be painful. • Notify physician if chills, dizziness, fever, headache, rash occur.

---

ribavirin

rye-ba-**vye**-rin
(Copegus, Rebetol, Ribasphere, Virazole)

BLACK BOX ALERT Pregnancy Category X. Significant teratogenic/embryocidal effects. Hemolytic anemia is significant toxicity, usually occurring within 1–2 wks. May worsen cardiac disease and lead to fatal or nonfatal MI. May interfere with safe and effective assisted ventilation.

Do not confuse ribavirin with riboflavin, rifampin, or Robaxin.

FIXED-COMBINATION(S)

With interferon alfa 2b (**Rebetron**). Individually packaged.

◆CLASSIFICATION

PHARMACOTHERAPEUTIC: Synthetic nucleoside. **CLINICAL:** Antiviral (see p. 71C).

ACTION

Inhibits replication of viral RNA, DNA, influenza virus RNA polymerase activity, interferes with expression of messenger RNA. **Therapeutic Effect:** Inhibits viral protein synthesis.

USES

Inhalation: Treatment of respiratory syncytial virus (RSV) infections (esp. in pts with underlying compromising conditions such as chronic lung disorders, congenital heart disease, recent transplant recipients). **Capsule/tablet/oral solution:** Treatment of chronic hepatitis C in pts with compensated hepatic disease. **OFF-LABEL:** Treatment of influenza A or B, West Nile virus. **Inhalation:** Treatment for respiratory syncytial virus (RSV) in adult hematopoietic stem cell or heart/lung transplant recipients.

PRECAUTIONS

Contraindications: Autoimmune hepatitis, creatinine clearance less than 50 ml/min, hemoglobinopathies (e.g., sickle cell anemia), hepatic decompensation, hypersensitivity to ribavirin products, men whose female partner is pregnant, women of childbearing age who do not use contraception reliably, pancreatitis, pregnancy, significant or unstable cardiac disease, concomitant use of didanosine. **Cautions: Inhalation:** Pts requiring assisted ventilation, COPD, asthma. **PO:** Cardiac or pulmonary disease, elderly, history of psychiatric disorders, renal impairment, pts with sarcoidosis. **Pregnancy Category X.**

INTERACTIONS

DRUG: Didanosine may increase risk of pancreatitis, peripheral neuropathy. May decrease effects of **didanosine. Nucleoside analogues (e.g., adefovir, didanosine, lamivudine, stavudine, zalcitabine, zidovudine)** may increase risk of lactic acidosis. **HERBAL:** None significant. **FOOD:** None known. **LAB VALUES:** None significant.

R

AVAILABILITY (Rx)

Capsules (Rebetol, Ribasphere): 200 mg. Powder for Aerosol (Virazole): 6 g. Powder for Solution, Nebulization (Virazole): 6 g. Solution, Oral (Rebetol): 40 mg/ml. Tablet (Copegus): 200 mg. (Ribasphere): 200 mg, 400 mg, 600 mg.

ADMINISTRATION/HANDLING

PO

• Capsules may be taken without regard to food. • Do not break, crush, open, or divide capsules. • Use oral solution in children 5 yrs or younger, those 25 kg or less, or those unable to swallow. • Give capsules with food when combined with peginterferon alfa-2b. • Tablets should be given with food.

Inhalation

◄ALERT► May be given via nasal or oral inhalation.
• Solution appears clear, colorless; is stable for 24 hrs at room temperature. • Discard solution for nebulization after 24 hrs. • Discard if discolored or cloudy. • Add 50–100 ml Sterile Water for Injection or Inhalation to 6-g vial. • Transfer to a flask, serving as reservoir for aerosol generator. • Further dilute to final volume of 300 ml, giving solution concentration of 20 mg/ml. • Use only aerosol generator available from manufacturer of drug. • Do not give concomitantly with other drug solutions for nebulization. • Discard reservoir solution when fluid levels are low and at least q24h. • Controversy exists over safety in ventilator-dependent pts; only experienced personnel should administer drug.

INDICATIONS/ROUTES/DOSAGE

Chronic Hepatitis C

PO (Capsule Combination with Interferon ALFA-2B): ADULTS, ELDERLY: 1,000–1,200 mg/day in 2 divided doses. CHILDREN WEIGHING 61 KG OR MORE: Use adult dosage. CHILDREN WEIGHING 50–60 KG: 400 mg twice a day. CHILDREN WEIGHING 37–49 KG: 200 mg in morning, 400 mg in evening. CHILDREN WEIGHING 24–36 KG: 200 mg twice a day.

PO (Capsules in Combination with Peginterferon ALFA-2B): ADULTS, ELDERLY: 800 mg/day (with food) in 2 divided doses.
PO (Tablets in Combination With Peginterferon ALFA-2B): ADULTS, ELDERLY: 800–1,200 mg/day in 2 divided doses.

Severe Lower Respiratory Tract Infection Caused by Respiratory Syncytial Virus (RSV)

Inhalation: CHILDREN, INFANTS: Use with Viratek small-particle aerosol generator at concentration of 20 mg/ml (6 g reconstituted with 300 ml Sterile Water for Injection) over 12–18 hrs/day for 3–7 days.

SIDE EFFECTS

Frequent (greater than 10%): Dizziness, headache, fatigue, fever, insomnia, irritability, depression, emotional lability, impaired concentration, alopecia, rash, pruritus, nausea, anorexia, dyspepsia, vomiting, decreased hemoglobin, hemolysis, arthralgia, musculoskeletal pain, dyspnea, sinusitis, flu-like symptoms. Occasional (10%–1%): Nervousness, altered taste, weakness.

ADVERSE EFFECTS/ TOXIC REACTIONS

Cardiac arrest, apnea, ventilator dependence, bacterial pneumonia, pneumonia, pneumothorax occur rarely. If treatment exceeds 7 days, anemia may occur.

NURSING CONSIDERATIONS

BASELINE ASSESSMENT

Obtain sputum specimens before giving first dose or at least during first 24 hrs of therapy. Assess respiratory status for baseline. PO: Obtain CBC with differential, pretreatment and monthly pregnancy test for women of childbearing age.

INTERVENTION/EVALUATION

Monitor Hgb, Hct, platelets, hepatic function tests, I&O, fluid balance carefully. Check hematology reports for anemia due to reticulocytosis when therapy exceeds 7 days. For ventilator-assisted pts,

R

watch for "rainout" in tubing and empty frequently; be alert to impaired ventilation/gas exchange due to drug precipitate. Assess skin for rash. Monitor B/P, respirations; assess lung sounds.

PATIENT/FAMILY TEACHING

• Report immediately any difficulty breathing, itching/swelling/redness of eyes, severe abdominal pain, bloody diarrhea, unusual bleeding/bruising. • Female pts should take measures to avoid pregnancy. • Male pts must use condoms during sexual activity.

rifabutin

rif-a-**bue**-tin
(Mycobutin)
Do not confuse rifabutin with rifampin.

◆CLASSIFICATION

PHARMACOTHERAPEUTIC: Antitubercular. **CLINICAL:** Antibacterial (antimycobacterial).

ACTION

Inhibits DNA-dependent RNA polymerase, an enzyme in susceptible strains of *Escherichia coli, Bacillus subtilis.* Broad-spectrum activity, including mycobacteria such as *Mycobacterium avium* complex (MAC). **Therapeutic Effect:** Prevents MAC disease.

PHARMACOKINETICS

Readily absorbed from GI tract. Protein binding: 85%. Widely distributed. Crosses blood-brain barrier. Extensive intracellular tissue uptake. Metabolized in liver. Excreted in urine; eliminated in feces. Unknown if removed by hemodialysis. **Half-life:** 16–69 hrs.

USES

Prevention of disseminated *Mycobacterium avium* complex (MAC) disease in those with advanced HIV infection. **OFF-LABEL:** Part of multidrug regimen for treatment of MAC. Prophylaxis for latent tuberculosis infection, part of multidrug regimen for treatment of active tuberculosis infection.

PRECAUTIONS

Contraindications: Hypersensitivity to other rifamycins (e.g., rifampin). **Cautions:** Renal/hepatic impairment.

⌛ LIFESPAN CONSIDERATIONS

Pregnancy/Lactation: Unknown if drug crosses placenta or is distributed in breast milk. **Pregnancy Category B. Children/Elderly:** No age-related precautions noted.

INTERACTIONS

DRUG: May decrease effectiveness of **oral contraceptives, clarithromycin, itraconazole.** May decrease concentration/effects of **non-nucleoside reverse transcriptase inhibitors (e.g., delavirdine, efavirenz, nevirapine), protease inhibitors (e.g., amprenavir, indinavir, ritonavir, saquinavir).** **HERBAL:** None significant. **FOOD:** **High-fat meals** may delay absorption. **LAB VALUES:** May increase serum alkaline phosphatase, AST, ALT.

AVAILABILITY (Rx)

Capsules: 150 mg.

ADMINISTRATION/HANDLING

PO

• Give without regard to food. Give with food if GI irritation occurs. • May mix with applesauce if pt is unable to swallow capsules whole.

INDICATIONS/ROUTES/DOSAGE

Prophylaxis of MAC Disease

PO: ADULTS, ELDERLY, CHILDREN 6 YRS AND OLDER: 300 mg once daily or 150 mg twice daily to reduce GI upset.

Concurrent use with efavirenz (no concomitant protease inhibitor), indinavir, nelfinavir: 150 mg/day when given

 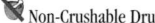

concurrently with nelfinavir or indinavir; 450–600 mg/day or 600 mg 3 times/wk when given concurrently with efavirenz.

Prevention of MAC
PO: ADULTS, ELDERLY: 300 mg once daily or 150 mg twice daily to reduce gastrointestinal upset. **Concurrent use of nelfinavir or indinavir:** 150 mg/day or 300 mg twice a wk. **Concurrent use of efavirenz:** 450–600 mg/day or 600 mg 3 times/wk. **CHILDREN, INFANTS:** 5 mg/kg once daily. **Maximum:** 300 mg once daily.

Dosage in Renal Impairment
Dosage is modified based on creatinine clearance. If creatinine clearance is less than 30 ml/min, reduce dosage by 50%.

SIDE EFFECTS

Frequent (30%): Red-orange or red-brown discoloration of urine, feces, saliva, skin, sputum, sweat, tears. **Occasional (11%–3%):** Rash, nausea, abdominal pain, diarrhea, dyspepsia, belching, headache, altered taste, uveitis, corneal deposits. **Rare (Less Than 2%):** Anorexia, flatulence, fever, myalgia, vomiting, insomnia.

ADVERSE EFFECTS/ TOXIC REACTIONS

Hepatitis, anemia, thrombocytopenia, neutropenia occur rarely.

NURSING CONSIDERATIONS

BASELINE ASSESSMENT
Obtain chest X-ray; sputum, blood cultures. Biopsy of suspicious node(s) must be done to rule out active tuberculosis. Obtain baseline CBC, serum hepatic function tests.

INTERVENTION/EVALUATION
Monitor serum hepatic function tests, platelet count, Hgb, Hct. Avoid IM injections, rectal temperatures, other trauma that may induce bleeding. Check temperature; notify physician of flu-like syndrome, rash, GI intolerance.

PATIENT/FAMILY TEACHING
• Urine, feces, saliva, sputum, perspiration, tears, skin may be discolored brown-orange. • Soft contact lenses may be permanently discolored. • Rifabutin may decrease efficacy of oral contraceptives; nonhormonal methods should be considered. • Avoid crowds, those with infection. • Report flu-like symptoms, nausea, vomiting, dark urine, unusual bruising/bleeding from any site, any visual disturbances.

rifampin

rif-**am**-pin
(Rifadin, Rofact ✦)
Do not confuse Rifadin with Rifater or Ritalin, or rifampin with ribavirin, rifabutin, Rifamate, rifapentine, rifaximin, or Ritalin.

FIXED-COMBINATION(S)

Rifamate: rifampin/isoniazid (an antitubercular): 300 mg/150 mg. **Rifater:** rifampin/isoniazid/pyrazinamide (an antitubercular): 120 mg/50 mg/300 mg.

◆CLASSIFICATION

PHARMACOTHERAPEUTIC: Semisynthetic agent. **CLINICAL:** Antibiotic, antitubercular, miscellaneous.

ACTION

Interferes with bacterial RNA synthesis by binding to DNA-dependent RNA polymerase, preventing attachment to DNA, thereby blocking RNA transcription. **Therapeutic Effect:** Bactericidal in susceptible microorganisms.

PHARMACOKINETICS

Well absorbed from GI tract (food delays absorption). Protein binding: 80%. Widely distributed. Metabolized in liver. Primarily eliminated by biliary system. Not removed by hemodialysis. **Half-life:**

3–5 hrs (increased in hepatic impairment).

USES

In conjunction with other antitubercular agents for initial treatment, re-treatment of active tuberculosis. Eliminates meningococci from nasopharynx of asymptomatic carriers. **OFF-LABEL:** Prophylaxis of *H. influenzae* type b infection, *Legionella* pneumonia, serious infections caused by *Staphylococcus* spp. (in combination with other agents).

PRECAUTIONS

Contraindications: Concomitant therapy with amprenavir, saquinavir, ritonavir; hypersensitivity to other rifamycins. **Cautions:** Hepatic impairment, active or treated alcoholism, porphyria. Concurrent medications associated with hepatotoxicity.

⧖ LIFESPAN CONSIDERATIONS

Pregnancy/Lactation: Crosses placenta. Distributed in breast milk. **Pregnancy Category C. Children/Elderly:** No age-related precautions noted.

INTERACTIONS

DRUG: Alcohol, hepatotoxic medications, ritonavir, saquinavir may increase risk of hepatotoxicity. May decrease effects of **digoxin, disopyramide, fluconazole, methadone, mexiletine, oral anticoagulants, oral antidiabetics, oral contraceptives, tacrolimus, tricyclic antidepressants, phenytoin, quinidine, tocainide, verapamil. HERBAL: St. John's wort** may decrease concentration. **FOOD: Food** decreases extent of absorption. **LAB VALUES:** May increase serum alkaline phosphatase, bilirubin, uric acid, AST, ALT.

AVAILABILITY (Rx)

Capsules (Rifadin): 150 mg, 300 mg. Injection, Powder for Reconstitution: 600 mg.

ADMINISTRATION/HANDLING

IV

Reconstitution • Reconstitute 600-mg vial with 10 ml Sterile Water for Injection

to provide concentration of 60 mg/ml. • Withdraw desired dose and further dilute with 0.9% NaCl or D₅W to concentration not to exceed 6 mg/ml.
Rate of Administration • For IV infusion only. Avoid IM, subcutaneous administration. • Avoid extravasation (local irritation, inflammation). • Infuse over 30 min to 3 hrs.
Storage • Reconstituted vial is stable for 24 hrs. • Once reconstituted vial is further diluted, it is stable for 4 hrs in D₅W or 24 hrs in 0.9% NaCl.

PO

• Preferably give 1 hr before or 2 hrs following meals with 8 oz of water (may give with food to decrease GI upset; will delay absorption). • For those unable to swallow capsules, contents may be mixed with applesauce, jelly. • Administer at least 1 hr before antacids, esp. those containing aluminum.

▦ IV INCOMPATIBILITY

Diltiazem (Cardizem).

▦ IV COMPATIBILITY

D₅W if infused within 4 hrs (risk of precipitation beyond this time period).

INDICATIONS/ROUTES/DOSAGE

Usual Dosage Range
ADULTS, ELDERLY: 600 mg once or twice daily. **CHILDREN, INFANTS:** 10–20 mg/kg/day in 1 or 2 divided doses. **Maximum:** 600 mg/day.

Tuberculosis (ACTIVE)
Note: A four-drug regimen is preferred for initial, empiric treatment.
PO, IV: ADULTS, ELDERLY: 10 mg/kg/day. **Maximum:** 600 mg/day. **CHILDREN:** 10–20 mg/kg/day in divided doses q12–24h. **Maximum:** 600 mg/day.

Prevention of Meningococcal Infections
PO, IV: ADULTS, ELDERLY: 600 mg q12h for 2 days. **CHILDREN 1 MO AND OLDER:** 20 mg/kg/day in divided doses q12–24h for 2 days. **Maximum:** 600 mg/dose. **IN-**

FANTS YOUNGER THAN 1 MO: 10 mg/kg/day in divided doses q12h for 2 days.

**Staphylococcal Infections
(Nasal Carriers)**
Note: Must be used with at least one other antistaphylococcal antibiotic.
PO, IV: ADULTS, ELDERLY: 600 mg once daily for 5–10 days. **CHILDREN:** 15 mg/kg/day in divided doses q12h for 5–10 days.

Staphylococcus Aureus Infections (in Combination with Other Anti-Infectives)
PO: ADULTS, ELDERLY: 600 mg once daily or 300–450 mg q12h. **NEONATES:** 5–20 mg/kg/day in divided doses q12h.

H. Influenzae Prophylaxis
PO: ADULTS, ELDERLY: 600 mg/day for 4 days. **CHILDREN 1 MO AND OLDER:** 20 mg/kg/day q24h for 4 days. **Maximum:** 600 mg. **CHILDREN YOUNGER THAN 1 MO:** 10 mg/kg/day q24h for 4 days.

SIDE EFFECTS

Frequent: Red-orange or red-brown discoloration of urine, feces, saliva, skin, sputum, sweat, tears. **Occasional (5%–3%):** Hypersensitivity reaction (flushing, pruritus, rash). **Rare (2%–1%):** Diarrhea, dyspepsia, nausea, oral candida (sore mouth, tongue).

ADVERSE EFFECTS/ TOXIC REACTIONS

Hepatotoxicity (risk is increased when rifampin is taken with isoniazid), hepatitis, blood dyscrasias, Stevens-Johnson syndrome, antibiotic-associated colitis occur rarely.

NURSING CONSIDERATIONS

BASELINE ASSESSMENT

Question for hypersensitivity to rifampin, rifamycins. Ensure collection of diagnostic specimens. Evaluate initial serum hepatic/renal function, CBC results.

INTERVENTION/EVALUATION

Assess IV site at least hourly during infusion; restart at another site at the first sign of irritation or inflammation. Monitor hepatic function tests, assess for hepatitis: jaundice, anorexia, nausea, vomiting, fatigue, weakness (hold rifampin, inform physician at once). Report hypersensitivity reactions promptly: any type of skin eruption, pruritus, flu-like syndrome with high dosage. Monitor daily pattern of bowel activity, stool consistency (potential for antibiotic-associated colitis). Monitor CBC results for blood dyscrasias, be alert for infection (fever, sore throat), unusual bruising/bleeding, unusual fatigue/weakness.

PATIENT/FAMILY TEACHING

• Preferably take on empty stomach with 8 oz of water 1 hr before or 2 hrs after meal (with food if GI upset). • Avoid alcohol. • Do not take **any** other medications without consulting physician, including antacids; must take rifampin at least 1 hr before antacid. • Urine, feces, sputum, sweat, tears may become red-orange; soft contact lenses may be permanently stained. • Notify physician of **any** new symptom, immediately for yellow eyes/skin, fatigue, weakness, nausea/vomiting, sore throat, fever, flu, unusual bruising/bleeding. • If taking oral contraceptives, check with physician (reliability may be affected).

rifaximin

rif-**ax**-i-min
(Xifaxan)
Do not confuse rifaximin with rifampin.

◆CLASSIFICATION

PHARMACOTHERAPEUTIC: Anti-infective. **CLINICAL:** Site-specific antibiotic.

ACTION

Inhibits bacterial RNA synthesis by binding to a subunit of bacterial DNA-dependent RNA polymerase. **Therapeutic Effect:** Bactericidal.

PHARMACOKINETICS

Less than 0.4% absorbed after PO administration. Primarily eliminated in feces; minimal excretion in urine. **Half-life:** 5.85 hrs.

USES

Treatment of traveler's diarrhea caused by noninvasive strains of *E. coli*. Reduction of risk for recurrence of overt hepatic encephalopathy. **OFF-LABEL:** Treatment of hepatic encephalopathy. Treatment of *C. difficile*–associated diarrhea.

PRECAUTIONS

Contraindications: Hypersensitivity to other rifamycin antibiotics. **Cautions:** Severe hepatic impairment.

⏳ LIFESPAN CONSIDERATIONS

Pregnancy/Lactation: Unknown if drug is distributed in breast milk. **Pregnancy Category C. Children:** Safety and efficacy not established in those younger than 12 yrs. **Elderly:** No age-related precautions noted.

INTERACTIONS

DRUG: None significant. **HERBAL:** None significant. **FOOD:** None known. **LAB VALUES:** None significant.

AVAILABILITY (Rx)

⚑ **Tablets:** 200 mg, 550 mg.

ADMINISTRATION/HANDLING

PO
• Give without regard to food. • Store at room temperature. • Do not break, crush, dissolve, or divide film-coated tablets.

INDICATIONS/ROUTES/DOSAGE

Traveler's Diarrhea
PO: ADULTS, ELDERLY, CHILDREN 12 YRS AND OLDER: 200 mg 3 times daily for 3 days.

Hepatic Encephalopathy
PO: ADULTS, ELDERLY: 550 mg 2 times a day.

SIDE EFFECTS

Occasional (11%–5%): Flatulence, headache, abdominal discomfort, rectal tenesmus, defecation urgency, nausea. **Rare (4%–2%):** Constipation, fever, vomiting.

ADVERSE EFFECTS/ TOXIC REACTIONS

Hypersensitivity reaction, superinfection occur rarely.

NURSING CONSIDERATIONS

BASELINE ASSESSMENT

Check baseline hydration status: skin turgor, mucous membranes for dryness, urinary status. Assess stool frequency, consistency.

INTERVENTION/EVALUATION

Encourage adequate fluid intake. Assess bowel sounds for peristalsis. Monitor daily pattern of bowel activity, stool consistency. Assess for GI disturbances, blood in stool.

PATIENT/FAMILY TEACHING

• Report if diarrhea worsens or if blood occurs in stool, fever develops within 48 hrs.

---

rilpivirine

ril-pi-**vir**-een
(Edurant)
Do not confuse rilpivirine with delavirdine, etravirine, or nevirapine.

FIXED-COMBINATION(S)

Complera: rilpivirine/emtricitabine (an antiretroviral)/tenofovir (an antiretroviral): 25 mg/200 mg/300 mg.

◆CLASSIFICATION

PHARMACOTHERAPEUTIC: Non-nucleoside reverse transcriptase inhibitor. **CLINICAL:** Antiretroviral (see p. 119C).

R

ACTION

Inhibits HIV-1 replication by noncompetitive inhibition of HIV-1 reverse transcriptase (RT). **Therapeutic Effect:** Interferes with HIV replication, slowing progression of HIV infection.

PHARMACOKINETICS

Readily absorbed after PO administration. Peak concentration: 4–5 hrs. Protein binding: 99.7%. Metabolized in liver. Excreted primarily in feces. **Half-life: 50 hrs.**

USES

Used in combination with at least two other antiretroviral agents for treatment of HIV-1 infection.

PRECAUTIONS

Contraindications: Concurrent use of carbamazepine, dexamethasone (greater than 1 dose), oxcarbazine, phenobarbital, phenytoin, proton pump inhibitors (see drug classification), rifabutin, rifampin, rifapentine, St. John's wort. **Cautions:** Severe depressive disorders, medications that increase risk of prolongation of QT interval (torsades de pointes).

⚥ LIFESPAN CONSIDERATIONS

Pregnancy/Lactation: Unknown if distributed in breast milk. HIV-infected mothers should not breastfeed infants due to risk of postnatal HIV transmission. **Pregnancy Category B. Children:** Safety and efficacy not established. **Elderly:** Caution due to higher risk of impaired renal/hepatic function.

INTERACTIONS

DRUG: CYP3A4 inducers (e.g., carbamazepine, oxcarbazepine, phenobarbital, phenytoin, proton pump inhibitors, rifabutin, rifampin, rifapentine) may significantly decrease effectiveness. **Antacids, H$_2$-receptor antagonists** may decrease plasma concentration. **CYP3A4 inhibitors (e.g., azole antifungal agents, macrolide antibiotics, protease inhibitors)** may

increase plasma concentration. **HERBAL: St. John's wort** may decrease concentration/effects. **FOOD: Grapefruit products** may increase potential for torsades de pointes. **LAB VALUES:** May increase serum creatinine, AST, ALT, bilirubin, cholesterol, triglycerides.

AVAILABILITY (Rx)

Tablets: 25 mg.

ADMINISTRATION/HANDLING

PO

• Give with a meal. Administer antacids 2 hrs before or 4 hrs after rilpivirine; H$_2$-receptor antagonist 12 hrs before or 4 hrs after rilpivirine.

INDICATIONS/ROUTES/DOSAGE

HIV Infection (in Combination with Other Antiretrovirals)
PO: ADULTS: 25 mg once daily with a meal.

SIDE EFFECTS

Occasional (3%): Headache, insomnia, rash. **Rare (1%):** Nausea, vomiting, abdominal pain, fatigue, dizziness, abnormal dreams.

ADVERSE EFFECTS/ TOXIC REACTIONS

Psychiatric disorders including depression, dysphoria, altered mood, suicidal ideation reported in 3% of pts. May prolong QT interval. May develop redistribution/accumulation of body fat (lipodystrophy) or immune reconstitution syndrome.

NURSING CONSIDERATIONS

BASELINE ASSESSMENT

Obtain CBC, serum chemistries, hepatic function test, lipid panel, CD4 count, viral load. Receive full medication history including herbal products. Question for history of prolonged QT interval, torsade de pointes, psychiatric disorder.

INTERVENTION/EVALUATION

Closely monitor for evidence of rash. Monitor lab tests, renal/hepatic function.

PATIENT/FAMILY TEACHING

• Offer emotional support. • Take with food (optimizes absorption). • Report any signs of depression, thoughts of suicide, decreased urine output, abdominal pain, yellowing of skin, darkened urine, clay-colored stools, chest tightness, difficulty breathing, palpitations. • Report any newly prescribed medications. • Rilpivirine does not cure HIV infection nor reduce risk of transmission to others. • Continue to practice safe sex with barrier methods or practice abstinence.

rimantadine

rye-**man**-ta-deen
(Flumadine)
Do not confuse Flumadine with fludarabine, flunisolide, or flutamide, or rimantadine with ranitidine or amantadine.

◆CLASSIFICATION

PHARMACOTHERAPEUTIC: Adamantane antiviral. **CLINICAL:** Antiviral agent.

ACTION

Exerts inhibitory effect early in viral replication cycle. May inhibit uncoating of virus. **Therapeutic Effect:** Prevents replication of influenza A virus.

PHARMACOKINETICS

Well absorbed following PO administration. Protein binding: 40%. Metabolized in liver. Excreted in urine. **Half-life:** 19–36 hrs.

USES

Adults: Prophylaxis, treatment of illness due to influenza A virus. **Children older than 1 yr:** Prophylaxis against influenza A virus.

PRECAUTIONS

Contraindications: Hypersensitivity to amantadine. **Cautions:** Hepatic disease, seizures, history of recurrent eczematoid dermatitis, uncontrolled psychosis, renal impairment, concomitant use of CNS stimulant medications, epilepsy.

⌛ LIFESPAN CONSIDERATIONS

Pregnancy/Lactation: Unknown if drug crosses placenta or is distributed in breast milk. **Pregnancy Category C. Children:** Safety and efficacy not established in infants. **Elderly:** May be more susceptible to CNS side effects.

INTERACTIONS

DRUG: Acetaminophen, aspirin may decrease concentration. **HERBAL:** None significant. **FOOD:** None known. **LAB VALUES:** None significant.

AVAILABILITY (Rx)

Tablets: 100 mg.

ADMINISTRATION/HANDLING

PO
• Give without regard to food.

INDICATIONS/ROUTES/DOSAGE

Treatment of Influenza A Virus
PO: ADULTS: 100 mg twice a day. **ELDERLY, DEBILITATED PTS, PTS WITH SEVERE HEPATIC/RENAL IMPAIRMENT:** 100 mg once a day.

Prevention of Influenza A Virus
PO: ADULTS, CHILDREN 10 YRS AND OLDER AND GREATER THAN 40 KG: 100 mg twice a day. **CHILDREN 10 YRS AND OLDER AND LESS THAN 40 KG:** 5 mg/kg/day in 2 divided doses. **CHILDREN YOUNGER THAN 10 YRS:** 5 mg/kg/day in 1 or 2 doses per day. **Maximum:** 150 mg.

SIDE EFFECTS

Occasional (3%–2%): Insomnia, nausea, nervousness, impaired concentration, dizziness. **Rare (Less Than 2%):** Vomiting, anorexia, dry mouth, abdominal pain, asthenia (loss of strength, energy), fatigue.

ADVERSE EFFECTS/
TOXIC REACTIONS

None known.

R

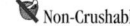

NURSING CONSIDERATIONS

INTERVENTION/EVALUATION

Assess for anxiety, nervousness; evaluate sleep pattern for insomnia. Provide assistance if dizziness occurs.

PATIENT/FAMILY TEACHING

• Avoid contact with those who are at high risk for influenza A (rimantadine-resistant virus may be shed during therapy). • Avoid tasks that require alertness, motor skills until response to drug is established. • Do not take aspirin, acetaminophen, compounds containing these drugs. May cause dry mouth.

---

riociguat

rye-oh-**sig**-ue-at
(Adempas)

BLACK BOX ALERT Do not administer during pregnancy. May cause fetal harm. Exclude pregnancy before and during treatment and at least 1 mo after discontinuation. Must use reliable form of birth control during therapy. Treatment for female pts is only available through restricted program called ADEMPAS Risk Evaluation and Mitigation Strategy (REMS).

◆CLASSIFICATION

PHARMACOTHERAPEUTIC: Soluble guanylate cyclase (sGC) stimulator. **CLINICAL:** Pulmonary vasodilator.

ACTION

Stimulates sGC, an enzyme in cardiopulmonary system and receptor for nitric oxide (NO). When sGC and NO bind, the enzyme catalyzes synthesis of cyclic guanosine monophosphate (cGMP), which is important in regulating vascular tone, proliferation, fibrosis, and inflammation. **Therapeutic Effect:** Produces vasodilation, improves exercise ability, slows clinical worsening of pulmonary arterial hypertension (PAH).

PHARMACOKINETICS

Readily absorbed following PO administration. Metabolized in liver. Protein binding: 95%. Peak plasma concentration: 1.5 hrs. Excreted in feces (53%), urine (40%). **Half-life:** 7–12 hrs.

USES

Treatment of adults with persistent/recurrent chronic thromboembolic pulmonary hypertension (CTEPH) World Health Organization group IV after surgical treatment or inoperable CTEPH to improve exercise capability and WHO functional class; or pulmonary arterial hypertension (PAH) (WHO group I) to improve exercise capability, improve WHO functional class, and delay clinical worsening.

PRECAUTIONS

Contraindications: Pregnancy (Category X). Concomitant use of aminophylline, nitrates or nitric oxide donors, phosphodiesterase (PDE) inhibitors. **Cautions:** Pulmonary edema with pulmonary veno-occlusive disease, anemia, autonomic dysfunction, baseline hypotension, HF, coronary artery disease (CAD), hepatic/renal impairment, hypovolemia, pulmonary edema, past hemorrhagic events.

⌛ LIFESPAN CONSIDERATIONS

Pregnancy/Lactation: May cause fetal harm. Must use reliable form of birth control during treatment. Recommend either intrauterine device (IUD) or oral contraceptive plus barrier methods. Unknown if distributed in breast milk. Must either discontinue drug or discontinue breastfeeding. **Pregnancy Category X. Children:** Safety and efficacy not established. **Elderly:** No age-related precautions noted.

INTERACTIONS

DRUG: Contraindicated with **aminophylline, nitrates or nitric oxide donors (e.g., isosorbide, nitroglycerin, nitroprusside), phosphodiesterase inhibitors (e.g., sildenafil, vardenafil)**; may cause severe symptomatic hypotension. **Antihypertensive medications** may increase hypotensive effects. Strong **CYP3A4 inhibitors (e.g., ketoconazole, itraconazole, ritonavir)** may increase concentration/effect. Strong **CYP3A inducers (e.g., rifampin, phenytoin), antacids** may decrease concentration/effect. **HERBAL: St. John's wort** may decrease concentration/effect. **FOOD:** None known. **LAB VALUES:** May decrease Hgb, Hct.

AVAILABILITY (Rx)

Tablets, Film-Coated: 0.5 mg, 1 mg, 1.5 mg, 2 mg, 2.5 mg.

ADMINISTRATION/HANDLING

PO
• Give without regard to meals. • Antacids should not be given within 1 hr of medication administration.

INDICATIONS/ROUTES/DOSAGE

Pulmonary Arterial Hypertension
PO: ADULTS/ELDERLY: Initially, 1 mg every 8 hrs (3 mg/day). May increase dose by 0.5 mg every 8 hrs at 2-wk increments (if systolic BP greater than 95 mm Hg and no signs/symptoms of hypotension). **Maximum:** 2.5 mg every 8 hrs (7.5 mg/day). Re-titrate dose for any treatment interruption greater than 3 days.

Dose Modification
Pts with Possible Hypotensive Reaction or Concomitant Use of Strong CYP and P-Glycoprotein Inhibitors:
Initial dose of 0.5 mg every 8 hrs and titrate accordingly.
Pts Who Smoke:
Consider titrating doses higher than 2.5 mg every 8 hrs. A decrease in dosage may be required for pts who quit smoking.
Hypotension Risk:
Gradually decrease dose by increments of 0.5 mg every 8 hrs.

SIDE EFFECTS

Frequent (27%–14%): Headache, dyspepsia, dizziness. **Occasional (14%–5%):** Nausea, diarrhea, hypotension, vomiting, constipation.

ADVERSE EFFECTS/ TOXIC REACTIONS

May cause severe symptomatic hypotension. Severe bleeding events including hematemesis, hemoptysis, intra-abdominal hemorrhage, subdural hematoma, vaginal hemorrhage reported in 2.4% of pts. May worsen cardiovascular status of pts with pulmonary veno-occlusive disease (PVOD). Gastritis and gastrointestinal reflux occurred in 21% and 5%, respectively. Other possible adverse effects including palpitations, epistaxis, dysphagia, abdominal distention, and peripheral edema reported.

NURSING CONSIDERATIONS

BASELINE ASSESSMENT

Obtain baseline vitals signs, CBC. Assess hydration status. Confirm negative pregnancy status before initiating treatment. Receive full medication history including herbal products. Question history of anemia, baseline hypotension, CAD, HF, hepatic/renal impairment, smoking, past hemorrhagic events, pulmonary disease.

INTERVENTION/EVALUATION

Monitor vital signs (esp. BP), CBC routinely. Monitor pregnancy status every mo during treatment and for at least 1 mo after discontinuation. Notify physician to obtain appropriate radiologic test if dyspnea occurs and screen for veno-occlusive disease or pulmonary embolism. Obtain EKG for palpitations, dyspnea. Offer antiemetics for nausea, vomiting. Encourage hydration. Immediately report altered mental status, CVA symptoms (aphagia, hemiplegia, homonymous hemianopsia [blindness of one half of vision on same side of both eyes]), hemorrhagic events.

PATIENT/FAMILY TEACHING

• May cause fetal harm. Immediately report suspected pregnancy. • Do not

R

breastfeed. • Do not have unprotected sexual intercourse if taking only oral hormonal birth control. Consult with gynecologist for appropriate birth control methods. • Do not take nitrates for chest pain or medications for erectile dysfunction (may cause low BP). • Do not take antacids within 1 hr of medication administration. • Go from lying to standing slowly (risk of orthostatic hypotension). • Report bleeding of any kind, changes in mental status, difficulty breathing, stroke-like symptoms. • Smokers may require lowered doses of medication if smoking cessation occurs.

---

risedronate

rize-droe-nate
(<u>Actonel</u>, Atelvia, Apo-Risedronate ✿, Novo-Risedronate ✿)
Do not confuse Actonel with Actos, or risedronate with alendronate.

FIXED-COMBINATION(S)

Actonel with Calcium: risedronate/calcium: 35 mg/6 × 500 mg.

◆CLASSIFICATION

PHARMACOTHERAPEUTIC: Bisphosphonate. **CLINICAL:** Calcium regulator (see p. 143C).

ACTION

Binds to bone hydroxyapatite, inhibits osteoclasts. **Therapeutic Effect:** Reduces bone turnover (number of sites at which bone is remodeled), bone resorption.

PHARMACOKINETICS

Rapidly absorbed following PO administration. Bioavailability decreased when administered with food. Protein binding: 24%. Not metabolized. Excreted unchanged in urine, feces. Not removed by hemodialysis. **Half-life:** 1.5 hrs (initial); 480 hrs (terminal).

USES

Actonel: Treatment of Paget's disease of bone (osteitis deformans). Treatment/prevention of postmenopausal, glucocorticoid-induced osteoporosis. Used to increase bone mass in men with osteoporosis. **Atelvia:** Treatment of osteoporosis in postmenopausal women.

PRECAUTIONS

Contraindications: Hypersensitivity to other bisphosphonates, including etidronate, tiludronate, alendronate; hypocalcemia; inability to stand or sit upright for at least 30 min; abnormalities of esophagus that delay esophageal emptying. **Cautions:** GI diseases (duodenitis, dysphagia, esophagitis, gastritis, ulcers [drug may exacerbate these conditions]), severe renal impairment (creatinine clearance less than 30 ml/min). **Pregnancy Category C.**

INTERACTIONS

DRUG: Antacids containing aluminum, calcium, magnesium; vitamin D may decrease absorption (avoid administration within 30 min of **risedronate**). **HERBAL:** None significant. **FOOD:** None known. **LAB VALUES:** None significant.

AVAILABILITY (Rx)

Tablets (Actonel): 5 mg, 30 mg, 35 mg, 150 mg. **Tablets, Delayed-Release (Atelvia):** 35 mg.

ADMINISTRATION/HANDLING

PO

Actonel: • Administer 30–60 min before any food, drink, other oral medications to avoid interference with absorption. • Give on empty stomach with full glass of plain water (not mineral water). • Pt must avoid lying down for at least 30 min after swallowing tablet (assists with delivery to stomach, reduces risk of esophageal irritation). • Give whole; do not crush, chew tablet.
Atelvia: • Take in morning immediately following breakfast with at least 4 oz water. • Remain upright for 30 min after taking dose.

INDICATIONS/ROUTES/DOSAGE

Paget's Disease
PO *(Actonel)*: **ADULTS, ELDERLY:** 30 mg/day for 2 mos. Retreatment may occur after 2-mo post-treatment observation period.

Prophylaxis, Treatment of Postmenopausal Osteoporosis
PO *(Actonel)*: **ADULTS, ELDERLY:** 5 mg/day or 35 mg once weekly or 150 mg once per mo.

Treatment of Postmenopausal Osteoporosis
PO *(Atelvia)*: **ADULTS, ELDERLY:** 35 mg once weekly.

Treatment of Male Osteoporosis
PO *(Actonel)*: **ADULTS, ELDERLY:** 35 mg once weekly.

Glucocorticoid-Induced Osteoporosis
PO *(Actonel)*: **ADULTS, ELDERLY:** 5 mg/day.

Dosage in Renal Impairment
Not recommended with creatinine clearance less than 30 ml/min.

SIDE EFFECTS

Frequent (30%): Arthralgia. **Occasional (12%–8%):** Rash, diarrhea, constipation, nausea, abdominal pain, dyspepsia, flu-like symptoms, peripheral edema. **Rare (5%–3%):** Bone pain, sinusitis, asthenia (loss of strength, energy), dry eye, tinnitus.

ADVERSE EFFECTS/ TOXIC REACTIONS

Overdose produces hypocalcemia, hypophosphatemia, significant GI disturbances, osteonecrosis of jaw.

NURSING CONSIDERATIONS

BASELINE ASSESSMENT

Assess symptoms of Paget's disease (bone pain, bone deformities). Hypocalcemia, vitamin D deficiency must be corrected before therapy begins. Obtain baseline laboratory studies, esp. serum electrolytes, renal function.

INTERVENTION/EVALUATION

Check serum electrolytes (esp. calcium, ionized calcium, phosphorus, alkaline phosphatase levels). Monitor I&O, BUN, creatinine in pts with renal impairment.

PATIENT/FAMILY TEACHING

• Expected benefits occur only when medication is taken with full glass (6–8 oz) of plain water, first thing in the morning and at least 30 min before first food, beverage, medication of the day. Any other beverage (mineral water, orange juice, coffee) significantly reduces absorption of medication. • Do not lie down for at least 30 min after taking medication (potentiates delivery to stomach, reduces risk of esophageal irritation). • Report swallowing difficulties, pain when swallowing, chest pain, new/worsening heartburn. • Consider weight-bearing exercises, modify behavioral factors (cigarette smoking, alcohol consumption). • Report jaw pain, incapacitating bone, joint, or muscle pain.

---

risperidone

TOP 200

ris-**per**-i-done
(Apo-Risperidone ✤, Novo-Risperidone ✤, Risperdal, Risperdal Consta, Risperdal M-Tabs)

BLACK BOX ALERT Increased risk of mortality in elderly pts with dementia-related psychosis, mainly due to pneumonia, HF.
Do not confuse Risperdal with Restoril, or risperidone with ropinirole.

◆CLASSIFICATION

PHARMACOTHERAPEUTIC: Benzisoxazole derivative. **CLINICAL:** Antipsychotic (see p. 67C).

ACTION

May antagonize dopamine, serotonin receptors. **Therapeutic Effect:** Suppresses psychotic behavior.

PHARMACOKINETICS

Well absorbed from GI tract; unaffected by food. Protein binding: 90%. Metabolized in liver. Primarily excreted in urine. **Half-life:** 3–20 hrs; metabolite, 21–30 hrs (increased in elderly). **Injection:** 3–6 days.

USES

(Oral): Treatment of schizophrenia, irritability/aggression associated with autistic disease in children. Treatment of acute mania associated with bipolar disorder. Short-term treatment of bipolar disorder in pediatric and adolescent pts. **(IM):** Management of schizophrenia, maintenance treatment of bipolar 1 disorder. **OFF-LABEL:** Tourette's syndrome. Psychosis/agitation associated with Alzheimer's dementia. Post-traumatic stress syndrome.

PRECAUTIONS

Contraindications: None known. **Cautions:** Renal/hepatic impairment, seizure disorders, cardiac disease, recent MI, breast cancer or other prolactin-dependent tumors, suicidal pts, pts at risk for aspiration pneumonia. Parkinson's disease, pts at risk for orthostatic hypotension, elderly, diabetes, decreased GI motility, urinary retention, BPH, xerostomia, visual problems, pts exposed to temperature extremes.

⧗ LIFESPAN CONSIDERATIONS

Pregnancy/Lactation: Unknown if drug crosses placenta or is distributed in breast milk. Breastfeeding not recommended. **Pregnancy Category C. Children:** Safety and efficacy not established. **Elderly:** More susceptible to postural hypotension. Age-related renal/hepatic impairment may require dosage adjustment.

INTERACTIONS

DRUG: Alcohol, other CNS depressants may increase CNS depression. **Carbamazepine** may decrease concentration. May decrease effects of **dopamine agonists, levodopa. Paroxetine, fluoxetine** may increase concentration, risk of extrapyramidal symptoms (EPS). **Antihypertensives, hypotension-producing medications** may increase hypotensive effect. **HERBAL: Gotu kola, kava kava, St. John's wort, valerian** may increase CNS depression. **FOOD:** None known. **LAB VALUES:** May increase serum prolactin. May cause EKG changes.

AVAILABILITY (Rx)

Injection, Powder for Reconstitution (Risperdal Consta): 12.5 mg, 25 mg, 37.5 mg, 50 mg. **Oral Solution (Risperdal):** 1 mg/ml. **Tablets (Risperdal):** 0.25 mg, 0.5 mg, 1 mg, 2 mg, 3 mg, 4 mg.

⬛ **Tablets (Orally Disintegrating [Risperdal M-Tabs]):** 0.25 mg, 0.5 mg, 1 mg, 2 mg, 3 mg, 4 mg.

ADMINISTRATION/HANDLING

◀**ALERT**▶ Do not administer via IV route.

IM

Reconstitution • Use only diluent and needle supplied in dose pack. • Prepare suspension according to manufacturer's directions. • May be given up to 6 hrs after reconstitution, but immediate administration is recommended. • If 2 min pass between reconstitution and injection, shake upright vial vigorously back and forth to resuspend solution.

Rate of Administration • Inject IM into upper outer quadrant of gluteus maximus or into deltoid muscle in upper arm.

Storage • Store at room temperature.

PO

• Give without regard to food. • May mix oral solution with water, coffee, orange juice, low-fat milk. Do not mix with cola, tea.

Orally Disintegrating Tablet
• Remove from blister pack immediately before administration. • Using gloves, place immediately on tongue. • Tablet dissolves in seconds. • Pt may swallow with or without liquid. • Do not split or chew.

INDICATIONS/ROUTES/DOSAGE

Psychotic Disorders
PO: ADULTS: Initially, 1 mg twice a day. May increase gradually (1–2 mg/day at intervals of at least 24 hrs) to target dose of 6 mg/day. **Range:** 4–8 mg/day. **Maintenance:** Target dose of 4 mg once a day (range: 2–8 mg/day). **ELDERLY:** Initially, 0.5 mg twice a day. May increase slowly at increments of no more than 0.5 mg twice a day. **Range:** 2–6 mg/day. **CHILDREN 13–17 YRS:** Initially, 0.5 mg/day (as single daily dose). May increase by 0.5–1 mg/day at intervals of greater than 24 hrs to recommended dose of 3 mg/day.
IM: ADULTS, ELDERLY: Initially, 12.5–25 mg q2wks. **Maximum:** 50 mg q2wks. Dosage adjustments should not be made more frequently than every 4 wks.

Bipolar Mania
PO: ADULTS, ELDERLY: Initially, 2–3 mg as a single daily dose. May increase by 1 mg/day at 24-hr intervals. **Range:** 1–6 mg/day.
PO: CHILDREN 10–17 YRS: Initially, 0.5 mg/day. May increase by 0.5 mg/day at intervals of greater than 24 hrs to recommended dose of 2.5 mg/day. **IM: ADULTS, ELDERLY:** 25 mg q2wks. **Maximum:** 50 mg q2wks. Dosage adjustments should not be made more frequently than every 4 wks.

Autism
CHILDREN 5 YRS AND OLDER WEIGHING MORE THAN 19 KG: Initially, 0.5 mg/day. May increase to 1 mg after 4 days. May further increase dose by 0.5 mg/day in greater than 2-wk intervals. **CHILDREN 5 YRS AND OLDER WEIGHING 15–19 KG:** Initially, 0.25 mg/day. May increase to 0.5 mg/day after 4 days. May further increase dose by 0.25 mg/day in greater than 2-wk intervals.

Dosage in Renal/Hepatic Impairment
Initial dosage for adults, elderly pts is 0.25–0.5 mg twice a day. Dosage is titrated slowly to desired effect.

SIDE EFFECTS

Frequent (26%–13%): Agitation, anxiety, insomnia, headache, constipation. **Occasional (10%–4%):** Dyspepsia, rhinitis, drowsiness, dizziness, nausea, vomiting, rash, abdominal pain, dry skin, tachycardia. **Rare (3%–2%):** Visual disturbances, fever, back pain, pharyngitis, cough, arthralgia, angina, aggressive behavior, orthostatic hypotension, breast swelling.

ADVERSE EFFECTS/ TOXIC REACTIONS

Rare reactions include tardive dyskinesia (characterized by tongue protrusion, puffing of the cheeks, chewing or puckering of mouth), neuroleptic malignant syndrome (marked by hyperpyrexia, muscle rigidity, altered mental status, irregular pulse or B/P, tachycardia, diaphoresis, cardiac arrhythmias, rhabdomyolysis, acute renal failure). Hyperglycemia, in some cases, life-threatening events such as ketoacidosis, hyperosmolar coma, death, has been reported.

NURSING CONSIDERATIONS

BASELINE ASSESSMENT
Serum renal/hepatic function tests should be performed before therapy begins. Assess behavior, appearance, emotional status, response to environment, speech pattern, thought content, baseline weight. Obtain fasting serum glucose value.

INTERVENTION/EVALUATION
Monitor B/P, heart rate, weight, hepatic function tests, EKG. Monitor for fine tongue movement (may be first sign of tardive dyskinesia, which may be irreversible). Monitor for suicidal ideation. Assess for therapeutic response (greater interest in surroundings, improved self-care, increased ability to concentrate, relaxed facial expression). Monitor for potential

R

♣ Canadian trade name   🐾 Non-Crushable Drug   🔲 High Alert drug neuroleptic malignant syndrome: fever, muscle rigidity, irregular B/P or pulse, altered mental status. Monitor fasting serum glucose periodically during therapy.

PATIENT/FAMILY TEACHING

• Avoid tasks that may require alertness, motor skills until response to drug is established (may cause dizziness/drowsiness). • Avoid alcohol. • Go from lying to standing slowly. • Report trembling in fingers, altered gait, unusual muscular/skeletal movements, palpitations, severe dizziness/ fainting, swelling/pain in breasts, visual changes, rash, difficulty breathing.

---

ritonavir

TOP 200

rit-**oh**-na-veer
(Norvir, Norvir SEC)

BLACK BOX ALERT Concurrent use with other medications (nonsedating antihistamines, sedative hypnotics, antiarrhythmics, ergot alkaloids) may result in potentially serious, life-threatening events.

Do not confuse Norvir with Norvasc, or ritonavir with Retrovir.

◆CLASSIFICATION

PHARMACOTHERAPEUTIC: Protease inhibitor. **CLINICAL:** Antiviral (see pp. 71C, 120C).

ACTION

Inhibits HIV-1 and HIV-2 proteases, rendering these enzymes incapable of processing polypeptide precursors leading to production of noninfectious, immature HIV particles. **Therapeutic Effect:** Slows HIV replication, reducing progression of HIV infection.

PHARMACOKINETICS

Well absorbed after PO administration (absorption increased with food). Protein binding: 98%–99%. Metabolized in liver. Primarily eliminated in feces. Unknown if removed by hemodialysis. **Half-life:** 2.7–5 hrs.

USES

Treatment of HIV infection in combination with other antiretroviral agents. May be used as "booster" for other protease inhibitors.

PRECAUTIONS

Contraindications: Due to potential serious and/or life-threatening drug interactions (e.g., arrhythmias, hematologic abnormalities, seizures), the following medications should not be given concomitantly with ritonavir: alfuzosin, amiodarone, dihydroergotamine, ergotamine, ergonovine, flecainide, lovastatin, methylergonovine, midazolam (oral), pimozide, propafenone, quinidine, sildenafil (when used for pulmonary arterial hypertension), simvastatin, St. John's wort, triazolam, voriconazole (when ritonavir dose 800 mg or greater/day). **Cautions:** Hepatic impairment, cardiomyopathy, ischemic heart disease, preexisting cardiac conduction abnormalities, pts with increased triglycerides, hemophilia A and B, diabetes, hepatitis B or C.

⌛ LIFESPAN CONSIDERATIONS

Pregnancy/Lactation: Breast-feeding not recommended (possibility of HIV transmission). **Pregnancy Category B. Children:** No age-related precautions noted in those older than 2 yrs. **Elderly:** None known.

INTERACTIONS

DRUG: See contraindications. May increase concentration of **clarithromycin, fluticasone, ketoconazole, protease inhibitors, sildenafil, statins.** May decrease concentration/effects of **methadone, phenytoin, warfarin. Rifampin** may decrease concentration/ effects. **HERBAL:** St. John's wort may decrease concentration/effects. **FOOD:** None known. **LAB VALUES:** May increase serum creatine kinase (CK), GGT, triglyc-

R

erides, uric acid, AST, ALT, glucose. May decrease Hgb, Hct, WBC, neutrophils.

AVAILABILITY (Rx)

Capsules: 100 mg. **Oral Solution:** 80 mg/ml.

 Tablets: 100 mg.

ADMINISTRATION/HANDLING

PO

• Store capsules in refrigerator. Store tablets, oral solution at room temperature. • Protect from light. • Give without regard to meals (preferably give with food). • Give tablets whole; do not cut, break, crush. • May improve taste of oral solution by mixing with chocolate milk, Ensure, Advera, Boost within 1 hr of dosing.

INDICATIONS/ROUTES/DOSAGE

Note: Not recommended as primary protease inhibitor in any regimen.

Treatment of HIV Infection
PO: ADULTS, CHILDREN 12 YRS AND OLDER: 600 mg twice daily. If nausea occurs at this dosage, give 300 mg twice daily for 1 day, then increase by 100 mg twice daily every 2–3 days to recommended dose of 600 mg twice daily. **CHILDREN 1 MO–11 YRS:** Initially, 250 mg/m²/dose twice daily. Increase by 50 mg/m²/dose q2–3days up to 350–400 mg/m²/dose. **Maximum:** 600 mg/dose twice daily.

Booster Therapy
PO: ADULTS, ELDERLY: 100–400 mg/day usually as 100–200 mg 1–2 times/day.

SIDE EFFECTS

Frequent: GI disturbances (abdominal pain, anorexia, diarrhea, nausea, vomiting), circumoral and peripheral paresthesia, altered taste, headache, dizziness, fatigue, asthenia (loss of strength, energy). **Occasional:** Allergic reaction, flu-like symptoms, hypotension. **Rare:** Diabetes mellitus, hyperglycemia.

ADVERSE EFFECTS/ TOXIC REACTIONS

Hepatitis, pancreatitis occur rarely.

NURSING CONSIDERATIONS

BASELINE ASSESSMENT

Pts beginning combination therapy with ritonavir and nucleosides may promote GI tolerance by beginning ritonavir alone, then subsequently adding nucleosides before completing 2 wks of ritonavir monotherapy. Obtain baseline laboratory testing, esp. hepatic function tests, triglycerides before beginning ritonavir therapy and at periodic intervals during therapy. Offer emotional support.

INTERVENTION/EVALUATION

Closely monitor for evidence of GI disturbances, neurologic abnormalities (particularly paresthesia). Monitor hepatic function tests, serum glucose, CD4 cell count, plasma levels of HIV RNA.

PATIENT/FAMILY TEACHING

• Continue therapy for full length of treatment. • Doses should be evenly spaced. • Ritonavir is not a cure for HIV infection, nor does it reduce risk of transmission to others. • Pts may continue to acquire illnesses associated with advanced HIV infection. • If possible, take ritonavir with food. • Taste of solution may be improved when mixed with chocolate milk, Ensure, Advera, Boost. • Inform physician of increased thirst, frequent urination, nausea, vomiting, abdominal pain.

rituximab TOP 200 HIGH ALERT

ri-**tux**-i-mab
(Rituxan)

BLACK BOX ALERT Profound, occasionally fatal infusion-related reactions reported during first 30–120 min of first infusion. Tumor lysis syndrome leading to acute renal failure may occur 12–24 hrs following first dose. Severe, some-

 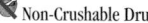

R

times fatal, mucocutaneous reactions resulting in multifocal leukoencephalopathy (PML) and death reported.

Do not confuse Rituxan with Remicade, or rituximab with bevacizumab or infliximab, brentuximab, ruxolitinib.

◆CLASSIFICATION

PHARMACOTHERAPEUTIC: Monoclonal antibody. **CLINICAL:** Antineoplastic (see p. 90C).

ACTION

Binds to CD20, the antigen found on surface of B lymphocytes, B-cell non-Hodgkin's lymphoma (NHL). **Therapeutic Effect:** Produces cytotoxicity, reduces tumor size.

PHARMACOKINETICS

Rapidly depletes B cells. **Half-life:** 59.8 hrs after first infusion, 174 hrs after fourth infusion.

USES

Treatment of relapsed or refractory low-grade or follicular B-cell non-Hodgkin's lymphoma (NHL). First-line treatment for diffuse large B-cell, CD20-positive, NHL. First-line treatment of previously untreated pts with follicular NHL in combination with cyclophosphamide, vincristine, and prednisolone (CVP therapy). Treatment of low-grade NHL in pts with stable disease or who achieve partial or complete response following CVP therapy, chronic lymphocytic leukemia (CLL), maintenance treatment for advanced follicular lymphoma in those responding to initial treatment of rituximab plus chemotherapy, moderate to severe rheumatoid arthritis (RA). In combination with glucocorticoids, treatment of Wegener's granulomatosis and microscopic polyangitis. **OFF-LABEL:** Treatment of autoimmune hemolytic anemia, chronic immune thrombocytopenic purpura (ITP), systemic autoimmune disease (other than rheumatoid arthritis), Burkitt's lymphoma, CNS lymphoma, Hodgkin's lymphoma.

PRECAUTIONS

Contraindications: Hypersensitivity to murine proteins. **Cautions:** Those with history of cardiac disease or pulmonary conditions, renal impairment. Pts at risk for developing tumor lysis syndrome.

⌛ LIFESPAN CONSIDERATIONS

Pregnancy/Lactation: Has potential to cause fetal B-cell depletion. Unknown if distributed in breast milk. Those with childbearing potential should use contraceptive methods during treatment and up to 12 mos following therapy. **Pregnancy Category C. Children:** Safety and efficacy not established. **Elderly:** No age-related precautions noted.

INTERACTIONS

DRUG: None known. **HERBAL: Echinacea** may decrease therapeutic effect. **Garlic, ginger, ginseng** may increase hypoglycemic effect. **FOOD:** None known. **LAB VALUES:** May increase creatinine, LDH. May decrease Hgb, Hct, neutrophils, platelets, B-cell counts, immunoglobulin concentrations.

AVAILABILITY (Rx)

Injection Solution: 10 mg/ml.

ADMINISTRATION/HANDLING
💧 IV

◄ALERT► Do not give by IV push or bolus.

Reconstitution • Dilute with 0.9% NaCl or D_5W to provide final concentration of 1–4 mg/ml into infusion bag.
Rate of Administration • Infuse at rate of 50 mg/hr. If no hypersensitivity or infusion-related reaction, may increase infusion rate in 50 mg/hr increments q30min to maximum 400 mg/hr. • Subsequent infusion can be given at 100 mg/hr and increased by 100 mg/hr increments q30min to maximum 400 mg/hr.
Storage • Refrigerate vials. • Diluted solution is stable for 24 hrs if refrigerated or at room temperature.

IV INCOMPATIBILITIES
Do not mix with any other medications.

INDICATIONS/ROUTES/DOSAGE
Note: Refer to specific protocols.

Non-Hodgkin's Lymphoma (NHL)
IV: ADULTS: 375 mg/m² once weekly for 4–8 wks. May administer a second 4-wk course.

Rheumatoid Arthritis
IV: ADULTS: 1,000 mg every 2 wks times 2 doses in combination with methotrexate. May repeat no sooner than 16 wks.

CLL
IV: ADULTS: 375 mg/m² in first cycle (on day prior to fludarabine/cyclophosphamide) and 500 mg/m² in cycles 2–6, administered every 28 days.

Wegener's Granulomatosis, Microscopic Polyangitis
IV: ADULTS: 375 mg/m² once weekly for 4 wks.

SIDE EFFECTS
Frequent (49%–10%): Fever, chills, nausea, asthenia (loss of strength, energy), headache, angioedema, hypotension, rash/pruritus. **Occasional (less than 10%):** Myalgia, dizziness, weakness, abdominal pain, throat irritation, vomiting, neutropenia, rhinitis, bronchospasm, urticaria.

ADVERSE EFFECTS/TOXIC REACTIONS
Hypersensitivity reaction produces hypotension, bronchospasm, angioedema. Arrhythmias may occur, particularly in pts with history of preexisting cardiac conditions.

NURSING CONSIDERATIONS

BASELINE ASSESSMENT
Pretreatment with acetaminophen and diphenhydramine before each infusion may prevent infusion-related effects. CBC should be obtained at regular intervals during therapy.

INTERVENTION/EVALUATION
Monitor for an infusion-related symptoms complex consisting mainly of fever, chills, rigors that generally occurs within 30 min–2 hrs of beginning first infusion. Slowing infusion resolves symptoms. Monitor renal/hepatic function, CBC, platelet count.

PATIENT/FAMILY TEACHING
• Report fever, sore throat, abdominal pain, yellowing of eyes/skin, unusual bruising/bleeding.

---

rivaroxaban

rye-va-**rox**-a-ban
(Xarelto)

BLACK BOX ALERT Epidural/spinal hematomas may occur in pts receiving neuraxial anesthesia or spinal puncture, resulting in long-term or permanent paralysis. Factors increasing risk of epidural/spinal hematoma include indwelling epidural catheters, concomitant drugs such as NSAIDs, platelet inhibitors, other anticoagulants; history of traumatic or repeated spinal or epidural punctures, history of spinal deformity or spinal surgery. Monitor for signs and symptoms of neurologic impairment. Consider benefits and risks before neuraxial intervention in anticoagulated pts or planned thromboprophylaxis. Increased risk of stroke may occur in pts with atrial fibrillation when discontinuing for reasons other than bleeding.
Do not confuse rivaroxaban with argatroban.

◆CLASSIFICATION
PHARMACOTHERAPEUTIC: Factor Xa inhibitor. **CLINICAL:** Anticoagulant (see p. 33C).

ACTION
Selectively blocks active site of factor Xa, a key factor in the intrinsic and extrinsic

 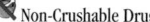

pathway of blood coagulation cascade. Prevents new clot formation, secondary thromboembolic complications. **Therapeutic Effect:** Inhibits blood coagulation.

PHARMACOKINETICS

Rapidly absorbed after PO administration. Peak plasma concentration: 2–4 hrs. Absorption dependent on site of drug release within GI tract. Avoid administration into small intestine due to reduced absorption. Protein binding: 92%–95%. Metabolized in liver. Excreted in urine (66%), feces (28%). **Half-life:** 5–9 hrs, 11–13 hrs (elderly).

USES

Prophylaxis of deep vein thrombosis (DVT) in pts undergoing knee or hip replacement surgery. Treatment of blood clots, DVT, pulmonary embolism (PE). Reduces risk/recurrence of thromboembolism/stroke in pts with nonvalvular atrial fibrillation/DVT/PE.

PRECAUTIONS

Contraindications: Active major bleeding. **Cautions:** Renal/hepatic impairment, pts at increased risk of bleeding (e.g., thrombocytopenia), stroke, uncontrolled hypertension. Concomitant use of CYP3A4 inducers or inhibitors.

⧗ LIFESPAN CONSIDERATIONS

Pregnancy/Lactation: Unknown if excreted in breast milk. **Pregnancy Category C. Children:** Safety and efficacy not established. **Elderly:** May be at increased risk for bleeding due to age-related renal impairment.

INTERACTIONS

DRUG: CYP3A4 inhibitors (e.g., ketoconazole, itraconazole, clarithromycin, erythromycin, fluconazole, ritonavir) may increase concentration, risk of bleeding. **Anticoagulants, antiplatelets, NSAIDs** may increase bleeding risk. **HERBAL: St. John's wort** may decrease effect. **FOOD: Grapefruit products** may increase risk of bleeding. **LAB VALUES:** May decrease platelets. May increase serum AST, ALT, bilirubin.

AVAILABILITY (Rx)

Tablets: 10 mg, 15 mg, 20 mg.

ADMINISTRATION/HANDLING

PO

• **DVT prophylaxis (knee, hip):** Give without regard to meals. • **Nonvalvular atrial fibrillation:** Give with evening meal. • **Treatment DVT/PE:** Give with food. • **Risk reduction DVT/PE:** Give with food.

INDICATIONS/ROUTES/DOSAGE

DVT Prophylaxis, Knee Replacement
PO: ADULTS: 10 mg daily for minimum 10–14 days. Initiate at least 6–10 hrs after surgery once hemostasis established. **CrCl less than 30 ml/min:** Avoid use.

DVT Prophylaxis, Hip Replacement
PO: ADULTS: 10 mg daily for 35 days. Initiate at least 6–10 hrs after surgery once hemostasis established. **CrCl less than 30 ml/min:** Avoid use.

Nonvalvular Atrial Fibrillation
PO: ADULTS: CrCl greater than 50 ml/min: 20 mg daily. **CrCl 15–50 ml/min:** 15 mg daily. **CrCl less than 15 ml/min:** Avoid use.

Recurrence of DVT/PE, Treatment of DVT/PE
PO: ADULTS, ELDERLY: 15 mg twice daily for 3 wks, then 20 mg once daily.

Reduce Risk of DVT/PE
PO: ADULTS, ELDERLY: 20 mg once daily.

SIDE EFFECTS

Rare (3%–1%): Wound secretion/oozing, extremity pain, muscle spasm, syncope, pruritus.

ADVERSE EFFECTS/ TOXIC REACTIONS

Increased risk of bleeding/hemorrhagic events including retroperitoneal hemorrhage, cerebral hemorrhage, subdural hematoma, epidural/spinal hematoma (esp. with epidural catheters, spinal trauma). Serious reactions including jaundice, cholestasis, cytolytic hepatitis, Stevens-Johnson syndrome, hypersensitivity reaction, anaphylaxis reported.

NURSING CONSIDERATIONS

BASELINE ASSESSMENT

Obtain CBC, serum chemistries, PT/INR, vital signs, urine pregnancy if applicable. Obtain EKG for pts with a history of atrial fibrillation. Question for history of bleeding disorders, recent surgery, spinal punctures, intracranial hemorrhage, bleeding ulcers, open wounds, anemia, renal/hepatic impairment. Receive full medication history including herbal products.

INTERVENTION/EVALUATION

Monitor CBC, serum chemistries, renal function, occult urine/stool. Be alert for complaints of abdominal/back pain, headache, confusion, weakness, vision change (may indicate hemorrhage). Question for increased menstrual bleeding/discharge. Assess peripheral pulses; skin for ecchymosis, petechiae. Check for excessive bleeding from minor cuts, scratches. Assess urine output for hematuria. Immediately report suspected pregnancy.

PATIENT/FAMILY TEACHING

• Do not take/discontinue any medication except on advice of physician. • Avoid alcohol, aspirin, NSAIDs. • Consult physician before surgery, dental work. • Use electric razor, soft toothbrush to prevent bleeding. • Report any unusual bleeding/bruising, spinal/epidural hematomas (e.g., tingling, numbness, muscular weakness). • Inform physician if pregnant or planning to become pregnant. • Avoid grapefruit products.

rivastigmine
TOP 200

riv-a-**stig**-meen
(Apo-Rivastigmine ✦, Exelon, Novo-Rivastigmine ✦)

◆CLASSIFICATION

PHARMACOTHERAPEUTIC: Cholinesterase inhibitor. **CLINICAL:** Anti-Alzheimer's dementia agent.

ACTION

Inhibits the enzyme acetylcholinesterase, increasing acetylcholine concentration at cholinergic synapses, enhancing cholinergic function. **Therapeutic Effect:** Slows progression of symptoms of Alzheimer's disease.

PHARMACOKINETICS

Rapidly, completely absorbed. Protein binding: 40%. Widely distributed throughout body. Rapidly, extensively metabolized. Primarily excreted in urine. **Half-life:** 1.5 hrs.

USES

Treatment of mild to moderate dementia of Alzheimer's or Parkinson's disease. **OFF-LABEL:** Severe dementia associated with Alzheimer's disease, Lewy body dementia.

PRECAUTIONS

Contraindications: Hypersensitivity to other carbamate derivatives (e.g., neostigmine). **Cautions:** Peptic ulcer disease, concurrent use of NSAIDs, sick sinus syndrome, bradycardia or supraventricular conduction defects, urinary obstruction, seizure disorders, asthma, COPD, pts with body weight less than 50 kg.

⌛ LIFESPAN CONSIDERATIONS

Pregnancy/Lactation: Unknown if distributed in breast milk. **Pregnancy Category B. Children:** Not indicated for use in this pt population. **Elderly:** No age-related precautions noted.

R

✦ Canadian trade name   ◆ Non-Crushable Drug   **HIGH ALERT** High Alert drug

INTERACTIONS

DRUG: May interfere with **anticholinergics** effects. May have additive effect with **bethanechol. NSAIDs** may increase GI effects, irritation. **HERBAL: Ginkgo biloba** may increase cholinergic effects. **FOOD:** None known. **LAB VALUES:** None known.

AVAILABILITY (Rx)

Oral Solution: 2 mg/ml. **Transdermal Patch:** 4.6 mg/24 hrs, 9.5 mg/24 hrs, 13.3 mg/24 hrs.

Capsules: 1.5 mg, 3 mg, 4.5 mg, 6 mg.

ADMINISTRATION/HANDLING

PO
• Give morning and evening doses with food. • Give capsule whole.

Oral Solution
• Using oral syringe provided by manufacturer, withdraw prescribed amount from container. • May be swallowed directly from syringe or mixed in small glass of water, cold fruit juice, soda (use within 4 hrs of mixing).

Transdermal Patch
• May apply the day following the last oral dose. • Apply to upper or lower back, upper arm, or chest. • Avoid reapplication to same spot of skin for 14 days. • Do not apply to red, irritated, or broken skin. • Avoid eye contact. • After removal, fold patch to press adhesive together and discard.

INDICATIONS/ROUTES/DOSAGE

Alzheimer's Disease
PO: ADULTS, ELDERLY: Initially, 1.5 mg twice daily. May increase at intervals of at least 2 wks to 3 mg twice daily, then 4.5 mg twice daily, and finally 6 mg twice daily. **Maximum:** 6 mg twice daily.

Parkinson's Disease
PO: ADULTS, ELDERLY: Initially, 1.5 mg twice daily. May increase at intervals of at least 4 wks to 3 mg twice daily, then 4.5 mg twice daily, and finally 6 mg twice daily. **Maximum:** 6 mg twice daily.

Transdermal: ADULTS, ELDERLY: Initially, 4.6 mg/24 hrs. May increase after 4 wks to 9.5 mg/24 hrs and then to 13.3 mg/24 hrs. Pts currently on oral rivastigmine, use 4.6 mg/24 hrs for those taking less than 6 mg/day and 9.5 mg/24 hrs for those taking 6–12 mg/day. Apply patch on next day following last oral dose.

SIDE EFFECTS

Frequent (47%–17%): Nausea, vomiting, dizziness, diarrhea, headache, anorexia. **Occasional (13%–6%):** Abdominal pain, insomnia, dyspepsia (heartburn, indigestion, epigastric pain), confusion, UTI, depression. **Rare (5%–3%):** Anxiety, drowsiness, constipation, malaise, hallucinations, tremor, flatulence, rhinitis, hypertension, flu-like symptoms, weight loss, syncope.

ADVERSE EFFECTS/ TOXIC REACTIONS

Overdose can produce cholinergic crisis, characterized by severe nausea/vomiting, increased salivation, diaphoresis, bradycardia, hypotension, respiratory depression, seizures.

NURSING CONSIDERATIONS

BASELINE ASSESSMENT

Obtain baseline vital signs. Assess history for peptic ulcer, urinary obstruction, asthma, COPD. Assess cognitive, behavioral, functional deficits.

INTERVENTION/EVALUATION

Monitor for cholinergic reaction: GI discomfort/cramping, feeling of facial warmth, excessive salivation, diaphoresis, lacrimation, pallor, urinary urgency, dizziness. Monitor for nausea, diarrhea, headache, insomnia.

PATIENT/ FAMILY TEACHING

• Take with meals (at breakfast, dinner). • Swallow capsule whole. Do not chew, crush, dissolve, or divide capsules. • Report nausea, vomiting, diarrhea, diaphoresis, increased salivary secretions, severe abdominal pain, dizziness.

rizatriptan
TOP 200

rye-za-**trip**-tan
(Apo-Rizatriptan ♣, Maxalt, Maxalt-MLT, Maxalt RPD ♣)

◆CLASSIFICATION

PHARMACOTHERAPEUTIC: Serotonin receptor agonist. **CLINICAL:** Antimigraine (see p. 65C).

ACTION

Binds selectively to vascular receptors, producing vasoconstrictive effect on cranial blood vessels. **Therapeutic Effect:** Relieves migraine headache.

PHARMACOKINETICS

Well absorbed after PO administration. Protein binding: 14%. Crosses blood-brain barrier. Metabolized by liver. Eliminated primarily in urine (82%), feces (12%). **Half-life:** 2–3 hrs.

USES

Treatment of acute migraine headache with or without aura.

PRECAUTIONS

Contraindications: Basilar or hemiplegic migraine, history of stroke; ischemic heart disease (including angina pectoris, history of MI, silent ischemia, and Prinzmetal's angina), uncontrolled hypertension, use within 24 hrs of ergotamine-containing preparations or another serotonin receptor agonist, MAOI use within 14 days. **Cautions:** Mild to moderate renal/hepatic impairment, dialysis pts, elderly; pt profile suggesting cardiovascular risks (e.g., hypertension, diabetes, hypercholesterolemia).

⧖ LIFESPAN CONSIDERATIONS

Pregnancy/Lactation: Unknown if drug is distributed in breast milk. **Pregnancy Category C. Children:** Safety and efficacy not established. **Elderly:** No age-related precautions noted.

INTERACTIONS

DRUG: Ergotamine-containing medications may produce vasospastic reaction. **Fluoxetine, fluvoxamine, paroxetine, sertraline** may produce hyperreflexia, incoordination, weakness. **MAOIs, propranolol** may dramatically increase concentration (avoid concurrent use). **HERBAL:** None significant. **FOOD: All foods** delay peak drug concentration by 1 hr. **LAB VALUES:** None known.

AVAILABILITY (Rx)

Tablets (Maxalt): 5 mg, 10 mg. **Tablets (Orally Disintegrating [Maxalt-MLT]):** 5 mg, 10 mg.

ADMINISTRATION/HANDLING

PO
• Orally disintegrating tablet is packaged in individual aluminum pouch. • Open packet with dry hands. • Place tablet onto tongue, allow to dissolve, swallow with saliva. Administration with water is not necessary.

INDICATIONS/ROUTES/DOSAGE

Acute Migraine Headache
PO: ADULTS OLDER THAN 18 YRS, ELDERLY: 5–10 mg. If significant improvement is not attained, dose may be repeated after 2 hrs. **Maximum:** 30 mg/24 hrs. (Use 5 mg/dose in pts taking propranolol with maximum of 15 mg/24 hrs.) **CHILDREN 6–17 YRS: 40 KG OR GREATER:** 10 mg as single dose. **LESS THAN 40 KG:** 5 mg as a single dose.

SIDE EFFECTS

Frequent (9%–7%): Dizziness, drowsiness, paresthesia, fatigue. **Occasional (6%–3%):** Nausea, chest pressure, dry mouth. **Rare (2%):** Headache; neck, throat, jaw pressure; photosensitivity.

ADVERSE EFFECTS/ TOXIC REACTIONS

Cardiac reactions (ischemia, coronary artery vasospasm, MI), noncardiac vasospasm-related reactions (hemorrhage, CVA) occur rarely, particularly in pts with hypertension, diabetes, strong family history of coronary artery disease; obesity; smokers; males older than 40 yrs; postmenopausal women.

NURSING CONSIDERATIONS

BASELINE ASSESSMENT

Question for history of peripheral vascular disease, renal/hepatic impairment. Question pt regarding onset, location, duration of migraine, possible precipitating symptoms.

INTERVENTION/EVALUATION

Monitor for evidence of dizziness. Assess for photophobia, phonophobia (sound sensitivity, nausea, vomiting), relief of migraine headache.

PATIENT/FAMILY TEACHING

• Take single dose as soon as symptoms of an actual migraine headache appear. • Medication is intended to relieve migraine, not to prevent or reduce number of attacks. • Avoid tasks that require alertness, motor skills until response to drug is established. • Report immediately if palpitations, pain/tightness in chest/throat, pain/weakness of extremities occurs. • Do not remove orally disintegrating tablet from blister pack until just before dosing. • Use protective measures (sunscreen, protective clothing) against exposure to UV light, sunlight.

roflumilast

roe-**floo**-mi-last
(Daliresp, Daxas ✦)

◆CLASSIFICATION

PHARMACOTHERAPEUTIC: Phosphodiesterase 4 (PDE4) inhibitor. **CLINICAL:** Anti-COPD agent (see p. 78C).

ACTION

Selectively inhibits PDE4, a major enzyme found in inflammatory cells and involved in pathogenesis of COPD. **Therapeutic Effect:** Slows progression of COPD.

PHARMACOKINETICS

Readily absorbed after PO administration. Maximum plasma concentration: 0.5–2 hrs. Protein binding: 99%. Metabolized in liver. Primarily excreted in urine (70%). **Half-life:** 17 hrs.

USES

◄**ALERT**► Not indicated as bronchodilator or relief of acute bronchospasm. Adjunct to bronchodilator therapy for treatment of severe COPD-associated chronic bronchitis.

PRECAUTIONS

Contraindications: Moderate to severe hepatic impairment. **Cautions:** Mild hepatic impairment, history of depression, suicidal ideation.

⧖ LIFESPAN CONSIDERATIONS

Pregnancy/Lactation: Unknown if distributed in breast milk. Not recommended for nursing mothers. **Pregnancy Category C. Children:** Safety and efficacy not established. **Elderly:** No age-related precautions noted.

INTERACTIONS

DRUG: CYP3A4 inducers (e.g., carbamazepine, phenobarbital, phenytoin, rifabutin, rifampin) may decrease efficacy. **CYP3A4 inhibitors (e.g., erythromycin, ketoconazole)** may increase concentration. **HERBAL:** None significant. **FOOD:** None known. **LAB VALUES:** None significant.

AVAILABILITY (Rx)

Tablets: 500 mcg.

ADMINISTRATION/HANDLING

PO
• Give without regard to food.

INDICATIONS/ROUTES/DOSAGE

Adjunct in Severe COPD
PO: ADULTS, ELDERLY: 500 mcg once daily.

SIDE EFFECTS

Occasional (10%–4%): Diarrhea, nausea, headache. **Rare (3%–2%):** Back pain, flu-like symptoms, insomnia, dizziness, decreased appetite, vomiting, abdominal pain, rhinitis, muscle spasm, tremor, dyspepsia.

ADVERSE EFFECTS/ TOXIC REACTIONS

Psychiatric events including worsening depression, suicidal ideation, anxiety reported in less than 2%. Moderate to severe weight loss may result in discontinuation.

NURSING CONSIDERATIONS

BASELINE ASSESSMENT

Assess vital signs, O₂ saturation, lungs sounds, body weight. Question for history of depression, anxiety, suicidal ideation, dehydration, COPD exacerbations, hepatic impairment. Assess plans of breast-feeding. Obtain full medication history.

INTERVENTION/EVALUATION

Monitor vital signs, O₂ saturation, psychiatric changes, body weight. Assess for dehydration if diarrhea occurs (skin turgor, mucous membranes, decreased urine output, dizziness, dry mouth).

PATIENT/FAMILY TEACHING

• Report changes in mood or behavior, thoughts of suicide, insomnia, anxiety. • Report any weight loss. • Increase fluid intake if dehydration suspected. • Worsening cough, fever, difficulty breathing may indicate exacerbation/infection. • Immediately notify physician if pregnancy is suspected.

romidepsin

roe-mi-**dep**-sin
(Istodax)
Do not confuse romidepsin with romiplostim.

◆CLASSIFICATION

PHARMACOTHERAPEUTIC: Histone deacetylase inhibitor. **CLINICAL:** Antineoplastic.

ACTION

Inhibits activity of specific enzymes that catalyze removal of acetyl groups of proteins, causing accumulation of acetylated histones. **Therapeutic Effect:** Induces cell cycle arrest, cell death.

PHARMACOKINETICS

Extensively metabolized. Protein binding: 92%–94%. **Half-life:** 3 hrs.

USES

Treatment of refractory cutaneous T-cell lymphoma (CTCL) or refractory peripheral T-cell lymphoma (PTCL).

PRECAUTIONS

Contraindications: None known. **Cautions:** Moderate or severe hepatic impairment, end-stage renal impairment, pre-existing cardiac disease, pts with QT interval prolongation, concomitant administration of medications prolonging QT interval. Avoid concomitant strong CYP3A4 inhibitors/inducers; caution with moderate CYP3A4 inhibitors or P-glycoprotein inhibitors.

⧖ LIFESPAN CONSIDERATIONS

Pregnancy/Lactation: May cause fetal harm. Unknown if distributed in breast milk. **Pregnancy Category D. Children:** Safety and efficacy not established. **Elderly:** No age-related precautions noted.

INTERACTIONS

DRUG: Coumarin-derivative antico-agulants prolong PT, INR. **Strong**

R

CYP3A4 inhibitors (atazanavir, clarithromycin, indinavir, itraconazole, ketoconazole, nefazodone, ritonavir) may increase concentration. Potent CYP3A4 inducers (carbamazepine, dexamethasone, phenobarbital, phenytoin, rifabutin, rifampin) may decrease concentration. HERBAL: St. John's wort may increase metabolism and decrease concentration. FOOD: Grapefruit products may increase concentration/effects. LAB VALUES: May decrease Hgb, Hct, WBC count, platelets, serum magnesium, calcium, potassium, sodium, albumin, phosphates. May increase serum glucose, AST, ALT, uric acid. May alter serum magnesium.

AVAILABILITY (Rx)

Injection, Powder for Reconstitution, 2-Vial Kit: 10 mg.

ADMINISTRATION/HANDLING

Reconstitution • Reconstitute powder with 2 ml of supplied diluent (80% propylene glycol, 20% dehydrated alcohol). • Swirl contents gently to dissolve powder. • Reconstituted solution provides 5 mg/ml. Further dilute in 500 ml 0.9% NaCl.

Rate of Administration • Infuse over 4 hrs.

Storage • Reconstituted solution is stable for at least 24 hrs at room temperature. • Solution appears clear, colorless. Discard if precipitate is present or solution is discolored.

INDICATIONS/ROUTES/DOSAGE

CTCL, PTCL

IV: ADULTS, ELDERLY: 14 mg/m^2 administered over 4 hrs on days 1, 8, and 15 of a 28-day cycle. Repeat cycles every 28 days if pt continues to benefit from and tolerates therapy.

SIDE EFFECTS

Frequent (57%–23%): Nausea, fatigue, vomiting, anorexia. Occasional (20%–7%): Diarrhea, fever, distorted sense of taste, constipation, hypotension, pruritus. Rare (4%–2%): Dermatitis, T-wave and ST-wave changes on EKG.

ADVERSE EFFECTS/ TOXIC REACTIONS

Infection is very common (47%), including sepsis, arrhythmias, acute respiratory distress syndrome, acute renal failure. Anemia occurs in 19% of pts, thrombocytopenia in 17%, neutropenia in 11%.

NURSING CONSIDERATIONS

BASELINE ASSESSMENT

Provide emotional support. Baseline PT, INR, CBC, serum chemistries, esp. potassium, sodium, calcium, magnesium, glucose, hepatic/renal function tests, EKG, should be obtained prior to therapy at baseline and routinely thereafter. Inform women of childbearing potential of risk to fetus if pregnancy occurs.

INTERVENTION/EVALUATION

Calculate daily absolute neutrophil count (ANC) using the formula: % neutrophils + % bands × WBC = ANC. Closely monitor hematologic, chemistry parameters, EKG. Diligently monitor for fever and obtain blood cultures times 2 if occurs. Provide antiemetics to control nausea/vomiting.

PATIENT/FAMILY TEACHING

• Diarrhea may cause dehydration, electrolyte depletion. • Do not have immunizations without physician's approval (lowers body's resistance). • Avoid contact with those who recently received live virus vaccine. • Avoid crowds, those with infection. • May reduce effectiveness of estrogen-containing contraceptives. • Report excessive nausea or vomiting, palpitations, chest pain, shortness of breath. Seek immediate medical attention if unusual bleeding occurs.

romiplostim

roe-mye-**ploe**-stim
(Nplate)
Do not confuse romiplostim with romidepsin.

◆CLASSIFICATION

PHARMACOTHERAPEUTIC: Recombinant fusion protein, thrombopoietin receptor agonist. **CLINICAL:** Hematologic agent.

ACTION

Binds and activates thrombopoietin (TPO) receptors on hematopoietic cells. **Therapeutic Effect:** Increases platelet production.

PHARMACOKINETICS

Concentration is dependent on dose and baseline platelet count. Peak concentration occurs in 7–50 hrs (median, 14 hrs). **Half-life:** 1–34 days (median, 3.5 days).

USES

Treatment of thrombocytopenia in pts with chronic immune (idiopathic) thrombocytopenic purpura (ITP) who have had an insufficient response to corticosteroids, immunoglobulins, or splenectomy.

PRECAUTIONS

Contraindications: None known. **Cautions:** Myelodysplastic syndrome, hematologic malignancy, pregnancy, hepatic impairment, renal impairment, history of cerebrovascular disease, concurrent anticoagulants or antiplatelet medication.

⌛ LIFESPAN CONSIDERATIONS

Pregnancy/Lactation: Studies suggest drug crosses placenta, is distributed in breast milk. **Pregnancy Category C. Children:** Safety and efficacy not established in those younger than 18 yrs. **Elderly:** Age-related renal, hepatic, cardiac abnormalities may require dosage adjustment.

INTERACTIONS

DRUG: **Anticoagulants/antiplatelets** may increase risk of bleeding. **HERBAL:** None significant. **FOOD:** None known. **LAB VALUES:** Increases platelet count.

AVAILABILITY (Rx)

Injection, Powder for Reconstitution: 250-mcg, 500-mcg single-use vial.

ADMINISTRATION/HANDLING

◀ ALERT ▶ Use syringe with 0.01-ml graduations for reconstitution.

Subcutaneous
Reconstitution • Reconstitute 0.72 ml Sterile Water for Injection to 250-mcg single-use vial for final concentration of 500 mcg/ml. • Reconstitute 1.2 ml Sterile Water for Injection to 500-mcg single-use vial for final concentration of 500 mcg/ml. • Gently swirl and invert vial to reconstitute; do not shake. • Dissolution takes less than 2 min. • Inject at abdomen, thigh, upper arm. • Do not inject at sites that are bruised, red, tender, or hard.
Storage • Refrigerate unreconstituted vial. • Reconstituted solution can be kept at room temperature or refrigerated for up to 24 hrs. • Protect reconstituted solution from light. • Do not use if discolored or particulate is present. • Discard unused portion.

INDICATIONS/ROUTES/DOSAGE

Thrombocytopenia
Subcutaneous: ADULTS, ELDERLY: Initially, 1 mcg/kg once weekly based on actual body weight. Adjust weekly doses by increments of 1 mcg/kg to achieve platelet count 50,000/mm^3 or greater and reduce risk of bleeding. **Maximum:** 10 mcg/kg weekly.

Dosage Adjustments

Platelet Count	Dose
Less than 50,000/mm^3	Increase by 1 mcg/kg
Greater than 200,000/mm^3 for 2 consecutive wks	Reduce by 1 mcg/kg
Greater than 400,000/mm^3	Hold dose

R

SIDE EFFECTS

Frequent (35%–26%): Headache, arthralgia. **Occasional (17%–6%):** Dizziness, insomnia, myalgia, extremity pain, abdominal pain, shoulder pain, paresthesia, dyspepsia.

ADVERSE EFFECTS/ TOXIC REACTIONS

Reticulin fiber deposits within the bone marrow, progressing to bone marrow fibrosis may occur. Worsening thrombocytopenia may be noted. Discontinuation of therapy may result in thrombocytopenia of greater severity than baseline, increasing risk of bleeding. Thromboembolic effects may occur. Increases risk of hematologic malignancies.

NURSING CONSIDERATIONS

BASELINE ASSESSMENT

Establish baseline CBC differential count prior to initiation, weekly during therapy and for 2 wks following discontinuation. Assess extent of RBC, WBC abnormalities.

INTERVENTION/EVALUATION

Monitor CBC differential count weekly during dose adjustment phase and then monthly following establishment of a stable dose.

PATIENT/FAMILY TEACHING

• Contact physician if bruising, bleeding occur. • Essential to receive drug therapy at scheduled times or risk of bleeding may occur.

ropinirole

roe-**pin**-i-role
(<u>Requip</u>, Requip XL)
Do not confuse ropinirole with Risperdal or risperidone.

◆CLASSIFICATION

PHARMACOTHERAPEUTIC: Dopamine agonist. **CLINICAL:** Antiparkinson agent (see p. 146C).

ACTION

Stimulates dopamine receptors in striatum. **Therapeutic Effect:** Relieves signs/symptoms of Parkinson's disease.

PHARMACOKINETICS

Rapidly absorbed after PO administration. Protein binding: 40%. Widely distributed. Extensively metabolized. Steady-state concentrations achieved within 2 days. Eliminated in urine. Unknown if removed by hemodialysis. **Half-life:** 6 hrs.

USES

Treatment of signs/symptoms of idiopathic Parkinson's disease. Treatment of moderate to severe primary restless legs syndrome (RLS).

PRECAUTIONS

Contraindications: None known. **Cautions:** History of orthostatic hypotension, cardiovascular or cerebrovascular disease, syncope, hallucinations (esp. in elderly), concurrent use of CNS depressants, preexisting dyskinesia, hepatic or severe renal dysfunction, major psychotic disorder.

⌛ LIFESPAN CONSIDERATIONS

Pregnancy/Lactation: Distributed in breast milk. Drug activity possible in breastfeeding infant. **Pregnancy Category C. Children:** Safety and efficacy not established. **Elderly:** No age-related precautions noted, but hallucinations may occur more frequently.

INTERACTIONS

DRUG: Ciprofloxacin may increase concentration. **Alcohol, CNS depressants** may increase CNS depressant effects. **HERBAL: Gotu kola, kava kava, St. John's wort, valerian** may increase CNS depression. **FOOD: All foods** delay

R

peak plasma levels by 1 hr but do not affect drug absorption. **LAB VALUES:** May increase serum alkaline phosphatase.

AVAILABILITY (Rx)

Tablets: 0.25 mg, 0.5 mg, 1 mg, 2 mg, 3 mg, 4 mg, 5 mg.

Tablets, Extended-Release: 2 mg, 4 mg, 6 mg, 8 mg, 12 mg.

ADMINISTRATION/HANDLING

PO

• May give without regard to meals. • Do not break, crush, dissolve, or divide extended-release tablets.

INDICATIONS/ROUTES/DOSAGE

Parkinson's Disease

PO *(Immediate-Release)*: **ADULTS, ELDERLY:** Initially, 0.25 mg 3 times a day based on individual pt response. Dosage should be titrated with weekly increments as noted: **Week 1:** 0.25 mg 3 times a day; total daily dose: 0.75 mg.
Week 2: 0.5 mg 3 times a day; total daily dose: 1.5 mg.
Week 3: 0.75 mg 3 times a day; total daily dose: 2.25 mg.
Week 4: 1 mg 3 times a day; total daily dose: 3 mg.
After week 4, may increase dose by 1.5 mg/day on weekly basis up to dose of 9 mg/day. May then further increase by 3 mg/day on weekly basis up to total dose of 24 mg/day.
(Extended-Release): Initially, 2 mg once daily for 1–2 wks. May increase by 2 mg/day at 1 wk or longer interval. **Maximum:** 24 mg/day.

Discontinuation Taper

Gradually taper over 7 days as follows: Decrease frequency from 3 times a day to twice a day for 4 days, then decrease from twice a day to once daily for remaining 3 days.

Restless Legs Syndrome

PO *(Immediate-Release)*: **ADULTS, ELDERLY:** 0.25 mg for days 1 and 2; 0.5 mg for days 3–7; 1 mg for wk 2; 1.5 mg for wk 3; 2 mg for wk 4; 2.5 mg for wk 5; 3 mg for wk 6; 4 mg for wk 7. Give all doses 1–3 hrs before bedtime.

SIDE EFFECTS

Frequent (60%–40%): Nausea, dizziness, extreme drowsiness. **Occasional (12%–5%):** Syncope, vomiting, fatigue, viral infection, dyspepsia, diaphoresis, asthenia (loss of strength, energy), orthostatic hypotension, abdominal discomfort, pharyngitis, abnormal vision, dry mouth, hypertension, hallucinations, confusion. **Rare (Less Than 4%):** Anorexia, peripheral edema, memory loss, rhinitis, sinusitis, palpitations, impotence.

ADVERSE EFFECTS/ TOXIC REACTIONS

Dyskinesia, impulsive/compulsive behavior (pathological gambling, hypersexuality, binge eating) occur rarely.

NURSING CONSIDERATIONS

BASELINE ASSESSMENT

Parkinson's disease: Assess signs/symptoms (e.g., tremor, gait). **Restless legs syndrome:** Assess frequency of symptoms, sleep pattern.

INTERVENTION/EVALUATION

Assess for clinical improvement, clinical reversal of symptoms (improvement of tremors of head/hands at rest, mask-like facial expression, shuffling gait, muscular rigidity). Assist with ambulation if dizziness occurs. Monitor B/P, daytime alertness.

R

PATIENT/FAMILY TEACHING

• Drowsiness, dizziness may be an initial response to drug. • Postural hypotension may occur more frequently during initial therapy. Go from lying to standing slowly. • Avoid tasks that require alertness, motor skills until response to drug is established. • If nausea occurs, take medication with food. • Hallucinations may occur, more so in the elderly than in younger pts with Parkinson's disease.

• Report occurrence of falling asleep during activities of daily living, new or worsening symptoms, changes in B/P, fainting, unusual urges. • Avoid alcohol.

rosiglitazone

roe-zi-**glit**-a-zone
(Avandia)

BLACK BOX ALERT May cause or exacerbate heart failure.
Do not confuse Avandia with Avalide or Avinza, or Avandaryl with Benadryl.

FIXED-COMBINATION(S)

Avandamet: rosiglitazone/metformin: 1 mg/500 mg, 2 mg/500 mg, 4 mg/500 mg, 2 mg/1 g, 4 mg/1 g. **Avandaryl:** rosiglitazone/glimepiride (an antidiabetic): 4 mg/1 mg, 4 mg/2 mg, 4 mg/4 mg.

◆CLASSIFICATION

PHARMACOTHERAPEUTIC: Thiazolidinedione. **CLINICAL:** Antidiabetic agent (see p. 45C).

ACTION

Improves target-cell response to insulin without increasing pancreatic insulin secretion. Decreases hepatic glucose output, increases insulin-dependent glucose utilization in skeletal muscle. **Therapeutic Effect:** Lowers serum glucose concentration.

PHARMACOKINETICS

Rapidly absorbed. Protein binding: 99%. Metabolized in liver. Excreted in urine (64%), feces (23%). Not removed by hemodialysis. **Half-life:** 3–4 hrs.

USES

Adjunct to diet/exercise to lower serum glucose in those with type 2 non–insulin-dependent diabetes mellitus (NIDDM). Used as monotherapy or in combination with metformin, sulfonylurea to improve glycemic control.

PRECAUTIONS

Contraindications: NYHA class III or IV HF. **Cautions:** Hepatic impairment, edematous pts, preexisting macular edema, diabetic retinopathy, pts at risk for cardiovascular events, anemia, premenopausal or anovulatory.

⌛ LIFESPAN CONSIDERATIONS

Pregnancy/Lactation: Unknown if drug crosses placenta or is distributed in breast milk. Not recommended in pregnant or breastfeeding women. **Pregnancy Category C. Children:** Safety and efficacy not established. **Elderly:** No age-related precautions noted.

INTERACTIONS

DRUG: Rifampin may decrease concentration/effects. **Gemfibrozil** may increase concentration, toxicity. **HERBAL: Garlic, ginger, ginseng** may cause hypoglycemia. **FOOD:** None known. **LAB VALUES:** May increase serum ALT, AST, cholesterol, HDL, LDL. May decrease Hgb, Hct.

AVAILABILITY (Rx)

Tablets: 2 mg, 4 mg, 8 mg.

ADMINISTRATION/HANDLING

PO
• Give without regard to meals.

INDICATIONS/ROUTES/DOSAGE

Diabetes Mellitus, Combination Therapy
PO *(with Sulfonylureas, Metformin)*: **ADULTS, ELDERLY:** Initially, 4 mg as single daily dose or in divided doses twice a day. May increase to 8 mg/day after 12 wks of therapy if fasting glucose level is not adequately controlled.

Diabetes Mellitus, Monotherapy
ADULTS, ELDERLY: Initially, 4 mg as single daily dose or in divided doses twice a day.

May increase to 8 mg/day after 12 wks of therapy.

SIDE EFFECTS

Frequent (9%): Upper respiratory tract infection. **Occasional (4%–2%):** Headache, edema, back pain, fatigue, sinusitis, diarrhea.

ADVERSE EFFECTS/ TOXIC REACTIONS

Hepatotoxicity occurs rarely. Increased risk of HF. May cause or worsen macular edema. May increase risk of fractures. Pts with ischemic heart disease are at high risk of MI.

NURSING CONSIDERATIONS

BASELINE ASSESSMENT

Obtain hepatic function test before initiation of therapy and periodically thereafter. Ensure follow-up instruction if pt, family do not thoroughly understand diabetes management, glucose-testing technique.

INTERVENTION/EVALUATION

Monitor Hgb, serum glucose, hepatic function tests, esp. AST, ALT. Assess for hypoglycemia (cool/wet skin, tremors, dizziness, anxiety, headache, tachycardia, numbness in mouth, hunger, diplopia), hyperglycemia (polyuria, polyphagia, polydipsia, nausea, vomiting, dim vision, fatigue, deep/rapid breathing). Be alert to conditions that alter glucose requirements (fever, increased activity/stress, trauma, surgical procedures).

PATIENT/ FAMILY TEACHING

• Diabetes mellitus requires lifelong control. • Prescribed diet, exercise are principal parts of treatment; do not skip/delay meals. • Wear medical alert identification. • Continue to adhere to dietary instructions, regular exercise program, regular testing of urine or blood glucose. • When taking combination drug therapy with a sulfonylurea or insulin, have source of glucose available to treat symptoms of low blood sugar. • Notify physician of rapid increase in weight, edema, shortness of breath, chest pain, abdominal pain, yellowing of skin/eyes.

---

rosuvastatin

roe-**soo**-va-**sta**-tin
(Apo-Rosuvastatin ♣, Crestor)
Do not confuse rosuvastatin with atorvastatin, lovastatin, nystatin, pitavastatin, or simvastatin.

◆CLASSIFICATION

PHARMACOTHERAPEUTIC: HMG-CoA reductase inhibitor. **CLINICAL:** Antihyperlipidemic (see p. 59C).

ACTION

Interferes with cholesterol biosynthesis by inhibiting conversion of the enzyme HMG-CoA to mevalonate, a precursor to cholesterol. **Therapeutic Effect:** Decreases LDL, VLDL, plasma triglyceride levels; increases HDL concentration.

PHARMACOKINETICS

Protein binding: 88%. Minimal hepatic metabolism. Primarily eliminated in feces. **Half-life:** 19 hrs (increased in severe renal dysfunction).

USES

Adjunct to diet therapy in pts with primary hyperlipidemia and mixed dyslipidemia; to decrease elevated total, LDL cholesterol, serum triglyceride levels; increases HDL. Adjunct to diet to slow progression of atherosclerosis in pts with elevated cholesterol. Treatment of primary dysbetalipoproteinemia, homozygous familial hypercholesterolemia (FH). Treatment of pts ages 10–17 yrs with heterozygous familial hypercholesterolemia (HeFH) to reduce elevated total cholesterol, LDL cholesterol, and apoli-

R

---

poprotein B. Primary prevention of cardiovascular disease (risk reduction of MI, stroke, arterial revascularization) without clinically evident CAD, but with multiple risk factors.

PRECAUTIONS

Contraindications: Active hepatic disease, breastfeeding, pregnancy, unexplained, persistent elevations of hepatic enzymes. **Cautions:** Anticoagulant therapy, history of hepatic impairment, substantial alcohol consumption, major surgery, renal impairment, renal failure, uncontrolled hypothyroidism, severe metabolic or endocrine disorders.

⏳ LIFESPAN CONSIDERATIONS

Pregnancy/Lactation: Contraindicated in pregnancy (suppression of cholesterol biosynthesis may cause fetal toxicity), lactation. Risk of serious adverse reactions in breastfeeding infants. **Pregnancy Category X. Children:** Safety and efficacy not established. **Elderly:** No age-related precautions noted.

INTERACTIONS

DRUG: Aluminum- and magnesium-containing antacids may decrease concentration/effects. Increased risk of myopathy with **cyclosporine, fibrate, gemfibrozil, niacin.** Increases concentrations of **estradiol, ethinyl, norgestrel.** Enhances anticoagulant effect of **warfarin. HERBAL:** None significant. **FOOD: Red yeast rice** contains 2.4 mg **lovastatin** per 600 mg rice. **LAB VALUES:** May increase serum alkaline phosphatase, bilirubin, creatinine phosphokinase, glucose, transaminases. May produce hematuria, proteinuria.

AVAILABILITY (Rx)

Tablets: 5 mg, 10 mg, 20 mg, 40 mg.

ADMINISTRATION/HANDLING

PO
• Give without regard to meals. May give at any time of day.

INDICATIONS/ROUTES/DOSAGE

Hyperlipidemia, Dyslipidemia, Atherosclerosis, Dysbetalipoproteinemia, Primary Prevention of Cardiovascular Disease
PO: ADULTS, ELDERLY: Usual starting dosage is 10 mg/day, with adjustments based on lipid levels; monitor q2–4wks until desired level is achieved. Lower starting dose of 5 mg is recommended in Asians. **Maximum:** 40 mg/day. **Range:** 5–40 mg/day.

FH
PO: ADULTS, ELDERLY: Initially, 20 mg/day. **Maximum:** 40 mg/day.

HeFH
PO: CHILDREN 10–17 YRS: Initially, 20 mg once daily. **Range:** 5–20 mg once daily.

Renal Impairment (Creatinine Clearance Less Than 30 ml/min)
PO: ADULTS, ELDERLY: 5 mg/day; do not exceed 10 mg/day.

Concurrent Cyclosporine Use
PO: ADULTS, ELDERLY: 5 mg/day maximum.

Concurrent Gemfibrozil, Atazanavir/Ritonavir, or Lopinavir/Ritonavir Therapy
PO: ADULTS, ELDERLY: 10 mg/day maximum.

SIDE EFFECTS

Generally well tolerated. Side effects are usually mild, transient. **Occasional (9%–3%):** Pharyngitis, headache, diarrhea, dyspepsia (heartburn, epigastric distress, indigestion), nausea, depression. **Rare (less than 3%):** Myalgia, asthenia (loss of strength, energy), back pain.

ADVERSE EFFECTS/ TOXIC REACTIONS

Potential for lens opacities. Hypersensitivity reaction, hepatitis, rhabdomyolysis occur rarely.

NURSING CONSIDERATIONS

BASELINE ASSESSMENT

Obtain dietary history, esp. fat consumption. Question for possibility of pregnancy before initiating therapy (Pregnancy Category X). Assess baseline lab results: serum cholesterol, triglycerides, hepatic function tests.

INTERVENTION/EVALUATION

Monitor serum cholesterol, triglycerides for therapeutic response. Lipid levels should be monitored within 2–4 wks of initiation of therapy or change in dosage. Monitor hepatic function tests at 12 wks following initiation of therapy, at any elevation of dose, and periodically (e.g., semiannually) thereafter. Monitor CPK if myopathy is suspected. Monitor daily pattern of bowel activity, stool consistency. Assess for headache, sore throat. Be alert for myalgia, weakness.

PATIENT/FAMILY TEACHING

• Use appropriate contraceptive measures (Pregnancy Category X). • Periodic lab tests are essential part of therapy. • Maintain appropriate diet (important part of treatment). • Report unexplained muscle pain, tenderness, weakness, esp. if associated with fever, malaise.

---

rufinamide

rue-**fin**-a-mide
(Banzel)

◆CLASSIFICATION

PHARMACOTHERAPEUTIC: Anticonvulsant. **CLINICAL:** Anticonvulsant.

ACTION

Modulates activity of sodium channels. Prolongs inactive state of the sodium channel in cortical neurons, limits sustained repetitive firing of sodium-dependent action potential, inhibiting excitatory neurotransmitter release. **Therapeutic Effect:** Exerts anticonvulsant activity.

PHARMACOKINETICS

Well absorbed following PO administration. Protein binding: 34%. Extensively metabolized. Eliminated in urine. **Half-life:** 6–10 hrs.

USES

Adjunctive therapy in treatment of seizures associated with Lennox-Gastaut syndrome in adults and children 4 yrs and older.

PRECAUTIONS

Contraindications: Familial short QT syndrome. **Cautions:** Other drugs that shorten QT interval, clinical depression, pts at high risk for suicide, mild to moderate hepatic impairment (not recommended in those with severe hepatic impairment).

⌛ LIFESPAN CONSIDERATIONS

Pregnancy/Lactation: May produce fetal skeletal abnormalities. May be distributed in breast milk. **Pregnancy Category C. Children:** Safety and efficacy not established in those younger than 4 yrs. **Elderly:** Age-related renal, hepatic, or cardiac impairment may require initiation of therapy at low end of dosing range.

INTERACTIONS

DRUG: May increase concentration of **phenobarbital, phenytoin.** May decrease concentration of **carbamazepine, lamotrigine. Valproate** may increase concentration. May decrease effect of **estradiol, norethindrone. Alcohol, CNS depressants** may increase CNS depressant effect. **HERBAL: Evening primrose** may decrease seizure threshhold. **FOOD:** None known. **LAB VALUES:** May decrease WBC count.

AVAILABILITY (Rx)

Oral Suspension: 40 mg/ml. **Tablets, Film-Coated:** 200 mg, 400 mg.

ADMINISTRATION/HANDLING

PO

• Give with food. • Film-coated tablets may be cut or crushed for dosing flexibility. • Shake oral suspension well before each dose; use bottle adapter and dosing syringes provided.

INDICATIONS/ROUTES/DOSAGE

Lennox-Gastaut Seizures

PO: ADULTS, ELDERLY: Initially, 400–800 mg/day, given in 2 equally divided doses. Dose should be increased by 400–800 mg/day every 2 days. **Maximum:** 3,200 mg/day, administered in 2 equally divided doses. **CHILDREN 4 YRS AND OLDER:** Treatment should be initiated at a daily dose of approximately 10 mg/kg/day, given in 2 equally divided doses. Increase by approximately 10-mg/kg increments every other day to a target dose of 45 mg/kg/day or 3,200 mg/day, whichever is less, administered in 2 equally divided doses. Renal impairment pts with creatinine clearance less than 30 ml/min do not require any dosage change.

SIDE EFFECTS

Children: Frequent (27%–11%): Headache, dizziness, fatigue, nausea, drowsiness, diplopia. **Occasional (6%–4%):** Tremor, nystagmus, blurred vision, vomiting. **Rare (3%):** Ataxia, upper abdominal pain, anxiety, constipation, dyspepsia, back pain, gait disturbance, vertigo.
Adults: Frequent (17%–7%): Lethargy, vomiting, headache, fatigue, dizziness, nausea. **Occasional (5%–4%):** Influenza, nasopharyngitis, anorexia, rash, ataxia, diplopia. **Rare (3%):** Bronchitis, sinusitis, psychomotor hyperactivity, upper abdominal pain, aggression, ear infection, inattention, pruritus.

ADVERSE EFFECTS/ TOXIC REACTIONS

Suicidal ideation or behavior occur rarely, noted as early as 1 wk after initiation of therapy and persisting for at least 24 wks. Shortening of the QT interval (up to 20 msec), hypersensitivity reaction (rash, fever, urticaria) have been noted. Abrupt withdrawal may precipitate seizure, status epilepticus.

NURSING CONSIDERATIONS

BASELINE ASSESSMENT

Review history of seizure disorder (intensity, frequency, duration, level of consciousness). Initiate seizure precautions.

INTERVENTION/EVALUATION

Provide safety measures as needed. Observe frequently for recurrence of seizure activity. Assess for clinical improvement (decrease in intensity, frequency of seizures). Assist with ambulation if drowsiness, lethargy occur. Question for evidence of headache.

PATIENT/FAMILY TEACHING

• Do not abruptly withdraw medication (may precipitate seizures). • Avoid tasks that require alertness, motor skills until response to drug is established. • Strict maintenance of drug therapy is essential for seizure control. • Avoid alcohol. • Female pts of childbearing age should be informed that concurrent use of rufinamide with hormonal contraceptives may render contraceptive less effective; nonhormonal forms of contraception are recommended. • Be alert for any unusual changes in mood/behavior (may increase risk of suicidal ideation/behavior).

ruxolitinib

rux-oh-**li**-ti-nib
(Jakafi)

◆CLASSIFICATION

PHARMACOTHERAPEUTIC: Kinase inhibitor. **CLINICAL:** Antineoplastic.

ACTION

Inhibits Janus-associated kinases (JAKs) JAK1 and JAK2, which mediate the signaling of cytokines and growth factor important for hematopoiesis and immune function. **Therapeutic Effect:** Reduces symptoms of myelofibrosis, including enlarged spleen.

PHARMACOKINETICS

Rapidly absorbed after PO administration. Widely distributed. Protein binding: 97%. Metabolized in liver. Excreted in urine (74%), feces (22%). **Half-life:** 3–5 hrs.

USES

Treatment of intermediate or high-risk myelofibrosis, including primary myelofibrosis, post-polycythemia vera myelofibrosis, post-essential thrombocythemia myelofibrosis.

PRECAUTIONS

Contraindications: None known. **Cautions:** Pts at risk for developing bacterial, fungal, or viral infections, renal impairment.

⌛ LIFESPAN CONSIDERATIONS

Pregnancy/Lactation: Unknown if distributed in breast milk. Not recommended in nursing mothers. Must either discontinue drug or discontinue breastfeeding. **Pregnancy Category C. Children:** Safety and efficacy not established. **Elderly:** No age-related precautions noted.

INTERACTIONS

DRUG: Strong CYP3A4 inhibitors (e.g., boceprevir, clarithromycin, cyclosporine, HIV protease inhibitors, itraconazole, ketoconazole) may increase concentration/effects. **HERBAL:** None known. **FOOD: Grapefruit products** may increase concentration. **LAB VALUES:** May decrease platelets, RBC, Hgb, Hct, WBC. May increase serum bilirubin, AST, ALT, cholesterol.

AVAILABILITY (Rx)

Tablets: 5 mg, 10 mg, 15 mg, 20 mg, 25 mg.

ADMINISTRATION/HANDLING

PO

• Give without regard to food.

FEEDING TUBE

• Suspend tablet in 40 ml water and stir for 10 min. • May administer suspension within 6 hrs after tablet has dispersed. • Flush with 75 ml water after administration.

INDICATIONS/ROUTES/DOSAGE

Myelofibrosis

PO: ADULTS: 20 mg twice daily if platelets greater than 200,000/mm^3 or 15 mg twice daily if platelets 100,000–200,000/mm^3. Dose reduction based on platelet response. **Maximum:** 25 mg twice daily.

Dosage in Renal Impairment

Creatinine clearance 15–59 ml/min	Platelets 100,000–150,000/mm^3	10 mg twice daily
Creatinine clearance 15–59 ml/min	Platelets less than 100,000/mm^3	Avoid use
End-stage renal disease (ESRD) on dialysis	Platelets 100,000–200,000/mm^3	15 mg after dialysis on days of dialysis
ESRD on dialysis	Platelets greater than 200,000/mm^3	20 mg after dialysis on days of dialysis
ESRD not requiring dialysis		Avoid use

Dosage in Hepatic Impairment

Hepatic impairment	Platelets 100,000–150,000/mm^3	10 mg twice daily
Hepatic impairment	Platelets less than 100,000/mm^3	Avoid use

SIDE EFFECTS

Frequent (23%–14%): Bruising, dizziness, vertigo, labyrinthitis, headache. **Occasional (9%–7%):** Weight gain, flatulence.

ADVERSE EFFECTS/ TOXIC REACTIONS

May cause severe thrombocytopenia (70%), anemia (96%), neutropenia (18%), which may improve with reduced

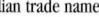 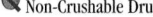

R

dose or temporarily withholding regimen. Anemic pts may require blood transfusions. Increased risk of developing opportunistic bacterial, mycobacterial, fungal, viral infections including herpes zoster, urinary tract infection, urosepsis, renal infection, pyuria. Increased risk of bleeding disorders including ecchymosis, hematoma, injection site hematoma, periorbital hematoma, petechiae, purpura.

NURSING CONSIDERATIONS

BASELINE ASSESSMENT

Obtain CBC, serum chemistries, renal function test, urinalysis, hepatic panel, cholesterol level. Assess recent vaccinations status. Receive full medication history including herbal products. Question for possibility of pregnancy, renal/hepatic impairment, HIV.

INTERVENTION/EVALUATION

Monitor CBC (every 2–4 wks until doses stabilized), serum chemistries, renal function test, cholesterol, hepatic panel. Obtain urinalysis with reflex culture for suspected UTI. Routinely assess vital signs, I&O, breath sounds, gait. Monitor temperature; be alert for fever, infectious process. Avoid IM injections, rectal temperatures, other traumas that induce bleeding. Assess skin for petechiae, hematoma, purpura.

PATIENT/FAMILY TEACHING

• Report any new bruising/bleeding, bloody stools or urine, fever, chills, rash, painful urination, suspected infection, fatigue, shortness of breath. • Do not breastfeed. • Avoid grapefruit products. • Open skin lesions, blisters may signal herpes infection. • Need to monitor CBC during treatment. If on dialysis, take only following dialysis.

R

salmeterol

TOP 200

sal-**met**-er-all
(Serevent Diskhaler ✤, Serevent Diskus)

BLACK BOX ALERT Long-acting beta₂-adrenergic agonists may increase risk of asthma-related deaths and asthma-related hospitalizations in pediatric and adolescents. Use only as adjuvant therapy. **Do not confuse salmeterol with Solu-Medrol, or Serevent with Atrovent, Combivent, Serentil, or Sinemet.**

FIXED-COMBINATION(S)

Advair Diskus: salmeterol/fluticasone (a corticosteroid): 50 mcg/100 mcg, 50 mcg/250 mcg, 50 mcg/500 mcg. **Advair HFA:** salmeterol/fluticasone (a corticosteroid): 21 mcg/45 mcg, 21 mcg/115 mcg, 21 mcg/230 mcg.

◆CLASSIFICATION

PHARMACOTHERAPEUTIC: Sympathomimetic (adrenergic agonist). **CLINICAL:** Bronchodilator (see pp. 77C, 78C).

ACTION

Stimulates beta₂-adrenergic receptors in lungs, resulting in relaxation of bronchial smooth muscle. **Therapeutic Effect:** Relieves bronchospasm, reducing airway resistance.

PHARMACOKINETICS

Route	Onset	Peak	Duration
Inhalation (asthma)	30–45 min	2–4 hrs	12 hrs
Inhalation (COPD)	2 hrs	3.25–4.75 hrs	12 hrs

Low systemic absorption; acts primarily in lungs. Protein binding: 95%. Metabolized in liver by hydroxylation. Primarily eliminated in feces. **Half-life:** 5.5 hrs.

USES

Maintenance therapy for asthma; prevention of exercise-induced bronchospasm, bronchospasm in pts with reversible obstructive airway disease including those with symptoms of nocturnal asthma. Long-term maintenance treatment of bronchospasm associated with COPD.

PRECAUTIONS

Contraindications: Status asthmaticus, acute episodes of asthma or COPD. Use without concurrent long-term asthma control medications (e.g., inhaled corticosteroids). **Cautions:** Not for acute symptoms; may cause paradoxical bronchospasm, severe asthma. Pts with cardiovascular disorders (coronary insufficiency, arrhythmias, hypertension), seizure disorders, diabetes, hyperthyroidism, hepatic impairment, hypokalemia.

⌛ LIFESPAN CONSIDERATIONS

Pregnancy/Lactation: Unknown if distributed in breast milk. **Pregnancy Category C. Children:** No age-related precautions in pts older than 4 yrs. **Elderly:** Lower dosages may be needed (may be more susceptible to tachycardia, tremors).

INTERACTIONS

DRUG: Beta-blockers reduce effect, may produce bronchospasm. **CYP3A4 inhibitors (e.g., ketoconazole, protease inhibitors)** may increase concentration, risk of QT prolongation. **MAOIs, tricyclic antidepressants** may increase concentration/effects, toxicity (wait 14 days after stopping MAOIs, tricyclic antidepressants before starting salmeterol). **HERBAL:** None significant. **FOOD:** None known. **LAB VALUES:** May decrease serum potassium. May increase serum glucose.

AVAILABILITY (Rx)

Powder for Oral Inhalation: 50 mcg/inhalation.

S

✤ Canadian trade name   Non-Crushable Drug   **HIGH ALERT** High Alert drug

ADMINISTRATION/HANDLING

Inhalation
• Shake container well, instruct pt to exhale completely through mouth; place mouthpiece between lips, holding inhaler upright. • Inhale deeply through mouth while fully depressing top of canister. Pt should hold breath as long as possible before exhaling slowly. • Allow at least 2 min before second dose (allows for deeper bronchial penetration). • Rinse mouth with water immediately after inhalation (prevents mouth/throat dryness).

INDICATIONS/ROUTES/DOSAGE

Maintenance and Prevention Therapy for Asthma
Inhalation *(Diskus)*: **ADULTS, ELDERLY, CHILDREN 4 YRS AND OLDER:** 1 inhalation (50 mcg) q12h.

Prevention of Exercise-Induced Bronchospasm
Inhalation *(Diskus)*: **ADULTS, ELDERLY, CHILDREN 4 YRS AND OLDER:** 1 inhalation at least 30 min before exercise. Additional doses should not be given for 12 hrs. Do not administer if already giving salmeterol twice daily.

Maintenance Therapy for COPD
Inhalation *(Diskus)*: **ADULTS, ELDERLY:** 1 inhalation (50 mcg) q12h.

SIDE EFFECTS

Frequent (28%): Headache. **Occasional (7%–3%):** Cough, tremor, dizziness, vertigo, throat dryness/irritation, pharyngitis. **Rare (less than 3%):** Palpitations, tachycardia, nausea, heartburn, GI distress, diarrhea.

ADVERSE EFFECTS/ TOXIC REACTIONS

May prolong QT interval (can precipitate ventricular arrhythmias). Hypokalemia, hyperglycemia may occur.

NURSING CONSIDERATIONS

BASELINE ASSESSMENT
Obtain baseline EKG and monitor for changes.

INTERVENTION/EVALUATION
Monitor rate, depth, rhythm, type of respiration; quality/rate of pulse, B/P. Assess lungs for wheezing, rales, rhonchi. Periodically evaluate serum potassium levels.

PATIENT/FAMILY TEACHING
• Not for relief of acute episodes. • Keep canister at room temperature (cold decreases effects). • Do not stop medication or exceed recommended dosage. • Notify physician promptly of chest pain, dizziness. • Wait at least 1 full min before second inhalation. • Administer dose 30–60 min before exercise when used to prevent exercise-induced bronchospasm. • Avoid excessive use of caffeine derivatives (coffee, tea, colas, chocolate).

saquinavir

sa-**kwin**-a-veer
(Invirase)
Do not confuse saquinavir with Sinequan.

◆CLASSIFICATION

PHARMACOTHERAPEUTIC: Protease inhibitor. **CLINICAL:** Antiretroviral (see pp. 71C, 120C).

ACTION

Inhibits HIV protease, rendering the enzyme incapable of processing polyprotein precursors needed to generate functional proteins in HIV-infected cells. **Therapeutic Effect:** Interferes with HIV replication, slowing progression of HIV infection.

PHARMACOKINETICS

Poorly absorbed after PO administration (absorption increased with high-calorie, high-fat meals). Protein binding: 99%. Metabolized in liver. Primarily eliminated in feces. Unknown if removed by hemodialysis. **Half-life:** 13 hrs.

USES

Treatment of HIV infection in combination with at least two other antiretroviral agents.

PRECAUTIONS

Contraindications: Concurrent use with alfuzosin, amiodarone, bepridil, dofetilide, ergot derivatives, flecainide, lidocaine, lovastatin, midazolam (oral), propafenone, quinidine, rifampin, ritonavir, sildenafil (when used for pulmonary arterial hypertension), simvastatin, trazodone, triazolam. Congenital or acquired QT prolongation, refractory hypokalemia or hypomagnesemia, concurrent medications that prolong QT interval, complete AV block (without pacemaker), severe hepatic impairment. **Cautions:** Preexisting conduction abnormalities, cardiovascular disease, mild to moderate hepatic impairment, hepatitis B or C, hemophilia, chronic alcoholism, cirrhosis, history of QT prolongation.

⌛ LIFESPAN CONSIDERATIONS

Pregnancy/Lactation: Breastfeeding not recommended (possibility of HIV transmission). **Pregnancy Category B. Children:** Safety and efficacy not established. **Elderly:** Age-related renal/hepatic/cardiac impairment may require dosage adjustment.

INTERACTIONS

DRUG: May increase concentration/effects of **atorvastatin, cyclosporine, tacrolimus, calcium channel-blocking agents, rifabutin, sildenafil, tadalafil, vardenafil.** May decrease concentration/effects of **efavirenz, methadone, oral contraceptives.** CYP3A4 inhibitors (e.g., **carbamazepine), phenobarbital, phenytoin, rifabutin** may decrease concentration/effects. **Delavirdine, atazanavir** may increase concentration, toxicity. **HERBAL: Garlic, St. John's wort** may decrease concentration/effects. **FOOD: High calorie, high fat meal** increases absorption. **Grapefruit products** may increase concentration (clinical significance unknown). **LAB VALUES:** May increase serum ALT, AST, amylase, creatine kinase, GGT, LDH, bilirubin, calcium, potassium, sodium, cholesterol, triglycerides. May decrease neutrophils, platelets, WBC count.

AVAILABILITY (Rx)

Capsules (Invirase): 200 mg. **Tablets (Invirase):** 500 mg.

ADMINISTRATION/HANDLING

PO
• Give within 2 hrs after a full meal. • Avoid grapefruit juice.

INDICATIONS/ROUTES/DOSAGE

Note: Do not initiate therapy if QT interval greater than 450 msec.

HIV Infection in Combination with Other Antiretrovirals
PO: ADULTS, ELDERLY: 1,000 mg (5 × 200 mg or 2 × 500 mg) twice a day in combination with ritonavir 100 mg twice a day.

SIDE EFFECTS

Occasional: Diarrhea, abdominal discomfort/pain, nausea, photosensitivity, stomatitis. **Rare:** Confusion, ataxia, asthenia (loss of strength, energy), headache, rash.

ADVERSE EFFECTS/ TOXIC REACTIONS

None known.

NURSING CONSIDERATIONS

BASELINE ASSESSMENT

Obtain baseline laboratory testing, esp. hepatic function tests, before beginning therapy and at periodic intervals during therapy. Offer emotional support. Obtain medication history.

S

INTERVENTION/EVALUATION

Monitor serum hepatic function tests, triglycerides, glucose, CD4 cell count, HIV RNA levels. Closely monitor for evidence of GI discomfort. Monitor daily pattern of bowel activity, stool consistency. Inspect mouth for signs of mucosal ulceration. Monitor serum chemistry tests for marked laboratory abnormalities. If serious or severe toxicities occur, interrupt therapy, contact physician.

PATIENT/FAMILY TEACHING

• Report persistent abdominal pain, nausea, vomiting. • Avoid exposure to sunlight, artificial light sources. • Continue therapy for full length of treatment. • Doses should be evenly spaced. • Saquinavir is not a cure for HIV infection, nor does it reduce risk of transmission to others. • Pts may continue to acquire illnesses associated with advanced HIV infection. • Take within 2 hrs after a full meal. • Avoid administration with grapefruit products.

---

sargramostim (granulocyte macrophage colony-stimulating factor, GM-CSF)

sar-gram-**o**-stim
(Leukine)
Do not confuse Leukine with leucovoran or Leukerin.

◆CLASSIFICATION

PHARMACOTHERAPEUTIC: Colony-stimulating factor. **CLINICAL:** Hematopoietic, antineutropenic agent.

ACTION

Stimulates proliferation/differentiation of hematopoietic cells to activate mature granulocytes and macrophages. **Therapeutic Effect:** Assists bone marrow in making new WBCs, increases their chemotactic, antifungal, antiparasitic activity. Increases cytoneoplastic cells, activates neutrophils to inhibit tumor cell growth.

PHARMACOKINETICS

Route	Onset	Peak	Duration
IV (increase WBCs)	7–14 days	N/A	1 wk

Detected in serum within 5 min after subcutaneous administration. **Peak serum levels:** 1–3 hrs. **Half-life: IV:** 1 hr; **Subcutaneous:** 3 hrs.

USES

Accelerates myeloid recovery in pts undergoing autologous or allogeneic bone marrow transplant or in pts who have undergone hematopoietic stem cell transplant following myeloablative chemotherapy. Prolongs survival in pts following bone marrow transplant in whom engraftment has been delayed or has failed. Enhances peripheral progenitor cell yield in autologous hematopoietic stem cell transplant. Shortens time to neutrophil recovery following induction chemotherapy of acute myelogenous leukemia (AML).

PRECAUTIONS

Contraindications: Concurrent (24 hrs preceding or following) myelosuppressive chemotherapy or radiation, excessive leukemic myeloid blasts in bone marrow or peripheral blood (greater than 10%), known hypersensitivity to yeast-derived products. **Cautions:** Preexisting HF, fluid retention; autoimmune, chronic inflammatory disease; hypertention; cardiovascular disease; pulmonary disease (hypoxia, pulmonary infiltrates); renal/hepatic impairment.

⌛ LIFESPAN CONSIDERATIONS

Pregnancy/Lactation: Unknown if drug crosses placenta or is distributed in breast milk. **Pregnancy Category C. Children:**

Safety and efficacy not established. **Elderly:** No age-related precautions noted.

INTERACTIONS

DRUG: None significant. **HERBAL:** None significant. **FOOD:** None known. **LAB VALUES:** May increase serum bilirubin, creatinine, hepatic enzymes. May decrease serum albumin.

AVAILABILITY (Rx)

Injection, Powder for Reconstitution: 250 mcg. Injection Solution: 500 mcg/ml.

ADMINISTRATION/HANDLING

 IV

Reconstitution • To 250-mcg vial, add 1 ml Sterile Water for Injection (preservative free) or Bactiostatic Water for Injection. Direct diluent to side of vial, gently swirl contents to avoid foaming; do not shake or vigorously agitate. • After reconstitution, further dilute in 25–50 ml 0.9% NaCl to a concentration of 10 mcg/ml or greater. If final concentration less than 10 mcg/ml, add 1 mg albumin/ml 0.9% NaCl to provide a final albumin concentration of 0.1% (e.g., 1 ml 5% albumin per 50 ml 0.9% NaCl).

◀**ALERT**▶ Albumin is added before addition of sargramostim (prevents drug adsorption to components of drug delivery system).

Rate of Administration • Give each single dose over 30 min, 2 hr, 6 hr, or continuous infusion.

Storage • Refrigerate powder, reconstituted solution, diluted solution for injection. • Do not shake. • Reconstituted solutions are clear, colorless. • Use within 6 hrs; discard unused portions. • Use 1 dose per vial; do not reenter vial.

🔃 IV INCOMPATIBILITIES

Amphotericin B complex (Abelcet, AmBisome, Amphotec), ondansetron (Zofran).

🔃 IV COMPATIBILITIES

Dexamethasone (Decadron), diphenhydramine (Benadryl), famotidine (Pep-

cid), granisetron (Kytril), heparin, metoclopramide (Reglan), promethazine (Phenergan).

INDICATIONS/ROUTES/DOSAGE

Neutrophil Recovery Following Chemotherapy in AML
IV Infusion: ADULTS, ELDERLY: 250 mcg/m²/day (as 4-hr infusion) starting approximately 4 days following completion of induction chemotherapy. Continue until ANC is greater than 1,500 cells/mm³ for 3 consecutive days to a maximum of 42 days.

Myeloid Recovery Following Bone Marrow Transplant (BMT)
IV Infusion: ADULTS, ELDERLY: Usual parenteral dosage: 250 mcg/m²/day (as 2-hr infusion). Begin 2–4 hrs after autologous bone marrow infusion and not less than 24 hrs after last dose of chemotherapy or last radiation treatment. Continue until ANC is over 1,500 cells/mm³ for 3 consecutive days. Discontinue if blast cells appear or underlying disease progresses.

Bone Marrow Transplant Failure, Engraftment Delay
IV Infusion: ADULTS, ELDERLY: 250 mcg/m²/day for 14 days. Infuse over 2 hrs. May repeat after 7 days off therapy if engraftment has not occurred. A third course with 500 mcg/m²/day for 14 days may be tried if engraftment still has not occurred.

Stem Cell Transplant, Mobilization of Peripheral Blood Progenitor Cells
IV, Subcutaneous: ADULTS: 250 mcg/m²/day (IV as 24-hr infusion). Continue until ANC is over 1,500 cells/mm³ for 3 consecutive days.

SIDE EFFECTS

Frequent: GI disturbances (nausea, diarrhea, vomiting, stomatitis, anorexia, abdominal pain), arthralgia or myalgia, headache, malaise, rash, pruritus. **Occasional:** Peripheral edema, weight gain, dyspnea, asthenia (loss of strength, en-

S

♣ Canadian trade name　　🟢 Non-Crushable Drug　　🔼 High Alert drug

ergy), fever, leukocytosis, capillary leak syndrome (fluid retention, irritation at local injection site, peripheral edema). **Rare:** Rapid/irregular heartbeat, thrombophlebitis.

ADVERSE EFFECTS/ TOXIC REACTIONS

Pleural/pericardial effusion occurs rarely after infusion.

NURSING CONSIDERATIONS

BASELINE ASSESSMENT

Obtain baseline pulmonary function testing, weight, vital signs. Obtain baseline chemistry studies (CBC with differential, serum renal/hepatic function tests).

INTERVENTION/EVALUATION

Monitor CBC with differential, serum renal/hepatic function, pulmonary function, vital signs, weight. Monitor for supraventricular arrhythmias during administration (particularly in pts with history of cardiac arrhythmias). Assess closely for dyspnea during and immediately following infusion (particularly in pts with history of lung disease). If dyspnea occurs during infusion, cut infusion rate by half. If dyspnea continues, stop infusion immediately. If neutrophil count exceeds 20,000 cells/mm³ or platelet count exceeds 500,000/mm³, stop infusion or reduce dose by half, based on clinical condition of pt. Blood counts return to normal or baseline 3–7 days after discontinuation of therapy.

saxagliptin TOP 200

sax-a-**glip**-tin
(Onglyza)
Do not confuse saxagliptin with sitagliptin or sumatriptan.

FIXED-COMBINATION(S)

Kombiglyze XR: saxagliptin/metformin (an antidiabetic): 2.5 mg/1,000 mg, 5 mg/500 mg, 5 mg/1,000 mg.

◆CLASSIFICATION

PHARMACOTHERAPEUTIC: DDP-4 inhibitor (gliptins). **CLINICAL:** Antidiabetic agent (see p. 44C).

ACTION

Slows the inactivation of incretin hormones by inhibiting DDP-4 enzyme. Incretin hormones increase insulin synthesis/release from pancreas and decrease glucagon secretion. **Therapeutic Effect:** Regulates glucose homeostasis.

PHARMACOKINETICS

Route	Onset	Peak	Duration
Oral	—	—	24 hrs

Rapidly absorbed following PO administration. Extensively metabolized (metabolite is active). Eliminated by both renal and hepatic pathways. **Half-life:** 2.5 hrs; metabolite, 3.1 hrs.

USES

Adjunctive treatment to diet and exercise to improve glycemic control in pts with type 2 diabetes mellitus as monotherapy or in combination with other antidiabetic agents.

PRECAUTIONS

Contraindications: None known. **Cautions:** Concurrent use of other glucose-lowering agents may increase risk of hypoglycemia, moderate to severe renal impairment, end-stage renal disease requiring hemodialysis, concurrent strong CYP3A4 inhibitors (e.g., clarithromycin).

⌛ LIFESPAN CONSIDERATIONS

Pregnancy/Lactation: Unknown if distributed in breast milk. **Pregnancy Category B. Children:** Safety and efficacy not established. **Elderly:** Age-related renal impairment may require dosage adjustment.

INTERACTIONS

DRUG: **CYP3A4 inhibitors (e.g., clarithromycin, itraconazole, ketoconazole)** may increase concentration. **CYP3A4 inducers (e.g., rifampin)** may decrease concentration. **HERBAL:** Herbal supplements that have hypoglycemic effects increase risk of hypoglycemia. **FOOD:** **Grapefruit products** may increase concentration. **LAB VALUES:** May slightly decrease WBCs, particularly lymphocyte count. May increase serum creatinine.

AVAILABILITY (Rx)

 Tablets, Film-Coated: 2.5 mg, 5 mg.

ADMINISTRATION/HANDLING

PO
• May give without regard to food. • Do not break, crush, dissolve, or divide film-coated tablets.

INDICATIONS/ROUTES/DOSAGE

Type 2 Diabetes Mellitus
PO: ADULTS OVER 18 YRS, ELDERLY: 2.5 or 5 mg once daily. **Moderate to Severe Renal Impairment (CrCl Less Than 50 ml/min):** 2.5 mg once daily. **Concurrent Strong CYP3A4 Inhibitors (e.g., ketoconazole):** 2.5 mg once daily. **Hemodialysis:** Give dose after dialysis.

SIDE EFFECTS

Occasional (7%): Headache. **Rare (3%–1%):** Peripheral edema, sinusitis, abdominal pain, gastroenteritis, vomiting, rash.

ADVERSE EFFECTS/ TOXIC REACTIONS

Lymphopenia, rash occur rarely. Upper respiratory tract infection, urinary tract infection occur in approximately 7% of pts.

NURSING CONSIDERATIONS

BASELINE ASSESSMENT

Check blood glucose concentration before administration. Discuss lifestyle to determine extent of learning, emotional needs. Ensure follow-up instruction if pt or family does not thoroughly understand diabetes management or glucose-testing technique.

INTERVENTION/EVALUATION

Assess for hypoglycemia (diaphoresis, tremors, dizziness, anxiety, headache, tachycardia, perioral numbness, hunger, diplopia, difficulty concentrating), hyperglycemia (polyuria, polyphagia, polydipsia, nausea, vomiting, dim vision, fatigue, deep, rapid breathing). Be alert to conditions that alter glucose requirements (fever, increased activity or stress, surgical procedures).

PATIENT/FAMILY TEACHING

• Diabetes mellitus requires lifelong control. Prescribed diet and exercise are principal parts of treatment; do not skip or delay meals. • Continue to adhere to dietary instructions, regular exercise program, regular testing of blood glucose. • When taking combination drug therapy or when glucose demands are altered (fever, infection, trauma, stress, heavy physical activity), have a source of glucose available to treat symptoms of hypoglycemia.

scopolamine

skoe-**pol**-a-meen
(Trans-Derm Scop, Transderm-V)

FIXED-COMBINATION(S)

Donnatal: scopolamine/atropine (anticholinergic)/hyoscyamine (anticholinergic)/phenobarbital (sedative): 0.0065 mg/0.0194 mg/0.1037 mg/16.2 mg.

◆CLASSIFICATION

PHARMACOTHERAPEUTIC: Anticholinergic. **CLINICAL:** Antinausea, antiemetic.

ACTION

Competitively inhibits action of acetylcholine at muscarinic receptors. Re-

S

duces excitability of labyrinthine receptors, depressing conduction in vestibular cerebellar pathway. **Therapeutic Effect:** Prevents motion-induced nausea/vomiting.

USES

Prevention of motion sickness, postop nausea/vomiting. **OFF-LABEL:** Breakthrough treatment of nausea/vomiting associated with chemotherapy.

PRECAUTIONS

Contraindications: Narrow-angle glaucoma, GI/GU obstruction, myasthenia gravis, paralytic ileus, tachycardia secondary to cardiac insufficiency, thyrotoxicosis. **Cautions:** Hepatic/renal impairment, cardiac disease (hypertension, heart failure), seizures, psychoses, coronary artery disease, prostatic hyperplasia, urinary retention, reflux esophagitis, ulcerative colitis, hyperthyroidism.

⧗ LIFESPAN CONSIDERATIONS

Pregnancy/Lactation: Crosses placenta; unknown if distributed in breast milk. **Pregnancy Category C. Children:** May be more susceptible to adverse effects. **Elderly:** Dizziness, hallucinations, confusion may require dosage adjustment.

INTERACTIONS

DRUG: Anticholinergics, antihistamines, tricyclic antidepressants may increase anticholinergic effects. **CNS depressants** may increase CNS depression. **HERBAL:** None significant. **FOOD: Grapefruit products** may increase concentration/effects. **LAB VALUES:** May interfere with gastric secretion test.

AVAILABILITY (Rx)

Transdermal System (Trans-Derm Scop): 1.5 mg.

ADMINISTRATION/HANDLING

Transdermal
• Apply patch to hairless area behind one ear. • If dislodged or on for more than 72 hrs, replace with fresh patch.

INDICATIONS/ROUTES/DOSAGE

Prevention of Motion Sickness
Transdermal: ADULTS: One system at least 4 hrs prior to exposure (best if 12 hrs before) and q72h as needed.

Postop Nausea/Vomiting
Transdermal: ADULTS, ELDERLY: 1 system no sooner than 1 hr before surgery and removed 24 hrs after surgery.

SIDE EFFECTS

Frequent (Greater Than 15%): Dry mouth, drowsiness, blurred vision. **Rare (5%–1%):** Dizziness, restlessness, hallucinations, confusion, difficulty urinating, rash.

ADVERSE EFFECTS/ TOXIC REACTIONS

None known.

NURSING CONSIDERATIONS

BASELINE ASSESSMENT
Obtain baseline hepatic function tests. Assess for use of other CNS depressants, drugs with anticholinergic action, history of narrow-angle glaucoma.

INTERVENTION/EVALUATION
Monitor serum hepatic/renal function tests. Observe for improvement of symptoms.

PATIENT/FAMILY TEACHING
• Avoid tasks requiring alertness, motor skills until response to drug is established (may cause drowsiness, disorientation, confusion). • Use only 1 patch at a time; do not cut. • Wash hands after administration.

selegiline

se-**le**-ji-leen
(Apo-Selegiline ❖, Eldepryl, Emsam, Novo-Selegiline ❖, Zelapar)
BLACK BOX ALERT Transdermal: Increased risk of suicidal thinking

and behavior in children, adolescents, young adults 18–24 yrs with major depressive disorder, other psychiatric disorders.

Do not confuse Eldepryl with Elavil or enalapril, selegiline with Salagen, sertraline, or Stelazine, or Zelapar with Zaleplon, Zemplar, or Zyprexa.

◆CLASSIFICATION

PHARMACOTHERAPEUTIC: MAOI. **CLINICAL:** Antiparkinson agent (see p. 146C).

ACTION

Irreversibly inhibits activity of monoamine oxidase type B (enzyme that breaks down dopamine), thereby increasing dopaminergic action. **Therapeutic Effect:** Relieves signs/symptoms of Parkinson's disease (tremor, akinesia, posture/equilibrium disorders, rigidity).

PHARMACOKINETICS

Route	Onset	Peak	Duration
PO	1 hr	—	24–72 hrs

Rapidly absorbed from GI tract. Crosses blood-brain barrier. Protein binding: 90%. Metabolized in liver. Primarily excreted in urine. **Half-life: PO:** 10 hrs. **Transdermal:** 18–25 hrs.

USES

Oral: Adjunct to levodopa/carbidopa in treatment of Parkinson's disease. **Transdermal:** Treatment of major depressive disorder (MDD). **OFF-LABEL:** Treatment of ADHD, early Parkinson's disease.

PRECAUTIONS

Contraindications: Concurrent use of meperidine. *Orally disintegrating tablet (additional):* Concurrent use of dextromethorphan, methadone, tramadol, oral selegine, other MAOIs. *Transdermal (additional):* Pheochromocytoma; concurrent use of bupropion, selective serotonin reuptake inhibitors (e.g., fluoxetine), dual serotonin/norepinephrine reuptake inhibitors (e.g., duloxetine), tricyclic antidepressants, buspirone, tramadol, methadone, dextromethorphan, St. John's wort, mirtazapine, cyclobenzaprine, oral selegine, other MAOIs, carbamazepine, oxcarbazepine. Elective surgery requiring general anesthesia, local anesthesia containing sympathomimetics; foods high in tyramine content. **Cautions:** Pts at high risk for suicide, depression, renal/hepatic impairment. **Transdermal:** Pts at risk for hypotension (cerebrovascular, cardiovascular disease, hypovolemia).

⌛ LIFESPAN CONSIDERATIONS

Pregnancy/Lactation: Unknown if drug crosses placenta or is distributed in breast milk. **Pregnancy Category C. Children:** Safety and efficacy not established. **Elderly:** No age-related precautions noted.

INTERACTIONS

DRUG: Fluoxetine, fluvoxamine, paroxetine, sertraline, venlafaxine may cause mania, serotonin syndrome (altered mental status, restlessness, diaphoresis, diarrhea, fever). **Meperidine** may cause potentially fatal reaction (e.g., excitation, diaphoresis, rigidity, hypertension/hypotension, coma, death). **Tricyclic antidepressants** may cause asystole, diaphoresis, hypertension, syncope, altered mental status, hyperpyrexia, seizures, tremors (wait 14 days between stopping selegiline and starting tricyclic antidepressants). **HERBAL: Kava kava, SAMe, St. John's wort, valerian** may increase risk of serotonin syndrome, excessive sedation. **FOOD: Tyramine-rich foods** may produce hypertensive reactions. **LAB VALUES:** None significant.

AVAILABILITY (Rx)

Capsules (Eldepryl): 5 mg. **Tablets (Eldepryl):** 5 mg. **Tablets (Orally Disintegrating [Zelapar]):** 1.25 mg. **Transdermal (Emsam):** 6 mg/24 hrs, 9 mg/24 hrs, 12 mg/24 hrs.

S

ADMINISTRATION/HANDLING

PO

• Give without regard to meals. • Avoid tyramine-containing foods, large quantities of caffeine-containing beverages.

PO (Orally Disintegrating Tablets)

• Give in morning before breakfast and without liquid. • Peel off backing with dry hands (do not push tablets through foil). • Immediately place on top of tongue, allow to disintegrate. • Avoid food, liquids for 5 min before and after taking selegiline.

Transdermal

• Apply to dry, intact skin on upper torso or thigh, outer surface of upper arm.

INDICATIONS/ROUTES/DOSAGE

Adjunctive Treatment of Parkinson's Disease

PO: ADULTS (ELDEPRYL): 10 mg/day in divided doses, such as 5 mg at breakfast and lunch, given concomitantly with each dose of carbidopa and levodopa. **ELDERLY:** Initially, 5 mg in the morning. May increase up to 10 mg/day. **ADULTS, ELDERLY (ZELAPAR):** Initially, 1.25 mg daily for at least 6 wks. May increase to 2.5 mg/day.

Major Depressive Disorder

Transdermal: ADULTS: Initially, 6 mg/24 hrs. May increase in 3 mg/24 hrs increments at minimum of 2 wks. **Maximum:** 12 mg/24 hrs. **ELDERLY:** 6 mg/24 hrs.

SIDE EFFECTS

Frequent (10%–4%): Nausea, dizziness, light-headedness, syncope, abdominal discomfort. **Occasional (3%–2%):** Confusion, hallucinations, dry mouth, vivid dreams, dyskinesia. **Rare (1%):** Headache, myalgia, anxiety, diarrhea, insomnia.

ADVERSE EFFECTS/ TOXIC REACTIONS

Symptoms of overdose may vary from CNS depression (sedation, apnea, cardiovascular collapse, death) to severe paradoxical reactions (hallucinations, tremor, sei-

zures). Impaired motor coordination, (loss of balance, blepharospasm [uncontrolled blinking], facial grimaces, feeling of heaviness in lower extremities), depression, nightmares, delusions, overstimulation, sleep disturbance, anger, hallucinations, confusion may occur.

NURSING CONSIDERATIONS

BASELINE ASSESSMENT

Obtain accurate medication history, diet history. Assess current state of mental health.

INTERVENTION/EVALUATION

Be alert to neurologic effects (headache, lethargy, mental confusion, agitation). Monitor for evidence of dyskinesia (difficulty with movement). Assess for clinical reversal of symptoms (improvement of tremors of head/hands at rest, mask-like facial expression, shuffling gait, muscular rigidity). Monitor for unusual behavior, worsening depression, suicidal ideation, especially at initiation of therapy or with changes in dosage.

PATIENT/FAMILY TEACHING

• Tolerance to feeling of light-headedness develops during therapy. • To reduce hypotensive effect, rise slowly from lying to sitting position, permit legs to dangle momentarily before standing. • Avoid tasks that require alertness, motor skills until response to drug is established. • Dry mouth, drowsiness, dizziness may be an expected response to drug. • Avoid alcohol during therapy. • Coffee, tea may help reduce drowsiness. • Notify physician of worsening depression, unusual behavior, thoughts of suicide. • Avoid tyramine-rich foods.

senna

sen-na
(Ex-Lax, Perdiem, Senexon, Senna-Gen, Senokot)

Do not confuse Perdiem with Pyridium, or Senokot with Depakote.

FIXED-COMBINATION(S)

Gentlax-S, Senokot-S: senna/docusate (a laxative): 8.6 mg/50 mg.

◆CLASSIFICATION

PHARMACOTHERAPEUTIC: GI stimulant. **CLINICAL:** Laxative.

ACTION

Direct effect on intestinal smooth musculature (stimulates intramural nerve plexi). **Therapeutic Effect:** Increases peristalsis, promotes laxative effect.

PHARMACOKINETICS

Route	Onset	Peak	Duration
PO	6–12 hrs	N/A	N/A
Rectal	0.5–2 hrs	N/A	N/A

Minimal absorption after PO administration. Hydrolyzed to active form by enzymes of colonic flora. Absorbed drug metabolized in the liver. Eliminated in feces via biliary system.

USES

Short-term use for constipation, to evacuate colon before bowel/rectal examinations.

PRECAUTIONS

Contraindications: Undiagnosed abdominal pain, appendicitis, intestinal obstruction or perforation, nausea, vomiting. **Cautions:** Prolonged use (longer than 1 wk) may lead to dependency, fluid and electrolyte imbalance, vitamin and mineral deficiency.

⏳ LIFESPAN CONSIDERATIONS

Pregnancy/Lactation: Unknown if distributed in breast milk. **Pregnancy Category C. Children:** Safety and efficacy not established in those younger than 6 yrs. **Elderly:** No age-related precautions noted; monitor for signs of dehydration, electrolyte loss.

INTERACTIONS

DRUG: May decrease transit time of concurrently administered **oral medications,** decreasing absorption. **HERBAL:** None significant. **FOOD:** None known. **LAB VALUES:** May increase serum glucose. May decrease serum potassium.

AVAILABILITY (OTC)

Syrup (Senokot): 8.8 mg/5 ml. **Tablets (Senexon, Senna-Gen, Senokot):** 8.6 mg. **(Ex-Lax, Perdiem):** 15 mg.

ADMINISTRATION/HANDLING

PO
• Give on an empty stomach (decreases time to effect). • Offer at least 6–8 glasses of water/day (aids stool softening). • Avoid giving within 1 hr of other oral medication (decreases drug absorption). • Syrup can be mixed with juice, milk, ice cream.

INDICATIONS/ROUTES/DOSAGE

Constipation
PO (Tablets): ADULTS, ELDERLY, CHILDREN 12 YRS AND OLDER: 2 tablets at bedtime. **Maximum:** 4 tablets twice daily. CHILDREN 6–11 YRS: 1 tablet at bedtime. **Maximum:** 2 tablets twice daily. CHILDREN 2–5 YRS: ½ tablet at bedtime. **Maximum:** 1 tablet twice daily.
PO (Syrup): ADULTS, ELDERLY, CHILDREN 12 YRS AND OLDER: 10–15 ml at bedtime. **Maximum:** 15 ml twice daily. CHILDREN 6–11 YRS: 5–7.5 ml at bedtime. **Maximum:** 7.5 ml twice daily. CHILDREN 2–5 YRS: 2.5–3.75 ml at bedtime. **Maximum:** 3.75 ml twice daily.

Bowel Evacuation
PO: ADULTS, ELDERLY, CHILDREN OLDER THAN 1 YR: 75 ml between 2 PM and 4 PM on day prior to procedure.

SIDE EFFECTS

Frequent: Pink-red, red-violet, red-brown, or yellow-brown discoloration of urine. **Occasional:** Some degree of abdominal discomfort, nausea, mild cramping, faintness.

S

ADVERSE EFFECTS/ TOXIC REACTIONS

Long-term use may result in laxative dependence, chronic constipation, loss of normal bowel function. Prolonged use/overdose may result in electrolyte, metabolic disturbances (e.g., hypokalemia, hypocalcemia, metabolic acidosis or alkalosis), vomiting, muscle weakness, persistent diarrhea, malabsorption, weight loss.

NURSING CONSIDERATIONS

INTERVENTION/EVALUATION

Encourage adequate fluid intake. Assess bowel sounds for peristalsis. Monitor daily pattern of bowel activity, stool consistency. Assess for GI disturbances. Monitor serum electrolytes in pts exposed to prolonged, frequent, excessive use of medication.

PATIENT/FAMILY TEACHING

• Urine may turn pink-red, red-violet, red-brown, yellow-brown (only temporary and not harmful). • Institute measures to promote defecation (increase fluid intake, exercise, high-fiber diet). • Laxative effect generally occurs in 6–12 hrs but may take 24 hrs. • Do not take other oral medication within 1 hr of taking senna (decreased effectiveness).

sertraline TOP 200

ser-tra-leen
(Apo-Sertraline ✦, PMS-Sertraline ✦, <u>Zoloft</u>)

BLACK BOX ALERT Increased risk of suicidal ideation and behavior in children, adolescents, young adults 18–24 yrs with major depressive disorder, other psychiatric disorders.

Do not confuse sertraline with selegiline, Serentil, or Serevent, or Zoloft with Zocor.

◆CLASSIFICATION

PHARMACOTHERAPEUTIC: Serotonin reuptake inhibitor. **CLINICAL:** Antidepressant, anxiolytic, obsessive-compulsive disorder adjunct (see p. 40C).

ACTION

Blocks reuptake of the neurotransmitter serotonin at CNS neuronal presynaptic membranes, increasing availability at postsynaptic receptor sites. **Therapeutic Effect:** Relieves depression, reduces obsessive-compulsive behavior, decreases anxiety.

PHARMACOKINETICS

Incompletely, slowly absorbed from GI tract; food increases absorption. Protein binding: 98%. Widely distributed. Metabolized in liver. Excreted in urine, feces. Not removed by hemodialysis. **Half-life:** 26 hrs.

USES

Treatment of major depressive disorders, panic disorder, obsessive-compulsive disorder (OCD), post-traumatic stress disorder (PTSD), premenstrual dysphoric disorder (PMDD), social anxiety disorder. **OFF-LABEL:** Eating disorders, generalized anxiety disorder (GAD), impulse control disorders, mild dementia-associated agitation in nonpsychotic pts, treatment of paraphilia/hypersexuality.

PRECAUTIONS

Contraindications: MAOI use within 14 days. Concurrent use of oral concentrate with disulfiram. **Cautions:** Seizure disorders, hepatic/renal impairment, suicidal pts, pts at risk for uric acid nephropathy, elderly, pts in third trimester of pregnancy.

⧗ LIFESPAN CONSIDERATIONS

Pregnancy/Lactation: Unknown if drug crosses placenta or is distributed in breast milk. **Pregnancy Category C. Children:** Children and adolescents are at increased risk for suicidal ideation and behavior or worsening of depression, esp. during the first few mos of therapy. **Elderly:** No age-related precautions noted, but lower initial dosages recommended.

INTERACTIONS

DRUG: May increase risk of bleeding with **aspirin, NSAIDs, warfarin.** May increase concentration, risk of toxicity of **highly protein-bound medications (e.g., digoxin, warfarin). MAOIs** may cause neuroleptic malignant syndrome, hypertensive crisis, hyperpyrexia, seizures, serotonin syndrome (diaphoresis, diarrhea, fever, mental changes, restlessness, shivering). May increase concentration, toxicity of **tricyclic antidepressants. HERBAL: Gotu kola, kava kava, St. John's wort, valerian** may increase CNS depression. **St. John's wort** may increase risk of serotonin syndrome. **FOOD:** None known. **LAB VALUES:** May increase total serum cholesterol, triglycerides, AST, ALT. May decrease serum uric acid.

AVAILABILITY (Rx)

Oral Concentrate: 20 mg/ml. **Tablets:** 25 mg, 50 mg, 100 mg.

ADMINISTRATION/HANDLING

PO
• Give with food, milk if GI distress occurs.
• Oral concentrate must be diluted before administration. Mix with 4 oz water, ginger ale, lemon/lime soda, or orange juice *only*. Give immediately after mixing.

INDICATIONS/ROUTES/DOSAGE

Depression
PO: ADULTS: Initially, 50 mg/day. May increase by 50 mg/day at 7-day intervals up to 200 mg/day. **ELDERLY:** Initially, 25 mg/day. May increase by 25–50 mg/day at 7-day intervals up to 200 mg/day.

Obsessive-Compulsive Disorder (OCD)
PO: ADULTS, CHILDREN 13–17 YRS: Initially, 50 mg/day with morning or evening meal. May increase by 50 mg/day at

7-day intervals up to 200 mg/day. **ELDERLY, CHILDREN 6–12 YRS:** Initially, 25 mg/day. May increase by 25–50 mg/day at 7-day intervals. **Maximum:** 200 mg/day.

Panic Disorder, Post-Traumatic Stress Disorder (PTSD), Social Anxiety Disorder (SAD)
PO: ADULTS, ELDERLY: Initially, 25 mg/day. May increase by 50 mg/day at 7-day intervals. Range: 50–200 mg/day. **Maximum:** 200 mg/day.

Premenstrual Dysphoric Disorder (PMDD)
PO: ADULTS: Initially, 50 mg/day. May increase up to 150 mg/day per menstrual cycle in 50-mg increments.

SIDE EFFECTS

Frequent (26%–12%): Headache, nausea, diarrhea, insomnia, drowsiness, dizziness, fatigue, rash, dry mouth. **Occasional (6%–4%):** Anxiety, nervousness, agitation, tremor, dyspepsia (heartburn, indigestion, epigastric pain), diaphoresis, vomiting, constipation, sexual dysfunction, visual disturbances, altered taste. **Rare (less than 3%):** Flatulence, urinary frequency, paresthesia, hot flashes, chills.

ADVERSE EFFECTS/ TOXIC REACTIONS

Serotonin syndrome (seizures, arrhythmias, high fever), neuroleptic malignant syndrome (muscle rigidity, cognitive changes), suicidal ideation have occurred.

NURSING CONSIDERATIONS

BASELINE ASSESSMENT

Assess appearance, behavior, speech patterns, level of interest, mood. For those on long-term therapy, serum hepatic/renal function tests, blood counts should be performed periodically.

INTERVENTION/EVALUATION

Assess mental status for depression, suicidal ideation (esp. at beginning of therapy or change in dosage), anxiety, social function, panic attack. Monitor daily

S

pattern of bowel activity, stool consistency. Assist with ambulation if dizziness occurs.

PATIENT/FAMILY TEACHING
• Dry mouth may be relieved by sugarless gum, sips of water. • Report headache, fatigue, tremor, sexual dysfunction. • Avoid tasks that require alertness, motor skills until response to drug is established (may cause dizziness, drowsiness). • Take with food if nausea occurs. • Inform physician if pregnancy occurs. • Avoid alcohol. • Do not take OTC medications without consulting physician. • Report worsening of depression, suicidal ideation.

---

sevelamer

TOP 200

se-**vel**-a-mer
(<u>Renagel</u>, <u>Renvela</u>)
Do not confuse Renagel with Reglan, Regonol, or Renvela, or sevelamer with Savella.

◆CLASSIFICATION
PHARMACOTHERAPEUTIC: Polymeric phosphate binder. **CLINICAL:** Antihyperphosphatemia agent.

ACTION
Binds with dietary phosphorus in GI tract, allowing phosphorus to be eliminated through normal digestive process, decreasing serum phosphorus level. **Therapeutic Effect:** Decreases incidence of hypercalcemic episodes in pts receiving calcium acetate treatment.

PHARMACOKINETICS
Not absorbed systemically. Unknown if removed by hemodialysis.

USES
Reduction of serum phosphorus in pts with chronic renal disease on hemodialysis.

PRECAUTIONS
Contraindications: Bowel obstruction, hypophosphatemia. **Cautions:** Dysphagia, severe GI tract motility disorders, major GI tract surgery, swallowing disorders.

⌛ LIFESPAN CONSIDERATIONS
Pregnancy/Lactation: Not distributed in breast milk. **Pregnancy Category C. Children:** Safety and efficacy not established. **Elderly:** No age-related precautions noted.

INTERACTIONS
DRUG: None significant. **HERBAL:** None significant. **FOOD:** None known. **LAB VALUES:** None significant.

AVAILABILITY (Rx)
Powder for Oral Suspension (Renvela): 0.8 g/pack, 2.4 g/pack.

 Tablets (Renagel): 400 mg, 800 mg. (Renvela): 800 mg.

ADMINISTRATION/HANDLING
PO
• Give with meals. • Space other medication by at least 1 hr before or 3 hrs after sevelamer. • Give tablets whole; do not break, crush, dissolve, or divide. • **Oral Suspension:** Mix 0.8 g with 30 ml water (2.4 g with 60 ml water). Stir vigorously to suspend (does not dissolve) just prior to drinking.

INDICATIONS/ROUTES/DOSAGE
◄ALERT► 667 mg calcium acetate equivalent to 800 mg sevelamer.

Hyperphosphatemia
PO: ADULTS, ELDERLY: 800–1,600 mg with each meal, depending on severity of hyperphosphatemia (5.5–7.4 mg/dl: 800 mg 3 times daily; 7.5–8.9 mg/dl: 1,200–1,600 mg 3 times daily; 9 mg/dl or greater: 1,600 mg 3 times daily). **Maintenance:** Based on serum phosphorus concentrations. Goal range: 3.5–5.5 mg/dl.

S

Serum Phosphorus Concentration	Dosage
Greater than 5.5 mg/dl	Increase by 400–800 mg per meal at 2-wk intervals
3.5–5.5 mg/dl	Maintain current dosage
Less than 3.5 mg/dl	Decrease by 400–800 mg per meal

SIDE EFFECTS

Frequent (20%–11%): Infection, pain, hypotension, diarrhea, dyspepsia, nausea, vomiting. **Occasional (10%–1%):** Headache, constipation, hypertension, increased cough.

ADVERSE EFFECTS/ TOXIC REACTIONS

Thrombosis occurs rarely.

NURSING CONSIDERATIONS

BASELINE ASSESSMENT

Obtain baseline serum phosphorus; assess for bowel obstruction.

INTERVENTION/EVALUATION

Monitor serum phosphorus, bicarbonate, chloride, calcium.

PATIENT/FAMILY TEACHING

• Take with meals, swallow tablets whole; do not chew, crush, dissolve, or divide tablets. • Report persistent headache, nausea, vomiting, diarrhea, hypotension.

---

sildenafil
TOP 200

sil-**den**-a-fil
(Apo-Sildenafil ✦, Revatio, <u>Viagra</u>)
Do not confuse Revatio with ReVia, sildenafil with silodosin, tadalafil, or vardenafil, or Viagra with Allegra or Vaniqa.

◆CLASSIFICATION

PHARMACOTHERAPEUTIC: Phosphodiesterase-5 enzyme (PDE5) inhibitor. **CLINICAL:** Erectile dysfunction adjunct.

ACTION

Inhibits type 5 cyclic guanosine monophosphate (a specific phosphodiesterase), a predominant isoenzyme of pulmonary vascular smooth muscle, corpus cavernosum of penis. **Therapeutic Effect:** Relaxes smooth muscle, increases blood flow, facilitating erection.

USES

Viagra: Treatment of male erectile dysfunction. **Revatio:** Treatment of pulmonary arterial hypertension (WHO Group I) to improve exercise ability. **OFF-LABEL:** Pulmonary hypertension (WHO II, III, IV); persistent pulmonary hypertension after left ventricular assist device placement.

PHARMACOKINETICS

Route	Onset	Peak	Duration
PO	1 hr	—	2–4 hrs

Rapidly absorbed. Protein binding: 96%. Metabolized in liver. Primarily eliminated in feces. **Half-life:** 4 hrs.

PRECAUTIONS

Contraindications: Concurrent use of nitrates in any form. Concurrent use of protease inhibitors when used for pulmonary arterial hypertension (Revatio). **Cautions:** Cardiac, hepatic/renal impairment; resting hypotension or hypertension; cardiovascular disease including HF, unstable angina; concurrent bosentan, other antihypertensive agents; anatomic deformation of penis; pts who may be predisposed to priapism (sickle cell anemia, multiple myeloma, leukemia). **Pregnancy Category B.**

INTERACTIONS

DRUG: Alpha-adrenergic blocking agents may increase symptomatic hy-

S

✦ Canadian trade name   🐄 Non-Crushable Drug   🔳 High Alert drug

potension. **Protease inhibitors** may increase concentration, toxicity. **Cimetidine, CYP3A4 inhibitors** (e.g., **erythromycin, itraconazole, ketoconazole**) may increase concentration. Potentiates hypotensive effects of **nitrates. HERBAL: St. John's wort** may decrease concentration. **FOOD: High-fat meals** delay maximum effectiveness by 1 hr. **Grapefruit products** may decrease blood pressure, increase heart rate. **LAB VALUES:** None known.

AVAILABILITY (Rx)

Injection, Solution: 0.8 mg/ml (12.5 ml). **Tablets: (Revatio):** 20 mg. **(Viagra):** 25 mg, 50 mg, 100 mg.

ADMINISTRATION/HANDLING

PO
• **Viagra:** May take approximately 1 hr before sexual activity but may be taken any time from 30 min–4 hrs before sexual activity. • Revatio may be given without regard to meals. • Give tablets at least 4–6 hrs apart.

 IV

• Give as bolus injection.

INDICATIONS/ROUTES/DOSAGE

Erectile Dysfunction
PO: ADULTS: 50 mg (30 min–4 hrs before sexual activity). Range: 25–100 mg. Maximum dosing frequency is once a day. **ELDERLY OLDER THAN 65 YRS, CREATININE CLEARANCE LESS THAN 30 ML/MIN:** Consider starting dose of 25 mg. **CONCURRENT PROTEASE INHIBITOR:** (Viagra) 25 mg q48h.

Pulmonary Arterial Hypertension
PO: ADULTS, ELDERLY: 20 mg 3 times daily taken 4–6 hrs apart.
IV: ADULTS, ELDERLY: 10 mg 3 times daily.

SIDE EFFECTS

Frequent: Headache (16%), flushing (10%). **Occasional (7%–3%):** Dyspepsia (heartburn, indigestion, epigastric pain), nasal congestion, UTI, abnormal vision, diarrhea. **Rare (2%):** Dizziness, rash.

ADVERSE EFFECTS/TOXIC REACTIONS

Prolonged erections (lasting over 4 hrs), priapism (painful erections lasting over 6 hrs) occur rarely. Sudden hearing decrease or loss; sudden loss of vision in one or both eyes has been reported.

NURSING CONSIDERATIONS

BASELINE ASSESSMENT
Viagra: Determine if pt has other medical conditions, including angina, cardiac disease, benign prostatic hyperplasia (BPH). Assess pt's baseline serum renal/hepatic function. **Revatio:** Obtain baseline ABGs; assess pulmonary function, cardiovascular status.

INTERVENTION/EVALUATION
Monitor pulse, B/P, oxygen saturation, PaO_2.

PATIENT/FAMILY TEACHING
• Sildenafil has no effect in absence of sexual stimulation. • Seek treatment immediately if erection lasts longer than 4 hrs. • Avoid nitrate drugs while taking sildenafil. • Inform pt that Revatio is not to be taken with Viagra or other PDE5 inhibitors. • Seek medical attention in event of sudden loss of vision or sudden decrease or loss of hearing (may be accompanied by tinnitus or dizziness).

silodosin

sil-oh-**doe**-sin
(Rapaflo)
Do not confuse Rapaflo with Rapamune.

◆CLASSIFICATION

PHARMACOTHERAPEUTIC: Alpha$_1$-adrenergic blocker. **CLINICAL:** Benign prostatic hyperplasia agent.

S

ACTION

Blocks alpha-adrenergic receptors. Produces vasodilation, decreases peripheral resistance, targets receptors around bladder neck, prostate. **Therapeutic Effect:** Relaxes smooth muscle, improves urinary flow.

PHARMACOKINETICS

Well absorbed following PO administration. Widely distributed. Protein binding: 97%. Metabolized in liver. Primarily excreted in feces with a lesser amount eliminated in urine. **Half-life:** 9–13 hrs.

USES

Treatment of signs and symptoms of benign prostatic hyperplasia.

PRECAUTIONS

Contraindications: Severe renal impairment (creatinine clearance less than 30 ml/min), severe hepatic impairment (Child-Pugh score equal to or less than 10), concurrent administration with ketoconazole, clarithromycin, itraconazole, ritonavir. **Cautions:** Moderate renal/hepatic impairment.

⌛ LIFESPAN CONSIDERATIONS

Pregnancy/Lactation: Not indicated for use in women. **Pregnancy Category B. Children:** Not indicated for this pt population. **Elderly:** No age-related precautions noted.

INTERACTIONS

DRUG: Other **alpha-adrenergic blocking agents (alfuzosin, doxazosin, prazosin, tamsulosin, terazosin)** may have additive effect. **Diltiazem, erythromycin, verapamil** may increase concentration. **CYP3A4 inhibitors (e.g., clarithromycin, itraconazole, ketoconazole, ritonavir)** significantly increase concentration (concurrent use contraindicated). **HERBAL:** None significant. **FOOD: Grapefruit, grapefruit juice** may increase risk of orthostatic hypotension. **LAB VALUES:** None significant.

AVAILABILITY (Rx)

🔖 **Capsules:** 4 mg, 8 mg.

ADMINISTRATION/HANDLING

PO

• Give with a meal. • Swallow whole; do not break, crush, dissolve, or divide capsule.

INDICATIONS/ROUTES/DOSAGE

Benign Prostatic Hyperplasia
PO: ADULTS, MILD RENAL IMPAIRMENT: 8 mg once daily, with a meal.

Moderate Renal Impairment (Creatinine Clearance 30–50 ml/min)
PO: ADULTS: 4 mg once daily, with a meal (contraindicated with creatinine clearance less than 30 ml/min).

SIDE EFFECTS

Frequent: (28%): Retrograde ejaculation. **Occasional (3%–2%):** Dizziness, diarrhea, orthostatic hypotension, headache, nasopharyngitis, nasal congestion. **Rare: (1% or Less):** Insomnia, sinusitis, abdominal pain, asthenia (loss of strength, energy).

ADVERSE EFFECTS/ TOXIC REACTIONS

First-dose syncope (orthostatic hypotension with sudden loss of consciousness) may occur shortly after giving initial dose. May be preceded by tachycardia (120–160 beats/min). Recovery occurs spontaneously.

NURSING CONSIDERATIONS

BASELINE ASSESSMENT

Obtain baseline renal/hepatic function tests. Give first dose at bedtime. If initial dose is given during daytime, assess B/P, pulse immediately before dose, and q15–30 min after (be alert to B/P fluctuations, postural hypotension).

INTERVENTION/EVALUATION

Assist with ambulation if dizziness occurs. Monitor renal/hepatic function. Monitor daily pattern of bowel activity, stool consistency.

S

♣ Canadian trade name Non-Crushable Drug 🔲 High Alert drug

PATIENT/FAMILY TEACHING

• Use caution when getting up from sitting or lying position. • Avoid tasks that require alertness, motor skills until response to drug is established. • Do not chew, crush, dissolve, or divide capsule.

silver sulfadiazine

sul-fa-**dye**-a-zeen
(Flamazine ✦, Silvadene, SSD, SSD AF, Thermazene)

◆ **CLASSIFICATION**

PHARMACOTHERAPEUTIC: Anti-infective. **CLINICAL:** Anti-bacterial burn preparation.

ACTION

Acts on cell wall/cell membrane in concentrations selectively toxic to bacteria. **Therapeutic Effect:** Produces bactericidal effect.

USES

Prevention, treatment of infection in second- and third-degree burns.

PRECAUTIONS

Contraindications: Premature neonates, infants younger than 2 mos. **Cautions:** Renal/hepatic impairment, G6PD deficiency. **Pregnancy Category B.**

INTERACTIONS

DRUG: Concurrent use may inactivate **collagenase, papain, sutilains. HERBAL:** None significant. **FOOD:** None known. **LAB VALUES:** None significant.

AVAILABILITY (Rx)

Topical Cream (Silvadene, SSD, SSD AF, Thermazene): 1% (10 mg/g).

ADMINISTRATION/HANDLING

Topical

• Apply to cleansed, debrided burns using sterile glove. • Keep burn areas covered with silver sulfadiazine cream at all times; reapply to areas where removed by pt activity. • Dressings may be ordered on individual basis.

INDICATIONS/ROUTES/DOSAGE

Usual Topical Dosage
Topical: ADULTS, ELDERLY, CHILDREN: Apply 1–2 times daily.

SIDE EFFECTS

Side effects characteristic of all sulfonamides may occur when systemically absorbed (extensive burn areas [over 20% of body surface]): anorexia, nausea, vomiting, headache, diarrhea, dizziness, photosensitivity, arthralgia. **Frequent:** Burning, stinging sensation at treatment site. **Occasional:** Brown-gray skin discoloration, rash, itching. **Rare:** Increased sensitivity of skin to sunlight.

ADVERSE EFFECTS/TOXIC REACTIONS

Hemolytic anemia, hypoglycemia, diuresis, peripheral neuropathy, Stevens-Johnson syndrome, agranulocytosis, disseminated lupus erythematosus, anaphylaxis, hepatitis, toxic nephrosis possible with significant systemic absorption. Fungal superinfections may occur. Interstitial nephritis occurs rarely.

NURSING CONSIDERATIONS

BASELINE ASSESSMENT

Determine initial CBC, serum renal/hepatic function test results.

INTERVENTION/EVALUATION

Monitor serum electrolytes, urinalysis, renal function, CBC if burns are extensive, therapy prolonged.

PATIENT/FAMILY TEACHING

• For external use only; may discolor skin.

simeprevir

sim-**e**-pre-vir
(Olysio)
Do not confuse simeprevir with sofosbuvir.

◆CLASSIFICATION

PHARMACOTHERAPEUTIC: Protease inhibitor. **CLINICAL:** Antiviral.

ACTION

Inhibits hepatitis C virus (HCV) protease needed for cleavage of HCV-encoded polyproteins by binding to active serine protease sites. **Therapeutic Effect:** Inhibits viral replication of hepatitis C virus.

PHARMACOKINETICS

Well absorbed after PO administration. Metabolized in liver. Protein binding: 99.9%. Peak plasma concentration: 4–6 hrs. Excreted primarily in feces (91%). Half-life: 10–13 hrs.

USES

Treatment of chronic hepatitis C virus (genotype 1), in combination with peginterferon alfa and ribavirin. Indicated for pts with compensated liver disease, including cirrhosis, who are previously untreated or who have failed previous interferon and ribavirin therapy.

PRECAUTIONS

◄**ALERT►** Safety and efficacy not established in moderate to severe hepatic impairment.
Contraindications: Pregnancy (Category X), breastfeeding, any contraindications to peginterferon alfa or ribavirin. **Cautions:** Pts of East Asian ancestry, sulfa allergy, or history of HIV, sunburns, concurrent use of moderate to strong CYP3A4 inhibitors or inducers.

⌛ LIFESPAN CONSIDERATIONS

Pregnancy/Lactation: Strictly avoid pregnancy. May cause birth defects or fetal demise. **Pregnancy Category C (X when used in ribavirin).** Women of child-bearing age must use two different forms of reliable of birth control during treatment and for at least 6 mos after discontinuation. Do not initiate therapy until negative pregnancy test confirmed. Unknown if distributed in breast milk. Breastfeeding contraindicated. **Children:** Safety and efficacy not established. **Elderly:** No age-related precautions noted. **Race:** Pts of East Asian ancestry may have increased risk of adverse reactions due to increased drug exposure/sensitivity.

INTERACTIONS

DRUG: May increase concentration/effects of **antiarrhythmics (e.g., amiodarone, quinidine), calcium channel blockers (e.g., felodipine, nifedipine), cyclosporine, digoxin, sedative/hypnotics (e.g., midazolam, triazolam), statins (e.g., atorvastatin, simvastatin), sildenafil, vardenafil.** May decrease concentration/effect of **sirolimus, tacrolimus. CYP3A4 inducers (e.g., carbamazepine, rifampin)** may decrease concentration/effect. **CYP3A4 inhibitors (e.g., itraconazole, fluconazole, clarithromycin, ritonavir)** may increase concentration/effect. **HERBAL: St. John's wort** may decrease concentration/effect. **Milk thistle (silybum marianum)** may increase concentration/effect. **FOOD:** None known. **LAB VALUES:** May increase serum alkaline phosphatase, bilirubin.

AVAILABILITY (Rx)

Capsules: 150 mg.

ADMINISTRATION/HANDLING

PO
• Administer with food. • Administer tablet whole; do not break, crush, or divide.

INDICATIONS/ROUTES/DOSAGE

◄**ALERT►** Must use in combination with peginterferon alfa and ribavirin. Not recommended as monotherapy. Dose reduction of simeprevir not recommended.

S

Chronic Hepatitis C
PO: ADULTS/ELDERLY: 150 mg daily with food for 12 wks (with peginterferon alfa and ribavirin).
Treatment Naïve, Prior Relapsers (Including Cirrhosis): Extend peginterferon alfa and ribavirin therapy for additional 12 wks after completing 12-wk triple therapy (24 wks total).
Prior Nonresponders (Including Cirrhosis): Extend peginterferon alfa and ribavirin therapy for additional 36 wks after completing 12-wk triple therapy (48 wks total).

Treatment Futility
If HCV RNA viral load greater than or equal to 25 IU/ml at wk 4, discontinue simeprevir, peginterferon alfa, and ribavirin. If HCV RNA viral load greater than or equal to 25 IU/ml at wk 12 or 24, discontinue peginterferon alfa and ribavirin (simeprevir already completed at wk 12). Discontinue therapy if serious adverse effects occur.

SIDE EFFECTS

Frequent (28%–22%): Rash, pruritus, nausea. **Occasional (16%–12%):** Myalgia, dyspnea.

ADVERSE EFFECTS/ TOXIC REACTIONS

Increased risk of thromboembolic events associated with peginterferon alfa. Dermatologic events/photosensitivity including generalized rash, erythema, eczema, maculopapular rash, dermatitis, skin exfoliation, rash erythematosus, urticaria, allergic dermatitis, cutaneous vasculitis, skin eruption, photodermatosis, sunburn reported. Mild to moderate dyspnea reported in 12% of pts. Pts of East Asian ancestry may have increased risk of photosensitivity.

NURSING CONSIDERATIONS

BASELINE ASSESSMENT

Obtain baseline vital signs, CBC, HCV-RNA level, complete metabolic panel, liver function test. Confirm hepatitis C genotype. Receive full history of home medications including herbal products. Screen for contraindications to peginterferon alfa and ribavirin. Confirm negative pregnancy test before initiating treatment. Question history of anemia, HIV, hepatitis B, liver transplantation, pulmonary disease, renal impairment. Conduct dermatologic exam, noting baseline skin characteristics, moles, lesions. Question if sunburn history.

INTERVENTION/EVALUATION

Assess vital signs routinely. Monitor CBC, HCV-RNA levels, electrolytes accordingly. Obtain urine pregnancy every mo and for 6 mos after discontinuation. Reinforce birth control compliance. Monitor international normalized ratio (INR) level if on warfarin. Monitor for bruising, dyspnea, hematuria, DVT, pulmonary embolism. Encourage nutritional intake and assess for anorexia, weight loss. Monitor for intrauterine device failures if applicable. Reinforce birth control compliance.

PATIENT/FAMILY TEACHING

• Treatment must be used in combination with peginterferon, ribavirin. Inform pts of side effects/contraindications of triple-medication regimen. Blood levels will be drawn routinely. • Report any newly prescribed medications. • Do not take herbal products. • Women of childbearing age must use two different forms of reliable birth control during treatment and for at least 6 mos after treatment. Do not breastfeed. Notify physician if female partner becomes pregnant. • Report difficulty breathing, weakness, dizziness, weight loss. • Avoid alcohol. • Take with meals. Do not use tanning beds. Limit sun exposure; use sun protective measures. Immediately report any changes to skin including rash, skin peeling, ulcers, or new moles/lesions.

simethicone

sye-**meth**-i-kone
(Gas-X, Mytab Gas, Ovol ✽, Phazyme)

Do not confuse simethicone with cimetidine.

FIXED-COMBINATION(S)

Mylanta, Extra Strength Maalox, Aludrox: simethicone/magnesium and aluminum hydroxide (antacids): 20 mg/200 mg/200 mg, 40 mg/400 mg/400 mg.

◆CLASSIFICATION

PHARMACOTHERAPEUTIC: Antiflatulent. **CLINICAL:** Antiflatulent.

ACTION

Changes surface tension of gas bubbles, allowing easier elimination of gas. **Therapeutic Effect:** Disperses, prevents formation of gas pockets in GI tract.

PHARMACOKINETICS

Does not appear to be absorbed from GI tract. Excreted unchanged in feces.

USES

Treatment of flatulence, gastric bloating, postop gas pain, when gas retention may be problem (i.e., peptic ulcer, spastic colon, air swallowing).

PRECAUTIONS

Contraindications: None known. **Cautions:** None known.

⌛ LIFESPAN CONSIDERATIONS

Pregnancy/Lactation: Unknown if drug crosses placenta or is distributed in breast milk. **Pregnancy Category C. Children/Elderly:** No age-related precautions noted.

INTERACTIONS

DRUG: None significant. **HERBAL:** None significant. **FOOD:** None known. **LAB VALUES:** None significant.

AVAILABILITY (OTC)

Capsules: 125 mg, 180 mg. **Oral Drops:** 40 mg/0.6 ml. **Tablets (Chewable):** 80 mg, 125 mg.

ADMINISTRATION/HANDLING

PO
• Give after meals and at bedtime as needed. • Chewable tablets are to be chewed thoroughly before swallowing. • Shake suspension well before using.

INDICATIONS/ROUTES/DOSAGE

Antiflatulent
PO: ADULTS, ELDERLY, CHILDREN 12 YRS AND OLDER: 40–250 mg after meals and at bedtime. **Maximum:** 500 mg/day. **CHILDREN 2–11 YRS:** 40 mg 4 times a day.
CHILDREN YOUNGER THAN 2 YRS: 20 mg 4 times a day.

SIDE EFFECTS

None known.

ADVERSE EFFECTS/TOXIC REACTIONS

None known.

NURSING CONSIDERATIONS

INTERVENTION/EVALUATION
Evaluate for therapeutic response (relief of flatulence, abdominal bloating).

PATIENT/FAMILY TEACHING
• Avoid carbonated beverages.• To reduce air swallowing, take after meals and at bedtime for best results.

---

simvastatin   TOP 200

sim-va-**sta**-tin
(Apo-Simvastatin ✤, Zocor)
Do not confuse simvastatin with atorvastatin, lovastatin, nystatin, pitavastatin, or pravastatin, or Zocor with Cozaar, Lipitor, Zoloft, or Zyrtec.

FIXED-COMBINATION(S)

Juvisync: simvastatin/sitagliptin (an antidiabetic agent): 10 mg/100 mg, 20 mg/100 mg, 40 mg/100 mg. **Simcor:**

S

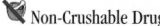

simvastatin/niacin (an antilipemic agent): 20 mg/500 mg, 40 mg/500 mg, 20 mg/750 mg, 20 mg/1,000 mg, 40 mg/1,000 mg. **Vytorin:** simvastatin/ezetimibe (a cholesterol absorption inhibitor): 10 mg/10 mg, 20 mg/10 mg, 40 mg/10 mg, 80 mg/10 mg.

◆CLASSIFICATION

PHARMACOTHERAPEUTIC: Hydroxymethylglutaryl-CoA (HMG-CoA) reductase inhibitor. **CLINICAL:** Antihyperlipidemic (see p. 59C).

ACTION

Interferes with cholesterol biosynthesis by inhibiting conversion of the enzyme HMG-CoA to mevalonate. **Therapeutic Effect:** Decreases LDL, cholesterol, VLDL, triglyceride levels; slight increase in HDL concentration.

PHARMACOKINETICS

Well absorbed from GI tract. Protein binding: 95%. Metabolized in liver. Primarily eliminated in feces. Unknown if removed by hemodialysis.

Route	Onset	Peak	Duration
PO (to reduce cholesterol)	3 days	14 days	N/A

USES

Secondary prevention of cardiovascular events in pts with hypercholesterolemia and coronary heart disease (CHD) or at high risk for CHD. Treatment of hyperlipidemias to reduce elevations in total serum cholesterol, LDL-C, apolipoprotein B, triglycerides, VLDL-C and increase HDL-C. Treatment of homozygous familial hypercholesterolemia. Treatment of heterozygous familial hypercholesterolemia in adolescents (10–17 yrs, females more than 1 yr postmenarche).

PRECAUTIONS

Contraindications: Active hepatic disease or unexplained, persistent elevations of hepatic function test results, pregnancy, breastfeeding, concurrent use of strong CYP3A4 inhibitors (e.g., erythromycin). **Cautions:** History of hepatic disease, diabetes, severe renal impairment, substantial alcohol consumption. Withholding or discontinuing simvastatin may be necessary when pt is at risk for renal failure secondary to rhabdomyolysis.

⧗ LIFESPAN CONSIDERATIONS

Pregnancy/Lactation: Contraindicated in pregnancy (suppression of cholesterol biosynthesis may cause fetal toxicity), lactation. Risk of serious adverse reactions in breastfeeding infants. **Pregnancy Category X. Children:** Safety and efficacy not established in children less than 10 yrs of age or in premenarcheal girls. **Elderly:** No age-related precautions noted.

INTERACTIONS

DRUG: Cyclosporine, CYP3A4 inhibitors (e.g., ketoconazole, erythromycin), amiodarone, calcium channel blockers, colchicine, fibrates, gemfibrozil, niacin, ranolazine may increase risk of acute renal failure, rhabdomyolysis. **HERBAL: St. John's wort** may decrease concentration. **FOOD: Grapefruit products** may increase concentration, toxicity. **Red yeast rice** contains 2.4 mg **lovastatin** per 600 mg rice. **LAB VALUES:** May increase serum creatine kinase (CK), transaminase.

AVAILABILITY (Rx)

Tablets: 5 mg, 10 mg, 20 mg, 40 mg, 80 mg.

ADMINISTRATION/HANDLING

PO
• Give without regard to meals. • Administer in evening for maximum efficacy.

INDICATIONS/ROUTES/DOSAGE

Note: Limit 80 mg dose to pts taking simvastatin longer than 12 months without evidence of myopathy.

Prevention of Cardiovascular Events, Hyperlipidemias
PO: ADULTS, ELDERLY: 20–40 mg once a day. Range: 5–80 mg/day. (80 mg not recommended).

Homozygous Familial Hypercholesterolemia
PO: ADULTS, ELDERLY: 40 mg once a day in evening.

Heterozygous Familial Hypercholesterolemia
PO: CHILDREN 10–17 YRS: 10 mg once a day in evening. Range: 10–40 mg/day.

Dosing Adjustment with Medications
Cyclosporine, gemfibrozil: Do not exceed 10 mg/day. **Amiodarone, amlodipine, ranolazine:** Do not exceed 20 mg/day. **Diltiazem, verapamil:** Do not exceed 10 mg/day.

Dosage In Renal Impairment
Creatinine clearance less than 30 ml/min: initially, 5 mg/day.

SIDE EFFECTS

Generally well tolerated. Side effects are usually mild and transient. **Occasional (3%–2%):** Headache, abdominal pain/cramps, constipation, upper respiratory tract infection. **Rare (less than 2%):** Diarrhea, flatulence, asthenia (loss of strength, energy), nausea/vomiting, depression.

ADVERSE EFFECTS/ TOXIC REACTIONS

Potential for lens opacities. Hypersensitivity reaction, hepatitis occur rarely. Myopathy (muscle pain, tenderness, weakness with elevated serum creatine kinase [CK], sometimes taking the form of rhabdomyolysis) has occurred.

NURSING CONSIDERATIONS

BASELINE ASSESSMENT

Obtain dietary history, esp. fat consumption. Question for possibility of pregnancy before initiating therapy (Pregnancy Category X). Question for history

of hypersensitivity to simvastatin. Assess baseline lab results: serum cholesterol, triglycerides, hepatic function tests.

INTERVENTION/EVALUATION

Monitor serum cholesterol, triglyceride lab results for therapeutic response. Monitor hepatic function tests. Monitor daily pattern of bowel activity, stool consistency. Assess for headache, myopathy.

PATIENT/FAMILY TEACHING

• Use appropriate contraceptive measures (Pregnancy Category X). • Periodic lab tests are essential part of therapy. • Maintain appropriate diet. Avoid grapefruit products. • Report unexplained muscle pain, tenderness, weakness.

---

sirolimus

sir-oh-**le**-mus
(Rapamune)

BLACK BOX ALERT Increased susceptibility to infection and potential for development of lymphoma. Not recommended for liver or lung transplant pts. Use only by physicians experienced in immunosuppressive therapy and management of transplant pts.
Do not confuse Rapamune with Rapaflo, or sirolimus with everolimus, pimecrolimus, tacrolimus, or temsirolimus.

◆CLASSIFICATION

PHARMACOTHERAPEUTIC: Immunosuppressant. **CLINICAL:** Immunosuppressant (see p. 123C).

ACTION

Inhibits T-lymphocyte proliferation induced by stimulation of cell surface receptors, mitogens, alloantigens, lymphokines. Prevents activation of enzyme target of rapamycin (TOR), a key regulatory kinase in cell cycle progression. **Therapeutic Effect:** Inhibits prolifera-

S

tion of T and B cells (essential components of immune response), prevents organ transplant rejection.

PHARMACOKINETICS

Rapidly absorbed from GI tract. Protein binding: 92%. Extensively metabolized in liver. Primarily eliminated in feces; minimal excretion in urine. **Half-life:** 57–63 hrs.

USES

Prophylaxis of organ rejection in pts after renal transplant in combination with cyclosporine and corticosteroids, including treatment of high immunologic risk in renal transplant recipient. **OFF-LABEL:** Immunosuppression in peripheral stem cell/bone marrow transplantation. Prophylaxis of organ rejection in heart transplant recipients. Treatment of soft tissue sarcoma. Treatment of refractory acute or chronic graft-vs-host disease.

PRECAUTIONS

Contraindications: None known. **Cautions:** Cardiovascular disease (HF, hypertension); pulmonary disease, hepatic impairment, renal impairment, hyperlipidemia, perioperative period due to increased chance of surgical complications from impaired wound and tissue healing.

⌛ LIFESPAN CONSIDERATIONS

Pregnancy/Lactation: Unknown if drug crosses placenta or is distributed in breast milk. **Pregnancy Category C. Children:** Safety and efficacy not established in those younger than 13 yrs. **Elderly:** No age-related precautions noted.

INTERACTIONS

DRUG: CYP3A4 inducers (e.g., **carbamazepine, phenobarbital, phenytoin, rifabutin, rifampin, rifapentine**) may decrease concentration/effects. **CYP3A4 inhibitors** (e.g., **clarithromycin, diltiazem, erythromycin, itraconazole, ketoconazole, verapamil, voriconazole**) may increase concentration, toxic-

ity. May increase concentration/effects of **cyclosporine. HERBAL: St. John's wort** may decrease concentration. **Cat's claw, echinacea** possess immunostimulant properties. **Garlic, ginger, ginseng** may increase hypoglycemia. **FOOD: Grapefruit products** may increase risk of myelotoxicity nephrotoxicity. **LAB VALUES:** May increase serum ALT, AST, alkaline phosphatase, LDH, BUN, creatine phosphate, cholesterol, triglycerides, creatinine. May alter WBC, serum glucose, calcium. May decrease Hgb, Hct.

AVAILABILITY (Rx)

Oral Solution: 1 mg/ml.

🔖 **Tablets:** 0.5 mg, 1 mg, 2 mg.

ADMINISTRATION/HANDLING

• Doses should be taken 4 hrs after cyclosporine. • Take consistently with or without food. • Do not break, crush, dissolve, or divide tablets. • Mix oral solution with only water or orange juice, stir vigorously, drink immediately.

INDICATIONS/ROUTES/DOSAGE

◄**ALERT**► Tablets and oral solution are not bioequivalent.

Prevention of Organ Transplant Rejection (Low to Moderate Risk)
PO: ADULTS, CHILDREN 13 YRS AND OLDER WEIGHING MORE THAN 40 KG: Loading dose: 6 mg. Maintenance: 2 mg/day. **ADULTS, CHILDREN 13 YRS AND OLDER WEIGHING LESS THAN 40 KG:** Loading dose: 3 mg/m². Maintenance: 1 mg/m²/day.

Prevention of Organ Transplant Rejection (High Risk)
PO: ADULTS: Loading dose: Up to 15 mg on day 1. Maintenance: 5 mg/day.

Dosage in Hepatic Impairment
Loading dose: No change. Maintenance dose: Mild to moderate impairment: reduce dose by 33%; severe impairment: reduce dose by 50%.

SIDE EFFECTS

Occasional: Hypercholesterolemia, hyperlipidemia, hypertension, rash. **High doses (5 mg/day):** Anemia, arthralgia, diarrhea, hypokalemia, thrombocytopenia. **Rare:** Peripheral edema.

ADVERSE EFFECTS/ TOXIC REACTIONS

Hepatotoxicity occurs rarely. Skin carcinoma (including basal cell, squamous cell, melanoma) has been observed.

NURSING CONSIDERATIONS

BASELINE ASSESSMENT

Obtain baseline serum hepatic profile. Assess for pregnancy, lactation. Question for medication usage (esp. cyclosporine, diltiazem, ketoconazole, rifampin). Determine if pt has chickenpox, herpes zoster, malignancy, infection.

INTERVENTION/EVALUATION

Monitor serum renal/hepatic function periodically. Monitor cholesterol, triglycerides, platelets, Hgb.

PATIENT/FAMILY TEACHING

• Avoid those with colds, other infections. • Avoid grapefruit products. • Avoid exposure to sunlight, artificial light sources. • Strict monitoring is essential in identifying, preventing symptoms of organ rejection. • Do not chew, crush, dissolve, or divide tablets.

---

sitagliptin   TOP 200 | HIGH ALERT

sit-a-**glip**-tin
(Januvia)
Do not confuse Januvia with Enjuvia, Jantoven, or Janumet, or sitagliptin with saxagliptin or sumatriptan.

FIXED-COMBINATION(S)

Janumet, Janumet XR: sitagliptin/metformin (an antidiabetic): 50 mg/500 mg, 50 mg/1,000 mg. **Juvisync:** sitagliptin/simvastatin (an antilipidemic agent): 100 mg/10 mg, 100 mg/20 mg, 100 mg/40 mg.

◆CLASSIFICATION

PHARMACOTHERAPEUTIC: DPP-4 inhibitors (gliptins). **CLINICAL:** Antidiabetic agent (see p. 44C).

ACTION

Slows inactivation of incretin hormones (involved in regulation of glucose homeostasis). **Therapeutic Effect:** Increases synthesis, postmeal release of insulin from pancreatic cells; lowers postmeal glucagon secretion leading to reduced glucose output from liver.

PHARMACOKINETICS

Route	Onset	Peak	Duration
PO	N/A	1–4 hrs	24 hrs

Rapidly absorbed following PO administration. Protein binding: 38%. Eliminated mainly in urine, with lesser amount excreted in feces. **Half-life:** 12 hrs.

USES

Adjunctive treatment to diet, exercise to improve glycemic control in pts with type 2 diabetes mellitus as monotherapy or in combination with other antidiabetic agents.

PRECAUTIONS

Contraindications: None known. **Cautions:** Type I diabetes, diabetic ketoacidosis, renal impairment, end-stage renal disease, history of pancreatitis, angioedema with other DPP-4 inhibitors. Concurrent use of other glucose-lowering agents may increase risk of hypoglycemia.

⧖ LIFESPAN CONSIDERATIONS

Pregnancy/Lactation: Unknown if distributed in breast milk. **Pregnancy Category B. Children:** Safety and efficacy not established. **Elderly:** No age-related precautions noted.

S

INTERACTIONS

DRUG: None known. **HERBAL:** None significant. **FOOD:** None known. **LAB VALUES:** May slightly increase WBCs, particularly neutrophil count. May increase serum creatinine.

AVAILABILITY (Rx)

Tablets (Film-Coated): 25 mg, 50 mg, 100 mg.

ADMINISTRATION/HANDLING

PO

• May give without regard to food. • Do not break, crush, dissolve, or divide film-coated tablets.

INDICATIONS/ROUTES/DOSAGE

Type 2 Diabetes
PO: ADULTS OVER 18 YRS, ELDERLY: 100 mg once daily.

Moderate Renal Impairment
Creatinine Clearance Equal to or Greater Than 30 ml/min to Less Than 50 ml/min: 50 mg once daily.

Severe Renal Impairment
Creatinine Clearance Less Than 30 ml/min: Dialysis: 25 mg once daily.

SIDE EFFECTS

Occasional (5% and greater): Headache, nasopharyngitis. Rare (3%–1%): Diarrhea, abdominal pain, nausea.

ADVERSE EFFECTS/ TOXIC REACTIONS

Hypersensitivity reactions including angioedema, Stevens-Johnson syndrome reported. Acute pancreatitis occurs rarely.

NURSING CONSIDERATIONS

BASELINE ASSESSMENT

Check serum glucose concentration before administration. Assess renal function. Discuss lifestyle to determine extent of learning, emotional needs. Ensure follow-up instruction if pt, family do not thoroughly understand diabetes management, glucose-testing technique.

INTERVENTION/EVALUATION

Monitor serum glucose, Hbg A1c, BUN, creatinine. Assess for hypoglycemia (diaphoresis, tremor, dizziness, anxiety, headache, tachycardia, perioral numbness, hunger, diplopia, difficulty concentrating), hyperglycemia (polyuria, polyphagia, polydipsia, nausea, vomiting, dim vision, fatigue, deep, rapid breathing). Be alert to conditions that alter glucose requirements (fever, increased activity, stress, trauma, surgical procedures).

PATIENT/FAMILY TEACHING

• Diabetes mellitus requires lifelong control. • Prescribed diet, exercise are principal part of treatment; do not skip, delay meals. • Continue to adhere to dietary instructions, regular exercise program, regular testing of serum glucose. • When taking combination drug therapy or when glucose demands are altered (fever, infection, trauma, stress, heavy physical activity), have source of glucose available to treat symptoms of hypoglycemia. • Report nausea, vomiting, anorexia, severe abdominal pain, pancreatitis.

sodium bicarbonate

soe-dee-um bye-**kar**-boe-nate (Neut)

◆CLASSIFICATION

PHARMACOTHERAPEUTIC: Alkalinizing agent. **CLINICAL:** Antacid electrolyte, urinary/systemic alkalinizer.

ACTION

Dissociates to provide bicarbonate ion. **Therapeutic Effect:** Neutralizes hydrogen ion concentration, raises blood, urinary pH.

PHARMACOKINETICS

Route	Onset	Peak	Duration
PO	15 min	N/A	1–3 hrs
IV	Immediate	N/A	8–10 min

Well absorbed following PO administration, sodium bicarbonate dissociates to sodium and bicarbonate ions. With increased hydrogen ion concentrations, bicarbonate ions combine with hydrogen ions to form carbonic acid, which then dissociates to CO_2, which is excreted by the lungs. Plasma concentration regulated by kidney (ability to form, excrete bicarbonate).

USES

Management of metabolic acidosis, antacid, alkalinization of urine, stabilizes acid-base status in cardiac arrest, life-threatening hyperkalemia. **OFF-LABEL:** Prevention of contrast-induced nephropathy.

PRECAUTIONS

Contraindications: Hypernatremia, unknown abdominal pain, excessive chloride loss, hypocalcemia, metabolic, respiratory alkalosis; severe pulmonary edema. **Cautions:** HF, edematous states, renal insufficiency, cirrhosis.

⧖ LIFESPAN CONSIDERATIONS

Pregnancy/Lactation: May produce hypernatremia, increase tendon reflexes in neonate or fetus whose mother is administered chronically high doses. May be distributed in breast milk. **Pregnancy Category C. Children:** No age-related precautions noted. Do not use as antacid in those younger than 6 yrs. **Elderly:** Age-related renal impairment may require dosage adjustment.

INTERACTIONS

DRUG: May increase concentration, toxicity of **quinidine, quinine.** May decrease effect of **lithium. HERBAL:** None significant. **FOOD: Milk, other dairy products** may result in milk-alkali syndrome. **LAB VALUES:** May increase serum, urinary pH.

AVAILABILITY

Injection Solution (Rx): 0.5 mEq/ml (4.2%), 1 mEq/ml (8.4%). **Tablets (OTC):** 325 mg, 650 mg.

ADMINISTRATION/HANDLING

 IV

◀ALERT▶ For direct IV administration in neonates or infants, use 0.5 mEq/ml concentration.

Reconstitution • May give undiluted.
Rate of Administration • For IV push, give up to 1 mEq/kg over 1–3 min for cardiac arrest. • For IV infusion, do not exceed rate of infusion of 1 mEq/kg/hr. • For children younger than 2 yrs, premature infants, neonates, administer by slow infusion, up to 10 mEq/min.
Storage • Store at room temperature.

PO
• Do not give other PO medication within 1–2 hrs of antacid administration. • Give 1–3 hrs after meals.

▦ IV INCOMPATIBILITIES

Amiodarone (Cordarone), ascorbic acid, calcium chloride, diltiazem (Cardizem), dobutamine (Dobutrex), dopamine (Intropin), hydromorphone (Dilaudid), magnesium sulfate, midazolam (Versed), norepinephrine (Levophed), ondansetron (Zofran).

▦ IV COMPATIBILITIES

Dexmedetomidine (Precedex), furosemide (Lasix), heparin, insulin, lidocaine, mannitol, milrinone (Primacor), morphine, phenylephrine (Neo-Synephrine), potassium chloride, propofol (Diprivan), vancomycin (Vancocin).

INDICATIONS/ROUTES/DOSAGE

◀ALERT▶ May give by IV push, IV infusion, or orally. Dose individualized based on severity of acidosis, laboratory values, pt age, weight, clinical conditions. Do not fully correct bicarbonate deficit during the first 24 hrs (may cause metabolic alkalosis).

S

Cardiac Arrest
◀**ALERT**▶ Routine use not recommended.
IV: ADULTS, ELDERLY: Initially, 1 mEq/kg. May repeat with 0.5 mEq/kg in 10 min one time during continued cardiopulmonary arrest. Use in postresuscitation phase is based on arterial blood pH, partial pressure of carbon dioxide in arterial blood ($PaCO_2$), base deficit calculation. **CHILDREN, INFANTS:** Initially, 0.5–1 mEq/kg. Repeat in 10 min one time, or as indicated by pt's acid-base status.

Metabolic Acidosis (Mild to Moderate)
IV: ADULTS, ELDERLY, CHILDREN: 2–5 mEq/kg over 4–8 hrs. May repeat based on acid-base status.

Prevention of Contrast-Induced Nephropathy
IV Infusion: ADULTS, ELDERLY: 154 mEq/L sodium bicarbonate in D_5W solution: 3 ml/kg/hr 1 hr immediately before contrast injection, then 1 ml/kg/hr during contrast exposure and for 6 hrs after procedure.

Metabolic Acidosis (Associated With Chronic Renal Failure)
PO: ADULTS, ELDERLY: Initially, 20–36 mEq/day in divided doses. Titrate to bicarbonate level of 18–20 mEq/L. **CHILDREN:** 1–3 mEq/kg/day.

Renal Tubular Acidosis (Distal)
PO: ADULTS, ELDERLY: 0.5–2 mEq/kg/day in 4–6 divided doses. **CHILDREN:** 2–3 mEq/kg/day in divided doses.

Renal Tubular Acidosis (Proximal)
PO: ADULTS, ELDERLY, CHILDREN: 5–10 mEq/kg/day in divided doses.

Urine Alkalinization
PO: ADULTS, ELDERLY: Initially, 4 g, then 1–2 g q4h. **Maximum:** 16 g/day (8g/day in adults older than 60 yrs). **CHILDREN:** 1–10 mEq/kg/day in divided doses q4–6h.

Antacid
PO: ADULTS, ELDERLY: 300 mg–2 g 1–4 times a day.

Hyperkalemia
IV: ADULTS, ELDERLY: 50 mEq over 5 min.

SIDE EFFECTS
Frequent: Abdominal distention, flatulence, belching.

ADVERSE EFFECTS/ TOXIC REACTIONS
Excessive, chronic use may produce metabolic alkalosis (irritability, twitching, paresthesia, cyanosis, slow or shallow respirations, headache, thirst, nausea). Fluid overload results in headache, weakness, blurred vision, behavioral changes, incoordination, muscle twitching, elevated B/P, bradycardia, tachypnea, wheezing, coughing, distended neck veins. Extravasation may occur at the IV site, resulting in tissue necrosis, ulceration.

NURSING CONSIDERATIONS

BASELINE ASSESSMENT
Assess for signs and symptoms of acidosis, alkalosis. Do not give PO medication within 1 hr of antacids.

INTERVENTION/EVALUATION
Monitor serum, urinary pH, CO_2 level, serum electrolytes, plasma bicarbonate levels. Watch for signs of metabolic alkalosis, fluid overload. Assess for clinical improvement of metabolic acidosis (relief from hyperventilation, weakness, disorientation). Monitor daily pattern of bowel activity, stool consistency. Monitor serum phosphate, calcium, uric acid levels. Assess for relief of gastric distress.

sodium chloride

so-dee-um **klor**-ide
(Muro 128, Nasal Moist, Ocean, SalineX)

◆CLASSIFICATION

PHARMACOTHERAPEUTIC: Salt. **CLINICAL:** Electrolyte, isotonic volume expander, ophthalmic adjunct, bronchodilator.

ACTION

Sodium is a major cation of extracellular fluid. **Therapeutic Effect:** Controls water distribution, fluid and electrolyte balance, osmotic pressure of body fluids; maintains acid-base balance.

PHARMACOKINETICS

Well absorbed from GI tract. Widely distributed. Primarily excreted in urine and, to a lesser degree, in sweat, tears, saliva.

USES

Parenteral: Source of hydration; prevention/treatment of sodium, chloride deficiencies (hypertonic for severe deficiencies). Prevention of muscle cramps, heat prostration occurring with excessive perspiration. **Nasal:** Restores moisture, relieves dry, inflamed nasal membranes. **Ophthalmic:** Therapy in reduction of corneal edema, diagnostic aid in ophthalmoscopic exam.

PRECAUTIONS

Contraindications: Fluid retention, hypernatremia, hypertonic uterus. **Cautions:** HF, renal impairment, cirrhosis, hypertension, edema. Do not use sodium chloride preserved with benzyl alcohol in neonates.

⏳ LIFESPAN CONSIDERATIONS

Pregnancy Category C. Children/Elderly: No age-related precautions noted.

INTERACTIONS

DRUG: May decrease effect of **lithium. HERBAL:** None significant. **FOOD:** None known. **LAB VALUES:** None significant.

AVAILABILITY

Injection (Concentrate) (Rx): 23.4% (4 mEq/ml). Injection Solution (Rx): 0.45%, 0.9%, 3%. Irrigation (Rx): 0.45%, 0.9%. Nasal Gel (Nasal Moist) (OTC): 0.65%. Nasal Solution (OTC): 0.4% (SalineX), 0.65% (Nasal Moist, Ocean). Ophthalmic Ointment (OTC [Muro 128]): 5%. Ophthalmic Solution (OTC [Muro 128]): 2%, 5%.

 Tablets (OTC): 1 g.

ADMINISTRATION/HANDLING

IV

• Hypertonic solutions (3% or 5%) are administered via large vein; avoid infiltration; do not exceed 100 ml/hr. • Vials containing 2.5–4 mEq/ml (concentrated NaCl) must be diluted with D_5W or $D_{10}W$ before administration.

PO

• Do not crush/break enteric-coated or extended-release tablets. • Administer with full glass of water.

Nasal

• Instruct pt to begin inhaling slowly just before releasing medication into nose. • Instruct pt to inhale slowly, then release air gently through mouth. • Continue technique for 20–30 sec.

Ophthalmic

• Place gloved finger on lower eyelid and pull out until pocket is formed between eye and lower lid. • Place prescribed number of drops (or ¼–½ inch of ointment) into pocket. • Instruct pt to close eye gently for 1–2 min so that medication will not be squeezed out of sac. • When lower lid is released, have pt keep eye open without blinking for at least 30 sec for solution; for ointment have pt close eye, roll eyeball around to distribute medication. • When using drops, apply gentle finger pressure to lacrimal sac at inner canthus for 1 min to minimize systemic absorption.

INDICATIONS/ROUTES/DOSAGE

◄**ALERT**► Dosage based on age, weight, clinical condition; fluid, electrolyte, acid-base balance status.

S

Usual Parenteral Dosage
IV: ADULTS, ELDERLY, CHILDREN: Determined by laboratory determinations (mEq). Dosage varies widely based on clinical conditions.

Usual Oral Dosage
PO: ADULTS, ELDERLY: 1–2 g 3 times a day.

Usual Nasal Dosage
Intranasal: ADULTS, ELDERLY, CHILDREN: 2–3 sprays as needed.

Usual Ophthalmic Dosage
Ophthalmic Solution: ADULTS, ELDERLY: Apply 1–2 drops q3–4h.
Ophthalmic Ointment: ADULTS, ELDERLY: Apply once a day or as directed.

SIDE EFFECTS

Frequent: Facial flushing. Occasional: Fever; irritation, phlebitis, extravasation at injection site. **Ophthalmic:** Temporary burning, irritation.

ADVERSE EFFECTS/ TOXIC REACTIONS

Too-rapid administration may produce peripheral edema, HF, pulmonary edema. Excessive dosage may produce hypokalemia, hypervolemia, hypernatremia.

NURSING CONSIDERATIONS

BASELINE ASSESSMENT
Obtain baseline serum electrolyte studies. Assess fluid balance (I&O, daily weight, lung sounds, edema).

INTERVENTION/EVALUATION
Monitor fluid balance (I&O, daily weight, lung sounds, edema), IV site for extravasation. Monitor serum electrolytes, acid-base balance, B/P. Hypernatremia associated with edema, weight gain, elevated B/P; hyponatremia associated with muscle cramps, nausea, vomiting, dry mucous membranes.

PATIENT/FAMILY TEACHING
• Temporary burning, irritation may occur upon instillation of eye medication.

• Discontinue eye medication and report severe pain, headache, rapid change in vision (peripheral, direct), sudden appearance of floating spots, acute redness of eyes, pain on exposure to light, double vision occurs.

sodium ferric gluconate complex

so-dee-um **fair**-ick **glu**-koe-nate com-plex
(Ferrlecit)

◆**CLASSIFICATION**
PHARMACOTHERAPEUTIC: Trace element. CLINICAL: Hematinic.

ACTION

Repletes total iron content in body. Replaces iron found in Hgb, myoglobin, specific enzymes; allows oxygen transport via Hgb. **Therapeutic Effect:** Prevents, corrects iron deficiency.

PHARMACOKINETICS

Half-life: 1 hr.

USES

Treatment of iron deficiency anemia in pts undergoing chronic hemodialysis who are receiving supplemental erythropoietin therapy. OFF-LABEL: Cancer/chemotherapy–associated anemia.

PRECAUTIONS

Contraindications: All anemias not associated with iron deficiency, hypersensitivity to iron products, hemochromatosis, hemolytic anemia, pts with iron overload. Cautions: Significant allergies, asthma, hepatic impairment, rheumatoid arthritis (RA).

⧗ LIFESPAN CONSIDERATIONS

Pregnancy/Lactation: Unknown if distributed in breast milk. **Pregnancy Cate-**

gory B. **Children:** Safety and efficacy not established. **Elderly:** No age-related precautions noted; lower initial dosages recommended.

INTERACTIONS

DRUG: May decrease absorption of **oral iron. HERBAL:** None significant. **FOOD:** None known. **LAB VALUES:** None significant.

AVAILABILITY (Rx)

Injection Solution: 12.5 mg/ml elemental iron.

ADMINISTRATION/HANDLING
 IV

Reconstitution • Must be diluted. • Test dose: Dilute 25 mg (2 ml) with 50 ml 0.9% NaCl. • Recommended dose: Dilute 125 mg (10 ml) with 100 ml 0.9% NaCl.
Rate of Administration • Infuse both test dose, recommended dose over 1 hr.
Storage • Store at room temperature. • Use immediately after dilution.

IV INCOMPATIBILITIES

Do not mix with any other medications.

INDICATIONS/ROUTES/DOSAGE

Iron Deficiency Anemia
IV Infusion: ADULTS, ELDERLY: 125 mg in 100 ml 0.9% NaCl infused over 1 hr. Minimum cumulative dose 1 g elemental iron given over 8 sessions at sequential dialysis treatments. May be given during dialysis session. **CHILDREN 6 YRS AND OLDER:** 1.5 mg/kg diluted in 25 ml 0.9% NaCl administered over 60 min at sequential dialysis sessions. **Maximum:** 125 mg/dose.

SIDE EFFECTS

Frequent (Greater Than 3%): Flushing, hypotension, hypersensitivity reaction. **Occasional (3%–1%):** Injection site reaction, headache, abdominal pain, chills, flu-like syndrome, dizziness, leg cramps, dyspnea, nausea, vomiting, diarrhea, myalgia, pruritus, edema.

ADVERSE EFFECTS/ TOXIC REACTIONS

Potentially fatal hypersensitivity reaction occurs rarely, characterized by cardiovascular collapse, cardiac arrest, dyspnea, bronchospasm, angioedema, urticaria. Rapid administration may cause hypotension associated with flushing, light-headedness, fatigue, weakness, severe pain in chest, back, groin.

NURSING CONSIDERATIONS

BASELINE ASSESSMENT

Do not give concurrently with oral iron form (excessive iron may produce excessive iron storage [hemosiderosis]). Be alert to pts with rheumatoid arthritis (RA), iron deficiency anemia (acute exacerbation of joint pain, swelling may occur).

INTERVENTION/EVALUATION

Monitor vital signs, lab tests, esp. CBC, serum iron concentrations (may not be accurate until 3 wks after administration). Monitor daily pattern of bowel activity, stool consistency.

PATIENT/FAMILY TEACHING

• Stools frequently become black with iron therapy (condition is harmless). Report to physician any red streaking, sticky consistency of stool, abdominal pain/cramping.

sodium polystyrene sulfonate

so-dee-um pol-ee-**stye**-reen
(Kayexalate, Kionex, PMS-Sodium Polystyrene Sulfonate ✤, SPS)
Do not confuse Kayexalate with Kaopectate.

◆CLASSIFICATION

PHARMACOTHERAPEUTIC: Cation exchange resin. **CLINICAL:** Antihyperkalemic.

S

ACTION

Releases sodium ions in exchange primarily for potassium ions. **Therapeutic Effect:** Moves potassium from blood into intestine to be expelled from the body.

PHARMACOKINETICS

Onset: 2–24 hrs. Eliminated only in feces.

USES

Treatment of hyperkalemia.

PRECAUTIONS

Contraindications: Hypokalemia, neonates with reduced GI motility, intestinal obstruction/perforation, any postoperative pt until normal bowel function resumes. **Cautions:** Severe HF, hypertension, edema.

⧗ LIFESPAN CONSIDERATIONS

Pregnancy/Lactation: Unknown if drug crosses placenta or is distributed in breast milk. **Pregnancy Category C. Children:** No age-related precautions noted. **Elderly:** Increased risk for fecal impaction.

INTERACTIONS

DRUG: Cation-donating antacids, laxatives (e.g., magnesium hydroxide) may decrease effect; may cause systemic alkalosis in pts with renal impairment. **HERBAL:** None significant. **FOOD:** None known. **LAB VALUES:** May decrease serum calcium, magnesium, potassium. May increase serum sodium.

AVAILABILITY (Rx)

Powder for Suspension (Kayexalate, Kionex): 15 g/4 level tsp (480 g). **Suspension (SPS):** 15 g/60 ml.

ADMINISTRATION/HANDLING

PO
• Shake suspension well prior to administration. • Do not mix with orange juice. • Chilling suspension will increase palatability.

Rectal
• After initial cleansing enema, insert large rubber tube into rectum well into sigmoid colon, tape in place. • Introduce suspension (with 100 ml sorbitol) via gravity. • Flush with 50–100 ml fluid and clamp. • Pt must retain for several hrs if possible. • Irrigate colon with non–sodium-containing solution to remove resin.

INDICATIONS/ROUTES/DOSAGE

Hyperkalemia
PO: ADULTS, ELDERLY: 60 ml (15 g) 1–4 times daily. **CHILDREN:** 1 g/kg/dose q6h.
Rectal: ADULTS, ELDERLY: 30–50 g as needed q6h. **CHILDREN:** 1 g/kg/dose q2–6h.

SIDE EFFECTS

Frequent: High dosage: Anorexia, nausea, vomiting, constipation. **High dosage in elderly:** Fecal impaction (severe stomach pain with nausea/vomiting). **Occasional:** Diarrhea, sodium retention (decreased urination, peripheral edema, increased weight).

ADVERSE EFFECTS/ TOXIC REACTIONS

Potassium deficiency may occur. Early signs of hypokalemia include confusion, delayed thought processes, extreme weakness, irritability, EKG changes (often associated with prolonged QT interval; widening, flattening, or inversion of T wave; prominent U waves). Hypocalcemia, manifested by abdominal/muscle cramps, occurs occasionally. Arrhythmias, severe muscle weakness may be noted.

NURSING CONSIDERATIONS

BASELINE ASSESSMENT

Does not rapidly correct severe hyperkalemia (may take hrs to days). Consider other measures in medical emergency (IV calcium, IV sodium bicarbonate/glucose/insulin, dialysis).

INTERVENTION/EVALUATION

Monitor serum potassium levels frequently. Assess pt's clinical condition, EKG (valuable in determining when treat-

S

ment should be discontinued). Also monitor serum magnesium, calcium levels. Monitor daily pattern of bowel activity, stool consistency (fecal impaction may occur in pts on high dosages, particularly in elderly).

sofosbuvir

soe-**fos**-bue-vir
(Sovaldi)
Do not confuse sofosbuvir with fosamprenavir or simeprevir.

◆**CLASSIFICATION**

PHARMACOTHERAPEUTIC: Nucleotide polymerase inhibitor. **CLINICAL:** Antiviral.

ACTION

Inhibits viral replication of viral-infected cells. Suppresses cell proliferation by interrupting polymerase activity, resulting in chain termination. **Therapeutic Effect:** Inhibits viral replication of hepatitis C virus.

PHARMACOKINETICS

Well absorbed after PO administration. Metabolized in liver. Protein binding: 61%–65%. Peak plasma concentration: 2–4 hrs. Excreted in urine (80%), feces (14%), expired air (2.5%). Approximately 18% of dose removed by dialysis. **Half-life:** 27 hrs.

USES

Treatment of chronic hepatitis C virus (HCV) infection, in combination with peginterferon alfa and/or ribavirin. Indicated for HCV genotype 1, 2, 3, or 4 infection, including pts with hepatocellular carcinoma that meet Milan criteria (awaiting liver transplantation), and pts with HCV/HIV-1 co-infection.

PRECAUTIONS

Contraindications: Pregnancy (Category X), breastfeeding, any contraindications

to peginterferon alfa or ribavirin. **Cautions:** Concurrent use of potent P-glycoprotein inducers (e.g., rifampin, St. John's wort) may decrease concentration/effects.

⧗ LIFESPAN CONSIDERATIONS

Pregnancy/Lactation: Strictly avoid pregnancy. May cause birth defects or fetal demise. **Pregnancy Category B (X when used in ribavirin).** Women of childbearing age must use two different forms of reliable birth control during treatment and for at least 6 mos after discontinuation. Do not initiate therapy until negative pregnancy test confirmed. Unknown if distributed in breast milk. Breastfeeding contraindicated. **Children:** Safety and efficacy not established in pts younger than 18 yrs. **Elderly:** No age-related precautions noted.

INTERACTIONS

DRUG: P-glycoprotein inducers (e.g., rifampin) may decrease concentration/effect. **HERBAL: St. John's wort** may decrease concentration/effect. **FOOD:** None known. **LAB VALUES:** May decrease Hgb, Hct, platelets, neutrophils, leukocytes. May increase serum ALT, AST, bilirubin, creatine kinase, lipase.

AVAILABILITY (Rx)

Tablets (Film-Coated): 400 mg.

ADMINISTRATION/HANDLING

PO
• Give without regard to meals.

INDICATIONS/ROUTES/DOSAGE

◀**ALERT**▶ Must use in combination with peginterferon alfa and/or ribavirin. Not recommended as monotherapy. Dose reduction of sofosbuvir not recommended.

Chronic Hepatitis C
PO: ADULTS/ELDERLY: (Genotype 1 or 4): 400 mg daily with food for 12 wks (with peginterferon alfa and ribavirin). If pt ineligible to receive peginterferon alfa, may consider extending ribavirin regimen

S

to 24 wks. If serious adverse reactions occur, consider dose reduction of peginterferon alfa and/or ribavirin. **(Genotype 2):** 400 mg daily with food for 12 wks (with ribavirin only). If serious adverse reactions occur, consider dose reduction of ribavirin. **(Genotype 3):** 400 mg daily with food for 24 wks (with ribavirin only). If serious adverse reaction occurs, consider dose reduction of ribavirin.

Ribavirin Dose Modification for Adverse Effects

History of Noncardiac Disease: Reduce ribavirin dose to 600 mg/day if Hgb less than 10 g/dl. Discontinue ribavirin if Hgb less than 8.5 g/dl. **History of Stable Cardiac Disease:** Reduce ribavirin dose to 600 mg/day if Hgb decreases greater than or equal to 2 g/dl during any 4-wk treatment period. Discontinue ribavirin if Hgb less than 12 g/dl despite 4 wks at reduced dose.

Chronic Hepatitis C with Hepatocellular Carcinoma (Awaiting Liver Transplantation)

PO: ADULTS/ELDERLY: 400 mg daily with food for 48 wks (with peginterferon alfa and ribavirin) or until liver transplantation occurs.

SIDE EFFECTS

(With ribavirin): Frequent (38%–22%): Fatigue, headache, nausea. **Occasional (15%–6%):** Insomnia, pruritus, irritability, diarrhea, rash, asthenia, anorexia, myalgia. **Rare (4%–2%):** Pyrexia, body aches, chills. **(With peginterferon alfa and ribavirin): Frequent (55%–29%):** Fatigue, headache, nausea, insomnia, pruritus. **Occasional (18%–14%):** Rash, anorexia, chills, body aches, diarrhea, myalgia, irritability, pyrexia. **Rare (3%):** Asthenia.

ADVERSE EFFECTS/ TOXIC REACTIONS

Increased risk of thromboembolic events associated with peginterferon alfa. Anemia may cause discontinuation of therapy. Severe depression, suicidal ideation occurs rarely.

NURSING CONSIDERATIONS

BASELINE ASSESSMENT

Obtain baseline vital signs, CBC, serum CPK, complete metabolic panel, liver function test, lipase level. Confirm hepatitis C genotype. Receive full history of home medications including herbal products. Screen for contraindications to peginterferon alfa/ribavirin. Confirm negative pregnancy test before initiating treatment. Question history of anemia, pancytopenia, dialysis, hepatitis B, HIV, liver transplantation, renal impairment, pancreatitis.

INTERVENTION/EVALUATION

Assess vital signs, O_2 saturation routinely. Monitor CBC routinely or with any dosage change. Obtain monthly pregnancy tests. Monitor for intrauterine device failures if applicable. Reinforce birth control compliance. Assess for anemia-related dizziness, exertional dyspnea, fatigue, weakness, syncope. Report decreases in Hgb, Hct, platelets, neutrophils. Monitor for acute infection (fever, diaphoresis, lethargy, oral mucosal changes, productive cough), bloody stools, bruising, DVT, hematuria, pulmonary embolism. Encourage nutritional intake; assess for anorexia, weight loss. Observe for signs of dyspnea or depression, suicidal ideation.

PATIENT/FAMILY TEACHING

• Blood levels will be drawn routinely. • Treatment must be used in combination with peginterferon, ribavirin. Inform pt of side effects/contraindications of multi-medication regimen. • Report any newly prescribed medications. • Do not take herbal products. • Women of childbearing age must use two different forms of reliable birth control during treatment and for at least 6 mos after treatment. Do not breastfeed. Notify physician if female partner becomes pregnant. • May alter taste of food or decrease appetite. • Report bloody stool/urine, increased bruising, difficulty breathing, weakness, dizziness, palpitation, weight loss. • Avoid alcohol. • Report signs of depression or suicidal ideation.

solifenacin

sol-i-**fen**-a-sin
(VESIcare)

◆ CLASSIFICATION

PHARMACOTHERAPEUTIC: Anticholinergic agent. **CLINICAL:** Urinary antispasmodic.

ACTION

Acts as direct antagonist at muscarinic acetylcholine receptors in cholinergically innervated organs. Reduces tonus (elastic tension) of smooth muscle in bladder, slows parasympathetic contractions. **Therapeutic Effect:** Decreases urinary bladder contractions, increases residual urine volume, decreases detrusor muscle pressure.

PHARMACOKINETICS

Well absorbed following PO administration. Protein binding: 98%. Metabolized in liver. Excreted in feces, urine. **Half-life:** 40–68 hrs.

USES

Treatment of overactive bladder with symptoms of urinary incontinence, urgency, frequency.

PRECAUTIONS

Contraindications: GI obstruction, uncontrolled narrow-angle glaucoma, urinary retention. **Cautions:** Bladder outflow obstruction, GI obstructive disorders, decreased GI motility, controlled narrow-angle glaucoma, renal/hepatic impairment, congenital or acquired QT prolongation.

⌛ LIFESPAN CONSIDERATIONS

Pregnancy/Lactation: Unknown if drug crosses placenta or is distributed is breast milk. **Pregnancy Category C. Children:** Safety and efficacy not established. **Elderly:** No age-related precautions noted.

INTERACTIONS

DRUG: CYP3A4 inhibitors (e.g., **keto-conazole, erythromycin, azole antifungals, clarithromycin**) may increase concentration/effects. **HERBAL: St. John's wort** may decrease concentration/effects. **FOOD: Grapefruit, grapefruit juice** may increase effects. **LAB VALUES:** None known.

AVAILABILITY (Rx)

Tablets: 5 mg, 10 mg.

ADMINISTRATION/HANDLING

PO
• Give without regard to food. Swallow tablets whole, with liquids.

INDICATIONS/ROUTES/DOSAGE

Overactive Bladder
PO: ADULTS, ELDERLY: 5 mg/day; if tolerated, may increase to 10 mg/day.

Dosage in Renal/Hepatic Impairment
Severe renal impairment (creatinine clearance less than 30 ml/min) or moderate hepatic impairment: Maximum dosage is 5 mg/day.

Dosage with CYP3A4 Inhibitors
Maximum: 5 mg/day.

SIDE EFFECTS

Frequent (11%–6%): Dry mouth, constipation, blurred vision. **Occasional (5%–3%):** UTI, dyspepsia (heartburn, indigestion, epigastric pain), nausea. **Rare (2%–1%):** Dizziness, dry eyes, fatigue, depression, edema, hypertension, epigastric pain, vomiting, urinary retention.

ADVERSE EFFECTS/ TOXIC REACTIONS

Angioneurotic edema, GI obstruction occur rarely. Overdose can result in severe anticholinergic effects.

S

❋ Canadian trade name   🦺 Non-Crushable Drug   **HIGH ALERT** High Alert drug

NURSING CONSIDERATIONS

BASELINE ASSESSMENT

Assess symptoms of overactive bladder before beginning the drug.

INTERVENTION/EVALUATION

Monitor I&O, anticholinergic effects, creatinine clearance. Assess for decrease in symptoms.

PATIENT/FAMILY TEACHING

• Avoid tasks requiring alertness, motor skills until response to drug is established. • Anticholinergic side effects include constipation, urinary retention, blurred vision, heat prostration in hot environment. • Use caution during exercise, exposure to heat.

---

somatropin

soe-ma-**troe**-pin
(Genotropin, Genotropin Miniquick, Humatrope, Norditropin, Nutropin, Nutropin AQ, Omnitrope, Saizen, Serostim, Zorbtive)
Do not confuse somatropin with sumatriptan.

◆CLASSIFICATION

PHARMACOTHERAPEUTIC: Polypeptide hormone. **CLINICAL:** Growth hormone.

ACTION

Stimulates cartilaginous growth areas of long bones; increases number, size of skeletal muscle cells; influences size of organs; increases RBC mass by stimulating erythropoietin. Influences metabolism of carbohydrates (decreases insulin sensitivity), fats (mobilizes fatty acids), minerals (retains phosphorus, sodium, potassium by promotion of cell growth), proteins (increases protein synthesis). **Therapeutic Effect:** Stimulates growth.

PHARMACOKINETICS

Well absorbed after subcutaneous, IM administration. Localized primarily in kidneys, liver. **Half-life: IV:** 20–30 min; **Subcutaneous, IM:** 3–5 hrs.

USES

Adults: Growth deficiency due to pituitary disease, hypothalamic disease, surgery, radiation, or trauma; AIDS-related wasting or cachexia; short bowel syndrome. **Children:** Long-term treatment of growth failure due to lack of or inadequate endogenous growth hormone secretion; chronic renal insufficiency; short stature associated with Turner's syndrome, Noonan's syndrome, or homeobox gene deficiency; idiopathic short stature. **OFF-LABEL:** Treatment of pediatric HIV pts with wasting/cachexia; HIV adipose redistribution syndrome.

PRECAUTIONS

Contraindications: Pts with Prader-Will syndrome with growth hormone deficiency who are severely obese or have severe respiratory impairment, Prader-Will syndrome without growth hormone deficiency; children with closed epiphyses; acute critical illness due to complications after open heart or abdominal surgery; multiple accidental trauma; acute respiratory failure; active neoplasia; diabetic retinopathy. **Cautions:** Diabetes mellitus; active malignancy; progression of active growing intracranial lesion or tumor.

⌛ LIFESPAN CONSIDERATIONS

Pregnancy/Lactation: Unknown if drug is distributed in breast milk. **Pregnancy Category B (Genotropin, Genotropin Miniquick, Omnitrope, Saizen, Serostim, Zorbtive);** C **(Humatrope, Norditropin, Nutropin, Nutropin AQ). Children/Elderly:** No age-related precautions noted.

INTERACTIONS

DRUG: Corticosteroids may inhibit growth response. **Oral estrogens** may decrease response to somatropin.

HERBAL: None significant. FOOD: None known. LAB VALUES: May increase serum alkaline phosphatase, inorganic phosphorus, parathyroid hormone. May decrease glucose tolerance. May slightly decrease thyroid function.

AVAILABILITY (Rx)

Injection, Powder for Reconstitution (Genotropin): 5 mg, 12 mg. (Genotropin Miniquick): 0.2 mg, 0.4 mg, 0.6 mg, 0.8 mg, 1 mg, 1.2 mg, 1.4 mg, 1.6 mg, 1.8 mg, 2 mg. (Humatrope): 6 mg, 12 mg, 24 mg. (Nutropin): 5 mg, 10 mg. (Omnitrope): 5.8 mg. (Saizen): 5 mg, 8.8 mg. (Serostim): 4 mg, 5 mg, 6 mg. (Zorbitive): 8.8 mg. Injection Solution: (Norditropin): 5 mg/1.5 ml, 10 mg/1.5 ml, 15 mg/1.5 ml. (Nutropin AQ): 5 mg/ml. (Omnitrope): 5 mg/1.5 ml, 10 mg/1.5 ml. (Norditropin FlexPro Pen): 5 mg/1.5 ml, 10 mg/1.5 ml, 30 mg/3 ml.

ADMINISTRATION/HANDLING

◄ALERT► Neonate: Benzyl alcohol as a preservative has been associated with fatal toxicity (gasping syndrome) in premature infants. Reconstitute with Sterile Water for Injection only. Use only 1 dose per vial. Discard unused portion.

Reconstitution

Genotropin, Genotropin Miniquick: Reconstitute with diluent provided.
Humatrope: Reconstitute with 1.5–5 ml diluent provided, swirl gently, do not shake.
Humatrope Cartridge: Dilute with solution provided with cartridge only.
Nutropin: Reconstitute each 5 mg with 1.5–5 ml diluent, swirl gently, do not shake.
Omnitrope: Reconstitute with diluents provided, swirl gently, do not shake.
Saigen: 5 mg: Reconstitute with 1–3 ml diluent provided, swirl gently, do not shake. 8.8 mg: Reconstitute with 2–3 ml diluent provided, swirl gently, do not shake.
Serostim: Reconstitute with Sterile Water for Injection.
Zorbitive: Reconstitute with 1–2 ml Bacteriostatic Water for Injection.

Storage

Long-term storage: Refrigerate all products except Zorbitive. Once reconstituted, Humatrope, Nutropin, Saigen, Zorbitive stable for 14 days, Genotrope for 21 days, Humatrope Cartridge for 28 days. **Genotropin Miniquick:** Refrigerate, use within 24 hrs.

INDICATIONS/ROUTES/DOSAGE

Growth Hormone Deficiency

Subcutaneous *(Genotropin, Omnitrope)*: ADULTS: 0.04 mg/kg weekly divided into 6–7 equal doses/wk. May increase at 4- to 8-wk intervals to maximum of 0.08 mg/kg/wk. CHILDREN: 0.16–0.24 mg/kg weekly divided into daily doses.

Subcutaneous *(Humatrope)*: ADULTS: 0.006 mg/kg once daily. May increase to maximum of 0.0125 mg/kg/day. CHILDREN: 0.18–0.3 mg/kg weekly divided into alternate-day doses or 6 doses/wk.

Subcutaneous *(Norditropin)*: ADULTS: 0.004 mg/kg/day. May increase after 6 wks up to 0.016 mg/kg/day. CHILDREN: 0.024–0.036 mg/kg/dose 6–7 times a wk.

Subcutaneous *(Nutropin)*: ADULTS: 0.006 mg/kg once daily. May increase to maximum of 0.025 mg/kg/day (younger than 35 yrs) or 0.0125/kg/day (35 yrs and older). CHILDREN: 0.3–0.7 mg/kg weekly divided into daily doses.

Subcutaneous *(Nutropin AQ)*: ADULTS: 0.006 mg/kg once daily. May increase to maximum of 0.0125 mg/kg/day.

Subcutaneous *(Saizen)*: ADULTS: 0.005 mg/kg/day. May increase up to 0.01 mg/kg/day after 4 wks. CHILDREN: 0.06 mg/kg 3 times a wk.

Chronic Renal Insufficiency

Subcutaneous *(Nutropin, Nutropin AQ)*: CHILDREN: 0.35 mg/kg weekly divided into daily doses.

Turner's Syndrome

Subcutaneous *(Humatrope, Nutropin, Nutropin AQ)*: CHILDREN: 0.375 mg/kg weekly divided into equal doses

S

3–7 times a wk. *(Genotropin)*: 0.33 mg/kg weekly divided into 6–7 doses.

AIDS-Related Wasting

Subcutaneous *(Serostim)*: **ADULTS WEIGHING MORE THAN 55 KG:** 6 mg once daily at bedtime. **ADULTS WEIGHING 45–55 KG:** 5 mg once daily at bedtime. **ADULTS WEIGHING 35–44 KG:** 4 mg once daily at bedtime. **ADULTS WEIGHING LESS THAN 35 KG:** 0.1 mg/kg once daily at bedtime.

Short Bowel Syndrome

Subcutaneous *(Zorbtive)*: **ADULTS:** 0.1 mg/kg/day. **Maximum:** 8 mg/day.

SIDE EFFECTS

Frequent: Otitis media, other ear disorders (with Turner's syndrome). **Occasional:** Carpal tunnel syndrome, gynecomastia, myalgia, peripheral edema, fatigue, asthenia (loss of strength, energy). **Rare:** Rash, pruritus, visual changes, headache, nausea, vomiting, injection site pain/swelling, abdominal pain, hip/knee pain.

ADVERSE EFFECTS/ TOXIC REACTIONS

Pancreatitis occurs rarely.

NURSING CONSIDERATIONS

BASELINE ASSESSMENT

Obtain baseline lab chemistries, thyroid function, serum glucose level.

INTERVENTION/EVALUATION

Monitor bone growth, growth rate in relation to pt's age. Monitor serum calcium, glucose, phosphorus levels; renal, parathyroid, thyroid function. Observe for decreased muscle wasting in AIDS pts.

PATIENT/FAMILY TEACHING

• Follow correct procedure to reconstitute drug for administration, safe handling/disposal of needles. • Regular follow-up with physician is important part of therapy. • Report development of severe headache, visual changes, pain in hip/knee, limping.

sorafenib

soe-**raf**-e-nib
(Nexavar)
Do not confuse Nexavar with Nexium, or sorafenib with imatinib or sunitinib.

◆CLASSIFICATION

PHARMACOTHERAPEUTIC: Multikinase inhibitor. **CLINICAL:** Antineoplastic (see p. 90C).

ACTION

Decreases tumor cell proliferation by interacting with multiple intracellular, cell surface kinases. **Therapeutic Effect:** Inhibits tumor growth.

PHARMACOKINETICS

Metabolized in liver. Protein binding: 99.5%. Eliminated mainly in feces, with lesser amount excreted in urine. **Half-life:** 25–48 hrs.

USES

Treatment of advanced renal cell carcinoma, unresectable hepatocellular carcinoma. Thyroid carcinoma refractory to radioactive iodine treatment. **OFF-LABEL:** Recurrent or metastatic angiosarcoma, resistant gastrointestinal stromal tumor.

PRECAUTIONS

Contraindications: Use in combination with carboplatin and paclitaxel in pts with squamous cell lung cancer. **Cautions:** Underlying or poorly controlled hypertension, pts with congenital long QT syndrome, medications that prolong QT interval, electrolyte imbalance, heart failure, bradyarrhythmias, concurrent use with strong CYP3A4 inducers.

⧖ LIFESPAN CONSIDERATIONS

Pregnancy/Lactation: May cause fetal harm. Adequate contraception should be used during therapy and for at least 2 wks after therapy completion. Unknown if distributed in breast milk. Breast-feeding not recommended. **Pregnancy Category D. Children:** Safety and efficacy not established. **Elderly:** No age-related precautions noted.

INTERACTIONS

DRUG: CYP3A4 inducers (e.g., **carbamazepine, dexamethasone, phenobarbital, phenytoin, rifampin**) may decrease concentration. **HERBAL: St. John's wort** may decrease concentration. **FOOD: High-fat meals** decrease effectiveness. **LAB VALUES:** May increase serum lipase, amylase, bilirubin, alkaline phosphatase, transaminases. May decrease serum phosphorus, lymphocytes, WBCs, Hgb, Hct.

AVAILABILITY (Rx)

Tablets: 200 mg (Nexavar).

ADMINISTRATION/HANDLING

PO

• Give 1 hr before or 2 hrs after eating (high-fat meal reduces effectiveness).
• Swallow tablet whole; do not break, crush, dissolve, or divide tablet.

INDICATIONS/ROUTES/DOSAGE

Renal Cell Carcinoma, Hepatocellular Carcinoma, Thyroid Carcinoma
PO: ADULTS, ELDERLY: 400 mg (2 tablets) twice daily without food.

Dosage in Renal Impairment

Creatinine Clearance	Dosage
40–59 ml/min	400 mg twice daily
20–39 ml/min	200 mg twice daily
Hemodialysis	200 mg once daily

Dosage in Hepatic Impairment
Bilirubin greater than 1 to 1.5 times ULN and/or AST greater than ULN: 400 mg twice daily. **Bilirubin greater than 1.5 to 3 times ULN and any AST:** 200 mg twice daily. **Albumin less than 2.5 g/dl (any bilirubin/AST):** 200 mg once daily.

SIDE EFFECTS

Frequent (43%–16%): Diarrhea, rash, fatigue, exfoliative dermatitis, alopecia, nausea, pruritus, hypertension, anorexia, vomiting. **Occasional (15%–10%):** Constipation, minor bleeding, dyspnea, sensory neuropathy, cough, abdominal pain, dry skin, weight loss, joint pain, headache. **Rare (9%–1%):** Acne, flushing, stomatitis, mucositis, dyspepsia (heartburn, indigestion, epigastric pain), arthralgia, myalgia, hoarseness.

ADVERSE EFFECTS/ TOXIC REACTIONS

Anemia, neutropenia, thrombocytopenia, leukopenia occur in less than 10% of pts. Pancreatitis, gastritis, erectile dysfunction occur occasionally. Hemorrhage, cardiac ischemia/infarction, hypertensive crisis occur rarely.

NURSING CONSIDERATIONS

BASELINE ASSESSMENT

Monitor B/P weekly during first 6 wks of therapy and routinely thereafter. CBC, serum chemistries including electrolytes, renal/hepatic function tests, chest X-ray should be performed before therapy begins and routinely thereafter.

INTERVENTION/EVALUATION

Determine serum amylase, lipase, phosphorus concentrations frequently during therapy. Monitor CBC for evidence of myelosuppression. Monitor for blood dyscrasias (fever, sore throat, signs of local infection, unusual bruising/bleeding from any site), symptoms of anemia (excessive fatigue, weakness). Monitor for signs of neuropathy (gait disturbances, fine motor control difficulties, numbness).

PATIENT/FAMILY TEACHING

• Report any episode of chest pain. • Do not have immunizations without physician's approval (drug lowers resistance). Avoid contact with those who have recently taken live virus vaccine. • Promptly report fever, sore throat, signs of local infection,

S

unusual bruising/bleeding from any site. • Swallow whole; do not chew, crush, dissolve, or divide tablet. • Avoid administration after high-fat meals.

sotalol

soe-ta-lol
(Apo-Sotalol ✤, Betapace, Betapace AF, Novo-Sotalol ✤, PMS-Sotalol ✤, Sorine)

BLACK BOX ALERT Initiation, titration to occur in a hospital setting with continuous EKG to monitor potential onset of life-threatening arrhythmias. Betapace should not be substituted for Betapace AF.
Do not confuse Betapace with Betapace AF, or sotalol with Stadol or Sudafed.

◆CLASSIFICATION

PHARMACOTHERAPEUTIC: Beta-adrenergic blocking agent. **CLINICAL:** Antiarrhythmic (see p. 19C).

ACTION

Prolongs cardiac action potential, effective refractory period, QT interval. Decreases heart rate, AV node conduction; increases AV node refractoriness. **Therapeutic Effect:** Produces antiarrhythmic activity.

PHARMACOKINETICS

Route	Onset	Peak	Duration
PO	1–2 hrs	2.5–4 hrs	8–16 hrs

Well absorbed from GI tract. Protein binding: None. Widely distributed. Primarily excreted unchanged in urine. Removed by hemodialysis. **Half-life:** 12 hrs (increased in elderly, renal impairment).

USES

Betapace, Sorine: Treatment of documented, life-threatening ventricular arrhythmias. **Betapace AF:** Maintain normal sinus rhythm in pts with symptomatic atrial fibrillation/flutter. **OFF-LABEL:** Fetal tachycardia, treatment of atrial fibrillation with hypertrophic cardiomyopathy.

PRECAUTIONS

Contraindications: Cardiogenic shock, congenital or acquired long QT syndrome, second- or third-degree heart block (unless functioning pacemaker is present), sinus bradycardia, uncontrolled cardiac failure. **Betapace AF** (additional): Baseline QT interval greater than 450 msec, bronchospastic conditions, creatinine clearance less than 40 ml/min, serum potassium less than 4 mEq/L, sick sinus syndrome. **Cautions:** Pts with history of ventricular tachycardia, ventricular fibrillation, cardiomegaly, compensated HF, diabetes mellitus, excessive prolongation of QT interval, hypokalemia, hypomagnesemia, renal impairment, within first 2 wks post MI, peripheral vascular disease, myasthenia gravis, psychiatric disease, bronchospastic disease. Concurrent use of digoxin, verapamil, diltiazem, history of severe anaphylaxis to allergens.

⌛ LIFESPAN CONSIDERATIONS

Pregnancy/Lactation: Crosses placenta. Distributed in breast milk. **Pregnancy Category B (D if used in second or third trimester). Children:** Safety and efficacy not established. **Elderly:** Age-related peripheral vascular disease may increase susceptibility to decreased peripheral circulation. Age-related renal impairment may require dosage adjustment.

INTERACTIONS

DRUG: Calcium channel blockers may increase effect on AV conduction, B/P. May mask symptoms of hypoglycemia, prolong hypoglycemic effects of **insulin, oral hypoglycemics. QT prolonging medications** may increase risk of prolonged QT interval. **HERBAL: Ephedra** may worsen arrhythmias. **FOOD:** None known. **LAB VALUES:** May increase BUN, serum glucose, alka-

S

line phosphatase, LDH, lipoprotein, AST, ALT, triglycerides, potassium, uric acid.

AVAILABILITY (Rx)

Tablets: 80 mg (Betapace, Betapace AF, Sorine), 120 mg (Betapace, Betapace AF, Sorine), 160 mg (Betapace, Betapace AF, Sorine), 240 mg (Sorine).

ADMINISTRATION/HANDLING

PO
• Give without regard to food. • Give at same time each day.

INDICATIONS/ROUTES/DOSAGE

Ventricular Arrhythmias
PO *(Betapace, Sorine)*: **ADULTS, ELDERLY:** Initially, 80 mg twice daily. May increase gradually at 2- to 3-day intervals. Range: 240–320 mg/day in 2–3 divided doses.

Atrial Fibrillation, Atrial Flutter
PO *(Betapace AF)*: **ADULTS, ELDERLY:** 80 mg twice daily. May increase up to 160 mg twice daily.

Dosage in Renal Impairment
Dosage interval is modified based on creatinine clearance.

BETAPACE, SORINE

Creatinine Clearance	Dosage
31–60 ml/min	24 hrs
10–30 ml/min	36–48 hrs
Less than 10 ml/min	Individualized

BETAPACE AF

Creatinine Clearance	Dosage
Greater than 60 ml/min	12 hrs
40–60 ml/min	24 hrs
Less than 40 ml/min	Contraindicated

SIDE EFFECTS

Frequent: Diminished sexual function, drowsiness, insomnia, asthenia (loss of strength, energy). **Occasional:** Depression, cold hands/feet, diarrhea, constipation, anxiety, nasal congestion, nausea, vomiting. **Rare:** Altered taste, dry eyes, pruritus, paresthesia of fingers, toes, scalp.

ADVERSE EFFECTS/ TOXIC REACTIONS

Bradycardia, HF, hypotension, bronchospasm, hypoglycemia, prolonged QT interval, torsade de pointes, ventricular tachycardia, premature ventricular complexes may occur.

NURSING CONSIDERATIONS

BASELINE ASSESSMENT

Pt must be on continuous cardiac monitoring upon initiation of therapy. Do not administer without consulting physician if pulse is 60 beats/min or less. Assess creatinine clearance before dosing.

INTERVENTION/EVALUATION

Diligently monitor for arrhythmias. Assess B/P for hypotension, pulse for bradycardia. Assess for HF: dyspnea, peripheral edema, jugular vein distention, increased weight, rales in lungs, decreased urinary output.

PATIENT/FAMILY TEACHING

• Do not discontinue, change dose without physician approval. • Avoid tasks requiring alertness, motor skills until response to drug is established (may cause drowsiness). • Periodic lab tests, EKGs are necessary part of therapy. • Report rapid heartbeat, chest pain, swelling of ankles/legs, difficulty breathing.

S

spironolactone

spir-**on**-oh-**lak**-tone
(Aldactone, Novo-Spiroton ✤)
BLACK BOX ALERT Has been shown to produce tumors in chronic toxicity studies.
Do not confuse Aldactone with Aldactazide.

FIXED-COMBINATION(S)

Aldactazide: spironolactone/hydro-chlorothiazide (a thiazide diuretic): 25 mg/25 mg, 50 mg/50 mg.

◆CLASSIFICATION

PHARMACOTHERAPEUTIC: Aldosterone antagonist. **CLINICAL:** Potassium-sparing diuretic, antihypertensive, antihypokalemic (see p. 105C).

ACTION

Interferes with sodium reabsorption by competitively inhibiting action of aldosterone in distal tubule, promoting sodium and water excretion, increasing potassium retention. **Therapeutic Effect:** Produces diuresis, lowers B/P.

PHARMACOKINETICS

Well absorbed from GI tract (absorption increased with food). Protein binding: 91%–98%. Metabolized in liver to active metabolite. Primarily excreted in urine. Unknown if removed by hemodialysis. **Half-life:** 78–84 min.

USES

Management of edema associated with excessive aldosterone secretion, hypertension; cirrhosis; hypokalemia, nephrotic syndrome; severe HF; primary hyperaldosteronism. **OFF-LABEL:** Treatment of edema, hypertension in children, female acne, female hirsutism.

PRECAUTIONS

Contraindications: Acute renal insufficiency, anuria, hyperkalemia. **Cautions:** Dehydration, hyponatremia, renal/hepatic impairment, concurrent use of supplemental potassium.

⧗ LIFESPAN CONSIDERATIONS

Pregnancy/Lactation: Active metabolite excreted in breast milk. Breastfeeding not recommended. **Pregnancy Category C (D if used in pregnancy-induced hypertension). Children:** No age-related precautions noted. **Elderly:** May be more susceptible to developing hyperkalemia. Age-related renal impairment may require dosage adjustment.

INTERACTIONS

DRUG: ACE inhibitors (e.g., captopril), potassium-containing medications, potassium supplements may increase risk of hyperkalemia. May increase half-life of **digoxin. NSAIDs** may decrease antihypertensive effect. **HERBAL:** Avoid **natural licorice** (possesses mineralocorticoid activity). **FOOD: Food** increases absorption. **LAB VALUES:** May increase urinary calcium excretion, BUN, serum glucose, creatinine, magnesium, potassium, uric acid. May decrease serum sodium.

AVAILABILITY (Rx)

Tablets: 25 mg, 50 mg, 100 mg.

ADMINISTRATION/HANDLING

PO
• Oral suspension containing crushed tablets in cherry syrup is stable for up to 30 days if refrigerated. • Drug absorption enhanced if taken with food. • Scored tablets may be crushed.

INDICATIONS/ROUTES/DOSAGE

Edema
PO: ADULTS, ELDERLY: 25–200 mg/day as single dose or in 2 divided doses. **CHILDREN:** 1–3.3 mg/kg/day in divided doses q6–12h. **Maximum:** 100 mg. **NEONATES:** 1–3 mg/kg/day in 1–2 divided doses.

Hypertension
PO: ADULTS, ELDERLY: 25–50 mg/day in 1–2 doses/day. **CHILDREN:** 1–3.3 mg/kg/day in divided doses q6–12h. **Maximum:** 100 mg.

Hypokalemia
PO: ADULTS, ELDERLY: 25–100 mg/day as single dose or in 2 divided doses.

Hirsutism
PO: ADULTS, ELDERLY: 50–200 mg/day as single dose or in 2 divided doses.

Primary Aldosteronism
PO: ADULTS, ELDERLY: 400 mg/day for 4 days up to 3–4 wks, then maintenance dose of 100–400 mg/day as single dose or in 2 divided doses. **CHILDREN:** 125–375 mg/m^2/day as single dose or in 2 divided doses.

HF
PO: ADULTS, ELDERLY: 12.5–25 mg/day adjusted based on pt response, evidence of hyperkalemia. **Maximum:** 50 mg.

Dosage in Renal Impairment
Dosage interval is modified based on creatinine clearance.

Creatinine Clearance	Dosage
31–50 ml/min	Decrease initial dose to 12.5 mg once daily
30 ml/min or less	Not recommended

SIDE EFFECTS

Frequent: Hyperkalemia (in pts with renal insufficiency, those taking potassium supplements), dehydration, hyponatremia, lethargy. **Occasional:** Nausea, vomiting, anorexia, abdominal cramps, diarrhea, headache, ataxia, drowsiness, confusion, fever. **Male:** Gynecomastia, impotence, decreased libido. **Female:** Menstrual irregularities (amenorrhea, postmenopausal bleeding), breast tenderness. **Rare:** Rash, urticaria, hirsutism.

ADVERSE EFFECTS/ TOXIC REACTIONS

Severe hyperkalemia may produce arrhythmias, bradycardia, EKG changes (tented T waves, widening QRS complex, ST segment depression). May proceed to cardiac standstill, ventricular fibrillation. Cirrhosis pts at risk for hepatic decompensation if dehydration, hyponatremia occurs. Pts with primary aldosteronism may experience rapid weight loss, severe fatigue during high-dose therapy.

NURSING CONSIDERATIONS

BASELINE ASSESSMENT

Weigh pt; initiate strict I&O. Evaluate hydration status by assessing mucous membranes, skin turgor. Obtain baseline serum electrolytes, renal/hepatic function, urinalysis. Assess for edema; note location, extent. Check baseline vital signs, note pulse rate/regularity.

INTERVENTION/EVALUATION

Monitor serum electrolyte values, esp. for increased potassium, BUN, creatinine. Monitor B/P. Monitor for hyponatremia: mental confusion, thirst, cold/clammy skin, drowsiness, dry mouth. Monitor for hyperkalemia: colic, diarrhea, muscle twitching followed by weakness/paralysis, arrhythmias. Obtain daily weight. Note changes in edema, skin turgor.

PATIENT/FAMILY TEACHING

• Expect increase in volume, frequency of urination. • Therapeutic effect takes several days to begin and can last for several days when drug is discontinued. This may not apply if pt is on a potassium-losing drug concomitantly (diet, use of supplements should be established by physician). • Report irregular or slow pulse, symptoms of electrolyte imbalance (see previous Intervention/Evaluation). • Avoid foods high in potassium, such as whole grains (cereals), legumes, meat, bananas, apricots, orange juice, potatoes (white, sweet), raisins. • Avoid alcohol. • Avoid tasks that require alertness, motor skills until response to drug is established (may cause drowsiness).

---

stavudine (d4T)

sta-vue-deen
(Zerit)
BLACK BOX ALERT Lactic acidosis, severe hepatomegaly with steatosis (fatty liver), pancreatitis have occurred. Fatalities reported.

S

Do not confuse Zerit with Zestril, Ziac, or Zyrtec.

◆CLASSIFICATION

PHARMACOTHERAPEUTIC: Nucleoside reverse transcriptase inhibitor. **CLINICAL:** Antiviral (see pp. 71C, 118C).

ACTION

Inhibits HIV reverse transcriptase by terminating viral DNA chain. Inhibits RNA-, DNA-dependent DNA polymerase, an enzyme necessary for HIV replication. **Therapeutic Effect:** Impedes HIV replication, slowing progression of HIV infection.

PHARMACOKINETICS

Rapidly, completely absorbed after PO administration. Undergoes intracellular phosphorylation. Excreted in urine. **Half-life:** 1–1.6 hrs (increased in renal impairment).

USES

Treatment of HIV infection in combination with at least two other agents.

PRECAUTIONS

Contraindications: None known. **Cautions:** History of peripheral neuropathy, renal/hepatic impairment, previous hypersensitivity to zidovudine, didanosine, or zalcitabine; preexisting bone marrow suppression.

⏳ LIFESPAN CONSIDERATIONS

Pregnancy/Lactation: Breastfeeding not recommended (possibility of HIV transmission). **Pregnancy Category C. Children:** No age-related precautions noted. **Elderly:** Information not available.

INTERACTIONS

DRUG: Zidovudine may have antagonistic antiviral effect. **HERBAL:** None significant. **FOOD:** None known. **LAB VALUES:** May increase serum alkaline phosphatase, ALT, AST, GGT, amylase, bilirubin.

AVAILABILITY (Rx)

Capsules: 15 mg, 20 mg, 30 mg, 40 mg. **Powder for Oral Solution:** 1 mg/ml.

ADMINISTRATION/HANDLING

PO
• Give without regard to meals.

INDICATIONS/ROUTES/DOSAGE

HIV Infection
PO: ADULTS, ELDERLY, CHILDREN WEIGHING 60 KG AND MORE: 40 mg q12h. **ADULTS, ELDERLY, CHILDREN WEIGHING 30–59 KG:** 30 mg q12h. **NEONATES 14 DAYS AND OLDER, INFANTS, CHILDREN WEIGHING LESS THAN 30 KG:** 1 mg/kg/dose q12h. **Maximum:** 30 mg q12h. **NEONATES 0–13 DAYS:** 0.5–1 mg/kg/dose q12h.

Dosage in Renal Impairment
Dosage and frequency are modified based on creatinine clearance and pt weight.

Creatinine Clearance	Weight 60 kg or More	Weight Less Than 60 kg
Greater than 50 ml/min	40 mg q12h	30 mg q12h
26–50 ml/min	20 mg q12h	15 mg q12h
10–25 ml/min	20 mg q24h	15 mg q24h

SIDE EFFECTS

Frequent (55%–14%): Headache, diarrhea, chills, fever, nausea, vomiting, myalgia, rash, asthenia (loss of strength, energy), insomnia, abdominal pain, anxiety, back pain, diaphoresis, arthralgia, malaise, depression. **Occasional:** Anorexia, weight loss, nervousness, dizziness, conjunctivitis, dyspepsia, dyspnea. **Rare:** Constipation, vasodilation, confusion, migraine, urticaria, abnormal vision.

ADVERSE EFFECTS/ TOXIC REACTIONS

Peripheral neuropathy (numbness, tingling, pain in hands/feet) occurs in 15%–21% of pts. Ulcerative stomatitis (erythema, ulcers of oral mucosa, glossitis, gingivitis), pneumonia, benign skin neoplasms occur occasionally. Pancreati-

S

tis, hepatomegaly, lactic acidosis have been reported.

NURSING CONSIDERATIONS

BASELINE ASSESSMENT

Obtain baseline laboratory testing, esp. serum hepatic function tests, before beginning stavudine therapy and at periodic intervals during therapy. Offer emotional support to pt, family. Question for history of peripheral neuropathy.

INTERVENTION/EVALUATION

Monitor for peripheral neuropathy (characterized by paresthesia in extremities). Symptoms resolve promptly if therapy is discontinued (symptoms may worsen temporarily after drug is withdrawn). If symptoms resolve completely, reduced dosage may be resumed. Assess for headache, nausea, vomiting, myalgia. Monitor skin for evidence of rash, signs of fever. Monitor daily pattern of bowel activity, stool consistency. Assess for myalgia, arthralgia, dizziness. Monitor sleep patterns. Assess eating pattern; monitor for weight loss. Check eyes for signs of conjunctivitis. Monitor CBC, Hgb, serum hepatic/renal function, CD4 cell count, HIV RNA levels.

PATIENT/FAMILY TEACHING

• Continue therapy for full length of treatment. • Doses should be evenly spaced. • Do not take any medications, including OTC drugs, without consulting physician. • Stavudine is not a cure for HIV infection, nor does it reduce risk of transmission to others. • Pt may continue to experience illnesses, including opportunistic infections. • Report tingling, burning, pain, numbness, abdominal discomfort, nausea, vomiting, fatigue, dyspnea, weakness.

Stribild

el-vye-**teg**-ra-veer/koe-**bis**-i-stat/
em-tri-**sit**-a-bine/ten-**oh**-foe-veer

(elvitegravir/cobicistat/
emtricitabine/tenofovir)

**Do not confuse elvitegravir/
cobicistat/emtricitabine/
tenofovir (Stribild) with emtri-
citabine/rilpivirine/tenofovir
(Complera), or efavirenz/
emtricitabine/tenofovir
(Atripla), or emtricitabine/
tenofovir (Truvada).**

BLACK BOX ALERT Serious, sometimes, fatal lactic acidosis and severe hepatomegaly with steatosis (fatty liver) have been reported. Severe exacerbations of hepatitis B virus (HBV) reported in pts coinfected with HIV-1 and HBV following discontinuation. If discontinuation occurs, monitor hepatic function for at least several months. Initiate anti-HBV therapy if warranted.

FIXED-COMBINATION(S)

Stribild: elvitegravir/cobicistat/emtricitabine/tenofovir: 150 mg/150 mg/200 mg/300 mg.

◆CLASSIFICATION

PHARMACOTHERAPEUTIC: Integrase inhibitor, reverse transcriptase inhibitor. **CLINICAL:** Combination antiretroviral agent.

ACTION

Elvitegravir inhibits catalytic activity of integrase, preventing integration into human DNA. Cobicistat inhibits CYP3A enzymes, enhancing elvitegravir exposure. Emtricitabine and fenofovir interfere with viral RNA-dependent DNA polymerase activities. **Therapeutic Effect:** Interferes with HIV replication, slowing progression of HIV infection.

PHARMACOKINETICS

Readily absorbed after oral administration. Peak concentration: 2–4 hrs. Protein binding: (elvitegravir, cobicistat) 98%, (emtricitabine) 4%, (tenofovir) 0.7%. Extensively metabolized in liver. Excreted primarily in feces, urine (vari-

S

ous). **Half-life:** (elvitegravir): 12.9 hrs, (cobicistat): 3.5 hrs.

USES

Treatment of HIV-1 infection in adults who are antiretroviral treatment naïve.

PRECAUTIONS

◄**ALERT**► Therapy not recommended in pts with creatinine clearance less than 70 ml/min, severe hepatic impairment, or suspected lactic acidosis.
Contraindications: Concurrent use with alfuzosin, ergot derivatives (e.g., ergotamine), lovastatin, nephrotoxic agents, other antiretrovirals, pimozide, rifampin, sildenafil (when used for pulmonary hypertension), simvastatin, St. John's wort; midazolam (oral), may produce extreme sedation and/or respiratory depression. **Cautions:** Renal impairment, mild to moderate hepatic impairment, pathologic fracture history, osteoporosis, osteopenia, preexisting cardiac conduction abnormalities, obesity.

⧖ LIFESPAN CONSIDERATIONS

Pregnancy/Lactation: Do not breastfeed infants because of risk for postnatal HIV transmission. Secreted in breast milk (see individual agents). **Pregnancy Category B. Children:** Safety and efficacy not established in pts younger than 18 yrs. **Elderly:** Increased risk of side effects/adverse reactions, osteopenia.

INTERACTIONS

DRUG: Antacids may decrease Stribild concentration. May increase concentration/effects of **antifungals (e.g., ketoconazole), atorvastatin, clarithromycin, colchicine, cyclosporine, PDE-5 inhibitors (e.g., sildenafil, tadalafil).** May alter effectiveness of **hormonal contraceptives. HERBAL: St. John's wort** may decrease effectiveness. **Red yeast** may increase risk for myopathy, rhabdomyolysis. **FOOD:** None known. **LAB VALUES:** May increase ALT/AST, amylase, bilirubin, BUN, 1,25-vitamin D, cholesterol, creatine kinase (CK), creatinine, serum glucose, parathyroid hormone, urine protein, triglycerides. May decrease creatinine clearance, neutrophils.

AVAILABILITY (Rx)

Tablets: (elvitegravir) 150 mg/(cobicistat) 150 mg/(emtricitabine) 200 mg/(tenofovir) 300 mg.

ADMINISTRATION/HANDLING

PO
• Give with food.

INDICATIONS/ROUTES/DOSAGE

◄**ALERT**► Supplementation of calcium and vitamin D may slow progression of bone density loss.

HIV Infection
PO: ADULTS/ELDERLY: One tablet daily with food.

Dosage in Renal Impairment
Discontinue if creatinine clearance less than 50 ml/min.

SIDE EFFECTS

Frequent (16%–12%): Nausea, asthenia, cough, diarrhea (loss of strength, energy). **Occasional (10%–4%):** Headache, vomiting, abnormal dreams, abdominal pain, depression, paresthesia, fatigue, dyspepsia, arthralgia, neuropathy, hyperpigmentation. **Rare (3%–1%):** Dizziness, eczema, insomnia, flatulence, somnolence, pruritus, urticaria.

ADVERSE EFFECTS/ TOXIC REACTIONS

May cause new or worsening renal failure including Fanconi's syndrome (nonabsorption of essential electrolytes, acids, buffers in renal tubules). May decrease bone mineral density, leading to pathologic fractures. May cause redistribution/accumulation of body fat (lipodystrophy). Fatal lactic acidosis and severe hepatomegaly with steatosis (fatty liver) reported. Pts coinfected with HBV may experience hepatic decompensation and/or failure if therapy discontinued. May induce immune recovery syndrome (inflammatory response to dormant opportunistic infections such as *Mycobacterium avium*, cytomegalovirus, PCP, tuberculosis, or acceleration of autoimmune disorders including Graves' disease, polymyositis, Guillain-Barré syndrome).

NURSING CONSIDERATIONS

BASELINE ASSESSMENT

Obtain baseline CBC, CMP, CD4$^+$ count, viral load, GFR, lipid panel, phosphate (with renal impairment), urine glucose, urine protein. Screen all pts for hepatitis B virus (HBV). Receive full medication history including herbal products. Question possibility of pregnancy.

INTERVENTION/EVALUATION

Monitor labs routinely. Obtain serum lactate level if lactic acidosis suspected. Monitor digoxin level if applicable. Assess for hepatic impairment (bruising, hematuria, jaundice, right upper abdominal pain, nausea, vomiting, weight loss). Monitor for immune recovery syndrome. Offer antiemetics if nausea occurs. Assess skin for urticaria, pruritus.

PATIENT/FAMILY TEACHING

• Offer emotional support. • Take with food (optimizes absorption). • Blood levels will be monitored routinely. • Report any signs of decreased urine output, abdominal pain, yellowing of skin or eyes, darkened urine, clay-colored stools, weight loss. • Report any newly prescribed medications. • Stribild does not cure HIV infection nor reduce risk for transmission. • Practice safe sex with barrier methods or abstinence. • Decreased bone density may lead to pathologic fractures. • As immune system strengthens, it may respond to dormant infections hidden within the body. • Report any new fever, chills, body aches, cough, night sweats, shortness of breath. • Antiretrovirals may cause excess body fat in upper back, neck, breast, trunk; and may cause decreased body fat in legs, arms, face.

sucralfate

soo-**kral**-fate
(Apo-Sucralfate ✦, Carafate, Novo-Sucralate ✦)
Do not confuse Carafate with Cafergot, or sucralfate with salsalate.

◆CLASSIFICATION

PHARMACOTHERAPEUTIC: Gastrointestinal agent. **CLINICAL:** Antiulcer.

ACTION

Forms ulcer-adherent complex with proteinaceous exudate (e.g., albumin) at ulcer site. Forms viscous, adhesive barrier on surface of intact mucosa of stomach, duodenum. **Therapeutic Effect:** Protects damaged mucosa from further destruction by absorbing gastric acid, pepsin, bile salts.

PHARMACOKINETICS

Minimally absorbed from GI tract. Eliminated in feces, with small amount excreted in urine. Not removed by hemodialysis.

USES

Short-term treatment (up to 8 wks) of duodenal ulcer. Maintenance therapy of duodenal ulcer after healing of acute ulcers. **OFF-LABEL:** Prevention, treatment of stress-related mucosal damage, esp. in acutely or critically ill pts; treatment of gastric ulcer; relief of GI symptoms associated with NSAIDs; treatment of gastroesophageal reflux disease (GERD). Esophagitis, treatment of stomatitis due to cancer chemotherapy (suspension); post-sclerotherapy for esophageal variceal bleeding.

PRECAUTIONS

Contraindications: None known. **Cautions:** Renal failure (due to accumulation of aluminum).

S

⧗ LIFESPAN CONSIDERATIONS

Pregnancy/Lactation: Unknown if drug crosses placenta or is distributed in breast milk. **Pregnancy Category B. Children:** Safety and efficacy not established. **Elderly:** No age-related precautions noted.

INTERACTIONS

DRUG: May decrease absorption of **digoxin, ketoconazole, levothyroxine, phenytoin, quinidine, quinolones (e.g., ciprofloxacin), ranitidine, tetracycline, theophylline.** **HERBAL:** None significant. **FOOD:** None known. **LAB VALUES:** None known.

AVAILABILITY (Rx)

Oral Suspension: 1 g/10 ml. **Tablets:** 1 g.

ADMINISTRATION/HANDLING

PO
• Administer 1 hr before meals and at bedtime. • Tablets may be crushed and dissolved in water. • Avoid antacids for 30 min before or after giving sucralfate. • Shake suspension well before using.

INDICATIONS/ROUTES/DOSAGE

Active Duodenal Ulcers
PO: ADULTS, ELDERLY: 1 g 4 times a day (before meals and at bedtime) or 2 g 2 times a day for up to 8 wks.

Maintenance Therapy of Duodenal Ulcers
PO: ADULTS, ELDERLY: 1 g twice a day.

SIDE EFFECTS

Frequent (2%): Constipation. **Occasional (less than 2%):** Dry mouth, backache, diarrhea, dizziness, drowsiness, nausea, indigestion, rash, urticaria, pruritus, abdominal discomfort.

ADVERSE EFFECTS/ TOXIC REACTIONS

Bezoars (compacted, undigestible material that does not pass into intestine) have been reported.

NURSING CONSIDERATIONS

INTERVENTION/EVALUATION
Monitor daily pattern of bowel activity, stool consistency.

PATIENT/FAMILY TEACHING
• Take medication on an empty stomach. • Antacids may be given as an adjunct but should not be taken for 30 min before or after sucralfate (formation of sucralfate gel is activated by stomach acid). • Dry mouth may be relieved by sour hard candy, sips of tepid water.

sucroferric oxyhydroxide

soo-krow-**fer**-ik ox-ee-hye-**drox**-ide (**Velphoro**)

◆CLASSIFICATION

PHARMACOTHERAPEUTIC: Polymeric phosphate binder. **CLINICAL:** Antihyperphosphatemia.

ACTION

Binds with dietary phosphorus in GI tract, allowing phosphorus to be eliminated through normal digestive process. **Therapeutic Effect:** Decreases serum phosphorus levels.

PHARMACOKINETICS

Not absorbed systemically. No physiologic process of metabolism/excretion.

USES

Reduction of serum phosphorus levels in pts with chronic renal disease on dialysis.

PRECAUTIONS

Contraindications: None known. **Cautions:** Significant gastric/hepatic disorders, history of hemochromatosis or other diseases with iron accumulation, peritoneal dialysis with peritonitis, recent major GI surgery.

S

⌛ LIFESPAN CONSIDERATIONS

Pregnancy/Lactation: Not distributed in breast milk. **Pregnancy Category B. Children:** Safety and efficacy not established. **Elderly:** No age-related precautions noted.

INTERACTIONS

DRUG: May decrease absorption/concentration of **alendronate, doxycycline, levothyroxine. HERBAL:** None significant. **FOOD:** None known. **LAB VALUES:** May decrease serum phosphorus.

AVAILABILITY (Rx)

Tablets (Chewable): 500 mg.

ADMINISTRATION/HANDLING

PO
• Give with meals. • Give other PO medications at least 1 hr before administration. • Instruct pt to chew tablet; do not swallow whole. • May crush if pt unable to chew.

INDICATIONS/ROUTES/DOSAGE

Hyperphosphatemia
PO: ADULTS/ELDERLY: Initially, 500 mg 3 times a day with meals (1,500 mg/day). May increase or decrease dose as early as 7 days by increments of 500 mg/day based on acceptable serum phosphorus levels. **Maximum Dose:** 3,000 mg/day (6 tablets/day).

SIDE EFFECTS

Frequent (26%–16%): Diarrhea, discolored feces. **Occasional (10%–2%):** Nausea, dysgeusia.

ADVERSE EFFECTS/ TOXIC REACTIONS

Severe hypophosphatemia may include muscle weakness, respiratory depression.

NURSING CONSIDERATIONS

BASELINE ASSESSMENT

Obtain baseline serum calcium, ionized calcium, phosphate level. Question history of gastric dysfunction, hemochromatosis, iron accumulation, peritoneal dialysis with peritonitis, or recent major GI surgery. Assess pt's ability to chew.

INTERVENTION/EVALUATION

Monitor serum calcium, ionized calcium, phosphate level. Encourage PO intake if diarrhea occurs. Obtain stool guaiac test if GI bleeding suspected. Offer antiemetics for nausea.

PATIENT/FAMILY TEACHING

• Tablets must be chewed or crushed; do not swallow whole. • Take with meals only. • Dark-colored stools are an expected side effect of treatment (due to iron content). • Dark-colored stools may mask GI bleeding. Report any clay- or maroon-colored feces.

TOP 200

sulfamethoxazole-trimethoprim

sul-fa-meth-**ox**-a-zole-trye-**meth**-oh-prim
(Apo-Sulfatrim ❖, Bactrim, Bactrim DS, Novo-Trimel ❖, Septra DS)
Do not confuse Bactrim with bacitracin or Bactroban.

FIXED-COMBINATION(S)

Bactrim, Septra: sulfa-methoxazole/trimethoprim: 5:1 ratio remains constant in all dosage forms (e.g., 400 mg/80 mg).

◆CLASSIFICATION

PHARMACOTHERAPEUTIC: Sulfonamide/folate antagonist. **CLINICAL:** Antibiotic.

ACTION

Blocks bacterial synthesis of essential nucleic acids. **Therapeutic Effect:** Bactericidal in susceptible microorganisms.

S

PHARMACOKINETICS

Rapidly, well absorbed from GI tract. Protein binding: 45%–60%. Widely distributed. Metabolized in liver. Excreted in urine. Minimally removed by hemodialysis. **Half-life:** sulfamethoxazole, 6–12 hrs; trimethoprim, 6–17 hrs (increased in renal impairment).

USES

Treatment of susceptible infections due to *S. pneumoniae, H. influenzae, E. coli, Klebsiella* spp., *Enterobacter* spp., *M. morganii, P. mirabilis, P. vulgaris, S. flexneri, Pneumocystis jiroveci* including acute or complicated and recurrent or chronic UTI, *Pneumocystis jiroveci* pneumonia (PCP), shigellosis, enteritis, otitis media, chronic bronchitis, traveler's diarrhea. Prophylaxis of PCP. **OFF-LABEL:** Chronic prostatitis, prophylaxis for UTI, MRSA infections.

PRECAUTIONS

Contraindications: Severe renal/hepatic impairment, pregnancy (at term), breastfeeding, hypersensitivity to trimethoprim or any sulfonamides, infants younger than 2 mos, megaloblastic anemia due to folate deficiency. **Cautions:** Those with G6PD deficiency, elderly, chronic alcoholics, malabsorption syndrome, asthma, thyroid dysfunction, concurrent anticonvulsant therapy.

⧗ LIFESPAN CONSIDERATIONS

Pregnancy/Lactation: Contraindicated during pregnancy at term and during lactation. Readily crosses placenta. Distributed in breast milk. May produce kernicterus in newborn. **Pregnancy Category C (D at term). Children:** Contraindicated in those younger than 2 mos; may increase risk of kernicterus in newborn. **Elderly:** Increased risk for severe skin reaction, myelosuppression, decreased platelet count.

INTERACTIONS

DRUG: May increase/prolong effects, increase adverse effects of **phenytoin, digoxin, oral hypoglycemics, warfarin.**
May increase effects of **methotrexate. HERBAL: Dong quai, St. John's wort** may increase photosensitization reaction. **FOOD:** None known. **LAB VALUES:** May increase BUN, serum creatinine, AST, ALT, bilirubin.

AVAILABILITY (Rx)

◀**ALERT**▶ All dosage forms have same 5:1 ratio of sulfamethoxazole (SMZ) to trimethoprim (TMP).
Injection Solution: SMZ 80 mg and TMP 16 mg per ml. **Oral Suspension:** SMZ 200 mg and TMP 40 mg per 5 ml. **Tablets (Bactrim):** SMZ 400 mg and TMP 80 mg. **Tablets (Double Strength [Bactrim DS, Septra DS]):** SMZ 800 mg and TMP 160 mg.

ADMINISTRATION/HANDLING

 IV

Reconstitution • For IV infusion (piggyback), dilute each 5 ml with 75–125 ml D_5W. • Do not mix with other drugs or solutions.
Rate of Administration • Infuse over 60–90 min. Must avoid bolus or rapid infusion. • Do not give IM. • Ensure adequate hydration.
Storage • IV infusion (piggyback) stable for 2 hrs (5 ml/75 ml D_5W), 4 hrs (5 ml/100 ml D_5W), 6 hrs (5 ml/125 ml D_5W). • Discard if cloudy or precipitate forms.

PO
• Store tablets, suspension at room temperature. • Administer on empty stomach with 8 oz water. • Give several extra glasses of water/day.

▨ IV INCOMPATIBILITIES

Fluconazole (Diflucan), foscarnet (Foscavir), midazolam (Versed), vinorelbine (Navelbine).

▨ IV COMPATIBILITIES

Dexmedetomidine (Precedex), diltiazem (Cardizem), heparin, hydromorphone (Dilaudid), lorazepam (Ativan), magnesium sulfate, morphine, nicardipine (Cardene).

INDICATIONS/ROUTES/DOSAGE

Usual Adult/Elderly Dosage Range
PO: One double-strength tablet q12–24h.
IV: 8–20 mg/kg/day as trimethoprim in divided doses q6–12h.

Usual Dosage Range, Children Older Than 2 Mos
Mild to Moderate Infection
PO: CHILDREN: 8–12 mg/kg/day as trimethoprim in divided doses q12h.

Severe Infections
PO: CHILDREN: 20 mg/kg/day as trimethoprim in divided doses q6h.
IV: CHILDREN: 8–12 mg/kg/day as trimethoprim in divided doses q6h.

Indication-Specific Dosing
Chronic Bronchitis
PO: ADULTS, ELDERLY: 1 double-strength or 2 single-strength tablets or 20 ml suspension q12h for 10–14 days.

***Pneumocystis jiroveci* Pneumonia (PCP)**
Prophylaxis
PO: ADULTS, ELDERLY: 1 double-strength tablet daily or 3 times a wk or 1 single-strength tablet daily. **CHILDREN 2 MOS AND OLDER:** 150 mg/m²/day as trimethoprim in 2 divided doses 3 times a wk on consecutive days.

PCP Treatment
PO, IV: ADULTS, ELDERLY, CHILDREN 2 MOS AND OLDER: 15–20 mg/kg/day as trimethoprim in 4 divided doses for 14–21 days.

Shigellosis
PO: ADULTS, ELDERLY: 1 double-strength tablet or 2 single-strength tablets or 20 ml suspension q12h for 5 days.
IV: ADULTS, CHILDREN: 8–10 mg/kg/day as trimethoprim in 2–4 divided doses for up to 5 days.

Otitis Media
PO: CHILDREN 2 MOS AND OLDER: 8 mg/kg/day trimethoprim q12h for 10 days.

UTI
PO: ADULTS, ELDERLY: 1 double-strength or 2 single-strength tablets or 20 ml suspension q12h for 3–14 days depending on severity. **CHILDREN 2 MOS AND OLDER:** 8 mg/kg/day as trimethoprim in 2 divided doses for 10 days.

Traveler's Diarrhea
PO: ADULTS, ELDERLY: 1 double-strength or 2 single-strength tablets or 20 ml suspension q12h for 5 days.

Dosage in Renal Impairment

Creatinine Clearance	Dosage
15–30 ml/min	50% of usual dosage
Less than 15 ml/min	Not recommended

SIDE EFFECTS

Frequent: Anorexia, nausea, vomiting, rash (generally 7–14 days after therapy begins), urticaria. **Occasional:** Diarrhea, abdominal pain, pain/irritation at IV infusion site. **Rare:** Headache, vertigo, insomnia, seizures, hallucinations, depression.

ADVERSE EFFECTS/ TOXIC REACTIONS

Rash, fever, sore throat, pallor, purpura, cough, shortness of breath may be early signs of serious adverse effects. Fatalities are rare but have occurred in sulfonamide therapy following Stevens-Johnson syndrome, toxic epidermal necrolysis, fulminant hepatic necrosis, agranulocytosis, aplastic anemia, other blood dyscrasias. Myelosuppression, decreased platelet count, severe dermatologic reactions may occur, esp. in the elderly.

NURSING CONSIDERATIONS

BASELINE ASSESSMENT

Obtain history for hypersensitivity to trimethoprim or any sulfonamide, sulfite sensitivity, bronchial asthma. Determine serum renal, hepatic, hematologic baselines.

S

INTERVENTION/EVALUATION

Monitor daily pattern of bowel activity, stool consistency. Assess skin for rash, pallor, purpura. Check IV site, flow rate. Monitor renal, hepatic, hematology reports. Assess I&O. Check for CNS symptoms (headache, vertigo, insomnia, hallucinations). Monitor vital signs at least twice a day. Monitor for cough, shortness of breath. Assess for overt bleeding, ecchymosis, edema.

PATIENT/FAMILY TEACHING

• Continue medication for full length of therapy. • Space doses evenly around the clock. • Take oral doses with 8 oz water and drink several extra glasses of water daily. • Report immediately any new symptoms, esp. rash, other skin changes, bleeding/bruising, fever, sore throat, diarrhea. • Avoid prolonged exposure to direct sunlight.

sulfasalazine

sul-fa-**sal**-a-zeen
(Alti-Sulfasalazine ✦, Azulfidine, Azulfidine EN-tabs, Salazopyrin ✦, Salazopyrin EN-Tabs ✦)
Do not confuse Azulfidine with Augmentin or azathioprine, or sulfasalazine with sulfadiazine or sulfisoxazole.

◆CLASSIFICATION

PHARMACOTHERAPEUTIC: Sulfonamide. **CLINICAL:** Anti-inflammatory.

ACTION

Inhibits prostaglandin synthesis, acting locally in colon. **Therapeutic Effect:** Decreases inflammatory response, interferes with GI secretion. Effect may be result of antibacterial action with change in intestinal flora.

PHARMACOKINETICS

Poorly absorbed from GI tract. Cleaved, absorbed in colon by intestinal bacteria, forming sulfapyridine and mesalamine (5-ASA). Widely distributed. Metabolized via colonic intestinal flora. Primarily excreted in urine. **Half-life:** 5.7–10 hrs.

USES

Treatment of mild to moderate ulcerative colitis, adjunctive therapy in severe ulcerative colitis, rheumatoid arthritis (RA), juvenile rheumatoid arthritis. **OFF-LABEL:** Treatment of ankylosing spondylitis, Crohn's disease, psoriasis, psoriatic arthritis.

PRECAUTIONS

Contraindications: Hypersensitivity to sulfa, salicylates; porphyria; GI or GU obstruction. **Cautions:** Severe allergies, bronchial asthma, impaired hepatic/renal function, G6PD deficiency, blood dyscrasias.

⧖ LIFESPAN CONSIDERATIONS

Pregnancy/Lactation: May produce infertility, oligospermia in men while taking medication. Readily crosses placenta; if given near term, may produce jaundice, hemolytic anemia, kernicterus in newborn. Distributed in breast milk. Pt should not breast-feed premature infant or those with hyperbilirubinemia or G6PD deficiency. **Pregnancy Category B (D if given near term). Children:** No age-related precautions noted in those older than 2 yrs. **Elderly:** No age-related precautions noted.

INTERACTIONS

DRUG: Hepatotoxic medications may increase risk of hepatotoxicity. **HERBAL: Dong quai, St. John's wort** may increase photosensitization. **FOOD:** None known. **LAB VALUES:** None significant.

AVAILABILITY (Rx)

Tablets (Azulfidine): 500 mg.

Tablets (Delayed-Release [Azulfidine EN-tabs]): 500 mg.

ADMINISTRATION/HANDLING

PO

• Space doses evenly (intervals not to exceed 8 hrs). • Administer after meals or with food. • Swallow enteric-coated tablets whole; do not break, crush, dissolve, or divide. • Give with 8 oz of water; encourage several glasses of water between meals.

INDICATIONS/ROUTES/DOSAGE

Ulcerative Colitis

PO: ADULTS, ELDERLY: Initially, 1 g 3–4 times a day in divided doses q4–6h. **Maximum:** 6 g/day. Maintenance: 2 g/day in divided doses at intervals less than or equal to q8h. **CHILDREN 2 YRS AND OLDER:** Initially, 40–60 mg/kg/day in 4–6 divided doses. **Maximum:** Initial Dose: 4 g/day. Maintenance: 30–50 mg/kg/day in 4 divided doses at intervals less than or equal to q8h. **Maximum:** Maintenance Dose: 2 g/day.

Rheumatoid Arthritis (RA)

PO: *(Delayed-Release Tablets):* **ADULTS, ELDERLY:** Initially, 0.5–1 g/day for 1 wk. Increase by 0.5 g/wk, up to 2 g/day in 2 divided doses. **Maximum:** 3 g/day.

Juvenile Rheumatoid Arthritis (JRA)

PO: *(Delayed-Release Tablets):* **CHILDREN:** Initially, 10 mg/kg/day. May increase by 10 mg/kg/day at weekly intervals. Range: 30–50 mg/kg/day. **Maximum:** 2 g/day.

Dosage in Renal Impairment

Not recommended.

Dosage in Hepatic Impairment

Avoid use.

SIDE EFFECTS

Frequent (33%): Anorexia, nausea, vomiting, headache, oligospermia (generally reversed by withdrawal of drug). **Occasional (3%):** Hypersensitivity reaction (rash, urticaria, pruritus, fever, anemia). **Rare (Less Than 1%):** Tinnitus, hypoglycemia, diuresis, photosensitivity.

ADVERSE EFFECTS/ TOXIC REACTIONS

Anaphylaxis, Stevens-Johnson syndrome, hematologic toxicity (leukopenia, agranulocytosis), hepatotoxicity, nephrotoxicity occur rarely.

NURSING CONSIDERATIONS

BASELINE ASSESSMENT

Question for hypersensitivity to medications. Check initial urinalysis, CBC, serum hepatic/renal function tests.

INTERVENTION/EVALUATION

Monitor I&O, urinalysis, renal function tests; ensure adequate hydration (minimum output 1,500 ml/24 hrs) to prevent nephrotoxicity. Assess skin for rash (discontinue drug, notify physician at first sign). Monitor daily pattern of bowel activity, stool consistency. (Dosage increase may be needed if diarrhea continues, recurs.) Monitor CBC closely; assess for and report immediately any hematologic effects (bleeding, ecchymoses, fever, pharyngitis, pallor, weakness, purpura). Monitor hepatic function tests; observe for jaundice.

PATIENT/FAMILY TEACHING

• May cause orange-yellow discoloration of urine, skin. • Space doses evenly around the clock. • Take after or with food with 8 oz of water; drink several glasses of water between meals. • Swallow enteric-coated tablets whole; do not chew, crush, dissolve, or divide tablets. • Continue for full length of treatment; may be necessary to take drug even after symptoms relieved. • Follow-up, lab tests are essential. • Inform dentist, surgeon of sulfasalazine therapy. • Avoid exposure to sun, ultraviolet light until photosensitivity determined (may last for mos after last dose).

sulindac

sul-**in**-dak

(Apo-Sulin ✤, Clinoril, Novo-Sundac ✤)

 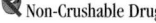

BLACK BOX ALERT Increased risk of serious cardiovascular thrombotic events, including myocardial infarction, CVA. Increased risk of severe GI reactions, including ulceration, bleeding, perforation of stomach, intestines.

Do not confuse Clinoril with Cleocin or Clozaril.

◆ CLASSIFICATION

PHARMACOTHERAPEUTIC: NSAID. **CLINICAL:** Anti-inflammatory, anti-gout (see p. 130C).

ACTION

Produces analgesic, anti-inflammatory effects by inhibiting prostaglandin synthesis. **Therapeutic Effect:** Reduces inflammatory response, intensity of pain.

PHARMACOKINETICS

Route	Onset	Peak	Duration
PO (antirheu-matic)	7 days	2–3 wks	N/A
Analgesic	1 hr	—	12–24 hrs

Well absorbed from GI tract. Protein binding: 93%–98%. Metabolized in liver to active metabolite. Primarily excreted in urine. Not removed by hemodialysis. **Half-life:** 7.8 hrs; metabolite, 16.4 hrs.

USES

Treatment of pain of rheumatoid arthritis (RA), osteoarthritis, ankylosing spondylitis, acute painful shoulder, bursitis, tendonitis, acute gouty arthritis. **OFF-LABEL:** Management of preterm labor.

PRECAUTIONS

Contraindications: Perioperative pain in setting of CABG surgery, history of hypersensitivity to aspirin, NSAIDs, history of asthma, urticaria. **Cautions:** Renal/hepatic impairment, renal lithiasis, history of GI tract disease, predisposition to fluid retention, concurrent anticoagulant use, HF, hypertension, GI bleeding, asthma.

⧖ LIFESPAN CONSIDERATIONS

Pregnancy/Lactation: Unknown if drug is distributed in breast milk. Avoid use during third trimester (may adversely affect fetal cardiovascular system: premature closure of ductus arteriosus). **Pregnancy Category C (D if used in third trimester near delivery). Children:** Safety and efficacy not established. **Elderly:** GI bleeding/ulceration more likely to cause serious adverse effects. Age-related renal impairment may increase risk of hepatic/renal toxicity; lower dosage recommended.

INTERACTIONS

DRUG: Antacids may decrease concentration. May decrease effects of **antihypertensives, diuretics. Aspirin, other salicylates** may increase risk of GI side effects, bleeding. May increase concentration/adverse effects of **cyclosporine.** May increase effects of **heparin, oral anticoagulants, thrombolytics.** May increase concentration, risk of toxicity of **lithium.** May increase risk of **methotrexate** toxicity. **HERBAL: Cat's claw, dong quai, evening primrose, feverfew, garlic, ginkgo, ginseng** possess antiplatelet activity, may increase bleeding. **FOOD:** None known. **LAB VALUES:** May increase serum alkaline phosphatase, AST, ALT, bleeding time.

AVAILABILITY (Rx)

Tablets: 150 mg, 200 mg.

ADMINISTRATION/HANDLING

PO
• Give with food, milk, antacids if GI distress occurs.

INDICATIONS/ROUTES/DOSAGE

Rheumatoid Arthritis (RA), Osteoarthritis, Ankylosing Spondylitis
PO: ADULTS, ELDERLY: Initially, 150 mg twice a day. May increase up to 400 mg/day.

Acute Shoulder Pain, Gouty Arthritis, Bursitis, Tendonitis
PO: ADULTS, ELDERLY: 200 mg twice a day for 7–14 days.

S

SIDE EFFECTS

Frequent (9%–4%): Diarrhea, constipation, indigestion, nausea, maculopapular rash, dermatitis, dizziness, headache. **Occasional (3%–1%):** Anorexia, abdominal cramps, flatulence.

ADVERSE EFFECTS/ TOXIC REACTIONS

Rare reactions with long-term use include peptic ulcer disease, GI bleeding, gastritis, nephrotoxicity (glomerular nephritis, interstitial nephritis, nephrotic syndrome), severe hepatic reactions (cholestasis, jaundice), severe hypersensitivity reactions (fever, chills, joint pain).

NURSING CONSIDERATIONS

BASELINE ASSESSMENT

Obtain baseline renal/hepatic function tests. Assess onset, type, location, duration of pain, fever, inflammation. Inspect affected joints for immobility, deformities, skin condition.

INTERVENTION/EVALUATION

Assist with ambulation if dizziness occurs. Monitor daily pattern of bowel activity, stool consistency. Assess for evidence of rash. Evaluate for therapeutic response (relief of pain, stiffness, swelling; increased joint mobility; reduced joint tenderness; improved grip strength). Monitor serum hepatic/renal function, CBC, platelets.

PATIENT/FAMILY TEACHING

• Therapeutic antiarthritic effect noted 1–3 wks after therapy begins. • Avoid aspirin, alcohol during therapy (increases risk of GI bleeding). • Take with food, milk if GI upset occurs. • Avoid tasks that require alertness, motor skills until response to drug is established (may cause dizziness).

sumatriptan

soo-ma-**trip**-tan

♣ Canadian trade name   🗲 Non-Crushable Drug   🔲 High Alert drug

(Alsuma, Apo-Sumatriptan ♣, Imitrex, Sumavel DosePro, Zecuity)
Do not confuse sumatriptan with saxagliptin, sitagliptin, somatropin, or zolmitriptan.

FIXED-COMBINATION(S)

Treximet: sumatriptan/naproxen (an NSAID): 85 mg/500 mg.

◆CLASSIFICATION

PHARMACOTHERAPEUTIC: Serotonin 5-HT$_1$ receptor agonist. **CLINICAL:** Antimigraine (see p. 65C).

ACTION

Binds selectively to vascular receptors, producing vasoconstrictive effect on cranial blood vessels. **Therapeutic Effect:** Relieves migraine headache.

PHARMACOKINETICS

Route	Onset	Peak	Duration
Nasal	15 min	N/A	24–48 hrs
PO	30 min	2 hrs	24–48 hrs
Subcutaneous	10 min	1 hr	24–48 hrs

Rapidly absorbed after subcutaneous administration. Absorption after PO administration is incomplete; significant amounts undergo hepatic metabolism, resulting in low bioavailability (about 14%). Protein binding: 10%–21%. Widely distributed. Undergoes first-pass metabolism in liver. Excreted in urine. **Half-life:** 2 hrs.

USES

PO, Subcutaneous, Intranasal, Transdermal: Acute treatment of migraine headache with or without aura. **Subcutaneous:** Treatment of cluster headaches.

PRECAUTIONS

Contraindications: Management of hemiplegic or basilar migraine, peripheral vascular disease, CVA, ischemic heart disease (including angina pectoris, history of MI, silent ischemia, Prinzmetal's angina), severe hepatic impairment, transient ischemic attack, uncontrolled hypertension, MAOI use within 14 days, use within 24 hrs of ergotamine preparations or another 5-HT₁ agonist. **Cautions:** Hepatic impairment, history of seizure disorder, controlled hypertension.

⌛ LIFESPAN CONSIDERATIONS

Pregnancy/Lactation: Unknown if distributed in breast milk. **Pregnancy Category C. Children:** Safety and efficacy not established. **Elderly:** No age-related precautions noted.

INTERACTIONS

DRUG: Ergotamine-containing medications may produce vasospastic reaction. **MAOIs** may increase concentration, half-life. **SSRIs** and **SNRI antidepressants** may increase risk of serotonin syndrome. **HERBAL:** None significant. **FOOD:** None known. **LAB VALUES:** None known.

AVAILABILITY (Rx)

Injection, Prefilled Autoinjector (Alsuma): 6 mg/0.5 ml. **Injection Solution (Imitrex):** 4 mg/0.5 ml, 6 mg/0.5 ml. **(Sumavel DosePro):** 6 mg/0.5 ml. **Nasal Spray (Imitrex Nasal):** 5 mg/0.1 ml, 20 mg/0.1 ml. **Tablets (Imitrex):** 25 mg, 50 mg, 100 mg. **Transdermal:** Delivers 6.5 mg over 4 hrs.

ADMINISTRATION/HANDLING

Subcutaneous
• Follow manufacturer's instructions for autoinjection device use. • Administer needleless (Sumavel DosePro) only to abdomen or thigh.

PO
• Swallow tablets whole. Do not split.
• Take with full glass of water.

Nasal
• Unit contains only one spray—do not test before use. • Instruct pt to gently blow nose to clear nasal passages. • With head upright, close one nostril with index finger, breathe out gently through mouth. • Have pt insert nozzle into open

nostril about ½ inch, close mouth and, while taking a breath through nose, release spray dosage by firmly pressing plunger. • Instruct pt to remove nozzle from nose and gently breathe in through nose and out through mouth for 10–20 sec; do not breathe in deeply.

Transdermal
• Apply to upper arm or thigh to dry, intact, nonirritated skin. • Do not cut patch. Do not bathe, shower, or swim while wearing patch.

INDICATIONS/ROUTES/DOSAGE

Acute Migraine Headache
PO: ADULTS, ELDERLY: 25–100 mg. Dose may be repeated after at least 2 hrs. **Maximum:** 100 mg/single dose; 200 mg/24 hrs.
Subcutaneous: ADULTS, ELDERLY: Up to 6 mg. **Maximum:** Up to two 6-mg injections/24 hrs (separated by at least 1 hr).
Intranasal: ADULTS, ELDERLY: 5–20 mg; may repeat in 2 hrs. **Maximum:** 40 mg/24 hrs.
Transdermal: ADULTS, ELDERLY: 6.5 mg (over 4 hrs). May repeat no sooner than 2 hrs after activation of first patch. **Maximum:** 2 patches in any 24-hr period.

SIDE EFFECTS

Frequent: PO (10%–5%): Tingling, nasal discomfort. **Subcutaneous (greater than 10%):** Injection site reactions, tingling, warm/hot sensation, dizziness, vertigo. **Nasal (greater than 10%):** Altered taste, nausea, vomiting. **Occasional: PO (5%–1%):** Flushing, asthenia (loss of strength, energy), visual disturbances. **Subcutaneous (10%–2%):** Burning sensation, numbness, chest discomfort, drowsiness, asthenia (loss of strength, energy). **Nasal (5%–1%):** Nasopharyngeal discomfort, dizziness. **Rare: PO (less than 1%):** Agitation, eye irritation, dysuria. **Subcutaneous (less than 2%):** Anxiety, fatigue, diaphoresis, muscle cramps, myalgia. **Nasal (less than 1%):** Burning sensation.

ADVERSE EFFECTS/ TOXIC REACTIONS

Excessive dosage may produce tremor, redness of extremities, reduced respirations, cyanosis, seizures, paralysis. Serious arrhythmias occur rarely, esp. in pts with hypertension, obesity, smokers, diabetes, strong family history of coronary artery disease. Serotonin syndrome may occur (agitation, confusion, hallucinations, hyper-reflexia, myoclonus, shivering, tachycardia).

NURSING CONSIDERATIONS

BASELINE ASSESSMENT

Question for history of peripheral vascular disease, renal/hepatic impairment, possibility of pregnancy. Question regarding onset, location, duration of migraine, possible precipitating symptoms.

INTERVENTION/EVALUATION

Evaluate for relief of migraine headache and resulting photophobia, phonophobia (sound sensitivity), nausea, vomiting.

PATIENT/FAMILY TEACHING

• Follow proper technique for loading of autoinjector, injection technique, discarding of syringe. • Do not use more than 2 injections during any 24-hr period and allow at least 1 hr between injections. • Report immediately if wheezing, palpitations, skin rash, facial swelling, pain/tightness in chest/throat occur.

---

sunitinib **HIGH ALERT**

soo-**nit**-in-ib
(Sutent)

BLACK BOX ALERT Hepatotoxicity may be severe and/or result in fatal liver failure.
Do not confuse sunitinib with imatinib or sorafenib.

◆CLASSIFICATION

PHARMACOTHERAPEUTIC: Tyrosine kinase inhibitor, vascular endothelial growth factor. **CLINICAL:** Antineoplastic (see p. 90C).

ACTION

Inhibitory action against multiple kinases, growth factor receptors, stem cell factor receptors, colony-stimulating factor receptors, glial cell-line neurotrophic factor receptors. **Therapeutic Effect:** Prevents tumor cell growth, produces tumor regression, inhibits metastasis.

PHARMACOKINETICS

Metabolized in liver. Protein binding: 95%. Excreted mainly in feces, with lesser amount eliminated in urine. **Half-life:** 40–60 hrs.

USES

Treatment of GI stromal tumor after disease progression while on or demonstrating intolerance to imatinib. Treatment of advanced renal cell carcinoma. Treatment of pancreatic neuroendocrine tumor (PNET). **OFF-LABEL:** Non-GI stromal tumor, soft tissue sarcomas, advanced thyroid cancer.

PRECAUTIONS

Contraindications: None known. **Cautions:** Cardiac abnormalities, bradycardia, electrolyte imbalance, bleeding tendencies, hypertension, history of prolonged QT interval, medications that prolong QT interval, concurrent use of strong CYP3A4 inducers or inhibitors, HF, impaired renal/liver function.

LIFESPAN CONSIDERATIONS

Pregnancy/Lactation: Has potential for embryotoxic, teratogenic effects. Breast-feeding not recommended. **Pregnancy Category D. Children:** Safety and efficacy not established. **Elderly:** No age-related precautions noted.

INTERACTIONS

DRUG: **CYP3A4 inhibitors** (e.g., ata-zanavir, **clarithromycin, indinavir, itra-conazole, ketoconazole, nefazodone,**

---

nelfinavir, ritonavir, saquinavir, voriconazole) may increase concentration, toxicity. CYP3A4 inducers (e.g., carbamazepine, dexamethasone, phenobarbital, phenytoin, rifabutin, rifampin, rifapentin) may decrease concentration/effects. HERBAL: St. John's wort may decrease concentration. FOOD: Grapefruit, grapefruit juice may increase concentration, potential for torsades, myelotoxicity. LAB VALUES: May increase serum alkaline phosphatase, bilirubin, amylase, lipase, creatinine, AST, ALT. May alter serum potassium, sodium, uric acid. May produce thrombocytopenia, neutropenia. May decrease serum phosphates, thyroid function levels.

AVAILABILITY (Rx)

Capsules: 12.5 mg, 25 mg, 50 mg.

ADMINISTRATION/HANDLING

PO

• Give without regard to food.

INDICATIONS/ROUTES/DOSAGE

GI Stromal Tumor, Renal Cell Carcinoma
PO: ADULTS, ELDERLY: 50 mg once daily for 4 wks, followed by 2 wks off of 6-wk cycle.

Pancreatic Neuroendocrine Tumor
PO: ADULTS, ELDERLY: 37.5 mg once daily continuously without a scheduled off-treatment period.

Dose Modification
PO: ADULTS, ELDERLY: Dosage increase or reduction in 12.5-mg increments is recommended based on safety and tolerability.

SIDE EFFECTS

Stromal tumor: Common (42%–30%): Fatigue, diarrhea, anorexia, abdominal pain, nausea, hyperpigmentation. **Frequent (29%–18%):** Mucositis/stomatitis, vomiting, asthenia (loss of strength, energy), altered taste, constipation, fever. **Occasional (15%–8%):** Hypertension, rash, myalgia, headache, arthralgia, back pain, dyspnea, cough. **Renal carcinoma: Common (74%–43%):** Fatigue, diarrhea, nausea, mucositis/stomatitis, dyspepsia (heartburn, indigestion, epigastric pain), altered taste. **Frequent (38%–20%):** Rash, vomiting, constipation, hyperpigmentation, anorexia, arthralgia, dyspnea, hypertension, headache, abdominal pain. **Occasional (18%–11%):** Limb pain, peripheral/periorbital edema, dry skin, hair color change, myalgia, cough, back pain, dizziness, fever, tongue pain, flatulence, alopecia, dehydration.

ADVERSE EFFECTS/TOXIC REACTIONS

Palmar-plantar erythrodysethesia syndrome (PPES) occurs occasionally (14%), manifested as blistering/rash/peeling of skin on palms of hands, soles of feet. Bleeding, decrease in left ventricular ejection fraction, deep vein thrombosis (DVT), pancreatitis, neutropenia, seizures occur rarely.

NURSING CONSIDERATIONS

BASELINE ASSESSMENT

Question possibility of pregnancy. Obtain baseline CBC, platelets, serum chemistries including electrolytes, renal/hepatic function tests (alkaline phosphatase, bilirubin, ALT, AST) before beginning therapy and prior to each treatment. Obtain baseline EKG, thyroid function tests.

INTERVENTION/EVALUATION

Assess eye area, lower extremities for early evidence of fluid retention. Offer antiemetics to control nausea, vomiting. Monitor daily pattern of bowel activity, stool consistency. Monitor CBC for evidence of neutropenia, thrombocytopenia; assess hepatic function tests for hepatotoxicity. Monitor for PPES.

PATIENT/FAMILY TEACHING

• Avoid crowds, those with known infection. • Avoid contact with anyone who recently received live virus vaccine. • Do not have immunizations without physician's approval (drug lowers resistance). • Avoid pregnancy; use effective contraceptive measures. • Promptly report fever, unusual bruising/bleeding from any site.

tacrolimus

tak-roe-li-mus
(Advagraf ✤, <u>Prograf</u>, Protopic)

BLACK BOX ALERT Increased susceptibility to infection and potential for development of lymphoma. Topical form associated with rare cases of malignancy. Topical form should be used only for short-term and intermittent treatment. Use in children less than 2 yrs of age not recommended. Use only 0.03% ointment for children 2–15 yrs of age.

Do not confuse Protopic with Protonix, or tacrolimus with everolimus, pimcrolimus, sirolimus, or temsirolimus.

◆CLASSIFICATION

PHARMACOTHERAPEUTIC: Immunologic agent. **CLINICAL:** Immunosuppressant (see p. 123C).

ACTION

Inhibits T-lymphocyte activation by binding to intracellular proteins, forming a complex, inhibiting phosphatase activity. **Therapeutic Effect:** Suppresses immunologically mediated inflammatory response; prevents organ transplant rejection.

PHARMACOKINETICS

Variably absorbed after PO administration (food reduces absorption). Protein binding: 99%. Metabolized in liver. Primarily eliminated in feces. Not removed by hemodialysis. **Half-life:** 21–61 hrs.

USES

PO/injection: Prophylaxis of organ rejection in pts receiving allogeneic liver, kidney, heart transplant. Should be used concurrently with adrenal corticosteroids. In heart and kidney transplants pts, should be used in conjunction with azathioprine or mycophenolate. **Topical:** Moderate to severe atopic dermatitis in immunocompetent pts. **OFF-LABEL:** Prevention of organ rejection in lung, small bowel recipients; prevention and treatment of graft-vs-host disease in allogeneic hematopoietic stem cell transplantation.

PRECAUTIONS

Contraindications: None known. **Cautions:** Hypersensitivity to HCO-60 polyoxyl 60 hydrogenated castor oil (used in solution for injection). Immunosuppressed pts, renal/hepatic impairment, concurrent use with cyclosporine (increases risk of nephrotoxicity). Concurrent use of strong CYP3A4 inhibitors or inducers. Pts at risk for pure red cell aplasia (e.g., concurrent use of mycophenolate). **Topical:** Exposure to sunlight.

⧗ LIFESPAN CONSIDERATIONS

Pregnancy/Lactation: Crosses placenta. Hyperkalemia, renal dysfunction noted in neonates. Distributed in breast milk. Breastfeeding not recommended. **Pregnancy Category C. Children:** May require higher dosages (decreased bioavailability, increased clearance). May make post-transplant lymphoproliferative disorder more common, esp. in pts younger than 3 yrs. **Elderly:** Age-related renal impairment may require dosage adjustment.

INTERACTIONS

DRUG: Aluminium-containing antacids may increase **tacrolimus** concentration. **CYP3A4 inhibitors (e.g., erythromycin, ketoconazole), protease inhibitors, calcium channel blockers** may increase concentration/effects. **CYP3A4 inducers (e.g., rifampin)** may decrease concentration/effects. May increase levels of **cyclosporine. HERBAL:** Echinacea, **St. John's wort** may decrease concentration/effects. **FOOD:** Food decreases rate/extent of absorption. **Grapefruit products** may increase concentration, toxicity (potential for nephrotoxicity). **LAB VALUES:** May increase serum glucose, BUN, creatinine, potassium, tri-

T

glycerides, cholesterol, bilirubin, amylase, AST, ALT. May decrease serum magnesium, Hgb, Hct, platelets. May alter leukocytes.

AVAILABILITY (Rx)

Capsules (Prograf): 0.5 mg, 1 mg, 5 mg.
Injection Solution (Prograf): 5 mg/ml.
Ointment (Protopic): 0.03%, 0.1%.

ADMINISTRATION/HANDLING

 IV

Reconstitution • Dilute with appropriate amount (250–1,000 ml, depending on desired dose) 0.9% NaCl or D_5W to provide concentration between 0.004 and 0.02 mg/ml.
Rate of Administration • Give as continuous IV infusion. • Continuously monitor pt for anaphylaxis for at least 30 min after start of infusion. • Stop infusion immediately at first sign of hypersensitivity reaction.
Storage • Store diluted infusion solution in glass or polyethylene containers and discard after 24 hrs. • Do not store in PVC container (decreased stability, potential for extraction).

PO
• Administer on empty stomach. • Do not give with grapefruit products or within 2 hrs of antacids.

Topical
• For external use only. • Do not cover with occlusive dressing. • Rub gently, completely onto clean, dry skin.

IV INCOMPATIBILITIES

Acyclovir.

IV COMPATIBILITIES

Calcium gluconate, dexamethasone (Decadron), diphenhydramine (Benadryl), dobutamine (Dobutrex), dopamine (Intropin), furosemide (Lasix), heparin, hydromorphone (Dilaudid), insulin, leucovorin, lorazepam (Ativan), morphine, nitroglycerin, potassium chloride.

INDICATIONS/ROUTES/DOSAGE

Prevention of Liver Transplant Rejection
PO: ADULTS, ELDERLY: 0.1–0.15 mg/kg/day in 2 divided doses 12 hrs apart. Begin oral therapy no sooner than 6 hrs post-transplant. **CHILDREN:** 0.15–0.2 mg/kg/day in 2 divided doses 12 hrs apart. Begin oral therapy no sooner than 6 hrs post-transplant.
IV: ADULTS, ELDERLY, CHILDREN: 0.03–0.05 mg/kg/day as continuous infusion.

Prevention of Kidney Transplant Rejection
PO: ADULTS, ELDERLY: 0.2 mg/kg/day (in combination with azathioprine) in 2 divided doses 12 hrs apart or 0.1 mg/kg/day in combination with mycophenolate. May be given within 24 hrs of transplant.
IV: ADULTS, ELDERLY: 0.03–0.05 mg/kg/day as continuous infusion.

Prevention of Heart Transplant Rejection
PO: ADULTS, ELDERLY: Initially, 0.075 mg/kg/day in 2 divided doses 12 hrs apart. Begin oral therapy no sooner than 6 hrs post-transplant (in combination with azathioprine or mycophenolate recommended).
IV: ADULTS, ELDERLY: 0.01 mg/kg/day as continuous infusion.

Atopic Dermatitis
Topical: ADULTS, ELDERLY, CHILDREN 2 YRS AND OLDER: Apply 0.03% or 0.1% ointment to affected area twice daily. Continue treatment for 1 wk after symptoms have resolved. If no improvement within 6 wks, re-examine to confirm diagnosis.

SIDE EFFECTS

Frequent (greater than 30%): Headache, tremor, insomnia, paresthesia, diarrhea, nausea, constipation, vomiting, abdominal pain, hypertension. **Occasional (29%–10%):** Rash, pruritus, anorexia, asthenia (loss of strength, energy), peripheral edema, photosensitivity.

ADVERSE EFFECTS/
TOXIC REACTIONS

Nephrotoxicity (characterized by increased serum creatinine, decreased

T

urinary output), neurotoxicity (tremor, headache, altered mental status), pleural effusion occur commonly. Thrombocytopenia, leukocytosis, anemia, atelectasis, sepsis, infection occur occasionally.

NURSING CONSIDERATIONS

BASELINE ASSESSMENT

Assess past medical history, esp. renal function; medication history, use of other immunosuppressants. Have aqueous solution of epinephrine 1:1,000, O_2 available at bedside before beginning IV infusion. Assess pt continuously for first 30 min following start of infusion and at frequent intervals thereafter.

INTERVENTION/EVALUATION

Closely monitor pts with renal impairment. Monitor lab values, esp. serum creatinine, potassium levels, CBC with differential, serum hepatic function tests. Monitor I&O closely. CBC should be performed weekly during first mo of therapy, twice monthly during second and third mos of treatment, then monthly throughout the first yr. Report any major change in pt assessment.

PATIENT/FAMILY TEACHING

• Take dose at same time each day. • Avoid crowds, those with infection. • Report decreased urination, chest pain, headache, dizziness, respiratory infection, rash, unusual bleeding/bruising. • Avoid exposure to sun, artificial light (may cause photosensitivity reaction). • Do not take within 2 hrs of taking antacids. Do not take with grapefruit products.

---

tadalafil

ta-**dal**-a-fil
(Adcirca, <u>Cialis</u>)
Do not confuse Adcirca with Advair or Advicor, or tadalafil with sildenafil or vardenafil.

◆CLASSIFICATION

PHARMACOTHERAPEUTIC: Phosphodiesterase inhibitor. **CLINICAL:** Erectile dysfunction adjunct.

ACTION

Inhibits phosphodiesterase type 5, the enzyme responsible for degrading cyclic guanosine monophosphate in corpus cavernosum of penis, pulmonary vascular smooth muscle; resulting in smooth muscle relaxation, increased blood flow. **Therapeutic Effect:** Facilitates erection, improves exercise ability.

PHARMACOKINETICS

Route	Onset	Peak	Duration
PO	60 min	—	36 hrs

Rapidly absorbed after PO administration. Protein binding: 94%. Metabolized in liver. Primarily eliminated in feces. Drug has no effect on penile blood flow without sexual stimulation. **Half-life:** 17.5 hrs.

USES

Cialis: Treatment of erectile dysfunction (ED). Treatment of benign prostatic hyperplasia (BPH). Simultaneous treatment of ED and BPH. **Adcirca:** Treatment of pulmonary arterial hypertension (PAH).

PRECAUTIONS

Contraindications: Concurrent use of nitrates in any form, severe hepatic impairment. **Cautions:** Concurrent use of alpha-adrenergic blockers, renal/hepatic impairment (not recommended in pts with severe hepatic impairment or cirrhosis), anatomical deformation of penis, pts who may be predisposed to priapism (sickle cell anemia, multiple myeloma, leukemia), left ventricular outflow obstruction (e.g., aortic stenosis), bleeding disorders, peptic ulcer, elderly, concurrent use of strong CYP3A4 inhibitors.

⌛ LIFESPAN CONSIDERATIONS

Pregnancy/Lactation: Pregnancy Category B. Children: Not indicated in this

T

 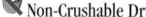

pt population. **Elderly:** No age-related precautions noted.

INTERACTIONS

DRUG: Alcohol increases risk of orthostatic hypotension. **Alpha-adrenergic blocks, other antihypertensive agents** may increase risk of hypotension. **Nitrates** contraindicated; may cause life-threatening hypotension. **CYP3A4 inhibitors (e.g., erythromycin, itraconazole, ketoconazole, ritonavir, saquinavir)** may increase concentration. **HERBAL: St. John's wort** may alter concentration/effects. **FOOD: Grapefruit products** may increase concentration, toxicity. **LAB VALUES:** May alter hepatic function levels, increase GGTP.

AVAILABILITY (Rx)

Tablets (Cialis): 2.5 mg, 5 mg, 10 mg, 20 mg. (Adcirca): 20 mg.

ADMINISTRATION/HANDLING

PO
• May give without regard to food. • Take at least 30 min before anticipated sexual activity. • Administer Adcirca dose once daily all at same time. Do not divide dosage.

INDICATIONS/ROUTES/DOSAGE

Erectile Dysfunction
PO: ADULTS, ELDERLY: Once daily dosing: 2.5 mg. **Range:** 2.5–5 mg based on tolerability. **Maximum:** 2.5 mg (with CYP3A4 inhibitors). As needed dosing: 10 mg at least 30 min prior to anticipated sexual activity. **Range:** 5–20 mg. No more than one dose/24 hr. **Maximum:** 10 mg (with CYP3A4 inhibitors) no more frequently than q72h.

BPH
PO: ADULTS, ELDERLY: (Cialis) 5 mg once daily. **With CYP3A4 inhibitors:** 2.5 mg once daily.

ED and BPH
PO: ADULTS, ELDERLY: (Cialis) 5 mg once daily. **With CYP3A4 inhibitors:** 2.5 mg once daily.

PAH
PO: ADULTS, ELDERLY: (Adcirca) 40 mg once daily.

Dosage in Renal Impairment
Erectile Dysfunction (Cialis)
Creatinine clearance 31–50 ml/min: As needed dosing: Starting dose is 5 mg before sexual activity once daily. **Maximum dose:** 10 mg no more frequently than once q48h. No dose adjustment for once daily dosing. **Creatinine clearance less than 31 ml/min:** Starting dose is 5 mg before sexual activity. Not to be given more often than q72h. Daily dosing not recommended.

PAH (Adcirca)
Creatinine clearance 31–80 ml/min: Initially, 20 mg daily. May increase to 40 mg based on tolerance. Avoid use if creatinine clearance less than 31 ml/min.

Dosage in Mild to Moderate Hepatic Impairment
Erectile dysfunction (Cialis)
Pts with Child-Pugh class A or B hepatic impairment should take no more than 10 mg once daily. Not recommended in severe hepatic impairment.

SIDE EFFECTS

Occasional: Headache, dyspepsia (heartburn, indigestion, epigastric pain), back pain, myalgia, nasal congestion, flushing, sudden hearing loss, visual field loss, postural hypotension.

ADVERSE EFFECTS/TOXIC REACTIONS

Prolonged erections (lasting over 4 hrs), priapism (painful erections lasting over 6 hrs) occur rarely. Angina, chest pain, MI have been reported.

NURSING CONSIDERATIONS

BASELINE ASSESSMENT
Assess cardiovascular status before initiating treatment for erectile dysfunction. Obtain baseline renal/hepatic function

tests. Screen for use of nitrate-based medications.

INTERVENTION/EVALUATION

Monitor B/P. Assess quality of sexual activity.

PATIENT/FAMILY TEACHING

• Has no effect in absence of sexual stimulation. • Seek treatment immediately if erection persists for over 4 hrs. • Report sudden decrease or loss of hearing or vision. • Avoid alcohol (may increase risk of postural hypotension). • Go from lying to standing slowly. • Do not ingest grapefruit products.

---

tamoxifen

tam-**ox**-i-fen
(Apo-Tamox ✤, Nolvadex-D ✤, Soltamox)

BLACK BOX ALERT Serious, possibly life-threatening stroke, pulmonary emboli, uterine malignancy (endometrial adenocarcinoma, uterine sarcoma) have occurred.
Do not confuse tamoxifen with pentoxifylline, tamsulosin, or temazepam.

◆CLASSIFICATION

PHARMACOTHERAPEUTIC: Nonsteroidal antiestrogen. **CLINICAL:** Antineoplastic (see p. 90C).

ACTION

Competes with estradiol for estrogen-receptor binding sites in breast, uterus, vaginal cells. **Therapeutic Effect:** Inhibits DNA synthesis, estrogen response.

PHARMACOKINETICS

Well absorbed from GI tract. Metabolized in liver. Primarily eliminated in feces by biliary system. **Half-life:** 7 days.

USES

Adjunct treatment in advanced breast cancer after primary treatment with surgery and radiation, reduce risk of breast cancer in women at high risk, reduce risk of invasive breast cancer in women with ductal carcinoma *in situ* (DCIS), metastatic breast cancer in women and men. **OFF-LABEL:** Induction of ovulation, treatment of desmoid tumors. Treatment of mastalgia, gynecomastia; ovarian, endometrial cancer; uterine sarcoma; precocious puberty in females; risk reduction in women with Paget's disease of breast.

PRECAUTIONS

Contraindications: Concomitant coumarin-type therapy when used in treatment of breast cancer in high-risk women, history of deep vein thrombosis (DVT) or pulmonary embolism (in high-risk women for breast cancer and in women with DCIS). **Cautions:** Leukopenia, thrombocytopenia, pregnancy, history of thromboembolic events, hyperlipidemia, concomitant drug therapy affecting CYP and Pgp (hepatic) metabolic pathways.

⌛ LIFESPAN CONSIDERATIONS

Pregnancy/Lactation: If possible, avoid use during pregnancy, esp. first trimester. May cause fetal harm. Unknown if distributed in breast milk. Breastfeeding not recommended. **Pregnancy Category D. Children:** Safe and effective in girls 2–10 yrs with McCune Albright syndrome, precocious puberty. **Elderly:** No age-related precautions noted.

INTERACTIONS

DRUG: May increase effects of **warfarin.** May decrease effects of **anastrozole. Cytotoxic agents** may increase risk of thromboembolic events. **Moderate/strong CYP2D6 inhibitors (e.g., fluoxetine, sertraline)** may decrease efficacy and increase risk of breast cancer. **HERBAL:** Avoid **black cohosh, dong quai** in estrogen-dependent tumors. **St. John's wort** may decrease concentration/effects. **FOOD:** None known. **LAB VALUES:** May increase serum cholesterol, calcium, triglycerides, hepatic enzymes.

AVAILABILITY (Rx)

Solution, Oral (Soltamox): 10 mg/5 ml.
Tablets: 10 mg, 20 mg.

ADMINISTRATION/HANDLING

PO
• Give without regard to food.

INDICATIONS/ROUTES/DOSAGE

Metastatic Breast Cancer (Males and Females)
PO: ADULTS, ELDERLY: 20–40 mg/day.
Give doses greater than 20 mg/day in divided doses. Duration is 5 yrs for premenopausal women and 2–3 yrs followed by an aromatase inhibitor to complete 5 yrs.

Prevention of Breast Cancer in High-Risk Women, Ductal Carcinoma *in Situ*, Adjunctive Treatment of Breast Cancer (Women)
PO: ADULTS, ELDERLY: 20 mg/day for 5 yrs.

SIDE EFFECTS

Frequent: Women (greater than 10%): Hot flashes, nausea, vomiting. **Occasional: Women (9%–1%):** Changes in menstruation, genital itching, vaginal discharge, endometrial hyperplasia, polyps. **Men:** Impotence, decreased libido. **Men and women:** Headache, nausea, vomiting, rash, bone pain, confusion, weakness, drowsiness.

ADVERSE EFFECTS/TOXIC REACTIONS

Retinopathy, corneal opacity, decreased visual acuity noted in pts receiving extremely high dosages (240–320 mg/day) for longer than 17 mos.

NURSING CONSIDERATIONS

BASELINE ASSESSMENT
Obtain estrogen receptor assay prior to therapy. Obtain baseline breast and gynecologic exams, mammogram results. CBC, serum calcium levels should be checked before and periodically during therapy.

INTERVENTION/EVALUATION
Be alert to increased bone pain; ensure adequate pain relief. Monitor I&O, weight. Observe for edema, esp. of dependent areas, signs and symptoms of DVT. Assess for hypercalcemia (increased urinary volume, excessive thirst, nausea, vomiting, constipation, hypotonicity of muscles, deep bone/flank pain, renal stones).

PATIENT/FAMILY TEACHING
• Report vaginal bleeding/discharge/itching, leg cramps, weight gain, shortness of breath, weakness. • May initially experience increase in bone, tumor pain (appears to indicate good tumor response). • Report persistent nausea, vomiting. • Nonhormonal contraceptives are recommended during treatment.

---

tamsulosin

tam-**sool**-o-sin
(<u>Flomax</u>, Ava-Tamsulosin ✦)
Do not confuse Flomax with Flonase, Flovent, Foltx, Fosamax, or Volmax, or tamsulosin with tamoxifen or terazosin.

FIXED-COMBINATION(S)

Jalyn: tamsulosin/dutasteride (an androgen hormone inhibitor): 0.4 mg/0.5 mg.

◆CLASSIFICATION

PHARMACOTHERAPEUTIC: Alpha$_1$-adrenergic blocker. **CLINICAL:** Benign prostatic hyperplasia agent.

ACTION

Targets receptors around bladder neck, prostate capsule. **Therapeutic Effect:** Relaxes smooth muscle, improves urinary flow, symptoms of prostatic hyperplasia.

PHARMACOKINETICS

Well absorbed, widely distributed. Protein binding: 94%–99%. Metabolized in liver. Primarily excreted in urine. Unknown if removed by hemodialysis. **Half-life:** 9–13 hrs.

USES

Treatment of symptoms of benign prostatic hyperplasia (BPH), alone or in combination with dutasteride (Avodart). **OFF-LABEL:** Treatment of bladder outlet obstruction or dysfunction. Facilitate expulsion of ureteral stones.

PRECAUTIONS

Contraindications: None known. **Cautions:** Concurrent use of phosphodiesterase (PDE5) inhibitors (sildenafil, tadalafil, vardenafil).

⌛ LIFESPAN CONSIDERATIONS

Pregnancy/Lactation: Not indicated for use in women. **Pregnancy Category B. Children:** Not indicated in this pt population. **Elderly:** No age-related precautions noted.

INTERACTIONS

DRUG: Other alpha-adrenergic blocking agents (e.g., doxazosin, prazosin, terazosin) may increase alpha-blockade effects. **Sildenafil, tadalafil, vardenafil** may cause symptomatic hypotension. **CYP3A4 inhibitors (e.g., ketoconazole)** may increase concentration. **HERBAL:** Avoid **saw palmetto** (limited experience with this combination). **Black cohosh, periwinkle** may increase hypotensive effect. **St. John's wort** may decrease concentration/effects. **FOOD: Grapefruit products** may increase potential for orthostatic hypotension. **LAB VALUES:** None known.

AVAILABILITY (Rx)

🔖 **Capsules:** 0.4 mg.

ADMINISTRATION/HANDLING

PO
• Give at same time each day, 30 min after the same meal. • Do not break, crush, dissolve, or open capsule.

INDICATIONS/ROUTES/DOSAGE

Benign Prostatic Hyperplasia (BPH)
PO: ADULTS: 0.4 mg once a day, approximately 30 min after same meal each day. May increase dosage to 0.8 mg if inadequate response in 2–4 wks.

SIDE EFFECTS

Frequent (9%–7%): Dizziness, drowsiness. **Occasional (5%–3%):** Headache, anxiety, insomnia, orthostatic hypotension. **Rare (less than 2%):** Nasal congestion, pharyngitis, rhinitis, nausea, vertigo, impotence.

ADVERSE EFFECTS/TOXIC REACTIONS

First-dose syncope (hypotension with sudden loss of consciousness) may occur within 30–90 min after initial dose. May be preceded by tachycardia (pulse rate of 120–160 beats/min).

NURSING CONSIDERATIONS

BASELINE ASSESSMENT

Assess history of prostatic hyperplasia (difficulty initiating urine stream, dribbling, sense of urgency, leaking). Question for sensitivity to tamsulosin, or use of other alpha-adrenergic blocking agents, warfarin. Obtain vital signs.

INTERVENTION/EVALUATION

Assist with ambulation if dizziness occurs. Monitor renal function, I&O, weight changes, peripheral edema, B/P. Monitor for first-dose syncope.

PATIENT/FAMILY TEACHING

• Take at same time each day, 30 min after the same meal. • Go from lying to standing slowly. • Avoid tasks that require alertness, motor skills until response to drug is established. • Do not break, chew, crush, open capsule.

T

tapentadol

ta-**pen**-ta-dol

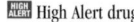

(Nucynta, Nucynta CR 🍁, Nucynta ER, Nucynta IR 🍁)

Do not confuse tapentadol with tramadol.

◆ CLASSIFICATION

PHARMACOTHERAPEUTIC: Centrally-acting synthetic analgesic. **CLINICAL:** Analgesic.

ACTION

Binds to and activates mu-opioid receptors in the central nervous system, increases norepinephrine by inhibiting its reabsorption into nerve cells. **Therapeutic Effect:** Produces analgesia.

PHARMACOKINETICS

Metabolized in liver. Primarily excreted in the urine. Widely distributed. Protein binding: 20%. **Half-life:** 4 hrs.

USES

Nucynta: Relief of moderate to severe acute pain in adults 18 yrs and older. **Nucynta ER:** Management of moderate to severe chronic pain when around-the-clock analgesic needed for extended period. Treatment of diabetic neuropathy pain.

PRECAUTIONS

Contraindications: Severe respiratory depression, acute or severe bronchial asthma; hypercapnia in uncontrolled settings, known or suspected paralytic ileus, concurrent use or ingestion within 14 days of MAOI use. **Cautions:** Respiratory disease or respiratory compromise (e.g., hypoxia, hypercapnia, or decreased respiratory reserve), asthma, COPD, severe obesity, sleep apnea syndrome, myxedema coma, CNS depression; pts with head injury, intracranial lesions, pancreatic or biliary disease, renal or hepatic impairment, history of seizures, conditions that increase risk of seizures; pts at risk for hypotension, adrenal insufficiency, hypothyroidism, prostatic hyperplasia/urinary stricture; concurrent use with serotonergic agents; elderly; debilitated or cachetic pts.

⏳ LIFESPAN CONSIDERATIONS

Pregnancy/Lactation: Unknown if drug crosses placenta or is distributed in breast milk. **Pregnancy Category C. Children:** Not recommended for use in this pt population. **Elderly:** Age-related renal impairment may increase risk of side effects.

INTERACTIONS

DRUG: Alcohol, CNS depressants may increase CNS depression, respiratory depression. **MAOIs, SSRIs (e.g., fluoxetine), tricyclic antidepressants (e.g., amitriptyline), triptans (e.g., sumatriptan)** may increase risk of serotonin syndrome. **HERBAL: Kava kava, St. John's wort, valerian** may increase CNS depression. **St. John's wort** may increase risk for serotonin syndrome. **FOOD:** None known. **LAB VALUES:** None significant.

AVAILABILITY (Rx)

Tablets: 50 mg, 75 mg, 100 mg.

🍁 Tablets, Extended-Release: 50 mg, 100 mg, 150 mg, 200 mg, 250 mg.

ADMINISTRATION/HANDLING

PO
• Give without regard to food. • Tablets may be crushed. • Give extended-release tablets whole; do not break, crush, dissolve, or divide.

INDICATIONS/ROUTES/DOSAGE

Note: Not recommended in severe renal or hepatic impairment.

Pain Control
PO: ADULTS, ELDERLY: Nucynta: 50–100 mg q4–6h as needed. **Maximum:** 600 mg/day. **Nucynta ER:** Initially, 50 mg twice daily (12 hr apart). May increase by 50 mg twice daily q3days to effective dose. **Range:** 100–250 mg twice daily.

Dosage in Hepatic Impairment
Immediate-Release: Moderate impairment: 50 mg q8h. **Maximum:** 3 doses/24 hrs. Extended-Release: Initially, 50 mg/day. **Maximum:** 100 mg/day.

SIDE EFFECTS

Frequent (greater than 10%): Nausea, dizziness, vomiting, sleepiness, headache.

ADVERSE EFFECTS/ TOXIC REACTIONS

Respiratory depression, serotonin syndrome have been reported.

NURSING CONSIDERATIONS

BASELINE ASSESSMENT

Assess onset, type, location, and duration of pain. Obtain vital signs before giving medication. If respirations are 12/min or lower, withhold medication, contact physician. Question history of hepatic impairment.

INTERVENTION/EVALUATION

Be alert for decreased respirations or B/P. Initiate deep breathing and coughing exercises, particularly in pts with impaired pulmonary function. Assess for clinical improvement and record onset of pain relief.

PATIENT/FAMILY TEACHING

• Avoid tasks that require alertness, motor skills until response to drug is established. • Avoid alcohol, CNS depressants. • Report nausea, vomiting, shortness of breath, difficulty breathing.

teduglutide

te-due-**gloo**-tide
(Gattex)
Do not confuse teduglutide with liraglutide or albiglutide, or Gattex with Gas-X.

◆CLASSIFICATION

PHARMACOTHERAPEUTIC: Human glucagon-like peptide-2. **CLINICAL:** Short bowel syndrome (short gut syndrome, short gut) agent.

ACTION

Analogue of naturally occurring peptide secreted by L cells of distal intestine, known to increase intestinal, portal blood flow, and inhibit gastric secretion. **Therapeutic Effect:** Improves intestinal absorption.

PHARMACOKINETICS

Degrades into small peptides, amino acids via catabolic pathway. Primarily excreted in urine. 86–89% bioavailability following subcutaneous injection. Peak plasma concentration: 3–5 hrs. **Half-life:** 1.3–2 hrs.

USES

Treatment of adults with short bowel syndrome (SBS) who are dependent on parenteral support.

PRECAUTIONS

Contraindications: None known. **Cautions:** Cardiovascular disease, HF, pts at increased risk for malignancy, biliary tract (gallbladder, pancreatic) disease, hypervolemia, stenosis, renal impairment.

⧗ LIFESPAN CONSIDERATIONS

Pregnancy/Lactation: Unknown if distributed in breast milk. **Pregnancy Category B. Children:** Safety and efficacy not established. **Elderly:** No age-related precautions noted.

INTERACTIONS

DRUG: May increase absorption of any **concomitant oral medication. HERBAL:** None significant. **FOOD:** None known. **LAB VALUES:** None significant.

AVAILABILITY (Rx)

Injection, Powder for Reconstitution: 5 mg (delivers maximum of 0.38 ml containing 3.8 mg teduglutide).

T

ADMINISTRATION/HANDLING

Subcutaneous

Reconstitution • If diluent syringe (contains 0.5 ml Sterile Water for Injection) has a white snap-off cap, snap or twist off white cap. • If diluent syringe has a gray screw top, unscrew top counter clockwise. • Push prefilled syringe into vial containing teduglutide. • After all diluent has gone into vial, remove syringe, needle and discard. • Allow vial to sit for 30 sec. • Gently roll vial for 15 sec (do not shake) and let stand for 2 min. • Withdraw prescribed dose, discard remaining fluid. • Use within 3 hrs following reconstitution. • Use abdomen, thighs, upper arms for injection. • Avoid injection sites where skin is tender, bruised, red, or hard.

Storage • Store kit in refrigerator. • Reconstituted solution should appear as a clear, colorless to light straw-colored liquid. • Discard if particulate is present. • Drug should be completely dissolved before solution is withdrawn from vial.

INDICATIONS/ROUTES/DOSAGE

Short Bowel Syndrome
Subcutaneous: ADULTS/ELDERLY: 0.05 mg/kg/day.

Moderate to Severe Renal Impairment
Subcutaneous: ADULTS/ELDERLY: 50% dose reduction.

SIDE EFFECTS

Frequent (30%–22%): Abdominal pain, nausea, injection site reactions. **Occasional (18%–14%):** Headache, abdominal distention, vomiting. **Rare (9%):** Flatulence, hypersensitivity, appetite disorders, sleep disturbances.

ADVERSE EFFECTS/
TOXIC REACTIONS

Upper respiratory tract infection occurs in 12% of pts. Fluid overload (hypervolemia) has been noted in 7% of pts. Potential for hypovolemia is increased in pts with cardiovascular disease, HF. Therapy increases risk for acceleration of neoplastic growth. Cholecystitis, cholangitis, cholelithiasis, pancreatitis has been reported.

BASELINE ASSESSMENT

Obtain baseline serum chemistries, hepatic function test, lipase, amylase. Colonoscopy (or alternate imaging) with removal of polyps should be completed within 5 mos prior to initiating treatment.

INTERVENTION/EVALUATION

Follow-up colonoscopy (or alternate imaging) is recommended at the end of 1 year. If no polyp is found, subsequent colonoscopies should be done no less frequently than every 5 years. If a polyp is found, adherence to current polyp follow-up guidelines is recommended. Discovery of intestinal obstruction, intestinal malignancy necessitates discontinuation of treatment. Subsequent laboratory assessments, hepatic functions tests are recommended every 6 mos. If clinically meaningful elevation is seen, further diagnostic workup is recommended as clinically indicated.

PATIENT/FAMILY TEACHING

• Teach proper use and administration of medication. • Be aware of need for any new supplies. • Instruct pt in preparation of medication and observe correct administration technique. • Report yellowing of skin or eyes, dark urine, changes in stool color or consistency, severe abdominal pain, nausea, vomiting, sudden weight gain, swelling, or difficulty breathing.

telaprevir

tel-**a**-pre-veer
(Incivek)
BLACK BOX ALERT Fatal and non-fatal skin reactions reported.
Do not confuse telaprevir with boceprevir or simeprevir.

◆CLASSIFICATION

PHARMACOTHERAPEUTIC: Protease inhibitor. **CLINICAL:** Antiviral.

ACTION

Inhibits hepatitis C virus (HCV) protease needed for cleavage of HCV-encoded polyproteins by binding to active serine protease sites. **Therapeutic Effect:** Inhibits viral replication of hepatitis C virus.

PHARMACOKINETICS

Well absorbed following PO administration. Peak concentration: 4–5 hrs. Protein binding: 59%–75%. Metabolized in liver. Excreted primarily in feces. Minimal removal by hemodialysis. **Half-life:** 9–11 hrs.

USES

Treatment of chronic hepatitis C genotype 1 in combination with peginterferon alfa and ribavirin in adults with compensated liver disease, including cirrhosis, who are previously untreated or who have failed previous interferon and ribavirin therapy.

PRECAUTIONS

◀ALERT▶ Safety and efficacy not established in decompensated cirrhosis, organ transplant, HIV, hepatitis B, previous failed therapies with protease inhibitors.
Contraindications: Pregnancy, male partners of pregnant women, drugs utilizing CYP3A for clearance (see drug interactions), any contraindications to peginterferon alfa or ribavirin. **Cautions:** Baseline anemia, moderate to severe hepatic impairment.

⧖ LIFESPAN CONSIDERATIONS

Pregnancy/Lactation: Strictly avoid pregnancy. May cause birth defects or fetal demise. **Pregnancy Category B (X when used with ribavirin).** Women of childbearing age must use 2 different forms of birth control: intrauterine device and barrier methods during treatment plus at least 6 mos after treatment. Hormonal contraceptives may have decreased effectiveness. Do not initiate therapy until negative pregnancy test confirmed. Unknown if drug crosses placenta or is distributed in breast milk. **Children:** Safety and efficacy not established. **Elderly:** No age-related precautions noted.

INTERACTIONS

DRUG: Contraindicated with **alfuzosin, atorvastatin, dihydroergotamine, ergonovine, ergotamine, lovastatin, methylergonovine, midazolam, pimozide, rifampin, sildenafil, simvastatin, tadalafil, triazolam.** May increase concentrations of **antiarrhythmics (amiodarone, digoxin, quinidine), antifungals (itraconazole, ketoconazole), calcium channel blockers (amlodipine, diltiazem, nicardipine), clarithromycin, colchicine, desipramine, dexamethasone, fluticasone, immunosuppressants, oral contraceptives, rifabutin, salmeterol, tadalafil, trazadone, vardenafil.** **HERBAL:** **St. John's wort** may decrease effectiveness. **FOOD:** **Low-fat meals** may decrease absorption. **LAB VALUES:** May decrease RBC, Hgb, Hct, neutrophils, leukocytes, platelets. May increase serum bilirubin, uric acid levels.

AVAILABILITY (Rx)

Tablets: 375 mg.

ADMINISTRATION/HANDLING

• Give with food containing approximately 20 grams of fat. Take approximately q7–9hr.

INDICATIONS/ROUTES/DOSAGE

Chronic Hepatitis C
PO: ADULTS, ELDERLY: 750 mg 3 times a day with food for 12 wks. Use triple therapy with peginterferon alfa, ribavirin. Duration based on response-guided therapy (RGT) guidelines.

Response-Guided Therapy Guidelines with HCV-RNA Level
Based on prior treatment and HCV-RNA results at wks 4 and 12. If level undetectable at 4 and 12 wks, continue only

T

peginterferon alfa, ribavirin for 12 more wks. If level detectable (1,000 international units/ml or less), continue peginterferon alfa, ribavirin for 36 wks.

Treatment Futility

Discontinue treatment if HCV-RNA viral load greater than or equal to 1,000 international units/ml at wks 4 and 12. If HCV-RNA detectable at wk 24, discontinue triple therapy.

Chronic Hepatitis C with Cirrhosis, or Poor Responders to Interferon

PO: ADULTS: 750 mg 3 times a day with food for 12 wks. Continue peginterferon alfa, ribavirin for 36 wks.

Dosage Modification

Do not reduce telaprevir dose during treatment. If adverse reaction or neutropenia occurs, recommend reduction/discontinuation of peginterferon and/or ribavirin. If Hgb less than 10 g/dl, reduce or interrupt ribavirin. If Hgb less than 8.5 g/dl, discontinue ribavirin.

SIDE EFFECTS

Frequent (56%–26%): Rash, fatigue, pruritus, nausea, diarrhea. **Occasional (13%–6%):** Vomiting, hemorrhoids, anorectal discomfort, dysgeusia, anal pruritus.

ADVERSE EFFECTS/ TOXIC REACTIONS

Increased risk of thromboembolic events associated with peginterferon, erythropoiesis-stimulating agent. Serious skin reactions including drug rash with eosinophilia, systemic symptoms, Stevens-Johnson syndrome reported. Simultaneous use of contraindicated medications may result in hypertension/hypotension, peripheral vasospasm/ischemia (ergot toxicity), arrhythmias, rhabdomyolysis (statins), hyperkalemia (oral contraception), visual abnormalities, syncope, increased sedation or respiratory depression (sedative/hypnotics), loss of virologic response.

NURSING CONSIDERATIONS

BASELINE ASSESSMENT

Assess vital signs, O_2 saturation. Obtain CBC, HCV-RNA level, serum chemistries, hepatic function test, TSH. Receive full medication history including vitamins, herbal products; screen for contraindications. Confirm negative pregnancy test before initiating treatment. Question history of anemia, HIV, hepatitis B.

INTERVENTION/EVALUATION

Assess vital signs, O_2 saturation routinely. Monitor CBC with differential (wks 4, 8, 12), and HCV-RNA levels (wks 4, 8, 12, 24), urine pregnancy every month and 6 mos after final treatment. Assess for anemia-related dizziness, exertional dyspnea, fatigue, weakness, syncope. Report decreases in Hgb, Hct, platelets, neutrophils. Check INR if on warfarin. Monitor for acute infection (fever, diaphoresis, lethargy, oral mucosal changes, productive cough), bloody stools, bruising, hematuria, DVT, pulmonary embolism. Encourage nutritional intake and assess for anorexia, weight loss. Monitor for intrauterine device failures if applicable. Reinforce birth control compliance. Obtain EKG for palpitations, tachycardia.

PATIENT/FAMILY TEACHING

• Must be used in combination with peginterferon, ribavirin. • Inform pt of side effects/contraindications of triple-medication regimen. • Blood levels will be drawn routinely. • Immediately report any newly prescribed medications. • Women of childbearing potential must use two different forms of birth control: intrauterine device plus barrier methods during treatment and for at least 6 mos after treatment. Hormonal birth control (oral, vaginal rings, injections) may be ineffective. Immediately notify physician if pregnancy occurs. • May alter taste of food or decrease appetite. • Report bloody stool/urine, increased bruising, difficulty breathing, weakness, dizziness, palpitations, weight loss. • Avoid alcohol. • Take with meals.

telavancin

tel-a-**van**-sin
(Vibativ)

BLACK BOX ALERT Pts with pre-existing renal impairment (CrCl less than 50 mL/min) who are treated for hospital-acquired pneumonia may have increased mortality risk when compared to vancomycin. May cause new or worsening renal impairment. May cause fetal harm (low birth weight, limb malformations). Women of childbearing potential should have pregnancy test before treatment; avoid use during pregnancy unless benefit to pt outweighs fetal risk.

Do not confuse telavancin with dalbavancin or oritavancin; or Vibativ with Vibra-Tabs or vigabatrin.

◆CLASSIFICATION

PHARMACOTHERAPEUTIC: Lipoglycopeptide antibacterial. **CLINICAL:** Antibiotic.

ACTION

Inhibits bacterial cell wall synthesis by blocking polymerization and cross-linking of peptidoglycan. Disrupts membrane potential and changes cell wall permeability. **Therapeutic Effect:** Bactericidal. Antibiotic.

PHARMACOKINETICS

Not metabolized in liver; pathway unspecified. Protein binding: 90%. Primarily excreted unchanged in urine. Not removed by hemodialysis. **Half-life:** 8–9 hrs.

USES

Treatment of complicated skin, soft tissue infections caused by gram-positive microorganisms, including methicillin-susceptible or methicillin-resistant *S. aureus*, vancomycin-susceptible *Enterococcus*. Treatment of hospital-acquired and ventilator-associated bacterial pneumonia caused by susceptible isolates of *S. aureus*.

PRECAUTIONS

Contraindications: Prior hypersensitivity reactions to telavancin. **Cautions:** Renal impairment, concurrent therapy with other nephrotoxic medications (NSAIDs, ACE inhibitors, aminoglycosides). Avoid use in pts with history of congenital QT syndrome, known prolongation of QT interval, uncompensated HF, severe left ventricular hypertrophy, or receiving treatment with other drugs known to prolong QT interval.

⧗ LIFESPAN CONSIDERATIONS

Pregnancy/Lactation: May cause fetal harm at regular dosage. Unknown if distributed in breast milk. **Pregnancy Category C. Children:** Safety and efficacy not established. **Elderly:** Age-related renal impairment may increase risk of nephrotoxicity; dosage adjustment recommended.

INTERACTIONS

DRUG: Telavancin may increase levels/effects of **dronedarone, nilotinib, pimozide, quinine, tetrabenazene, thioridazine, ziprasidone. Ciprofloxacin** may increase levels/effect. **HERBAL:** None significant. **FOOD:** None known. **LAB VALUES:** May alter serum potassium. May increase serum bilirubin, AST, ALT, BUN, creatinine, PT, aPTT, INR. May decrease Hgb, Hct, WBC count.

AVAILABILITY (Rx)

Injection, Powder for Reconstitution: 250-mg, 750-mg single-dose vial.

ADMINISTRATION/HANDLING

IV

◀ALERT▶ Give by intermittent IV infusion (piggyback). Do not give by IV push (may result in hypotension).

Reconstitution • 250-mg vial: Reconstitute with 15 ml Sterile Water for Injection, D₅W, or 0.9% NaCl to provide concentration of 15 mg/ml (total volume approximately 17 ml). • **750-mg vial:** Reconstitute with 45 ml Sterile Water for Injection, D₅W, or 0.9% NaCl to provide concentration of 15 mg/ml

T

(total volume approximately 50 ml).
• Prior to administration, further dilute with D_5W or 0.9% NaCl to final concentration of 0.6–8 mg/ml. • Do not shake.
Rate of Administration • Infuse over at least 60 min.
Storage • Discard if particulate is present. • Following reconstitution, drug is stable for 4 hrs at room temperature or 72 hrs if refrigerated in vial or infusion bag.

🔲 IV INCOMPATIBILITY

Amphotericin, colistimethate, levofloxacin (Levaquin), micafungin (Mycomine).

🔲 IV COMPATIBILITY

Azithromycin, caspofungin, cefepime, ceftazidine, ceftriaxone, ciprofloxacin, doripenem, doxycycline, gentamicin, ertapenem, fluconazole, meropenem, tobramycin, pantoprazole, piperacillin-tazobactam, tigecycline.

INDICATIONS/ROUTES/DOSAGE

Usual Parenteral Dosage
IV Infusion: ADULTS, ELDERLY: 10 mg/kg once every 24 hrs for 7–21 days. Duration based on severity, infection site, and clinical progress of pt.

Dosage in Renal Impairment

Creatinine Clearance	Dosage
50 ml/min or greater	10 mg/kg every 24 hrs
30–49 ml/min	7.5 mg/kg every 24 hrs
10–29 ml/min	10 mg/kg every 48 hrs

SIDE EFFECTS

Frequent (33%–27%): Taste disturbance (metallic or soapy), nausea. **Occasional (14%–6%):** Vomiting, foamy urine, diarrhea, dizziness, pruritus. **Rare (4%–2%):** Rigors, rash, infusion site pain, anorexia, infusion site erythema.

ADVERSE EFFECTS/ TOXIC REACTIONS

Nephrotoxicity (acute kidney injury, acute tubular necrosis, renal failure); diarrhea due to *C. difficile* may occur. "Red-man syndrome" characterized by erythema on face, neck, upper torso; tachycardia, hypotension, myalgia, angioedema may occur from too-rapid rate of infusion.

NURSING CONSIDERATIONS

BASELINE ASSESSMENT

Obtain pregnancy test prior to treatment. Obtain baseline serum BUN, creatinine, creatinine clearance prior to initiating therapy, every 48–72 hrs, and after treatment is completed. Obtain culture and sensitivity tests before giving first dose (therapy may begin before results are known).

INTERVENTION/EVALUATION

Monitor renal function tests, I&O. Assess skin for rash. Avoid rapid infusion ("red-man syndrome"). Monitor daily pattern of bowel activity, stool consistency. Obtain C-Diff PCR test if diarrhea occurs.

PATIENT/FAMILY TEACHING

• Use effective contraception during treatment. • Report rash, signs/symptoms of nephrotoxicity, diarrhea. • Routine lab tests are important part of total therapy.

telmisartan

tel-mi-**sar**-tan
(Micardis)
BLACK BOX ALERT May cause fetal injury, mortality if used during second or third trimester of pregnancy.

FIXED-COMBINATION(S)

Micardis HCT: telmisartan/hydrochlorothiazide (a diuretic): 40 mg/12.5 mg, 80 mg/12.5 mg. **Twynsta:** telmisartan/amlodipine (a calcium channel blocker): 40 mg/5 mg, 40 mg/10 mg, 80 mg/5 mg, 80 mg/10 mg.

◆CLASSIFICATION

PHARMACOTHERAPEUTIC: Angiotensin II receptor antagonist. **CLINICAL:** Antihypertensive (see p. 11C).

ACTION

Blocks vasoconstrictor and aldosterone-secreting effects of angiotensin II, inhibiting binding of angiotensin II to AT_1 receptors. **Therapeutic Effect:** Causes vasodilation, decreases peripheral resistance, decreases B/P.

PHARMACOKINETICS

Route	Onset	Peak	Duration
PO (reduce B/P)	1–2 hrs	—	24 hrs

Rapidly, completely absorbed after PO administration. Protein binding: greater than 99%. Metabolized in liver. Excreted in feces. Unknown if removed by hemodialysis. **Half-life:** 24 hrs.

USES

Treatment of hypertension alone or in combination with other antihypertensives. Reduces risk of stroke, MI, death in pts 55 yrs of age or older with cardiovascular abnormalities (e.g., coronary artery disease, high-risk diabetes mellitus).

PRECAUTIONS

Contraindications: Concurrent use with aliskiren in pts with diabetes. **Cautions:** Hypovolemia, hepatic/renal impairment, renal artery stenosis (unilateral, bilateral), biliary obstructive disease, significant aortic/mitral stenosis. Concurrent use with ramipril not recommended.

⧗ LIFESPAN CONSIDERATIONS

Pregnancy/Lactation: May cause fetal harm. Unknown if drug is distributed in breast milk. **Pregnancy Category C (D if used in second or third trimester). Children:** Safety and efficacy not established. **Elderly:** No age-related precautions noted.

INTERACTIONS

DRUG: NSAIDs may decrease antihypertensive effect. May increase **digoxin** concentration, risk of toxicity. **HERBAL: Ephedra, ginger, licorice, ginseng, yohimbe** may worsen hypertension. **Black cohosh, periwinkle** may increase antihypertensive effect. **FOOD:** None known. **LAB VALUES:** May increase serum BUN, creatinine, uric acid, cholesterol. May decrease Hgb, Hct.

AVAILABILITY (Rx)

Tablets: 20 mg, 40 mg, 80 mg.

ADMINISTRATION/HANDLING

PO
• Give without regard to meals.

INDICATIONS/ROUTES/DOSAGE

Hypertension
PO: ADULTS: 40 mg once daily. **ELDERLY:** 20 mg once daily. **Range:** 20–80 mg/day.

Cardiovascular Risk Reduction
PO: ADULTS, ELDERLY: 80 mg once daily.

SIDE EFFECTS

Occasional (7%–3%): Upper respiratory tract infection, sinusitis, back/leg pain, diarrhea. **Rare (1%):** Dizziness, headache, fatigue, nausea, heartburn, myalgia, cough, peripheral edema.

ADVERSE EFFECTS/ TOXIC REACTIONS

Overdosage may manifest as hypotension, tachycardia; bradycardia occurs less often.

NURSING CONSIDERATIONS

BASELINE ASSESSMENT

Obtain B/P, apical pulse immediately before each dose, in addition to regular monitoring (be alert to fluctuations). If excessive reduction in B/P occurs, place pt in supine position, feet slightly elevated. Assess medication history (esp. diuretics). Question for history of hepatic/renal impairment, renal artery stenosis. Obtain

T

BUN, serum creatinine, Hgb, Hct, vital signs (particularly B/P, pulse rate).

INTERVENTION/EVALUATION

Monitor B/P, pulse, serum electrolytes, renal function. Monitor for hypotension when initiating therapy.

PATIENT/FAMILY TEACHING

• Avoid tasks that require alertness, motor skills until response to drug is established (possible dizziness effect). • Maintain proper hydration. • Avoid pregnancy. • Inform physician as soon as possible if pregnancy occurs. • Report any sign of infection (sore throat, fever). • Avoid excessive exertion during hot weather (risk of dehydration, hypotension).

---

temazepam

te-**maz**-e-pam
(Apo-Temazepam ✦, Novo-Temazepam ✦, PMS-Temazepam ✦, Restoril)
Do not confuse Restoril with Risperdal, Vistaril, or Zestril, or temazepam with flurazepam, lorazepam, or clonazepam.

◆ CLASSIFICATION

PHARMACOTHERAPEUTIC: Benzodiazepine **(Schedule IV). CLINICAL:** Sedative-hypnotic (see p. 148C).

ACTION

Enhances action of inhibitory neurotransmitter gamma-aminobutyric acid (GABA), resulting in CNS depression. **Therapeutic Effect:** Induces sleep.

PHARMACOKINETICS

Well absorbed from GI tract. Protein binding: 96%. Widely distributed. Crosses blood-brain barrier. Metabolized in liver. Primarily excreted in urine. Not removed by hemodialysis. **Half-life:** 9.5–12.4 hrs.

USES

Short-term treatment of insomnia (5 wks or less). Reduces sleep-induction time, number of nocturnal awakenings; increases length of sleep. **OFF-LABEL:** Treatment of anxiety, depression, panic attacks.

PRECAUTIONS

Contraindications: Angle-closure glaucoma, CNS depression, pregnancy, breast-feeding, severe, uncontrolled pain, sleep apnea. **Cautions:** Mental impairment, pts with drug dependence potential.

⧖ LIFESPAN CONSIDERATIONS

Pregnancy/Lactation: Crosses placenta. May be distributed in breast milk. Chronic ingestion during pregnancy may produce withdrawal symptoms, CNS depression in neonates. **Pregnancy Category X. Children:** Not recommended in those younger than 18 yrs. **Elderly:** Use small initial doses with gradual dosage increases to avoid ataxia, excessive sedation.

INTERACTIONS

DRUG: Alcohol, other CNS depressants may increase CNS depression. **HERBAL: St. John's wort** may decrease concentration. **Gotu kola, kava kava, St. John's wort, valerian** may increase CNS depression. **FOOD:** None known. **LAB VALUES:** None significant.

AVAILABILITY (Rx)

Capsules: 7.5 mg, 15 mg, 22.5 mg, 30 mg.

ADMINISTRATION/HANDLING

PO
• Give without regard to meals. • Capsules may be emptied and mixed with food.

INDICATIONS/ROUTES/DOSAGE

Insomnia
PO: ADULTS, CHILDREN 18 YRS AND OLDER: 15–30 mg at bedtime. **ELDERLY, DEBILITATED:** 7.5–15 mg at bedtime.

SIDE EFFECTS

Frequent: Drowsiness, sedation, rebound insomnia (may occur for 1–2 nights after

---

drug is discontinued), dizziness, confusion, euphoria. **Occasional:** Asthenia (loss of strength, energy), anorexia, diarrhea. **Rare:** Paradoxical CNS excitement, restlessness (particularly in elderly, debilitated pts).

ADVERSE EFFECTS/ TOXIC REACTIONS

Abrupt or too-rapid withdrawal may result in pronounced restlessness, irritability, insomnia, hand tremor, abdominal/ muscle cramps, vomiting, diaphoresis, seizures. Overdose results in drowsiness, confusion, diminished reflexes, respiratory depression, coma. **Antidote:** Flumazenil (see Appendix K for dosage).

NURSING CONSIDERATIONS

BASELINE ASSESSMENT

Question for possibility of pregnancy before initiating therapy (Pregnancy Category X). Assess B/P, pulse, respirations immediately before administration. Raise bed rails. Provide environment conducive to sleep (back rub, quiet environment, low lighting). Assess mental status, sleep patterns.

INTERVENTION/EVALUATION

Assess elderly or debilitated pts for paradoxical reaction, particularly during early therapy. Monitor respiratory, cardiovascular, mental status. Evaluate for therapeutic response: decrease in number of nocturnal awakenings, increase in length of sleep.

PATIENT/FAMILY TEACHING

• Avoid alcohol, other CNS depressants. • May cause daytime drowsiness. • Avoid tasks that require alertness, motor skills until response to drug is established. • Take approximately 30 min before bedtime. • Inform physician if pregnant or planning to become pregnant.

---

temozolomide   HIGH ALERT

tem-oh-**zoe**-loe-myde
(Temodal ✦, Temodar)

Do not confuse Temodar with Tambocor.

◆CLASSIFICATION

PHARMACOTHERAPEUTIC: Imidazotetrazine derivative. **CLINICAL:** Antineoplastic (see p. 90C).

ACTION

Acts as prodrug and is converted to highly active cytotoxic metabolite. Cytotoxic effect is associated with methylation of DNA. **Therapeutic Effect:** Inhibits DNA replication, causing cell death.

PHARMACOKINETICS

Rapidly, completely absorbed after PO administration. Protein binding: 15%. Peak plasma concentration: 1 hr. Penetrates blood-brain barrier. Eliminated in urine (38%), feces (19%). **Half-life:** 1.6–1.8 hrs.

USES

Treatment of adults with refractory anaplastic astrocytoma; newly diagnosed glioblastoma multiforme (concomitantly with radiotherapy, then as maintenance therapy). **OFF-LABEL:** Malignant glioma, metastatic melanoma, metastatic CNS lesions, cutaneous T-cell lymphomas, advanced neuroendocrine tumors, soft tissue sarcoma, pediatric neuroblastoma.

PRECAUTIONS

Contraindications: Hypersensitivity to dacarbazine. **Cautions:** Severe renal/hepatic impairment, pregnancy.

⌛ LIFESPAN CONSIDERATIONS

Pregnancy/Lactation: May cause fetal harm. May produce malformation of external organs, soft tissue, skeleton. If possible, avoid use during pregnancy. Unknown if drug is distributed in breast milk. **Pregnancy Category D. Children:** Safety and efficacy not established. **Elderly:** Those older than 70 yrs may experience higher risk of developing grade 4 neutropenia, grade 4 thrombocytopenia.

T

✦ Canadian trade name   Non-Crushable Drug   **HIGH ALERT** High Alert drug

INTERACTIONS

DRUG: Medications causing blood dyscrasias (altering blood cell counts) may increase leukopenic, thrombocytopenic effects. **Valproic acid** may decrease oral clearance. **Bone marrow depressants** may increase myelosuppression. **Live virus vaccines** may potentiate virus replication, increase vaccine side effects, decrease pt's antibody response to vaccine. **HERBAL: Echinacea** may decrease effects. **FOOD: All foods** decrease rate, extent of drug absorption. **LAB VALUES:** May decrease Hgb, neutrophil, platelet, WBC count, lymphocytes.

AVAILABILITY (Rx)

Capsules: 5 mg, 20 mg, 100 mg, 140 mg, 180 mg, 250 mg. **Injection, Powder for Reconstitution:** 100 mg.

ADMINISTRATION/HANDLING

 IV

• Reconstitute each 100-mg vial with 41 ml Sterile Water for Injection to provide concentration of 2.5 mg/ml. • Swirl gently; do not shake. • Do NOT further dilute. • Infuse over 90 min. • Stable for 14 hrs (includes infusion time).

PO
• Food reduces rate, extent of absorption; increases risk of nausea, vomiting. • For best results, administer at bedtime. • Give capsule whole with glass of water. Do not break, open, or crush capsules.

INDICATIONS/ROUTES/DOSAGE

Anaplastic Astrocytoma
IV Infusion, PO: ADULTS, ELDERLY: Initially, 150 mg/m²/day for 5 consecutive days of 28-day treatment cycle. Subsequent doses of 100–200 mg/m²/day based on platelet count, absolute neurophil count (ANC) during previous cycle. **ANC greater than 1,500 per microliter and platelets more than 100,000 per microliter: Maintenance:** 200 mg/m²/day for 5 days q4wks. Continue until disease progression is observed. Minimum: 100 mg/m²/day for 5 days q4wks.

Glioblastoma Multiforme
IV Infusion, PO: ADULTS, ELDERLY: 75 mg/m² daily for 42 days. **Maintenance: (Cycle 1):** 150 mg/m² once daily for 5 days followed by 23 days without treatment. **(Cycles 2–6):** May increase to 200 mg/m² once daily for 5 days followed by 23 days without treatment if ANC greater than 1,500/mm³, platelets greater than 100,000/mm³, and nonhematologic toxicity with previous cycle.

SIDE EFFECTS

Frequent (53%–33%): Nausea, vomiting, headache, fatigue, constipation, seizure. **Occasional (16%–10%):** Diarrhea, asthenia (loss of strength, energy), fever, dizziness, peripheral edema, incoordination, insomnia. **Rare (9%–5%):** Paresthesia, drowsiness, anorexia, urinary incontinence, anxiety, pharyngitis, cough.

ADVERSE EFFECTS/ TOXIC REACTIONS

Myelosuppression is characterized by neutropenia and thrombocytopenia, with elderly and women showing higher incidence of developing severe myelosuppression. Usually occurs within first few cycles; is not cumulative. Nadir occurs in approximately 26–28 days, with recovery within 14 days of nadir. May increase occurrence of pneumocystis carinii pneumonia, myelodysplastic syndrome including myeloid leukemia, or secondary malignancies.

NURSING CONSIDERATIONS

BASELINE ASSESSMENT
Obtain baseline CBC. Before dosing, ANC must be greater than 1,500/mm³ and platelet count greater than 100,000/mm³. Potential for nausea, vomiting readily controlled with antiemetic therapy.

INTERVENTION/EVALUATION

Obtain CBC on day 22 (21 days after first dose) or within 48 hrs of that day, and weekly, until ANC is greater than 1,500/mm³ and platelet count is greater than 100,000/mm³. Monitor for hematologic toxicity (fever, sore throat, signs of local infection, unusual bruising/bleeding from any site), symptoms of anemia (excessive fatigue, weakness).

PATIENT/FAMILY TEACHING

• To reduce nausea/vomiting, take on an empty stomach. • Promptly report fever, sore throat, signs of local infection, unusual bruising/bleeding from any site, or difficulty breathing. • Avoid crowds, those with infection. • Do not have immunizations without physician's approval. • Avoid pregnancy.

---

temsirolimus HIGH ALERT

tem-sir-oh-**li**-mus
(Torisel)
Do not confuse temsirolimus with everolimus, sirolimus, or tacrolimus.

◆CLASSIFICATION

PHARMACOTHERAPEUTIC: Kinase inhibitor. **CLINICAL:** Antineoplastic (see p. 90C).

ACTION

Prevents activation of mTOR (mammalian target of rapamycin), preventing tumor cell division. **Therapeutic Effect:** Inhibits tumor cell growth, produces tumor regression.

PHARMACOKINETICS

Metabolized in liver. Eliminated primarily in feces. **Half-life:** 17 hrs.

USES

Treatment of advanced renal cell carcinoma.

PRECAUTIONS

Contraindications: Moderate-severe hepatic impairment; bilirubin greater than 1.5 times the upper limit of normal (ULN). **Cautions:** Hypersensitivity to sirolimus, mild hepatic impairment, diabetes mellitus, hyperlipidemia. Concurrent use with other medication that may cause angioedema (e.g., ACE inhibitors).

LIFESPAN CONSIDERATIONS

Pregnancy/Lactation: May cause fetal harm. Unknown if distributed in breast milk. **Pregnancy Category D. Children:** Safety and efficacy not established. **Elderly:** No age-related precautions noted.

INTERACTIONS

DRUG: CYP3A4 inhibitors (e.g., atazanavir, clarithromycin, itraconazole, ketoconazole, nefazodone, ritonavir) may increase concentration. **CYP3A4 inducers (e.g., carbamazepine, dexamethasone, phenobarbital, phenytoin, rifampin)** may decrease concentration. **FOOD: Grapefruit products** may increase plasma concentration. **HERBAL: St. John's wort** may decrease plasma concentration. Herbs with hypoglycemic properties **(e.g., garlic, ginger, ginseng)** may increase risk for hypoglycemia. **LAB VALUES:** May increase serum bilirubin, alkaline phosphatase, AST, creatinine, glucose, cholesterol, triglycerides. May decrease WBCs, neutrophils, Hgb, platelets, serum phosphorus, potassium.

AVAILABILITY (Rx)

Injection Solution Kit: 25 mg/ml supplied with 1.8-ml diluent vial.

ADMINISTRATION/HANDLING

 IV

Reconstitution • Inject 1.8 ml of diluent into vial. • The vial contains an overfill of 0.2 ml (30 mg/1.2 ml). • Due to the overfill, the drug concentration of resulting solution will be 10 mg/ml. • A total volume of 3 ml will be obtained,

 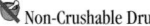
T

including the overfill. • Mix well by inverting the vial. Allow sufficient time for air bubbles to subside. • Mixture must be injected rapidly into 250 ml 0.9% NaCl. • Invert bag to mix; avoid excessive shaking (may cause foaming).

Rate of Administration • Administer through an in-line filter not greater than 5 microns; infuse over 30–60 min. • Final diluted infusion solution should be completed within 6 hrs from the time drug solution and diluent mixture is added to the 250 ml 0.9% NaCl.

Storage • Refrigerate kit. • Reconstituted solution appears clear to slightly turbid, colorless to yellow, and free from visible particulates. • The 10 mg/ml drug solution/diluent mixture is stable for up to 24 hrs at room temperature. • Solutions diluted for infusion (in 250 ml 0.9% NaCl) must be infused within 6 hrs of preparation.

⚑ IV INCOMPATIBILITIES

Both acids and bases degrade solution; combinations of temsirolimus with agents capable of modifying solution pH should be avoided.

INDICATIONS/ROUTES/DOSAGE

◀ALERT▶ Pretreat with IV diphenhydramine 25–50 mg, 30 min before infusion.

Renal Cancer
IV: ADULTS/ELDERLY: 25 mg once weekly. Treatment should continue until disease progresses or unacceptable toxicity occurs.

SIDE EFFECTS

Common (51%–32%): Asthenia (loss of strength, energy), rash, mucositis, nausea, edema (facial edema, peripheral edema), anorexia. **Frequent (28%–20%):** Generalized pain, dyspnea, diarrhea, cough, fever, abdominal pain, constipation, back pain, impaired taste. **Occasional (19%–8%):** Weight loss, vomiting, pruritus, chest pain, headache, nail disorder, insomnia, nosebleed, dry skin, acne, chills, myalgia.

ADVERSE EFFECTS/ TOXIC REACTIONS

UTI occurs in 15% of pts, hypersensitivity reaction in 9%, pneumonia in 8%, upper respiratory tract infection, hypertension, conjunctivitis in 7%.

NURSING CONSIDERATIONS

BASELINE ASSESSMENT

Question possibility of pregnancy. Obtain baseline CBC, serum chemistries, hepatic and renal function tests routinely thereafter.

INTERVENTION/EVALUATION

Offer antiemetics to control nausea, vomiting. Monitor daily pattern of bowel frequency, stool consistency. Assess skin for evidence of rash, edema. Monitor CBC, particularly Hgb, platelets, neutrophil count; hepatic function tests (AST, ALT, total bilirubin), renal function tests. Monitor for shortness of breath, fatigue, hypertension. Assess oropharynx for stomatitis, mucositis.

PATIENT/FAMILY TEACHING

• Avoid crowds, those with known infection. • Avoid contact with anyone who recently received live virus vaccine. • Do not have immunizations without physician's approval (drug lowers body resistance). • Promptly report fever, unusual bruising/bleeding from any site.

---

tenecteplase

ten-**eck**-te-plase
(TNKase)
Do not confuse TNKase with tPA.

◆CLASSIFICATION

PHARMACOTHERAPEUTIC: Tissue plasminogen activator. **CLINICAL:** Thrombolytic (see p. 34C).

ACTION

Produced by recombinant DNA that binds to fibrin and converts plasminogen to plasmin. Initiates fibrinolysis by degrading fibrin clots, fibrinogen, other plasma proteins. **Therapeutic Effect:** Exerts thrombolytic action (dissolves clots).

PHARMACOKINETICS

Extensively distributed to tissues. Completely eliminated by hepatic metabolism. **Half-life:** 90–130 min.

USES

Management of ST-elevation myocardial infarction (STEMI) for lysis of thrombi to restore perfusion and reduce mortality.

PRECAUTIONS

Contraindications: Active internal bleeding, cerebral aneurysm, AV malformation, bleeding diathesis, history of CVA, intracranial or intraspinal surgery or trauma within past 2 mos, intracranial neoplasm, severe uncontrolled hypertension. **Cautions:** Recent major surgery, GI or GU bleeding, trauma, acute pericarditis, subacute bacterial endocarditis, pregnancy, severe hepatic impairment, hemorrhagic ophthalmic conditions, concurrent use of anticoagulant, elderly.

LIFESPAN CONSIDERATIONS

Pregnancy/Lactation: Unknown if distributed in breast milk. **Pregnancy Category C. Children:** Safety and efficacy not established. **Elderly:** May have increased risk of intracranial hemorrhage, stroke, major bleeding; caution advised.

INTERACTIONS

DRUG: Anticoagulants (e.g., heparin, warfarin), aspirin, dipyridamole, glycoprotein IIb/IIIa inhibitors increase risk of bleeding. **HERBAL:** Herbs with anticoagulant or antiplatelet properties (**e.g., cat's claw, dong quai, evening primrose, feverfew, garlic, ginkgo biloba, ginseng, red clover**) may increase risk of bleeding. **FOOD:** None known. **LAB VALUES:** Decreases

plasminogen, fibrinogen levels during infusion, decreasing clotting time (confirms presence of lysis). May decrease Hgb, Hct.

AVAILABILITY (Rx)

Injection, Powder for Reconstitution: 50 mg.

ADMINISTRATION/HANDLING

IV

Reconstitution • Add 10 ml Sterile Water for Injection without preservative to vial to provide concentration of 5 mg/ml. • Gently swirl until dissolved. Do not shake. • If foaming occurs, leave vial undisturbed for several min.
Rate of Administration • Administer as IV push over 5 sec.
Storage • Store at room temperature. • If possible, use immediately, but may refrigerate up to 8 hrs after reconstitution. • Appears as colorless to pale yellow solution. • Do not use if discolored or contains particulates. • Discard after 8 hrs.

IV INCOMPATIBILITIES

Do not mix with dextrose-containing solutions or any other medications.

INDICATIONS/ROUTES/DOSAGE

◀ALERT▶ Give as single IV bolus over 5 sec. Precipitate may occur when given in IV line containing dextrose. Flush line with saline before and after administration.

Acute MI
IV: ADULTS: Dosage is based on pt's weight. Treatment should be initiated as soon as possible after onset of symptoms.

Weight (kg)	(mg)	(ml)
90 or more	50	10
80–less than 90	45	9
70–less than 80	40	8
60–less than 70	35	7
Less than 60	30	6

SIDE EFFECTS

Frequent: Bleeding (minor, 21.8%; major, 4.7%).

ADVERSE EFFECTS/ TOXIC REACTIONS

Bleeding at internal sites, including intracranial, retroperitoneal, GI, GU, respiratory sites, may occur. Lysis of coronary thrombi may produce atrial or ventricular arrhythmias, stroke.

NURSING CONSIDERATIONS

BASELINE ASSESSMENT

Obtain baseline B/P, apical pulse. Record weight. Evaluate 12-lead EKG, cardiac enzymes, serum electrolytes. Assess Hgb, Hct, platelet count, thrombin time, aPTT, PT, fibrinogen level before therapy is instituted. Type and hold blood. Screen for contraindications (e.g., history of CVA, bleeding of any kind, uncontrolled hypertension).

INTERVENTION/EVALUATION

Monitor continuous EKG for arrhythmias, B/P, pulse, respirations q15min until stable, then hourly or per protocol. Check peripheral pulses, heart and lung sounds. Monitor for chest pain relief; notify physician of continuation/recurrence (note location, type, intensity). Assess for overt or occult blood in any body substance. Monitor aPTT per protocol. Maintain B/P. Avoid any trauma that might increase risk of bleeding (e.g., injections, shaving). Assess neurologic status with vital signs.

tenofovir   TOP 200

ten-**oh**-foe-veer
(Viread)

BLACK BOX ALERT Lactic acidosis, severe hepatomegaly with steatosis (fatty liver), including fatalities, have occurred.

FIXED-COMBINATION(S)

Atripla: tenofovir/efavirenz/emtricitabine (antiretroviral agents): 300 mg/600 mg/200 mg. **Complera:** tenofovir/emtricitabine/rilpivirine (antiretroviral agents): 300 mg/200 mg/25 mg. **Stribild:** tenofovir/elvitegravir (an integrase inhibitor)/cobicistat (a pharmacokinetic enhancer)/emtricitabine (a nucleoside reverse transcriptase inhibitor): 300 mg/150 mg/150 mg/200 mg. **Truvada:** tenofovir/emtricitabine (an antiretroviral agent): 300 mg/200 mg.

◆CLASSIFICATION

PHARMACOTHERAPEUTIC: Nucleotide analogue (reverse transcriptase inhibitor). **CLINICAL:** Antiviral (see pp. 71C, 119C).

ACTION

Inhibits HIV reverse transcriptase by being incorporated into viral DNA, resulting in DNA chain termination. **Therapeutic Effect:** Slows HIV replication, reduces HIV RNA levels (viral load).

PHARMACOKINETICS

Bioavailability in fasted pts is approximately 25%. High-fat meals increase bioavailability. Protein binding: 0.7%–7.2%. Excreted in urine. Removed by hemodialysis. **Half-life:** 17 hrs.

USES

Treatment of HIV-1 infection in combination with at least two other antiretroviral agents. Treatment of chronic hepatitis B in pts with hepatic disease.

PRECAUTIONS

Contraindications: None known. **Cautions:** Hepatic/renal impairment, concomitant strong CYP3A4 inhibitors/inducers, elderly.

⧖ LIFESPAN CONSIDERATIONS

Pregnancy/Lactation: Unknown if drug crosses placenta or is distributed in breast milk. **Pregnancy Category B. Children:** Safety and efficacy not established. **Elderly:** No age-related precautions noted.

INTERACTIONS

DRUG: May increase **didanosine** concentration. May decrease concentrations of **atazanavir, indinavir, lamivudine, lopinavir, ritonavir. HERBAL:** None significant. **FOOD: High-fat food** increases bioavailability. **LAB VALUES:** May increase serum ALT, AST, creatinine, glucose (urine), phosphate (urine), protein (urine). May decrease neutrophils.

AVAILABILITY (Rx)

Tablets: 150 mg, 200 mg, 250 mg, 300 mg. **Oral Powder:** 40 mg per 1 g of oral powder.

ADMINISTRATION/HANDLING

PO

• May be given without regard to meals.
• Give oral powder with food.

INDICATIONS/ROUTES/DOSAGE

Hepatitis B
PO: ADULTS, ELDERLY, CHILDREN 12 YRS AND OLDER (WEIGHT 35 KG OR GREATER): 300 mg once daily.

HIV (in Combination with Other Antiretroviral Agents)
PO: ADULTS, ELDERLY, CHILDREN 12 YRS AND OLDER (WEIGHT 35 KG OR GREATER): 300 mg once daily. **CHILDREN 2 YRS AND OLDER (WEIGHT LESS THAN 35 KG):** 8 mg/kg/dose once daily. **Maximum:** 300 mg/day.

Dosage in Renal Impairment

Creatinine Clearance	Dosage
30–49 ml/min	300 mg q48h
10–29 ml/min	300 mg q72–96h
Hemodialysis	300 mg q7days or after approximately 12 hrs of dialysis

SIDE EFFECTS

Occasional: GI disturbances (diarrhea, flatulence, nausea, vomiting).

ADVERSE EFFECTS/ TOXIC REACTIONS

Lactic acidosis, hepatomegaly with steatosis (excess fat in liver) occur rarely; may be severe.

NURSING CONSIDERATIONS

BASELINE ASSESSMENT

Obtain baseline laboratory testing, esp. serum hepatic/renal function tests, triglycerides and at periodic intervals during therapy. Offer emotional support.

INTERVENTION/EVALUATION

Closely monitor for evidence of GI discomfort. Monitor daily pattern of bowel activity, stool consistency. Monitor CBC, reticulocyte count, serum hepatic/renal function, CD4 cell count, HIV, RNA plasma levels.

PATIENT/FAMILY TEACHING

• Continue therapy for full length of treatment. • Tenofovir is not a cure for HIV infection, nor does it reduce risk of transmission to others. • Take with a high-fat meal (increases absorption). • Inform physician if persistent abdominal pain, nausea, vomiting occurs.

---

terazosin

ter-**ay**-zoe-sin
(Apo-Terazosin ♣, Hytrin ♣)

◆CLASSIFICATION

PHARMACOTHERAPEUTIC: Alpha-adrenergic blocker. **CLINICAL:** Antihypertensive, benign prostatic hyperplasia agent (see p. 61C).

ACTION

Blocks alpha-adrenergic receptors. Produces vasodilation, decreases peripheral resistance, targets receptors around bladder neck, prostate. **Therapeutic Effect:** In hypertension, decreases B/P. In benign prostatic hyperplasia (BPH), relaxes smooth muscle, improves urine flow.

T

♣ Canadian trade name   🗡 Non-Crushable Drug   🔲 High Alert drug

PHARMACOKINETICS

Rapidly, completely absorbed from GI tract. Protein binding: 90%–94%. Metabolized in liver. Primarily eliminated in feces via biliary system; excreted in urine. Not removed by hemodialysis. **Half-life:** 9.2–12 hrs.

USES

Treatment of mild to moderate hypertension. Used alone or in combination with other antihypertensives. Treatment of benign prostatic hyperplasia (BPH). **OFF-LABEL:** Pediatric hypertension.

PRECAUTIONS

Contraindications: None known. **Cautions:** Pts with cataracts or undergoing corrective cataract surgery.

⌛ LIFESPAN CONSIDERATIONS

Pregnancy/Lactation: Unknown if drug crosses placenta or is distributed in breast milk. **Pregnancy Category C. Children:** Safety and efficacy not established. **Elderly:** No age-related precautions noted but may be more sensitive to hypotensive effects.

INTERACTIONS

DRUG: NSAIDs, sympathomimetics may decrease hypotensive effects. **Hypotensive medications (e.g., antihypertensives, diuretics)** may increase effects. **HERBAL: Ephedra, ginseng, yohimbe** may worsen hypertension. **Garlic** may increase antihypertensive effect. **FOOD:** None known. **LAB VALUES:** May decrease Hgb, Hct, serum albumin, total protein, WBC count.

AVAILABILITY (Rx)

Capsules: 1 mg, 2 mg, 5 mg, 10 mg.

ADMINISTRATION/HANDLING

PO

• Give without regard to food. • Administer first dose at bedtime (minimizes risk of fainting due to "first-dose syncope").

INDICATIONS/ROUTES/DOSAGE

◄ALERT► If medication has been discontinued for several days, retitrate initially using 1-mg dose at bedtime.

Mild to Moderate Hypertension
PO: ADULTS, ELDERLY: Initially, 1 mg at bedtime. Slowly increase dosage to desired levels. **Range:** 1–5 mg/day as single or 2 divided doses. **Maximum:** 20 mg.

Benign Prostatic Hyperplasia (BPH)
PO: ADULTS, ELDERLY: Initially, 1 mg at bedtime. May increase up to 10 mg/day. If no response with 10 mg after 4–6 wks, may increase to 20 mg/day.

SIDE EFFECTS

Frequent (9%–5%): Dizziness, headache, fatigue. **Rare (Less Than 2%):** Peripheral edema, orthostatic hypotension, myalgia, arthralgia, blurred vision, nausea, vomiting, nasal congestion, drowsiness.

ADVERSE EFFECTS/ TOXIC REACTIONS

First-dose syncope (hypotension with sudden loss of consciousness) generally occurs 30–90 min after initial dose of 2 mg or more, too-rapid increase in dosage, or addition of another antihypertensive agent to therapy. First-dose syncope may be preceded by tachycardia (pulse rate of 120–160 beats/min).

NURSING CONSIDERATIONS

BASELINE ASSESSMENT

Assess history of prostatic hyperplasia (difficulty initiating urine stream, dribbling, sense of urgency, leaking). Give first dose at bedtime. If initial dose is given during daytime, pt must remain recumbent for 3–4 hrs. Assess B/P, pulse immediately before each dose and q15–30min until stabilized (be alert to B/P fluctuations).

INTERVENTION/EVALUATION

Monitor pulse diligently (first-dose syncope may be preceded by tachycardia).

Assist with ambulation if dizziness occurs. Assess for peripheral edema. Monitor B/P, GU function.

PATIENT/FAMILY TEACHING

• Noncola carbonated beverage, unsalted crackers, dry toast may relieve nausea. • Nasal congestion may occur. • Full therapeutic effect may not occur for 3–4 wks. • Avoid tasks requiring alertness, motor skills until response to drug is established. • Go from lying to standing slowly. • Report dizziness, palpitations. • Avoid alcohol.

---

terbinafine

ter-bin-a-feen
(Apo-Terbinafine ✦, Lamisil, Lamisil AT, Terbinex)
Do not confuse Lamisil with Lamictal, or terbinafine with terbutaline.

◆ CLASSIFICATION

PHARMACOTHERAPEUTIC: Synthetic allylamine antifungal. **CLINICAL:** Antifungal (see p. 50C).

ACTION

Inhibits the enzyme squalene epoxidase, thereby interfering with fungal biosynthesis. **Therapeutic Effect:** Results in death of fungal cells.

PHARMACOKINETICS

Well absorbed following PO administration. Protein binding: 99%. Metabolized in liver. Primarily excreted in urine; minimal elimination in feces. **Half-life:** PO, 36 hrs; topical, 22–26 hrs.

USES

Systemic: Treatment of onychomycosis (fungal disease of nails due to dermatophytes). Treatment of tinea capitis. **Topical:** Treatment of tinea cruris (jock itch), tinea pedis (athlete's foot), tinea corporis (ringworm), tinea versicolor.

PRECAUTIONS

Contraindications: None known. **Cautions:** Preexisting hepatic or renal impairment (creatinine clearance 50 ml/min or less), sensitivity to allylamine antifungals (e.g., butenafine).

⬙ LIFESPAN CONSIDERATIONS

Pregnancy/Lactation: Distributed in breast milk. **Pregnancy Category B. Children:** Safety and efficacy not established. **Elderly:** Age-related renal impairment may require dosage adjustment.

INTERACTIONS

DRUG: Alcohol, other hepatotoxic medications may increase risk of hepatotoxicity. **Hepatic enzyme inducers (e.g., rifampin)** may increase clearance. **Hepatic enzyme inhibitors (e.g., cimetidine, fluconazole)** may decrease clearance. **HERBAL:** None significant. **FOOD:** None known. **LAB VALUES:** May increase serum hepatic enzymes (AST, ALT).

AVAILABILITY (Rx)

Cream (Lamisil AT): 1%. **Oral Granules (Lamisil):** 125 mg/packet. **Tablets (Lamisil, Terbinex):** 250 mg. **Topical Solution (Lamisil, Lamisil AT):** 1%.

ADMINISTRATION/HANDLING

• Tablets may be given without regard to food. • Granules should be sprinkled on a spoonful of nonacidic food (e.g., mashed potatoes). Instruct pt to swallow without chewing.

INDICATIONS/ROUTES/DOSAGE

Tinea Pedis
Topical: ADULTS, ELDERLY, CHILDREN 12 YRS AND OLDER: Apply twice daily until signs/symptoms significantly improve; not to exceed 4 wks.

Tinea Cruris, Tinea Corporis
Topical: ADULTS, ELDERLY, CHILDREN 12 YRS AND OLDER: Apply 1–2 times daily until signs/symptoms significantly improve; not to exceed 4 wks.

T

Onychomycosis
PO: ADULTS, ELDERLY, CHILDREN 12 YRS AND OLDER: 250 mg/day for 6 wks (fingernails) or 12 wks (toenails).

Tinea Versicolor
Topical Solution: ADULTS, ELDERLY: Apply to the affected area twice daily for 7 days.

Systemic Mycosis
PO: ADULTS, ELDERLY: 250–500 mg/day for up to 16 mos.

Tinea Capitis
PO: CHILDREN 4 YRS AND OLDER: (Use granules). **WEIGHING GREATER THAN 35 KG:** 250 mg once daily. **WEIGHING 25–35 KG:** 187.5 mg once daily. **WEIGHING LESS THAN 25 KG:** 125 mg once daily.

SIDE EFFECTS

Frequent (13%): PO: Headache. **Occasional (6%–3%): PO:** Abdominal pain, flatulence, urticaria, visual disturbance. **Rare: PO:** Diarrhea, rash, dyspepsia (heartburn, indigestion, epigastric pain), pruritus, altered taste, nausea. **Topical:** Irritation, burning, pruritus, dryness.

ADVERSE EFFECTS/ TOXIC REACTIONS

Hepatobiliary dysfunction (including cholestatic hepatitis), serious skin reactions, severe neutropenia occur rarely. Ocular lens, retinal changes have been noted.

NURSING CONSIDERATIONS

BASELINE ASSESSMENT
Serum hepatic function tests should be obtained in pts receiving treatment for longer than 6 wks.

INTERVENTION/EVALUATION
Check for therapeutic response. Discontinue medication, notify physician if local reaction occurs (irritation, redness, swelling, pruritus, oozing, blistering, burning).

Monitor serum hepatic function in pts receiving treatment for longer than 6 wks.

PATIENT/FAMILY TEACHING
• Keep areas clean, dry; wear light clothing to promote ventilation. • Avoid topical cream contact with eyes, nose, mouth, other mucous membranes. • Rub well into affected, surrounding area. • Do not cover with occlusive dressing. • Report rash, dark urine, abdominal pain, anorexia, yellowing of skin.

terbutaline

ter-**bue**-ta-leen
(Brethine, Bricanyl ✦)
Do not confuse Brethine with methergine, or terbutaline with terbinafine.

◆CLASSIFICATION

PHARMACOTHERAPEUTIC: Sympathomimetic (adrenergic agonist). **CLINICAL:** Bronchodilator, premature labor inhibitor.

ACTION

Stimulates beta$_2$-adrenergic receptors, resulting in relaxation of uterine, bronchial smooth muscle. **Therapeutic Effect:** Relieves uterine contractions. Relieves bronchospasm, reduces airway resistance.

PHARMACOKINETICS

Partially absorbed in GI tract following PO administration. Protein binding: 14%–25%. Metabolized in liver. Excreted in urine (30%–50%), feces (unspecified). **Half-life:** 11–16 hrs.

USES

Symptomatic relief of reversible bronchospasm due to bronchial asthma, bronchitis, emphysema. **OFF-LABEL:** Delays premature labor in pregnancies between 20 and 34 wks.

PRECAUTIONS

Contraindications: Cardiac arrhythmias associated with tachycardia, tachycardia caused by digoxin toxicity. **Injection:** Prolonged prevention or management of preterm labor. **Oral:** Prevention or treatment of preterm labor. **Cautions:** Cardiac impairment, diabetes mellitus, hypertension, hyperthyroidism, history of seizures.

LIFESPAN CONSIDERATIONS

Pregnancy/Lactation: Crosses placenta; distributed in breast milk. **Pregnancy Category B. Children:** Safety and efficacy not established in pts younger than 6 yrs. **Elderly:** Increased risk of tremors, tachycardia due to sympathomimetic sensitivity.

INTERACTIONS

DRUG: May decrease effects of **beta-blockers. Digoxin, sympathomimetics** may increase risk of arrhythmias. **MAOIs** may increase risk of hypertensive crisis. **Tricyclic antidepressants** may increase cardiovascular effects. **HERBAL: Ephedra, yohimbe** may cause CNS stimulation. **FOOD:** None known. **LAB VALUES:** May decrease serum potassium. May increase serum glucose.

AVAILABILITY (Rx)

Injection Solution: 1 mg/ml. **Tablets:** 2.5 mg, 5 mg.

ADMINISTRATION/HANDLING

🖦 IV

• May administer undiluted, direct IV over 5–10 min or continuous infusion diluted in D$_5$W or 0.9% NaCl.

Subcutaneous

• Do not use if solution appears discolored. • Inject subcutaneously into lateral deltoid region.

PO

• Give without regard to food (give with food if GI upset occurs). • Tablets may be crushed.

INDICATIONS/ROUTES/DOSAGE

Bronchospasm

PO: ADULTS, ELDERLY, CHILDREN 15 YRS AND OLDER: Initially, 2.5 mg 3–4 times a day. **Maintenance:** 2.5–5 mg 3 times a day q6h while awake. **Maximum:** 15 mg/day. **CHILDREN 12–14 YRS:** 2.5 mg 3 times a day. **Maximum:** 7.5 mg/day. **CHILDREN YOUNGER THAN 12 YRS:** Initially, 0.05 mg/kg/dose q8h. May increase up to 0.15 mg/kg/dose. **Maximum:** 5 mg/24 hr.

Subcutaneous: ADULTS, CHILDREN 12 YRS AND OLDER: Initially, 0.25 mg. Repeat in 15–30 min for 3 doses. Total dose of 0.75 mg should not be exceeded. **CHILDREN YOUNGER THAN 12 YRS:** 0.005–0.01 mg/kg/dose to a maximum of 0.4 mg/dose q15–20min for 3 doses. May repeat q2–6h as needed.

Preterm Labor

◄ **ALERT** ► IV form should be used with caution in pregnancy; do not administer for longer than 48–72 hrs.

IV: ADULTS: Acute: 2.5–10 mcg/min. May increase gradually q15–20min up to 17.5–30 mcg/min. **Subcutaneous:** 0.25 mg q20min–3 hrs.

Dosage in Renal Impairment

Creatinine Clearance	Dosage
10–50 ml/min	50% of normal
Less than 10 ml/min	Avoid use

SIDE EFFECTS

Frequent (38%–23%): Tremor, anxiety. **Occasional (11%–10%):** Drowsiness, headache, nausea, heartburn, dizziness. **Rare (3%–1%):** Flushing, asthenia (loss of strength, energy), oropharyngeal dryness, irritation (with inhalation therapy).

ADVERSE EFFECTS/ TOXIC REACTIONS

Too-frequent or excessive use may lead to decreased drug effectiveness and/or severe, paradoxical bronchoconstriction. Excessive sympathomimetic stimulation may cause palpitations, extrasystoles, tachycardia, chest pain, slight increase in

T

 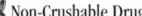

B/P followed by a substantial decrease, chills, diaphoresis, skin blanching.

NURSING CONSIDERATIONS

BASELINE ASSESSMENT

Bronchospasm: Offer emotional support (high incidence of anxiety due to difficulty in breathing, sympathomimetic response to drug). **Preterm labor:** Assess baseline maternal pulse, B/P, frequency and duration of contractions, fetal heart rate.

INTERVENTION/EVALUATION

Bronchospasm: Monitor rate, depth, rhythm, type of respiration; quality, rate of pulse. Assess lung sounds for rhonchi, wheezing, rales. Monitor ABGs. Observe lips, fingernails for cyanosis (blue or dusky color in light-skinned pts; gray in dark-skinned pts). Observe for clavicular retractions, hand tremor. Evaluate for clinical improvement (quieter, slower respirations, relaxed facial expression, cessation of clavicular retractions). **Preterm labor:** Monitor for frequency, duration, strength of contractions. Diligently monitor maternal and fetal heart rate.

PATIENT/FAMILY TEACHING

• Report persistent palpitations, chest pain, muscle tremor, dizziness, headache, flushing, breathing difficulties. • May cause nervousness, anxiety, shakiness. • Avoid excessive use of caffeine derivatives (chocolate, coffee, tea, cola, cocoa).

---

teriflunomide

ter-i-**floo**-noe-myde
(Aubagio)
Do not confuse teriflunomide with leflunomide.

> **BLACK BOX ALERT** May result in major birth defects (Pregnancy Category X). Pregnancy must be excluded before initiating therapy, and must be avoided during treatment or prior to completion of an accelerated elimination procedure. Severe hepatic injury may occur. Do not initiate with acute/chronic liver disease or ALT greater than 2 times upper limit of normal.

◆CLASSIFICATION

PHARMACOTHERAPEUTIC: Pyrimidine synthesis inhibitor, immunomodulatory agent. **CLINICAL:** Multiple sclerosis agent.

ACTION

Inhibits pyrimidine synthesis, exhibiting anti-inflammatory and antiproliferative properties. **Therapeutic Effect:** May slow progression of multiple sclerosis.

PHARMACOKINETICS

Well absorbed following PO administration. Peak concentration: 1–4 h. Protein binding: greater than 99%. Metabolized by hydrolysis. Excreted through renal, biliary system. **Half-life:** 18–19 days.

USES

Treatment of relapsing forms of multiple sclerosis.

PRECAUTIONS

Contraindications: Pregnant women or women of childbearing potential who are not using reliable contraception, severe hepatic impairment, concurrent use of leflunomide. **Cautions:** Concomitant neurotoxic medications, diabetes, pulmonary disease, severe immunodeficiency or bone marrow dysplasia, history of significant hematologic abnormalities, uncontrolled infection, history of new/recurrent infections, pts older than 60 yrs.

⧗ LIFESPAN CONSIDERATIONS

May produce embryo-fetal toxicity. Pregnancy contraindicated. Avoid breastfeeding. Detected in human semen. **Pregnancy Category X. Children:** Safety and efficacy not established in those younger than 18 yrs of age. **Elderly:** No age-related precautions noted.

INTERACTIONS

DRUG: May increase concentration/effects of **CYP2C8 substrates (e.g., repaglinide, paclitaxel, pioglitazone, or rosiglitazone), oral contraceptives.** May decrease concentration/effects of **warfarin, CYP1A2 substrates (e.g., duloxetine, tizanidine). HERBAL:** None significant. **FOOD:** None known. **LAB VALUES:** May increase serum potassium, AST, ALT, alkaline phosphatase, bilirubin. May decrease WBCs, neutrophil count.

AVAILABILITY (Rx)

Tablets: 7 mg, 14 mg.

ADMINISTRATION/HANDLING

PO
• Give without regard to food.

INDICATIONS/ROUTES/DOSAGE

Multiple Sclerosis
PO: ADULTS, ELDERLY: 7 mg or 14 mg once daily.

SIDE EFFECTS

Frequent (19%–6%): Headache, diarrhea, nausea, alopecia, paresthesia, upper abdominal pain. **Occasional (4%–3%):** Hypertension, oral herpes, anxiety, hypertension, toothache, musculoskeletal pain. **Rare (2%–1%):** Seasonal allergy, sciatica, burning sensation, carpal tunnel syndrome, blurred vision, acne, pruritus, myalgia, abdominal distention, conjunctivitis.

ADVERSE EFFECTS/ TOXIC REACTIONS

Influenza occurs in 12% of pts, upper respiratory infection with sinusitis, bronchitis, in 9%. Cystitis, sinusitis, viral gastroenteritis may occur. Neutropenia, leukopenia occur rarely.

NURSING CONSIDERATIONS

BASELINE ASSESSMENT

Because of high potential for birth defects/fetal death, female pts must avoid pregnancy (Pregnancy Category X). Obtain baseline PPD for latent TB. Obtain CBC, hepatic function test results prior to treatment, and for 6 mos thereafter. Obtain baseline pregnancy test. Assess limitations for activities of daily living due to multiple sclerosis.

INTERVENTION/EVALUATION

Monitor for signs/symptoms of infection. Treatment should not be initiated if pt has active infection; discontinuation of treatment must be considered. If drug-induced hepatic impairment, peripheral neuropathy, severe skin reaction occur, discontinue medication, begin accelerated elimination procedure (cholestyramine or charcoal for 11 days).

PATIENT/FAMILY TEACHING

• Women of childbearing potential must be counseled regarding fetal risk, use of reliable contraceptives confirmed, possibility of pregnancy excluded (Pregnancy Category X). • May take without regard to food.

---

teriparatide

ter-i-**par**-a-tide
(Forteo)
BLACK BOX ALERT Increased risk of osteosarcoma; risk dependent on dose and duration.

◆CLASSIFICATION

PHARMACOTHERAPEUTIC: Synthetic hormone. **CLINICAL:** Osteoporosis agent (see p. 143C).

ACTION

Acts on bone to mobilize calcium; acts on kidney to reduce calcium clearance, increase phosphate excretion. **Therapeutic Effect:** Increases rate of release of calcium from bone into blood; stimulates new bone formation.

T

PHARMACOKINETICS

Extensively absorbed following subcutaneous injection. Metabolized in liver. Excreted in urine. **Half-life: 1 hr.**

USES

Treatment of postmenopausal women with osteoporosis who are at increased risk for fractures. Treatment of men with primary or hypogonadal osteoporosis who are at high risk for fractures. High-risk pts include those with a history of osteoporotic fractures, who have failed previous osteoporosis therapy, or were intolerant of previous osteoporosis therapy. Treatment of glucocorticoid-induced osteoporosis in men and women.

PRECAUTIONS

Contraindications: None known. **Cautions:** Conditions that increase risk of osteosarcoma (e.g., Paget's disease, unexplained elevations of alkaline phosphatase level, open epiphyses, prior skeletal radiation therapy, implant therapy), hypercalcemia, hypercalcemic disorders (e.g., hyperparathyroidism), bone metastases, history of skeletal malignancies, metabolic bone diseases other than osteoporosis, cardiac disease, renal/hepatic impairment, pts at risk for orthostasis, active or recent urolithiasis.

⌛ LIFESPAN CONSIDERATIONS

Pregnancy/Lactation: Unknown if drug crosses placenta or is distributed in breast milk. **Pregnancy Category C. Children:** Safety and efficacy not established. **Elderly:** No age-related precautions noted.

INTERACTIONS

DRUG: None significant. **HERBAL:** None significant. **FOOD:** None known. **LAB VALUES:** May increase serum calcium (transient).

AVAILABILITY (Rx)

Injection Solution: 250 mcg/ml (3 ml) delivers 20 mcg/dose.

ADMINISTRATION/HANDLING

Subcutaneous
• Refrigerate, but minimize time out of refrigerator. Do not freeze; discard if frozen. • Administer into thigh, abdominal wall.

INDICATIONS/ROUTES/DOSAGE

Osteoporosis
Subcutaneous: ADULTS, ELDERLY: 20 mcg once daily into thigh, abdominal wall.

SIDE EFFECTS

Occasional: Leg cramps, nausea, dizziness, headache, orthostatic hypotension, tachycardia.

ADVERSE EFFECTS/ TOXIC REACTIONS

Angina pectoris has been reported.

NURSING CONSIDERATIONS

BASELINE ASSESSMENT

Check urinary, serum calcium, ionized calcium levels, serum parathyroid hormone levels.

INTERVENTION/EVALUATION

Monitor bone mineral density, urinary/serum calcium levels, serum parathyroid hormone levels. Observe for symptoms of hypercalcemia. Monitor B/P for hypotension, pulse for tachycardia.

PATIENT/FAMILY TEACHING

• Go from lying to standing slowly. • Report persistent symptoms of hypercalcemia (nausea, vomiting, constipation, lethargy, asthenia [loss of strength, energy]).

testosterone   TOP 200

tes-**tos**-te-rone
(Andriol , Androderm, <u>AndroGel</u>, Andropository , Axiron, Delatestryl, Depotest , Depo-Testoster-

one, Everone ♣, FIRST-Testosterone, FIRST-Testosterone MC,
Fortesta, Striant, Testim, Testopel)
BLACK BOX ALERT Virilization in
children and women may occur following secondary exposure to testosterone gel.
**Do not confuse testosterone
with testolactone, Testoderm
with Estraderm.**

◆ **CLASSIFICATION**

PHARMACOTHERAPEUTIC: Androgen. **CLINICAL:** Sex hormone.

ACTION

Promotes growth, development of male
sex organs, maintains secondary sex characteristics in androgen-deficient males.
Therapeutic Effect: Relieves androgen
deficiency.

PHARMACOKINETICS

Well absorbed after IM administration.
Protein binding: 98%. Metabolized in
liver. Primarily excreted in urine. Unknown if removed by hemodialysis.
Half-life: 10–100 min.

USES

Injection: Androgen replacement therapy in treatment of delayed male puberty,
male hypogonadism, inoperable female
breast cancer. **Pellet:** Androgen replacement therapy in treatment of delayed
male puberty, male hypogonadism. **Buccal, topical gel, topical solution,
transdermal:** Male hypogonadism. **OFF-
LABEL:** Androgen deficiency in men with
AIDS wasting.

PRECAUTIONS

Contraindications: Breastfeeding, severe
cardiac impairment, hypercalcemia,
pregnancy, prostate or breast cancer in
males, severe hepatic/renal disease. **Cautions:** Renal/hepatic/cardiac dysfunction,
diabetes.

⧗ LIFESPAN CONSIDERATIONS

Pregnancy/Lactation: Contraindicated
during lactation. **Pregnancy Category X.
Children:** Safety and efficacy not established; use with caution. **Elderly:** May
increase risk of hyperplasia, stimulate
growth of occult prostate carcinoma.

INTERACTIONS

DRUG: May decrease serum glucose, requiring **insulin** adjustments. **HERBAL: St.
John's wort** may decrease concentration/
effects. **FOOD:** None known. **LAB VALUES:**
May increase Hgb, Hct, LDL, serum alkaline phosphatase, bilirubin, calcium, potassium, sodium, AST. May decrease HDL.

AVAILABILITY (Rx)

Gel, Topical (AndroGel, Testim): 1%,
1.62%. **Injection (Cypionate [Depo-Tes-
tosterone]):** 100 mg/ml, 200 mg/ml. **(Enanthate [Delatestryl]):** 200 mg/ml. **Muco-
adhesive, for Buccal Application (Striant):**
30 mg. **Pellet, for Subcutaneous Implantation (Testopel):** 75 mg. **Solution (Metered
Dose Pump [Axiron]):** 30 mg/activation.
Transdermal System (Androderm): 2 mg/
day or 4 mg/day.

ADMINISTRATION/HANDLING

IM
• Give deep in gluteal muscle. • Do not
give IV. • Warming or shaking redis-
solves crystals that may form in long-
acting preparations. • Wet needle of syringe may cause solution to become
cloudy; this does not affect potency.

Buccal
(Striant): • Apply to gum area (above
incisor tooth). • Hold firmly in place for
30 sec to ensure adhesion. Instruct pt to
not chew or swallow. • Not affected by
food, toothbrushing, gum, chewing, alcoholic beverages. • Remove before placing new system.

Transdermal
(Androderm): • Apply to clean, dry
area on skin on back, abdomen, upper

T

arms, thighs. • Do not apply to bony prominences (e.g., shoulder) or oily, damaged, irritated skin. Do not apply to scrotum. • Rotate application site with 7-day interval to same site.

Transdermal Gel

(AndroGel, Testim): • Apply (morning preferred) to clean, dry, intact skin of shoulder, upper arms (AndroGel 1% may also be applied to abdomen). • Upon opening packet(s), squeeze entire contents into palm of hand, immediately apply to application site. • Allow to dry. • Do not apply to genitals. **(Fortesta):** Apply to skin of front and inner thighs.

Topical Solution

(Axiron): • Apply using applicator to axilla at same time each morning. • Avoid washing site for 2 hrs after application.

INDICATIONS/ROUTES/DOSAGE

Male Hypogonadism
IM: ADULTS: 50–400 mg q2–4wks or 75–100 mg/wk or 150–200 mg q2wks. **ADOLESCENTS:** Initiation of pubertal growth: 25–75 mg q3–4wks, titrate q6–9mos to 100–150 mg. **Duration:** 3–4yrs. **Maintenance Virilizing Dose:** 100 mg/m²/dose twice a mo.
Subcutaneous *(Pellets):* **ADULTS:** 150–450 mg q3–6mos.
Topical Gel *(Fortesta):* 40 mg once daily in morning. **Range:** 10–70 mg.
Topical Solution *(Axiron):* **ADULTS, ELDERLY:** 60 mg once daily (1 pump activation of 30 mg to each axilla). **Range:** 30–120 mg.
Transdermal Patch *(Androderm):* **ADULTS, ELDERLY:** Start therapy with 4 mg/day patch applied at night. Apply patch to abdomen, back, thighs, upper arms. Dose adjustment based on testosterone levels.
Transdermal Gel *(AndroGel):* **ADULTS, ELDERLY:** **(AndroGel 1%):** Initial dose of 5 g delivers 50 mg testosterone and is applied once daily to abdomen, shoulders, upper arms. May increase to 7.5 g,

then to 10 g, if necessary. **(AndroGel 1.62%):** Initial dose of 40.5 mg applied once daily in the morning to shoulder and upper arms. May increase to 81 mg. Further adjustments based on testosterone levels.
Transdermal Gel *(Testim):* **ADULTS, ELDERLY:** Initial dose of 5 g delivers 50 mg testosterone and is applied once daily to the shoulders, upper arms. May increase to 10 g (100 mg testosterone).
Buccal *(Striant):* **ADULTS, ELDERLY:** 30 mg q12h.

Delayed Male Puberty
IM *(Cypionate or enanthate):* **ADOLESCENTS:** 50–200 mg q2–4wks for limited duration.
Subcutaneous *(Pellets):* **ADULTS:** 150–450 mg q3–6mos.

Breast Carcinoma
IM *(Testosterone Cypionate, Testosterone Ethanate):* **ADULTS:** 200–400 mg q2–4wks.

SIDE EFFECTS

Frequent: Gynecomastia, acne. **Females:** Hirsutism, amenorrhea, other menstrual irregularities; deepening of voice; clitoral enlargement (may not be reversible when drug is discontinued). Occasional: Edema, nausea, insomnia, oligospermia, priapism, male-pattern baldness, bladder irritability, hypercalcemia (in immobilized pts, those with breast cancer), hypercholesterolemia, inflammation/pain at IM injection site. **Transdermal:** Pruritus, erythema, skin irritation. Rare: Polycythemia (with high dosage), hypersensitivity.

ADVERSE EFFECTS/ TOXIC REACTIONS

Peliosis hepatitis (presence of blood-filled cysts in parenchyma of liver), hepatic neoplasms, hepatocellular carcinoma have been associated with prolonged high-dose therapy. Anaphylactic reactions occur rarely.

NURSING CONSIDERATIONS

BASELINE ASSESSMENT

Establish baseline weight, B/P, Hgb, Hct. Check serum hepatic function, electrolytes, cholesterol. Wrist X-rays may be ordered to determine bone maturation in children.

INTERVENTION/EVALUATION

Weigh daily, report weekly gain of more than 5 lb; evaluate for edema. Monitor I&O. Monitor B/P. Assess serum electrolytes, cholesterol, Hgb, Hct (periodically for high dosage), hepatic function test results, radiologic exam of wrist, hand (when using in prepubertal children). With breast cancer or immobility, check for hypercalcemia (lethargy, muscle weakness, confusion, irritability). Ensure adequate intake of protein, calories. Assess for virilization. Monitor sleep patterns. Check injection site for redness, swelling, pain.

PATIENT/FAMILY TEACHING

• Regular visits to physician and monitoring tests are necessary. • Do not take any other medication without consulting physician. • Maintain diet high in protein, calories. • Food may be better tolerated in small, frequent feedings. • Weigh daily, report 5 lb/wk gain. • Report nausea, vomiting, acne, pedal edema. • **Females:** Promptly report menstrual irregularities, hoarseness, deepening of voice. • **Males:** Report frequent erections, difficulty urinating, gynecomastia.

tetracycline

tet-ra-**sye**-kleen
(Apo-Tetra ✦, Nu-Tetra ✦)

FIXED-COMBINATION(S)

Pylera: tetracycline/bismuth/metronidazole (an anti-infective): 125 mg/140 mg/125 mg.

◆CLASSIFICATION

PHARMACOTHERAPEUTIC: Tetracycline. **CLINICAL:** Antibiotic.

ACTION

Inhibits bacterial protein synthesis by binding to ribosomes. **Therapeutic Effect:** Bacteriostatic.

PHARMACOKINETICS

Readily absorbed from GI tract. Protein binding: 30%–60%. Widely distributed. Excreted in urine; eliminated in feces through biliary system. Not removed by hemodialysis. **Half-life:** 6–11 hrs (increased in renal impairment).

USES

Treatment of susceptible infections due to *Rickettsiae, M. pneumoniae, C. trachomatis, C. psittaci, H. ducreyi, Yersinia pestis, Francisella tularensis, Vibrio cholerae, Brucella* spp.; treatment of susceptible infections due to gram-negative organisms including inflammatory acne vulgaris, Lyme disease, mycoplasma disease, *Legionella*, Rocky Mountain spotted fever, chlamydial infection in pts with gonorrhea. Part of multidrug regimen of *H. pylori* eradication to reduce risk of duodenal ulcer recurrence.

PRECAUTIONS

Contraindications: None known. **Cautions:** Sun, ultraviolet light exposure (severe photosensitivity reaction). Renal, hepatic impairment. Avoid use during tooth development (children 8 yrs or younger). Do not use during pregnancy.

⌧ LIFESPAN CONSIDERATIONS

Pregnancy/Lactation: Readily crosses placenta. Distributed in breast milk. Avoid use in women during last half of pregnancy. **Pregnancy Category D. Children:** Not recommended in those 8 yrs or younger; may cause permanent staining of teeth, enamel hypoplasia, decreased linear skeletal growth rate. **Elderly:** No age-related precautions noted.

INTERACTIONS

DRUG: May decrease effect of **oral contraceptives. Antacids, calcium or iron supplements, laxatives containing magnesium** may form nonabsorbable, undigestable complexes. **HERBAL: Dong quai, St. John's wort** may increase risk of photosensitivity. **FOOD: Dairy products** inhibit absorption. **LAB VALUES:** May increase BUN, serum alkaline phosphatase, amylase, bilirubin, AST, ALT.

AVAILABILITY (Rx)

Capsules: 250 mg, 500 mg.

ADMINISTRATION/HANDLING

PO
• Give with full glass of water 1 hr before or 2 hrs after meals. • Avoid antacids, dairy products within 3 hrs of tetracycline.

INDICATIONS/ROUTES/DOSAGE

◀**ALERT**▶ Space doses evenly around the clock.

Usual Dosage
PO: ADULTS, ELDERLY: 250–500 mg q6–12h. **CHILDREN 8 YRS AND OLDER:** 25–50 mg/kg/day in 4 divided doses. **Maximum:** 3 g/day.

H. Pylori Infection
PO: ADULTS, ELDERLY: 500 mg 2–4 times a day (in combination with at least one other antibiotic and an acid-suppressing agent [proton pump inhibitor or H_2 antagonist]).

Dosage in Renal Impairment
Dosage interval is modified based on creatinine clearance.

Creatinine Clearance	Dosage
50–80 ml/min	Usual dose q8–12h
10–49 ml/min	Usual dose q12–24h
Less than 10 ml/min	Usual dose q24h

SIDE EFFECTS

Frequent: Dizziness, light-headedness, diarrhea, nausea, vomiting, abdominal cramps, photosensitivity (may be severe). **Occasional:** Pigmentation of skin, mucous membranes; anal/genital pruritus; stomatitis; discoloration of teeth.

ADVERSE EFFECTS/ TOXIC REACTIONS

Superinfection (esp. fungal), anaphylaxis, elevated ICP may occur. Bulging fontanelles occur rarely in infants.

NURSING CONSIDERATIONS

BASELINE ASSESSMENT
Question for history of allergies, esp. tetracyclines, sulfite.

INTERVENTION/EVALUATION
Assess skin for rash. Monitor daily pattern of bowel activity, stool consistency. Monitor food intake, tolerance. Be alert for superinfection (diarrhea, stomatitis, anal/genital pruritus). Monitor B/P, level of consciousness (potential for ICP).

PATIENT/FAMILY TEACHING
• Continue antibiotic for full length of treatment. • Space doses evenly. • Take oral doses on empty stomach (1 hr before or 2 hrs after food, beverages). • Avoid antacids, dairy products within 3 hrs of tetracycline. • Drink full glass of water with capsules; avoid bedtime doses. • Report diarrhea, rash, other new symptoms. • Protect skin from sun, ultraviolet light exposure. • Consult physician before taking any other medication. • Avoid tasks that require alertness, motor skills until response to drug is established (may cause dizziness, light-headedness).

thalidomide

thal-**id**-o-myde
(Thalomid)
BLACK BOX ALERT Significant risk of severe birth defects, fetal death, even with one dose. Increased risk

of deep vein thrombosis, pulmonary embolism in multiple myeloma pts. Two methods of contraception must be used 4 wks before, during, and after therapy.

Do not confuse thalidomide with flutamide or lenalidomide.

◆CLASSIFICATION

PHARMACOTHERAPEUTIC: Immuno-modulator. **CLINICAL:** Immunosuppressive agent.

ACTION

Has sedative, anti-inflammatory, immunosuppressive activity. Action may be due to selective inhibition of production of tumor necrosis factor-alpha. **Therapeutic Effect:** Reduces muscle wasting in HIV pts; reduces local and systemic effects of leprosy.

PHARMACOKINETICS

Protein binding: 55%–66%. Metabolized by nonenzymatic hydrolysis in plasma. Excreted in urine. **Half-life:** 5–7 hrs.

USES

Treatment of leprosy, newly diagnosed multiple myeloma. **OFF-LABEL:** Graft-vs-host reactions following bone marrow transplantation, refractory Crohn's disease, recurrent aphthous stomatitis in HIV pts, maintenance therapy of multiple myeloma.

PRECAUTIONS

Contraindications: Women of childbearing potential, pts unable to comply with S.T.E.P.S. program (including males), pregnancy. **Cautions:** History of seizures, neurologic disorders, constipation, HIV infection, cardiovascular disease.

⌛ LIFESPAN CONSIDERATIONS

Pregnancy/Lactation: Contraindicated in women who are or may become pregnant and who are not using two required types of birth control or who are not continuously abstaining from heterosexual sexual contact. Can cause severe birth defects, fetal death. Unknown if distributed in breast milk. **Pregnancy Category X. Children:** Safety and efficacy not established in pts younger than 12 yrs. **Elderly:** No age-related precautions noted.

INTERACTIONS

DRUG: **Alcohol, other CNS depressants** may increase sedative effects. **Medications associated with peripheral neuropathy (e.g., isoniazid, lithium, metronidazole, phenytoin)** may increase peripheral neuropathy. May decrease effect of **oral contraceptives. Carbamazepine, phenytoin** may decrease concentration. **HERBAL:** **Cat's claw, echinacea** possess immunostimulant properties. **FOOD:** None known. **LAB VALUES:** None significant.

AVAILABILITY (Rx)

Capsules: 50 mg, 100 mg, 150 mg, 200 mg.

ADMINISTRATION/HANDLING

◀ALERT▶ Thalidomide may be prescribed only by licensed prescribers who are registered in the S.T.E.P.S. program and understand the risk of teratogenicity if thalidomide is used during pregnancy.

• Administer thalidomide with water at least 1 hr after evening meal and, if possible, at bedtime due to risk of drowsiness.

INDICATIONS/ROUTES/DOSAGE

AIDS-Related Muscle Wasting, Aphthous Stomatitis
PO: ADULTS: 200 mg twice daily for 5 days, then 200 mg once daily for up to 8 wks.

Leprosy
PO: ADULTS, ELDERLY: Initially, 100–300 mg/day as single bedtime dose, at least 1 hr after evening meal. Continue until active reaction subsides, then reduce dose q2–4wks in 50-mg increments.

Multiple Myeloma
PO: ADULTS, ELDERLY: 200 mg once daily, preferably at bedtime, with dexametha-

T

sone 40 mg on days 1–4, 9–12, 17–20 of
each 28-day cycle.

SIDE EFFECTS

Frequent: Drowsiness, dizziness, mood
changes, constipation, dry mouth, peripheral neuropathy. **Occasional:** Increased appetite, weight gain, headache,
loss of libido, edema of face/limbs, nausea, alopecia, dry skin, rash, hypothyroidism.

ADVERSE EFFECTS/ TOXIC REACTIONS

Neutropenia, peripheral neuropathy,
thromboembolism occur rarely.

NURSING CONSIDERATIONS

BASELINE ASSESSMENT

Assess for hypersensitivity to thalidomide.
Assess for pregnancy 24 hrs before beginning therapy (contraindicated). Determine use of other medications (many
interactions).

INTERVENTION/EVALUATION

Monitor WBC, nerve conduction studies,
HIV viral load. Observe for signs/symp-
toms of peripheral neuropathy. Perform
pregnancy tests on women of childbearing potential weekly during the first 4
wks of use, then at 4-wk intervals in
women with regular menstrual cycles or
q2wks in women with irregular menstrual cycles.

PATIENT/FAMILY TEACHING

• Avoid tasks requiring alertness, motor
skills until response to drug is established. • Avoid use of alcohol, other
drugs causing drowsiness. • Pregnancy
tests must be obtained within 24 hrs before starting thalidomide, then q2–4wks
in women of childbearing age. • Discontinue and report symptoms of peripheral
neuropathy. • Male pts should always use
a latex condom during any sexual contact.

theophylline

thee-**off**-i-lin
(Elixophyllin, Theo-24, Uniphyl ✦)

◆**CLASSIFICATION**

PHARMACOTHERAPEUTIC: Xanthine
derivative. **CLINICAL:** Bronchodilator.

ACTION

Directly relaxes smooth muscle of bronchial airways and pulmonary blood vessels. **Therapeutic Effect:** Relieves bronchospasm, increases vital capacity.

USES

Symptomatic relief, prevention of bronchial asthma, reversible bronchospasm
due to chronic bronchitis, emphysema,
or chronic obstructive pulmonary disease (COPD).

PRECAUTIONS

Contraindications: None known. **Cautions:** Cardiac disease, hypertension,
hyperthyroidism, peptic ulcer, tachyarrhythmias, underlying seizure disorder.
Pregnancy Category C.

INTERACTIONS

DRUG: Phenytoin, rifampin may increase metabolism. **Cimetidine, ciprofloxacin, clarithromycin, erythromycin, norfloxacin** may increase concentration, toxicity. **Smoking** may decrease
concentration. **HERBAL:** None significant.
**FOOD: Charcoal-broiled foods, high-
protein/low-carbohydrate diet** may
decrease serum level. **LAB VALUES:** None
significant.

AVAILABILITY (Rx)

Capsules (Extended-Release [Theo-24]):
100 mg, 200 mg, 300 mg, 400 mg. **Elixir
(Elixophyllin):** 80 mg/15 ml. **Infusion
(Theophylline):** 400 mg/500 ml.

🍁 **Tablets, Extended-Release:** 100 mg, 200
mg, 300 mg, 450 mg, 600 mg.

ADMINISTRATION/HANDLING

IV

Rate of Administration • Do not exceed flow rate of 1 ml/min (25 mg/min) for either piggyback or infusion. • Administer loading dose over 20–30 min. • Use infusion pump or microdrip to regulate IV administration.
Storage • Store at room temperature. • Discard if solution contains precipitate.

PO

• Give with food to prevent GI distress. • Do not crush/break controlled-release, extended-release forms. • Extended-release capsules may be opened and sprinkled on soft food. Pt cannot chew beads.

IV INCOMPATIBILITIES

Amiodarone (Cordarone), ciprofloxacin (Cipro), dobutamine (Dobutrex), ondansetron (Zofran).

IV COMPATIBILITIES

Aztreonam (Azactam), ceftazidime (Fortaz), dexmedetomidine (Precedex), diphenhydramine (Benadryl), fluconazole (Diflucan), heparin, morphine, potassium chloride, propofol (Diprivan).

INDICATIONS/ROUTES/DOSAGE

Doses are based on ideal body weight.

Acute Symptoms (Loading Dose)
IV, PO: ADULTS, CHILDREN: 5 mg/kg orally (4.6 mg/kg IV). If theophylline is given within 24 hrs, loading dose not recommended without obtaining serum theophylline concentration.

Acute Symptoms (Maintenance Dose)
IV: ADULTS OLDER THAN 60 YRS: 0.3 mg/kg/hr. **Maximum:** 400 mg/day. **ADULTS 16–60 YRS:** 0.4 mg/kg/hr. **Maximum:** 900 mg/day. **CHILDREN 12–16 YRS (NONSMOKERS):** 0.5 mg/kg/hr. **Maximum:** 900 mg/day. **CHILDREN 12–16 YRS (SMOKERS):** 0.7 mg/kg/hr. **CHILDREN 9–11 YRS:** 0.7 mg/kg/hr. **CHILDREN 1–8 YRS:** 0.8 mg/kg/hr. **INFANTS (6–52 WKS):**

$(0.008 \times$ age in wks$) + 0.21$. **(4 WKS TO LESS THAN 6 WKS):** 1.5 mg/kg/dose q12h.

Chronic Conditions
PO *(Extended-Release)*: **ADULTS, CHILDREN 45 KG OR GREATER:** Initially, 300–400 mg/day once daily. **Maintenance:** 400–600 mg/day. **CHILDREN 1 YR AND OLDER, LESS THAN 45 KG:** Initially, 10–14 mg/kg/day (**maximum:** 300 mg/day). **Maintenance:** Up to 20 mg/kg/day. (**maximum:** 600 mg/day).
Oral Solution: ADULTS, CHILDREN 45 KG OR GREATER: Initially, 300 mg/day in divided doses q6–8h. **Maintenance:** 400–600 mg/day. **CHILDREN 1 YR AND OLDER, LESS THAN 45 KG:** Initially, 10–14 mg/kg/day (**maximum:** 300 mg) in divided doses q4–6h. **Maintenance:** Up to 20 mg/kg/day (**maximum:** 600 mg). **CHILDREN LESS THAN 1 YR:** Total daily dose = $[(0.2 \times$ age in wks$) + 5] \times$ (wgt in kg). Frequency based on age. **27–52 WKS:** Divide in 4 equal doses q6h. **LESS THAN 27 WKS:** Divide in 3 equal doses q8h.

SIDE EFFECTS

Frequent: Altered smell (during IV administration), restlessness, tachycardia, tremor. **Occasional:** Heartburn, vomiting, headache, mild diuresis, insomnia, nausea.

ADVERSE EFFECTS/ TOXIC REACTIONS

Too-rapid IV administration may produce marked hypotension with accompanying syncope, light-headedness, palpitations, tachycardia, hyperventilation, nausea, vomiting, angina-like pain, seizures, ventricular fibrillation, cardiac standstill.

NURSING CONSIDERATIONS

BASELINE ASSESSMENT

Offer emotional support (high incidence of anxiety due to difficulty in breathing and sympathomimetic response to drug). Peak serum concentration should be drawn 1 hr following IV dose, 1–2 hrs

T

---

after immediate-release dose, 3–8 hrs after extended-release dose. Draw trough level just before next dose.

INTERVENTION/EVALUATION

Monitor rate, depth, rhythm, type of respiration; quality/rate of pulse. Assess lung sounds for rhonchi, wheezing, rales. Monitor ABGs. Observe lips, fingernails for cyanosis. Observe for clavicular retractions, hand tremor. Evaluate for clinical improvement (quieter, slower respirations, relaxed facial expression, cessation of clavicular retractions). Monitor serum theophylline levels (**therapeutic serum level range: 10–20 mcg/ml**).

PATIENT/FAMILY TEACHING

• Increase fluid intake (decreases lung secretion viscosity). • Avoid excessive caffeine derivatives (chocolate, coffee, tea, cola, cocoa). • Smoking, charcoal-broiled food, high-protein/low-carbohydrate diet may decrease serum theophylline level. • Report nausea, vomiting, persistent headache, palpitations.

---

thiamine (vitamin B₁)

thy-a-min
(Betaxin ✦)
Do not confuse thiamine with Thorazine.

◆CLASSIFICATION

PHARMACOTHERAPEUTIC: Water-soluble vitamin. **CLINICAL:** Vitamin B complex (see p. 157C).

ACTION

Combines with adenosine triphosphate in liver, kidneys, leukocytes to form thiamine diphosphate, a coenzyme necessary for carbohydrate metabolism. **Therapeutic Effect:** Prevents, reverses thiamine deficiency.

PHARMACOKINETICS

Rapidly and completely absorbed from GI tract, primarily in duodenum, after IM administration. Widely distributed. Primarily excreted in urine.

USES

Prevention/treatment of thiamine deficiency (e.g., beriberi, Wernicke's encephalopathy syndrome, peripheral neuritis associated with pellagra, alcoholic pts with altered sensorium), metabolic disorders.

PRECAUTIONS

Contraindications: None known. **Cautions:** Wernicke's encephalopathy.

⌛ LIFESPAN CONSIDERATIONS

Pregnancy/Lactation: Crosses placenta. Unknown if drug is distributed in breast milk. **Pregnancy Category A (C if used in doses above recommended daily allowance). Children/Elderly:** No age-related precautions noted.

INTERACTIONS

DRUG: None significant. **HERBAL:** None significant. **FOOD:** None known. **LAB VALUES:** None significant.

AVAILABILITY

Injection Solution (Vitamin B₁): 100 mg/ml. **Tablets (OTC):** 50 mg, 100 mg, 250 mg, 500 mg.

ADMINISTRATION/HANDLING

◄**ALERT**► IV, IM administration used only in acutely ill or those unresponsive to PO route (GI malabsorption syndrome). IM route preferred to IV use. Give by IV push, or add to most IV solutions and give as infusion.

PO
• May take without regard to food.

▦ IV INCOMPATIBILITY

None known.

IV COMPATIBILITIES

Famotidine (Pepcid), multivitamins, folic acid magnesium.

INDICATIONS/ROUTES/DOSAGE

Dietary Supplement
PO: ADULTS, ELDERLY: 1–2 mg/day. **CHILDREN:** 0.5–1 mg/day. **INFANTS:** 0.3–0.5 mg/day.

Thiamine Deficiency (Beriberi)
PO: ADULTS, ELDERLY: 5–30 mg/dose IM or IV 3 times/day (if critically ill), then 5–30 mg/day orally, as a single dose or in 3 divided doses, for 1 mo. **CHILDREN:** 10–25 mg IM or IV (if critically ill) or 10–50 mg/dose orally every day for 2 wks, then 5–10 mg/day for 1 mo.

Alcohol Withdrawal Syndrome
IV, IM: ADULTS, ELDERLY: 100 mg/day for several days, then **PO:** 50–100 mg/day.

Metabolic Disorders
PO: ADULTS: 10–20 mg/day.

Wernicke's Encephalopathy
IV: ADULTS, ELDERLY: Initially, 100 mg then **IV/IM:** 50–100 mg/day until consuming a regular, balanced diet.

SIDE EFFECTS

Frequent: Pain, induration, tenderness at IM injection site.

ADVERSE EFFECTS/ TOXIC REACTIONS

IV administration may result in rare, severe hypersensitivity reaction marked by feeling of warmth, pruritus, urticaria, weakness, diaphoresis, nausea, restlessness, tightness in throat, angioedema, cyanosis, pulmonary edema, GI tract bleeding, cardiovascular collapse.

NURSING CONSIDERATIONS

INTERVENTION/EVALUATION

Monitor EKG readings, lab values for erythrocyte activity. Assess for clinical improvement (improved sense of well-being, weight gain). Observe for reversal of deficiency symptoms (**neurologic:** altered mental status, peripheral neuropathy, hyporeflexia, nystagmus, ophthalmoplegia, ataxia, muscle weakness; **cardiac:** venous hypertension, bounding arterial pulse, tachycardia, edema).

PATIENT/FAMILY TEACHING

• Discomfort may occur with IM injection. • Foods rich in thiamine include pork, organ meats, whole grain and enriched cereals, legumes, nuts, seeds, yeast, wheat germ, rice bran. • Urine may appear bright yellow.

---

thioridazine

thy-o-**rid**-a-zeen

BLACK BOX ALERT Dose-related prolongation of QT interval may cause arrhythmias, sudden death.
Do not confuse thioridazine with thiothixene or Thorazine.

◆CLASSIFICATION

PHARMACOTHERAPEUTIC: Phenothiazine. **CLINICAL:** Antipsychotic, sedative, antidyskinetic (see p. 67C).

ACTION

Blocks dopamine at postsynaptic receptor sites. Possesses strong anticholinergic, sedative effects. **Therapeutic Effect:** Suppresses behavioral response in psychosis; reduces locomotor activity, aggressiveness.

PHARMACOKINETICS

Absorption may be erratic. Protein binding: Very high. Metabolized in liver. Excreted in urine. **Half-life:** 21–24 hrs.

USES

Treatment of refractory schizophrenic pts. **OFF-LABEL:** Treatment of behavioral problems in children, schizophrenia/psychoses in children, dementia, depressive

T

---

neurosis, psychosis/agitation related to Alzheimer's dementia.

PRECAUTIONS

Contraindications: Severe CNS depression, coma, severe heart disease. Concurrent use of medication inhibiting metabolism of thioridazine, concurrent use of drugs that prolong QT interval, severe CNS depression, pts known to have genetic defect leading to reduced levels of activity of CYP2D6. **Cautions:** Seizures, decreased GI motility, urinary retention, benign prostatic hypertrophy, visual problems, Parkinson's disease, pts at risk for pneumonia, pts at risk for orthostatic hypotension, hemodynamic instability; severe cardiac, hepatic, renal disease.

⌛ LIFESPAN CONSIDERATIONS

Pregnancy/Lactation: Drug crosses placenta; is distributed in breast milk. **Pregnancy Category C. Children:** Increased risk for development of extrapyramidal symptoms (EPS), neuromuscular symptoms, esp. dystonias. **Elderly:** Prone to anticholinergic effects (dry mouth, EPS, orthostatic hypotension, sedation).

INTERACTIONS

DRUG: **Fluoxetine, paroxetine, fluvoxamine, propranol** may increase concentration/effects by inhibiting metabolism (Contraindicated). **Medications causing QT interval prolongation (e.g., erythromycin, procainamide, quinidine)** may lengthen QT interval. **HERBAL:** **Gotu kola, kava kava, St. John's wort, valerian** may increase CNS depression. **Dong quai, St. John's wort** may increase photosensitization. **FOOD:** None known. **LAB VALUES:** May cause EKG changes. **Therapeutic serum level:** 0.2–2.6 mcg/ml; **toxic serum level:** not established.

AVAILABILITY (Rx)

Tablets: 10 mg, 25 mg, 50 mg, 100 mg.

ADMINISTRATION/HANDLING

PO
• May give without regard to food.• Do not take antacid within 2 hrs of administration.

INDICATIONS/ROUTES/DOSAGE

Psychosis
PO: ADULTS, ELDERLY, CHILDREN 12 YRS AND OLDER: Initially, 25–100 mg 3 times daily; dosage increased gradually. **Maximum:** 800 mg/day in 2–4 divided doses. **Maintenance:** 20–200 mg 2–4 times/ day. **CHILDREN 2–11 YRS:** Initially, 0.5–3 mg/kg/day in 2–3 divided doses. **Maximum:** 3 mg/kg/day.

SIDE EFFECTS

Generally well tolerated with only mild, transient side effects. **Occasional:** Drowsiness during early therapy, dry mouth, blurred vision, lethargy, constipation, diarrhea, nasal congestion, peripheral edema, urinary retention. **Rare:** Ocular changes, altered skin pigmentation (in pts taking high doses for prolonged periods), photosensitivity, darkening of urine.

ADVERSE EFFECTS/ TOXIC REACTIONS

Prolonged QT interval may produce torsade de pointes, a form of ventricular tachycardia, sudden death.

NURSING CONSIDERATIONS

BASELINE ASSESSMENT

Assess behavior, appearance, emotional status, response to environment, speech pattern, thought content.

INTERVENTION/EVALUATION

Assess for extrapyramidal symptoms. Monitor EKG, CBC, B/P, serum potassium, hepatic function, eye exams. Monitor for fine tongue movement (may be early sign of tardive dyskinesia). Supervise suicidal-risk pt closely during early therapy (as depression lessens, energy level improves, increasing suicide potential). Assess for therapeutic response (interest in surroundings, improvement in self-care, increased ability to concentrate, relaxed facial expression). **Therapeutic serum level:** 0.2–2.6 mcg/ml; **toxic serum level:** not established.

PATIENT/FAMILY TEACHING

• Full therapeutic effect may take up to 6 wks. • Urine may darken. • Do not abruptly withdraw from long-term drug therapy. • Report visual disturbances. • Sugarless gum, sips of water may relieve dry mouth. • Drowsiness generally subsides during continued therapy. • Avoid tasks that require alertness, motor skills until response to drug is established. • Avoid alcohol. • Avoid exposure to sunlight, artificial light.

---

thiotepa `HIGH ALERT`

thye-oh-**tep**-a
(Thioplex)
Do not confuse thiotepa with thioguanine.

◆CLASSIFICATION

PHARMACOTHERAPEUTIC: Alkylating agent. **CLINICAL:** Antineoplastic (see p. 91C).

ACTION

Inhibits DNA, RNA protein synthesis by cross-linking with DNA, RNA strands, preventing cell growth. Cell cycle–phase nonspecific. **Therapeutic Effect:** Produces cell death.

PHARMACOKINETICS

Incompletely absorbed from GI tract. Metabolized in liver. Excreted in urine. **Half-life:** 2.3–2.4 hrs.

USES

Treatment of superficial tumors of bladder; palliative treatment of adenocarcinoma of breast or ovary; control of pleural, pericardial, or peritoneal effusions caused by metastatic tumors. **OFF-LABEL:**

Intrathecal treatment of leptomeningeal metastases.

PRECAUTIONS

Contraindications: None known. **Cautions:** Hepatic/renal impairment, bone marrow dysfunction.

LIFESPAN CONSIDERATIONS

Pregnancy/Lactation: May cause fetal harm. Unknown if drug is distributed in breast milk. **Pregnancy Category D. Children:** Safety and efficacy not established. **Elderly:** No age-related precautions noted.

INTERACTIONS

DRUG: Bone marrow depressants may increase myelosuppression. **Live virus vaccines** may potentiate virus replication, increase vaccine side effects, decrease pt's antibody response to vaccine. **HERBAL:** Avoid **black cohosh, dong quai** in estrogen-dependent tumors. **St. John's wort** may increase photosensitization. **Echinacea** may decrease effects. **FOOD:** None known. **LAB VALUES:** May increase serum uric acid.

AVAILABILITY (Rx)

Injection, Powder for Reconstitution: 15 mg.

ADMINISTRATION/HANDLING

◄ALERT► May be carcinogenic, mutagenic, teratogenic. Handle with extreme caution during preparation/administration.

 IV

◄ALERT► Give by IV, intrapleural, intraperitoneal, intrapericardial, or intratumor injection; intravesical instillation.
Reconstitution • Reconstitute 15-mg vial with 1.5 ml Sterile Water for Injection to provide concentration of 10 mg/ml. Shake solution gently; let stand to clear. • May further dilute with 0.9% NaCl at concentration 1 mg/ml or greater. • For intravesical lavage, dilute in 30–60 ml Sterile Water for Injection or 0.9% NaCl.
Rate of Administration • Withdraw reconstituted drug through 0.22-micron

---

T

filter before administration. • For IV push, give over 1–2 min at concentration of 10 mg/ml. • Give IV infusion over 10–60 min. • For intravesical lavage, instill directly into bladder and retain for at least 2 hrs.

Storage • Refrigerate unopened vials. • Reconstituted solution appears clear to slightly opaque; is stable for 28 days if refrigerated (7 days at room temperature). Discard if solution appears grossly opaque or precipitate forms.

🔲 IV INCOMPATIBILITIES

Cisplatin (Platinol-AQ), filgrastim (Neupogen), vinorelbine (Navelbine).

🔲 IV COMPATIBILITIES

Allopurinol (Aloprim), bumetanide (Bumex), calcium gluconate, carboplatin (Paraplatin), cyclophosphamide (Cytoxan), dexamethasone (Decadron), diphenhydramine (Benadryl), doxorubicin (Adriamycin), etoposide (VePesid), fluorouracil, gemcitabine (Gemzar), granisetron (Kytril), heparin, hydromorphone (Dilaudid), leucovorin, lorazepam (Ativan), magnesium sulfate, morphine, ondansetron (Zofran), paclitaxel (Taxol), potassium chloride, vinblastine (Velban), vincristine (Oncovin).

INDICATIONS/ROUTES/DOSAGE

◀ALERT▶ Dosage individualized based on clinical response, tolerance to adverse effects. When used in combination therapy, consult specific protocols for optimum dosage, sequence of drug administration.

Ovarian, Breast Cancer
IV: ADULTS, ELDERLY: Initially, 0.3–0.4 mg/kg every 1–4 wks. Maintenance dose adjusted weekly based on blood counts.

Control of Effusions
Intracavitary Injection: ADULTS, ELDERLY: 0.6–0.8 mg/kg (or 30–60 mg) every 1–4 wks.

Bladder Cancer
Intravesical: 60 mg in 30–60 ml 0.9% NaCl retained for 2 hrs once weekly for 4 wks.

SIDE EFFECTS

Occasional: Pain at injection site, headache, dizziness, urticaria, rash, nausea, vomiting, anorexia, stomatitis. **Rare:** Alopecia, cystitis, hematuria (following intravesical administration).

ADVERSE EFFECTS/ TOXIC REACTIONS

Hematologic toxicity (leukopenia, anemia, thrombocytopenia, pancytopenia) may occur due to bone marrow depression. Although WBC count falls to its lowest point 10–14 days after initial therapy, bone marrow effect may not be evident for 30 days. Stomatitis, ulceration of intestinal mucosa may occur.

NURSING CONSIDERATIONS

BASELINE ASSESSMENT

Obtain hematologic tests at least weekly during therapy and for 3 wks after therapy is discontinued.

INTERVENTION/EVALUATION

Interrupt therapy if WBC falls below 3,000/mm^3, platelet count below 150,000/mm^3, WBC or platelet count declines rapidly. Monitor serum uric acid levels, hematology tests. Assess for stomatitis. Monitor for hematologic toxicity: infection (fever, sore throat, signs of local infection), unusual bruising/bleeding from any site, symptoms of anemia (excessive fatigue, weakness). Assess skin for rash, urticaria.

PATIENT/FAMILY TEACHING

• Maintain strict oral hygiene. • Do not have immunizations without physician's approval (drug lowers resistance). • Avoid crowds, those with infection. • Promptly report fever, sore throat, signs of local infection, unusual bruising/bleeding from any site.

thiothixene

thy-oh-**thix**-een
(Navane)

BLACK BOX ALERT Elderly pts with dementia related psychosis are at increased risk for death.

Do not confuse Navane with Norvasc or Nubain, or thiothixene with fluoxetine or thioridazine.

◆CLASSIFICATION

PHARMACOTHERAPEUTIC: Thioxanthene derivative. **CLINICAL:** Antipsychotic (see p. 67C).

ACTION

Blocks postsynaptic dopamine receptor sites in brain. Has alpha-adrenergic blocking effects, depresses release of hypothalamic, hypophyseal hormones. **Therapeutic Effect:** Suppresses psychotic behavior.

PHARMACOKINETICS

Well absorbed from GI tract after IM administration. Widely distributed. Metabolized in liver. Primarily excreted in urine. Unknown if removed by hemodialysis. **Half-life:** 34 hrs.

USES

Symptomatic management of schizophrenia. **OFF-LABEL:** Psychosis (children), psychosis/agitation related to Alzheimer's dementia. Rapid tranquilization. Dementia behavior in elderly.

PRECAUTIONS

Contraindications: Blood dyscrasias, circulatory collapse, CNS depression, coma. **Cautions:** Seizures, cardiovascular disease, cerebrovascular disease, narrow-angle glaucoma, renal/hepatic impairment, myasthenia gravis, Parkinson's disease, seizure disorder, pts with underlying QT prolongation, decreased GI motility, paralytic ileus, urinary retention, BPH, visual problems, pts at risk for orthostatic hypotension, pneumonia.

⏳ LIFESPAN CONSIDERATIONS

Pregnancy/Lactation: Drug crosses placenta; distributed in breast milk. **Pregnancy Category C. Children:** May develop neuromuscular or extrapyramidal symptoms (EPS), esp. dystonias. **Elderly:** More prone to orthostatic hypotension, anticholinergic effects (e.g., dry mouth), sedation, EPS.

INTERACTIONS

DRUG: Alcohol, other CNS depressants may increase CNS, respiratory depression, hypotensive effects. **Extrapyramidal symptoms (EPS)–producing medications** may increase risk of EPS. **CYP3A4 inducers (e.g., carbamazepine)** may decrease concentration/effects. **HERBAL: Kava kava, gotu kola, St. John's wort, valerian** may increase CNS depression. **FOOD:** None known. **LAB VALUES:** May decrease serum uric acid.

AVAILABILITY (Rx)

Capsules: 1 mg, 2 mg, 5 mg, 10 mg.

ADMINISTRATION/HANDLING

PO
• Give with food or water.

INDICATIONS/ROUTES/DOSAGE

Mild to Moderate Psychosis
PO: ADULTS, ELDERLY, CHILDREN 12 YRS AND OLDER: 2 mg 3 times daily up to 20–30 mg/day.

Severe Psychosis
PO: ADULTS, ELDERLY, CHILDREN 12 YRS AND OLDER: Initially, 5 mg twice daily. May increase gradually up to 60 mg/day.

Rapid Tranquilization of Agitated Pt
PO: ADULTS, ELDERLY: 5–10 mg q30–60min. Average total dose: 15–30 mg.

SIDE EFFECTS

Frequent: Transient drowsiness, dry mouth, constipation, blurred vision, na-

T

---

sal congestion. **Occasional:** Diarrhea, peripheral edema, urinary retention, nausea. **Rare:** Ocular changes, altered skin pigmentation (in those taking high doses for prolonged periods), photosensitivity, hypotension, dizziness, syncope.

ADVERSE EFFECTS/ TOXIC REACTIONS

Most common extrapyramidal reaction is akathisia, characterized by motor restlessness, anxiety. Akinesia (marked by rigidity, tremor, increased salivation, mask-like facial expression, reduced voluntary movements) occurs less frequently. Dystonias, including torticollis (neck muscle spasm), opisthotonos (rigidity of back muscles), oculogyric crisis (rolling back of eyes), occur rarely. Tardive dyskinesia, characterized by tongue protrusion, puffing of cheeks, chewing/puckering of mouth, occurs rarely but may be irreversible. Elderly female pts have greater risk of developing this reaction. Grand mal seizures may occur in epileptic pts. Neuroleptic malignant syndrome occurs rarely.

NURSING CONSIDERATIONS

BASELINE ASSESSMENT

Assess behavior, appearance, emotional status, response to environment, speech pattern, thought content.

INTERVENTION/EVALUATION

Supervise suicidal-risk pt closely during early therapy (as depression lessens, energy level improves, increasing suicide potential). Monitor B/P for hypotension. Assess for peripheral edema. Monitor daily pattern of bowel activity, stool consistency. Prevent constipation. Observe for extrapyramidal symptoms (EPS), tardive dyskinesia; monitor for potentially fatal, rare neuroleptic malignant syndrome. Assess for therapeutic response (interest in surroundings, improvement in self-care, increased ability to concentrate, relaxed facial expression).

PATIENT/FAMILY TEACHING

• Full therapeutic effect may take up to 6 wks. • Report visual disturbances. • Sugarless gum, sips of water may relieve dry mouth. • Drowsiness generally subsides during continued therapy. • Avoid tasks that require alertness, motor skills until response to drug is established. • Avoid alcohol, other CNS depressants. • Avoid exposure to direct sunlight, artificial light.

tiagabine

tye-**a**-ga-bine
(Gabitril)
Do not confuse tiagabine with tizanidine.

◆CLASSIFICATION

PHARMACOTHERAPEUTIC: Anticonvulsant. **CLINICAL:** Anticonvulsant (see p. 37C).

ACTION

Blocks reuptake in presynaptic neurons of gamma-aminobutyric acid (GABA), the major inhibitory neurotransmitter in the CNS, in the presynaptic neurons, increasing GABA levels at postsynaptic neurons. **Therapeutic Effect:** Inhibits seizures.

USES

Adjunctive therapy for treatment of partial seizures in adults and children 12 yrs or older.

PHARMACOKINETICS

Rapidly absorbed from GI tract. Protein binding: 96%. Metabolized in liver. Primarily eliminated in feces. **Half-life:** 2–5 hrs.

PRECAUTIONS

Contraindications: None known. **Cautions:** Hepatic impairment. Concurrent use of alcohol, other CNS depressants may cause seizures. Pts at risk for suicidal behavior/thoughts.

⌛ LIFESPAN CONSIDERATIONS

Pregnancy/Lactation: May produce teratogenic effects. Distributed in breast milk. **Pregnancy Category C. Children:** Safety and efficacy not established in pts younger than 12 yrs. **Elderly:** Age-related hepatic impairment may require dosage adjustment.

INTERACTIONS

DRUG: Carbamazepine, phenobarbital, phenytoin may increase clearance. May alter effects of **valproic acid.** **HERBAL: Evening primrose** may decrease seizure threshold. **St. John's wort** may decrease concentration. **Gotu kola, kava kava, St. John's wort, valerian** may increase CNS depression. **FOOD:** None known. **LAB VALUES:** None significant.

AVAILABILITY (Rx)

Tablets: 2 mg, 4 mg, 12 mg, 16 mg.

ADMINISTRATION/HANDLING

• Give with food.

INDICATIONS/ROUTES/DOSAGE

Partial Seizures
PO: ADULTS, ELDERLY: Initially, 4 mg once daily. May increase by 4–8 mg/day at weekly intervals. **Maximum:** 56 mg/day in 2–4 divided doses. **CHILDREN 12–18 YRS:** Initially, 4 mg once daily. May increase by 4 mg at wk 2 and by 4–8 mg at weekly intervals thereafter. **Maximum:** 32 mg/day in 2–4 divided doses.

SIDE EFFECTS

Frequent (34%–20%): Dizziness, asthenia (loss of strength, energy), drowsiness, nervousness, confusion, headache, infection, tremor. **Occasional:** Nausea, diarrhea, abdominal pain, impaired concentration.

ADVERSE EFFECTS/ TOXIC REACTIONS

Overdose characterized by agitation, confusion, hostility, weakness. Full recovery occurs within 24 hrs of discontinuation.

NURSING CONSIDERATIONS

BASELINE ASSESSMENT

Review history of seizure disorder (intensity, frequency, duration, LOC). Observe frequently for recurrence of seizure activity. Initiate seizure precautions.

INTERVENTION/EVALUATION

For pts on long-term therapy, serum hepatic/renal function tests, CBC should be performed periodically. Assist with ambulation if dizziness occurs. Assess for clinical improvement (decrease in intensity, frequency of seizures). Monitor for depression, unusual behavior, suicidal ideation or thoughts.

PATIENT/FAMILY TEACHING

• Go from lying to standing slowly. • Avoid tasks that require alertness, motor skills until response to drug is established. • Avoid alcohol. • Report worsening seizure activity, thoughts of suicide, increased depression.

ticagrelor

tye-**ka**-grel-or
(Brilinta)

BLACK BOX ALERT May cause significant, sometimes fatal bleeding. Do not use with active bleeding or history of intracranial bleeding. Do not initiate in pts planning urgent coronary artery bypass graft (CABG) surgery. Discontinue at least 5 days prior to any surgery. Suspect bleeding in any pt who is hypotensive and has had recent percutaneous coronary intervention (PCI), CABG, or other surgical procedures. If possible, manage bleeding without discontinuing therapy to decrease risk of cardiovascular events. Aspirin maintenance doses greater than 100 mg/day may reduce effectiveness and should be strictly avoided.

T

♣ Canadian trade name   🚫 Non-Crushable Drug   📶 High Alert drug

◆CLASSIFICATION

PHARMACOTHERAPEUTIC: P2Y$_{12}$ platelet inhibitor. **CLINICAL:** Antiplatelet (see p. 34C).

ACTION

Reversibly inhibits platelet P2Y$_{12}$ ADP receptor to prevent signal transduction and platelet activation. **Therapeutic Effect:** Prevents platelet aggregation.

PHARMACOKINETICS

Readily absorbed after PO administration. Protein binding: 99%. Metabolized in liver. Primarily excreted in feces (58%), urine (26%). **Half-life:** 7–9 hrs.

USES

Reduction of thrombolytic cardiovascular events in conjunction with aspirin in pts with acute coronary syndrome (ACS) including unstable angina (UA), non-ST elevation myocardial infarction (STEMI), or STEMI. **OFF-LABEL:** Initial treatment of UA, non-STEMI in pts with allergy to aspirin or major GI intolerance to aspirin.

PRECAUTIONS

Contraindications: History of intracranial hemorrhage, active pathologic bleeding, severe hepatic impairment. **Cautions:** Moderate hepatic impairment, renal impairment, history of hyperuricemia or gouty arthritis. Pts at increased risk of bradycardia; concurrent use of strong CYP3A4 inhibitors or inducers. Recommend holding dose 5 days before planned surgery if applicable.

⏳ LIFESPAN CONSIDERATIONS

Pregnancy/Lactation: Unknown if distributed in breast milk. Must either discontinue breastfeeding or discontinue drug therapy. **Pregnancy Category C. Children:** Safety and efficacy not established. **Elderly:** No age-related precautions noted.

INTERACTIONS

DRUG: Aspirin greater than 100 mg/day may decrease effectiveness. **CYP3A4 in-** hibitors (e.g., **atazanavir, clarithromycin, itraconazole, ketoconazole, nefazodone, ritonavir, saquinavir**) may increase concentration/effects. **CYP3A4 inducers** (e.g., **carbamazepine, dexamethasone, phenobarbital, phenytoin, rifampin**) may decrease concentration/effects. **Anticoagulants, antiplatelets, NSAIDs** may increase risk of bleeding. May increase concentration of **digoxin, simvastatin, lovastatin.** **HERBAL: St. John's wort** may decrease effectiveness. **Fenugreek, feverfew, flaxseed, garlic, ginger, ginkgo biloba, ginseng, omega-3, red clover** with anticoagulant/antiplatelet activity may increase risk of bleeding. **FOOD: Grapefruit products** may increase potential for bleeding. **LAB VALUES:** May increase uric acid, creatinine.

AVAILABILITY (Rx)

Tablets: 90 mg.

ADMINISTRATION/HANDLING

PO
• Give without regard to meals.

INDICATIONS/ROUTES/DOSAGE

Acute Coronary Syndrome
PO: ADULTS: 180 mg once, then 90 mg twice daily. Give with aspirin 325 mg once (loading dose), then maintain with aspirin 75–100 mg daily.

SIDE EFFECTS

Occasional (13%–7%): Dyspnea, headache. **Rare (5%–3%):** Cough, dizziness, nausea, diarrhea, back pain, fatigue.

ADVERSE EFFECTS/ TOXIC REACTIONS

Life-threatening events including intracranial bleeding, epistaxis, intrapericardial bleeding with cardiac tamponade, hypovolemic shock requiring vasopressive support, or blood transfusion reported. Pts with history of sick sinus syndrome, second- or third-degree AV block, bradycardic syncope have increased risk of bradycardia. May induce episodes of atrial fibrillation, hypotension, hypertension. Gynecomastia reported in less than 1% of men.

NURSING CONSIDERATIONS

BASELINE ASSESSMENT

Obtain CBC, serum chemistries, hepatic and renal function test, digoxin level if applicable. Question for history of bleeding, stomach ulcers, colon polyps, head trauma, cardiac arrhythmias, unstable angina, recent MI, hepatic impairment, hypertension, stroke. Receive full medication history including herbal products. Question for history of COPD, chronic bronchitis, emphysema, asthma, exertional dyspnea.

INTERVENTION/EVALUATION

Routinely screen for bleeding. Assess skin for bruising, hematoma. Monitor renal function, uric acid, digoxin levels if applicable. Report hematuria, epistaxis, coffee-ground emesis, black/tarry stools. Monitor EKG for chest pain, shortness of breath, syncope.

PATIENT/FAMILY TEACHING

• It may take longer to stop bleeding during therapy. • Do not vigorously blow nose. • Use soft toothbrush, electric razor to decrease risk of bleeding. • Immediately report bloody stool, urine, or nosebleeds. • Report all newly prescribed medications. • Inform physician of any planned dental procedures or surgeries.

---

ticlopidine   HIGH ALERT

tye-**klo**-pye-deen
(Apo-Ticlopidine , Novo-
Ticlopidine)

BLACK BOX ALERT Risk of neutropenia, agranulocytosis, thrombotic thrombocytopenia purpura, aplastic anemia.

◆CLASSIFICATION

PHARMACOTHERAPEUTIC: Aggregation inhibitor. **CLINICAL:** Antiplatelet (see p. 34C).

ACTION

Inhibits release of adenosine diphosphate from activated platelets, preventing fibrinogen from binding to glycoprotein IIb/IIIa receptors on surface of activated platelets. **Therapeutic Effect:** Inhibits platelet aggregation, thrombus formation.

PHARMACOKINETICS

Route	Onset	Peak
PO (platelet inhibition)	6 hrs	3–5 days

Rapidly absorbed following PO administration. Protein binding: 98%. Metabolized in liver. Primarily excreted in urine; partially eliminated in feces. **Half-life:** 13 hrs.

USES

To reduce risk of stroke in pts who have experienced stroke-like symptoms (transient ischemic attacks) or with history of thrombotic stroke. **OFF-LABEL:** Prevention of postop deep vein thrombosis (DVT), protection of aortocoronary bypass grafts, reduction of graft loss after renal transplant, diabetic microangiopathy, ischemic heart disease.

PRECAUTIONS

Contraindications: Active pathologic bleeding (e.g., bleeding peptic ulcer, intracranial bleeding), hematopoietic disorders (neutropenia, thrombocytopenia), presence of hemostatic disorder, severe hepatic impairment. **Cautions:** Pts at increased risk for bleeding, mild to moderate hepatic/renal disease, concurrent treatment with anticoagulants.

⧖ LIFESPAN CONSIDERATIONS

Pregnancy/Lactation: Unknown if drug crosses placenta or is distributed in breast milk. **Pregnancy Category B. Children:** Safety and efficacy not established. **Elderly:** No age-related precautions noted.

INTERACTIONS

DRUG: Aspirin, heparin, NSAIDs, oral anticoagulants, thrombolytics may increase risk of bleeding. May increase concentration, risk of toxicity of **phenytoin, theophylline. HERBAL:** Cat's claw, dong quai, evening primrose, feverfew, garlic, ginger, ginkgo biloba, ginseng possess antiplatelet activity, may increase risk of bleeding. **FOOD: All foods** increase bioavailability. **LAB VALUES:** May increase serum cholesterol, alkaline phosphatase, bilirubin, AST, ALT triglycerides. May prolong bleeding time. May decrease neutrophil, platelet counts.

AVAILABILITY (Rx)

Tablets: 250 mg.

ADMINISTRATION/HANDLING

PO

• Give with food or just after meals (bioavailability increased, GI discomfort decreased).

INDICATIONS/ROUTES/DOSAGE

Prevention of Stroke
PO: ADULTS, ELDERLY: 250 mg twice a day.

SIDE EFFECTS

Frequent (13%–5%): Diarrhea, nausea, dyspepsia (heartburn, indigestion, epigastric pain, bloating). **Rare (2%–1%):** Vomiting, flatulence, pruritus, dizziness.

ADVERSE EFFECTS/
TOXIC REACTIONS

Neutropenia occurs in approximately 2% of pts. Thrombotic thrombocytopenia purpura, agranulocytosis, hepatitis, cholestatic jaundice, tinnitus occur rarely.

NURSING CONSIDERATIONS

BASELINE ASSESSMENT

Drug should be discontinued 10–14 days before surgery if antiplatelet effect is not desired.

INTERVENTION/EVALUATION

Monitor daily pattern of bowel activity, stool consistency. Assist with ambulation if dizziness occurs. Observe, monitor neurologic status for changes. Assess skin for flushing, rash. Observe for signs of bleeding. Monitor CBC, serum hepatic/renal function tests.

PATIENT/FAMILY TEACHING

• Take with food to decrease GI symptoms. • Periodic blood tests are essential. • Report fever, sore throat, chills, unusual bleeding.

tigecycline

tye-gee-**sye**-kleen
(Tygacil)

♦**CLASSIFICATION**
PHARMACOTHERAPEUTIC: Glycylcycline. **CLINICAL:** Antibiotic.

ACTION

Blocks protein synthesis by binding to ribosomal receptor sites of bacterial cell wall. **Therapeutic Effect:** Bacteriostatic effect.

PHARMACOKINETICS

Extensive tissue distribution, minimally metabolized. Eliminated by biliary/fecal route (59%), urine (33%). Protein binding: 71%–89%. **Half-life:** Single dose: 27 hrs; following multiple doses: 42 hrs.

USES

Treatment of susceptible infections due to *E. coli, E. faecalis, S. aureus, S. agalactiae, S. anginosus* group (includes *S. anginosus, S. intermedius, S. constellatus), S. pyogenes, B. fragilis, Citrobacter freundii, E. cloacae, K. oxytoca, K. pneumoniae, B. thetaiotaomicron, B. uniformis, B. vulgatus, C. perfringens, Peptostreptococcus micros* including complicated skin/skin structure infections, complicated intra-abdominal infections, community-acquired bacterial pneumonia.

PRECAUTIONS

Contraindications: None known. **Cautions:** Hypersensitivity to tetracyclines, last half of pregnancy, hepatic impairment, intestinal perforation.

⧗ LIFESPAN CONSIDERATIONS

Pregnancy/Lactation: May cause fetal harm. May be distributed in breast milk. Permanent discoloration of the teeth (brown-gray) may occur if used during tooth development. **Pregnancy Category D.** **Children:** Safety and efficacy not established in pts younger than 18 yrs. **Elderly:** No age-related precautions noted.

INTERACTIONS

DRUG: May decrease effects of **oral contraceptives** may be decreased. May increase concentration of **warfarin;** increase bleeding time. **HERBAL:** None significant. **FOOD:** None known. **LAB VALUES:** May increase serum alkaline phosphatase, amylase, BUN, bilirubin, glucose, LDH, ALT, AST. May decrease Hgb, WBCs, thrombocytes, serum potassium, protein.

AVAILABILITY (Rx)

Injection, Powder for Reconstitution (Tygacil): 50-mg vial.

ADMINISTRATION/HANDLING

 IV

Reconstitution • Add 5.3 ml 0.9% NaCl or D₅W to each 50-mg vial. • Swirl gently to dissolve. • Resulting solution is 10 mg/ml. • Immediately withdraw 5 ml reconstituted solution and add to 100 ml 0.9% NaCl or D₅W bag for infusion (final concentration should not exceed 1 mg/ml).
Rate of Administration • Administer over 30–60 min every 12 hrs. • May be given through a dedicated line or by Y-site piggyback. If same line is used for sequential infusion of several different drugs, line should be flushed before and after infusion of tigecycline with either 0.9% NaCl or D₅W.

Storage • Reconstituted solution is stable for up to 6 hrs at room temperature or up to 24 hrs if refrigerated. • Reconstituted solution appears yellow to red-orange. • Discard if solution is discolored (green, black) or precipitate forms.

▦ IV INCOMPATIBILITIES

Amphotericin B, methylprednisolone, voriconazole.

▦ IV COMPATIBILITIES

Amikacin, azithromycin, aztreonam, cefepime, ceftazidime, ciprofloxacin, doripenem, ertapenem, fluconazole, gentamicin, linezolid, piperacillin-tazobactam, potassium chloride, telavancin, tobramycin, vancomycin.

INDICATIONS/ROUTES/DOSAGE

Systemic Infections
IV: ADULTS OVER 18 YRS, ELDERLY: Initially, 100 mg, followed by 50 mg every 12 hrs for 5–14 days.

Dosage in Severe Hepatic Impairment
IV: ADULTS OVER 18 YRS, ELDERLY: Initially, 100 mg, followed by 25 mg every 12 hrs.

SIDE EFFECTS

Frequent (29%–13%): Nausea, vomiting, diarrhea. **Occasional (7%–4%):** Headache, hypertension, dizziness, increased cough, delayed healing. **Rare (3%–2%):** Peripheral edema, pruritus, constipation, dyspepsia (heartburn, indigestion, epigastric pain), asthenia (loss of strength, energy), hypotension, phlebitis, insomnia, rash, diaphoresis.

ADVERSE EFFECTS/ TOXIC REACTIONS

Dyspnea, abscess, pseudomembranous colitis (abdominal cramps, severe watery diarrhea, fever) ranging from mild to life-threatening may result from altered bacterial balance in GI tract.

T

NURSING CONSIDERATIONS

BASELINE ASSESSMENT

Obtain baseline hepatic function test. Question for history of allergies, esp. tetracyclines, before therapy.

INTERVENTION/EVALUATION

Monitor daily pattern of bowel activity, stool consistency. Be alert for superinfection: fever, anal/genital pruritus, oral mucosal changes (ulceration, pain, erythema). Nausea, vomiting may be controlled by antiemetics. Monitor tigecycline therapeutic levels.

PATIENT/FAMILY TEACHING

• Report diarrhea, rash, mouth soreness, other new symptoms.

tiludronate

tye-**loo**-dro-nate
(Skelid)

◆ CLASSIFICATION

PHARMACOTHERAPEUTIC: Bone resorption inhibitor. **CLINICAL:** Calcium regulator.

ACTION

Inhibits functioning osteoclasts through disruption of cytoskeletal ring structure, inhibition of osteoclastic proton pump. **Therapeutic Effect:** Inhibits bone resorption.

PHARMACOKINETICS

Well absorbed following PO administration. Protein binding: 90%. Minimally metabolized in liver. Excreted in urine. **Half-life:** 150 hrs.

USES

Treatment of Paget's disease of bone (osteitis deformans) in pts having a level of serum alkaline phosphatase (SAP) at least twice upper limit of normal, or are symptomatic, or at risk for future complications.

PRECAUTIONS

Contraindications: Inability to stand or sit upright for at least 30 min. **Cautions:** GI disease (e.g., dysphagia, symptomatic esophageal disease), severe renal impairment, impending invasive dental procedures (risk of osteonecrosis of jaw).

⧗ LIFESPAN CONSIDERATIONS

Pregnancy/Lactation: Unknown if drug crosses placenta or is distributed in breast milk. **Pregnancy Category C. Children:** Safety and efficacy not established. **Elderly:** No age-related precautions noted.

INTERACTIONS

DRUG: Antacids containing aluminum or magnesium, calcium, salicylates may interfere with absorption. **HERBAL:** None significant. **FOOD:** None known. **LAB VALUES:** None significant.

AVAILABILITY (Rx)

Tablets: 200 mg.

ADMINISTRATION/HANDLING

PO
• Must take with 6–8 oz plain water.
• Do not give within 2 hrs of food intake.
• Pt must not lie down for at least 30 min following administration. • Avoid giving aspirin, calcium supplements, mineral supplements, antacids within 2 hrs of tiludronate administration.

INDICATIONS/ROUTES/DOSAGE

Paget's Disease
PO: ADULTS, ELDERLY: 400 mg once a day for 3 mos. Not recommended in pts with creatinine clearance less than 30 ml/min.

SIDE EFFECTS

Frequent (9%–6%): Nausea, diarrhea, generalized body pain, back pain, headache. **Occasional (Less Than 6%):** Rash, dyspepsia (heartburn, indigestion, epigastric pain), vomiting, rhinitis, sinusitis, dizziness.

T

ADVERSE EFFECTS/ TOXIC REACTIONS

Dysphagia, esophagitis, esophageal ulcer, gastric ulcer occur rarely.

NURSING CONSIDERATIONS

BASELINE ASSESSMENT

Assess if pt is using other medications (esp. aluminum, magnesium, calcium, salicylates). Determine baseline renal function. Assess for GI disease.

INTERVENTION/EVALUATION

Monitor serum osteocalcin, alkaline phosphatase, adjusted calcium, urinary hydroxyproline to assess effectiveness of medication.

PATIENT/FAMILY TEACHING

• Take with 6–8 oz water. • Avoid other medication for 2 hrs before or after taking tiludronate. • Check with physician if calcium, vitamin D supplements are necessary.

---

timolol   HIGH ALERT

tim-oh-lol
(Apo-Timol ✦, Betimol, Istalol, PMS-Timolol ✦, Timoptic, Timoptic GFS, Timoptic Ocudose, Timoptic-XE)
Do not confuse Timoptic with Betoptic or Viroptic.

FIXED-COMBINATION(S)

Combigan: timolol/brimonidine (an alpha₂ agonist): 0.5%/0.2%. **Cosopt:** timolol/dorzolamide (a carbonic anhydrase inhibitor): 0.5%/2%.

◆CLASSIFICATION

PHARMACOTHERAPEUTIC: Beta-adrenergic blocker. **CLINICAL:** Antiglaucoma (see p. 53C, 74C).

ACTION

Blocks beta₁-, beta₂-adrenergic receptors. **Therapeutic Effect:** Reduces intraocular pressure (IOP) by reducing aqueous humor production.

PHARMACOKINETICS

Route	Onset	Peak	Duration
Ophthalmic	30 min	1–2 hrs	12–24 hrs

Systemic absorption may occur with ophthalmic administration.

USES

Ophthalmic: Reduces IOP in management of open-angle glaucoma, aphakic glaucoma, ocular hypertension, secondary glaucoma.

PRECAUTIONS

Contraindications: Bronchial asthma, cardiogenic shock, HF (unless secondary to tachyarrhythmias), COPD, second- or third-degree heart block, sinus bradycardia. **Cautions:** Diabetes mellitus, arterial obstruction, history of severe anaphylaxis to allergens.

⌛ LIFESPAN CONSIDERATIONS

Pregnancy/Lactation: Distributed in breast milk; not for use in breastfeeding women due to potential for serious adverse effect on breastfeeding infant. Avoid use during first trimester. May produce bradycardia, apnea, hypoglycemia, hypothermia in infant during delivery; low birth-weight infants. **Pregnancy Category C. Children:** Safety and efficacy not established. **Elderly:** Age-related peripheral vascular disease increases susceptibility to decreased peripheral circulation.

INTERACTIONS

DRUG: Diuretics, other antihypertensives may increase hypotensive effect. May mask symptoms of hypoglycemia, prolong hypoglycemic effects of **insulin, oral hypoglycemics. HERBAL:** None known. **FOOD:** None known. **LAB VALUES:** May increase antinuclear antibody titer (ANA), serum LDH, alkaline phosphatase, BUN, bilirubin, creatinine, potas-

 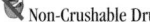

sium, uric acid, AST, ALT, triglycerides, lipoproteins.

AVAILABILITY (Rx)

Ophthalmic Gel (Timoptic-XE): 0.25%, 0.5%. Ophthalmic Solution (Betimol, Istalol, Timoptic, Timoptic Ocudose): 0.25%, 0.5%.

ADMINISTRATION/HANDLING

Ophthalmic

◄ALERT► When using gel, invert container, shake once prior to each use. • Place gloved finger on lower eyelid and pull out until pocket is formed between eye and lower lid. • Place prescribed number of drops or amount of prescribed gel into pocket. • Instruct pt to close eye gently so that medication will not be squeezed out of sac. • Apply gentle finger pressure to the lacrimal sac at inner canthus for 1 min following instillation (lessens risk of systemic absorption).

INDICATIONS/ROUTES/DOSAGE

Reduction of Intraocular
Pressure (IOP)
Ophthalmic: ADULTS, ELDERLY, CHILDREN: 1 drop of 0.25% solution in affected eye(s) twice daily. May be increased to 1 drop of 0.5% solution in affected eye(s) twice daily. When IOP is controlled, dosage may be reduced to 1 drop once daily. If pt is switched to timolol from another antiglaucoma agent, administer concurrently for 1 day. Discontinue other agent on following day. Ophthalmic *(Timoptic XE)*: ADULTS, ELDERLY: 1 drop/day (0.25% or 0.5%). Ophthalmic *(Istalol)*: ADULTS, ELDERLY: Apply 1 drop (0.5%) once daily in the morning.

SIDE EFFECTS

Frequent: Eye irritation, visual disturbances. Occasional: Nasal congestion, nausea. Rare: Altered taste, dry eyes, pruritus, numbness of fingers, toes, scalp.

ADVERSE EFFECTS/ TOXIC REACTIONS

Ophthalmic overdose may produce bradycardia, hypotension, bronchospasm, acute cardiac failure.

NURSING CONSIDERATIONS

BASELINE ASSESSMENT
Screen for contraindications.

INTERVENTION/EVALUATION

Assess pulse for quality, rate, rhythm. Monitor pulse for irregular rate, bradycardia. Monitor EKG for cardiac arrhythmias, particularly PVCs. Monitor daily pattern of bowel activity, stool consistency. Monitor heart rate, B/P, serum hepatic/renal function, IOP (ophthalmic preparation).

PATIENT/FAMILY TEACHING

• Instill drops correctly following guidelines. • Transient stinging, discomfort may occur upon instillation.

---

tinzaparin   HIGH ALERT

tin-**zap**-a-rin
(Innohep)

◆CLASSIFICATION

PHARMACOTHERAPEUTIC: Low molecular weight heparin. CLINICAL: Anticoagulant (see p. 32C).

ACTION

Inhibits factor Xa. Causes less inactivation of thrombin, inhibition of platelets, bleeding than with standard heparin. Does not significantly influence bleeding time, PT, aPTT. Therapeutic Effect: Produces anticoagulation.

PHARMACOKINETICS

Well absorbed after subcutaneous administration. Partially metabolized. Pri-

---

marily eliminated in urine. **Half-life:** 3–4 hrs.

USES

Treatment of acute symptomatic deep vein thrombosis (DVT) with or without pulmonary embolism, when given in conjunction with warfarin. Prophylaxis of DVT following hip/knee replacement surgery, general surgery. Prevent clotting in indwelling IV lines and extracorporeal circuit during hemodialysis.

PRECAUTIONS

Contraindications: Active major bleeding, heparin-induced thrombocytopenia (current or past history). Acute or subacute endocarditis, hemophilia, major clotting disorders; uncontrolled severe hypertension; diabetic or hemorrhagic retinopathy; injury/surgery involving brain, spinal cord, eyes, or ears. **Cautions:** Conditions with increased risk of hemorrhage (e.g., bacterial endocarditis, bleeding disorders, severe uncontrolled hypertension, recent GI bleeding), renal impairment, hepatic impairment, history of thrombocytopenia or platelet defects, elderly.

⚕ LIFESPAN CONSIDERATIONS

Pregnancy/Lactation: Use with caution, particularly during last trimester, immediate postpartum period (increased risk of maternal hemorrhage). Unknown if distributed in breast milk. **Pregnancy Category B. Children:** Safety and efficacy not established. **Elderly:** May be more susceptible to bleeding.

INTERACTIONS

DRUG: Anticoagulants, NSAIDs, platelet aggregation inhibitors may increase risk of bleeding. **HERBAL: Cat's claw, dong quai, evening primrose, feverfew, garlic, ginkgo biloba, ginseng, horse chestnut, red clover** may increase risk of bleeding. **FOOD:** None known. **LAB VALUES:** May increase serum AST, ALT.

AVAILABILITY (Rx)

Injection Solution: 10,000 anti-Xa international units/ml, 20,000 anti-Xa international units/ml.

ADMINISTRATION/HANDLING

◀**ALERT**▶ Do not mix with other injections or infusions. Do not give IM.

Subcutaneous
• Parenteral form appears clear and colorless to pale yellow. • Store at room temperature.

INDICATIONS/ROUTES/DOSAGE

Deep Vein Thrombosis (DVT), PE
Subcutaneous: ADULTS, ELDERLY: 175 anti-Xa international units/kg once a day. **Maximum:** 18,000 anti-Xa international units/day. Continue for at least 6 days and until pt is sufficiently anticoagulated with warfarin (international normalized ratio [INR] of 2 or more for 2 consecutive days). Use with caution in pts with creatinine clearance 50 ml/min or less.

DVT Prophylaxis
Subcutaneous: ADULTS, ELDERLY: 75 anti-Xa international units/kg once daily for 7–10 days.

Anticoagulant During Hemodialysis (HD)
IV: ADULTS, ELDERLY: 2,250 international units for HD 4 hrs or less; 4,500 international units for HD longer than 4 hrs.

SIDE EFFECTS

Frequent (16%): Injection site reaction (e.g., inflammation, oozing, nodules, skin necrosis). **Rare (Less Than 2%):** Nausea, asthenia (loss of strength, energy), constipation, epistaxis.

ADVERSE EFFECTS/ TOXIC REACTIONS

Overdose may lead to bleeding complications ranging from local ecchymoses to major hemorrhage. **Antidote:** Dose of protamine sulfate (1% solution) should

T

be equal to dose of tinzaparin injected. 1 mg protamine sulfate neutralizes 100 units of tinzaparin. Second dose of 0.5 mg protamine sulfate per 100 units tinzaparin may be given if aPTT tested 2–4 hrs after initial infusion remains prolonged.

NURSING CONSIDERATIONS

BASELINE ASSESSMENT
Obtain baseline CBC. Determine baseline B/P.

INTERVENTION/EVALUATION
Periodically monitor CBC, platelet count. Assess for any sign of bleeding: bleeding at surgical site, hematuria, blood in stool, bleeding from gums, petechiae, bruising, bleeding from injection sites. Administer only subcutaneously.

PATIENT/FAMILY TEACHING
• May have tendency to bleed easily, use precautions (e.g., use electric razor, soft toothbrush). • Report chest pain, unusual bleeding/bruising, pain, numbness, tingling, swelling in joints, injection site reaction (oozing, nodules, inflammation).

tiotropium

TOP 200

tye-oh-**trope**-ee-yum
(Spiriva)
Do not confuse Spiriva with Inspra, or tiotropium with ipratropium.

◆CLASSIFICATION
PHARMACOTHERAPEUTIC: Anticholinergic. **CLINICAL:** Bronchodilator (see p. 75C).

ACTION
Binds to recombinant human muscarinic receptors at smooth muscle, resulting in long-acting bronchial smooth muscle re-laxation. **Therapeutic Effect:** Relieves bronchospasm.

PHARMACOKINETICS
Binds extensively to tissue. Protein binding: 72%. Metabolized by oxidation. Excreted in urine. **Half-life:** 5–6 days.

USES
Long-term maintenance treatment of bronchospasm associated with COPD, including chronic bronchitis, emphysema, and for reducing COPD exacerbations.

PRECAUTIONS
Contraindications: History of hypersensitivity to ipratropium. **Cautions:** Narrow-angle glaucoma, prostatic hypertrophy, bladder neck obstruction, moderate to severe renal impairment, history of hypersensitivity to atropine, myasthenia gravis.

⌛ LIFESPAN CONSIDERATIONS
Pregnancy/Lactation: Unknown if distributed in breast milk. **Pregnancy Category C. Children:** Safety and efficacy not established. **Elderly:** Higher frequency of dry mouth, constipation, UTI noted with increasing age.

INTERACTIONS
DRUG: Concurrent administration with **anticholinergics (e.g., ipratropium)** may increase adverse effects. **HERBAL:** None significant. **FOOD:** None known. **LAB VALUES:** None significant.

AVAILABILITY (Rx)
Powder for Inhalation: 18 mcg/capsule (in blister packs).

ADMINISTRATION/HANDLING
Inhalation
• Open dustcap of HandiHaler by pulling it upward, then open mouthpiece. • Place capsule in center chamber and firmly close mouthpiece until a click is heard, leaving the dustcap open. • Hold

HandiHaler device with mouthpiece upward, press piercing button completely in once, and release. • Instruct pt to breathe out completely before breathing in slowly and deeply but at rate sufficient to hear the capsule vibrate. • Have pt hold breath as long as it is comfortable until exhaling slowly. • Instruct pt to repeat once again to ensure full dose is received.

Storage • Store at room temperature. Do not expose capsules to extreme temperature, moisture. • Do not store capsules in HandiHaler device. • Use immediately once foil is peeled back or removed.

INDICATIONS/ROUTES/DOSAGE

COPD (Maintenance Treatment, Reduction of COPD Exacerbations)
Inhalation: ADULTS, ELDERLY: 18 mcg (1 capsule)/day via HandiHaler inhalation device.

SIDE EFFECTS

Frequent (16%–6%): Dry mouth, sinusitis, pharyngitis, dyspepsia, UTI, rhinitis. **Occasional (5%–4%):** Abdominal pain, peripheral edema, constipation, epistaxis, vomiting, myalgia, rash, oral candidiasis.

ADVERSE EFFECTS/ TOXIC REACTIONS

Angina pectoris, depression, flu-like symptoms, glaucoma, increased intraocular pressure occur rarely.

NURSING CONSIDERATIONS

BASELINE ASSESSMENT
Offer emotional support (high incidence of anxiety due to difficulty in breathing, sympathomimetic response to drug). Auscultate lung sounds.

INTERVENTION/EVALUATION
Monitor rate, depth, rhythm, type of respiration; quality, rate of pulse. Assess lung sounds for rhonchi, wheezing, rales. Monitor ABGs. Observe for clavicular retractions, hand tremor. Evaluate for clini-

cal improvement (quieter, slower respirations, relaxed facial expression, cessation of clavicular retractions).

PATIENT/FAMILY TEACHING
• Increase fluid intake (decreases lung secretion viscosity). • Do not use more than 1 capsule for inhalation at any one time. • Rinsing mouth with water immediately after inhalation may prevent mouth/throat dryness, thrush. • Avoid excessive use of caffeine derivatives (chocolate, coffee, tea, cola, cocoa). • Report eye pain/discomfort, blurred vision, visual halos.

tipranavir

tye-**pran**-a-veer
(Aptivus)

BLACK BOX ALERT May cause hepatitis (including fatalities), hepatic dysfunction. Intracranial hemorrhage has occurred.

◆ CLASSIFICATION

PHARMACOTHERAPEUTIC: Antiretroviral. **CLINICAL:** Protease inhibitor (see p. 120C).

ACTION

Prevents virus-specific processing of polyproteins, HIV-1 infected cells. **Therapeutic Effect:** Prevents formation of mature viral cells.

PHARMACOKINETICS

Incompletely absorbed following PO administration. Protein binding: 98%–99%. Metabolized in liver. Eliminated in feces (82%), urine (4%). **Half-life:** 6 hrs.

USES

Treatment of HIV infection in combination with ritonavir and other antiretroviral agents (limited to highly treatment experienced or multi–protease inhibitor resistance).

T

PRECAUTIONS

Contraindications: Moderate to severe hepatic impairment, concurrent use of tipranavir/ritonavir with alfuzosin, amiodarone, bepridil, dihydroergotamine, ergonovine, ergotamine, flecainide, lovastatin, methylergonovine, midazolam (oral), propafenone, quinidine, rifampin, sildenafil (pulmonary arterial hypertension), simvastatin, St. John's wort, triazolam, voriconazole. **Cautions:** Hemophilia, known sulfonamide allergy, mild hepatic impairment, pts at increased risk for bleeding from trauma, surgery, concurrent antiplatelet/anticoagulant therapy.

⌛ LIFESPAN CONSIDERATIONS

Pregnancy/Lactation: Unknown if drug crosses placenta or is distributed in breast milk. **Pregnancy Category C. Children:** Safety and efficacy not established. **Elderly:** Age-related hepatic impairment may require dosage adjustment.

INTERACTIONS

DRUG: May interfere with metabolism of **amiodarone, bepridil, ergotamine, midazolam, oral contraceptives. Carbamazepine, phenobarbital, phenytoin, rifampin** may decrease concentration. May increase concentration of **colchicine, HMG-CoA reductase inhibitors, fluoxetine, paroxetine, sertraline. HMG-CoA reductase inhibitors** may increase risk of myopathy including rhabdomyolysis. **HERBAL: St. John's wort** may lead to loss of virologic response, potential resistance to tipranavir. **FOOD: High-fat meals** may increase bioavailability. **LAB VALUES:** May increase serum cholesterol, triglycerides, amylase, ALT, AST. May decrease WBC count.

AVAILABILITY (Rx)

Capsules: 250 mg. **Oral Solution:** 100 mg/ml.

ADMINISTRATION/HANDLING

PO
• May take without regard to food. When taken with ritonavir tablets, must be taken with meals. • Store unopened bottles of capsules in refrigerator. • Do not freeze/refrigerate oral solution. • Once bottle is opened, capsules may be stored at room temperature for 60 days. Use oral solution within 60 days after opening.

INDICATIONS/ROUTES/DOSAGE

Note: Must be taken with ritonavir.

HIV Infection
PO: ADULTS, ELDERLY: 500 mg (2 capsules) administered with 200 mg of ritonavir twice a day. **CHILDREN 2–18 YRS:** 14 mg/kg with 6 mg/kg ritonavir twice daily. **Maximum:** 500 mg with 200 mg ritonavir twice daily.

SIDE EFFECTS

Frequent (11%): Diarrhea. **Occasional (7%–2%):** Nausea, fever, fatigue, headache, depression, vomiting, abdominal pain, weakness, rash. **Rare (Less Than 2%):** Abdominal distention, anorexia, flatulence, dizziness, insomnia, myalgia.

ADVERSE EFFECTS/ TOXIC REACTIONS

Bronchitis occurs in 3% of pts. Anemia, neutropenia, thrombocytopenia, diabetes mellitus, hepatic failure, hepatitis, peripheral neuropathy, pancreatitis occur rarely.

NURSING CONSIDERATIONS

BASELINE ASSESSMENT

Obtain baseline hepatic function tests before beginning therapy and at periodic intervals during therapy. Offer emotional support. Obtain full medication history.

INTERVENTION/EVALUATION

Closely monitor for evidence of GI discomfort. Monitor daily pattern of bowel activity, stool consistency. Assess skin for

T

evidence of rash. Monitor serum chemistry tests for marked laboratory abnormalities, particularly hepatic profile, CD4 cell count, HIV, RNA plasma levels. Assess for opportunistic infections (onset of fever, oral mucosa changes, cough, other respiratory symptoms).

PATIENT/FAMILY TEACHING

• Eat small, frequent meals to offset nausea, vomiting. • Continue therapy for full length of treatment. • Doses should be evenly spaced. • Tipranavir is not a cure for HIV infection, nor does it reduce risk of transmission to others. • Pt may continue to experience illnesses, including opportunistic infections. • Diarrhea can be controlled with OTC medication.

---

tizanidine

tye-**zan**-i-deen
(Apo-Tizanidine ✦, Zanaflex, Zanaflex Capsules)
Do not confuse tizanidine with tiagabine.

◆CLASSIFICATION

PHARMACOTHERAPEUTIC: Skeletal muscle relaxant. **CLINICAL:** Antispastic (see p. 152C).

ACTION

Increases presynaptic inhibition of spinal motor neurons mediated by alpha$_2$-adrenergic agonists, reducing facilitation to postsynaptic motor neurons. **Therapeutic Effect:** Reduces muscle spasticity.

PHARMACOKINETICS

Metabolized in liver. Primarily excreted in urine. **Half-life:** 2 hrs.

USES

Acute and intermittent management of muscle spasticity (spasms, stiffness, rigidity), spasticity associated with mul-

tiple sclerosis or spinal cord injury. **OFF-LABEL:** Acute low back pain, tension headaches.

PRECAUTIONS

Contraindications: Concurrent use with ciprofloxacin or fluvoxamine. **Cautions:** Renal/hepatic disease, hypotension, cardiac disease, psychiatric disorders. Avoid concurrent administration of oral contraceptives. **Pregnancy Category C.**

INTERACTIONS

DRUG: Alcohol, other CNS depressants may increase CNS depressant effects. **Antiarrhythmics, cimetidine, oral contraceptives, acyclovir** may increase risk of bradycardia, hypotension, or **CNS** depression. **HERBAL: Gotu kola, kava kava, St. John's wort, valerian** may increase CNS depression. **Black cohosh, hawthorn, periwinkle** may increase hypotensive effect. **FOOD:** None known. **LAB VALUES:** May increase serum alkaline phosphatase, AST, ALT.

AVAILABILITY (Rx)

Capsules: 2 mg, 4 mg, 6 mg. **Tablets:** 2 mg, 4 mg.

ADMINISTRATION/HANDLING

PO
• Capsules may be opened and sprinkled on food. • May give without regard to food. • Administration should be consistent and not switched between giving with or without food.

INDICATIONS/ROUTES/DOSAGE

Muscle Spasticity
PO: ADULTS, ELDERLY: Initially, 2–4 mg, gradually increased in 2- to 4-mg increments q6–8h. **Maximum:** 3 doses/day or 36 mg/24 hrs.

Dosage in Renal Impairment
May require dose reduction/less frequent dosing. **Creatinine clearance less than 25 ml/min:** Reduce dose by 50%.

T

✦ Canadian trade name   🔴 Non-Crushable Drug   🔲 High Alert drug

Dosage in Hepatic Impairment
Avoid use if possible. If used, monitor for adverse effects (e.g., hypotension).

SIDE EFFECTS

Frequent (49%–41%): Dry mouth, drowsiness, asthenia (loss of strength, energy). **Occasional (16%–4%):** Dizziness, UTI, constipation. **Rare (3%):** Nervousness, amblyopia, pharyngitis, rhinitis, vomiting, urinary frequency.

ADVERSE EFFECTS/ TOXIC REACTIONS

Hypotension may be associated with bradycardia, orthostatic hypotension, and, rarely, syncope. Risk of hypotension increases as dosage increases; hypotension is noted within 1 hr after administration.

NURSING CONSIDERATIONS

BASELINE ASSESSMENT

Record onset, type, location, duration of muscular spasm. Check for immobility, stiffness, swelling. Obtain baseline serum hepatic function tests, alkaline phosphatase, total bilirubin.

INTERVENTION/EVALUATION

Assist with ambulation at all times. For those on long-term therapy, serum hepatic/renal function tests should be performed periodically. Evaluate for therapeutic response (decreased intensity of skeletal muscle pain/tenderness, improved mobility, decrease in spasticity). Go from lying to standing slowly.

PATIENT/FAMILY TEACHING

• Avoid tasks that require alertness, motor skills until response to drug is established. • Avoid sudden changes in posture. • May cause hypotension, sedation, impaired coordination. • Avoid alcohol.

tobramycin

toe-bra-**mye**-sin

(AK-Tob, PMS-Tobramycin ✹, TOBI, Tobrex)

BLACK BOX ALERT May cause neurotoxicity, nephrotoxicity, ototoxicity. Ototoxicity usually is irreversible. Increased risk of neuromuscular blockade, including respiratory paralysis, particularly when given after anesthesia or muscle relaxants.

Do not confuse tobramycin with vancomycin, or Tobrex with TobraDex.

FIXED-COMBINATION(S)

TobraDex: tobramycin/dexamethasone (a steroid): 0.3%/0.1% per ml or per g. **Zylet:** tobramycin/loteprednol: 0.3%/0.5%.

◆CLASSIFICATION

PHARMACOTHERAPEUTIC: Aminoglycoside. **CLINICAL:** Antibiotic (see p. 22C).

ACTION

Irreversibly binds to protein on bacterial ribosomes. **Therapeutic Effect:** Interferes with protein synthesis of susceptible microorganisms.

PHARMACOKINETICS

Rapid, complete absorption after IM administration. Protein binding: less than 30%. Widely distributed (does not cross blood-brain barrier; low concentrations in CSF). Excreted unchanged in urine. Removed by hemodialysis. **Half-life:** 2–4 hrs (increased in renal impairment, neonates; decreased in cystic fibrosis, febrile or burn pts).

USES

Treatment of susceptible infections due to *P. aeruginosa*, other gram-negative organisms including skin/skin structure, bone, joint, respiratory tract infections; postop, burn, intra-abdominal infections; complicated UTI; septicemia; meningitis. **Ophthalmic:** Superficial eye infections: blepharitis, conjunctivitis, keratitis, corneal ulcers. **Inhalation:** Bronchopulmonary infec-

T

tions *(Pseudomonas aeruginosa)* in pts with cystic fibrosis.

PRECAUTIONS

Contraindications: Hypersensitivity to other aminoglycosides (cross-sensitivity) and their components, pregnancy. **Cautions:** Renal impairment, preexisting auditory or vestibular impairment, concomitant use of neuromuscular blocking agents, myasthenia gravis, hypocalcemia.

⏳ LIFESPAN CONSIDERATIONS

Pregnancy/Lactation: Drug readily crosses placenta; distributed in breast milk. May cause fetal nephrotoxicity. Ophthalmic form should not be used in breastfeeding mothers and only when specifically indicated in pregnancy. **Pregnancy Category D (B for ophthalmic form). Children:** Immature renal function in neonates, premature infants may increase risk of toxicity. **Elderly:** Age-related renal impairment may increase risk of toxicity; dosage adjustment recommended.

INTERACTIONS

DRUG: Nephrotoxic medications (e.g., NSAIDs, IV contrast), ototoxic medications (e.g., bumetanide, furosemide) may increase risk of nephrotoxicity, ototoxicity. **Neuromuscular blockers (e.g., cisatracurium, vercuronium)** may increase neuromuscular blockade. **HERBAL:** None significant. **FOOD:** None known. **LAB VALUES:** May increase BUN, serum bilirubin, creatinine, alkaline phosphatase, LDH, AST, ALT. May decrease serum calcium, magnesium, potassium, sodium. Therapeutic peak serum level: 5–20 mcg/ml; therapeutic trough serum level: 0.5–2 mcg/ml. Toxic peak serum level: greater than 20 mcg/ml; toxic trough serum level: greater than 2 mcg/ml.

AVAILABILITY (Rx)

Infusion, Premix: 80 mg/100 ml. **Inhalation Powder (TOBI Podhaler):** 28 mg in a capsule. **Injection, Powder for Reconstitution:** 1.2 g. **Injection, Solution:** 10 mg/ml, 40 mg/ml. **Ointment, Ophthalmic (Tobrex):** 0.3%. **Solution, Nebulization (TOBI):** 60 mg/ml. **Solution, Ophthalmic (AK-Tob, Tobrex):** 0.3%.

ADMINISTRATION/HANDLING

◀**ALERT**▶ Coordinate peak and trough lab draws with administration times.

 IV

Reconstitution • Dilute with 50–100 ml D_5W or 0.9% NaCl. Amount of diluent for infants, children depends on individual need.

Rate of Administration • Infuse over 30–60 min.

Storage • Store vials at room temperature. • Solutions may be discolored by light or air (does not affect potency). • Reconstituted solution stable for 24 hrs at room temperature or 96 hrs if refrigerated.

IM

• To minimize discomfort, give deep IM slowly. • Less painful if injected into gluteus maximus rather than lateral aspect of thigh.

Inhalation

• Refrigerate. • May store at room temperature up to 28 days after removing from refrigerator. • Do not use if cloudy or contains particulates. • **Podhaler:** • Pt must not swallow capsules. • Doses should be as close as possible to 12 hrs apart and not less than 6 hrs apart. • Use Podhaler device supplied.

Ophthalmic

• Place gloved finger on lower eyelid, pull out until pocket is formed between eye and lower lid. • Place correct number of drops (¼–½ inch ointment) into pocket. • **Solution:** Apply digital pressure to lacrimal sac for 1–2 min (minimizes drainage into nose/throat, reducing risk of systemic effects). • **Ointment:** Instruct pt to close eye for 1–2 min, rolling eyeball (increases contact area of drug to eye). • Remove excess solution/ointment around eye with tissue.

T

▓ IV INCOMPATIBILITIES

Amphotericin B complex (Abelcet, AmBisome, Amphotec), heparin, indomethacin (Indocin), piperacillin-tazobactam (Zosyn), propofol (Diprivan), sargramostim (Leukine, Prokine).

▓ IV COMPATIBILITIES

Amiodarone (Cordarone), calcium gluconate, cefepime, ceftaroline, ceftazidime, dexmedetomidine (Precedex), diltiazem (Cardizem), furosemide (Lasix), hydromorphone (Dilaudid), insulin, linezolid (Zyvox), magnesium sulfate, midazolam (Versed), morphine, nicardipine (Cardene), tigecycline (Tygacil).

INDICATIONS/ROUTES/DOSAGE

◄ALERT► Space parenteral doses evenly around the clock. Dosage based on ideal body weight. Peak, trough levels determined periodically to maintain desired serum concentrations (minimizes risk of toxicity). Recommended peak level: 4–10 mcg/ml; trough level: 0.5–2 mcg/ml.

Usual Parenteral Dosage
IV: ADULTS, ELDERLY: 3–7.5 mg/kg/day in 3 divided doses. Once-daily dosing: 4–7 mg/kg every 24 hrs. **CHILDREN 5 YRS AND OLDER:** 2–2.5 mg/kg/dose q8h. **CHILDREN YOUNGER THAN 5 YRS:** 2.5 mg/kg/dose q8h. **NEONATES LESS THAN 1 KG (14 DAYS OR YOUNGER):** 5 mg/kg/dose q48h; **(15–28 DAYS):** 4–5 mg/kg/dose q24–48hrs. **1–2 KG (7 DAYS OR YOUNGER):** 5 mg/kg/dose q48h; **(8–28 DAYS):** 4–5 mg/kg/dose q24–48hrs. **GREATER THAN 2 KG (7 DAYS OR YOUNGER):** 4 mg/kg q24h; **(8–28 DAYS):** 4 mg/kg q12–24hrs.

Usual Ophthalmic Dosage
Ophthalmic Ointment: ADULTS, ELDERLY, CHILDREN 2 MOS AND OLDER: Apply ½ inch to conjunctiva q8–12h (q3–4h for severe infections).
Ophthalmic Solution: ADULTS, ELDERLY, CHILDREN 2 MOS AND OLDER: 1–2 drops in affected eye q4h (2 drops/hr for severe infections).

Usual Inhalation Dosage (Cystic Fibrosis)
Inhalation High Dose: ADULTS, CHILDREN 6 YRS AND OLDER: 300 mg q12h 28 days on, 28 days off. **Podhaler:** Four 28-mg capsules twice daily for 28 days.

Dosage in Renal Impairment
Dosage and frequency modified based on degree of renal impairment, serum drug concentration. After loading dose of 1–2 mg/kg, maintenance dose and frequency are based on serum creatinine levels, creatinine clearance.

Creatinine Clearance	Dosing Interval
41–60 ml/min	q12h
21–40 ml/min	q24h
10–20 ml/min	q48h
Less than 10 ml/min	q72h
Hemodialysis	Loading dose 2–3 mg/kg then 1–2 mg/kg q48–72h
Continuous renal replacement therapy	Loading dose 2–3 mg/kg then 1–2.5 mg/kg q24–48h

SIDE EFFECTS

Occasional: IM: Pain, induration. **IV:** Phlebitis, thrombophlebitis. **Topical:** Hypersensitivity reaction (fever, pruritus, rash, urticaria). **Ophthalmic:** Tearing, itching, redness, eyelid swelling. **Rare:** Hypotension, nausea, vomiting.

ADVERSE EFFECTS/ TOXIC REACTIONS

Nephrotoxicity (acute kidney injury, acute tubular necrosis, renal failure) may be reversible if drug is stopped at first sign of symptoms. Irreversible ototoxicity (dizziness, ringing/roaring in ears, hearing loss), neurotoxicity (headache, dizziness, lethargy, tremor, visual disturbances) occur occasionally. Risk increases with higher dosages or prolonged therapy or if solution is applied directly to mucosa. Superinfections, particularly fungal infections, may result from bacterial imbalance with any administration route. Anaphylaxis may occur.

NURSING CONSIDERATIONS

BASELINE ASSESSMENT

Dehydration must be treated before beginning parenteral therapy. Question for history of allergies, esp. aminoglycosides, sulfite (and parabens for topical, ophthalmic routes). Establish baseline for hearing acuity. Obtain baseline lab tests, esp. renal function.

INTERVENTION/EVALUATION

Monitor I&O (maintain hydration), urinalysis, renal function. Monitor results of peak/trough blood tests. **Therapeutic serum level:** peak: 5–20 mcg/ml; trough: 0.5–2 mcg/ml. **Toxic serum level:** peak: greater than 20 mcg/ml; trough: greater than 2 mcg/ml. Be alert to ototoxic, neurotoxic symptoms. Evaluate IV site for phlebitis (heat, pain, red streaking over vein). Assess for rash. Be alert for superinfection, particularly anal/genital pruritus, changes of oral mucosa, diarrhea. When treating pts with neuromuscular disorders, assess respiratory response carefully. **Ophthalmic:** Assess for redness, swelling, itching, tearing.

PATIENT/FAMILY TEACHING

• Report any hearing, visual, balance, urinary problems, even after therapy is completed. • **Ophthalmic:** Blurred vision, tearing may occur briefly after application. • Report persistent tearing, redness, irritation.

---

tocilizumab

toe-si-**liz**-oo-mab
(Actemra)

BLACK BOX ALERT Tuberculosis, serious, invasive fungal infections, other opportunistic infections have occurred. Test for tuberculosis prior to and during treatment, regardless of initial result.

◆CLASSIFICATION

PHARMACOTHERAPEUTIC: Interleukin (IL)-6 receptor inhibitor. **CLINICAL:** Rheumatoid arthritis agent.

ACTION

Binds to IL-6 receptors, inhibiting signals of proinflammatory cytokines. **Therapeutic Effect:** Inhibits/slows structural joint damage, improves physical function.

PHARMACOKINETICS

Distributed in steady state of plasma and tissue compartments. Undergoes biphasic elimination from circulation. **Half-life:** 11–13 days.

USES

Treatment of moderate to severe rheumatoid arthritis (inhibits and slows structural joint damage, improves physical function). Used for inadequate response to prior tumor necrosis factor (TNF) antagonist therapy. May be used as monotherapy or in combination with methotrexate or other disease-modifying antirheumatic drugs (DMARDs). Treatment of active systemic juvenile idiopathic arthritis (SJIA) in pts 2 yrs of age and older. Treatment of polyarticular juvenile idiopathic arthritis (PJIA) in pts 2 yrs and older.

PRECAUTIONS

Contraindications: None known. **Cautions:** Platelet count equal to or less than 100,000/mm³, ANC less than 2,000/mm³, AST/ALT greater than 1.5 times upper limit of normal (ULN) prior to treatment. History of opportunistic infections (bacterial, mycobacterial, invasive fungal, viral, protozoal), esp. tuberculosis, histoplasmosis, aspergillosis, candidiasis, coccidioidomycosis, listeriosis, pneumocystosis; preexisting or recent-onset CNS demyelinating disorders, including multiple sclerosis; pts with chronic or recurrent infection or who have been exposed to tuberculosis; hematologic cytopenia, hepatic impairment, perforation. Avoid live vaccinations.

T

⌛ LIFESPAN CONSIDERATIONS

Pregnancy/Lactation: Unknown if distributed in breast milk. **Pregnancy Category C. Children:** Safety and efficacy not established. **Elderly:** Cautious use due to increased risk of serious infections, malignancy.

INTERACTIONS

DRUG: Anakinra, abatacept, corticosteroids, methotrexate may increase risk of infection. **Live vaccines** not recommended. May decrease effects of **lovastatin, simvastatin, oral contraceptives, phenytoin, warfarin. HERBAL: Echinacea** may alter levels/effects. **FOOD:** None known. **LAB VALUES:** May increase serum ALT, AST (up to 48% of pts), lipids. May decrease platelets, neutrophils.

AVAILABILITY (Rx)

Injection Solution: 20 mg/ml (80 mg/4 ml, 200 mg/10 ml, 400 mg/20 ml). **Syringe for Subcutaneous Administration:** 162 mg/0.9 ml.

ADMINISTRATION/HANDLING

◀ **ALERT** ▶ Do not infuse IV push or bolus.

 IV

Reconstitution • Dilute in 100 ml 0.9% NaCl (50 ml 0.9% NaCl for SJIA pts weighing less than 30 kg). • Prior to mixing, withdraw and discard volume of NaCl equal to volume of patient-dosed solution. • Invert bag to avoid foaming. • Inject solution and dilute for mixture that equals 50 ml or 100 ml in NaCl bag. **Rate of Administration** • Infuse over 1 hr.
Storage • Refrigerate vials; do not freeze. • Solution must be at room temperature before administration, but not for longer than 24 hrs. • Protect from light until time of use. • Solution appears colorless. Discard solution if appears cloudy, discolored, or contains particulate.

INDICATIONS/ROUTES/DOSAGE

Note: Do not infuse concomitantly in same IV line with other drugs.

Moderate to Severely Active Rheumatoid Arthritis
IV Infusion: ADULTS, ELDERLY: 4 mg/kg every 4 wks initially. May increase to 8 mg/kg every 4 wks. **Maximum:** 800 mg per dose.
Subcutaneous: ADULTS, ELDERLY (100 KG OR GREATER): 162 mg/wk. **(LESS THAN 100 KG):** 162 mg every other wk. May increase to every wk based on clinical response.

Dosage Modification
Hepatic enzyme levels greater than ULN.

Lab Value	Recommendation
1–3 times ULN	Dose modify concomitant DMARDs or reduce dose to 4 mg/kg until ALT/AST normalized
Greater than 3–5 times ULN	Interrupt treatment until ALT/AST less than 3 times ULN, then follow guidelines for 1–3 times ULN
Greater than 5 times ULN	Discontinue treatment

SJIA
IV: CHILDREN MORE THAN 30 KG: 8 mg/kg q2wks. **CHILDREN 30 KG OR LESS:** 12 mg/kg q2wks.

PJIA
IV: CHILDREN MORE THAN 30 KG: 8 mg/kg q4wks. **CHILDREN 30 KG OR LESS:** 10 mg/kg q4wks.

SIDE EFFECTS

Occasional (8%–6%): Upper respiratory tract infection, nasopharyngitis, headache, hypertension. **Rare (5%–3%):** Infusion reaction, dizziness, bronchitis, rash, oral ulceration.

ADVERSE EFFECTS/ TOXIC REACTIONS

Up to 48% of pts experience elevated ALT, AST. Neutropenia, thrombocytopenia occur in 4% of pts. Serious infections, including sepsis, pneumonia, tuberculosis, invasive fungal infections, hepatitis B have occurred. Anaphylactic reaction, rash, pruritus, urticaria, bronchospasm, swelling, dyspnea occur in less than 0.2% of pts; hypersensitivity reactions (hypertension, headaches, flushing) occur more frequently. Increased risk of lymphoma, melanoma. New onset or exacerbation of CNS demyelinating disorders, including multiple sclerosis. Risk of gastric perforation with concomitant use of NSAIDs, corticosteroids.

NURSING CONSIDERATIONS

BASELINE ASSESSMENT

Evaluate pt for active tuberculosis and test for latent infection prior to initiating treatment and periodically during therapy. Induration of 5 mm or greater with tuberculin skin testing should be considered a positive test result when assessing for latent tuberculosis. Antifungal therapy should be considered for pts who reside or travel to regions where mycoses are endemic. Do not initiate therapy during an active infection. Viral reactivation can occur in cases of herpes zoster, HIV. Assess baseline lab results (hepatic enzymes, cholesterol, triglycerides, platelets, neutrophils) q4–8wks during treatment. Pts should report history of diverticulitis, weakened immune system, HIV, hepatic disease, GI bleeding, coughing up blood, diarrhea, weight loss, cancer, prior cancer treatment, use of NSAIDs, glucocorticosteroids.

INTERVENTION/EVALUATION

Monitor hepatitis B carriers during and several months following therapy. If reactivation occurs, consider interrupting treatment. Monitor pts for signs/symptoms of tuberculosis regardless of baseline PPD. Discontinue treatment if pt develops acute infection, opportunistic infection, or sepsis and initiate appropriate antimicrobial therapy. Monitor warfarin, theophylline, cyclosporine levels for therapeutic ranges. Modify, interrupt, or discontinue treatment if AST/ALT is 1–5 times ULN.

PATIENT/FAMILY TEACHING

• Inform pt that therapy may lower immune system response. • Detail any concomitant immunosuppressive therapy, methotrexate. • Report any history of HIV, fungal infections, hepatitis B, multiple sclerosis, hemoptysis, tuberculosis, or close relatives with active tuberculosis. • Report any travel plans to possible endemic areas. • Report signs/symptoms of stomach pain to evaluate risk of gastric perforation or history of taking NSAIDs, corticosteroids, methotrexate. • Pt will need blood levels drawn q4–8wks during treatment along with routine tuberculosis screening. • Seek immediate medical attention if adverse reaction occurs. • Do not receive live vaccines during therapy. • Notify physician if pregnant or planning on becoming pregnant. • During treatment, report any signs of liver problems, such as stomach pains, yellowing of skin/eyes, dark-amber urine, clay-colored or bloody stools, fatigue, reduced appetite, coffee ground emesis. • Pt must adhere to strict dosing schedule. • Decreased platelet count may lead to risk of bleeding.

tofacitinib

toe-fa-**sye**-ti-nib
(Xeljanz)
Do not confuse tofacitinib with tipifarnib or Xeljanz with Xeloda.

BLACK BOX ALERT Increased risk for developing bacterial, viral, invasive fungal, other opportunistic infections including tuberculosis, cryptococcosis, pneumocystosis that may lead to hospitalization or death; infections often occurred in combination with other immunosuppressants (methotrexate, corticosteroids). Test for latent tuberculosis prior to treatment and during treatment, regardless of initial result. Malignancies including lymphoma, nonmelanoma skin cancer reported. Increased rate of Epstein-Barr virus–associated post-transplant lymphoproliferative disorder observed in renal transplant pts who are treated with tofacitinib and other immunosuppressive therapy drugs.

◆CLASSIFICATION

PHARMACOTHERAPEUTIC: Janus kinase (JAK) inhibitor. **CLINICAL:** Antirheumatic agent.

ACTION

Inhibits JAK enzymes which are involved in stimulating hematopoiesis and immune cell functioning. **Therapeutic Effect:** Reduces inflammation, tenderness, swelling of joints; slows or prevents progressive joint destruction in rheumatoid arthritis (RA).

PHARMACOKINETICS

Rapidly absorbed following PO administration. Protein binding: 40%. Peak concentration: 30–60 min. Metabolized in liver. Eliminated primarily in urine. **Half-life:** 3 hrs.

USES

Treatment of adult pts with moderate to severe active rheumatoid arthritis with previous inadequate response or intolerance to methotrexate. May be used as monotherapy or in combination with methotrexate or other nonbiologic disease-modifying antirheumatic drugs (DMARDs). Do not use in combination with other biologic DMARDs or with potent immunosuppressants (e.g., azathioprine, cyclosporine).

PRECAUTIONS

◄ALERT► Do not initiate treatment in pts with baseline active infection (systemic/localized), severe hepatic impairment, lymphocytes less than 500/mm³, ANC less than 1,000/mm³, Hgb less than 9 g/dL. **Contraindications:** None known. **Cautions:** Pts exposed to TB, history of serious opportunistic infections, conditions that predispose to infections (e.g., diabetes), pts at risk for GI perforation (e.g., diverticulitis), pts who resided or traveled in areas where TB is endemic, moderate to severe renal impairment, elderly, hepatic impairment, history of anemia, hyperlipidemia, hepatitis.

⧗ LIFESPAN CONSIDERATIONS

Pregnancy/Lactation: Not recommended in nursing mothers. Must either discontinue drug or discontinue breastfeeding. Unknown if distributed in breast milk. **Pregnancy Category C. Children:** Safety and efficacy not established. **Elderly:** Increased risk for serious infections, malignancy.

INTERACTIONS

DRUG: May alter effects of **live virus vaccines. Immunosuppressants (e.g., azathioprine, cyclosporine)** may increase risk for added immunosuppression, infection. **CYP3A4 inhibitors (e.g., ketoconazole), CYP2C19 inhibitors (e.g., fluconazole)** may increase concentration/effects. **CYP3A4 inducers (e.g., rifampin, phenytoin)** may decrease concentration/effects. **HERBAL: St. John's wort** may decrease concentration/effect. **FOOD:** None known. **LAB VALUES:** May increase AST/ALT, bilirubin, lipids, creatinine. May decrease Hgb, neutrophils, lymphocytes.

AVAILABILITY (Rx)

Tablets, Film-Coated: 5 mg.

ADMINISTRATION/HANDLING

PO
• Give without regard to food.

INDICATIONS/ROUTES/DOSAGE

Moderate to Severe Rheumatoid Arthritis
PO: ADULTS/ELDERLY: 5 mg twice daily.

Dose Modification
Reduce to 5 mg once daily for any of the following: moderate to severe renal impairment, moderate hepatic impairment, concurrent use of potent CYP3A4 inhibi-

tors, concurrent use of one or more moderate CYP3A4 or potent CYP2C19 inhibitors.

Lymphopenia
Interrupt treatment until lymphocytes greater than or equal to 500/mm³. Discontinue if lymphocytes less than 500/mm³ after repeat testing.

Neutropenia
Interrupt treatment until neutrophils greater than 1,000/mm³. Discontinue if neutrophils less than 500/mm³ after repeat testing.

Anemia
Interrupt treatment until Hgb greater than or equal to 9 g/dL or baseline Hgb decreases less than or equal to 2 g/dL after repeat testing.

Hepatotoxicity
Interrupt treatment until diagnosis of drug-induced hepatic injury has been excluded.

SIDE EFFECTS

Rare (4%–2%): Upper respiratory tract infection, diarrhea, nasopharyngitis, headache, hypertension.

ADVERSE EFFECTS/ TOXIC REACTIONS

Neutropenia, lymphopenia may increase risk for infection. Serious infections may include aspergillosis, BK virus, cellulitis, coccidioidomycosis, cryptococcus, cytomegalovirus, esophageal candidiasis, histoplasmosis, invasive fungal infections, listeriosis, pneumocystosis, pneumonia, tuberculosis, UTI, sepsis. Increased risk for various malignancies. May induce viral reactivation of hepatitis B or C, herpes zoster, HIV. Epstein-Barr virus–associated post-transplant lymphoproliferative disorder reported in 2% of pts with renal transplant. Increased risk for GI perforation.

NURSING CONSIDERATIONS

BASELINE ASSESSMENT
Obtain vital signs, CBC, serum chemistries, renal and hepatic function test, lipid panel, urine pregnancy test results. Evaluate for active tuberculosis (TB) and test for latent infection prior to and during treatment. Induration of 5 mm or greater with purified protein derivative (PPD) is considered positive result when assessing for latent TB. Question possibility of pregnancy or breastfeeding. Screen for history/comorbidities. Obtain full medication history including vitamins, herbal products.

INTERVENTION/EVALUATION
Obtain CBC every 4–8 wks, then every 3 mos, lipid panel 4–8 wks after initiation; hepatic function panel if hepatic impairment suspected. Monitor for TB regardless of baseline PPD. Consider discontinuation if pt develops acute infection, opportunistic infection, sepsis; initiate appropriate antimicrobial therapy. Immediately report any hemorrhaging, melena, abdominal pain, hemoptysis (may indicate GI perforation).

PATIENT/FAMILY TEACHING
• Blood levels will be monitored routinely. • Therapy will lower immune system response. • Do not receive live virus vaccines. • Other immunosuppressant drugs may increase risk for infection. • Expect routine TB screening. • Fever, cough, burning with urination, body aches, chills, skin changes may indicate infection. • Report history of HIV, recent infections, hepatitis B or C, TB or close relatives who have active TB. • Report any travel plans to possible endemic areas. • Notify physician if pregnant or planning pregnancy. • Do not breastfeed. • Immediately report bleeding of any kind. • Yellowing of skin or eyes, right upper quadrant abdominal pain, bruising, clay-colored stool, dark urine may indicate liver problem. • Avoid grapefruit products.

T

tolterodine

tol-**ter**-oh-deen
(Detrol, <u>Detrol LA</u>, Unidet ✦)
Do not confuse Detrol with Ditropan, or tolterodine with fesoterodine.

◆CLASSIFICATION

PHARMACOTHERAPEUTIC: Muscarinic receptor antagonist. **CLINICAL:** Antispasmodic.

ACTION

Exhibits potent antimuscarinic activity by interceding via cholinergic muscarinic receptors, thereby inhibiting urinary bladder contraction. **Therapeutic Effect:** Decreases urinary frequency, urgency.

PHARMACOKINETICS

Immediate-release form rapidly, well absorbed after PO administration. Protein binding: 96%. Metabolized in liver. Primarily excreted in urine. Unknown if removed by hemodialysis. **Half-life:** Immediate-release: 2–10 hrs. Extended-release: 7–18 hrs.

USES

Treatment of overactive bladder in pts with symptoms of urinary frequency, urgency, incontinence.

PRECAUTIONS

Contraindications: Gastric retention, uncontrolled narrow-angle glaucoma, urinary retention. **Cautions:** Renal impairment, clinically significant bladder outflow obstruction (risk of urinary retention), GI obstructive disorders (e.g., pyloric stenosis [risk of gastric retention]), treated narrow-angle glaucoma, myasthenia gravis, prolonged QT interval (congenital/medications), hepatic impairment.

⧗ LIFESPAN CONSIDERATIONS

Pregnancy/Lactation: Unknown if drug is distributed in breast milk. Breastfeeding not recommended. **Pregnancy Category C.**

Children: Safety and efficacy not established. **Elderly:** No age-related precautions noted.

INTERACTIONS

DRUG: CYP3A4 inhibitors (e.g., clarithromycin, erythromycin, itraconazole, ketoconazole) may increase concentration. **Fluoxetine** may inhibit metabolism. **HERBAL: St. John's wort** may decrease concentration/effects. **FOOD:** None known. **LAB VALUES:** None known.

AVAILABILITY (Rx)

Tablets (Detrol): 1 mg, 2 mg.

✦ **Capsules (Extended-Release [Detrol LA]):** 2 mg, 4 mg.

ADMINISTRATION/HANDLING

PO

• May give without regard to food. • Do not crush, dissolve, open extended-release capsules; give whole.

INDICATIONS/ROUTES/DOSAGE

Overactive Bladder
PO: ADULTS, ELDERLY (IMMEDIATE-RELEASE): 1–2 mg twice a day. **(WITH CYP3A4 INHIBITORS):** 1 mg twice a day. **(EXTENDED-RELEASE):** 2–4 mg once a day **(WITH CYP3A4 INHIBITORS):** 2 mg once daily.

Dosage in Severe Renal/Hepatic Impairment
PO: ADULTS, ELDERLY (IMMEDIATE-RELEASE): 1 mg twice a day. **(EXTENDED-RELEASE):** 2 mg once a day.

SIDE EFFECTS

Frequent (40%): Dry mouth. **Occasional (11%–4%):** Headache, dizziness, fatigue, constipation, dyspepsia (heartburn, indigestion, epigastric pain), upper respiratory tract infection, UTI, dry eyes, abnormal vision (accommodation problems), nausea, diarrhea. **Rare (3%):** Drowsiness, chest/back pain, arthralgia, rash, weight gain, dry skin.

ADVERSE EFFECTS/ TOXIC REACTIONS

Overdose can result in severe anticholinergic effects, including abdominal cramps, facial warmth, excessive salivation/lacrimation, diaphoresis, pallor, urinary urgency, blurred vision, prolonged QT interval.

NURSING CONSIDERATIONS

BASELINE ASSESSMENT

Assess degree of overactive bladder (urinary urgency, frequency, incontinence).

INTERVENTION/EVALUATION

Assist with ambulation if dizziness occurs. Question for visual changes. Monitor incontinence, postvoid residuals.

PATIENT/FAMILY TEACHING

• May cause blurred vision, dry eyes/mouth, constipation. • Report any confusion, altered mental status. • Avoid tasks that require alertness, motor skills until response to drug is established.

tolvaptan

tol-**vap**-tan
(Samsca)

BLACK BOX ALERT Osmotic demyelination (dysphagia, lethargy, slurred speech or inability to speak, seizures, coma, death) may occur with too-rapid correction of hyponatremia; slow rate of correction is essential. Should be initiated and reinitiated only in a hospital where serum sodium is monitored closely.

◆CLASSIFICATION

PHARMACOTHERAPEUTIC: Vasopressin antagonist. **CLINICAL:** Hyponatremia adjunct.

ACTION

Promotes excretion of free water (without loss of serum electrolytes), resulting in net fluid loss, increased urine output, decreased urine osmolarity and increase in serum sodium concentration. **Therapeutic Effect:** Restores normal serum sodium levels.

PHARMACOKINETICS

Readily absorbed following oral administration. Metabolized in liver. Protein binding: 99%. Eliminated entirely by nonrenal routes. **Half-life:** 5 hrs.

USES

Treatment of symptomatic hypervolemic or euvolemic hyponatremia resistant to correction with fluid restriction, including pts with HF, cirrhosis, and syndrome of inappropriate antidiuretic hormone (SIADH).

PRECAUTIONS

Contraindications: Hypovolemic hyponatremia, concurrent use with strong CYP3A4 inhibitors (clarithromycin, indinavir, itraconazole, ketoconazole, nefazodone, nelfinavir, ritonavir, saquinavir), pts with urgent need to raise sodium level, inability to sense or respond to thirst, pts who are anuric. **Cautions:** Hyperkalemia, concurrent use of medications that increase serum potassium, GI bleeding in pts with cirrhosis, dehydration, hypovolemia, concurrent use with hypertonic saline.

⧗ LIFESPAN CONSIDERATIONS

Pregnancy/Lactation: Systemic exposure to fetus likely. Potential for decreased neonatal viability, delayed growth/development. Unknown if distributed in breast milk. **Pregnancy Category C. Children:** Safety and efficacy not established. **Elderly:** No age-related precautions noted.

INTERACTIONS

DRUG: CYP3A4 inhibitors (e.g., clarithromycin, diltiazem, erythromycin, fluconazole, itraconazole, ketoconazole, nefazodone, saquinavir, verapamil) may increase levels, effects. **CYP3A4 inducers** (e.g., carbamazepine, phenytoin, rifabutin, rifampin) may reduce concentration. **Cyclosporine** may increase concentration. **HERBAL: St. John's wort** may reduce concentration. **FOOD: Grapefruit products** may increase absorption, concentration. **LAB VALUES:** May increase serum potassium, magnesium. May alter serum glucose.

AVAILABILITY (Rx)

Tablets: 15 mg, 30 mg, 60 mg.

ADMINISTRATION/HANDLING

• Give without regard to meals.

INDICATIONS/ROUTES/DOSAGE

Usual Dosage
PO: ADULTS, ELDERLY: 15 mg once daily. Increase dose to 30 mg once daily, after at least 24 hrs (**maximum:** 60 mg once daily), to achieve desired level of serum sodium.

SIDE EFFECTS

Frequent (16%–13%): Thirst, dry mouth. **Occasional (11%–4%):** Increase in urine output/urgency, asthenia (loss of strength, energy), nausea, constipation, hyperglycemia, anorexia.

ADVERSE EFFECTS/ TOXIC REACTIONS

Dysphagia, lethargy, slurred speech or inability to speak, affective changes, spastic quadriparesis, seizures, coma, death may occur with too-rapid correction of hyponatremia.

NURSING CONSIDERATIONS

BASELINE ASSESSMENT

Initiate only in hospital setting with serum sodium monitoring. Obtain baseline serum sodium, hepatic enzyme levels, BUN, creatinine, CBC. Assess for increased pulse rate, poor skin turgor, nausea, diarrhea (signs of hyponatremia).

INTERVENTION/EVALUATION

During initiation and titration, frequently monitor for changes in serum electrolytes and volume. Avoid fluid restriction during first 24 hrs of therapy. Monitor for improvement in signs/symptoms of hyponatremia, hypernatremia (flushing, edema, restlessness, dry mucous membranes, fever).

PATIENT/FAMILY TEACHING

• Continue ingesting fluids in response to thirst. • Report urinary changes, loss of strength, unusual fatigue. • Report immediately symptoms of osmotic demyelination (e.g., trouble speaking/swallowing, confusion, mood changes, trouble controlling body movements, seizures).

topiramate

toe-**peer**-a-mate
(Apo-Topiramate ❖, Novo-Topiramate ❖, <u>Topamax</u>, Trokendi XR)
Do not confuse Topamax or topiramate with Tegretol, Tegretol XR, or Toprol XL.

◆CLASSIFICATION

PHARMACOTHERAPEUTIC: Carbonic anhydrase inhibitor. **CLINICAL:** Anticonvulsant (see p. 37C).

ACTION

Blocks repetitive, sustained firing of neurons by enhancing ability of gamma-aminobutyric acid (GABA) to induce influx of chloride ions into neurons; may block sodium channels. **Therapeutic Effect:** Decreases seizure activity.

PHARMACOKINETICS

Rapidly absorbed after PO administration. Protein binding: 15%–41%. Metabolized in liver. Primarily excreted unchanged in urine. Removed by hemodialysis. **Half-life:** 21 hrs.

USES

Adjunctive therapy for treatment of partial-onset seizures and primary generalized tonic-clonic seizures; initial monotherapy in partial or primary generalized tonic-clonic seizures; seizures associated with Lennox-Gastaut syndrome (LGS). Prevention of migraine headache. **Trokendi XR:** Initial monotherapy in pts 10 yrs or older with partial-onset or primary generalized tonic-clonic seizures, adjunctive therapy in pts 6 yrs or older with partial-onset or primary generalized tonic-clonic seizures and seizures associated with LGS. **OFF-LABEL:** Neuropathic pain, diabetic neuropathy, cluster headaches, infantile spasms.

PRECAUTIONS

Contraindications: None known. **Cautions:** Sensitivity to topiramate or sulfa, hepatic/renal impairment, pts who are high risk for suicide, respiratory impairment.

⏳ LIFESPAN CONSIDERATIONS

Pregnancy/Lactation: Unknown if distributed in breast milk. **Pregnancy Category C. Children:** No age-related precautions noted in those older than 2 yrs. **Elderly:** Age-related renal impairment may require dosage adjustment.

INTERACTIONS

DRUG: Alcohol, other CNS depressants may increase CNS depression. **Carbamazepine, phenytoin, valproic acid** may decrease concentration/effects. **Carbonic anhydrase inhibitors** may increase risk of kidney stone formation and severity of metabolic acidosis. May decrease effectiveness of **oral contraceptives. HERBAL: Evening primrose** may decrease seizure threshold. **FOOD:** None known. **LAB VALUES:** May reduce serum bicarbonate, increase AST, ALT.

AVAILABILITY (Rx)

Capsules (Sprinkle): 15 mg, 25 mg.
🔪 **Tablets:** 25 mg, 50 mg, 100 mg, 200 mg. 🔪 **Capsules, Extended-Release (Trokendi XR):** 25 mg, 50 mg, 100 mg, 200 mg.

ADMINISTRATION/HANDLING

PO

• Do not break or crush tablets (bitter taste). • Give without regard to meals. • Capsules may be swallowed whole or contents sprinkled on teaspoonful of soft food and swallowed immediately; do not chew. • **Trokendi XR:** • Give whole. Do not sprinkle on food, chew, or crush.

INDICATIONS/ROUTES/DOSAGE

Adjunctive Treatment of Partial-Onset Seizures, Lennox-Gastaut Syndrome (LGS), Tonic-Clonic Seizures
PO: ADULTS, ELDERLY, CHILDREN 17 YRS AND OLDER: Initially, 25–50 mg for 1 wk. May increase by 25–50 mg/day at weekly intervals. **Usual maintenance dose:** 100–200 mg twice daily. **Maximum:** 1,600 mg/day. **CHILDREN 2–16 YRS:** Initially, 1–3 mg/kg/day to maximum of 25 mg at night for 1 wk. May increase by 1–3 mg/kg/day at weekly intervals given in 2 divided doses. **Maintenance:** 5–9 mg/kg/day in 2 divided doses. **ADULTS, ELDERLY: (Trokendi XR) (Partial-Onset, LGS):** Initially, 25–50 mg once daily. Increase by 25–50 mg at weekly intervals, up to 200–400 mg/day. **(Generalized Tonic-Clonic):** Initially, 25–50 mg/day. Increase by 25–50 mg/day at weekly intervals, up to 400 mg/day. **CHILDREN 6 YRS AND OLDER:** Initially, 1–3 mg/kg once daily. May increase by 1–3 mg/kg at 2-wk intervals up to 5–9 mg/kg once daily.

Monotherapy with Partial-Onset, Tonic-Clonic Seizures
PO: ADULTS, ELDERLY, CHILDREN 10 YRS AND OLDER: Initially, 25 mg twice a day. Increase at weekly intervals up to 400 mg/day according to the following schedule: Wk 1, 25 mg twice a day. Wk 2, 50 mg twice a day. Wk 3, 75 mg twice a day. Wk 4, 100 mg twice a day. Wk 5, 150 mg twice a day. Wk 6, 200 mg twice a day. **CHILDREN 2–9 YRS:** Initially, 25 mg/day. Then 25 mg 2 times/day week 2; then increase by 25–50 mg/day at weekly intervals up to minimum dose. **ADULTS, ELDERLY, CHILDREN 10 YRS OR OLDER: (Trokendi XR):** Initially, 50 mg

T

once daily. Increase by 50 mg/day at weekly intervals for first 4 wks, then by 100 mg/day for wks 5 and 6, up to 400 mg/day.

Wgt.	Minimum	Maximum
11 kg or less	150 mg/day in 2 divided doses	250 mg/day in 2 divided doses
12–22 kg	200 mg/day in 2 divided doses	300 mg/day in 2 divided doses
23–31 kg	200 mg/day in 2 divided doses	350 mg/day in 2 divided doses
32–38 kg	250 mg/day in 2 divided doses	350 mg/day in 2 divided doses
39 or more kg	250 mg/day in 2 divided doses	400 mg/day in 2 divided doses

Migraine Prevention
PO: ADULTS, ELDERLY: Initially, 25 mg/day. May increase by 25 mg/day at 7-day intervals up to a total daily dose of 100 mg/day in 2 divided doses.

Dosage in Renal Impairment
Reduce drug dosage by 50% and titrate more slowly in pts who have creatinine clearance less than 70 ml/min.

SIDE EFFECTS

Frequent (30%–10%): Drowsiness, dizziness, ataxia, nervousness, nystagmus, diplopia, paresthesia, nausea, tremor. **Occasional (9%–3%):** Confusion, breast pain, dysmenorrhea, dyspepsia (heartburn, indigestion, epigastric pain), depression, asthenia (loss of strength, energy), pharyngitis, weight loss, anorexia, rash, musculoskeletal pain, abdominal pain, difficulty with coordination, sinusitis, agitation, flu-like symptoms. **Rare (3%–2%):** Mood disturbances (e.g., irritability, depression), dry mouth, aggressive behavior, impaired heat regulation.

ADVERSE EFFECTS/ TOXIC REACTIONS

Psychomotor slowing, impaired concentration, language problems (esp. word-finding difficulties), memory disturbances occur occasionally. Metabolic acidosis, suicidal ideation occur rarely.

NURSING CONSIDERATIONS

BASELINE ASSESSMENT

Seizures: Review history of seizure disorder (intensity, frequency, duration, level of consciousness). Initiate seizure precautions. Provide quiet, dark environment. Question for sensitivity to topiramate, pregnancy, use of other anticonvulsant medication (esp. carbamazepine, valproic acid, phenytoin). **Migraine:** Assess pain location, duration, intensity. Assess renal function.

INTERVENTION/EVALUATION

Observe frequently for recurrence of seizure activity. Assess for clinical improvement (decrease in intensity/frequency of seizures). Monitor renal function tests, hepatic function tests. Assist with ambulation if dizziness occurs.

PATIENT/FAMILY TEACHING

• Avoid tasks that require alertness, motor skills until response to drug is established (may cause dizziness, drowsiness, impaired concentration). • Drowsiness usually diminishes with continued therapy. • Avoid use of alcohol, other CNS depressants. • Do not abruptly discontinue drug (may precipitate seizures). • Strict maintenance of drug therapy is essential for seizure control. • Do not break tablets (bitter taste). • Maintain adequate fluid intake (decreases risk of renal stone formation). • Report blurred vision, eye pain. • Report suicidal ideation, depression, unusual behavior. • Use caution with activities that may increase core temperature (exposure to extreme heat, dehydration). • Instruct pt to use alternative/additional means of contraception (topiramate decreases effectiveness of oral contraceptives).

topotecan

toe-poe-**tee**-kan
(Hycamtin)

BLACK BOX ALERT Must be administered by personnel trained in administration/handling of chemotherapeutic agents. Potent immunosuppressant; severe neutropenia (absolute neutrophil count [ANC] less than 500 cells/mm³) occurs in 60% of pts.

Do not confuse Hycamtin with Hycomine, Mycamine, or topotecan with irinotecan.

◆CLASSIFICATION

PHARMACOTHERAPEUTIC: DNA topoisomerase inhibitor. **CLINICAL:** Antineoplastic (see p. 91C).

ACTION

Interacts with topoisomerase I, an enzyme that relieves torsional strain in DNA by inducing reversible single-strand breaks. Prevents religation of DNA strand, resulting in damage to double-strand DNA, cell death. **Therapeutic Effect:** Produces cytotoxic effect.

PHARMACOKINETICS

Hydrolyzed to active form after IV administration. Protein binding: 35%. Excreted in urine. **Half-life:** 2–3 hrs (increased in renal impairment).

USES

Treatment of metastatic carcinoma of ovary after failure of initial or recurrent chemotherapy. Treatment of sensitive, relapsed small cell lung cancer. Treatment of late-stage cervical cancer. **OFF-LABEL:** Treatment of central nervous system lesions/lymphoma, Ewing's sarcoma, rhabdomyosarcoma, neuroblastoma.

PRECAUTIONS

Contraindications: Baseline neutrophil count less than 1,500 cells/mm³ and platelet count less than 100,000/mm³, breastfeeding, pregnancy, severe myelosuppression. **Cautions:** Mild myelosuppression, hepatic/renal impairment.

⧗ LIFESPAN CONSIDERATIONS

Pregnancy/Lactation: May cause fetal harm. Avoid pregnancy; breastfeeding not recommended. **Pregnancy Category D. Children:** Safety and efficacy not established. **Elderly:** Age-related renal impairment may require dosage adjustment.

INTERACTIONS

DRUG: Live virus vaccines may potentiate virus replication, increase vaccine side effects, decrease pt's antibody response to vaccine. **Other bone marrow depressants** may increase risk of myelosuppression. **HERBAL: Echinacea** may decrease effectiveness. **FOOD:** None known. **LAB VALUES:** May increase serum bilirubin, AST, ALT, alkaline phosphatase. May decrease RBC, leukocyte, neutrophil, platelet counts, Hgb, Hct.

AVAILABILITY (Rx)

Injection, Powder for Reconstitution: 4 mg (single-dose vial). **Injection, Solution:** 1 mg/ml (4 ml).

 Capsule: 0.25 mg, 1 mg.

ADMINISTRATION/HANDLING

◀ALERT▶ Because topotecan may be carcinogenic, mutagenic, teratogenic, handle drug with extreme care during preparation/administration.

PO
• May take with or without food. • Swallow whole; do not crush, break, divide capsule. • Do not take replacement dose if vomiting occurs.

⧗ IV

Reconstitution • Reconstitute each 4-mg vial with 4 ml Sterile Water for Injection. • Further dilute with 50–100 ml 0.9% NaCl or D₅W.

Rate of Administration • Administer as IV infusion over 30 min or by continu-

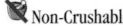

ous infusion over 24 hrs. • Extravasation associated with only mild local reactions (erythema, ecchymosis).
Storage • Store vials at room temperature in original cartons. • Reconstituted vials diluted for infusion stable at room temperature, ambient lighting for 24 hrs, or 7 days if refrigerated.

⊞ IV INCOMPATIBILITIES

Dexamethasone (Decadron), 5-fluorouracil, mitomycin (Mutamycin).

⊞ IV COMPATIBILITIES

Carboplatin (Paraplatin), cisplatin (Platinol AQ), cyclophosphamide (Cytoxan), doxorubicin (Adriamycin), etoposide (VePesid), gemcitabine (Gemzar), granisetron (Kytril), ondansetron (Zofran), paclitaxel (Taxol), palonosetron (Aloxi), vincristine (Oncovin).

INDICATIONS/ROUTES/DOSAGE

◄ALERT► Do not give topotecan if baseline neutrophil count is less than 1,500 cells/mm^3 and platelet count is less than 100,000/mm^3.

Ovarian Carcinoma, Small Cell Lung Cancer
IV: ADULTS, ELDERLY: 1.5 mg/m^2/day over 30 min for 5 consecutive days, beginning on day 1 of 21-day course. Minimum of 4 courses recommended. If severe neutropenia (neutrophil count less than 1,500/mm^3) occurs during treatment, reduce dose for subsequent courses by 0.25 mg/m^2 or administer filgrastim (G-CSF) no sooner than 24 hrs after last dose of topotecan.
PO *(Small Cell Lung Cancer)*: **ADULTS, ELDERLY:** 2.3 mg/m^2/day for 5 days; repeat q21days (dose rounded to nearest 0.25 mg).

Cervical Cancer
IV: ADULTS, ELDERLY: 0.75 mg/m^2/day for 3 days (followed by cisplatin 50 mg/m^2 on day 1 only). Repeat q21days (baseline neutrophil count greater than 1,500/mm^3 and platelet count greater than 100,000 mm^3).

Dosage in Renal Impairment
No dosage adjustment is necessary in pts with mild renal impairment (creatinine clearance 40–60 ml/min). For moderate renal impairment (creatinine clearance 20–39 ml/min), give 0.75 mg/m^2.

SIDE EFFECTS

Frequent (77%–21%): Nausea, vomiting, diarrhea, total alopecia, headache, dyspnea. **Occasional (9%–3%):** Paresthesia, constipation, abdominal pain. **Rare:** Anorexia, malaise, arthralgia, asthenia (loss of strength, energy), myalgia.

ADVERSE EFFECTS/ TOXIC REACTIONS

Severe neutropenia (absolute neutrophil count [ANC] less than 500 cells/mm^3) occurs in 60% of pts (develops at median of 11 days after day 1 of initial therapy). Thrombocytopenia (platelet count less than 25,000/mm^3) occurs in 26% of pts. Severe anemia (RBC count less than 8 g/dl) occurs in 40% of pts (develops at median of 15 days after day 1 of initial therapy).

NURSING CONSIDERATIONS

BASELINE ASSESSMENT

Offer emotional support. Assess CBC with differential before each dose. Myelosuppression may precipitate life-threatening hemorrhage, infection, anemia. If platelet count drops, minimize trauma to pt (e.g., IM injections, pt positioning). Premedicate with antiemetics on day of treatment, starting at least 30 min before administration.

INTERVENTION/EVALUATION

Assess for bleeding, signs of infection, anemia. Monitor hydration status, I&O, serum electrolytes (diarrhea, vomiting are common side effects). Monitor CBC with differential, Hgb, platelets for evidence of myelosuppression. Monitor renal/hepatic function tests. Assess response to medication; provide interventions (e.g., small, frequent meals; antiemetics for nausea/ vomiting). Question for complaints of headache. Assess breathing pattern for evidence of dyspnea.

PATIENT/FAMILY TEACHING

• Hair loss is reversible but new hair may have different color, texture. • Diarrhea may cause dehydration, electrolyte depletion. • Antiemetic and antidiarrheal medications may reduce side effects. • Notify physician if diarrhea, vomiting, persistent fever, bruising/bleeding, yellowing of eyes/skin occur. • Do not have immunizations without physician's approval (drug lowers resistance). • Avoid contact with those who have recently received live virus vaccine.

---

toremifene

tor-**em**-i-feen
(Fareston)
BLACK BOX ALERT May prolong QT interval.

◆CLASSIFICATION

PHARMACOTHERAPEUTIC: Nonsteroidal antiestrogen. **CLINICAL:** Antineoplastic (see p. 91C).

ACTION

Binds to estrogen receptors on tumors, producing complex that decreases DNA synthesis, inhibits estrogen effects. **Therapeutic Effect:** Blocks growth-stimulating effects of estrogen in breast cancer.

PHARMACOKINETICS

Well absorbed after PO administration. Protein binding: greater than 99%. Metabolized in liver. Eliminated in feces. **Half-life:** Approximately 5 days.

USES

Treatment of metastatic breast cancer in postmenopausal women with estrogen receptor–positive or estrogen receptor unknown. **OFF-LABEL:** Treatment of desmoid tumors (soft tissue sarcoma).

PRECAUTIONS

Contraindications: Long QT syndrome, uncorrected hypokalemia or hypomagnesemia. **Cautions:** Preexisting endometrial hyperplasia, leukopenia, thrombocytopenia, hepatic impairment, history of thromboembolic disease, HF, electrolyte abnormalities.

⏳ LIFESPAN CONSIDERATIONS

Pregnancy/Lactation: Unknown if distributed in breast milk. **Pregnancy Category D. Children:** Safety and efficacy not established. Not prescribed in this pt population. **Elderly:** No age-related precautions noted.

INTERACTIONS

DRUG: Medications that prolong QT interval (e.g., amiodarone, levofloxacin) may increase risk of QT prolongation. **CYP3A4 inducers (e.g., carbamazepine, phenobarbital, phenytoin)** may decrease concentration. May increase risk of bleeding with **warfarin**. **CYP3A4 inhibitors (e.g., ketoconazole, clarithromycin)** may increase concentration/toxicity. **HERBAL: St. John's wort** may decrease concentration. **FOOD: Grapefruit juice** may increase concentration/effects. **LAB VALUES:** May increase serum alkaline phosphatase, bilirubin, calcium, AST.

AVAILABILITY (Rx)

Tablets: 60 mg.

ADMINISTRATION/HANDLING

PO
• Give without regard to food.

INDICATIONS/ROUTES/DOSAGE

Breast Cancer
PO: ADULTS: 60 mg/day as a single dose until disease progression is observed.

SIDE EFFECTS

Frequent (35%–9%): Hot flashes, diaphoresis, nausea, vaginal discharge, dizziness, dry eyes. **Occasional (5%–2%):**

T

Edema, vomiting, vaginal bleeding. **Rare:** Fatigue, depression, lethargy, anorexia.

ADVERSE EFFECTS/ TOXIC REACTIONS

Ocular toxicity (cataracts, glaucoma, decreased visual acuity), hypercalcemia may occur.

NURSING CONSIDERATIONS

BASELINE ASSESSMENT

Estrogen receptor assay should be done before beginning therapy. CBC, serum calcium levels should be checked before and periodically during therapy.

INTERVENTION/EVALUATION

Assess for hypercalcemia (increased urinary volume, excessive thirst, nausea, vomiting, constipation, hypotonicity of muscles, deep bone/flank pain, renal stones). Monitor RBC, Hgb, Hct, leukocyte, platelet counts, serum calcium, hepatic function tests.

PATIENT/FAMILY TEACHING

• May have initial flare of symptoms (bone pain, hot flashes) that will subside. • Report vaginal bleeding/discharge/itching, leg cramps, weight gain, shortness of breath, weakness. • Report persistent nausea/vomiting. • Nonhormone contraceptives are recommended during treatment.

torsemide

tor-se-myde
(Demadex)
Do not confuse torsemide with furosemide.

◆CLASSIFICATION

PHARMACOTHERAPEUTIC: Loop diuretic. **CLINICAL:** Antihypertensive, antiedema (see p. 104C).

ACTION

Enhances excretion of sodium, chloride, potassium, water at ascending limb of loop of Henle. Reduces plasma, extracellular fluid volume. **Therapeutic Effect:** Produces diuresis; lowers B/P.

PHARMACOKINETICS

Route	Onset	Peak	Duration
PO, IV (diuresis)	30–60 min	1–2 hrs	6–8 hrs

Rapidly, well absorbed from GI tract. Protein binding: 97%–99%. Metabolized in liver. Primarily excreted in urine. Not removed by hemodialysis. **Half-life:** 2–4 hrs.

USES

Treatment of hypertension either alone or in combination with other antihypertensives. Edema associated with HF, renal disease, hepatic disease.

PRECAUTIONS

Contraindications: Anuria, other sulfonylureas. **Cautions:** Pts with cirrhosis.

⧗ LIFESPAN CONSIDERATIONS

Pregnancy/Lactation: Unknown if drug is distributed in breast milk. **Pregnancy Category B. Children:** Safety and efficacy not established. **Elderly:** No age-related precautions noted.

INTERACTIONS

DRUG: NSAIDs, aspirin may increase risk of renal impairment. May increase risk of **digoxin** toxicity associated with torsemide-induced hypokalemia. May increase risk of **lithium** toxicity. **Other hypokalemia-causing medications** may increase risk of hypokalemia. **HERBAL: Ephedra, ginseng, yohimbe, licorice** may worsen hypertension. **Black cohosh** may increase antihypertensive effect. **FOOD:** None known. **LAB VALUES:** May increase BUN, serum creatinine, uric acid. May decrease serum calcium, chloride, magnesium, potassium, sodium.

AVAILABILITY (Rx)

Injection Solution: 10 mg/ml. **Tablets:** 5 mg, 10 mg, 20 mg, 100 mg.

ADMINISTRATION/HANDLING

 IV

Rate of Administration

◀ **ALERT** ▶ Flush IV line with 0.9% NaCl before and following administration. • May give undiluted as IV push over minimum of 2 min. • For continuous IV infusion, dilute with 0.9% or 0.45% NaCl or D₅W and infuse over 24 hrs. • Too-rapid IV rate, high dosages may cause ototoxicity; administer IV rate **slowly**.

Storage • Store at room temperature. IV infusion stable for 24 hrs at room temperature.

PO

• Give without regard to food. Give with food to avoid GI upset, preferably with breakfast (prevents nocturia).

▦ IV COMPATIBILITY

Milrinone (Primacor).

INDICATIONS/ROUTES/DOSAGE

Hypertension

PO: ADULTS, ELDERLY: Initially, 2.5–5 mg/day. May increase to 10 mg/day if no response in 4–6 wks. If no response, add additional antihypertensive. **Range:** 2.5–10 mg/day.

Edema Associated with HF

PO, IV: ADULTS, ELDERLY: Initially, 10–20 mg/day. May increase by approximately doubling dose until desired therapeutic effect is attained. **Maximum dose:** PO: 200 mg; IV: 100–200 mg.

Chronic Renal Failure

PO, IV: ADULTS, ELDERLY: Initially, 20 mg/day. May increase by approximately doubling dose until desired therapeutic effect is attained. **Maximum dose:** PO: 200 mg; IV: 100–200 mg.

Hepatic Cirrhosis

PO: ADULTS, ELDERLY: Initially, 5 mg/day given with aldosterone antagonist or potassium-sparing diuretic. May increase by approximately doubling dose until desired therapeutic effect is attained. **Maximum single dose:** 40 mg.

SIDE EFFECTS

Frequent (10%–4%): Headache, dizziness, rhinitis. **Occasional (3%–1%):** Asthenia (loss of strength, energy), insomnia, nervousness, diarrhea, constipation, nausea, dyspepsia (heartburn, indigestion, epigastric pain), edema, EKG changes, pharyngitis, cough, arthralgia, myalgia. **Rare (Less Than 1%):** Syncope, hypotension, arrhythmias.

ADVERSE EFFECTS/ TOXIC REACTIONS

Ototoxicity may occur with too-rapid IV administration or with high doses; must be given slowly. Overdose produces acute, profound water loss; volume/electrolyte depletion; dehydration; decreased blood volume; circulatory collapse.

NURSING CONSIDERATIONS

BASELINE ASSESSMENT

Check serum electrolyte levels, esp. potassium. Obtain baseline weight; check for edema. Assess for rales in lungs, signs of HF.

INTERVENTION/EVALUATION

Monitor B/P, serum electrolytes (esp. potassium), I&O, weight. Notify physician of any hearing abnormality. Note extent of diuresis. Assess lungs for rales. Check for signs of edema, particularly of dependent areas. Although less potassium is lost with torsemide than with furosemide, assess for signs of hypokalemia (change of muscle strength, tremor, muscle cramps, altered mental status, cardiac arrhythmias).

PATIENT/FAMILY TEACHING

• Take medication in morning to prevent nocturia. • Expect increased urinary vol-

T

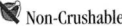

ume, frequency. • Report palpitations, muscle weakness, cramps, nausea, dizziness. • Do not take other medications (including OTC drugs) without consulting physician. • Eat foods high in potassium such as whole grains (cereals), legumes, meat, bananas, apricots, orange juice, potatoes (white, sweet), raisins.

---

tramadol

TOP 200

tram-a-dol
(ConZip, Ralivia ER❋, Rybix ODT, Ryzolt, Tridural❋, Ultram, Ultram ER)
Do not confuse tramadol with tapentadol, Toradol, Trandate or Ultram with Ultracet.

FIXED-COMBINATION(S)

Ultracet: tramadol/acetaminophen (a non-narcotic analgesic): 37.5 mg/ 325 mg.

◆CLASSIFICATION

PHARMACOTHERAPEUTIC: Centrally acting synthetic opioid analgesic. **CLINICAL:** Analgesic.

ACTION

Binds to μ-opioid receptors, inhibits reuptake of norepinephrine, serotonin. Reduces intensity of pain stimuli incoming from sensory nerve endings. **Therapeutic Effect:** Reduces pain.

PHARMACOKINETICS

Route	Onset	Peak	Duration
PO	Less than 1 hr	2–3 hrs	9 hrs

Rapidly, almost completely absorbed after PO administration. Protein binding: 20%. Metabolized in liver (reduced in pts with advanced cirrhosis). Primarily excreted in urine. Minimally removed by hemodialysis. **Half-life:** 6–7 hrs.

USES

Management of moderate to moderately severe pain. **Extended-Release:** Around-the-clock management of moderate to moderately severe pain for extended period.

PRECAUTIONS

Contraindications: Acute alcohol intoxication, concurrent use of centrally acting analgesics, hypnotics, opioids, psychotropic drugs, hypersensitivity to opioids. **ConZip, Ryzolt:** (Additional) Severe/ acute bronchial asthma, hypercapnia, significant respiratory depression. **Caution:** CNS depression, anoxia, advanced hepatic cirrhosis, respiratory depression, elevated ICP, history of seizures or risk for seizures, hepatic/renal impairment, acute abdominal conditions, opioid-dependent pts, head injury, myxedema, hypothyroidism, hypoadrenalism, pregnancy. Avoid use in pts who are suicidal or addiction prone, emotionally disturbed, depressed, heavy alcohol users.

⧗ LIFESPAN CONSIDERATIONS

Pregnancy/Lactation: Crosses placenta. Distributed in breast milk. **Pregnancy Category C. Children:** Safety and efficacy not established. **Elderly:** Age-related renal impairment may require dosage adjustment.

INTERACTIONS

DRUG: Alcohol, other CNS depressants may increase CNS, depression. **Carbamazepine** decreases concentration/effects. **CYP2D6 inhibitors (e.g., paroxetine), CYP3A4 inhibitors (e.g., erythromycin), triptans, selective serotonin reuptake inhibitors (SSRIs), tricyclic antidepressants** may increase risk of seizures, risk of serotonin syndrome. **HERBAL: Gotu kola, kava kava, St. John's wort, valerian** may increase CNS depression. **St. John's wort** may increase risk of serotonin syndrome. **FOOD:** None known. **LAB VALUES:** May increase serum creatinine, AST, ALT. May decrease Hgb. May cause proteinuria.

AVAILABILITY (Rx)

Tablets (Immediate-Release) (Ultram): 50 mg. **Capsule (Variable-Release):** ConZip: 100 mg (25 mg immediate/75 mg extended), 200 mg (50 mg immediate/150 mg extended), 300 mg (50 mg immediate/250 mg extended).

▼ **Tablets (Extended-Release) (Ryzolt, Ultram ER):** 100 mg, 200 mg, 300 mg.
▼ **Tablets, Orally Disintegrating (Rybix):** 50 mg.

ADMINISTRATION/HANDLING

PO
• Give without regard to meals but consistently with or without meals. • Do not break, crush, dissolve, or divide; give extended-release tablets whole.

ODT
• Remove from foil blister, place on tongue. • May take with or without water. • Do not break, crush, or divide tablet.

INDICATIONS/ROUTES/DOSAGE

Moderate to Moderately Severe Pain
PO *(Immediate-Release)*: **ADULTS, ELDERLY:** 50–100 mg q4–6h. **Maximum:** 400 mg/day for pts 75 yrs and younger; 300 mg/day for pts older than 75 yrs.
PO *(Extended-Release)*: **ADULTS, ELDERLY:** 100–300 mg once a day (titrate to desired effect).

Dosage in Renal Impairment
Immediate-Release: For pts with creatinine clearance less than 30 ml/min, increase dosing interval to q12h. **Maximum:** 200 mg/day. Do not use extended-release.

Dosage in Hepatic Impairment
Immediate-Release: Dosage is decreased to 50 mg q12h. Do not use extended-release with severe hepatic impairment.

SIDE EFFECTS

Frequent (25%–15%): Dizziness, vertigo, nausea, constipation, headache, drowsiness. **Occasional (10%–5%):** Vomiting, pruritus, CNS stimulation (e.g., nervousness, anxiety, agitation, tremor, euphoria, mood swings, hallucinations), asthenia (loss of strength, energy), diaphoresis, dyspepsia (heartburn, indigestion, epigastric pain), dry mouth, diarrhea. **Rare (less than 5%):** Malaise, vasodilation, anorexia, flatulence, rash, blurred vision, urinary retention/frequency, menopausal symptoms.

ADVERSE EFFECTS/TOXIC REACTIONS

Seizures reported in pts receiving tramadol within recommended dosage range. May have prolonged duration of action, cumulative effect in pts with hepatic/renal impairment, serotonin syndrome (agitation, hallucinations, tachycardia, hyperreflexia).

NURSING CONSIDERATIONS

BASELINE ASSESSMENT
Assess onset, type, location, duration of pain. Assess drug history, esp. carbamazepine, analgesics, CNS depressants, MAOIs. Review past medical history, esp. epilepsy, seizures. Assess renal/hepatic function lab values.

INTERVENTION/EVALUATION
Monitor pulse, B/P, renal/hepatic function. Assist with ambulation if dizziness, vertigo occurs. Dry crackers, cola may relieve nausea. Palpate bladder for urinary retention. Monitor daily pattern of bowel activity, stool consistency. Sips of water may relieve dry mouth. Assess for clinical improvement, record onset of relief of pain.

PATIENT/FAMILY TEACHING
• May cause dependence. • Avoid alcohol, OTC medications (analgesics, sedatives). • May cause drowsiness, dizziness, blurred vision. • Avoid tasks requiring alertness, motor skills until response to drug is established. • Report severe constipation, difficulty breathing, excessive sedation, seizures, muscle weakness, tremors, chest pain, palpitations.

trametinib

tra-**me**-ti-nib
(Mekinest)
Do not confuse trametinib with imatinib or tipifarnib.

◆ CLASSIFICATION

PHARMACOTHERAPEUTIC: Kinase inhibitor. **CLINICAL:** Antineoplastic.

ACTION

Inhibits BRAF kinase gene mutation, a main cause of tumor cell growth, in the absence of growth factors that are normally required for proliferation. **Therapeutic Effect:** Inhibits tumor cell growth and metastasis.

PHARMACOKINETICS

Rapidly absorbed after PO administration. Protein binding: 97.4%. Peak plasma concentration: 1.5 hrs. Metabolized in liver. Excreted in feces (80%), urine (20%). **Half-life:** 3.9–4.8 days.

USES

Used as a single agent or in combination with dabrafenib for treatment of unresectable or metastatic melanoma with BRAF V600E or V600L mutations, as detected by FDA-approved test. Single-agent regimen is not indicated in pts who have received prior BRAF-inhibitor therapy.

PRECAUTIONS

Contraindications: None known. **Cautions:** Diabetes mellitus, cardiomyopathy, HF, COPD, dehydration, electrolyte imbalance, glaucoma, hepatic/renal impairment, hypertension, prolonged QT syndrome; history of deep vein thrombosis (DVT), pulmonary embolism (PE), gastric ulcers, hemorrhoids, hemorrhoidal/intracranial/nasal/rectal/urinary/vaginal bleeding.

⧗ LIFESPAN CONSIDERATIONS

Pregnancy/Lactation: Avoid pregnancy. May cause fetal harm. Must use effective nonhormonal contraception during treatment and for at least 4 wks after discontinuation (intrauterine device, barrier methods). Unknown if distributed in breast milk. Must either discontinue breastfeeding or discontinue treatment. **Pregnancy Category D. Children:** Safety and efficacy not established. **Elderly:** May have increased risk of adverse effects, skin lesions, primary malignancies. **Males:** May decrease sperm count.

INTERACTIONS

DRUG: SINGLE REGIMEN: Azithromycin, antiarrhythmics, antipsychotics, fluoroquinolones may prolong QT interval; may cause bradycardic arrhythmias. May decrease effectiveness of **hormonal contraceptives. COMBINATION REGIMEN: Antacids, H$_2$-receptors blockers, proton pump inhibitors, carbamazepine, phenytoin, rifampin** may decrease concentration/effect. **Clarithromycin, gemfibrozil, ketoconazole** may increase concentration/effect. May decrease effectiveness of **insulin, oral hypoglycemics. HERBAL: St. John's wort** may decrease concentration/effect. **FOOD: High-fat meals** may decrease absorption/effect. **LAB VALUES: SINGLE REGIMEN:** May increase serum alkaline phosphatase, ALT, AST. May decrease serum albumin, Hgb, Hct. **COMBINATION REGIMEN:** May increase serum alkaline phosphatase, ALT, AST, bilirubin, calcium, creatinine, glucose, GGT, potassium. May decrease Hgb, Hct, leukocytes, lymphocytes, neutrophils, platelets, serum albumin, calcium, magnesium, phosphorus, potassium, sodium.

AVAILABILITY (Rx)

Tablets: 0.5 mg, 1 mg, 2 mg.

ADMINISTRATION/HANDLING

PO
• Administer at least 1 hr before or 2 hrs after meal.

INDICATIONS/ROUTES/DOSAGE

Melanoma
PO: ADULTS/ELDERLY: 2 mg once daily (or in combination with dabrafenib 150 mg

twice daily). Continue until disease progression or unacceptable toxicity occurs.

Dose Reduction Schedule
Trametinib Regimen: FIRST DOSE REDUCTION: 1.5 mg once daily. **SECOND DOSE REDUCTION:** 1 mg once daily. Discontinue if unable to tolerate 1-mg dose.
Dabrafenib Combination Regimen: FIRST DOSE REDUCTION: 100 mg twice daily. **SECOND DOSE REDUCTION:** 75 mg twice daily.
THIRD DOSE REDUCTION: 50 mg twice daily. Discontinue if unable to tolerate 50-mg dose.

Dose Modification
Based on Common Terminology Criteria for Adverse Events (CTCAE) grading 1–4.
Cardiac: ASYMPTOMATIC DECREASE IN LEFT VENTRICULAR EJECTION FRACTION (LVEF) GREATER THAN 10% FROM BASELINE: Withhold trametinib up to 4 wks. If LVEF improved, resume at lower dose level. Discontinue if not improved. Do not modify dabrafenib dose. **SYMPTOMATIC HF OR DECREASE IN LVEF GREATER THAN 20% FROM BASELINE:** Discontinue trametinib. Withhold dabrafenib until improved, then resume at lower dose level. **CUTANEOUS EVENTS: INTOLERABLE GRADE 2 SKIN TOXICITY OR GRADE 3–4 TOXICITY:** Withhold both regimens for up to 3 wks. If improved, resume both at lower dose level. Discontinue both regimens if not improved. **FEBRILE EVENTS: FEVER OF 101.3°F–104°F:** Do not modify trametinib dose. Withhold dabrafenib until fever resolved, then resume at either same dose or lower dose level.
FEVER GREATER THAN 104°F OR FEVER COMPLICATED BY DEYDRATION, HYPOTENSION, RENAL FAILURE: Withhold trametinib until resolved, then resume at either same dose or lower dose level. Withhold dabrafenib until resolved, then resume at either lower dose level or discontinue.
New Primary Malignancies: CUTANEOUS: No changes required for either regimen. **NONCUTANEOUS:** Do not change trametinib dose. Discontinue dabrafenib in pts who develop RAS mutation-positive malignancies.
Nonspecific Adverse Reactions: INTOLERABLE GRADE 2 OR ANY GRADE 3: Withhold both regimens until resolved to grade 0–1, then resume at lower dose level. Discontinue both regimens if not improved. **FIRST OCCURRENCE OF ANY GRADE 4 REACTIONS:** Withhold both regimens until resolved to grade 0–1, then resume at lower dose level or discontinue.
Ocular Toxicities: GRADE 2–3 RETINAL PIGMENT EPITHELIAL DETACHMENTS: Withhold trametinib up to 3 wks. If improved to grade 0–1, resume at lower dose level. Discontinue if not improved. Do not modify dabrafenib. **RETINAL VEIN OCCLUSION:** Discontinue trametinib. Do not modify dabrafenib.
UVEITIS OR IRITIS: Do not modify trametinib. Withhold dabrafenib for up to 6 wks. If improved to grade 0–1, then resume at same dose level. Discontinue if not improved.
Pulmonary: INTERSTITIAL LUNG DISEASE: Discontinue trametinib. Do not modify dabrafenib.
Venous Thromboembolism: UNCOMPLICATED (DVT) OR (PE): Withhold trametinib for up to 3 wks. If improved to grade 0–1, then resume at lower dose level. Discontinue if not improved. Do not modify dabrafenib. **LIFE-THREATENING PE:** Discontinue both regimens.

SIDE EFFECTS

Single Regimen:
Frequent (57%–32%): Rash, diarrhea, lymphedema, peripheral edema. **Occasional (19%–10%):** Dermatitis acneiform, hypertension, stomatitis, mouth ulceration, mucosal ulceration, abdominal pain, dry skin, pruritus, paronychia, folliculitis, cellulitis, dizziness, dysgeusia, blurred vision, dry eye.
Combination Regimen:
Frequent (71%–40%): Pyrexia, chills, fatigue, rash, nausea, vomiting. **Occasional (36%–11%):** Diarrhea, abdominal pain, peripheral edema, headache, cough, arthralgia, night sweats, myalgia, constipation, decreased

appetite, back pain, dry skin, insomnia, dermatitis acneiform, dizziness, muscle spasm, extremity pain, actinic keratosis, erythema, oral/throat pain, urinary tract infection, pruritus, dry mouth, dehydration.

ADVERSE EFFECTS/ TOXIC REACTIONS

Primary malignancies including basal or squamous cell carcinoma, keratoacanthoma, pancreatic adenocarcinoma, glioblastoma (brain cancer) reported. DVT, PE reported in 9% of pts. May increase cell proliferation of wild-type BRAF melanoma or new malignant melanomas. Serious, sometimes fatal intracranial or gastric bleeding occurred in 5% of pts. Other hemorrhagic events may include conjunctival/gingival/rectal/hemorrhoidal/vaginal bleeding; epistaxis (nosebleed), melena (bloody stools). Cardiomyopathy, HF, decreased LVEF reported in 7%–9% of pts. Ocular (eye) toxicities such as retinal vein occlusion, retinal detachment, vision loss, glaucoma, uveitis, iritis reported. Cough, dyspnea, hypoxia, pleural effusion, infiltrates may indicate interstitial lung disease (ILD). Serious febrile reactions may lead to renal failure, severe dehydration, hypotension, rigors. Skin toxicities including palmar-plantar erythrodysesthesia syndrome (PPES), papilloma have occurred. Hyperglycemia reported in 2%–5% of pts. Other effects may include hypertension, rhabdomyolysis. May prolong QT interval of cardiac cycle.

NURSING CONSIDERATIONS

BASELINE ASSESSMENT

Obtain baseline CBC, serum metabolic panel (with liver function test), magnesium, phosphate, ionized calcium, capillary glucose level, vital signs. Obtain BRAF V600E mutation history, negative pregnancy status, ophthalmologic exam with visual acuity, echocardiogram, EKG before initiating treatment. Assess skin for moles, lesions, papillomas. Question current breastfeeding status. Receive full medication history including herbal products. Question any history as listed in PRECAUTIONS.

INTERVENTION/EVALUATION

Offer emotional support. Monitor CBC, serum electrolytes, capillary blood glucose, stool characteristics routinely. Monitor for signs of hyperglycemia (thirst, polyuria, confusion, dehydration). Assess skin for new lesions, toxicities every 2 mos during treatment and at least 6 mos after discontinuation. Obtain LVEF by echocardiogram 1 mo after initiation, then every 2–3 mos; ophthalmologic exam with any vision changes. Immediately report any altered mental status, bleeding events, vision changes, eye pain/swelling/infection, fever, urinary changes. Screen for bleeding of any kind. If dyspnea or leg swelling occurs, contact physician and initiate appropriate medical therapy (may require oxygen therapy, EKG, or radiologic test to rule out DVT, PE, or ILD).

PATIENT/FAMILY TEACHING

• Blood work, cardiac function tests, eye exams will be performed routinely. • Treatment may lead to heart failure, vision changes, lung complications, difficulty breathing, fever, skin toxicities (such as severe rash, peeling), high blood pressure, severe diarrhea. • Report bloody stools/urine, heavy menstruation, or nosebleeds. • Do not breastfeed. • Avoid pregnancy; nonhormonal contraception should be used during treatment and up to 4 wks after treatment. • Take medication at least 1 hr before or at least 2 hrs after meal (food reduces absorption). • Report any increased urination, thirst, confusion (may indicate high blood sugar); chest pain, eye pain, fever, leg swelling, new skin moles or lesions, vision changes. • Minimize sunlight exposure. • Males may experience a decreased sperm count. • Report any newly prescribed medications.

tranylcypromine

tran-il-**sip**-roe-meen
(Parnate)

BLACK BOX ALERT Increased risk of suicidal ideation and behavior in children, adolescents, young adults 18–24 yrs with major depressive disorder, other psychiatric disorders.

◆CLASSIFICATION

PHARMACOTHERAPEUTIC: MAOI. **CLINICAL:** Antidepressant (see p. 39C).

ACTION

Inhibits activity of the enzyme monoamine oxidase at CNS storage sites, leading to increasing levels of neurotransmitters epinephrine, norepinephrine, serotonin, dopamine at neuronal receptor sites. **Therapeutic Effect:** Relieves depression.

USES

Treatment of depression without melancholia.

PRECAUTIONS

Contraindications: Concurrent use of antihistamines, antihypertensives, antiparkinson drugs, bupropion, buspirone, CNS depressants, MAOIs, SSRIs or SNRIs, sympathomimetics, excessive use of caffeine. Pheochromocytoma, uncontrolled hypertension, cerebrovascular defects, history of headache, history of hepatic disease or abnormal hepatic function tests, foods high in tyramine. **Cautions:** Pts at high risk for suicide, glaucoma, hyperthyroidism, diabetes, hypotension, history of substance abuse, acute alcoholism, renal impairment, pts at risk for seizures.

⌛ LIFESPAN CONSIDERATIONS

Pregnancy/Lactation: Crosses placenta. Minimally distributed in breast milk. **Pregnancy Category C. Children:** Not recommended for this pt population (increased risk of suicidal ideation). **Elderly:** In-

creased risk of drug toxicity may require dosage adjustment.

INTERACTIONS

DRUG: **Alcohol, other CNS depressants** may increase CNS depressant effects. **Buspirone** may increase risk of hypertension. **Caffeine-containing medications** may increase risk of cardiac arrhythmias, hypertension. **Carbamazepine, cyclobenzaprine, other MAOIs, maprotiline** may precipitate hypertensive crisis. **Dopamine, tryptophan** may cause sudden, severe hypertension. **Fluoxetine, trazodone, tricyclic antidepressants** may cause serotonin syndrome, neuroleptic malignant syndrome. May increase effects of **insulin, oral antidiabetics. Meperidine, other opioid analgesics** may produce serotonin syndrome. **HERBAL:** **Valerian, St. John's wort, SAMe, kava kava** may increase risk of serotonin syndrome or excessive sedation. **FOOD:** **Foods containing pressor amines (aged cheese, caffeine, red wine), tyramine** may cause sudden, severe hypertension. **LAB VALUES:** None significant.

AVAILABILITY (Rx)

Tablets: 10 mg.

ADMINISTRATION/HANDLING

◄ALERT► At least 14 days must elapse between tranylcypromine and selective serotonin reuptake inhibitors (SSRIs). Avoid foods containing tryptophan and caffeine; tyramine-containing foods/beverages (e.g., aged cheese, air-dried or cured meats, fava, soy sauce, soybean condiments, tap/draft beer).

INDICATIONS/ROUTES/DOSAGE

Depression
PO: ADULTS, ELDERLY: Initially, 10 mg twice daily. May increase by 10 mg/day at 1- to 3-wk intervals up to 60 mg/day in divided doses. **Usual effective dose:** 30 mg/day.

SIDE EFFECTS

Frequent: Orthostatic hypotension, restlessness, GI upset, insomnia, dizziness,

T

✤ Canadian trade name   Non-Crushable Drug   **HIGH ALERT** High Alert drug lethargy, weakness, dry mouth, peripheral edema. **Occasional:** Flushing, diaphoresis, rash, urinary frequency, increased appetite, transient impotence. **Rare:** Visual disturbances.

ADVERSE EFFECTS/ TOXIC REACTIONS

Hypertensive crisis occurs rarely, marked by severe hypertension, occipital headache radiating frontally, neck stiffness/soreness, nausea, vomiting, diaphoresis, fever/chills, clammy skin, dilated pupils, palpitations, tachycardia, bradycardia, constricting chest pain. Intracranial bleeding may be associated with severe hypertension.

NURSING CONSIDERATIONS

BASELINE ASSESSMENT

Perform baseline serum hepatic/renal function tests. Assess sensitivity to tranylcypromine. Assess for other medical conditions, esp. alcoholism, HF, pheochromocytoma, arrhythmias, cardiovascular disease, hypertension, suicidal tendencies. Question for other medications, including CNS depressants, meperidine, other antidepressants.

INTERVENTION/EVALUATION

Assess appearance, behavior, speech pattern, level of interest, mood. Supervise suicidal-risk pt closely during early therapy (as depression lessens, energy level improves, increasing suicide potential). Monitor for occipital headache radiating frontally, neck stiffness/soreness (may be first signal of impending hypertensive crisis). Monitor B/P diligently for hypertension. Assess skin, temperature for fever. Discontinue medication immediately if palpitations, frequent headaches occur. Monitor weight.

PATIENT/FAMILY TEACHING

• Take second daily dose no later than 4 PM to avoid insomnia. • Antidepressant relief may be noted during first wk of therapy; maximum benefit noted within 3 wks. • Notify physician of worsening depression, unusual behavior, suicidal thoughts or ideation. • Report headache, neck stiffness/soreness immediately. • Go from lying to standing slowly. • Avoid foods that require bacteria/molds for their preparation/preservation, those that contain tyramine (e.g., cheese, sour cream, beer, wine, pickled herring, liver, figs, raisins, bananas, avocados, soy sauce, yeast extracts, yogurt, papaya, broad beans, meat tenderizers), excessive amounts of caffeine (coffee, tea, chocolate), OTC cold/allergy preparations, weight reduction medications.

---

trastuzumab

tras-**too**-zoo-mab
(<u>Herceptin</u>)

BLACK BOX ALERT Anaphylactic reaction, infusion reaction, acute respiratory distress syndrome have been associated with fatalities. Reduction in left ventricular ejection fraction, severe heart failure may result in thrombus formation, stroke, cardiac death. Exposure during pregnancy may result in pulmonary hypoplasia, skeletal malformations, neonatal death.

◆CLASSIFICATION

PHARMACOTHERAPEUTIC: Monoclonal antibody. **CLINICAL:** Antineoplastic (see p. 91C).

ACTION

Binds to *HER2* protein, overexpressed in 25%–30% of primary breast cancers, inhibiting proliferation of tumor cells. **Therapeutic Effect:** Inhibits growth of tumor cells, mediates antibody-dependent cellular cytotoxicity.

PHARMACOKINETICS

Half-life: 5.8 days (range: 1–32 days).

USES

Treatment of *HER2* overexpressing breast cancer (adjuvant), metastatic breast cancer, metastatic gastric or gastroesophageal junction adenocarcinoma (in pts without prior treatment). **OFF-LABEL:** Treatment of *HER2*–positive metastatic breast cancer in pts who have not received prior anti-*HER2* therapy or in pts whose cancer has progressed on prior trastuzumab therapy (in combination with lapatinib).

PRECAUTIONS

Contraindications: None known. **Cautions:** Preexisting cardiac disease or dysfunction, pulmonary disease, or extensive pulmonary tumor involvement.

⌛ LIFESPAN CONSIDERATIONS

Pregnancy/Lactation: Unknown if distributed in breast milk. **Pregnancy Category D. Children:** Safety and efficacy not established. **Elderly:** Age-related cardiac dysfunction may require dosage adjustment.

INTERACTIONS

DRUG: None significant. **HERBAL:** None significant. **FOOD:** None known. **LAB VALUES:** None significant.

AVAILABILITY (Rx)

Injection, Powder for Reconstitution: 440 mg.

ADMINISTRATION/HANDLING
 IV

Reconstitution • Reconstitute with 20 ml Bacteriostatic Water for Injection to yield concentration of 21 mg/ml. • Add calculated dose to 250 ml 0.9% NaCl (do not use D_5W). • Gently mix contents in bag.
Rate of Administration • Do not give IV push or bolus. • Give loading dose (4 mg/kg) over 90 min. Give maintenance infusion (2 mg/kg) over 30 min.
Storage • Refrigerate. • Reconstituted solution appears colorless to pale yellow.

• Reconstituted solution in vial is stable for 28 days if refrigerated after reconstitution with Bacteriostatic Water for Injection (if using Sterile Water for Injection without preservative, use immediately; discard unused portions). • Solution diluted in 250 ml 0.9% NaCl stable for 24 hrs if refrigerated.

🏥 IV INCOMPATIBILITIES

Do not mix with D_5W or any other medications.

INDICATIONS/ROUTES/DOSAGE

Breast Cancer (Adjuvant)
IV: ADULTS, ELDERLY: (with concurrent paclitaxel or docetaxel): Initially, 4 mg/kg as 90-min infusion, then 2 mg/kg weekly as 30-min infusion for 12 wks followed 1 wk later (when concurrent chemotherapy completed) by 6 mg/kg infusion over 30–90 min q3wks for total therapy duration of 52 wks. **(with docetaxel/carboplatin):** Initially, 4 mg/kg as 90-min infusion, then 2 mg/kg weekly as 30-min infusion for a total of 18 wks, followed 1 wk later (when concurrent chemotherapy completed) by 6 mg/kg infused over 30–90 min q3wks for total therapy duration of 52 wks.

Breast Cancer (Metastatic)
IV: ADULTS, ELDERLY: Initially, 4 mg/kg as 90-min infusion, then 2 mg/kg as 30-min infusion weekly until disease progression.

Stomach Cancer
IV: ADULTS, ELDERLY: Initially, 8 mg/kg over 90 min, then 6 mg/kg over 30–90 min q3wks until disease progression.

Dosage Adjustment in Cardiotoxicity
Left ventricular ejection fraction (LVEF) 16% or greater decrease from baseline WNL (within normal limits) or LVEF below normal limits and 10% or greater decrease from baseline: Hold treatment for 4 wks. Repeat LVEF q4wks. Resume therapy if LVEF returns to normal limits in 4–8 wks and remains at 15% or less decrease from baseline.

T

SIDE EFFECTS

Frequent (Greater Than 20%): Pain, asthenia (loss of strength, energy), fever, chills, headache, abdominal pain, back pain, infection, nausea, diarrhea, vomiting, cough, dyspnea. **Occasional (15%–5%):** Tachycardia, HF, flu-like symptoms, anorexia, edema, bone pain, arthralgia, insomnia, dizziness, paresthesia, depression, rhinitis, pharyngitis, sinusitis. **Rare (Less Than 5%):** Allergic reaction, anemia, leukopenia, neuropathy, herpes simplex.

ADVERSE EFFECTS/ TOXIC REACTIONS

Cardiomyopathy, ventricular dysfunction, HF occur rarely. Pancytopenia may occur.

NURSING CONSIDERATIONS

BASELINE ASSESSMENT

Evaluate left ventricular function. Obtain baseline echocardiogram, EKG, multigated acquisition (MUGA) scan. Obtain CBC at baseline and at regular intervals during therapy.

INTERVENTION/EVALUATION

Frequently monitor for deteriorating cardiac function. Assess for asthenia (loss of strength, energy). Assist with ambulation if asthenia (loss of strength, energy) occurs. Monitor for fever, chills, abdominal pain, back pain. Offer antiemetics if nausea, vomiting occur. Monitor daily pattern of bowel activity, stool consistency.

PATIENT/FAMILY TEACHING

• Do not have immunizations without physician's approval (lowers resistance). • Avoid contact with those who have recently taken oral polio vaccine. • Avoid crowds, those with infection.

---

trazodone

TOP 200

traz-o-done
(Apo-Trazodone 🍁,
Novo-Trazodone 🍁, Oleptro,
PMS-Trazodone 🍁)

BLACK BOX ALERT Increased risk of suicidal ideation and behavior in children, adolescents, young adults 18–24 yrs with major depressive disorder, other psychiatric disorders.
Do not confuse trazodone with tramadol or ziprasidone.

◆ **CLASSIFICATION**

PHARMACOTHERAPEUTIC: Serotonin reuptake inhibitor. **CLINICAL:** Antidepressant (see pp. 15C, 41C).

ACTION

Blocks reuptake of serotonin at neuronal presynaptic membranes, increasing its availability at postsynaptic receptor sites. **Therapeutic Effect:** Relieves depression.

PHARMACOKINETICS

Well absorbed from GI tract. Protein binding: 85%–95%. Metabolized in liver. Primarily excreted in urine. Unknown if removed by hemodialysis. **Half-life:** 5–9 hrs.

USES

Treatment of depression. **OFF-LABEL:** Hypnotic, potential augmenting agent for antidepressants.

PRECAUTIONS

Contraindications: None known. **Cautions:** Cardiac disease, arrhythmias, cerebrovascular disease, hepatic/renal impairment, high risk of suicide, concurrent or recent MAOI use. Conditions predisposing to priapism (e.g., sickle cell anemia); concurrent use of CYP3A4 inhibitors/inducers, antihypertensives; history of seizure disorder, elderly.

⧗ LIFESPAN CONSIDERATIONS

Pregnancy/Lactation: Drug crosses placenta; minimally distributed in breast milk. **Pregnancy Category C. Children:** Safety and efficacy not established in those younger than 6 yrs. **Elderly:** More likely to experience sedative, hypotensive effects; lower dosage recommended.

INTERACTIONS

DRUG: CYP3A4 inhibitors (e.g., ritonavir, ketoconazole) increase concentration/effects. May increase concentration of **digoxin, phenytoin. HERBAL: Gotu kola, kava kava, St. John's wort, valerian** may increase CNS depression and serotonin syndrome. **FOOD:** None known. **LAB VALUES:** May decrease WBC, neutrophil counts.

AVAILABILITY (Rx)

Tablets: 50 mg, 100 mg, 150 mg, 300 mg.
 Tablets: (Extended-Release [Oleptro]): 150 mg, 300 mg.

ADMINISTRATION/HANDLING

PO

• Give shortly after snack, meal (reduces risk of dizziness). • Tablets may be crushed. • Do not break, crush, or dissolve extended-release tablets. Give whole or break in half along score line. • Best taken at bedtime.

INDICATIONS/ROUTES/DOSAGE

◄ALERT► Therapeutic effect may take up to 6 wks to occur.

Depression
PO: ADULTS: Initially, 150 mg/day in 3 equally divided doses. Increase by 50 mg/day at 3- to 7-day intervals until therapeutic response is achieved. **Maximum:** 600 mg/day. **ELDERLY:** Initially, 25–50 mg at bedtime. May increase by 25–50 mg every 3–7 days. **Range:** 75–150 mg/day. **TABLETS (EXTENDED-RELEASE):** Initially, 150 mg once daily. May increase by 75 mg q3days. **Maximum:** 375 mg/day. **ADOLESCENTS 13–18 YRS:** Initially, 25–50 mg/day. May increase to 100–150 mg/day in divided doses. **CHILDREN 6–12 YRS:** Initially, 1.5–2 mg/kg/day in divided doses. May increase gradually to 6 mg/kg/day in 3 divided doses.

SIDE EFFECTS

Frequent (9%–3%): Drowsiness, dry mouth, light-headedness, dizziness, headache,

blurred vision, nausea, vomiting. **Occasional (3%–1%):** Nervousness, fatigue, constipation, myalgia/arthralgia, mild hypotension. **Rare:** Photosensitivity reaction.

ADVERSE EFFECTS/ TOXIC REACTIONS

Priapism, altered libido, retrograde ejaculation, impotence occur rarely. Appears to be less cardiotoxic than other antidepressants, although arrhythmias may occur in pts with preexisting cardiac disease.

NURSING CONSIDERATIONS

BASELINE ASSESSMENT

Assess mental status, mood, behavior. For those on long-term therapy, serum hepatic/renal function tests, blood counts should be performed periodically. Elderly are more likely to experience sedative, hypotensive effects.

INTERVENTION/EVALUATION

Monitor for suicidal ideation (esp. at beginning of therapy or dosage change). Assess appearance, behavior, speech pattern, level of interest, mood. Monitor WBC, neutrophil count, hepatic enzymes. Assist with ambulation if dizziness, light-headedness occurs.

PATIENT/FAMILY TEACHING

• Immediately discontinue medication, consult physician if priapism occurs. • May take after meal, snack. • May take at bedtime if drowsiness occurs. • Change positions slowly to avoid hypotensive effect. • Tolerance to sedative, anticholinergic effects usually develops during early therapy. • Avoid tasks that require alertness, motor skills until response to drug is established. • Photosensitivity to sun may occur. • Dry mouth may be relieved by sugarless gum, sips of water. • Report visual disturbances, worsening depression, suicidal ideation, unusual changes in behavior. • Do not abruptly discontinue medication. • Avoid alcohol.

T

✤ Canadian trade name   Non-Crushable Drug   High Alert drug

treprostinil

tre-**pros**-tin-il
(Remodulin, Tyvaso)

◆CLASSIFICATION

PHARMACOTHERAPEUTIC: Aggregation inhibitor, vasodilator. **CLINICAL:** Antiplatelet.

ACTION

Directly dilates pulmonary, systemic arterial vascular beds, also inhibits platelet aggregation. **Therapeutic Effect:** Reduces symptoms of pulmonary arterial hypertension associated with exercise.

PHARMACOKINETICS

Rapidly, completely absorbed after subcutaneous infusion. Protein binding: 91%. Metabolized by liver. Excreted mainly in urine, with lesser amount eliminated in feces. **Half-life:** 2–4 hrs.

USES

Injection: Treatment of pulmonary arterial hypertension (PAH) in pts with NYHA class II–IV symptoms to decrease exercise associated symptoms; diminish clinical deterioration when transitioning from epoprostenol (Flolan). **Inhalation:** Treatment of PAH in pts with NYHA class III symptoms to increase walk distance.

PRECAUTIONS

Contraindications: None known. **Cautions:** Hepatic/renal impairment, pts older than 65 yrs, pts with significant underlying lung disease (e.g., COPD); low systemic arterial pressure; concomitant use of anticoagulants or antiplatelets, CYP2C8 inducers (e.g., rifampin), CYP2C8 inhibitors (e.g., gemfibrozil).

⌛ LIFESPAN CONSIDERATIONS

Pregnancy/Lactation: Unknown if distributed in breast milk. **Pregnancy Category B. Children:** Safety and efficacy not established. **Elderly:** Consider dose selection carefully because of increased incidence of diminished organ function, concurrent disease, other drug therapy.

INTERACTIONS

DRUG: Anticoagulants, aspirin, heparin, thrombolytics may increase risk of bleeding. **CYP2C8 inhibitors (e.g., gemfibrozil)** may increase concentration/effects. **CYP2C8 inducers (e.g., rifampin)** may decrease concentration/effects. **HERBAL:** None significant. **FOOD:** None known. **LAB VALUES:** None significant.

AVAILABILITY (Rx)

Injection Solution (Remodulin): 1 mg/ml, 2.5 mg/ml, 5 mg/ml, 10 mg/ml. **Solution for Oral Inhalation (Tyvaso):** 0.6 mg/ml (2.9-ml ampoule) delivers 6 mcg per inhalation.

ADMINISTRATION/HANDLING

Inhalation

• Use only with supplied inhalation system. Refer to product information. Give undiluted. • Wait 1 min before inhaling next dose (allows for deeper bronchial penetration). • Administer 4 times daily 4 hrs apart, during waking hrs.

Reconstitution • Dilute with either Sterile Water for Injection or 0.9% NaCl to final volume of 50 ml or 100 ml.

Rate of Administration • Give as continuous IV infusion via indwelling central venous catheter.

Storage • Store unopened vials at room temperature. • Diluted solutions stable for 48 hrs at room temperature.

Subcutaneous

Reconstitution • Intended to be administered without further dilution using an appropriately designed infusion pump. • To avoid potential interruptions in drug delivery, pt must have immediate access to backup infusion pump, subcutaneous infusion sets.

Rate of Administration • Give as continuous subcutaneous infusion via subcutaneous catheter, using infusion pump

designed for subcutaneous drug delivery.
Storage • Store unopened vials at room temperature.

INDICATIONS/ROUTES/DOSAGE

Pulmonary Arterial Hypertension (PAH)
Continuous Subcutaneous Infusion, IV Infusion: ADULTS, ELDERLY: Initially, 1.25 ng/kg/min. Reduce infusion rate to 0.625 ng/kg/min if initial dose cannot be tolerated. Increase infusion rate in increments of no more than 1.25 ng/kg/min per wk for first 4 wks, then no more than 2.5 ng/kg/min per wk for duration of infusion. **Inhalation: ADULTS, ELDERLY:** 3 breaths (18 mcg) per treatment session. Reduce to 1 or 2 breaths if 3 breaths are not tolerated. Increase by 3 breaths at 1- to 2-wk intervals. Titrate to target dose of 9 breaths (54 mcg) per treatment session.

Hepatic Impairment (Mild to Moderate)
IV/Subcutaneous: ADULTS, ELDERLY: Decrease initial dose to 0.625 ng/kg/min based on ideal body weight; increase cautiously.

SIDE EFFECTS

IV: Frequent: Infusion site pain, erythema, induration, rash. **Occasional:** Headache, diarrhea, jaw pain, vasodilation, nausea. **Rare:** Dizziness, hypotension, pruritus, edema. **Inhalation: Common (54%–25%):** Cough, headache, throat irritation. **Occasional (19%–6%):** Nausea, flushing, syncope.

ADVERSE EFFECTS/ TOXIC REACTIONS

Abrupt withdrawal, sudden large reductions in dosage may result in worsening of pulmonary arterial hypertension symptoms. Inhalation may produce symptomatic hypotension.

NURSING CONSIDERATIONS

INTERVENTION/EVALUATION

Monitor for dyspnea, fatigue, decreased activity, symptoms of excessive dose (e.g., headache, nausea, vomiting). Monitor for changes in B/P.

PATIENT/FAMILY TEACHING

• Delivery occurs via self-inserted subcutaneous catheter using ambulatory subcutaneous pump; carefully follow instructions for drug administration. • Follow guidelines for care of subcutaneous catheter, troubleshooting infusion pump problems. • Avoid skin or eye contact with Tyvaso (rinse immediately with water).

---

tretinoin

tret-i-noyn
(Atralin, Avita, Refissa, Rejuva-A ✦, Renova, Retin-A, Retin-A Micro, Tretin X, Vesanoid ✦)

BLACK BOX ALERT High risk for teratogenicity; major fetal abnormalities, spontaneous abortions. Pts with acute promyelocytic leukemia (APL) are at severe risk for reactions (fever, dyspnea, acute respiratory distress syndrome [pulmonary infiltrates, pleural effusions, pericardial effusions]), edema, hepatic, renal, and/or multiorgan failure; 40% develop leukocytosis.

Do not confuse tretinoin with isotretinoin, phenytoin or triamcinolone.

FIXED-COMBINATION(S)

With octyl methoxycinnamate and oxybenzone, moisturizers, and SPF-12, a sunscreen **(Retin-A Regimen Kit).**

◆CLASSIFICATION

PHARMACOTHERAPEUTIC: Retinoid. **CLINICAL:** Antiacne, transdermal, antineoplastic (see p. 91C).

ACTION

Antiacne: Decreases cohesiveness of follicular epithelial cells. Increases turnover of follicular epithelial cells. **Therapeutic Effect:** Causes expulsion of blackheads. Bacterial skin counts are not altered. **Transdermal:** Exerts effects on growth/differentiation of epithelial cells. **Thera-**

peutic Effect: Alleviates fine wrinkles, hyperpigmentation. **Antineoplastic:** Induces maturation, decreases proliferation of acute promyelocytic leukemia (APL) cells. **Therapeutic Effect:** Repopulation of bone marrow, blood by normal hematopoietic cells.

PHARMACOKINETICS

Topical: Minimally absorbed. **PO:** Well absorbed following PO administration. Protein binding: greater than 95%. Metabolized in liver. Primarily excreted in urine. **Half-life:** 0.5–2 hrs.

USES

Topical: Treatment of acne vulgaris, photodamaged skin, some skin cancers. **PO:** Induction of remission in pts with acute promyelocytic leukemia (APL). **OFF-LABEL (PO):** Maintenance therapy in APL, combination therapy (arsenic trioxide) for remission induction in APL.

PRECAUTIONS

Contraindications: Sensitivity to parabens (used as preservative in gelatin capsule). **Extreme Caution: Topical:** Eczema, sun exposure. **Cautions: Topical:** Those with considerable sun exposure in their occupation, hypersensitivity to sun. **PO:** Elevated serum cholesterol/triglycerides, concurrent use of antifibrinolytic agents.

⚠ LIFESPAN CONSIDERATIONS

Pregnancy/Lactation: Topical: Use during pregnancy only if clearly necessary. Unknown if distributed in breast milk; exercise caution in breastfeeding mother. **Topical: Pregnancy Category C. PO:** Teratogenic, embryotoxic effect. **Pregnancy Category D. Children/Elderly:** Safety and efficacy not established.

INTERACTIONS

DRUG: TOPICAL: Retinoids (e.g., acitretin, oral tretinoin) may increase drying, irritative effects. **PO: Tetracyclines** may increase risk of pseudotumor cerebri, intracranial hypertension. **Aminocaproic**

acid may increase risk of thrombotic complications. **CYP3A4 inducers (e.g., phenobarbital, rifampin)** may decrease concentration/effects. **CYP3A4 inhibitors (e.g., ketoconazole)** may increase concentration, risk of toxicity. **HERBAL: St. John's wort** may decrease concentration/effects. **Dong quai, St. John's wort** may increase photosensitization. **Vitamin A** supplementation may increase vitamin A toxicity. **FOOD:** None known. **LAB VALUES: PO:** Leukocytosis occurs commonly (40%). May elevate serum hepatic function tests, cholesterol, triglycerides.

AVAILABILITY (Rx)

Cream: 0.02% (Renova), 0.025% (Avita, Retin-A, Tretin X), 0.05% (Refissa, Retin-A, Tretin X), 0.1% (Retin-A). **Gel:** 0.01% (Retin-A, Tretin X), 0.025% (Avita, Retin-A, Tretin X), 0.04% (Retin-A Micro), 0.1% (Retin-A Micro).

✇ Capsules: (Vesanoid): 10 mg.

ADMINISTRATION/HANDLING

PO
• Do not crush/break capsule. • Administer with a meal.

Topical
• Thoroughly cleanse area before applying tretinoin. • Lightly cover only affected area. Liquid may be applied with fingertip, gauze, cotton; do not rub onto unaffected skin. • Keep medication away from eyes, mouth, angles of nose, mucous membranes. • Wash hands immediately after application.

INDICATIONS/ROUTES/DOSAGE

Acne
Topical: ADULTS, CHILDREN 12 YRS AND OLDER: Apply once daily at bedtime or on alternate days.

Remission Induction in Acute Promyelocytic Leukemia (APL)
PO: ADULTS: 45 mg/m²/day given as 2–3 evenly divided doses until complete remission is documented. Discontinue

T

therapy 30 days after complete remission or after 90 days of treatment, whichever comes first.

Remission Maintenance in APL

PO: ADULTS, ELDERLY: 45 mg/m²/day in 2 divided doses for 15 days q3mos for 2 yrs. **CHILDREN:** 25 mg/m²/day in 2 divided doses for 15 days q3mos for 2 yrs.

SIDE EFFECTS

Topical: Temporary change in pigmentation, photosensitivity. Local inflammatory reactions (peeling, dry skin, stinging, erythema, pruritus) are to be expected and are reversible with discontinuation of tretinoin. **Frequent: PO (87%–54%):** Headache, fever, dry skin/oral mucosa, bone pain, nausea, vomiting, rash. **Occasional: PO (26%–6%):** Mucositis, earache or feeling of fullness in ears, flushing, pruritus, diaphoresis, visual disturbances, hypotension/hypertension, dizziness, anxiety, insomnia, alopecia, skin changes. **Rare (Less Than 6%):** Altered visual acuity, temporary hearing loss.

ADVERSE EFFECTS/ TOXIC REACTIONS

PO: Retinoic acid syndrome (fever, dyspnea, weight gain, abnormal chest auscultatory findings [pulmonary infiltrates, pleural/pericardial effusions], episodic hypotension) occurs commonly (25%), as does leukocytosis (40%). Syndrome generally occurs during first month of therapy (sometimes after first dose). High-dose steroids (dexamethasone 10 mg IV) at first suspicion of syndrome reduce morbidity, mortality. Pseudotumor cerebri may be noted, esp. in children (headache, nausea, vomiting, visual disturbances). **Topical:** Possible tumorigenic potential when combined with ultraviolet radiation.

NURSING CONSIDERATIONS

BASELINE ASSESSMENT

PO: Inform women of childbearing potential of risk to fetus if pregnancy occurs. Instruct on need for use of 2 reliable forms of contraceptives concurrently during therapy and for 1 mo after discontinuation of therapy, even in infertile women. Pregnancy test should be obtained within 1 wk before institution of therapy. Obtain initial serum hepatic function tests, cholesterol, triglyceride levels.

INTERVENTION/EVALUATION

PO: Monitor serum hepatic function tests, hematologic, coagulation profiles, cholesterol, triglycerides. Monitor for signs/symptoms of pseudotumor cerebri in children.

PATIENT/FAMILY TEACHING

• **Topical:** Avoid exposure to sunlight, tanning beds; use sunscreens, protective clothing. • Protect affected areas from wind, cold. • If skin is already sunburned, do not use drug until fully healed. • Keep tretinoin away from eyes, mouth, angles of nose, mucous membranes. • Do not use medicated, drying, abrasive soaps; wash face no more than 2–3 times a day with gentle soap. • Avoid use of preparations containing alcohol, menthol, spice, lime (e.g., shaving lotions, astringents, perfume). • Mild redness, peeling are expected; decrease frequency or discontinue medication if excessive reaction occurs. • Nonmedicated cosmetics may be used; however, cosmetics must be removed before tretinoin application. • Improvement noted during first 24 wks of therapy. • **Antiacne:** Therapeutic results noted in 2–3 wks; optimal results in 6 wks. **Oral:** • Avoid tasks requiring motor skills, alertness until response to drug is established. • Avoid alcohol. • Avoid exposure to sunlight, tanning beds. • Report persistent vomiting, diarrhea, unusual bleeding/bruising, acute abdominal pain, vision changes, or if pregnancy is suspected.

triamcinolone

trye-am-**sin**-oh-lone

triamcinolone acetonide

(Kenalog, Kenalog-10, Kenalog-40, <u>Nasacort AQ</u>, Triderm)

triamcinolone hexacetonide

(Aristospan)

Do not confuse Nasacort with Nasalcrom.

FIXED-COMBINATION(S)

Myco-II, Mycolog II, Myco-Triacet: triamcinolone/nystatin (an antifungal): 0.1%/100,000 units/g.

◆CLASSIFICATION

PHARMACOTHERAPEUTIC: Adrenocortical steroid. **CLINICAL:** Antiinflammatory (see pp. 3C, 100C, 102C).

ACTION

Inhibits accumulation of inflammatory cells at inflammation sites, phagocytosis, lysosomal enzyme release, synthesis/release of mediators of inflammation. **Therapeutic Effect:** Prevents/suppresses cell-mediated immune reactions. Decreases/prevents tissue response to inflammatory process.

USES

Nasal inhalation: Seasonal, perennial rhinitis. **Intra-articular:** Acute gouty arthritis, bursitis, tenosynovitis, epicondylitis, rheumatoid arthritis, synovitis of osteoarthritis. **Intralesional:** Alopecia areata, discoid lupus erythematosus, keloids, lichen plaques, psoriatic plaques. **Topical:** Relief of inflammation, pruritus associated with corticoid-responsive dermatoses.

PRECAUTIONS

Contraindications: Systemic fungal infections, cerebral malaria, serious infections. **IM:** Idiopathic thrombocytopenic purpura. **Topical:** Local fungal, viral, bacterial infections. **Cautions:** Administration of live virus vaccines, following acute MI, elderly, hepatic impairment, myasthenia gravis, pts at risk for osteoporosis/seizures/GI disease, history of tuberculosis (may reactivate disease), hypothyroidism, cirrhosis, HF, hypertension, renal insufficiency, diabetes. Prolonged therapy should be discontinued slowly. **Pregnancy Category C (D if used in first trimester).**

INTERACTIONS

DRUG: Amphotericin, diuretics may worsen hypokalemia. May increase risk of **digoxin** toxicity (due to hypokalemia). May decrease effects of **insulin, oral hypoglycemics**. Hepatic enzyme **inducers (e.g., phenytoin, rifampin)** may decrease effects. May reduce response to **vaccines** due to inhibition of antibody response. **HERBAL: Echinacea** may decrease effect. **FOOD:** None known. **LAB VALUES:** May increase serum glucose, lipid, amylase, sodium. May decrease serum calcium, potassium, thyroxine.

AVAILABILITY (Rx)

Cream: 0.025%, 0.1%. **Injection, Suspension (Kenalog-10):** 10 mg/ml. **(Kenalog-40):** 40 mg/ml. **Ointment:** 0.025%, 0.1%, 0.5%. **Paste, Oral, Topical:** 0.1%. **Suspension, Spray Nasal Inhalation (Nasacort AQ):** 55 mcg/inhalation.

ADMINISTRATION/HANDLING

Topical
• Gently cleanse area before application.
• Use occlusive dressings only as ordered.
• Apply sparingly, rub into area thoroughly.

INDICATIONS/ROUTES/DOSAGE

Triamcinolone Hexacetonide
Intralesional: Up to 0.5 mg/square inch. Range: 2–48 mg.
Intra-Articular: Average dose: 2–20 mg q3–4 wks.

Triamcinolone Acetonide
Intra-Articular: ADULTS, ELDERLY: Initially: 2–20 mg/day. Doses can be adjusted between 20–80 mg as needed.

Rhinitis
Intranasal: ADULTS, ELDERLY, CHILDREN 12 YRS AND OLDER: Initially, 220 mcg/day as 2 sprays in each nostril once daily. Maintenance: 110 mcg/day as 1 spray in each nostril once daily. **CHILDREN 6–11 YRS:** Initially, 110 mcg/day as 1 spray in each nostril once daily. **Maximum:** 2 sprays in each nostril once daily. **CHILDREN 2–5 YRS:** 110 mcg/day as 1 spray in each nostril once daily.

Usual Topical Dosage
Topical: ADULTS, ELDERLY, CHILDREN: 2–3 times a day. May give 1–2 times a day or as intermittent therapy.

SIDE EFFECTS

Frequent: Insomnia, dry mouth, heartburn, nervousness, abdominal distention, diaphoresis, acne, mood swings, increased appetite, facial flushing, delayed wound healing, increased susceptibility to infection, diarrhea, constipation. **Occasional:** Headache, edema, change in skin color, frequent urination. **Rare:** Tachycardia, allergic reaction (rash, urticaria), altered mental status, hallucinations, depression. **Topical:** Allergic contact dermatitis.

ADVERSE EFFECTS/ TOXIC REACTIONS

Long-term therapy: Muscle wasting (arms, legs), osteoporosis, spontaneous fractures, amenorrhea, cataracts, glaucoma, peptic ulcer, HF. **Abrupt withdrawal following long-term therapy:** Anorexia, nausea, fever, headache, arthralgia, rebound inflammation, fatigue, weakness, lethargy, dizziness, orthostatic hypotension. Anaphylaxis occurs rarely with parenteral administration. Sudden discontinuation may be fatal. Blindness has occurred rarely after intralesional injection around face, head.

NURSING CONSIDERATIONS

BASELINE ASSESSMENT

Question for hypersensitivity to any corticosteroids. Obtain baselines for height, weight, B/P, serum glucose, electrolytes.

INTERVENTION/EVALUATION

Oral inhalation, intranasal: Check mucous membranes for signs of fungal infection. Monitor growth in children. Monitor B/P.

PATIENT/FAMILY TEACHING

• Report if condition being treated persists or worsens. • Avoid exposure to chickenpox or measles. • Avoid alcohol. • **Inhalation:** Do not take for acute asthma attack. • Rinse mouth to decrease risk of mouth soreness. • Report oropharyngeal lesions or soreness (stomatitis). • **Nasal:** Report unusual cough/ spasm, persistent nasal bleeding, burning, infection.

triamterene

trye-**am**-ter-een
(Dyrenium)

BLACK BOX ALERT Hyperkalemia risk, potentially fatal if uncorrected; increased incidence in renal impairment, diabetes (even without evidence of diabetic nephropathy), elderly, severely ill pts.
Do not confuse Dyrenium with Pyridium, or triamterene with trimipramine.

FIXED-COMBINATION(S)

Dyazide, Maxzide: triamterene/ hydrochlorothiazide (a diuretic): 37.5 mg/25 mg, 50 mg/25 mg, 75 mg/50 mg.

◆CLASSIFICATION

PHARMACOTHERAPEUTIC: Potassium-sparing diuretic. **CLINICAL:** Antiedema agent, antihypertensive (see p. 105C).

T

ACTION

Inhibits sodium, potassium, ATPase. Interferes with sodium/potassium exchange in distal tubule, cortical collecting tubule, collecting duct. Increases sodium, decreases potassium excretion. Increases magnesium, decreases calcium loss. **Therapeutic Effect:** Produces diuresis, lowers B/P.

PHARMACOKINETICS

Route	Onset	Peak	Duration
PO	2–4 hrs	N/A	7–9 hrs

Incompletely absorbed from GI tract. Widely distributed. Metabolized in liver. Primarily eliminated in feces via biliary route. **Half-life:** 1.5–2.5 hrs (increased in renal impairment).

USES

Treatment of edema, hypertension. Decreases potassium excretion caused by kaliuretic diuretics.

PRECAUTIONS

Contraindications: Drug-induced or preexisting hyperkalemia, progressive or severe renal disease, severe hepatic disease. **Cautions:** Hepatic/renal impairment, history of renal calculi, diabetes mellitus, gouty arthritis.

⧗ LIFESPAN CONSIDERATIONS

Pregnancy/Lactation: Drug crosses placenta; distributed in breast milk. Breastfeeding not recommended. **Pregnancy Category B (D if used in pregnancy-induced hypertension). Children:** Safety and efficacy not established. **Elderly:** May be at increased risk for developing hyperkalemia.

INTERACTIONS

DRUG: ACE inhibitors (e.g., captopril), cyclosporine, potassium-containing medications, potassium supplements may increase risk of hyperkalemia. May decrease clearance, increase risk of toxicity of **lithium**. NSAIDs may decrease antihypertensive

effect. **HERBAL:** None significant. **FOOD:** None known. **LAB VALUES:** May increase urinary calcium excretion, BUN, serum glucose, calcium, magnesium, creatinine, potassium, uric acid. May decrease serum sodium.

AVAILABILITY (Rx)

Capsules: 50 mg, 100 mg.

ADMINISTRATION/HANDLING

PO
• Give with food if GI disturbance occurs.

INDICATIONS/ROUTES/DOSAGE

Edema, Hypertension
PO: ADULTS, ELDERLY: 25–100 mg/day as single dose or in 2 divided doses. **Maximum:** 300 mg/day. **CHILDREN:** 1–2 mg/kg/day as single dose or in 2 divided doses. **Maximum:** 3–4 mg/kg/day or 300 mg/day.

SIDE EFFECTS

Occasional: Fatigue, nausea, diarrhea, abdominal pain, leg cramps, headache. **Rare:** Anorexia, asthenia (loss of strength, energy), rash, dizziness.

ADVERSE EFFECTS/ TOXIC REACTIONS

May result in hyponatremia (drowsiness, dry mouth, increased thirst, lack of energy), severe hyperkalemia (irritability, anxiety, heaviness of legs, paresthesia, hypotension, bradycardia, EKG changes [tented T waves, widening QRS complex, ST segment depression]), particularly in those with renal impairment, diabetes, elderly, severely ill. Agranulocytosis, nephrolithiasis, thrombocytopenia occur rarely.

NURSING CONSIDERATIONS

BASELINE ASSESSMENT

Obtain baseline B/P. Assess baseline serum electrolytes, particularly check for hypokalemia. Assess serum renal/hepatic function tests. Assess for edema (note location, extent), skin turgor, mucous membranes for hydration status. Assess muscle strength, mental status. Note skin temperature, moisture. Obtain baseline weight. Initiate strict I&O. Note pulse rate, regularity.

INTERVENTION/EVALUATION

Monitor B/P, vital signs, serum electrolytes (particularly potassium), I&O, weight. Watch for changes from initial assessment (hyperkalemia may result in muscle strength changes, tremor, muscle cramps), altered mental status (orientation, alertness, confusion), cardiac arrhythmias. Weigh daily. Note extent of diuresis. Assess lung sounds for rhonchi, wheezing.

PATIENT/FAMILY TEACHING

• Take medication in morning. • Expect increased urinary volume, frequency. • Therapeutic effect takes several days to begin and can last for several days when drug is discontinued. • Avoid prolonged exposure to sunlight. • Report severe, persistent weakness, headache, dry mouth, nausea, vomiting, fever, sore throat, unusual bleeding/bruising. • Avoid excessive intake of food high in potassium, salt substitutes.

---

trifluoperazine

trye-floo-oh-**per**-a-zeen
(Apo-Trifluoperazine ✦, Novo-Trifluzine ✦, PMS-Trifluoperazine ✦)

BLACK BOX ALERT Elderly pts with dementia-related psychosis are at increased risk for death.
Do not confuse trifluoperazine with triflupromazine or trihexyphenidyl.

◆CLASSIFICATION

PHARMACOTHERAPEUTIC: Phenothiazine derivative. **CLINICAL:** Antipsychotic, antianxiety (see p. 67C).

ACTION

Blocks dopamine at postsynaptic receptor sites. Possesses strong extrapyrami-dal, antiemetic effects, weak anticholinergic, sedative effects. **Therapeutic Effect:** Suppresses behavioral response in psychosis; reduces locomotor activity, aggressiveness.

PHARMACOKINETICS

Readily absorbed following PO administration. Protein binding: 90%–99%. Metabolized in liver. Excreted in urine. **Half-life:** 24 hrs.

USES

Treatment of schizophrenia, generalized nonpsychotic anxiety. **OFF-LABEL:** Psychotic disorders, behavioral symptoms associated with dementia behavior, psychosis/agitation related to Alzheimer's dementia.

PRECAUTIONS

Contraindications: Severe CNS depression, bone marrow suppression, blood dyscrasias, severe hepatic disease, coma. **Cautions:** Seizure disorder, severe cardiac/renal disease, pts at risk for pneumonia, hypotensive episodes, decreased GI motility, urinary retention, BPH, visual problems, narrow-angle glaucoma, myasthenia gravis, Parkinsons disease, elderly.

⌛ LIFESPAN CONSIDERATIONS

Pregnancy/Lactation: Drug crosses placenta; is distributed in breast milk. **Pregnancy Category C. Children:** Safety and efficacy not established in those younger than 2 yrs. **Elderly:** Higher risk of sedative, anticholinergic, extrapyramidal, hypotensive effects.

INTERACTIONS

DRUG: Alcohol, other CNS depressants may increase CNS, respiratory depression, hypotensive effects. **Extrapyramidal symptom (EPS)–producing medications** may increase extrapyramidal symptoms. **Hypotensive agents** may increase hypotension. **MAOIs, tricyclic antidepressants** may increase anticholinergic, sedative effects. **HERBAL: Gotu kola, kava kava, St. John's wort, valerian**

T

✦ Canadian trade name   ● Non-Crushable Drug   **HIGH ALERT** High Alert drug

may increase CNS depression. **Dong quai, St. John's wort** may increase photosensitization. **FOOD:** None known. **LAB VALUES:** May cause EKG changes.

AVAILABILITY (Rx)

Tablets: 1 mg, 2 mg, 5 mg, 10 mg.

ADMINISTRATION/HANDLING

PO

• May give with food to decrease GI effects. • Do not take within 2 hrs of any antacids.

INDICATIONS/ROUTES/DOSAGE

Schizophrenia
PO: ADULTS, ELDERLY, CHILDREN 12 YRS AND OLDER: Initially, 2–5 mg 1–2 times a day. **Range:** 15–20 mg/day. **Maximum:** 40 mg/day. **CHILDREN 6–11 YRS:** Initially, 1 mg 1–2 times a day. **Maintenance:** Up to 15 mg/day.

Nonpsychotic Anxiety
PO: ADULTS, ELDERLY: 1–2 mg 2 times/ day. **Maximum:** 6 mg/day. Therapy should not exceed 12 wks.

SIDE EFFECTS

Frequent: Hypotension, dizziness, syncope (occur frequently after first injection, occasionally after subsequent injections, rarely with oral form). **Occasional:** Drowsiness during early therapy, dry mouth, blurred vision, lethargy, constipation, diarrhea, nasal congestion, peripheral edema, urinary retention. **Rare:** Ocular changes, altered skin pigmentation (in those taking high doses for prolonged periods), photosensitivity.

ADVERSE EFFECTS/ TOXIC REACTIONS

Extrapyramidal symptoms appear to be dose-related (particularly high doses) and are divided into 3 categories: akathisia (inability to sit still, tapping of feet); parkinsonian symptoms (mask-like face, tremors, shuffling gait, hypersalivation); acute dystonias: torticollis (neck muscle spasm), opisthotonos (rigidity of back muscles),

oculogyric crisis (rolling back of eyes). Dystonic reaction may produce diaphoresis, pallor. Tardive dyskinesia (tongue protrusion, puffing of cheeks, chewing/puckering of the mouth) occurs rarely (may be irreversible). Abrupt withdrawal after long-term therapy may precipitate nausea, vomiting, gastritis, dizziness, tremors. Blood dyscrasias, particularly agranulocytosis, mild leukopenia may occur. May lower seizure threshold.

NURSING CONSIDERATIONS

BASELINE ASSESSMENT

Assess behavior, appearance, emotional status, response to environment, speech pattern, thought content.

INTERVENTION/EVALUATION

Monitor B/P for hypotension. Assess for EPS. Monitor WBC for blood dyscrasias. Monitor for fine tongue movement (may be early sign of tardive dyskinesia); tremor; gait changes; abnormal movement in trunk, neck, extremities. Supervise suicidal-risk pt closely during early therapy (as depression lessens, energy level improves, increasing suicide potential). Monitor target behaviors. Assess for therapeutic response (interest in surroundings, improvement in self-care, increased ability to concentrate, relaxed facial expression).

PATIENT/FAMILY TEACHING

• Do not take antacids within 2 hrs of tri-fluoperazine. • Avoid alcohol. • Avoid excessive exposure to sunlight, artificial light. • Avoid tasks that require alertness, motor skills until response to drug is established (may cause drowsiness). • Rise slowly from lying or sitting position (prevents hypotension).

trihexyphenidyl

trye-hex-ee-**fen**-i-dil
(PMS-Trihexyphenidyl)

Do not confuse trihexiphenidyl with trifluoperazine.

◆CLASSIFICATION

PHARMACOTHERAPEUTIC: Anticholinergic. **CLINICAL:** Antiparkinson agent.

ACTION

Blocks central cholinergic receptors (aids in balancing cholinergic and dopaminergic activity). **Therapeutic Effect:** Decreases salivation, relaxes smooth muscle.

USES

Adjunctive treatment for all forms of Parkinson's disease, including postencephalitic, arteriosclerotic, idiopathic types. Controls symptoms of drug-induced extrapyramidal symptoms (EPS).

PRECAUTIONS

Contraindications: None known. **Cautions:** Glaucoma, renal/hepatic impairment, cardiovascular disease, prostatic hyperplasia, obstructive diseases of GI tract, excessive activity during hot weather, exercise. **Pregnancy Category C.**

INTERACTIONS

DRUG: Alcohol, CNS depressants may increase sedative effect. **Amantadine, anticholinergics, MAOIs** may increase anticholinergic effects. **HERBAL:** None significant. **FOOD:** None known. **LAB VALUES:** None significant.

AVAILABILITY (Rx)

Elixir: 2 mg/5 ml. **Tablets:** 2 mg, 5 mg.

ADMINISTRATION/HANDLING

PO

• Administer with food, water to decrease GI irritation.

INDICATIONS/ROUTES/DOSAGE

Parkinsonism
PO: ADULTS, ELDERLY: Initially, 1 mg on first day. May increase by 2 mg/day at 3- to 5-day intervals up to 6–10 mg/day (12–15 mg/day in pts with postencephalitic parkinsonism).

Drug-Induced Extrapyramidal Symptoms
PO: ADULTS, ELDERLY: Initially, 1 mg/day. **Range:** 5–15 mg/day in 3–4 divided doses.

SIDE EFFECTS

◀**ALERT**▶ Those older than 60 yrs tend to develop mental confusion, disorientation, agitation, psychotic-like symptoms. **Frequent:** Drowsiness, dry mouth. **Occasional:** Blurred vision, urinary retention, constipation, dizziness, headache, muscle cramps. **Rare:** Skin rash, seizures, depression.

ADVERSE EFFECTS/ TOXIC REACTIONS

Hypersensitivity reaction (eczema, pruritus, rash, cardiac arrhythmias, photosensitivity) may occur. Overdosage may vary from CNS depression (sedation, apnea, cardiovascular collapse, death) to severe paradoxical reaction (hallucinations, tremor, seizures).

NURSING CONSIDERATIONS

INTERVENTION/EVALUATION

Be alert to neurologic effects (headache, lethargy, mental confusion, agitation). Monitor elderly closely for paradoxical reaction. Assess for clinical reversal of symptoms (improvement of tremor of head/hands at rest, mask-like facial expression, shuffling gait, muscular rigidity).

PATIENT/FAMILY TEACHING

• Take after meals or with food. • Do not stop medication abruptly. • Inform physician if GI effects, palpitations, eye pain, rash, fever, heat intolerance occur. • Avoid alcohol, other CNS depressants. • May cause dry mouth, drowsiness. • Avoid tasks that require alertness, motor skills until response to drug is established. • Difficulty urinating, constipation may occur (inform physician if they persist).

T

---

trimethoprim

trye-**meth**-oh-prim
(Apo-Trimethoprim ✢, Primsol)

FIXED-COMBINATION(S)

Bactrim, Septra: trimethoprim/sulfamethoxazole (a sulfonamide): 16 mg/80 mg/ml (injection), 40 mg/200 mg/5 ml (suspension), 80 mg/400 mg, 160 mg/800 mg (tablets).

◆CLASSIFICATION

PHARMACOTHERAPEUTIC: Folate antagonist. **CLINICAL:** Antibacterial.

ACTION

Blocks bacterial biosynthesis of nucleic acids, proteins by interfering with metabolism of folinic acid. **Therapeutic Effect:** Bacteriostatic.

PHARMACOKINETICS

Rapidly, completely absorbed from GI tract. Protein binding: 42%–46%. Widely distributed, including to CSF. Metabolized in liver. Primarily excreted in urine. Moderately removed by hemodialysis. **Half-life:** 8–10 hrs (increased in renal impairment, newborns; decreased in children).

USES

Treatment of UTI caused by susceptible strains of *E. coli, P. mirabilis, K. pneumoniae.* Treatment of acute otitis media due to *H. influenzae, S. pneumoniae.* **OFF-LABEL:** Treatment of pneumonia caused by *Pneumocystis jiroveci.*

PRECAUTIONS

Contraindications: Megaloblastic anemia due to folic acid deficiency. **Cautions:** Renal/hepatic impairment, pts with folic acid deficiency.

⌛ LIFESPAN CONSIDERATIONS

Pregnancy/Lactation: Drug readily crosses placenta; is distributed in breast milk. **Pregnancy Category C. Children:** Safety and efficacy not established. **Elderly:** No age-related precautions noted. May increase incidence of thrombocytopenia.

INTERACTIONS

DRUG: Folate antagonists (e.g., methotrexate) may increase risk of megaloblastic anemia. May increase levels/side effects of **phenytoin. HERBAL:** None significant. **FOOD:** None known. **LAB VALUES:** May increase BUN, serum bilirubin, creatinine, AST, ALT.

AVAILABILITY (Rx)

Oral Solution (Primsol): 50 mg/5 ml. **Tablets:** 100 mg.

ADMINISTRATION/HANDLING

PO
• Space doses evenly to maintain constant therapeutic level. • Give without regard to meals (if GI upset occurs, give with food).

INDICATIONS/ROUTES/DOSAGE

UTI
PO: ADULTS, ELDERLY, CHILDREN 12 YRS AND OLDER: 100 mg q12h or 200 mg once daily for 10–14 days. **CHILDREN YOUNGER THAN 12 YRS:** 4–6 mg/kg/day in 2 divided doses for 10 days.

Otitis Media
PO: CHILDREN, 6 MOS AND OLDER: 10 mg/kg/day in divided doses q12h for 10 days. **Maximum:** 400 mg/day.

***Pneumocystis jiroveci* Pneumonia (PCP)**
ADULTS, ELDERLY, CHILDREN 12 YRS AND OLDER: 15–20 mg/kg/day in 3 divided doses for 21 days in combination with dapsone.

Dosage in Renal Impairment
Dosage and frequency are modified based on creatinine clearance.

Creatinine Clearance	Dosage
Greater than 30 ml/min	No change
15–30 ml/min	50 mg q12h
Less than 15 ml/min	Avoid use

SIDE EFFECTS

Occasional: Nausea, vomiting, diarrhea, decreased appetite, abdominal cramps, headache. **Rare:** Hypersensitivity reaction (pruritus, rash), methemoglobinemia (bluish fingernails, lips, skin; fever; pale skin; sore throat; asthenia [loss of strength, energy]), photosensitivity.

ADVERSE EFFECTS/ TOXIC REACTIONS

Stevens-Johnson syndrome, erythema multiforme, exfoliative dermatitis, anaphylaxis occur rarely. Hematologic toxicity (thrombocytopenia, neutropenia, leukopenia, megaloblastic anemia) more likely to occur in elderly, debilitated, alcoholics, those with renal impairment or receiving prolonged high dosage.

NURSING CONSIDERATIONS

BASELINE ASSESSMENT
Assess hematology baseline reports, serum renal function tests.

INTERVENTION/EVALUATION
Assess skin for rash. Evaluate food tolerance. Monitor serum hematology reports, renal/hepatic function test results. Check for developing signs of hematologic toxicity (pallor, fever, sore throat, malaise, bleeding/bruising).

PATIENT/FAMILY TEACHING
• Space doses evenly. • Complete full length of therapy (10–14 days). • May take on empty stomach or with food if stomach upset occurs. • Avoid sun, ultraviolet light; use sunscreen, wear protective clothing. • Immediately report pallor, fatigue, sore throat, bruising/ bleeding, discoloration of skin, fever, rash.

triptorelin

trip-toe-**rel**-in
(Trelstar, Trelstar Depot, Trelstar LA)

◆**CLASSIFICATION**
PHARMACOTHERAPEUTIC: Gonadotropin-releasing hormone analogue. **CLINICAL:** Antineoplastic.

ACTION

Through a negative feedback mechanism, inhibits gonadotropin hormone secretion. Circulating levels of luteinizing hormone (LH), follicle-stimulating hormone (FSH), testosterone, estradiol rise initially, then subside with continued therapy. **Therapeutic Effect:** Suppresses growth of abnormal prostate tissue.

USES

Treatment of advanced prostate cancer (alternate to orchiectomy or estrogen administration). **OFF-LABEL:** Treatment of endometriosis, precocious puberty, uterine sarcoma.

PRECAUTIONS

Contraindications: Hypersensitivity to luteinizing hormone-releasing hormone (LHRH), LHRH agonists, pregnancy. **Cautions:** None known.

⧖ LIFESPAN CONSIDERATIONS

Pregnancy/Lactation: Unknown if distributed in breast milk. **Pregnancy Category X. Children:** Safety and efficacy not established. **Elderly:** No age-related precautions noted.

INTERACTIONS

DRUG: None significant. **HERBAL:** None significant. **FOOD:** None known. **LAB VALUES:** May alter serum pituitary-gonadal function test results. May cause transient increase in serum testosterone, usually during first wk of treatment.

T

AVAILABILITY (Rx)

Injection, Powder for Reconstitution (Trelstar Depot): 3.75 mg. Injection, Powder for Reconstitution (Trelstar LA): 11.25 mg, 22.5 mg.

ADMINISTRATION/HANDLING

IM

• Reconstitute with 2 ml Sterile Water for Injection. • Administer into large muscle mass, esp. gluteus muscle, alternating injection sites.

INDICATIONS/ROUTES/DOSAGE

Prostate Cancer
IM *(Trelstar Depot)*: **ADULTS, ELDERLY:** 3.75 mg once q4wks.
IM *(Trelstar LA)*: **ADULTS, ELDERLY:** 11.25 mg q12wks, 22.5 mg q24wks.

SIDE EFFECTS

Frequent (Greater Than 5%): Hot flashes, skeletal pain, headache, impotence. **Occasional (5%–2%):** Insomnia, vomiting, leg pain, fatigue. **Rare (Less Than 2%):** Dizziness, emotional lability, diarrhea, urinary retention, UTI, anemia, pruritus.

ADVERSE EFFECTS/ TOXIC REACTIONS

Bladder outlet obstruction, skeletal pain, hematuria, spinal cord compression with weakness, paralysis of lower extremities may occur.

NURSING CONSIDERATIONS

INTERVENTION/EVALUATION

Obtain serum testosterone, prostate-specific antigen (PSA), prostatic acid phosphatase (PAP) levels periodically during therapy. Serum testosterone, PAP levels should increase during first wk of therapy. Testosterone level then should decrease to baseline level or less within 2 wks, PAP level within 4 wks. Monitor pt closely for worsening signs and symptoms of prostatic cancer, esp. during first wk of therapy (due to transient increase in testosterone).

PATIENT/FAMILY TEACHING

• Do not miss monthly injections. • May experience increased skeletal pain, blood in urine, urinary retention initially (subsides within 1 wk). • Hot flashes may occur. • Report tachycardia, persistent nausea/vomiting, numbness of arms/legs, pain/swelling of breasts, difficulty breathing, infection at injection site.

trospium

tro-spee-um
(Sanctura, Sanctura XR, Trosec ✦)

◆CLASSIFICATION

PHARMACOTHERAPEUTIC: Anticholinergic. **CLINICAL:** Antispasmotic.

ACTION

Antagonizes effect of acetylcholine on muscarinic receptors, producing para-sympatholytic action. **Therapeutic Effect:** Reduces smooth muscle tone in bladder.

PHARMACOKINETICS

Minimally absorbed after PO administration. Protein binding: 50%–85%. Distributed in plasma. Excreted in feces (82%), urine (6%). **Half-life:** 20 hrs.

USES

Treatment of overactive bladder with symptoms of urge urinary incontinence, urgency, urinary frequency.

PRECAUTIONS

Contraindications: Gastric retention, uncontrolled narrow-angle glaucoma, urinary retention. **Cautions:** Decreased GI motility, renal/hepatic impairment, obstructive GI disorders, ulcerative colitis, intestinal atony, myasthenia gravis, controlled narrow-angle glaucoma, significant bladder obstruction, Alzheimer's disease, hot weather/exercise, elderly.

⧗ LIFESPAN CONSIDERATIONS

Pregnancy/Lactation: Unknown if drug crosses placenta or is distributed in breast milk. **Pregnancy Category C. Children:** Safety and efficacy not established. **Elderly:** Higher incidence of dry mouth, constipation, dyspepsia, UTI, urinary retention in those 75 yrs and older.

INTERACTIONS

DRUG: Other anticholinergic agents increase severity, frequency of side effects, may alter absorption of other drugs due to anticholinergic effects on GI motility. **Morphine, procainamide, tenofovir, vancomycin** may increase concentration. **HERBAL:** None significant. **FOOD: High-fat meals** may reduce absorption. **LAB VALUES:** None significant.

AVAILABILITY (Rx)

🔖 Tablets (Sanctura): 20 mg. 🔖 Capsules, Extended-Release (Sanctura XR): 60 mg.

ADMINISTRATION/HANDLING

PO

• Store at room temperature. • Give at least 1 hr before meals or on an empty stomach. • Do not crush, break tablet, extended-release capsule; swallow whole. • Administer tablets at bedtime, capsules in morning with full glass of water, 1 hr before eating.

INDICATIONS/ROUTES/DOSAGE

Overactive Bladder

PO: ADULTS: 20 mg twice daily. **ELDERLY 75 YRS AND OLDER:** 20 mg once daily at bedtime. **Extended-release:** 60 mg once daily.

Dosage in Renal Impairment

For pts with creatinine clearance less than 30 ml/min, dosage reduced to 20 mg once daily at bedtime. Extended-release not recommended.

SIDE EFFECTS

Frequent (20%): Dry mouth. **Occasional (10%–4%):** Constipation, headache. **Rare (Less Than 2%):** Fatigue, upper abdominal pain, dyspepsia (heartburn, indigestion, epigastric pain), flatulence, dry eyes, urinary retention.

ADVERSE EFFECTS/TOXIC REACTIONS

Overdose may result in severe anticholinergic effects, characterized by nervousness, restlessness, nausea, vomiting, confusion, diaphoresis, facial flushing, hypertension, hypotension, respiratory depression, irritability, lacrimation. Supraventricular tachycardia and hallucinations occur rarely.

NURSING CONSIDERATIONS

BASELINE ASSESSMENT

Assess for presence of dysuria, urinary urgency, frequency, incontinence.

INTERVENTION/EVALUATION

Monitor for symptomatic relief. Monitor I&O; palpate bladder for retention. Monitor daily pattern of bowel activity, stool consistency. Dry mouth may be relieved by sips of tepid water.

PATIENT/FAMILY TEACHING

• Report nausea, vomiting, diaphoresis, increased salivary secretions, palpitations, severe abdominal pain.

T

ustekinumab

yoo-ste-**kin**-ue-mab
(Stelara)
**Do not confuse Stelara with
Aldara, or ustekinumab with in-
fliximab or rituximab.**

◆ CLASSIFICATION

PHARMACOTHERAPEUTIC: Monoclonal antibody. **CLINICAL:** Antipsoriasis
agent.

ACTION

Strongly binds with cellular components
involved in responses to inflammation
and immune system, thereby decreasing
likelihood of aggravating psoriatic eruptions. **Therapeutic Effect:** Significantly
slows growth, migration of circulating
total lymphocytes (predominant in psoriatic lesions).

PHARMACOKINETICS

Following subcutaneous injections, clearance is affected by body weight, is not affected by gender or race. Degraded into
small peptides and amino acids via catabolic pathways. Serum concentration
reaches steady state at 28 wks. **Half-life:**
10–126 days.

USES

Treatment of adults 18 yrs or older with
moderate to severe plaque psoriasis who
are candidates for systemic therapy or
phototherapy. Treatment of active psoriatic arthritis alone or in combination
with methotrexate.

PRECAUTIONS

Contraindications: None known. **Cautions:** History of chronic infection, recurrent infection, active tuberculosis, prior
malignancy, renal/hepatic impairment.
Avoid use of live vaccines.

⧗ LIFESPAN CONSIDERATIONS

Pregnancy/Lactation: Unknown if distributed in breast milk. **Pregnancy Category B. Children:** Not indicated for use
in this pt population. **Elderly:** Age-related increased incidence of infection
requires cautious use.

INTERACTIONS:

DRUG: Immunosuppressive agents
increase risk of infection. **Live virus
vaccine** decreases immune response.
Abciximab, trastuzumab may increase
concentration/effects. **HERBAL: Echinacea** may decrease concentration/effects.
FOOD: None known. **LAB VALUES:** May
increase lymphocyte count.

AVAILABILITY (Rx)

Injection Solution: 45 mg/0.5 ml.

ADMINISTRATION/HANDLING

Subcutaneous
• Do not inject into areas where skin is
tender, bruised, erythematous, indu-
rated. • Administer into thigh, abdomen,
buttocks, upper arm. • Refrigerate unopened vial. • Solution appears colorless
to light yellow. Discard if solution contains more than a few small translucent
or white particles or is cloudy.

INDICATIONS/ROUTES/DOSAGE

Plaque Psoriasis
**Subcutaneous: ADULTS,   ELDERLY
WEIGHING 100 KG OR LESS:** Initially, 45 mg,
then 45 mg 4 wks later, followed by 45
mg every 12 wks. **WEIGHING MORE THAN
100 KG:** Initially, 90 mg, then 90 mg 4 wks
later, followed by 90 mg every 12 wks.

Psoriatic Arthritis
Subcutaneous: ADULTS, ELDERLY: Initially, 45 mg repeated in 4 wks followed
by 45 mg q12wks. **PTS WITH COEXISTENT
MODERATE TO SEVERE PLAQUE PSORIASIS
WEIGHING MORE THAN 100 KG:** Initially, 90
mg repeated in 4 wks, then 90 mg
q12wks.

SIDE EFFECTS

Occasional (8%–4%): Nasopharyngitis, upper respiratory tract infection, headache. **Rare (3%–1%):** Fatigue, diarrhea, back pain, dizziness, pruritus, injection site erythema, myalgia, depression.

ADVERSE EFFECTS/ TOXIC REACTIONS

Worsening of psoriasis, thrombocytopenia, malignancies, serious infections (cellulitis, diverticulitis, gastroenteritis, pneumonia, osteomyelitis, UTI, postoperative wound infection) have been noted. Reversible posterior leukoencephalopathy syndrome (headache, seizures, confusion, visual disturbances) occurs rarely.

NURSING CONSIDERATIONS

BASELINE ASSESSMENT

Pts should not receive live vaccines during treatment, 1 yr prior to initiating treatment, or 1 yr following discontinuation of treatment. Inform pt of duration of treatment and required monitoring procedures. Assess skin prior to therapy; document extent and location of psoriasis lesions. Test pt for tuberculosis infection prior to initiating treatment.

INTERVENTION/EVALUATION

Closely monitor for signs/symptoms of active tuberculosis during and after treatment. Assess skin throughout therapy for evidence of improvement of psoriasis lesions. Monitor for worsening of lesions.

PATIENT/FAMILY TEACHING

• If appropriate, pt may self-inject after proper training in preparation and injection technique. • Inform physician if signs of infection occurs. • If new diagnosis of malignancy occurs, inform physician of current treatment with ustekinumab.

U

valacyclovir

val-a-**sye**-kloe-veer
(Apo-Valacyclovir ✢, <u>Valtrex</u>)
**Do not confuse valacyclovir with
acyclovir or valganciclovir, or
Valtrex with Valcyte.**

◆CLASSIFICATION

PHARMACOTHERAPEUTIC: Antiviral.
CLINICAL: Antiherpetic agent (see
p. 71C).

ACTION

Converted to acyclovir triphosphate, becoming part of viral DNA chain. **Therapeutic Effect:** Interferes with DNA synthesis, replication of herpes simplex
virus (HSV), varicella-zoster virus (VZV).

PHARMACOKINETICS

Rapidly absorbed after PO administration.
Protein binding: 13%–18%. Rapidly converted by hydrolysis to active compound
acyclovir. Widely distributed to tissues,
body fluids (including CSF). Primarily
eliminated in urine. Removed by hemodialysis. **Half-life:** (acyclovir) 2.5–3.3 hrs
(increased in renal impairment).

USES

Treatment of herpes zoster (shingles)
in immunocompetent adults. Treatment
of initial and recurrent genital herpes in
immunocompetent adults. Prevention of
recurrent genital herpes and reduction of
heterosexual transmission of genital herpes. Suppression of genital herpes in
HIV-infected pts. Treatment of cold sores,
chickenpox in immunocompetent children. **OFF-LABEL:** Prophylaxis and treatment of cancer-related HSV, VZV.

PRECAUTIONS

Contraindications: Hypersensitivity to or
intolerance of acyclovir, valacyclovir, or
their components. **Cautions:** Renal impairment, concurrent use of nephrotoxic
agents.

⌛ LIFESPAN CONSIDERATIONS

Pregnancy/Lactation: May cross placenta. May be distributed in breast milk.
Pregnancy Category B. Children: Safety
and efficacy not established. **Elderly:**
Age-related renal impairment may require dosage adjustment.

INTERACTIONS

**DRUG: Nephrotoxic medications (e.g.,
ACE inhibitors, aminoglycosides, IV
contrast media)** may increase risk of
nephrotoxicity, renal impairment. **HERBAL:**
None significant. **FOOD:** None known. **LAB
VALUES:** None significant.

AVAILABILITY (Rx)

Caplets: 500 mg, 1,000 mg. **Tablets:** 500
mg, 1,000 mg.

ADMINISTRATION/HANDLING

PO
• Give without regard to meals. • If GI
upset occurs, give with meals.

INDICATIONS/ROUTES/DOSAGE

Herpes Zoster (Shingles)
PO: ADULTS, ELDERLY: 1 g 3 times a day
for 7 days.

Herpes Simplex (Cold Sores)
PO: ADULTS, ELDERLY: 2 g twice a day for
1 day (separate by 12 hrs).

Initial Episode of Genital Herpes
PO: ADULTS, ELDERLY: 1 g twice a day for
10 days.

Recurrent Episodes of Genital Herpes
PO: ADULTS, ELDERLY: 500 mg twice a day
for 3 days.

**Suppressive Therapy of Genital Herpes in
HIV-Infected Pts**
PO: ADULTS, ELDERLY: 500 mg twice a day.

Prevention of Genital Herpes
PO: ADULTS, ELDERLY: 500–1,000 mg/day.

Genital Herpes

Creatinine Clearance	Initial Episode	Recurrent Episode	Suppressive Therapy
10–29 ml/min	1 g q24h	500 mg q24h	500 mg q24–48h
Less than 10 ml/min	500 mg q24h	500 mg q24h	500 mg q24–48h

Chickenpox

PO: CHILDREN 2–17 YRS: 20 mg/kg/dose 3 times/day for 5 days. **Maximum:** 1 g/dose.

Dosage in Renal Impairment

Dosage and frequency are modified based on creatinine clearance. **HD:** Give dose postdialysis.

Cold Sores/Herpes Zoster

Creatinine Clearance	Herpes Zoster	Cold Sores
30–49 ml/min	1 g q12h	1 g q12h × 2 doses
10–29 ml/min	1 g q24h	500 mg q12h × 2 doses
Less than 10 ml/min	500 mg q24h	500 mg as single dose

SIDE EFFECTS

Frequent: Herpes zoster (17%–10%): Nausea, headache. **Genital herpes (17%):** Headache. **Occasional: Herpes zoster (7%–3%):** Vomiting, diarrhea, constipation (50 yrs and older), asthenia (loss of strength, energy), dizziness (50 yrs and older). **Genital herpes (8%–3%):** Nausea, diarrhea, dizziness. **Rare: Herpes zoster (3%–1%):** Abdominal pain, anorexia. **Genital herpes (3%–1%):** Asthenia (loss of strength, energy), abdominal pain.

ADVERSE EFFECTS/ TOXIC REACTIONS

Neutropenia, thrombocytopenia, renal failure occur rarely.

NURSING CONSIDERATIONS

BASELINE ASSESSMENT

Question for history of allergies, particularly to valacyclovir, acyclovir. Tissue cultures for herpes zoster, herpes simplex should be obtained before giving first dose (therapy may proceed before results are known). Assess medical history, esp. HIV infection, bone marrow or renal transplantation, renal/hepatic impairment.

INTERVENTION/EVALUATION

Evaluate cutaneous lesions. Monitor serum renal/hepatic function tests, CBC, urinalysis. Provide analgesics, comfort measures for herpes zoster (esp. exhausting to elderly). Encourage fluids. Keep pt's fingernails short, hands clean.

PATIENT/FAMILY TEACHING

• Drink adequate fluids. • Do not touch lesions with fingers to avoid spreading infection to new site. • **Genital herpes:** Continue therapy for full length of treatment. • Space doses evenly. • Avoid sexual intercourse during duration of lesions to prevent infecting partner. • Valacyclovir does not cure herpes. • Notify physician if lesions recur or do not improve. • Pap smears should be done at least annually due to increased risk of cervical cancer in women with genital herpes. • Initiate treatment at first sign of recurrent episode of genital herpes or herpes zoster (early treatment within first 24–48 hrs is imperative for therapeutic results).

valganciclovir

val-gan-**sye**-kloe-veer
(Valcyte)

BLACK BOX ALERT May adversely affect spermatogenesis, fertility. Risk for granulocytopenia, anemia, thrombocytopenia.

Do not confuse Valcyte with Valium or Valtrex, or valganciclovir with valacyclovir.

◆CLASSIFICATION

PHARMACOTHERAPEUTIC: Synthetic nucleoside. **CLINICAL:** Antiviral (see p. 71C).

ACTION

Competes with viral DNA esterases, is incorporated directly into growing viral DNA chains. **Therapeutic Effect:** Interferes with DNA synthesis, viral replication.

PHARMACOKINETICS

Well absorbed, rapidly converted to ganciclovir by intestinal mucosal cells and hepatocytes. Widely distributed including CSF, ocular tissue. Slowly metabolized intracellularly. Primarily excreted in urine. Removed by hemodialysis. **Half-life:** Ganciclovir: 4 hrs (increased in renal impairment).

USES

Adults: Treatment of cytomegalovirus (CMV) retinitis in AIDS. Prevention of CMV disease in high-risk renal, cardiac, renal-pancreas transplant pts. **Children:** Prevention of CMV disease in high-risk renal and cardiac transplant pts.

PRECAUTIONS

Contraindications: Hypersensitivity to acyclovir, ganciclovir. **Cautions:** Extreme caution in children because of long-term carcinogenicity, reproductive toxicity. Renal impairment, concurrent nephrotoxic medications, preexisting bone marrow suppression or cytopenias, history of cytopenic reactions to other drugs, elderly (at greater risk for renal impairment).

⧖ LIFESPAN CONSIDERATIONS

Pregnancy/Lactation: Effective contraception should be used during therapy; valganciclovir should not be used during pregnancy. Avoid breastfeeding; may be resumed no sooner than 72 hrs after last dose of valganciclovir. **Pregnancy Category C. Children:** Safety and efficacy not established in those younger than 12 yrs. **Elderly:** Age-related renal impairment may require dosage adjustment.

INTERACTIONS

DRUG: Bone marrow depressants may increase myelosuppression. May increase risk of toxicity of **didanosine, mycophenolate. Probenecid** may decrease renal clearance, increase concentration. **Zidovudine (AZT)** may increase risk of hematologic toxicity. **HERBAL:** None significant. **FOOD: All foods** maximize drug bioavailability. **LAB VALUES:** May decrease creatinine clearance, platelet count, neutrophils, Hgb, Hct. May increase serum creatinine.

AVAILABILITIES (Rx)

Powder for Oral Solution: 50 mg/ml (100 ml).

⧫ **Tablets:** 450 mg.

ADMINISTRATION/HANDLING

PO

• Do not break, crush tablets; give whole (potential carcinogen). • Avoid contact with skin. • Wash skin with soap, water if contact occurs. • Give with food. • Store oral suspension in refrigerator. Discard after 49 days.

INDICATIONS/ROUTES/DOSAGE

Cytomegalovirus (CMV) Retinitis
PO: ADULTS: Initially, 900 mg (two 450-mg tablets) twice daily for 21 days. **Maintenance:** 900 mg once daily.

Prevention of CMV After Transplant
PO: ADULTS, ELDERLY: 900 mg once daily beginning within 10 days of transplant and continuing until 100 days (heart, kidney, or pancreas transplant) or 200 days (kidney transplant) post-transplant. **CHILDREN 4 MOS–16 YRS:** Once daily based on body surface area (BSA) and creatinine clearance (CrCl) using formula: (Dose = 7 × BSA × CrCl). **Maximum:** 900 mg/day.

Dosage in Renal Impairment
Dosage and frequency are modified based on creatinine clearance.

Creatinine Clearance	Induction Dosage	Maintenance Dosage
60 ml/min or higher	900 mg twice daily	900 mg once daily
40–59 ml/min	450 mg twice daily	450 mg once daily
25–39 ml/min	450 mg once daily	450 mg every 2 days
10–24 ml/min	450 mg every 2 days	450 mg twice a wk

SIDE EFFECTS

Frequent (16%–9%): Diarrhea, neutropenia, headache. **Occasional (8%–3%):** Nausea. **Rare (Less Than 3%):** Insomnia, paresthesia, vomiting, abdominal pain, fever.

ADVERSE EFFECTS/ TOXIC REACTIONS

Hematologic toxicity, including severe neutropenia (most common), anemia, thrombocytopenia, leukopenia, aplastic anemia, pancytopenia, bone marrow suppression may occur. Retinal detachment occurs rarely. Overdose may result in renal toxicity. May decrease sperm production, fertility.

NURSING CONSIDERATIONS

BASELINE ASSESSMENT

Obtain baseline CBC, serum chemistries, renal function, urinalysis. Receive full medication history.

INTERVENTION/EVALUATION

Monitor I&O, ensure adequate hydration (minimum 1,500 ml/24 hrs). Diligently evaluate CBC for decreased WBCs, Hgb, Hct, platelets, changes in urinary characteristics, consistency. Question pt regarding vision, therapeutic improvement, complications.

PATIENT/FAMILY TEACHING

• Valganciclovir provides suppression, not cure, of CMV retinitis. • Frequent blood tests are necessary during therapy because of toxic nature of drug. • Ophthalmologic exam q4–6wks during treatment is advised. • Report any new symptom promptly. • May temporarily or permanently inhibit sperm production in men, suppress fertility in women. • Barrier contraception should be used during and for 90 days after therapy (mutagenic potential). • Avoid handling broken/crushed tablets, oral solution. • Report fever, chills, unusual bleeding/bruising; urinary changes.

valproic acid

val-**pro**-ick **as**-id
(Apo-Divalproex ✤, Depacon, Depakene, <u>Depakote</u>, <u>Depakote ER</u>, Depakote Sprinkle, Novo-Divalproex ✤, Stavzor)

BLACK BOX ALERT Embryo, fetal neural tube defects (spina bifida) have occurred. Life-threatening pancreatitis, complete hepatic failure have occurred.

Do not confuse Depakene with Depakote.

◆ CLASSIFICATION

PHARMACOTHERAPEUTIC: Carboxylic acid derivative. **CLINICAL:** Anticonvulsant, antimanic, antimigraine (see p. 37C).

ACTION

Directly increases concentration of inhibitory neurotransmitter gamma-aminobutyric acid (GABA). **Therapeutic Effect:** Produces anticonvulsant effect, stabilizes mood, prevents migraine headache.

PHARMACOKINETICS

Well absorbed from GI tract. Protein binding: 80%–90%. Metabolized in liver. Primarily excreted in urine. Not removed by hemodialysis. **Half-life:** 9–16 hrs (may be increased in hepatic impairment, elderly, children younger than 18 mos).

USES

Treatment of simple and complex absence (petit mal) seizures (monotherapy

V

preferred due to unpredictable interactions, increased risk of hepatotoxicity). Adjunctive therapy of multiple seizures (**Stavzor**). Treatment of manic episodes with bipolar disorders, complex partial seizures. Prophylaxis of migraine headaches. **OFF-LABEL:** Refractory status epilepticus, diabetic neuropathy.

PRECAUTIONS

Contraindications: Active hepatic disease, urea cycle disorders. **Cautions:** History of hepatic disease, bleeding abnormalities, pts at high risk for suicide, elderly.

LIFESPAN CONSIDERATIONS

Pregnancy/Lactation: Drug crosses placenta; is distributed in breast milk. **Pregnancy Category D. Children:** Increased risk of hepatotoxicity in pts younger than 2 yrs. **Elderly:** No age-related precautions, but lower dosages recommended.

INTERACTIONS

DRUG: Carbapenems (e.g., meropenem), CYP3A4 inducers (e.g., carbamazepine, phenytoin) may decrease concentration/effects. May alter effects of **warfarin.** May increase concentration of **lamotrigine. Topiramate** may increase risk of elevated serum ammonia levels. **HERBAL: Evening primrose** may decrease seizure threshold. **FOOD:** None known. **LAB VALUES:** May increase serum LDH, bilirubin, AST, ALT. **Therapeutic serum level:** 50–100 mcg/ml; **toxic serum level:** greater than 100 mcg/ml.

AVAILABILITY (Rx)

Capsules (Depakene): 250 mg. **Capsules, Sprinkle (Depakote Sprinkle):** 125 mg. **Injection, Solution (Depacon):** 100 mg/ml. **Syrup (Depakene):** 250 mg/5 ml.
Capsules, Delayed-Release (Stavzor): 125 mg, 250 mg, 500 mg. **Tablets, Delayed-Release (Depakote):** 125 mg, 250 mg, 500 mg. **Tablets, Extended-Release (Depakote ER):** 250 mg, 500 mg.

ADMINISTRATION/HANDLING

IV

Reconstitution • Dilute each single dose with at least 50 ml D₅W, 0.9% NaCl, or lactated Ringer's.
Rate of Administration • Infuse over 60 min at rate of 20 mg/min or less. **•** Alternatively, single doses of up to 45 mg/kg given over 5–10 min (1.5–6 mg/kg/min).
Storage • Store vials at room temperature. **•** Diluted solutions stable for 24 hrs. **•** Discard unused portion.

PO

• May give without regard to food. Do not mix oral solution with carbonated beverages (may cause mouth/throat irritation). **•** May sprinkle capsule (Depakote Sprinkle) contents on applesauce and give immediately (do not chew sprinkle beads). **•** Give delayed-release/extended-release tablets whole. Do not crush, break, open delayed-release capsule (Stavzor). **•** Regular-release and delayed-release formulations usually given in 2–4 divided doses/day. Extended-release formulation (Depakote ER) usually given once daily.

IV INCOMPATIBILITIES

None known.

IV COMPATIBILITIES

Cefepime, ceftazidime.

INDICATIONS/ROUTES/DOSAGE

Seizures
PO: ADULTS, ELDERLY, CHILDREN 10 YRS AND OLDER: Initially, 10–15 mg/kg/day in 1–3 divided doses. May increase by 5–10 mg/kg/day at weekly intervals up to 30–60 mg/kg/day. **Usual adult dosage:** 1,000–2,500 mg/day. *(Stavzor):* Initially, 10–15 mg/kg/day, may increase by 5–10 mg/kg/day at 1-wk intervals to achieve desired response. **Maximum:** 60 mg/kg/day.
IV: ADULTS, ELDERLY, CHILDREN: Same frequency as oral dose.

V

Manic Episodes

PO *(Depakote)*: ADULTS, ELDERLY: Initially, 750–1,500 mg/day in divided doses. **Maximum:** 60 mg/kg/day.

PO *(Extended-Release [Depakote ER])*: Initially, 25 mg/kg/day once daily. **Maximum:** 60 mg/kg/day. *(Delayed-Release [Stavzor])*: Initially, 750 mg/day in divided dose. Titrate to lowest therapeutic dose. **Maximum:** 60 mg/kg/day.

Prevention of Migraine Headaches

PO *(Extended-Release [Depakote ER])*: ADULTS, ELDERLY: Initially, 500 mg/day for 7 days. May increase up to 1,000 mg/day.

PO *(Delayed-Release [Depakote])*: ADULTS, ELDERLY: 250 mg twice a day. May increase up to 1,000 mg/day. *(Stavzor)*: 250 mg twice a day. May increase to 1,000 mg/day.

SIDE EFFECTS

Frequent: Epilepsy: Abdominal pain, irregular menses, diarrhea, transient alopecia, indigestion, nausea, vomiting, tremors, fluctuations in body weight. **Mania (22%–19%):** Nausea, drowsiness. **Occasional: Epilepsy:** Constipation, dizziness, drowsiness, headache, skin rash, unusual excitement, restlessness. **Mania (12%–6%):** Asthenia (loss of strength, energy), abdominal pain, dyspepsia (heartburn, indigestion, epigastric distress), rash. **Rare: Epilepsy:** Mood changes, diplopia, nystagmus, spots before eyes, unusual bleeding/bruising.

ADVERSE EFFECTS/ TOXIC REACTIONS

Hepatotoxicity may occur, particularly in first 6 mos of therapy. May be preceded by loss of seizure control, malaise, weakness, lethargy, anorexia, vomiting rather than abnormal serum hepatic function test results. Blood dyscrasias may occur.

NURSING CONSIDERATIONS

BASELINE ASSESSMENT

Anticonvulsant: Review history of seizure disorder (intensity, frequency, duration, level of consciousness). Initiate safety measures, quiet dark environment. CBC should be performed before and 2 wks after therapy begins, then 2 wks following maintenance dose. Obtain baseline hepatic function tests. **Antimanic:** Assess behavior, appearance, emotional status, response to environment, speech pattern, thought content. **Antimigraine:** Question pt regarding onset, location, duration of migraine, possible precipitating symptoms.

INTERVENTION/EVALUATION

Monitor serum hepatic function tests, bilirubin, ammonia, CBC. **Anticonvulsant:** Observe frequently for recurrence of seizure activity. Monitor serum hepatic function tests, CBC. Assess skin for ecchymoses, petechiae. Monitor for clinical improvement (decrease in intensity/frequency of seizures). **Antimanic:** Question for suicidal ideation. Assess for therapeutic response (interest in surroundings, increased ability to concentrate, relaxed facial expression). **Antimigraine:** Evaluate for relief of migraine headache and resulting photophobia, phonophobia, nausea, vomiting. **Therapeutic serum level:** 50–100 mcg/ml; **toxic serum level:** greater than 100 mcg/ml.

PATIENT/ FAMILY TEACHING

• Do not abruptly discontinue medication after long-term use (may precipitate seizures). • Strict maintenance of drug therapy is essential for seizure control. • Drowsiness usually disappears during continued therapy. • Avoid tasks that require alertness, motor skills until response to drug is established. • Avoid alcohol. • Carry identification card, bracelet that notes anticonvulsant therapy. • Report nausea, vomiting, lethargy, altered mental status, weakness, loss of appetite, abdominal pain, yellowing of skin, unusual bruising/bleeding. • Report if seizure control worsens, suicidal ideation (depression, unusual changes in behavior, suicidal thoughts) occurs.

V

✤ Canadian trade name   🗡 Non-Crushable Drug   🔲 High Alert drug

valsartan

val-**sar**-tan
(Diovan)

BLACK BOX ALERT May cause fetal injury, mortality if used during second or third trimester of pregnancy. **Do not confuse Diovan with Zyban, or valsartan with losartan or Valstar.**

FIXED-COMBINATION(S)

Diovan HCT: valsartan/hydrochlorothiazide (a diuretic): 80 mg/12.5 mg, 160 mg/12.5 mg, 160 mg/25 mg, 320 mg/12.5 mg, 320 mg/25 mg. **Exforge:** valsartan/amlodipine (a calcium channel blocker): 160 mg/5 mg, 160 mg/10 mg, 320 mg/5 mg, 320 mg/10 mg. **Exforge HCT:** valsartan/amlodipine (a calcium channel blocker)/hydrochlorothiazide (a diuretic): 160 mg/5 mg/12.5 mg, 160 mg/5 mg/25 mg, 160 mg/10 mg/12.5 mg, 160 mg/10 mg/25 mg, 320 mg/10 mg/25 mg. **Valturna:** valsartan/aliskiren (a direct renin inhibitor): 160 mg/150 mg, 320 mg/300 mg.

◆ CLASSIFICATION

PHARMACOTHERAPEUTIC: Angiotensin II receptor antagonist. **CLINICAL:** Antihypertensive (see p. 11C, 62C).

ACTION

Potent vasodilator. Blocks vasoconstrictor, aldosterone-secreting effects of angiotensin II, inhibiting binding of angiotensin II to AT_1 receptors. **Therapeutic Effect:** Produces vasodilation, decreases peripheral resistance, decreases B/P.

PHARMACOKINETICS

Poorly absorbed after PO administration. Food decreases peak plasma concentration. Protein binding: 95%. Me-tabolized in liver. Eliminated in feces (83%), urine (13%). Unknown if removed by hemodialysis. **Half-life:** 6 hrs.

USES

Treatment of hypertension alone or in combination with other antihypertensives. Treatment of HF. Reduce mortality in high-risk pts (left ventricular failure/dysfunction) following MI.

PRECAUTIONS

Contraindications: Concomitant use with aliskiren in pts with diabetes. **Cautions:** Concurrent use of potassium-sparing diuretics or potassium supplements, mild to severe hepatic impairment, unstented bilateral/unilateral renal artery stenosis, renal impairment, significant aortic/mitral stenosis.

⧖ LIFESPAN CONSIDERATIONS

Pregnancy/Lactation: May cause fetal harm. Unknown if distributed in breast milk. **Pregnancy Category C (D if used in second or third trimester). Children:** Safety and efficacy not established. **Elderly:** No age-related precautions noted.

INTERACTIONS

DRUG: **NSAIDs** may decrease antihypertensive effect. **Potassium-sparing drugs, potassium supplements** may increase serum potassium. **Diuretics** may produce additive hypotensive effects. **HERBAL:** **Ginger, ginseng, licorice** may worsen hypertension. **Black cohosh, periwinkle** may increase antihypertensive effects. **FOOD:** None known. **LAB VALUES:** May increase serum bilirubin, AST, ALT, BUN, creatinine, potassium. May decrease Hgb, Hct, WBC.

AVAILABILITY (Rx)

Tablets: 40 mg, 80 mg, 160 mg, 320 mg.

ADMINISTRATION/HANDLING

PO
• Give without regard to meals.

INDICATIONS/ROUTES/DOSAGE

Hypertension

PO: ADULTS, ELDERLY: Initially, 80–160 mg/day in pts who are not volume depleted. **Maximum:** 320 mg/day. **CHILDREN 6–16 YRS:** Initially, 1.3 mg/kg once a day (**Maximum:** 40 mg). May increase up to 2.7 mg/kg once a day (**Maximum:** 160 mg/day).

HF

PO: ADULTS, ELDERLY: Initially, 40 mg twice a day. May increase up to 160 mg twice a day. **Maximum:** 320 mg/day.

Post-MI

PO: ADULTS, ELDERLY: May initiate 12 hrs or longer following MI. Initially, 20 mg twice a day. May increase within 7 days to 40 mg twice a day. May further increase up to target dose of 160 mg twice a day.

SIDE EFFECTS

Rare (2%–1%): Insomnia, fatigue, heartburn, abdominal pain, dizziness, headache, diarrhea, nausea, vomiting, arthralgia, edema.

ADVERSE EFFECTS/ TOXIC REACTIONS

Overdosage may manifest as hypotension, tachycardia. Bradycardia occurs less often. Viral infection, upper respiratory tract infection (cough, pharyngitis, sinusitis, rhinitis) occur rarely.

NURSING CONSIDERATIONS

BASELINE ASSESSMENT

Obtain B/P, apical pulse immediately before each dose, in addition to regular monitoring (be alert to fluctuations). If excessive reduction in B/P occurs, place pt in supine position, feet slightly elevated. Question for possibility of pregnancy. Assess medication history (esp. diuretic). Question for history of hepatic/renal impairment, renal artery stenosis, history of severe HF. Obtain baseline chemistries, blood counts.

INTERVENTION/EVALUATION

Maintain hydration (offer fluids frequently). Assess for evidence of upper respiratory infection. Monitor serum electrolytes, renal/hepatic function tests, Hgb, Hct, urinalysis, B/P, pulse. Observe for symptoms of hypotension.

PATIENT/ FAMILY TEACHING

• Take measures to avoid pregnancy • Inform physician as soon as possible if pregnancy occurs. • Report any sign of infection (sore throat, fever). • Do not stop taking medication. • Report swelling of extremities, chest pain, palpitations.

vancomycin

van-koe-**mye**-sin
(<u>Vancocin</u>)
Do not confuse vancomycin with clindamycin, gentamicin, tobramycin, or Vibramycin.

◆CLASSIFICATION

PHARMACOTHERAPEUTIC: Tricyclic glycopeptide antibiotic. **CLINICAL:** Antibiotic.

ACTION

Binds to bacterial cell walls, altering cell membrane permeability, inhibiting RNA synthesis. **Therapeutic Effect:** Bactericidal.

PHARMACOKINETICS

PO: Poorly absorbed from GI tract. Primarily eliminated in feces. **Parenteral:** Widely distributed (except CSF). Protein binding: 10%–50%. Primarily excreted unchanged in urine. Not removed by hemodialysis. **Half-life:** 4–11 hrs (increased in renal impairment).

USES

Systemic: Treatment of infections caused by staphylococcal, streptococcal spp. bacteria. **PO:** Treatment of antibiotic colitis,

---

❦ Canadian trade name   🍷 Non-Crushable Drug   🟥**HIGH ALERT** High Alert drug pseudomembranous colitis, antibiotic-associated diarrhea produced by *C. difficile* staphylococcal enterocolitis. **OFF-LABEL:** Treatment of infections caused by gram-positive organisms in pts with serious allergies to beta-lactam antibiotics; treatment of beta-lactam-resistant gram-positive infections.

PRECAUTIONS

Contraindications: None known. **Cautions:** Renal impairment; concurrent therapy with other ototoxic, nephrotoxic medications.

⌛ LIFESPAN CONSIDERATIONS

Pregnancy/Lactation: Drug crosses placenta. Unknown if distributed in breast milk. **Pregnancy Category C (injection), B (PO).** **Children:** Close monitoring of serum levels recommended in premature neonates, young infants. **Elderly:** Age-related renal impairment may increase risk of ototoxicity, nephrotoxicity; dosage adjustment recommended.

INTERACTIONS

DRUG: Aminoglycosides, amphotericin B, cisplatin may increase risk of ototoxicity, nephrotoxicity of parenteral vancomycin. **HERBAL:** None significant. **FOOD:** None known. **LAB VALUES:** May increase BUN. **Therapeutic peak serum level:** (Not routinely obtained) 20–40 mcg/ml; **therapeutic trough serum level:** 10–20 mcg/ml. **Toxic peak serum level:** greater than 40 mcg/ml; **toxic trough serum level:** greater than 20 mcg/ml.

AVAILABILITY (Rx)

Capsules (Vancocin): 125 mg, 250 mg. **Infusion (Premix [Vancocin HCl]):** 500 mg/100 ml, 1 g/200 ml. **Injection, Powder for Reconstitution (Vancocin HCl):** 500 mg, 750 mg, 1 g.

ADMINISTRATION/HANDLING

 IV

◀ **ALERT** ▶ Give by intermittent IV infusion (piggyback) or continuous IV infusion. Do not give IV push (may result in exaggerated hypotension or "red man" syndrome).

Reconstitution • For intermittent IV infusion (piggyback), reconstitute each 500-mg vial with 10 ml Sterile Water for Injection (20 ml for 1-g vial) to provide concentration of 50 mg/ml. • Further dilute with D_5W or 0.9% NaCl to final concentration not to exceed 5 mg/ml.

Rate of Administration • Administer over 60 min or longer (30 min for each 500 mg recommended). • Monitor B/P closely during IV infusion.

Storage • Reconstituted vials are stable for 14 days at room temperature or if refrigerated. • Diluted solutions are stable for 14 days if refrigerated or 7 days at room temperature. • Discard if precipitate forms.

PO

• May give with food. • Powder for injection may be reconstituted and diluted for oral administration.

🔀 IV INCOMPATIBILITIES

Albumin, amphotericin B complex (Abelcet, AmBisome, Amphotec), aztreonam (Azactam), cefazolin (Ancef), cefotaxime (Claforan), cefoxitin (Mefoxin), ceftazidime (Fortaz), ceftriaxone (Rocephin), cefuroxime (Zinacef), foscarnet (Foscavir), heparin, nafcillin (Nafcil), piperacillin and tazobactam (Zosyn).

🔀 IV COMPATIBILITIES

Amiodarone (Cordarone), calcium gluconate, dexmedetomidine (Precedex), diltiazem (Cardizem), hydromorphone (Dilaudid), insulin, lorazepam (Ativan), magnesium sulfate, midazolam (Versed), morphine, nicardipine (Cardene), potassium chloride, propofol (Diprivan).

INDICATIONS/ROUTES/DOSAGE

Usual Parenteral Dosage
IV: ADULTS, ELDERLY: 10–20 mg/kg/dose q8–12h. Dosage requires adjustment in renal impairment. **CHILDREN OLDER THAN 1 MO:** 10–15 mg/kg/dose q6h. **NEONATES:**

15 mg/kg q24h up to 10–15 mg/kg/dose q6–8h.

Staphylococcal Enterocolitis, Antibiotic-Associated Pseudomembranous Colitis Caused by *Clostridium difficile*
PO: ADULTS, ELDERLY: 125–250 mg 4 times a day for 7–10 days. **CHILDREN:** 40 mg/kg/day in 3–4 divided doses for 7–10 days. **Maximum:** 2 g/day.

Dosage in Renal Impairment
After loading dose, subsequent dosages and frequency are modified based on creatinine clearance, severity of infection, and serum concentration of drug.

SIDE EFFECTS

Frequent: PO: Bitter/unpleasant taste, nausea, vomiting, mouth irritation (with oral solution). **Rare: Parenteral:** Phlebitis, thrombophlebitis, pain at peripheral IV site, dizziness, vertigo, tinnitus, chills, fever, rash, necrosis with extravasation. **PO:** Rash.

ADVERSE EFFECTS/ TOXIC REACTIONS

Nephrotoxicity (acute kidney injury, acute tubular necrosis, renal failure), ototoxicity (temporary or permanent hearing loss) may occur. "Red man syndrome" or "red neck syndrome" is common adverse reaction characterized by pruritus, urticaria, erythema, angioedema, tachycardia, hypotension, myalgia, maculopapular rash (usually appears on face, neck, upper torso). Cardiovascular toxicity (cardiac depression, arrest) occurs rarely. Onset usually occurs within 30 min of start of infusion, resolves within hrs following infusion. May result from too-rapid rate of infusion.

NURSING CONSIDERATIONS

BASELINE ASSESSMENT
Avoid other ototoxic, nephrotoxic medications if possible. Obtain culture, sensitivity test before giving first dose (therapy may begin before results are known).

INTERVENTION/EVALUATION
Monitor serum renal function tests, I&O. Assess skin for rash. Check hearing acuity, balance. Monitor B/P carefully during infusion. Evaluate IV site for phlebitis (heat, pain, red streaking over vein). Obtain vancomycin peak/trough level as ordered by physician or pharmacist. **Therapeutic serum level: peak:** 20–40 mcg/ml; **trough:** 10–20 mcg/ml. **Toxic serum level: peak:** greater than 40 mcg/ml; **trough:** greater than 20 mcg/ml.

PATIENT/ FAMILY TEACHING
• Continue therapy for full length of treatment. • Doses should be evenly spaced. • Report tinnitus (ringing in the ears), hearing loss, changes in urinary frequency or consistency. • Lab tests are important part of total therapy.

vandetanib

van-**det**-a-nib
(Caprelsa)

BLACK BOX ALERT Can prolong QT interval (torsade de pointes and sudden cardiac death reported). Do not use in pts with hypokalemia, hypocalcemia, hypomagnesemia, congenital long QT syndrome. Electrolyte imbalances must be corrected prior to initiating therapy. If medication that prolongs QT interval is needed, more frequent EKG monitoring is recommended. EKGs should be obtained during wks 2–4 and wks 8–12 after starting therapy and 3 mos thereafter. Any dose reduction or interruption related to QT prolongation greater than 2 wks must have frequent EKG monitoring as noted above. Only prescribers and pharmacies certified with restricted distribution program are able to prescribe and dispense.

◆CLASSIFICATION

PHARMACOTHERAPEUTIC: Tyrosine kinase inhibitor. **CLINICAL:** Antineoplastic (see p. 91C).

V

✤ Canadian trade name   🍴 Non-Crushable Drug   **HIGH ALERT** High Alert drug

ACTION

Inhibits epidermal growth factor (EGF)-stimulated receptor tyrosine kinase phosphorylation in tumor cells and endothelial cells. Inhibits cell migration, proliferation, survival, and angiogenesis (new blood vessel formation). **Therapeutic Effect:** Inhibits thyroid tumor cell growth and metastasis.

PHARMACOKINETICS

Slowly absorbed following PO administration. Peak concentration: 4–10 hrs. Metabolized in liver. Protein binding: 90%. Excreted in feces (44%), urine (25%). **Half-life:** 19 days.

USES

Treatment of symptomatic or progressive medullary thyroid cancer in pts with unresectable locally advanced or metastatic disease.

PRECAUTIONS

Contraindications: Congenital long QT syndrome. **Cautions:** Pregnancy, concurrent medications that prolong QT interval, strong CYP3A4 inducers, thyroid, cerebrovascular disease, bradyarrhythmias, moderate to severe renal/hepatic impairment, hypertension, uncompensated HF, history of torsade de pointes.

⧗ LIFESPAN CONSIDERATIONS

Pregnancy/Lactation: May cause fetal harm. Avoid pregnancy. Must use effective contraception during treatment and for at least 4 mos after treatment. Unknown if distributed in breast milk. **Pregnancy Category D. Children:** Safety and efficacy not established. **Elderly:** No age-related precautions noted.

INTERACTIONS

DRUG: **Medications prolonging QT interval** (e.g., **azithromycin, amiodarone, clarithromycin, erythromycin, ciprofloxacin, haloperidol**) may increase risk of QT prolongation. **CYP3A4 inducers** (e.g., **carbamazepine, oxcarbazepine, phenytoin, rifampin**) may decrease concentration/effects. **HERBAL:** **St. John's wort** may decrease effectiveness. **FOOD:** **Grapefruit products** may increase risk of torsades, myelotoxicity. **LAB VALUES:** May decrease WBC, Hgb, neutrophils. May increase serum bilirubin, AST, ALT, creatinine, urine protein. May alter serum calcium, glucose, magnesium, potassium.

AVAILABILITY (Rx)

Tablets: 100 mg, 300 mg.

ADMINISTRATION/HANDLING

PO

• Give without regard to food. • Do not crush. • May disperse in 2 oz of non-carbonated water and stir for 10 min until tablet is evenly dispersed (will not completely dissolve). May administer dispersion immediately. Can be given via feeding tube. • Direct contact of crushed tablets with skin or mucous membranes should be strictly avoided. If contact occurs, wash thoroughly.

Storage • Contact pharmacy to properly discard out-of-date tablets.

INDICATIONS/ROUTES/DOSAGE

Thyroid Cancer
PO: ADULTS, ELDERLY: 300 mg once daily.

Dosage in Renal Impairment
(Creatinine clearance less than 50 ml/min): 200 mg once daily.

Dosage Adjustment for QT Prolongation or Toxicity
Interrupt therapy until resolved or improved, then restart at 100–200 mg once daily.

SIDE EFFECTS

Frequent (57%–21%): Diarrhea/colitis, rash, dermatitis acneiform/acne, nausea, headache, fatigue, anorexia, abdominal pain. **Occasional (15%–10%):** Dry skin, vomiting, asthenia (loss of strength, energy), photosensitivity, insomnia, nasopharyngitis, dyspepsia, cough, pruritus, weight decrease, depression.

ADVERSE EFFECTS/ TOXIC REACTIONS

Prolonged QT interval resulting in torsade de pointes, ventricular arrhythmias, sudden cardiac death have been reported. Frequent diarrhea may result in electrolyte imbalances. Severe skin reactions, including Stevens-Johnson syndrome, have been noted. Interstitial lung disease (ILD) or pneumonitis reported (may result in respiratory-related death). Consider ILD in pts with hypoxia, pleural effusion, cough, dyspnea. Ischemic cerebrovascular events have been reported. Life-threatening events including hypertensive crisis, reversible posterior leukoencephalopathy syndrome (RPLS) have been noted. Adverse reactions resulting in death included respiratory failure/arrest, aspiration pneumonia, cardiac failure, sepsis, GI bleeding.

NURSING CONSIDERATIONS

BASELINE ASSESSMENT

Obtain CBC with differential, serum chemistries, magnesium, ionized calcium, TSH, UA, EKG, vital signs. Obtain negative urine pregnancy before therapy. Question for history of congenital long QT syndrome, HF, arrhythmias, hepatic/renal impairment, seizures, CVA, hemorrhagic events, HTN. Obtain full medication history including contraception. Perform full head-to-toe exam including visual acuity, thorough skin assessment.

INTERVENTION/EVALUATION

Monitor blood levels including electrolytes esp. during episodes of diarrhea. EKG during wks 2–4, wks 8–12, then every 3 mos thereafter. Obtain EKG for palpitations, chest pain, hypokalemia, hyperkalemia, hypocalcemia, bradycardia, ventricular arrhythmias, syncope. Report any respiratory changes including dyspnea, cough (may indicate ILD). Reversible posterior leukoencephalopathy syndrome should be considered in pts with seizures, headache, visual disturbances, confusion, altered mental status. Ophthalmologic exams including slit lamp recommended in pts with visual disturbances.

PATIENT/FAMILY TEACHING

• Blood levels, EKGs will be routinely monitored. • Strictly avoid pregnancy. Contraception should be taken during treatment and 4 mos after discontinuation. • Changes in mental status, seizures, headache, blurry vision, trouble speaking, one-sided weakness may indicate stroke, high blood pressure crisis, or life-threatening brain swelling. Immediately report any newly prescribed medications. • Do not take herbal products. • Limit exposure to sunlight. • Report any yellowing of skin or eyes, abdominal pain, bruising, black/tarry stools, dark urine, decreased urine output, skin changes. • Report palpitations, chest pain, shortness of breath, dizziness, fainting (may indicate arrhythmia).

vardenafil

var-**den**-a-fil
(Levitra, Staxyn)
Do not confuse Levitra with Kaletra or Lexiva, or vardenafil with sildenafil or tadalafil.

◆CLASSIFICATION

PHARMACOTHERAPEUTIC: Phosphodiesterase inhibitor. **CLINICAL:** Erectile dysfunction adjunct.

ACTION

Inhibits phosphodiesterase type 5 (PDE5), the enzyme responsible for degrading cyclic guanosine monophosphate in corpus cavernosum of penis, resulting in smooth muscle relaxation, increased blood flow. **Therapeutic Effect:** Facilitates penile erection.

PHARMACOKINETICS

Rapidly absorbed after PO administration. Extensive tissue distribution. Protein binding: 95%. Metabolized in liver. Excreted in feces (91%–95%), urine

V

(2%–6%). Drug has no effect on penile blood flow without sexual stimulation.
Half-life: 4–5 hrs.

USES

Treatment of erectile dysfunction.

PRECAUTIONS

Contraindications: Concurrent use of nitrates in any form. **Cautions:** Renal/hepatic impairment, left ventricular outflow obstruction, cardiac disease, elderly, prolonged QT interval, anatomical deformation of penis, pts who may be predisposed to priapism (sickle cell anemia, multiple myeloma, leukemia), concurrent use with alpha-adrenergic blockers, CYP3A4 inhibitors, elderly.

⧗ LIFESPAN CONSIDERATIONS

Pregnancy/Lactation: Not indicated for use in women, newborns. **Pregnancy Category B. Children:** Not indicated for use in children. **Elderly:** No age-related precautions noted, but initial dose should be 5 mg.

INTERACTIONS

DRUG: Alpha-adrenergic blockers (e.g., alfuzosin, doxazosin, prazosin, tamsulosin, terazosin), nitrates may significantly lower B/P. **CYP3A4 inhibitors (e.g., erythromycin, indinavir, itraconazole, ketoconazole, ritonavir)** may increase concentration. **HERBAL:** None significant. **FOOD:** High-fat meals delay maximum effectiveness. **Grapefruit products** may increase concentration, risk of toxicity. **LAB VALUES:** May increase creatinine kinase, GGTP. May alter AST, ALT.

AVAILABILITY (Rx)

Tablets (Levitra): 2.5 mg, 5 mg, 10 mg, 20 mg.

⧬ **Tablets, Orally Disintegrating (Staxyn):** 10 mg.

ADMINISTRATION/HANDLING

PO
• May take approximately 1 hr before sexual activity. • May give without regard to food.

Orally Disintegrating
• Take 1 hr before sexual activity. • Take without regard to meals. • Place on tongue, do not crush, split. • Do not take with liquid.

INDICATIONS/ROUTES/DOSAGE

Erectile Dysfunction
PO: ADULTS: 10 mg approximately 1 hr before sexual activity. Dose may be increased to 20 mg or decreased to 5 mg, based on pt tolerance. **Maximum dosing frequency:** Once daily. **ELDERLY OLDER THAN 65 YRS:** 5 mg. **Orally disintegrating tablet:** 10 mg 1 hr prior to sexual activity.

Dosage in Moderate Hepatic Impairment
PO: For pts with Child-Pugh class B hepatic impairment, dosage is 5 mg 1 hr before sexual activity. ODT not recommended.

Dosage with Concurrent Ritonavir, Fosamprenavir/Ritonavir, Lopinavir/Ritonavir, Tipranavir
PO: ADULTS: 2.5 mg in 72-hr period.

Dosage with Concurrent Atazanavir, Clarithromycin, Ketoconazole (at 400 mg/day), Itraconazole (at 400 mg/day), Indinavir, Saquinavir, Fosamprenavir/Nelfinavir
PO: ADULTS: 2.5 mg in 24-hr period.

Dosage with Concurrent Ketoconazole (at 200 mg/day), Itraconazole (at 200 mg/day), Erythromycin
PO: ADULTS: 5 mg in 24-hr period.

SIDE EFFECTS

Occasional: Headache, flushing, rhinitis, indigestion, sudden hearing loss. **Rare (Less Than 2%):** Dizziness, changes in color vision, blurred vision, postural hypotension.

ADVERSE EFFECTS/ TOXIC REACTIONS

Prolonged erections (lasting over 4 hrs), priapism (painful erections lasting over 6 hrs) occur rarely.

V

NURSING CONSIDERATIONS

BASELINE ASSESSMENT

Assess cardiovascular status, medication history (esp. alpha-adrenergic blockers, nitrates) before initiating treatment for erectile dysfunction.

INTERVENTION/EVALUATION

Monitor B/P. Assess quality of sexual activity.

PATIENT/FAMILY TEACHING

• Has no effect in absence of sexual stimulation. • Seek treatment immediately if erection persists for over 4 hrs. • Avoid grapefruit juice. • Report sudden decrease or loss of hearing or vision. • Do not take nitrates for chest pain.

---

varenicline
TOP 200

var-**en**-i-kleen
(Champix ✤, Chantix)

BLACK BOX ALERT Risk of psychiatric symptoms and suicidal behavior. Agitation, hostility, depressed mood have been reported.

◆CLASSIFICATION

PHARMACOTHERAPEUTIC: Selective partial nicotine agonist. **CLINICAL:** Smoking deterrent (see p. 156C).

ACTION

Binds to acetylcholine receptors, producing agonist activity, preventing nicotine from binding to specific receptors. Blocks ability of nicotine to stimulate central dopamine system, believed to be mechanism underlying reinforcement/reward experienced with smoking. **Therapeutic Effect:** Decreases desire to smoke.

PHARMACOKINETICS

Completely absorbed following PO administration. Absorption unaffected by food, time of day dosing. Maximum plasma concentration: 3–4 hrs; steady-state condition: within 4 days. Protein binding: 20%. Minimal metabolism. Removed by hemodialysis. Primarily excreted unchanged in urine. **Half-life:** 24 hrs.

USES

Aid to smoking cessation treatment.

PRECAUTIONS

Contraindications: None known. **Cautions:** Renal impairment, history of suicidal ideation, bipolar disorder, depression, schizophrenia.

⌛ LIFESPAN CONSIDERATIONS

Pregnancy/Lactation: Unknown if distributed in breast milk. **Pregnancy Category C. Children:** Not recommended. **Elderly:** Age-related renal impairment may require dosage adjustment.

INTERACTIONS

DRUG: Cimetidine may increase effect. **HERBAL:** None significant. **FOOD:** None known. **LAB VALUES:** None significant.

AVAILABILITY

🔖 **Tablets (Film-Coated):** 0.5 mg, 1 mg.

ADMINISTRATION/HANDLING

• Give with food and with full glass of water. • Do not break, crush, dissolve, or divide film-coated tablets.

INDICATIONS/ROUTES/DOSAGE

◀ALERT▶ Therapy should start 1 wk before stopping smoking.

Smoking Deterrent
PO: ADULTS, ELDERLY: Days 1–3: 0.5 mg once daily. **Days 4–7:** 0.5 mg twice daily. **Day 8–end of treatment:** 1 mg twice daily. Therapy should last for 12 wks. Pts who have successfully stopped smoking at the end of 12 wks should continue with an additional 12 wks of treatment to increase likelihood of long-term abstinence.

Severe Renal Impairment *(creatinine clearance less than 30 ml/min):*

V

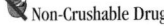

0.5 mg once daily. **Maximum:** 0.5 mg twice daily.

End-Stage Renal Disease, Undergoing Hemodialysis: Maximum: 0.5 mg once daily.

SIDE EFFECTS

Frequent (30%–13%): Nausea, insomnia, headache, abnormal dreams. **Occasional (8%–5%):** Constipation, abdominal discomfort, fatigue, dry mouth, flatulence, altered taste, dyspepsia (heartburn, indigestion, epigastric pain), vomiting, anxiety, depression, irritability. **Rare (3%–1%):** Drowsiness, rash, increased appetite, lethargy, nightmares, gastroesophageal reflux disease, rhinorrhea, agitation, mood swings.

ADVERSE EFFECTS/ TOXIC REACTIONS

Abrupt withdrawal may cause irritability, sleep disturbances in 3% of pts. Hypertension, angina pectoris, arrhythmia, bradycardia, coronary artery disease, gingivitis, anemia, lymphadenopathy occur rarely. May cause bizarre behavior, suicidal ideation.

NURSING CONSIDERATIONS

BASELINE ASSESSMENT

Screen, evaluate for coronary heart disease (history of MI, angina pectoris), cardiac arrhythmias, suicidal ideation.

INTERVENTION/EVALUATION

Discontinue use if cardiovascular symptoms occur or worsen. Monitor for psychiatric symptoms (changes in behavior, mood, level of interest, appearance).

PATIENT/FAMILY TEACHING

• Initiate treatment 1 wk before quit smoking date. • Take with food and with full glass of water. • With twice-daily dosing, take 1 tablet in morning, 1 in evening. • Report persistent nausea, insomnia. • Report change in behavior, mood, level of interest, appearance.

vasopressin

vay-soe-**pres**-in
(Pitressin, Pressyn ✸, Pressyn AR ✸)
Do not confuse Pitressin with Pitocin.

◆CLASSIFICATION

PHARMACOTHERAPEUTIC: Posterior pituitary hormone. **CLINICAL:** Vasopressor, antidiuretic.

ACTION

Increases reabsorption of water by renal tubules. Directly stimulates smooth muscle in GI tract. **Therapeutic Effect:** Causes peristalsis, vasoconstriction.

PHARMACOKINETICS

Route	Onset	Peak	Duration
IV	N/A	N/A	0.5–1 hr
IM, sub-cutaneous	1–2 hrs	N/A	2–8 hrs

Distributed throughout extracellular fluid. Metabolized in liver, kidney. Primarily excreted in urine. **Half-life:** 10–20 min.

USES

Adjunct in treatment of acute massive GI hemorrhage or esophageal varices. Prevention/control of polydipsia, polyuria, dehydration in pts with neurogenic diabetes insipidus or differential diagnosis of diabetes insipidus. Treatment of pulseless arrest ventricular fibrillation or tachycardia and vasodilatory shock with hypotension unresponsive to fluids or exogenous catecholamines.

PRECAUTIONS

Contraindications: None known. **Cautions:** Seizures, migraine, asthma, vascular disease, renal/cardiac disease, goiter (with cardiac complications), arteriosclerosis, nephritis.

V

⧖ LIFESPAN CONSIDERATIONS

Pregnancy/Lactation: Caution in giving to breastfeeding women. **Pregnancy Category C. Children/Elderly:** Caution due to risk of water intoxication/hyponatremia.

INTERACTIONS

DRUG: Alcohol, demeclocycline, lithium, norepinephrine may decrease antidiuretic effect. **Carbamazepine, chlorpropamide, clofibrate** may increase antidiuretic effect. **HERBAL:** None significant. **FOOD:** None known. **LAB VALUES:** None significant.

AVAILABILITY (Rx)

Injection Solution: 20 units/ml (0.5 ml, 1 ml).

ADMINISTRATION/HANDLING

🖐 IV

Reconstitution • Dilute with D_5W or 0.9% NaCl to concentration of 0.1–1 unit/ml (usual concentration: 100 units/500 ml D_5W).
Rate of Administration • Give as IV infusion.
Storage • Store at room temperature.

IM, Subcutaneous
• Give with 1–2 glasses of water to reduce side effects.

🔲 IV INCOMPATIBILITIES

Furosemide (Lasix), phenytoin (Dilantin).

🔲 IV COMPATIBILITIES

Amiodarone, argatroban, diltiazem (Cardizem), dobutamine (Dobutrex), dopamine (Intropin), heparin, insulin, milrinone (Primacor), nitroglycerin, norepinephrine (Levophed), pantoprazole (Protonix), phenylephrine.

INDICATIONS/ROUTES/DOSAGE

Pulseless Arrest
IV: ADULTS, ELDERLY: 40 units as one-time bolus.

Diabetes Insipidus
◀ALERT▶ May be administered intranasally by nasal spray or on cotton pledgets; dosage is individualized.
IV Infusion: ADULTS, CHILDREN: 0.5 milliunits/kg/hr. May double dose q30min. **Maximum:** 10 milliunits/kg/hr.
IM, Subcutaneous: ADULTS, ELDERLY: 5–10 units 2–4 times a day. **Range:** 5–60 units/day. **CHILDREN:** 2.5–10 units, 2–4 times a day.

GI Hemorrhage
IV Infusion: ADULTS, ELDERLY: Initially, 0.2–0.4 unit/min progressively increased to 0.8 unit/min. **CHILDREN:** 0.002–0.005 unit/kg/min. Titrate as needed. **Maximum:** 0.01 unit/kg/min.

Vasodilatory Shock
IV Infusion: ADULTS, ELDERLY: Initially, 0.01–0.04 units/min. Titrate to desired effect.

SIDE EFFECTS

Frequent: Pain at injection site (with vasopressin tannate). **Occasional:** Abdominal cramps, nausea, vomiting, diarrhea, dizziness, diaphoresis, pale skin, circumoral pallor, tremors, headache, eructation, flatulence. **Rare:** Chest pain, confusion, allergic reaction (rash, urticaria, pruritus, wheezing, difficulty breathing, facial/peripheral edema), sterile abscess (with vasopressin tannate).

ADVERSE EFFECTS/ TOXIC REACTIONS

Anaphylaxis, MI, water intoxication have occurred. Elderly, very young are at higher risk for water intoxication.

NURSING CONSIDERATIONS

BASELINE ASSESSMENT

Establish baselines for weight, B/P, pulse, serum electrolytes, Hgb, Hct, urine specific gravity.

V

INTERVENTION/EVALUATION

Monitor I&O closely, restrict intake as necessary to prevent water intoxication. Weigh daily if indicated. Check B/P, pulse twice daily. Monitor serum electrolytes, Hgb, Hct, urine specific gravity. Evaluate injection site for erythema, pain, abscess. Report side effects to physician for dose reduction. Be alert for early signs of water intoxication (drowsiness, listlessness, headache). Observe for evidence of GI bleeding. Withhold medication, report immediately any chest pain, allergic symptoms.

PATIENT/FAMILY TEACHING

• Promptly report headache, chest pain, shortness of breath, other symptoms. • Stress importance of I&O. • Avoid alcohol.

---

vemurafenib

vem-ue-**raf**-e-nib
(Zelboraf)

◆CLASSIFICATION

PHARMACOTHERAPEUTIC: Threonine kinase inhibitor. **CLINICAL:** Antineoplastic.

ACTION

Inhibits BRAF serine-threonine kinase gene mutation, a main cause of tumor cell proliferation in the absence of growth factors normally required for proliferation. **Therapeutic Effect:** Exhibits antitumor effects.

PHARMACOKINETICS

Readily absorbed after PO administration. Protein binding: 99%. Minimally metabolized in liver. Primarily excreted in feces (94%). **Half-life:** 57 hrs. Range: 30–120 hrs.

USES

Treatment of unresectable or metastatic melanoma with BRAF mutation as detected by FDA-approved test.

PRECAUTIONS

Contraindications: None known. **Cautions:** Prolonged QT syndrome, concurrent use of medications that prolong QT interval, hepatic impairment, uncorrected electrolyte imbalance.

⌛ LIFESPAN CONSIDERATIONS

Pregnancy/Lactation: Avoid pregnancy. May cause fetal harm. Must use effective contraception during treatment and for at least 2 mos after discontinuation. Unknown if distributed in breast milk. Must either discontinue breastfeeding or discontinue therapy. **Children:** Safety and efficacy not established. **Elderly:** May have increased risk of adverse reactions, side effects.

INTERACTIONS

DRUG: Antiarrhythmics (**amiodarone, procainamide, quinidine, sotalol**), **azithromycin, barbiturates, ciprofloxacin, dexamethasone, fluconazole, haloperidol, phenothiazines, phenytoins, trazodone, tricyclic antidepressants, vardenafil, voriconazole** may prolong QT interval. **CYP3A4 inhibitors** (**e.g., atazanavir, clarithromycin, itraconazole, ketoconazole, phenobarbital, rifampin**) may alter concentration. May increase bleeding effect with **warfarin**. **HERBAL:** None significant. **FOOD:** None known. **LAB VALUES:** May increase serum alkaline phosphatase, AST, ALT, gamma-glutamyl transferase (GGT), bilirubin.

AVAILABILITY (Rx)

▧ **Film-Coated Tablets:** 240 mg.

ADMINISTRATION/HANDLING

PO
• Give without regard to food. • Do not break, crush, dissolve, or divide tablets. • Give with full glass of water.

INDICATIONS/ROUTES/DOSAGE

Note: Management of adverse drug reactions may require dose reduction, treatment interruption, or discontinuation.

V

Melanoma
PO: ADULTS, ELDERLY: 960 mg twice daily (in morning and evening about 12 hrs apart).

Dosage Modification
Based on adverse reaction criteria (grades 1–4). Interrupt therapy and reduce to 720 mg twice daily. Further reduction to 480 mg twice daily if more severe adverse reaction occurs. Discontinue treatment if repeated higher grades occur.

SIDE EFFECTS

Frequent (53%–33%): Arthralgia, alopecia, fatigue, rash, nausea. **Occasional (28%–11%):** Diarrhea, hyperkeratosis, headache, pruritus, pyrexia, dry skin, extremity pain, anorexia, vomiting, peripheral edema, erythema, dysgeusia, myalgia, constipation, asthenia (loss of strength, energy). **Rare (8%–5%):** Maculopapular rash, actinic keratosis, musculoskeletal pain, back pain, cough, papular rash.

ADVERSE EFFECTS/ TOXIC REACTIONS

Cutaneous squamous cell carcinoma (cuSCC) and keratocanthomas reported in 24% of pts. Pts at increased risk of cuSCC include elderly, pts with prior skin cancer, chronic sun exposure. Hypersensitivity reactions including erythema, hypotension, anaphylaxis reported. Mild to severe photosensitivity were reported. Serious dermatologic reactions include Stevens-Johnson syndrome, epidermal necrolysis. Ophthalmologic reactions including uveitis reported. Increased LFTs may lead to discontinuation.

NURSING CONSIDERATIONS

BASELINE ASSESSMENT

Obtain serum chemistries, renal function test, magnesium, ionized calcium, EKG, PT/INR if taking warfarin. Assess skin for moles, lesions, papilloma and perform full dermatologic exam. Obtain baseline ophthalmologic exam, visual acuity. Assess medication history for QT-prolonging drugs. Obtain negative urine pregnancy before initiating treatment.

INTERVENTION/EVALUATION

Monitor EKG 15 days after initiation, then monthly for first 3 mos, then every 3 mos thereafter. Routinely assess skin and for 6 mos after discontinuation. Immediately report any new skin lesions. Obtain EKG for palpitations, chest pain, hypokalemia, hyperkalemia, hypocalcemia, bradycardia, ventricular arrhythmias, syncope. Monitor PT/INR while pt is on warfarin. Pruritus, difficulty breathing, erythema, hypotension may indicate anaphylaxis.

PATIENT/FAMILY TEACHING

• Blood levels, EKG, eye examinations are routinely ordered. • Strictly avoid pregnancy. Contraception should be used during treatment and 2 mos after discontinuation. • Avoid sunlight exposure. • Report any skin changes including new warts, sores, reddish bumps that bleed or do not heal, change in mole size or color. • Report any yellowing of skin or eyes, abdominal pain, bruising, black/tarry stools, dark urine, decreased urine output, skin changes. • Report palpitations, chest pain, shortness of breath, dizziness, fainting (may indicate arrhythmia).

---

venlafaxine

TOP 200

ven-la-**fax**-een
(Effexor, Effexor XR)

BLACK BOX ALERT Increased risk of suicidal ideation and behavior in children, adolescents, young adults 18–24 yrs with major depressive disorder, other psychiatric disorders.

◆CLASSIFICATION

PHARMACOTHERAPEUTIC: Phenethylamine derivative. **CLINICAL:** Antidepressant (see pp. 15C, 41C).

V

♣ Canadian trade name   Non-Crushable Drug   High Alert drug

ACTION

Potentiates CNS neurotransmitter activity by inhibiting reuptake of serotonin, norepinephrine, and, to lesser degree, dopamine. **Therapeutic Effect:** Relieves depression.

PHARMACOKINETICS

Well absorbed from GI tract. Protein binding: 25%–30%. Metabolized in liver. Primarily excreted in urine. Not removed by hemodialysis. **Half-life:** 3–7 hrs; metabolite, 9–13 hrs (increased in hepatic/renal impairment).

USES

Treatment of depression. Treatment of generalized anxiety disorder (GAD), social anxiety disorder (SAD). Treatment of panic disorder, with or without agoraphobia. **OFF-LABEL:** Treatment of ADHD, obsessive-compulsive disorder (OCD), hot flashes, neuropathic pain, post-traumatic stress disorder (PTSD), migraine prophylaxis.

PRECAUTIONS

Contraindications: Use of MAOIs within 14 days. **Cautions:** Seizure disorder, renal/hepatic impairment, suicidal pts, recent MI, mania, volume-depleted pts, narrow-angle glaucoma, HF, hyperthyroidism, abnormal platelet function. Pts with increased intraocular pressure, elderly.

⧖ LIFESPAN CONSIDERATIONS

Pregnancy/Lactation: Unknown if distributed in breast milk. **Pregnancy Category C. Children:** Children, adolescents are at increased risk for suicidal ideation and behavior, worsening depression, esp. during first few mos of therapy. **Elderly:** No age-related precautions noted.

INTERACTIONS

DRUG: CYP3A4 inhibitors (e.g., ketoconazole) may increase concentration/effects. **MAOIs** may cause neuroleptic malignant syndrome, autonomic instability (including rapid fluctuations of vital signs), extreme agitation, hyperthermia, altered mental status, myoclonus, rigidity, coma. **Triptans, selegiline, SSRIs, trazodone, tricyclic antidepressants** may increase risk of serotonin syndrome. May increase risk of bleeding with **NSAIDs, aspirin, warfarin. HERBAL: Gotu kola, kava kava, St. John's wort, valerian** may increase CNS depression. **St. John's wort** may increase risk of serotonin syndrome. **FOOD:** None known. **LAB VALUES:** May increase serum cholesterol CPK, LDH, prolactin, GGT.

AVAILABILITY (Rx)

Tablets (Effexor): 25 mg, 37.5 mg, 50 mg, 75 mg, 100 mg.

❦ **Capsules (Extended-Release [Effexor XR]):** 37.5 mg, 75 mg, 150 mg. ❦ **Tablets (Extended-Release):** 37.5 mg, 75 mg, 150 mg, 225 mg.

ADMINISTRATION/HANDLING

PO

• Give with food. • Scored tablet may be crushed. • Do not break, crush, dissolve, or divide extended-release tablets. • May open capsule, sprinkle on applesauce. Give immediately without chewing and follow with full glass of water.

INDICATIONS/ROUTES/DOSAGE

Depression

PO *(Immediate-Release):* **ADULTS, ELDERLY:** Initially, 75 mg/day in 2–3 divided doses with food. May increase by 75 mg/day at intervals of 4 days or longer. **Maximum:** 375 mg/day in 3 divided doses.
PO *(Extended-Release):* **ADULTS, ELDERLY:** 37.5–75 mg/day as single dose with food. May increase by 75 mg/day at intervals of 4 days or longer. **Maximum:** 225 mg/day.

Generalized Anxiety Disorder (GAD)

PO *(Extended-Release):* **ADULTS, ELDERLY:** Initially, 37.5–75 mg/day. May increase by 75 mg/day at 4-day intervals up to 225 mg/day.

Panic Disorder

PO *(Extended-Release):* Initially, 37.5 mg/day. May increase to 75 mg after 7 days followed by increases of 75 mg/day at 7-day intervals up to 225 mg/day.

Social Anxiety Disorder (SAD)
PO: ADULTS, ELDERLY: 75 mg once daily.

Dosage in Renal/Hepatic Impairment
Expect to decrease venlafaxine dosage by 50% in pts with moderate hepatic impairment, 25% in pts with mild to moderate renal impairment, 50% in pts on dialysis (withhold dose until completion of dialysis). When discontinuing therapy, taper dosage slowly over 2 wks.

SIDE EFFECTS

Frequent (greater than 20%): Nausea, drowsiness, headache, dry mouth. **Occasional (20%–10%):** Dizziness, insomnia, constipation, diaphoresis, nervousness, asthenia (loss of strength, energy), ejaculatory disturbance, anorexia. **Rare (less than 10%):** Anxiety, blurred vision, diarrhea, vomiting, tremor, abnormal dreams, impotence.

ADVERSE EFFECTS/ TOXIC REACTIONS

Sustained increase in diastolic B/P of 10–15 mm Hg occurs occasionally. Serotonin syndrome (agitation, confusion, hallucinations, hyper-reflexia), neuroleptic malignant syndrome (muscular rigidity, fever, cognitive changes), suicidal ideation have occurred.

NURSING CONSIDERATIONS

BASELINE ASSESSMENT
Obtain initial weight, B/P. Assess appearance, behavior, speech pattern, level of interest, mood.

INTERVENTION/EVALUATION
Monitor signs/symptoms of depression, B/P, weight. Assess sleep pattern for evidence of insomnia. Check during waking hours for drowsiness, dizziness, anxiety; provide assistance as necessary. Assess appearance, behavior, speech pattern, level of interest, mood for therapeutic response. Monitor for suicidal ideation

(esp. at initiation of therapy or changes in dosage).

PATIENT/ FAMILY TEACHING
• Take with food to minimize GI distress. • Do not increase, decrease, suddenly stop medication. • Avoid tasks that require alertness, motor skills until response to drug is established. • Inform physician if breastfeeding, pregnant, or planning to become pregnant. • Avoid alcohol. • Report worsening depression, suicidal ideation, unusual changes in behavior.

verapamil

ver-**ap**-a-mil
(Apo-Verap ✦, Calan, Calan SR, Chronovera ✦, Covera-HS, Isoptin SR, Novo-Veramil SR ✦, Verelan, Verelan PM)
Do not confuse Calan with Covera-HS or Verelan with Voltaren.

FIXED-COMBINATION(S)

Tarka: verapamil/trandolapril (an ACE inhibitor): 240 mg/1 mg, 180 mg/2 mg, 240 mg/2 mg, 240 mg/4 mg.

◆CLASSIFICATION

PHARMACOTHERAPEUTIC: Calcium channel blocker. **CLINICAL:** Antihypertensive, antianginal, antiarrhythmic, hypertrophic cardiomyopathy therapy adjunct (see pp. 19C, 63C, 80C).

ACTION

Inhibits calcium ion entry across cardiac, vascular smooth-muscle cell membranes, dilating coronary arteries, peripheral arteries, arterioles. **Therapeutic Effect:** Decreases heart rate, myocardial contractility; slows SA, AV conduction. Decreases total peripheral vascular resistance by vasodilation.

V

✦ Canadian trade name   Non-Crushable Drug   High Alert drug

PHARMACOKINETICS

Well absorbed from GI tract. Protein binding: 90% (60% in neonates). Metabolized in liver. Primarily excreted in urine. Not removed by hemodialysis. **Half-life: (single dose):** 2–8 hrs, **(multiple doses):** 4.5–12 hrs.

USES

Parenteral: Management of supraventricular tachyarrhythmias (SVT), temporary control of rapid ventricular rate in atrial flutter/fibrillation. **PO:** Treatment of hypertension, angina pectoris, supraventricular tachyarrhythmias (SVT), atrial fibrillation/flutter (rate control). **OFF-LABEL:** Treatment of bipolar disorder (manic manifestations), hypertrophic cardiomyopathy.

PRECAUTIONS

Contraindications: Atrial fibrillation/flutter in presence of accessory bypass tract (e.g., Wolff-Parkinson-White, Lown-Ganong-Levine syndromes), severe left ventricular dysfunction, cardiogenic shock, second- or third-degree heart block (except with pacemaker), hypotension, sick sinus syndrome (except with pacemaker). **IV (additional):** IV beta-blocking agents, ventricular tachycardia. **Cautions:** Renal/hepatic impairment, concomitant use of beta-blockers and/or digoxin, myasthenia gravis, hypertrophic cardiomyopathy.

⏳ LIFESPAN CONSIDERATIONS

Pregnancy/Lactation: Drug crosses placenta; distributed in breast milk. Breastfeeding not recommended. **Pregnancy Category C. Children:** No age-related precautions noted. **Elderly:** Age-related renal impairment may require dosage adjustment.

INTERACTIONS

DRUG: Beta-adrenergic blockers may have additive negative effects on heart rate, AV conduction, or contractility. **Statins** may increase risk of myopathy, rhabdomyolysis. May increase concentration of **cyclosporine, carbamazepine.** May in-

crease **digoxin** concentration. **CYP3A4 inducers (e.g., rifampin)** may decrease concentration/effects. **HERBAL: St. John's wort** may decrease concentration/effects. **Ephedra, ginseng, ginger, licorice, yohimbe, black cohosh, periwinkle** may worsen hypertension. **FOOD: Grapefruit, grapefruit juice** may increase concentration. **LAB VALUES:** EKG may show prolonged PR interval. **Therapeutic serum level:** 0.08–0.3 mcg/ml; **toxic serum level:** N/A.

AVAILABILITY (Rx)

Caplets (Sustained-Release [Calan SR]): 120 mg, 180 mg, 240 mg. **Injection Solution:** 2.5 mg/ml. **Tablets (Calan):** 40 mg, 80 mg, 120 mg.

 Capsules (Extended-Release [Verelan PM]): 100 mg, 200 mg, 300 mg. **Capsules (Extended-Release):** 120 mg, 180 mg, 240 mg. **Capsules (Sustained-Release [Verelan]):** 120 mg, 180 mg, 240 mg, 360 mg. **Tablets (Extended-Release [Covera-HS]):** 180 mg, 240 mg. **Tablets (Sustained-Release [Isoptin SR]):** 120 mg, 180 mg, 240 mg.

ADMINISTRATION/HANDLING

💧 IV

Reconstitution • May give undiluted.
Rate of Administration • Administer IV push over 2 min for adults, children; give over 3 min for elderly. • Continuous EKG monitoring during IV injection is required for children, recommended for adults. • Monitor EKG for rapid ventricular rate, extreme bradycardia, heart block, asystole, prolongation of PR interval. Notify physician of any significant changes. • Monitor B/P q5–10min. • Pt should remain recumbent for at least 1 hr after IV administration.
Storage • Store vials at room temperature.

PO

• Do not give with grapefruit, grapefruit juice. • Non–sustained-release tablets may be given without regard to food. • Give extended-release, sustained-release tablets whole; do not break, crush, dissolve, or divide. • Sustained-release capsules (Verelan, Verelan PM) may be opened and sprinkled on applesauce, then swallowed immediately (do not chew).

🔳 IV INCOMPATIBILITIES

Albumin, amphotericin B complex (Abelcet, AmBisome, Amphotec), nafcillin (Nafcil), propofol (Diprivan), sodium bicarbonate.

🔳 IV COMPATIBILITIES

Amiodarone (Cordarone), calcium chloride, calcium gluconate, dexamethasone (Decadron), digoxin (Lanoxin), dobutamine (Dobutrex), dopamine (Intropin), furosemide (Lasix), heparin, hydromorphone (Dilaudid), lidocaine, magnesium sulfate, metoclopramide (Reglan), milrinone (Primacor), morphine, multivitamins, nitroglycerin, norepinephrine (Levophed), potassium chloride, potassium phosphate, procainamide (Pronestyl), propranolol (Inderal).

INDICATIONS/ROUTES/DOSAGE

Supraventricular Tachyarrhythmias (SVT)
IV: ADULTS, ELDERLY: Initially, 2.5–5 mg over 2 min. May give 5–10 mg 30 min after initial dose. **Maximum total dose:** 20–30 mg. **CHILDREN 1–15 YRS:** 0.1–0.3 mg/kg over 2 min. **Maximum initial dose:** 5 mg. May repeat in 30 min. **Maximum second dose:** 10 mg.

Angina, Unstable Angina, Chronic Stable Angina
PO: ADULTS (IMMEDIATE-RELEASE): Initially, 80–120 mg 3 times a day. For elderly pts, those with hepatic dysfunction, 40 mg 3 times a day. Titrate to optimal dose. **Maintenance:** 240–480 mg/day in 3–4 divided doses. Usual range: 80–160 mg 3 times/day. **(EXTENDED-RELEASE) (Covera-HS):** Initially, 180 mg at bedtime. May increase at weekly intervals to 240 mg/day, 360 mg/day, up to 480 mg/day.

Hypertension
PO (Immediate-Release): ADULTS, ELDERLY: 80 mg 3 times a day. Range: 80–320 mg/day in 2 divided doses.
PO (Sustained-Release [Calan SR, Isoptin SR]): ADULTS, ELDERLY: Initially, 120–180 mg once daily. May increase at weekly intervals to 240 mg once daily, then 180 mg twice daily. **Maximum:** 240 mg twice daily.
[Verelan]: Initially, 120–180 mg once daily. May increase dose at weekly intervals to 240 mg/day, then 360 mg/day, then 480 mg/day maximum.
PO (Extended-Release [Covera-HS]): ADULTS, ELDERLY: Initially, 180 mg once daily at bedtime. May increase at weekly intervals to 240 mg/day, then 360 mg/day, then 480 mg/day maximum.
PO (Extended-Release [Verelan PM]): ADULTS, ELDERLY: Initially, 100–200 mg once daily at bedtime. May increase dose at weekly intervals to 300 mg once daily, then 400 mg once daily maximum.

Chronic Atrial Fibrillation (Rate Control), SVT
PO (Immediate-Release): ADULTS, ELDERLY: 240–480 mg/day in 3–4 divided doses. **Usual range:** 120–360 mg/day.

Dosage for Renal Impairment
Creatinine clearance less than 10 ml/min: Give 50%–75% normal dose.

SIDE EFFECTS

Frequent (7%): Constipation. **Occasional (4%–2%):** Dizziness, light-headedness, headache, asthenia (loss of strength, energy), nausea, peripheral edema, hypotension. **Rare (less than 1%):** Bradycardia, dermatitis, rash.

ADVERSE EFFECTS/ TOXIC REACTIONS

Rapid ventricular rate in atrial flutter/ fibrillation, marked hypotension, extreme bradycardia, HF, asystole, second- or third-degree AV block occur rarely. **Antidote:** Glucagon 5–10 mg over 1 min, then infuse 1–10 mg over 1 hour.

NURSING CONSIDERATIONS

BASELINE ASSESSMENT

Record onset, type (sharp, dull, squeezing), radiation, location, intensity, duration of anginal pain, precipitating factors (exertion, emotional stress). Check B/P for hypotension, pulse for bradycardia immediately before giving medication.

INTERVENTION/EVALUATION

Assess pulse for quality, rate, rhythm. Monitor B/P. Monitor EKG for cardiac changes, particularly prolongation of PR interval. Notify physician of any significant EKG interval changes. Assist with ambulation if dizziness occurs. Assess for peripheral edema behind medial malleolus (sacral area in bedridden pts). For those taking oral form, monitor daily pattern of bowel activity, stool consistency. **Therapeutic serum level:** 0.08–0.3 mcg/ml; **toxic serum level:** N/A.

PATIENT/FAMILY TEACHING

• Do not abruptly discontinue medication. • Compliance with therapy regimen is essential to control anginal pain. • Go from lying to standing slowly. • Avoid tasks that require alertness, motor skills until response to drug is established. • Limit caffeine. • Avoid or limit alcohol. • Report continued, persistent angina pain, irregular heartbeats, shortness of breath, swelling, dizziness, constipation, nausea, hypotension. • Avoid grapefruit products.

vilazodone

vil-**az**-oh-done
(Viibyrd)

BLACK BOX ALERT Increased risk of suicidal ideation and behavior in children, adolescents, and young adults 18–24 yrs of age with major depressive disorder, other psychiatric disorders.

◆CLASSIFICATION

PHARMACOTHERAPEUTIC: Serotonin reuptake receptor inhibitor. **CLINICAL:** Antidepressant (see p. 41C).

ACTION

Enhances serotonergic activity in CNS by selectively inhibiting reuptake of serotonin. **Therapeutic Effect:** Relieves depression.

PHARMACOKINETICS

Readily absorbed from GI tract. Peak concentration: 4–5 hrs. Widely distributed. Protein binding: 96%–99%. Metabolized in liver. **Half-life:** 25 hrs.

USES

Treatment of depression exhibited as persistent, prominent dysphoria (occurring nearly every day for at least 2 wks) manifested by 4 of 8 symptoms: change in appetite, change in sleep pattern, increased fatigue, impaired concentration, feelings of guilt or worthlessness, loss of interest in usual activities, psychomotor agitation or retardation, suicidal tendencies.

PRECAUTIONS

Contraindications: Pts either currently receiving MAOIs or within 14 days of stopping or starting a MAOI. **Cautions:** Concurrent use of NSAIDs, aspirin, or other drugs that affect coagulation; history of seizures; pts at risk for suicide; history of bipolar disorder, mania, hypomania; hepatic impairment; concomitant CNS depressants; strong or moderate CYP3A4 inhibitors; elderly.

⌛ LIFESPAN CONSIDERATIONS

Pregnancy/Lactation: Unknown if drug crosses placenta or is excreted in breast milk. **Pregnancy Category C. Children:** Safety and efficacy not established. **Elderly:** No age-related precautions noted.

INTERACTIONS

DRUG: Aspirin, NSAIDs, warfarin may increase risk of bleeding. Strong **CYP3A4**

inhibitors (e.g., ketoconazole, nefazodone, ritonavir) increase concentration. **Almotriptan, buspirone, eletriptan, naratriptan, SNRIs (e.g., venlafaxine), SSRIs (e.g., sertraline), sumatriptan, tramadol, tryptophan** may increase risk of serotonin syndrome. **HERBAL: St. John's wort** may increase risk of serotonin syndrome. **FOOD:** None known. **LAB VALUES:** None significant.

AVAILABILITY (Rx)

Tablets: 10 mg, 20 mg, 40 mg.

ADMINISTRATION/HANDLING

PO
• Give with food (administration without food can result in inadequate drug concentration, may diminish effectiveness).

INDICATIONS/ROUTES/DOSAGE

Depression
PO: ADULTS, ELDERLY: Initially, 10 mg once daily for 7 days, followed by 20 mg once daily for an additional 7 days, and then increased to 40 mg once daily. **Note:** When discontinuing treatment, reduce dose gradually.

Concomitant Moderate/Strong CYP3A4 Inhibitors
PO: ADULTS, ELDERLY: 20 mg/day.

SIDE EFFECTS

Frequent (28%–23%): Diarrhea, nausea. **Occasional (9%–3%):** Dizziness, dry mouth, insomnia, vomiting, decreased libido, abnormal dreams, fatigue, sweating. **Rare (2%):** Dyspepsia (heartburn, GI upset), flatulence, paresthesia, restlessness, arthralgia, abnormal orgasm, delayed ejaculation, increased appetite, palpitations, tremor.

ADVERSE EFFECTS/ TOXIC REACTIONS

Serotonin syndrome (agitation, confusion, hallucinations, hyper-reflexia), neuroleptic malignant syndrome (fever, muscular rigidity, cognitive changes).

NURSING CONSIDERATIONS

BASELINE ASSESSMENT
Assess behavior, appearance, emotional status, response to environment, speech pattern, thought content, risk of suicide.

INTERVENTION/EVALUATION
Monitor B/P, heart rate, weight. Monitor for suicidal ideation (esp. at initiation of therapy or changes in dosage). Assess for therapeutic response (greater interest in surroundings, improved self-care, increased ability to concentrate, relaxed facial expression).

PATIENT/FAMILY TEACHING
• Avoid tasks that may require alertness, motor skills until response to drug is established (may cause dizziness). • Take with food. • Do not suddenly stop taking medication; withdraw gradually. • Use caution when changing position from lying or sitting to standing. Report suicidal ideation, signs of mania/hypomania. Avoid alcohol.

---

*vinBLAStine

vin-**blas**-teen
(Velban)

BLACK BOX ALERT Must be administered by personnel trained in administration/handling of chemotherapeutic agents. Fatal if given intrathecally (ascending paralysis, death). Vesicant; avoid extravasation.
Do not confuse vinblastine with vincristine or vinorelbine.

◆CLASSIFICATION
PHARMACOTHERAPEUTIC: Vinca alkaloid. **CLINICAL:** Antineoplastic (see p. 91C).

 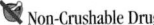

ACTION

Binds to microtubular protein of mitotic spindle, causing metaphase arrest. **Therapeutic Effect:** Inhibits cell division.

PHARMACOKINETICS

Does not cross blood-brain barrier. Protein binding: 99%. Metabolized in liver. Primarily eliminated in feces by biliary system. **Half-life:** 24.8 hrs.

USES

Treatment of disseminated Hodgkin's disease, non-Hodgkin's lymphoma, advanced stage of mycosis fungoides, advanced testicular carcinoma, Kaposi's sarcoma, Letterer-Siwe disease, breast carcinoma, choriocarcinoma. **OFF-LABEL:** Treatment of bladder, ovarian cancer; non–small-cell lung cancer; soft tissue sarcoma, melanoma.

PRECAUTIONS

Contraindications: Bacterial infection, significant granulocytopenia (unless a result of disease being treated). **Cautions:** Hepatic impairment, severe leukopenia, neurotoxicity, recent exposure to radiation therapy, chemotherapy, ischemic heart disease, preexisting pulmonary disease.

⌛ LIFESPAN CONSIDERATIONS

Pregnancy/Lactation: If possible, avoid use during pregnancy, esp. during first trimester. Breastfeeding not recommended. **Pregnancy Category D. Children/Elderly:** No age-related precautions noted.

INTERACTIONS

DRUG: May decrease concentration/anticonvulsant effects of **phenytoin. CYP3A4 inhibitors (e.g., erthromycin)** may increase level/toxicity. **Bone marrow depressants** may increase myelosuppression. **Live virus vaccines** may potentiate virus replication, increase vaccine side effects, decrease pt's antibody response to vaccine. **HERBAL: St. John's wort** may decrease concentra-

tion. Avoid **black cohosh, dong quai** in estrogen-dependent tumors. **FOOD:** None known. **LAB VALUES:** May increase serum uric acid.

AVAILABILITY (Rx)

Injection, Powder for Reconstitution: 10 mg. **Injection Solution:** 1 mg/ml.

ADMINISTRATION/HANDLING

◀**ALERT**▶ May be carcinogenic, mutagenic, teratogenic. Handle with extreme care during preparation and administration. Give by IV injection. Leakage from IV site into surrounding tissue may produce extreme irritation. Avoid eye contact with solution (severe eye irritation, possible corneal ulceration may result). If eye contact occurs, immediately irrigate eye with water.

 IV

Reconstitution • Reconstitute 10-mg vial with 10 ml 0.9% NaCl preserved with phenol or benzyl alcohol to provide concentration of 1 mg/ml. May further dilute in 50 ml D₅W or 0.9% NaCl.
Rate of Administration • Inject into tubing of running IV infusion or directly into vein over 1 min (IV infusion over 5–15 min). • Do not inject into extremity with impaired, potentially impaired circulation caused by compression or invading neoplasm, phlebitis, varicosity. • Rinse syringe, needle with venous blood before withdrawing needle (minimizes possibility of extravasation). • Extravasation may result in cellulitis, phlebitis. Large amount of extravasation may result in tissue sloughing. If extravasation occurs, give local injection of hyaluronidase, apply warm compresses.
Storage • Refrigerate unopened vials. • Solution appears clear, colorless. • Following reconstitution, solution is stable for 30 days if refrigerated. • Discard if solution is discolored or precipitate forms.

🖥 IV INCOMPATIBILITIES

Furosemide (Lasix).

Seneca LIBRARIES

Customer name: Huiling Su
Customer ID: *****8137
Messages

Items that you have signed out

Title:
 Saunders nursing drug handbook /
 Barbara B. Hodgson, Robert J. Kizior.
ID: 0134112127532
Due: March-22-16
Messages:

Total items: 1
Account balance: $0.00
08/03/2016 3:54 PM
Checked out: 1
Overdue: 0
Hold requests: 0
Ready for collection: 0
Messages:

Thank you for using Seneca Libraries
SelfCheck (NH1)

🔲 IV COMPATIBILITIES

Allopurinol (Aloprim), cisplatin (Platinol AQ), cyclophosphamide (Cytoxan), doxorubicin (Adriamycin), etoposide (VePesid), 5-fluorouracil, gemcitabine (Gemzar), granisetron (Kytril), heparin, leucovorin, methotrexate, ondansetron (Zofran), paclitaxel (Taxol), vinorelbine (Navelbine).

INDICATIONS/ROUTES/DOSAGE

◀ALERT▶ Dosage individualized based on clinical response, tolerance to adverse effects. When used in combination therapy, consult specific protocols for optimum dosage, sequence of drug administration.

Usual Dosage
IV: ADULTS, ELDERLY: 3.7–7.4 mg/m² q7days. **Maximum:** 18.5 mg/m². **CHILDREN:** 2.5–6 mg/m² q7–14days. **Maximum:** 12.5 mg/m²/wk.

Dosage in Hepatic Impairment
Direct serum bilirubin concentration greater than 3 mg/dl: Reduce dose by 50%.

SIDE EFFECTS

Frequent: Nausea, vomiting, alopecia. **Occasional:** Constipation, diarrhea, rectal bleeding, headache, paresthesia (occur 4–6 hrs after administration, persist for 2–10 hrs), malaise, asthenia (loss of strength, energy), dizziness, pain at tumor site, jaw/face pain, depression, dry mouth. **Rare:** Dermatitis, stomatitis, phototoxicity, hyperuricemia.

ADVERSE EFFECTS/ TOXIC REACTIONS

Hematologic toxicity manifested most commonly as leukopenia, less frequently as anemia. WBC reaches its nadir 4–10 days after initial therapy, recovers within 7–14 days (high dosage may require 21-day recovery period). Thrombocytopenia is usually mild and transient, with recovery occurring in few days. Hepatic insufficiency may increase risk of toxicity. Acute shortness of breath, broncho-spasm may occur, particularly when administered concurrently with mitomycin.

NURSING CONSIDERATIONS

BASELINE ASSESSMENT

Nausea, vomiting easily controlled by antiemetics. Discontinue therapy if WBC, platelet counts fall abruptly (unless drug is clearly destroying tumor cells in bone marrow). Obtain CBC weekly or before each dosing.

INTERVENTION/EVALUATION

If WBC falls below 2,000/mm³, assess diligently for signs of infection. Assess for stomatitis; maintain strict oral hygiene. Monitor for hematologic toxicity: infection (fever, sore throat, signs of local infection), unusual bruising/bleeding from any site, symptoms of anemia (excessive fatigue, weakness). Monitor daily pattern of bowel activity, stool consistency. Avoid constipation.

PATIENT/FAMILY TEACHING

• Immediately report any pain/burning at injection site during administration. • Pain at tumor site may occur during or shortly after injection. • Do not have immunizations without physician approval (drug lowers resistance). • Avoid crowds, those with infection. • Promptly report fever, sore throat, signs of local infection, unusual bruising/bleeding from any site. • Hair loss is reversible, but new hair growth may have different color, texture. • Report persistent nausea/vomiting. • Avoid constipation by increasing fluids, bulk in diet, exercise as tolerated.

---

*vinCRIStine

vin-**cris**-teen
(Marqibo, Vincasar PFS)
BLACK BOX ALERT Must be administered by personnel trained in administration/handling of chemotherapeutic agents. Fatal if given

---

 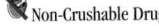
V

intrathecally (ascending paralysis, death). Vesicant; avoid extravasation. Marqibo and Vincasar are not interchangeable. **Do not confuse vincristine with vinblastine.**

◆CLASSIFICATION

PHARMACOTHERAPEUTIC: Vinca alkaloid. **CLINICAL:** Antineoplastic (see p. 91C).

ACTION

Binds to microtubular protein of mitotic spindle, causing metaphase arrest. **Therapeutic Effect:** Inhibits cell division.

PHARMACOKINETICS

Does not cross blood-brain barrier. Protein binding: 75%. Metabolized in liver. Primarily eliminated in feces by biliary system. **Half-life:** 24 hrs. Marqibo: 45 hrs.

USES

Vincasar: Treatment of acute lymphocytic leukemia (ALL), Hodgkin's lymphoma, advanced non-Hodgkin's lymphomas, neuroblastoma, rhabdomyosarcoma, Wilms tumor. **Marqibo:** Relapsed Philadelphia chromosome negative (Ph⁻) ALL. **OFF-LABEL:** Treatment of multiple myeloma, chronic lymphocytic leukemia (CLL), brain tumors, small cell lung cancer, ovarian germ cell tumors.

PRECAUTIONS

Contraindications: Demyelinating form of Charcot-Marie-Tooth syndrome. Intrathecal administration. **Caution:** Hepatic impairment, pts receiving radiation therapy through ports (including liver), neurotoxicity, preexisting neuromuscular disease, hepatobiliary dysfunction, elderly.

⌛ LIFESPAN CONSIDERATIONS

Pregnancy/Lactation: If possible, avoid use during pregnancy, esp. first trimester. May cause fetal harm. Breastfeeding not recommended. **Pregnancy Category D.**

Children: No age-related precautions noted. **Elderly:** More susceptible to neurotoxic effects.

INTERACTIONS

DRUG: May decrease concentration/anticonvulsant effects of **phenytoin. Itraconazole** may increase severity of neuromuscular side effects. **Live virus vaccines** may potentiate virus replication, increase vaccine side effects, decrease pt's antibody response to vaccine. **HERBAL: St. John's wort, echinacea** may decrease concentration. **FOOD:** None known. **LAB VALUES:** May increase serum uric acid.

AVAILABILITY (Rx)

Injection Solution: 1 mg/ml. Marqibo: Kit for IV administration containing 5 mg/31 ml vincristine.

ADMINISTRATION/HANDLING
 IV

◀**ALERT**▶ May be carcinogenic, mutagenic, teratogenic. Handle with extreme care during preparation and administration. Give by IV injection. Use extreme caution in calculating, administering vincristine. Overdose may result in serious or fatal outcome.

Reconstitution • May give undiluted or diluted in 25–50 ml D₅W or 0.9% NaCl. **Rate of Administration** • Inject dose into tubing of running IV infusion or directly into vein over 1 min. May be administered as 5–10 min infusion (preferred). • Do not inject into extremity with impaired, potentially impaired circulation caused by compression or invading neoplasm, phlebitis, varicosity. • Extravasation produces stinging, burning, edema at injection site. Terminate injection immediately, locally inject hyaluronidase, apply heat (disperses drug, minimizes discomfort, cellulitis).

Storage • Refrigerate unopened vials. • Solution appears clear, colorless. • Discard if solution is discolored or precipitate forms.

IV INCOMPATIBILITIES

Furosemide (Lasix), idarubicin (Idamycin).

IV COMPATIBILITIES

Allopurinol (Aloprim), cisplatin (Platinol AQ), cyclophosphamide (Cytoxan), cytarabine (Ara-C, Cytosar), doxorubicin (Adriamycin), etoposide (VePesid), 5-fluorouracil, gemcitabine (Gemzar), granisetron (Kytril), leucovorin, methotrexate, ondansetron (Zofran), paclitaxel (Taxol), vinorelbine (Navelbine).

INDICATIONS/ROUTES/DOSAGE

Usual Dosage

IV: ADULTS, ELDERLY: 1.4 mg/m², frequency may vary based on protocol. **CHILDREN WEIGHING MORE THAN 10 KG:** 1.5–2 mg/m², frequency may vary based on protocol. **CHILDREN WEIGHING LESS THAN 10 KG:** 0.05 mg/kg once weekly. **Maximum:** 2 mg.

Hepatic Impairment

Bilirubin	Dosage
Bilirubin greater than 3 mg/dl	50% of normal

ALL (Marqibo)

IV: ADULTS, ELDERLY: 2.25 mg/m² q7days. Infuse over 1 hr.

SIDE EFFECTS

Expected: Peripheral neuropathy (occurs in nearly every pt; first clinical sign is depression of Achilles tendon reflex). **Frequent:** Peripheral paresthesia, alopecia, constipation/obstipation (upper colon impaction with empty rectum), abdominal cramps, headache, jaw pain, hoarseness, diplopia, ptosis/drooping of eyelid, urinary tract disturbances. **Occasional:** Nausea, vomiting, diarrhea, abdominal distention, stomatitis, fever. **Rare:** Mild leukopenia, mild anemia, thrombocytopenia.

ADVERSE EFFECTS/ TOXIC REACTIONS

Acute shortness of breath, bronchospasm may occur, esp. when administered concurrently with mitomycin. Prolonged or high-dose therapy may produce foot/wrist drop, difficulty walking, slapping gait, ataxia, muscle wasting. Acute uric acid nephropathy may occur.

NURSING CONSIDERATIONS

BASELINE ASSESSMENT

Obtain baseline CBC, hepatic function studies. Offer pt/family emotional support.

INTERVENTION/EVALUATION

Monitor serum uric acid levels, renal/hepatic function studies, CBC. Assess Achilles tendon reflex. Monitor daily pattern of bowel activity, stool consistency. Monitor for ptosis, diplopia, blurred vision. Question pt regarding urinary changes.

PATIENT/FAMILY TEACHING

• Immediately report any pain/burning at injection site during administration. • Hair loss is reversible, but new hair growth may have different color/texture. • Report persistent nausea/vomiting. • Report signs of peripheral neuropathy (burning/numbness of bottom of feet, palms of hands). • Report fever, sore throat, unusual bleeding/bruising, shortness of breath.

vinorelbine

vin-oh-**rel**-been
(Navelbine)

BLACK BOX ALERT Must be administered by personnel trained in administration/handling of chemotherapeutic agents. Fatal if given intrathecally (ascending paralysis, death). Extravasation produces thrombophlebitis, local tissue necrosis. May produce severe granulocytopenia.

Do not confuse vinorelbine with vinblastine or vincristine.

◆CLASSIFICATION

PHARMACOTHERAPEUTIC: Vinca alkaloid. **CLINICAL:** Antineoplastic (see p. 92C).

ACTION

Interferes with mitotic microtubule assembly. **Therapeutic Effect:** Prevents cellular division.

PHARMACOKINETICS

Widely distributed after IV administration. Protein binding: 80%–90%. Metabolized in liver. Primarily eliminated in feces by biliary system. **Half-life:** 28–43 hrs.

USES

Single agent or in combination with cisplatin for treatment of unresectable, advanced, non–small-cell lung cancer (NSCLC). **OFF-LABEL:** Treatment of metastatic breast cancer, cervical carcinoma, ovarian carcinoma, malignant pleural mesothelioma, soft tissue sarcoma.

PRECAUTIONS

Contraindications: Granulocyte count before treatment of less than 1,000 cells/mm³. **Cautions:** Compromised marrow reserve due to prior chemotherapy/radiation therapy; hepatic impairment, neurotoxicity; neuropathy, pulmonary impairment.

☒ LIFESPAN CONSIDERATIONS

Pregnancy/Lactation: If possible, avoid use during pregnancy, esp. during first trimester. May cause fetal harm. Unknown if distributed in breast milk. Breastfeeding not recommended. **Pregnancy Category D. Children:** Safety and efficacy not established. **Elderly:** No age-related precautions noted.

INTERACTIONS

DRUG: Bone marrow depressants may increase risk of myelosuppression. **Cisplatin** significantly increases risk of granulo-cytopenia. **Live virus vaccines** may potentiate virus replication, increase vaccine side effects, decrease pt's antibody response to vaccine. **Mitomycin** may produce an acute pulmonary reaction. **Paclitaxel** may increase neuropathy. **CYP3A4 inhibitors (e.g., ketoconazole)** may increase concentration/effect. **HERBAL: St. John's wort** may decrease concentration. **FOOD:** None known. **LAB VALUES:** May increase serum bilirubin, alkaline phosphatase, AST, ALT.

AVAILABILITY (Rx)

Injection Solution: 10 mg/ml (1-ml, 5-ml vials).

ADMINISTRATION/HANDLING

◆ IV

◀**ALERT**▶ IV needle, catheter must be correctly positioned before administration. Leakage into surrounding tissue produces extreme irritation, local tissue necrosis, thrombophlebitis. Handle drug with extreme care during administration; wear protective clothing per protocol. If solution comes in contact with skin/mucosa, immediately wash thoroughly with soap, water.

Reconstitution • Must be diluted and administered via syringe or IV bag. SYRINGE DILUTION • Dilute calculated vinorelbine dose with D₅W or 0.9% NaCl to concentration of 1.5–3 mg/ml. IV BAG DILUTION • Dilute calculated vinorelbine dose with D₅W, 0.45% or 0.9% NaCl, 5% dextrose and 0.45% NaCl, Ringer's or lactated Ringer's to concentration of 0.5–2 mg/ml.

Rate of Administration • Administer diluted vinorelbine over 6–10 min into side port of free-flowing IV closest to IV bag followed by flushing with 75–125 ml of one of the solutions. • If extravasation occurs, stop injection immediately; give remaining portion of dose into another vein.

Storage • Refrigerate unopened vials. • Protect from light. • Unopened vials are stable at room temperature for 72 hrs. • Do not administer if particulate has formed. • Diluted vinorelbine may be used for up to 24 hrs under normal room light when stored in polypropylene syringes or polyvinyl chloride bags at room temperature.

🏵 IV INCOMPATIBILITIES

Acyclovir (Zovirax), allopurinol (Aloprim), amphotericin B (Fungizone), amphotericin B complex (Abelcet, AmBisome, Amphotec), ampicillin (Omnipen), cefazolin (Ancef), ceftriaxone (Rocephin), cefuroxime (Zinacef), 5-fluorouracil (5-FU), furosemide (Lasix), ganciclovir (Cytovene), methylprednisolone (Solu-Medrol), sodium bicarbonate.

🏵 IV COMPATIBILITIES

Calcium gluconate, carboplatin (Paraplatin), cisplatin (Platinol AQ), cyclophosphamide (Cytoxan), cytarabine (ARA-C, Cytosar), dacarbazine (DTIC), daunorubicin (Cerubidine), dexamethasone (Decadron), diphenhydramine (Benadryl), doxorubicin (Adriamycin), etoposide (VePesid), gemcitabine (Gemzar), granisetron (Kytril), hydromorphone (Dilaudid), idarubicin (Idamycin), methotrexate, morphine, ondansetron (Zofran), vinblastine (Velban), vincristine (Oncovin).

INDICATIONS/ROUTES/DOSAGE

◀ALERT▶ Dosage adjustments should be based on granulocyte count obtained on the day of treatment, as follows:

Granulocyte Count (cells/mm³) on Day of Treatment	Dosage
1,500 or higher	100% of starting dose
1,000–1,499	50% of starting dose
Less than 1,000	Do not administer

NSCLC Monotherapy
IV Injection: ADULTS, ELDERLY: 30 mg/m² administered weekly over 6–10 min.

NSCLC Combination Therapy with Cisplatin
IV Injection: ADULTS, ELDERLY: 25–30 mg/m² every wk.

Dosage in Hepatic Impairment

Bilirubin	Dosage
2 mg/dl or less	100% of dose
2.1–3 mg/dl	50% of dose
Greater than 3 mg/dl	25% of dose

SIDE EFFECTS

Frequent (35%–12%): Asthenia (loss of strength, energy), nausea, constipation, erythema, pain, vein discoloration at injection site, fatigue, peripheral neuropathy manifested as paresthesia, hyperesthesia, diarrhea, alopecia. **Occasional (10%–5%):** Phlebitis, dyspnea, loss of deep tendon reflexes. **Rare:** Chest pain, jaw pain, myalgia, arthralgia, rash.

ADVERSE EFFECTS/ TOXIC REACTIONS

Bone marrow depression is manifested mainly as granulocytopenia (may be severe). Other hematologic toxicities (neutropenia, thrombocytopenia, leukopenia, anemia) increase risk of infection, bleeding. Acute shortness of breath, severe bronchospasm occur infrequently, particularly in pts with preexisting pulmonary dysfunction.

NURSING CONSIDERATIONS

BASELINE ASSESSMENT
Review medication history. Assess hematology (RBC, Hgb, Hct, platelet count, differential) values before giving each dose. Granulocyte count should be at least 1,000 cells/mm³ before vinorelbine administration. Granulocyte nadirs occur 7–10 days following dosing. Do not give hematologic growth factors within 24 hrs before administration of chemotherapy or earlier than 24 hrs following cytotoxic chemotherapy. Advise women of childbearing potential to avoid pregnancy during drug therapy.

V

INTERVENTION/EVALUATION

Diligently monitor injection site for swelling, redness, pain. Frequently monitor for myelosuppression during and following therapy (infection [fever, sore throat, signs of local infection], unusual bleeding/bruising, anemia [excessive fatigue, weakness]). Monitor pts developing severe granulocytopenia for evidence of infection, fever. Crackers, dry toast, sips of cola may help relieve nausea. Monitor daily pattern of bowel activity, stool consistency. Question for tingling, burning, numbness of hands/feet (peripheral neuropathy). Pt complaint of "walking on glass" is sign of hyperesthesia.

PATIENT/FAMILY TEACHING

• Immediately report redness, swelling, pain at injection site. • Avoid crowds, those with infection. • Do not have immunizations without physician's approval. • Promptly report fever, signs of infection, unusual bruising/bleeding from any site, difficulty breathing. • Avoid pregnancy. • Hair loss is reversible, but new hair growth may have different color, texture.

---

vismodegib

vis-moe-**deg**-ib
(Erivedge)

BLACK BOX ALERT May result in embryo-fetal death or severe birth defects including missing digits, midline defects, irreversible malformations due to embryotoxic and teratogenic properties. Verify pregnancy status prior to initiation. Advise use of effective contraception in female pts. Advise male pts of potential exposure risk through seminal fluid.

◆CLASSIFICATION

PHARMACOTHERAPEUTIC: Hedgehog pathway inhibitor. **CLINICAL:** Antineoplastic (see p. 92C).

ACTION

An inhibitor of Hedgehog pathway, binding to and inhibiting smoothened, a transmembrane protein involved in hedgehog signal transduction. **Therapeutic Effect:** Inhibits tumor cell growth and metastasis of basal cell carcinoma.

PHARMACOKINETICS

Metabolized in liver. Protein binding: 99%. Excreted in feces (82%), urine (4%). **Half-life:** 4 days (daily dosing), 12 days (single dose).

USES

Treatment of adult pts with metastatic basal cell carcinoma, locally advanced basal cell carcinoma with recurrence after surgery, or pts who are not candidates for surgery or radiation.

PRECAUTIONS

◄**ALERT**► Do not donate blood products for at least 7 mos after discontinuation.
Contraindications: None known. **Cautions:** None known.

⌛ LIFESPAN CONSIDERATIONS

Pregnancy/Lactation: May cause fetal harm. Not recommended in nursing mothers. Must either discontinue drug or discontinue breastfeeding. Unknown if distributed in breast milk. Contraception recommended during treatment and up to 7 mos after discontinuation. **Pregnancy Category D. Children:** Safety and efficacy not established. **Elderly:** Safety and efficacy not established.

INTERACTIONS

DRUG: P-glycoprotein **inhibitors (e.g., clarithromycin, erythromycin)** may increase concentration/effect. **Antacids, H₂ blockers, proton pump inhibitors** may decrease concentration/effect. **HERBAL:** None significant. **FOOD:** None known. **LAB VALUES:** May decrease potassium, sodium, GFR. May increase serum BUN, creatinine.

V

AVAILABILITY (Rx)

Capsules: 150 mg.

ADMINISTRATION/HANDLING

PO

• Give without regard to food. • Give whole. Do not crush, dissolve, open capsule.

INDICATIONS/ROUTES/DOSAGE

Advanced Basal Cell Carcinoma
PO: ADULTS/ELDERLY: 150 mg once daily.

SIDE EFFECTS

Frequent (71%–40%): Muscle spasm, alopecia, dysgeusia, weight loss, fatigue. **Occasional (30%–11%):** Nausea, amenorrhea, diarrhea, anorexia, constipation, vomiting, arthralgia, loss of taste.

ADVERSE EFFECTS/
TOXIC REACTIONS

May cause spontaneous abortion, fetal demise, birth defects. Azotemia (renal impairment) reported in 2% of pts.

NURSING CONSIDERATIONS

BASELINE ASSESSMENT

Obtain negative pregnancy test (urine/serum) before initiation, BMP. Question current breastfeeding status. Assess skin, moles for other possible malignancies.

INTERVENTION/EVALUATION

Obtain STAT human chorionic gonadotropin (HCG) level if pregnancy suspected, BMP if electrolyte imbalance or renal impairment suspected. Offer emotional support. Encourage PO intake if diarrhea occurs. Offer antiemetics for nausea/vomiting. Report oliguria, dark or concentrated urine.

PATIENT/FAMILY TEACHING

• Avoid pregnancy. • May cause birth defects or miscarriage. • Do not breastfeed. • Male pts must use condoms with spermicide during sexual activity, despite history of vasectomy. • Female pts must use contraception for at least 7 mos after stopping treatment. • Immediately report suspected pregnancy. • Do not donate blood for at least 7 mos after stopping treatment. • Swallow capsules whole; do not crush, open, or chew. • Hair loss is an expected side effect. • Strictly monitor menstrual cycle. • Report dark-colored urine or decreased urine output despite hydration.

---

vitamin A

vite-a-min A
(Aquasol A)
Do not confuse Aquasol A with Anusol.

◆CLASSIFICATION

PHARMACOTHERAPEUTIC: Fat-soluble vitamin. **CLINICAL:** Nutritional supplement (see p. 157C).

ACTION

May act as cofactor in biochemical reactions. **Therapeutic Effect:** Essential for normal function of retina, visual adaptation to darkness, bone growth, testicular and ovarian function, embryonic development; preserves integrity of e

PHARMACOKINETICS

Rapidly absorbed from GI tra
pancreatic lipase, protein, o
present. Transported in blood to liver, where it is metabolized; stored in parenchymal hepatic cells, then transported in plasma as retinol, as needed. Excreted primarily in bile and, to lesser extent, in urine.

USES

Treatment and prevention of vitamin A deficiency (biliary tract, pancreatic disease, sprue, colitis, hepatic cirrhosis, celiac disease, regional enteritis, extreme dietary inadequacy, partial gastrectomy, cystic fibrosis), dietary supplement. **OFF-LABEL:** Treatment of xerophthalmia

V

---

caused by vitamin A deficiency. Prevent complications in children with measles.

PRECAUTIONS

Contraindications: Hypervitaminosis A, pregnancy (dose exceeding RDA). **Cautions:** None significant.

⌛ LIFESPAN CONSIDERATIONS

Pregnancy/Lactation: Crosses placenta. Distributed in breast milk. **Pregnancy Category A (X if used in doses above recommended daily allowance). Children/Elderly:** Caution with higher dosages.

INTERACTIONS

DRUG: Oral contraceptives may increase concentration. **HERBAL:** None significant. **FOOD:** None known. **LAB VALUES:** None significant.

AVAILABILITY (Rx)

Injection Solution (Aquasol A): 50,000 units/ml. **Tablets:** 10,000 units, 15,000 units.

📷 **Capsules:** 10,000 units, 25,000 units.

ADMINISTRATION/HANDLING

◀ **ALERT** ▶ IM administration used only in acutely ill or pts unresponsive to oral ⬚ I malabsorption syndrome).

⬚ M injection in adults, if dosage is ⬚ ⬚ 0,000 international units), may give in deltoid muscle; if dosage is over 1 ml, give in large muscle mass. Anterolateral thigh is site of choice for infants, children younger than 7 mos.

PO

• Do not crush, break capsules. • Give with food or milk.

INDICATIONS/ROUTES/DOSAGE

Severe Vitamin A Deficiency
IM: ADULTS, ELDERLY, CHILDREN 8 YRS AND OLDER: 100,000 units/day for 3 days, then 50,000 units/day for 14 days followed by oral supplementation: 10,000–20,000

units once daily for 2 mos. **CHILDREN 1–7 YRS:** 17,500–35,000 units/day for 10 days followed by oral supplementation: 5,000–10,000 units once daily for 2 mos. **INFANTS YOUNGER THAN 1 YR:** 7,500–15,000 units/day for 10 days followed by oral supplementation: 5,000–10,000 units once daily for 2 mos.

Malabsorption Syndrome
PO: ADULTS, ELDERLY, CHILDREN 8 YRS AND OLDER: 10,000–50,000 units/day.

SIDE EFFECTS

None known.

ADVERSE EFFECTS/ TOXIC REACTIONS

Chronic overdose produces malaise, nausea, vomiting, drying/cracking of skin/lips, inflammation of tongue/gums, irritability, alopecia, night sweats. Bulging fontanelles have occurred in infants.

NURSING CONSIDERATIONS

INTERVENTION/EVALUATION

Closely supervise for overdosage symptoms during prolonged daily administration over 25,000 international units. Monitor for therapeutic serum vitamin A levels (80–300 international units/ml).

PATIENT/FAMILY TEACHING

• Foods rich in vitamin A include cod, halibut, tuna, shark (naturally occurring vitamin A found only in animal sources). • Avoid taking mineral oil, cholestyramine (Questran) while taking vitamin A.

vitamin D (vitamin D analogues)

calcitriol

kal-si-**trye**-ole
(Calcijex ✦, Rocaltrol, Vectical)

V

doxercalciferol

dock-sir-kal-**sih**-fer-al
(Hectorol)

ergocalciferol

er-goe-kal-**sih**-fer-al
(Drisdol)

paricalcitol

par-i-kal-si-tol
(Zemplar)

◆ CLASSIFICATION

PHARMACOTHERAPEUTIC: Fat-soluble vitamin. **CLINICAL:** Vitamin D analogue (see p. 158C).

ACTION

Calcitriol: Stimulates calcium transport in intestines, resorption in bones, and tubular reabsorption in kidney; suppresses parathyroid hormone (PTH) secretion/synthesis. **Doxercalciferol:** Regulates blood calcium levels, stimulates bone growth, suppresses PTH secretion/synthesis. **Ergocalciferol:** Promotes active absorption of calcium and phosphorus, increasing serum levels to allow bone mineralization; mobilizes calcium and phosphate from bone, increases reabsorption of calcium and phosphate by renal tubules. **Paricalcitol:** Suppresses PTH secretion/synthesis. **Therapeutic Effect:** Essential for absorption, utilization of calcium, phosphate, control of PTH levels.

PHARMACOKINETICS

Calcitriol: Rapidly absorbed. Protein binding: 99.9%. Metabolized to active metabolite (ergocalciferol). Primarily excreted in feces/urine. **Half-life:** 5–8 hrs. **Doxercalciferol:** Metabolized in liver. **Half-life:** 32–37 hrs. **Ergocalciferol:** Metabolized in liver. **Paricalci-**tol: Readily absorbed. Protein binding: 99.8%. Metabolized in liver. Primarily excreted in feces. **Half-life:** 5–7 hrs.

USES

Calcitriol: Manage hypocalcemia in pts on chronic renal dialysis, secondary hypoparathyroidism in chronic kidney disease (CKD), manage hypocalcemia in hypoparathyroidism. **(Topical):** Treatment of mild to moderate plaque psoriasis. **Doxercalciferol:** Treatment of secondary hyperparathyroidism in CKD. **Ergocalciferol:** Treatment of refractory rickets, hypophosphatemia, hypoparathyroidism, dietary supplement. **Paricalcitol: (Intravenous):** Treatment/prevention of secondary hyperparathyroidism associated with stage 5 CKD. **(PO):** Treatment/prevention of secondary hyperparathyroidism associated with stage 3 and 4 CKD and stage 5 CKD pts on hemodialysis or peritoneal dialysis. **OFF-LABEL:** **Calcitriol:** Vitamin D-dependent rickets. **Ergocalciferol:** Prevention/treatment of vitamin D deficiency in pts with CKD, osteoporosis prevention.

PRECAUTIONS

Contraindications: Vitamin D toxicity, hypercalcemia. **Cautions:** Pts with malabsorption syndrome. Concurrent use with digoxin.

⧖ LIFESPAN CONSIDERATIONS

Pregnancy/Lactation: Unknown if drug crosses placenta. Infant risk cannot be excluded. **Pregnancy Category: (Calcitriol):** A (C if used in doses above recommended daily allowance). **(Doxercalciferol):** B. **(Ergocalciferol):** A (C if used in doses above recommended daily allowance). **(Paricalcitol):** C. **Children/Elderly:** No age-related precautions noted.

INTERACTIONS

DRUG: Magnesium-containing antacids may increase risk of hypermagnesemia. **Calcium-containing products, concurrent vitamin D (or**

V

derivatives) may increase risk of hypercalcemia. May increase **digoxin** toxicity due to hypercalcemia (may cause arrhythmias). **HERBAL:** None significant. **FOOD:** None known. **LAB VALUES:** May increase serum cholesterol, calcium, magnesium, phosphate, ALT, AST, BUN, creatinine.

AVAILABILITY (Rx)

Calcitriol
Capsules, Softgel (Rocaltrol): 0.25 mcg, 0.5 mcg. **Injection Solution:** 1 mcg/ml. **Oral Solution (Rocaltrol):** 1 mcg/ml.

Doxercalciferol
Capsules, Softgel (Hectorol): 0.5 mcg, 1 mcg, 2.5 mcg. **Injection Solution (Hectorol):** 2 mcg/ml.

Ergocalciferol
Capsules (Drisdol): 50,000 units (1.25 mg). **Liquid, Oral (Drisdol):** 8,000 units/ml (200 mcg/ml). **Tablets:** 400 units.

Paricalcitol
Capsules, Gelatin (Zemplar): 1 mcg, 2 mcg, 4 mcg. **Injection Solution (Zemplar):** 2 mcg/ml.

ADMINISTRATION/HANDLING

Calcitriol
PO
• May take without regard to food.

 IV
• May give as IV bolus at end of dialysis.

Doxercalciferol
PO
• May take without regard to food.

 IV
• May give as IV bolus via catheter at end of dialysis.

Ergocalciferol
PO
• May take without regard to food.

Paricalcitol
PO
• May take without regard to food. • For 3 times/wk dosing, give no more frequently than every other day.

 IV
• Give bolus anytime during dialysis.
• Do not give more frequently than every other day.

INDICATIONS/ROUTES/DOSAGE

Calcitriol
Hypocalcemia on Chronic Renal Dialysis
PO: ADULTS, ELDERLY: (ROCALTROL): Initially, 0.25 mcg/day or every other day. May increase by 0.25 mcg/day at 4- to 8-wk intervals. **Range:** 0.5–1 mcg/day.
IV: ADULTS, ELDERLY: 1–2 mcg 3 times/wk. Adjust dose at 2- to 4-wk intervals. Range: 0.5–4 mcg 3 times/wk.

Hypocalcemia in Hypoparathyroidism
PO: ADULTS, CHILDREN 6 YRS AND OLDER: **(ROCALTROL):** Initially, 0.25 mcg/day. May increase at 2- to 4-wk intervals. Range: 0.5–2 mcg/day. **CHILDREN 1–5 YRS:** 0.25–0.75 mcg once daily. **CHILDREN YOUNGER THAN 1 YR:** 0.04–0.08 mcg/kg once daily. **NEONATES:** 1 mcg once daily first 5 days of life.

Secondary Hyperparathyroidism Associated with Moderate to Severe CKD Not on Dialysis
PO: ADULTS, ELDERLY, CHILDREN 3 YRS AND OLDER: (ROCALTROL): Initially, 0.25 mcg/day. May increase to 0.5 mcg/day. **CHILDREN YOUNGER THAN 3 YRS:** Initially, 0.01–0.015 mcg/kg/day.

Doxercalciferol
Secondary Hyperparathyroidism (Dialysis)
PO: ADULTS, ELDERLY: Initial dose (intact parathyroid hormone [iPTH] greater than 400 pg/ml): 10 mcg 3 times/wk at dialysis. Dose titrated to lower iPTH to 150–300 pg/ml, with dosage adjustments made at 8-wk intervals. **Maximum:** 20 mcg 3 times/wk.

IV: **ADULTS, ELDERLY:** Initial dose (iPTH greater than 400 pg/ml): 4 mcg 3 times/wk after dialysis, given as bolus dose. Dose titrated to lower iPTH to 150–300 pg/ml, with dosage adjustments made at 8-wk intervals. **Maximum:** 18 mcg/wk.

Secondary Hyperparathyroidism (Predialysis)
PO: **ADULTS, ELDERLY:** Initially, 1 mcg/day. Titrate dose to lower iPTH to 35–70 pg/ml for stage 3 CKD and 70–110 pg/ml for stage 4 CKD. **Maximum:** 3.5 mcg/day.

Ergocalciferol
Dietary Supplement
PO: **ADULTS, ELDERLY, CHILDREN:** 10 mcg (400 units)/day. **NEONATES:** 10–20 mcg (400–800 units)/day.

Hypoparathyroidism
PO: **ADULTS, ELDERLY:** 625 mcg–5 mg (25,000–200,000 units)/day (with calcium supplements). **CHILDREN:** 1.25–5 mg (50,000–200,000 units)/day (with calcium supplements).

Nutritional Rickets, Osteomalacia
PO: **ADULTS, ELDERLY, CHILDREN:** 25–125 mcg (1,000–5,000 units)/day for 8–12 wks. **ADULTS, ELDERLY (WITH MALABSORPTION SYNDROME):** 250–7,500 mcg (10,000–300,000 units)/day. **CHILDREN (WITH MALABSORPTION SYNDROME):** 250–625 mcg (10,000–25,000 units)/day.

Vitamin D–Dependent Rickets
PO: **ADULTS, ELDERLY:** 250 mcg–1.5 mg (10,000–60,000 units)/day. **CHILDREN:** 75–125 mcg (3,000–5,000 units)/day. **Maximum:** 1,500 mcg (60,000 units)/day.

Vitamin D–Resistant Rickets
PO: **ADULTS, ELDERLY, CHILDREN:** 300 mcg–12.5 mg (12,000–500,000 units)/day.

Hypophosphatemia
PO: **ADULTS, ELDERLY:** 250–1,500 mcg (10,000–60,000 units)/day with phosphate supplements. **CHILDREN:** 1,000–2,000 mcg (40,000–80,000 units)/day with phosphate supplements.

Plaque Psoriasis
Topical: **ADULTS, ELDERLY:** Apply to affected area twice daily.

Paricalcitol
Secondary Hyperparathyroidism in Stage 5 CKD
IV: **ADULTS, ELDERLY, CHILDREN 5 YRS AND OLDER:** Initially, 0.04–0.1 mcg/kg given as bolus dose no more frequently than every other day at any time during dialysis. May increase by 2–4 mcg every 2–4 wks. Dose is based on serum iPTH levels.

Secondary Hyperparathyroidism in Stages 3 and 4 CKD
Note: Initial dose based on baseline serum iPTH levels. Dose adjusted q2wks based on iPTH levels relative to baseline.
PO: **ADULTS, ELDERLY: (iPTH 500 PG/ML OR LESS):** 1 mcg/day or 2 mcg 3 times/wk. **(iPTH GREATER THAN 500 PG/ML):** 2 mcg/day or 4 mcg 3 times/wk.

SIDE EFFECTS

Frequencies not defined. **Calcitriol:** Cardiac arrhythmias, headache, pruritus, hypercalcemia, polydipsia, abdominal pain, metallic taste, nausea, vomiting, myalgia, soft tissue calcification. **Doxercalciferol:** Edema, pruritus, nausea, vomiting, headache, dizziness, dyspnea, malaise, hypercalcemia. **Ergocalciferol:** Hypercalcemia, hypervitaminosis D, decreased renal function, soft tissue calcification, bone demineralization, nausea, constipation, weight loss. **Paricalcitol:** Edema, nausea, vomiting, hypercalcemia.

ADVERSE EFFECTS/ TOXIC REACTIONS

Early signs of overdose manifested as weakness, headache, drowsiness, nau-

V

---

sea, vomiting, dry mouth, constipation, muscle/bone pain, metallic taste. Later signs of overdose evidenced by polyuria, polydipsia, anorexia, weight loss, nocturia, photophobia, rhinorrhea, pruritus, disorientation, hallucinations, hyperthermia, hypertension, cardiac dysrhythmias.

NURSING CONSIDERATIONS

BASELINE ASSESSMENT
Obtain baseline serum calcium, ionized calcium, phosphorus, alkaline phosphatase, creatinine, iPTH.

INTERVENTION/EVALUATION
Monitor serum, urinary calcium levels, serum phosphate, magnesium, BUN, creatine, alkaline phosphatase determinations (therapeutic calcium level: 9–10 mg/dl), iPTH measurements. Estimate daily dietary calcium intake. Encourage adequate fluid intake. Monitor for signs/symptoms of vitamin D intoxication.

PATIENT/FAMILY TEACHING
• Adequate calcium intake should be maintained. • Dietary phosphorus may need to be restricted (foods high in phosphorus include beans, dairy products, nuts, peas, whole-grain products). • Oral formulations may cause hypersensitivity reactions. Avoid excessive doses. • Report signs/symptoms of hypercalcemia (headache, weakness, drowsiness, nausea, vomiting, dry mouth, constipation, metallic taste, muscle or bone pain). • Maintain adequate hydration. • Avoid changes in diet or supplemental calcium intake (unless directed by health care professional). • Avoid magnesium-containing antacids in pts with renal failure.

vitamin E

vite-a-min E
(Aquasol E, E-Gems, Key-E, Key-E Kaps)

Do not confuse Aquasol E with Anusol or Aquasol A.

◆CLASSIFICATION
PHARMACOTHERAPEUTIC: Fat-soluble vitamin. **CLINICAL:** Nutritional supplement (see p. 158C).

ACTION
Prevents oxidation of vitamins A and C, protects fatty acids from attack by free radicals, protects RBCs from hemolysis by oxidizing agents. **Therapeutic Effect:** Prevents/treats vitamin E deficiency.

PHARMACOKINETICS
Variably absorbed from GI tract (requires bile salts, dietary fat, normal pancreatic function). Primarily concentrated in adipose tissue. Metabolized in liver. Primarily eliminated by biliary system.

USES
Prevention/treatment of vitamin E deficiency.

PRECAUTIONS
Contraindications: None known. **Cautions:** None known.

⌛ LIFESPAN CONSIDERATIONS
Pregnancy/Lactation: Unknown if drug crosses placenta or is distributed in breast milk. **Pregnancy Category A (C if used in doses above recommended daily allowance). Children/Elderly:** No age-related precautions noted in normal dosages.

INTERACTIONS
DRUG: May increase effects of **warfarin.** May increase concentration of **cyclosporine. HERBAL:** None significant. **FOOD:** None known. **LAB VALUES:** None significant.

AVAILABILITY (OTC)
🗇 **Capsules:** 100 units, 200 units, 400 units, 600 units, 1,000 units. 🗇 **Tablets:** 100 units, 200 units, 400 units, 500 units.

ADMINISTRATION/HANDLING

PO
- Do not crush, break tablets/capsules.
- Give without regard to food.

INDICATIONS/ROUTES/DOSAGE

Vitamin E Deficiency
PO: ADULTS, ELDERLY: 60–75 units/day. **CHILDREN:** 1 unit/kg/day. Patients with cystic fibrosis, beta-thalassemia, sickle cell anemia may require higher maintenance doses.

SIDE EFFECTS

Rare: Contact dermatitis, sterile abscess.

ADVERSE EFFECTS/ TOXIC REACTIONS

Chronic overdose may produce fatigue, weakness, nausea, headache, blurred vision, flatulence, diarrhea.

NURSING CONSIDERATIONS

PATIENT/FAMILY TEACHING
- Swallow tablets/capsules whole; do not crush, chew. • Toxicity consists of blurred vision, diarrhea, dizziness, nausea, headache, flu-like symptoms. • Consume foods rich in vitamin E, including vegetable oils, vegetable shortening, margarine, leafy vegetables, milk, eggs, meat.

---

vitamin K

vite-a-min K

phytonadione (vitamin K₁)

(AquaMEPHYTON ✦, Konakion ✦, Mephyton)
Do not confuse Mephyton with melphalan or methadone.

◆ CLASSIFICATION

PHARMACOTHERAPEUTIC: Fat-soluble vitamin. **CLINICAL:** Nutritional supplement, antidote (drug-induced hypoprothrombinemia), antihemorrhagic.

ACTION

Promotes hepatic formation of coagulation factors II, VII, IX, X. **Therapeutic Effect:** Essential for normal clotting of blood.

PHARMACOKINETICS

Readily absorbed from GI tract (duodenum) after IM, subcutaneous administration. Metabolized in liver. Excreted in urine; eliminated by biliary system. Onset of action (increased coagulation factors): **PO:** 6–10 hrs; **IV:** 1–2 hrs. Peak effect (INR values return to normal): **PO:** 24–48 hrs; **IV:** 12–14 hrs.

USES

Prevention, treatment of hemorrhagic states in neonates. Antidote for hemorrhage induced by oral anticoagulants, hypoprothrombinemic states due to vitamin K deficiency. Hypoprothrombinemia caused by malabsorption or inability to synthesize vitamin K.

PRECAUTIONS

Contraindications: None known. **Cautions:** Newborns (esp. premature): Risk of hemolysis, jaundice, hyperbilirubinemia.

☒ LIFESPAN CONSIDERATIONS

Pregnancy/Lactation: Crosses placenta. Distributed in breast milk. **Pregnancy Category C. Children/Elderly:** No age-related precautions noted.

INTERACTIONS

DRUG: May decrease effects of **oral anticoagulants. HERBAL:** None significant. **FOOD:** None known. **LAB VALUES:** None significant.

AVAILABILITY (Rx)

Injection Solution: 1 mg/0.5 ml, 10 mg/ml. **Tablets (Mephyton):** 5 mg.

V

ADMINISTRATION/HANDLING

 IV

◄ALERT► Restrict to emergency use only.

Reconstitution • May dilute with 0.9% NaCl or D_5W immediately before use. Do not use other diluents. • Discard unused portions.

Rate of Administration • Administer slow IV at rate of 1 mg/min. • Monitor continuously for hypersensitivity, anaphylactic reaction during and immediately following IV administration.

Storage • Store at room temperature.

IM, Subcutaneous

• Inject into anterolateral aspect of thigh, deltoid region.

PO

• Scored tablets may be crushed. • May give without regard to food.

IV INCOMPATIBILITY

None known.

IV COMPATIBILITIES

Heparin, potassium chloride, sodium bicarbonate.

INDICATIONS/ROUTES/DOSAGE

◄ALERT► PO/subcutaneous route preferred; IV/IM use restricted to emergent situations.

Oral Anticoagulant Overdose
PO, IV, Subcutaneous: ADULTS, ELDERLY: 2.5–10 mg/dose. May repeat in 12–48 hrs if given orally, in 6–8 hrs if given by IV or subcutaneous route. **CHILDREN:** 0.5–5 mg depending on need for further anticoagulation, severity of bleeding.

Hemorrhagic Disease of Newborn
IM, Subcutaneous: NEONATE: Treatment: 1 mg/dose/day. May increase to 2 mg. **Prophylaxis:** 0.5–1 mg within 1 hr of birth.

SIDE EFFECTS

◄ALERT► PO/subcutaneous administration less likely to produce side effects than IV/IM routes.

Occasional: Pain, soreness, swelling at IM injection site, pruritic erythema (with repeated injections), facial flushing, altered taste.

ADVERSE EFFECTS/ TOXIC REACTIONS

Newborns (esp. premature infants) may develop hyperbilirubinemia. Severe reaction (cramp-like pain, chest pain, dyspnea, facial flushing, dizziness, rapid/weak pulse, rash, diaphoresis, hypotension progressing to shock, cardiac arrest) occurs rarely, immediately after IV administration.

NURSING CONSIDERATIONS

INTERVENTION/EVALUATION

Monitor PT, international normalized ratio (INR) routinely in pts taking anticoagulants. Assess skin for ecchymoses, petechiae. Assess gums for gingival bleeding, erythema. Assess urine for hematuria. Assess Hct, platelet count, urine/stool culture for occult blood. Assess for decrease in B/P, increase in pulse rate, complaint of abdominal/back pain, severe headache (may be evidence of hemorrhage). Question for increase in amount of discharge during menses. Assess peripheral pulses. Check for excessive bleeding from minor cuts, scratches.

PATIENT/FAMILY TEACHING

• Discomfort may occur with parenteral administration. • **Adults:** Use electric razor, soft toothbrush to prevent bleeding. • Report any sign of red or dark urine, black or red stool, coffee-ground vomitus, red-speckled mucus from cough. • Do not use any OTC medication without physician approval (may interfere with platelet aggregation). • Consume foods rich in vitamin K_1, including leafy green vegetables, meat, cow's milk, vegetable oil, egg yolks, tomatoes.

voriconazole

vor-i-**kon**-a-zole
(Vfend)
**Do not confuse voriconazole
with fluconazole.**

◆CLASSIFICATION

PHARMACOTHERAPEUTIC: Triazole
derivative. **CLINICAL:** Antifungal (see
p. 48C).

ACTION

Inhibits synthesis of ergosterol (vital component of fungal cell wall formation). **Therapeutic Effect:** Damages fungal cell wall membrane.

PHARMACOKINETICS

Rapidly, completely absorbed after PO administration. Widely distributed. Protein binding: 58%. Metabolized in liver. Primarily excreted as metabolite in urine. **Half-life:** Variable, dose dependent.

USES

Treatment of invasive aspergillosis, esophageal candidiasis. Treatment of serious fungal infections caused by *Scedosporium apiospermum, Fusarium* spp. Treatment of candidemia in non-neutropenic pts. Treatment of disseminated *Candida* infections of skin and viscera. **OFF-LABEL:** Fungal infection prophylaxis in moderate- to high-risk neutropenic cancer pts, empiric therapy for persistent neutropenic fever. Empiric treatment of fungal meningitis or osteoarticular infections.

PRECAUTIONS

Contraindications: Concurrent administration of carbamazepine, ergot alkaloids, pimozide, quinidine (may cause prolonged QT interval, torsade de pointes), rifabutin, rifampin, ritonavir, sirolimus, St. John's wort. **Cautions:** Severe renal/hepatic impairment, hypersensitivity to other azole antifungal agents. Pts at risk for acute pancreatitis.

⌛ LIFESPAN CONSIDERATIONS

Pregnancy/Lactation: May cause fetal harm. **Pregnancy Category D. Children:** Safety and efficacy not established in those younger than 12 yrs. **Elderly:** No age-related precautions noted.

INTERACTIONS

DRUG: May increase concentration, risk of toxicity of **alprazolam, calcium channel blockers, cyclosporine, efavirenz, ergot alkaloids, HMG-CoA reductase inhibitors (e.g., lovastatin), methadone, midazolam, protease inhibitors (e.g., amprenavir, saquinavir), rifabutin, sirolimus, tacrolimus, triazolam, warfarin. Carbamazepine, rifabutin, rifampin, ritonavir** may decrease concentration/effect. **HERBAL: St. John's wort** may significantly decrease concentration. **FOOD: Grapefruit products** may increase concentration. **LAB VALUES:** May increase serum alkaline phosphatase, ALT, AST, bilirubin, creatinine. May decrease potassium.

AVAILABILITY (Rx)

Injection, Powder for Reconstitution: 200 mg. **Powder for Oral Suspension:** 200 mg/5 ml. **Tablets:** 50 mg, 200 mg.

ADMINISTRATION/HANDLING

 IV

Reconstitution • Reconstitute 200-mg vial with 19 ml Sterile Water for Injection to provide concentration of 10 mg/ml. Further dilute with 0.9% NaCl or D₅W to provide concentration of 0.5–5 mg/ml. **Rate of Administration** • Infuse over 1–2 hrs at a rate not to exceed 3 mg/kg/hr. **Storage** • Store powder for injection at room temperature. • Use reconstituted solution immediately. • Do not use after 24 hrs when refrigerated.

PO
• Give 1 hr before or 1 hr after a meal.
• Do not mix oral suspension with any other medication or flavoring agent.

• Shake suspension for about 10 sec before use.

IV INCOMPATIBILITY

Tigecycline (Tygacil).

IV COMPATIBILITY

Anidulafungin, caspofungin, ceftaroline, doripenem.

INDICATIONS/ROUTES/DOSAGE

Invasive Aspergillosis
IV: ADULTS, ELDERLY, CHILDREN 12 YRS AND OLDER: Initially, 6 mg/kg q12h for 2 doses, then 4 mg/kg q12h, then oral maintenance dose. **(LESS THAN 40 KG):** 100 mg q12h (**maximum:** 300 mg/day). **(40 KG OR GREATER):** 200 mg q12h (**maximum:** 400 mg/day). **CHILDREN 3–11 YRS OF AGE:** Initially, 6–8 mg/kg (**maximum:** 400 mg) q12h for 2 doses, then 7 mg/kg (**maximum:** 200 mg) q12h.
Or orally: Initially, 8 mg/kg (**maximum:** 400 mg) q12h for 2 doses, then 7 mg/kg (**maximum:** 200 mg) q12h.

Candidemia, Other Deep Tissue Candida Infections
IV: ADULTS, ELDERLY, CHILDREN 12 YRS AND OLDER: Initially, 6 mg/kg q12h for 2 doses, then 3–4 mg/kg q12h, then oral maintenance dose. **(LESS THAN 40 KG):** 100 mg q12h (**maximum:** 300 mg/day). **(40 KG OR GREATER):** 200 mg q12h (**maximum:** 600 mg/day).

Esophageal Candidiasis
PO: ADULTS, ELDERLY WEIGHING 40 KG OR MORE: 200 mg q12h for minimum of 14 days, then at least 7 days following resolution of symptoms. **Maximum:** 600 mg/day. **ADULTS, ELDERLY WEIGHING LESS THAN 40 KG:** 100 mg q12h for minimum of 14 days, then at least 7 days following resolution of symptoms. **Maximum:** 300 mg/day.

Dosage in Pts Receiving Phenytoin
IV: Increase maintenance dose to 5 mg/kg q12h.

PO: Increase 200 mg q12h to 400 mg q12h (pts weighing 40 kg or more) or 100 mg q12h to 200 mg q12h (pts weighing less than 40 kg).

Dosage in Pts Receiving Cyclosporine, Omeprazole
Reduce cyclosporine dose by 50%. Reduce omeprazole by 50% in pts maintained on 40 mg or more per day.

Dosage in Pts Receiving Efavirenz
Increase dose to 400 mg q12h and reduce efavirenz to 300 mg/day.

Dosage in Hepatic Impairment
Mild to Moderate: Reduce maintenance dose by 50%.
Severe: Use only if benefits outweigh risks. Monitor closely for toxicity.

SIDE EFFECTS

Frequent (20%–6%): Abnormal vision, fever, nausea, rash, vomiting. **Occasional (5%–2%):** Headache, chills, hallucinations, photophobia, tachycardia, hypertension.

ADVERSE EFFECTS/ TOXIC REACTIONS

Hepatotoxicity (jaundice, hepatitis, hepatic failure), acute renal failure have occurred in severely ill pts.

NURSING CONSIDERATIONS

BASELINE ASSESSMENT

Obtain baseline serum hepatic/renal function tests. Receive full medication history and screen for interactions.

INTERVENTION/EVALUATION

Monitor serum hepatic/renal function tests. Monitor visual function (visual acuity, visual field, color perception) for drug therapy lasting longer than 28 days.

PATIENT/FAMILY TEACHING

• Take at least 1 hr before or 1 hr after a meal. • Avoid grapefruit products. • Avoid driving at night. • Notify physician of visual changes (blurred vision, photophobia, yellowing of skin/eyes). • Avoid performing hazardous tasks if changes in vision occur. • Avoid direct sunlight. • Women of childbearing potential should use effective contraception.

---

vorinostat

vor-**in**-o-stat
(Zolinza)
Do not confuse vorinostat with Votrient.

◆CLASSIFICATION

PHARMACOTHERAPEUTIC: Histone deacetylase inhibitor. **CLINICAL:** Antineoplastic (see p. 92C).

ACTION

Inhibits activity of specific enzymes that catalyze removal of acetyl groups of proteins, causing accumulation of acetylated histones. **Therapeutic Effect:** Induces cell arrest.

PHARMACOKINETICS

Protein binding: 71%. Metabolized to inactive metabolites. Excreted in urine. **Half-life:** 2 hrs.

USES

Treatment of cutaneous manifestations in pts with cutaneous T-cell lymphoma (CTCL) with progressive, persistent, or recurrent disease, on or following two systemic therapies.

PRECAUTIONS

Contraindications: Severe hepatic impairment. **Cautions:** History of deep vein thrombosis (DVT), diabetes mellitus, mild to moderate hepatic impairment, preexisting hypokalemia, hypomagnesemia, pts with history of QT prolongation or medications that prolong QT interval.

⌛ LIFESPAN CONSIDERATIONS

Pregnancy/Lactation: May cause fetal harm. Unknown if distributed in breast milk. **Pregnancy Category D. Children:** Safety and efficacy not established. **Elderly:** No age-related precautions noted.

INTERACTIONS

DRUG: May increase effect of **warfarin. Valproic acid** increases risk of GI bleeding, thrombocytopenia. **HERBAL:** None significant. **FOOD:** None known. **LAB VALUES:** May decrease serum calcium, potassium, sodium, phosphate, platelet count. May increase serum glucose, creatinine, urine protein.

AVAILABILITY (Rx)

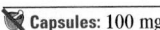 **Capsules:** 100 mg.

ADMINISTRATION/HANDLING

PO
• Do not break, crush, dissolve, or divide capsules. • Give with food. • Maintain adequate hydration during treatment.

INDICATIONS/ROUTES/DOSAGE

Cutaneous T-Cell Lymphoma (CTCL)
PO: ADULTS, ELDERLY: 400 mg once daily with food. Dosage adjustment for toxicity: Dose may be reduced to 300 mg once daily with food. May be further reduced to 300 mg once daily with food for 5 consecutive days each wk.

SIDE EFFECTS

Frequent (50%–24%): Fatigue, diarrhea, nausea, altered taste, anorexia. **Occasional (21%–11%):** Weight decrease, muscle spasms, alopecia, dry mouth, chills, vomiting, constipation, dizziness, peripheral edema, headache, pruritus, cough, fever.

ADVERSE EFFECTS/ TOXIC REACTIONS

Thrombocytopenia occurs in 25% of pts, anemia in 15%. Pulmonary embolism

V

 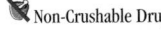

occurs in 4% of pts. Deep vein thrombosis (DVT) occurs rarely.

NURSING CONSIDERATIONS

BASELINE ASSESSMENT

Baseline PT, international normalized ratio (INR), CBC, serum chemistry tests, esp. serum potassium, calcium, magnesium, glucose, creatinine should be obtained prior to therapy and every 2 wks during first 2 mos of therapy and monthly thereafter. Inform women of childbearing potential of risk to fetus if pregnancy occurs.

INTERVENTION/EVALUATION

Monitor platelet count, PT, INR, monitor serum electrolytes, CBC q2wks for 2 mos, then monthly. Monitor signs/symptoms of DVT. Encourage fluid intake, approximately 2 L/day input. Assess for evidence of dehydration. Provide antiemetics to control nausea/vomiting. Monitor daily pattern of bowel activity, stool consistency.

PATIENT/FAMILY TEACHING

• Drink at least 2 L/day of fluids to prevent dehydration. • Report persistent vomiting, diarrhea. • Report shortness of breath, pain in any extremity.

vortioxetene

vor-tye-**ox**-e-teen
(Brintellix)
Do not confuse vortioxetene with fluoxetine, paroxetine, or venlafaxine.

BLACK BOX ALERT Antidepressants have an increased risk of suicidal ideation and behavior in children, adolescents, and young adults. Monitor closely for worsening or emergence of suicidal thoughts and behaviors. Advise families to monitor closely and communicate concerns with prescriber. Not evaluated for use in pediatric pts.

◆CLASSIFICATION

PHARMACOTHERAPEUTIC: Selective serotonin reuptake inhibitor (SSRI). **CLINICAL:** Antidepressant.

ACTION

Blocks reuptake of neurotransmitter serotonin at CNS presynaptic membranes, increasing availability at postsynaptic receptor sites. **Therapeutic Effect:** Relieves depression.

PHARMACOKINETICS

Readily absorbed following PO administration. Metabolized in liver, primarily through oxidation. Protein binding: 98%. Peak plasma concentration: 7–11 hrs. Steady state reached within 2 wks. Excreted in urine (59%), feces (26%). **Half-life:** 66 hrs.

USES

Treatment of major depressive disorder.

PRECAUTIONS

Contraindications: Prior hypersensitivity reaction to drug. Monoamine oxidase inhibitors (MAOIs). Do not use MAOIs within 21 days of stopping vortioxetene; do not use vortioxetene within 14 days of stopping an MAOI. Concomitant use of linezolid or intravenous methylene blue. **Cautions:** History of angioedema (tongue swelling), dehydration, hyponatremia, pts at risk for bleeding, elderly, prior suicidal behaviors, or questionable history or undiagnosed bipolar disorder.

⏳ LIFESPAN CONSIDERATIONS

Pregnancy/Lactation: May cause fetal harm when administered in third trimester. Unknown if distributed in breast milk. Exposed neonates are at increased risk of apnea, cyanosis, prolonged hospitalization, pulmonary hypertension, seizures, serotonin syndrome. **Pregnancy Category C. Children:** Safety and efficacy not established in pediatric population. **Elderly:** May have increased risk of dehydration, hyponatremia.

INTERACTIONS

DRUG: **Strong CYP inducers (e.g., carbamazepine, phenytoin, rifampin)** may decrease concentration/effect. **Strong CYP2D6 inhibitors (e.g., bupropion, fluoxetine, paroxetine)** may increase concentration/effect. **MAOIs** contraindicated; may cause malignant hyperthermia, hypertensive crisis, hyperreflexia, seizures, serotonin syndrome. **Serotonergic drugs (e.g., buspirone, fentanyl, linezolid, tramadol, tricyclic antidepressants, triptans)** may increase risk of serotonin syndrome. **Anticoagulants, antiplatelets, NSAIDs** may increase risk of bleeding. **Diuretics** may increase risk of hyponatremia. **HERBAL:** St. John's wort may increase risk of serotonin syndrome. **FOOD:** None known. **LAB VALUES:** May decrease serum sodium.

AVAILABILITY (Rx)

Tablets (Immediate-Release): 5 mg, 10 mg, 15 mg, 20 mg.

ADMINISTRATION/HANDLING

PO

• Give without regard to meals. May administer with milk or food if GI upset occurs.

INDICATIONS/ROUTES/DOSAGE

Major Depressive Disorder
PO: ADULTS/ELDERLY: Initially, 10 mg once daily. May increase to 20 mg as tolerated. **Discontinuation:** If pt is receiving 15-mg or 20-mg dose, reduce dose to 10 mg for 7 days prior to discontinuation.

Dose Modification
Concomitant Use of Strong CYP2D6 Inhibitors: Reduce dose by half of intended therapy. **Maximum:** 10 mg once daily. **Concomitant Use of Strong CYP Inducers:** If co-administered for more than 14 days, consider increasing vortioxetene dose. **Maximum:** Do not exceed more than 3 times original dose.

SIDE EFFECTS

Frequent (32%–22%): Nausea, sexual dysfunction. **Occasional (10%–3%):** Diarrhea, dizziness, dry mouth, constipation, vomiting, flatulence, abnormal dreams, pruritus.

ADVERSE EFFECTS/TOXIC REACTIONS

Life-threatening serotonin syndrome may include mental status changes (agitation, hallucinations, delirium, coma), autonomic instability (tachycardia, labile blood pressure, dizziness, sweating, flushing, hyperthermia), neuromuscular symptoms (tremor, rigidity, myoclonus [localized muscle twitching], hyperactive reflexes, incoordination), seizures, GI symptoms (nausea, vomiting, diarrhea). May increase risk of bleeding events such as ecchymosis, hematoma, epistaxis (nosebleed), petechiae. Mania/hypomania may indicate baseline bipolar disorder. Syndrome of inappropriate antidiuretic hormone (SIADH), also known as water intoxication or dilutional hyponatremia, may induce seizures, coma, or death. Angioedema, dyspnea, rash may indicate allergic reaction. May increase risk of suicidal ideation and behavior once treatment is therapeutic. May alter sexual drive, ease of arousal, ease of reaching orgasm, or cause erectile dysfunction in men or decreased lubrication in women.

NURSING CONSIDERATIONS

BASELINE ASSESSMENT

Obtain baseline electrolytes. Note serum sodium level. Assess appearance, behavior, speech pattern, level of interest, mood. Screen for history of bipolar disorder, bleeding events, SIADH, prior allergic reactions to drug class. Receive full medication history including herbal products.

INTERVENTION/EVALUATION

Monitor serum sodium levels. Screen for signs of SIADH (confusion, seizures).

V

Offer emotional support. Assess mental status for depression, suicidal ideation (esp. during first few mo of therapy or with dosage change), anxiety, social function. Monitor daily pattern of bowel activity, stool consistency. Assist with ambulation if dizziness occurs. Monitor pt for symptoms of serotonin syndrome, mania/hypomania. Offer antiemetic for nausea, vomiting. Monitor for allergic reactions.

PATIENT/FAMILY TEACHING

• Dry mouth may be relieved with sugarless gum, sips of water. • Report neurologic changes: confusion, excessive talking, hallucinations, headache, hyperactivity, insomnia, racing thoughts, seizure-like activity, tremors; sexual dysfunction; fever; or any type of allergic reaction • Avoid tasks that require alertness, motor skills until response to drug is established (may cause dizziness, drowsiness). • Take with food if nausea occurs. • Report pregnancy. • Avoid alcohol. • Do not take OTC medications such as aspirin or ibuprofen without consulting physician. • Immediately report thoughts of suicide, self-destructive behavior, or violence. • Sexual dysfunction such as inability to reach orgasm, difficulty maintaining an erection, or lack of sexual drive may occur.

warfarin

`TOP 200` `HIGH ALERT`

war-far-in
(Apo-Warfarin ♣, <u>Coumadin</u>,
Jantoven, Novo-Warfarin ♣)

BLACK BOX ALERT May cause major or fatal bleeding. Risk factors include history of GI bleeding, hypertension, cerebrovascular disease, heart disease, malignancy, trauma, anemia, renal insufficiency, age 65 yrs and older, high anticoagulation factor (INR greater than 4). Consider cardiac/hepatic function, age, nutritional status, concurrent medications, risk of bleeding when dosing warfarin. Genetic variations have been identified as factors associated with dosage and bleeding risk. Genotyping tests are available. **Do not confuse Coumadin with Kemadrin, or Jantoven with Janumet or Januvia.**

◆CLASSIFICATION

PHARMACOTHERAPEUTIC: Coumarin derivative. **CLINICAL:** Anticoagulant (see p. 33C).

ACTION

Interferes with hepatic synthesis of vitamin K–dependent clotting factors, resulting in depletion of coagulation factors II, VII, IX, X. **Therapeutic Effect:** Prevents further extension of formed existing clot; prevents new clot formation, secondary thromboembolic complications.

PHARMACOKINETICS

Route	Onset	Peak	Duration
PO	1.5–3 days	5–7 days	2–5 days

Well absorbed from GI tract. Protein binding: 99%. Metabolized in liver. Primarily excreted in urine. Not removed by hemodialysis. **Half-life:** 20–60 hrs.

USES

Prophylaxis, treatment of venous thrombosis, pulmonary embolism, and thromboembolic disorders. Prophylaxis, treatment of thromboembolic complications associated with cardiac valve replacement or atrial fibrillation. Reduces risk of death, recurrent MI, stroke, embolization after MI. **OFF-LABEL:** Treatment adjunct in transient ischemic attacks.

PRECAUTIONS

Contraindications: Hemorrhagic tendencies (e.g., cerebral aneurysms), surgery of eye or CNS, neurosurgical procedures, open wounds, severe hypertension, spinal puncture procedures, uncontrolled bleeding, ulcers, unreliable or noncompliant pt, unsupervised senile or psychotic pt, blood dyscrasias, pericarditis or pericardial effusion, pregnancy (except in women with mechanical heart valves at high risk for thromboembolism), bacterial endocarditis, threatened abortion. **Cautions:** Active tuberculosis, acute infection, diabetes, heparin-induced thrombocytopenia, pts at risk for hemorrhage, necrosis, gangrene, moderate to severe hepatic, renal impairment, moderate to severe hypertension, thyroid disease.

⌛ LIFESPAN CONSIDERATIONS

Pregnancy/Lactation: Contraindicated in pregnancy (fetal, neonatal hemorrhage, intrauterine death). Crosses placenta; distributed in breast milk. **Pregnancy Category X. Children:** More susceptible to effect. **Elderly:** Increased risk of hemorrhage; lower dosage recommended.

INTERACTIONS

DRUG: Amiodarone, azole antifungals, cimetidine, disulfiram, fluvoxamine, sulfamethoxazole-trimethoprim, levothyroxine, metronidazole, NSAIDs, omeprazole, platelet aggregation inhibitors, salicylates, thrombolytic agents, thyroid hormones may increase effect. **Griseofulvin, hepatic enzyme inducers** (e.g., rifampin), vitamin K may decrease effects. **Alcohol** may enhance anticoagulant effect. **HERBAL: Cat's claw, dong quai, evening primrose, feverfew, garlic, ginger, ginkgo biloba, ginseng** possess antiplatelet activity,

W

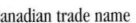 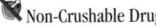

may increase risk of bleeding. **Ginseng, St. John's wort** may decrease effect. **FOOD:** None known. **LAB VALUES:** None known.

AVAILABILITY (Rx)

Tablets (Coumadin, Jantoven): 1 mg, 2 mg, 2.5 mg, 3 mg, 4 mg, 5 mg, 6 mg, 7.5 mg, 10 mg.

ADMINISTRATION/HANDLING

PO
• Scored tablets may be crushed. • Give without regard to food. Give with food if GI upset occurs. • Give at same time each day.

INDICATIONS/ROUTES/DOSAGE

◄**ALERT**► Initial dosing must be individualized.

Anticoagulant
PO: ADULTS, ELDERLY: Initially, 2–5 mg/ daily for 2 days **OR** 5–10 mg daily for 1–2 days, adjusting the dose based on INR results. **Usual maintenance dose:** 2–10 mg/day, but may vary outside these guidelines. **CHILDREN:** Initially, 0.05–0.2 mg/kg/day. **Maximum:** 10 mg. Maintenance: Adjust based on INR.

SIDE EFFECTS

Occasional: GI distress (nausea, anorexia, abdominal cramps, diarrhea). **Rare:** Hypersensitivity reaction (dermatitis, urticaria), esp. in those sensitive to aspirin.

ADVERSE EFFECTS/ TOXIC REACTIONS

Bleeding complications ranging from local ecchymoses to major hemorrhage may occur. **Antidote:** Vitamin K. Amount based on INR, significance of bleeding. Range: 2.5–10 mg given orally or slow IV infusion (see Appendix K for dosage).

Hepatotoxicity, blood dyscrasias, necrosis, vasculitis, local thrombosis occur rarely.

NURSING CONSIDERATIONS

BASELINE ASSESSMENT

Cross-check dose with coworker. Determine INR before administration and daily following therapy initiation. When stabilized, follow with INR determination q4–6wks. Obtain genotyping prior to initiating therapy if available.

INTERVENTION/EVALUATION

Monitor INR reports diligently. Assess Hct, platelet count, AST, ALT, urine/stool for occult blood. Be alert to complaints of abdominal/back pain, severe headache (may be sign of hemorrhage). Decrease in B/P, increase in pulse rate may be sign of hemorrhage. Question for increase in amount of menstrual discharge. Assess peripheral pulses; skin for ecchymoses, petechiae. Check for excessive bleeding from minor cuts, scratches. Assess gums for erythema, gingival bleeding.

PATIENT/ FAMILY TEACHING

• Take medication at same time each day. • Do not take, discontinue any other medication except on advice of physician. • Avoid alcohol, aspirin, drastic dietary changes. • Do not change from one brand to another. • Consult with physician before surgery, dental work. • Urine may become red-orange. • Avoid, minimize significant bodily trauma. • Notify physician if bleeding, bruising, red or brown urine, black stools occur. • Use electric razor, soft toothbrush to prevent bleeding. • Report coffee-ground vomitus, blood-tinged mucus from cough. • Do not use any OTC medication without physician approval (may interfere with platelet aggregation).

W

zafirlukast

za-**fir**-loo-kast
(Accolate)
**Do not confuse Accolate with
Accupril, Accutane, or Aclovate.**

◆CLASSIFICATION

PHARMACOTHERAPEUTIC: Leukotriene receptor antagonist. **CLINICAL:** Antiasthma (see p. 78C).

ACTION

Binds to leukotriene receptors, inhibiting bronchoconstriction due to sulfur dioxide, cold air, specific antigens (grass, cat dander, ragweed). **Therapeutic Effect:** Reduces airway edema, smooth muscle constriction; alters cellular activity associated with inflammatory process.

PHARMACOKINETICS

Rapidly absorbed after PO administration (food reduces absorption). Protein binding: 99%. Metabolized in liver. Primarily excreted in feces. Unknown if removed by hemodialysis. **Half-life:** 10 hrs.

USES

Prophylaxis, chronic treatment of bronchial asthma in adults and children 5 yrs and older.

PRECAUTIONS

Contraindications: Hepatic impairment. **Cautions:** Concomitant warfarin therapy.

⌛ LIFESPAN CONSIDERATIONS

Pregnancy/Lactation: Drug is distributed in breast milk. Do not administer to breastfeeding women. **Pregnancy Category B. Children:** Safety and efficacy not established in pts younger than 5 yrs. **Elderly:** No age-related precautions noted.

INTERACTIONS

DRUG: Erythromycin, theophylline may decrease concentration/effect. **Aspirin** may increase concentration/effect. Increases effect of **warfarin** (increases INR). **HERBAL:** None significant. **FOOD: Food** decreases bioavailability by 40%. **LAB VALUES:** None significant.

AVAILABILITY (Rx)

Tablets: 10 mg, 20 mg.

ADMINISTRATION/HANDLING

PO
• Give 1 hr before or 2 hrs after meals.

INDICATIONS/ROUTES/DOSAGE

Bronchial Asthma
PO: ADULTS, ELDERLY, CHILDREN 12 YRS AND OLDER: 20 mg twice daily. **CHILDREN 5–11 YRS:** 10 mg twice daily.

SIDE EFFECTS

Frequent (13%): Headache. **Occasional (3%):** Nausea, diarrhea. **Rare (Less Than 3%):** Generalized pain, asthenia (loss of strength, energy), myalgia, fever, dyspepsia (heartburn, indigestion, epigastric pain), vomiting, dizziness.

ADVERSE EFFECTS/ TOXIC REACTIONS

Concurrent administration of inhaled corticosteroids increases risk of upper respiratory tract infection.

NURSING CONSIDERATIONS

BASELINE ASSESSMENT

Obtain medication history. Assess serum hepatic function lab values.

INTERVENTION/EVALUATION

Monitor rate, depth, rhythm, type of respiration; quality, rate of pulse. Assess lung sounds for rhonchi, wheezing, rales. Monitor serum hepatic function tests.

PATIENT/FAMILY TEACHING

• Increase fluid intake (decreases lung secretion viscosity). • Take as prescribed, even during symptom-free periods. • Do not use for acute asthma episodes. • Do not alter, stop other asthma medications.

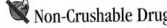

◆ Canadian trade name   Non-Crushable Drug   **HIGH ALERT** High Alert drug

Z

• Do not breastfeed. • Report nausea, jaundice, abdominal pain, flu-like symptoms, worsening of asthma.

zaleplon

zal-e-plon
(Sonata)
Do not confuse zaleplon with zolpidem.

◆CLASSIFICATION

PHARMACOTHERAPEUTIC: Nonbenzodiazepine. **(Schedule IV).** CLINICAL: Hypnotic (see p. 149C).

ACTION

Enhances action of inhibitory neurotransmitter gamma-aminobutyric acid (GABA). **Therapeutic Effect:** Induces sleep.

PHARMACOKINETICS

Rapidly, almost completely absorbed following PO administration. Protein binding: 45%–75%. Metabolized in liver. Primarily excreted in urine. Partially eliminated in feces. **Half-life:** 1 hr.

USES

Short-term treatment of insomnia (7–10 days). Decreases sleep onset time (no effect on number of nocturnal awakenings, total sleep time).

PRECAUTIONS

Contraindications: None known. **Cautions:** Mild to moderate hepatic impairment (avoid use in severe impairment), depression, history of drug dependence, elderly, compromised respiratory function, depression, risk for suicide.

⌛ LIFESPAN CONSIDERATIONS

Pregnancy/Lactation: Unknown if drug crosses placenta; distributed in breast milk. **Pregnancy Category C. Children:** Safety and efficacy not established.

Elderly: May be more sensitive to zaleplon effects.

INTERACTIONS

DRUG: **Alcohol, other CNS depressants** may increase CNS depression. **Cimetidine** may increase concentration/effect. **CYP3A4 inducers (e.g., carbamazepine, phenobarbital, phenytoin, rifampin)** may decrease concentration. HERBAL: **St. John's wort** may decrease levels/effect. **Gotu kola, kava kava, St. John's wort, valerian** may increase CNS depression. FOOD: **High-fat, heavy meals** may delay onset of sleep by approximately 2 hrs. LAB VALUES: None significant.

AVAILABILITY (Rx)

Capsules: 5 mg, 10 mg.

ADMINISTRATION/HANDLING

PO
• Give immediately before bedtime.
• Giving drug with or immediately after high-fat meal results in slower absorption. • Capsules may be emptied and mixed with food.

INDICATIONS/ROUTES/DOSAGE

Insomnia
PO: ADULTS: 10 mg at bedtime. Range: 5–20 mg. ELDERLY: 5 mg at bedtime. **Maximum:** 10 mg.

Dosage in Hepatic Impairment
Mild to moderate: 5 mg. Severe: Not recommended.

SIDE EFFECTS

Expected: Drowsiness, sedation, mild rebound insomnia (on first night after drug is discontinued). **Frequent (28%–7%):** Nausea, headache, myalgia, dizziness. **Occasional (5%–3%):** Abdominal pain, asthenia (loss of strength, energy), dyspepsia (heartburn, indigestion, epigastric pain), eye pain, paresthesia. **Rare (2%):** Tremor, amnesia, hyperacusis (acute sense of hearing), fever, dysmenorrhea.

Z

ADVERSE EFFECTS/ TOXIC REACTIONS

May produce altered concentration/ behavior changes, impaired memory. Taking medication while ambulating may result in hallucinations, impaired coordination, dizziness, light-headedness. Overdose results in drowsiness, confusion, diminished reflexes, coma.

NURSING CONSIDERATIONS

BASELINE ASSESSMENT

Provide for safety; raise bed rails. Provide environment conducive to sleep (back rub, quiet environment, low lighting).

INTERVENTION/EVALUATION

Assess sleep pattern.

PATIENT/FAMILY TEACHING

• Take right before bedtime or when in bed and not falling asleep. • Avoid tasks requiring alertness, motor skills until response to drug is established. • Do not exceed prescribed dosage. • Do not take with or immediately after a high-fat or heavy meal. • Rebound insomnia may occur when drug is discontinued after short-term therapy. • Avoid alcohol, other CNS depressants.

zanamivir

zan-**am**-i-veer
(Relenza)

◆ CLASSIFICATION

PHARMACOTHERAPEUTIC: Antiviral. **CLINICAL:** Anti-influenza (see p. 71C).

ACTION

Appears to inhibit influenza virus enzyme neuraminidase, essential for viral replication. **Therapeutic Effect:** Prevents viral release from infected cells.

PHARMACOKINETICS

Systemically absorbed, approximately 4%–17%. Protein binding: less than 10%. Not metabolized. Partially excreted unchanged in urine. **Half-life:** 2.5–5.1 hrs.

USES

Treatment of uncomplicated acute illness due to influenza virus A and B in adults, children 7 yrs and older who have been symptomatic for less than 2 days. Prevention of influenza A and B in adults and children 5 yrs and older.

PRECAUTIONS

Contraindications: None known. **Cautions:** COPD, asthma, severe renal/hepatic impairment.

⌛ LIFESPAN CONSIDERATIONS

Pregnancy/Lactation: Unknown if drug crosses placenta or is distributed in breast milk. **Pregnancy Category C. Children:** Safety and efficacy not established in those younger than 7 yrs. **Elderly:** No age-related precautions noted.

INTERACTIONS

DRUG: None significant. **HERBAL:** None significant. **FOOD:** None known. **LAB VALUES:** None significant.

AVAILABILITY (Rx)

Powder for Inhalation: 5 mg/blister.

ADMINISTRATION/HANDLING

Inhalation
• Instruct pt to use Diskhaler device provided, exhale completely; then, holding mouthpiece 1 inch away from lips, inhale and hold breath as long as possible before exhaling. • Rinse mouth with water immediately after inhalation (prevents mouth/throat dryness). • Store at room temperature.

INDICATIONS/ROUTES/DOSAGE

Treatment of Influenza Virus
Inhalation: ADULTS, ELDERLY, CHILDREN 7 YRS AND OLDER: 2 inhalations (one 5-mg blister per inhalation for total dose of 10

mg) twice daily (approximately 12 hrs apart) for 5 days.

Prevention of Influenza Virus
Inhalation: ADULTS, ELDERLY, CHILDREN 5 YRS AND OLDER: 2 inhalations (10 mg) once daily for duration of exposure period (10 days for household exposure, 28 days for community exposure).

SIDE EFFECTS

Occasional (3%–2%): Diarrhea, sinusitis, nausea, bronchitis, cough, dizziness, headache. **Rare (Less Than 1.5%):** Malaise, fatigue, fever, abdominal pain, myalgia, arthralgia, urticaria.

ADVERSE EFFECTS/ TOXIC REACTIONS

May produce neutropenia. Bronchospasm may occur in those with history of COPD, bronchial asthma.

NURSING CONSIDERATIONS

BASELINE ASSESSMENT

Pts requiring an inhaled bronchodilator at same time as zanamivir should use the bronchodilator before zanamivir administration.

INTERVENTION/EVALUATION

Provide assistance if dizziness occurs. Monitor daily pattern of bowel activity, stool consistency.

PATIENT/FAMILY TEACHING

• Follow manufacturer guidelines for use of delivery device. • Avoid contact with those who are at high risk for influenza. • Continue treatment for full 5-day course. • Doses should be evenly spaced. • In pts with respiratory disease, an inhaled bronchodilator should be readily available.

zidovudine

zye-**doe**-vue-deen
(Apo-Zidovudine ✤, Novo-AZT ✤, Retrovir)

BLACK BOX ALERT Neutropenia, severe anemia may occur. Lactic acidosis, severe hepatomegaly with steatosis (fatty liver), including fatalities, have occurred. Symptomatic myopathy, myositis associated with prolonged use.
Do not confuse Retrovir with acyclovir or ritonavir.

FIXED-COMBINATION(S)

Combivir: zidovudine/lamivudine (an antiviral): 300 mg/150 mg. **Trizivir:** zidovudine/lamivudine/abacavir (an antiviral): 300 mg/150 mg/300 mg.

◆CLASSIFICATION

PHARMACOTHERAPEUTIC: Nucleoside reverse transcriptase inhibitors. **CLINICAL:** Antiviral (see pp. 71C, 118C).

ACTION

Interferes with viral RNA-dependent DNA polymerase, an enzyme necessary for viral HIV replication. **Therapeutic Effect:** Slows HIV replication, reducing progression of HIV infection.

PHARMACOKINETICS

Rapidly, completely absorbed from GI tract. Protein binding: 25%–38%. Metabolized in liver. Crosses blood-brain barrier and is widely distributed, including to CSF. Primarily excreted in urine. Minimal removal by hemodialysis. **Half-life:** 0.5–3 hrs (increased in renal impairment).

USES

Treatment of HIV infection in combination with at least two other antiretroviral agents. Prevention of maternal/fetal HIV transmission. **OFF-LABEL:** Prophylaxis in health care workers at risk for acquiring HIV after occupational exposure.

PRECAUTIONS

Contraindications: Life-threatening allergic reactions to zidovudine or its components. **Cautions:** Bone marrow compromise, renal/hepatic dysfunction, decreased hepatic blood flow.

⏳ LIFESPAN CONSIDERATIONS

Pregnancy/Lactation: Unknown if drug crosses placenta or is distributed in breast milk. Unknown if fetal harm or effects on fertility can occur. **Pregnancy Category C. Children:** No age-related precautions noted. **Elderly:** Information not available.

INTERACTIONS

DRUG: Bone marrow depressants, ganciclovir may increase myelosuppression. May be antagonistic with **doxorubicin.** Hematologic toxicities may occur with **interferon alfa. HERBAL:** None significant. **FOOD:** None known. **LAB VALUES:** May increase mean corpuscular volume (MCV).

AVAILABILITY (Rx)

Capsules (Retrovir): 100 mg. **Injection Solution (Retrovir):** 10 mg/ml. **Syrup (Retrovir):** 50 mg/5 ml. **Tablets:** 300 mg.

ADMINISTRATION/HANDLING

💧 IV

Reconstitution • Must dilute before administration. • Remove calculated dose from vial and add to D₅W to provide concentration no greater than 4 mg/ml.
Rate of Administration • Infuse over 1 hr. May infuse over 30 min in neonates.
Storage • After dilution, IV solution is stable for 24 hrs at room temperature; 48 hrs if refrigerated. • Use within 8 hrs if stored at room temperature or 24 hrs if refrigerated to minimize potential for microbial-contaminated solution. • Do not use if solution is discolored or precipitate forms.

PO

• Keep capsules in cool, dry place. Protect from light. • Food, milk do not affect GI absorption. • Space doses evenly around the clock. • Pt should maintain an upright position when given medication to prevent esophageal ulceration.

💧 IV INCOMPATIBILITY

None known.

💧 IV COMPATIBILITIES

Dexamethasone (Decadron), dobutamine (Dobutrex), dopamine (Intropin), heparin, lorazepam (Ativan), morphine, potassium chloride.

INDICATIONS/ROUTES/DOSAGE

HIV Infection
PO: ADULTS, ELDERLY, CHILDREN OLDER THAN 12 YRS: 200 mg q8h or 300 mg q12h. **CHILDREN 12 YRS AND YOUNGER:** 160 mg/m²/dose (**maximum:** 200 mg)q8h or 240 mg/m² q12h (**maximum:** 300 mg). **FULL-TERM NEONATES:** 4 mg/kg/dose q12h. **PREMATURE NEONATES:** 2–4 mg/kg/dose q12h based on gestation at birth.
IV: ADULTS, ELDERLY, CHILDREN OLDER THAN 12 YRS: 1 mg/kg/dose q4h around the clock. **CHILDREN 12 YRS AND YOUNGER:** 120 mg/m²/dose q6h. **Maximum:** 160 mg/dose. **FULL-TERM NEONATES:** 3 mg/kg/dose q12h. **PREMATURE NEONATES:** 1.5–2.3 mg/kg/dose q12h based on gestation at birth.

Prevention of Maternal/Fetal HIV Transmission
PO: ADULTS: 200 mg 3 times/day, or 300 mg 2 times/day. Begin at 14–34 wks' gestation and continue until start of labor.
IV (During Labor and Delivery): 2 mg/kg loading dose, then IV infusion of 1 mg/kg/hr until umbilical cord clamped. **NEONATAL:** Begin 6–12 hrs after birth and continue for first 6 wks of life. Use IV route only until oral therapy can be administered.
PO: FULL-TERM INFANTS: 4 mg/kg/dose q12h (IV: 3 mg/kg/dose q12h). **INFANTS 30–34 WKS' GESTATION:** 2 mg/kg/dose q12h; increase to 3 mg/kg/dose at 2 wks of age (IV: 1.5 mg/kg/dose q12h; increase to 2.3 mg/kg/dose at 2 wks of age). **INFANTS LESS THAN 30 WKS' GESTATION:** 2 mg/kg/dose q12h; increase to 3 mg/kg/dose at 4 wks of age (IV: 1.5 mg/kg/dose q12h; increase to 2.3 mg/kg/dose at 4 wks of age).

♣ Canadian trade name   🐄 Non-Crushable Drug   ⬛ High Alert drug

Z

Dosage in Renal Impairment
Creatinine clearance less than 15 ml/min, including hemodialysis or peritoneal dialysis: 100 mg PO or 1 mg/kg IV q6–8h.

SIDE EFFECTS

Expected (46%–42%): Nausea, headache. **Frequent (20%–16%):** Abdominal pain, asthenia (loss of strength, energy), rash, fever, acne. **Occasional (12%–8%):** Diarrhea, anorexia, malaise, myalgia, drowsiness. **Rare (6%–5%):** Dizziness, paresthesia, vomiting, insomnia, dyspnea, altered taste.

ADVERSE EFFECTS/ TOXIC REACTIONS

Anemia (occurring most commonly after 4–6 wks of therapy), granulocytopenia are particularly significant in pts with pretherapy low baselines. Neurotoxicity (ataxia, fatigue, lethargy, nystagmus, seizures) may occur.

NURSING CONSIDERATIONS

BASELINE ASSESSMENT

Avoid drugs that are nephrotoxic, cytotoxic, myelosuppressive; may increase risk of toxicity. Obtain specimens for viral diagnostic tests before starting therapy (therapy may begin before results are obtained). Check hematology reports for accurate baseline.

INTERVENTION/EVALUATION

Monitor CBC, MCV, reticulocyte count, CD4 cell count, HIV RNA plasma levels. Check for bleeding. Assess for headache, dizziness. Monitor daily pattern of bowel activity, stool consistency. Evaluate skin for acne, rash. Be alert to development of opportunistic infections (fever, chills, cough, myalgia). Monitor I&O, serum renal/hepatic function tests. Check for insomnia.

PATIENT/FAMILY TEACHING

• Doses should be evenly spaced around the clock. • Zidovudine is not a cure for HIV infection, nor does it reduce risk of transmission to others. Acts to reduce symptoms and slows or arrests progress of disease. • Do not take any medications without physician's approval. • Bleeding from gums, nose, rectum may occur and should be reported to physician immediately. • Blood counts are essential because of bleeding potential. • Dental work should be done before therapy or after blood counts return to normal (often wks after therapy has stopped). • Inform physician if muscle weakness, difficulty breathing, headache, inability to sleep, unusual bleeding, rash, signs of infection occur.

---

ziprasidone   TOP 200

zi-**prah**-si-done
(<u>Geodon</u>, Zeldox ✦)

BLACK BOX ALERT Increased risk of mortality in elderly pts with dementia-related psychosis, mainly due to pneumonia, HF.
Do not confuse Ziprasidone with trazodone.

◆CLASSIFICATION

PHARMACOTHERAPEUTIC: Piperazine derivative. **CLINICAL:** Antipsychotic (see p. 68C).

ACTION

Antagonizes alpha-adrenergic, dopamine, histamine, serotonin receptors; inhibits reuptake of serotonin, norepinephrine. **Therapeutic Effect:** Diminishes symptoms of schizophrenia, depression.

PHARMACOKINETICS

Well absorbed after PO administration. Food increases bioavailability. Protein binding: 99%. Metabolized in liver. Eliminated in feces. Not removed by hemodialysis. **Half-life: PO:** 7 hrs; **IM:** 2–5 hrs.

USES

Treatment of schizophrenia, acute agitation in pts with schizophrenia, acute bi-

Z

polar mania, mania. Maintenance treatment of bipolar disorder as adjunct to lithium or valproic acid. **OFF-LABEL:** Tourette's syndrome, psychosis/agitation related to Alzheimer's dementia.

PRECAUTIONS

Contraindications: Conditions associated with risk of prolonged QT interval, congenital long QT syndrome, concurrent use of other QT prolongation medications. Uncompensated HF. Recent MI. **Cautions:** Pts with bradycardia, hypokalemia, hypomagnesemia may be at greater risk for torsade de pointes (atypical ventricular tachycardia). History of MI or unstable heart disease, seizures; pts at risk for aspiration, pneumonia, hepatic impairment. Pts at high risk for suicide, hypotensive episodes, breast cancer, or other prolactin-dependent tumors.

⌛ LIFESPAN CONSIDERATIONS

Pregnancy/Lactation: Unknown if drug crosses placenta or is distributed in breast milk. **Pregnancy Category C. Children:** Safety and efficacy not established. **Elderly:** No age-related precautions noted.

INTERACTIONS

DRUG: Alcohol, other CNS depressants may increase CNS depression. **Carbamazepine** may decrease concentration. **Ketoconazole** may increase concentration. **Medications causing prolongation of QT interval (e.g., amiodarone, dofetilide, sotalol)** may increase effects on cardiac conduction leading to malignant arrhythmias (e.g., torsade de pointes). **HERBAL: Gotu kola, kava kava, St. John's wort, valerian** may increase CNS depression. **St. John's wort** may decrease concentration. **FOOD: All foods** enhance bioavailability. **LAB VALUES:** May prolong QT interval. May increase serum glucose, prolactin levels.

AVAILABILITY (Rx)

Capsules: 20 mg, 40 mg, 60 mg, 80 mg.
Injection, Powder for Reconstitution: 20 mg.

ADMINISTRATION/HANDLING

IM
• Store vials at room temperature; protect from light. • Reconstitute each vial with 1.2 ml Sterile Water for Injection to provide concentration of 20 mg/ml. • Reconstituted solution stable for 24 hrs at room temperature or 7 days if refrigerated.

PO
• Give with food (increases bioavailability).

INDICATIONS/ROUTES/DOSAGE

◀ALERT▶ Dosage greater than 80 mg twice daily are not recommended in most pts.

Schizophrenia
PO: ADULTS, ELDERLY: Initially, 20 mg twice daily with food. Titrate at intervals of no less than 2 days. **Maintenance:** 20–100 mg twice daily.

Acute Agitation (Schizophrenia)
IM: ADULTS, ELDERLY: 10 mg q2h or 20 mg q4h. **Maximum:** 40 mg/day.

Acute Mania in Bipolar Disorder
PO: ADULTS, ELDERLY (Acute): Initially, 40 mg twice daily. May increase to 60–80 mg twice daily on second day of treatment. **Maintenance:** 40–80 mg twice daily.

Adjunct to Lithium Valproate in Bipolar Disorder
PO: ADULTS, ELDERLY: 40–80 mg twice daily.

SIDE EFFECTS

Frequent (30%–16%): Headache, drowsiness, dizziness. **Occasional:** Rash, orthostatic hypotension, weight gain, restlessness, constipation, dyspepsia (heartburn, indigestion, epigastric pain). **Rare:** Hyperglycemia, priapism.

ADVERSE EFFECTS/ TOXIC REACTIONS

Prolongation of QT interval (as seen on EKG) may produce torsade de pointes, a

Z

form of ventricular tachycardia. Pts with bradycardia, hypokalemia, hypomagnesemia are at increased risk.

NURSING CONSIDERATIONS

BASELINE ASSESSMENT

Assess pt's behavior, appearance, emotional status, response to environment, speech pattern, thought content. EKG should be obtained to assess for QT prolongation before instituting medication. Blood chemistry for serum magnesium, potassium should be obtained before beginning therapy and routinely thereafter.

INTERVENTION/EVALUATION

Assess for therapeutic response (greater interest in surroundings, improved self-care, increased ability to concentrate, relaxed facial expression). Monitor weight.

PATIENT/FAMILY TEACHING

• Avoid tasks that require alertness, motor skills until response to drug is established. • Avoid alcohol.

---

zoledronic acid   [TOP 200]

zoe-le-**dron**-ik **as**-id
(Aclasta ✦, Reclast, <u>Zometa</u>)
Do not confuse Zometa with Zofran or Zoladex.

◆CLASSIFICATION

PHARMACOTHERAPEUTIC: Bisphosphonate. **CLINICAL:** Calcium regulator, bone resorption inhibitor (see p. 143C).

ACTION

Inhibits resorption of mineralized bone, cartilage; inhibits increased osteoclastic activity, skeletal calcium release induced by stimulatory factors released by tumors. **Therapeutic Effect:** Increases urinary calcium, phosphorus excretion; decreases serum calcium, phosphorus levels.

USES

Zometa: Treatment of hypercalcemia of malignancy, bone metastases of solid tumors. Treatment of multiple myeloma. **Reclast:** Treatment and prevention of postmenopausal osteoporosis, glucocorticoid-induced osteoporosis, treatment of Paget's disease. Treatment of osteoporosis in men to increase bone mass. **OFF-LABEL:** Prevention of bone loss associated with aromatase inhibitor therapy in postmenopausal women with breast cancer or androgen deprivation therapy in men with prostate cancer.

PRECAUTIONS

Contraindications: Hypersensitivity to other bisphosphonates, including alendronate, etidronate, pamidronate, risedronate, tiludronate. Creatinine clearance less than 35 ml/min, evidence of acute renal impairment, hypocalcemia (Reclast). **Cautions: (Oncology Indications)** History of aspirin-sensitive asthma, renal impairment. **(Non-Oncology Indications)** Hypoparathyroidism, malabsorption syndrome.

LIFESPAN CONSIDERATIONS

Pregnancy/Lactation: Unknown if drug crosses placenta or is distributed in breast milk. **Pregnancy Category D. Children:** Safety and efficacy not established. **Elderly:** Age-related renal impairment may require dosage adjustment.

INTERACTIONS

DRUG: Loop diuretics (e.g., furosemide) may increase risk for hypocalcemia. **Nephrotoxic drugs** may increase risk for nephrotoxicity. **HERBAL:** None significant. **FOOD:** None known. **LAB VALUES:** May decrease serum magnesium, calcium, phosphate.

AVAILABILITY (Rx)

Injection Solution (Zometa): 4 mg/5 ml vial, 4 mg/100 ml single-use ready-to-use bottle. **(Reclast):** 5 mg diluted in 100 ml ready-to-infuse solution.

Z

ADMINISTRATION/HANDLING

◀ **ALERT** ▶ Pt should be adequately re-hydrated before administration of zole-dronic acid.

 IV (Zometa)

Reconstitution • Further dilute Zometa with 100 ml 0.9% NaCl or D_5W.
Rate of Administration • Adequate hydration is essential in conjunction with zoledronic acid. • Administer as IV infusion over not less than 15 min (increases risk of deterioration in renal function).
Storage • Store intact vials at room temperature. • Infusion of solution must be completed within 24 hrs.

 IV (Reclast)

• Administer as IV infusion over not less than 15 min. • Follow infusion with a 10-ml 0.9% NaCl flush of IV line.

IV INCOMPATIBILITIES

Do not mix with other medications.

INDICATIONS/ROUTES/DOSAGE

Hypercalcemia (Zometa)
IV Infusion: ADULTS, ELDERLY: 4 mg IV infusion given over no less than 15 min. Retreatment may be considered, but at least 7 days should elapse to allow for full response to initial dose.

Multiple Myeloma, Bone Metastases of Solid Tumors (Zometa)
IV: ADULTS, ELDERLY: 4 mg q3–4wks.

Paget's Disease (Reclast)
IV: ADULTS, ELDERLY: 5 mg as a single dose. Data about retreatment not available.

Osteoporosis Treatment (Reclast)
IV: ADULTS, ELDERLY: 5 mg once yearly.

Treatment/Prevention of Glucocorticoid-Induced Osteoporosis (Reclast)
IV: ADULTS, ELDERLY: 5 mg once yearly.

Prevention of Postmenopausal Osteoporosis (Reclast)
IV: ADULTS, ELDERLY: 5 mg once q2yrs.

Dosage in Renal Impairment
Reclast: **Creatinine clearance less than 35 ml/min:** Not recommended.
Zometa:

Creatinine Clearance	Dosage
50–60 ml/min	3.5 mg
40–49 ml/min	3.3 mg
30–39 ml/min	3 mg
Less than 30 ml/min	Not recommended

SIDE EFFECTS

Frequent (44%–26%): Fever, nausea, vomiting, constipation. **Occasional (15%–10%):** Hypotension, anxiety, insomnia, flu-like symptoms (fever, chills, bone pain, myalgia, arthralgia). **Rare:** Conjunctivitis.

ADVERSE EFFECTS/ TOXIC REACTIONS

Renal toxicity may occur if IV infusion is administered in less than 15 min.

NURSING CONSIDERATIONS

BASELINE ASSESSMENT

Prior to initiation, obtain dental exam for pts at risk for osteonecrosis. Establish baseline serum electrolytes, creatinine.

INTERVENTION/EVALUATION

Monitor serum renal function, CBC, Hgb, Hct. Assess vertebral bone mass (document stabilization, improvement). Monitor serum calcium, phosphate, magnesium, creatinine levels. Assess for fever. Monitor food intake, daily pattern of bowel activity, stool consistency. Check I&O, BUN, serum creatinine in pts with renal impairment.

zolmitriptan

zole-mi-**trip**-tan
(<u>Zomig</u>, Zomig Rapimelt ✦,
Zomig-ZMT)
Do not confuse zolmitriptan with sumatriptan.

✦ Canadian trade name   🐗 Non-Crushable Drug   🔲 High Alert drug

◆CLASSIFICATION

PHARMACOTHERAPEUTIC: Serotonin receptor agonist. **CLINICAL:** Antimigraine (see p. 65C).

ACTION

Binds selectively to vascular receptors, producing vasoconstrictive effect on cranial blood vessels. **Therapeutic Effect:** Relieves migraine headache.

PHARMACOKINETICS

Well absorbed after PO administration. Protein binding: 25%. Metabolized in liver. Eliminated in urine (60%), feces (30%). **Half-life:** 2.8–3.7 hrs.

USES

Treatment of acute migraine attack with or without aura.

PRECAUTIONS

Contraindications: Arrhythmias associated with conduction disorders (e.g., Wolff-Parkinson-White syndrome), basilar or hemiplegic migraine, coronary artery disease, ischemic heart disease (including angina pectoris, history of MI, silent ischemia, Prinzmetal's angina), uncontrolled hypertension, use within 24 hrs of ergotamine-containing preparations or another serotonin receptor agonist, MAOI used within 14 days. Additional for nasal spray: Cerebrovascular syndromes (e.g., stroke), peripheral vascular disease. **Cautions:** Mild to moderate renal/hepatic impairment, pt profile suggesting cardiovascular risks (e.g., hypertension, hypercholesterolemia, smoker, obesity, diabetes).

⊠ LIFESPAN CONSIDERATIONS

Pregnancy/Lactation: Unknown if drug is distributed in breast milk. **Pregnancy Category C. Children:** Safety and efficacy not established in those younger than 12 yrs. **Elderly:** No age-related precautions noted.

INTERACTIONS

DRUG: Ergotamine-containing medications may produce vasospastic reaction. **Fluoxetine, fluvoxamine, paroxetine, sertraline** may produce hyperreflexia, incoordination, weakness. **MAOIs** may dramatically increase concentration. **HERBAL:** None significant. **FOOD:** None known. **LAB VALUES:** None significant.

AVAILABILITY (Rx)

Nasal Spray (Zomig): 5 mg/0.1 ml. **Tablets (Zomig):** 2.5 mg, 5 mg.

🐾 **Tablets (Orally Disintegrating [Zomig-ZMT]):** 2.5 mg, 5 mg.

ADMINISTRATION/HANDLING

PO
• Give without regard to food. Tablets may be broken.

Orally Disintegrating Tablet
• Give whole; do not break, crush, cut.
• Place on pts tongue, allow to dissolve.
• Not necessary to administer with liquid.

Nasal
• Instruct pt to clear nasal passages as much as possible before use. • With head upright, pt should close one nostril with index finger, breathe out gently through mouth. • Instruct pt to insert nozzle into open nostril about ½ inch, close mouth, and while taking a breath through nose, release spray dosage by firmly pressing plunger. • Have pt remove nozzle from nose, gently breathe in through nose and out through mouth for 15–20 sec. Tell pt to avoid breathing in deeply.

INDICATIONS/ROUTES/DOSAGE

Acute Migraine Attack
PO: ADULTS, ELDERLY, CHILDREN OLDER THAN 18 YRS: Initially, 2.5 mg or less (may break tablet). If headache returns, may repeat dose after 2 hrs. **Maximum:** 10 mg/24 hrs.

Z

Orally Disintegrating Tablet: ADULTS, ELDERLY: 2.5 mg at onset of migraine headache. If headache returns, may repeat dose after 2 hrs. **Maximum:** 10 mg/24 hrs.

Intranasal: ADULTS, ELDERLY: 5 mg (1 spray). If headache returns, may repeat dose after 2 hrs. **Maximum:** 10 mg/24 hrs.

SIDE EFFECTS

Frequent (8%–6%): PO: Dizziness; paresthesia, neck/throat/jaw pressure; drowsiness. **Nasal:** Altered taste, paresthesia. **Occasional (5%–3%): PO:** Warm/hot sensation, asthenia (loss of strength, energy), chest pressure. **Nasal:** Nausea, drowsiness, nasal discomfort, dizziness, asthenia (loss of strength, energy), dry mouth. **Rare (2%–1%):** Diaphoresis, myalgia.

ADVERSE EFFECTS/ TOXIC REACTIONS

Cardiac events (ischemia, coronary artery vasospasm, MI), noncardiac vasospasm-related reactions (hemorrhage, stroke) occur rarely, particularly in pts with hypertension, diabetes, strong family history of coronary artery disease; pts who are obese; smokers; males older than 40 yrs; postmenopausal women.

NURSING CONSIDERATIONS

BASELINE ASSESSMENT

Question for history of peripheral vascular disease, coronary artery disease, renal/hepatic impairment, MAOI use. Question pt regarding onset, location, duration of migraine, possible precipitating factors.

INTERVENTION/EVALUATION

Monitor for evidence of dizziness. Monitor B/P, esp. in pts with hepatic impairment. Assess for relief of migraine headache, migraine potential for photophobia, phonophobia (sound sensitivity, light sensitivity, nausea, vomiting).

PATIENT/FAMILY TEACHING

• Take single dose as soon as symptoms of actual migraine attack appear. • Medica-

tion is intended to relieve migraine, not to prevent or reduce number of attacks. • Lie down in quiet dark room for additional benefit after taking medication. • Avoid tasks that require alertness, motor skills until response to drug is established. • Report chest pain; palpitations; tightness in throat; edema of face, lips, eyes; rash; easy bruising; blood in urine or stool; pain or numbness in arms or legs.

---

zolpidem

TOP 200

zole-pi-dem
(Ambien, Ambien CR, Edluar, Intermezzo, Sublinox ✦, Zolpimist)
Do not confuse Ambien with ativan, or zolpidem with zaleplon.

◆CLASSIFICATION

PHARMACOTHERAPEUTIC: Nonbenzodiazepine **(Schedule IV). CLINICAL:** Sedative-hypnotic (see p. 149C).

ACTION

Enhances action of inhibitory neurotransmitter gamma-aminobutyric acid (GABA). **Therapeutic Effect:** Induces sleep with fewer nightly awakenings, improves sleep quality.

PHARMACOKINETICS

Route	Onset	Peak	Duration
PO	30 min	N/A	6–8 hrs

Rapidly absorbed from GI tract. Protein binding: 92%. Metabolized in liver; excreted in urine. Not removed by hemodialysis. **Half-life:** 1.4–4.5 hrs (increased in hepatic impairment).

USES

Ambien, Edluar, Zolpimist: Short-term treatment of insomnia (with difficulty of sleep onset). **Ambien CR:** Treatment of insomnia (with difficulty of sleep onset and/or sleep maintenance).

Intermezzo: Treatment of insomnia characterized by middle-of-the-night awakening followed by difficulty returning to sleep.

PRECAUTIONS

Contraindications: None known. **Cautions:** Hepatic/renal impairment, pts with depression, history of drug dependence, sleep apnea, COPD, respiratory disease, myasthenia gravis, debilitated pts.

⌛ LIFESPAN CONSIDERATIONS

Pregnancy/Lactation: Unknown if drug crosses placenta or is distributed in breast milk. **Pregnancy Category C. Children:** Safety and efficacy not established. **Elderly:** More likely to experience falls or confusion; decreased initial doses recommended. Age-related hepatic impairment may require dosage adjustment.

INTERACTIONS

DRUG: Alcohol, other **CNS depressants** may increase CNS depression. **HERBAL:** Gotu kola, kava kava, valerian may increase CNS depression. **St. John's wort** may decrease concentration/effect. **FOOD:** None known. **LAB VALUES:** None significant.

AVAILABILITY (Rx)

Oral Solution (Zolpimist): 5 mg/actuation. **Tablets (Ambien):** 5 mg, 10 mg. **Tablets (Sublingual [Edluar]):** 5 mg, 10 mg. **(Intermezzo):** 1.75 mg, 3.5 mg.

Tablets (Extended-Release [Ambien CR]): 6.25 mg, 12.5 mg.

ADMINISTRATION/HANDLING

PO
• For faster sleep onset, do not give with or immediately after a meal. • Do not break, crush, dissolve, or divide Ambien CR tablets; give whole. • Edluar sublingual tablets to be placed under tongue and allowed to disintegrate. Do not swallow or administer with water. • Spray Zolpimist directly into mouth over tongue.

INDICATIONS/ROUTES/DOSAGE

Insomnia
PO, Spray, Sublingual (Edluar, Zolpimist): **ADULTS:** (males) 10 mg, (females) 5 mg immediately before bedtime. **ELDERLY, DEBILITATED:** 5 mg immediately before bedtime.

(Intermezzo): **ADULTS, ELDERLY:** 1.75 mg (females) 3.5 mg (males) taken once in middle of night with 4 or more hrs of expected sleep yet to come.

PO   (Extended-Release):   ADULTS: (males) 12.5 mg, (females) 6.25 mg immediately before bedtime. **ELDERLY, DEBILITATED:** 6.25 mg immediately before bedtime.

Dosage in Hepatic Impairment
PO: (Immediate-Release   Tablet, Spray, Sublingual Tablet): 5 mg. **(Extended-Release Tablet):** 6.25 mg. **(Intermezzo):** 1.75 mg.

SIDE EFFECTS

Occasional (7%): Headache. **Rare (less than 2%):** Dizziness, nausea, diarrhea, muscle pain, sleepwalking.

ADVERSE EFFECTS/ TOXIC REACTIONS

Overdose may produce severe ataxia (clumsiness, unsteadiness), bradycardia, diplopia, severe drowsiness, nausea, vomiting, difficulty breathing, unconsciousness. Abrupt withdrawal following long-term use may produce weakness, facial flushing, diaphoresis, vomiting, tremor. Drug tolerance/dependence may occur with prolonged use of high dosages.

NURSING CONSIDERATIONS

BASELINE ASSESSMENT
Assess B/P, pulse, respirations, mental status, sleep patterns. Raise bed rails, provide call light. Provide environment conducive to sleep (back rub, quiet environment, low lighting).

INTERVENTION/EVALUATION
Monitor sleep pattern of pt. Evaluate for therapeutic response to insomnia: de-

crease in number of nocturnal awakenings, increase in length of sleep. Monitor daytime alertness, respiratory rate, behavior profile.

PATIENT/FAMILY TEACHING

• Do not abruptly discontinue medication after long-term use. • Avoid alcohol and tasks that require alertness, motor skills until response to drug is established. • Tolerance, dependence may occur with prolonged use of high dosages. • Do not break, chew, crush, dissolve, or divide Ambien CR tablets; swallow whole.

zonisamide

zoe-**nis**-a-mide
(Zonegran)
Do not confuse Zonegran with Sinequan, or zonisamide with lacosamide.

◆CLASSIFICATION

PHARMACOTHERAPEUTIC: Succinimide. **CLINICAL:** Anticonvulsant (see p. 38C).

ACTION

May stabilize neuronal membranes, suppress neuronal hypersynchronization by blocking sodium, calcium channels. **Therapeutic Effect:** Reduces seizure activity.

PHARMACOKINETICS

Well absorbed after PO administration. Metabolized in liver. Extensively bound to RBCs. Protein binding: 40%. Primarily excreted in urine. **Half-life:** 63 hrs (plasma), 105 hrs (RBCs).

USES

Adjunctive therapy in treatment of partial seizures in adults, children older than 16 yrs with epilepsy. **OFF-LABEL:** Bipolar disorder.

PRECAUTIONS

Contraindications: Allergy to sulfonamides. **Cautions:** Renal/hepatic impairment, pts at high risk for suicide or metabolic acidosis (e.g., severe respiratory disease).

⌛ LIFESPAN CONSIDERATIONS

Pregnancy/Lactation: Unknown if distributed in breast milk. **Pregnancy Category C. Children:** Safety and efficacy not established in pts younger than 16 yrs. **Elderly:** No age-related precautions noted, but lower dosages recommended.

INTERACTIONS

DRUG: Alcohol, other CNS depressants may increase sedative effect. **CYP3A4 inducers (e.g., carbamazepine, phenobarbital, phenytoin, valproic acid)** may increase metabolism, decrease effect. **HERBAL:** None significant. **FOOD:** None known. **LAB VALUES:** May increase BUN, serum creatinine.

AVAILABILITY (Rx)

▼ **Capsules:** 25 mg, 50 mg, 100 mg.

ADMINISTRATION/HANDLING

PO
• May give with or without food. • Do not crush, break capsules. Give capsules whole. • Do not give to pts allergic to sulfonamides.

INDICATIONS/ROUTES/DOSAGE

Note: Do not use if creatinine clearance is less than 50 ml/min.

Partial Seizures
PO: ADULTS, ELDERLY, CHILDREN OLDER THAN 16 YRS: Initially, 100 mg/day. May increase to 200 mg/day after 2 wks. Further increases to 300 mg/day and 400 mg/day can be made with minimum of 2 wks between adjustments. **Range:** 100–600 mg/day.

SIDE EFFECTS

Frequent (17%–9%): Drowsiness, dizziness, anorexia, headache, agitation, irri-

---

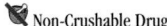

Z

tability, nausea. **Occasional (8%–5%):** Fatigue, ataxia, confusion, depression, impaired memory/concentration, insomnia, abdominal pain, diplopia, diarrhea, speech difficulty. **Rare (4%–3%):** Paresthesia, nystagmus, anxiety, rash, dyspepsia (heartburn, indigestion, epigastric pain), weight loss.

ADVERSE EFFECTS/ TOXIC REACTIONS

Overdose characterized by bradycardia, hypotension, respiratory depression, coma. Leukopenia, anemia, thrombocytopenia occur rarely.

NURSING CONSIDERATIONS

BASELINE ASSESSMENT

Review history of seizure disorder (intensity, frequency, duration, LOC). Initiate seizure precautions. Serum hepatic function tests, CBC should be performed before therapy begins and periodically during therapy.

INTERVENTION/EVALUATION

Observe frequently for recurrence of seizure activity. Assess for clinical improvement (decrease in intensity, frequency of seizures). Assist with ambulation if dizziness occurs.

PATIENT/FAMILY TEACHING

• Strict maintenance of drug therapy is essential for seizure control. • Avoid tasks that require alertness, motor skills until response to drug is established. • Avoid alcohol. • Report if rash, back/abdominal pain, blood in urine, fever, sore throat, ulcers in mouth, easy bruising occur. • Notify physician of worsening depression, unusual behavior, suicidal ideation.

Z

CALCULATION OF DOSES

Frequently, dosages ordered do not correspond exactly to what is available and must be calculated.

RATIO/PROPORTION:

A pt is to receive 65 mg of a medication. It is available as 80 mg/2 ml. What volume (ml) needs to be administered to the patient?

STEP 1: Set up ratio.

$$\frac{80 \text{ mg}}{2 \text{ ml}} = \frac{65 \text{ mg}}{x \text{ (ml)}}$$

STEP 2: Cross multiply and divide each side by the number with x to determine volume to be administered.

$$80 \text{ mg} \times (x) \text{ ml} = 65 \text{ mg} \times 2 \text{ ml}$$
$$80 \text{ x} = 130$$
$$x = \frac{130}{80} = 1.625 \text{ ml}$$

CALCULATIONS IN MICROGRAMS PER KILOGRAM PER MINUTE (mcg/kg/min):

A 63-year-old pt (weight 165 lb) is to receive medication A at a rate of 8 mcg/kg/min. Given a solution containing medication A in a concentration of 500 mg/250 ml, at what rate (ml/hr) would you infuse this medication?

STEP 1: Convert to same units. In this problem, the dose is expressed in mcg/kg; therefore, convert weight to kg (2.2 lb = 1 kg) and drug concentration to mcg/ml (1 mg = 1,000 mcg).

$$165 \text{ lb divided by } 2.2 = 75 \text{ kg}$$
$$\frac{500 \text{ mg}}{250 \text{ ml}} = \frac{2 \text{ mg}}{\text{ml}} = \frac{2,000 \text{ mcg}}{\text{ml}}$$

STEP 2: Number of mcg/hr.

$$(75 \text{ kg}) \times 8 \text{ mcg/kg/min} = 600 \text{ mcg/min or } 36,000 \text{ mcg/hr}$$

STEP 3: Number of ml/hr.

$$36,000 \text{ mcg/hr divided by } 2,000 \text{ mcg/ml} = 18 \text{ ml/hr}$$

CONTROLLED DRUGS (UNITED STATES)

Schedule I: Medications having no legal medical use. These substances may be used for research purposes with proper registration (e.g., heroin, LSD).

Schedule II: Medications having a legitimate medical use but are characterized by a very high abuse potential and/or potential for severe physical and psychic dependency. Emergency telephone orders for limited quantities of these drugs are authorized, but the prescriber must provide a written, signed prescription order (e.g., morphine, amphetamines).

Schedule III: Medications having significant abuse potential (less than Schedule II). Telephone orders are permitted (e.g., opiates in combination with other substances such as acetaminophen).

Schedule IV: Medications having a low abuse potential. Telephone orders are permitted (e.g., benzodiazepines, propoxyphene).

Schedule V: Medications having the lowest abuse potential of the controlled substances. Some Schedule V products may be available without a prescription (e.g., certain cough preparations containing limited amounts of an opiate).

Appendix C

FDA PREGNANCY CATEGORIES

◄ALERT► Medications should be used during pregnancy only if clearly needed.

A: Adequate and well-controlled studies have failed to show a risk to the fetus in the first trimester of pregnancy (also, no evidence of risk has been seen in later trimesters). Possibility of fetal harm appears remote.

B: Animal reproduction studies have failed to show a risk to the fetus, and there are no adequate/well-controlled studies in pregnant women.

C: Animal reproduction studies have shown an adverse effect on the fetus, and there are no adequate/well-controlled studies in humans. However, the benefits may warrant use of the drug in pregnant women despite potential risks.

D: There is positive evidence of human fetal risk based on data from investigational or marketing experience or from studies in humans, but the potential benefits may warrant use of the drug despite potential risks (e.g., use in life-threatening situations in which other medications cannot be used or are ineffective).

X: Animal or human studies have shown fetal abnormalities and/or there is evidence of human fetal risk based on adverse reaction data from investigational or marketing experience where the risks of using the medication clearly outweigh potential benefits.

CHRONIC WOUND CARE

Introduction

A chronic wound is one that has not healed completely after 4–6 wks. The most common chronic wounds include pressure ulcers (also called *decubitus ulcers* or *bedsores),* diabetic ulcers (diabetes causes neuropathy, which inhibits the perception of pain and may cause repeated injury), and venous ulcers, primarily occurring in legs, most likely affecting the elderly.

Causes of chronic wounds include the following:
- **Diseases:** Diabetes, cancer, liver/kidney conditions may slow the healing process
- **Poor blood supply/oxygen:** Decreased blood flow may be due to low blood pressure, blocked or narrow blood vessels; low oxygen may be due to heart or lung disease
- **Repeated trauma:** May be due to swelling, increased pressure in tissues, constant pressure on the wound area
- **Impaired immune system:** May be due to radiation, poor nutrition, medications (e.g., steroids)
- **Infection or presence of foreign objects:** May delay wound healing

Treatment

Treatment is based on the severity of the wound, the location of the wound, and whether other areas are affected. Staging of ulcers and other chronic wounds is common practice and relates to the depth and severity of the wound.

Stage 1: Wound is seen as nonblanching redness of intact skin
Stage 2: Ulcer extends through the epidermis or dermis
Stage 3: Ulcer extends through the full thickness of the skin into the subcutaneous tissue, creating a crater
Stage 4: Tissue necrosis with muscle, bone, or underlying structural damage

Treatment of chronic wounds involves maintaining appropriate moisture levels, preventing/treating infections, debridement (removal of necrotic or fibrous tissue, which may include surgical debridement for pts with sepsis or advancing cellulitis), cleansing the wound, eliminating or minimizing pain, and protecting the surrounding skin.

During the healing process, wounds progress through three, sometimes overlapping, phases:
- **Inflammatory phase:** Redness, heat, pain, swelling
- **Proliferative phase:** Migration of fibroblasts into the wound, cellular proliferation, granulation
- **Maturation phase:** New collagen production, deposition and migration of epithelial cells

Products used for treatment of chronic wounds include antimicrobials, debriding agents, dressings, and wound cleansers. **Note:** Papain-containing products are no longer available. These products have historically been marketed without approval. Also, adverse events with use of these products raise serious safety concerns (reported to produce hypersensitivity reactions, anaphylactic reactions, hypotension, tachycardia). Pts allergic to latex may be allergic to papaya, the source of papain.

Wound Care Products

Description	General Uses	Comments
Alginate dressings: Spun fibers of brown seaweed that act as ion exchange mechanisms to absorb serous fluid or exudate, forming a gel-like covering that conforms to the shape of the wound. Facilitate autolytic debridement and maintain a moist wound environment. **Products:** AlgiDERM, Curasorb, Sorbsan. Available as ropes, pads.	Abrasions/lacerations/skin tears Arterial/venous ulcers Deep and tunneling wounds Diabetic ulcers Pressure ulcers Second-degree burns Odorous wounds Contaminated and infected wounds	Good for moderately to heavily exudative wounds and hemorrhagic wounds Can be left in place until soaked with exudate Requires a secondary dressing (e.g., transparent film, foam, hydrocolloids) Do not moisten prior to use Nonadhesive, nonocclusive Contraindicated in third-degree burns; not recommended for dry or minimally exudative wounds
Collagenase ointment: Sterile enzymatic debriding ointment that possesses the ability to digest collagen in necrotic tissue. **Products:** Santyl.	Eschar or necrotic tissue in wound bed Diabetic foot ulcer Pressure ulcers, stages 2–4 Varicose ulcers	Can be used for infected wounds Gauze is used as a secondary dressing Discontinue when granulation tissue is present Optimal pH for enzymatic action is 6–8 Avoid acidic agents for cleansing; avoid detergents and agents containing heavy metal (e.g., mercury or silver), which may adversely affect enzymatic activity
Trypsin, castor oil, Peru balsam: Trypsin is a mild debriding agent that helps shed damaged skin cells. **Castor oil** acts as a lubricant to protect tissue. **Peru balsam** increases blood flow to a wound area, reduces wound odor. **Products:** Granulex, Xenaderm. Available as gel, ointment, spray.	Eschar or necrotic tissue in wound bed Pressure ulcers, stages 1–4 Varicose ulcers	Can be used for infected wounds Avoid concurrent use of silver-containing products (may reduce efficacy) Promotes healing and relieves pain caused by bed sores and other skin ulcers
Hydrophilic polyurethane foam: Also called open cell foam dressings. Sheets of foamed solutions of polymers containing variably sized open cells that can hold wound exudate away from wound bed. Maintains moist wound environment. **Products:** Biopatch, Curafoam, Flexzan. Available as sheets in a wide variety of formulations.	Moderate to heavy exudative wounds with or without a clean granular wound bed Diabetic ulcers, pressure ulcers, venous stasis ulcers Draining surgical incisions Superficial burns Tube and drain sites	Contraindicated for use in third-degree burns Not recommended for wounds with little to no exudate or when tunneling is present Good for cavitating wounds Highly absorbent, semi-occlusive dressing Usual dressing change is up to 3 times per wk

Description	General Uses	Comments
Hydrocolloids: Formulations of elastomeric, adhesive, and gelling agents; the most common absorbent ingredient is carboxymethylcellulose. Most hydrocolloids are backed with a semi-occlusive film layer. The wound side of the dressing is adhesive, adhering to a moist surface as well as to dry skin but not to the moist wound bed. As wound fluid is absorbed, the hydrocolloid forms a viscous gel in the wound bed, enhancing a moist wound environment. **Products:** Aquacel, Curaderm, DuoDerm. Available as dressings, granules, patches, paste.	Minimal to moderate exudate in partial and full thickness wounds Cuts and abrasions First- and second-degree burns Pressure ulcers Stasis ulcers	Not for wounds producing heavy exudate, infected wounds, dry eschar-covered wounds May provide pain relief Good for chronic wounds that are epithelializing Can be left in place for up to 7 days Contraindicated for third-degree burns
Hydrogels: Glycerin- or water-based dressings designed to hydrate the wound. May absorb small amounts of exudate. **Products:** Curasol, Tegaderm, Flexderm, Vigilon. Available as gel, sheets, gauze.	Partial and full thickness wounds Dry to minimal exudate Cuts and abrasions First- and second-degree burns Pressure ulcers Stasis ulcers	Not for wounds producing moderate to heavy exudate Not for infected wounds May provide pain relief Good for wounds that are debriding Good for keeping a dry wound moist Can be left in place for 1–3 days
Iodine compounds: Cadexomer iodine: Iodine is complexed with a polymeric cadexomer starch vehicle, forming a topical gel or paste. The cadexomer moiety absorbs exudate and debris and releases iodine for antimicrobial activity. **Products:** Iodosorb, Iodoflex. Available as gel, dressing, ointment, powder.	Chronic nonhealing, exuding wounds including pressure or leg ulcers and exuding, infected wounds	Requires use of a secondary dressing Contraindicated in pts with iodine sensitivity, Hashimoto's thyroiditis, nontoxic nodular goiter, children Dressing to be changed when it turns white, indicating that the iodine has been depleted
Silver compounds Silver sulfadiazine cream: Silver possesses bactericidal properties. Has been shown to reduce bacterial density, vascular margination, migration of inflammatory cells. Enhances rate of re-epithelialization.	Prevent infection in second- and third-degree burns Prevent or treat infection in chronic wounds	May have cytotoxic effects that could delay wound healing Allergic reactions may occur Use should be limited to a 2- to 4-wk period Bacteria may become resistant with prolonged use Avoid use with collagenase- or trypsin-containing debriding agents

(continued)

Description	General Uses	Comments
Transparent film dressings: Polyurethane sheets coated on one side with an adhesive that is inactivated by moisture and will not adhere to a moist surface such as the wound bed. Have no absorbent capacity and are impermeable to fluids and bacteria but are semipermeable to oxygen and water vapor. **Products:** Bioclusive, CarraFilm, Tegaderm HP. Available in a variety of sizes and features.	Prophylaxis on high-risk intact skin Superficial wounds with minimal or no exudate Eschar-covered wounds when autolysis is indicated Clean, closed surgical incisions Pressure ulcers, stage 1 or 2 Second-degree burns	Prevents wound desiccation and contamination by bacteria Contraindicated in third-degree burns Promotes autolysis of necrotic tissue in the wound; maintains moist environment Avoid in arterial ulcers and infected wounds requiring frequent monitoring Do not use as primary dressing on wounds with depth or tunneling May provide pain relief Leave in place for up to 7 days or until fluid leaks
Becaplermin gel: Recombinant formulation of platelet-derived growth factor that promotes cell mitogenesis and protein synthesis for granulation tissue granulation. **Products:** Regranex.	Diabetic foot ulcers that extend into subcutaneous tissue or beyond	Usually applied daily Adequate blood supply and absence of necrotic tissue are needed for efficacy Repeated use (3 or more tubes) may increase risk of cancer-related death Use cautiously in pts with known malignancy

DRUGS OF ABUSE

Substance	Brand/ Street Names	Administered	Effects of Intoxication	Potential Health Consequences
Amphetamine	*Dexedrine;* bennies, black beauties, hearts, speed, truck drivers, uppers	Injection, smoked, snorted	Increased heart rate, blood pressure, body temperature, metabolism; increased energy, mental alertness; tremors; reduced appetite; irritability; anxiety; panic; violent behavior; psychosis	Weight loss, insomnia, cardiac or cardiovascular complications, stroke, seizures, addiction, tremor, irritability
Barbiturates	*Nembutal, Seconal, Phenobarbital;* barbs, reds, phennies, yellow, yellow jackets	Injection, oral	Reduction of pain and anxiety; feeling of well-being; lowered inhibitions; slowed pulse/breathing; lowered blood pressure; poor concentration; sedation, drowsiness	Confusion, fatigue; impaired coordination, memory, judgment; respiratory depression or arrest; addiction; depression; unusual excitement; fever; irritability; slurred speech; dizziness
Benzodiazepines	*Ativan, Librium, Valium, Xanax;* candy, downers, tranks	Oral	Reduction of pain and anxiety; feeling of well-being; lowered inhibitions; slowed pulse/breathing; lowered blood pressure; poor concentration; sedation, drowsiness	Confusion, fatigue; impaired coordination, memory, judgment; respiratory depression or arrest; addiction; dizziness
Cocaine	Blow, bump, candy, coke, crack, rack, snow, toot	Injection, smoked, snorted	Increased heart rate, blood pressure, body temperature, metabolism; increased energy, mental alertness; tremors; reduced appetite; irritability; anxiety; panic; violent behavior; psychosis	Weight loss, insomnia, cardiac or cardiovascular complications, stroke, seizures, addiction, nasal damage from snorting, rapid or irregular heartbeat, headaches, malnutrition

(continued)

Substance	Brand/ Street Names	Administered	Effects of Intoxication	Potential Health Consequences
Codeine	*Fiorinal with codeine, Tylenol with codeine;* Captain Cody, schoolboy, loads, pancakes and syrup	Injection, oral	Pain relief, euphoria, drowsiness	Respiratory depression and arrest, nausea, confusion, constipation, sedation, unconsciousness, coma, tolerance, addiction
Dextromethorphan	Found in some cough and cold medications; robotripping, poor man's PCP, velvet, Robo, Triple C	Oral	Impaired motor function, feeling of being separated from one's body and environment; euphoria; slurred speech; confusion; dizziness; distorted visual perceptions	
Flunitrazepam	*Rohypnol;* forget-me pill, Mexican Valium, roofies, roofinol, rope, rophies	Oral, snorted	Sedation, muscle relaxation, confusion, memory loss, dizziness, impaired coordination, reduced pain/anxiety, feeling of well-being	Addiction; confusion, fatigue, memory loss, respiratory depression
GHB	Georgia home boy, grievous bodily harm, liquid ecstasy, soap, scoop, goop, liquid X	Oral	Drowsiness, nausea, headache, disorientation, loss of coordination, memory loss	Unconsciousness, seizures, coma, confusion, nausea, vomiting, headache
Heroin	Smack, horse, brown sugar, dope, junk, white horse, China white	Injection, smoked, snorted	Euphoria, drowsiness, impaired coordination, dizziness, confusion, nausea, sedation, feeling of heaviness in the body, slowed breathing	Constipation, confusion, sedation, respiratory depression, coma, addiction

Substance	Brand/ Street Names	Administered	Effects of Intoxication	Potential Health Consequences
Hydrocodone	*Vicodin, Lortab*	Oral	Pain relief, euphoria, drowsiness	Respiratory depression and arrest, nausea, confusion, constipation, sedation, unconsciousness, coma, tolerance, addiction
Inhalants	Solvents (paint thinner, glues), nitrites (laughing gas, snappers, poppers)	Inhaled through nose or mouth	Stimulation, loss of inhibition, headache, nausea or vomiting, slurred speech, loss of motor coordination, wheezing	Cramps, muscle weakness, depression, memory impairment, damage to cardiovascular and nervous systems, unconsciousness, sudden death
Ketamine	*Ketalar;* cat Valium, Special K, vitamin K	Injection, snorted, smoked	Increased heart rate and blood pressure, impaired motor function, feelings of being separated from one's body and environment; at high doses: delirium, depression, respiratory depression or arrest; death	Memory loss, numbness, nausea/vomiting, anxiety, tremors, respiratory depression
LSD	Acid, cubes, microdot, yellow sunshine, blue heaven	Oral, absorbed through mouth tissues	Altered states of perception and feeling; hallucinations; nausea; increased body temperature, heart rate, blood pressure; loss of appetite; sweating; sleeplessness; numbness; dizziness; weakness; tremors; impulsive behavior; rapid shifts in emotion	Flashbacks, hallucinogen persisting perception disorder

(continued)

Substance	Brand/ Street Names	Administered	Effects of Intoxication	Potential Health Consequences
Marijuana	Blunt, ganja, grass, joint, Mary Jane, pot, reefer, sinsemilla, skunk, weed	Oral, smoked	Euphoria, relaxation, slowed reaction time, impaired balance and coordination, increased heart rate and appetite, impaired learning and memory, anxiety, panic attacks, psychosis	Cough, impaired memory and learning, anxiety, panic attacks, frequent respiratory infections, possible mental health decline, addiction
MDMA	Ecstasy, Adam, clarity, Eve, lover's speed, peace, uppers	Injection, oral, snorted	Mild hallucinogenic effects, increased tactile sensitivity, empathic feelings, lowered inhibition, anxiety, chills, sweating, teeth clenching, muscle cramping	Reduced appetite, irregular heartbeat, heart failure, impaired memory, hyperthermia, addiction
Mescaline	Buttons, cactus, peyote	Oral, smoked	Altered states of perception and feeling; hallucinations; nausea; increased body temperature, heart rate, blood pressure; loss of appetite; sweating; sleeplessness; numbness; dizziness; weakness; tremors; impulsive behavior; rapid shifts in emotion	Loss of appetite, nausea, weakness, chronic mental disorders
Methamphetamine	Desoxyn; meth, ice, crank, crystal, go fast, speed	Oral, injection, smoked, snorted	Increased heart rate, blood pressure, body temperature, metabolism; increased energy, mental alertness; tremors; reduced appetite; irritability; anxiety; panic; violent behavior; psychosis	Weight loss, insomnia, cardiac or cardiovascular complications, stroke, seizures, addiction, severe dental problems, behavior/memory loss, impaired memory and learning, tolerance, addiction

Substance	Brand/ Street Names	Administered	Effects of Intoxication	Potential Health Consequences
Methylphenidate	*Ritalin;* JIF, MPH, Skippy, smart drug, vitamin R	Injection, oral, snorted	Increase or decrease in blood pressure; psychotic episodes	Digestive problems, loss of appetite, weight loss, reduced appetite, rapid irregular heartbeat, heart failure, seizures, stroke
Morphine	*Roxanol, Duramorph;* M, Miss Emma, monkey, white stuff	Injection, oral, smoked	Pain relief, euphoria, drowsiness	Respiratory depression and arrest, nausea, confusion, constipation, sedation, unconsciousness, coma, tolerance, addiction
Oxycodone	*OxyContin, Percodan;* oxycotton, oxycet, hillbilly heroin, percs	Injection, oral	Pain relief, euphoria, drowsiness	Respiratory depression and arrest, nausea, confusion, constipation, sedation, unconsciousness, coma, tolerance, addiction
PCP	*Phencyclidine;* angel dust, boat, hog, love boat, peace pill	Injection, oral, smoked	Impaired motor function, feelings of being separated from one's body and environment, analgesia, psychosis, aggression, violence, slurred speech, loss of coordination, hallucinations	Memory loss, loss of appetite, panic, aggression, violence
Psilocybin	Magic mushrooms, purple passion, little smoke	Oral	Altered states of perception and feeling, hallucinations, nausea, nervousness, paranoia, panic	Chronic mental disorders

EQUIANALGESIC DOSING

Guidelines for equianalgesic dosing of commonly used analgesics are presented in the following table. The dosages are approximate to 10 mg of morphine intramuscularly. These guidelines are for the management of acute pain in the opioid-naïve pt. Dosages may vary for the opioid-tolerant pt and for the management of chronic pain. Dosing adjustments for renal or hepatic insufficiency may also be necessary. Clinical response is the criterion that must be applied for each pt with titration to desired response.

Name	Equianalgesic Oral Dose	Equianalgesic Parenteral Dose (IV, IM, Subcutaneous)
Codeine	200 mg	100–130 mg
Fentanyl	Not available	0.1 mg (100 micrograms)
Hydrocodone	30–45 mg	Not available
Hydromorphone (Dilaudid)	7.5–8 mg	1.5–2 mg
Hydromorphone (Dilaudid) (Controlled-Release)	7.5 mg	N/A
Meperidine (Demerol)	300 mg	75 mg
Methadone (Dolophine)	10–20 mg	10 mg
Morphine	30 mg	10 mg
Oxycodone (OxyContin)	20–30 mg	Not available
Oxymorphone	10 mg	1 mg
Oxymorphone (Extended-Release)	10 mg	N/A

Appendix G

HERBALS: COMMON NATURAL MEDICINES

The use of herbal therapies is increasing in the United States. Because of the rise in the use of herbal therapy, the following is presented to provide some basic information on some of the more popular herbs. Please note this is not an all-inclusive list, which is beyond the scope of this handbook.

Name	Uses	Comments
Aloe vera	Orally: osteoarthritis, inflammatory bowel diseases (e.g., ulcerative colitis), fever, itching, inflammation. Topically: burns, wound healing, psoriasis, sunburn, frostbite, cold sores.	Well tolerated. Orally can cause abdominal pain, cramps; topically can cause burning, itching, contact dermatitis. May lower blood glucose levels and have additive effects with antidiabetic medications.
Bilberry	Orally: improve visual acuity (e.g., night vision, cataracts), atherosclerosis, chronic fatigue syndrome. Topically: mild inflammation of mouth and throat mucous membranes.	Can inhibit platelet aggregation, increase risk of bleeding when combined with antiplatelet or anticoagulant medications (e.g., aspirin, clopidogrel, enoxaparin, warfarin). May lower blood glucose.
Bitter orange	Orally: appetite stimulant, dyspepsia. Topically: inflammation of the eyelid, conjunctiva, retina.	May cause hypertension, cardiovascular toxicity. May increase concentration/effects of midazolam; concurrent use with MAOIs may increase blood pressure (avoid use); combination with caffeine can increase blood pressure, heart rate.
Black cohosh	Orally: symptoms of menopause, premenstrual syndrome (PMS), dysmenorrhea, dyspepsia. Topically: acne, mole, and wart removal; improve skin appearance.	Can cause GI upset, rash, headache, dizziness, increased weight, cramping, breast tenderness, vaginal spotting/bleeding. May decrease effects of cisplatin; may increase risk of hepatic damage with hepatotoxic medications.
Capsicum (cayenne pepper)	Orally: dyspepsia, flatulence, diarrhea, cramps, toothache, hyperlipidemia. Topically: pain of shingles, osteoarthritis, rheumatoid arthritis, postherpetic neuralgia, diabetic neuralgia, trigeminal neuralgia.	Orally can cause upper abdominal discomfort (e.g., gas, bloating, nausea, diarrhea, belching); topically can cause burning, stinging, erythema. May increase effects/adverse effects of antiplatelet medications.
Chamomile	Prepared as a tea and used as a mild sedative, relaxant, and sleeping aid; used for indigestion, itching, and inflammation.	Large amounts may cause vomiting.

(continued)

Name	Uses	Comments
Chastberry	Orally: menstrual irregularities (e.g., dysmenorrhea, amenorrhea, metrorrhagia).	Can cause GI upset, headache, diarrhea, nausea, itching, urticaria, rash, insomnia, increased weight, irregular menstrual bleeding. Can interfere with efficacy of oral contraceptives, hormone replacement therapy.
Clove (clove oil)	Orally: dyspepsia, expectorant, diarrhea, halitosis, flatulence, nausea, vomiting. Topically: toothache, mouth and throat inflammation.	Topically can cause tissue irritation, allergic dermatitis.
Co-enzyme Q-10	Heart failure, angina, diabetes, hypertension.	Can cause GI side effects (e.g., nausea, vomiting, diarrhea, appetite suppression, heartburn, epigastric discomfort). Can decrease blood pressure and have an additive effect with antihypertensive medications; may reduce anticoagulant effects of warfarin.
Cranberry	Prevention/treatment of urinary tract infections, neurogenic bladder, urinary deodorizer in incontinence.	Large amounts can cause GI upset, diarrhea. Greater than 1,000 ml daily can increase risk of uric acid, kidney stone formation.
DHEA	Slow or reverse aging, weight loss, metabolic syndrome, increase immune and cognitive function.	At high dose can cause acne, hirsutism, hair loss, voice deepening, insulin resistance, altered menstrual pattern. May interfere with antiestrogen effects of anastrozole, letrozole, or other aromatase inhibitors; may overcome estrogen receptor antagonist activity of tamoxifen in estrogen receptor positive cancer cells.
Dong quai	Dysmenorrhea, premenstrual syndrome, menopausal symptoms.	May cause photosensitivity and photodermatitis. May increase effect/risk of bleeding with antiplatelet and anticoagulant medications (e.g., aspirin, warfarin).
Echinacea	Treat/prevent common cold, other upper respiratory tract infections.	Can cause GI effects (e.g., nausea, abdominal pain, diarrhea, vomiting). Stimulates immune function—may exacerbate autoimmune diseases (e.g., multiple sclerosis, rheumatoid arthritis, systemic lupus erythematosis).

Name	Uses	Comments
Eucalyptus	Orally: infections, fever, dyspepsia, expectorant for coughs. Topically: inflammation of respiratory tract mucous membranes, rheumatoid arthritis, nasal stuffiness.	Orally: GI effects (e.g., nausea, vomiting, diarrhea). Topically (prolonged exposure/large amounts): agitation, drowsiness, muscle weakness, ataxia.
Evening primrose oil	Premenstrual syndrome, endometriosis, symptoms of menopause (e.g., hot flashes).	May increase risk of bruising/bleeding with antiplatelet/anticoagulant medications (e.g., aspirin, clopidogrel, enoxaparin, warfarin).
Feverfew	Orally: fever, headaches, prevention of migraines, menstrual irregularities. Topically: toothaches, antiseptic.	Orally: GI effects (e.g., heartburn, nausea, diarrhea, constipation, abdominal pain, bloating, flatulence). Topically: contact dermatitis. May have additive effects, increase risk of bleeding with antiplatelet medications.
Fish oil	Hyperlipidemia, hypertriglyceridemia, hypertension, stroke, depression, rheumatoid arthritis, osteoporosis, psoriasis, Crohn's disease.	Can cause a fishy aftertaste, halitosis, heartburn, dyspepsia, nausea, loose stools, rash. May have additive effect with antihypertensive medication.
Garlic	Hypertension, hyperlipidemia, age-related vascular changes, atherosclerosis, chronic fatigue syndrome, menstrual disorders.	Dose-related effects including breath/body odor, mouth and GI burning/irritation, heartburn, flatulence, nausea, vomiting, diarrhea. May increase effects of antiplatelets (e.g., aspirin, clopidogrel, enoxaparin), anticoagulants (e.g., warfarin); may decrease effects of oral contraceptives, cyclosporine, protease inhibitors, and NNRTIs.
Ginger	Motion sickness, morning sickness, dyspepsia, rheumatoid arthritis, osteoarthritis, loss of appetite, migraine headache.	At high doses of 5 g/day may cause abdominal discomfort, heartburn, diarrhea, irritant effect in mouth and throat. May increase risk of bleeding with antiplatelet medications and anticoagulants (e.g., aspirin, clopidogrel, enoxaparin, warfarin).
Ginkgo	Dementia (including Alzheimer's), vascular dementia, mixed dementia.	Mild GI upset, headache, dizziness, constipation, palpitations, allergic skin reactions. Decreases platelet aggregation; may increase risk of bleeding with antiplatelet and anticoagulants (e.g., aspirin, clopidogrel, enoxaparin, warfarin).

(continued)

Name	Uses	Comments
Ginseng	Increases resistance to environmental stress, improves well-being, boosts energy, aphrodisiac.	May cause insomnia, vaginal bleeding, headache, hypertension, hypotension. May decrease platelet aggregation (use caution with antiplatelet or anticoagulant medications).
Glucosamine	Osteoarthritis, glaucoma, temporomandibular joint arthritis.	May cause mild GI effects (e.g., nausea, heartburn, diarrhea, constipation). May increase risk of bleeding with anticoagulants (e.g., warfarin).
Gotu kola	Reduce fatigue, anxiety, depression, improve memory and intelligence.	May cause GI upset, nausea, drowsiness. May cause additive sedative effects/side effects with CNS depressants (e.g., clonazepam, lorazepam, zolpidem).
Grapefruit	Hyperlipidemia, atherosclerosis, weight loss and obesity.	May increase concentrations/effects of benzodiazepines, calcium channel blockers, carbamazepine, carvedilol, clomipramine, cyclosporine, estrogens, lovastatin, simvastatin, atorvastatin.
Green tea	Improve cognitive performance and mental alertness.	Can cause nausea, vomiting, abdominal bloating, dyspepsia, flatulence, diarrhea. Higher doses can cause dizziness, insomnia, fatigue, agitation. May increase effects of amphetamines, caffeine.
Kava kava	Anxiety disorders, stress, ADHD, insomnia, restlessness.	GI upset, headache, dizziness, drowsiness, enlarged pupils and disturbances of oculomotor equilibrium and accommodation, dry mouth, allergic skin reactions. May increase drowsiness, motor reflex depression with alcohol, benzodiazepines, other CNS depressants.
L-carnitine	Treatment of primary L-carnitine deficiency, acute myocardial infarction, supplement to total parenteral nutrition, L-carnitine deficiency in those requiring hemodialysis.	Can cause nausea, vomiting, abdominal cramps, heartburn, gastritis, diarrhea, body odor, seizures.

Name	Uses	Comments
Licorice	Gastric and duodenal ulcers, sore throat, bronchitis, dyspepsia, cough, osteoarthritis.	Excessive ingestion can cause pseudohyperaldosteronism with sodium and water retention, hypokalemia, alkalosis. May lead to hypertension, edema, arrhythmias. May reduce effect of antihypertensive medication therapy.
Melatonin	Jet lag, insomnia, shift-work disorder.	Can cause daytime drowsiness, headache, dizziness. May increase effect of antiplatelets, anticoagulants (e.g., aspirin, clopidogrel, enoxaparin, warfarin). May cause additive sedation with CNS depressants (e.g., alcohol, benzodiazepines).
Milk thistle	Liver disorders, chronic inflammatory liver disease, hepatic cirrhosis, chronic hepatitis.	Can cause nausea, diarrhea, dyspepsia, flatulence, abdominal bloating, anorexia.
Peppermint	Common cold, cough, inflammation of mouth and pharynx, sinusitis, fever, cramps of upper GI tract, dyspepsia, flatulence.	Can cause heartburn, nausea, vomiting, allergic reactions including flushing and headache. May increase concentration/effects of cyclosporine.
Red yeast	Maintain desirable cholesterol levels in healthy people; reduce cholesterol in hyperlipidemia; indigestion; diarrhea; improve blood circulation.	Can cause abdominal discomfort, heartburn, flatulence, dizziness. May increase risk of myopathy with cyclosporine, gemfibrozil, or niacin; may increase risk of liver damage with alcohol.
SAMe	Depression, anxiety, heart disease, fibromyalgia, osteoarthritis, tendonitis, dementia, Alzheimer's disease, Parkinson's disease.	Higher doses can cause flatulence, nausea, vomiting, diarrhea, constipation, headache, mild insomnia, anorexia, sweating, dizziness, nervousness. May have additive adverse effects with MAOIs including hypertension, hyperthermia, agitation, confusion, coma. May have additive serotonergic effects and serotonin syndrome-like effects (e.g., agitation, tremors, tachycardia, diarrhea, hyperreflexia, shivering, diaphoresis) with antidepressants.
Saw palmetto	Symptoms of benign prostatic hyperplasia (BPH).	Can cause dizziness, headache, GI complaints (e.g., nausea, vomiting, constipation, diarrhea). May increase effect of antiplatelets, anticoagulants (e.g., aspirin, clopidogrel, enoxaparin, warfarin).

(continued)

Name	Uses	Comments
St. John's wort	Depression, anxiety, heart palpitations; mood disturbances associated with menopause, ADHD, OCD, SAD.	Can cause insomnia, vivid dreams, restlessness, agitation, irritability, GI discomfort, diarrhea, fatigue, dry mouth, dizziness, headache. May decrease effect of alprazolam, amitriptyline, oral contraceptives, cyclosporine, imatinib, irinotecan, NNRTIs, phenytoin, protease inhibitors, tacrolimus, warfarin. May cause additive serotonergic effects with antidepressants, paroxetine, sertraline, tramadol.
Valerian	Insomnia, anxiety-associated restlessness, sleeping disorders.	Can cause headache, excitability, insomnia, gastric discomfort, dry mouth, vivid dreams, morning drowsiness. May have additive sedative effects with alcohol, benzodiazepines, other CNS depressants.
Yohimbe	Aphrodisiac, impotence, exhaustion, angina, hypertension, diabetic neuropathy, postural hypotension.	Can cause excitation, tremors, insomnia, anxiety, hypertension, tachycardia, dizziness, irritability, headache, fluid retention, rash, nausea, vomiting. High doses can cause respiratory depression. May have additive effects with MAOIs. Tyramine-containing foods increase risk of hypertensive crisis.

LIFESPAN, CULTURAL ASPECTS, AND PHARMACOGENOMICS OF DRUG THERAPY

LIFESPAN

Drug therapy is unique to pts of different ages. Age-specific competencies involve understanding the development and health needs of the various age groups. Pregnant pts, children, and elderly people represent different age groups with important considerations during drug therapy.

CHILDREN

In pediatric drug therapy, drug administration is guided by the age of the child, weight, level of growth and development, and height. The dosage ordered is to be given either by kilogram of body weight or by square meter of body surface area, which is based on the height and weight of the child. Many dosages based on these calculations must be individualized based on pediatric response.

If the oral route of administration is used, often syrup or chewable tablets are given. Additionally, sometimes medication is added to liquid or mixed with foods. Remember to never force a child to take oral medications because choking or emotional trauma may ensue.

If an intramuscular injection is ordered, the vastus lateralis muscle in the midlateral thigh is used because the gluteus maximus is not developed until walking occurs and the deltoid muscle is too small. For intravenous medications, administer very slowly in children. If given too quickly, high serum drug levels will occur with the potential for toxicity.

PREGNANCY

Women of childbearing years should be asked about the possibility of pregnancy before any drug therapy is initiated. Advise a woman who is either planning a pregnancy or believes she may be pregnant to inform her physician immediately. During pregnancy, medications given to the mother pass to the fetus via the placenta. Teratogenic (fetal abnormalities) effects may occur. Breastfeeding while the mother is taking certain medications may not be recommended due to the potential for adverse effects on the newborn.

The choice of drug ordered for pregnant women is based on the stage of pregnancy because the fetal organs develop during the first trimester. Cautious use of drugs in women of reproductive age who are sexually active and who are not using contraceptives is essential to prevent the potential for teratogenic or embryotoxic effects. Refer to the different pregnancy categories (found in Appendix C) to determine the relative safety of a medication during pregnancy.

ELDERLY

Elderly people are more likely to experience an adverse drug reaction owing to physiologic changes (e.g., visual, hearing, mobility changes, chronic diseases) and cognitive changes (short-term memory loss or alteration in the thought process) that may lead to multiple medication dosing. In chronic disease states such as hypertension, glaucoma, asthma, or arthritis, the daily ingestion of multiple medications increases the potential for adverse reactions and toxic effects.

Decreased renal or hepatic function may lower the metabolism of medications in the liver and reduce excretion of medications, thus prolonging the half-life of the drug and the potential for toxicity. Dosages in elderly people should initially be smaller than for the general adult population and then slowly titrated based on pt response and therapeutic effect of the medication.

CULTURE

The term *ethnopharmacology* was first used to describe the study of medicinal plants used by indigenous cultures. More recently, it is being used as a reference to the action and effects of drugs in people from diverse racial, ethnic, and cultural backgrounds. Although there are insufficient data from investigations involving people from diverse backgrounds that would provide reliable information on ethnic-specific responses to all medications, there is growing evidence that modifications in dosages are needed for some members of racial and ethnic groups. There are wide variations in the perception of side effects by pts from diverse cultural backgrounds. These differences may be related to metabolic differences that result in higher or lower levels of the drug, individual differences in the amount of body fat, or cultural differences in the way individuals perceive the meaning of side effects and toxicity. Nurses and other health care providers need to be aware that variations can occur with side effects, adverse reactions, and toxicity so that pts from diverse cultural backgrounds can be monitored.

Some cultural differences in response to medications include the following:

African Americans: Generally, African Americans are less responsive to beta blockers (e.g., propranolol [Inderal]) and angiotensin-converting enzyme (ACE) inhibitors (e.g., enalapril [Vasotec]).

Asian Americans: On average, Asian Americans have a lower percentage of body fat, so dosage adjustments must be made for fat-soluble vitamins and other drugs (e.g., vitamin K used to reverse the anticoagulant effect of warfarin).

Hispanic Americans: Hispanic Americans may require lower dosages and may experience a higher incidence of side effects with tricyclic antidepressants (e.g., amitriptyline).

Native Americans: Alaskan Eskimos may suffer prolonged muscle paralysis with the use of succinylcholine when administered during surgery.

There has been a desire to exert more responsibility over one's health and, as a result, a resurgence of self-care practices. These practices are often influenced by folk remedies and the use of medicinal plants. In the United States, there are several major ethnic population subgroups (white, black, Hispanic, Asian, and Native Americans). Each of these ethnic groups has a wide range of practices that influence beliefs and interventions related to health and illness. At any given time, in any group, treatment may consist of the use of traditional herbal therapy, a combination of ritual and prayer with medicinal plants, customary dietary and environmental practices, or the use of Western medical practices.

African Americans

Many African Americans carry the traditional health beliefs of their African heritage. Health denotes harmony with nature of the body, mind, and spirit, whereas illness is seen as disharmony that results from natural causes or divine punishment. Common practices to the art of healing include treatments with herbals and rituals known empirically to restore health. Specific forms of healing include using home remedies, obtaining medical advice from a physician, and seeking spiritual healing.

Examples of healing practices include the use of hot baths and warm compresses for rheumatism, the use of herbal teas for respiratory illnesses, and the use of kitchen condiments in folk remedies. Lemon, vinegar, honey, saltpeter, alum, salt, baking soda, and Epsom salt are common kitchen ingredients used. Goldenrod, peppermint, sassafras, parsley, yarrow, and rabbit tobacco are a few of the herbals used.

Hispanic Americans

The use of folk healers, medicinal herbs, magic, and religious rituals and ceremonies are included in the rich and varied customs of Hispanic Americans. This ethnic group believes that God is responsible for allowing health or illness to occur. Wellness may be viewed as good luck, a reward for good behavior, or a blessing from God. Praying, using herbals and spices, wearing religious objects such as medals, and maintaining a balance in diet and physical activity are methods considered appropriate in preventing evil or poor health.

Hispanic ethnopharmacology is more complementary to Western medical practices. After the illness is identified, appropriate treatment may consist of home remedies (e.g., use of vegetables and herbs), use of over-the-counter patent medicines, and use of physician-prescribed medications.

Asian Americans

For Asian Americans, harmony with nature is essential for physical and spiritual well-being. Universal balance depends on harmony among the elemental forces: fire, water, wood, earth, and metal. Regulating these universal elements are two forces that maintain physical and spiritual harmony in the body: the *yin* and the *yang*. Practices shared by most Asian cultures include meditation, special nutritional programs, herbology, and martial arts.

Therapeutic options available to traditional Chinese physicians include prescribing herbs, meditation, exercise, nutritional changes, and acupuncture.

Native Americans

The theme of total harmony with nature is fundamental to traditional Native American beliefs about health. It is dependent on maintaining a state of equilibrium among the physical body, the mind, and the environment. Health practices reflect this holistic approach. The method of healing is determined traditionally by the medicine man, who diagnoses the ailment and recommends the appropriate intervention.

Treatment may include heat, herbs, sweat baths, massage, exercise, diet changes, and other interventions performed in a curing ceremony.

European Americans

Europeans often use home treatments as the front-line interventions. Traditional remedies practiced are based on the magical or empirically validated experience of ancestors. These cures are often practiced in combination with religious rituals or spiritual ceremonies.

Household products, herbal teas, and patent medicines are familiar preparations used in home treatments (e.g., saltwater gargle for sore throat).

PHARMACOGENOMICS

Traditionally, medications are prescribed using a "one size fits all" philosophy. In general, the genetic makeup is similar in all humans, regardless of race or sex. However, people inherit variations in their genes, which can affect the way a person responds to a medication.

A genetic variation may make a medication stay in the body longer, causing serious side effects, or a variation may make the medication less potent.

For example, two people taking the same cancer medication may have very different responses. One may have severe, life-threatening side effects, whereas the second may have few, if any, side effects. The drug may shrink a tumor in one person but not in another.

Pharmacogenomics examines how a person's genetic makeup affects response to medications. Although widespread application still lies in the future, pharmacogenomics has the potential to personalize medical therapies. Physicians eventually will be able to prescribe medications based on an individual's genotype, thereby maximizing effectiveness and minimizing side effects. A few tests are available today.

Cytochrome P450 genotyping test. Cytochrome (CYP) 450 enzymes CYP2D6 and CYP2C19 are involved in the metabolism of many cardiovascular, antidepressant, and antipsychotic agents. More than 1% of the human population has a genetic variation that affects CYP2D6 and CYP2C19. These patients may eliminate drugs metabolized by the CYP2D6 and CYP2C19 enzyme systems "normally" (extensive metabolizers), too quickly (ultra-rapid metabolizers), too slowly (intermediate metabolizers), or not at all (poor metabolizers). Clinical effect would be a greater likelihood of adverse reactions in people who are poor metabolizers and a greater likelihood of treatment failure in people who are rapid metabolizers. Poor metabolizers include 5%–10% Caucasians, whereas rapid metabolizers include 10% Spaniards and 39% Ethiopians.

Thiopurine methyltransferase test. An enzyme called thiopurine methyltransferase (TPMT) breaks down a type of chemotherapy medication called thiopurine (e.g., mercaptopurine, thioguanine, azathioprine), which is used in the treatment of some leukemias and autoimmune disorders. Some people have genetic variations that prevent them from producing this enzyme, resulting in the buildup of thiopurine levels in the body and leading to severe toxic reactions, including profound myelosuppression, with normal doses. Data on the frequency of occurrence in specific population groups are not available.

UGT1A1 TA repeat genotype test. This test, commonly known as the UFT1A1 test, detects a variation in a gene that affects the UGT1A1 enzyme. This enzyme determines how the body breaks down irinotecan (Camptosar), a chemotherapy medication used in the treatment of colorectal cancer. A deficiency of this enzyme allows the medication to build up to toxic levels, possibly causing bone marrow suppression, gastrointestinal toxicities, infection, and death. Deficiency of this enzyme occurs in 16% of Chinese and 40% of European and East Indian individuals.

Dihydropyrimidine dehydrogenase test. The medication 5-fluorouracil (5-FU) and its related compounds (e.g., capecitabine) are commonly used chemotherapy medications. Some people have a genetic variation that results in a decrease in the dihydropyrimidine dehydrogenase enzyme, which is responsible for breaking down 5-FU. As a result of the deficiency, some people may develop severe or even fatal reactions to 5-FU. This deficiency occurs in 0.9% of Caucasians.

By utilizing the information provided by pharmacogenomic testing, drug therapy is changing to a more individualized approach. Anticipated benefits of pharmacogenomics include creation of better vaccines, safer medications targeted to specific diseases, and more appropriate dosing of medications at the onset of therapy. Ultimately, we may see a decrease in health care costs due to more efficient clinical trials, reduced adverse drug reactions, and less time needed to find effective therapy for patients.

Appendix I

NORMAL LABORATORY VALUES

HEMATOLOGY/COAGULATION

Test	Normal Range
Activated partial thromboplastin time (aPTT)	25–35 sec
Erythrocyte count (RBC count)	M: 4.5–5.5 million cells/mm³ F: 4.0–4.9 million cells/mm³
Hematocrit (HCT, Hct)	M: 41%–50% F: 36%–44%
Hemoglobin (Hb, Hgb)	M: 13.5–16.5 g/dl F: 12.0–15.0 g/dl
Leukocyte count (WBC count)	4.5–10.0 thousand cells/mm³

Leukocyte differential count
  Basophils
  Eosinophils
  Lymphocytes
  Monocytes
  Neutrophils—bands
  Neutrophils—segmented
	
	0%–0.75%
	1%–3%
	25%–33%
	3%–7%
	3%–5%
	54%–62%

Mean corpuscular hemoglobin (MCH)	26–34 pg/cell
Mean corpuscular hemoglobin concentration (MCHC)	31%–37% Hb/cell
Mean corpuscular volume (MCV)	80–100 fL
Partial thromboplastin time (PTT)	60–85 sec
Platelet count (thrombocyte count)	100–450 thousand/mm³
Prothrombin time (PT)	11–13.5 sec
RBC count (see Erythrocyte count)	

CLINICAL CHEMISTRY (SERUM PLASMA, URINE)

Test	Normal Range
Alanine aminotransferase (ALT)	8–36 units/L 8–78 units/L (children 0–2 mos)
Albumin	3.2–5 g/dl
Alkaline phosphatase	33–131 (adults 25–60 yrs) 51–153 (adults older than 60 yrs)
Amylase	30–110 units/L
Aspartate aminotransferase (AST)	5–35 units/L
Bilirubin (direct)	0–0.3 mg/dl
Bilirubin (total)	0.1–1.2 mg/dl
BUN	7–20 mg/dl
Calcium, ionized	2.24–2.46 mEq/L

continued

Test	Normal Range
Calcium (total)	8.6–10.3 mg/dl
Carbon dioxide (CO_2) total	23–30 mEq/L
Chloride	95–108 mEq/L

Cholesterol (total)
   HDL cholesterol
   LDL cholesterol
	Less than 200 mg/dl
	40–60 mg/dl
	Less than 160 mg/dl

Creatinine	0.5–1.4 mg/dl
Creatinine clearance	M: 80–125 ml/min/1.73 m^2 F: 75–115 ml/min/1.73 m^2

Creatine kinase (CK) isoenzymes
   CK-BB
   CK-MB (cardiac)
   CK-MM (muscle)
	
	0%
	0%–3.9%
	96%–100%

Creatine phosphokinase (CPK)	8–150 units/L
Ferritin	13–300 ng/ml
Glucose (preprandial)	Less than 115 mg/dl
Glucose (fasting)	60–110 mg/dl
Glucose (nonfasting, 2 hrs postprandial)	Less than 120 mg/dl
Hemoglobin A_{1c}	Less than 8
Iron	66–150 mcg/dl
Iron-binding capacity, total (TIBC)	250–420 mcg/dl
Lactate dehydrogenase (LDH)	56–194 units/L
Lipase	23–208 units/L
Magnesium	1.6–2.5 mg/dl
Osmolality	289–308 mOsm/kg
Oxygen saturation	90–95 (arterial) 40–70 (venous)
pH	7.35–7.45 (arterial) 7.32–7.42 (venous)
Phosphorus, inorganic	2.8–4.2 mg/dl
Potassium	3.5–5.2 mEq/L
Protein (total)	6.5–7.9 g/dl
Sodium	134–149 mEq/L
Thyroid-stimulating hormone (TSH)	0.7–6.4 milliunits/L (adults 20 yrs or younger) 0.4–4.2 milliunits/L (adults 21–54 yrs) 0.5–8.9 milliunits/L (adults 55–87 yrs)
Transferrin	Greater than 200 mg/dl
Triglycerides (TG)	45–155 mg/dl
Urea nitrogen	7–20 mg/dl
Uric acid	M: 2–8 mg/dl F: 2–7.5 mg/dl

CYTOCHROME P450 (CYP) ENZYMES

Most drugs are eliminated from the body, at least in part, by being changed chemically to a less lipid-soluble product (i.e., metabolized) and thus more likely to be excreted from the body via the kidney or bile. Drugs may go through two different metabolic processes: phase 1 and phase 2 metabolism.

In phase 1 metabolism, hepatic microsomal enzymes found in the endothelium of liver cells metabolize drugs via hydrolysis and oxidation and reduction reactions. These chemical reactions make the drug more water soluble. In phase 2 metabolism, large water-soluble substances (e.g., glucuronic acid, sulfate) are attached to the drug, forming inactive, or significantly less active, water-soluble metabolites. Phase 2 processes include glucuronidation, sulfation, conjugation, acetylation, and methylation.

Virtually any of the phase 1 and phase 2 enzymes can be inhibited, and some of these enzymes can be induced by drugs. Inhibiting the activity of metabolic enzymes results in increased concentrations of the drug (substrate), whereas inducing metabolic enzymes results in decreased concentrations of the drug (substrate).

The term "cytochrome P450" (CYP enzymes) refers to a family of more than 100 enzymes in the human body that modulate various physiologic functions. First identified in the 1950s, the CYP enzyme system contains two large subgroups: steroidogenic and xenobiotic enzymes. Only the xenobiotic group is involved in the metabolism of drugs. The xenobiotic group includes four major enzyme families: CYP1, CYP2, CYP3, and CYP4. The primary role of these families is the metabolism of drugs. These families are further subdivided into subfamilies designated by a capital letter and given a specific enzyme number (1, 2, 3, etc.) according to the similarity in amino acid sequence it shares with other enzymes (e.g., CYP1A2).

The key CYP450 enzymes include CYP1A2, CYP2C9, CYP2C19, CYP2D6, and CYP3A4 and may be responsible for metabolism of 75% of all drugs, with the CYP3A subfamily responsible for nearly half of this activity.

The CYP enzymes are found in the endoplasmic reticulum of cells in a variety of human tissue but are primarily concentrated in the liver and intestine. CYP enzymes can be both inhibited and induced, leading to increased or decreased serum concentration of the drug (along with its effects).

The following tables of CYP substrates, inhibitors, and inducers provide a perspective on drugs that are affected by, or affect, cytochrome P450 (CYP) enzymes. **CYP substrate** includes drugs reported to be metabolized, at least in part, by one or more CYP enzymes. **CYP inhibitor** includes drugs reported to inhibit one or more CYP enzymes. **CYP inducer** contains drugs reported to induce one or more CYP enzymes.

P450 ENZYMES: SUBSTRATES, INHIBITORS, INDUCERS

CYP1A2 ENZYME

CYP1A2 SUBSTRATES	CYP1A2 INHIBITORS	CPY1A2 INDUCERS
Caffeine	Cimetidine (Tagamet)	Barbiturates
Clozapine (Clozaril)	Ciprofloxacin (Cipro)	Carbamazepine (Tegretol)
Mirtazapine (Remeron)	Fluvoxamine	Rifampin (Rifadin)
Olanzapine (Zyprexa)	Zileuton (Zyflo)	Smoking
Ramelteon (Rozerem)		
Ropinirole (Requip)		
Tizanidine (Zanaflex)		

- CYP1A2 enzyme is increasingly involved in drug interactions.
- More potent inhibitors include cimetidine, ciprofloxacin, and fluvoxamine.
- Smoking is the most important inducer, but rifampin and barbiturates also can increase enzyme activity.
- Example of reaction: Tizanidine plasma concentrations increased more than 30-fold when the inhibitor fluvoxamine was given concurrently.

CYP2C9 ENZYME

CYP2C9 SUBSTRATES	CYP2C9 INHIBITORS	CYP2C9 INDUCERS
Candesartan (Atacand)	Amiodarone (Cordarone)	Barbiturates
Celecoxib (Celebrex)	Clopidogrel (Plavix)	Carbamazepine (Tegretol)
Diclofenac (Voltaren)	Fluconazole (Diflucan)	Rifampin (Rifadin)
Glipizide (Glucotrol)	Metronidazole (Flagyl)	St. John's wort
Glyburide (DiaBeta)	Sulfamethoxazole	
Ibuprofen (Advil, Motrin)	Valproic acid (Depakote)	
Irbesartan (Avapro)		
Meloxicam (Mobic)		
Warfarin (Coumadin)		

- More potent inhibitors include amiodarone, metronidazole, and sulfamethoxazole.
- All of the inducers can substantially increase enzyme activity.
- Both warfarin and oral hypoglycemics are of serious concern with regard to drug interactions. Substrates warranting attention include warfarin and oral hypoglycemics.

CYP2C19 ENZYME

CYP2C19 SUBSTRATES	CYP2C19 INHIBITORS	CYP2C19 INDUCERS
Citalopram (Celexa)	Cimetidine (Tagamet)	Barbiturates
Diazepam (Valium)	Clopidogrel (Plavix)	Carbamazepine (Tegretol)
Escitalopram (Lexapro)	Esomeprazole (Nexium)	Rifampin (Rifadin)
Omeprazole (Prilosec)	Fluconazole (Diflucan)	St. John's wort
Pantoprazole (Protonix)	Fluvoxamine	
Sertraline (Zoloft)	Modafinil (Provigil)	

- Inhibition by itself does not frequently cause adverse effects compared with other CYP enzymes because many of the substrates do not have serious toxicity.
- Inhibition or induction of the enzyme nonetheless may result in an adverse drug interaction.
- Racial background is important in the likelihood of being deficient in this enzyme (e.g., 3%–5% of Caucasians and 12%–23% of Asians are poor metabolizers of this enzyme).

CYP2D6 ENZYME

CYP2D6 SUBSTRATES	CYP2D6 INHIBITORS	CYP2D6 INDUCERS
Amitriptyline (Elavil)	Amiodarone (Cordarone)	See comment below
Atomoxetine (Strattera)	Bupropion (Wellbutrin)	
Duloxetine (Cymbalta)	Fluoxetine (Prozac)	
Fluoxetine (Prozac)	Paroxetine (Paxil)	
Metoclopramide (Reglan)		
Metoprolol (Lopressor)		
Paroxetine (Paxil)		
Risperidone (Risperdal)		
Tamoxifen (Nolvadex)		
Tolterodine (Detrol)		
Tramadol (Ultram)		
Venlafaxine (Effexor)		

- Potent inhibitors include fluoxetine and paroxetine.
- Evidence suggests that this enzyme is not very susceptible to enzyme induction.
- Genetics, rather than drug therapy, accounts for most ultra-rapid metabolizers (e.g., Greeks, Portuguese, Saudis, and Ethiopians have high enzyme activity).

CYP3A4 ENZYME

CYP3A4 SUBSTRATES	CYP3A4 INHIBITORS	CYP3A4 INDUCERS
Alfuzosin (Uroxatral)	Amiodarone (Cordarone)	Carbamazepine (Tegretol)
Alprazolam (Xanax)	Clarithromycin (Biaxin)	Efavirenz (Sustiva)
Budesonide (Entocort EC)	Diltiazem (Cardizem)	Phenobarbital
Carbamazepine (Tegretol)	Erythromycin (Ery-Tab)	Rifampin (Rifadin)
Cyclosporine (Neoral)	Fluconazole (Diflucan)	St. John's wort
Fluticasone (Flovent)	Fluoxetine (Prozac)	
Lovastatin (Mevacor)	Itraconazole (Spoiranox)	
Repaglinide (Prandin)	Ketoconazole (Nizoral)	
Sildenafil (Viagra)	Verapamil (Calan, Isoptin)	
Simvastatin (Zocor)		
Tadalafil (Cialis)		

- This enzyme metabolizes about half of all medications on the market.
- Drug toxicity of CYP3A4 substrates due to inhibition of CYP3A4 is relatively common.
- This enzyme is very sensitive to induction, tending to lower plasma concentrations of substrates, resulting in reduced efficacy of the substrate.
- Most potent inhibitors include clarithromycin, itraconazole, and ketoconazole.
- Rifampin is a potent inducer and may reduce serum concentrations of substrates by as much as 90%.

Appendix K

POISON ANTIDOTE CHART

Poisoning Agent	Antidote	Dosage
Acetaminophen	Acetylcysteine (Acetadote, Mucomyst)	PO: ADULTS, CHILDREN: Loading dose: 140 mg/kg, then 70 mg/kg q4h for a total of 18 doses. Total dose delivered: 1,330 mg/kg. IV: ADULTS, CHILDREN: Loading dose: 150 mg/kg over 60 min, then 50 mg/kg over 4 hrs, then 100 mg/kg over 16 hrs. Total dose delivered: 300 mg/kg.
Anticholinergic agents (e.g., atropine)	Physostigmine	IM/IV/SUBCUTANEOUS: ADULTS: Initially, 0.5–2 mg, then repeat q20min until response occurs or adverse effects occur. Repeat 1–4 mg q30–60min as life-threatening symptoms recur. IV: CHILDREN (Reserve for life-threatening situation only): 0.01–0.03 mg/kg/dose. May repeat after 15–20 min to maximum total dose of 2 mg, or until response occurs or adverse cholinergic effects occur.
Arsenic	Dimercaprol (BAL in oil)	Mild Poisoning IM: ADULTS, CHILDREN: 2.5 mg/kg/dose q6h for 2 days, then q12h for 1 day, then once daily for 10 days. Severe Poisoning IM: ADULTS, CHILDREN: 3 mg/kg/dose q4h for 2 days, then q6h for 1 day, then q12h for 10 days.
Benzodiazepines (e.g., midazolam)	Flumazenil (Romazicon)	IV: ADULTS: 0.2 mg over 30 sec. May give 0.3-mg dose after 30 sec if desired LOC not obtained. Additional doses of 0.5 mg can be given over 30 sec at 1-min intervals up to cumulative dose of 3 mg. CHILDREN: 0.01 mg/kg (**maximum:** 0.2 mg) with repeat doses of 0.01 mg/kg (**maximum:** 0.2 mg) given every minute to maximum total cumulative dose of 1 mg.
Beta blockers (e.g., propranolol)	Glucagon	IV: ADULTS: 5–10 mg over 1 min, followed by infusion of 1–10 mg/hr.
Calcium channel blockers (e.g., verapamil)	Glucagon	IV: ADULTS: 5–10 mg over 1 min, followed by infusion of 1–10 mg/hr.

Poisoning Agent	Antidote	Dosage
Carbamate pesticides	Atropine	IV: ADULTS: Initially, 1–5 mg doubled q5min until signs of muscarinic excess abate. IV INFUSION: ADULTS: 0.5–1 mg/hr. IM: ADULTS (Mild symptoms): 2 mg. If severe symptoms develop after first dose, 2 additional doses should be repeated in 10 min. (Severe symptoms): Immediately administer three 2-mg doses. IV: CHILDREN: 0.02–0.05 mg/kg q10–20min until atropine effect observed, then q1–4h for at least 24 hrs. IM: 0.5–2 mg/dose based on weight (0.5 mg: 15–40 lb, 1 mg: 41–90 lb, 2 mg: greater than 90 lb). (Mild symptoms): 1 injection. (Severe symptoms): 2 additional injections given in rapid succession 10 min after receiving first injection.
Digoxin (Lanoxin)	Digoxin immune FAB (Digibind)	**ADULTS** Unknown amount of ingestion: 800 mg IV infusion if acute ingestion, 240 mg IV infusion if chronic ingestion. **Dosing for Ingestion of Single Large Dose** Dose (in no. of vials) = (Total digitalis body load in mg)/(0.5 mg of digitalis bound per vial). Total digitalis body load in mg = (No. of tablets/capsules ingested) $\times$ (mg strength of tablet/capsule) $\times$ (bioavailability of tablet/capsule). Digoxin tablets and elixir are 80% bioavailable. Digoxin capsules and injection are 100% bioavailable. **Dosing Based on Serum Level** Digoxin: Dose (in no. of vials) = (Serum digoxin level in ng/mL) $\times$ (weight in kg)/(100). Digitoxin: Dose (in no. of vials) = (Serum digitoxin level in ng/mL) $\times$ (weight in kg)/(1,000). **CHILDREN** **Dosing for Ingestion of Single Large Dose** Dose (in no. of vials) = (Total digitalis body load in mg)/(0.5 mg of digitalis bound per vial). Total digitalis body load in mg = (No. of tablets/capsules ingested) $\times$ (mg strength of tablet/capsule) $\times$ (bioavailability of tablet/capsule). Digoxin tablets and elixir are 80% bioavailable. Digoxin capsules and injection are 100% bioavailable. WEIGHING 20 kg or less: Dilution of reconstituted vial to 1 mg/ml may be desirable for doses of 3 mg or less. Dose (in no. of mg) = Dose (in no. of vials) $\times$ 38 mg/vial. Dose (in no. of vials) = (Serum digoxin level in ng/ml) $\times$ (weight in kg)/(100).

(continued)

Poisoning Agent	Antidote	Dosage
Ethylene glycol	Fomepizole (Antizol)	IV: ADULTS, CHILDREN: Loading dose 15 mg/kg, then 10 mg/kg q12h for 4 doses, then 15 mg/kg q12h thereafter until ethylene glycol levels reduced to less than 20 mg/dl and patient is asymptomatic with normal pH.
Extravasation vasoconstrictive agents (e.g., dopamine)	Phentolamine (Regitine)	ADULTS, CHILDREN: Infiltrate area with small amount of solution made by diluting 5–10 mg in 10 ml 0.9% NaCl within 12 hrs of extravasation. In general, do not exceed 0.1–0.2 mg/kg (5 mg total).
Heparin	Protamine	IV: ADULTS, CHILDREN: Dosage is determined by most recent dosage of heparin or low molecular weight heparin (LWH): 1 mg protamine neutralizes 90–115 units of heparin and 1 mg (100 units) of LWH. **Maximum dose:** 50 mg.
Iron	Deferoxamine (Desferal)	Acute IM: ADULTS: Initially, 1,000 mg, then 500 mg q4h for 2 doses. Additional doses of 0.5 g q4–12h. **Maximum:** 6 g/24 hrs. CHILDREN 3 YRS AND OLDER: 90 mg/kg/dose q8h (not to exceed 1 g/dose). **Maximum:** 6 g/24 hrs. IV: ADULTS, CHILDREN: 15 mg/kg/hr. **Maximum:** 6 g/24 hrs. Chronic IM: ADULTS: 500–1,000 mg/day. IV: ADULTS, CHILDREN: 15 mg/kg/hr. **Maximum:** 12 g/24 hrs.
Isoniazid	Pyridoxine (vitamin B_6)	IV: ADULTS, CHILDREN: Total dose of pyridoxine equal to amount of isoniazid ingested as first dose of 1–4 g IV, then 1 g IM q30min until total dose completed. If not known, give 5 g at rate of 1 g/min. May repeat q5–10min.
Lead	Calcium EDTA	Symptomatic Treat for 3–5 days; give in conjunction with dimercaprol. IM: ADULTS, CHILDREN: 167 mg/m^2 every 4 hrs. IV: ADULTS, CHILDREN: 1 g/m^2 as 8- to 24-hr infusion or divided q12h. Lead Encephalopathy Treat for 5 days; give concurrently with dimercaprol. IM: ADULTS, CHILDREN: 250 mg/m^2 every 4 hrs. IV: ADULTS, CHILDREN: 50 mg/kg/day as 24-hr continuous infusion.
Lead	Dimercaprol (BAL in oil)	Mild IM: ADULTS, CHILDREN: Loading dose 4 mg/kg, then 3 mg/kg/dose q4h for 2–7 days. Begin calcium EDTA with second dose. Severe and Lead Encephalopathy IM: ADULTS, CHILDREN: 4 mg/kg/dose q4h for 3–5 days. Begin calcium EDTA with second dose.

Poisoning Agent	Antidote	Dosage
Lead	Succimer (Chemet)	PO: ADULTS, CHILDREN: 10 mg/kg/dose q8h for 5 days, then q12h for 14 days. **Maximum:** 500 mg/dose. Note: For children younger than 5 yrs, dose based on mg/m^2.
Methanol	Fomepizole (Antizol)	IV: ADULTS, CHILDREN: Loading dose 15 mg/kg, then 10 mg/kg q12h for 4 doses, then 15 mg/kg q12h thereafter until ethylene glycol levels reduced to less than 20 mg/dl and patient is asymptomatic with normal pH.
Opioids (e.g., morphine)	Naloxone (Narcan)	IV/IM/SUBCUTANEOUS: ADULTS: 0.4–2 mg/dose. May repeat every 2–3 min as needed. Therapy may need to be reassessed if no response is seen after cumulative dose of 10 mg. CHILDREN (5 YRS OR OLDER or WEIGHING 20 KG OR GREATER): 2 mg/dose IV/IM/SUBCUTANEOUS. May repeat every 2–3 min as needed. Therapy may need to be reassessed if no response is seen after cumulative dose of 10 mg. CHILDREN (WEIGHING LESS THAN 20 KG): 0.1 mg/kg/dose. May repeat every 2–3 min as needed.
Organophosphate pesticides	Atropine	IV: ADULTS: Initially, 1–5 mg doubled q5min until signs of muscarinic excess abate. IV INFUSION: ADULTS: 0.5–1 mg/hr. IM: ADULTS (Mild symptoms): 2 mg. If severe symptoms develop after first dose, 2 additional doses should be repeated in 10 min. (Severe symptoms): Immediately administer three 2-mg doses. IV: CHILDREN: 0.02–0.05 mg/kg q10–20min until atropine effect observed, then q1–4h for at least 24 hrs. IM: 0.5–2 mg/dose based on weight (0.5 mg: 15–40 lb, 1 mg: 41–90 lb, 2 mg: greater than 90 lb). (Mild symptoms): 1 injection. (Severe symptoms): 2 additional injections given in rapid succession 10 min after receiving first injection.
Organophosphate pesticides	Pralidoxime (Protopam)	IM/IV: ADULTS: 1–2 g. Repeat in 1–2 hrs if muscle weakness has not been relieved, then at 10- to 12-hr intervals if cholinergic signs recur. CHILDREN: 20–50 mg/kg/dose. Repeat in 1–2 hrs if muscle weakness is not relieved, then at 10- to 12-hr intervals if cholinergic signs recur.
Warfarin (Coumadin)	Phytonadione (vitamin K)	PO/IV/SUBCUTANEOUS: ADULTS: 2.5–10 mg/dose. May repeat in 12–48 hrs if given PO, 6–8 hrs if given by IV or subcutaneous route. CHILDREN: 0.5–5 mg depending on need for further anticoagulation, severity of bleeding.

Appendix L

PREVENTING MEDICATION ERRORS AND IMPROVING MEDICATION SAFETY

Medication safety is a high priority for the health care professional. Prevention of medication errors and improved safety for the pt are important, esp. in today's health care environment when today's pt is older and sometimes sicker and the drug therapy regimen can be more sophisticated and complex.

A medication error is defined by the National Coordinating Council for Medication Error Reporting and Prevention (NCC MERP) as "any preventable event that may cause or lead to inappropriate medication use or pt harm while the medication is in the control of the health care professional, pt, or consumer."

Most medication errors occur as a result of multiple, compounding events as opposed to a single act by a single individual.

Use of the wrong medication, strength, or dose; confusion over sound-alike or look-alike drugs; administration of medications by the wrong route; miscalculations (esp. when used in pediatric pts or when administering medications intravenously); and errors in prescribing and transcription all can contribute to compromising the safety of the pt. The potential for adverse events and medication errors is definitely a reality and is potentially tragic and costly in both human and economic terms.

Health care professionals must take the initiative to create and implement procedures to prevent medication errors from occurring and implement methods to reduce medication errors. The first priority in preventing medication errors is to establish a multidisciplinary team to improve medication use. The goal for this team would be to assess medication safety and implement changes that would make it difficult or impossible for mistakes to reach the pt. Some important criteria in making improved medication safety successful include the following:

- Promote a nonpunitive approach to reducing medication errors.
- Increase the detection and the reporting of medication errors, near misses, and potentially hazardous situations that may result in medication errors.
- Determine root causes of medication errors.
- Educate about the causes of medication errors and ways to prevent these errors.
- Make recommendations to allow organization-wide, system-based changes to prevent medication errors.
- Learn from errors that occur in other organizations and take measures to prevent similar errors.

Some common causes and ways to prevent medication errors and improve safety include the following:

Handwriting: Poor handwriting can make it difficult to distinguish between two medications with similar names. Also, many drug names sound similar, esp. when the names are spoken over the telephone, poorly enunciated, or mispronounced.

- Take time to write legibly.
- Keep phone or verbal orders to a minimum to prevent misinterpretation.
- Repeat back orders taken over the telephone.
- When ordering a new or rarely used medication, print the name.

- Always specify the drug strength, even if only one strength exists.
- Express dosages for oral liquids only in metric weights or volumes (e.g., mg or ml), not by teaspoon or tablespoon.
- Print generic and brand names of look-alike or sound-alike medications.

Zeros and decimal points: Hastily written orders can present problems even if the name of the medication is clear.

- Never leave a decimal point "naked." Place a zero before a decimal point when the number is less than a whole unit (e.g., use 0.25 mg or 250 mcg, **not** .25 mg).
- Never have a trailing zero following a decimal point (e.g., use 2 mg, **not** 2.0 mg).

Abbreviations: Errors can occur because of a failure to standardize abbreviations. Establishing a list of abbreviations that should never be used is recommended.

- Never abbreviate unit as "U"; spell out "unit."
- Do not abbreviate "once daily" as OD or QD or "every other day" as QOD; spell it out.
- Do not use D/C, as this may be misinterpreted as either discharge or discontinue.
- Do not abbreviate drug names; spell out the generic and/or brand names.

Ambiguous or incomplete orders: These types of orders can cause confusion or misinterpretation of the writer's intention. Examples include situations when the route of administration, dose, or dosage form has not been specified.

- Do not use slash marks—they may be read as the number one (1).
- When reviewing an unusual order, verify the order with the person writing the order to prevent any misunderstanding.
- Read over orders after writing.
- Encourage that the drug's indication for use be provided on medication orders.
- Provide complete medication orders—do not use "resume preop" or "continue previous meds."
- Provide the age and, when appropriate, the weight of the pt.

High-alert medications: Medications in this category have an increased risk of causing significant pt harm when used in error. Mistakes with these medications may or may not be more common but may be more devastating to the pt if an error occurs. A list of high-alert medications can be obtained from the Institute for Safe Medication Practices (ISMP) at www.ismp.org.

Technology available today that can be used to address and help solve potential medication problems or errors includes the following:

- Electronic prescribing systems—This refers to computerized prescriber order entry systems. Within these systems is the capability to incorporate medication safety alerts (e.g., maximum dose alerts, allergy screening). Additionally, these systems should be integrated or interfaced with pharmacy and laboratory systems to provide drug–drug and drug–disease interactions alerts and include clinical order screening capability.
- Bar codes—These systems are designed to use bar-code scanning devices to validate identity of pts, verify medications administered, document administration, and provide safety alerts.
- "Smart" infusion pumps—These pumps allow users to enter drug infusion protocols into a drug library along with predefined dosage limits. If a dosage is outside the limits established, an alarm is sounded and drug delivery is halted, informing the clinician that the dose is outside the recommended range.

- Automated dispensing systems; point-of-use dispensing system—These systems should be integrated with information systems, esp. pharmacy systems.
- Pharmacy order entry system—This should be fully integrated with an electronic prescribing system with the capability of producing medication safety alerts. Additionally, the system should generate a computerized medication administration record (MAR), which would be used by the nursing staff while administering medications.

Medication reconciliation: Medication errors generally occur at transition points in the pt's care (admission, transfer from one level of care to another [e.g., critical care to general care area], and discharge). Incomplete documentation can account for up to 60% of potential medication errors. Therefore, it becomes necessary to accurately and completely reconcile medication across the continuum of care. This includes the name, dosage, frequency, and route of medication administration.

Medication reconciliation programs are a process of identifying the most accurate list of all medications a pt is taking and using this list to provide correct medications anywhere within the health care system. The focus is on not only compiling a list but using the list to reduce medication errors and provide quality pt care.

Additional Strategies to Reduce Medication Errors

The Institute for Safe Medication Practices (ISMP), FDA, and other agencies have identified high-risk areas associated with medication errors. They include the following:

At-risk population: At-risk populations primarily include pediatric and geriatric pts. For both, this risk is due to altered pharmacokinetic parameters with little published information regarding medication use in these groups. Additionally, in the pediatric population, the risk is due to the need for calculating doses based on age and weight, lack of available dosage forms, and concentrations for smaller children.

In a USP report, more than one-third of medication errors reaching the pt occurred in pts 65 yrs of age and older. Almost 40% of people 60 yrs and older take at least five medications. More than 50% of fatal hospital medication errors involve seniors. In the senior population, age-related physiologic changes (e.g., decreased renal function, reduced muscle mass) increase the risk for adverse events.

Avoid abbreviations and nomenclature: The confusion caused by abbreviations has prompted the ISMP to develop a list of abbreviations that should be avoided (see back cover of handbook).

Recognize prescription look-alike and sound-alike medications: The ISMP has developed an extensive list of confused drug names (see www.jointcommission.org). See individual monographs for **DO NOT CONFUSE** information.

Focus on high alert medications: High alert medications are medications that bear a heightened risk of causing significant pt harm if incorrectly used. High alert medications in the handbook have a colored background for the entire monograph.

Look for duplicate therapies and interactions: Drug interactions and duplicate therapies can increase risk of adverse reactions. Refer to individual monographs for significant interaction information (drug, herbal, food).

Report errors to improve process: This action plays an important role in preventing further errors. The intent is to identify system failures that can be altered to prevent further errors.

PARENTERAL FLUID ADMINISTRATION

Replacing fluids in the body is based on body fluid needs. Water comprises approximately 60% of the adult body. Approximately 40% is intracellular fluid and 20% is extracellular fluid, of which 15% is interstitial (tissues) and 5% is intravascular. The walls separating these compartments are porous, allowing water to move freely between them. Small particles such as sodium and chloride can pass through the walls, but larger molecules such as proteins and starches usually are unable to pass through the walls.

Hydrostatic and osmotic pressures are forces that move water and regulate the body's water. Intravenous fluid manipulates these two pressures. Hydrostatic pressure reflects the weight and volume of water. The greater the volume, the higher the blood pressure.

Effects of Osmotic Pressure: *Osmosis* is the diffusion of water across a semipermeable membrane from an area of high concentration to an area of low concentration (water moves into the compartment of higher concentration of particles, or solute). This is similar to the action of a sponge soaking up water. This pull is referred to as *osmotic pressure.* It is the number of particles in each compartment that keeps water where it is supposed to be. By administering fluids with more (or fewer) particles than blood plasma, fluid is pulled into the compartment where it is needed the most.

How do we know where the water is needed? To assess water balance, measure the *osmolality* of blood plasma (number of particles [osmoles] in a kilogram of fluid). *Osmolarity* is the number of particles in a liter of fluid. Normal serum osmolality is approximately 300 milliosmoles (mOsm) per liter.

Crystalloids are made of substances that form crystals (e.g., sodium chloride) and are small, so easy movement between compartments is possible. Crystalloids are categorized by their tonicity (a synonym for osmolality). An isotonic solution has the same number of particles (osmolality) as plasma and will not promote a shift of fluids into or out of cells. Examples of isotonic crystalloid solutions are 0.9% sodium chloride and lactated Ringer's solution. Dextrose 5% in water is another isotonic crystalloid. However, it is quickly metabolized, and the fluid quickly becomes hypotonic. Hypotonic solutions (e.g., D_5W, 0.45% sodium chloride) are a good source of free water, causing a shift out of the vascular bed and into cells by way of osmosis. Hypotonic solutions are given to correct cellular dehydration and hypernatremia. Hypertonic solutions have more particles than body water and pull water back into the circulation, which can shrink cells.

Sodium Chloride
Uses
- Extracellular fluid replacement when chloride loss is greater than or equal to sodium loss
- Treatment of metabolic alkalosis in the presence of fluid loss; chloride ions cause a compensatory decrease of bicarbonate ions
- Sodium depletion, extracellular fluid volume deficit with sodium deficit
- Initiation and termination of blood transfusion, preventing hemolysis of RBCs (occurs with dextrose in water solutions)

Side Effects/Abnormalities
- Hypernatremia
- **Acidosis:** 0.9% sodium chloride contains one-third more chloride ions than is present in extracellular fluid; excess chloride ions cause loss of bicarbonate, resulting in acidosis

- **Hypokalemia:** Increased potassium excretion at the same time extracellular fluid is increasing, which further decreases potassium concentration in extracellular fluid
- Circulatory overload

Dextrose (Glucose)
Effects
- Provides calories for essential energy
- Improves hepatic function because it is converted into glycogen
- Spares body protein, preventing unnecessary breakdown of protein tissue
- Prevents ketosis
- Stored in the liver as glycogen, causing a shift of potassium from extracellular to intracellular fluid compartment

Uses
- Dehydration
- Hyponatremia
- Hyperkalemia
- Vehicle of drug delivery and nutrition

Note: Once infused, dextrose is rapidly metabolized to water and carbon dioxide, becoming hypotonic rather than isotonic.

Side Effects/Abnormalities
- Dehydration: Osmotic diuresis occurs if dextrose is given faster than the pt's ability to metabolize it
- Hypokalemia (see Effects)
- Hyperinsulinism due to rapid infusion of hypertonic solution
- Water intoxication due to an imbalance based on increase in extracellular fluid volume from water alone

Selected Parenteral Fluids

Solution	Comments
Dextrose 5% in water (D$_5$W)	Supplies approximately 170 cal/L and free water to aid in renal excretion of solutes Avoid excessive volumes in pts with increased antidiuretic hormone activity or to replace fluids in hypovolemic pts
0.9% Sodium chloride (0.9% NaCl)	Isotonic fluid commonly used to expand extracellular fluid in presence of hypovolemia Can be used to treat mild metabolic alkalosis
0.45% Sodium chloride (0.45% NaCl)	Hypotonic solution that provides sodium, chloride, and free water; sodium and chloride allow kidneys to select and retain needed amounts Free water is desirable as aid to kidneys in elimination of solutes
3% Sodium chloride	Used only to treat severe hyponatremia
Lactated Ringer's solution	Isotonic solution that contains sodium, potassium, calcium, and chloride in approximately the same concentrations as found in plasma Used to treat hypovolemia, burns, and fluid loss as bile or diarrhea

General Index

A

abacavir, 1–2
5-aminosalicylic acid,
   753–755
5-ASA, 753–755
5-FU, 502–504
Abacavir, 69C–70C,
   117C–120C
Abacavir/lamivudine,
   117C–120C
abatacept, 2–4
abciximab, 4–6, 32C–34C
Abelcet, 64–66, 47C–48C
Abenol, 8–11
Abilify Discmelt, 80–82
Abilify Maintena, 80–82
Abilify, 80–82, 66C–68C
abiraterone, 6–8, 81C–92C
Abraxane, 910–912
Absorica, 648–650
Abstral, 481–485
acarbose, 43C–45C
Accolade, 75C–78C
Accolate, 1291–1292
AccuNeb, 29–31, 75C–78C
Accupril, 1025–1027,
   9C–10C, 61C–62C
Accuretic, 572–574,
   1025–1027
Accutane, 648–650
Acebutolol, 17C–18C,
   72C–74C
Aceon, 9C–10C
Acephen, 8–11
Acetadote, 12–15
acetaminophen, 8–11
Acetazolam, 11–12
acetazolamide, 11–12
acetylcysteine, 12–15
acetylsalicylic acid, 89–91
Acilac, 666–668
Aciphex, 1029–1030, 147C
Aclasta, 1298–1299
aclidinium, 15–16,
   75C–78C
Aclovate, 101C–102C
Actemra, 1203–1205
Actimmune, 631–632
Actiq, 481–485
Activase, 46–48, 32C–34C

Activella, 449–452
Actonel with Calcium,
   1060–1061
Actonel, 1060–1061,
   142C–143C
Actoplus Met, 758–760,
   962–964
Actos, 962–964, 43C–45C
Acular, 660–662
Acuvail, 660–662
acyclovir, 16–19, 69C–70C
Adalat CC, 849–851,
   61C–62C
Adalat XL, 849–851
Adalat, 79C–80C
adalimumab, 19–21
Adasuve, 66C–68C
Adavgraf, 1143–1145
Adcetris, 155–157, 81C–92C
Adcirca, 1145–1147
Adderall, 351–352
Adderall-XR, 351–352
adefovir, 21–22, 69C–70C
Adempas, 1058–1060
Adenocard, 22–24
Adenoscan, 22–24
adenosine, 22–24
ado-trastuzumab, 24–26
Adoxa, 399–401
Adrenalin, 426–428
Adriamycin, 396–399,
   81C–92C
Adrucil, 502–504, 81C–92C
Advair Diskus, 510–513,
   1085–1086, 75C–78C
Advair HFA, 510–513,
   1085–1086, 75C–78C
Advair, 510–513
Advate, 74–76
Advicor, 725–727, 843–845
Advil, 594–596, 129C–130C
Advil Children's, 594–596
Advil Cold, 1016–1017
Advil Infants', 594–596
Advil Junior, 594–596
Advil Migraine, 594–596
Advil PM, 373–375
Aerius, 338–339
afatinib, 26–27
Afeditab CR, 849–851

Afinitor Disperz, 463–465
Afinitor, 463–465, 81C–92C
Afrin, 4C
Aggrastat, 32C–34C
Aggrenox, 89–91, 377–378
AHF, 74–76
Airomir, 29–31
AK-Dilate, 956–958
Akne-Mycin, 442–444
AK-Pred, 141C
AK-Tob, 1200–1203
Alamast, 140C
Alavert Allergy and Sinus,
   718–719
Alavert, 718–719
Alaway, 140C–141C
albumin, human, 27–29
Albuminar-25, 27–29
Albuminar-5, 27–29
AlbuRx, 27–29
Albutein, 27–29
albuterol, 29–31, 75C–78C
Albuterol/ipratropium,
   75C–78C
Alcaftadine, 139C
Alclometasone, 101C–102C
Aldactazide, 572–574,
   1125–1127
Aldactone, 1125–1127,
   103C–105C
aldesleukin, 632–634,
   81C–92C
Aldomet, 61C–62C
Aldoril, 572–574
alemtuzumab, 31–33,
   81C–92C
alendronate, 33–35,
   142C–143C
Alertec, 805–806
Aleve, 828–831
alfuzosin, 35–36
Alimta, 937–938, 81C–92C
Alinia, 855–856
aliskiren, 36–37, 61C–62C
Alkeran IV, 746–748
Alkeran, 746–748, 81C–92C
Allegra, 489–490, 54C–55C
Allegra Children's Allergy
   ODT, 489–490
Allegra-D, 1016–1017

---

italics – classification name   **bold page #** – main drug entry

---

italics – classification name   **bold page #** – main drug entry

---

bold – generic drug name   regular type – trade name

---

bold – generic drug name

regular type – trade name

1352   General Index

Follitropin beta, 107C–109C
Folotyn, 978–980
fondaparinux, 517–519,
  32C–34C
Foradil Aerolizer, 519–520
Foradil, 75C–78C
Forfivo XL, 165–167
formoterol, 519–520,
  75C–78C
Formoterol/budesonide,
  75C–78C
Formoterol/Mometasone,
  75C–78C
Formulex, 358–359
Fortamet, 758–760
Fortaz, 223–225, 23C–25C
Forteo, 1171–1172, 143C
Fortesta, 1172–1175
Fortical, 176–177, 143C
Fosamax, 32, 142C–143C
Fosamax Plus D, 32
fosamprenavir, 520–522,
  117C–120C
fosaprepitant, 77–79
foscarnet, 522–524,
  66C–68C
Foscavir, 522–524, 66C–68C
fosinopril, 524–526,
  9C–10C
fosphenytoin, 526–527,
  35C–38C
Fosrenol, 674–675
Fragmin, 310–312, 32C–34C
Frova, 527–529, 64C
frovatriptan, 527–529,
  64C
fulvestrant, 529–530,
  81C–92C
Fungizone, 64–66
Fungoid, 49C–50C
Furadantin, 856–857
furosemide, 530–532,
  103C–105C
Fuzeon, 418–419,
  117C–120C
Fycompa, 946–948

G

gabapentin, 533–535,
  35C–38C
Gabitril, 1186–1187,
  35C–38C
galantamine, 535–536
Gammagard Liquid, 611–613
Gammagard S/D, 611–613
Gammaplex, 611–613

Gamunex-C, 611–613
ganciclovir, 536–538,
  66C–68C
Garamycin, 22C
Garlic, 1317–1322
Gas-X, 1104–1105
Gattex, 1151–1152
Gaviscon, 734
Gazyva, 870–871
gefitinib, 539–540,
  81C–92C
Gelnique, 902–904
Gelusil, 734
gemcitabine, 540–542,
  81C–92C
gemfibrozil, 542–544,
  56C–58C
gemifloxacin, 544–545,
  26C
Gemzar, 540–542, 81C–92C
Genahist, 373–375
Genaphed, 1016–1017
Generlac, 666–668
Gengraf, 299–302
Genotropin, 1120–1122
Genotropin Miniquick,
  1120–1122
Gentak, 545–548
gentamicin, 545–548, 22C
Gen-Timolol, 1193–1194
Gentlax-S, 1094–1096
Geodon, 1296–1298,
  66C–68C
Gianvi, 94C–98C
Gilenya, 495–496
Gilotrif, 26–27
Ginger, 1317–1322
Ginkgo, 1317–1322
Ginseng, 1317–1322
GlucaGen Diagnostic Kit,
  552–554
glatiramer, 548–549
Gleevec, 605–607, 81C–92C
Gliadel Wafer, 198–200
glimepiride, 549–550,
  43C–45C
glipizide, 551–552,
  43C–45C
GlucaGen, 552–554
glucagon, 552–554
Glucagon Emergency Kit,
  552–554
GlucoNorm, 1044–1046
Glucophage, 758–760,
  43C–45C
Glucophage XR, 758–760

Glucosamine, 1317–1322
Glucotrol, 551–552,
  43C–45C
Glucotrol XL, 551–552
Glucovance, 554–555,
  758–760
Glumetza, 758–760
glyburide, 554–555,
  43C–45C
Glycon, 758–760
Glynase Pres-Tab, 554–555
Glyset, 43C–45C
GM-CSF, 1088–1090
golimumab, 555–558
GoLYTELY, 970–971
Gonal-F, 107C–109C
goserelin, 558–559,
  81C–92C, 107C–109C
Gotu kola, 1317–1322
Gralise, 533–535
granisetron, 559–561
Granisol, 559–561
**granulocyte macrophage
  colony-stimulating
  factor, 1088–1090**
Grapefruit, 1317–1322
Green tea, 1317–1322
Grifulvin V, 561–562
griseofulvin, 561–562
Gris-PEG, 561–562
guaifenesin, 562–563
guanfacine, 563–565

H

H_2 *antagonists, 110C–111C*
Habitrol, 847–849
Halaven, 437–438
Halcyon, 148C–149C
Haldol Decanoate, 566–568
Haldol, 566–568, 66C–68C
Haley's MO, 734
Halfprin, 89–91
Halobetasol, 101C–102C
haloperidol, 566–568,
  66C–68C
Hectorol, 1276
Helidac, 142–143, 780–782
*Hematinic preparations,
  111C–112C*
Hemofil M, 74–76
Hepalean, 568–570
Hepalean Leo, 568–570
heparin, 568–570,
  32C–34C
Hep-Lock, 568–570
Hepsera, 21–22, 69C–70C

---

bold – generic drug name   regular type – trade name

---

bold – generic drug name

regular type – trade name

---

bold – generic drug name   regular type – trade name

1364   General Index

---

bold – generic drug name   regular type – trade name

---

italics – classification name   **bold page #** – main drug entry

---

bold – generic drug name

regular type – trade name

COMMONLY USED ABBREVIATIONS

ABG(s)—arterial blood gas(es)
ACE—angiotensin-converting enzyme
ADHD—attention-deficit hyperactivity disorder
AIDS—acquired immunodeficiency syndrome
ALT—alanine aminotransferase, serum
ANC—absolute neutrophil count
aPTT—activated partial thromboplastin time
AST—aspartate aminotransferase, serum
AV—atrioventricular
bid—twice per day
B/P—blood pressure
BSA—body surface area
BUN—blood urea nitrogen
CBC—complete blood count
Ccr—creatinine clearance
CNS—central nervous system
CO—cardiac output
COPD—chronic obstructive pulmonary disease
CPK—creatine phosphokinase
CSF—cerebrospinal fluid
CT—computed tomography
CVA—cerebrovascular accident
D_5W—dextrose 5% in water
dl—deciliter
DNA—deoxyribonucleic acid
EEG—electroencephalogram
EKG—electrocardiogram
esp.—especially
g—gram
GGT—gamma glutamyl transpeptidase
GI—gastrointestinal
GU—genitourinary
H_2—histamine
Hct—hematocrit
HDL—high-density lipoprotein
HF—heart failure
Hgb—hemoglobin
HIV—human immunodeficiency virus
HMG-CoA—3-hydroxy-3-methylglutaryl-coenzyme A (HMG-CoA) reductase inhibitors (statins)
hr/hrs—hour/hours
HTN—hypertension
I&O—intake and output
ICP—intracranial pressure
ID—intradermal
IgA—immunoglobulin A

IM—intramuscular
IOP—intraocular pressure
IV—intravenous
K—potassium
kg—kilogram
LDH—lactate dehydrogenase
LDL—low-density lipoprotein
LOC—level of consciousness
MAC—*Mycobacterium avium* complex
MAOI—monoamine oxidase inhibitor
mcg—microgram
mEq—milliequivalent
mg—milligram
MI—myocardial infarction
min—minute(s)
mo/mos—month/months
N/A—not applicable
Na—sodium
NaCl—sodium chloride
NG—nasogastric
NSAID(s)—nonsteroidal anti-inflammatory drug(s)
OD—right eye
OS—left eye
OTC—over the counter
OU—both eyes
PCP—*Pneumocystis jiroveci* pneumonia
PO—orally, by mouth
prn—as needed
PSA—prostate-specific antigen
pt/pts—patient/patients
PT—prothrombin time
PTCA—percutaneous transluminal coronary angiography
q—every
qid—four times daily
RBC—red blood cell count
REM—rapid eye movement
RNA—ribonucleic acid
SA—sinoatrial node
sec—second(s)
SSRI—selective serotonin reuptake inhibitor
tbsp—tablespoon
tid—three times daily
TNF—tumor necrosis factor
tsp—teaspoon
UTI—urinary tract infection
VLDL—very-low-density lipoprotein
WBC—white blood cell count
wk/wks—week/weeks
yr/yrs—year/years